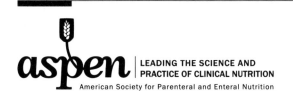

LEADING THE SCIENCE AND
PRACTICE OF CLINICAL NUTRITION

American Society for Parenteral and Enteral Nutrition

THE ASPEN ADULT NUTRITION SUPPORT CORE CURRICULUM
Third Edition

EDITOR-IN-CHIEF

Charles M. Mueller, PhD, RDN, CDN, CNSC
Department of Nutrition and Food Studies
New York University
New York, NY

SECTION EDITORS

Linda M. Lord, NP, CNSC, ACNP-BC
University of Rochester Medical Center
Rochester, NY

Mary Marian, DCN, RDN, CSO, FAND
Department of Nutritional Sciences, University of Arizona
Tucson, AZ

Stephen A. McClave, MD, FASPEN, FASGE, FACN, AGAF
University of Louisville School of Medicine
Louisville, KY

Sarah J. Miller, PharmD, BCNSP
University of Montana School of Pharmacy
Missoula, MT

AMERICAN SOCIETY FOR PARENTERAL AND ENTERAL NUTRITION

The American Society for Parenteral and Enteral Nutrition (ASPEN) is a scientific society whose members are healthcare professionals—physicians, dietitians, nurses, pharmacists, other allied health professionals, and researchers—dedicated to ensuring that every patient receives safe, efficacious, and high-quality patient care.

ASPEN's mission is to improve patient care by advancing the science and practice of clinical nutrition and metabolism.

NOTE: This publication is designed to provide accurate authoritative information with regard to the subject matter covered. It is sold with the understanding that the publisher is not engaged in rendering medical or other professional advice. Trademarked commercial product names are used only for education purposes and do not constitute endorsement by ASPEN.

This publication does not constitute medical or professional advice, and should not be taken as such. To the extent the information published herein may be used to assist in the care of patients, this is the result of the sole professional judgment of the attending health professional whose judgment is the primary component of quality medical care. The information presented herein is not a substitute for the exercise of such judgment by the health professional.

Print ISBN: 978-1-889622-31-6
eBook ISBN: 978-1-889622-32-3

Printed in the United States

5 6 7 8 9 10

Contents

Contributors

Karen S. Allen, MD
Clinical Assistant Professor of Medicine
University of Oklahoma Health Sciences Center
Oklahoma City, OK

Natalia Bailey, MS, RD, CD
Registered Dietitian
Harborview Medical Center
Oregon Health and Science University School of
    Medicine
Seattle, WA

Albert Barrocas, MD, FACS, FASPEN
Vice President, Chief Medical Officer
Wellstar Atlanta Medical Center
Atlanta, GA

Matthew V. Benns, MD
Department of Surgery, Division of Trauma and
    Critical Care
University of Louisville School of Medicine
Louisville, KY

Neal Bhutiani, MD
Department of Surgery, Division of Trauma and
    Critical Care
University of Louisville School of Medicine
Louisville, KY

Kim K. Birtcher, PharmD, MS, BCPS (AQ
    Cardiology), CDE, CLS
Clinical Professor
University of Houston College of Pharmacy

Clinical Pharmacist
Kelsey-Seybold Clinic, Cardiology Department
Houston, TX

John C. Brown, PhD
Professor Emeritus
Department of Molecular Biosciences
University of Kansas
Lawrence, KS

Christan Bury, MS, RD, LD, CNSC
Advance Practice I Clinical Dietitian ICU
Cleveland Clinic
Cleveland, OH

Todd W. Canada, PharmD, BCNSP, BCCCP, FASHP,
    FTSHP
University of Texas MD Anderson Cancer Center
Division of Pharmacy
Houston, TX

Panna A. Codner, MD, FACS
Associate Professor of Surgery
Medical College of Wisconsin
Milwaukee, WI

Tina Colaizzo-Anas, PhD, RD-AP, CDN, CNSC, FAND
Associate Professor and Director, Dietitian Education
    Program
SUNY-Buffalo State
Buffalo, NY

Bryan R. Collier, DO, FACS, CNSC
Associate Professor of Surgery, Section Chief and
    Medical Director of Trauma, Section Chief
    of Surgical Critical Care, Director of Surgical
    Nutrition
Virginia Tech Carilion School of Medicine
Carilion Roanoke Memorial Hospital
Roanoke, VA

Gail A.M. Cresci, PhD, RD, LD, CNSC
Full Staff
Pediatric, Lerner Research, Digestive Disease, and
    Surgery Institutes
Cleveland Clinic
Cleveland, OH

Jennifer Doley, MBA, RD, CNSC, FAND
Regional Clinical Nutrition Manager and Dietetic
    Internship Director
Morrison Healthcare at Carondelet St. Mary's Hospital
Tucson, AZ

Kathryn Drogan, MS, NP, ANP-BC
Nurse Practitioner
Adult Nutrition Support Services
University of Rochester Medical Center
Rochester, NY

Miriam Erick, MS, RD, LDN, CDE
Senior Dietitian
Department of Nutrition
Brigham and Women's Hospital
Boston, MA

David C. Evans, MD, FACS, PNS
Associate Professor of Surgery
Medical Director, Level 1 Trauma Center and
    Nutrition Support Service
The Ohio State University
Columbus, OH

Phyllis J. Famularo, DCN, RD, CSG, LDN, FAND
Senior Manager, Nutrition Services
Sodexo
Gaithersburg, MD

John C. Fang, MD
Freston Takeda Professor of Medicine
Chief, Division of Gastroenterology, Hepatology,
    and Nutrition
University of Utah Health
Salt Lake City, UT

David Frankenfield, MS, RD
Manager
Nutrition Support Dietitian
Department of Clinical Nutrition
PennState Health Milton S. Hershey Medical Center
Hershey, PA

Marianne Galang, RD, LD, CSO
Clinical Dietitian, Advanced Practice 1
Digestive Disease Institute, Center for Human
    Nutrition
Cleveland Clinic
Cleveland, OH

Jane Gervasio, PharmD, BCNSP, FCCP
Chair and Professor of Pharmacy Practice
Butler University College of Pharmacy and Health
    Sciences
Indianapolis, IN

Jeanette M. Hasse, PhD, RD, LD, FADA, CNSC
Transplant Nutrition Manager
Baylor University Medical Center
Simmons Transplant Institute
Dallas, TX

Jimmi Hatton Kolpek, PharmD, FCCP, FCCM, FNAP
Professor Pharmacy Practice and Science
University of Kentucky College of Pharmacy
Lexington, KY

Eileen Hendrickson, RPh, PharmD, MBA
Director of Pharmacy
Cleveland Clinic Infusion Pharmacy at Home
Cleveland, OH

Thomas J. Herron, MD
Assistant Professor in Surgery
Division of Acute Care Surgery
University of South Florida
Tampa, FL

Peggy Hipskind, MA, RD, LD
Advanced Practice II Clinical Dietitian
Cleveland Clinic
Cleveland, OH

Mary Hise, PhD, RDN, CNSC
Senior Director
Global Medical Affairs
Nutrition Baxter Healthcare

Leah A. Hoffman, PhD, RD, LD, CNSC
Assistant Professor
Department of Nutritional Sciences
University of Oklahoma Health Sciences Center
Oklahoma City, OK

Ryan T. Hurt, MD, PhD
Associate Professor of Medicine and Director of
    Home Parenteral Enteral Nutrition
Mayo Clinic
Rochester, MN

Kristin M. Izzo, MS, RD, LD, CNSC
Nutrition Support Clinician
Center for Gut Rehabilitation and Transplant
    Program
Cleveland Clinic Center for Human Nutrition
Cleveland, OH

Rachael Janas, RD, CNSC

Andrea K. JeVenn, MEd, RD, LD, CNSC
Advance Practice Dietitian I, Nutrition Support Team
Center for Human Nutrition
Cleveland Clinic
Cleveland, OH

Kellie Jones, MD
Department of Medicine, Section of Pulmonary and
    Critical Care
University of Oklahoma Health Sciences Center
Oklahoma City, OK

Matthew R. Kappus, MD
Assistant Professor
Transplant Hepatology and Gastroenterology
Duke University
Durham, NC

Dong Wook Kim, MD, PNS
Assistant Professor
Boston University School of Medicine
Boston Medical Center
Boston, MA

Merin Kinikini, DNP, FNP, RD, CNSC
Nurse Practitioner
Outpatient/Inpatient Metabolic Nutrition Support
    Service
Intermountain Medical Center
Murray, UT

Rachelle Kirsch, RD, LD, CNSC
Clinical Dietitian
Baylor University Medical Center Trauma/Surgical ICU
Dallas, TX

Denise Konrad, RD, CNSC
Nutrition Support Clinician, Home Nutrition
    Support Service
Digestive Disease Institute
Cleveland Clinic
Cleveland, OH

Csaba P. Kovesdy, MD
Fred Hatch Professor of Medicine and Director,
    Clinical Outcomes and Clinical Trials Program
Division of Nephrology
University of Tennessee Health Science Center

Nephrology Section Chief
Memphis VA Medical Center
Memphis, TN

Michelle Kozeniecki, MS, RD, CNSC
Lead Clinical Dietitian
Froedtert Hospital
Milwaukee, WI

Kristine Krueger, MD
Professor of Medicine
Chief of Academic and Clinical Affairs, Division of
    Gastroenterology, Hepatology, and Nutrition
University of Louisville School of Medicine
Louisville, KY

Vanessa J. Kumpf, PharmD, BCNSP
Clinical Specialist, Nutrition Support
Vanderbilt University Medical Center
Nashville, TN

Berkeley N. Limketkai, MD, PhD
Clinical Assistant Professor
Stanford University School of Medicine
Stanford, CA

Pei-Ra Ling, MD
Senior Research Scientist
Feihe Nutrition Laboratory, Center for the Study of
    Nutrition Medicine
Department of Surgery
Beth Israel Deaconess Medical Center
Boston, MA

Linda M. Lord, NP, CNSC, ACNP-BC
Nurse Practitioner
Adult Nutrition Support Service
University of Rochester Medical Center
Rochester, NY

Barbara Magnuson Woodward, PharmD, CNSC
Nutrition Support Service, Coordinator
University of Kentucky Healthcare

Associate Professor
UK College of Pharmacy
Lexington, KY

Ainsley M. Malone, MS, RD, LD, CNSC, FAND,
   FASPEN
Nutrition Support Dietitian
Mt. Carmel West Hospital

Clinical Practice Specialist
American Society for Parenteral and Enteral Nutrition
Columbus, OH

Mary Marian, DCN, RDN, CSO, FAND
Assistant Professor of Practice and Director, Didactic
   Program in Dietetics
College of Agriculture and Life Sciences
Department of Nutritional Sciences
University of Arizona

Nutrition Consultant, AZ Oncology
Tucson, AZ

Robert G. Martindale, MD, PhD
Professor of Surgery, Chief of General and
   Gastrointestinal Surgery, and Medical Director for
   Hospital Nutritional Services
Oregon Health and Sciences University
Portland, OR

Laura E. Matarese, PhD, RDN, LDN, FADA, CNSC,
   FASPEN, FAND
Professor of Medicine
Brody School of Medicine
East Carolina University
Greenville, NC

Kristen Mathieson, MBA, RD, CDN
Senior Dietitian
NewYork-Presbyterian Hospital
New York, NY

Todd Mattox, PharmD, BCNSP
Critical Care/Nutrition Support Pharmacy Specialist
Moffitt Cancer Center
Tampa, FL

Stephen A. McClave, MD, FASPEN, FASGE, FACN, AGAF
Professor of Medicine
Division of Gastroenterology, Hepatology, and
   Nutrition
University of Louisville School of Medicine
Louisville, KY

Karen C. McCowen, MD
Associate Professor of Medicine
University of California San Diego
San Diego, CA

Liam McKeever, MS, PhD, RDN
Clinical Instructor
University of Illinois at Chicago
Chicago, IL

Valentina Medici, MD
Associate Professor
Department of Internal Medicine, Division of
   Gastroenterology and Hepatology
University of California Davis
Sacramento, CA

Keith R. Miller, MD
Department of Surgery, Division of Trauma and
   Critical Care
University of Louisville School of Medicine
Louisville, KY

Jay M. Mirtallo, MSc, RPh, BCNSP, FASHP, FASPEN
Professor of Clinical Pharmacy
College of Pharmacy, Division of Pharmacy Practice
   and Science
The Ohio State University
Columbus, OH

Ronelle Mitchell, MA, RD, CNSC
Nutrition Support Clinician, Home Nutrition
   Support Service
Digestive Disease Institute, Cleveland Clinic
Cleveland, OH

Kris M. Mogensen, MS, RD-AP, LDN, CNSC
Team Leader Dietitian Specialist
Department of Nutrition
Brigham and Women's Hospital
Boston, MA

Gerard E. Mullin, MD
Associate Professor of Medicine
The Johns Hopkins University School of Medicine
Baltimore, MD

Manpreet S. Mundi, MD
Associate Professor of Medicine
Division of Endocrinology
Mayo Clinic
Rochester, MN

Antoinette M. Neal, BSN, RN, CRNI, VA-BC, CNSC
Clinical Infusion Nurse
Cleveland Clinic Connected Care at Home Infusion
  Pharmacy
Cleveland, OH

Douglas R. Oyler, PharmD, BCCCP
Clinical Pharmacist
Trauma/Acute Care Surgery
University of Kentucky Healthcare
Lexington, KY

Lena B. Palmer, MD, MSCR
Medical Director of Clinical Nutrition, Associate
  Professor of Medicine
Division of Gastroenterology and Nutrition
Loyola University Chicago
Stritch School of Medicine
Maywood, IL

Sam Pappas, MD
Department of Surgery
Loyola University Chicago
Stritch School of Medicine
Chicago, IL

Jayshil J. Patel, MD
Associate Professor of Medicine
Medical College of Wisconsin
Milwaukee, WI

Rina Patel, PharmD, BCNSP
Clinical Pharmacy Specialist—Critical Care/
  Nutrition Support
University of Texas MD Anderson Cancer Center
Houston, TX

Wendy Phillips, MS, RD, CNSC, CLE, FAND
Division Director of Clinical Nutrition
Morrison Healthcare
St. George, UT

Mary Ellen Posthauer, RDN, CD, LD, FAND
President
MEP Healthcare Dietary Services, Inc.
Evansville, IN

Susan Roberts, MS, RDN, LD, CNSC
Area Director of Clinical Nutrition and Dietetic
  Internship Director
Baylor University Medical Center/Aramark Healthcare
Houston, TX

Carol J. Rollins, MS, RD, CNSC, PharmD, BCNSP,
  FASPEN
Clinical Professor
College of Pharmacy
University of Arizona
Tucson, AZ

David S. Rubin, MD
Medical Director
Circle Care Center
Norwalk, CT

Kathryn Ruf, PharmD, BCPS
Pharmacy Clinical Coordinator, Surgery/Trauma
University of Kentucky Healthcare
Lexington, KY

Mardeli Saire Mendoza, MD
Gastroenterology Staff
Overton Brooks VAMC
Shreveport, LA

Menaka Sarav, MD
Clinical Assistant Professor
University of Chicago Pritzker School of Medicine
Division of Nephrology and Hypertension,
  NorthShore University HealthSystem
Evanston, IL

Denise Baird Schwartz, MS, RD, FADA, FAND, FASPEN
Bioethics Committee Member
Providence Saint Joseph Medical Center
Burbank, CA

Sorana Segal-Maurer, MD
Director
The Dr. James J. Rahal Jr. Division of Infectious Diseases
NewYork-Presbyterian
Queens, Flushing, NY

Associate Professor of Clinical Medicine
Weill Cornell Medical College
Cornell University
New York, NY

David S. Seres, MD, FASPEN, PNS
Director of Medical Nutrition, Associate Clinical Ethicist, and Associate Professor of Medicine
Institute of Human Nutrition
Columbia University Medical Center
NewYork-Presbyterian Hospital
New York, NY

Michael Sprang, MD
Assistant Professor of Medicine
Loyola University Medical Center
Maywood, IL

Maria Szeto, MS, RD
Registered Dietitian
Mackenzie Health
Richmond Hill, ON, Canada

Anne M. Tucker, PharmD, BCNSP
Clinical Pharmacy Specialist—Critical Care/ Nutrition Support
University of Texas MD Anderson Cancer Center
Houston, TX

Amber Verdell, PharmD, BCPS, BCNSP
Assistant Professor, Pharmacy Practice
West Coast University School of Pharmacy
Los Angeles, CA

E. Annelie M. Vogt, DCN, RD, LDN, CSO, CNSC
Doctor of Clinical Nutrition
Medstar Washington Hospital Center—Washington Cancer Institute
Washington, DC

Renee Walker, MS, RD, LD, CNSC
Clinical Pharmacy Specialist—Critical Care/ Nutrition Support
Michael E. DeBakey Veteran Affairs Medical Center
Houston, TX

Peter Wasserman, BSc, MA
Metabolic Support Clinician and Research Associate
Infectious Disease Division, Department of Medicine
NewYork-Presbyterian Queens

Senior Lecturer in Medicine
Weill Cornell Medical College
New York, NY

Joseph West, MD
University of Oklahoma Health Sciences Center
Department of Internal Medicine
Oklahoma City, OK

Valaree Williams, MS, RDN, CSO, FAND
Clinical Dietitian
University of Colorado Health Cancer Center
Aurora, CO

Lorraine S. Young, MS, RD, LDN, CNSC
Clinical Nutrition Manager, Boston Medical Center
Instructor of Medicine, Boston University School of Medicine
Boston, MA

Rena Zelig, DCN, RD, CDE, CSG
Assistant Professor, Department of Nutritional Sciences
Director, Master of Science in Clinical Nutrition Program
School of Health Professions
Rutgers University
Newark, NJ

Reviewers

Denise Andersen, MS, RDN, LD, CLC
Business Consultant, Private Practice
St. Paul, MN

Albert Barrocas, MD, FACS, FASPEN
Vice President, Chief Medical Officer
Wellstar Atlanta Medical Center
Atlanta, GA

Bruce R. Bistrian, MD, PhD
Chief, Clinical Nutrition, Beth Israel Deaconess
    Medical Center
Professor of Medicine, Harvard Medical School
Boston, MA

Michelle Bratton, RDN, CSO
Clinical Nutritionist
University of Arizona Cancer Center
Tucson, AZ

Britta D. Brown, MS, RD, LD, CNSC
Clinical Dietitian
Hennepin County Medical Center
Minneapolis, MN

Jennifer Burris, PhD, RD, CNSC, CDE, CSSD, CSG
Adjunct Faculty
California State University Los Angeles
Los Angeles, CA

Phila Callahan, RN, CNSC
Nutrition Support Nurse
Christiana Care Health Services
Newark, DE

Lingtak-Neander Chan, PharmD, BCNSP, CNSC, FACN
Professor of Pharmacy and Interdisciplinary Faculty
    in Nutritional Sciences
University of Washington, Seattle
Seattle, WA

Pam Charney, PhD, RD
Program Chair, Healthcare Informatics
Bellevue College
Bellevue, WA

Panna A. Codner, MD, FACS
Associate Professor of Surgery
Medical College of Wisconsin
Milwaukee, WI

Bryan Collier, DO, FACS, CNSC
Section Chief of Trauma and Surgical Critical Care,
    Director of Surgical Nutrition, Carilion Clinic,
    Carilion Roanoke Memorial Hospital
Associate Professor of Surgery, Virginia Tech Carilion
    School of Medicine
Roanoke, VA

Charlene Compher, PhD, RD, CNSC, LDN, FASPEN
Professor of Nutrition Science
University of Pennsylvania School of Nursing
Philadelphia, PA

Robert DeChicco, MS, RD, LD, CNSC
Manager, Nutrition Support Team
Cleveland Clinic
Cleveland, OH

Karrie Derenski, PharmD, BCNSP, CNSC
Pharmacy Clinical Supervisor, Coordinator
 Metabolic Support, Director of PGY2 Critical Care
 Pharmacy Residency
CoxHealth
Springfield, MO

Sara R. DiCecco, MS, RDN, LD
Clinical Dietitian
Mayo Clinic Rochester
Rochester, MN

Roland Dickerson, PharmD, BCNSP
Professor of Clinical Pharmacy
University of Tennessee College of Pharmacy
Memphis, TN

Becky Dorner, RDN, LD, FAND
President
Becky Dorner and Associates, Inc.
Dunedin, FL

Lindsay Dowhan, MS, RD, CSO, LD, CNSC
Advanced Practice Nutrition Support Clinician,
 Center for Gut Rehab and Transplant
Cleveland Clinic
Cleveland, OH

John W. Drover, MD, FRCSC, FACS, CCPE
Professor
Queen's University
Kingston, ON, Canada

Sinead Duggan, PhD
Postdoctoral Research Fellow
Department of Surgery, Trinity College
Dublin, Ireland

Kristen Dwinnells, MA, RDN, LDN, CNSC
Clinical Dietitian Specialist
Hospital of the University of Pennsylvania
Philadelphia, PA

Arlene A. Escuro, MS, RD, LD, CNSC
Advanced Practice Dietitian
Cleveland Clinic
Cleveland, OH

Eric H. Frankel, MSE, PharmD, BCNSP
Co-owner/Consultant, West Texas Clinical Pharmacy
 Associates, Inc., Lubbock, TX
Clinical Pharmacist, Benewah Community Hospital,
 St. Maries, ID

Thomas Frazier, MD
Medical Director of Endoscopy and Nutrition, Three
 Rivers Medical Center
Assistant Clinical Professor, University of Louisville
Louisa, KY

Michele M. Gottschlich, PhD, RD, CSP, CCRP
Clinical Research Scientist, Shriners Hospital for
 Children
Adjunct Associate Professor, Department of Surgery,
 University of Cincinnati
Cincinnati, OH

Linda Griffith, PhD, RD
Registered Dietitian/Consultant
FNR Associates Consulting
Overland Park, KS

Kathleen M. Gura, PharmD, BCNSP, FASHP, FPPAG,
 FASPEN
Manager, Pharmacy Clinical Research Programs
Clinical Specialist, Gastroenterology/Nutrition
Boston Children's Hospital
Boston, MA

Cindy Hamilton, MS, RD, LD, FAND
Director, Nutrition, Center for Human Nutrition
Cleveland Clinic
Cleveland, OH

Leslie A. Hamilton, PharmD, BCPS, BCCCP
Associate Professor of Clinical Pharmacy
University of Tennessee Health Science Center
 College of Pharmacy
Knoxville, TN

Mary Harris, PhD, RDN
Professor of Nutrition/Didactic Program Director
Department of Food Science and Human Nutrition
Colorado State University
Fort Collins, CO

Lillian Harvey Banchik, MD, FACS, CNSC
Department of Surgery
North Shore University Hospital
Manhasset, NY

Jeanette M. Hasse, PhD, RD, LD, FADA, CNSC
Transplant Nutrition Manager
Baylor University Medical Center, Simmons
    Transplant Institute
Dallas, TX

Leslie A. Hourigan, MS, RD, CNSC
Clinical Nutrition Manager
Brooke Army Medical Center
San Antonio, TX

Carol Ireton-Jones, PhD, RD, LD, CNSC, FASPEN,
    FAND
Nutrition Therapy Specialist/Consultant
Carrollton, TX

Khursheed N. Jeejeebhoy, MBBS, PhD, FRCP, FRCPC
Emeritus Professor of Medicine, University of
    Toronto
Physician and Director, Home Parenteral Nutrition,
    St. Michael's Hospital Toronto
Toronto, ON, Canada

Donald F. Kirby, MD, FACP, FACN, FACG, AGAF,
    CNSC, CPNS
Director, Center for Human Nutrition
Cleveland Clinic
Cleveland, OH

Mark G. Klang, MS, PhD, RPh, BCNSP
Core Manager, Research Pharmacy
Memorial Sloan Kettering Cancer Center
New York, NY

Donald P. Kotler, MD
Chief, Division of Gastroenterology
Jacobi Medical Center
Bronx, NY

Elizabeth Krzywda, APNP
Nurse Practitioner
Medical College of Wisconsin Surgical Oncology
Milwaukee, WI

Cynthia C. Lowen, RD, LD, CNSC, CCRP
Clinical Instructor, University of Louisville
    Department of Medicine
Medical Scientific Liaison, Nestlé Health Science
Louisville, KY

Ainsley M. Malone, MS, RD, LD, CNSC, FAND, FASPEN
Nutrition Support Dietitian, Mt. Carmel West
    Hospital
Clinical Practice Specialist, American Society for
    Parenteral and Enteral Nutrition
Columbus, OH

Laura E. Matarese, PhD, RDN, LDN, FADA, CNSC,
    FASPEN, FAND
Professor of Medicine
Brody School of Medicine, East Carolina University
Greenville, NC

Theresa Mayes, RD, CSP, LD, CCRC
Clinical Dietitian
Cincinnati Children's Hospital Medical Center
Cincinnati, OH

Carol McGinnis, DNP, APRN-CNS, CNSC
Clinical Nurse Specialist/Nutrition Support
Sanford USD Medical Center
Sioux Falls, SD

Robin B. Mendelsohn, MD
Assistant Attending Physician
Memorial Sloan Kettering Cancer Center
New York, NY

Gayle Minard, MD, FACS
Professor of Surgery
University of Tennessee Health Science Center
Memphis, TN

Julie O'Sullivan Maillet, PhD, RDN, FADA, FASAHP
Professor, Nutritional Sciences
School of Health Professions
Rutgers, the University of New Jersey
Newark, NJ

Douglas Oyler, PharmD, BCCCP
Clinical Pharmacist, Trauma/Acute Care Surgery
University of Kentucky Healthcare
Lexington, KY

Domingo Pinero, PhD
Clinical Associate Professor, Director of
    Undergraduate Studies
Department of Nutrition and Food Studies
New York University
New York, NY

Steven Plogsted, PharmD, BCNSP, CNSC
Nutrition Support Pharmacist
Nationwide Children's Hospital
Columbus, OH

Mary Rath, BS, RD, LD, CNSC
Nutrition Support Dietitian
Cleveland Clinic
Cleveland, OH

Carol Rees Parrish, MS, RD
Nutrition Support Specialist
University of Virginia Health System, Digestive
    Health Center
Charlottesville, VA

Mary Russell, MS, RDN, LDN, FAND
Senior Manager, US Nutrition Medical Affairs
Baxter Healthcare Corporation
Deerfield, IL

Marcia Ryder, PhD, MS, RN
Research Scientist
Ryder Science, Inc.
Nashville, TN

Douglas L. Seidner, MD, AGAF, FACG, FASPEN,
    CNSC
Associate Professor of Medicine
Director, Vanderbilt Center for Human Nutrition
Vanderbilt School of Medicine, Vanderbilt
    University Medical Center
Nashville, TN

Janet J. Skates, RD, LDN, FADA
Nutrition Consultant
Kingsport, TN

Ezra Steiger, MD, FACS
Professor of Surgery, Cleveland Clinic Lerner College
    of Medicine
Nutrition Support Team, Intestinal Rehab and
    Transplant Program, Digestive Disease Institute,
    Cleveland Clinic
Cleveland, OH

David E. St-Jules, PhD, RD
Assistant Professor
Center for Healthful Behavior Change, Division of
    Health and Behavior, Department of Population
    Health
New York University School of Medicine
New York, NY

Beth E. Taylor, DCN, RD-AP, CNSC, FCCM
Clinical Nutrition Research/Education Specialist
Barnes-Jewish Hospital
St. Louis, MO

Cameo Tynan, MS, RD, CNSC
Clinical Dietitian
University of Colorado Hospital
Aurora, CO

Charles W. Van Way, III, MD
Emeritus Professor of Surgery, University of
    Missouri, Kansas City, School of Medicine
Director of Metabolic Support, Truman Medical
    Center
Kansas City, MO

Renee Walker, MS, RD, LD, CNSC, FAND
Dietitian
Michael E. DeBakey Veteran Affairs Medical Center
Houston, TX

Susan Whiting, PhD
Distinguished Professor of Nutrition
University of Saskatchewan
Saskatoon, SK, Canada

Kate Willcutts, DCN, RDN, CNSC
Co-manager, Clinical Nutrition
University of Virginia Hospital
Charlottesville, VA

Abby Wood, RDN, CSO, LD, CNSC
Clinical Dietitian—Oncology
Baylor Scott and White Healthcare—T Boone
    Pickens Cancer Hospital
Dallas, TX

Jennifer A. Wooley, MS, RD, CNSC
Clinical Nutrition Specialist
GE Healthcare
Madison, WI

Daniel Dante Yeh, MD
Massachusetts General Hospital
Boston, MA

Yong Ming Yu, MD, PhD
Researcher, Department of Surgery
Massachusetts General Hospital and Shriners
    Hospital for Children, Harvard Medical School
Boston, MA

Ayman M. AL-Qaaneh, PhD, RPh, BCNSP, PPTC
Manager
Johns Hopkins Aramco Healthcare
Dhahran, Saudia Arabia

Foreword

The American Society for Parenteral and Enteral Nutrition (ASPEN), an interdisciplinary society leading the science and practice of clinical nutrition, presents *The ASPEN Adult Nutrition Support Core Curriculum*, 3rd edition. This comprehensive book addresses the principles of nutrition support and nutrition support recommendations for selected medical and surgical conditions. Professional and management issues, including home nutrition support, ethics, quality improvement, evidence-based practice, and guideline development, also are discussed.

Since the last edition, new practice guidelines and research have advanced nutrition support and created greater awareness of the importance of nutrition care across the continuum of care. For example, ASPEN has updated recommendations for safe practices in enteral nutrition and the appropriate use of parenteral nutrition, and new research has demonstrated the association of malnutrition with high rates of readmission, longer hospital stays, and increased healthcare costs. This edition includes this information, among many other topics, and is a valuable resource for clinicians at all levels who aim to advance and apply this knowledge to their nutrition practice and/or prepare for recertification in nutrition support.

We are grateful for the leadership of editor-in-chief, Charles M. Mueller, PhD, RDN, CDN, CNSC, and the section editors, Linda M. Lord, NP, CNSC, ACNP-BC, Mary Marian, DCN, RDN, CSO, FAND, Stephen A. McClave, MD, FASPEN, FASGE, FACN, AGAF, and Sarah J. Miller, PharmD, BCNSP. These individuals bring a wealth of expertise in nutrition support clinical practice, research, and education. A diverse group of respected authors and reviewers have ensured that chapters feature up-to-date content that is aligned with current guidelines and recommendations from ASPEN and other medical societies. This diversity reflects the importance of collaboration of clinicians from multiple disciplines to provide high-quality nutrition care.

M. Molly McMahon, MD
President, American Society for Parenteral and
    Enteral Nutrition

and

Professor of Medicine
Division of Endocrinology, Diabetes, Metabolism,
    and Nutrition
Mayo Clinic
Rochester, MN

Preface

The *ASPEN Adult Nutrition Support Core Curriculum*, third edition, is the progeny of previous editions of the *Core Curriculum*, previous dietetics and nursing core curriculums, and a selection of case-based study guides published by American Society for Parenteral and Enteral Nutrition (ASPEN) pharmacists. Over the years, the *Core Curriculum* has become a practice reference for professionals, a textbook for students, and a study guide for certification and board examinations. The original version, published in 2001, *The Science and Practice of Nutrition Support, A Case-Based Core Curriculum*, represented ASPEN's commitment to interdisciplinary organizational, educational, and practice models integrated into a single text for all nutrition support professionals.[1] The content of the 2001 text was gleaned from a systematic analysis of content outlines for the MD, RD, and RN National Board of Nutrition Support Certification (NBNSC) examinations and the pharmacy certification in nutrition support offered by the Board of Pharmacy Specialists. In 2008, NBNSC replaced individual professional certifications in nutrition support with 1 credential (and 1 exam) for all professions, Certified Nutrition Support Clinician (CNSC). This change was based on the ASPEN interdisciplinary model and was confirmed as the best approach to nutrition support practice certification by a practice survey of ASPEN members.[2] Subsequently, the content of the single exam was confirmed by a second audit of practice,[3] with continuing audits planned for every 5 years thereafter. *Core Curriculum* editors have similarly adopted the interdisciplinary model as the basis for the curriculum's contents, with the range of nutrition support professions fully represented among its authors.

When the first edition of the *Adult Core Curriculum* was published in 2007,[4] the ASPEN Board of Directors proposed that a 3-volume curriculum—pediatric, adult, and older adult—be developed. *The A.S.P.E.N. Pediatric Nutrition Support Core Curriculum*[5] was first published in 2010 and revised in 2015.[6] A core curriculum for the older adult has not been published, but the *Adult Core Curriculum* includes a chapter (Chapter 36) titled Nutrition Support for Older Adults.

The text of this new edition is organized into 4 sections. Part I lays the foundation by providing an overview of nutrient intake digestion and absorption and reviewing specific nutrition requirements and dynamics for energy, carbohydrate, pre- and probiotics, protein, fat, fluid, and micronutrients. Part II surveys enteral and parenteral feeding methods and pharmacotherapeutic considerations. Part III logically progresses to nutrition support during specific states and disorders. Finally, Part IV covers specific management and professional issues including home care, ethics, quality improvement, and evidence-based practice.

The general organization of content in the chapters in Part III is consistent with the previous editions. These chapters on nutrition support for specific states begin with evidence-based, didactic background information about the core science. Each chapter in this part discusses relevant nutrition assessment issues, including the determination of nutrient requirements, and covers the appropriate route of nutrition support, including oral diet considerations. Chapters also identify monitoring concerns and potential treatment complications, and, finally, outcomes relevant to the specific state are addressed. The chapters offer practice recommendations where appropriate, and these recommendations are consistent with the most recent ASPEN clinical guidelines.

Each of the 41 chapters in the third edition has been fully revised to reflect current knowledge and practice. Recognized content experts authored and reviewed every chapter. Among the notable updates in this edition are expanded discussion of the following:

- Malnutrition screening and assessment
- Gut microbiota
- Innovations in enteral access devices, enteral and parenteral formulations, and lipid injectable emulsions
- Surgical alterations of the gastrointestinal tract and potential complications
- Quality improvement in clinical practice
- Evidence-based medicine and the derivation of clinical guidelines

Every chapter in the book features at least one Practice Scenario, a feature introduced in the second edition. Each Practice Scenario asks and answers a clinical question elucidated by a scenario and provides a rationale for the answer. The goal of the scenarios is to provide readers with specific examples of clinical decision-making that extend practical understanding of text content.

The ASPEN Adult Nutrition Support Core Curriculum, third edition, represents the best efforts of nutrition support practitioners applying their expertise and ASPEN's collective resources to provide a comprehensive text based on scientific evidence. The editors, authors, reviewers, and ASPEN staff who worked to bring you this edition hope that the text will become a centerpiece of your practice and professional growth.

Charles M. Mueller, PhD, RDN, CDN, CNSC
Editor-in-Chief

References

1. Gottschlich MM, ed. *The Science and Practice of Nutrition Support: A Case-based Core Curriculum.* Dubuque, IA: American Society for Parenteral and Enteral Nutrition and Kendall Hunt Publishers; 2001.
2. Schwartz DB, Mirtallo JM, Matarese LE. Practice audit of nutrition support certification. *Nutr Clin Pract.* 2008;23(3):329–340.
3. Matarese LE, Chinn RN, Hertz NR, et al. Practice analysis of nutrition support professionals: evidence-based multidisciplinary nutrition support certification examination. *JPEN J Parenter Enteral Nutr.* 2012;6(6):663–670. doi:10.1177/0148607111435330.
4. Gottschlich MM, ed. *The A.S.P.E.N. Adult Nutrition Support Core Curriculum: A Case-Based Approach—The Adult Patient.* Silver Spring, MD. American Society for Parenteral and Enteral Nutrition; 2007.
5. Corkins MR, ed. *The A.S.P.E.N. Pediatric Nutrition Support Core Curriculum.* Silver Spring, MD: American Society for Parenteral and Enteral Nutrition; 2010.
6. Corkins MR, ed. *The A.S.P.E.N. Pediatric Nutrition Support Core Curriculum.* 2nd ed. Silver Spring, MD: American Society for Parenteral and Enteral Nutrition; 2015.

Acknowledgments

This text represents the effort and hard work of many professional volunteers and ASPEN staff over a period of a year and a half from start to finish. The editors, authors, and reviewers are all volunteers. In some cases, volunteerism has been equivalent to a part-time job (the editors); in other cases (the authors and reviewers), it has involved hours of work to hone drafts for publication.

I could not have completed my duties as editor-in-chief without the assistance of our 4 associate editors, each representing their profession and drawing from their experience in their respective roles in the practice of nutrition support. As associate editors, Mary Marian, Linda Lord, Sarah Miller, and Stephen McClave were the first line of editorial expertise for the authors and reviewers. They also worked with me and the ASPEN publications staff to develop consensus on the content and presentation of the third edition. Mary Marian, representing dietetics, has a long history in nutrition support practice that is well known to most readers, as well as editorial expertise and an impressive record of volunteerism for our profession. She was a delight to work with and did double duty as first author for Chapter 33, Cancer, and coauthor for Chapter 21, Wound Healing. I was thrilled to recruit Linda Lord to represent nursing expertise in nutrition support for this edition. Linda has long exemplified professional generosity as an ASPEN volunteer and author, and she was a coauthor in this edition for Chapter 13, Complications of Enteral Nutrition, and Chapter 7, Fluids, Electrolytes, and Acid-Base Disorders. Sarah Miller served again as our pharmacy editor. Her editorial eye is as keen as any I know of, and her work ethic never flags. As he did for the previous edition, Stephen McClave recruited numerous physician authors—including several new contributors—to provide a fresh perspective from the highest level of clinical practice. In addition to his editorial skills, Steve applied his expertise in the derivation of evidence-based practice guidelines as first author for Chapter 41 and his clinical expertise as coauthor of Chapter 28, Pancreatitis. As in the past, Steve's sense of humor and self-deprecating manner helped the team maintain realistic expectations and focus on the project. Each of these associate editors has advanced ASPEN's mission by working on this text, as well as by serving on ASPEN committees and taskforces and, in Steve's case, acting as president of the organization. Throughout the revision process, the editors left their egos at the door, and the work at hand was the singular focus. To Mary, Linda, Sarah, and Steve, I owe my unqualified gratitude and thanks.

I also want to thank Catherine Wattenberg, director of publications for ASPEN, who oversaw the production of the third edition, and our managing editor, Elizabeth Nishiura. Catherine patiently supported the editors and authors as they did their best to stay on the production schedule, offering encouragement all along the way. Elizabeth provided expertise and experience in the publication of medical texts that was apparent in all facets of the process from peer review to copy editing and the sticky business of permissions citations. She was an invaluable resource to the editors, authors, and reviewers.

Finally, on behalf of the editors and ASPEN staff, I would like to thank the authors and reviewers who shared their expertise in the spirit of altruism. There would be no *Core Curriculum* without them. If I may speak for my fellow editors, our reward is the professional enrichment we derive from working with such a stellar cohort of healthcare professionals.

Charles M. Mueller, PhD, RDN, CDN, CNSC
Editor-in-Chief

BASICS OF NUTRITION AND METABOLISM

1 Nutrient Intake, Digestion, Absorption, and Excretion

Tina Colaizzo-Anas, PhD, RD-AP, CDN, CNSC, FAND

CONTENTS

Objectives

1. Use information on the regulation of appetite to manage transitional feeding regimens.
2. Apply knowledge of the physiology of gastrointestinal (GI) motility to planning enteral nutrition (EN) regimens for patients with altered GI motility.
3. Understand mechanisms of digestion and the absorption of various nutrients.
4. Associate the functions of each component of the GI system with their effects on nutrient digestion and absorption and implications for nutrition support.

Test Your Knowledge Questions

1. Which of the following practices is most likely to succeed in improving oral nutrient intake in patients with a prolonged history of weight loss due to poor intake, nausea, and depressed appetite?
   A. Providing a high-energy oral liquid supplement 3 times daily
   B. Offering 6 small, low-fat meals daily
   C. Ordering fiber-supplemented snacks 3 times daily
   D. Planning primarily solid meals and limiting fluids
2. Which of the following statements explains why fermentable fiber is a beneficial addition to enteral formulas?
   A. Colonic bacteria act on the fiber to produce short-chain fatty acids (SCFAs) that provide an energy source to the intestinal mucosa.
   B. Colonic bacteria act on the fiber to produce SCFAs, which, in turn, exert trophic effects on the intestinal mucosa.
   C. Fermentable fiber may help control diarrhea by slowing gastric emptying.
   D. All of the above.
3. Which of the following nutrients is added to rehydration liquids to promote water absorption in patients with diarrhea?
   A. Sodium and glucose
   B. Amino acids
   C. Long-chain fatty acids
   D. Alcohol

Test Your Knowledge Answers

1. The correct answer is **B**. When patients experience a prolonged negative energy balance, the stomach's adaptive accommodation function declines; therefore, patients may not be able to consume their goal nutrient targets in 3 regular-sized meals because of a feeling of fullness.[1] Eating 6 small meals may be a more realistic option. To address nausea, measures should be taken to prevent slowing of gastric emptying, which could potentiate nausea. These measures may include limiting high-fat foods.[2,3] Providing high-energy or high-fiber supplements initially may not be the best recommendation because, like fat, energy density and fiber content can slow gastric emptying.[2-4] Answer D is not a good choice because providing fluids, not limiting them, facilitates gastric emptying.[2]
2. The correct answer is **D**. Although more confirming evidence is needed, the addition of fermentable fibers to enteral formulas likely has multiple beneficial effects, both in the healthy gut and in the malfunctioning gut. Fermentable fibers (eg, pectin, gums, fructooligosaccharides [FOS]) are metabolized by colonic bacteria to produce SCFAs. SCFAs have multiple benefits for the colonic mucosa. These benefits include providing a significant source of energy for and exerting trophic effects on the intestinal lining.[4,5] However, fiber is not recommended for patients with diarrhea caused by *Clostridium difficile* pseudomembranous colitis (PMC) or during low-flow states.
3. The correct answer is **A**. Sodium is the nutrient that is added to rehydration liquids to promote glucose and water absorption in patients with diarrhea. The presence of sodium in the lumen of the small intestine facilitates the absorption of glucose. When more sodium is absorbed, more water from the lumen of the intestines is absorbed. For this reason, oral rehydration fluids used to treat sodium and water losses from diarrhea contain sodium chloride (NaCl) and glucose.[6]

Background

Knowledge of the GI system (gut), including its anatomy, physiology, and pathology, is central to applying methods of nutrition support. The GI tract is the organ system that allows us to regulate appetite; ingest, digest, and absorb nutrients, phytochemicals, and other food components; and excrete indigestible components of the food we consume. This organ system also serves as one of the body's largest defenses against pathogens as well as a vehicle for delivery of nutrients and substances that modulate the immune and neurological responses. The following discussion will address each of these roles of the GI system.

Nutrient Intake and Appetite

Appetite is measured collectively in terms of hunger, satiation, and satiety. When the stomach is empty, one would describe the associated sensation as *hunger*. When a person indicates after a meal that he or she may be "full," the sensation of *satiation* is being described. Finally, when one describes the duration with which they feel satiated after a meal, the description is referring to *satiety*.[7]

Blundell and Stubbs have proposed that the physiology of appetite is the physiology of feeding behavior,[1] but an expanded view is described in the following discussion. The physiology of feeding behavior integrates both the physiology of the central nervous system (CNS) and peripheral nervous system with hormone metabolism. The human appetite system is a redundant system, which means there are overlapping subsystems within it, each of which individually may not be necessary for the system to function normally.[1,8] This redundancy allows feeding behavior to vary in terms of meal size, meal frequency, and food composition.

The human appetite system can sense changes in its internal (eg, metabolism of pregnancy) and external (eg, ambient temperature) environments and interacts with other biological systems related to motivation and behavior.[1] A physiological tendency toward overconsumption has evolved and is, therefore, primed to respond to energy and nutrient deficits. The human appetite system exists within an equilibrium of energy balance in which energy intake normally equals energy expenditure, except when body weight increases or decreases to a new equilibrium. Nonetheless, adults in the United States gain an average of 0.2 to 2.0 kg per year.[9]

As previously suggested, food intake normally adjusts to maintain body weight or undo changes in weight. When individuals lose weight because of illness, they often regain weight spontaneously during recovery. Likewise, after individuals intentionally lose weight while on weight-reduction diets, many regain the lost weight. This sort of weight adjustment also occurs in animals.[10]

The triggers that influence food intake include satiety signals and hunger signals. Overconsumption is likely influenced more strongly by hunger signals than satiety signals. The evidence for the influence of hunger signals on food intake relates to data describing the course of prolonged negative energy balance and significant loss of lean body tissue. However, it is not clear whether the hunger signals in prolonged negative energy balance are the same signals that control day-to-day feeding behavior. Data that describe how these signals influence meal size, frequency, and composition are continuing to emerge.[1,11]

Taste is an aspect of food that influences feeding behavior in a way that is distinct from hunger or satiation signals. Whereas textbooks have traditionally stated that certain areas of the tongue have taste buds for 5 specific qualities of food (sweet, salty, sour, bitter, umami), most areas of the tongue can sense all 5 qualities.[12,13] Individuals who experience the most intense taste sensations are called "supertasters." It was once thought that supertasters' extraordinary taste sensations were limited to bitterness, but it is now widely accepted that these individuals perceive unusually strong tastes in general. Supertasters often have strong aversions or preferences for vegetables, sweets, salty food, and alcoholic beverages that differ from the aversions and preferences of nonsupertasters. Accordingly, supertasters may have disease risks that are different from the norm. For example, because supertasters often consume foods that are lower in fat and sugar, they have a reduced risk for cardiovascular disease. Alternatively, the risk for colon cancer may be higher for supertasters because they consume fewer vegetables.[13]

Food intake behavior can be described within 3 phases, each of which is under control of the parasympathetic nervous system: the cephalic phase, the postingestive phase, and the postabsorptive phase. The cephalic phase often is a conditioned response to the sight or smell of food. The postingestive phase mediates satiation signals that are produced by mechanical distention of the gut or the chemical effect of food on gut hormone secretion. Signals mediating the postabsorptive phase are stimulated by nutrient entry into the portal vein or by nutrient concentrations in the plasma or brain.[7]

Neurohormonal Influences on Feeding Responses

Neural and hormonal regulation of GI function is complex. Neuroendocrine cells in the GI tract secrete more than 30 GI hormone peptides.[14] The mechanisms of action of hormone peptides include activity as blood-borne hormones, neurotransmitters, or local growth factors.[14] Neural and hormonal signals that influence food intake are integrated in the brain, primarily in the arcuate nucleus (ARC) of the hypothalamus and the brainstem. In the ARC, orexigenic (appetite-stimulating) cells express the neurotransmitters, neuropeptide Y (NPY) and agouti-related peptide (AgRP), and anorexigenic (appetite-suppressing) cells express proopiomelanocortin (POMC) and cocaine and amphetamine–regulated transcript (CART). POMC is a natural opioid. ARC signals regulate activity in the paraventricular nucleus (PVN) of the hypothalamus.[15] NPY messenger ribonucleic acid increases in the hypothalamus during feeding and decreases during satiety. The effects of NPY may be redundant as gene knock-out animals exhibit no significant changes in feeding.[1]

Major inputs influencing appetite regulation include short-term signals related to meal ingestion that are transmitted by the "gut-brain axis," signals associated with energy stores that are mediated by leptin, and signals deriving from lean body mass. A fourth system influencing appetite regulation is the circadian rhythm, which will not be discussed in this chapter.[15] The gut-brain axis reflects energy balance via a signaling system between the GI tract and the hypothalamus and brainstem. Both neural (vagal) and gut hormones transmit the signals. The major orexigenic gut hormone is ghrelin, and anorexigenic gut hormones include glucagon-like peptide-1 and -2 (GLP-1, GLP-2), oxyntomodulin (OXM), peptide tyrosine-tyrosine (PYY), pancreatic polypeptide (PP), cholecystokinin (CCK), and others.[7,16,17] Gut- and fat-derived hormones—ghrelin, leptin, insulin, and PYY—are involved in feedback regulation of feeding through signals affecting hunger, satiety, and energy needs.[18] POMC and AgRP expression are regulated by insulin and leptin.[19] GLP-1, OXM, and PYY are secreted by the distal gut. PP is secreted by the PP cells of the islet of Langerhans in the pancreas. PYY and PP increase in response to feeding. GLP-1 binds GLP-1 receptors in the pancreatic islet cell, heart, lungs, ARC, and PVN. PYY inhibits NPY and activates POMC. Increased GLP-1, OXM, PYY, and PP all result in decreased food intake. GLP-1 also delays gastric empyting[15] (Table 1-1). Insulin, as well as these gut-derived hormones, affects neural signals in the brain related to acute changes in energy levels. Insulin, along with leptin, inhibits the same neural circuits (dopaminergic) that are stimulated by ghrelin.[18] Ghrelin is a gastric-synthesized polypeptide that stimulates growth hormone secretion and results in increased food intake. Blood levels are decreased when food is eaten and increase during fasting. Ghrelin increases food intake by stimulating the ARC of the hypothalamus.

CCK exerts its effects on appetite by crossing the blood-brain barrier to reduce hypothalamic levels of NPY. The same intestinal cells that produce CCK also produce PYY and a precursor protein to glucagon, GLP-1, GLP-2, OXM, and glicentin. Most of the hormones secreted by these intestinal L cells result in satiation, decreased GI motility, and reduced food

intake and appetite.[14] CCK has been shown to reduce meal size specifically, rather than meal frequency—that is, it seems to be involved in satiation (bringing a meal to an end).[1] PYY has strong effects on satiety and is released in response to energy, glucose, fat, and protein loads. GLP-1 in humans is the strongest stimulator of insulin secretion and decreases gastric emptying.[14] PYY (secreted in the small intestine and colon), gastrin-releasing peptide (GRP), glucagon, somatostatin, and CCK have all been proposed to decrease food intake.[10]

Luminal nutrients or factors often stimulate epithelial cell secretion of gut hormones that trigger vagal responses related to appetite regulation and gastric emptying and secretion. These hormones include CCK, GLP-1, PYY, and 5-hydroxytryptamine (5-HT). For example, luminal glucose stimulates the release of 5-HT.[20] Glucose is also proposed to regulate food intake through its utilization by the neurons in the satiety center. A possible mechanism may be related to low neuronal glucose utilization: when neuronal activity decreases, satiety decreases,

TABLE 1-1 Gut Hormones and Peptides Influencing Food Intake

Hormone	Site of Secretion	Stimulated by	Mechanism of Action	Effect
GLP-1	Distal gut	• Food intake proportional to energy intake	• Binds GLP-1 receptors in pancreatic islet cells, heart, lungs, and brain (ARC and PVC)	• Reduces appetite and energy intake • Delays gastric emptying • Enhances postprandial insulin release
OXM	L cells of the distal gut	• Food intake	• Agonist at glucagon receptor • Undefined neural effects	• Reduces food intake • Increases energy expenditure
PYY	L cells of the distal gut	• Food intake (released in proportion to energy, fat, and protein intake)	• Y receptors found throughout the CNS and on vagal afferents • NPY inhibition • POMC activation • Associated with increased activity of OFC	• Reduces food intake
PP	Pancreatic polypeptide cells of the islets of Langerhans in the pancreas	• Food intake • Vagal stimulation	• Enters CNS via diffusion in the brain stem and ARC	• Reduces food intake
CCK	L cells of the gut, nerves in distal ileum and colon, neurons in the brain	• Dietary protein and fat • Gastric acid	• Reduces hypothalamic NPY	• Inhibits gastric emptying • Reduces food intake
Leptin	Large amounts from the gastric mucosa; white adipose tissue	• Food deprivation is associated with low levels	• Low levels influence ARC • Possibly decreases gene expression of NPY and increases activity of POMC-secreting neurons	• Low levels increase energy intake and decrease energy expenditure
Ghrelin	Stomach	• Food intake decreases levels • Fasting increases levels	• Stimulates ARC via receptors • Stimulates GH secretion	• Increases food intake

ARC, arcuate nucleus; CCK, cholecystokinin; CNS, central nervous system; GH, growth hormone; GLP-1, glucagon-like peptide-1; NPY, neuropeptide Y; OFC, orbitofrontal cortex; OXM, oxyntomodulin; POMC, proopiomelanocortin; PP, pancreatic polypeptide; PVC, paraventricular nucleus; PYY, peptide-tyrosine-tyrosine.

and hunger ensues.[10] *Hunger* can be defined as the intrinsic desire for food. Conversely, when glucose utilization is high, the feeding center is inhibited and hunger abates.[10] A decrease in blood glucose is currently considered to be a biomarker for satiety and signals the onset of meal initiation.[21]

Luminal contents also affect neuronal activity by direct action on vagal afferents and through stretch receptors and nutrient chemoreceptors.[18,20] Examples of these luminal factors include glutamate, SCFAs, and lipopolysaccharide.[20] Vagal signals are channeled through the brain stem and then coordinated with appetite regulation via the ARC. End neural signaling in the brain affects "learning about (food) rewards, attending to food rewards, valuation of stimuli in the environment, processing information about energy stores and gastrointestinal contents. Reward pathways motivate food intake and pleasure associated with eating."[18]

Generally speaking, appetite is regulated in 2 areas of the hypothalamus, a lateral "feeding center" and a medial "satiety center." When the feeding center is stimulated, animals eat. Conversely, when the feeding center is damaged, severe, fatal anorexia can result. When the satiety center is stimulated, animals stop eating. Alternatively, when lesions occur in the satiety center, overeating occurs. Some evidence suggests that the satiety center functions by transiently inhibiting the feeding center after food is ingested.[10] When animals gain weight because of lesions in the satiety center, their intake plateaus (after a period of weight gain) and increased weight is thus maintained.

Leptin is an adipose tissue–derived hormone that acts on the hypothalamus to decrease food intake and increase energy expenditure. It provides feedback on the body's fat stores. Serum leptin levels increase in proportion to percentage of body fat. Leptin was originally found in white adipose tissue, but it is also expressed in a variety of other tissues, including the gastric mucosa, which secretes large amounts.[22] Low levels of leptin associated with food deprivation result in increased energy intake and decreased energy expenditure.[23] The reduction of leptin levels during starvation occurs in obese as well as normal weight individuals.[24] However, in obese individuals, leptin levels affect not only the ARC but also centers of the brain that regulate smell, taste, and learning the rewarding aspects of food.[23] The mechanism for the action of leptin on the ARC is to bind receptors on neurons that coexpress NPY, AgRP, POMC, and CART.[24,25] The net result leads to anorexia and weight loss.[24]

In addition to biological influences on food intake, environmental and cognitive events play major roles in what and when we eat. Factors including convenience, price, nutrition-related beliefs, availability, brand image, and cultural and social influences all serve as determinants of food intake.

Resting Metabolic Rate, Fat-Free Mass, and Appetite

As discussed previously, control of appetite generally involves signals from adipose tissue, GI peptide hormones, and neurohormonal interactions. Recent studies have definitively demonstrated a strong, positive correlation in obese individuals between fat-free mass (which includes water, protein, and mineral components of body composition) and meal size and food intake. Alternatively, fat mass inhibits food intake in lean individuals. These data point to a new frontier in the study of appetite regulation, a frontier that integrates the influence of fat and fat-free mass and resting metabolic rate with GI signals on the control of appetite.[11] The implications of this model of appetite control for hospitalized patients, who often experience significant loss of lean body mass (ie, muscle mass) due to catabolic illness, are unknown.

Dietary Influences on Feeding Responses

Diet composition plays a role in feeding responses. Some research suggests that high-fat diets promote higher energy intake.[26,27] However, other studies have demonstrated increased energy intake when the carbohydrate density of the diet was increased.[28] Still others have shown that an isocaloric meal that is higher in fiber and protein than a control meal results in lower energy intake and decreased hunger scores.[29] Similarly, studies on the effect of sweetness on appetite and the effect of fat on satiety show conflicting results. However, evidence suggests that all 3 major macronutrients exert effects on satiety to different extents. Protein seems to be more satiating than carbohydrate, which is more satiating than fat. In multiple studies, protein has been shown to significantly increase subjective feelings of satiety[30-32] and decrease hunger.[33] Furthermore, certain proteins have been shown to increase satiety more than others. For example, whey protein has had a significantly stronger influence on satiety than casein.[34] A randomized trial with parallel design found that higher protein diets (18% of energy) and associated increased satiety may increase the rate of weight maintenance in humans after they lose 50% of body weight.[35] Despite the variability in research findings, it seems that dietary fat content is a risk factor for weight gain.[1]

While the influences of macronutrients on appetite control are well-established notions, the role of fiber,[36] especially resistant starch (RS2), is becoming clearer. RS2 is found in native starch granules in produce such as maize, raw potatoes, and green bananas. Human dietary studies with RS2 have documented its satiety value with associated decreases in food intake.[37,38] The effect of fiber on appetite was also demonstrated when enteral formula was used as the sole source of nutrition. EN supplemented with pea fiber and FOS resulted in increased satiety and feelings of fullness.[39]

In addition to energy value or nutrient content, food weight and volume can be important variables influencing food intake.[1,40] Gastric distention triggers receptors and vagal afferents, leading to a feeling of fullness and reduced food intake.[40] Weight and volume influence intrameal satiation more than postingestive (between-meal) satiety.[41] Viscosity has an inverse effect on hunger.[42]

Gastric distention, stomach size, and aging also influence food intake. Gastric distention decreases food intake. Contractions of an empty stomach lead to increased food intake. Furthermore, stomach size can also influence the amount of food eaten, and its size is related to the amount of food habitually eaten. For this reason, during nutrition rehabilitation of undernourished patients, small frequent meals should be initiated to increase nutrient intake until a time when patients can increase their food intake comfortably at a single sitting.[1] Under normal circumstances, the stomach delivers metered amounts of nutrients to the duodenum, often on the basis of the amount of energy intake. Subsequently, satiety signals arise from the small intestine as well as the stomach. In fact, the satiating influence of fat is, in part, mediated via signals in the small intestine.[1] This role of the small intestine has been shown specifically when corn oil is infused directly into the jejunum or ileum, bypassing the stomach. Furthermore, products of fat digestion have been shown to influence the development of nausea more than products of carbohydrate or protein digestion do.[40] These findings regarding macronutrient composition, fiber content, food volume, and viscosity may have implications for the design of transitional feeding regimens. When the oral diet is resumed, patient intakes may respond more favorably to food or supplements that are lower in fat or fiber.

Finally, aging is associated with decreased appetite and food intake, probably because of decreased basal hunger rather than increased meal satiety.[43] If the nutrition assessment suggests the need for an enteral supplement, the nutrition support team should consider using a liquid supplement rather than a solid one. In a controlled feeding trial, liquids attenuated postprandial decline in hunger more than solids with resultant higher energy intake.[44]

Pharmacological Interventions to Improve Appetite

Clinicians often need to encourage patients who have decreased appetites associated with illness, surgery, or emotional distress to increase their food intake. In some instances, pharmacological intervention may be offered to stimulate appetite.

Megestrol acetate has been studied in cancer, human immunodeficiency virus infection, and acquired immunodeficiency syndrome (AIDS).[45] However, additional studies may be needed to prove the safety and efficacy of megestrol. The drug has been associated with adverse GI effects (eg, nausea, vomiting, gas, and diarrhea) in 5% of patients with AIDS and 1% to 4% of patients in general.[45] Adverse effects of megestrol have also been documented in other major organ systems (eg, pulmonary, cardiovascular, and genitourinary).[45]

Medical marijuana has been proposed as an appetite stimulant. However, outcome data are conflicting.[46]

Microbiome Influences on Appetite

The human microbiome produces many chemicals, especially SCFAs, that enter the general circulation to reach targets including the enteric nervous system (ENS) and the brain. SCFAs can cross the blood-brain barrier and influence neurotransmitter synthesis.[14] SCFAs also modulate the 5-HT and PYY secretion in the gut. The interaction of the gut microbiome with GI hormones and the brain affects satiety.[14] Interestingly, one way in which fiber (eg, guar gum and FOS) exerts its satiating effects is through CCK.[20]

Gastrointestinal Motility

The assimilation of nutrients occurs as a result of 3 general and distinct processes: (1) the movement of food throughout the GI tract; (2) the digestion of food; and (3) the absorption of nutrients. Each of the structures of the GI tract has specific

functions regarding these 3 processes. The roles of each of the structures of the GI tract are outlined in the following discussion.

Neural and Hormonal Control of Motility

Normal GI motility is important for optimal digestion and absorption. Each section of the GI tract is structured to handle food of a specific physical character and viscosity and has motor activities that support its specialized function. For example, the esophagus transports small chunks of food, whereas the stomach stores, digests, and grinds solid food into small particles and controls the emptying of food into the small bowel. Sphincters separate sections of the GI tract and act as one-way valves in the forward direction. They control both the direction of movement and the amount moved through the GI tract.[47] For example, the lower esophageal sphincter (LES) relaxes in response to swallowing. Between meals, the LES is closed to prevent reflux of gastric contents into the esophagus,[48] which protects the esophageal mucosa from the erosive effects of gastric acid. Chronic acid damage to the esophagus by gastric reflux can result in morphologic changes that, when untreated, can eventually lead to Barrett's esophagus and an increased risk of esophageal cancer. The closed tone of the LES is under neural control.

GI motility follows 2 patterns: one in the interdigestive period and the other in the postprandial period. The interdigestive period involves a 4-phase pattern of contractions referred to as the *migratory motor complex* (MMC). The third phase of the MMC is the phase that propels residual food through the GI tract. In the postprandial phase, continuous contractions propel food through the stomach and small intestine. As the movements of the gut propel food forward through the GI tract, mixing movements combine food with GI secretions (see the "Small Intestine Motility" section later in this chapter for a description of mixing movements). Peristalsis is the basic propulsive movement.[47,49] When the gut wall is stretched by its contents, peristalsis occurs in all parts of the GI tract from the esophagus to rectum. The stretch stimulus causes a release of serotonin leading to smooth muscle contraction.[48] Layers of smooth muscle underlie a layer of connective tissue called the *lamina propria*, which is adjacent to the single layer of epithelial cells lining the luminal walls of the GI tract.[8] Other stimuli for peristalsis are chemical or physical irritation of the epithelial lining of the gut. Strong parasympathetic stimulation leads to strong peristalsis.[49] Peristaltic waves in the esophagus and gastric emptying are stimulated by the vagus nerve.[47]

Myogenic, neural, and hormonal factors regulate GI motility. Myogenic control of GI motility is mediated by smooth muscle. Smooth muscle in the GI tract is normally in a polarized state in which the outside of the cell is positively charged relative to the inside of the cell. Contraction of the muscle is associated with depolarization. Conversely, inhibition of contraction is associated with a hyperpolarized state. The depolarized state results from the transfer of positively charged ions (primarily calcium [Ca^{2+}] with some sodium [Na^+] ions) into the cell, the exit of negatively charged chloride (Cl^-) ions out of the cell, and the inhibition of potassium (K^+) transfer out of the cell. Hyperpolarization, the state of a muscle cell in which its membrane potential is more negative, is accompanied by an increase of K^+ or decrease of Cl^- transfer out of the cell. The hyperpolarized state inhibits Ca^{2+} channels, preventing Ca^{2+} entry into cells. The actions of hormones and neurotransmitters alter intracellular Ca^{2+} concentrations to influence muscle contraction and subsequent GI motility.[47,49]

GI muscle fibers are depolarized in response to (1) stretching of the muscle fiber, (2) acetylcholine released by parasympathetic neurons, and (3) gut hormones. GI muscle fibers are hyperpolarized in response to (1) norepinephrine or epinephrine and (2) sympathetic nerves that secrete norepinephrine.[49]

The neural control of smooth muscle is executed by the ENS, an intrinsic nervous system that innervates the GI tract from the esophagus to anus. The ENS can function autonomously, but it is connected to the CNS via parasympathetic and sympathetic fibers. Generally, the sympathetic nervous system modulates the activity of the ENS with inhibitory signals. The parasympathetic nervous system stimulates motility via the ENS.[8,49]

The ENS is organized into the myenteric (Auerbach's) plexus and the submucosal (Meissner's) plexus. GI movement is controlled by the myenteric plexus. The submucosal plexus controls GI secretions and blood flow. The fibers of the parasympathetic neural network that innervate the esophagus, stomach, pancreas, small intestine, and first half of the large intestine are in the vagus nerve. The sympathetic neural fibers arise from the spinal cord and innervate the entire gut. Norepinephrine is the predominant neurotransmitter secreted by the sympathetic nerve endings.[49]

The neurotransmitters of the ENS include acetylcholine; norepinephrine and serotonin; γ-aminobutyrate; adenosine triphosphate (ATP); nitric oxide (NO) and carbon monoxide (CO); dopamine; CCK; substance P; vasoactive intestinal peptide (VIP); somatostatin; leu-enkephalin; and met-enkephalin.[8,49] Acetylcholine is generally excitatory in action (increases muscular activity), whereas norepinephrine exerts inhibitory effects. Epinephrine, which is secreted by the adrenal medullae, is also inhibitory.[49]

Afferent sensory nerve fibers in the ENS are also involved in the neural control of the gut. Sensory stimuli include irritation of the mucosa, excessive distention, or chemical stimuli. Sensory signals are transmitted to the spinal cord, brain stem, or brain medulla, many via afferent fibers of the vagus nerve. These signals are followed by vagal reflexes to the gut.[49]

Although the predominant role of GI hormones is to regulate GI secretions, GI hormones also influence GI motility. See Table 1-2,[8,14,49,50] which summarizes the actions of intestinal

TABLE 1-2 Gastrointestinal Hormones Affecting Gastrointestinal Secretions and Motility

Hormone	Stimuli for Secretion	Sites of Secretion	Actions
Gastrin	Protein, GI distention, gastric-releasing peptide	G cells of the antrum, duodenum, and jejunum	Stimulates gastric acid secretion and mucosal growth; promotes gastric emptying
Cholecystokinin	Protein, fat, acid	I cells of the duodenum, jejunum, and ileum	Stimulates pancreatic enzyme secretion, gallbladder contraction, and growth of exocrine pancreas; inhibits gastric emptying
Secretin	Acid	S cells of the duodenum, jejunum, and ileum	Stimulates pepsin, pancreatic and biliary bicarbonate secretion, and growth of exocrine pancreas; inhibits gastric emptying and gastric acid secretion
GIP	Protein, fat, carbohydrate	K cells of the duodenum and jejunum	Stimulates insulin release and secretion; inhibits gastric acid secretion and emptying
Motilin	Fat; acid; gastric distention; bile acids; serotonin; low pH in duodenum	M cells of the duodenum and jejunum, stomach, colon	Stimulates gastric motility and intestinal motility
VIP	GI distention	Nerves of the GI tract	Stimulates secretion of electrolytes and water secretion; inhibits gastric acid
Somatostatin	Acid	Pancreas, GI mucosa, hypothalamus	Inhibits secretion of gastrin, VIP, GIP, secretin, motilin, exocrine pancreatic secretion, gallbladder contraction, gastric acid secretion, and gastric motility
Serotonin (5-HT)	Luminal contents including glucose and SCFAs, GI distention	Nerve fibers of the enteric nervous system	Increases intestinal motility
PYY	Fat	Jejunum	Inhibits gastric acid secretion and gastric motility

5-HT, 5-hydroxytryptamine; GI, gastrointestinal; GIP, gastric inhibitory peptide; PYY, peptide-tyrosine-tyrosine; SCFA, short-chain fatty acid; VIP, vasoactive intestinal peptide.
Source: Data are from references 8, 14, 49, and 50.

hormones, their stimuli for secretion, and the sites of secretion. The actions include modulating gastric emptying and the rate of small intestinal transit.[49]

Gastric Motility

To understand the stomach's role in motility, digestion, and absorption, it is helpful to review relevant aspects of its anatomy and physiology (Figure 1-1). The cardia is the portion of the stomach just distal to the esophagus. Located between the esophagus and the stomach is the LES. At the distal end of the stomach, the pyloric sphincter is positioned between the stomach and the duodenum. The fundus is the uppermost portion of the stomach. Above the fundus is the diaphragm. The body of the stomach begins at the horizontal plane of the junction between the stomach and esophagus, the gastroesophageal junction. The antrum, the lower 25% to 30% of the stomach, begins where the lesser curvature of the stomach turns to the right.[2]

The motor functions of the stomach make significant contributions to digestion of food. These contributions include storing food, mixing food with gastric secretions, and emptying the semifluid mixture (chyme) into the duodenum.[51] Gastric tone is regulated in multiple ways. Intragastric pressure falls in response to the vagal nerve–mediated swallowing reflex and in response to gastric distention by the presence of food. The latter is accomplished by stretch receptors in the gastric wall. Biochemical mediators of proximal gastric relaxation principally include NO and VIP in addition to dopamine, gastrin, CCK, secretin, GRP, and glucagon. Decreases in gastric tone result from duodenal distention, colonic distention, and ileal perfusion with glucose.[2,43] A relaxed stomach can accommodate a volume of 0.8 to 1.5 liters. Mixing waves of constriction lead into powerful peristaltic waves that propel the chyme

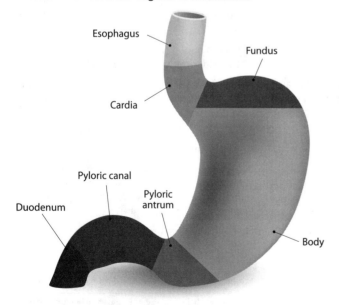

FIGURE 1-1 Anatomical Regions of the Stomach

Esophagus
Fundus
Cardia
Pyloric canal
Pyloric antrum
Duodenum
Body

Credit: Stock illustration ID:467010940. iStock.com/ttsz.

toward the pylorus, which ultimately leads to intense peristalsis in the stomach antrum and subsequent gastric emptying.[51]

Gastric emptying is regulated by the volume of food, gastrin, enteric gastric nervous reflexes from the duodenum, ghrelin (secreted by the stomach and duodenum),[14] and hormonal feedback from the duodenum. Increased food volume leads to increased gastric distention, the release of gastrin, and the reduction of ghrelin. Gastrin has an independent effect on stimulating gastric emptying as well as intestinal motility, while ghrelin's stimulatory effects on gastric emptying are reduced.[14,52] Three types of inhibitory reflexes arise from the duodenum: (1) from the ENS, (2) from the sympathetic neural fibers, and (3) from the inhibitory fibers of the vagus nerve. These inhibitory reflexes are stimulated by (1) duodenal distention, (2) irritation of the duodenal mucosa, (3) pH less than 3.5 or 4.0, (4) high osmolality, and (5) the presence of breakdown products of protein and fat digestion.[51]

Hormonal feedback from the duodenum has an inhibitory effect on gastric emptying. Dietary fat is the strongest stimulus for hormones of the duodenum and jejunum (eg, CCK). These intestinal hormones act specifically on the pyloric pump and pyloric sphincter. Other probable hormones inhibiting gastric emptying include secretin and gastric inhibitory peptide (GIP).[51]

The tone of proximal stomach influences liquid emptying, whereas the distal stomach is involved in solid emptying. Liquids empty more quickly than solids.[53] The average half-emptying time of water or isotonic saline is 12 minutes. In other words, if one drinks 300 mL of water, 150 mL will enter the duodenum in about 12 minutes (range 10 to 65 minutes).[53] The emptying time for liquids changes when the composition of the liquid changes. The rate of emptying amounts to about 200 kcal/h for liquids up to 1 molar concentration. Duodenal osmoreceptors, secretin, and VIP regulate liquid emptying. The half-emptying time of solids is about 45 to 110 minutes.[53] The rate of solids emptying is influenced significantly by meal particle size, energy content, and fat content.[28] As mentioned previously, the swallowing reflex influences gastric tone. When the swallowing mechanism is bypassed, as in nasogastric (NG) tube feeding, the rate of gastric emptying is faster.

Gastric motility can influence positioning of nasoduodenal tubes. Often the goal during nasoduodenal intubation for enteral feeding is for peristalsis of the stomach to carry the tube tip through the pylorus. In situations in which the tip fails to pass, prokinetic agents may be used to increase gastric emptying. Because the duodenal mucosa possesses sensory receptors that are associated with neurohumoral reflexes that influence gastric emptying, gastric emptying time after feeding tube placement may decrease significantly if feeding tubes are placed in the jejunum, bypassing the duodenum.[47]

Meal nutrient composition influences the rate of gastric emptying. Emptying may be slowed by increasing the energy content, fat content, viscosity, fiber content, or osmolality of a meal.[2,4] These effects are mediated by duodenal osmoreceptors, glucoreceptors, and pH receptors via neurohumoral routes.[2,4] Consideration of these factors may be useful in planning medical nutrition therapy for patients who experience nausea (an unpleasant sensation felt in the upper abdomen that is associated with the desire to vomit[54]). Limiting foods high in fat or fiber is recommended to reduce nausea associated with cancer.[3] Carbohydrate-rich foods leave the stomach in a few hours; protein-rich foods empty later; fat is the slowest macronutrient to empty.[48]

Small Intestine Motility

The amount of chyme that enters the intestine from the stomach is determined by feedback inhibition signaled by duodenal distention, acidity, osmolar changes, and the presence of products of carbohydrate, protein, and fat digestion. Movements of the small intestine can be characterized as mixing contractions and propulsive contractions. Mixing contractions (also known as *segmentation contractions*) are elicited when the small intestine is distended by chyme. Segmentation contractions promote a bidirectional flow of chyme, which allows chyme to mix with pancreatic, intestinal, and biliary digestive juices and prolongs its contact with intestinal cells in order for absorption to occur. Typically, the rate of mixing contractions is 2 or 3 per minute or maximally 12 per minute. Propulsive movements of the small intestine (peristalsis) move in the direction of the anus at a rate of 0.5 to 2.0 cm/sec. Hence, the average time that it takes for chyme to travel from the pylorus to the ileocecal valve is 3 to 5 hours.[51]

Intestinal peristalsis is regulated by neural and hormonal controls. Neural control is partly initiated when chyme stretches the intestinal wall. Additionally, when the stomach is stretched, a gastroenteric reflex initiates intestinal peristalsis.[51,52]

Hormonal control of intestinal peristalsis includes both inhibitory and stimulatory signals. The stimulatory hormones include gastrin, CCK, insulin, motilin, and serotonin. Inhibitory hormones include secretin and glucagon.[51] When chyme reaches the end of the terminal ileum, its passage into the cecum is metered by constrictions of the ileocecal sphincter. After a meal, peristalsis increases in the ileum in response to a gastroileal reflex. The volume of chyme that empties into the cecum is approximately 1500 to 2000 mL/d.[51]

Colorectal Motility

The motor activities of the colon mix, store, concentrate, and eliminate food residues. The ascending colon receives liquid contents through the ileocecal valve. The ileocecal valve prevents backflow of fecal contents into the small intestine. As food residues move through the transverse colon to the descending colon, luminal contents become more solid.[47] This fact has implications for understanding the consistency of stool in ascending colostomies vs descending colostomies. The stool from an ascending colostomy is likely to be more liquid than stool from a descending colostomy. As in the stomach and the small intestine, the movements of the colon are mixing and propulsive movements. The mixing movements of the colon result in maximum exposure of feces to the mucosal surface, allowing absorption of fluid and other substances. This concentrating action of the colon results in expulsion of only 80 to 200 mL feces daily. Chyme requires as many as 8 to 15 hours to move from the ileocecal valve through the colon.[51]

Mass movements from the cecum to the sigmoid colon occur 1 to 3 times daily, and are most common during the first hour after eating breakfast. Mass movements occur in response to distention of the stomach and duodenum, which trigger gastrocolic and duodenocolic reflexes. These contractions may occur with or without defecation.[51] Normally, the rectum is empty. Mass movements in the colon propel food residue into the rectum. Distention of the rectum results in the urge to defecate with associated reflex relaxation of the internal and external anal sphincters. Both sphincters contract under voluntary control.[38] In addition, gastric distention by food can stimulate rectal relaxation (gastrocolic reflex) and, subsequently, the urge to defecate.[47,51] The normal frequency for bowel movements in developed countries is every 1 to 3 days.[47]

The motility of the colon is more complex than the motility of the small intestine. A variety of contractions occur and controlled by colonic MMC and nonmigrating motor complexes. Colon surgery can disrupt neural plexus, and colon motility is the last to recover following GI surgery.

Abnormalities of Gastrointestinal Motility

Small Bowel Obstruction

Motility of the small bowel is often prohibited by mechanical obstruction or postoperative ileus. Each year, small bowel obstructions caused by adhesions associated with previous abdominal surgeries (including GI and gynecological procedures) lead to more than 300,000 hospitalizations.[55] Intraabdominal adhesions account for up to 75% of cases of small bowel obstruction. Management of this condition is discussed in Practice Scenario 1-1.[56,57]

Practice Scenario 1-1

Question: What medical nutrition therapy should be offered to a patient who has reobstruction of the small intestine after surgery (lysis of adhesions) for small bowel obstruction?

Scenario: A 59-year-old man was in a normal state of health until he presented acutely with a history of vomiting, abdominal distention, and hyperactive bowel sounds. He was 170 cm tall and weighed 80 kg. Laboratory findings suggested hypovolemia, hemoconcentration, and electrolyte abnormalities. Past medical history included surgical reduction of an umbilical hernia 5 years prior to admission. Physical examination provided no evidence of hernias in the inguinal or femoral areas, and stools were negative for gross or occult blood. An abdominal series showed dilated small bowel loops greater than 3 cm, air-fluid levels, and limited air in the colon. A computed tomography scan documented findings of a discrete transition zone with dilation of bowel proximally, decompression of bowel distally, intraluminal contrast that did not pass beyond the transition zone, and a colon with only a small amount of gas or fluid. A diagnosis of small bowel obstruction was made. Isotonic intravenous fluids and prophylactic broad-spectrum antibiotics were started. The stomach was decompressed via nasogastric (NG) tube. On hospital Day 4 the patient underwent an exploratory laparotomy with lysis of adhesions. Postoperatively, his NG tube output increased to 1500 mL, and he redeveloped abdominal distention.

Intervention: The patient was kept on bowel rest and *nil per os* (NPO), and on hospital Day 7 he was assessed for parenteral nutrition (PN).

Answer: Given the patient's normal nutrition status on admission, the best nutrition intervention is no initial intervention. After surgery, the stomach and colon may normally require approximately 48 hours for the return of peristalsis and bowel function. The small bowel takes less time for peristalsis to return (24 hours on average).[56] However, this patient had increasing abdominal distention and increased NG tube output, suggesting reobstruction of the small intestine. Obstruction in the early postoperative period occurs in 0.7% of patients.[56] Given that the patient's period of NPO extended beyond 7 days, PN was appropriate to decrease risk of malnutrition-associated complications.[57]

Rationale: Ideally, when feasible, oral nutrition or enteral nutrition (EN) should be provided postoperatively within 24 hours of surgery for optimal patient outcomes. Failure to initiate EN in the immediate postoperative period can delay return of bowel function. To promote tolerance of oral intake or EN, patient management should include adequate resuscitation and optimal management of fluids, electrolytes, acid-base balance, and glucose control. The enteral route was not feasible in this patient because of the continued obstruction. PN would not have been the best option during the initial period of NPO, because PN has been associated higher infection morbidity in previously well-nourished patients compared with standard care. In a previously well-nourished patient, PN should be considered only after 7 days of NPO. (See Chapter 14.)

Postoperative Ileus

Postoperative ileus, the temporary loss of GI motility,[58] is the most common cause of delayed discharge after abdominal surgery. Although ileus is a common complication of abdominal surgery, it can also accompany infection and inflammation, electrolyte imbalances, and the use of certain drugs (especially sedatives, opioid analgesics, α_2-adrenergic receptor agonists, and catecholamine vasopressors). Potential etiologies or contributing factors include opiate use, sympathetic hyperactivity, altered spinal-intestinal neural reflexes, changes in hormone expression and secretion, hypomagnesemia, hypokalemia, and local and systemic inflammation. Symptoms include nausea, vomiting, abdominal distention, and delayed passage of flatus and stool. On average, after abdominal surgery, the small intestine regains peristalsis within 24 hours (or sooner), and motility of the stomach and colon returns between 48 and 72 hours.[56] Because motility resumes quickly within the small bowel, early EN can often be initiated successfully within 6 hours after surgery.[49] Treatment of ileus includes NG suction, intravenous fluids and electrolytes, and minimal use of sedatives.[59] In some situations, transpyloric feeding may be feasible. PN is warranted if EN is not possible for 7 days.[57]

Chronic Intestinal Pseudo-Obstruction

Chronic intestinal pseudo-obstruction (CIP) is a motility disorder of peristalsis. CIP most often affects the small bowel, but it can occur at any point in the GI tract.[60] CIP has been classified as primary, secondary, or idiopathic with 3 histological types: neuropathies, myopathies, and mesenchymopathies. Secondary causes of CIP include collagen vascular and endocrine diseases, neurologic diseases, medication-related effects, and a wide variety of other diseases and conditions.[60] Colonic pseudo-obstructions can develop in patients as a complication of narcotic use, bed rest, or disease. Mechanical obstruction is absent in pseudo-obstruction, but the presence of a massively dilated bowel can prevent normal bowel function. Treatment includes fluid and electrolyte management, nutrition rehabilitation, treatment of infections, symptom management (nausea, pain, vomiting, and bloating), and discontinuation of narcotics, anticholinergics, or other medications that are associated with ileus.

Symptoms of CIP depend on the area of the GI tract that is affected. Pain is often chronic. Decompression of the distended sections of the GI tract with intermittent NG suction, rectal tubes, or endoscopy may be necessary.[60] Some patients require a decompressive gastrostomy or small intestinal resections.[56] CIP can predispose patients to small intestinal bacterial overgrowth (SIBO) with associated diarrhea and steatorrhea.[60,61] Colonic CIP may lead to significant constipation. Treatment of CIP often consists of palliation of symptoms including nausea and vomiting with antiemetics and/or prokinetics,[60] provision of intravenous hydration or PN, nocturnal cyclic EN when possible, and, when necessary, withholding of oral intake of food. For patients who can consume an oral diet (which is the preferred mode of nutrition), small, frequent meals that are low in fat and fiber are recommended, as well as emphasis on liquid forms of energy and protein.[60] A daily vitamin and mineral supplement should be recommended, and if the patient has SIBO, emphasis should be placed on fat-soluble and B_{12} vitamins. Elemental diets with medium-chain triglycerides (MCTs) may be considered if the patient does not tolerate polymeric nutrients. Because of the progressive nature of CIP, many patients require PN.[60] Patients who develop severe complications of PN may be considered for small bowel transplantation.[60]

Diarrhea

Diarrhea, which refers to an increased frequency and liquidity of stool, can be defined many ways.[62] The most common definitions are 2 to 3 liquid stools or more than 250 mL liquid stool per day.[57] The discharge of diarrhea can be explosive, nocturnal, bacterial, viral, protozoan, osmotic, bloody, chronic, acute, voluminous, fatty, or secretory. Etiologies can range from infection to malabsorption.[63] Watery diarrhea can occur with fecal impaction or obstructing tumor.[64] Antibiotic-associated diarrhea (AAD) is very common in patients taking antibiotics.[65] A recent meta-analysis of AAD treated with probiotics suggests that use of probiotics reduced risk of AAD in adults but not in elderly people. Patients with *Clostridium difficile* infections were excluded in this study.[65] See Chapter 4 for further discussion of probiotic use.

With diarrhea, when transit time is rapid, large amounts of sodium, potassium, and water pass through the colon, which may lead to severe fluid and electrolyte abnormalities, fluid loss, dehydration, hypovolemia, and, if untreated, hypovolemic shock and cardiovascular collapse.[48] Other serious consequences of diarrhea include increased risk of pressure ulcers, compromised nutrition status, and increased length of hospital stay.[62]

When evaluating diarrhea, a left shift with increased white blood cells (WBCs) on a complete blood count may indicate an infectious process. Decreased hemoglobin may indicate anemia from blood loss. Serum sodium and blood urea nitrogen may be increased from dehydration, and serum sodium and serum potassium may be decreased due to losses. Blood pH may reflect an acidosis related to hyperchloremia or alkalosis related to dehydration. Stool cultures should be ordered to rule out infectious etiologies, and tests for *C. difficile* toxins A and B should be ordered if the patient had received antibiotics or chemotherapy in recent weeks. Sigmoidoscopy is indicated with bloody diarrhea or when PMC or ulcerative colitis is suspected. PMC refers to the intestinal inflammation that is accompanied by presence of pseudomembranes on the intestinal mucosa.[66] Most cases of PMC involve the colon (the small intestine is rarely involved), and all cases are related to *C. difficile* infection. The etiology of up to 20% of cases of AAD is *C. difficile* infection.[67]

Symptoms of PMC include diarrhea, abdominal pain, fever, elevated WBC count, and history of recent use of antibiotics. PMC can lead to life-threatening colitis, which can progress to toxic megacolon and subsequent perforation.[68] When abdominal pain is present or obstruction is suspected, imaging studies may include abdominal radiographs to screen for toxic megacolon and bowel ischemia.[64] Antiperistaltic agents should be used with caution in patients suspected of having infectious diarrhea or antibiotic-associated colitis.[64] With infectious diarrhea, slowing GI motility may increase risk for bacterial translocation. For severe or refractory diarrhea, bowel rest may be recommended.

Evidence-based diet recommendations for infectious diarrhea have not been established, especially in individuals who have severe dysmotility. However, anecdotal information suggests initial refeeding with caffeine-free clear liquids advanced to a low-lactose, low-fat, low-fiber diet. As diarrhea resolves, foods may be added back according to individual tolerances. Oral rehydration fluids may be used to restore fluid and electrolyte balance and control diarrhea. The World Health Organization has published a standard recipe for an oral rehydration solution: 2.6 g NaCl, 13.5 g anhydrous glucose, 1.5 g potassium chloride, 2.9 g trisodium citrate, and 1 liter water.[69] Commercial rehydration solutions as well as homemade recipes using commercial sport drinks (eg, Gatorade) and salt or salt and sugar are also options. Intravenous fluids should be provided if oral intake is less than estimated fluid needs. PN should be reserved for patients who do not tolerate an oral diet or EN. The use of probiotics with lactobacilli or as yogurt with live cultures has been suggested when diarrhea is related to antibiotic therapy, but safety data may be lacking. Some have recommended banana flakes, apple powder, or other pectin sources to thicken the consistency of stools.[70] See Practice Scenario 1-2 for an example of medical nutrition therapy for PMC.

Practice Scenario 1-2

Question: What enteral medical nutrition therapy would you offer to a patient with severe diarrhea related to *Clostridium difficile* pseudomembranous colitis (PMC)?

Scenario: A 56-year-old man was admitted to the hospital for evaluation of crampy abdominal pain and severe diarrhea. The patient had a history of chronic immunosuppression following renal transplantation 3 years prior to admission, gastroesophageal reflux disease, and dyslipidemia. His medications included prednisone, tacrolimus, mycophenolate mofetil, and ranitidine. For 4 weeks prior to admission, he was diagnosed with sinusitis and treated with a 10-day course of oral trimethoprim-sulfamethoxazole. Several days after completion of his antibiotic, the patient developed crampy abdominal pain and fever. He reported 10 to 12 watery stools per day without blood or mucus. On admission, he had a temperature of 102°F, moderate right-lower quadrant tenderness, and a white blood cell count of 27,000 cells/mcL; a stool gram stain showed many leukocytes and fecal flora. A computed tomography scan showed right colon thickening but no abscess. Stool specimens for enteric pathogens and *C. difficile* toxins were obtained, and empiric therapy with 500 mg metronidazole orally every 6 hours and 250 mg levofloxacin intravenously every 24 hours was begun. A colonoscopy was performed to evaluate for cytomegalovirus or other opportunistic causes of colitis, and it showed numerous whitish plaques and friable erythematous mucosa consistent with PMC. All subsequent stool cultures for enteric pathogens and viruses were negative. Colon biopsies were negative for viral inclusions. *C. difficile* toxins were found in stool. A diagnosis of *C. difficile* PMC was made, levofloxacin was discontinued, and therapy was switched from oral metronidazole to 125 mg vancomycin orally every 6 hours. Nutrition assessment data included body mass index, 28; percentage of weight loss after rehydration with intravenous fluids, 3% in 1 month; and percentage of usual body weight, 97%. Electrolytes had normalized by the time the nutrition assessment was done.

Intervention: The patient was kept *nil per os* until the diarrhea improved on the vancomycin therapy, about 4 days.

Answer: The patient was started on caffeine-free clear liquids and was advanced to a low-lactose, low-fat, low-fiber diet.

Rationale: While evidence-based diet recommendations for PMC diarrhea have not been established, the goal is to initiate nutrition through the gastrointestinal (GI) tract as early as possible to limit gut mucosa atrophy. Caffeine-free clear liquids are recommended initially to eliminate the stimulatory effects of caffeine on GI motility. A low-lactose, low-fat, low-fiber diet addresses likely transient nutrient intolerances associated with suspected loss of brush border enzymes related to diarrhea. American Society for Parenteral and Enteral Nutrition guidelines do not support the use of supplemental fiber in patients with *C. difficile* diarrhea. Intravenous fluids should be provided if oral fluid intake does not keep up with losses. Parenteral nutrition would not be offered to this patient because he was not severely malnourished on admission and nutrient intake could be resumed in fewer than 7 days. Probiotics may be supplemented as lactobacillus or as yogurt with live cultures, but the evidence base for this practice is weak.

Soluble fermentable fiber is recommended as an addition to standard enteral formula to control noninfectious diarrhea when other causes have been ruled out. Colonic bacteria ferment fibers (eg, FOS, inulin, pectin, guar gum, psyllium) to form SCFAs. SCFAs, particularly butyrate, are the major energy sources for colonocytes. SCFAs help to control diarrhea by stimulating the uptake of water and electrolytes by colonocytes.[57] Furthermore, fiber slows gastric emptying and binds bile acids. Additional clinical studies are needed to delineate the specific benefits of fiber supplementation in enterally fed patients with diarrhea.[4,71] Current American Society for Parenteral and Enteral Nutrition (ASPEN) guidelines support the use of soluble fiber–containing or small peptide formulations in enterally fed patients with noninfectious diarrhea who are hemodynamically stable.[57] These guidelines also state that insoluble fiber should be avoided in critically ill patients. In patients who are at risk for bowel ischemia, both soluble and insoluble fiber should be avoided.[57] See Chapter 13 for a full discussion of the evaluation and management of diarrhea in patients receiving EN.

Gastroparesis

Gastroparesis refers to a pathological delay in gastric emptying in the absence of obstruction. Its symptoms include fullness after eating and early satiety, and it is often associated with nausea, vomiting, bloating, and abdominal pain. At times, symptoms can result in inadequate nutrient intake. The causes of gastroparesis include diabetes mellitus (at least 25% of cases[72]), complications of surgery, renal disease, collagen disease, drugs, malignancy, hypothyroidism, and possible idiopathic reasons.[72] The autonomic neuropathy of prolonged uncontrolled diabetes results in gastroparesis that may affect 50% of patients with diabetes, with a smaller percentage of these patients reporting symptoms. Controlling blood glucose in patients with diabetic gastroparesis is challenging, with the potential of resultant diabetic ketoacidosis or hypoglycemia.

A nuclear medicine gastric emptying study is the test of choice for diagnosing gastroparesis as well as for assessing response to treatment. Prokinetic agents such as metoclopramide[73] and domperidone can alleviate gastroparesis as well as symptoms of nausea. Low-dose erythromycin can also be used as a promotility agent.[73]

Postsurgical gastroparesis occurs in 2% to 3% of cases after surgeries for gastric outlet obstruction or vagotomy. When medical treatments fail, surgical intervention (a near-total gastrectomy and Roux-en-Y gastrojejunostomy) is offered. Practice Scenario 1-3 addresses a patient who has failed dietary intervention for diabetic gastroparesis.[74]

Practice Scenario 1-3

Question: What nutrition intervention is recommended for a patient with gastroparesis who has failed to respond to dietary interventions?

Scenario: A 42-year-old man was admitted with nausea, vomiting, and abdominal pain. He had a 25-year history of type 1 diabetes, diabetic retinopathy, and gastroparesis previously confirmed by a solid-phase nuclear medicine gastric emptying scan. He also had a history of peripheral neuropathy and reflux esophagitis. His diabetes was treated with lispro insulin. Other medications included 20 mg famotidine twice daily. He had been treated with a low-fat, low-fiber diet and promotility agents including metoclopramide. In the previous year, he had 5 similar admissions. On admission, he was made *nil per os* (NPO) to control vomiting, which was exacerbated by eating. Nutrition assessment data included weight, 70 kg; body mass index, 22; and percentage of weight loss, 5% in 6 months. Electrolytes and hemoglobin were concentrated and suggestive of dehydration. While the patient was NPO, his elevated blood glucose was addressed with sliding-scale insulin. His glycated hemoglobin (A1C) was 7.6%, indicating less than optimal glucose control.

Intervention: Intravenous feedings were initiated, and a nasogastric (NG) tube was placed to suction. When the patient demonstrated low NG tube output, a duodenal feeding tube was placed under fluoroscopy. The tip was positioned in the second portion of the duodenum. A 1 kcal/mL enteral standard feeding formula was initiated at 20 mL/h and advanced every 12 hours by 20 mL/h increments to a goal of 1.3-times basal energy expenditure and 1.2 g protein per kg body weight. Serum electrolytes with magnesium and phosphorus were obtained daily to monitor for refeeding syndrome. The patient was transitioned to a trial of cycled nighttime feedings and demonstrated good tolerance of this regimen with no evidence of abdominal distention, nausea, or vomiting.

Answer: The patient was offered the option of a percutaneous endoscopic jejunostomy tube placement for long-term intestinal feedings at night. An oral diet of small amounts of low-fat, low-fiber foods with liquids as tolerated was recommended to address his desire to eat. Given that lispro is a short-acting insulin, a longer-acting insulin was ordered to control glucose levels during nighttime feedings.

Rationale: The clinical history indicated that this patient was an oral diet failure. His good response to nighttime, cycled intestinal feedings suggested that he could be a candidate for a jejunostomy tube for long-term feeding. Jejunal feedings bypass the stomach and obviate the potential of formula intolerance associated with delayed gastric emptying.[74] The recommendation of small amounts of low-fat, low-fiber foods taken with fluids may be made to address psychosocial need to eat.

Dietary treatments for gastroparesis include small, frequent meals, drinking fluids with meals, limiting dietary fat and fiber,[75] maintaining good glucose control, and, when necessary, feeding past the pylorus. Guidelines for the treatment of gastroparesis recommend consultation with a dietitian and frequent intake of small meals that are low in fat and soluble fiber.[73]

Constipation

Constipation is a group of syndromes characterized by infrequent and/or difficult bowel movements (eg, frequency of fewer than 3 bowel movements per week, hard stools, excessive straining, prolonged time spent on the toilet, a sense of incomplete evacuation, and abdominal discomfort or bloating). Risk factors include advanced age, low-fiber and low-fluid diet, sedentary lifestyle, and polypharmacy (especially drugs with anticholinergic effects such as antidepressants, narcotics, antipsychotics; calcium and aluminum antacids; and calcium channel blockers). Conditions that are associated with constipation include diabetes mellitus, hypothyroidism, hypercalcemia, dehydration, neurologic disorders, anorectal disease, and collagen vascular/muscular diseases.[76] Treatment includes gradually increasing fiber in the diet to 25 to 30 g/d, with the fiber goal individualized to an amount that promotes regularity. Fluids should be provided orally (up to 1.5 to 2.0 L/d[77,78]) or via PN or tube feedings and flushes. (See Chapter 7 for more information on fluids.) When nonpharmacological approaches fail, first-line medication treatments are the hydrophilic colloids (psyllium, bran methylcellulose, and polycarbophil), stool softeners, and osmotic laxatives (polyethylene glycol, lactulose, sorbitol, and magnesium salts). Second-line medications include stimulants (senna/docusate, bisacodyl/docusate, or casanthranol/docusate) and lubricants (mineral oil). Mineral oil has the disadvantages of binding fat-soluble vitamins and, if aspiration occurs, could cause a lipoid pneumonia.[76] When constipation is severe, osmotic laxatives may sometimes be combined with suppositories or enemas to loosen stools from a proximal as well as a distal approach.

Dumping Syndrome

Dumping syndrome is a group of symptoms that develop after gastric surgery and are related to increased gastric emptying following vagotomy and bypass or destruction of the pylorus. Dumping syndrome can also occur with too rapid infusion of EN through a small-bore feeding tube. Dumping syndrome is accompanied by both GI symptoms and vasomotor symptoms. GI symptoms include a feeling of fullness after eating, crampy abdominal pain, nausea, vomiting, and explosive diarrhea. Vasomotor symptoms include diaphoresis, weakness, dizziness, flushing, and palpitations. Weight loss and food fear may develop. Symptoms can be classified as early or late dumping. Early is defined as within 30 to 60 minutes of eating. Late occurs 2 to 3 hours after eating and usually is limited to vasomotor symptoms. GI symptoms are related to the rapid emptying of hyperosmolar chyme into the small intestine from the stomach, eliciting an osmotic diuresis into the intestinal lumen and subsequent distention. Vasomotor symptoms are related to the rapid delivery of glucose to the upper small intestine, which results in peripheral and splanchnic vasodilation. Rapid delivery of glucose to the small

intestine precipitates an increased serum insulin release followed by hypoglycemia and vasomotor symptoms. Dietary modification (see subsequent discussion) controls dumping in most patients. Octreotide, a somatostatin analogue, may be used in patients with severe dumping or in those in whom dietary treatment fails to slow intestinal transit time.[79]

Dietary treatment of dumping syndrome involves slow introduction of solid food, elimination of simple sugars, frequent small meals, and no liquids with meals. Patients are advised to lie down after eating and consider adding functional fibers to delay gastric emptying. The initial postoperative clear liquid diet should not include simple sugars. Dairy products should be restricted initially because temporary lactose intolerance may occur. Liquid multivitamin/multimineral supplements and vitamin B_{12} injections may be warranted in patients who have undergone a gastric resection.[79]

Enhanced Recovery After Surgery Protocols and Gastrointestinal Motility

Enhanced Recovery After Surgery (ERAS) protocols for perioperative care are relatively new approaches that aim to enable early mobilization and feeding and ultimately improve nutrition status and decrease length of stay after surgery.[80] ERAS protocols are usually multimodal in their design and may include preoperative exercise, smoking and alcohol cessation, minimal starvation, oral preoperative carbohydrate intake, preoperative antibiotics, intraoperative management strategies, and early EN and mobilization postoperatively, among other interventions.[81] In a study by Boelens et al, early oral intake or EN reduced the incidence of ileus and facilitated the return to normal GI motility.[82] In this study, the primary endpoint was first defecation. Others have argued that a more meaningful endpoint may be diet tolerance, because that is a common discharge criterion.[49] See Chapter 24 for a more detailed discussion of ERAS protocols.

Gastrointestinal Secretions

Before a comprehensive discussion of digestion and absorption can be commenced, a thorough understanding of GI secretions must be established. Secretions in the GI tract serve 2 primary functions: to supply digestive enzymes and to supply lubricating mucus. Mucus facilitates passage of food through the GI tract and prevents damage to the mucosa. GI secretions are often stimulated by the presence of food, which in turn stimulates the ENS and autonomic nervous system. Likewise, GI hormones contribute to the regulation of volume and type of secretions.[83]

Saliva

Digestion begins in the mouth, and the role of saliva is a topic of ongoing investigation. Saliva is secreted by parotid, submandibular, and sublingual glands. It includes mucin for lubrication and ptyalin (α-amylase), an enzyme for starch digestion, as well as immunoglobulin A (IgA) and lysozyme from protection against oral bacteria.[8,83] Additional components of saliva that may play a role in innate immunity include histamines, defensins, cytokines, growth factors, hormones, and mucins. Saliva has important antibacterial, antiviral, and antifungal roles; for these reasons, anticipation of the clinical consequences of conditions that result in low saliva production may be important.[24]

Humans secrete approximately 1000 to 1500 mL/d.[8] Regulation of saliva secretion is primarily under parasympathetic control.[8,24,83] Saliva is secreted in response to food in the mouth, stomach, or upper intestine. Conditioned secretion occurs with the sight, smell, and thought of food.[8,83]

Stretch and chemical receptors mediate the stimulatory influences of saliva in the stomach via parasympathetic neurons that end on parietal cells. Additionally, the salivary glands are innervated by nerve fibers that contain substance P and VIP, which regulate saliva secretion. Substance P and VIP work together with leptin, ghrelin, NPY, AgRP, and CCK to modulate salivation.[24] Hyposalivation, which often occurs in obesity via increased leptin and decreased ghrelin, can lead to alterations in taste perception, chewing and swallowing problems, and intolerance of spicy foods. Consequentially, it can encourage dietary choices that compromise nutrition status and increase the risk for dental plaque and periodontal disease. Dental hygiene and topical fluoride treatments are especially critical for patients with low saliva production.[24] In addition to obese patients, populations at risk for xerostomia include older adults, patients with Sjogren's syndrome, those undergoing radiotherapy or chemotherapy for cancer, and those with hormone disorders and infections.[24,84] Saliva stimulants and substitutes as well as topical treatments have been proposed as interventions for dry mouth.[84]

Gastric Secretions

Each day, the gastric glands secrete approximately 2500 mL of gastric secretions, which include hydrochloric acid. Gastric secretions derive from mucus-secreting cells, oxyntic glands (gastric glands), and pyloric glands.[83] Mucus is secreted to protect the gastric lining and duodenum from hydrochloric acid.[2] Oxyntic glands are made up of 3 kinds of cells: mucus-producing cells; peptic (or chief) cells, which secrete pepsinogen and gastric lipase; and parietal cells, which secrete hydrogen chloride (HCl) and intrinsic factor.[8,83] Parietal cells are located in the body and fundus.[8,83] The hydrogen potassium ATPs in the membranes of parietal cells pump the hydrogen ion (H^+) against its concentration gradient. When these cells are stimulated, more hydrogen potassium ATPs move to the cell membrane where H^+ is exchanged for K^+. The pH of the gastric acid is approximately 0.8.[83]

Intrinsic factor, required for the absorption of vitamin B_{12}, is secreted by the same cells that secrete HCl. Therefore, when the parietal cells of the stomach are destroyed (as in chronic gastritis), achlorhydria (the absence of acid) develops in addition to pernicious anemia and vitamin B_{12} deficiency caused by loss of intrinsic factor.[2]

Biochemical stimulants for acid secretion are gastrin, histamine via H_2 receptors, and acetylcholine released by parasympathetic stimulation. Gastrin is secreted in the antrum of the stomach in response to the presence of luminal oligopeptides, gastric distention, and GRP (bombesin), which is an enteric

nerve neurotransmitter.[8] Gastrin travels through the blood to reach parietal cells and enterochromaffin-like (ECL) cells. ECL cells release histamine, which stimulates parietal cell secretion. An additional layer of stimulation of parietal cell secretion is provided by enteric nerve endings in the fundus.[8] Gastrin secretion is inhibited by gastric pH and somatostatin, which is released by D cells in the antrum.[8] Both histamine-secreting ECL cells and somatostatin-secreting D cells are found in the fundus and the body.

As mentioned previously, peptide products of protein digestion stimulate gastrin production, which can augment acid secretion. The presence of carbohydrate, protein, or fat in the duodenum inhibits gastric acid and pepsin secretion as well as gastric motility. Caffeine and alcohol stimulate gastrin[14] and acid production.

Acetylcholine also stimulates pepsinogen and mucus secretion. Pepsinogen is hydrolyzed in the presence of HCl to its active form, pepsin, a protein digestive enzyme.[83] Somatostatin inhibits the secretion of pepsinogens.[2]

Peptic ulcers develop when the gastric lining's protective barrier against irritation and autodigestion is compromised. Treatment involves suppression of gastric acid production. Proton-pump inhibitor drugs exert their effects on acid suppression by interfering with hydrogen potassium ATP activity. H_2-receptor antagonist drugs block histamine stimulation of acid production. H_2-blocking drugs can reduce basal acid secretion by 75% to 90%.

Gastric juices are secreted in 3 phases. In the first phase, the cephalic phase, acid is secreted via vagal stimulation in response to the thought, sight, smell, and/or taste of food. The vagus nerve releases acetylcholine, which stimulates the ECL cells and parietal cells. The cephalic phase accounts for 30% of the volume of acid secretion. The gastric phase of secretion begins when food arrives in the stomach. In the gastric phase, amino acids and peptides stimulate the G cells in the antrum to produce gastrin, which enters the general circulation and stimulates parietal cells as an endocrine hormone. Gastric distention also leads to acid secretion via a reflex involving the vagus nerve. Antral distention, in particular, stimulates gastrin secretion, which acts on ECL cells to release histamine. The gastric phase of acid secretion accounts for 60% of the volume of acid secreted.[83]

The final phase of gastric secretion is the intestinal phase. Food in the duodenum continues to stimulate small amounts of gastric secretions, likely related to the small amount of gastrin that is secreted by the duodenal mucosa. The intestinal phase accounts for approximately 10% of gastric acid secretion.[83]

Gastric secretions are inhibited by signals from the intestines in multiple ways. Paradoxically, food in the small intestine not only stimulates gastrin release (which increases secretions) but also initiates a reverse enterogastric reflex that inhibits gastric secretions. Secondly, the presence of acid, fat, products of protein digestion, hyper- or hypotonic fluids, or irritants in the proximal small bowel stimulate the secretion of intestinal hormones. These gastric secretion–inhibiting hormones include secretin, GIP, VIP, and somatostatin. Overall, the presence of carbohydrate, protein, or fat in the duodenum inhibits gastric acid and pepsin secretion and gastric motility.

During the interdigestive period, gastric secretions can increase in response to emotional stimuli and reach a level high enough to contribute to the development of peptic ulcers.[83]

Biliary Secretion

Liver-derived bile is central to the digestion and absorption of fat because of its role as an emulsifier and its role in aiding absorption of digested fat into the intestinal mucosa. Bile is comprised of water, bile salts, bile pigments, cholesterol, lecithin, fatty acids, and electrolytes. Bile salts are sodium and potassium salts of bile acids, which are metabolites of cholesterol. The 2 principal bile acids are cholic acid and chenodeoxycholic acid, which are formed in the liver. Colonic bacteria convert cholic acid to deoxycholic acid and chenodeoxycholic acid to lithocholic acid, the secondary bile acids (which are formed after deconjugation and dehydroxylation). Deoxycholate is absorbed. For the most part, lithocholic acid is excreted in the stool.[8,48]

Bile pigments include bilirubin and biliverdin, which are responsible for the yellow color of bile. Bilirubin is a waste product of the breakdown of hemoglobin. In pathological conditions when bilirubin accumulates in the blood, skin, sclera, and mucous membranes, it imparts a yellow color; this condition is called *jaundice*. Jaundice often can be detected when total plasma bilirubin exceeds 2 mg/dL. The brown color of stools derives from pigments formed by colonic bacteria action on bile pigments. Stools become white when bile acids are prevented from entering the colon (eg, biliary obstruction).[48]

Bile production is stimulated by the vagus nerve and by secretin. Bile drains from the liver continually into canaliculi, interlobular septa, and, eventually, the right and left hepatic ducts. The right and left hepatic ducts form the common bile duct, which eventually leads to the sphincter of Oddi in the duodenum.[48] Because the sphincter of Oddi remains closed between meals, bile is directed to the gallbladder. The gallbladder contracts after a meal, especially if that meal is high in fat. The sphincter of Oddi then relaxes (opens), and bile flows into the duodenum.[47] Relaxation of the sphincter of Oddi is mediated by the action of CCK, which also stimulates the gallbladder to contract.[48] CCK secretion is stimulated by the presence of fat in the duodenum.[8]

Bile is concentrated in the gallbladder where water is absorbed. Approximately 500 mL of bile is secreted per day.[1,8] On the average, 90% to 95% of bile salts are reabsorbed in the terminal ileum. Reabsorbed bile salts and bile pigments are transported to the liver via the portal vein and then are reexcreted in the bile. This process is called *enterohepatic circulation*.[1,8] The role of bile salts in the digestion of fat is to act as emulsifiers along with phospholipids and monoglycerides. Without bile, up to 50% of ingested fat can appear in the feces; in contrast, under normal circumstances, nearly 100% of fat is absorbed.[1]

Pancreatic Secretions

The pancreas has a variety of functions important to digestion. Pancreatic secretions are produced in response to the presence of chyme in the proximal small bowel. The composition of the pancreatic juice is determined partially by the composition of the chyme. Digestive enzymes are produced in glandular-like cells that secrete the enzymes in zymogen granules via exocytosis into pancreatic ducts.[8,83] Small pancreatic ducts drain into a large central duct that empties into the common bile duct. About 1500 mL of alkaline, bicarbonate-rich pancreatic juice is secreted daily into the duodenum through the sphincter of Oddi. Pancreatic secretions, along with intestinal secretions and bile, neutralize gastric acid (pH ranges from 1 to 4) to raise the pH of duodenal contents to between 6 and 7. Pancreatic juice contains enzymes for digestion of the 3 major macronutrients: carbohydrate (pancreatic amylase), protein (pancreatic proteases), and fat (pancreatic lipase, cholesterol esterase, and phospholipase). Pancreatic proteases (trypsin, chymotrypsin, and carboxypolypeptidase, proelastase, collagenase) are released as inactive proenzymes. The brush border enzyme enteropeptidase (enterokinase) converts trypsinogen to the active enzyme trypsin. Trypsin then converts chymotrypsinogen into chymotrypsin and autocatalyzes trypsinogen to produce more trypsin. Under normal circumstances, the pancreas releases small amounts of enzymes into the general blood circulation. However, in acute pancreatitis, serum levels of amylase and lipase rise dramatically and are useful in making a diagnosis.[8,52,83] (See Chapter 28 for further information on pancreatitis.)

Secretion of pancreatic juice, particularly high-volume, enzyme-poor, bicarbonate-rich secretions, is stimulated by secretin. CCK promotes the secretion of low-volume, enzyme-rich pancreatic juice from acinar cells. Acinar cells are also stimulated by the vagus nerve and the parasympathetic and enteric nervous systems via acetylcholine.[48,52,83] In addition, neuropeptide substance P and VIP stimulate secretion of pancreatic enzymes and bicarbonate respectively.[52] Somatostatin inhibits pancreatic secretion.[52]

It is important to remember that in the fasting state without any EN, gastric secretions can amount to 500 to 1000 mL/d, and biliary and pancreatic secretions can be up to 1000 to 2000 mL/d.[85] This fact underscores the importance of continued peristalsis during periods of *nil per os*.

Small and Large Bowel Secretions

Digestion that began in the mouth and stomach is completed in the small intestine, and products of digestion, vitamins, and minerals are absorbed. The small intestine has 3 regions: the duodenum, the jejunum, and the ileum. The duodenum becomes the jejunum at the ligament of Treitz. The lower 60% of the small bowel that is distal to the ligament of Treitz is designated as the ileum. Between the ileum and the colon is the ileocecal valve. The length of the small bowel can vary from approximately 12 to 20 feet (approximately 350 to 600 cm). When colonic pressure increases, the ileocecal valve shuts. Conversely, when ileal pressure increases or when food exits the stomach (gastroileal reflex), the ileocecal valve opens. When the ileocecal valve is resected, small bowel contents enter the colon quickly and some malabsorption occurs, but the amount may not be significant.[48]

Small bowel secretions begin in the proximal duodenum where Brunner glands secrete mucus, which protects the duodenum from gastric acid. A total of 9 liters of fluid enter the small intestine each day: 2 liters from dietary sources and 7 liters of GI secretions; however, only 1 to 2 liters of fluid normally enter the colon and an average of 200 mL of stool is lost daily.[8,48]

To optimize the surface area for absorption, the epithelial lining of the small bowel is folded into finger-like projections called *villi*.[8,48] Each villus contains capillaries and a lymphatic vessel (lacteal). At the edge of the epithelium of the villi are microvilli that make up the brush border. The so-called brush border enzymes are on the outer layer of the cell membranes of these mucosal cells, which are also called *enterocytes*.[48] An unstirred layer is located between the brush border and intestinal lumen, and solutes must traverse it to be absorbed. These substances pass into the enterocytes and then exit via basolateral membrane.[6]

Positioned between the villi are the crypts of Lieberkühn. Lining both the crypts and the villi is an epithelial layer containing goblet cells and enterocytes. The goblet cells secrete mucus throughout the small intestine. Enterocytes secrete large amounts of water (approximately 1800 mL/d) and electrolytes, and reabsorb water and electrolytes along with products of digestion. Interestingly, the digestive enzymes that are produced by enterocytes are not secreted into the watery secretions. Small bowel enzymes (eg, peptidases, sucrase, maltase, isomaltase, lactase, and intestinal lipase) digest while nutrients are being absorbed through the epithelium.[8,83]

Undifferentiated stem cells are formed in the crypts of Lieberkühn. Subsequently, they migrate up the villi, undergo apoptosis (programmed cell death), and are sloughed off into the lumen of the small bowel and exit through the stool. The highly proliferative lining of the small bowel turns over every 2 to 5 days.[8,48] The loss of the sloughed cells translates into a loss of about 30 g protein per day.[48] The small bowel mucosa is particularly susceptible to damage by chemotherapeutic agents that target mitotic cells because it is such a highly proliferating tissue.

The large bowel continues to secrete mucus from crypts of Lieberkühn. Again, the mucus serves to protect the mucosa. Furthermore, mucus in the colon provides an adherent medium for holding feces together. When the large bowel becomes irritated, the mucosa can secrete large volumes of water and electrolytes, which serves to dilute and "wash" the irritant out of the colon.[83]

Nutrient Effects on Gastrointestinal Hormone Secretion

Luminal nutrients have important effects on the secretion of GI hormones. For example, glucose stimulates the secretion of 5-HT, GIP, GLP-1, and PYY. Likewise, fat and protein stimulate the release of CCK.

Digestion

Digestion of Carbohydrate

Starches (glucose polymers) and disaccharides must be digested before they are absorbed. The digestion of starch begins in the mouth with the action of salivary α-amylase (Table 1-3).[8] When food enters the stomach, the action of salivary α-amylase is gradually inhibited by gastric acid. Starch digestion continues in the more alkaline small intestine where pancreatic α-amylase hydrolyzes α (1-4) linkages to form the oligosaccharides maltose and maltotriose, larger polymers, and α-dextrins (glucose polymers of average chain length of 8 glucose molecules). Brush border enzymes are then responsible for further digestion of the oligosaccharides, including isomaltase, maltase, and sucrase. Sucrase hydrolyzes sucrose into the monosaccharides glucose and fructose. Another brush border enzyme, lactase, catalyzes the hydrolysis of lactose to the monosaccharides galactose and glucose. When there is a deficiency of brush border oligosaccharidases, diarrhea, bloating, and flatulence may occur. Undigested oligosaccharides are osmotically active and cause a shift of water into the intestinal lumen. The osmotic pressure exerted by luminal contents increases further when colonic bacteria act on remaining oligosaccharides and increase the number of osmotically active particles. Flatulence and bloating are perpetuated because of the formation of CO_2 and H_2 from bacterial fermentation of undigested/unabsorbed carbohydrates in the intestine and colon.[6]

Deficiency of the lactase enzyme is common in African Americans, Native Americans, Asians, and individuals of Mediterranean descent; in these populations, 70% to 100% are deficient and require low-lactose diets, supplemental oral lactase, or lactase-treated food products. Often, people with lactase deficiency tolerate yogurt with live bacterial cultures because the bacteria produce lactase enzyme.

Acquired disorders of brush border enzyme deficiency—which typically occur after a bout of gastroenteritis or protracted diarrhea with resultant small bowel villous atrophy—are usually transient, resolve in a short period of time, and may be addressed temporarily by a low-lactose diet. Additional information regarding carbohydrate absorption is found in Chapter 3.

Digestion of Protein

Protein digestion begins in the stomach with the action of pepsin (Table 1-3). In an acid environment, pepsin hydrolyzes the bonds involving aromatic amino acids. This cleavage produces polypeptides of various sizes. When the partially digested chyme enters the alkaline environment of the duodenum, pepsin is inactivated. At this point, trypsin, chymotrypsin, and proelastase—the endopeptidases—hydrolyze internal bonds of the polypeptides. Pancreatic carboxypeptidases—the exopeptidases—hydrolyze the carboxy terminal amino acids of the polypeptides. Most protein digestion results from hydrolysis by pancreatic enzymes. Free amino acids and di- and tripeptides are cleaved off by intestinal polypeptidases and dipeptidases in the brush border. They are then carried into the interior of the enterocyte where di-and tripeptides are digested to amino acids.[86]

The small intestine digests and absorbs 95% to 98% of the protein in its lumen. Bacteria in the colon digest some of the remaining protein, producing ammonia. Ammonia is absorbed and transported to the liver. The rate of ammonia absorption depends on the size of the bacterial population of the colon and the colonic pH. When the number of bacteria

TABLE 1-3 Principle Digestive Enzymes

Source	Enzyme	Activator	Substrate	Catalytic Function or Products
Salivary glands	Salivary α-amylase	Cl⁻	Starch	Hydrolyze α (1-4) linkages, producing α-limit dextrins, maltotriose, and maltose
Stomach	Pepsins (pepsinogens)	HCl	Proteins and polypeptides	Cleave peptide bonds adjacent to aromatic amino acids
	Gastric lipase		Triglycerides	Fatty acids and glycerol
Exocrine pancreas	Trypsin (trypsinogen)	Enteropeptidase	Proteins and polypeptides	Cleave peptide bonds on the carboxyl side of basic amino acids (arginine or lysine)
	Chymotrypsins	Trypsin	Proteins and polypeptides	Cleave peptide bonds on the carboxyl side of aromatic amino acids
	Elastase (proelastase)	Trypsin	Elastin, some other proteins	Cleave bonds on the carboxyl side of aliphatic amino acids
	Carboxypeptidase A and B (procarboxypeptidase A and B)	Trypsin	Proteins and polypeptides	Cleave carboxylterminal amino acids that have aromatic or branched aliphatic side chains (A) or basic side chains (B)
	Colipase	Trypsin	Fat droplets	Binds pancreatic lipase to oil droplets in the presence of bile acids
	Pancreatic lipase		Triglycerides	Monoglycerides and fatty acids
	Cholesterol ester hydrolase	Cholesterol esters	Cholesterol	Cholesterol
	Pancreatic α-amylase	Cl⁻	Starch	Same as salivary α-amylase
	Ribonuclease		RNA	Nucleotides
	Deoxyribonuclease		DNA	Nucleotides
	Phospholipase A_2 (prophospholipase A_2)	Trypsin	Phospholipids	Fatty acids, lysophopholipids
Intestinal mucosa	Enteropeptidase	Trypsinogen	Trypsinogen	Trypsin
	Aminopeptidases		Polypeptides	Cleave amino terminal amino acid from peptide
	Carboxypeptidases		Polypeptides	Cleave carboxyl terminal amino acid from peptide
	Endopeptidases		Polypeptides	Cleave between residues in mid portion of peptide
	Dipeptidases		Dipeptides	Two amino acids
	Maltase		Maltose, maltotriose	Glucose
	Lactase		Lactose	Galactose and glucose
	Sucrase		Sucrose; also, maltose and maltotriose, α-limit dextrins	Fructose and glucose
	Isomaltase		Maltotriose	Glucose
	Nuclease and related enzymes		Nucleic acids	Pentoses and purine and pyrimidine bases
Cytoplasm of mucosal cells	Various peptidases		Di-, tri-, and tetrapeptides	Amino acids

Cl⁻, chloride; DNA, deoxyribonucleic acid; HCl, hydrogen chloride; RNA, ribonucleic acid.

Source: Reprinted with permission from reference 8: Barrett KE, Barman SM, Boitano S, and Brooks H. Overview of gastrointestinal function and regulations. In: *Ganong's Review of Medical Physiology*. 25th ed. New York: McGraw-Hill Lange Medical; 2016. Copyright © McGraw-Hill Education.

is reduced (eg, after antibiotic administration) or the colonic pH is low (eg, after lactulose administration), the amount of ammonia absorbed decreases.[54] Ammonia absorption may be clinically relevant during GI bleeding and in the setting of liver disease, where it may contribute to the development of hepatic encephalopathy. During starvation or during periods of prolonged bowel rest, the peptidase activity of the brush border declines.[6]

Digestion of Fat

Fat digestion begins in the mouth and stomach through the actions of lingual lipase and gastric lipase, respectively (Table 1-3). The contribution of gastric lipase is small, but lingual lipase hydrolyzes up to 10% of dietary fat. Most fat digestion occurs in the duodenum by pancreatic lipase.[86]

The first major step of fat digestion occurs in the duodenum where bile emulsifies fat globules into smaller globules to increase the surface area on which water-soluble lipase enzymes may act. The major sites of action of pancreatic lipase are on the 1- and 3-bonds of triacylglycerols. For this reason, the primary products of digestion by pancreatic lipase are 2-monoglycerides and free fatty acids.[6,86] Hydrolysis by pancreatic lipase is highly reversible; therefore, the next step in fat digestion, the formation of micelles by bile salts, is critical to keep the products of digestion separated. Subsequently, the bile salt micelles transport the monoglycerides and free fatty acids to the brush border where they are absorbed and the micelles are returned to the chyme.[85]

Two other types of pancreatic enzymes are involved in fat digestion. Cholesterol ester hydrolase hydrolyzes cholesterol esters, and phospholipases A_2 and B_2 hydrolyze phospholipids. Again, micelles are required for transport to the brush border.[86] In a setting of pancreatic insufficiency, fat is maldigested and patients have fatty, bulky, clay-colored stools.

Digestion of Nucleic Acids

Ribonuclease and deoxyribonuclease from the pancreas hydrolyze ribonucleic acid and deoxyribonucleic acid to form mononucleotides. Nucleotides are further cleaved to nucleosides and phosphoric acid by enzymes on the surface of mucosal cells. Finally, nucleosides are cleaved into purines and pyrimidines that are absorbed by active transport.[6]

Absorption

As noted earlier, the small intestine is presented with approximately 9 liters of fluid to absorb daily, of which 2 liters are dietary fluid and 7 liters are secretions. The small intestine absorbs all but 1.5 liters of this fluid. The rest passes through the ileocecal valve to the colon. Central to the process of absorption are the highly specialized anatomy, histology, and arrangement of the cells and structures of the small intestine.[86] Nutrients enter a single cell layer of epithelial cells in which uptake of nutrients is controlled.[8]

The architecture of the small intestinal mucosa and villi maximizes the potential surface area for absorption. The absorptive area of the small intestine is approximately the same area as a tennis court. The stomach, on the other hand, does not have the same maximized surface area. Accordingly, the only substances that are absorbed in the stomach in appreciable amounts are alcohol and aspirin (water is also absorbed here to some degree).[86] The efficiency of absorption is remarkable: 85% of carbohydrate, 66% to 95% of protein, and nearly all fat are absorbed before they could enter the large bowel.[87]

Mechanisms of Absorption

A variety of mechanisms affect the movement of nutrients from the lumen of the intestine across the mucosal membranes into the cytoplasm. Water is transported by diffusion and obeys the laws of osmosis, which are concentration dependent. Other absorbed substances may move by either passive or active transport or facilitated diffusion. Passive transport is accomplished by diffusion of solutes according to their electrochemical gradients. Transport by passive diffusion may occur across cell membranes or between cells. Negatively charged chloride ions, for example, diffuse along an electrochemical gradient to "follow" positively charged sodium ions. Active transport is an energy-requiring mechanism that may be used against an electrochemical gradient.

Active transport is limited to movement across cell membranes. Ions such as Na^+ are actively transported from the chyme through the brush border into the cytoplasm. Na^+ may be cotransported with amino acids or glucose by carrier proteins or may be exchanged with H^+.[86] Endocytosis is a process in which the cell membrane engulfs particles into cells (eg, whole protein allergens). Facilitated diffusion is the movement of nutrients across a semipermeable membrane in conjunction with transport proteins.[56]

Carbohydrate Absorption

Monosaccharides are absorbed rapidly before reaching the terminal ileum. Glucose and galactose are absorbed via the sodium-glucose transporter 1 (SGLT1), which simultaneously transports sodium and glucose or galactose. When intraluminal glucose concentrations are high, glucose is also absorbed via facilitated glucose transporter type 2 (GLUT2). GLUT2 also transports fructose out of enterocytes across the basolateral membrane.[52]

As mentioned previously, glucose and sodium share common cotransporters. High concentrations of Na^+ in the chyme increase glucose transport. Low concentrations of Na^+ decrease glucose absorption. Na^+ moves into mucosal cells along its concentration gradient and brings glucose along. The active transport of Na^+ out of the cell provides the energy for glucose transport. The transport of Na^+ out of the cell maintains the concentration gradient needed for Na^+ to shuttle more glucose into the mucosal cells.[52]

Galactose is transported by the same SGLT1 transporter as glucose, whereas the absorption of fructose is independent of Na^+ and glucose. Fructose transport into the mucosal cells is accomplished by facilitated diffusion by GLUT5. From the mucosal cells, these molecules pass into the capillaries, which drain into the portal vein.[6]

Amino Acid Absorption

Amino acid transport can be categorized into processes that require Na^+ and cotransporters and those that are do not require Na^+.[6,52] Amino acid transport can also be categorized by different active transport systems—for example, neutral, basic, and acidic amino acids each have separate transport mechanisms.[6]

Peptides are absorbed more rapidly than free amino acids and are likely to be the primary means for amino acid absorption.[52] Di- and tripeptide absorption via the peptide transporter 1 system into enterocytes requires the comovement of H^+.[52] Absorption of longer-chain peptides is limited.[6] Up to 99% of protein consumed is absorbed before the distal jejunum is reached. Nearly all the protein in stools is from cellular debris or of bacterial origin.[6]

Clinically significant protein deficiencies secondary to enterocyte amino acid transport abnormalities are very unusual. Protein absorption defects can be inherited or acquired. An example of such a defect is Hartnup syndrome, which may present as a pellagra-like syndrome.[88] Additional information regarding amino acid absorption is found in Chapter 6.

Lipid Absorption

As discussed above, lipids are presented to the brush border membrane for absorption in the form of micelles. Bile salts arrange into micelles whose hydrophilic portions face out while their hydrophobic portions face toward the center where lipids collect. Monoglycerides and free fatty acids are transported to the brush border of the intestine, where they diffuse directly into the interior of the epithelial cells.[86] Fatty acids are absorbed by protein-independent mechanisms and protein-dependent fatty acid transport proteins that are produced by the intestine. Neither model requires energy.[52] Once inside enterocytes, fatty acids and cholesterol are reesterified into triglycerides and cholesterol esters. Additional cholesterol and phospholipids, together with protein, envelope these reesterified products to form chylomicrons. The chylomicrons exit enterocytes and enter the lymphatic circulation. Normally, around 95% to 97% of fat is absorbed when fat intake is moderate.[48,86] Most of the cholesterol that is absorbed is packaged into chylomicrons. Nonabsorbable soy-based sterols reduce cholesterol absorption and are recommended as a serum cholesterol–lowering intervention.[48]

Vitamin Absorption

Generally, vitamins are absorbed from the small intestine via passive diffusion and active transport.[52] Like fatty acids, fat-soluble vitamins are transported to the brush border within micelles. Absorption usually occurs via passive diffusion or, in the case of vitamin A, by a carotenoid transporter.[52] Fat-soluble vitamin absorption depends on normal fat digestion and absorption because fat-soluble vitamins are carried away from the sites of absorption when fat is malabsorbed. Water-soluble vitamins often require Na^+ cotransporters for absorption. Exceptions include vitamin B_{12} and folic acid. Folate is absorbed via a proton-coupled folate transporter.[52]

Vitamin B_{12} requires a unique mechanism for absorption. Vitamin B_{12} is released from food and binds to R proteins in saliva and gastric secretions. R proteins release vitamin B_{12}, and it subsequently binds intrinsic factor, a glycoprotein that is secreted by the parietal cells of the stomach. The intrinsic factor–vitamin B_{12} complex is taken up by receptors in the distal ileum by endocytosis.[52] Intracellularly, vitamin B_{12} is transferred to transcobalamin for transport in the portal vein.[52] Loss of parietal cells for any reason (eg, gastrectomy, chronic gastritis) or loss of distal ileum may lead to vitamin B_{12} deficiency and requires B_{12} supplementation by monthly injections, high-dose oral administration, or nasal sprays.[48]

Vitamin K and some B vitamins may be produced by colonic bacteria and are absorbed, sometimes in significant amounts.[52] Additional information regarding vitamin absorption is found in Chapter 8.

Water, Mineral, and Electrolyte Absorption

Although a small amount of water can be absorbed in the stomach, the small bowel and colon are primarily responsible for water absorption. Water movement drives to equalize the osmotic pressure between the plasma and intestinal contents. Sodium moves in and out of the small bowel along its concentration gradient. Na^+ facilitates the absorption of glucose, some amino acids, and bile acids.[8] For this reason, oral rehydration fluids used to treat Na^+ and water losses from diarrhea contain NaCl and glucose.[6]

Water, Na^+, and other minerals are absorbed in the colon. Sodium is actively transported, and water follows via osmosis. Potassium and bicarbonate are secreted into the colon, potassium along its electrochemical gradient. Enough potassium may be secreted into the colon to lead to significant hypokalemia associated with ileal or colonic losses caused by diarrhea. Potassium is also actively transported from the colon.

Calcium and iron absorption are dependent on body stores. The amount of Ca^{2+} absorbed is dependent on 1,25-dihydroxycholecalciferol. Calcium absorption is inhibited by phosphates and oxalates, which form insoluble salts with Ca^{2+}. Protein facilitates both calcium and magnesium absorption.

Only 3% to 6% of dietary iron is absorbed under conditions of iron sufficiency. Its absorption is inhibited by phytates in cereal, phosphates, and oxalates. These compounds form insoluble compounds with iron. Iron is absorbed in the ferrous form. Because most dietary iron is in the ferric form, it must be reduced to the ferrous form. This form may be absorbed by an iron transporter, divalent metal transporter 1, in the brush border. When iron complexes with ascorbic acid, the reduction of the ferric form to the ferrous form is facilitated. Heme iron is absorbed through a different mechanism. Heme complexes with a transport protein in the mucosal cells and is transferred into the cytoplasm. There, HO_2, a type of heme oxygenase, dissociates the iron from the heme.[6] Additional information regarding trace element absorption is found in Chapter 8.

Substances that are not absorbed remain in the feces and are subsequently eliminated. Feces also contain inorganic material, fiber, water, and bacteria. Bacteria comprises 30% of the dry weight of fecal matter. Because fecal contents include material other than food residue, the passage of feces continues during prolonged bowel rest when patients are restricted from consuming food.[6]

Medium-Chain Triglyceride Absorption

MCTs are triglycerides with fatty acids that have chain lengths of 8 to 12 carbons. Because they are water soluble, MCTs do not require the formation of micelles or the action of bile salts. Medium-chain fatty acids are hydrolyzed and pass through enterocytes directly into the portal circulation. MCTs may be used as an energy supplement in patients who maldigest or malabsorb fat.

Short-Chain Fatty Acid Absorption and the Microbiome

SCFAs, 2- to 5-carbon fatty acids, are produced in the colon by the action of bacteria on fermentable dietary fiber. The types of SCFAs formed include acetate, propionate, and butyrate. Once absorbed by the colon mucosal cells, SCFAs are metabolized and serve as an energy source for active transport and other cellular processes of colonic cells. Other effects of SCFAs include increased sodium and water absorption; trophic effects on mucosal cells of the colon; inhibition of cholesterol synthesis by in the liver; improvement of colonic and splanchnic circulation; enhancement of immunity through stimulation of the production of macrophages, T helper lymphocytes, neutrophils and antibodies,; and acidification of colonic pH, which lowers the solubility of bile acids and their subsequent conversion to cytotoxic bile acids and inhibits the growth of pathogenic bacteria.[48,52,87] See Chapter 4 for a more complete discussion of the gut microbiome.

Gastrointestinal (Splanchnic) Blood Circulation

The network of arteries, veins, and minor blood vessels in the GI tract is referred to as *splanchnic circulation*. Relatively speaking, the GI tract is a blood-rich area of the body. At rest, 25% of cardiac output is delivered to the splanchnic circulation. This amount is similar to the amount delivered to the kidneys, and more than the amount that is delivered to any other vascular bed, including skeletal muscle. At rest, the splanchnic organs consume 30% of total body oxygen, making the oxygen consumption in splanchnic circulation greater than that of any other area of the body. The demand for oxygen is determined by the large mass of the tissue that is supplied by the splanchnic circulation as well as the high energy demands of absorption, GI secretion, and GI mixing and propulsion. The distribution of the splanchnic blood flow varies disproportionately among organs, with nearly half being supplied to the small intestine.[89]

During feeding, splanchnic blood flow increases 40% to 60% and oxygen demand in the splanchnic-supplied organs increases up to 30%. These facts become important when dealing with states of low splanchnic blood flow, which will be discussed subsequently. All blood in the GI tract, including the spleen and pancreas, flows to the liver via the portal vein.[8,49] In the liver, blood encounters reticuloendothelial system (RES) cells in the lining of liver blood vessels (sinusoids). The RES is a system of macrophages that clears the blood of bacteria and other particulate matter to prevent systemic infection before blood leaves the liver. Blood exits the liver by way of the hepatic vein, which leads to the vena cava.[49]

Blood is delivered to the small intestine by the superior and inferior mesenteric arteries, which branch off the aorta. The celiac artery supplies the stomach. Splanchnic blood vessels branch progressively down to arterioles that supply individual villi lining the intestines. Arterioles empty into venules in each villus with the flow of arterioles opposite in direction to the venules. Normally, 80% of the oxygen in the arterioles may diffuse out into the venules without reaching the tip of the villus. Although this shunting of oxygen is not normally harmful, it can become harmful in low-flow states such as circulatory collapse. In circulatory collapse, the oxygen deprivation in the tips of the villi can result in an ischemic death of the villi, leading to decreased absorptive capacity.[49]

Alterations in Digestion/Absorption: Starvation, Bowel Rest, Mucosal Atrophy, and Low-Flow States

Mucosal atrophy occurs during starvation, stress, PN, and bowel rest.[71] Complete bowel rest results in gut mucosal atrophy that becomes apparent in as little as a few days. PN cannot prevent this change. After 1 week of a protein-deficient diet, the microvilli shorten. This finding suggests that the bowel mucosa requires luminal nutrients to supply its nutrient needs.[90] The need for luminal nutrition contributes to the rationale for the ASPEN guideline that recommends that EN be initiated for critically ill patients within 24 to 48 hours when oral intake is not possible. The role of EN in maintaining gut mucosa integrity is related to EN relationship to action in maintaining tight junctions and stimulating blood flow and release of trophic agents (eg, CCK, gastrin, and bile salts). EN also supports the production of IgA from B cells and plasma cells.[57]

Glutamine is a principal metabolic fuel for intestinal cells,[4] and its absence may directly contribute to mucosal atrophy that accompanies bowel rest. Atrophic changes during bowel rest have been reduced by glutamine-enriched PN.[91] "Trickle" enteral feeding (ie, 10 to 20 mL/h or 10 to 20 kcal/h) can prevent mucosal atrophy in low- to moderate-risk patients, but it will not achieve desired EN clinical outcomes in high-risk patients. Higher risk patients may need to receive more than 50% to 65% of goal energy from nutrition support to prevent increases in gut mucosa permeabilitiy.[57]

Severe metabolic stress that accompanies sepsis or trauma may lead to shock and associated hypoperfusion of the gut splanchnic circulation. In this setting, peristalsis may be decreased or absent, patients may require bowel rest, and, consequently, mucosal atrophy may occur. ASPEN clinical guidelines[57] advise that EN be withheld in patients with hypoperfused gut when patients are being initiated on catecholamines, when catecholamine doses are increasing, or when patients require a high level of hemodynamic support including high-dose catecholamines (eg, norepinephrine, phenylephrine, epinephrine, dopamine) to maintain cellular perfusion. EN is withheld to avoid ischemic bowel. These patients usually have a mean arterial blood pressure of less than 50 mmHg. Patients on stable, low doses of pressors may be given EN, but they must be monitored closely for signs of intolerance, which could signal development of gut ischemia. Signs of intolerance include abdominal distention, increasing NG tube output or gastric residual volumes, decreased passage of stool, increasing metabolic acidosis, and/or base deficit.[57]

Immunity and the Gut

The GI tract is exposed to many beneficial and pathogenic microorganisms and antigens. A variety of immune defenses operate in the gut. Immune cells including T and B lymphocytes, plasma cells, natural killer cells, macrophages, and other cells are present throughout the gut. The lymphoid tissue in the mucosa is called *mucosa-associated lymphoid tissue*; *gut-associated lymphoid tissue* (GALT) refers to lymphoid tissue located in nonmucosal layers of the gut.[52] In the small intestine, in addition to immune cells, many proteolytic and lipolytic enzymes secreted by the pancreas degrade pathogens. Mucin, which is produced by the enterocytes, limits the proliferation of bacteria. Additionally, peristalsis acts to propel pathogens out of the gut. Finally, tight junctions between epithelial cells provide a barrier against translocation of pathogens from the lumen into the systemic circulation.[92]

The GALT is one of the largest components of the immune system. Gut epithelial cells and their mucus layer provide defense by trapping pathogens. When the epithelial cells are sloughed off, they are excreted along with the pathogens in the feces. As an additional defense, intraepithelial cytolytic T lymphocytes are positioned between epithelial cells. The lamina propria (a layer of connective tissue that, together with the epithelium, comprises the mucosa) houses many different types of immune cells, including B cells, T helper cells, mast cells, and eosinophils. The B cells secrete IgA into the lumen of the gut. Mast cells and eosinophils are involved in allergic and hypersensitivity reactions and target parasites. Also present are M cells, which transport antigens to dendritic cells and macrophages and serve as antigen-presenting cells to T cells in the GALT. This process, in turn, results in the production of IgA by plasma cells in the mucosa. Lymphocytes are then activated, enter the lymphatic circulation, and eventually enter the systemic circulation via the thoracic duct.[92]

The GALT depends on luminal nutrition to maintain its integrity. In patients receiving EN, the GALT atrophies when nutrition is withheld for extended periods. Furthermore, in conditions associated with severe metabolic stress, bacteria from the lumen of the gut migrate across the gut barriers and into the mesenteric lymph nodes and beyond. This bacterial translocation has been implicated as an etiologic factor for septic complications and multiple organ failure.[52,92] Because EN helps to maintain tight junctions between epithelial cells and hence reduces the risk of increased permeability during metabolic stress, ASPEN guidelines recommend that EN be initiated within 24 to 48 hours in critically ill patients in whom oral is inadequate.[57] See Chapter 10 for an expanded discussion of the benefits of early EN.

Summary

When providing nutrition support, clinicians must consider the complex physiological and environmental factors that influence nutrient intake and GI function. Navigating the neurohormonal control of GI function and diverse environmental signals in the context of patient illness is a formidable clinical challenge. Appetite, intake, digestion, and absorption are both positively and negatively influenced by the interaction of food components with the systems innervating the GI tract, with hormone-secreting cells, and with the gut microbiome. Our challenge is to identify and implement clinical interventions that can capitalize on these interactions in a way that supports optimal nutrition status and desired patient outcomes.

References

1. Blundell JE, Stubbs J. Diet composition and the control of food intake in humans. In: Bray GA, Bouchard C, eds. *Handbook of Obesity: Etiology and Pathophysiology*. New York: Marcel Dekker; 2004:427–460.
2. Dempsey DT. Stomach. In: Brunicardi FC, ed. *Schwartz's Principles of Surgery*. 8th ed. New York: McGraw-Hill Medical; 2005:933–996.
3. Dietitians of Canada and American Dietetic Association. Cancer. In: *Manual of Clinical Dietetics*. 6th ed. Chicago, IL: American Dietetic Association and Dietitians of Canada; 2000:236–252.
4. Marino PL. Enteral nutrition. In: Marino PL, ed. *The ICU Book*. 2nd ed. Baltimore, MD: Williams & Wilkins; 1998:737–754.
5. Gottschlich MM. Early and perioperative nutrition support. In: Matarese L, Gottschlich MM, eds. *Contemporary Nutrition Support Practice: A Clinical Guide*. 2nd ed. Philadelphia, PA: Saunders; 2003:276–289.
6. Digestion and absorption. In: Ganong WF. *Review of Medical Physiology*. 22nd ed. New York: McGraw-Hill Lange Medical; 2005: 467–478.
7. Corfe BM, Harden CJ, Bull M, Garaiova I. The multifactorial interplay of diet, the microbiome and appetite control: current knowledge and future challenges. *Proc Nutr Soc*. 2015;74(3):235–244.
8. Barrett KE, Barman SM, Boitano S, Brooks H. Overview of gastrointestinal function and regulations. In: *Ganong's Review of Medical Physiology*. 25th ed. New York: McGraw-Hill Lange Medical; 2016.
9. Kant AK, Graubard BL, Schatzkin A, Ballard-Barbash R. Proportion of energy intake from fat and subsequent weight change in the NHANES epidemiological follow-up study. *Am J Clin Nutr*. 1995;61:11–17.
10. Central regulation of visceral function. In: Ganong WF. *Review of Medical Physiology*. 22nd ed. New York: McGraw-Hill Lange Medical; 2005:232–255.
11. Blundell JE, Finlayson G, Gibbons C, Caudwell P, Hopkins M. The biology of appetite control: do resting metabolic rate and fat-free mass drive energy intake? *Physiol Behav*. 2015;152:473–478.
12. Carpenter GH. The secretion, components, and properties of saliva. *Annu Rev Food Sci Technol*. 2013;4:267–276.
13. Baroshuk LM, Snyder DJ. Taste. In: Pfaff DW, ed. *Neuroscience in the 21st Century: From Basic to Clinical*. New York: Springer; 2013: 781–813.
14. Reinehr T, Roth CL. The gut sensor as regulator of body weight. *Endocrine*. 2015;49:35–50.
15. Cegla J, Tan TM, Bloom SR. Gut-brain cross-talk in appetite regulation. *Curr Opin Clin Nutr Metab Care*. 2010;13(5):588–593.
16. Chaudhri OB, Field BCT, Bloom SR. Gastrointestinal satiety signals. *Int J Obes*. 2008;32(Suppl 7):S28–S31.

17. Zac-Vargheses S, Tan T, Sloom SR. Hormonal interactions between gut and brain. *Discov Med.* 2010;10(55):543–552.

18. Blumenthal DM, Gold MS. Neurobiology of food addiction. *Curr Opin Clin Nutr Metab Care.* 2010;13:359–365.

19. Sasaki T, Kitamura T. Roles of FoxO1 and Sirt1 in the central regulation of food intake. *Endocrine J.* 2010;57(11):939–946.

20. Dockray GJ. Enteroendocrine cell signaling via the vagus nerve. *Curr Opin Pharm.* 2013;13:954–958.

21. de Graaf C, Blom WA, Smeets PA, et al. Biomarkers of satiation and satiety. *Am J Clin Nutr.* 2004;79:946–961.

22. Cammisotto PG, Levy E, Bukowiecki LJ. Bendayan M. Cross-talk between adipose and gastric leptins for the control of food intake and energy metabolism. *Prog Hist Cytochem.* 2010;45(3):143–200.

23. Zheng H, Lenard NR, Shi AC, Berhoud HR. Appetite control and energy balance regulation in the modern world; reward-driven brain overrides repletion signals. *Int J Obes* 2009;33(Suppl 2):S8–S13.

24. Ueda H, Yagi T, Amitani H, et al. The roles of salivary secretion, brain-peptides, and oral hygiene in obesity. *Obes Res Clin Pract.* 2013;7(5):e321–e329.

25. Higuchi H, Hasegawa A, Yamaguchi T. Transcriptional regulation of neuropeptide Y gene by leptin and its effect on feeding. *J Pharmacol Sci.* 2005;98:225–231.

26. Feinle-Bisset C. Modulation of hunger and satiety: hormones and diet. *Curr Opin Clin Nutr Metab Care.* 2014;458–464.

27. Lissner L, Levitsky DA, Strupp BJ, et al. Dietary fat and the regulation of energy intake in human subjects. *Am J Clin Nutr.* 1987;46:886–892.

28. Stubbs RJ, Johnstone AM, Harbron CG, Reid C. Covert manipulation of the energy density of high-carbohydrate diets; effect on ad libitum food intake in "pseudo free-living" humans. *Int J Obes.* 1998;819:11–22.

29. Poortvliet PC, Berube-Parent S, Drapeau V, et al. Effects of a healthy meal course on spontaneous energy intake, satiety and palatability. *Br J Nutr.* 2007;97(3):584–590.

30. Halton TL, Hu FB. The effects of high protein diets on thermogenesis, satiety, and weight loss. *J Am Coll Nutr.* 2004; 23(5):373–385.

31. St-Onge MP, Rubiano F, DeNino WF, et al. Added thermogenic and satiety effects of a mixed nutrient vs a sugar-only beverage. *Int J Obes Rel Metab Dis.* 2004;28(2):248–253.

32. Lejeune MP, Westerterp KR, Adam TC, Luscombe-Marsh ND, Westerterp-Plantenga MS. Ghrelin and glucagon-like peptide 1 concentrations, 24-h satiety, and energy and substrate metabolism during a high-protein diet and measured in a respiration chamber. *Am J Clin Nutr.* 2006;83(1):89–94.

33. Nickols-Richardson SM, Coleman MD, Volpe JJ, Hosig KW. Perceived hunger is lower and weight loss is greater in overweight premenopausal women consuming a low-carbohydrate/high-protein vs high-carbohydrate/low-fat diet. *J Am Diet Assoc.* 2005;105(9):1433–1437.

34. Hall WL, Millward DJ, Long SJ, Morgan LM. Casein and whey exert different effects on plasma amino acid profiles, gastrointestinal hormone secretion and appetite. *Br J Nutr.* 2003;89(2):239–248.

35. Westerterp-Plantenga MS, Lejeune MP, Nijs I, van Ooijen M, Kovacs EM. High protein intake sustains weight maintenance after body weight loss in humans. *Int J Obes Rel Metab Dis.* 2004;28(1):57–64.

36. Lyly M, Liukkonen KH, Salmenkallio-Marttila M, et al. Fibre in beverages can enhance perceived satiety. *Eur J Nutr.* 2009;48(4):251–258.

37. Willis HJ, Eldridge AL, Beiseigel J, Thomas W, Slavin JL. Greater satiety response with resistant starch and corn bran in human subjects. *Nutr Res.* 2009;29(2):100–105.

38. Bodinham CL, Frost GS, Robertson MD. Acute ingestion of resistant starch reduces food intake in healthy adults. *Br J Nutr.* 2010;103(6):917–922.

39. Whelan K, Efthymiou L, Judd PA, Preedy VR, Taylor MA. Appetite during consumption of enteral formula as a sole source of nutrition: the effect of supplementing pea-fibre and fructo-oligosaccharides. *Br J Nutr.* 2006;96(2):350–356.

40. Blundell JI, Stubbs J. Diet composition and the control of food intake in humans. In: Bray GA, Bouchard C, eds. *Handbook of Obesity: Etiology and Pathophysiology.* New York: Marcel Dekker; 2004:427-460.

41. Stubbs J, Ferres S, Horgan G. Energy density foods: effects on energy intake. *Crit Rev Food Sci Nutr.* 2004;40(Suppl 6):S481–S515.

42. Mattes RD, Rothacker D. Beverage viscosity is inversely related to postprandial hunger in humans. *Physiol Behav.* 2001;74(4–5):551–557.

43. Sturm K, MacIntosh CG, Parker BA, et al. Appetite, food intake, and plasma concentrations of cholecystokinin, ghrelin, and other gastrointestinal hormones in undernourished older women and well-nourished young and older women. *J Clin Endocrin Metabol.* 2003;88(8):3747–3755.

44. Stull AJ, Apolzan JW, Thalacker-Mercer AE, Iglay HB, Campbell WW. Liquid and solid meal replacement products differentially affect postprandial appetite and food intake in older adults. *J Am Diet Assoc.* 2008;108(7):1226–1230.

45. Megestrol acetate. In: McElvoy GK. *AHFS Drug Information 2016.* 58th ed. Bethesda, MD: American Society of Health-System Pharmacists; 2016. http://hubnet.buffalo.edu:2062/Document.aspx?fxId=1&docId=335. Accessed January 31, 2017.

46. Parmar JR, Forrest BD, Freeman RA. Medical marijuana patient counseling points for health care professionals based on trends in the medical uses efficacy, and adverse effects of cannabis-based pharmaceutical drugs. *Admin Pharm.* 2016;12:638–654.

47. Goyal RG. Alimentary tract motor function. In: Stein JH. *Internal Medicine.* 5th ed. St. Louis, MO: Mosby; 1998:1976–1980.

48. Regulation of GI function. In: Ganong WF. *Review of Medical Physiology.* 22nd ed. New York: McGraw-Hill Lange Medical; 2005:479–514.

49. General principles of gastrointestinal function—motility, nervous control, and blood circulation. In: Hall JE. *Guyton and Hall Textbook of Medical Physiology.* 12th ed. Philadelphia, PA: Elsevier; 2010:753–762.

50. Peeters TL. Gastro intestinal hormones and gut motility. *Curr Opin Endocrinol Diabetes Obes.* 2015;22:9–13.

51. Propulsion and mixing of food in the alimentary tract. In: Hall JE. *Guyton and Hall Textbook of Medical Physiology.* 12th ed. Philadelphia, PA: Elsevier; 2010:763–772.

52. Gropper SS, Smith JL. *Advanced Nutrition and Human Metabolism.* 7th ed. Belmont, CA: Wadsworth Cengage Learning; 2018.

53. Fischbach F. *Manual of Laboratory and Diagnostic Tests.* 7th ed. Philadelphia, PA: Lippincott Williams & Wilkins; 2004: 674.

54. McCallum RW, Soykan I. Nausea, vomiting, and anorexia. In: Stein JH. *Internal Medicine.* 5th ed. St. Louis, MO: Mosby; 1998: 2025–2030.

55. Ray NF, Denton WG, Thamer M, et al. Abdominal adhesiolysis: inpatient care and expenditures in the United States in 1994. *J Am Coll Surg.* 1998;186:1–9.

56. Whang EE, Ashley SW, Zinner MJ. Small intestine. In: Brunicardi FC. *Schwartz's Principles of Surgery.* 8th ed. New York: McGraw-Hill Medical; 2005:1017–1054.

57. McClave SA, Taylor BE, Martindale RG, et al. Guidelines for the provision and assessment of nutrition support therapy in the adult critically ill patient: Society of Critical Care Medicine

(SCCM) and the American Society for Parenteral and Enteral Nutrition (A.S.P.E.N.). *JPEN J Parenter Enteral Nutr.* 2016; 40(2):159–211.

58. Carroll J, Alavi K. Pathogenesis and management of ileus. *Clin Colon Rectal Surg.* 2009;22(1):047–050.

59. Acute abdomen and surgical gastroenterology: abdominal pain. In: Beers MH, Berkow R, eds. *The Merck Manual of Diagnosis and Therapy.* 18th ed. New York: Wiley; 2006:94–108.

60. Gabbard SL, Lacy BE. Chronic intestinal pseudo-obstruction. *Nutr Clin Pract.* 2013;28(3):307–316.

61. Tan SA, Sarosi GA. Gastrointestinal motility disorders. In: Mulholland MW, Lillemoe KD, Doherty GM, et al, eds. *Greenfield's Surgery Scientific Principles and Practice.* 5th ed. Philadelphia, PA: Lippincott Williams & Wilkins; 2011:1027–1038.

62. de Brito-Ashurst I, Preiser JC. Diarrhea in critically ill patients: the role of enteral feeding. *JPEN J Parenter Enteral Nutr.* 2016; 40(7):913–923.

63. Diarrhea. In: *Stedman's Medical Dictionary.* Baltimore, MD: Lippincott Williams & Wilkins; 2016. STAT!Ref Online Electronic Medical Library. http://hubnet.buffalo.edu:2062/Splash.aspx?SessionId=2541E96HQYVBQUQF. Accessed January 27, 2017.

64. Abel C, Grimes JA. Diarrhea. In: Domino FJ, ed. *5-Minute Clinical Consult.* 19th ed. Philadelphia, PA: Lippincott Williams & Wilkins; 2011:394–397.

65. Jafarnejad S, Shab-Bidar S, Speakman JR, et al. Probiotics reduce the risk of antibiotic-associated diarrhea in adults (18–64) but not the elderly (>65 years): a meta-analysis. *Nutr Clin Pract.* 2016;31(4):502–513.

66. Ros PR, Buetow PC, Pantograg-Brown L, et al. Pseudomembranous colitis. *Radiology.* 1996;198(1):1–9.

67. Kelly CP, Pothoulakis C, LaMont JT. *Clostridium difficile* colitis. *N Engl J Med.* 1994;330(4):257–262.

68. Kawamoto S, Horton KM, Fishman EK. Pseudomembranous colitis: spectrum of imaging findings with clinical and pathologic correlation. *Radiographics.* 1999;19(4):887–897.

69. World Health Organization. Oral rehydration salts: production of the new ORS. 2006. http://apps.who.int/iris/bitstream/10665/69227/1/WHO_FCH_CAH_06.1.pdf?ua=1&ua=1. Accessed February 6, 2017.

70. Academy of Nutrition and Dietetics. Diarrhea. In: *Nutrition Care Manual.* Chicago, IL: Academy of Nutrition and Dietetics. https://www.nutritioncaremanual.org/client_ed.cfm?ncm_client_ed_id=20. Accessed September 30, 2016.

71. Slavin J. Dietary fiber. In: Matarese L, Gottschlich MM, eds. *Contemporary Nutrition Support Practice: A Clinical Guide.* 2nd ed. Philadelphia, PA: Saunders; 2003:173–187.

72. Jung HK, Choung RS, Locke R. The incidence, prevalence, and outcomes of patients with gastroparesis in Olmsted County, Minnesota from 1996–2006. *Gastroenterology.* 2009;136(4):1225–1233.

73. Camilleri M, Parkman HP, Shafi MA, Abell TL, Gerson L. Clinical guideline: management of gastroparesis. *Am J Gastroenterol.* 2013;108:18–37.

74. American College of Gastroenterology. Clinical guideline: management of gastroparesis. Agency for Healthcare Research and Quality National Guideline Clearinghouse. https://www.guideline.gov/summaries/summary/43612. Accessed September 30, 2016.

75. Wytiaz V, Homko C, Duffy F, Schey R, Parkman HP. Foods provoking and alleviating symptoms in gastroparesis: patient experiences. *Dig Dis Sci.* 2015;60(4):1052–1058.

76. Baldor RA. Constipation. In: Domino FJ, ed. *5-Minute Clinical Consult.* 19th ed. Philadelphia, PA: Lippincott Williams & Wilkins; 2011:306–307.

77. Academy of Nutrition and Dietetics. Constipation nutrition therapy. In: *Nutrition Care Manual.* Chicago, IL: Academy of Nutrition and Dietetics. https://www.nutritioncaremanual.org/client_ed.cfm?ncm_client_ed_id=41. Accessed September 30, 2016.

78. Academy of Nutrition and Dietetics. Constipation. In: *Nutrition Care Manual.* Chicago, IL: Academy of Nutrition and Dietetics. https://www.nutritioncaremanual.org/topic.cfm?ncm_category_id=1&lv1=5522&lv2=145248&ncm_toc_id=145248&ncm_heading=&. Accessed September 30, 2016.

79. Academy of Nutrition and Dietetics. Gastric surgery. In: *Nutrition Care Manual.* Chicago, IL: Academy of Nutrition and Dietetics. https://www.nutritioncaremanual.org/topic.cfm?ncm_category_id=1&lv1=5522&lv2=19309&ncm_toc_id=19309&ncm_heading=&. Accessed September 30, 2016.

80. Miller TE, Thacker JK, White WD, et al. Reduced length of hospital stay in colorectal surgery after an enhanced recovery protocol. *Anesth Analg.* 2014;118(5) 1052–1061.

81. Nanavati AJ, Nagral S, Prabhakar S. Fast track surgery in India. *Natl Med J India.* 2014;27:79–83.

82. Boelens PG, Heesakkers FF, Luyer MD, et al. Reduction of postoperative ileus by early enteral nutrition in patients undergoing major rectal surgery: prospective randomized, controlled trial. *Ann Surg.* 2014;259(4):649–655.

83. Secretory functions of the alimentary tract. In: Hall JE. *Guyton and Hall Textbook of Medical Physiology.* 12th ed. Philadelphia, PA: Elsevier; 2010:773–788.

84. Furness S, Worthington HV, Bryan G, Birchenough S, McMillan R. Interventions for the management of dry mouth: topical therapies. *Cochrane Database Syst Rev.* http://onlinelibrary.wiley.com/doi/10.1002/14651858.CD008934.pub2/full. Accessed September 30, 2016.

85. Warren J, Bhalla V, Cresci G. Postoperative diet advancement: surgical dogma vs evidence-based medicine. *Nutr Clin Pract.* 2011; 26(2):115–125.

86. Hall JE. Digestion and absorption in the gastrointestinal tract. In: Hall JE. *Guyton and Hall Textbook of Medical Physiology.* 12th ed. Philadelphia, PA: Elsevier; 2010:788–798.

87. Krajmalnik-Brown R, Ilhan ZE, Kang DW, DiBaise JK. Effects of gut microbes on nutrient absorption and energy regulation. *Nutr Clin Pract.* 2012;27(2):201–214.

88. Jepson JB. Hartnup's disease. In: Stanbury JB, Wyngarten JB, Fredriksno DS, eds. *The Metabolic Basis of Inherited Disease.* 4th ed. New York: McGraw-Hill; 1978:1563–1574.

89. Johnson LR. *Essential Medical Physiology.* 2nd ed. Philadelphia, PA: Lippincott-Raven; 1998.

90. Bragg LE, Thompson JS, Rikkers LF. Influence of nutrient delivery on gut structure and function. *Nutrition.* 1991;7(4):237–243.

91. Young LS, Stoll S. Proteins and amino acids. In: Matarese LE, Gottschlich MM, eds. *Contemporary Nutrition Support Practice: A Clinical Guide.* 2nd ed. Philadelphia, PA: Saunders; 2003:94–104.

92. Kimchi ET, Gusani NJ, Kaifi JT. Anatomy and physiology of the small intestines. In: Mulholland MW, Lillemoe KD, Doherty GM, Maier RV, Simeone DM, Upchurch GR, eds. *Greenfield's Surgery Scientific Principles and Practice.* 5th ed. Philadelphia, PA: Lippincott Williams & Wilkins; 2011:738–748.

2 Energy

David Frankenfield, MS, RD

CONTENTS

Acknowledgments: Jennifer Wooley, MS, RD, CNSC, was the coauthor of this chapter for the second edition.

Objectives

1. Compare energy metabolism during health and illness.
2. Identify evidence-based methods for calculating resting metabolic rate (RMR).
3. Review methods to measure energy expenditure.

Test Your Knowledge Questions

1. Which of the following is the largest component of total energy expenditure (TEE)?
   A. RMR
   B. Thermogenic effect of digestion
   C. Physical activity
   D. Metabolic stress
2. Which of the following is the most commonly used method for assessing energy expenditure?
   A. Indirect calorimetry (IC)
   B. Predictive equations
   C. The reverse Fick equation
   D. Doubly labeled water
3. Which parameter is measured when using IC?
   A. Heat loss
   B. Catabolic rate
   C. Gas exchange
   D. Free energy balance
4. You are determining the energy intake target for a 53-year-old, critically ill, male patient who is about to start enteral feeding. He is 170 cm in height and weighs 150 kg. His body mass index (BMI) is 51.9 and his ideal body weight is 70 kg. Body temperature is 37.3 degrees Celsius and minute ventilation is 12.5 L/min. Based on the 2016 American Society for Parenteral and Enteral Nutrition (ASPEN) guideline[1] for calculating a goal energy intake for such a critically ill patient, what energy value would you use as the basis for the feeding plan?
   A. 1750 kcal/d (25 kcal per kg ideal body weight)
   B. 1225 kcal/d (70% of the calculated 25 kcal per kg ideal body weight)
   C. 2250 kcal/d (25 kcal per kg adjusted body weight)
   D. 2615 kcal/d (Penn State equation)

Test Your Knowledge Answers

1. The correct answer is **A**. The thermogenic effect of digestion is generally thought to contribute no more than 10% to TEE.[2] Activity contributes 5% to 30% to TEE.[2] With the exceptions of burn (see Chapter 24) and sepsis (see Chapter 23), metabolic stress contributes less than 50% to TEE. However, in almost all situations, RMR constitutes 60% to 75% of TEE.[3]
2. The correct answer is **B**. Most nutrition support feeding regimens are based on predictive equations used to assess energy expenditure.[4] The measurement of energy expenditure via IC is more accurate than predictive equations but is underused because the equipment is expensive to purchase and operate, and because some patients cannot be measured for various technical and physiological reasons.

3. The correct answer is **C**. Indirect calorimeters measure respiratory gas exchange (the difference between inspired and expired oxygen and carbon dioxide).[5] If proper testing conditions are observed, respiratory gas exchange is equivalent to metabolic gas exchange (the consumption of oxygen and production of carbon dioxide [CO_2] at the cellular level). Gas exchange data are converted to RMR using the Weir equation.[6]
4. The correct answer is **A**. The ASPEN guideline states that the goal intake for all classes of obesity should not exceed 65% to 70% of target energy expenditure as measured by IC.[1] For class III obesity (BMI equal to or greater than 40), an intake of 22 to 25 kcal per kg ideal body weight is recommended. The Penn State equation (answer D) has been validated as being among the most accurate ways of calculating energy expenditure up to a BMI of at least 80.[7,8] However, answer D is incorrect if following the ASPEN guideline because that guideline emphasizes the kcal/kg method. The patient has class III obesity; therefore, ideal body weight would be used for the calculation, making answer C incorrect because it uses adjusted body weight. Answer B is incorrect because the guideline already factors the 30% reduction in the energy calculation into the standard; therefore, if the energy expenditure were calculated and then multiplied by 70%, the effect would be to reduce the energy intake target to about 50% of expenditure.

Background

Acquisition and transformation of energy are among the most basic characteristics of life.[9] Living things must be capable of consuming chemical energy from the environment, converting it to cellular components, and transforming it to a form that can power work. Energy transformations (metabolism) are necessary for living things to maintain homeostasis and perform the other activities associated with life. In humans, energy metabolism has evolved into a series of interrelated and complex biochemical processes by which humans consume fuels from the environment, convert them to tissue or oxidize them to release energy to perform work, and ultimately convert the fuels to heat, water, and CO_2, all of which are dissipated back to the environment.

This chapter reviews energy metabolism in healthy subjects as the framework for understanding the alterations in energy metabolism during malnutrition and illness. The energy prescription is a fundamental aspect of the nutrition support regimen. Therefore, emphasis in this chapter is placed on evidence-based methods for determining the energy expenditure of those patients who are unable to meet their needs orally and therefore require nutrition support therapy.

Overview of Energy Metabolism

The basic fuels of the body are carbohydrate, protein, and fat (ethanol can also be oxidized). Glucose is used preferentially after meals, whereas fat is stored for later oxidation. Protein generally is used for structural and functional, rather than oxidative, purposes; however, during routine protein turnover, some is oxidized. (See Chapters 3, 5, and 6.) When energy is not available in the form of food, the body cannibalizes its own tissues as an endogenous energy source. This catabolic process is hormonally driven and is reversible by feeding. The maintenance of an endogenous source of glucose supply while limiting protein loss is of primary importance, and the body has complex mechanisms to create and store glucose if dietary intake is interrupted.[10,11] Over time, further metabolic adaptations provide alternate fuels for oxidative pathways that substitute for and recycle glucose and that access the large store of energy in the adipose tissue. These changes decrease protein catabolism and allow conservation of the body protein mass while providing enough energy to maintain core body functions.[12–14]

Components of Energy Expenditure

TEE can be divided into 3 major components in healthy, well-nourished adults: basal metabolic rate (BMR) or RMR, energy required for the thermogenic effect of digestion, and energy expenditure associated with physical activity. Tissue synthesis is an energy-consuming process, and illness may cause an alteration in rest, thermogenesis, and physical activity.

Basal or Resting Metabolic Rate

The terms BMR and RMR sometimes cause confusion, partly because they have distinct but similar definitions, and partly because some authors use the terms interchangeably. BMR is metabolic rate measured in a fasting state, immediately upon awakening and before any physical activity is undertaken.[2,3] RMR also is measured in a fasted state,[2,3] but some movement (dressing, walking) is allowed before testing. A rest time of 20 to 30 minutes is necessary for recovery from this level of activity.[2,15] Once this rest period is provided, the difference between RMR and BMR is small, with RMR being slightly higher. Because BMR is a more cumbersome measurement (requiring confinement in a metabolic ward or laboratory), most studies of human metabolism are made in a resting rather than a basal state. In many nutrition support patients, even the less restrictive RMR standard of measurement is not obtained because the patients are fed continuously and thus are never in a fasted state. Instead, the resting definition is modified to include the metabolic effect of feeding.[3,16]

Even in the most physically active individuals and the most hypermetabolic patients, RMR accounts for the largest portion of TEE (60% to 75%). RMR is determined largely by body size and body composition.[17,18] Sex and age also affect RMR (RMR is lower in females and in the elderly).[18,19] Some of the sex and age effects are indirect, being a result of the amount or composition of the fat-free mass rather than related to biological sex differences or age effects per se.[18,19] Composition of the fat-free mass might also explain some observed racial differences in RMR.[19–21]

Thermogenic Effect of Digestion

The digestion of macronutrients following the consumption of a meal leads to an increase in metabolic rate referred to as the *thermogenic effect of digestion*. This still ill-defined phenomenon was originally thought to be specific to protein (hence, its original name, "specific dynamic action").[5] The presence,

magnitude, and duration of the thermogenic effect of digestion seem to be influenced by numerous factors. Diet factors include the size and composition of the meal and the time of day the meal is eaten.[2] Other factors include age, smoking, stress, and caffeine use.[2] In general, a 5% to 10% increase in TEE is ascribed to the thermogenic effect of digestion.[13,22] However, Heymsfield and associates[23] have demonstrated in healthy people that if feeding is delivered as a continuous infusion of liquid formula via gastric feeding tube, the thermogenic effect of digestion is not induced. This finding is pertinent to the nutrition support population; the same seems to be true for critically ill patients being fed continuously, although the data are limited. Frankenfield and Ashcraft[24] found only a 1% difference in RMR between fed and unfed patients with brain injuries (1982 ± 249 kcal/d vs 2002 ± 425 kcal/d).

Physical Activity

Physical activity is the most variable and difficult to predict portion of TEE. In nonhospitalized adults, the amount of energy expended on physical activity is a function of the duration and vigor of exercise and nonexercise movement and work, and can be influenced by conscious and unconscious factors.[25,26] For critically ill patients, care activities, such as bathing, turning, wound care, and chest physiotherapy, can substantially raise the metabolic rate. However, these activities are short-lived and their cumulative effect on TEE is usually small. Typical activity in critically ill patients has been measured at about 5% to 10% above rest.[27–29] In hospitalized patients who are ambulatory, agitated, or fidgeting, energy expended in physical activity might be considerably higher than 10%.

Tissue Synthesis

In nutrition repletion, pregnancy, and childhood, energy requirements increase to support tissue growth.[30] Tissue synthesis is a high-energy activity. Not only is the newly synthesized tissue composed of fuel (protein and fat), but the synthesis of the new tissue from individual amino acids, fatty acids, and glucose is an energy-requiring reaction.[30,31] Wound repair may be thought of in a similar way but on a smaller scale.[31]

Illness

Hypermetabolism is often noted in people who are chronically or acutely ill.[7,32–35] Taylor has reviewed many studies of RMR in chronic illness.[32] A common finding in these studies is that the mean increase in RMR is 10% above the healthy resting level. This mean value sits right on the upper edge of the range of "normal" (±10% of the predicted healthy level) and indicates that RMR is not elevated in about 50% of chronically ill patients, whereas it is elevated in the other 50%.

A limited number of studies of RMR have been carried out in acutely ill, spontaneously breathing patients. Gariballa and Forster[33] reported that the Harris-Benedict equation for RMR in healthy people approximated the measured RMR in a group of such patients; however, the equation accurately predicted the measured RMR in only 47% of the cases, meaning that the other 53% were either hypermetabolic or hypometabolic

TABLE 2-1 Rates and Degrees of Hypermetabolism and Hypometabolism in Healthy; Acutely Ill; and Critically Ill, Mechanically Ventilated Patients

Group (Reference)	N	% Obese	Mean Resting Metabolic Rate Increase (% of Mifflin–St. Jeor)	Percentage of Measurements >10% Above Mifflin–St. Jeor	Maximum Above Mifflin–St. Jeor	Percentage of Measurements <10% Above Mifflin–St. Jeor	Maximum Below Mifflin–St. Jeor
Healthy (35)	337	46	1.01	11	1.45	6.8	0.83
Acutely ill (38)	56	35	1.17	60	1.54	3.5	0.77
Critically ill (7)	202	47	1.23	74	2.14	1.5	0.75

(the authors did not describe the distribution). Weijs and colleagues[34] measured the RMR of a group of inpatients and found that the Mifflin–St. Jeor equation for healthy people accurately estimated the RMR in 50% of the cases. Frankenfield and Ashcraft[35] found a similar accuracy rate for the Mifflin–St. Jeor equation (42%), with a mean elevation in RMR of 17% above Mifflin–St. Jeor equation value.

The RMR of critically ill patients has been measured more extensively than the RMR for perhaps any other group.[3] RMR equations for healthy people (primarily Harris-Benedict or Mifflin–St. Jeor) are routinely found to be inaccurate in most critically ill patients, with the direction of the error indicating that most critically ill patients are hypermetabolic. Most metabolic studies of the critically ill group patients by disease type (eg, trauma, surgery, sepsis); however, a clear hierarchy in the degree of hypermetabolism by illness type has not emerged, perhaps because it is the inflammatory response to the illness—rather than the illness itself—that determines the RMR. Thus, a febrile surgical patient may have a higher RMR than an afebrile trauma patient. Frankenfield and colleagues[36] found that differences in the RMRs of trauma, surgery, and medical critical care patients were eliminated when the impact of body temperature was controlled. Raurich et al[37] likewise found no differences in RMRs among trauma, surgical, and medical patients when RMR was measured at body temperatures between 36 and 38 degrees Celsius.

Table 2-1 shows how measured RMR compares with comparative standards for healthy people in (1) healthy individuals;[38] (2) acutely ill, spontaneously breathing patients;[35] and (3) critically ill, mechanically ventilated patients.[7] In healthy adults, 11% have measured RMR above the expected rate. In acutely ill patients, this figure increases to 60%. In mechanically ventilated, critically ill patients, the measured RMR exceeds the healthy comparative standard 74% of the time. Hypometabolism is rare in all 3 groups but notably less so in ill patients than in healthy people. The maximum increase in RMR is higher in the critically ill than in the healthy or acutely ill groups.

Overview of Methods to Determine Energy Expenditure

Measurement of Energy Expenditure

A foundational goal of nutrition support is to preserve lean body mass and maintain immune function while avoiding complications related to under- or overfeeding. Despite the availability of more than 200 predictive equations to estimate energy expenditure, predicting the needs of an individual critically ill patient is difficult. Measurement of RMR is the most reliable method of determining energy needs.[2,3,16]

Direct Calorimetry

Direct calorimetry measures heat and chemical energy released from the body. Because the fuel energy used by the body is ultimately transformed to heat, heat release is considered a direct measurement of metabolic rate. Urine is also collected and measured to account for the small amount of chemical energy lost in urea excretion in urine. Direct calorimeters are sophisticated machines consisting of a living space or chamber thermally isolated from the outside, with equipment to extract and measure the heat released into the air of the chamber from the subject residing within.[5] Experiments can last for days, and this method allows for the partitioning of energy expended at rest, in sleep, and during physical activity (which is sometimes tracked using a radar system inside the chamber). Direct calorimetry is most appropriate in the study of healthy subjects done in research and academic environments. The technique is not practical in the patient care because the individual must remain alone in the chamber over an extended time without caregivers or medical equipment (both of which produce heat).

Indirect Calorimetry

Among the first metabolic observations of living things was that they consumed some substance from the atmosphere.[5] It was found later that this substance was oxygen and that, furthermore, CO_2 was produced. In the late 19th and early 20th centuries, some direct calorimeters were outfitted with equipment to measure gas exchange simultaneously with the measurement of heat. These "respiration calorimeters" were used to deduce the ratios of gas exchange to heat production and to prove the equivalence of the 2 processes—the measurement of gas exchange was shown to be an indirect but accurate reflection of energy expenditure.[5] Ignoring the energy loss from urea excretion in urine was found not to significantly alter the accuracy of the IC measurement;[6] for this reason, urine is usually not collected when IC is conducted.

Indirect calorimeters have many advantages over direct calorimeters in terms of smaller size, lower cost, easier measurement and maintenance, shorter measurement periods, and minimal interruption of patient care. Subjects do not need to be isolated inside of room-size chambers as long as their respiratory gases can be completely captured for approximately 30 minutes. IC is now considered a gold standard method for measuring RMR in research and clinical settings, even in critically ill patients not breathing atmospheric air. Numerous brands of IC devices are commercially available. Most consist of sensors for measuring oxygen and CO_2 concentrations in inspired and expired air, a device for measuring exhaled minute volume, and a computer system to calculate parameters and manage data.[5]

Ventilator-Derived Measurement of Carbon Dioxide Production

Stapel et al[39] have described a method for calculating the volume of CO_2 production (VCO_2) from the end tidal CO_2 and expired gas volumes measured by some commercially available mechanical ventilators. VCO_2 is calculated as the breath-by-breath exhaled volume multiplied by the fraction of expired CO_2, averaged over a minute, and then aggregated to a 24-hour period. The theoretical respiratory quotient (RQ) of the macronutrient intake is then calculated from the actual fuel intake (or assumed to be approximately 0.85). Oxygen consumption (VO_2) is calculated from the algebraic manipulation of the RQ equation and combined with the Weir equation to calculate RMR, as follows:[6]

$$VO_2 = VCO_2/RQ$$

$$RMR = (VO_2 \times 3.91) + (VCO_2 \times 1.1) + 1.44$$

where RMR is measured in kcal/d, and VO_2 and VCO_2 are measured in mL/min.

Two advantages of this system are that (1) the monitoring is continuous and results in a measure of TEE rather than RMR, and (2) facilities do not need to purchase a separate indirect calorimeter. However, the functionality is probably not included in the ventilator's basic software package and thus would need to be purchased separately. The idea of measuring just VCO_2 and calculating VO_2 and RMR by assuming an RQ is not new.[5] Harris and Benedict relate a similar method in their classic monograph (measuring VCO_2 and assuming an RQ to calculate RMR).[40]

Reverse Fick Equation

Oxygen consumption can be estimated using the Fick principles derived from oxygen content differences in arterial and mixed venous blood multiplied by cardiac output measurements from pulmonary artery catheters.[41] Placement of a pulmonary artery catheter is highly invasive, and the oxygen consumption measurements are poorly correlated with IC oxygen consumption ($R^2 = 0.30$) and biased toward underestimation.[42] Therefore, the Fick equation is not useful for clinical assessment of energy expenditure.

Doubly Labeled Water

The doubly labeled water technique is another option for assessing energy expenditure. This method administers a sta-

ble isotope of water (^2H_2O) to the patient and measures its disappearance rate over time (days).[43] Disappearance of ^2H is proportional to water turnover, whereas the disappearance of ^{18}O is proportional to water turnover plus VCO_2 production. The difference between the 2 disappearance rates is the VCO_2. VO_2 is not measured; instead, it is computed from the "food quotient" (FQ), which is the sum of the CO_2 produced from all food eaten divided by the sum of the oxygen consumed during oxidation of all food eaten. From FQ and measured VCO_2, VO_2 can be computed: $VCO_2/FQ = VO_2$. Alternately, an RQ can be assumed and VO_2 computed as $VCO_2/RQ = VO_2$. The doubly labeled water technique of measuring metabolic rate is useful in field research, but it is not generally used in clinical care.

Mathematical Equations

Given the significant cost and limited availability of measurement equipment, the predominant method of determining RMR in nutrition support patients is calculation.[4,16] Many equations exist for this purpose. Not all have been tested for validity, and few of those that have been tested are considered accurate enough for general use.[44] Even the accurate equations have a significant error rate and magnitude. Most equations take advantage of correlations between body size and composition and energy use to determine RMR. Some calculation methods for sick or injured patients use an equation for healthy people multiplied by various stress factors, which are based on the type of illness or injury.[3,44] Other equations are specific to patients with illnesses or injuries and use body size and physiological variables such as body temperature, heart rate, respiratory rate, or minute volume to capture the hypermetabolism that often occurs in patients.[3,44]

Application of Methods to Determine Energy Requirements

Indirect Calorimetry

When operating an indirect calorimeter, the fundamental concept to bear in mind is that it provides a respiratory measurement and certain conditions must prevail for the respiratory measurement of gas exchange to be equivalent to metabolic gas exchange. The best way to ensure such conditions is to follow an evidence-based protocol as strictly as possible.[2,3,16] These protocols indicate that to conduct a useful IC measurement, the clinician must pay attention to the selection and preparation of the patient and environment; the measurement must meet certain quality criteria; and the overall situation of the patient and the overall care plan must be kept in mind when results are interpreted.[2,3,16]

Indications for Indirect Calorimetry

There is no absolute indication for IC. All indications are relative. For example, it has been demonstrated that the metabolic rate of an underweight critically ill or acutely ill patient is more likely to be inaccurately predicted than the metabolic rate of a normal weight or obese patient.[8] Therefore, it would seem

TABLE 2-2 Relative Indications for Indirect Calorimetry

- Body mass index <20.5
- Body mass index >80
- Concern about overfeeding in a patient with unexplained high ventilator requirement or who for an unknown reason cannot be liberated from the ventilator
- Unwanted weight loss over time not explained by volume status in a patient who regularly receives nearly 100% of target feeding
- Massive tissue loss from amputation
- Preadmission fluid overload (ascites, volume resuscitation, "third spacing") without a reliable report of body weight at proper hydration

reasonable that a low BMI is a good indication for measurement of the energy expenditure. However, predictive energy equations are accurate about 50% of the time in underweight patients; therefore, if such a patient is receiving a calculated energy load that does not seem to be causing respiratory distress or further weight loss, then an IC measurement may not be needed. The decision to measure expenditure will nearly always be subjective, must be based on individual circumstances, and ideally is a decision of a multidisciplinary team (physician, dietitian, respiratory therapist, and nurse). Table 2-2 lists selected relative indications for IC.

Contraindications for Indirect Calorimetry

There are several absolute contraindications for IC. Again, recalling that IC is a respiratory measurement that under proper conditions is equivalent to metabolism, any factor that violates these conditions is a contraindication to IC (Table 2-3).[16] Furthermore, if RMR is the desired value to be measured (and it usually is), then any factor that prevents the patient from being at rest or cooperating with the device operator is also a contraindication.

Patient Preparation

Before IC is used, mechanically ventilated patients must be checked for recent ventilator changes (within the past 30

TABLE 2-3 Contraindications for Indirect Calorimetry

- Air leak (chest tubes, cuff leak, any other leak in ventilator circuit, leaks around face masks, canopies, etc)
- Extracorporeal membrane oxygenation
- Hemodialysis (during and for several hours afterward)
- For mechanically ventilated patients, a fraction of inspired oxygen >60%
- For spontaneously breathing patients:
  - Reliance on any supplemental oxygen (cannula, face mask, etc)
  - Inability to cooperate with the measurement
  - Claustrophobia or any anxiety about the measurement

minutes)[16,28] and recent nursing care involving patient movement or pain (within the past 30 minutes).[28] For spontaneously breathing patients, the operator needs to check that the patient is not claustrophobic and does not have other anxiety about the measurement, that there is no supplemental oxygen in use, and that the patient has not been out of bed or received care in the past 30 minutes.

In healthy people, the definition of a resting state includes fasting. In patients who are being continuously fed by nonvolitional means, the fasting requirement is suspended, partly because it is more accurate to capture the effect,[3,16] but also because it is unclear if a thermogenic effect is even present.[23,24] For patients eating food by mouth, IC should be conducted after a 7-hour fast,[2] and for ill patients being bolus fed, IC should not be conducted until 4 hours after the feeding.[2]

Environmental Factors

Although there are scant data to support the concept, it is logical that external stimulation of the patient should be minimal if RMR is to be measured.[2,3,16] For example, patients should avoid reading,[45] conversation, administration of care, and stimulation by family members before and during the test. Generally, the level of ambient light is reduced, although the level of light has not been proven to affect results. Ambient noise should probably be kept to a minimum—music increases RMR in conscious patients.[45] In patients who are heavily sedated, comatose, or medically paralyzed, these precautions are probably less important than for a patient who is fully aware of his/her surroundings. Nursing care can increase RMR;[25-28] therefore, patients should not be measured within about 30 minutes of such activities. It is not known if 30 minutes of rest time is necessary in heavily sedated critically ill patients.[3]

Room temperature should be controlled to the extent possible. At low ambient temperature (less than 20 degrees Celsius [68 degrees Fahrenheit]), the body will make adaptations to minimize heat loss (vasoconstriction) and increase heat production (shivering and nonshivering thermogenesis) to maintain body temperature.[2,3,16] The result is an increase in metabolic rate.[46-48] If the room temperature cannot be increased, use of blankets to raise the temperature of the air immediately around the patient will prevent these metabolic adaptations.[46] At ambient temperature greater than body temperature, the body will give off heat to the environment to keep itself cool, thus increasing metabolic rate.[49]

Measurement Procedure

If all environmental and patient conditions are met, the IC measurement can be started. The step-by-step measurement procedure varies from device to device. The procedure instructions from the manufacturer should be scrupulously followed every time the indirect calorimeter is used. In addition to device configuration, these instructions include proper warm-up time and calibration of the device instruments for measuring gas volumes and concentrations.

Measurement times can vary between 10 and 30 minutes.[2,3,16] The first 5 minutes of measurement are typically discarded as a time for the patient to become acclimated to

FIGURE 2-1 Measurement Times for Indirect Calorimetry

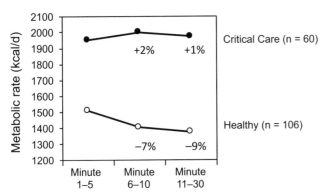

Change in metabolic rate recording in the first 5-minute "discard" period in a group of critically ill, mechanically ventilated patients (closed circles) and a group of spontaneously breathing healthy volunteers (open circles). The difference between the first 5 minutes and the remainder of the test is minimal for the critically ill group but significantly different for the healthy group. Therefore, discarding the first 5 minutes of test results is important for measurements of spontaneously breathing people being measured with indirect calorimetry, but may be less so for mechanically ventilated patients. Source: Data collected by author.

the procedure. Discarding these early data is vital in conscious patients who are aware that a measurement is being conducted, and especially in patients being measured with canopy or facemask air collection systems, but it is probably not as important for sedated patients in whom the device connections are made at the ventilator rather than the nose or mouth (Figure 2-1). A period of steady state is then sought as a precaution against respiratory artifact destroying the correlation between respiratory and metabolic gas exchange. Various steady-state definitions have been validated.[2,16] Most require some limit in the minute-to-minute variation in VO_2 and VCO_2 over a defined time period (eg, 10% coefficient of variation over 10 minutes of measurement).

Measurement Interpretation

When interpreting data, the first steps are to note whether resting conditions prevailed during the measurement and whether a steady-state period was achieved. If these conditions were met, then the 2 measured gas parameters, VO_2 and VCO_2, are used to calculate the metabolic rate using the modified Weir equation:[6]

$$RMR = [(VO_2 \times 3.94) + (VCO_2 \times 1.11)] \times 1.44$$

where RMR is measured in kcal/d and VO_2 and VCO_2 are measured in mL/min.

The modified version of the Weir equation differs from the full equation in that it ignores the small energy loss in the form of urea excretion. Although a small error (1% to 2%) results from this omission, using the modification means urea nitrogen does not need to be measured to complete the IC study.

RQ can be calculated as the ratio of VCO_2 to VO_2. The metabolic range of RQ is somewhere between 0.67 and 1.3. Although each macronutrient fuel has its own RQ signature

when oxidized in isolation (eg, in a bomb calorimeter), the macronutrients are oxidized simultaneously in a living system, making interpretation of the RQ much less straightforward. The metabolic interpretation of RQ greater than 1 is net fat synthesis and is often taken as an indicator of overfeeding. However, published reports have noted RQ values greater than 1 in patients who were not being overfed and RQ less than 1 in patients who were being overfed.[2,16] What then is the proper interpretation of RQ? Brandi[50] wrote a remarkable paper on the effect of respiratory artifact on gas exchange measures. He produced a wide excursion in RQ by introducing respiratory artifact (creating a large and not physiological 35% change in minute ventilation by increasing or decreasing the tidal volume in patients whose clinical condition did not call for such a change). Importantly, this artificial change in minute ventilation did not significantly alter VO_2 or RMR (about 2%), but it did change the apparent VCO_2 (about 12%) and therefore RQ (about 16%). Thus, it is possible to produce a valid measure of RMR even when RQ and VCO_2 recordings are altered by respiratory rather than metabolic factors. Clearly, a metabolic interpretation of RQ in mechanically ventilated patients can therefore be unreliable, and RQ should not be used to assess the feeding state of individual patients. The main use of RQ should be to determine whether egregious error might be present, especially if the RQ is outside the physiological range of 0.67 to 1.3. Notably, the large respiratory artifact made by Brandi[50] increased the RQ to 1.02 or decreased it to 0.73 from a baseline of 0.88—changes within the physiological range.

Measurement Frequency

IC measurements in critically ill, mechanically ventilated patients have a useful life of 3 or 4 days, after which the measurement needs to be repeated or calculation methods substituted.[51] IC studies repeated weekly are no more accurate over time than predictive equations (Figure 2-2).[51] The necessary frequency of measurement for acutely ill spontaneously breathing patients is not known.

Predictive Energy Expenditure Equations for Healthy Individuals

In most instances when a nutrition support regimen is being formulated, measured RMR is not available and the clinician must rely on an estimate of the energy requirement. Equations for predicting RMR have been available since at least 1916.[52] The original purpose of the equations was to develop a standard against which to test whether an RMR measurement fell within the normal range (analogous to determining the laboratory standard for serum sodium concentration in a human being). Over the decades, standard calculations have proliferated and their use has evolved to their current purpose of calculating energy prescriptions.

Harris-Benedict Equation

In 1916, Dubois may have produced the first standard metabolic equations.[52] These formulas predate the now more famous Harris-Benedict equation[41] by 3 years but have almost

FIGURE 2-2 Accuracy Over Time for Measured and Calculated Resting Metabolic Rate

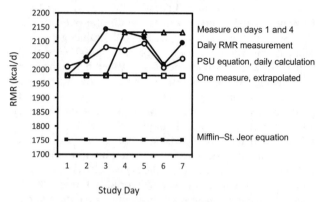

Measure on days 1 and 4
Daily RMR measurement
PSU equation, daily calculation
One measure, extrapolated

Mifflin–St. Jeor equation

Study Day

Cumulative measured resting metabolic rate (RMR) was 14,548 ± 2,344 kcal/d. Penn State (PSU) equation recalculated daily was 1.7% ± 5.9% below cumulative daily measurement and was more accurate than a single measurement extrapolated over the 7 days (4.1% ± 11.2% below cumulative daily measurement). Measurements conducted every 3 or 4 days are more accurate than the PSU equation (0.5% ± 4.8% above cumulative daily measurement).
Source: Data collected by author, based on reference 51.

been forgotten. The Harris-Benedict equation has now also mostly transitioned from a clinical tool to a historical landmark. This equation is remarkable for 3 reasons. First is its longevity, being published in 1919. Second, it represents the first use of regression techniques in physiology.[53] Third, after being initially received with some skepticism, it established linear rather than allometric scaling for calculating resting metabolism, although the argument over which approach is best continues today.[54] The term *allometric* describes a change in one biological parameter that is not linear with another (eg, a curve).

Benedict himself recognized that the Harris-Benedict equation tended to overestimate the true RMR,[55] and this observation has been documented in subsequent validation studies.[45,56–59] A 2003 evidence review by the American Dietetic Association (ADA, now known as Academy of Nutrition and Dietetics [AND]) indicates that other equations are more reliable than the Harris-Benedict,[44] and use of the Harris-Benedict equation has since waned. Notably, most of the descriptive studies of metabolism in illness have used the Harris-Benedict equation as the base calculation; therefore, most of the stress factors currently in use today likely need to be recalculated (or abandoned).

Mifflin–St. Jeor Equation

In 1990, Mifflin and colleagues published a study proposing new predictive equations for RMR.[59] In this study, the investigators measured the RMR of 247 women and 251 men, ages 19 to 78 years. Roughly half of the subjects were obese, with a maximum BMI of 42. Fat-free mass was also measured and found to be the strongest single predictor of RMR ($R^2 = 0.64$). However, the combination of body weight, height, age, and sex were found to correlate better than fat-free mass ($R^2 =$

0.71), and, being easier quantities to obtain, this combination of factors was chosen to construct the predictive equation. In this way, the Mifflin–St. Jeor equation resembles the Harris-Benedict equation. Mifflin and associates obtained the highest correlation when the obese and nonobese subjects were combined into a single sex-specific equation, as follows:

Men: RMR = 5 + (10 × W) + (6.25 × H) – (5 × A)

Women: RMR = –161 + (10 × W) + (6.25 × H) – (5 × A)

where RMR is measured in kcal/d; W is weight (kg); H is height (cm); and A is age (years).

Whether the combining of obese and nonobese people into one equation is successful because of a statistical artifact (ie, error spread over a wider range of measured values will raise the correlation coefficient) or because it fits physiological reality is debatable, but the Mifflin–St. Jeor equation has been shown to be valid in both men and women, including people with BMI greater than the BMI in the original sample (42).[38,60] The ADA systematic review found more favorable evidence for the Mifflin–St. Jeor equation than for any other,[44] although the accuracy rate of Mifflin–St. Jeor falls somewhat when applied to obese people (75% in people with BMI 30 or higher compared with 87% in people with BMI less than 30) and not every study shows the Mifflin–St. Jeor equation to be the most accurate.[60–62] Because of this evidence analysis, the AND recommends the Mifflin–St. Jeor equation in the current edition of *Nutrition Care Manual*.[63]

Livingston Equation

Livingston and Kohlstadt[54] resurrected the linear vs allometric scaling argument with the publication of a new predictive equation in 2005. This equation was calculated from a database of the Harris-Benedict data, the Owen data,[57,58] and the authors' measurements from 327 additional patients (total N = 670). The equations are simplified in that they use only weight and age, but the computation is made slightly more complex by the presence of a power function:

Men: RMR = (293 × W^0.4330) – (5.92 × A)

Women: RMR = (248 × W^0.4356) – (5.09 × A)

where RMR is measured in kcal/d; W is weight (kg); and A is age (years).

Livingston and Kohlstadt[54] included a validation sample of 767 individual RMR determinations obtained from the Institute of Medicine. This validation study indicated that the Livingston and Mifflin–St. Jeor equations performed about the same in a mixed sample of obese and nonobese individuals. Weijs[60] found the same result, with the Livingston and Mifflin–St. Jeor equations both accurately predicting RMR in 79% of a sample of overweight and obese Americans. (Interestingly, these equations were not as successful at predicting RMR in a sample overweight and obese Dutch.[60]) Frankenfield[38] found the Livingston and Mifflin–St. Jeor equations predicted RMR with similar accuracy in nonobese people (88% vs 87%) but that Mifflin–St. Jeor was more accurate in obesity (75% vs

FIGURE 2-3 Difference in the Relationship Between Metabolic Rate and Body Weight When Scaled Allometrically vs Linearly

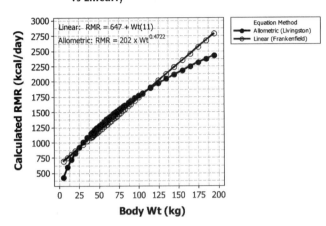

The difference is small enough that the allometric scale nearly matches the linear between body weights of 25 and 150 kg. RMR, resting metabolic rate; Wt, weight. Source: Allometric equation published in Livingston and Kohlstadt.[54] Linear equation based on data from Frankenfield et al.[64] Reprinted with permission from reference 65: Frankenfield DC, Ashcraft CM. Estimating energy needs in nutrition support patients. *JPEN J Parenter Enteral Nutr.* 2011;35:563–570.

69%), including the most severely obese population (68% vs 57% accuracy) in which a curve should have been most advantageous. The allometric scaling of the Livingston equation may have been to slight advantage in people with BMI less than 20 (85% vs 80% accuracy), again in a range of BMI where a curve should be advantageous (Figure 2-3).[54,64,65]

Predictive Equations for Critically Ill Patients

The 2 earliest and possibly still most common ways to predict RMR in critically ill patients are to use a ratio of kcal to kg of body weight or to calculate healthy RMR (with Harris-Benedict or Mifflin–St. Jeor) and multiply by a stress factor. The kcal/kg method continues to be promulgated by organizations such as ASPEN.[1] Other organizations such as AND have recommended population-specific regression equations, such as the Penn State equations, based on the strength of evidence analysis.[66]

Ratio Method

The kcal/kg ratio calculation has simplicity in its favor, but it is not an accurate way to predict RMR in the critically ill. Part of this inaccuracy stems from the very simplicity of the method, which does not consider the effect of age or sex on the RMR and does not account for variation due to altered physiology, except in a subjective way—the clinician can select a kcal/kg ratio from a range of values, but there is no basis for making the selection. The effect of obesity is captured in the ASPEN method[1] by changing the kcal/kg range or the mass used for the calculation (ideal body weight, rather than actual body weight, is used for patients with BMI greater than 50). Validation studies of kcal/kg ratio calculations usually show an accuracy rate of less than 50%.[44]

Ireton-Jones Equation

The Ireton-Jones equation was one of the first to approach metabolic rate prediction in the critically ill without adding a stress factor to a healthy RMR equation. However, the calculation uses static and categorical variables and so cannot account for dynamic changes in RMR:[67] The equation is as follows:

$$RMR = 1784 - (11 \times A) + (5 \times W) + (244 \times S) + (239 \times T) + (804 \times B)$$

where RMR is measured in kcal/d; A is age (years); W is actual body weight (kg); S is sex (male = 1, female = 0); T is diagnosis of trauma (present = 1, absent = 0); and B is diagnosis of burn (present = 1, absent = 0).

Validation studies have shown that this equation has a low accuracy rate in mechanically ventilated, critical care patients.[7,68-70] The AND Evidence Analysis Library for critical care nutrition does not recommend the use of the Ireton-Jones equation.[3]

Swinamer Equation

The Swinamer equation[68] is an early example of an equation that used dynamic physiological variables in addition to body size to predict RMR in critically ill patients. The advantage of using such variables as body temperature, respiratory rate, and tidal volume is that, as these variables change from day to day, they can reflect day-to-day changes in RMR that equations based on static variables cannot. The Swinamer equation is as follows:

$$RMR = (BSA \times 941) - (A \times 6.3) + (Temp \times 104) + (RR \times 24) + (VT \times 804) - 4243$$

where RMR is measured in kcal/d; BSA is body surface area (m²); A is age (years); Temp is body temperature (degrees Celsius); RR is respiratory rate (breaths/min); and VT is tidal volume (L).

The Swinamer equation has been found to accurately predict RMR in about 55% of patients and to cause large error (more than 15% above measured RMR) 30% of the time.[7] In the AND systematic review, the equation was not recommended for use because of this high error rate.[3]

Penn State Equation

The Penn State equation was first published in 1998 and revised twice based on subsequent validation studies.[71] Like the Swinamer equation, it combines variables that relate RMR to body size and composition (ie, the Mifflin–St. Jeor equation) with dynamic physiological variables to capture day-to-day variation in the RMR. The Penn State equation is as follows:[72]

$$RMR = (Mifflin\text{–}St.\ Jeor \times 0.96) + (V_E \times 32) + (T_{max} \times 167) - 6212$$

where RMR and Mifflin–St. Jeor estimates are measured in kcal/d; T_{max} is maximum body temperature in the previous 24 hours (degrees Celsius); and V_E is minute ventilation (L/min).

Numerous validation studies have been conducted on this equation,[7,8,24,51,73-78] and it has been recommended for use by AND.[3] Since the AND recommendation was made, the equation has been demonstrated to be accurate in morbidly obese patients (80% accuracy up to a BMI of at least 80), patients with brain injuries (72% accuracy), and patients in barbiturate coma (73% accuracy). Accuracy rates are lower in patients with low BMI (63% accuracy when BMI is less than 20.5) and patients with cystic fibrosis (58% accuracy; most of these patients had very low BMI, which might be the underlying reason for the low accuracy rate). In a study of serial RMR measurements, the equation was more accurate if recalculated daily than a single RMR measurement extrapolated for 7 days. Measurement of RMR was more accurate than the equation only when measurement was repeated every 3 or 4 days.[51] (See Figure 2-2.)

Not all research studies show the Penn State equation to be valid. In a study by De Waele and associates,[76] correlation between measured RMR and the Penn State equation was low; also, the mean difference between the 2 values (−265 kcal); and the limit of agreement (−872 to 340 kcal/d) were both large. The study did not report the accuracy rate. Two cautionary aspects of this study are worthy of mention because they could explain the result. The first is that the measured RMR seems low (1571 ± 424 kcal/d or 8% above the calculated Mifflin–St. Jeor value),[76] compared with the original Penn State equation validation work (2000 ± 534 kcal/d or 23% above calculated Mifflin–St. Jeor),[7] but the indirect calorimeter used in the De Waele study (the Vmax Encore) tends to measure RMR lower than the Deltatrac (the device used in the original Penn State equation work).[79] The second is that the Penn State equation value may have been miscalculated in the De Waele study. Based on reported mean height, weight, age, sex, body temperature, and minute ventilation, the mean Penn State equation value should have been 1697 kcal/d rather than the reported 2106 kcal/d. Considering both of these factors together, it is possible that the RMR measurement should have been higher and the RMR estimate should have been lower in the De Waele study, resulting in better agreement with the Penn State calculations than was reported.

Ratzlaff and colleagues tested the Penn State equation for validity in mechanically ventilated cardiothoracic surgery patients and reported the equation accuracy to be 11% compared with measured RMR.[77] Insufficient descriptive data were included in the paper to recreate the Penn State equation calculation; however, given that this was a retrospective study, it is possible that the incorrect body weight, body temperature, or minute ventilation was used in the computation. The measured RMR in this study is a greater concern. The mean RMR was 2406 ± 587 kcal/d, and the device used was the Medgraphics Ultima.[77] Sundstrom et al[80] have shown that measurements from the Medgraphics Express, a similar device from the same manufacturer and using similar, if not the same, technology, differed markedly from Deltatrac measurements in the same patients (2876 ± 656 kcal/d vs 1749 ± 389 kcal/d). As stated previously, the Deltatrac was the device used in the original Penn State equation work. It is therefore quite possible that the IC data were out of phase in the Ratzlaff study.[73] By comparison to the 2406 kcal/d value

recorded, measured RMR in the other validation studies of the Penn State equation were 2000 kcal/d,[7] 1571 kcal/d,[76] and 2029 kcal/d.[78]

In a third study in which the Penn State equation (and numerous other predictive equations) failed to predict RMR, de Góes and associates measured RMR in critically ill patients with acute kidney injury using a Quark RMR indirect calorimeter.[78] Measurements were conducted before renal replacement therapy was initiated, and measured RMR was similar to the Penn State equation validation study[7] but with a higher standard deviation (2029 ± 760 kcal/d vs 2000 ± 533 kcal/d). Nine equations were tested. Of these 9, 8 were also tested by Frankenfield and colleagues in 2009.[7] In every equation except 1, the accuracy rate was higher in the Frankenfield paper. For example, the Penn State equation accuracy was 33% in de Góes vs 67% in Frankenfield, and the accuracy rates for the Ireton-Jones equation were 27% and 46%, respectively.[7,78] Possible reasons for the discrepancies between the 2 studies include differences in the equipment used and the types of patients studied. In 2013, Sundstrom and coauthors found the Quark RMR device used in the de Góes study to be accurate;[80] however, in subsequent work (2016), Sundstrom et al noted a bias of about 10%, with a tendency for the Quark to measure higher than the Deltatrac.[81] Patients in the study by de Góes et al had acute kidney injury, and their pulmonary gas exchange values therefore may not have fully represented metabolic gas exchange. More importantly, the de Góes paper originated in Brazil, and it may be that the base RMR in this population is poorly represented by the Mifflin–St. Jeor equation, which, if true, would make the Penn State equation also inaccurate.[62] The Mifflin–St. Jeor equation underestimated RMR by a mean of 14% in healthy Brazilians, and the Penn State equation, which uses the Mifflin–St. Jeor equation, underestimated RMR by a mean of 5% in critically ill Brazilians.[62]

Predictive Equations for Acutely Ill Patients

Much research has been focused on describing and predicting the RMR of mechanically ventilated, critically ill patients. However, this research cannot necessarily be used to guide energy assessment in nutrition support patients who are spontaneously breathing. Certainly, any equation that contains minute ventilation or tidal volume as a variable cannot be used in these patients because those variables are not measured. Two equations have been proposed for spontaneously breathing, acutely ill patients, and these equations have recently undergone validation testing. The first of these equations is from Ireton-Jones:[67]

$$RMR = (W \times 25) - (A \times 11) - (OB \times 609) + 629$$

where RMR is measured in kcal/d; W is actual weight (kg); A is age (years); and OB is presence of obesity (1 = yes; 0 = no).

The second equation is from Frankenfield and Ashcraft and is based on the validation data for the Penn State equation absent the minute ventilation variable:[65]

$$RMR = (\text{Mifflin–St. Jeor} \times 0.94) + (T_{max} \times 186) - 6597$$

where RMR is measured in kcal/d; Mifflin–St. Jeor (kcal/d) is calculated using actual body weight; and T_{max} is maximum body temperature in the previous 24 hours (degrees Celsius).

These equations were tested in a group of 55 acutely ill, spontaneously breathing hospitalized patients receiving nutrition support.[35] The modified Penn State equation was accurate 71% of the time compared with 44% of the time for the Ireton-Jones equation. Similar to the Penn State equation for mechanically ventilated, critically ill patients, the predictions using the Penn State equation for spontaneously breathing patients failed more often in underweight patients (accuracy rate 47%) than in normal weight (76% accuracy rate) or obese patients (84% accuracy rate).

Measurements from Mechanical Ventilators

Stapel and coauthors[39] conducted a validation study of RMR calculated from ventilator-derived VCO_2 vs IC with a Deltatrac. Several equations also were included in the validation study (Harris-Benedict, 25 kcal per kg body weight, Faisy, and Penn State). Two error thresholds were evaluated. The VCO_2 method was accurate to within 10% of measured values in 61% of patients compared with 40% for the ratio method and 54% for the Penn State equation. For a 15% error threshold, the VCO_2 method was accurate 79% of the time, the ratio method 56% of the time, and the Penn State equation 75% of the time.

Nutrition Support Therapy and Energy Requirements

The human body requires a constant supply of energy to maintain homeostasis. If this energy is not supplied by food, the body must catabolize itself to meet the deficit. The body can do this for a time without suffering impairment, but function will eventually be compromised by the resulting tissue loss. The length of time before compromise depends on the patient's nutrition status, the size of the energy deficit, and the body compartment being catabolized. The critical deficit may be reached sooner in (1) malnourished patients (because they start with a reduced tissue reserve), (2) hypermetabolic patients (because they create larger daily deficits), and (3) in cases where inflammatory response favors catabolism of protein over fat. One of the goals of nutrition support is to minimize this energy deficit while avoiding overfeeding. The degree of precision required for the energy prescription is still debated by researchers and practicing clinicians. However, in general, an accurate assessment of energy demand is an important part of the nutrition care of the patient receiving nutrition support. Practice Scenario 2-1 addresses several questions related to energy assessment in a critically ill, obese, older man receiving nutrition support.[1,82]

Practice Scenario 2-1

Scenario: A 73-year-old man was admitted to the critical care unit with respiratory failure related to pneumonia. The condition progressed to acute respiratory distress syndrome, and the patient was also in septic shock. He had a spontaneous pneumothorax for which he received a chest tube, which developed an air leak. His previous medical history included diabetes mellitus and congestive heart failure. Since he was intubated and expected to remain so for at least 3 days, a feeding tube was placed, a low-rate tube feeding was started, and a nutrition support consult was ordered.

When reviewing the chart, the dietitian noted a current body weight of 165 kg and a height of 178 cm, which would suggest the body mass index (BMI) to be 52.1. However, intake/output records indicated a large volume resuscitation for the septic shock, and the physician note indicated +4 edema in all extremities. Clearly, the current body weight of 165 kg was skewed by volume overload. Fortunately, the patient had been followed in one of the hospital clinics for his chronic conditions, which meant that his electronic health record contained a preadmission history of measured body weights. This record indicated that his body weight fluctuated due to water retention from his congestive heart failure, but the nadir was 120 kg for a BMI of 37.9. The dietitian went to the bedside and observed that the recorded height of 178 cm seems to be accurate. The dietitian also observed obvious edema, as noted by the physician, which explained the discrepancy in body weight between the value recorded in clinic and the value recorded in the critical care unit. Therefore, 120 kg and 178 cm were taken as the patient's true weight and height. His Nutrition Risk Screening score was 4 (0 points for nutrition, 3 points for disease state, 1 point for age).[82] Current vital signs were maximum body temperature 37.8 degrees Celsius, heart rate 110 beats/min, and minute ventilation 11.5 L/min. His fraction of inspired oxygen was 70%, and his arterial blood gas was 7.33/50/90/33 (respiratory acidosis not yet compensated). He was sedated with fentanyl and receiving norepinephrine to support his blood pressure.

Question 1: Should indirect calorimetry (IC) be used in this scenario? Why or why not?

Answer 1: In this case, fluid overload masked the patient's true body weight. The rationale for measuring resting metabolic rate (RMR) with IC would be that current body weight was grossly different from his dry weight, which would interfere with calculating the RMR. However, the dietitian had a way of determining the dry weight. The patient had severe obesity but his dry weight and BMI were not in the range that would categorically invalidate prediction equations for his RMR. Therefore, there would be no strict indication to conduct an IC measurement.

Question 2: Would IC be feasible for this patient?

Answer 2: No. The patient had an air leak from his chest tube and his fraction of inspired oxygen was too high for an open-circuit indirect calorimeter to function accurately.

Question 3: What body weight should be used for calculating RMR? What values would result?

Answer 3: Current BMI was greater than 50, and the American Society for Parenteral and Enteral Nutrition (ASPEN) guidelines[1] suggest using ideal body weight for RMR calculation in this weight class. However, his dry weight BMI was 37.9; therefore, actual body weight would be used. The ASPEN guidelines[1] suggest 11 to 14 kcal per kg body weight, which would mean his calculated

RMR would be 1320 to 1680 kcal/d. The Penn State equation result would be 2335 kcal/d. One reason for the discrepancy between the 2 values is that the ASPEN standard is modified to represent 65% to 70% of the theoretical true RMR if measured with IC.

Question 4: Two weeks later, the patient remained on the ventilator despite attempts to liberate him from it. Fraction of inspired oxygen decreased to 50%, and the chest tube had been removed. His minute ventilation was unexpectedly high (20.3 L/min). He was febrile (body temperature 38.5 degrees Celsius), and his body weight was 125 kg. The dietitian had set the energy intake goal at 2725 kcal/d, but the critical care team wondered whether overfeeding might explain his high minute ventilation. Would IC now be appropriate?

Answer 4: At this point, IC would be more clearly indicated. The critical care team had no explanation for his elevated minute ventilation and failure to wean from the ventilator. Although his current body weight was now close to his usual dry weight, it was likely that the patient lost tissue mass during his past 2 weeks of illness so that his new true dry body weight could be below his baseline weight of 120 kg. If the estimate of dry body weight were too high, the Penn State equation would overestimate his energy demand, leading to overfeeding. Measurement of his RMR would quickly determine whether his RMR were lower than expected. The IC data could furthermore be used to determine dead space ventilation, which could help the team determine why his minute ventilation was so high.

Question 5: The patient's IC results were RMR 2500 kcal/d, respiratory quotient 0.84, oxygen consumption 370 mL/min, volume of carbon dioxide production (VCO_2) 302 mL/min, and minute ventilation 20.1 L/minute. The arterial blood gas was 7.36/50/120/40 (compensated respiratory acidosis). Analyze and interpret these data.

Answer 5: The measured RMR was 11% lower than the predicted RMR, which indicates that the patient was being slightly overfed. The degree of overfeeding would not likely be the cause for the patient's continued ventilator dependence or high minute ventilation.

With the available data, the patient's dead space fraction (Vd/Vt) could be calculated. He had a partial pressure of carbon dioxide ($PaCO_2$) of 50 torr and a mixed expiratory CO_2 ($FeCO_2$) concentration of 1.50% calculated from the IC data. Barometric pressure read from the indirect calorimeter was 747 mmHg, and the pressure of water vapor was assumed to be 47 mmHg. Therefore, his partial pressure of mixed expiratory carbon dioxide ($PeCO_2$) was 9.8 torr, and his dead space fraction was 80%. The mathematical steps for this calculation are as follows:

$$FeCO_2 = VCO_2/Ve = (302/20100) = 0.0150$$

$$PeCO_2 = (\text{Barometric Pressure} - 47) \times FECO_2$$
$$= (747 - 47) \times 0.0150) = 9.8$$

$$Vd/Vt = (PaCO_2 - PeCO_2)/PaCO_2 = (50 - 9.8)/50$$
$$= 0.80$$

where VCO_2 is volume of CO_2 production (mL/min); Ve is expired volume (mL/min); and $PeCO_2$ is measured in torr.

Even in the absence of an arterial blood gas, his ventilatory equivalent (Ve/VCO$_2$, the liters of minute volume required to remove 1 liter of carbon dioxide) was high (66.6 L/L), indicating that his problem was not metabolic in nature.

Question 6: Eventually, the patient was liberated from the ventilator. He was not cleared by the speech pathologist to start an oral diet, so he remained on tube feeding. His body weight decreased to 110 kg, there was no sign of edema, and he was up and walking frequently. Maximum body temperature was 36.5 degrees Celsius. At this point, what would be his energy requirement?

Answer 6: The patient's Mifflin–St. Jeor equation value was 1850 kcal/d at his new dry weight, and his RMR calculated by the Penn State equation for spontaneously breathing people was 1930 kcal. This RMR was only 4% above his Mifflin–St. Jeor value, indicating that the patient was no longer hypermetabolic. There was probably no thermogenic effect of feeding since he remained on a continuous feeding infusion; however, the energy goal might need adjustment for movement (walking) of about 10%, bringing his total energy requirement to 2125 kcal/d.

References

1. McClave SA, Taylor BE, Martindale RG, et al. Guidelines for the provision and assessment of nutrition support therapy in the adult critically ill patient: Society of Critical Care Medicine (SCCM) and American Society for Parenteral and Enteral Nutrition (ASPEN). *JPEN J Parenter Enteral Nutr.* 2016;40:159–211.
2. Fullmer S, Benson-Davies S, Earthman CP, et al. Evidence Analysis Library review of best practices for performing indirect calorimetry in healthy and non-critically ill individuals. *J Acad Nutr Diet.* 2015;115:1417–1446.
3. Academy of Nutrition and Dietetics Evidence Analysis Library. Critical illness. Measuring resting metabolic rate (RMR) in the critically ill guideline (2013). https://wwwandeal.org/topic.cfm ?menu=5299&cat= 5017. Accessed June 17, 2016.
4. Heyland DK, Cahill N, Day AG. Optimal amount of calories for critically ill patients: depends on how you slice the cake! *Crit Care Med.* 2011;39:2619–2626.
5. Frankenfield DC. On heat, respiration and calorimetry. *Nutrition.* 2010;26:939–950.
6. Weir JB. New methods for calculating metabolic rate with special reference to protein metabolism. *J Physiol.* 1949;109:1–14.
7. Frankenfield DC, Coleman A, Alam S, Cooney RN. Analysis of estimation methods for resting metabolic rate in critically ill adults. *JPEN J Parenter Enteral Nutr.* 2009;33:27–36.
8. Frankenfield DC, Ashcraft CM, Galvan DA. Prediction of resting metabolic rate in critically ill patients at the extremes of body mass index. *JPEN J Parenter Enteral Nutr.* 2012;37:361–367.
9. Koshland DE. The seven pillars of life. *Science.* 2002;295: 2215–2216.
10. Hellerstein MK, Neese RA, Linfoot P, et al. Hepatic gluconeogenic fluxes and glycogen turnover during fasting in humans: a stable isotope study. *J Clin Invest.* 1997;100:1305–1319.
11. Nurjhan N, Bucci A, Perriello G, et al. Glutamine: a major gluconeogenic precursor and vehicle for interorgan carbon transport in man. *J Clin Invest.* 1995;95:272–277.
12. Chandra RK. 1990 McCollum Award Lecture. Nutrition and immunity: lessons from the past and new insights into the future. *Am J Clin Nutr.* 1991;53:1087–1101.

13. Reichard GA, Haff AC, Skutches CL, et al. Plasma acetone metabolism in the fasting human. *J Clin Invest.* 1979;63:619–626.

14. Owen OE, Smalley KJ, D'Alessio DA, et al. Protein, fat, and carbohydrate requirements during starvation: anaplerosis and cataplerosis. *Am J Clin Nutr.* 1998;68:12–34.

15. Frankenfield DC, Coleman A. Recovery to resting metabolic state after walking. *J Am Diet Assoc.* 2009;109:1914–1916.

16. Compher CW, Frankenfield DC, Keim N, Roth-Yousey L. Best practice methods to apply to measurement of resting metabolic rate. *J Am Diet Assoc.* 2006;106:881–903.

17. Wang Z, Heshka S, Gallagher D, et al. Resting energy expenditure–fat-free mass relationship: new insights provided by body composition modeling. *Am J Physiol Endocrinol Metab.* 2000;279: E539–E545.

18. Muller MJ, Bosy-Westphal A, Kutzner D, Heller M. Metabolically active components of fat-free mass and resting energy expenditure in humans: recent lessons from imaging technologies. *Obes Rev.* 2002;3:113–122.

19. Javed F, He Q, Davidson LE, et al. Brain and high metabolic rate organ mass: contribution to resting energy expenditure beyond fat free mass. *Am J Clin Nutr.* 2010;91:907–912.

20. Gallagher D, Albu J, He Q, et al. Small organs with high metabolic rate explain lower resting energy expenditure in African American than in white adults. *Am J Clin Nutr.* 2006;83:1062–1067.

21. Fukagawa NK, Bandini LG, Young JB. Effect of age on body composition and resting metabolic rate. *Am J Physiol.* 1990;259: E233–E238.

22. Kinabo JL, Durnin JV. Thermic effect of food in man: effect of meal composition and energy content. *Br J Nutr.* 1990;64:37–44.

23. Heymsfield SB, Hill JO, Evert M, Casper K, Digirolamo M. Energy expenditure during continuous intragastric infusion of fuel. *Am J Clin Nutr.* 1987;45:526–533.

24. Frankenfield DC, Ashcraft CM. Description and prediction of resting metabolic rate after stroke and traumatic brain injury. *Nutrition.* 2012;28:906–911.

25. Drenowatz C, Grieve GL, DeMello MM. Change in energy expenditure and physical activity in response to aerobic and resistance exercise programs. *SpringerPlus.* 2015;4:798. doi:10.1186/ s40064-015-1594-2.

26. Villablanca PA, Alegria JR, Mookadam F, et al. Nonexercise activity thermogenesis in obesity management. *Mayo Clin Proc.* 2015;90:509–519.

27. Weissman C, Kemper M, Damask MC, et al. Effect of routine intensive care interactions on metabolic rate. *Chest.* 1984;86:815–818.

28. Swinamer DL, Phang PT, Jones RL, Grace M, Garner King E. Twenty-four hour energy expenditure in critically ill patients. *Crit Care Med.* 1987;15:637–643.

29. Frankenfield DC, Wiles CE, Bagley S, et al. Relationships between resting and total energy expenditure in injured and septic patients. *Crit Care Med.* 1994;22:1796–1804.

30. Malina RM, Bouchard C, Bar-Or O. *Growth, Maturation, and Physical Activity,* 2nd ed. Champaign, IL: Human Kinetics; 2004.

31. Apell SP, Neidrauer M, Papazoglou ES, Pizziconi V. Physics of wound healing I. Energy considerations. Online arXiv:1212.3778. December 16, 2012. https://arxiv.org/abs/1212.3778. Accessed January 7, 2017.

32. Taylor SJ. *Energy and Nitrogen Requirements in Disease States.* London, UK: Smith-Gordon; 2007.

33. Gariballa S, Forster S. Energy expenditure of acutely ill hospitalized patients. *Nutr J* (online) 2006;5:1–5. doi:10.1186/1475-2891-5-9.

34. Weijs PMJ, Kruizenga HM, van Dijk, et al. Validation of predictive equations for resting energy expenditure in adult outpatients and inpatients. *Clin Nutr.* 2008;27:150–157.

35. Frankenfield DC, Ashcraft CM. Toward the development of predictive equations for resting metabolic rate in acutely ill spon-

taneously breathing patients. *JPEN J Parenter Enteral Nutr.* 2016 (online ahead of print). doi:10.1177/0148607116657647.

36. Frankenfield DC, Smith JS, Cooney RN, Blosser SA, Sarson GY. Relative association of fever and injury with hypermetabolism in critically ill patients. *Injury.* 1997;28:617–621.

37. Raurich JM, Ibanez J, Marse P, Riera M, Homar X. Resting energy expenditure during mechanical ventilation and its relationship with type of lesion. *JPEN J Parenter Enteral Nutr.* 2007;31:58–62.

38. Frankenfield DC, Bias and accuracy of resting metabolic rate equations in non-obese and obese adults. *Clin Nutr.* 2013;32:976–982.

39. Stapel SN, De Grooth HJS, Alimohamad H, et al. Ventilator-derived carbon dioxide production to assess energy expenditure in critically ill patients: proof of concept. *Crit Care.* 2015; 19:370–380.

40. Harris JA, Benedict FG. *A Biometric Study of Basal Metabolism in Man.* Publication no. 279. Washington, DC: Carnegie Institute; 1919.

41. Brandi LS, Grana M, Mazzanti T, et al. Energy expenditure and gas exchange measurements in post-operative patients: thermodilution vs. indirect calorimetry. *Crit Care Med.* 1992;20:1273–1283.

42. Ogawa AM, Shikora SA, Burke LM, et al. The thermodilution technique for measuring resting energy expenditure does not agree with indirect calorimetry for the critically ill patient. *JPEN J Parenter Enteral Nutr.*1998;22:347–351.

43. Schoeller DA, Van Santen E. Measurement of energy expenditure in free-living humans by using doubly labeled water. *J Nutr.* 1988;118:1278–1289.

44. Frankenfield DC, Roth-Yousey L, Compher C. Comparison of predictive equations for resting metabolic rate in healthy nonobese and obese individuals, a systematic review. *J Am Diet Assoc.* 2005;105:775–789.

45. Snell B, Fullmer S, Eggert D. Reading and listening to music increase resting energy expenditure during an indirect calorimetry test. *J Acad Nutr Diet.* 2014;114:1939–1942.

46. van Ooijen AMJ, Lichtenbelt VM, van Steenhoven AA, et al. Seasonal changes in metabolic and temperature responses to cold air in humans. *Physiol Behav.* 2004;82:545–553.

47. Kasiwazaki H, Dejima Y, Suzuki T. Influence of upper and lower thermoneutral room temperatures (20 degrees C and 25 degrees C) on fasting and post-prandial resting metabolism under different outdoor temperatures. *Eur J Clin Nutr.* 1990;44:405–413.

48. Claessens-Van Ooijen AMJ, Westerterp KR, Wouters L, et al. Heat production and body temperature during cooling and rewarming in overweight and lean men. *Obesity.* 2006;14:1914–1920.

49. Charkoudian N. Skin blood flow in adult human thermoregulation. How it works, when it does not, and why. *Mayo Clin Proc.* 2003;78:603–612.

50. Brandi LS, Bertolini R, Santini L, Cavani S. Effects of ventilator resetting on indirect calorimetry measurement in the critically ill surgical patient. *Crit Care Med.* 1999;27:531–539.

51. Frankenfield DC, Ashcraft CM, Galvan DA. Longitudinal prediction of metabolic rate in critically ill patients. *JPEN J Parenter Enteral Nutr.* 2012;36:700–712.

52. Gephart FC, Dubois EF. The basal metabolism of normal adults with special reference to surface area. Clinical Calorimetry Paper XIII. *Arch Intern Med.* 1916;17:902–914.

53. Frankenfield DC, Muth E, Rowe WA. The Harris-Benedict studies of human basal metabolism: history and limitations. *J Am Diet Assoc.* 1998;98:439–445.

54. Livingston EH, Kohlstadt I. Simplified resting metabolic rate—predicting formulas for normal-sized and obese individuals. *Obes Res.* 2005;13:1255–1262.

55. Benedict FG. Basal metabolism data on normal men and women (series II) with some considerations on the use of prediction standards. *Am J Physiol.* 1928;85:607–620.

56. Robertson JD, Reid DD. Standard for the basal metabolism of normal people in Britain. *Lancet.* 1952;1:940–943.

57. Owen OE, Kavle E, Owen RS, et al. A reappraisal of caloric requirements in healthy women. *Am J Clin Nutr.* 1986;44:1-19.

58. Owen OE, Holup JL, D'Alessio DA, et al. A reappraisal of the caloric requirements of men. *Am J Clin Nutr.* 1987;46:875-885.

59. Mifflin MD, St. Jeor ST, Hill LA, et al. A new predictive equation for resting energy expenditure in healthy individuals. *Am J Clin Nutr.* 1990;51:241-247.

60. Weijs PJM. Validity of predictive equations for resting energy expenditure in US and Dutch overweight and obese class I and II adults aged 18-65 y. *Am J Clin Nutr.* 2008;88:959-970.

61. Melzer K, Laurie K, Genton L, et al. Comparison of equations for estimating resting metabolic rate in healthy subjects over 70 years of age. *Clin Nutr.* 2007;26:498-505.

62. de Oliveira EP, Orsatti FL, Teixeira O, et al. Comparison of predictive equations for resting energy expenditure in overweight and obese adults. *J Obes.* 2011;2011:534714.

63. Academy of Nutrition and Dietetics. Nutrition Care Manual. Calculators. https://www.nutritioncaremanual.org/calculators.cfm ?ncm_category_id=10&ncm_heading=. Accessed August 29, 2016.

64. Frankenfield DC, Rowe WA, Smith JS, Cooney RN. Validation of several established equations for resting metabolic rate in obese and nonobese people. *J Am Diet Assoc.* 2003;103:1152-1159.

65. Frankenfield DC, Ashcraft CM. Estimating energy needs in nutrition support patients. *JPEN J Parenter Enteral Nutr.* 2011;35:563-570.

66. Frankenfield DC, Hise M, Malone A, Russell M, Gradwell E, Compher C. Prediction of resting metabolic rate in critically ill adult patients: results of a systematic review of the evidence. *J Am Diet Assoc.* 2007;107:1552-1561.

67. Ireton-Jones CS, Turner WW, Liepa GU, Baxter CR. Equations for estimation of energy expenditure of patients with burns with special reference to ventilator status. *J Burn Care Rehabil.* 1992;13:330-333.

68. Swinamer DL, Grace MG, Hamilton SM, et al. Predictive equation for assessing energy expenditure in mechanically ventilated critically ill patients. *Crit Care Med.* 1990;18:657-661.

69. Flancbaum L, Choban PS, Sambucco S, et al. Comparison of indirect calorimetry, the Fick method, and prediction equations in estimating the energy requirements of critically ill patients. *Am J Clin Nutr.* 1999;69:461-466.

70. MacDonald A, Hildebrandt L. Comparison of formulaic equations to determine energy expenditure in the critically ill patient. *Nutrition.* 2003;19:233-239.

71. Frankenfield DC. Energy dynamics. In: Matarese LE, Gottschlich MM, eds. *Contemporary Nutrition Support Practice. A Clinical Guide.* Philadelphia, PA: Saunders; 1998:79-98.

72. Frankenfield DC, Smith JS, Cooney RN. Validation of two approaches to predicting resting metabolic rate in critically ill patients. *JPEN J Parenter Enteral Nutr.* 2004;28:259-264.

73. Frankenfield DC. Validation of an equation for resting metabolic rate in older obese, critically ill patients. *JPEN J Parenter Enteral Nutr.* 2011;35:264-269.

74. Ashcraft CM, Frankenfield DC. Energy expenditure during barbiturate coma. *Nutr Clin Pract.* 2013;28:603-608.

75. Frankenfield DC, Ashcraft CM, Drasher TL, Reid EK, Vender RL. Characteristics of resting metabolic rate in critically ill, mechanically ventilated adults with cystic fibrosis. *JPEN J Parenter Enteral Nutr.* 2015 (online ahead of print). doi:10.1177/0148607115617152.

76. De Waele E, Opsomer T, Honore PM, et al. Measured versus calculated resting energy expenditure in critically ill patients. Do mathematics match the gold standard? *Minerva Anestesiol.* 2015;5:272-282.

77. Ratzlaff R, Nowak D, Gordillo D, et al. Mechanically ventilated, cardiothoracic surgical patients have significantly different energy requirements comparing indirect calorimetry and the Penn State equations. *JPEN J Parenter Enteral Nutr.* 2016;40:959-965.

78. de Góes CR, Berbel-Bufarah MN, Sanches AC, et al. Poor agreement between predictive equations of energy expenditure and measured energy expenditure in critically ill acute kidney injury patients. *Ann Nutr Metab.* 2016;68:276-284.

79. Frankenfield DC, Ashcraft CM, Wood C, Chinchilli VM. Validation of an indirect calorimeter using n-of-1 methodology. *Clin Nutr.* 2016;35:163-168.

80. Sundstrom M, Tjader I, Rooyackers O, Wernerman J. Indirect calorimetry in mechanically ventilated patients. A systematic comparison of three instruments. *Clin Nutr.* 2013;32:118-121.

81. Rehal Sundstrom M, Fiskaare E, Tjader I, et al. Measuring energy expenditure in the intensive care unit: a comparison of indirect calorimetry by E-sCOVX and QuarkRMR with Deltatrac II in mechanically ventilated critically ill patients. *Crit Care.* 2016;20:54. doi:10.1186/s13054-016-1232-6.

82. Kondrup J, Rasmussen HH, Hamberg O, Stanga Z; Ad Hoc ESPEN Working Group. Nutrition Risk Screening (NRS 2002): a new method based on an analysis of controlled clinical trials. *Clin Nutr.* 2003;22:321-336.

3 Carbohydrates

Karen C. McCowen, MD, and Pei-Ra Ling, MD

CONTENTS

Objectives

1. Understand the basic structures of carbohydrates and their digestion and absorption.
2. Describe glucose metabolism inside cells.
3. Analyze how different hormones and organs help maintain appropriate plasma glucose concentrations during fasting and fed states.
4. Identify factors that determine carbohydrate requirements.
5. Understand structure and function of fructose and fiber.

Test Your Knowledge Questions

1. Which of the following is true about the net chemical reaction of glucose catabolism?
   A. Pyruvate is the final product.
   B. Oxygen is required for adenosine triphosphate (ATP) synthesis.
   C. Both water and carbon dioxide (CO_2) are produced.
   D. CO_2 is produced but water is not.
   E. Water is produced but CO_2 is not.

2. Which of the following incorrectly pairs a metabolic process with its site of occurrence?
   A. Glycolysis and cytosol
   B. Tricarboxylic acid (TCA) cycle and mitochondrial membrane
   C. ATP phosphorylation and cytosol and mitochondria
   D. Electron transport chain and mitochondrial membrane
   E. Oxidative decarboxylation of pyruvate and mitochondria
3. Which of the following is least likely to occur during oxygen debt?
   A. Buildup of lactic acid
   B. Buildup of pyruvate
   C. Decrease in pH
   D. Increased fatigue
   E. Shortage of ATP

Test Your Knowledge Answers

1. The correct answer is **C**. Pyruvate is the final product of glycolysis. When pyruvate leaves the cytoplasm and enters the mitochondria, it loses CO_2. The acetyl group then transfers to coenzyme A (CoA) and forms acetyl-CoA. In aerobic conditions, pyruvate can be further oxidized during cell respiration. In anaerobic conditions, pyruvate can be broken down into lactate. Both metabolic pathways can produce ATP. After all energy has been released from the glucose moiety, CO_2 and water are the final products.
2. The correct answer is **B**. The TCA cycle is the metabolic reaction of cell respiration, which occurs inside the eukaryotic mitochondrion (not on the mitochondrial membrane). Glycolysis occurs in the cytoplasm. ATP phosphorylation occurs both during glycolysis (in the cytoplasm) and the TCA cycle (in the mitochondrion). The electron transport chain is a carrier mechanism within the inner mitochondrion. The oxidative decarboxylation of pyruvate occurs in the mitochondrion.
3. The correct answer is **B**. Under anaerobic conditions, pyruvate accepts a hydrogen atom from nicotinamide adenine dinucleotide plus hydrogen (NADH), forming nicotinamide adenine dinucleotide (NAD^+) and lactic acid. At physiological pH, lactic acid is dissociated into lactate and protons. Thus, the local pH decreases. Using this pathway, only 2 ATPs can be generated. A shortage of ATP is possible, leading to muscle fatigue.

Background

Carbohydrate is a class of organic compounds composed of carbon, hydrogen, and oxygen with a 1:2:1 molar ratio of carbon to hydrogen to oxygen. Carbohydrate is a major energy source in human nutrition. Theoretically, oxidation of 1 g carbohydrate yields 4 kcal. When carbohydrate is hydrated in solution as dextrose and oxidized, 3.4 kcal/g results. Humans can store carbohydrate as glycogen in liver and muscle (and, to a lesser extent, in other body systems) for later use. In addition to their role as an energy source, some carbohydrates, such as sucrose (table sugar), are sweetening agents, whereas others are components of dietary fibers, such as in vegetables. Fiber is a form of carbohydrate that is a remnant of plant cells that resists digestion by small intestinal enzymes in humans. Fibers do not provide energy or nutrients by normal digestive processes in the small bowel, but they can be fermented by bacteria under anaerobic conditions in the large bowel (see Chapter 4 for discussion of the gut microbiome).

Classification and Structure of Carbohydrates

Carbohydrates can be classified as either simple or complex. Simple carbohydrates include monosaccharides (1 sugar unit) and disaccharides (2 sugar units). A common name for simple carbohydrates is *sugar*. Monosaccharides are water soluble and have low molecular weight. Glucose, galactose, and fructose are examples of monosaccharides. Glucose and galactose contain a ring with 6 carbon atoms. Fructose also contains 6 carbons, although the ring structure contains 4 carbons (Figure 3-1). Sucrose (1 glucose and 1 fructose), maltose (2 glucose moieties), and lactose (1 glucose and 1 galactose) are 3 common disaccharides.

Multiple units of monosaccharides and disaccharides can be joined together to form polysaccharides (ie, complex carbohydrates). Complex carbohydrates are water insoluble and have high molecular weights. Polysaccharides containing

FIGURE 3-1 Chemical Structures of Monosaccharides

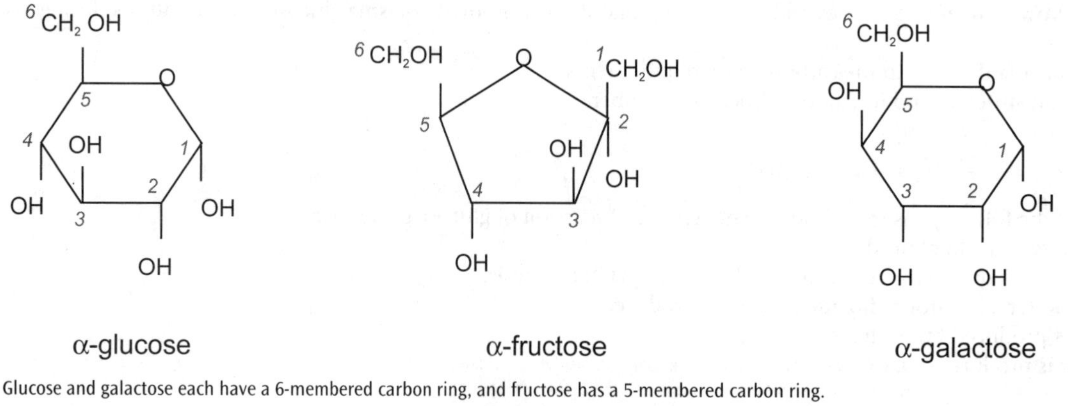

Glucose and galactose each have a 6-membered carbon ring, and fructose has a 5-membered carbon ring.

fewer than 10 glucose units are called *oligosaccharides*. Starch, glycogen, and some fibers (eg, cellulose) are polysaccharides that contain hundreds to many thousands of monosaccharides (usually glucose) connected by straight and/or branched chains.

Plants store glucose as starch. The structure of starch resembles that of glycogen, but starch has longer and less frequent branches. In starch (Figure 3-2), the straight chains are called *amylose* (about 15% to 20% of the total starch), and branched chains are denoted *amylopectin* (80% to 85% of the total starch). Amylose is the inner, water-soluble component of starch, whereas amylopectin is a nearly insoluble substance derived from the outer part of starch granules.

Plant foods contain fiber mainly as a component of their cell walls. Polysaccharide plant fibers are important in the human diet, with cellulose being of particular significance—it helps the gastrointestinal (GI) tract function properly. Other types of plant fibers include pectin and lignin.

The structural polysaccharides in plant cells contain different kinds of simple sugars with various degrees of branching. Unlike starch and glycogen, cellulose has no side chains linking glucose units; instead, it is a long, straight, and rigid molecule. Humans cannot digest cellulose because they lack the enzymes needed to break down the linkages in the molecule.

Fiber may be classified as either *soluble* or *insoluble*, based on the degree of dispersion in hot water. Soluble fibers can be partially digested in the large bowel, whereas insoluble fibers are not.

Digestion and Absorption of Carbohydrates

Food in its natural state contains different types of carbohydrates. The end products of digestion of dietary carbohydrates are the monosaccharides: glucose, fructose, and galactose. The process of carbohydrate digestion begins in the mouth where foods are mechanically broken into smaller pieces and mixed with saliva.[1] Salivary amylase acts on the interior α-1,4 linkages of amylose and amylopectin (Figure 3-2) and breaks the polysaccharides into small intermediate forms. In the gut, these molecules are further broken down by pancreatic amylase and by other intestinal enzymes to disaccharides (ie, maltose). Subsequently, the enzyme maltase digests these disaccharides into glucose, galactose, and fructose (Figure 3-3). Small amounts of glucose are absorbed directly through the oral mucosa, but most monosaccharides are absorbed in the small intestine.

Sodium-glucose transporter 1 (SGLT1)—a protein in the apical membrane of the enterocyte—cotransports either

FIGURE 3-2 Chemical Structures of Starch

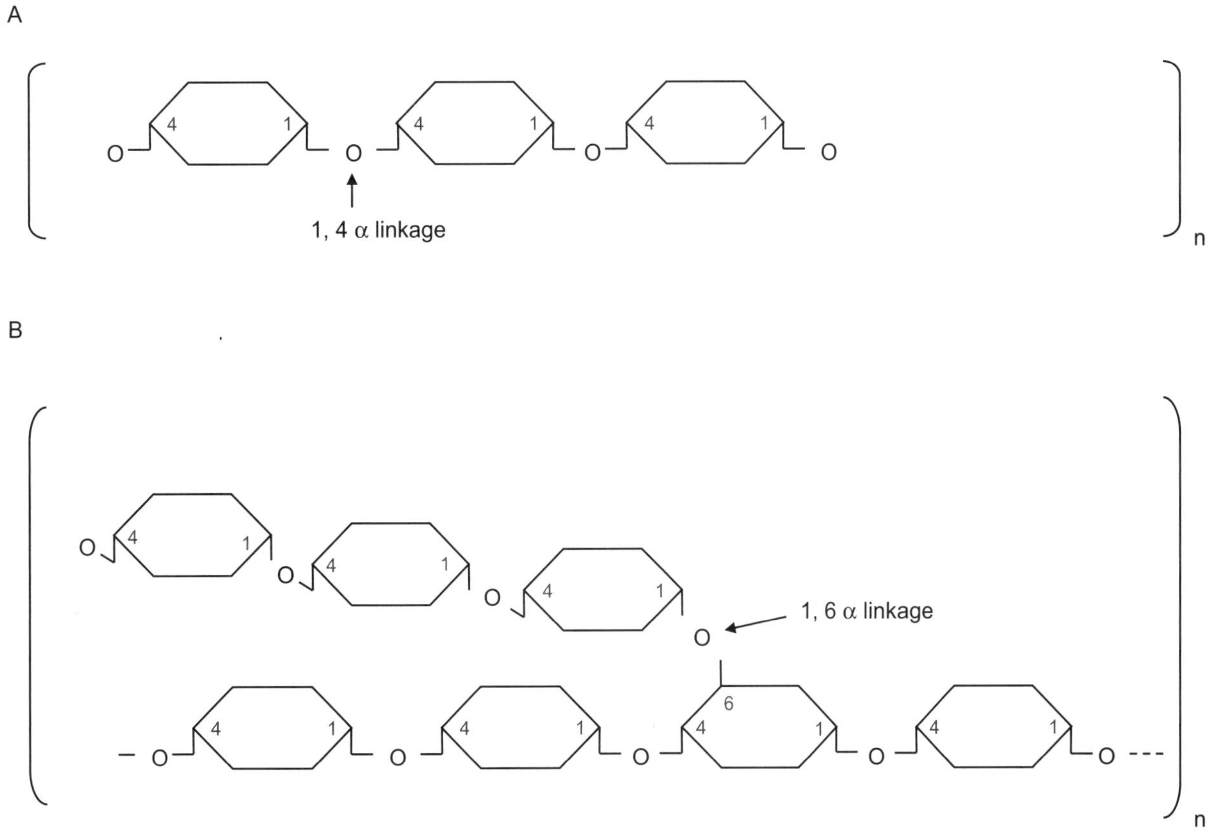

Starch is a mixture of amylose and amylopectin. (A) Amylose has a linear structure of glucose units linked by bonds with α-1,4 configuration. (B) Amylopectins contain branched structures with α-1,6 bonds at the branch points.

FIGURE 3-3 Intestinal Digestion of Dietary Carbohydrates

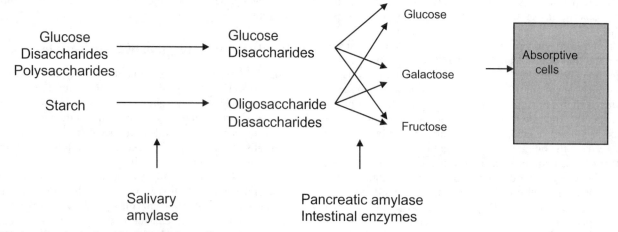

Carbohydrate digestion begins with salivary amylase and is completed in the small intestine with formation of monosaccharides that are readily absorbed.

glucose or galactose with sodium from the intestinal lumen into the enterocyte. This process requires energy provided by hydrolysis of ATP and is, therefore, called *an active transport system*. Another energy-dependent pump, the ATP-dependent sodium-potassium pump, which is present in the basolateral membrane of the enterocyte, maintains a low intracellular sodium concentration in the enterocyte and an electronegative cell interior, which favors sodium movement across the apical cell membrane from the lumen into the cell (Figure 3-4). Oral rehydration therapy makes use of this cotransport for salt-losing diarrheal states. In these states, the mechanism for absorbing sodium in the intestinal wall is hindered, and oral intake of saline solution alone is therefore not beneficial. However, if glucose is added to the correct amount of saline, glucose transporters (SGLT1) must absorb sodium (and water) along with the glucose.

Fructose is transported through a special protein called *glucose transporter 5* (GLUT5), which also is present in the apical membrane. Fructose, as well as glucose and galactose, is also exported into the bloodstream through a different glucose transport protein called *glucose transporter 2* (GLUT2), which is located in the basolateral membrane of the enterocyte (Figure 3-4).

Transporters cannot carry larger carbohydrate moieties across membranes. Therefore, starch and disaccharides must be digested to monosaccharides for absorption.

Insoluble fiber is poorly broken down and thus increases the bulk of the stool, rather than contributing to the energy load. Soluble fiber is fermented by bacteria in the colon to produce short-chain fatty acids (SCFAs), which can be absorbed into the bloodstream. See Chapter 4 for further discussion of SCFAs.

In the bloodstream, most absorbed compounds pass first through the liver. In the fed state, the liver removes two-thirds of the glucose from the portal vein blood. Fructose and galactose are almost totally removed by the liver. The increase in blood glucose following a meal is a component in the process that stimulates release of insulin from the pancreatic islets.

However, a complex cascade of neural and GI signals that prepares the pancreas for insulin release begins when food intake is anticipated, and it is enhanced by every step in the digestive process. Glucose can enter many tissues through mass action down its concentration gradient, even in the absence of insulin or exercise. Insulin and muscle contraction promote glucose uptake by cells, mostly muscle and adipose cells, which reduces the blood glucose concentration toward its basal state.

Carbohydrate Metabolism

Movement of Glucose into Cells—Glucose Transporters

Shifting glucose into cells occurs by means of 2 classes of glucose transport proteins located in the plasma membrane that serve as channels for glucose. One class, the sodium-dependent glucose transporters (such as SGLT1), is involved in the active, ATP-dependent absorption of glucose from the intestinal lumen into cells. These transport proteins also function in the reabsorption of filtered glucose in the proximal tubule of the kidney.[2]

Cell membrane glucose transporters in the second class are called *facilitative transporters*. They function as passive diffusion channels (ie, channels dependent on the gradient of glucose concentration between extra- and intracellular compartments) and do not require sodium or ATP. Many different types of facilitative glucose transporters are present in different tissues.[2]

Glucose transporter 1 (GLUT1) is widely distributed, with particularly high concentrations in endothelial and glial cells of the brain. The endothelial cells lining the microvessels of the brain comprise a major part of the blood-brain barrier. GLUT1 transports glucose and galactose, but not fructose.

GLUT2 is mainly located in the liver, small intestine, and kidney. In hepatocytes, GLUT2 has a low affinity but high capacity for glucose, allowing quick equilibration of intra- and extracellular glucose concentrations across the membrane during fasting and fed states. In the small intestine, GLUT2 is

FIGURE 3-4 Intestinal Absorption of Dietary Carbohydrates

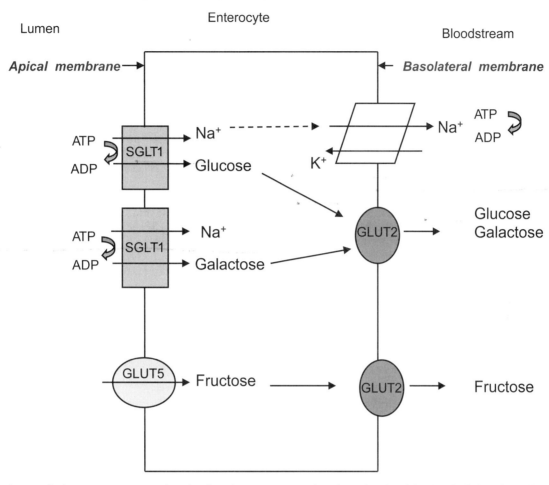

Glucose and galactose enter enterocytes through sodium-glucose transporter 1 (SGLT1), an adenosine triphosphate (ATP)–dependent active transporter. Fructose is transported by glucose transporter 5 (GLUT5). Glucose, galactose, and fructose are all exported into the bloodstream through the facilitation of glucose transporter 2 (GLUT2), located in the basolateral membrane of the enterocyte. The ATP-dependent sodium (Na^+)–potassium (K^+) pump located in the basolateral membrane maintains sodium concentration within the cell. ADP, adenosine diphosphate.

important in the transepithelial transport of the absorbed glucose, as described previously. In the kidney, GLUT2 transports the reabsorbed glucose back into the bloodstream from proximal tubular epithelia. In the beta cells of the pancreas, the transport of glucose by GLUT2 serves as part of the glucose-sensing apparatus that controls insulin release.

Glucose transporter 3 (GLUT3) seems to be present in all tissues, but its highest concentration is in the neuronal membranes of the brain. GLUT3 controls the rate of glucose entry into neuronal cells, which is different from the action of GLUT1 in the brain in the transportation of glucose across the blood-brain barrier.

Glucose transporter 4 (GLUT4) is the major insulin-regulated glucose transporter in adipose (brown and white) and muscle (skeletal and cardiac) tissues. GLUT4 is primarily located in intracellular vesicles of these tissues but can be translocated to the cell surface in response to a rise in plasma insulin concentrations (or muscle contraction). A rise

in circulating insulin results in as much as a 15- to 20-fold increase in GLUT4 on the cell surface of insulin-sensitive cells within minutes, allowing glucose uptake into cells.[3] A dysregulation of GLUT4 translocation in response to insulin is a key defect contributing to the development of type 2 diabetes mellitus and stress hyperglycemia, although the precise molecular mechanisms remain to be elucidated.[4] The movement of GLUT4 from vesicles to the cell surface requires ATP. In contrast, action of the other members of this glucose transport family is not sensitive to the prevailing insulin concentrations. GLUT5 is primarily located in the apical membrane of the jejunum and is the main transporter of fructose from the lumen to the enterocytes.

To date, 14 transporters have been described in the facilitative transporter class. The functions of the more recently discovered transporters are less well established.[5]

Once glucose enters cells, the carbon skeleton is broken down through a series of enzymatic reactions, and the energy stored in the carbon–carbon bonds is released. This energy is used for synthesis of other substrates and for a variety of metabolic functions.

The net chemical reaction of glucose catabolism results in an equal number of moles of CO_2 and oxygen, creating a respiratory quotient of 1. This reaction is expressed in the following formula:

$$C_6H_{12}O_2 + 6O_2 \rightarrow 6CO_2 + 6H_2O + Energy$$

Glycolysis

Glycolysis is the process of breakdown of a glucose (6-carbon) molecule into pyruvate (3-carbon) molecules with the release of energy (Figure 3-5).[6] The glycolytic pathway is an anaerobic process occurring in the cytoplasm and is catalyzed by specific enzymes at each step of the reaction. The net reaction of glycolysis is:

$$\text{1 Glucose + 2 ADP + 2 Inorganic Phosphate + 2 NAD}^+$$
$$\rightarrow \text{2 Pyruvate + 2 ATP + 2 NADH + 2 H}^+ + \text{2 H}_2\text{O}$$

During the degradation of glucose, adenosine diphosphate (ADP) and inorganic phosphate combine to form ATP, and the cell uses the coenzyme NAD^+ to shuttle energy between reactions. After a series of reactions, 2 types of activated energy carrier molecules are produced: ATP and NADH. During glycolysis, the formation of ATP depends directly on the dehydration of glucose. This process is called *substrate level phosphorylation*. During the formation and degradation of ATP, energy is stored in and released from cells. Approximately 7 kcal are released per mole of ATP. In addition, 2 molecules of NADH are formed from NAD^+ after hydrogen atoms from glucose are received.

Glycolysis releases only a small fraction of the initial energy stored in the glucose molecule, and most of the energy is still present within the chemical bonds of the pyruvate. Pyruvate can be oxidized under aerobic conditions for maximum

FIGURE 3-5 Glycolytic Pathway

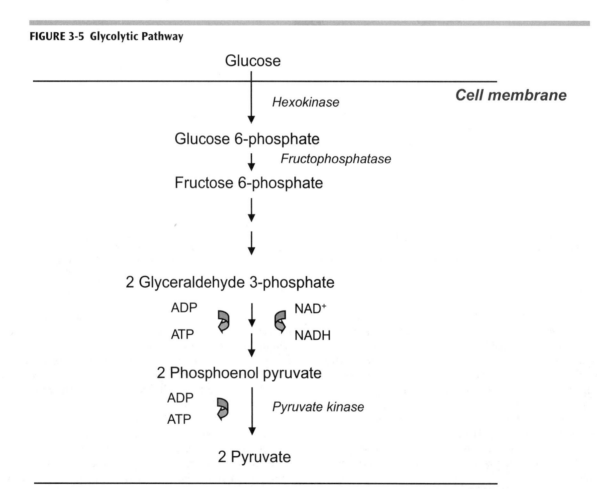

Glycolysis is an anaerobic process occurring in the cytosol and a key reaction of metabolism. It supplies energy (in the form of 2 ATP/1 glucose, substrate phosphorylation) and the reduced form of NADH, and it converts carbohydrates into pyruvate. The pathways are shown as they occur in the liver. Each arrow may represent 1 or more steps in this pathway. The 3 major enzymes are glucokinase, phosphofructokinase, and pyruvate kinase. ADP, adenosine diphosphate; ATP, adenosine triphosphate; NAD$^+$, nicotinamide adenine dinucleotide; NADH, nicotinamide adenine dinucleotide plus hydrogen.

energy production. During anaerobic glycolysis, pyruvate is reduced to lactate, with production of fewer moles of ATP.

In the liver, fructose and galactose also can enter the glycolytic pathway. However, additional enzymes are required to phosphorylate fructose to fructose 1,6-phosphate, and convert galactose to glucose 1-phosphate before glycolysis.

Cell Respiration—Tricarboxylic Acid Cycle

Under aerobic conditions, pyruvate is transported into the mitochondrial matrix and undergoes a decarboxylation process by which a CO_2 is released and 1 molecule of ATP is generated. The remaining 2 carbons (the acetyl group) then transfer to CoA to form acetyl-CoA. The TCA cycle begins with the combination of the 2-carbon acetyl group from acetyl-CoA with a 4-carbon compound, oxaloacetate, to form citrate. A series of 7 complicated reactions follows (Figure 3-6). With the complete oxidation of glucose, 2 molecules of CO_2 are released and 1 molecule of oxaloacetate is regenerated to be used in subsequent turns of the TCA cycle. During the TCA cycle, electrons are transferred to NAD$^+$ and flavin adenine dinucleotide, producing their reduced forms of NADH and reduced flavin adenine dinucleotide, respectively. These coenzymes then transport the electrons to oxygen via the electron transport chain (a series of carrier molecules in the inner mitochondrial membrane), which leads to the release of free energy for the synthesis of

more ATP, a process termed *oxidative phosphorylation*. Oxidative phosphorylation seems to generate 32 molecules of ATP, although there is some controversy about the exact number. Thus, the TCA cycle yields the energy stored in glucose much more efficiently than glycolysis. Mature erythrocytes do not possess mitochondria; therefore, glucose is never oxidized to water and CO_2. Instead, pyruvate is reduced to lactate. The TCA cycle is also known as the *Krebs cycle* or the *citric acid cycle*.

To sum up, the oxidation of 1 glucose molecule produces 4 molecules of ATP via substrate phosphorylation (2 from glycolysis and 2 from pyruvate decarboxylation) plus 32 molecules via oxidative phosphorylation, for a total of 36 molecules of ATP.

Pyruvate-Lactate Pathway

Under anaerobic conditions, pyruvate accepts a hydrogen atom from NADH, forming NAD$^+$ and lactic acid. At physiological pH, lactic acid will be in the form of lactate and protons. Thus, the local hydrogen ion concentration in the muscle increases. Using this pathway, 2 ATPs can be generated per molecule of pyruvate.

In most animals and humans, muscle can function for short periods under anaerobic conditions when the energy needs exceed oxygen supply. When lactate accumulates, buffering capacity can be exhausted, and intracellular pH drops

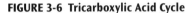

FIGURE 3-6 Tricarboxylic Acid Cycle

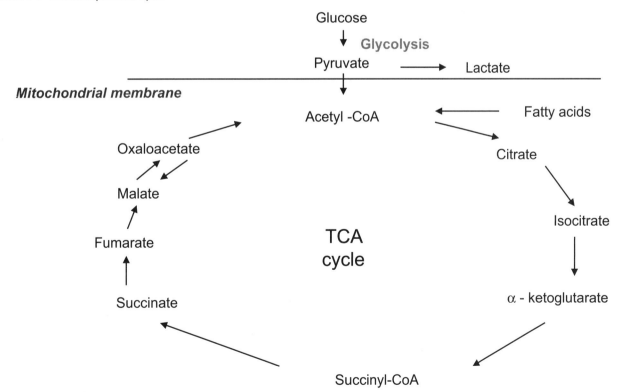

The tricarboxylic acid (TCA) cycle operates only under aerobic conditions and occurs inside of mitochondria. It plays a major role in energy metabolism and also provides intermediates for the synthesis of amino acids and fatty acids. The pathways are shown as they occur in the liver. Each arrow may represent 1 or more steps in this pathway. The oxidative phosphorylation in the respiratory chain produces 32 adenosine triphosphate. CoA, coenzyme A.

in active muscle, which inhibits glycolysis. When the oxygen supply is restored, the lactate can be converted back to pyruvate, and the pH returns toward normal. Oxidative glycolysis predominates again. Although this pathway is an inefficient method of glucose catabolism, it allows some organisms to survive under anaerobic conditions.

Gluconeogenesis

Gluconeogenesis is the endogenous formation of glucose. This step is important to maintain plasma glucose concentration in the normal range during fasting and allows constant provision of energy for metabolic needs. Gluconeogenesis occurs mainly in the liver, but it can also occur in the kidney and small intestine under some conditions.[7,8] The pathways of gluconeogenesis are not simply the reverse reactions of glycolysis. There are 4 distinctive, irreversible reactions (Figure 3-7): (1) Pyruvate is carboxylated in mitochondria to oxaloacetate; (2) the formed oxaloacetate is phosphorylated in the cytosol to phosphoenolpyruvate; (3) special phosphatases hydrolyze fructose 1,6-bisphosphate; and (4) special phosphatases hydrolyze glucose 6-phosphate.

During fasting or carbohydrate deprivation, amino acids and fat can provide carbon for gluconeogenesis. All amino acids except lysine and leucine are eligible sources because they can be catabolized to pyruvate, oxaloacetate, or precursors of these. Alanine is the most preferred contributor to gluconeogenesis in the liver. Glycerol derived from hydrolysis

FIGURE 3-7 Gluconeogenic Pathway

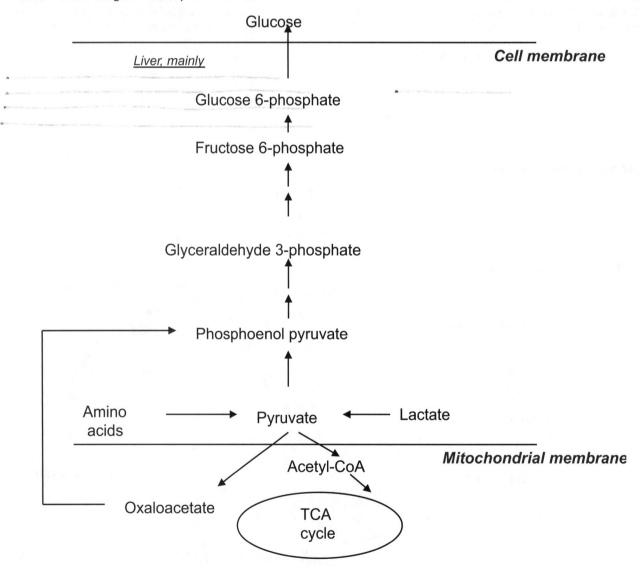

In humans and animals, the formation of glucose takes place primarily in the liver (as shown here; each arrow may represent 1 or more steps in this pathway). The kidney and small intestine are also sites of gluconeogenesis. Most steps in the gluconeogenesis reaction are a reversal of the respective steps in the glycolysis reaction, with the favored step in the direction of glucose synthesis. CoA, coenzyme A; TCA, tricarboxylic acid.

of triacylglycerols in fat cells can also be used for gluconeogenesis because glycerol can be phosphorylated to glycerol 3-phosphate, a glycolytic intermediate. In addition, fatty acids can be oxidized and transported into the mitochondria and converted to acetyl-CoA. Although oxidation of fatty acids produces large amounts of energy, 2 carbons are lost as CO_2 in the TCA cycle. For this reason, gluconeogenesis does not lead to the net conversion of fatty acids to carbohydrate.

Gluconeogenesis and glycolysis are strictly controlled by intracellular signals and are constantly coordinated with each other through hormonal regulation. In general, gluconeogenesis and glycolysis do not take place simultaneously in the same cell. Glycolysis occurs under fed conditions, whereas gluconeogenesis occurs under starved conditions.

Three major enzymes, glucokinase, phosphofructokinase, and pyruvate kinase, control the rate of glycolysis and gluconeogenesis. Locally, cells trap glucose by phosphorylation via the enzyme glucokinase, which prevents free glucose diffusing back to the bloodstream. The product of this reaction, glucose 6-phosphate, inhibits glucokinase, which ensures that free glucose does not accumulate within cells. Phosphofructokinase, a rate-limiting enzyme of glycolysis, is inhibited when ATP is plentiful. This step prevents further breakdown of glucose and allows the cell to divert glucose to be stored as glycogen for later use. When ATP is limited, phosphofructokinase is activated. Pyruvate kinase, the enzyme that converts phosphoenolpyruvate to pyruvate, also is maximally activated under these conditions, optimizing pyruvate entry to the TCA cycle and allowing maximal ATP production. In addition, a hormone-activated cyclic adenosine monophosphate (cAMP) cascade regulates the activities of these enzymes.

Glycogenesis and Glycogenolysis

As noted earlier, the body stores carbohydrate as glycogen. In general, only small quantities of ingested glucose are polymerized into glycogen, with the most glucose being oxidized as described previously. Glycogen is present in small amounts in most body tissues, but it is mainly found in the liver and skeletal muscle. Heart muscle has no glycogen reserves.

In a 70-kg healthy person, the liver contains approximately 100 g glycogen, which has the potential to provide 390 kcal. Skeletal muscle contains about 300 to 400 g glycogen, yielding less than 1560 kcal, suggesting that an adult stores enough glycogen for about a day of normal activities. Because glycogen is stored with water, this depot is somewhat bulky and, therefore, an inefficient storage method. Fat is anhydrous and provides a concentrated energy source, so most energy reserves are in adipose tissue.

Liver glycogen can be catabolized to provide glucose for use by the whole body. In contrast, skeletal muscle glycogen can only provide glucose to the muscle cells themselves. Myocytes do not have glucose 6-phosphatase; therefore, glucose 6-phosphate is the final product in the skeletal muscle and enters glycolysis inside the myocytes. Glucose 6-phosphatase also is present in the kidney and has recently been discovered in the small intestine; therefore, the kidney and possibly the small intestine may help control glucose homeostasis. The kidney may contribute 20% or more of whole body glucose

production during fasting (discussed below). The formation of glycogen is called *glycogenesis*, whereas glycogen breakdown is called *glycogenolysis*. Glycogen synthesis and glycogenolysis are relatively simple biochemical processes that are regulated according to cellular needs via the rate-limiting enzymes glycogen synthase and glycogen phosphorylase, respectively. Usually, activation of glycogen synthase occurs only after the inactivation of glycogen phosphorylase in hepatocytes.[9] Three key elements contribute to this glucose-sensing system in the liver. First, glucose 6-phosphatase is not inhibited by its product glucose 6-phosphate, which means that glucose 6-phosphate can be readily converted to glycogen if glucose 6-phosphate is in excess inside the cells. Second, insulin, glucagon, and epinephrine have hormonal influences. Finally, the concentration of glucose itself can increase or inhibit the formation of glycogen by modulating phosphorylation of glycogen synthase and glycogen phosphorylase. In response to feeding and a rise in plasma glucose concentrations, insulin advances glycogen synthesis through regulation of the activities of glycogen synthase and glycogen phosphorylase, so that glycogenesis is promoted, and glycogenolysis is inhibited. In response to a fall in blood glucose, pancreatic islets release the hormone glucagon, which has many functions opposite to those of insulin and is usually associated with increased production of glucose. Epinephrine is a hormone released from the adrenal medulla, usually during stress or shock, which also promotes breakdown of glycogen stores to provide energy for the fight-or-flight response. Both glucagon and epinephrine activate a cascade of second messengers through cAMP formation inside cells. The cAMP cascade leads to the phosphorylation and activation of glycogen phosphorylase, even if levels of cellular ATP and glucose 6-phosphate are high. As a result, glucose 1-phosphate in hepatocytes may be converted to glucose 6-phosphate and dephosphorylated, allowing glucose release to the bloodstream in times of need. Insulin antagonizes the glucagon- and epinephrine-induced cAMP cascades. With these hormonal interactions, the needs of the organism take precedence over the needs of the cell.

As Gerich and colleagues have described,[10] the contribution of gluconeogenesis in the kidney increases as the duration of fasting lengthens. Two parts of the kidney are involved. The renal medulla is the primary site in the kidney for glucose uptake and use, whereas renal gluconeogenesis mostly (perhaps exclusively) involves the renal cortex. Enzyme distribution along the nephron leads to this functional partition. In the renal cortex, cells do not synthesize significant amounts of glycogen but gluconeogenic enzymes are present. Glucose-phosphorylating and glycolytic enzyme activity occur in the renal medulla; however, the renal medulla does not have gluconeogenic enzymes such as glucose-6-phosphatase.[10]

In humans, the primary substrates to gluconeogenesis are lactate, glutamine, alanine, and glycerol. Alanine is preferred over glutamine as an amino acid substrate in the liver, and lactate and glutamine are the most important substrates for gluconeogenesis in the kidneys.[10]

Formation of Precursors for Other Metabolites

The precursors used to synthesize numerous physiologically significant molecules are formed via glycolysis and the TCA cycle. For example, the synthesis of nucleotides depends on glucose 6-phosphate. Pyruvate is a precursor of alanine. Acetyl-CoA can be used for synthesis of triglycerides, and citrate from the TCA cycle is used for the synthesis of cholesterol. Other intermediates from the TCA cycle are the precursors of some amino acids. For example, oxaloacetate and α-ketoglutarate are the precursors of aspartate and glutamate.

Fructose Metabolism

Excess consumption of fructose (usually as high-fructose corn syrup) has been linked to a number of serious metabolic outcomes, such as diabetes, fatty liver, and dyslipidemia. Acute ingestion of fructose provides substrates for both glycogen and fat synthesis, after intracellular phosphorylation. A diet that is chronically high in fructose upregulates the GLUT5 transporter and hepatic enzymes of lipogenesis. Human studies demonstrate that insulin resistance worsens after both short- and long-term excess fructose feeding.[11]

Plasma Glucose Homeostasis

Plasma glucose concentrations are normally maintained in the range of 70 to 120 mg/dL. This level provides constant nutrition for the tissues and organs in which metabolic function is regulated primarily by the extracellular glucose concentration.

Glucose Regulation During Fasting and Fed States

The liver contributes to glucose homeostasis during fasting and fed states. If the blood glucose concentration level is adequate (ie, the fed state), the liver metabolizes glucose to fill energy reserves (Figure 3-8). Glucose is metabolized readily to produce ATP, pyruvate, and acetyl-CoA. The latter can be

converted to triglycerides and exported in the form of lipoprotein to adipose tissues. During the fed state, very little glucose is metabolized through the TCA cycle in the liver. The elevated insulin concentration triggered by the rise in blood glucose, in parallel with a very low plasma glucagon concentration, is the primary signal for the metabolic pathways that consume glucose in hepatocytes.[6]

If blood glucose is lower (ie, the fasting state), the liver prioritizes the generation of glucose to maintain blood glucose concentrations (Figure 3-9). Therefore, glucose 6-phosphate is converted to glucose inside hepatocytes and exported to the bloodstream via GLUT2. In the early fasting state, glycogen is an important source of glucose 6-phosphate. Because the hepatic glycogen store is limited, the next source is gluconeogenesis from lactate, amino acids, and glycerol. The primary signal for homeostasis in the fasting state is elevated glucagon concentrations in concert with low plasma insulin.[6]

After 24 hours of fasting, glucose utilization is substantially reduced in most tissues and organs because the supply of glucose is reduced and circulating insulin concentration has declined. Higher glucagon concentrations promote fatty acid oxidation. Fat tissue becomes the main energy source for nearly all tissues. After 14 days of fasting, adipose tissue can provide more than 90% of daily energy requirements. Glycerol is transported to hepatocytes and enters the gluconeogenic pathway. When fatty acid oxidation rates are elevated, acetyl-CoA is generated in amounts that exceed the capacity of the TCA cycle. Acetyl-CoA is diverted into ketogenesis. Acetoacetate, 1-hydroxybutyrate, and acetone (the 3 ketones formed) are measurable in blood when formed in excess. The rate of ketogenesis is determined by the supply of fatty acids and the regulation of fatty acid oxidation, which is promoted by lower circulating insulin concentrations. In addition, protein catabolism also contributes to gluconeogenesis. In the early phases

FIGURE 3-8 Glucose Metabolism in the Liver in the Fed State

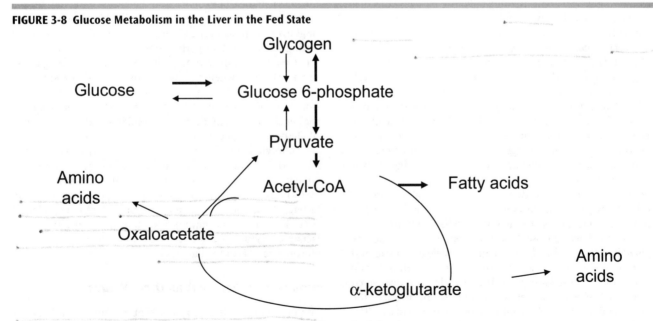

Each arrow may represent 1 or more steps in this pathway. The heavy arrow indicates stimulation. CoA, coenzyme A.

FIGURE 3-9 Glucose Metabolism in the Liver in the Fasting State

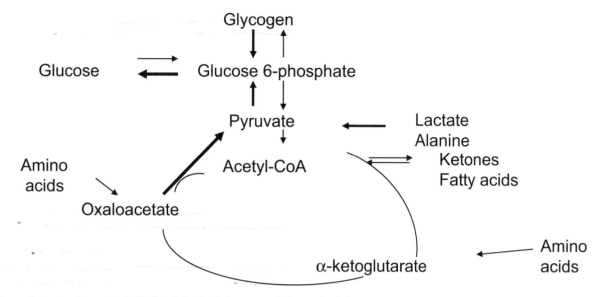

Each arrow may represent 1 or more steps in this pathway. The heavy arrow indicates stimulation. CoA, coenzyme A.

of fasting, ketones fuel the heart and musculoskeletal system, while the available glucose fuels the brain. After 1 to 2 weeks of starvation, the brain is able to adapt and use ketones as a source of energy. This metabolic fuel switch helps preserve the protein mass in prolonged fasting, as fat stores can be used in preference to protein stores.

Two other conditions, diabetes mellitus and a high-fat, low-carbohydrate diet, often lead to deficient intracellular glucose supplies. In diabetes, glucose entry into insulin-sensitive cells is impaired, related either to deficient insulin concentrations or resistance to insulin action. Similarly, in carbohydrate-restricted diets, the insulin level is relatively low, the glucagon level is elevated, fat is plentiful, and ketone production is enhanced. The brain adapts to metabolize ketones in low-carbohydrate diets, which has been shown in studies to reduce the frequency of seizures in children with epilepsy.[12]

Hormonal Regulation

Multiple hormones, including insulin, glucagon, glucocorticoids, catecholamines, and growth hormone, interact to regulate blood glucose. Normally, pancreatic beta cells secrete insulin following a meal in response to increased circulating glucose concentration (typically 90 mg/dL or greater). Compared with the response to an equivalent intravenous glucose infusion, the insulin secretory response to an oral glucose load is much greater because incretins such as glucose-dependent insulinotropic peptide, cholecystokinin, and glucagon-like peptide 1 increase the direct effect of glucose on beta cells. In individuals who do not have diabetes, this incretin effect is responsible for at least half of insulin release following oral glucose. However, in patients with type 2 diabetes, the pancreatic response to incretins is blunted, leading to reduced insulin release following oral glucose.[13]

During fasting, blood glucose levels fall and insulin secretion decreases accordingly. Under these conditions, pancreatic alpha cells become active and deliver glucagon to the bloodstream. Stress, infection, or exercise also can stimulate glucagon secretion. Insulin suppresses glucagon release independent of blood glucose. In response to fasting, increased glucagon stimulates the formation of glucose and its movement from the liver to the bloodstream. Muscle proteolysis is also stimulated by glucagon, which results in amino acid precursors used in hepatic gluconeogenesis. Hormonal regulation of renal gluconeogenesis is predominantly by epinephrine, and not by glucagon, an effect that Gerich and colleagues note "is consistent with the rich autonomic innervation of the kidney."[10] In these ways, hormonal regulatory mechanisms coordinate glucose metabolism to maintain glucose homeostasis during fasting and feeding.

Insulin is glycogenic, antigluconeogenic, antilipolytic, and antiketotic in its actions. It favors storage of absorbed nutrients and is, therefore, an anabolic hormone. In contrast, glucagon is glycogenolytic, gluconeogenic, lipolytic, and ketogenic in its actions. Thus, glucagon mobilizes energy storage and is a catabolic hormone.

Diabetes Mellitus

Diabetes mellitus is defined as hyperglycemia (elevated plasma glucose concentrations) caused by deficiency of the action of insulin. Hyperglycemia is the result of the increased production of glucose through gluconeogenesis and glycogen degradation, plus reduction in glucose uptake by cells. There are 2 common types of diabetes: (1) absolute insulin deficiency due to autoimmune pancreatic beta cell destruction (type 1 diabetes), and (2) relative insulin deficiency (type 2 diabetes).

Compared with patients with type 1 diabetes, those with type 2 diabetes have milder hyperglycemia and rarely experience ketoacidosis. Most people with type 2 diabetes are overweight or obese. A core defect in type 2 diabetes is insensitivity of liver, muscle, and adipose cells to the prevailing insulin concentrations, and inability of the beta cell to release sufficient insulin to overcome the resistance. The symptoms of type 2 diabetes are usually less pronounced than the symptoms of type 1 diabetes and develop at a slower pace. Diabetes may also develop during pregnancy because of increased placental hormones, which cause marked insulin resistance, usually in the third trimester. Gestational diabetes goes away when the pregnancy ends, but women who have had gestational diabetes have a greater risk of developing type 2 diabetes. See Practice Scenario 3-1 for a discussion of gestational diabetes and Chapter 34 for detailed information on diabetes mellitus.

Practice Scenario 3-1

Question: What should be done if a pregnant patient with gestational diabetes loses weight?

Scenario: LR was a 30-year-old primigravid woman with a pre-pregnancy body mass index of 30 and a 25-pound weight gain during the first 28 weeks of pregnancy. She was diagnosed with gestational diabetes and counseled regarding self-monitoring of blood glucose and her diet. LR reduced her carbohydrate intake to 20 g at lunch and 20 g at dinner. She avoided carbohydrate completely at breakfast because of hyperglycemia particularly at that meal. With this approach, her postprandial glucose values remained in the acceptable range of 130 to 140 mg/dL. However, the carbohydrate restriction led to LR to lose 3 pounds per week over the next 2 weeks.

Intervention: LR's obstetrician asked her to test her urine for ketones before each meal and at bedtime for 3 days and encouraged her to continue diet counseling, where LR was counseled to increase her carbohydrate intake.

Answer: Ketosis and weight loss were caused by carbohydrate avoidance, which is a strategy tried by many women diagnosed with gestational diabetes. Although urine assays for ketones are poor markers of serum ketones, they can serve to reinforce to a patient the importance of balanced carbohydrate nutrition in pregnancy. With liberalized carbohydrate intake, LR may require exogenous insulin and education on the same.

Rationale: Self-starvation during this scenario results from a misguided effort to avoid hyperglycemia. Adequate carbohydrate intake in this patient may cause hyperglycemia. If hyperglycemia occurs, it is appropriately managed with insulin injections before meals and at bedtime. Very low carbohydrate intake leads to decreases in plasma insulin and elevations in circulating glucagon, which permit glycogenolysis, gluconeogenesis, and lipolysis, and increase beta oxidation of fatty acids. This results in ketogenesis. Ketone production during pregnancy leads to ketone transfer across the placenta to the fetus and has been associated with reductions in intelligence quotient in the offspring. Weight loss during pregnancy is controversial, but it is probably acceptable if limited, slow, and not associated with ketone production.

Stress Hyperglycemia

Stress hyperglycemia indicates an elevation of the blood glucose in response to the inflammation of illness. Historically, it was usually defined as a plasma glucose concentration greater than 200 mg/dL.[14,15] Prior to 2001, control of such hyperglycemia in hospitalized patients was not a clinical priority, and even blood glucose levels greater than 200 mg/dL were often left untreated. Subsequently, a series of randomized clinical trials (RCTs) addressed the question of whether interventions to maintain normal glycemic levels were beneficial in hospitalized patients and brought into question what the true definition of stress hyperglycemia should be. The debate has not been fully resolved, although many experts consider blood glucose levels greater than 180 mg/dL to be abnormally elevated for hospitalized patients.[15] This state of hyperglycemia can be aggravated by nutrition support, particularly by the parenteral route. Hyperglycemia varies from mild to severe and disappears when the stress is over. During periods of illness and trauma, there is increased production of stress hormones such as epinephrine and cortisol, accompanied by an elevation in growth hormone and glucagon. These counterregulatory hormones oppose insulin action, causing increased glucose production by the liver (may exceed 500 g glucose per day) and decreased utilization of glucose in peripheral tissues. This hormonal milieu is also responsible for increased protein breakdown from muscle and enhanced fatty acid oxidation, which is viewed as a metabolic adaptation to provide fuels for heightened demands. Acute and chronic disease and injury also increase production of cytokines such as tumor necrosis factor-α, interleukin-1, and interleukin-6, which further contribute to hyperglycemia through stimulation of counterregulatory hormone release and suppression of insulin action.[16,17] See Chapters 24 and 34 for additional information on hyperglycemia and glycemic control.

Role of Fiber in Clinical Nutrition

Most Western diets contain inadequate fiber, largely because processed food intake tends to be high and fruit and vegetable intake is insufficient. However, no disease syndrome is associated with a fiber-deficient diet.[18] Constipation is the most easily recognized effect of fiber deficiency, although high-fiber diets can produce bloating and excessive gas.

In the upper digestive tract, fibers may increase satiety. High doses of fiber tend to delay gastric emptying, whereas lower doses do not show a significant effect. Gastric emptying may be delayed because of the increased viscosity of gastric contents, which reduces pyloric flow. In a patient with diabetes, increased time to empty the stomach may lead to a smaller peak postprandial glucose concentration.[19]

Under anaerobic conditions in the large intestine, dietary fibers are broken to their component sugars and fermentation by bacteria occurs. The amount of resistance of fibers to digestion varies substantially, with soluble fibers undergoing the most complete breakdown. SCFAs (butyrate, propionate, and acetate) result from this metabolism. They are absorbed by colonic epithelia, where butyrate may also be metabolized. These SCFAs then enter the portal vein and are transferred to the liver or, eventually, to the systemic circulation. The biological relevance of SCFA metabolism is not understood (see Chapter 4 for additional information).

Putative health claims for the benefits of fiber in a variety of primarily bowel disorders remain unproven in large RCTs.[20] Fibers that resist degradation and fermentation add bulk, as well as water, to the stool. In some human trials, the addition of fiber to tube feeding for ill patients has been associated with less diarrhea and firmer stools; however, not all studies have been concordant.[21,22] Use of a high-fiber diet in ambulatory patients to relieve constipation, while theoretically sensible, has not been consistently shown to improve bowel function.[23,24]

The role of fiber to improve glucose control in patients with diabetes is better established, although the overall effect is not large and compliance with higher fiber diets over long periods of time is suboptimal.[25,26] In a crossover RCT of 13 adults with type 2 diabetes, a 50-g fiber diet for 6 weeks was associated with lower 24-hour insulin and glucose concentrations compared with a 24-g fiber diet. Cholesterol, triglycerides, and very-low-density lipoproteins were all reduced in parallel with the high-fiber diet.[27] A meta-analysis of high-quality prospective RCTs of high- vs low-fiber intakes in patients with diabetes (total N = 605 participants) showed a benefit to lower glycated hemoglobin (0.5%) and fasting plasma glucose (–10 mg/dL) in the high-fiber group.[28]

In the Nurses' Health Study, epidemiologists followed more than 7800 women with diabetes for many years.[29] Whole grain and bran intake were associated with lowering of all-cause and cardiovascular mortality. Other large observational studies have largely concurred. In a cohort followed for 7 years, low dietary fiber intake at baseline was associated with a higher risk of developing diabetes.[30] The authors questioned whether the noted inverse association between dietary fiber and inflammatory markers (C-reactive protein and interleukin-6) might have etiologic relevance. Another potential mediator of the fiber effect is magnesium, which may improve insulin sensitivity. In a cohort study of Hawaiian patients without diabetes, the risk of developing diabetes was reduced by 10% in those with the highest intake of either grain fiber or magnesium, and these 2 intakes were highly correlated.[31] In general, recent reviews concur that dietary fiber supplementation in patients with diabetes is associated with improved glucose metabolism.[25,32]

Dietary fiber has been proposed as a protective factor against colorectal carcinoma as well as adenoma.[33] In some epidemiologic studies, fiber consumption is inversely proportional to risk of colonic neoplasia incidence or recurrence.[33,34] However, other studies have reached different conclusions. For example, the Nurses' Health Study noted no relationship between fiber intake and the risk of colorectal tumors.[35] In addition, intervention studies using higher fiber diet (such as the Women's Health Initiative) do not confirm protection.[36]

The mechanism whereby fiber lowers cardiovascular disease rates, both in patients with diabetes and those without, is thought to relate to favorable changes in plasma lipid profiles. Meta-analyses have shown that soluble fiber has been associated with improvements in total cholesterol as well as low-density lipoprotein cholesterol.[37,38] High-density lipoprotein cholesterol is usually not influenced by fiber intake. Fiber could reduce lipids by many possible mechanisms, including the binding of fibers in the gut to compounds such as sterols

that might otherwise be included in cholesterol metabolism, improvements in insulin sensitivity, or impact of hepatic metabolism of SCFAs on liver production of lipid particles.

The Health and Medicine Board (formerly Institute of Medicine) of the National Academies of Science, Engineering, and Medicine recommends that adults consume 20 to 35 g dietary fiber per day.[39] The Dietary Reference Intake (DRI) for fiber for adults is 14 g per 1000 kcal ingested (ie, about 25 g/d for women and 38 g/d for men).[39] The DRI is based on epidemiologic and clinical data about the cardioprotective effects of fiber consumption. In the United States, many people do not meet the DRI for dietary fiber. Among adults, intake of dietary fiber is typically 12 to 18 g. The latest Dietary Guidelines for Americans recommend a healthy eating pattern, rather than goals for the ingestion of specific nutrients, although it is unclear how this guideline will affect behavior.[40]

Carbohydrate Requirements

Healthy Adults

The Recommended Dietary Allowances for carbohydrate reflect the brain's need for glucose.[39] A minimum of 50 g carbohydrate per day is required to avoid ketone production. In a healthy adult, endogenous glucose production, from glycogen or gluconeogenesis, is approximately 2 mg/kg/min following an overnight fast, suggesting that a 70-kg individual can endogenously provide approximately 200 g glucose per day.[41] In the nonfed (postabsorptive) state, glycogenolysis in the liver accounts for about half of glucose production; the other half is from gluconeogenesis.

Different carbohydrate-containing foods have varying effects on blood glucose levels following oral ingestion. Glycemic index and glycemic load are 2 methods to classify foods by their effects on glucose levels.[42] Glycemic index assigns values to carbohydrate-containing foods according to their rapidity of digestion and absorption. Glycemic index is the area under the curve for the increase in blood glucose during the 2 hours following ingestion of 50 g of food, as compared with ingestion of 50 g of reference food (either white bread or glucose).[42,43] A food with a low glycemic index causes a smaller rise in blood glucose than one with a higher glycemic index. The glycemic index of food is strongly influenced by the ratio of amylose to amylopectin: Foods with a higher ratio, such as legumes, tend to have lower glycemic index values. Glycemic load quantifies the glucose response to total carbohydrate intake, taking into account the glycemic index and the quantity of carbohydrate ingested.[42] A table of glycemic index and glycemic load values for many foods is published in reference 42.

In theory, manipulating carbohydrate intakes according to the values of glycemic index and glycemic load might limit postprandial blood glucose concentrations and, hence, insulin excursions. This approach to meal planning might be desirable as adjunctive therapy for diabetes, dyslipidemia, and weight control. However, practical application of glycemic index and glycemic load is not straightforward. In general, given the same amount of protein and fat in a meal, higher GI foods will elicit a higher glycemic response than lower GI foods, but the physical forms of a food (such as juice vs whole fruit), methods of cooking (different cooking times), and the consumption of other foods within the same meal all influence the body's glycemic response to a specific food item.[44] In addition, age and gender often cause variations in hormonal release in response to food. The effects of glycemic load from a previous meal also can alter blood glucose response to the current meal.[45] Thus, no standard value of glycemic index is recommended for any medical conditions.

Exercise

The carbohydrate needs of exercise depend on both duration and intensity. A muscle at rest or during low-intensity exercise (ie, less than 25% maximal oxygen consumption [VO_{2max}]) primarily uses fatty acids to spare glucose for the brain. With increasing workloads, glucose becomes more important as fuel. For example, during moderate exercise (ie, less than 65% VO_{2max}), approximately 60% of the energy is provided by glucose (50% from glycogen, 10% from plasma glucose).[46] Muscle contains limited glycogen; therefore, additional glucose is supplied by liver glycogen breakdown. Extremely hard (ie, approximately 80% VO_{2max}) or prolonged physical work (eg, running a marathon) can potentially exhaust glycogen stores. In one research protocol, simply rinsing the mouth with a carbohydrate-containing drink increased sports performance in comparison with placebo. The mechanism behind this finding is hypothesized to be a neurological signal that can modify motor output.[47]

Carbohydrate loading (eg, 10 to 12 g carbohydrate per kilogram of body mass per day in the 36 to 48 hours before exercise) may provide optimal stores of muscle glycogen, improve performance, and reduce fatigue in individuals engaging in exercise for more than 90 minutes. Carbohydrate loading does not seem to provide a benefit for individuals engaged in moderate-intensity cycling or running for shorter periods of time.[48]

After exercise, individuals must consume adequate amounts of carbohydrate to refill glycogen stores in muscle and liver. Studies in athletes have suggested that individuals should ingest 50 to 100 g of carbohydrate immediately after exercise, and then eat a high-carbohydrate meal 2 hours later.[49] When protein and carbohydrate are consumed together in the immediate postexercise phase, insulin responses are augmented, and glycogen restorage is enhanced. To have enough carbohydrate available before and during exercise, and replenish carbohydrate stores after exercise, individuals who are very active may require up to 9 to 10 g carbohydrate per kilogram of body mass per day. Studies have also shown that consumption of 30 to 60 g carbohydrate per hour during sustained intensive exercise attenuated the usual increases in exercise-induced stress hormone release and immune depression.[50] Therefore, a low-carbohydrate diet is not advisable for athletes, particularly for those who perform high-intensity anaerobic exercise and resistance training.

Illness and Injury

The characteristic hypermetabolic response to illness and injury (inflammatory metabolism) involves negative nitrogen balance, insulin resistance, hyperglycemia, and fatty acid oxidation and mobilization. Provision of energy (carbohydrate or fat) is required to minimize protein degradation and lipolysis in all forms of illness and injury.[51] However, the clearance rate of endogenous and exogenous circulating lipid is decreased during illness, leading to the development of hypertriglyceridemia and hepatic fat accumulation. Thus, carbohydrate should be considered the primary energy source for these patients.[52] On the other hand, the capacity for glucose oxidation is also impaired during illness. In burn patients, glucose oxidation rates slow significantly if dextrose is given intravenously at a rate greater than 5 mg/kg/min.[53] In addition, patients, receiving parenteral nutrition who are fed glucose intravenously at rates in excess of 4 mg/kg/min have a substantial incidence of hyperglycemia.[14] Carbohydrate utilization and requirements in specific disease and trauma conditions are reviewed extensively in the chapters in Part III of this textbook.

Summary

Carbohydrate metabolism is relevant to diverse areas of medical care and research, and it is a pivotal part of a prevalent chronic disease, diabetes mellitus. Much information about carbohydrates has already been well defined; however, as the fields of obesity and exercise science evolve, our knowledge of carbohydrate metabolism will expand.

References

1. Gray GM. Carbohydrate digestion and absorption: role of the small intestine. *N Engl J Med.* 1975;292:1225–1230.
2. Pessin JE, Bell SI. Mammalian facilitative glucose transporter family: structure and molecular regulation. *Annu Rev Physiol.* 1992;54:911–930.
3. Simpson IA, Cushman SW. Hormonal regulation of mammalian glucose transport. *Annu Rev Biochem.* 1986;55:1059–1089.
4. Kotani K, Peroni OD, Minokoshi Y, et al. GLUT4 glucose transporter deficiency increases hepatic lipid production and peripheral lipid utilization. *J Clin Invest.* 2004;114:1666–1675.
5. Mueckler M, Thorens B. The SLC2 (GLUT) family of membrane transporters. *Mol Aspects Med.* 2013;34:121–138.
6. Berg JM, Tymoczko JL, Stryer L, eds. *Biochemistry.* 8th ed. New York: W.H. Freeman; 2015.
7. Mithieux G, Gautier-Stein A. Intestinal glucose metabolism revisited. *Diabetes Res Clin Pract.* 2014;105:295–301.
8. Ekberg K, Landau BR, Wajngot A, et al. Contributions by kidney and liver to glucose production in the postabsorptive state and after 60 h of fasting. *Diabetes.* 1999;48:292–298.
9. Stalmans W, De Wulf H, Hue L, et al. The sequential inactivation of glycogen phosphorylase and activation of glycogen synthetase in liver after administration of glucose to mice and rats. The mechanism of hepatic threshold to glucose. *Eur J Biochem.* 1974;41:117–134.
10. Gerich JE, Meyer C, Woerle HJ, Stumvoll M. Renal gluconeogenesis: its importance in human glucose homeostasis. *Diabetes Care.* 2001;24:382–391.
11. Herman MA, Samuel VT. The sweet path to metabolic demise: fructose and lipid synthesis. *Trends Endocrinol Metab.* 2016;27(10):719–730.
12. Sharma S, Jain P. The ketogenic diet and other dietary treatments for refractory epilepsy in children. *Ann India Acad Neurol.* 2014;17(3):253–258. doi:10.4103/0972-2327.138471.

13. Ahrén B. Incretin dysfunction in type 2 diabetes: clinical impact and future perspectives. *Diabetes Metab.* 2013;39:195–201.

14. McCowen KC, Malhotra A, Bistrian BR. Stress-induced hyperglycemia. *Crit Care Clin.* 2001;17:107–124.

15. Kavanagh BP, McCowen KC. Clinical practice. Glycemic control in the ICU. *N Engl J Med.* 2010;363:2540–2546.

16. Ling PR, Smith RJ, Bistrian BR. Hyperglycemia enhances cytokine production and oxidative responses to a low but not high dose of endotoxin in rats. *Crit Care Med.* 2005;33:1084–1089.

17. McCowen KC, Ling PR, Ciccarone A, et al. Sustained endotoxemia leads to marked down-regulation of early steps in the insulin signaling cascade. *Crit Care Med.* 2001;29:839–846.

18. Otles S, Ozgoz S. Health effects of dietary fiber. *Acta Sci Pol Technol Aliment.* 2014;13:191–202.

19. Jenkins DJ, Jenkins AL. Dietary fiber and the glycemic response. *Proc Soc Exp Biol Med.* 1985;180:422–431.

20. Anderson JW, Baird P, Davis RH, et al. Health benefits of dietary fiber. *Nutr Rev.* 2009;67:188–205.

21. Shimoni Z, Averbuch Y, Shir E, et al. The addition of fiber and the use of continuous infusion decrease the incidence of diarrhea in elderly tube-fed patients in medical wards of a general regional hospital: a controlled clinical trial. *J Clin Gastroenterol.* 2007;41:901–905.

22. Frankenfield DC, Beyer PL. Dietary fiber and bowel function in tube-fed patients. *J Am Diet Assoc.* 1991;91:590–596, 599.

23. Maffei HV, Vicentini AP. Prospective evaluation of dietary treatment in childhood constipation: high dietary fiber and wheat bran intake are associated with constipation amelioration. *J Pediatr Gastroenterol Nutr.* 2011;52:55–59.

24. Badiali D, Corazziari E, Habib FI, et al. Effect of wheat bran in treatment of chronic nonorganic constipation. A double-blind controlled trial. *Dig Dis Sci.* 1995;40:349–356.

25. Wolfram T, Ismail-Beigi F. Efficacy of high-fiber diets in the management of type 2 diabetes mellitus. *Endocr Pract.* 2011;17:132–142.

26. Vuksan V, Rogovik AL, Jovanovski E, et al. Fiber facts: benefits and recommendations for individuals with type 2 diabetes. *Curr Diab Rep.* 2009;9:405–411.

27. Chandalia M, Garg A, Lutjohann D, et al. Beneficial effects of high dietary fiber intake in patients with type 2 diabetes mellitus. *N Engl J Med.* 2000;342:1392–1398.

28. Silva FM, Kramer CK, de Almeida JC, et al. Fiber intake and glycemic control in patients with type 2 diabetes mellitus: a systematic review with meta-analysis of randomized controlled trials. *Nutr Rev.* 2013;71:790–801.

29. He M, van Dam RM, Rimm E, et al. Whole-grain, cereal fiber, bran, and germ intake and the risks of all-cause and cardiovascular disease-specific mortality among women with type 2 diabetes mellitus. *Circulation.* 2010;121:2162–2168.

30. Wannamethee SG, Whincup PH, Thomas MC, et al. Associations between dietary fiber and inflammation, hepatic function, and risk of type 2 diabetes in older men: potential mechanisms for the benefits of fiber on diabetes risk. *Diabetes Care.* 2009;32:1823–1825.

31. Hopping BN, Erber E, Grandinetti A, et al. Dietary fiber, magnesium, and glycemic load alter risk of type 2 diabetes in a multiethnic cohort in Hawaii. *J Nutr.* 2010;140:68–74.

32. Bajorek SA, Morello CM. Effects of dietary fiber and low glycemic index diet on glucose control in subjects with type 2 diabetes mellitus. *Ann Pharmacother.* 2010;44:1786–1792.

33. Sansbury LB, Wanke K, Albert PS, et al. The effect of strict adherence to a high-fiber, high-fruit and -vegetable, and low-fat eating pattern on adenoma recurrence. *Am J Epidemiol.* 2009;170:576–584.

34. Kunzmann AT, Coleman HG, Huang WY, et al. Dietary fiber intake and risk of colorectal cancer and incident and recurrent adenoma in the Prostate, Lung, Colorectal, and Ovarian Cancer Screening Trial. *Am J Clin Nutr.* 2015;102(4):881–890. doi:10.3945/ajcn.115.113282.

35. Fuchs CS, Giovannucci EL, Colditz GA, et al. Dietary fiber and the risk of colorectal cancer and adenoma in women. *N Engl J Med* 1999;340:169–176.

36. Beresford SA, Johnson KC, Ritenbaugh C, et al. Low-fat dietary pattern and risk of colorectal cancer: the Women's Health Initiative randomized controlled dietary modification trial. *JAMA.* 2006;295:643–654.

37. Brown L, Rosner B, Willett WW, et al. Cholesterol-lowering effects of dietary fiber: a meta-analysis. *Am J Clin Nutr.* 1999;69:30–42.

38. Talati R, Baker WL, Pabilonia MS, et al. The effects of barley-derived soluble fiber on serum lipids. *Ann Fam Med.* 2009;7:157–163.

39. Health and Medicine Division, National Academies of Sciences, Engineering, and Medicine. Dietary Reference Intakes tables and application. http://www.nationalacademies.org/hmd/Activities/Nutrition/SummaryDRIs/DRI-Tables.aspx. Accessed April 3, 2017.

40. US Department of Agriculture. Dietary Guidelines for Americans 2015–2020. https://www.choosemyplate.gov/dietary-guidelines. Accessed April 3, 2017.

41. Chandramouli V, Ekberg K, Schumann WC, et al. Quantifying gluconeogenesis during fasting. *Am J Physiol.* 1997;273:E1209–E1215.

42. Foster-Powell K, Holt SH, Brand-Miller JC. International table of glycemic index and glycemic load values: 2002. *Am J Clin Nutr.* 2002;76(1):5–56.

43. Jenkins DJ, Wolever TM, Taylor RH, et al. Glycemic index of foods: a physiological basis for carbohydrate exchange. *Am J Clin Nutr.* 1981;34:362–366.

44. Fernandes G, Velangi A, Wolever TM. Glycemic index of potatoes commonly consumed in North America. *J Am Diet Assoc.* 2005;105:557–562.

45. Granfeldt Y, Wu X, Bjorck I. Determination of glycemic index: some methodological aspects related to the analysis of carbohydrate load and characteristics of the previous evening meal. *Eur J Clin Nutr.* 2005;60:104–112.

46. Holloszy JO, Kohrt WM. Regulations of carbohydrate and fat metabolism during and after exercise. *Annu Rev Nutr.* 1996;16:121–138.

47. Jeukendrup A, Chambers ES. Oral carbohydrate sensing and exercise performance. *Curr Opin Clin Nutr Metab Care.* 2010;13:447–451.

48. Beck KL, Thomson JS, Swift RJ, von Hurst PR. Role of nutrition in performance enhancement and postexercise recovery. *Open Access J Sports Med.* 2015;11:259–267.

49. Hargreaves M. Carbohydrate and exercise. *J Sports Sci.* 1991;9:17–28.

50. Gleeson M, Nieman DC, Pedersen BK. Exercise, nutrition and immune function. *J Sports Sci.* 2004;22:115–125.

51. Blackburn GL, Wollner S, Bistrian BR. Nutrition support in the intensive care unit: an evolving science. *Arch Surg.* 2010;145:533–538.

52. Bistrian BR. Fat versus carbohydrate feeding in the critically ill. *Crit Care Med.* 2001;29:1475–1476.

53. Wolfe RR, Allsop JR, Burke JF. Glucose metabolism in man: responses to intravenous glucose. *Metabolism.* 1979;28:210–220.

4 Gut Microbiota

Gail A.M. Cresci, PhD, RD, LD, CNSC, and Kristin M. Izzo, MS, RD, LD, CNSC

CONTENTS

Objectives

1. Present an overview of the complexity of the human gut microbiota and the factors that influence its development and balance.
2. Provide working definitions for *probiotic* and *prebiotic*.
3. Review available evidence for the application of probiotics and prebiotics in clinical practice relating to common nutrition therapy issues.

Test Your Knowledge Questions

1. Which of the following statements best describes the human gut microbiota?
   A. The human gut microbiota is established by the age of 3 years and few factors influence it.
   B. Trillions of bacteria currently comprise the human gut microbiota.
   C. The human gut microbiota is highly dependent on the host for survival but provides little benefit to the host.
   D. The human gut microbiota is not influenced by the mode of infant delivery.

2. Which of the following statements best describes a probiotic?
   A. A probiotic is a live organism used to make yogurt.
   B. A probiotic is a "live nonpathogenic organism (bacteria or yeast) which when administered in adequate amounts confers a health benefit on the host."
   C. Probiotics are on the Generally Recognized As Safe (GRAS) list and therefore can be safely provided to all humans receiving nutrition support therapy.
   D. The mechanisms of probiotics are well known, making probiotic therapy a great addition to nutrition support therapy.
3. Which of the following statements best describes a prebiotic?
   A. All fibers are considered prebiotics.
   B. Prebiotics are synthetic compounds.
   C. Prebiotics are dietary polysaccharides that escape digestion by the host enzymes, are fermented by the gut microbiota, and influence the gut microbiota pattern in a beneficial manner.
   D. All prebiotics are fermented to yield the same short-chain fatty acids (SCFAs).

Test Your Knowledge Answers

1. The correct answer is **B**. Humans are sterile in utero and are first colonized depending on the mode of delivery. The gut microbiota development increases as the diet increases in complexity. The colonization of gut microbiota is influenced primarily by undigested polysaccharides that ferment to produce SCFAs. The SCFAs serve many biological functions in the host's body. The gut microbiota also has many other positive benefits to the host.
2. The correct answer is **B**. While the starter cultures used to make yogurt, *Lactobacillus bulgaricus* and *Streptococcus thermophilus,* are on the GRAS list and therefore considered safe for human consumption, they are not probiotics. There are specific criteria that a bacterium must meet to be considered a probiotic. The mechanisms of action of probiotics are still being researched, but what is known is that each strain of bacteria behaves differently, particularly in different environments. Therefore, a general application of probiotic therapy for nutrition support patients is not recommended.
3. The correct answer is **C**. Prebiotics are naturally occurring substances, predominantly dietary polysaccharides, which escape digestion by the host enzymes. They reach the distal intestine where they are fermented by the host gut microbiota to yield SCFAs and beneficially influence the gut microbiota pattern. Prebiotics are commonly thought of as dietary fiber; however, not all fibers are fermentable, and not all fermentable polysaccharides yield the same molar ratios of SCFAs.

Overview of the Gut Microbiota

The *gut microbiome,* a phrase coined by the molecular biologist Joshua Lederberg in 2001, is defined as the totality of microorganisms and their collective genetic material present in the intestine. The gut microbiota comprises all the microorganisms—commensal, symbiotic, and pathogenic—residing in the intestine. While mucosal surfaces of humans are colonized with bacteria, most bacteria reside within the gastrointestinal (GI) tract.[1] An estimated 800 different bacterial species with more than 7000 strains and approximately 100 trillion total bacteria are present in the human gut; these bacteria are predominantly anaerobic bacteria based on the sequencing of the highly conserved 16S region of ribosomal ribonucleic acid RNA (rRNA).[2] rRNA, the RNA component of the ribosome, provides a mechanism for decoding messenger RNA into amino acids and interacts with transfer RNAs during translation. Bacterial ribosomes contain about 60% rRNA and 40% protein by weight and consist of 2 subunits of unequal size; the larger subunit has a sedimentation coefficient of 50S whereas the sedimentation coefficient of the smaller one is 30S. The 30S subunit contains 1 molecule of 16S rRNA and 21 proteins. Multiple sequences of 16S rRNA can exist within a single bacterium.[3] The density of bacteria is 10^8 colony-forming units (CFUs) per mL in the distal small intestine and 10^{11} to 10^{12} CFU/mL in the colon. In comparison, low densities of bacteria (10^2 CFU per mL luminal contents) are located in the proximal intestinal tract (ie, stomach, duodenum, and jejunum). This lower density is due to the acidic gastric environment, presence of bile, and peristalsis.[2]

The human host has a mutualistic relationship with its gut microbiota. The gut microbiota plays a role in energy balance,[4–7] metabolism of xenobiotics,[8,9] resistance to pathogen colonization,[10,11] and the maturation of the intestinal and immune systems.[12,13] A *xenobiotic* is a chemical that is found in an organism but is not normally produced or expected to be present within it.

Recent studies have challenged the traditional understanding that the human GI tract is sterile until the birthing process. Although further study is needed, there is increasing evidence that microorganisms inhabit the placenta, amniotic fluid, and umbilical cord; thus, by swallowing amniotic fluid in utero, the fetus begins to colonize the developing GI tract.[14] Colonization continues with the birthing process, with the gut microbiota of newborns closely resembling the microbes encountered during birth. The colonization of neonates differs among those born vaginally compared to those born via cesarean section (C-section). The primary flora of vaginally delivered babies includes *Lactobacillus, Prevotella,* or *Sneathia* spp. In contrast to vaginally delivered neonates, babies delivered by C-section harbor bacterial communities that resemble those of the skin, comprising *Staphylococcus, Corynebacterium,* and *Propionibacterium* spp.[15,16] Analysis of these communities finds that they do not resemble the mother's flora more closely than those of other women's flora, indicating that the baby is in contact with microbes from humans other than the mother.[17] Because babies delivered by C-section do not receive that first vaginal maternal inoculum, their development of the GI microbiota is affected,[18,19] which may explain the increased vulnerability these babies have to certain pathogens.[17] Compared to vaginally delivered babies, C-section–delivered babies have higher incidences of atopic diseases,[20] allergies and asthma,[21,22] and skin infection with methicillin-resistant *Staphylococcus aureus* (among hospitals in the United States, 64% to 82% of readmissions of babies diagnosed with MRSA were delivered by C-section).[23]

While the newborn's gut microbiota is comprised of relatively few species and lineages, diversity rapidly increases within the first few years of life.[24,25] The exact reason for the increase in diversity is unknown, but it is hypothesized to be from (1) an enlarging intestinal tract that provides a larger habitat for more bacteria, (2) increased exposure to environmental bacteria, and/or (3) dietary changes.[17] Breastfeeding has been shown to enrich vaginally acquired, lactic acid–producing bacteria in the baby's intestine.[26] Breast milk contains bifidobacteria, with *Bifidobacterium longum* the most widely found species followed by *B. animalis*, *B. bifidum*, and *B. catenulatum*; all are *Bifidobacterium* species that may promote healthy microbiota development.[27]

Advancing the diet from simple solid foods (eg, rice cereal) to one including more complex plant polysaccharides (eg, peas) changes the relative ratio of bacterial phyla in the GI tract from an unstable community dominated by Actinobacteria and Proteobacteria to a stable mixture dominated by Firmicutes and Bacteroidetes, like that of an adult-like microbiota.[24] Analysis of the gut microbiota from African and Italian children found that African children had an increased abundance and diversity of Bacteroidetes.[28] This raises the possibility that the gut microbiota is adapted by local diets, and that the gut microbiota can adapt via genomic changes to changes in the host's diet; this adaption can be achieved by incorporating genes from bacteria in the environment.[29]

The composition of the gut microbiota among human family members tends to be more similar than the composition in unrelated individuals,[30] and the same bacterial strains can be shared among family members.[31–33] The gut microbiota pattern varies geographically with the host,[28] as well as with age—the gut microbiota in older adults varies from that found in younger adults.[34–36] Organisms have defined life spans and play different roles throughout their life span. Nature has created biological clocks to monitor the position of an individual in the aging spectrum; these clocks are phylogenetically deep and well conserved.[37] One type of clock includes bifunctional genes, which are genes beneficial to young individuals but costly in aging individuals.[38] Subsets of endogenous microbiota may have bifunctional genes,[17] and there is evidence for selection of microbes that coevolve with their host.[39]

These familial, geographic, and age-related variations in microbiota could have an impact on drug and nutrient metabolism, making it even more important to perform drug and nutrition trials in age- and location-matched populations to avoid the effects of differences in the metabolic capabilities of the human gut microbiota.[34] The variations also could influence outcomes after probiotic supplements are taken. Species that are beneficial to the young age group (eg, *Lactobacillus* and *Bifidobacterium*) might be harmful to older adults. These issues are important topics for study. In addition to diet, age, and geographical residence of the host, the gut microbiota can be altered by other factors such as medications and both physiological and psychological stress.[39]

Gut Dysbiosis

Attempts have been made to define a "core microbiome," as it is speculated that deviation from a core structure may lead to pathological states.[30] Because levels of interindividual variation are high, a conserved core microbiome structure is difficult to identify; however, community function may be conserved within this variation.[40] Both human and animal studies have increased our understanding of the delicate symbiosis between the gut microbiota and the host. Disruption of this mutual tolerance, or *gut dysbiosis*, may have a significant role in modulating host physiology. Environmental influences such as diet, exercise, and early life exposures can significantly affect the composition of the microbiota, potentially creating dysbiosis, which is associated with several autoimmune and metabolic diseases, including inflammatory bowel disease (IBD), type 2 diabetes, irritable bowel syndrome, metabolic syndrome, obesity, and cancer. The exact mechanisms of gut dysbiosis are uncertain, but, in most cases, they are linked with inflammation and alterations in immune responses and metabolism.[14]

Gut Microbiota in Select Patient Populations

Obesity

The gut microbiota has genetic and metabolic attributes that may play a role in human obesity. By analyzing the bacterial 16S rRNA gene, scientists have gained a better understanding of variations in the gut microbiota of lean vs obese animals and humans. The gut microbiota of obese individuals exhibits less taxonomic richness and potentially diminished metabolic capacity than the microbiota of lean individuals. In a mouse model colonized with the human gut microbiota, the mice became obese when their diet was manipulated from a high-carbohydrate diet to a high-fat "Western" diet; this change in diet also provided a rapid switch of the microbe community.[41] When this modified gut microbiota was transferred to germ-free mice known to be lean, they adapted the obese phenotype. In humans, analysis of the gut microbiota of lean vs obese adults has yielded conflicting results. The first study analyzing stool samples of obese vs matched lean individuals showed a shift in bacterial phyla (lower Bacteroidetes and more Firmicutes).[42] When the human subjects lost weight by following a fat-restricted or carbohydrate-restricted low-calorie diet, the ratio of Bacteroidetes to Firmicutes approached a lean-type profile after 52 weeks.[42] However, later work by other investigators indicates that the ratio of Bacteroidetes to Firmicutes is not altered in obese humans,[43] that more Bacteroidetes were detected in obese humans compared to normal-weight humans,[44] and that surgical manipulation via gastric bypass surgery decreased Firmicutes.[44] Discrepancies in the results could be related to variations in the methodologies used for bacterial analysis among the studies.[45] A large study identifying 3 robust clusters, referred to as *enterotypes*, identified in people from different countries and continents did not reveal any correlation between body mass index (BMI) and Firmicutes/Bacteroidetes ratio.[46] A set of 3 gene modules have been strongly correlated with the host's BMI; 2 are adenosine triphosphatase complexes, and this finding supports a conceptual link between gut microbiota capacity for energy harvest and obesity in a host.[46] Evidence indicates that the microbiota of obese individuals exhibits less taxonomic richness and potentially diminished metabolic capacity than the microbiota of lean individuals.[30,47,48]

Inflammatory Bowel Disease

The underlying etiology of IBD remains unknown. A central hypothesis is that commensal gut bacteria generate an autoimmune response contributing to mucosal inflammation. Compared with the microbiota in the general population, the microbiota of individuals with IBD varies widely in number and diversity. In areas of inflammation, notably fewer Firmicutes, Bacteroidetes, and *Clostridium* are detected and the proportion of Proteobacteria and Actinobacteria bacterial counts increases.[49] This finding is concerning because the diminished phyla contribute to the production of SCFAs and, in particular, butyrate, which is important for intestinal health.

Curative therapies for IBD are yet to be found. Current therapies for induction and maintenance of remission include immunosuppressive drugs (eg, corticosteroids, methotrexate) and anti-inflammatory drugs (eg, antitumor necrosis factor).[50] Because approximately 30% to 50% of patients with IBD are nonresponders to these medications and require surgical intervention, alternative therapies are needed—and the concept of shifting the gut microbiota back to a "healthy" balance seems like a promising option. In a variety of cohort studies, fecal microbiota transplant (FMT) has provided therapeutic effects that alter the composition of gut microbiota and enhance the diversity and proliferation of beneficial bacteria. The shift in microbiota composition post-FMT provides ulcerative colitis (UC) patients with the opportunity to more adequately defend against pathogenic bacteria and subsequent inflammatory complications.[51]

The standard surgical treatment to help manage refractory UC, UC with dysplasia, or familial adenomatous polyposis (FAP), is reconstructive proctocolectomy with the creation of an ileal-pouch anal anastomosis (IPAA). This formed pouch takes place of the removed rectum and often has associated complications, including increased stool, urgent stool, rectal bleeding, incontinence, or fever. Additionally, endoscopic findings show that postsurgical patients are at risk for mucosal edema, granulation, decreased vasculature, and ulceration. Approximately 50% of individuals with UC who have undergone IPAA creation will experience acute pouchitis; in contrast, only a few patients who underwent the same procedure to address underlying FAP develop pouchitis. Of note, the risk of acute pouchitis seems to be related to the individual's genetic predisposition and altered gut microbiota of the conduit eliciting an immune response rather than the reconstruction itself.[52]

Small Intestinal Bacterial Overgrowth

Arising from a variety of underlying disease states, notably short-gut syndrome, small intestinal bacterial overgrowth (SIBO) is characterized by an increase in bacteria in the small intestine, which usually has a very low bacterial load. Clinical symptoms of SIBO include chronic diarrhea, foamy or frothy stool, nausea, vomiting, foul-smelling stool, bloating, and constipation. While definitive therapies for SIBO are not available, typical treatment includes broad-spectrum antibiotics, which can further alter the composition of the gut

microbiota. In pilot studies, probiotic supplementation along with antibiotic regimens has shown promise, with reduction in clinical symptoms of chronic diarrhea, abdominal distention, pain, bloating, and belching. In one study, patients with SIBO supplemented with probiotics post–antibiotic therapy showed greater reduction in posttreatment hydrogen breath tests, suggesting more effective eradication of bacterial overgrowth, when compared with controls.[53]

Critical Illness

Critically ill patients are at risk for developing infections, and most patients receive antibiotics, which contribute to gut dysbiosis. Additionally, the therapies used to treat critically ill patients and the metabolic conditions these patients have can negatively alter the gut microbiota. Critical illness can cause redistribution of splanchnic perfusion, resulting in intestinal hypoperfusion, gut ischemia, and mucosal injury. Disruption of the intestinal barrier, an altered gut immune system, and dysfunctional metabolic activities of commensal bacteria make the intestine a major contributor to systemic infections.[54] Negative shifts in gut microbiota have been demonstrated within 6 hours of a metabolic insult, prior to provision of antibiotics, with alterations not returning to baseline patterns during the hospital stay.[55] A recent (2016) prospective study including several institutions demonstrates significant differences in the microbiome, including the gut microbiota, in critically ill patients compared with the microbiome of a healthy population, as demonstrated by analysis of fecal, oral, and skin sample collections.[56] This rapidly occurring dysbiosis increased in magnitude throughout the length of stay in the intensive care unit (ICU).

Probiotics

The literal definition derived from Greek for *probiotic* is "for life." The Food and Agriculture Organization of the United Nations and the World Health Organization (FAO/WHO) have defined probiotics as "live non-pathogenic organisms (bacteria or yeast) which when administered in adequate amounts confer a health benefit on the host."[57] Currently, the US regulatory framework does not include a definition of probiotics, nor has the federal government established any rules or regulations specific to probiotics. This lack of regulation is concerning because a product can be called a "probiotic" without having substantiated evidence demonstrating that it meets the minimum criteria set forth in guidelines issued by the FAO/WHO.[57]

Not all bacteria or live cultures found in foods and/or supplements can be characterized as probiotics. According to FAO/WHO, an organism must meet very strict criteria to be considered a probiotic (Table 4-1).[57] Ideally, the live, viable organism with strain identification must be able to survive the proximal GI tract environment and reach the distal intestine. There it must function and/or adhere to the gut epithelial tissue, have a beneficial impact on the gut microbiota pattern, and be scientifically proven to exert a positive health effect. Lastly, the organism should be safe for human consumption.[57] Even though conventional yogurt is a food rich in protein and

TABLE 4-1 Probiotic Criteria

- Strain identification
- Human origin
- Live microorganism
- Viable
- Safe for human consumption
- Survive proximal gastrointestinal tract
- Reach distal intestine and colon
- Function/adhere to gut epithelial tissue
- Colonize distal gut, affecting microbiome composition
- Scientifically proven health benefits

Source: Data are from reference 57.

calcium, the 2 starter cultures used to produce it, *Streptococcus thermophilus* and *Lactobacillus bulgaricus*, are not probiotics because they do not meet all probiotic criteria. Additionally, while other yogurt cultures may possibly be probiotic, scientific evidence must indicate that the yogurt product in question has high amounts of the probiotic strains and has demonstrated health benefits. These standards should also be applied to probiotic supplements.

To appropriately identify a probiotic, one should look at the genus, species, and strain names (eg, *Bifidobacterium* [genus] *lactis* [species] Bb-12 [strain]). Most manufacturers do not include this information in their labeling of products such as yogurts or other fermented milk foods and supplements. Often, manufacturers have not conducted research on the specific probiotic strain used in their fermented milk product or supplement; instead, companies typically generalize health claims from the other research sources for the genus and/or species included in the product. This lack of specific information poses a challenge for the clinician and the consumer regarding whether the product confers a health benefit.

Mechanisms of Action

Elie Metchnikoff, a Russian Nobel Prize winner of the 20th century, was the first to propose beneficial effects of probiotics among aging Eastern Europeans. He hypothesized that proteolytic microbes in the colon produced toxic substances responsible for the aging process and proposed that consumption of fermented milk would coat the colon with *Lactobacillus*, thus decreasing luminal pH, suppressing proteolytic bacteria, and slowing the aging process.[58] Recent advances in the field are beginning to sort out how probiotics exert their beneficial effects. Probiotic strains do not all exert the same mechanisms of action; instead, there is considerable interstrain diversity. Therefore, properties of one probiotic should not be extrapolated to another. One also cannot assume that probiotic actions in vitro reflect mechanisms of action in vivo or that the same probiotic strain exerts the same mechanism of action in different metabolic environments of the host, such as an ambulatory care setting vs an intensive care setting.

Probiotic strains may have multiple activities (Table 4-2) and therefore may be influential at various times.[59] Various probiotics exert their predominant action in the lumen, at

the mucosal surface, by engagement with the mucosal innate immune response, or by action beyond the gut with stimulation of the acquired immune response.[60] For example, the probiotic *Lactobacillus salivarius* UCC118 provided protective luminal action by producing an antimicrobial, bacteriocin, against *L. monocytogenes*. The same probiotic was effective in protecting against salmonella infection but by a different mechanism.[61] The luminal actions of probiotics can also cause metabolic alterations of commensal resident microbiota. For example, inoculation of germ-free mice with probiotic bacteria resulted in marked changes in gene expression within the resident commensal microbiome.[62]

Some probiotics have been shown to have action at the mucosal surface. These effects include induction of mucins (MUC2 and MUC3),[63] with the resultant enhanced mucus layer overlying the gut epithelial lining then serving as an antibacterial shield that prevents the binding of enteric pathogens to mucosal surfaces and increases the clearance of pathogens from the gut.[64] Additionally, mucin-producing cells secrete trefoil factors in response to microbial pathogens, which act together with mucins to prevent their binding to mucosal surfaces.[65] Certain probiotics may also enhance gut integrity and its barrier function by preventing changes in tight junction proteins (eg, occludins, claudins) and enhancing the tight junction transepithelial electrical resistance.[66]

Some probiotics express pathogen-associated molecular patterns capable of engaging with the same pattern-recognition receptors used by pathogens; therefore, probiotics have the means to protect the mucosal surface by competitive exclusion.[66] Some probiotics have exhibited the ability to stimulate

TABLE 4-2 Probiotic Proposed Mechanisms of Action

Colonization resistance:
- Competitive exclusion

Intestinal barrier function maintenance:
- Maintain tight junctions
- Reduce macromolecular permeability and bacterial translocation

Enhancement of gut microbiome pattern:
- Enhance ratio of commensal bacteria

Modulation of inflammatory and immunoregulatory signaling:
- NF-κB
- Interleukin-10
- Toll-like receptor(s) innate/adaptive immune modulation

Increased mucin regulatory genes and mucin production:
- Defensin production
- Engagement with dendritic cells
- Immunoglobulin (IgA, IgG, IgM) production

Metabolic effects:
- Nutrient metabolism
- Bacteriocins
- Decrease luminal pH
- Quorum sensing

NF-κB, nuclear factor kappa–light-chain-enhancer of activated B cells.

the innate and acquired immune system via induction of regulatory T-cell function.[67] The secretion of anti-inflammatory (eg, interleukin-10) and proinflammatory (eg, interleukin-12) cytokines by immune cells can be affected in a strain-specific manner by some probiotic strains.[59] Some probiotics have also been able to activate specific gut opioid and cannabinoid receptors, thus having the potential to modulate visceral pain.[68]

Probiotic Sources

A challenge to clinicians is finding a commercially available probiotic product that has scientific evidence of its benefit to patients. Many probiotic strains reported in the literature are not commercially available products, limiting the clinician's ability to readily translate scientific evidence into clinical practice. Additionally, most manufacturers do not disclose the strain specificity or quantity of viable organisms (CFU) for

products, thus further confounding the clinical application. Table 4-3 lists a select number of commercially available probiotic products.

Prebiotics

The primary food sources for commensal microbiota are undigested polysaccharides and sloughed proteins. A prebiotic is defined as "a selectively fermented ingredient that allows specific changes, both in the composition and/or activity in the GI microbiota, that confer benefits upon host well-being and health."[69] An ingredient must meet necessary criteria to be considered a prebiotic (Table 4-4).[70] To selectively stimulate the growth and activity of the gut microbiota in a beneficial manner, a prebiotic must be resistant to the host's gastric acidity and digestive enzymes and must be fermented in the distal intestine (ileum and colon) by the commensal anaerobic gut

TABLE 4-3 Select Commercially Available Probiotics

Strain(s)	Initial Product	Supplier	Year Introduced
Lactobacillus casein strain Shirota	Yakult	Yakult	1935
Streptococcus thermophiles *Lactobacillus bulgaricus* *Lactobacillus acidophilus* *Bifidus*	Yogurt	Stoneyfield	1973
Bifidobacterium longum BBS36	Bifidus milk	Moringa Milk Products	1977
Bifidobacterium breve strain Yakult	Mil-Mil (Bifiene)	Yakult	1978
Bifidobacterium lactis BB-12	Yogurt	Chr. Hansen	1988
Lactobacillus rhamnosus GG	Gefilus	Valio	1990
Lactobacillus casei DN-114-001 (*Lactobacillus casei Immunitas*)	Actimel (DanActive)	Danone	1994
Lactobacillus johnsonii La-1	LC1	Nestlé	1994
Lactobacillus plantarum 299v	ProViva	Probi	1994
Bifidobacterium animalis DN-173-010 (*Bifidus regularis*)	BIO (Activia)	Danone	1995
Lactobacillus gasseri LG21	LG21	Meiji Milk Products	2000
Bifidobacterium lactis HN-019	Supplement	Danisco	2001
Lactobacillus casei KW2110	Yogurt	Kirin Holdings	2003
Lactobacillus casei F19	Cultura	Arla Foods	2004
Streptococcus thermophilus *Bifidobacterium breve* *Bifidobacterium lactis* *Bifidobacterium infantis* *Lactobacillus acidophilus* *Lactobacillus plantarum* *Lactobacillus para casei* *Lactobacillus helveticus*	VSL#3	Sigma-Tau HealthScience	2000
Escherichia coli Nissle 1917[a]	Mutaflor	Ardeypharm GmbH	1971
Bacillus clausii[a]	Enterogermina	Sanofi Aventis	1999

[a]Not manufactured in the United States.

TABLE 4-4 Prebiotic Characteristics

Three necessary criteria of ingredients:
- Must be resistant to gastric acidity, to hydrolysis by mammalian enzymes, and to GI absorption
- Must be fermented in the GI tract by gut microbiota
- Must be selective in the stimulation of the gut microbiota growth and/or activity that contribute to health and well-being

Not available to all bacterial species in gut microbiome

Simple, naturally occurring or synthetic sugars:
- Lactobacilli and bifidobacteria are considered indicator organisms:
  - Inulin (chicory, leeks, onion, garlic, artichoke, asparagus): DP 10–60
  - Inulin-type fructans (oligofructose or fructooligosaccharide): DP_{max} 10 via partial hydrolysis of inulin or synthetically from monomers
  - Transgalactooligosaccharides
  - Enzymatic synthesis based on lactose
  - Lactulose

DP, degree of polymerization; GI, gastrointestinal.
Source: Data are from reference 70.

microbiota.[70] Demonstration of prebiotic activity of an ingredient is difficult; therefore, an ingredient may have prebiotic effects but not yet be called a prebiotic because there is insufficient evidence to prove the ingredient meets the necessary criteria.

Prebiotics are simple, naturally occurring or synthetic sugars that vary with their degree of polymerization. A prebiotic is not available to all bacterial species that inhabit GI ecosystems. *Lactobacillus* and *Bifidobacterium* are considered indicator organisms because currently known prebiotics stimulate the composition or activity of these organisms, but not necessarily others, in the gut microbiota.

Upon reaching the distal intestine (ileum and colon), prebiotics are fermented by endogenous anaerobic bacteria and SCFAs; gases (carbon dioxide, hydrogen, and methane) are produced; endogenous bacterial cell mass is increased; and endogenous bacterial enzyme activities are altered. This process decreases intraluminal pH, thereby favoring the predominance of beneficial bacteria (eg, bifidobacteria, lactobacilli, and nonpathogenic *Escherichia coli*) and decreasing *Bacteroidaceae*.[71] As with a high-fiber diet, ingestion of prebiotics (5 to 20 g/d) can produce unwanted symptoms such as flatulence, bloating, abdominal pain, eructation, and borborygmi,[72] with a wide individual variation found. The stoichiometry of fermentation differs for carbohydrates of differing chain lengths and monosaccharide composition, degree of polymerization, and branching, with slower fermentation associated with longer chain length. Prebiotics can also affect bowel function, resulting in a laxative effect through stimulation of microbial growth and increased bacterial cell mass, leading to stimulation of peristalsis by increased bowel content.[72] However, the effect on bowel function is small, and well-controlled studies are needed to measure an effect. The type of prebiotic influences fecal stool weight. Fibers from grains tend to increase

stool weight the most, whereas inulin has little effect (1 g inulin increases stool weight by <1 g).[72a] Prebiotic inulin-type fructans significantly increase the absorption of both calcium and magnesium in growing animals and in adolescents when added to the diet.[73] In pubertal adolescents, a mixed short- and long-degree of polymerization inulin-type fructan product (8 g/d) provided daily for 8 weeks significantly increased calcium absorption and enhanced bone mineralization. These effects may be modulated by genetic factors, including specific vitamin D–receptor gene polymorphisms.[73]

Prebiotics are fermented by endogenous commensal gut microbiota producing SCFAs, predominantly acetate, propionate, and butyrate.[74] Prebiotics do not all yield equal amounts and the same types of SCFAs.[74] SCFAs are known to serve several biological functions, including ion transport (eg, sodium, bicarbonate); modulation of intracellular pH and cell volume; provision of a metabolic cellular fuel source; and regulation of cellular proliferation, differentiation, and gene expression.[75] Butyrate in particular contributes to differentiation of epithelial cells, enhances water and electrolyte absorption, modulates immune function, exerts anti-inflammatory effects, and possesses tumor-suppressor effects in the colon through its role as an inhibitor of histone deacetylases and as a ligand for butyrate transporters and receptors.[76,77]

Synbiotics

A *synbiotic* is a physical combination of prebiotics and probiotics. Often, candidates for probiotic therapy have inadequate dietary intake of prebiotics and/or their commensal microbiome is altered. Therefore, providing a prebiotic or a probiotic alone may not produce a beneficial effect. A synbiotic product may have the advantage of providing substrate (prebiotic) for a potentially beneficial probiotic, which in turn benefits the host (patient).[78] Additionally, a synbiotic might maximize the viability and beneficial function of the probiotic before utilization and later as a therapeutic agent in the host GI tract.[79]

Prebiotic and Probiotic Applications

Potential Candidates for Prebiotic or Probiotic Use

Prebiotics and probiotics may be beneficial for individuals with poor diets, older adults, patients experiencing stress, and those who are taking medications that alter gut microbial balance. Potential health benefits vary depending on the type, timing, and dosing of the probiotic and/or prebiotic.

Type, Timing, and Dosing

When considering probiotic or prebiotic supplementation, the clinician must investigate the optimal strain for the clinical condition of interest and identify supportive research with evidence for justified and cost-effective usage. This research can be challenging because the literature covers a variety of probiotic strains and doses that are not commercially available. Additionally, diverse patient populations, study designs, and small sample sizes have limited the ability of analysts to make evidence-based recommendations. Further confusion arises because of uncertainty about how probiotic strains behave in various metabolic environments and clinical conditions, the synergy with strain combinations, or when probiotic strains are combined with various prebiotics.[80] Nevertheless, the clinician must adhere to the precept that *a probiotic, identified by strain, should only be provided to a patient with a clinical condition in which the probiotic strain has research evidence to support its use.* As has been noted previously, probiotics are live viable organisms and may behave differently in various metabolic and environmental milieus. Therefore, providing a probiotic strain without careful consideration of the evidence could potentially lead to adverse effects.

It is speculated based on current literature that the optimal dose for probiotic and prebiotic effect, although condition-specific, is approximately 10^9 to 10^{12} CFU/d for a probiotic and 5 to 20 g/d for a prebiotic. Dosing schedules vary from 1 or 2 times daily to 3 or 4 times per week. Probiotic colonization is transient; therefore, continued dosing may be necessary to maintain a treatment effect for some conditions (eg, *C. difficile* remission).[59]

Safety Issues

Common, safe probiotic species include many bifidobacteria (eg, *B. bifidum*, *B. longum,* and *B. infantis*) as well as many lactic acid bacteria (LAB). Used in foods for many years, LAB are considered harmless. They fall under the Medical Food and Supplement Act and are afforded GRAS status. LAB that grow as adventitious microflora or are added to foods as cultures do not pose a health risk to healthy humans. Several strains of LAB species have been isolated from the human GI tract and administered to humans without reported adverse effects. These include *Lactobacillus reuteri*, *L. plantarum,* and *L. casei* (subspecies *rhamnosus*). However, although probiotics are normal commensals of mammalian microbiota and are generally thought to be without pathological potential, individual patients may be susceptible to opportunistic infections via normal microbiota. In case reports, adverse effects seen when probiotics were administered have included sepsis (bacteremia, fungemia), bowel ischemia, and mortality, most of which occurred in patients who had underlying medical conditions.[81–84] Other potential theoretical risks are deleterious metabolic activities related to altered polysaccharide fermentation, lipid metabolism, and glucose homeostasis; immune deviation or excessive immune stimulation; and microbial resistance.[81]

Contraindications

Whereas prebiotic use does not seem to be contraindicated except for patients who are hemodynamically unstable, probiotic use in certain patient populations may not be safe. Studies investigating probiotic benefits typically include strict exclusion criteria that are often not considered by practitioners when using a probiotic in clinical practice. In a review of 92 cases of invasive *Saccharomyces* infections, treatment with antibiotic therapy and existing intravenous catheters were identified as the most frequent predisposing factors.[83] *Lacto-*

bacillus has been isolated in the blood of patients with short-gut syndrome, leukemia, mitral regurgitation, and cardiac surgery.[81] Risk factors for developing infectious complications associated with the use of probiotics include the presence of a central venous catheter, immunocompromised status, administration of the probiotic directly into the small intestine, concomitant administration of broad-spectrum antibiotics in which the probiotic is resistant, cardiac valvular disease, and intestinal barrier compromise.[81,84]

Restoring the Gut Microbiota: What Is the Evidence?

Many clinical conditions can alter the gut microbiota, making attempts to correct imbalances attractive. Interventions aimed at preventing or correcting gut dysbiosis have been investigated in a variety of clinical conditions, including diarrhea, allergy, IBD, critical illness, and surgery.

Antibiotic-Associated Diarrhea

Antibiotic-associated diarrhea (AAD) is a common adverse effect of antibiotic therapy. With AAD, the pathogenic bacteria in the gut microbiota outnumber the beneficial by 10 to 1.[85] Disturbing the normal gut microbiota is believed to predispose the host to pathogenic bacterial colonization.[86] Approximately 25% to 30% of cases of AAD in hospitalized patients involve *Clostridium difficile*.[87] *C. difficile* infection can be debilitating and has a high recurrence rate; it can cause pseudomembranous lesions in the colonic mucosa, causing severe inflammation.[85] Fluoroquinolones are the antibiotics most likely to cause AAD/*C. difficile*–associated disease (CDAD). AAD typically begins 4 to 9 days following antibiotic cessation, but it can occur up to 8 weeks later. Other risk factors for AAD/CDAD include severe illness, advanced age, presence of a nasogastric tube, provision of medications to raise gastric pH, GI surgery or manipulation, immunocompromised status, and extended hospital stay.[85] The most effective treatment of AAD/CDAD is to stop use of the inciting antibiotic. *C. difficile* identified by a positive stool culture is typically treated with metronidazole initially, with correction of fluid and electrolyte imbalance as needed. The treatment is repeated in patients that fail initial treatment; if they relapse again, they are then treated with oral vancomycin. Relapses may occur within 1 to 2 weeks of discontinuing antibiotic treatment. Relapse is believed to be caused by the survival of *C. difficile* spores that later germinate producing vegetative forms and critical illness.[85]

In theory, providing probiotics in patients receiving antibiotics to prevent gut dysbiosis and recolonize the gut colony with commensal bacteria makes sense. In the past few decades, several strain-specific organisms have been researched in the prevention and treatment of AAD/CDAD. These include *Bifidobacterium*, *Lactobacillus paracasei* subspecies, including *L. GG* (LGG), *L. casei*, *L. plantarum* 299v, *Enterococcus faecium*, *Saccharomyces boulardii*, *S. cerevisiae*, *Bacillus clausii*, *Clostridium butyricum,* and *L. acidophilus*.[85] Details on individual studies are presented elsewhere.[85] Probiotic therapy recommendations to prevent and/or treat AAD/CDAD are elusive because of the heterogeneity in choices of probiotics, lack of criteria for diagnosing CDAD, variation in the definition of diarrhea, and variations in probiotic dosing, timing, and duration. However, in a meta-analysis of 2810 patients, probiotic provision along with antibiotic therapy showed promise toward alleviating AAD, but not CDAD.[88] *Saccharomyces boulardii*, LGG, and probiotic mixtures seemed to exhibit the best protection from AAD. *S. boulardii* significantly reduced *C. difficile* recurrence in patients who were also receiving high-dose oral vancomycin (Practice Scenario 4-1).[85,88,89]

Practice Scenario 4-1

Question: When would the use of a probiotic be appropriate for a tube-fed patient with new onset of diarrhea?

Scenario: A 72-year-old woman residing in a long-term care facility for 3 weeks after being discharged from an acute care facility following a stroke is receiving enteral nutrition via a percutaneous endoscopic gastrostomy and develops diarrhea. Her tube feeding is a fiber-containing standard isotonic formula. She has been receiving her goal volume for 2 weeks with good tolerance until 2 days ago, when she was noted to have excessive, watery, foul-smelling diarrhea. In review of her medical record, she finished a 10-day course of antibiotics 5 days prior to this onset of diarrhea.

Intervention: The nutrition support clinician is consulted to change the enteral formula because it is suspected of causing this patient to have diarrhea. The clinician reviews the medical record and notes the previously mentioned information. She rules out osmotic diarrhea from feeds or medications. Noting that the onset of diarrhea was within 7 days of stopping a fluoroquinolone antibiotic, the clinician suspects antibiotic-associated diarrhea/*Clostridium difficile*–associated diarrhea (AAD/CDAD). She recommends that a stool culture be obtained and analyzed for *C. difficile*. It comes back positive for *C. difficile*. Metronidazole is ordered for 10 days at 500 mg 3 times per day. The clinician also recommends providing *Saccharomyces boulardii* throughout the course of metronidazole and for 14 days after its cessation.

Answer: Often, enteral formula is blamed as causing diarrhea in patients. In this case, the patient was receiving an isotonic formula in the stomach and had been tolerating it for several weeks. Medications provided for enterally fed stable patients are often liquid but may contain sorbitol or sugar, which can induce an osmotic load in the gut and cause gastrointestinal intolerance and diarrhea, but this patient was not receiving these types of medications. Antibiotics, particularly fluoroquinolones, are most likely to start the downward spiral of AAD/CDAD.[85] The onset of this type of diarrhea typically will occur 4 to 9 days following the cessation of antibiotics.[85] This patient's course of antibiotics was completed 7 days before the onset of diarrhea, so the clinician reasonably suspected that she might be experiencing AAD/CDAD and had a stool culture ordered to confirm the diagnosis.

Rationale: This patient was positive for *C. difficile* in her stool sample. In addition to treatment with metronidazole, certain probiotics have been shown to be effective in decreasing the duration and symptoms of AAD/CDAD as well as reducing the recurrence of CDAD, with *S. boulardii* having the best outcomes against *C. difficile*.[88,89] Providing the probiotic during the course of antibiotics and then for 14 more days helps to maintain and re-establish commensal microbiota that are altered negatively during the antibiotic therapy.

FMT is the process by which a homogenized stool sample from a healthy donor is administered into the GI tract of an individual. Some refer to FMT as the "optimal probiotic." FMT has been shown to eliminate recurrent and refractory *C. difficile* infection and re-establish a healthy colony in certain patients.[90] Because of FMT's cure rate for refractory *C. difficile* infection, researchers are now exploring its potential to treat other causes of gut dysbiosis.

Critical Illness

The modulating effects of prebiotic, probiotic, and synbiotic supplementation on infections and infectious complications have been extensively evaluated in animal studies and clinical trials. Like the studies of AAD, the clinical trials focused on critical illness are heterogeneous; they vary not only in patient populations and underlying diseases but also regarding probiotic strains and combinations, dosage, duration, delivery method, supplemental feeding, concomitant therapies, and outcome measurements. Multiple systematic reviews and meta-analyses have been performed to determine probiotic, prebiotic, and synbiotic efficacy in critically ill patients. Because of the study heterogeneity and varying primary study outcomes, the results of these reviews vary according to which studies were included in the analysis.

For example, a systematic review of adult patients in the ICU found no evidence to support use of prebiotics, probiotics, or synbiotics in adult patients in the ICU.[91] In this analysis, randomized controlled trials including 8 studies of approximately 1000 total patients were reviewed for evidence that these supplements can affect rates of nosocomial infection, length of ICU stay, hospital mortality, or incidence of pneumonia. The supplements used in the studies varied and included *Lactobacillus plantarum* 299v (2 trials), synbiotic (6 trials), Synbiotic 2000 (lactobacilli, pediacocci, *Leuconostoc* plus prebiotics; 2 trials), and *L. plantarum* plus fiber (1 trial). Other trials used different combinations and doses of both prebiotics and probiotics. Patient populations included liver transplant (1 trial), abdominal surgery (2 trials), and general ICU (5 trials).

A recent (2016) systematic review and meta-analysis evaluated 30 randomized controlled trials (N = 2972 patients) that analyzed clinical outcomes associated with providing a probiotic or a synbiotic.[92] The primary outcome was overall number of new infections, and secondary outcomes included mortality, ICU and hospital length of stay, and diarrhea. Subgroup analyses were performed to determine a role of other key factors, such as probiotic specificity and patient mortality risk, on the effect of probiotics on outcomes. Although probiotics did not affect mortality, length of stay, or diarrhea, probiotic use was associated with a reduction in infections (relative risk [RR] = 0.80; 95% confidence interval [CI], 0.68–0.95; P = 0.009). Additionally, the incidence of ventilator-associated pneumonia was reduced (RR = 0.74; 95% CI, 0.61–0.90; P = 0.002).

The 2016 guidelines for nutrition support in critically ill patients by the American Society for Parenteral and Enteral Nutrition (ASPEN) and the Society of Critical Care Medicine (SCCM) state that the use of identified probiotics species and strains seems to be safe in general ICU patients, but they should be used only for the select medical and surgical patient populations for which randomized controlled trials have documented safety and outcome benefit (eg, ventilator-associated pneumonia, liver transplantation).[93] Currently, no recommendation is available for the routine use of probiotics across the general population of ICU patients.[93] For patients with severe acute pancreatitis receiving early enteral feeding, a probiotic is suggested; however, no specific dose or strain is known.[93]

Necrotizing Enterocolitis

Probiotic supplementation in preterm infants has significantly reduced risk for stage II or higher necrotizing enterocolitis (NEC) and all-cause mortality; decreased time to achieve full feeds; reduced hospital length of stay, feeding intolerance, duration of indirect hyperbilirubinemia; and increased weight and growth velocity.[94] One meta-analysis found that the combination of *Lactobacillus acidophilus* and *Bifidobacterium bifidum* was associated with a lower incidence of NEC in preterm infants compared with other strains used individually or as combinations of strains.[94] However, the evidence for optimal individual strains or combination of strains and dosage of probiotics is not consistent enough to make specific recommendations about which types of probiotic supplementation provide a benefit to neonates at risk for GI complications. There were no noted adverse events related to outcomes associated with probiotic supplementation in the reviewed trials.[94] Randomized controlled studies are now investigating the use of synbiotics to reduce the incidence and severity of NEC. Further studies to indicate specific probiotic strains and doses for prevention of NEC are warranted.

Inflammatory Bowel Disease

Ulcerative Colitis and Pouchitis

Currently, investigations aim to identify the effectiveness of individual probiotic strains and doses in patients with IBD. Derikx and colleagues[49] determined that *Escherichia coli* Nissle 1917 and VSL#3 were used in most trials to test the efficacy of probiotics to influence time to remission and recurrence rates in patients with active UC were (Table 4-3). The review concluded that *E. coli* Nissle 1917 (5–50 × 10^9 CFU/d) was equally as effective as traditional therapies; however, results do not indicate *E. coli* Nissle 1917 as a viable stand-alone therapy. In UC patients, VSL#3 (3.6–9 × 10^{12} CFU/d) was effective in reducing time to remission and recurrence of remission.[49] Other probiotic trials include *Lactobacillus* and *Bifidobacterium* strains. Endoscopic improvement was seen in one trial utilizing *B. breve* (3 × 10^9 CFU/d) in conjunction with the prebiotic

galactooligosaccharide (5.5 g/d).[49] Although results of these studies have shown promise, larger randomized placebo-controlled studies are needed.[49]

Crohn's Disease

In theory, prebiotics and probiotics should influence the composition and function of gut microbiota and provide a therapeutic effect in patients with Crohn's disease; however, evidence for the effectiveness of prebiotics and probiotics in patients with this condition remains inconclusive. The use of inulin has shown some potential for prebiotic effects in small trials, but larger, well-powered studies have not exhibited significant benefits for the use of prebiotics in active Crohn's disease. To date, probiotics and prebiotics that have been investigated have not shown significant benefits in patients regarding induction or maintenance of remission or in preventing recurrence of active Crohn's disease.[95]

Pouchitis

Probiotic supplementation in patients with an IPAA creation has aimed to modify the conduit microflora in an attempt to treat the active pouchitis, prevent recurrence, or, even more importantly, prevent the initial onset (see Practice Scenario 4-2). Administration of prophylactic probiotic supplementation (VSL#3) in postoperative restorative proctocolectomy patients has been evaluated for effectiveness in preventing initial onset of acute pouchitis.[52] The rate of pouchitis-free survival for at least 1 year was 90% in patients who received VSL#3 directly after surgery compared with 60% in control groups (P <0.05). Compared with placebos, VSL#3 was effective in reducing patient's time to remission in episodes of active acute pouchitis and in delaying remission when taken in rotation with antibiotic regimes.[52]

Practice Scenario 4-2

Question: How would you manage a patient with ulcerative colitis and a newly created ileal pouch who is receiving parenteral nutrition (PN)?

Scenario: A 33-year-old man is admitted for abdominal pain and bloody stools negative for *Clostridium difficile*. His past medical history includes underlying ulcerative colitis since he was 8 years old, which has required multiple bowel resections and corticosteroids use over the course of several years. Prior to this admission, the patient had oily and foamy chronic diarrhea with a distinct foul odor and was diagnosed with small intestinal bacterial overgrowth (SIBO) and treated with antibiotic cycling. Following a thorough evaluation, the patient undergoes a restorative proctocolectomy with creation of an ileal-pouch anal anastomosis (IPAA) with a loop ileostomy and a remaining small bowel length of greater than 200 cm. The surgeon orders a consult for PN because of the IPAA creation and high ostomy output. The plan is to discharge the patient home with PN for 3 months and then schedule stomal closure and resume use of the ileal pouch in place of the previous rectum. Given the patient's complicated medical history and the initiation of PN, what are the most appropriate interventions for the clinician to recommend in this situation?

Intervention: Begin daily VSL#3 immediately after surgery. Provide oral rehydration solution and a diet high in starch and low in simple sugars once the oral diet is advanced.

Answer: Typically, corticosteroids and/or antibiotics are indicated for treatment of inflammation in this situation, whereas measures for prevention of future onset of inflammation are not necessarily implemented. PN is indicated because of the patient's high outputs, malabsorption, and poor nutrition status, but PN will further compromise the diversity of the gut microbiota. The patient's history of SIBO, altered gut immune function, and new ileal pouch make it appropriate to begin VSL#3 daily immediately after surgery, with a plan to continue the same probiotic daily at home. Additionally, the patient should receive education regarding oral rehydration solutions to prevent dehydration as well as dietary choices to prevent increased ostomy output while optimizing nutrition status when weaned from PN.

Rationale: The patient is at risk for onset of acute pouchitis and SIBO. The effectiveness of VSL#3 in preventing the onset of acute pouchitis in this patient population has been demonstrated. The patient's past and current medical and nutrition status warrant VSL#3 administration immediately after surgery and on discharge as a primary intervention to prevent the onset of acute pouchitis and preserve gut integrity. The benefits of this daily regimen outweigh the costs of potential complications and readmission.

Clinical Evidence with Prebiotic Provision

Multiple clinical issues complicate attempts to confirm the efficacy of prebiotic use in clinical practice. The gut microbiome is complex, and multiple physiological processes may play a role in treatment effect. These processes include changes in pH, microbe-microbe interactions, host-microbe interactions, antibiotic activities, and metabolic activities. Knowledge of an individual's presupplemented microbiota pattern and prebiotic dietary consumption is necessary to detect a change with supplementation. In people who normally consume a high-fiber diet, studies noted little effect with additional (prebiotic) supplementation.[71,74,75] Because data on the state of the gut microbiota and prebiotic intake before supplementation are challenging to collect, most study is in vitro. For example, batch culture studies use fecal slurries incubated with various polysaccharides for defined time periods after which an output reading is done to determine which bacteria genus is most affected.[70] Other models include continuous culture systems inoculated with fecal slurries to resemble the proximal colon. The best in vivo model uses germ-free rodents inoculated with various prebiotics and/or probiotics to evaluate pattern changes in the gut microbiota. In summary, challenges with human studies include variance in the host's prior diet composition with prebiotics and identifying whether a treatment effect was related to the prebiotic or changes in host-microbe interactions, metabolic milieu, or microbe-microbe interactions.[70]

Prebiotic Therapy and Enteral Nutrition

Diarrhea is a common occurrence in patients receiving enteral nutrition (EN) and can be attributed to many factors, including metabolic stress, hyperosmolar formulas or medications, antibiotics, enteropathogenic colonization, and variable colonic responses to enteral feeding. EN is associated with alterations in the gut microbiota, which can lead to decreased production of SCFAs. SCFAs are involved with water and electrolyte absorption.[74]

The data on the use of prebiotics to prevent diarrhea during EN are limited. Available studies report fiber-containing formulas with additional but unspecified quantities of fructooligosaccharides (FOS) and a compound with uncertain prebiotic characteristics provide a positive effect on diarrhea.[96] A 2015 meta-analysis of 8 studies did not find an effect of prebiotics—including soy polysaccharide, partially hydrolyzed guar gum psyllium, oat, soy fiber, FOS, inulin, banana flakes, and galactomannan—on diarrhea incidence.[96] However, a review of trials testing guar gum or partially hydrolyzed guar gum noted a decrease in the incidence of diarrhea in patients receiving EN.[97] Overall, results in that review found that fiber had a positive effect on the incidence of diarrhea in patients receiving EN (odds ratio [OR] = 0.47; 95% CI, 0.29–0.77; P = 0.02), particularly in stable patients (OR = 0.31; 95% CI, 0.19–0.51; P <0.01), but not in critically ill patients (OR = 0.89; 95% CI, 0.41–1.92; P = 0.77). Despite its manipulative effect on bifidobacteria concentrations and SCFA in healthy humans, prebiotic supplementation in EN does not consistently decrease the incidence of diarrhea.

Despite the difficulty in assessing true prebiotic effects in humans, the ASPEN/SCCM 2016 guidelines for nutrition support in critically ill patients suggest that a fermentable soluble fiber additive (eg, FOS, inulin) be considered for routine use in all hemodynamically stable medical ICU and surgical ICU patients receiving a standard enteral formulation. The guidelines suggest 10 to 20 g of a fermentable soluble fiber supplement be given in divided doses over 24 hours as adjunctive therapy if there is evidence of diarrhea.[93]

References

1. Hooper L, Midtvedt T, Gordon JI. How host-microbial interactions shape the nutrient environment of the mammalian intestine. *Annu Rev Nutr.* 2002;22:283–307.
2. Ley R, Peterson DA, Gordon JI. Ecological and evolutionary forces shaping microbial diversity in the human intestine. *Cell.* 2006;124:837–848.
3. Dethlefsen L, Huse S, Sogin ML, Relman DA. The pervasive effects of an antibiotic on the human gut microbiota, as revealed by deep 16S rRNA sequencing. *PLoS Biology* 2008;6:e280.
4. Backhed F, Ding H, Wang T, et al. The gut microbiota as an environmental factor that regulates fat storage. *Proc Natl Acad Sci U S A.* 2004;101:1518–1523.
5. Backhed F, Manchester J, Semenkovich CF, et al. Mechanisms underlying the resistance to diet-induced obesity in germ-free mice. *Proc Natl Acad Sci U S A.* 2007;104:979–984.
6. Samuel BS, Shaito A, Motoike T, et al. Effects of the gut microbiota on host adiposity are modulated by the short-chain fatty acid binding G protein-coupled receptor, Gpr41. *Proc Natl Acad Sci U S A.* 2008;105:16727–16772.

7. Martens EC, Chiang H, Gordon JI. Mucosal glycan foraging enhances fitness and transmission of a saccharolytic human gut bacterial symbiont. *Cell Host Microbe.* 2008;4:447–457.

8. Swann J, Wang Y, Abecia L, et al. Gut microbiome modulates the toxicity of hydrazine: a metabonomic study. *Mol Biosyst.* 2009;5:351–355.

9. Nicholson JK, Holmes E, Wilson ID. Gut microorganisms, mammalian metabolism, and personalized health care. *Nat Rev Microbiol.* 2005;3:431–438.

10. Boullier S, Nougayrède J, Marches O, et al. Genetically engineered enteropathogenic *Escherichia coli* strain elicits a specific immune response and protects against a virulent challenge. *Microbes Infect.* 2003;5:857–867.

11. Wells C. Relationship between intestinal microecology and the translocation of intestinal bacteria. *Antonie Van Leeuwenhoek.* 1990;58:87–93.

12. Mazmanian S, Liu Ch, Tzianabos AO, et al. An immunomodulatory molecule of symbiotic bacteria directs maturation of the host immune system. *Cell.* 2005;122:107–118.

13. Are A, Aronsson L, Wang S, et al. *Enterococcus faecalis* from newborn babies regulate endogenous PPAR-gamma activity and IL-10 levels in colonic epithelial cells. *Proc Natl Acad Sci U S A.* 2008;105:1943–1948.

14. Cresci G, Bawden E. Gut microbiome: what we do and don't know. *Nutr Clin Pract.* 2015;30:734–746.

15. Dominguez-Bello M, Costello, EK, Contreras M, et al. Delivery mode shapes the acquisition and structure of the initial microbiota across multiple body habitats in newborns. *Proc Natl Acad Sci U S A.* 2010;107:11971–119715.

16. Mackie RI, Sighir A, Gaskins HR. Developmental microbial ecology of the neonatal gastrointestinal tract. *Am J Clin Nutr.* 1999;69(suppl):S1035–S1045.

17. Dominguez-Bello MG, Blaser M, Ley R, Knight R. Development of the human gastrointestinal microbiota and insights from high throughput sequencing. *Gastroenterology.* 2011;140:1713–1719.

18. Biasucci G, Benebati B, Morelli L, et al. Cesarean delivery may affect the early biodiversity of intestinal bacteria. *J Nutr.* 2008;138(suppl):S1796–S1800.

19. Biasucci G, Rubini M, Riboni S, et al. Mode of delivery affects the bacterial community of the newborn gut. *Early Human Dev.* 2010;86(Suppl 1):13–15.

20. Penders J, Thijs C, van den Brandt PA, et al. Gut microbiota composition and development of atopic manifestations in infancy: the KOALA Birth Cohort Study. *Gut.* 2007;56:661–667.

21. Bager P, Wohlfhahrt J, Westergaard T. Caesarean delivery and risk of atopy and allergic disease: meta-analyses. *Clin Exp Allergy.* 2008;38:634–642.

22. Negele K, Heinrish J, Borte M, et al. Mode of delivery and development of atopic disease during the first 2 years of life. *Pediatr Allergy Immunol.* 2004;15:48–54.

23. Watson J, Jones R, Cortes C, et al. Community-associated methicillin-resistant *Staphylococcus aureus* infection among healthy newborns—Chicago and Los Angeles County, 2004. *JAMA.* 2004;296:36–38.

24. Koenig J, Spor A, Scalfone N, et al. Microbes and Health Sackler Colloquium: succession of microbial consortia in the developing infant gut microbiome. *Proc Natl Acad Sci U S A.* 2011;108(Suppl 1):4578–4585.

25. Palmer C, Bik EM, DiGiulio DB, et al. Development of the human infant intestinal microbiota. *PLoS Biol.* 2007;5:e177.

26. Zivkovic A, German JB, Lebrilla CB, et al. Microbes and Health Sackler Colloquium: human milk glycobiome and its impact on the infant gastrointestinal microbiota. *Proc Natl Acad Sci U S A.* 2011;108(Suppl 1):4653–4658.

27. Cani P, Lecuort E, Dewulf EM, et al. Gut microbiota fermentation of prebiotics increases satietogenic and incretin gut peptide production with consequences for appetite sensation and glucose response after a meal. *Am J Clin Nutr.* 2009;90:1236–1243.

28. De Filippo C, Cavalieri D, Di Paola M, et al. Impact of diet in shaping gut microbiota revealed by a comparative study in children from Europe and rural Africa. *Proc Natl Acad Sci U S A.* 2010;107:14691–14696.

29. Hehemann J, Correc G, Barbeyron T, et al. Transfer of carbohydrate active enzymes from marine bacteria to Japanese gut microbiota. *Nature.* 2010;464:908–912.

30. Turnbaugh P, Hamady M, Yatsunenko T, et al. A core gut microbiome in obese and lean twins. *Nature.* 2009;457:480–484.

31. Vaishampayan P, Kuehl JV, Froula JL, et al. Comparative metagenomics and population dynamics of the gut microbiota in mother and infant. *Genome Biol Evol.* 2010;6:53–66.

32. Falush D, Wirth T, Linz B, et al. Traces of human migrations in *Helicobacter pylori* populations. *Science.* 2003;299:1582–1585.

33. Moodley Y, Linz B, Yamaoka Y, et al. The peopling of the Pacific from a bacterial perspective. *Science.* 2009;323:527–530.

34. Rajilic-Stojanovic M, Heilig HG, Molenaar D, et al. Development and application of the human intestinal tract chip, a phylogenetic microarray: analysis of universally conserved phylotypes in the abundant microbiota of young and elderly adults. *Environ Microbiol.* 2009;11:1736–1751.

35. Claesson MJ, Cusack S, O'Sullivan O, et al. Composition, variability, and temporal stability of the intestinal microbiota of the elderly. *Proc Natl Acad Sci U S A.* 2011;108(Suppl 1):4680–4687.

36. Biagi E, Nylund L, Candela M, et al. Through ageing, and beyond: gut microbiota and inflammatory status in seniors and centenarians. *PLoS One.* 2010;5:e10667.

37. Harley C. Telomere loss: mitotic clock or genetic time bomb? *Mutat Res.* 1991;256:271–282.

38. Williams G. Pleiotropy, natural selection and the evolution of senescence. *Evolution.* 1957;11:398–411.

39. Ley R, Lozupone CA, Hamady M, et al. Worlds within worlds: evolution of the vertebrate gut microbiota. *Nat Rev Microbiol.* 2008;6:776–788.

40. Qin J, Li R, Raes J, et al. A human gut microbial gene catalogue established by metagenomic sequencing. *Nature.* 2010; 464:59–65.

41. Turnbaugh P, Ridaura VK, Faith JJ, et al. The effect of diet on the human gut microbiome: a megagenomic analysis in humanized gnotobiotic mice. *Sci Transl Med.* 2009;1(6ra):14.

42. Ley R, Turnbaugh PJ, Klein S, et al. Microbial ecology: human gut microbes associated with obesity. *Nature.* 2006;444:1022–1023.

43. Duncan S, Lobley GE, Holtrop G, et al. Human colonic microbiota associated with diet, obesity and weight loss. *Int J Obes (Lond).* 2008;32:1720–1724.

44. Zhang H, DiBaise JK, Zuccolo A, et al. Human gut microbiota in obesity and after gastric bypass. *Proc Natl Acad Sci U S A.* 2009; 106:2365–2370.

45. Hoyles L, McCartney AL. What do we mean when we refer to Bacteroidetes populations in the human gastrointestinal microbiota? *FEMS Microbiol Lett.* 2009;299:175–183.

46. Arumugam M, Raes J, Pelletier E, et al. Enterotypes of the human gut microbiome. *Nature.* 2011;473:174–180.

47. Greenblum S, Turnbaugh PJ, Borenstein E. Metagenomic systems biology of the human gut microbiome reveals topological shifts associated with obesity and inflammatory bowel disease. *Proc Natl Acad Sci U S A.* 2012;109:594–599.

48. Kovatcheva-Datchary P, Arora T. Nutrition, the gut microbiome and the metabolic syndrome: EBSCO host. *Best Pract Res Clin Gastroenterol.* 2013;27:59–72.

49. Derikx L, Dieleman L, Hoentjen F. Probiotics and prebiotics in ulcerative colitis. *Best Pract Res Clin Gastroenterol*. 2016;30:55–71.

50. Sandborn WJ. The present and future of inflammatory bowel disease. *Gastroenterol Hepatol*. 2016;12(7):438–441.

51. Shi Y, Dong Y, Huang W, Zhu D, Mao H, Su P. Fecal microbiota transplantation for ulcerative colitis: a systematic review and meta-analysis. *PLoS One*. 2016;11(6):e0157259.

52. Lichtenstein L, Avni-Biron I, Ben-Bassat O, The current place of probiotics and prebiotics in the treatment of pouchitis. *Best Pract Res Clin Gastroenterol*. 2016;30:73–80.

53. Chen WC, Quigley EMM. Probiotics, prebiotics & synbiotics in small intestinal bacterial overgrowth: opening up a new therapeutic horizon! *Indian J Med Res*. 2014;140(5):582–584.

54. Mittal R, Coopersmith CM. Redefining the gut as the motor of critical illness. *Trends Mol Med*. 2014;20:214–223.

55. Hayakawa M, Asahara T, Henzan N, et al. Dramatic changes of the gut flora immediately after severe and sudden insults. *Dig Dis Sci*. 2011;56:2361–2365.

56. McDonald D, Ackermann G, Khailova L, et al. Extreme dysbiosis of the microbiome in critical illness. *mSphere*. 2016;1(4): e00199–e00116.

57. Food and Agriculture Organization, World Health Organization. *Guidelines for the Evaluation of Probiotics in Food*. London, ON, Canada: Food and Agriculture Organization and World Health Organization; 2001. http://who.int/foodsafety/fs_management/en/probiotic_guidelines.pdf. Accessed September 27, 2016.

58. Gordon S. Elie Metchnikoff: father of natural immunity. *Eur J Immunol*. 2008;38:3257–3264.

59. Sherman P, Ossa JC, Johnson-Henry K. Unraveling mechanisms of action of probiotics. *Nutr Clin Pract*. 2009;24:10–14.

60. Shanahan F. Probiotics in perspective. *Gastroenterology*. 2010;139: 1808–1812.

61. Corr S, Li Y, Riedel CU, et al. Bacteriocin production as a mechanism for the anti-infective activity of *Lactobacillus salivarius* UCC118. *Proc Natl Acad Sci U S A*. 2007;104:7617–7621.

62. Sonnenburg J, Chen CTL, Gordon JI. Genomic and metabolic studies of the impact of probiotics on a model gut symbiont and host. *PLoS Biol*. 2006;4:2213–2226.

63. Mack D, Michail S, Wei S, McDougall L, Hollingsworth MA. Probiotics inhibit enteropathogenic *E. coli* adherence in vitro by inducing intestinal mucin gene expression. *Am J Physiol*. 1999; 276:G941–G950.

64. Linden S, Sutten P, Karlsson NG, et al. Mucins in the mucosal barrier to infection. *Mucosal Immunol*. 2008;1:183–197.

65. Clyne M, Dillon P, Daly S, et al. *Helicobacter pylori* interacts with the human single-domain trefoil protein TFF1. *Proc Natl Acad Sci U S A*. 2004;101:7409–7414.

66. Lebeer S, Vanderleyden J, De Keersmaecker SCJ. Host interactions of probiotic bacterial surface molecules: comparison with commensals and pathogens. *Nat Rev Microbiol*. 2010;8:171–184.

67. O'Mahony C, Scully P, O'Mahony D, et al. Commensal-induced regulatory T cells mediate protection against pathogen-stimulated NF-kB activation. *PLoS Pathogens*. 2008;4:e1000112.

68. Rousseaux C, Thuru X, Gelot A, et al. *Lactobacillus acidophilus* modulates intestinal pain and induces opioid and cannabinoid receptors. *Nat Med*. 2007;13:35–37.

69. Gibson GR, Probert HM, Van Loo J, et al. Dietary modulation of the human colonic microbiota: updating the concept of prebiotics. *Nutr Res Rev*. 2004;17:259–275.

70. Roberfroid M, Gibson GR, Hoyles L, et al. Prebiotic effects: metabolic and health benefits. *Br J Nutr*. 2010;104(Suppl 2):S1–S63.

71. Damaskos D, Kolios G. Probiotics and prebiotics in inflammatory bowel disease: microflora "on the scope." *Br J Clin Pharm*. 2008;65:453–467.

72. Cummings J, Macfarlane GT. Gastrointestinal effects of prebiotics. *Br J Nutr*. 2002;87(Suppl 2):S145–S151.

72a. Slavin J. Fiber and prebiotics: mechanisms and health benefits. *Nutrients*. 2013;5(4):1417–1435.

73. Abrams S, Griffin IJ, Hawthorne KM, et al. A combination of prebiotic short and long-chain inulin-type fructans enhances calcium absorption and bone mineralization in young adolescents. *Am J Clin Nutr*. 2005;82:471–476.

74. Cummings JH, Macfarlane GT, Englyst HN. Prebiotic digestion and fermentation. *Am J Clin Nutr*. 2001;73(suppl):415S–420S.

75. Topping D, Clifton PM. Short-chain fatty acids and human colonic function: roles of resistant starch and nonstarch polysaccharides. *Physiol Rev*. 2001;81:1031–1064.

76. Thangaraju M, Cresci G, Itagaki S, et al. Sodium-coupled transport of the short-chain fatty acid butyrate by SLC5A8 and its relevance to colon cancer. *J Gastrointest Surg*. 2008;12:1773–1782.

77. Thangaraju M, Cresci G, Liu K, et al. GPR109A is a G-protein coupled receptor for the bacterial fermentation product butyrate and functions as a tumor suppressor in colon. *Cancer Research*. 2009;69:2826–2832.

78. Kolida S, Gibson GR., Synbiotics in health and disease. *Annu Rev Food Sci Technol*. 2011;2:373–393.

79. Bengmark S. Bacteria for optimal health. *Nutrition*. 2000;16: 611–615.

80. Worthington M, Ranz R. Use of probiotics in critically ill patients. *Support Line*. 2009;31(4):8–17.

81. Boyle R, Robins-Browne R, Tang M. Probiotic use in clinical practice: what are the risks? *Am J Clin Nutr*. 2006;83:1256–1264.

82. Besselink M, Van Santvoort HC, Buskens E, et al. Probiotic prophylaxis in predicted severe acute pancreatitis: a randomized double-blind, placebo-controlled trial. *Lancet*. 2008;371:651–659.

83. Enache-Angoulvant A, Hennequin C. Invasive Saccharomyces infection: a comprehensive review. *Clin Infect Dis*. 2005;41: 1559–1568.

84. Doron S, Snydman DR. Risk and safety of probiotics. *Clin Infect Dis*. 2015;60(Suppl 2):S129–S134.

85. Rohde C, Bartolini V, Jones N. The use of probiotics in the prevention and treatment of antibiotic-associated diarrhea with special interest in *Clostridium difficile*–associated diarrhea. *Nutr Clin Pract*. 2009;24:33–40.

86. Asha N, Tompkins D, Wolcox MH. Comparative analysis of prevalence, risk factors, and molecular epidemiology of antibiotic associated diarrhea due to *Clostridium difficile, Clostridium perfringens*, and *Staphylococcus aureus*. *J Clin Microbiol*. 2006; 44:2785–2791.

87. Mehmet C, Bulent B, Ismail A, et al. Prophylactic *Saccharomyces boulardii* in the prevention of antibiotic-associated diarrhea: a prospective study. *Med Sci Monit*. 2006;12:119–122.

88. McFarland L. Meta-analysis of probiotics for the prevention of antibiotic associated diarrhea and the treatment of *Clostridium difficile* disease. *Am J Gastroenterol*. 2006;101:812–822.

89. Surawicz C, McFarland LV, Greenberg RN, et al. The search for a better treatment for recurrent *Clostridium difficile* disease: use of high-dose vancomycin with *Saccharomyces boulardii*. *Clin Infect Dis*. 2000;31:1012–1017.

90. Wage ZK, Yang YS, Chen Ye, et al. Intestinal microbiota pathogenesis and fecal microbiota transplantation for inflammatory bowel disease. *World J Gastroenterol*. 2014;20:14805–14820.

91. Watkinson PJ, Barber VS, Dark P, Young JD. The use of pre-, pro-, and synbiotics in adult intensive care unit patients: systematic review. *Clin Nutr*. 2007; 26:182–192.

92. Manzanares W, Lemieux M, Langlois PL, Wischmeyer PE. Probiotic and synbiotic therapy in critical illness: a systematic review and meta-analysis. *Crit Care*. 2016;20:262.

93. McClave S, Taylor B, Martindale R, et al; Society of Critical Care Medicine (SCCM) and American Society for Parenteral and Enteral Nutrition (A.S.P.E.N.). Guidelines for the provision and assessment of nutrition support therapy in the adult critically ill patient. *JPEN J Parenter Enteral Nutr.* 2016;40:159–211.

94. Johnson-Henry KC, Abrahamsson TR, Wu RU, Sherman PM. Probiotics, prebiotics, and synbiotics for the prevention of necrotizing enterocolitis. *Adv Nutr.* 2016;7:928–937.

95. Lichtenstein L, Avni-Biron I, Ben-Bassat O. Probiotics and prebiotics in Crohn's disease therapies. *Best Pract Res Clin Gastroenterol.* 2016;30:81–88.

96. Zaman MK, Chin KF, Rai V, et al. Fiber and prebiotic supplementation in enteral nutrition: a systematic review and meta-analysis. *World J Gastroenterol.* 2015;21:5372–5381.

97. Quartarone G. Role of PHGG as a dietary fiber: a review article. *Minerva Gastroenterol Dietol.* 2013;59:329–340.

5 Lipids

Mary Hise, PhD, RD, CNSC, and John C. Brown, PhD

CONTENTS

Objectives

1. Describe the nomenclature, route of delivery, and requirements for lipids in the diet of healthy individuals and in formulations for those who require specialized nutrition support.
2. Identify the lipid components in enteral and parenteral formulations.
3. Discuss the clinical effects and biological activity of fatty acids in specialized nutrition support.

Test Your Knowledge Questions

1. What are some of the possible ramifications of activation of the enzyme, phospholipase A$_2$?
   A. Cyclooxygenase (COX)–dependent, eicosanoid-mediated inflammatory reactions
   B. Enzymatic degradation of resolvins and protectins
   C. Desaturation of linoleic acid within lipids
   D. Chylomicron maturation
2. How might propofol, when provided to patients within a 10% (w/v) lipid injectable emulsion (ILE), increase risk of hypertriglyceridemia? (Refer to the section on "Parenteral Delivery and Metabolism of Lipid Injectable Emulsions" for an explanation of this new terminology to replace *intravenous fat emulsion* [IVFE]).
   A. Propofol causes acute uptake of triglycerides (TGs) by the microvilli of the small intestine.
   B. Propofol is known to activate the release of TGs from adipose tissue.
   C. The increased presence of liposomes in the propofol ILE may interfere with chylomicron and pseudo-chylomicron metabolism.
   D. The presence of sedative in the ILE prevents phospholipid formation, which results in an increased level of TGs in the blood.
3. Which ionized form of a short-chain fatty acid (SCFA; up to 6 carbons in length) is thought to be the most important to colonic health and why?
   A. Myristate
   B. Caproate
   C. Butyrate
   D. Valerate

Test Your Knowledge Answers

1. The correct answer is **A**. Arachidonic acid (AA), common to membrane phospholipids, usually occupies the *sn*-2 position within lipids and is almost always found at this position within the important membrane phospholipid phosphatidylinositol. During membrane cell signaling events, a possible outcome is the activation of phospholipase A$_2$, the enzyme that acts on membrane phospholipids to release fatty acids from the *sn*-2 position. Release of AA sets in motion subsequent intracellular metabolic activity via the COX pathway that leads to the synthesis of the 2-series of prostaglandins, including prostaglandin E$_2$ (PGE$_2$), and thromboxanes, including thromboxane A$_2$.
2. The correct answer is **C**. Hypertriglyceridemia may be caused by interference with chylomicron and pseudo-chylomicron metabolism as a result of the presence of liposomes within the ILE. Liposomes are formed during the emulsification process when parenteral ILE is produced. These liposomes are usually metabolized in a manner similar to the metabolism of pseudo-chylomicrons, but their presence may lead to the formation of a spherical bilayer of phospholipid and cholesterol known as *lipoprotein-X*. This lipoprotein inhibits both lipoprotein lipase and hepatic lipase enzymatic activity, and thus can interfere with the proper metabolism of the TGs that are part of

the structure of chylomicrons and pseudo-chylomicrons. This interference and the accumulation of endogenous cholesterol can subsequently lead to an increase in circulating TGs and cholesterol. Because 10% (w/v) ILE contains a greater number of liposomes relative to 20% (w/v) ILE as a result of the relative ratio of phospholipid emulsifier to oil, the former formulation places the patient at greater risk for hypertriglyceridemia.
3. The correct answer is **C**. SCFAs such as acetate, propionate, and butyrate are primarily produced in the colon by bacteria and can serve as important energy sources for colonic tissue. Butyrate in particular is thought to modify inflammatory activity and promote colon health. For example, when applied directly to the colon, butyrate can attenuate the inflammatory activity seen in ulcerative colitis. In addition, the fermentation of carbohydrate (fiber) and the production of SCFAs in the colon, especially butyrate production, appear to act as antitumorigenic stimuli.

Background

Lipids are biological substances that are soluble in organic solvents, such as methanol and chloroform, but insoluble in water. Lipids include waxes, various oils, sterols, fats, TGs, and individual components known as *fatty acids*. TGs, through the contribution of their fatty acid components, serve as major dietary sources of energy. Also, certain lipids provide much of the critical structural and metabolically functional components of all biological membranes. Because of these properties, lipids and the fatty acids that comprise part of their structure contribute significantly to a broad range of cellular functions needed for the maintenance and biological activity of healthy living cells (Figure 5-1). For example, the structure of membrane lipids can include the fatty acids AA, eicosapentaenoic acid (EPA), and docosahexaenoic acid (DHA). These particular fatty acids are critically important to proper development as well as inflammatory and other physiologic processes. For example, the metabolic products of AA, EPA, and DHA include (1) inflammatory mediators (eicosanoids such as prostaglandins, leukotrienes, and thromboxanes); (2) gene regulators; (3) substances that assist in the resolution of an inflammatory response (eicosanoids such as protectins, resolvins, and lipoxins); and (4) substances that regulate overall lipid metabolism.[1-5] Furthermore, AA, EPA, DHA, and other fatty acids contribute to membrane fluidity, membrane and intracellular cell signals, and modulation of apoptotic pathways.[6] This chapter focuses on general lipid structure, fatty acid biochemistry and nomenclature, lipid metabolism, and the clinical aspects of lipid provision in enteral nutrition (EN) and parenteral nutrition (PN).

General Lipid Structure

The basic TG structure consists of a glycerol backbone and various fatty acids attached in ester linkage at the carbon-1 (*sn*-1), carbon-2 (*sn*-2), and carbon-3 (*sn*-3) positions. TGs are the most abundant lipids in the body, but they do not serve as components of membranes. Instead, these substances serve as an energy reserve for cells via the enzyme-dependent release,

FIGURE 5-1 The Varied Roles of Fatty Acids in Cell Structure and Function

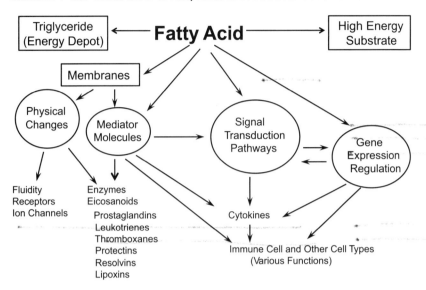

Fatty Acid Biochemistry and Nomenclature

Each fatty acid is comprised of several carbon, many hydrogen, and 2 oxygen atoms. All fatty acids consist of a chain of carbon atoms linked together by covalent bonds. Each carbon atom within the chain has 1 or more hydrogen atoms attached. A methyl (CH_3–) group is at one end of the chain, and, at the opposite end of the chain is an acidic carboxyl (–COOH) group. Thus, the representative overall structure for every fatty acid is CH_3–$(CH_2)_x$–COOH.

Fatty acids are classified in several ways. One classification groups fatty acids based on the number of carbon atoms within the hydrocarbon chain. A given fatty acid is classified as short chain (2 to 4 carbons), medium chain (6 to 12 carbons), long chain (14 to 18 carbons), or very long chain (20 or more carbons). For example, acetic acid, found in vinegar, CH_3–COOH, a 2-carbon fatty acid, and caprylic acid, CH_3–$(CH_2)_6$–COOH, an 8-carbon fatty acid, represent a SCFA and a medium-chain fatty acid (MCFA), respectively. The length of the hydrocarbon chain conveys unique physical and chemical properties to fatty acids, and, these properties are reflected in the lipids of which these fatty acids are a part. Because a 2-carbon unit, acetyl-coenzyme A (acetyl-CoA), is used for fatty acid synthesis, almost all fatty acids consist of an even number of carbon atoms.

Another fatty acid classification is based on the number of hydrogen atoms present on each carbon atom within the molecule. If all hydrogen atoms that could be present are present, the fatty acid is said to be *saturated*. Acetic acid and caprylic acid are saturated fatty acids. Alternatively, if some hydrogen atoms are missing, the fatty acid is said to be *unsaturated*. The degree of unsaturation among such fatty acids varies. Some fatty acids may have 2, 4, or more hydrogen atoms missing. If adjacent carbon atoms within the chain are missing hydrogen atoms, there will be a double bond instead of a single bond at that position. Thus, for unsaturated fatty acids, 1 or more double bonds may be present within the hydrocarbon chain. The greater the number of double bonds, the greater the degree of unsaturation is. This configuration, like chain length, provides various physical and chemical properties to the "behavior" of such a fatty acid. The absence of hydrogen atoms does not occur by chance. It is generated by specific enzymatically catalyzed chemical reactions. The enzymatically catalyzed removal of hydrogen atoms occurs in pairs, with 1 hydrogen atom removed from each of 2 adjacent carbon atoms within the carbon chain. This desaturation of the molecule is an oxidation reaction that results in the subsequent formation of a double bond between the 2 adjacent carbons. The enzymes that perform the oxidation reaction that removes hydrogen atoms are known as *desaturases*. In humans, there are 4 desaturase enzymes. Each desaturase is identified by the numerical position of the first carbon of the pair of carbons involved in the chain, numbered from the carboxyl end, which has a hydrogen

distribution, and oxidation of fatty acids. When stored as fat in tissues (eg, adipose), energy-dense TGs provide by weight approximately 6-fold the energy available from the same weight of stored carbohydrate such as glycogen. Compared with a gram of carbohydrate, a gram of fat stored in tissues has more recoverable energy because (1) TGs have a lower intrinsic level of oxidation than carbohydrate, and (2) the weight contribution of water common to carbohydrates and proteins is missing from lipids. TGs circulate to a limited extent within the bloodstream but are more significantly stored within adipose tissue. In contrast to circulating and stored TGs, the major constituents of the membrane lipid bilayer are compound lipids known as *phosphoglycerides*. Similar to TGs, 2 carbon positions on the glycerol backbone, *sn*-1 and *sn*-2, are esterified by fatty acids; however, the third available position, *sn*-3, is occupied by a phosphate group in phosphoester linkage (known as *1,2-diacylphosphoglycerides*). The most abundant phospholipids found within membranes also have a polar group of some kind, such as ethanolamine, serine, or choline, attached to the phosphate moiety. As a consequence, membrane lipids are amphipathic (or amphiphilic ["loving both"]), meaning that they simultaneously possess both hydrophobic and hydrophilic characteristics. This amphipathic property allows lipid bilayer membrane formation. Thermodynamic forces induced by interaction of the polar aqueous environment external to and within cells with the hydrocarbon portions (tails) of the 2 fatty acids within each phospholipid results in formation of linear rows of phospholipids in opposing leaflets. The linear rows of polar groups face outward (aqueous environment outside the cell) on the external leaflet and inward (aqueous environment inside the cell) on the internal leaflet of the bilayer. Hydrophobic or other amphipathic molecules such as sterols and proteins may be embedded within the lipid bilayer. For example, cholesterol, itself an amphipathic molecule and the precursor of steroid hormones, is an integral constituent of animal cell membranes.

atom removed and a double bond formed by the enzyme in question. These enzymes are: Δ^4-, Δ^5-, Δ^6-, and, Δ^9-desaturases. The Greek letter Delta (Δ) followed by a superscript numeral identifies the numerical position of the first carbon of the double bond pair. For example, Δ^4-desaturase acts on the fourth carbon atom in the chain, removing a hydrogen atom from and generating a double bond between carbons 4 and 5. Similarly, Δ^9-desaturase removes hydrogen atoms and forms a double bond between carbons 9 and 10 in the sequence. A fatty acid that contains only 1 double bond is known as a *monounsaturated fatty acid* (MUFA), whereas a fatty acid with a minimum of 2 double bonds is known as a *polyunsaturated fatty acid* (PUFA). The most abundant fatty acid in humans, oleic acid, an 18-carbon fatty acid that has a single double bond located between carbon atoms 9 and 10, is formed by desaturation of the saturated 18-carbon fatty acid, stearic acid, by Δ^9-desaturase. Similarly, the presence of 3 or more double bonds within an unsaturated fatty acid is known as a *highly unsaturated fatty acid*. These desaturases remove hydrogens from the same "side" of adjacent carbon atoms, forming what is known as a *cis double bond*.

The removal of hydrogen atoms on the same "side" (cis) of adjacent carbon atoms and introduction of a single, cis double bond between the 2 carbon atoms, results in significant bending of the fatty acid chain, by approximately 30°. Consequently, 2 cis double bonds may result in an approximate 60° bend in the molecule. This property of unsaturated fatty acids has important ramifications with respect to individual lipid characteristics and, consequently, the physical and functional characteristics of membranes. If 2 or more saturated fatty acids are next to each another within a leaflet of a lipid bilayer, the carbon atoms in adjacent long chains within the leaflet can interact with relative ease via hydrophobic bonding and pack more closely. Conversely, the bending of unsaturated fatty acid molecules does not allow adjacent lipids to interact so closely. As a result, membrane fluidity and responsiveness to stimuli vary relative to the amount of saturated vs unsaturated fatty acids present. As the number of unsaturated fatty acids among membrane lipids increases, the fluidity of the membrane increases, with the converse being true if more saturated fatty acids are present.

Table 5-1 presents the various nomenclatures that may be used to identify some of the more common biological fatty acids. Each of these systems may identify the total number of carbons and number of double bonds present; some classifications also denote the numerical position of any double bond that may be present.

One system uses the uppercase Greek letter Delta (Δ). In this system, the carboxyl group of each fatty acid is considered to occupy the first (numerical "1") position. For example, the polyunsaturated 18-carbon fatty acid, linoleic acid, contains 2 double bonds, 1 between the number 9 and 10 carbons, and 1 between the number 12 and 13 carbon atoms. Thus, this fatty acid is designated as $18:2\Delta^{9,12}$.

Linoleic acid is known chemically as *9,12-octadecadienoic acid*. "Octa" signifies 8 carbons, "deça" signifies 10 carbons (ie, 18 carbons total), and "dienoic" (or "diene") refers to the 2 double bonds within the acid. A "trienoic" (or "triene") fatty acid contains 3 double bonds.

An additional system of nomenclature used for PUFAs identifies different fatty acid families based on the last, relative to the carboxyl group, double-bond location. These fatty acid families are members of the ω (or *n*) series. In this system, the last double bond that occurs relative to the carboxyl group is designated with the last letter in the Greek alphabet, omega (ω). However, in this instance, the numerical position of this double bond is numbered relative to the terminal methyl (C_H3) group within the molecule. Thus, linoleic acid is denoted as an ω-6 fatty acid family member because the last double-bonded carbon atom occurs 6 carbon atoms from and including the methyl terminus of the hydrocarbon chain. One may also denote these fatty acids by substituting the italicized English letter *n* for ω. When the *n* series designation is applied, a combinatorial system is used. Thus, linoleic acid is denoted as $18:2n$-6 (ω-6 or *n*-6 family member).

Humans can synthesize all fatty acids necessary for life except for linoleic acid and α-linolenic acid. Humans cannot synthesize these 2 fatty acids because the specific desaturase enzymes that can introduce a double bond past position 9–10 within a given fatty acid are absent, which prevents the de novo synthesis of linoleic and α-linolenic fatty acids. Thus, the synthesis by elongation and subsequent desaturation of longer-chained fatty acids necessary for life is prohibited. Absence of the necessary desaturase enzymes means that all human unsaturated fatty acids are synthesized from palmitoleic ($16:1\Delta^9$ [$16:1n$-7]), oleic ($18:1\Delta^9$ [$18:1n$-9]), linoleic ($18:2\Delta^{9,12}$ [$18:2n$-6]), or α-linolenic ($18:3\Delta^{9,12,15}$ [$18:3n$-3]) acids. Consequently, both linoleic and α-linolenic acids must be obtained via the diet, and each serves as a critical precursor for the synthesis of other necessary long-chain unsaturated fatty acids, such as AA and DHA. In this regard, it is important to note that the efficiency of conversion of linoleic acid to AA, and α-linolenic acid to DHA is suboptimal in the critically ill or malnourished patient.

Enteral Delivery and Metabolism of Dietary Lipids

In the typical Western diet, about 35% of ingested food is in the form of fat and TGs comprise 90% of all ingested dietary lipids within the fat. Various oils, the animal fat in meat or dairy, and plant TGs in seeds (nuts) and vegetables contribute in varying amounts to fat intake. Depending on the source, the TGs within the lipid fraction may contain different proportions of saturated and unsaturated fatty acids of different chain lengths. The TGs in animal fat contain more saturated fatty acids, whereas certain plant TGs may contain more unsaturated fatty acids. The human diet may also contain about 2 to 3 g of the charged phosphoglyceride, phosphatidylcholine, per day. Bile, discussed later in the chapter, provides about 12 g of phosphatidylcholine per day to the intestinal lumen.[7,8]

Without a mechanism to "solubilize" these substances, humans could not physiologically use TGs for energy, development, or cellular structure. Sophisticated systems allow these enterally ingested substances to be broken down, absorbed, reassembled, and transported throughout the body. When TGs are exposed to the environments of the digestive system, the presence of bile acids is initially important to making them

TABLE 5-1 Fatty Acid Nomenclature

Common Name	Chemical Name	No. of Double Bonds	No. of Carbon Atoms	Scientific Δ Double Bond Numbering	n and ω Numbering
Butyric acid	Butanoic acid	0	4	4:0	NA
Caproic acid	Hexanoic acid	0	6	6:0	NA
Caprylic acid	Octanoic acid	0	8	8:0	NA
Capric acid	Decanoic acid	0	10	10:0	NA
Lauric acid	Dodecanoic acid	0	12	12:0	NA
Myristic acid	Tetradecanoic acid	0	14	14:0	NA
Palmitic acid	Hexadecanoic acid	0	16	16:0	NA
Palmitoleic acid	9-hexadecenoic acid	1	16	$16:1\Delta^9$	$16:1n\text{-}7\ \omega\text{-}7$
Stearic acid	Octadecanoic acid	0	18	18:0	NA
Oleic acid	9-octadecenoic acid	1	18	$18:1\Delta^9$	$18:1n\text{-}9\ \omega\text{-}9$
Vaccenic acid	11-octadecenoic acid	1	18	$18:1\Delta^{11}$	$18:1n\text{-}7\ \omega\text{-}7$
Linoleic acid	9,12-octadecadienoic acid	2	18	$18:2\Delta^{9,12}$	$18:2n\text{-}6\ \omega\text{-}6$
α-Linolenic acid	9,12,15-octadecatrienoic acid	3	18	$18:3\Delta^{9,12,15}$	$18:3n\text{-}3\ \omega\text{-}3$
γ-Linolenic acid	6,9,12-octadecatrienoic acid	3	18	$18:3\Delta^{6,9,12}$	$18:3n\text{-}6\ \omega\text{-}6$
Dihomo-γ-linolenic acid	8,11,14-eicosatrienoic acid	3	20	$20:3\Delta^{8,11,14}$	$20:3n\text{-}6\ \omega\text{-}6$
Arachidic acid	Eicosanoic acid	0	20	20:0	NA
Gadoleic acid	9-eicosenoic acid	1	20	$20:1\Delta^9$	$20:1n\text{-}9\ \omega\text{-}11$
"Mead" acid	5,8,11-eicosatrienoic acid	3	20	$20:3\Delta^{5,8,11}$	$20:3n\text{-}9\ \omega\text{-}9$
Arachidonic acid	5,8,11,14-eicosatetraenoic acid	4	20	$20:4\Delta^{5,8,11,14}$	$20:4n\text{-}6\ \omega\text{-}6$
Eicosapentaenoic acid	5,8,11,14,17-eicosapentaenoic acid	5	20	$20:5\Delta^{5,8,11,14,17}$	$20:5n\text{-}3\ \omega\text{-}3$
Behenic acid	Docosanoic acid	0	22	22:0	NA
Erucic acid	13-docosenoic acid	1	22	$22:1\Delta^{13}$	$22:1n\text{-}9\ \omega\text{-}9$
Docosahexaenoic acid	4,7,10,13,16,19-docosahexaenoic acid	6	22	$22:6\Delta^{4,7,10,13,16,19}$	$22:6n\text{-}3\ \omega\text{-}3$
Lignoceric acid	Tetracosanoic acid	0	24	24:0	NA

NA, not applicable.

available for use. Bile is produced and secreted by the liver and stored in the gall bladder, and enters the small intestine via the bile duct into the duodenum. Bile is about 92% water and 6% bile acids (bile salts), plus a few other components, such as phosphatidylcholine, cholesterol, and some fatty acids. Bile salts are derivatives of cholesterol and contain either a glycine (glycocholic acid) or taurine (taurocholic acid) molecule conjugated to the cholesterol derivative cholic acid. Glycine is the simplest amino acid. Although often identified as an amino acid, taurine (made from the sulfur-containing amino acid cysteine), is not an amino acid (no carboxyl group); instead, it is a naturally occurring sulfonic acid.

Bile salts are amphipathic. This characteristic is important with respect to their subsequent interaction with TGs as TGs enter the digestive tract and appear within the lumen of the small intestine. Bile salts are effectively detergents, as they interact directly with TGs within the aqueous environment of the small intestine to form an emulsion (ie, a system that involves small, mostly spherical globules known as *micelles*, comprised of hydrophobic regions oriented internally, with polar or charged groups facing externally, which interact with the polar aqueous system). Why does the emulsion form and remain stable in aqueous systems? Briefly, in an aqueous system, there is a fair amount of thermodynamic disorder (ie, entropy). If a hydrophobic molecule is introduced into such a polar system, a possible outcome would be for water molecules to structurally surround each hydrophobic molecule. This action, were it to occur, would substantially structure the water molecules. This result is not thermodynamically favored; it requires energy input. Consequently, hydrophobic molecules in water (or any polar environment) will cluster into large droplets or regions that exclude water, with water molecules structured only around the surfaces of the large globules. This action results in a much more ultimately disordered system, which favors entropy, and is therefore more thermo-dynamically stable. In the presence of a detergent such as bile salts (which are not truly dissolved), the lipid molecules occupy very small regions surrounded by detergent molecules and can form a stable emulsion. Therefore, with the detergent-like activity of bile salts, amphipathic TGs form mostly spherical globules with water structured only around the surface of the globule (micelle). These micelles, then, are the form of TG and bile salt emulsions that one finds within the lumen of the small intestine.

The emulsification process and micelle formation make TGs and fatty acid esters available for hydrolysis by intestinal lipases and esterases. This activity is critical for metabolism of long-chain TGs. Ingested glycerol and individual fatty acids of up to 10 carbons in length can be absorbed directly via the villi of the intestinal mucosa and can enter the bloodstream through available capillaries. Medium-chain TG (MCT) lipid emulsions can be directly absorbed without requiring either bile salts for emulsification or energy for uptake. Such MCFAs and glycerol can be directly transported to the liver by lipid carrier proteins. However, long-chain TGs require bile salts for both enzymatic digestion and formation of micelles. Enzymatic activity at the micelle-aqueous interface by lipases preferentially releases fatty acids, first from the *sn*-3 position, and then, the *sn*-1 position, from the TGs. These actions result in a mixture of free fatty acids, in addition to the glycerol molecule with 1 fatty acid attached (a monoglyceride) or 2 fatty acids attached (a diglyceride) in ester linkage.

The major lipase activity within the duodenum involves 2 components, colipase and pancreatic lipase (triacylglycerol lipase), which are both secreted by the pancreas. Colipase is generated from a procolipase by the action of trypsin within the duodenum. This small protein of approximately 10,000 Da specifically binds to pancreatic lipase to form a complex that, in association with the micelle, becomes enzymatically active. This complex, via colipase, binds to the lipid-water interface (polar region) of the micelle. Binding of this complex to the micelle initiates a conformational change in the lipase that alters the structure of the enzyme, allows binding to the hydrophobic region of the micelle, and allows hydrolysis of the embedded TGs to occur. Once bound, the lipase acts on the TGs at the *sn*-3 position, which releases the fatty acid at that position and forms a 1,2-diglyceride. Then, further enzymatic activity releases the fatty acid from the *sn*-1 position, which leaves a monoglyceride. In addition to this activity, the enzyme phospholipase A$_2$ secreted by the pancreas (also activated by trypsin action on prophospholipase A$_2$), interacts with phosphatidylcholine and removes the fatty acid at *sn*-2 to generate lysophosphatidylcholine (which requires bile acids for enzymatic activity). The final result of the lipid hydrolysis of the micelles is, therefore, the generation of free fatty acids released from positions 1 and 3; 1,2-diglycerides; 2-monoglycerides; and lysophosphatidylcholine molecules within the lumen.

The micelles that contain a mixture of free fatty acids and the different mono- and diglycerides interact with and are absorbed by the microvilli of the epithelial cells of the small intestine (intestinal mucosal enterocytes). After absorption by the microvilli, the fatty acids and glycerides within the micelles dissociate, diffuse across the epithelial cell membranes, and enter the cytoplasm.

The bile salts are destined to return to the liver via the superior mesenteric and portal veins after reabsorption by the small intestine enterocytes. Inside the cytoplasm, the absorbed free fatty acids, mono- and diglycerides, and endogenous fatty acids previously synthesized by these cells are used for reesterification to form TGs. In this environment, the TGs combine with phospholipids (about 85%), cholesterol esters, and apolipoprotein B-48 (apoB-48) to form immature chylomicrons.

Immature chylomicrons are released by exocytosis from the enterocytes into the lymphatic system. After circulating through the lymphatic system, the immature chylomicrons eventually encounter the bloodstream via the emptying of the thoracic duct into the left subclavian vein. Within the blood, these immature chylomicrons mature through interaction with high-density lipoprotein (HDL), where a donation occurs. The HDL provides the apolipoproteins apoC-II and apoE to form a mature chylomicron—the largest lipoprotein particle to circulate.

Acquisition of the various apolipoproteins that occurs in the blood allows the chylomicron to interact with various tissues. The main classes of apolipoproteins include A, B, C, D, and E. The various lipoprotein classes may have subclasses, such as apoA-I and apoA-IV, apoB-48, apoC-I, or apoC-II. These proteins function in lipid transport, as a cofactor necessary for a particular lipase activity and/or as a structure necessary for a circulating lipoprotein particle to associate with a cell surface receptor. Lipids are delivered in the form of chylomicrons primarily to the liver and to cells that comprise adipose tissue. These chylomicrons also specifically deliver lipids, via appropriate lipoprotein–cell-surface receptor binding, to the heart, skeletal muscle, and other organs. Indeed, the major energy source used continuously by the heart, resting muscle, and long-term exercised muscle tissue, is lipid.

As lipoproteins circulate through the bloodstream and interact with various tissues, the enzyme lipoprotein lipase within the membranes of the capillary endothelial cells hydrolyzes the TGs to free fatty acids and glycerol, which are absorbed by the different tissues. Over time, the hydrolysis of the chylomicron TG core results in smaller-sized circulating chylomicron enriched in cholesterol and proteins. This form of the chylomicron, known as a *remnant*, is eventually degraded by the liver via specific liver tissue receptors, and thus removed from the circulation. Endogenously (liver) synthesized cholesterol and TGs are converted within the liver to very low-density lipoprotein (VLDL), which is then secreted into the bloodstream. Within the blood, the gradual enzymatic degradation of VLDL, first to intermediate-density lipoprotein (IDL) and finally to low-density lipoprotein (LDL), occurs. TGs released by this process enter the tissues, and the LDL particles subsequently bind to specific membrane receptors and deliver cholesterol to the tissues. A portion of IDL may bind to the liver and, through the action of hepatic lipase, be remodeled to release LDL into the blood. A portion of LDL may also be taken up by the liver, the proteins degraded and cholesterol released. The return of cholesterol and various lipids from tissues to the liver is accomplished via HDLs. Thus, while LDL delivers cholesterol to the tissues, HDL scavenges this substance from the tissues and returns the material to the liver, where conversion of cholesterol to bile acids takes place. Loss of bile acids through intestinal transport effectively removes cholesterol from the tissues. For these reasons, LDLs are euphemistically known as "bad" cholesterol and HDLs as "good" cholesterol. Any free fatty acids in the blood that are generated by mobilization of lipid stores and conversion to fatty acids and glycerol by lipase activity bind to albumin and circulate through the bloodstream and eventually reach the tissues that demand an energy source.[7,8]

Parenteral Delivery and Metabolism of Lipid Injectable Emulsions

Terminology

In this edition of the *Core Curriculum*, the term *lipid injectable emulsion* (ILE) replaces the term *intravenous fat emulsion* (IVFE). This change in terminology has been recommended by the American Society for Parenteral and Enteral Nutrition (ASPEN) to agree with the US Pharmacopeia terminology and, for patient safety, to avoid confusion between the abbreviation IVFE and the abbreviation for intravenous iron (IVFe).

Types of Lipid Injectable Emulsions

ILEs are oil-in-water emulsions consisting of 1 or more TG–containing oils, glycerin, and a phospholipid emulsifier. Commercial parenteral ILE are provided in TG concentrations of 10%, 20%, and 30% (w/v). These emulsions may also contain other lipid-soluble substances such as vitamin E, vitamin K, phytosterols (plant cholesterol–like substances), and cholesterol. Table 5-2 lists selected oils present in commercially available parenteral emulsions.

Structure and Metabolism

The parenteral ILEs listed in Table 5-2 are each structurally designed such that the chylomicron-like particles (micelles) within each emulsion resemble natural chylomicrons with respect to size, core TGs, and a monolayer of phospholipid. Like natural chylomicrons, these spherical pseudo-chylomicrons are, on average, 200 to 500 nm in diameter and have a central TG core surrounded by a phospholipid (emulsifier) envelope.[9] In natural chylomicrons, the types of core TGs reflect dietary intake, whereas pseudo-chylomicrons contain a TG core that consists of specific commercial oils (see Table 5-2). Also, whereas natural chylomicrons enter the circulation bearing apolipoproteins and further acquire additional apolipoproteins from HDL, pseudo-chylomicrons enter the circulation with no apolipoproteins but rapidly acquire them from HDL.[10]

Emulsifying agents, such as egg phosphatide, have a detergent-like action and are added to ILEs to provide a barrier that prevents coalescence of the oil droplets of the emulsion. However, the necessary addition of an emulsification agent can cause a potentially undesirable structure known as a *liposome* to form. Liposomes, spherical byproducts of the emulsifier used in the emulsification process, are less than 70 nm in diameter and consist primarily of a phospholipid bilayer that surrounds a trapped aqueous phase. Metabolism of each of these entities requires several stages, and the process begins immediately upon entrance into the bloodstream.

Pseudo-chylomicrons behave very similarly to natural chylomicrons with respect to their metabolism. Once in the circulation, pseudo-chylomicrons acquire apolipoproteins and endogenous cholesterol, and, through cell membrane and

TABLE 5-2 Fat Composition of Selected Lipid Emulsions

Emulsion Product	Lipid, %	Energy, kcal/L	Glycerol, g/L	Egg Phosphatide, g/L	Oil Content, g/L			
					Soybean Oil	Olive Oil	MCT Oil	Fish Oil
ClinOleic, Clinolipid	20	2000	22.5	12	40	160	—	—
Intralipid 30%	30	3000	17.0	12	300	—	—	—
Intralipid 20%	20	2000	22.5	12	200	—	—	—
Ivelip	20	2000	25	12	200	—	—	—
Lipofundin MCT	20	1908	25	12	100	—	100	—
Lipofundin N	20	2008	25	12	200	—	—	—
Lipoplus	20	1910	25	12	80	—	100	20
Lipovenoes	20	2000	25	12	200	—	—	—
Nutrilipid	20	2000	25	12	200	—	—	—
Omegaven	10	1120	25	12	—	—	—	100
Smoflipid	20	2000	25	12	60	50	60	30
Structolipid	20	1960	22	12	64% (w/w) LCT	—	36% (w/w) MCT	—

LCT, long-chain triglyceride; MCT, medium-chain triglyceride.

other lipoprotein interactions, exchange phospholipids. These dynamically changing pseudo-chylomicrons are efficiently transported in the circulation and engage tissue cell membranes. Cellular interaction (smooth and cardiac muscle and adipose tissue) exposes the pseudo-chylomicron to lipoprotein lipase activity, the result of which is the release of fatty acids from the TG core and movement of free fatty acids into the cells. The degradation of the pseudo-chylomicrons in this manner ultimately results in the appearance of small, TG-poor pseudo-chylomicrons that are known as *remnants*. Like natural chylomicron remnants, pseudo-chylomicron remnants are removed by the liver. Similarly, liposomes acquire apolipoproteins and undergo, in general, metabolic consequences similar to those of pseudo-chylomicrons.

Dysfunction of this system can lead to hypercholesterolemia and/or hyperlipidemia. These conditions may involve any of the lipoproteins discussed previously. When TGs alone are involved, the condition is known as *hypertriglyceridemia*. For example, an abnormal lipoprotein known as *lipoprotein-X* can form from liposomes present in the circulation. Recall that liposomes are the product of emulsifiers that are added to the lipid emulsion. Lipoprotein-X is essentially a spherical bilayer of phospholipid and cholesterol. This abnormal protein, identified in obstructive jaundice and in congenital lecithin-cholesterol acyltransferase deficiency, inhibits lipase activity (both lipoprotein lipase and hepatic lipase) toward natural chylomicrons and pseudo-chylomicrons.[11,12] Consequently, a high concentration of lipoprotein-X in the circulation can inhibit lipid metabolism and lead to hypercholesterolemia or hypertriglyceridemia.[6,9] The relative number of liposomes within an ILE and, therefore, the potential for lipoprotein-X to form depend on the oil content. Thus, a 10% (w/v) emulsion will contain a larger number of liposomes than a 20% (w/v) emulsion, because of the relative ratio of phospholipid emulsifier to oil. And, although most commercial ILEs are available as 20% (w/v) formulations, ILEs used as vehicles for intravenous (IV) drug delivery (eg, propofol) are usually 10% (w/v) ILE (see Practice Scenario 5-1). Consequently, lipoprotein-X may still form under certain circumstances, and clinicians should consider this risk over the long term or when high amounts of such ILEs have been provided. In the absence of careful monitoring, hypertriglyceridemia, a condition indicated by elevated plasma TG levels, is a possible adverse effect of provision of lipids in PN. It occurs when the body cannot clear TGs from plasma lipids via oxidation and/or storage in adipose tissue, and it may be caused when the supply of lipids into the bloodstream exceeds lipoprotein lipase activity or, as described previously, when lipoprotein lipase activity is reduced.[13-15]

Hypertriglyceridemia is associated with various clinical and metabolic problems, such as sepsis, renal failure, and pancreatitis.[16] Consequently, whenever ILEs are used, clinicians should consistently monitor patients for the threshold plasma TG level above which the exogenously administered lipids cannot be efficiently metabolized.

Fatty Acid β-Oxidation

The degradation (ie, catabolism) of fatty acids—whether saturated or unsaturated, or even-chain or odd-chain—proceeds by oxidative pathways. As previously addressed, the oxidation of fatty acids (and/or lipids) releases substantially more energy than does oxidation of carbohydrate. Cells can use this available energy to help meet the enormous energy demands required for various metabolic processes. The oxidation of fatty acids is, therefore, critically important to meeting energy demands. The most common pathway of oxidative degradation of fatty acids is known as β-*oxidation*. The β-oxidation of even-chain fatty acids yields several molecules (equal to one-half the total number of carbons) of the 2-carbon compound acetyl-CoA. For example, complete β-oxidation of the 16-carbon saturated fatty acid palmitic acid would yield 8 moles of acetyl-CoA per mole of palmitic acid. Similarly, oxidation of odd-chain fatty acids yields several molecules of acetyl-CoA and 1 molecule of propionyl coenzyme A (propionyl-CoA) (last oxidation step). Acetyl-CoA can directly enter the citric acid (Krebs) cycle, whereas propionyl-CoA is first converted to succinyl coenzyme A (succinyl-CoA), which also can directly enter the citric acid cycle. An example of the substantial energy yield afforded by this oxidative process is the net synthesis of 129 moles of adenosine-5′-triphosphate per mole of palmitic acid (aerobic respiration coupled to oxidative phosphorylation) upon the complete β-oxidation of this fatty acid. For β-oxidation to proceed, free fatty acids in the cytoplasm must first be transported into the mitochondrial matrix. Generally, fatty acids of up to 10 carbons in length may simply cross the mitochondrial membranes and reach the mitochondrial matrix without the requirement for special transport mechanisms. The first step in the β-oxidation of these molecules is the thioester linkage of coenzyme A (CoA) to the fatty acid by an acyl-CoA synthetase. Acyl-CoA synthetase enzymes are classified by their chain-length specificity. In contrast to the unrestricted movement of SCFAs into the mitochondrial matrix, long-chain fatty acids (LCFAs) must be shuttled across the membranes by specific carrier and translocase mechanisms that require L-carnitine. The first step in this translocation process is the covalent connection of the fatty acids to CoA by acyl-CoA synthetases. These enzymes are located within the outer membranes of mitochondria. Once the fatty acid is activated in the mitochondrial outer membrane by addition of CoA, the acyl-CoA products enter the intermembrane space and are transported to the mitochondrial matrix by a specific L-carnitine shuttle system. When the fatty acid–CoA derivative reaches the inner membrane surface, the fatty acid is transferred from CoA in ester linkage to the hydroxyl group of carnitine and subsequently translocated across the inner membrane to the matrix region. Before release from the inner membrane, the fatty acid–carnitine derivative associates with an enzyme that transfers the fatty acid from carnitine to CoA and the fatty acid–CoA derivative is released to the matrix. Carnitine is subsequently transported back across the inner membrane to the intermembrane space, and there it can again participate in subsequent shuttles of CoA-activated fatty acids to the mitochondrial matrix. Once in the matrix, the fatty acid–CoA derivative is acted upon by several enzymes that progress down the length of the fatty acid from the carboxyl group to the last methyl group to oxidize the fatty acid by 2 carbon lengths at a time (acetyl-CoA is produced). Each round of oxidation yields a remaining fatty acid that is

2 carbons shorter than the previous molecule. This activity repeats, round after round, until the entire fatty acid has been oxidatively degraded to several molecules of acetyl-CoA (or, in the case of odd-numbered fatty acids, several molecules of acetyl-CoA and 1 molecule of propionyl-CoA). Unsaturated fatty acids undergo identical enzymatic conversion, except that additional enzymatic steps cope with a double bond. The double bond is essentially shifted in position, which allows a 2-carbon segment to be oxidized and released as acetyl-CoA.

Lipid Recommendations for Individuals Requiring Specialized Nutrition Support

Patients receiving specialized nutrition support require a mixed substrate of carbohydrate and lipids to meet metabolic and energy needs, but the ideal amount of lipids to administer is unknown. Lipid recommendations usually exceed quantities necessary to prevent essential fatty acid deficiency (EFAD). Higher levels of lipids are used because (1) lipids provide the highest energy yield among fuel substrates; (2) the oxidative metabolism of lipid produces less carbon dioxide than similar glucose loads; and (3) specific fatty acids may potentially modify immune and inflammatory responses.

Patients who receive enteral or parenteral lipid formulations may be at risk for EFAD if insufficient quantities of linoleic acid and α-linolenic acid are provided. Reports have suggested that providing between 1% and 4% of total energy as linoleic acid is sufficient to prevent EFAD.[17,18] The requirement for α-linolenic acid is lower (0.25% to 0.5% of total energy).[18,19] A variety of plant oils have been used as the lipid source to provide essential fatty acids for patients requiring specialized nutrition support (Table 5-3).[20] As shown in Table 5-3, soybean and corn oil

TABLE 5-3 Comparison of Dietary Fatty Acids in Common Oils

| Dietary Fat | Breakdown of Fatty Acid Content, %[a] | | | |
	Saturated Fatty Acids	Linoleic Acid	α-Linolenic Acid	Monounsaturated Fatty Acid
Canola oil	6	22	10	62
Safflower oil	10	77	Trace	13
Sunflower oil	11	69	0	20
Corn oil	13	61	0	25
Olive oil	14	8	1	77
Soybean oil	15	54	7	24
Palm oil	45	12	1	37
Palm kernel oil	52	10	1	11
Coconut oil	92	2	0	6
Cod liver oil[b]	23	1	1	47

[a]Normalized to 100%.
[b]Cod liver oil has approximately 27% eicosapentaenoic acid and docosahexaenoic acid.
Adapted with permission of McGraw-Hill Education from reference 20: Wardlaw GM. *Perspectives in Nutrition.* 4th ed. New York: McGraw-Hill; 1999. Permission conveyed through Copyright Clearance Center, Inc.

are rich sources of linoleic acid that contain, respectively, 54% and 61% of this fatty acid. Soybean and canola oils are each good sources of α-linolenic acid that provide 7% and 10%, respectively, of this essential fatty acid (EFA).

Enteral Nutrition Recommendations

To meet EFA requirements, commercial enteral formulas include a variety of oils, including corn, soybean, safflower, and canola oils (Table 5-4). There is no absolute recommendation for a given enteral formula's lipid content; consequently, as demonstrated by Table 5-4, the lipid content of common enteral formulas varies widely. Among commercial enteral formulas, elemental products generally provide the least amount of fat. In contrast, polymeric enteral products often provide more than 25% of energy in the form of fat, and this percentage increases as formulas are concentrated into more energy-dense solutions. Current enteral fat recommendations are driven primarily by disease state and must be considered in context with the quantity and kind(s) of lipids provided. Chapters in Part III of this book discuss disease-specific lipid recommendations.

Parenteral Nutrition Recommendations

Two 100% soybean oil–based emulsions are currently available in the United States for IV use. In each of these emulsions, linoleic acid provides approximately 55% to 60% of total energy and approximately 3% to 4% of total energy is from α-linolenic acid.

A newer generation alternative ILE, Smoflipid, has recently become commercially available in the United States. Like all alternative ILEs, this emulsion is designed to meet EFA requirements and is composed of a blend of soybean oil, olive oil, fish oil, and MCTs. Another blended, alternative ILE, ClinOleic/Clinolipid, composed of soybean and olive oils is approved but not commercially available in the United States. The amount of EFAs in the alternative emulsions may vary significantly when compared with soybean oil–based ILEs; consequently, the blended oils must be balanced to provide sufficient concentrations of EFAs. These newer generation ILEs reduce the soybean oil portion of the emulsion with the intention of lowering potential inflammatory mediators that may be associated with higher levels of linoleic acid. To prevent inadequate EFA dosing, the EFA content of alternative ILEs that contain significantly lower soybean oil should be identified before they are administered. Compared with soybean oil, Smoflipid and ClinOleic/Clinolipid contain approximately 67.0% to 66.2% less linoleic acid, respectively.

To meet EFA requirements in adult PN patients with 100% soybean oil–based ILEs, a variety of lipid regimens may be prescribed. Often, 500 mL of a 20% ILE may be given weekly.[21] Given the lower concentration of linoleic acid found in Smoflipid and ClinOleic/Clinolipid, the lipid dosage for patients receiving either of these products should be calculated based on their energy requirements and whether any other sources of lipids are provided. The 2016 critical care guidelines from ASPEN and the Society of Critical Care Medicine (SCCM) suggest that when using soybean oil emulsion as

TABLE 5-4 Fat Composition of Selected Enteral Formulas

Formula	% of Energy	Source	g/L	Linoleic Acid, g/L	MCTs, g/L	n-3 Fatty Acids, g/L
Compleat	34	Canola oil	40	8.6	0	2.6
Diabetisource AC	44	Canola oil, refined fish oil (anchovy, sardine)	58.8	10	0	6.2
Fibersource HN	29	Canola oil, MCTs	40	6.6	8.0	2.7
Glucerna 1.0 Cal	49	High-oleic safflower and canola oils	54.5	7.8	0	0.7
Glucerna 1.2 Cal	45	High-oleic safflower and canola oils	60.0	10.25	0	2.52
Glucerna 1.5 Cal	45	High-oleic safflower and canola oils	75.0	12.8	0	3.15
Glytrol	42	Canola oil, high-oleic safflower oil, MCTs	47.6	6.8	9.6	1.8
Impact	25	Palm kernel oil, refined fish oil (anchovy, sardine), high-linoleic safflower oil, high-oleic sunflower oil	28.0	3.0	0	2.5
Impact Peptide 1.5	38	MCTs, refined fish oil (anchovy, sardine), canola oil, soybean oil	63.6	8.3	31.6	6.1
Isosource 1.5 Cal	35	Canola oil, MCTs	59.2	9.7	12.0	4.0
Isosource HN	29	Canola oil, MCTs	40.0	6.5	8.0	2.7
Jevity 1 Cal	29	Canola oil, corn oil, MCTs, soy lecithin	34.7	10.0	6.6	1.5
Jevity 1.2 Cal	29	Canola oil, corn oil, MCTs, soy lecithin	39.3	11.2	7.9	2.0
Jevity 1.5 Cal	29.4	Canola oil, corn oil, MCTs, soy lecithin	49.8	13.5	9.5	2.6
Nepro with Carb Steady	48	High-oleic safflower and canola oils	95.8	14.5	0.0	2.5
Novasource Renal	45	Canola oil	100.0	20.3	0.0	8.4
Nutren 1.0	30	Canola oil, MCTs	34.0	5.8	6.8	2.4
Nutren 1.0 Fiber	30	Canola oil, MCTs	34.0	5.9	6.8	2.4
Nutren 1.5	35	Canola oil, MCTs	60.0	10.0	12.0	4.1
Nutren 2.0	41	MCTs, canola oil	92.0	9.8	46	4.0
Nutren Pulmonary	56	MCTs, canola oil, corn oil	94.8	15.8	40	3.9
NutriHep	12	MCTs, canola oil, corn oil	21.2	2.0	14.8	0.5
Osmolite 1 Cal	29	Canola oil, corn oil, MCTs, soy lecithin	34.7	9.5	6.9	1.8
Osmolite 1.2 Cal	29	Canola oil, high-oleic safflower oil, MCTs, soy lecithin	39.3	5.4	7.5	1.3
Osmolite 1.5 Cal	29	Canola oil, high-oleic safflower oil, MCTs, soy lecithin	49.1	6.7	9.8	1.5
Oxepa	55.2	Canola oil, MCTs, marine oil, borage oil, soy lecithin	93.8	15.9	23.5	11.7
Peptamen	33	MCTs, soybean oil	39.0	5.2	27.6	0.7
Peptamen with Prebio	35	MCTs, soybean oil	40	5.2	28	0.7
Peptamen 1.5	33	MCTs, soybean oil	56.0	6.6	40	0.8
Peptamen 1.5 with Prebio	34	MCTs, soybean oil	56	6.6	40	0.8
Peptamen AF	40	MCTs, refined fish oil (anchovy, sardine), soybean oil	54	6.3	28	3.8
Peptamen Intense VHP	34	MCTs, refined fish oil (anchovy, sardine), high-linoleic safflower oil, soybean oil	38.0	4.4	18	2.3
Perative	25	Canola oil, MCTs, corn oil, soy lecithin	37.3	6.8	14.9	1.2
Pivot 1.5	30	Marine oil/MCT structured lipid, soy oil, canola oil, soy lecithin	50.8	10.6	9.4	6.9
Promote	23	Soy oil, MCTs, safflower oil, soy lecithin	26.0	11.7	4.7	1.3

TABLE 5-4 Fat Composition of Selected Enteral Formulas *(continued)*

Formula	% of Energy	Source	g/L	Linoleic Acid, g/L	MCTs, g/L	*n*-3 Fatty Acids, g/L
Promote with Fiber	25	Soy oil, MCTs, safflower oil, soy lecithin	28.2	12.2	4.7	1.3
Pulmocare	55.1	Canola oil, MCTs, corn oil, high-oleic safflower oil, soy lecithin	93.3	18.4	18.7	4.8
RenalCal	36	MCTs, canola oil, corn oil	82	6.2	60	1.4
Replete	30	Canola oil, MCTs	34.0	5.6	6.8	2.4
Replete Fiber	30	Canola oil, MCTs	34.0	5.6	6.8	2.3
Suplena with Carb Steady	48	High-oleic safflower oil, canola oil	95.8	16.1	0.0	3.1
Tolerex	2	Safflower oil	2	1.2	0.0	0.0
TwoCal HN	40.1	High-oleic safflower oil, MCTs, canola oil, soy lecithin	90.5	10.1	16.9	1.1
Vital 1.0 Cal	33	Canola oil/MCT structured lipid, canola oil, MCTs, DATEM	38.1	3.5	18	1.6
Vital 1.5 Cal	33	Canola oil/MCT structured lipid, canola oil, MCTs, DATEM	57.1	5.5	27	2.5
Vital AF 1.2 Cal	39	Marine oil/MCT structured lipid, MCTs, canola oil, soy oil, DATEM	53.9	6.3	24	7.3
Vital High Protein	20	MCTs, marine oil, corn oil	23.2	0.95	11.6	4.2
Vivonex Plus	6	Soybean oil	6.7	4	0.0	0.5
Vivonex RTF	10	Soybean oil, MCTs	11.6	3.6	4.8	0.5
Vivonex T.E.N.	3	Safflower oil	3	2.2	0.0	0.0

DATEM, diacetyl tartaric acid esters of mono- and diglycerides; MCT, medium-chain triglyceride.

the sole IV fat source, the ILE should be held for the first week or given at a maximum of 100 g/wk if there is a concern or risk for EFAD.[22] European guidelines suggest that most patients on long-term home PN with chronic intestinal failure without ongoing metabolic complications can be safely treated with provision of no more than 1 g of IV soybean-based lipid emulsion per kg per day.[23]

PN lipid dosing depends on energy expenditure, the patient's clinical status, body weight, tolerance, ability to metabolize the lipid emulsion, and consideration of additional energy given to the patient.[24] Before starting the infusion, clinicians should obtain the patient's serum TG levels to establish the baseline value. In adult patients requiring PN, ILEs should not exceed 2.5 g lipid per kg per day.[25] In critically ill patients requiring PN, the recommendations are more consistently conservative, with some data supporting less than 1 g lipid per kg per day.[25-27] These recommendations for lipid provision are based on evidence that the potential for metabolic adverse reactions associated with rapid infusion and excessive amounts of parenteral lipids may be reduced while simultaneously improving capacity for lipid clearance (see Practice Scenario 5-1).[28] Additional recommendations for ILEs include limiting the infusion rate so it does not exceed 0.11 g/kg/h

to prevent potential adverse reactions or toxicities associated with rapid infusion.[29]

Practice Scenario 5-1

Question: What strategies can prevent adverse metabolic outcomes when propofol is used concomitantly with nutrition support?

Scenario: A 62-year-old woman (height, 157 cm; weight, 50 kg; body mass index, 20.3) with a past medical history of alcohol abuse and chronic obstructive pulmonary disease was involved in a motor vehicle collision. After being admitted to the hospital, the patient underwent an exploratory laparotomy, which found blunt hepatic trauma and mesentery injuries. The nutrition assessment provided a Nutrition Risk in Critically ill (NUTRIC) score (without the interleukin-6 value) of 6, and indirect calorimetry was used to determine that the patient's resting energy expenditure was 1550 kcal/d, with a respiratory quotient of 0.79. The initial diet order was for trophic enteral feeding (polymeric formula 30% lipid). On postoperative Day 3, the patient's clinical condition declined. She required vasopressor administration and was in respiratory failure. Physical examination showed that her abdomen was firm and distended. A kidney, ureter, and bladder x-ray was consistent with postoperative ileus. Since admission, the patient received a continuous infusion of propofol (Diprivan 1%, Fresenius Kabi, USA) for sedation. Sedation was problematic because the patient was experiencing alcohol withdrawal, and the propofol dose was subsequently increased to a relatively constant 15 mL/h (30 mg/kg/h), providing 36 g of fat (396 kcal) per 24 hours. The patient's serum electrolytes were within normal limits. Her serum triglyceride (TG) level was 331 mg/dL on Day 5 and 550 mg/dL on Day 7.

Intervention: On Day 4 of admission, clinicians determined that the patient had failed trophic enteral feedings, and her diet order was changed to a 3-in-1 parenteral nutrition (PN) prescription containing 20 g of a 20% lipid injectable emulsion (ILE).

Answer: Propofol alone was providing 26% of the patient's energy requirements (0.72 g lipid per kg body weight). Current propofol administration alone provided an acceptable level of lipid dose for this patient (less than 1 g/kg/d). With the addition of 20 g of a 20% ILE as part of the PN prescription, this patient would receive 1.12 g fat per kg per day. Because of the elevated serum TG level and potential variation in propofol administration, clinicians should monitor the patient's serum TG concentration frequently (eg, twice per week). To lower the total fat dose and possibly improve TG clearance, lipids should be removed from the PN solution. Recommendations for acceptable serum TG levels are less than 250 mg/dL 4 hours after ILE infusion for "piggybacked" lipids and less than 400 mg/dL for continuous ILE infusion.[50] The patient should be started on hypocaloric, fat-free PN (equal to or less than 20 kcal/kg/d) because her nutrition risk is high (NUTRIC score = 6).

Rationale: The patient was at significant risk for hypertriglyceridemia and/or fat overload syndrome because of her critical illness and propofol infusion. Fat overload syndrome, a rare complication of ILE infusion, may occur when the dose or rate of lipid infusion exceeds the body's lipid clearance capacity. The presence of the higher concentration of phospholipids in 10% ILE (used as the drug vehicle for propofol) may result in an increase in lipoprotein-X particles that compete with TG-rich particles for lipoprotein lipase. This competition for lipase activity may lead to decreased TG hydrolysis, with the concomitant result of an increase in circulating TGs.

Manifestations of Essential Fatty Acid Deficiency in Patients Receiving Specialized Nutrition Support

In 1929, Burr and Burr documented EFAD in animals,[30] but it was not identified in humans until the development of PN 4 decades later. In the early 1970s and 1980s, biochemical and clinical manifestations of deficiencies of both linoleic and α-linolenic fatty acids were observed in patients requiring PN for extended periods of time (2 to 4 weeks).[31-34] The most notable clinical change associated with linoleic acid deficiency is a dry, scaly skin rash. However, other clinical symptoms have been noted, including increased susceptibility to infection, impaired wound healing, and immune dysfunction.[35-37]

Biochemical changes that occur in response to linoleic acid deficiency are manifested by a decrease in linoleic acid and AA (tetraenoic acid) levels and an increase in the mead acid (triene acid, 20:3n-9) level. Mead acid is primarily produced in humans in the absence of EFAs. A triene:tetraene ratio greater than 0.2 (Holman index) has been used to identify the presence of EFAD.[38] The time required to exhibit an EFAD in adults varies depending on the individual's underlying disease and nutrition status. EFAD may occur rapidly in patients receiving continuous fat-free PN administration because of elevated insulin levels that prevent adipose tissue lipolysis. EFAD may typically be seen in patients after 4 weeks of fat-free PN, although clinical signs may be detected earlier (eg, between 10 and 20 days).[24,32,39] Hypocaloric fat-free PN or a cyclic feeding schedule of fat-free PN may extend the period of time before the patient exhibits EFAD. It is thought that when PN is cycled or hypocaloric PN is provided, EFAs are mobilized and enter the circulation as a result of increased lipolysis of endogenous fat stores in response to a reduction in serum insulin concentration. In addition, hypocaloric feeding prevents the risk of hepatic dysfunction that may occur if the energy deficit (caused by the removal of lipids) is corrected by increasing the energy from dextrose or protein to maintain energy requirements. When ILEs are contraindicated, short-term hypocaloric, fat-free PN has been shown to be safe and appropriate for the critically ill patient (see Practice Scenario 5-2).[22,40,41]

Practice Scenario 5-2

Question: How can essential fatty acid deficiency (EFAD) be prevented when a lipid-free parenteral nutrition (PN) regimen is initiated in the intensive care unit (ICU)?

Scenario: A 57-year-old woman (height, 167 cm; weight, 82 kg; body mass index, 29.4) was admitted to the ICU of a regional hospital with respiratory failure related to pneumonia. Patient had a history of type 1 diabetes and hypertriglyceridemia. Her estimated energy requirement was 2100 kcal/d and her estimated protein requirement was 110 g/d. On hospital Day 2, polymeric enteral feeding was started at 15 mL/h. On hospital Day 3, the patient exhibited clinical signs of feeding intolerance, which was confirmed by x-ray as an ileus. Enteral feeding was discontinued, but the patient's condition worsened as the day progressed, and severe sepsis was diagnosed. On hospital Day 7, the patient's condition had stabilized, and her organ systems and metabolic parameters were improving. The following laboratory data were documented:
- Serum glucose: 167 to 255 mg/dL (range during hospitalization)
- Serum triglycerides (TGs): Day 3: 499 mg/dL; Day 4: 563 mg/dL; Day 7: 479 mg/dL

Intervention: On hospital Day 7, a fat-free, hypocaloric PN prescription formula (1700 kcal, 90 g protein) was initiated.

Answer: A decision to hold PN during the acute phase of severe sepsis was made for this patient.[22] In this case, in light of elevated TGs, to prevent excessive glucose administration, and to improve the possibility of mobilizing essential fatty acids (EFAs) from endogenous lipid stores, a fat-free hypocaloric feeding regimen was initiated at 80% of estimated needs.[41] After approximately 14 days of not receiving any lipid, or when clinical signs and symptoms indicate the possibility of EFAD, plasma fatty acid profiles should be obtained (Holman index) to assess the patient for EFAD.

Rationale: Patients should be monitored for EFAD if all sources of lipids are removed from the diet for more than 2 to 4 weeks. The dosing of lipid injectable emulsions (ILEs) depends on energy expenditure, the patient's clinical status, body weight, tolerance, and ability to metabolize lipids. Providing 2% to 4% of the energy requirement as linoleic acid may correct EFA insufficiency. Clinicians should calculate the linoleic acid dose from 100% soybean ILE or an alternative ILE to ensure adequate dosing of EFAs. Initiation of low-dose or trophic enteral feeding may also be used to offset risk of EFAD. A polymeric enteral formula containing soybean oil and a mixture of other high-linoleic oils may be used. Generally, a polymeric enteral formula that provides 10% to 15% of the patient's total energy requirements will supply adequate EFAs. However, when the patient is at high risk for fat malabsorption, or when enteral feeding is interrupted or stopped for a significant period (14 days) with no other lipid source provided, the linoleic acid dose and EFAD risk should be evaluated.

When the diet is deficient of only α-linolenic acid, eicosatrienoic acid levels remain within normal range, and no rash is detectable. Clear evidence of α-linolenic acid deficiency was first reported in a 1982 case study by Holman and colleagues of a 6-year-old girl who had been maintained on PN solution lacking α-linolenic acid.[31] The observed symptoms of deficiency were primarily neurological abnormalities, including numbness, paresthesia, blurred vision, and difficulties in walking.

Several years later, α-linolenic acid deficiency was reported in elderly nursing home residents who were receiving intragastric feeding of an elemental formula that did not contain α-linolenic acid.[42] With the addition of α-linolenic acid to these elderly patients' nutrition regimen, clinical symptoms disappeared.

Interestingly, Heird and Lapillonne[43] reported that the metabolites of either linoleic acid metabolism (ie, γ-linolenic acid [GLA], dihomo-γ-linolenic acid [DGLA], and AA) or α-linolenic acid metabolism (ie, EPA and DHA) may correct the clinical symptoms of EFAD. Also, more recent data suggest that fish oil lipid emulsion alone may satisfy the EFA requirements for humans. In studies of children who received fish oil monotherapy, none of the patients expressed biochemical parameters or other indications of EFAD after 3 years or more of treatment.[44] However, it is unknown whether linoleic acid and α-linolenic acid, per se, have specific functional properties that cannot be met by provision of their fatty acid metabolites.

Evidence suggests that the risk of EFAD is increased in some patients who require home PN solutions.[45-47] Evaluation of the EFA status of home PN patients has revealed alterations in fatty acid profiles (decreases in linoleic acid plasma levels, increases in AA plasma levels, and an increase in the AA:linoleic acid ratio) and biochemical signs associated

with EFAD.[46-49] ILEs may not be required or provided for all patients receiving home PN, and data are insufficient to recommend the optimal amount of EFAs required for these patients. Home PN patients may be at risk for adverse events because of the amount of dietary fat consumed, the degree of intestinal inefficiency, the frequency of ILE provided in the PN solution, and the availability of endogenous lipid stores. Ling and colleagues[48] have demonstrated that linoleic acid provided at 3.2% of total energy with a daily average of 0.24 ± 0.13 g fat per kg is sufficient to prevent the development of EFAD in home PN patients. Others have reported that a weekly minimum of 1.0 g fat per kg of body weight or 500 mL of 20% ILE weekly may be necessary to correct or avoid biochemical alterations associated with EFAD.[46,50]

Recently, Gramlich and associates[51] described 3 cases in which EFAD was suspected in patients on alternative ILEs to be a potential cause of abnormal liver enzymes. The fatty acid profiles revealed reduced linoleic acid and elevated mead acid levels, which may suggest EFAD; however, when the patients were further examined using the triene:tetrane ratio, this index remained well below the level that would indicate EFAD. In these case reports, it is important to note that the diagnosis of EFAD was made by the observation of reduced linoleic acid levels and elevated mead acid levels. With alternate ILEs in which the amount of linoleic acid may be reduced, the fatty acid profile should be interpreted cautiously. ILEs with high concentrations of ω-9 fatty acids may result in higher conversion of mead acid. Serum fatty acid profiles may reflect linoleic acid levels that are low but remain adequate for prevention of EFAD. Reduced linoleic acid composition of alternative ILEs could result in false-positives for EFAD if the definitive diagnosis of a triene:tetraene ratio greater than 0.2 is not used. The 3 patient cases demonstrated daily averages of (1) 11.4 g linoleic acid (4.7% of total energy); (2) 13 g linoleic acid (7% of total energy); and (3) 7.54 g linoleic acid (3.7% of total energy); the reported energy values were based on energy intake or calculated requirements.[51]

Eicosanoid Biosynthesis: ω-6 and ω-3 Fatty Acids

Fatty acids are indirectly involved as metabolic precursors for eicosanoids, lipid substances that can profoundly affect platelet aggregation, neurotransmitter release, vascular function, infection responses, inflammatory activity, and immune system activity.[52-54] Eicosanoids contain 20 carbons and include prostaglandins, leukotrienes, thromboxanes, prostacyclins, lipoxins, resolvins, and protectins (neuroprotectins). Consequently, under certain conditions, these byproducts of fatty acid metabolism can have far-ranging and potentially detrimental effects. Members of the ω-6 and ω-3 series of fatty acids (AA and EPA, respectively) are the precursors for the intracellular synthesis of inflammatory eicosanoids. The most common dietary sources of ω-6 fatty acids are plants such as soybean, safflower, and corn. Plant dietary sources of ω-3 fatty acids are found in canola oil, flax seed, and leafy vegetables. Fish such as tuna, sardines, and salmon are also sources of ω-3 fatty acids. AA may be ingested in the diet via intake of meat or organ tissue. This lipid is also synthesized when dietary linoleic acid is desaturated by the enzyme Δ6-desaturase to form GLA (18:3n-6), which in turn is converted by elongation enzyme 2-carbon addition to form DGLA (20:3n-6). This compound is desaturated by Δ5-desaturase to form, in the final reaction of this pathway, AA. The ω-3 fatty acid, α-linolenic acid (18:3n-3), is the EFA that is the precursor of EPA and DHA, although the enzymatic conversion of α-linolenic acid to EPA and DHA is inefficient. Although EPA and DHA may be somewhat enzymatically interconvertible (alternate pathways may exist), the most efficient source of EPA and DHA is via the diet. Both EPA and DHA are critical to development of proper eyesight and brain function, and EPA is the precursor of the less biologically active inflammatory mediators of the 3-series prostaglandins and 5-series leukotrienes eicosanoid series. Other anti-inflammatory prostaglandins and clot-inhibiting thromboxanes of the 1-series, however, may be synthesized from DGLA (ω-6), one of the intermediates in the AA synthesis pathway.

AA, common to membrane phospholipids, usually occupies the sn-2 position and is almost always found at this position within the important membrane phospholipid phosphatidylinositol. During membrane cell signaling events, a possible outcome is the activation of phospholipase A2, the enzyme that acts on membrane phospholipids to release fatty acids from the sn-2 position.[55] Release of AA sets in motion subsequent intracellular metabolic activity via the COX pathway that leads to the synthesis of the 2-series of prostaglandins, including PGE$_2$, and thromboxanes, including thromboxane A$_2$. AA is initially converted to prostaglandin H$_2$ by the enzymes COX-1 and COX-2. Subsequently, prostaglandin H$_2$, as substrate for prostaglandin synthesis, is converted to the various prostaglandins that include PGD$_2$, PGE$_2$, PGF$_{2\alpha}$, PGI$_2$, and 15-d-PGJ$_2$. The enzyme COX-1 is generally thought to be constitutively expressed in almost all bodily tissues and is involved in many bodily "housekeeping" activities. The enzyme COX-2, on the other hand, is an inducible enzyme that is directly involved in inflammation.[56,57] Entrance of AA into the lipoxygenase pathway leads to the synthesis of the 4-series leukotrienes that include LTB$_4$. The 2-series of prostaglandins and thromboxanes are powerful inflammatory mediators that can induce significantly detrimental inflammatory effects. For example, PGE$_2$ has been extensively studied and is a known immunosuppressant.[58–60] In contrast, ω-6 fatty acid–derived 1-series prostaglandins and thromboxanes and ω-3 fatty acid–derived 3-series prostaglandins and thromboxanes and 5-series leukotrienes (via COX-1 and COX-2 and lipoxygenases) are less immunosuppressive and less inflammatory. For example, thromboxane A$_2$ strongly stimulates platelet aggregation and vasoconstriction. In contrast, platelets fail to aggregate and vasoconstriction is mild at best in the presence of thromboxane A$_3$.[61,62]

Additionally, ω-3 fatty acids are competitive inhibitors of 2- and 4-series eicosanoid formation from AA, and thus their physiological availability directly influences synthesis of these substances.[63] Because of these desirable consequences, provision of ω-6 fatty acids such as GLA and DGLA in addition to the ω-3 fatty acid EPA in the diet may serve to attenuate inflammatory events.[64] For example, dietary supplementation with fish oil can result in a lower chemotactic activity displayed by neutrophils and monocytes, and in vitro exposure

of endothelial cells, macrophages, or lymphocytes to fish oil ω-3 fatty acids can lower adhesion molecule expression by these cells.[65]

AA, EPA, and DHA are also the precursors of novel anti-inflammatory eicosanoids (ie, lipoxins, resolvins, and protectins) that contribute to the active resolution of an inflammatory response. Lipoxins are metabolic derivatives of AA that are generated during an inflammatory response and serve as powerful anti-inflammatory mediators. For example, lipoxin A$_4$ inhibits LTB$_4$-stimulated neutrophil chemotaxis through specific receptor signaling, and simultaneously attracts monocytes to apoptotic cells generated as a result of inflammation.[66–68] Resolvins of the E-series, generated from EPA, modify inflammation by, for example, inhibiting polymorphonuclear leukocyte transmigration and protecting the large bowel in colitis. Among other activities, resolvins of the D-series, generated from DHA, protect kidney tissue from ischemic injury. Protectins such as PD$_1$ are substances derived from DHA that also play an active role in resolution of an inflammatory response. When these same substances are produced in neural tissue, they are known as *neuroprotectins* (eg, NPD$_1$) to denote the tissue of origin. These substances, like lipoxin A$_4$, inhibit neutrophil migration. In addition, protectins reduce the tissue damage caused by stroke and, among several other inflammation-resolution activities, help to protect the liver from inflammatory damage.[69] Although these substances are clearly critical to physiological processes, their specific role(s) in the clinical aspects of EN and PN remain to be determined.

The Clinical Impact of Specific Fatty Acids in Enteral Nutrition

ω-3 Fatty Acids

Research on Cardiovascular and Cerebrovascular Disease Risk

Considerable research has been done on the potential cardiovascular and cerebrovascular benefits of supplementation with ω-3 fatty acids. Earlier studies suggested that dietary supplementation with both EPA and DHA may reduce cardiac-associated mortality.[70,71] In addition, initial evidence indicated that the levels of all-cause mortality, stroke, and cardiovascular disease (CVD) among individuals examined throughout the world were inversely related to the level of long-chain ω-3 fatty acid dietary intake.[72] However, more recent data offer significantly different conclusions with respect to the effect of EPA and DHA dietary supplementation on CVD. Although increased dietary intake of these ω-3 fatty acids effectively lowers circulating TG levels, a known risk factor for CVD, DHA supplementation increased LDL cholesterol levels.[73,74] Also, even when ω-3 supplementation has been associated with improvements in CVD risk factors, it has failed to demonstrate benefit relative to CVD reduction. Indeed, examination and analysis of over 20 years of randomized trials and other studies of ω-3 dietary supplementation (total N = more than 83,000 participants), the overall conclusion is that ω-3 supplementation does not lower time to death from cardiovascular causes, hospital admission related to cardiovascular causes, cardiovascular endpoints, postoperative atrial fibrillation, all-cause mortality, sudden death, myocardial infarction, or stroke.[75-80]

When considering the implications of the research on ω-3 fatty acid supplementation described here, clinicians should be aware that treatment guidelines have recently been revised to reflect evolving views of serum cholesterol levels as risk factors for disease. In November 2013, a joint task force for the American College of Cardiology and American Heart Association[81] released new guidelines for the treatment of blood cholesterol that no longer recommend treatment target goals for LDL cholesterol and non-HDL cholesterol, factors that have historically been evaluated in studies of ω-3 fatty acids and disease risk, including some of the research noted here. These new treatment guidelines are controversial.[82]

A systematic review and meta-analysis of data that represented almost 800,000 individuals found that fish consumption, although moderate in effect, was significantly associated with reduced cerebrovascular events. In contrast, long-chain ω-3 fatty acids measured as circulating biomarkers in observational studies or as supplements in primary and secondary prevention trials were not statistically associated with cerebrovascular events.[83] Consequently, fish may offer cardiovascular benefits beyond that assumed for the ω-3 fatty acids the fish provide.

Supplementation in Critical Illness

The 2016 ASPEN/SCCM guidelines for nutrition support therapy in critical illness recommend that clinicians avoid the routine use of (1) all specialty formulas in critically ill patients in a medical ICU and (2) all disease-specific formulas in the surgical ICU.[22] Specifically, the guidelines state that immune-modulating enteral formulations of arginine with other agents—including EPA, DHA, glutamine, and nucleic acid—should not be used routinely in the medical ICU; furthermore, these products and other similar formulations (eg, fish oil with or without arginine) should not be administered to severely septic patients.[22]

The ASPEN/SCCM guidelines further state that a recommendation cannot currently be made regarding the routine use of an enteral formulation characterized by an anti-inflammatory lipid profile (eg, ω-3 fish oils, borage oil) and antioxidants in patients with acute respiratory distress syndrome (ARDS) or severe acute lung injury, given the significant amount of conflicting data.[22] Other recent investigations, reviews, and meta-analyses reiterate the lack of consistent evidence regarding the routine use of these enteral formulations in patients with ARDS and support the current lack of recommendation.[84-86]

The ASPEN/SCCM guidelines recommend formulations that contain fish oil and arginine be considered in severe trauma patients and further recommend the use of either arginine-containing immune-modulating formulations or EPA/DHA supplementation with standard enteral formula in patients with traumatic brain injury (TBI).[22] In a 2016 review of experimental animal studies, Trépanier and colleagues concluded that provision of ω-3 PUFA in the form of DHA ameliorates inflammatory mediators in TBI.[87] In a retrospective analysis of 240 patients with isolated TBI, Painter et al showed that

tube-fed patients who received enteral immune-enhancing formula (with arginine, glutamine, EPA, and DHA), when compared with those receiving a standard enteral formula, had fewer cases of bacteremia (P <0.05) and higher posttreatment prealbumin levels in Weeks 2 and 3 of treatment (P = 0.006 and P = 0.04, respectively).[88] However, patients who received the immune-enhancing formula remained longer in the ICU (P = 0.02) and spent more days on mechanical ventilation (P = 0.001). The hospital length of stay and mortality were not significantly different between the 2 groups.[88]

The ASPEN/SCCM guidelines recommend that an immune-modulating formula (containing both arginine and fish oils) be routinely used in the surgical ICU for postoperative patients who require EN.[22] Recent studies and analyses support the use of such formulas.[89,90] In summary, there is support for the consideration (severe trauma) or routine use (TBI and surgical ICU) of enteral regimens that use immune-enhancing formulations.

ω-9 Fatty Acids

Diets containing oils high in ω-9 fatty acids (primarily, oleic acid within olive oil) have been reported to be beneficial for health because they lower cholesterol and TG levels without the negative effects of lipid peroxidation.[91] A recent study with more than 7000 subjects showed that the risk of stroke may be significantly reduced when a diet high in olive oil is used intensively.[92] Because high-oleic oils are stable and have a favorable fatty acid profile, they are often used in enteral formulas (Table 5-4). Enteral formulas using engineered sunflower and safflower oils may have an average oleic acid content greater than 70%, which is comparable to the oleic acid content in olive oil.[93] Historically, polymeric formulas with high to moderate oleic acid content have been examined in research studies of Crohn's disease with mixed results, which may be partially explained by the source and amount of oleic acid used (synthetic trioleate vs olive oil) and the contribution of other fatty acids, such as high linoleic content, in the enteral formulations.[94,95]

Short-Chain Fatty Acids

SCFAs play an integral role in colonic health. These fatty acids occur naturally in foods (butter, milk) but only in modest concentrations. The primary source of SCFAs is the large intestine via bacterial anaerobic fermentation of nondigestible dietary carbohydrates and fiber polysaccharides. Fermentation of these carbohydrate compounds produces the following SCFAs: acetate (2C), propionate (3C), and butyrate (4C). SCFAs are absorbed and metabolized primarily by the colon and, to a lesser degree, by liver, muscle, and brain tissue. The functions of SCFAs are diverse and include (1) a primary energy source for colonocytes, (2) stimulation of water and sodium absorption in the colon, and (3) trophic effects to the intestinal mucosa.[96,97] Butyrate has been shown to be the most important SCFA in regulation and maintenance of colonic tissue. An important role of butyrate may be to modify inflammatory activity by inhibiting the release of the transcription factor, nuclear factor κ–light-chain-enhancer, of activated B cells.[98] In addition, butyrate has been shown to exhibit antitumorigenic effects on cancer cell lines and has been identified with gene regulation involving processes of cellular apoptosis, proliferation, and differentiation.[99,100] Daly and colleagues[101] demonstrated that many of the butyrate-responsive genes are deregulated in colon carcinoma tissue as an apparent result of downregulation of cellular expression of the butyrate transporter. The data suggest that a reduction in transport of butyrate into the luminal membrane may contribute to sequential genetic alterations that lead to initiation of colorectal cancer.

More recent research has additionally established that levels of butyrate-producing bacteria are reduced in patients with type 2 diabetes, and concentrations of fecal SCFAs are also reduced in patients with severe systematic inflammatory response syndrome (SIRS) when compared with heathy controls.[101,102] Further studies of butyrate and other SCFAs may provide important insights into how gut microbes may contribute to or attenuate disease progression and offer additional approaches for therapeutic intervention. (See Chapter 4 for additional information on gut microbiota.)

Medium-Chain Triglycerides

MCTs are saturated and are 6 to 12 carbons in length. These fatty acids were developed commercially in the 1950s and are among the first medical foods derived as an alternative to plant oils and other conventional fats. This lipid product is isolated primarily from plants high in MCTs, such as palm kernel and coconut oils. The MCT product does not provide EFAs and has an energy density of 8.3 kcal/g. Compared with long-chain TGs (LCTs), MCTs are significantly different with respect to absorption, metabolism, and physiological functions. Ingestion of saturated LCTs from palm kernel and coconut oils is thought to contribute to coronary heart disease via an increase in LDL cholesterol,[103,104] but the effect of saturated MCTs from the same sources on LDL cholesterol levels is not clear—in some reports, LDL cholesterol levels increased[105] and in others, they decreased.[106] In many of these studies, the contributions and specific effects of MCTs alone are difficult to separate from other confounders.[107–109]

MCTs are smaller and more water soluble than LCTs. Liberation of fatty acids through hydrolysis of MCTs in the intestinal lumen is significantly faster relative to LCTs, and absorption of MCFAs is more rapid when compared with LCFAs. The absorptive rate of MCTs may be faster because they do not require the presence of bile or pancreatic lipases for absorption and are transported directly to the liver via the portal vein (bypassing the traditional LCT pathway). Once in the liver, MCTs are used primarily as an energy source. In comparison to LCTs, MCTs are not stored to any significant degree in adipose tissue, nor do they affect the reticuloendothelial system. Because MCTs are ketogenic, these TGs may provide a useful energy source for enterocytes, lymphocytes, and cells of other tissues in hypermetabolically stressed patients. Oxidation of MCTs is less affected by glucose and insulin than LCTs.[110] In addition, oxidation of LCTs can be impaired by slow elimination rates from the plasma or by the requirement of carnitine for intracellular transport. In contrast, the metabolism of MCTs is a carnitine-independent system for transport into the

mitochondria.[111] Because of these metabolic differences, MCTs may be beneficial in attenuating inflammatory stress conditions. The metabolic characteristics of MCTs increase their role as an important lipid source for individuals with impaired and dysfunctional gastrointestinal tracts. For example, MCTs may be beneficial for individuals who have defects of fat digestion and absorption (eg, patients with pancreatitis), as well as those individuals with malabsorption secondary to intestinal resections, inflammatory bowel disease, chylous ascites, or autoimmune enteropathies.

Many enteral products have been designed with MCTs as a significant lipid component to maximize the absorption, metabolism, and tolerance of these products for use in various disease and metabolic conditions (Table 5-4).

Structured Lipids

First developed in the mid-1980s,[112–115] structured lipids are "designer" TG molecules that are specifically synthesized in the laboratory via chemical and/or enzymatic methodology or, more recently, via genetic engineering.[116] The resulting TG mixture contains a randomly esterified pattern of MCTs and LCTs that can contain within the same TG molecule both MCFAs and LCFAs. In structured lipids, the MCFAs are predominantly 8 or 10 carbons in length and usually are esterified at the sn-1 and sn-3 positions, and the LCFA usually is esterified at the sn-2 position on the glycerol backbone of the structured lipid. Usually, the LCFAs are predominantly members of the ω-3 family, such as GLA, EPA, or DHA. As previously stated, the enzymatic activities of gastric and pancreatic lipases predominantly catalyze the release of fatty acids at the sn-1 and sn-3 positions from the glycerol backbone of the structured lipid. This catalysis results in formation of 2-LCFA-monoacylglycerols and, for sn-2 MCFA structured lipids, free MCFAs. In physical mixtures of LCTs and MCTs, this activity results in 2-monoacylglycerols and a mixture of MCFAs and LCFAs.

Unlike pancreatic lipase, gastric lipase does not require bile salts for enzymatic activity and is more efficiently catalytic against the acyl-MCFA in MCFA-esterified TGs.[117] As previously discussed, these more rapidly liberated MCFAs do not require bile salts for absorption, readily enter the portal system for transport, and enter mitochondria independently of the carnitine membrane transport pathway. Consequently, structured lipids offer a defined mechanism to rapidly deliver MCFAs and to provide a more rapid availability of EPA and DHA with, as one result, the entire attendant array of nutritionally positive aspects of these substances. Investigators have demonstrated that fatty acids located at the sn-2 position on the glycerol backbone are preferentially absorbed,[118,119] and, in structured lipids, both EPA and DHA esterified at the sn-2 position are, indeed, more readily absorbed.[120] Furthermore, in experimental animal studies of intestinally injured rats, structured lipids prepared with MCTs and fish oils (containing a range of LCFAs from 18:3n-3 to 22:n-6) infused gastrically were absorbed more quickly in comparison to the physical mixture of the fish oil and MCTs emulsion.[121] Selected human[122,123] and experimental animal EN studies[124–126] have demonstrated various physiological benefits associated with the use of structured lipids, including better fatty acid absorption, lower infection rates, and improved hepatic, renal, and immune function.

Structured lipids are approved for inclusion in certain enteral formulas used in the United States and elsewhere. In addition, PN formulas that contain structured lipids are approved for use in Europe.

The Clinical Impact of Specific Fatty Acids in Parenteral Nutrition

ω-6 Fatty Acids

In the United States, two 100% soybean oil–based lipid emulsions are currently available for use in PN. Soybean oil–based ILEs contain large quantities of linoleic acid. Exclusive provision of soybean oil–based ILEs may therefore greatly exceed dietary recommendations (ie, Dietary Reference Intakes) for ω-6 fatty acids. Fatty acids of the ω-6 family influence the immune system by alteration of membrane structure and function, by modulation of immune function through AA metabolites, and by stimulation of inflammatory cytokines. IV soybean oil emulsions have been shown to depress immune function in both in vitro and ex vivo studies. These types of emulsions have been shown to decrease the cellular immune response in several in vitro studies at varying lipid concentrations. Depression of immunoglobulin M and immunoglobulin A levels, decreases in lymphocyte proliferation, depression of natural killer cell activity, and depression of neutrophil chemotactic motility have been reported with use of soybean oil–based emulsions.[127-131] However, the most significant factor of these in vitro studies seems to be a dose-related response associated with increased immunosuppression in response to increased lipid concentrations. Well-designed, prospective, randomized clinical trials (RCTs) evaluating the effects of soybean oil–based ILEs upon infections and other clinical outcomes are needed.

In a small, prospective, randomized study (N = 57) by Battistella et al,[132] trauma patients who received PN with soybean ILE had more infections, longer ventilation time, and a longer hospital stay compared with patients receiving lipid-free PN. Unfortunately, this study did not administer equivalent amounts of energy to the patients. McCowen and associates[133] performed a randomized study of PN with and without soybean ILE in 40 critically ill patients and found that while infections were more common in the group receiving soybean ILE, the difference was not statistically significant (53% vs 29%; P = 0.2). However, the nutrition regimens used in this study were not isocaloric. Another randomized study by Muller and colleagues[134] followed patients administered PN for 10 days prior to surgery for gastrointestinal cancer. In this study, 46 patients received soybean ILE plus glucose and 66 patients received glucose only; all patients received similar amounts of amino acids.[134] Mortality and major complications affecting the site of operation were significantly higher in the group receiving ILE-containing PN compared with the lipid-free PN group (P <0.05). The study results are, however, confounded by the high energy intake and large amount of lipid (50% of energy) administered to the patients. The quantity of energy and amount of lipid within the ILE used in the study exceeded

2016 ASPEN/SCCM guidelines recommendations. The largest trial to evaluate soybean ILE and infection was performed in patients who had bone marrow transplants.[135] Patients were randomly assigned to low-dose (6% to 8% of energy; n = 259) or standard-dose (25% to 30% of energy; n = 253) ILE-based PN. Investigators found no association between lipid dose within the ILE and first infection. Similar numbers of patients in each group developed bacterial and fungal infections. Data also showed no difference between groups for engraftment or graft-vs-host disease, relapse, or survival. In another, very small study, 15 malnourished patients with advanced gastric or esophageal cancer received 2 weeks of preoperative and 1 week of postoperative isocaloric and isonitrogenous PN with and without soybean-based ILE.[136] Postoperative infections (13 vs 15; 87.5% vs 85.7%) and hospital length of stay (21 vs 23.7 days) were similar between groups. Overall, the clinical data regarding soybean oil–based ILE and infections are contradictory and no clear relationship between the use of soybean oil–based ILE and infections has been established.

The 2016 ASPEN/SCCM guidelines suggest withholding or limiting 100% soybean oil–based ILE during the first week following initiation of PN in the critically ill patient to a maximum of 100 g/wk, if EFAD is a concern. The ASPEN/SCCM task force deemed the quality of the evidence for this recommendation to be very low, and task force members were relatively divided (64% agreement) whether the recommendation should be (1) simply to withhold 100% soybean oil–based ILE or (2) to withhold or limit it to 100 g/wk.[22]

ω-3 Fatty Acids

A number of earlier clinical trials and studies investigated the impact of ILEs that contain fish oil on clinical outcomes among adult patients.[137-156] A few of these studies showed that perioperative ω-3 fatty acid treatment seemed to improve outcomes.[153,156] However, many other investigations of various outcomes among hospitalized patients had inconsistent findings. The lack of consistent results may potentially be explained by analysis limitations,[139] study design limitations,[142] and/or the heterogeneity and complexity of the patient populations in the studies with respect to types of illness, trauma, and/or surgery.

Recent studies suggest use of fish oil and/or other ω-3 fatty acid–containing emulsions may improve outcomes and may lower inflammation as assessed by liver function. In an investigation that included 451 patients distributed among several groups that received either soybean oil–based, olive oil–based, or fish oil PN emulsion, clinical outcomes were significantly improved in the ω-3 and ω-9 groups. When the soybean oil–based ILE group was compared to the fish oil–based ILE group, the times to discontinuation of mechanical ventilation (P = 0.05) and to ICU discharge alive (P = 0.001) were significantly shorter in the fish oil group. Comparison of patients receiving olive oil–based and soybean oil–based ILEs led to a similar result. The olive oil–based ILE group were terminated from mechanical ventilation sooner (P = 0.02), and had a shorter time to ICU discharge alive (P <0.001).[157] In a small (60 patients) RCT, Hall and colleagues[158] showed that, based on a sequential organ failure assessment (SOFA) score,[159] parenteral ω-3 treatment via fish oil administration significantly reduced new organ dysfunction in septic patients.[158] Furthermore, a prospective, double-blind RCT compared the efficacy and safety of an ω-3 fatty acid–enriched MCT/LCT ILE and an MCT/LCT ILE in 99 elective surgery patients with gastric and colorectal cancer.[160] Although no differences were observed between groups in proinflammatory markers, the ω-3–enriched group had significantly lower TG, free fatty acid, and HDL levels. Gong and associates[161] demonstrated a significant decrease 7 days postsurgery in white blood cell count, alanine aminotransferase (ALT), aspartate transaminase (AST), total bilirubin, and prothrombin time in hepatectomy patients who received 100 mL of a 10% fish oil emulsion per day, for 5 days. Another RCT that examined 63 hepatectomy patients with hepatitis type B virus–associated hepatocellular carcinoma, found that fish oil supplementation led to significantly better liver function as well as significantly fewer infectious complications and shorter length of hospital stay.[162] Lastly, a randomized, double-blind, multicenter investigation of 73 intestinal failure patients receiving long-term PN compared a completely soybean-based ILE to an alternative soybean oil–MCT–olive oil–fish oil blend ILE. After 4 weeks of treatment, the latter ILE led to significantly lower ALT, AST, and total bilirubin values.[163]

However, the results of several recent systematic reviews and meta-analyses are substantially less definitive with respect to the influence of ω-3 fatty acid–enriched alternative ILEs on clinical outcomes. A meta-analysis of 6 RCTs that involved 306 patients compared ILEs with soybean oil only, a soybean oil–MCT–olive oil–fish oil blend, and a soybean oil–olive oil blend. It found no significant differences in adverse events and lengths of hospital stay among the trials, whereas both soybean oil–MCT–olive oil–fish oil blend and soybean oil–olive oil blend ILEs similarly lowered liver enzymes relative to soybean oil alone. However, the quality of evidence from the trials that evaluated these ILEs was considered to be moderate to low.[164]

A systematic review of statistically aggregated results from 12 RCTs showed that when alternative lipid ILEs were used to spare soybean oil exposure, trends to lower mortality ($P = 0.20$), duration of mechanical ventilation ($P = 0.09$), and ICU length of stay ($P = 0.13$) were observed.[165] However, compared with soybean oil alone, alternative lipid emulsions had no effect on infectious complications ($P = 0.35$).[165]

Manzanares and colleagues published a systematic review and meta-analysis of parenteral fish oil lipid emulsion studies in critically ill patients that involved statistically aggregated results from 6 RCTs and 390 patients.[166] This analysis found that emulsions that contained fish oil led to a trend toward reduced mortality ($P = 0.08$) and shorter duration of mechanical ventilation ($P = 0.17$), but, as found in the previous analysis,[165] the fish oil emulsions had no effect upon infections ($P = 0.35$).[166] In contrast to the previous analysis, no significant effect on ICU length of stay was found ($P = 0.84$).[166]

A systematic review and meta-analysis of statistically aggregated results from 10 RCTs that examined the effect of fish oil lipid emulsion treatment among 733 patients also led predominantly to only trends, at best, in positive outcomes. There were no significant reductions in mortality ($P = 0.46$); days on mechanical ventilation ($P = 0.14$); hospital length of stay ($P = 0.19$); or ICU length of stay ($P = 0.37$).[167] However, a significant reduction in infectious complications among patients treated with fish oil–containing ILE was found ($P = 0.02$).[167]

Although the evidence discussed here is inconclusive, both the US and Canadian guidelines currently suggest that clinicians can consider the use of non–soybean oil–based ILEs in critical illness. The 2016 ASPEN/SCCM guidelines[22] state that alternative ILEs may provide outcome benefit over soybean oil–based ILEs; however, a recommendation was not made at the time because of the lack of availability of these products in the United States. Members of the ASPEN/SCCM task force suggested that if such ILE formulations become available in the United States, their use be considered in critically ill patients who are appropriate candidates for PN.[22]

Since the publication of the ASPEN/SCCM guidelines, an alternative ILE (Smoflipid; a soybean oil, MCT, olive oil, and fish oil emulsion) has become commercially available in the United States, and another alternative ILE (Clinolipid; a soybean oil and olive oil emulsion) has been approved for use. Clinicians should note that the package inserts for these emulsions provide qualifying statements about their effects upon clinical outcomes. The package insert for the ILE with the soybean oil–MCT–olive oil–fish oil blend states that "the omega-6:omega-3 fatty acid ratio and medium chain triglycerides in Smoflipid have not been shown to improve clinical outcomes compared to other intravenous lipid emulsions." Similarly, the package insert for the ILE with the soybean oil–olive oil blend states that "the omega-3:omega-6 fatty acid ratio in Clinolipid has not been shown to improve clinical outcomes compared to other intravenous lipid emulsions."

ω-9 Fatty Acids

Commercial ILEs with high olive oil content have been developed to reduce ω-6 fatty acid content and thus the risk associated with in vivo oxidative stress and the potential for a proinflammatory environment. When compared with soybean oil–based ILEs, olive oil–based ILEs are less inhibitory of various neutrophil responses, including human neutrophil viability,[168] phagocytic activity,[169,170] inflammatory cytokine production,[169,171] and oxidative burst induction.[169,172] Studies generally demonstrate a greater immune-neutral effect of olive oil–based emulsions when compared with soybean oil–based ILEs. However, well-designed RCTs are needed to examine the effect of olive oil–based ILEs on clinical outcomes.

Observational survey studies and meta-analysis subgroup examinations have demonstrated clinical benefits of olive oil–based vs soybean oil–based ILEs.[157,165] However, in a double-blind RCT of 100 ICU patients, Umpierrez and associates[173] found no differences in clinical outcomes, including rates of infectious and noninfectious complications, between olive oil–based ILE and soybean oil–based ILE.

Recently, Jia and colleagues compared olive oil–based and soybean oil–based ILEs in the largest prospective, randomized, open-label multicenter study to date (N = 458).[174] In this study of surgical patients, the safety and efficacy of a PN regimen including olive oil–based ILE in a multichamber bag and a soybean oil–based ILE PN compounded regimen were compared. The olive oil–based ILE regimen was proven to be effective (noninferior to soybean oil ILE regimen), was well tolerated, and resulted in a significant decrease in infections relative to the soybean oil–based PN (P <0.01).[174] It should be noted that, in studies comparing compounded PN with multichamber PN, rates of bloodstream infections are higher in the compounded group.[175] However, in the trial by Jia et al,[174] there were no differences in bloodstream infections between groups, and most of the infections identified were from pulmonary, incision site, and urinary tract infections.

In a double-blind, prospective RCT, 94 esophageal cancer surgical patients who received either an MCT/LCT or olive oil–based ILE in combination with EN were examined for clinical outcomes.[176] In this study, no differences were observed between groups with respect to ICU length of stay (P = 0.619), hospital length of stay (P = 0.544), total infectious complications (P = 0.533), or, hospital mortality (P = 0.613).

Short-Chain Fatty Acids

Much of the recent nutrition support research has focused on the role of butyrate to alter the gut lumen environment and influence intestinal adaptation in short bowel syndrome. In investigational animal models of PN, the addition of butyrate has been shown to prevent PN-associated mucosal atrophy and improve epithelial surface proliferation.[177] Similarly, in a study that examined calorically matched mice allowed to feed ad libitum (controls), treated with standard PN (amino acids, glucose, micronutrients), or treated with standard PN with added butyrate, the addition of butyrate significantly restored the number of Peyer's patch lymphocytes and immunoglobulin A levels that were reduced in standard PN mice (P <0.05); also, the PN with butyrate treatment restored gut morphology with respect to recovery of crypt and villous height lost as a result of standard PN treatment (P <0.05).[178] Tappenden and colleagues[179,180] have shown that incorporation of SCFA in PN solutions may modulate the transport capacity of glucose and other nutrients and may further improve intestinal adaptation by the upregulation of glucagon-like peptide 2. Notably, levels of butyrate-producing bacteria are reduced in patients with type 2 diabetes and, as previously discussed, concentrations of fecal SCFAs are also reduced in patients with severe SIRS when compared with heathy controls.[102,181] Greater understanding of alterations of the gut microbiota associated with butyrate, and perhaps other SCFAs, may provide insights into how the gut microbiota contribute to disease progression and whether this area may become an important focus for therapeutic intervention. (See Chapter 4 for additional information on gut microbiota.)

Medium- and Long-Chain Triglycerides

Although MCTs are more commonly added to enteral formulas, they have been used in PN mixtures. LCTs and MCTs may be physically mixed to generate an emulsion that simultaneously provides both LCTs and MCTs in varying ratios and percentages, or LCTs may be interesterified either chemically or enzymatically with MCTs to create structured lipids (as discussed earlier in the chapter). Physical mixtures of LCTs and MCTs (50:50 w/w mixture) have been used in PN solutions for years in Europe and other nations outside of the United States.

These ILEs may provide benefit by (1) providing a better oxidized energy source, (2) improving nitrogen balance (attenuating protein catabolism in stress), and (3) providing rapid clearance of lipid from the blood. In addition, patients who receive MCT-LCT emulsions have been shown to have a fatty acid profile (extracted from cellular phospholipids) that is closer to normal when compared with individuals who receive soybean oil–based ILEs.[182] Additionally, emulsions that contain MCTs may provide a more stable lipid emulsion relative to LCT emulsions, because MCT emulsions have decreased susceptibility to peroxidation. However, the use of MCTs in PN may increase the risk of metabolic acidosis and may lead to a lower level of glucose oxidation relative to LCTs alone[6]— possibilities that are particularly important to consider when treating critically ill patients. Nonetheless, the use of MCTs in nutrition seems to be a viable alternative for some patients.

In 2016, Wu and coauthors published a systematic review and meta-analysis of 21 clinical trials that examined the use of structured lipids in 1135 intent-to-treat surgical or critically ill patients.[183] The trials investigated various clinical parameters and clinical outcomes in patients who received either a structured lipid, MCT-LCT PN emulsion (structured lipid group), or a physically mixed, MCT-LCT PN emulsion (MCT/LCT group). The analysis revealed significantly better protein management (P <0.00001) and higher values for prealbumin (P <0.000001) and albumin (P <0.0001) in the structured lipid group. However, plasma TGs values were significantly lower in the structured lipid group relative to the MCT/LCT group (P <0.0001). A trend that almost achieved significance was shorter hospital length of stay in the structured lipid group (P = 0.05). The authors of the analysis concluded that administration of the structured lipid PN emulsion improved nitrogen balance, was more protective of the liver, more efficiently eliminated TGs, and resulted in a strong trend toward a shorter hospital length of stay.[183]

Phytosterols and Vitamin E in Parenteral Nutrition

Plant-based ILEs provide EFAs and a rich energy source to hospitalized and home PN patients. However, prolonged use of these ILEs can carry risks, including the risk for parenteral nutrition–associated liver disease (PNALD), particularly among infants.[184] PNALD encompasses many liver dysfunctions, such as cholestasis (the most common in children), steatosis (the most common in adults), and cirrhosis, that may progress in rare instances to complete liver failure. One possible explanation for these liver disorders is the presence of phytosterols within the lipid emulsion. Phytosterols, the most common of which are campesterol, sitosterol, and stigmasterol, are plant analogues of cholesterol and are found in all currently available plant-based ILE formulations.[185] There is evidence that these compounds, because of their structural similarity to cholesterol, interfere with bile synthesis and transport and thus interfere with bile acid homeostasis. This effect, coupled with the high concentrations of peroxidation-sensitive PUFAs in plant-based ILE that could lead to free radical damage of liver cells, may possibly explain subsequent liver dysfunction.

In animal studies, soybean oil–based emulsions and purified individual phytosterols, particularly stigmasterol, seem to be dominant contributors to the disruption of bile synthesis and secretion, with the subsequent induction of cholestasis.[186] Investigators have explored the possibility that the suspected harmful effects of phytosterols could be ameliorated (1) through use of fish oil that does not contain phytosterols or (2) by adding an antioxidant such as vitamin E (specifically α-tocopherol) to plant-based ILE. To date, the data are conflicting. A mouse study by El Kasmi et al[187] clearly showed that, in contrast to mice that received a soy-based PN emulsion, mice that were given fish oil–based PN did not exhibit PNALD. Furthermore, liver damage and cholestasis were dependent on the presence of phytosterols (stigmasterol in particular) and occurred when phytosterols were added to a fish oil–based PN emulsion. In this instance, the presence of high concentrations of ω-3 fatty acids in the fish oil emulsion did not protect the animals from the effect(s) of added stigmasterol. A more recent examination of the effect of phytosterols in mice by Harris et al[188] suggests that gut microbiota may contribute to, in the authors' terminology, parenteral nutrition–associated liver injury (PNALI), perhaps through interactions of the microbiome with phytosterols. Harris and associates[188] showed that the mouse gut microbiome was altered in mice demonstrating PNALI. Specifically, use of soybean-based PN resulted in PNALI and additionally led to increased appearance of the Erysipelotrichaceae taxa of bacteria in the colonic microbiota. Removal of soybean-based PN attenuated PNALI and significantly reduced the level of Erysipelotrichaceae bacteria. Addition of stigmasterol to fish oil–based PN resulted in the reappearance of Erysipelotrichaceae bacteria at a rate equivalent to that for soybean-based PN animals and again resulted in PNALI.[188] In contrast to these data, Ng et al found no evidence for PNALD in preterm piglets similarly treated with soybean-based ILE–equivalent phytosterols concentrations added to a fish oil emulsion.[189]

In addition to the possible effects of phytosterols on liver function, PUFAs may be involved in lipid peroxidation that in turn causes liver cell damage and, ultimately, aberrant liver function. To counter this problem, antioxidants, such as vitamin E, may be important. A form of vitamin E may be added to fish oil emulsions; additionally, vitamin E can be found naturally in plant oils used in various ILE formulations.[190,191] The 8 isoforms of vitamin E are α-, β-, γ-, and δ-tocopherol and α-, β-, γ-, and δ-tocotrienol, all of which are fat soluble and all of which can act equivalently as an antioxidant. For humans, however, only α-tocopherol is biologically active. The enzymatically synthesized natural form of α-tocopherol present in plants, and, therefore, within the oil derived from them, is known as *RRR-α-tocopherol*. The RRR designation refers to the R orientation of the attached methyl group at each of the 3 chiral centers at carbons 2 (ring), 4′, and 8′ (side chain) of the molecule. One may also use synthetic vitamin E, which is known as all-rac-α-tocopherol (all-racemic-α-tocopherol). Because of chemical instead of enzymatic synthesis, *all-rac-α*-tocopherol has 8 stereoisomers of α-tocopherol (RRR, RRS, RSR, RSS, SRR, SRS, SSR, SSS); only the 4 with R chirality at the 2 (ring) position, known as *2R-α-tocopherol*, have biological activity in humans (2, 4′, and 8′ positions yield: RRR, RRS, RSR, RSS). All 8 of the stereoisomers, however, have equivalent antioxidant activity.

Studies that examined the influence of vitamin E on the occurrence of PNALD have led to conflicting results. In addition to studying the effect of phytosterols on PNALD, Ng et al[189] examined the effect of α-tocopherol on the occurrence of PNALD through addition of RRR-α-tocopherol to soybean-based ILE at a concentration that matched the biological equivalents of RRR-α-tocopherol concentration already present in the fish oil emulsion. Under this condition, addition of vitamin E ameliorated PNALD in preterm piglets. However, a similar study by Muto and coauthors[192] found that addition of vitamin E—in this instance *all-rac-α-tocopherol acetate*—to soybean-based ILE, had no effect upon cholestasis, level of inflammation, or level of oxidative stress in neonatal, term piglets.

Although data are conflicting regarding the ameliorating effect of vitamin E on PNALD, the many animal studies and human data extensively reviewed by Zaloga[186] are consistent with the hypothesis that higher phytosterol exposure is associated with PNALD and, reduction of soybean-based ILE and/or use of fish oil that does not contain any phytosterols can reduce the incidence of PNALD. Appropriately designed and powered RCTs to investigate this critically important area are needed.

Conclusion

Various enteral and ILE formulations provide numerous options for treating critically ill patients, but data are insufficient to recommend specific enteral or ILE formulations for many conditions (eg SIRS, ARDS), situations (eg, surgery, trauma), or patient populations (eg, adults, preterm or term infants). Because the appropriate selection of enteral and ILE formulations can save lives, it is critical that well-designed and adequately powered studies of the use of these formulations remain a goal of the medical and scientific community.

References

1. Serhan CN. Resolvins and protectins: novel lipid mediators in anti-inflammation and resolution. *Scand J Food Nutr*. 2006;50 (suppl 2):68–78.
2. Le HD, Meisel JA, de Meijer VE, Gura KM, Puder M. The essentiality of arachidonic acid and docosahexaenoic acid. *Prostaglandins Leukot Essent Fatty Acids*. 2009;81:165–170.
3. Deckelbaum RJ, Worgall TS, Seo T. Fatty acids and gene expression. *Am J Clin Nutr*. 2006;83(suppl):1520S–1525S.
4. Kopecky J, Rossmeisl M, Flachs P, et al. Symposium on "Frontiers in adipose tissue biology" n-3 PUFA: bioavailability and modulation of adipose tissue function. *Proc Nutr Soc*. 2009;68:361–369.
5. Minihane AM. Nutrient gene interactions in lipid metabolism. *Curr Opin Clin Nutr Metab Care*. 2009;12:357–363.
6. Wanten GJA, Calder PC. Immune modulation by parenteral lipid emulsions. *Am J Clin Nutr*. 2007;85:1171–1184.
7. Rhoads RA. Lipid digestion and absorption. In: Rhoads RA, Bell DR, eds. *Medical Physiology: Principles for Clinical Medicine*. 4th ed. Baltimore, MD: Wolters Kluwer; 2012.
8. Voet D, Voet JG, Pratt CW. Lipid digestion, absorption and transport. In: *Fundamentals of Biochemistry*. 2nd ed. Hoboken, NJ: John Wiley and Sons; 2006.
9. Ferezou J, Bach AC. Structure and metabolic fate of triacylglycerol and phospholipid-rich particles of commercial parenteral fat emulsions. *Nutrition*. 1999;15:44–50.

10. Whittaker JS, Allard JP, Freeman HJ. Nutrition in gastrointestinal disease. In: Thomson ABR, Shaffer EA, eds. *First Principles of Gastroenterology: The Basis of Disease and an Approach to Management*. 5th ed. Toronto, Canada: Janssen-Ortho; 2009:49–78.

11. Seidel D, Alaupovic P, Furman RH, et al. A lipoprotein characterizing obstructive jaundice 1. Method for quantitative separation and identification of lipoproteins in jaundiced subjects. *J Clin Invest*. 1969;48:1211–1223.

12. Torsvik H, Berg K, Magnani HN, et al. Identification of the abnormal cholestatic lipoprotein (LP-X) in familial lecithin: cholesterol acyltransferase deficiency. *FEBS Lett*. 1972;24:165–168.

13. Miles JM, Park Y, Harris WS. Lipoprotein lipase and triglyceride-rich lipoprotein metabolism. *Nutr Clin Pract*. 2001;16:273–279.

14. Goulet O. Lipid emulsions: dosage and monitoring. *Education and Critical Practice Program. 23rd ESPEN Congress Munich*. 2001:87–93.

15. Rader DJ, Rosas S. Management of selected lipid abnormalities. Hypertriglyceridemia, low HDL cholesterol, lipoprotein(a), in thyroid and renal diseases, and post-transplantation. *Med Clin N Am*. 2000;84:43–61.

16. Llop J, Sabin P, Garau M, et al. The importance of clinical factors in parenteral nutrition-associated hypertriglyceridemia. *Clin Nutr*. 2003;22:577–583.

17. Wiese HF, Hansen AE, Adam DJ. Essential fatty acids in infant nutrition. I. Linoleic acid requirement in terms of serum di-, tri- and tetraenoic acid levels. *J Nutr*. 1958;66:345–360.

18. Bistrian BR. Clinical aspects of essential fatty acid metabolism: Jonathan Rhoads Lecture. *JPEN J Parenter Enteral Nutr*. 2003;27:168–175.

19. Sardesai VM. The essential fatty acids. *Nutr Clin Pract*. 1992;7:179–186.

20. Wardlaw GM. *Perspectives in Nutrition*. 4th ed. New York: McGraw-Hill; 1999.

21. Seidner DL, Mascioli EA, Istfan NW, et al. Effects of long-chain triglyceride emulsions on reticuloendothelial system function in humans. *JPEN J Parenter Enteral Nutr*. 1989;13:614–619.

22. McClave SA, Taylor BE, Martindale RG, et al. Guidelines for the provision and assessment of nutrition support therapy in the adult critically ill patient: Society of Critical Care Medicine (SCCM) and American Society for Parenteral and Enteral Nutrition (A.S.P.E.N.). *JPEN J Parenter Enteral Nutr*. 2016;40:159–211.

23. Pironi L, Arends J, Bozzetti F, et al. ESPEN guidelines on chronic intestinal failure in adults. *Clin Nutr*. 2016;35:247–307.

24. Mirtallo J, Canada T, Johnson D, et al. Safe practices for parenteral nutrition. *JPEN J Parenter Enteral Nutr*. 2004;28(suppl):S39–S70.

25. A.S.P.E.N. Board of Directors and the Clinical Guideline Task Force. Guidelines for the use of parenteral and enteral nutrition in adult and pediatric patients. *JPEN J Parenter Enteral Nutr*. 2002;26(suppl):1SA–138SA.

26. Delafosse B, Viale JP, Tissot S, et al. Effects of glucose-to-lipid ratio and type of lipid on substrate oxidation rate in patients. *Am J Physiol*. 1994;267:E775–E780.

27. Battistella FD, Widergren JT, Anderson JT, et al. A prospective, randomized trial of intravenous fat emulsion administration in trauma victims requiring total parenteral nutrition. *J Trauma*.1997;43:52–60.

28. A.S.P.E.N. Board of Directors. Guidelines for the use of parenteral and enteral nutrition in adult and pediatric patients. *JPEN J Parenter Enteral Nutr*. 1993;17(4 Suppl):1SA–52SA.

29. Klein S, Miles JM. Metabolic effects of long-chain and medium-chain triglyceride emulsions in humans. *JPEN J Parenter Enteral Nutr*. 1994;18:396–397.

30. Burr GO, Burr MD. A new deficiency disease produced by the rigid exclusion of fat from the diet. *J Biol Chem*. 1929;82:345–367.

31. Holman RT, Johnson SB, Hatch TF. A case of human linolenic acid deficiency involving neurological abnormalities. *Am J Clin Nutr*. 1982;35: 617–623.

32. Wene JD, Connor WE, Den Besten L. The development of essential fatty acid deficiency in healthy men fed fat-free diets intravenously and orally. *J Clin Invest*. 1975;56:127–134.

33. Richardson TJ, Sgoutas D. Essential fatty acid deficiency in four adult patients during total parenteral nutrition. *Am J Clin Nutr*. 1975;28:258–263.

34. Fleming CR, Smith LM, Hodges RE. Essential fatty acid deficiency in adults receiving total parenteral nutrition. *Am J Clin Nutr*. 1976;29:976–983.

35. Cederholm TE, Berg AB, Johansson EK, et al. Low levels of essential fatty acids are related to impaired delayed skin hypersensitivity in malnourished chronically ill elderly people. *Eur J Clin Invest*. 1994;24:615–620.

36. Hulsey TK, O'Neill JA, Neblett WR, et al. Experimental wound healing in essential fatty acid deficiency. *J Pediatr Surg*. 1980;15:505–508.

37. Dupont J, Dowd MK. Eicosanoid synthesis as a functional measurement of essential fatty acid requirement. *J Am Coll Nutr*. 1990;9:272–276.

38. Holman RT, Smythe L, Johnson S. Effect of sex and age on fatty acid composition of human serum lipids. *Am J Clin Nutr*. 1979;32:2390–2399.

39. Dickerson RN, Rosato EF, Mullen JL. Net protein anabolism with hypocaloric parenteral nutrition in obese stressed patients. *Am J Clin Nutr*. 1986;44:747–755.

40. Leung N, O'Brien T, McMahon MM. Parenteral feeding in a patient with hypertriglyceridemia and increased liver enzyme levels. *Endocr Pract*. 1999;5:194–197.

41. McClave SA, Martindale RG, Vanek VW, et al. Guidelines for the provision and assessment of nutrition support therapy in the adult critically ill patient: Society of Critical Care Medicine (SCCM) and American Society for Parenteral and Enteral Nutrition (A.S.P.E.N.). *JPEN J Parenter Enteral Nutr*. 2009;33:277–316.

42. Bjerve KS, Mostad I, Thoresen L. Alpha-linolenic acid deficiency in patients on long-term gastric tube feeding: estimation of linolenic acid and long-chain unsaturated n-3 fatty acid requirement in man. *Am J Clin Nutr*. 1987;15:897–904.

43. Heird WC, Lapillonne A. The role of essential fatty acids in development. *Annu Rev Nutr*. 2005;25:549–571.

44. Nandivada P, Fell GL, Mitchell PD, et al. Long-term fish oil lipid emulsion use in children with intestinal failure-associated liver disease. *JPEN J Parenter Enteral Nutr*. 2016(Mar 9);pii: 0148607116633796. Epub ahead of print.

45. Jeppesen PB, Hoy CE, Mortensen PB. Differences in essential fatty acid requirements by enteral and parenteral routes of administration in patients with fat malabsorption. *Am J Clin Nutr*. 1999;70:78–84.

46. Abushufa R, Reed P, Weinkove C, et al. Essential fatty acid status in patients on long-term home parenteral nutrition. *JPEN J Parenter Enteral Nutr*. 1995;19:286–290.

47. Jeppesen PB, Hoy CE, Mortensen PB. Essential fatty acid deficiency in patients receiving home parenteral nutrition. *Am J Clin Nutr*. 1998;68:126–133.

48. Ling PR, Ollero M, Khaodhiar L, et al. Disturbances in essential fatty acid metabolism in patients receiving long-term home parenteral nutrition. *Dig Dis Sci*. 2002;47:1679–1685.

49. Pironi L, Belluzzi A, Miglioli M. Low levels of essential fatty acids in the red blood cell membrane phospholipid fraction of long term home parenteral nutrition patients. *JPEN J Parenter Enteral Nutr*. 1996;20:377–378.

50. Mascioli EA, Lopes SM, Champagne C, et al. Essential fatty acid deficiency and home total parenteral nutrition patients. *Nutrition*. 1996;12:245–249

51. Gramlich L, Meddings L, Alberda C, et al. Essential fatty acid deficiency in 2015: the impact of novel intravenous lipid emulsions. *JPEN J Parenter Enteral Nutr.* 2015;39(1 Suppl):61S–66S.

52. Gottschlich MM. Selection of optimal lipid sources in enteral and parenteral nutrition. *Nutr Clin Pract.* 1992;7:152–165.

53. Goetzl EJ, An S, Smith WL. Specificity of expression and effects of eicosanoid mediators in normal physiology and human diseases. *FASEB J.* 1995;9:1051–1058.

54. Phipps RP, Stein SH, Roper RL. A new view of prostaglandin-E regulation of the immune response. *Immunol Today.* 1991;12:349–352.

55. Janniger CK, Racis SP. The arachidonic acid cascade: an immunologically based review. *J Med.* 1987;18:69–80

56. Smith WL, Meade EA, DeWitt DL. Pharmacology of prostaglandin endoperoxide synthase isozymes-1 and -2. *Ann N Y Acad Sci.* 1994;714:136–142.

57. O'Banion MK. Cyclooxygenase-2: molecular biology, pharmacology and neurobiology. *Crit Rev Neurobiol.* 1999;13:45–82.

58. Choudhry MA, Ahmed Z, Sayeed MM. PGE(2)-mediated inhibition of T-cell p59 (fyn) is independent of cAMP. *Am J Physiol.* 1999;277:C302–C309.

59. Choudhry MA, Hockberger PE, Sayeed MM. PGE2 suppresses mitogen-induced Ca^{2+} mobilization in T cells. *Am J Physiol.* 1999;277:R1741–R1748.

60. Cosme R, Lublin D, Takafuji V, et al. Prostanoids in human colonic mucosa: effects of inflammation on PGE(2) receptor expression. *Hum Immunol.* 2000;61:684–696.

61. Herold PM, Kinsella JE. Fish oil consumption and decreased risk of cardiovascular disease: a comparison of findings from animal and human feeding trials. *Am J Clin Nutr.* 1986;43:566–598.

62. Dyerberg J, Bang HO, Stoffersen E, et al. Eicosapentaenoic acid and prevention of thrombosis and atherosclerosis? *Lancet.* 1978;2:117–119.

63. Palombo JD, DeMichele SJ, Boyce PJ, et al. Metabolism of dietary alpha-linolenic acid vs. eicosapentaenoic acid in rat immune cell phospholipids during endotoxemia. *Lipids.* 1998;33:1099–1105.

64. Fan YY, Chapkin RS. Importance of dietary γ-linolenic acid in human health and nutrition. *J Nutr.* 1998;128:1411–1414.

65. Calder PC. Omega-3 fatty acids and inflammatory processes. *Nutrients.* 2010;2:355–374.

66. Maddox JF, Serhan, CN. Lipoxin A4 and B4 are potent stimuli for human monocyte migration and adhesion: selective inactivation by dehydrogenation and reduction. *J Exp Med.* 1996;183:137–146.

67. Serhan CN, Fiore S, Brezinski DA, Lynch S. Lipoxin A4 metabolism by differentiated HL-60 cells and human monocytes: conversion to novel 15-oxo and dihydro products. *Biochemistry.* 1993;32:6313–6319.

68. Serhan CN. Lipoxins and aspirin-triggered 15-epi-lipoxin biosynthesis: an update and role in anti-inflammation and proresolution. *Prostaglandins Other Lipid Mediat.* 2002;68-69:433–455.

69. Amiram A, Serhan CN. Resolvins and protectins in the termination program of acute inflammation. *Trends Immunol.* 2007;28:176–183.

70. Schmidt EB, Arnesen H, Christensen JH, et al. Marine n-3 polyunsaturated fatty acids and coronary heart disease. Part II. *Thromb Res.* 2005;115:257–262.

71. Kris-Etherton PM, Harris WS, Appel LJ, et al. Fish consumption, fish oil, omega-3 fatty acids, and cardiovascular disease. *Circulation.* 2002;106:2747–2757.

72. Hibbeln JR, Nieminen LR, Blasbalg TL, et al. Healthy intakes of n-3 and n-6 fatty acids: estimations considering worldwide diversity. *Am J Clin Nutr.* 2006;83(suppl):1483S–1493S.

73. Mozaffarian D, Wu JH. Omega-3 fatty acids and cardiovascular disease: effects on risk factors, molecular pathways, and clinical events. *J Am Coll Cardiol.* 2011;58:2047–2067.

74. Jacobson TA, Glickstein SB, Rowe JD, et al. Effects of eicosapentaenoic acid and docosahexaenoic acid on low-density lipoprotein cholesterol and other lipids: a review. *J Clin Lipidol.* 2012;6(1):5–18.

75. Mohebi-Nejad A, Bikdeli B. Omega-3 supplements and cardiovascular diseases. *Tanaffos.* 2014;13:6–14.

76. Rizos EC, Ntzani EE, Bika E, et al. Association between omega-3 fatty acid supplementation and risk of major cardiovascular disease events: a systematic review and meta-analysis. *JAMA.* 2012;308:1024–1033.

77. Kotwal S, Jun M, Sullivan D, et al. Omega 3 fatty acids and cardiovascular outcomes: systematic review and meta-analysis. *Circ Cardiovasc Qual Outcomes.* 2012;5:808–818.

78. Mozaffarian D, Marchioli R, Macchia A, et al. Fish oil and postoperative atrial fibrillation: the Omega-3 Fatty Acids for Prevention of Postoperative Atrial Fibrillation (OPERA) randomized trial. *JAMA.* 2012;308:2001–2011.

79. Kowey PR, Reiffel JA, Ellenbogen KA, et al. Efficacy and safety of prescription omega-3 fatty acids for the prevention of recurrent symptomatic atrial fibrillation: a randomized controlled trial. *JAMA.* 2010;304:2363–2372.

80. Roncaglioni MC, Tombesi M, Avanzini F, et al. Risk and Prevention Study Collaborative Group. n-3 fatty acids in patients with multiple cardiovascular risk factors. *N Engl J Med.* 2013;368:1800–1808.

81. Stone NJ, Robinson J, Lichtenstein AH, et al. 2013 ACC/AHA guideline on the treatment of blood cholesterol to reduce atherosclerotic cardiovascular risk in adults: a report of the American College of Cardiology/American Heart Association Task Force on Practice Guidelines. *Circulation.* Epub Nov. 12, 2013. doi:10.1161/01.cir.0000437738.63853.7a.

82. Raymond C, Cho L, Rocco M, et al. New guidelines for reduction of blood cholesterol: was it worth the wait? *Cleve Clin J Med.* 2014;81:11–19.

83. Chowdhury R, Stevens S, Gorman D, et al. Association between fish consumption, long chain omega 3 fatty acids, and risk of cerebrovascular disease: systematic review and meta-analysis. *BMJ.* 2012;345:e6698.

84. de Acilu MG, Leal S, Caralt B, et al. The role of omega-3 polyunsaturated fatty acids in the treatment of patients with acute respiratory distress syndrome: a clinical review. *Biomed Res Int.* 2015;2015:653750. doi:10.1155/2015/653750.

85. Zhu D, Zhang Y, Li S, et al. Enteral omega-3 fatty acid supplementation in adult patients with acute respiratory distress syndrome: a systematic review of randomized controlled trials with meta-analysis and trial sequential analysis. *Intensive Care Med.* 2014;40:504–512.

86. Kagan I, Cohen J, Stein M, et al. Preemptive enteral nutrition enriched with eicosapentaenoic acid, gamma-linolenic acid and antioxidants in severe multiple trauma: a prospective, randomized, double-blind study. *Intensive Care Med.* 2015;41:460–469.

87. Trépanier MO, Hopperton KE, Orr SK, et al. n-3 polyunsaturated fatty acids in animal models with neuroinflammation: an update. *Eur J Pharmacol.* 2016;785:187–206.

88. Painter TJ, Rickerds J, Alban RF. Immune enhancing nutrition in traumatic brain injury—a preliminary study. *Int J Surg.* 2015;21:70–74.

89. Chow O, Barbul A. Immunonutrition: role in wound healing and tissue regeneration. *Adv Wound Care (New Rochelle).* 2014;3:46–53.

90. Chevrou-Séverac H, Pinget C, Cerantola Y, et al. Cost-effectiveness analysis of immune-modulating nutritional support for gastrointestinal cancer patients. *Clin Nutr.* 2014;33:649–654.

91. Miller M, Stone NJ, Ballantyne C, et al. Triglycerides and cardiovascular disease: a scientific statement from the American Heart Association. *Circulation.* 2011;123:2292–2333.

92. Samieri C, Féart C, Proust-Lima C, et al. Olive oil consumption, plasma oleic acid, and stroke incidence: the Three-City Study. *Neurology*. 2011;77:418–425.

93. Corbett P. Research in the area of high oleic oils. *Plant Biotechnol Inst Bull*. 2002;1:3.

94. Gassull MA, Fernández-Bañares F, Cabré E, et al. European Group on Enteral Nutrition in Crohn's Disease. Fat composition may be a clue to explain the primary therapeutic effect of enteral nutrition in Crohn's disease: results of a double blind randomised multicentre European trial. *Gut*. 2002;51:164–168.

95. Gonzailez-Huix F, de Leon R, Fernandez-Baniares F, et al. Polymeric enteral diets as primary treatment of active Crohn's disease: a prospective steroid controlled trial. *Gut*. 1993;34:778–782.

96. Rombeau JL, Kripke SA. Metabolic and intestinal effects of short chain fatty acids. *JPEN J Parenter Enteral Nutr*. 1990;14(suppl):181S–185S.

97. Cook SI, Sellin JH. Review article: short chain fatty acids in health and disease. *Aliment Pharmacol Ther*. 1998;12:499–507.

98. Segain JP, Raingeard de la Bletiere D, Bourreille A, et al. Butyrate inhibits inflammatory responses through NFkappaB inhibition: implications for Crohn's disease. *Gut*. 2000;47:397–403.

99. Miller SJ. Cellular and physiological effects of short-chain fatty acids. *Mini Rev Med Chem*. 2004;4:839–845.

100. Daly K, Cuff MA, Fung F, et al. The importance of colonic butyrate transport to the regulation of genes associated with colonic tissue homeostasis. *Biochem Soc Trans*. 2005;33:733–735.

101. Arora T, Bäckhed F. The gut microbiota and metabolic disease: current understanding and future perspectives. *J Intern Med*. 2016(Apr 12). Epub ahead of print. doi:10.1111/joim.12508.

102. Yamada T, Shimizu K, Ogura H, et al. Rapid and sustained long-term decrease of fecal short-chain fatty acids in critically ill patients with systemic inflammatory response syndrome. *JPEN J Parenter Enteral Nutr*. 2015;39:569–577.

103. Institute of Medicine. *Dietary Reference Intakes: Energy, Carbohydrate, Fiber, Fat, Fatty Acids, Cholesterol, Protein, and Amino Acids*. Washington, DC: National Academies Press; 2005.

104. Ascherio A, Katan MB, Zock PL, et al. Trans fatty acids and coronary heart disease. *N Engl J Med*. 1999;340:1994–1998.

105. Tholstrup T, Ehnholm C, Jauhiainen M, et al. Effects of medium-chain fatty acids and oleic acid on blood lipids, lipoproteins, glucose, insulin, and lipid transfer protein activities. *Am J Clin Nutr*. 2004;79:564–569.

106. St-Onge MP, Lamarche B, Mauger JF, et al. Consumption of a functional oil rich in phytosterols and medium-chain triglyceride oil improves plasma lipid profiles in men. *J Nutr*. 2003;133:1815–1820.

107. Hayes KC. Medium-chain triacylglycerols may not raise cholesterol. *Am J Clin Nutr*. 2000;72:1583.

108. Tsai YH, Park S, Kovacic J, et al. Mechanisms mediating lipoprotein responses to diets with medium-chain triglyceride and lauric acid. *Lipids*. 1999;34:895–905.

109. Hayes KC, Lindsey S, Pronczuk A, et al. Fatty acid modulation of lipoprotein metabolism by natural triglycerides in hamsters: lipoprotein turnover and hepatic mRNA abundance. In: Christophe A, ed. *Structurally Modified Food Fats: Synthesis, Biochemistry, and Use*. Champaign, IL: AOCS Press;1998:170–181.

110. McGarry JD, Foster DW. The regulation of ketogenesis from octanoic acids. The role of the tricarboxylic acid cycle and fatty acid synthesis. *J Biol Chem*. 1971;246:1149–1159.

111. Bohles H, Akcetin Z, Lehnert W. The influence of intravenous medium and long-chain triglycerides and carnitine on the excretion of dicarboxylic acids. *JPEN J Parenter Enteral Nutr*. 1987;11:46–48.

112. Bach AC, Babayan VK. Medium-chain triglycerides: an update. *Am J Clin Nutr*. 1982;36:950–962.

113. Mok KT, Maiz A, Yamazaki K, et al. Structured medium-chain and long-chain triglyceride emulsions are superior to physical mixtures in sparing body protein in the burned rat. *Metabolism*. 1984;33:910–915.

114. Babayan VK. Medium chain triglycerides and structured lipids. *Lipids*. 1987;22:417–420.

115. Lee KT, Akoh CC. Structured lipids: synthesis and applications. *Food Rev Int*. 1998;14:17–34.

116. Osborn HT, Akoh CC. Structured lipids novel fats with medical, nutraceutical and food applications. *Compr Rev Food Sci Food Safety*. 2002;1:93–103.

117. Phan CT, Tso P. Intestinal lipid absorption and transport. *Front Biosci*. 2001;6:299–319.

118. Jensen MM, Christensen MS, Hoy CE. Intestinal absorption of octanoic, decanoic, and linoleic acids: effect of triglyceride structure. *Ann Nutr Metab*. 1994;38:104–116.

119. Stein J. Chemically defined structured lipids: current status and future directions in gastrointestinal diseases. *Int J Colorectal Dis*.1999;14:79–85.

120. Christensen MS, Hoy CE, Becker CC, et al. Intestinal absorption and lymphatic transport of eicosapentaenoic (EPA), docosahexaenoic (DHA), and decanoic acids: dependence on intramolecular triacylglycerol structure. *Am J Clin Nutr*. 1995;61:56–61.

121. Tso P, Lee T, Demichele SJ. Lymphatic absorption of structured triglycerides vs. physical mix in a rat model of fat malabsorption. *Am J Physiol*. 1999;277:G333–G340.

122. Swails WS, Kenler AS, Driscoll DF, et al. Effect of fish oil structured lipid-based diet on prostaglandin release from mononuclear cells in cancer patients after surgery. *JPEN J Parenter Enteral Nutr*. 1997;21:266–274.

123. Kenler AS, Swails WS, Driscoll DF, et al. Early enteral feeding in postsurgical cancer patients. Fish oil structured lipid-based polymeric formula versus a standard polymeric formula. *Ann Surg*. 1996;223:316–333.

124. Lee KT, Akoh CC, Flatt WP, et al. Nutritional effects of enzymatically modified soybean oil with caprylic acid versus physical mixture analogue in obese Zucker rats. *J Agric Food Chem*. 2000;48:5696–5701.

125. Mu H, Hoy CE. Effects of different medium-chain fatty acids on intestinal absorption of structured triacylglycerols. *Lipids*. 2000;35:83–89.

126. Straarup EM, Hoy CE. Structured lipids improve fat absorption in normal and malabsorbing rats. *J Nutr*. 2000;130:2802–2808.

127. Salo M. Inhibition of immunoglobulin synthesis in vitro by intravenous lipid emulsion (Intralipid). *JPEN J Parenter Enteral Nutr*. 1990;14:459–462.

128. Ladisch S, Poplack DG, Blaese RM. Inhibition of human lymphoproliferation by intravenous lipid emulsion. *Clin Immunol Immunopathol*. 1982;25:196–202.

129. Granato D, Blum S, Rossle C, et al. Effects of parenteral lipid emulsions with different fatty acid composition on immune cell functions in vitro. *JPEN J Parenter Enteral Nutr*. 2000;24:113–118.

130. Loo LS, Tang JP, Kohl S. Inhibition of cellular cytotoxicity of leukocytes for herpes simplex virus-infected cells in vitro and in vivo by Intralipid. *J Infect Dis*. 1982;146:64–70.

131. Kohelet D, Peller S, Arbel E, Goldberg M. Preincubation with intravenous lipid emulsion reduces chemotactic motility of neutrophils in cord blood. *JPEN J Parenter Enteral Nutr*. 1990;14:472–473.

132. Battistella FD, Widergren JT, Anderson JT, et al. A prospective randomized trial of intravenous fat emulsion administration in trauma victims requiring total parenteral nutrition. *J Trauma*.1997;43:52–58.

133. McCowen KC, Friel C, Sternberg J, et al. Hypocaloric total parenteral nutrition: effectiveness in prevention of hyperglycemia and

infectious complications: a randomized clinical trial. *Crit Care Med.* 2000;28:3606–3611.

134. Muller JM, Keller HW, Brenner U, et al. Indications and effects of preoperative parenteral nutrition. *World J Surg.* 1986;10:53–63.

135. Lenssen P, Bruemmer BA, Bowden RA, et al. Intravenous lipid dose and incidence of bacteremia and fungemia in patients undergoing bone marrow transplantation. *Am J Clin Nutr.* 1998;67:927–933.

136. Dionigi P, Dionigi R, Prati U, et al. Effect of Intralipid on some immunological parameters and leukocyte functions in patients with esophageal and gastric cancer. *Clin Nutr.* 1985;4:229–234.

137. Berger MM, Tappy L, Revelly JP, et al. Fish oil after abdominal aorta aneurysm surgery. *Eur J Clin Nutr.* 2008;62:1116–1122.

138. Friesecke S, Lotze C, Köhler J, et al. Fish oil supplementation in the parenteral nutrition of critically ill medical patients: a randomised controlled trial. *Intensive Care Med.* 2008;34:1411–1420.

139. Grimm H, Mertes N, Goeters C, et al. Improved fatty acid and leukotriene pattern with a novel lipid emulsion in surgical patients. *Eur J Nutr.* 2006;45:55–60.

140. Grimminger F, Mayser P, Papavassilis C, et al. A double-blind, randomized, placebo-controlled trial of n-3 fatty acid based lipid infusion in acute, extended guttate psoriasis. Rapid improvement of clinical manifestations and changes in neutrophil leukotrienes profile. *Clin Invest.* 1993;71:634–643.

141. Heller AR, Rössel T, Gottschlich B, et al. Omega-3 fatty acids improve liver and pancreas function in postoperative cancer patients. *Int J Cancer.* 2004;111:611–616.

142. Heller AR, Rössler S, Litz RJ, et al. Omega-3 fatty acids improve the diagnosis-related clinical outcome. *Crit Care Med.* 2006;34:972–979.

143. Katz DP, Manner T, Furst P, et al. The use of an intravenous fish oil emulsion enriched with omega-3 fatty acids in patients with cystic fibrosis. *Nutrition.* 1996;12:334–339.

144. Klek S, Kulig J, Szczepanik AM, et al. The clinical value of parenteral immunonutrition in surgical patients. *Acta Chir Belg.* 2005;105:175–179.

145. Leeb BF, Sautner J, Andel I, et al. Intravenous application of omega-3 fatty acids in patients with active rheumatoid arthritis. The ORA-1 trial. An open pilot study. *Lipids.* 2006;41:29–34.

146. Liang B, Wang S, Ye YJ, et al. Impact of postoperative omega-3 fatty acid-supplemented parenteral nutrition on clinical outcomes and immunomodulations in colorectal cancer patients. *World J Gastroenterol.* 2008;14:2434–2439.

147. Mayer K, Fegbeutel C, Hattar K, et al. Omega-3 vs. omega-6 lipid emulsions exert differential influence on neutrophils in septic shock patients: impact on plasma fatty acids and lipid mediator generation. *Intensive Care Med.* 2003;29:1472–1481.

148. Mayser P, Mayer K, Mahloudjian M, et al. A double-blind, randomized, placebo-controlled trial of n-3 versus n-6 fatty acid-based lipid infusion in atopic dermatitis. *JPEN J Parenter Enteral Nutr.* 2002;26:151–158.

149. Mayser P, Mrowietz U, Arenberger P, et al. Omega 3 fatty acid-based lipid infusion in patients with chronic plaque psoriasis: results of a double-blind, randomized, placebo-controlled, multicenter trial. *J Am Acad Dermatol.* 1998;38:539–547. (Erratum in *J Am Acad Dermatol.* 1998;39:421.)

150. Mertes N, Grimm H, Fürst P, et al. Safety and efficacy of a new parenteral lipid emulsion (Smoflipid) in surgical patients: a randomized, double-blind, multicenter study. *Ann Nutr Metab.* 2006;50:253–259.

151. Sabater J, Masclans JR, Sacanell J, et al. Effects on hemodynamics and gas exchange of omega-3 fatty acid-enriched lipid emulsion in acute respiratory distress syndrome (ARDS): a prospective, randomized, double-blind, parallel group study. *Lipids Health Dis.* 2008;7:39.

152. Senkal M, Geier B, Hannemann M, et al. Supplementation of omega-3 fatty acids in parenteral nutrition beneficially alters phospholipid fatty acid pattern. *JPEN J Parenter Enteral Nutr.* 2007;31:12–17.

153. Tsekos E, Reuter C, Stehle P, et al. Perioperative administration of parenteral fish oil supplements in a routine clinical setting improves patient outcome after major abdominal surgery. *Clin Nutr.* 2004;23:325–330.

154. Wang X, Li W, Li N, et al. Omega-3 fatty acids-supplemented parenteral nutrition decreases hyperinflammatory response and attenuates systemic disease sequelae in severe acute pancreatitis: a randomized and controlled study. *JPEN J Parenter Enteral Nutr.* 2008;32:236–241.

155. Weiss G, Meyer F, Matthies B, et al. Immunomodulation by perioperative administration of n-3 fatty acids. *Brit J Nutr.* 2002;87(Suppl 1):S89–S94.

156. Wichmann MW, Thul P, Czarnetzki HD, et al. Evaluation of clinical safety and beneficial effects of a fish oil containing lipid emulsion (Lipoplus, MLF541): data from a prospective, randomized, multicenter trial. *Crit Care Med.* 2007;35:700–706.

157. Edmunds CE, Brody RA, Parrott JS, et al. The effects of different IV fat emulsions on clinical outcomes in critically ill patients. *Crit Care Med.* 2014;42:1168–1177.

158. Hall TC, Bilku DK, Al-Leswas D, et al. A randomized controlled trial investigating the effects of parenteral fish oil on survival outcomes in critically ill patients with sepsis. *JPEN J Parenter Enteral Nutr.* 2015;39:301–312

159. Vincent JL, Moreno R, Willatts S, et al. The SOFA (Sepsis-related Organ Failure Assessment) score to describe organ dysfunction/failure. On behalf of the Working Group on Sepsis-Related Problems of the European Society of Intensive Care Medicine. *Intensive Care Med.* 1996;22:707–710.

160. Ma CJ, Wu JM, Tsai HL, et al. Prospective double-blind randomized study on the efficacy and safety of an n-3 fatty acid enriched intravenous fat emulsion in postsurgical gastric and colorectal cancer patients. *Nutr J.* 2015;14:9–20.

161. Gong Y, Liu Z, Liao Y, et al. Effectiveness of ω-3 polyunsaturated fatty acids based lipid emulsions for treatment of patients after hepatectomy: a prospective clinical trial. *Nutrients.* 2016;8:357–364.

162. Wu Z, Qina J, Pu L. Omega-3 fatty acid improves the clinical outcome of hepatectomized patients with hepatitis B virus (HBV)-associated hepatocellular carcinoma. *J Biomed Res* 2012;26:395–399.

163. Klek S, Chambrier C, Singer P, et al. Four-week parenteral nutrition using a third generation lipid emulsion (Smoflipid)—a double-blind, randomised, multicentre study in adults. *Clin Nutr.* 2013;32:224–231.

164. Tian H, Yao X, Zeng R, et al. Safety and efficacy of a new parenteral lipid emulsion (SMOF) for surgical patients: a systematic review and meta-analysis of randomized controlled trials. *Nutr Rev.* 2013;71:815–821.

165. Manzanares W, Dhaliwal R, Jurewitsch B, et al. Alternative lipid emulsions in the critically ill: a systematic review of the evidence. *Intensive Care Med.* 2013;39:1683–1694.

166. Manzanares W, Dhaliwal R, Jurewitsch B. Parenteral fish oil lipid emulsions in the critically ill: a systematic review and meta-analysis. *JPEN J Parenter Enteral Nutr.* 2014;38:20–28.

167. Manzanares W, Langlois PL, Dhaliwal R, et al. Intravenous fish oil lipid emulsions in critically ill patients: an updated systematic review and meta-analysis. *Critical Care.* 2015;19:167–181.

168. Cury-Boaventura MF, Gorjão R, de Lima TM, et al. Effect of olive oil-based emulsion on human lymphocyte and neutrophil death. *JPEN J Parenter Enteral Nutr.* 2008;32:81–87.

169. Buenestado A, Cortijo J, Sanz MJ, et al. Olive oil-based lipid emulsion's neutral effects on neutrophil functions and leuko-

cyte: endothelial cell interactions. *JPEN J Parenter Enteral Nutr.* 2006;30:286–296.

170. Versleijen MW, Roelofs HM, te Morsche RH, et al. Parenteral lipids impair pneumococcal elimination by human neutrophils. *Eur J Clin Invest.* 2010;40:729–734.

171. Haase B, Faust K, Heidemann M, et al. The modulatory effect of lipids and glucose on the neonatal immune response induced by *Staphylococcus epidermidis. Inflamm Res.* 2011;60:227–232.

172. Jüttner B, Kröplin J, Coldewey SM, et al. Unsaturated long-chain fatty acids induce the respiratory burst of human neutrophils and monocytes in whole blood. *Nutr Metab.* 2008;5:19.

173. Umpierrez GE, Spiegelman R, Zhao V, et al. A double-blind, randomized clinical trial comparing soybean oil-based versus olive oil-based lipid emulsions in adult medical-surgical intensive care unit patients requiring parenteral nutrition. *Crit Care Med.* 2012;40:1792–1798.

174. Jia ZY, Yang J, Xia Y, et al; OliClinomel N4 Study Group. Safety and efficacy of an olive oil-based triple-chamber bag for parenteral nutrition: a prospective, randomized, multi-center clinical trial in China. *Nutr J.* 2015;14:119–133.

175. Pontes-Arruda A, Dos Santos MC, Martins LF, et al. Influence of parenteral nutrition delivery system on the development of bloodstream infections in critically ill patients: an international, multicenter, prospective, open-label, controlled study—EPICOS study. *JPEN J Parenter Enteral Nutr.* 2012;36:574–586.

176. Wang WP, Yan XL, Ni YF, et al. Effects of lipid emulsions in parenteral nutrition of esophageal cancer surgical patients receiving enteral nutrition: a comparative analysis. *Nutrients.* 2013;6:111–123.

177. Bartholome AL, Albin DM, Baker DH, et al. Supplementation of total parenteral nutrition with butyrate acutely increases structural aspects of intestinal adaptation after an 80% jejunoileal resection in neonatal piglets. *JPEN J Parenter Enteral Nutr.* 2004;28:210–223.

178. Murakoshi S, Fukatsu K, Omata J, et al. Effects of adding butyric acid to PN on gut-associated lymphoid tissue and mucosal immunoglobulin A levels. *JPEN J Parenter Enteral Nutr.* 2011;35:465–472.

179. Tappenden KA, Albin DM, Bartholome AL, et al. Glucagon-like peptide-2 and short-chain fatty acids: a new twist to an old story. *J Nutr.* 2003;133:3717–3720.

180. Tappenden KA. Emerging therapies for intestinal failure. *Arch Surg.* 2010;145:528–532.

181. Arora T, Bäckhed F. The gut microbiota and metabolic disease: current understanding and future perspectives. *J Intern Med.* 2016(Apr 12). Epub ahead of print. doi:10.1111/joim.12508.

182. Martin-Pena G, Culebras JM, De P, et al. Effects of 2 lipid emulsions (LCT versus MCT/LCT) on the fatty acid composition of plasma phospholipid: a double-blind randomized trial. *JPEN J Parenter Enteral Nutr.* 2002;26:30–41.

183. Wu GH, Zaniolo O, Schuster H, et al. Structured triglycerides versus physical mixtures of medium- and long-chain triglycerides for parenteral nutrition in surgical or critically ill adult patients: Systematic review and meta-analysis. *Clin Nutr.* 2016(Jan 21). Epub ahead of print. doi:10.1016/j.clnu.2016.01.004.

184. Nandivada P, Fell GL, Gura KM, Puder M. Lipid emulsions in the treatment and prevention of parenteral nutrition–associated liver disease in infants and children. *Am J Clin Nutr.* 2016;103 (suppl):629S–634S.

185. Xu Z, Harvey KA, Pavlina T, et al. Steroidal compounds in commercial parenteral lipid emulsions. *Nutrients.* 2012;4:904–921.

186. Zaloga GP. Phytosterols, lipid administration, and liver disease during parenteral nutrition. *JPEN J Parenter Enteral Nutr.* 2015;39 (suppl):39S–60S.

187. El Kasmi KC, Anderson AL, Devereaux MW, et al. Phytosterols promote liver injury and Kupffer cell activation in parenteral nutrition-associated liver disease. *Sci Transl Med.* 2013;5: 206ra137. doi:10.1126/scitranslmed.3006898.

188. Harris JK, El Kasmi KC, Anderson AL, et al. Specific microbiome changes in a mouse model of parenteral nutrition-associated liver injury and intestinal inflammation. *PLoS One.* 2014;9:e110396.

189. Ng K, Stoll B, Chacko S, et al. Vitamin E in new generation lipid emulsions protects against parenteral nutrition-associated liver disease in parenteral nutrition-fed pre-term pigs. *JPEN J Parenter Enteral Nutr.* 2016;40:656–671.

190. Xu Z, Harvey KA, Pavlina TM, et al. Tocopherol and tocotrienol homologs in parenteral lipid emulsions. *Eur J Lipid Sci Technol.* 2015;117:15–22.

191. Grilo EC, Costa PN, Gurgel CS, et al. Alpha-tocopherol and gamma-tocopherol concentration in vegetable oils. *Food Sci Technol Campinas.* 2014;34:379–385.

192. Muto M, Lim D, Soukvilay A, et al. Supplemental parenteral vitamin E into conventional soybean lipid emulsion does not prevent parenteral nutrition-associated liver disease in full-term neonatal piglets. *JPEN J Parenter Enteral Nutr.* 2015(Oct 12). pii:0148607115561030. Epub ahead of print.

6 Protein

Lorraine S. Young, MS, RD, LDN, CNSC, and Dong Wook Kim, MD, PNS

CONTENTS

Acknowledgments: Laurel Kearns, RD, MS, CNSC, LDN, Sandra Schoepfel, RD, RN, CNSC, LDN, and Nicole Caron Clark, RD, MS, CNSC, LDN, coauthored this chapter for the second edition. The authors also gratefully acknowledge the assistance of Jiseok Park, MD.

Objectives

1. Compare the available methods to determine protein and amino acid utilization.
2. Contrast normal, starvation, and injury protein metabolism.
3. Identify the "conditionally essential" amino acids, and explain in what conditions they become essential.
4. Identify the most clinically useful method for assessing protein status.

Test Your Knowledge Questions

1. Which of the following statements is true relating to hydrochloric acid (HCl) and protein digestion?
   A. HCl aids in the conversion of pepsin to pepsinogen.
   B. HCl denatures protein structures to make them more susceptible to enzymatic action.
   C. HCl is secreted by the parietal cells within the duodenum in response to dietary proteins.
   D. HCl's release is stimulated by the hormone insulin.
2. During protein metabolism, branched-chain amino acids (BCAAs):
   A. Are extracted primarily by the liver after a protein-containing meal.
   B. Are released by the skeletal muscle at a higher rate than other amino acids.
   C. Serve as the primary fuel sources for the enterocytes.
   D. Produce oxidative wastes during metabolism within the skeletal muscle, which are removed by alanine and glutamine.
3. Proteins perform all the following physiological functions *except:*
   A. Provide a major source of energy.
   B. Maintain acid-base balance.
   C. Contribute to immune defense.
   D. Serve as a mode of transport for substances.
4. The rate of protein turnover in catabolic, critically ill patients:
   A. Does not change.
   B. Decreases.
   C. Increases.
   D. Is not affected by nutrition support.

Test Your Knowledge Answers

1. The correct answer is **B**. Denaturing protein structures, making them more susceptible to enzymatic action, is a primary role of HCl. HCl plays several roles in protein digestion, including conversion of the proenzyme pepsinogen to its active form pepsin. HCl is secreted by the parietal cells within the stomach, not the duodenum. HCl secretion is stimulated by gastrin, not insulin.
2. The correct answer is **D**. Nitrogen end products produced during BCAA oxidation within the skeletal muscle are removed by the nitrogen carriers alanine and glutamine. BCAAs are extracted primarily by the skeletal muscle, with minimal extraction by the liver. BCAAs are primarily oxidized in the skeletal muscle (not the enterocytes) and are released from the muscle at a lower rate than other amino acids.

3. The correct answer is **A**. Carbohydrates and fats are the major energy source in the human diet. Protein is not preferentially used as a source of energy in health. Protein is used as the body's primary buffer to maintain acid-base balance. All cells of the immune system (ie, white blood cells, macrophages, and so on) are made up of proteins. Proteins are the primary carriers for substances such as minerals, vitamins, and hormones.
4. The correct answer is **C**. Protein turnover rates increase dramatically in critical illness. Nutrition support will improve protein synthesis somewhat, but it has little effect on protein degradation.

Introduction

Proteins are an essential component of all living organisms and are important components of body mass and structure. The word *protein* is derived from the Greek *protos* ("first"); as the name suggests, protein is clearly thought of as the most important macronutrient in the body. A thorough knowledge of how proteins are used by the healthy body and the changes in protein metabolism that occur with injury and disease is essential in nutrition support practice.

Amino Acids and Peptides

Amino Acids

Amino acids play central roles both as building blocks of proteins and as intermediates in metabolism. The "nutritional value" of dietary protein is closely related to the in vivo biochemical processes of the metabolism or use of individual amino acids released from the dietary proteins after digestion. The 20 amino acids found within proteins convey a vast array of chemical versatility. The content and sequence of the amino acids of a specific protein are determined by the sequence of the bases in the gene that encodes that protein through complex transcription, translation, and posttranslational modifications. The chemical properties of a protein's amino acids and their spatial configurations in a protein determine their biological activity. Proteins not only catalyze most of the reactions in living cells; they control virtually all cellular processes.[1] Understanding amino acid structure and properties is key to understanding protein structure and properties.

Dietary proteins are important sources of amino acids. Some amino acids are considered nutritionally essential (indispensable) because they cannot be physiologically synthesized in the human body. Our bodies cannot manufacture them, so they must be obtained exogenously. There are also nonessential (dispensable) amino acids, which are synthesized from available carbon and nitrogen precursors. In addition, there are a few amino acids that can be manufactured by the body under normal circumstances but become "conditionally essential" under certain clinical conditions, meaning the demand exceeds what can be produced. For example, tyrosine is a nonessential amino acid that is normally synthesized from the essential amino acid phenylalanine. However, tyrosine becomes conditionally essential if inadequate phenylalanine is provided, or if, under certain clinical conditions, the tyrosine converted from phenylalanine cannot meet the body's requirements. Other examples of conditionally essential amino acids include cysteine, glutamine, histidine, and taurine.

The classification of an amino acid as essential or nonessential is based on whether the amino acid can be synthesized in the body under physiological conditions. Humans can produce 11 of the 20 amino acids that are the building blocks of proteins. The others must be supplied exogenously. Muscle protein is catabolized when the exogenous essential amino acid requirement for even a single amino acid is not met. Unlike fat and starch, excessive amino acids are not stored for later use. Therefore, amino acids must be consumed from exogenous sources or the body must accelerate the breakdown of its own proteins.

The nutritionally essential amino acids are phenylalanine, isoleucine, leucine, lysine, methionine, threonine, tryptophan, valine, and histidine; the latter is essential primarily in infants and children. Foods of animal origin, such as meat, poultry, fish, eggs, and dairy products, are the richest sources of the essential amino acids. Plant sources of protein are often deficient in one or more of the essential amino acids. It was once believed that all the essential amino acids had to be "balanced" at each meal for vegetarians to obtain adequate amounts of protein. For example, it was thought that grains and beans had to be consumed at the same meal. However, more recent research has indicated that consuming a proper mixture of amino acids is important, but it is not necessary to consume all types at the same meal.[2]

The distinctions between essential and nonessential amino acids are not always clearly delineated in all physiological and pathophysiological conditions. The labels "indispensable" and "dispensable" were originally defined not only in dietary terms but also in relation to the role of amino acids in supporting protein deposition and growth. Reeds[3] has examined these labels as they apply to amino acids from 3 different perspectives. The first perspective comes from a traditional nutrition-focused view that some amino acids are absolute dietary necessities if normal growth is to be maintained. The second perspective comes from a metabolism-focused view that there may be significant limitations on the synthesis of some amino acids, thereby rendering potential limitations to growth. In addition, a consideration of in vivo amino acid metabolism leads to the definition of a third class of amino acids, termed *conditionally essential*, whose synthesis can be carried out by mammals but is limited by a variety of factors. These factors include the dietary supply of the appropriate precursors and the maturity and health of the individual. Finally, from a functional perspective, all amino acids, including nonessential and conditionally essential amino acids, are essential to optimize physiological function.[3]

Peptides

Peptides are composed of amino acids linked together chemically by peptide bonds. The link between one amino acid residue and the next is an amide bond and is sometimes referred to as a *peptide bond*. The peptide bond always involves a single covalent link between the α-carboxy (oxygen-bearing carbon) of one amino acid and the amino nitrogen of a second amino acid. In the formation of a peptide bond from 2 amino acids,

a molecule of water is eliminated. An amide bond is somewhat shorter than a typical carbon-nitrogen single bond and has a partial double-bond character because the participating carbon atom is double-bonded to an oxygen atom and the nitrogen has a lone pair of electrons available for bonding. Dipeptides are 2 amino acids bonded together, whereas 3 amino acids bonded together by peptide bonds are called *tripeptides*. Polypeptides consist of 10 or more amino acids bonded together by peptide bonds and an intermediate string between 4 and 10 amino acids is an oligopeptide.

Peptides differ from proteins, which are also long chains of amino acids, by virtue of their size. Traditionally, peptide chains that are short enough to be made synthetically from the constituent amino acids are called *peptides*, rather than proteins. In essence, a peptide is a small protein.[4]

The gastrointestinal (GI) tract produces a variety of chemical transmitters (GI peptides) that are involved in GI motility, secretion, absorption, growth, and development.[5] Dietary protein, for example, is digested in the GI tract to free amino acids and peptides by the action of gastric acid and enzymatic hydrolysis. Multiple amino acid transport systems exist for absorption of the amino acids (see Chapter 1). The cells that produce GI peptides are dispersed throughout the GI tract, and regulatory peptides are found in the esophagus, stomach, small and large bowel, and the pancreas. Although GI peptides are typically thought of as hormones, not all peptides act via the traditional endocrine pathway by which they are secreted into the bloodstream and act at a distant site. Many of the peptides in the GI tract are also found in the enteric nervous system and the central nervous system. GI peptides can act on the same cells from which they are released, on neighboring cells via classic endocrine mechanisms, and on cells following their release from nerves.[6] Table 6-1 lists the secretory sites, targets, and functions of the nutritionally important GI peptides.

Functions and Structure of Proteins

Functions of Proteins

Proteins are the most abundant organic molecules in cells and are fundamental to cell structure and function. All proteins are constructed from the same basic set of 20 amino acids, covalently linked in characteristic sequences. Because each of these amino acids has a distinctive side chain that lends it chemical individuality, this group of 20 building-block molecules may be regarded as the "alphabet" of protein structure. All proteins contain carbon, hydrogen, oxygen, and nitrogen. Some contain sulfur, and others contain phosphorus, iron, zinc, and copper.

The roles of protein are versatile. Table 6-2 lists some of the many important roles proteins play in the body.[7] Newer research reveals increasingly complex roles for protein and amino acids in regulation of body composition and bone health, GI function and bacterial flora, glucose homeostasis, cell signaling, and satiety.[8]

Structure of Proteins

To understand protein function, one must understand protein structure. Two classes of strong bonds (peptide and disulfide)

TABLE 6-1 Gastrointestinal Peptides and Their Functions

Peptide	Secretory Sites	Main Target Sites	Functions
Gastrin	G cell (pyloric antrum, duodenum, and pancreas)	Parietal cell	Acid secretion, gastric contraction
Secretin	S cell (duodenum)	Pancreas	Water and bicarbonate secretion
Cholecystokinin	I cell (duodenum and jejunum)	Pancreas, gallbladder	Pancreatic enzyme secretion, gallbladder contraction
Gastric inhibitory peptide	K cell (duodenum and jejunum)	Pancreas	Insulin secretion
Glucagon-like peptide-1	L cell (small intestine)	Pancreas	Insulin secretion
Glucagon-like peptide-2	L cell (small intestine)	Small intestine	Intestinal growth (crypt cell)
Peptide YY	L cell (small intestine)	Brain stem	Slowing the gastric emptying, reducing appetite
Somatostatin	Delta cell (pyloric antrum), hypothalamus	GI tract, pituitary gland	Suppressing the release of GI hormones

GI, gastrointestinal.

TABLE 6-2 Functions of Proteins and Amino Acids

- *Growth, maintenance, and movement:* Proteins form integral parts of most body structures, such as skin, tendons, membranes, muscles, organs, and bones. As such, they support the growth and repair of body tissues.
- *Enzymes:* Proteins facilitate chemical reactions.
- *Hormones:* Some, but not all, hormones are made of protein. They function as messengers and signals and regulate body processes.
- *Immunity:* Antibodies, cytokines, and chemokines are proteins involved in immunological processes. Proteins regulate gene transcription and translation through mTOR signaling pathway.
- *Fluid and electrolyte balance:* Proteins help maintain fluid volume and the composition of body fluids.
- *Acid-base balance:* Proteins help maintain the acid-base balance of body fluids by acting as buffers.
- *Transportation and storage:* Proteins transport substances, such as lipids, vitamins, minerals, and oxygen, throughout the body. Some proteins, such as ferritin, store a specific micronutrient, such as iron.

mTOR, mammalian target of rapamycin.

and 3 classes of weak bonds (hydrogen, hydrophobic, and electrostatic or salt) stabilize most protein structures. Protein structure is broken down into the following 4 levels:

- *Primary structure* refers to the "linear" sequence of amino acids in the polypeptide chain(s) and the location of disulfide bonds, if these are present. In contrast, the higher orders of protein structure (secondary, tertiary, and quaternary) involve mainly noncovalent interactions.
- *Secondary structure* refers to "local" ordered structure brought about via hydrogen bonding mainly within the peptide backbone. The most common secondary structure elements in proteins are the alpha (α) helix and the beta-13 sheet (sometimes called "13-pleated sheet").
- *Tertiary structure* refers to the "global" folding of a single polypeptide chain. Hydrogen bonding involving groups from both the peptide backbone and the side chains is important in stabilizing tertiary structure. Disulfide bonds between cysteine residues stabilize the tertiary structure of some proteins.

- *Quaternary structure* refers to the stable association of multiple polypeptide chains resulting in an active unit united by forces other than covalent bonds (not peptide or disulfide bonds). The forces that stabilize these aggregates are hydrogen bonds and electrostatic (or salt) bonds formed between residues on the surfaces of the polypeptide chains. The protein structure is formed through the processes of translation and posttranslational modification. The configuration of a protein determines the physical property and the function of the protein. Taking enzyme protein as an example, the configuration of an enzyme protein determines the catalytic ability of the individual enzyme.

Transport Proteins

Transport proteins in plasma bind and carry specific molecules or ions from one organ to another. Some transport proteins are not attached to membranes; instead, they move via bodily fluids, carrying nutrients and other molecules. Some examples of proteins acting as transport proteins include hemoglobin carrying oxygen from the lungs to the cells, lipoproteins transporting lipids around the body, and special proteins that carry vitamins (eg, retinol-binding protein), minerals (eg, albumin), or hormones (eg, prealbumin). Other kinds of transport proteins are present in cell membranes and are adapted to bind and transport glucose, amino acids, and other nutrients across the membranes into cells. Iron transport provides a good illustration of these proteins' specificity and precision. Dietary iron is mainly absorbed in the duodenum and proximal jejunum, where it may be stored bound to ferritin or transported into circulation. As iron is transported by an export protein from the cell into circulation, it is attached to the carrier protein transferrin, which is necessary to transport the iron to other tissues such as bone marrow or other storage sites where it is stored as ferritin or hemosiderin. During periods of physiological need, iron is incorporated into proteins such as those in the red blood cells and muscles that assist in oxygen transport and use. Since plasma proteins play such important roles in directly transporting substrates (such as minerals) as well as metabolic mediators (such as various hormones and growth factors), the dynamic status of plasma proteins is closely related to the delivery of the protein-bound substrates and the functions of these metabolic mediators.

Protein Signaling

Amino acids and proteins also have important functions as signaling molecules modulating the process of protein synthesis. The *target of rapamycin* is a protein kinase initially discovered in yeast, and it is the major signaling pathway regulating messenger ribonucleic acid translation. It is involved in the control of cell growth and proliferation and is activated by hormones and growth factors as well as amino acids, specifically leucine, and cellular energy status. Research on the mammalian target of rapamycin–signaling pathway may help identify the mechanisms involved in the longevity associated with energy restriction observed in certain species. Research on this topic may also have implications for the regulation of cancer cell growth, as well as our understanding of the role of muscle protein turnover in critical illness.

Digestion and Absorption

Protein and its amino acid components enter the GI tract via both endogenous and exogenous routes. Endogenous sources include desquamated mucosal cells, digestive enzymes, and other glycoproteins such as mucus. Exogenous sources (ie, dietary protein) in the form of meat, poultry, fish, milk products, grains, legumes, and vegetables provide both energy and amino acids essential to the body in roles, as previously described.[8]

As exogenous proteins travel through the GI tract, they are digested into peptides and free amino acids through a series of hydrolytic reactions and feedback mechanisms (Figure 6-1). Minimal protein digestion occurs within the mouth or esophagus. However, once proteins reach the stomach, HCl is released by the parietal cells of the stomach. HCl release may be stimulated by the hormone gastrin, the neurotransmitter acetylcholine from vagal nerve stimulation, the neuropep-

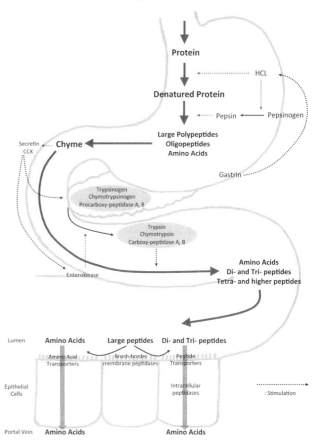

FIGURE 6-1 Schemata of Digestion and Absorption of Proteins

CCK, cholecystokinin; HCL, hydrochloric acid.

tide gastrin-releasing peptide, or the amine histamine.[8] HCl denatures protein structures to make them more susceptible to enzymatic action and converts pepsinogen, an inactive proenzyme or zymogen released by the stomach's chief cells, to its active form, pepsin (see Chapter 1). Pepsin in turn may activate other pepsinogen molecules or hydrolyze specific peptide bonds into the end products of large polypeptides, oligopeptides, and free amino acids.[9]

This mixture, known as *acid chyme*, next passes into the duodenum and small intestine where most protein digestion takes place. The end products within the acid chyme stimulate the secretion of the hormones secretin and cholecystokinin (CCK), which in turn travel through the bloodstream to the acinar cells of the pancreas to stimulate the release of alkaline pancreatic juices. Secretin and CCK also stimulate the release of digestive proenzymes trypsinogen, procarboxypeptidases, chymotrypsinogen, and proelastase (Table 6-3). While deactivating pepsin, the higher pH of the duodenum is now optimal for the activity of the pancreatic enzymes. By releasing proteolytic enzymes initially in their inactive form, the enzyme-forming cells are protected from self-digestion.

Enterokinase (also known as *enteropeptidase*) is an enzyme secreted from the brush border of the small intestine, also in response to secretin and CCK. Enterokinase serves to activate

TABLE 6-3 Selected Enzymes Responsible for the Digestion of Protein

Zymogen	Enzyme or Activator	Enzyme	Site of Activity
Pepsinogen	HCl or pepsin	Pepsin	Stomach
Trypsinogen	Enteropeptidase trypsin	Trypsin	Intestine
Chymotrypsinogen	Trypsin	Chymotrypsin	Intestine
Procarboxy-peptidases	Trypsin	Carboxypeptidase A, B Aminopeptidases	Intestine

HCl, hydrochloric acid.

trypsinogen into trypsin, which in turn converts many of the other proenzymes into their respective enzymatic forms for ongoing protein hydrolysis.[9] At this point, endogenous protein sources from sloughing mucosal cells or other secretory proteins are also recycled through the digestive process to form the general pool of amino acids. The presence of protein within the gut signals further enzyme secretions. When most of the protein has been digested, the presence of unbound trypsin acts as a feedback mechanism to turn off further secretion of trypsinogen by the pancreas.[10] At this point, the byproducts of pancreatic protease digestion, free amino acids and peptides of 2 to 6 amino acid components, now enter the final phases of digestion. The brush border of the small intestine produces a variety of peptidases, which allow peptide digestion to continue through the distal small intestine and ileum.[8,11,12]

The end products of protein digestion (eg, free amino acids, dipeptides, and tripeptides) are now ready for absorption within the small intestine. The absorption of intact proteins may occur through leaks in cell junctions to a lesser extent, which accounts for the immune response associated with food allergies.[10,13] However, most amino acids are absorbed in the proximal small intestine, leaving less than 1% of dietary protein to be excreted in the feces.[8,10] Through both sodium-dependent and sodium-independent active transport systems, amino acids pass from the lumen of the small intestine into the enterocyte. The various amino acid carrier systems have an affinity for specific amino acids.[14] The rate of amino acid absorption may vary depending on the chemical properties of the amino acid. Essential (indispensable) amino acids are absorbed faster than nonessential (dispensable) amino acids. Methionine and the BCAAs leucine, isoleucine, and valine are the most rapidly absorbed.[15] Competition can occur between amino acids for transport by a carrier system.

The active transport of dipeptides and tripeptides across the brush border membrane of the enterocyte also involves a competition for transporters but uses different carrier systems than those of the free amino acids. In fact, peptide absorption occurs more rapidly than an equivalent mixture of free amino acid.[16,17] It is estimated that 67% of dietary protein is absorbed as dipeptides and tripeptides, with the remaining 33% absorbed as free amino acids[10,18,19] Once inside the enterocyte, these peptides are converted to free amino acids by peptide hydrolases. The final phase of amino acid absorption occurs across the basolateral membrane of the entero-

cyte by diffusion or active transport into the portal circulation (Figure 6-1).

Hydrolyzed Enteral Formulas

The use of peptide-based enteral formulas for patients with impaired GI function and malabsorption remains controversial. The GI tract has a large reserve capacity for digestive and absorptive processes with a multitude of intestinal folds, villi, and microvilli increasing its surface area. Malabsorption of some nutrients may not be manifested until 90% of organ function is impaired, such as in exocrine pancreatic disease.[20,21] Peptide length may also play a role in effectiveness of GI absorption, with dipeptides and tripeptides being most readily absorbed. A meta-analysis of elemental (free amino acids) versus polymeric (intact protein) formulas did not show an advantage with the former for patients with Crohn's disease.[22,23] Free amino acid formulas also have a higher osmolality, are less palatable, and cost more, further limiting their application in the clinical setting.[8]

Protein Synthesis, Turnover, and Breakdown

Protein Synthesis

The human body contains an estimated 10,000 to 50,000 different kinds of proteins. Each protein has a specific function, and that function is determined during protein synthesis. Protein synthesis is a fundamental process for all living organisms. The liver is the major site of amino acid metabolism. The sequence of amino acids in each protein determines its configuration, which supports a specific function. If a genetic error alters the amino acid sequence of a protein, or if a mistake is made in copying the sequence, an altered protein will result, sometimes with dramatic consequences. Because proteins are composed of amino acids, the information necessary for their production resides in the cellular nucleus as deoxyribonucleic acid (DNA). The instructions for protein synthesis are transmitted by genetic information received at conception. There are 5 major stages in protein synthesis, each requiring multiple components. A brief outline of the different stages follows:[24]

- *Stage 1: Activation of amino acids:* To inform a cell of the sequence of amino acids for a needed protein, a stretch of DNA serves as a template for making a strand of RNA that carries a code, which lists in order the amino acids that will be needed to make a given protein. Each messenger RNA strand copies exactly the instructions for making a protein that the cell needs.

- *Stage 2: Initiation of the polypeptide chain:* The messenger RNA leaves the nucleus through the nuclear membrane. DNA remains inside the nucleus. The messenger RNA, bearing the code for the polypeptide to be made, attaches itself to the protein-making machinery of the cell in the cytosol, the ribosomes.
- *Stage 3: Elongation:* Another form of RNA, *transfer RNA*, collects amino acids from the cell fluid. Each transfer RNA carries its amino acids to the messenger RNA, which dictates the sequence in which the amino acids will be attached to form the protein strands. Thus, the messenger RNA ensures that the amino acids are arranged in the correct sequence.
- *Stage 4: Termination and release:* As the amino acids are lined up in the right sequence and the ribosome moves along the messenger, an enzyme bonds one amino acid after another to the growing protein strand. The transfer RNA is freed to return for more amino acids. When all the amino acids have been attached, the completed protein is released.
- *Stage 5: Folding and processing:* Finally, the messenger RNA is degraded. To achieve its native biologically active form, the polypeptide must undergo folding into its proper 3-dimensional conformation. Before or after folding, the new polypeptide may undergo processing by enzymatic action to remove initiating amino acids; to introduce phosphate, methyl, carboxyl, or other groups into certain amino acid residues; or to attach oligosaccharides or prosthetic groups. Between 40 and 100 amino acids can be rapidly added to a growing protein strand in a cell. The completed protein strand is released (stage 4), the messenger is degraded, and the transfer RNA is freed to return for another load of amino acids.

Measurement of Protein Turnover and Breakdown

Protein turnover is the measurement of protein synthesis and breakdown rates. Protein turnover constantly occurs in the body with all proteins participating at varying rates. The amino acids liberated during protein turnover contribute to the free amino acid pool. There is constant flux of amino acids between muscle and organs, and the turnover rate of individual proteins varies depending on the function of the protein. For example, peptides and hormones have relatively high rates of synthesis and degradation in contrast to structural or plasma proteins. In a normal 24-hour period, dietary intake matches nitrogen output; thus, protein breakdown matches synthesis. This process is altered by disease and certain physiological states as well as changes in nutrient intake.[25] Typically, daily protein intake provides approximately 25% of total nitrogen turnover in the body, with other sources coming from muscle, the viscera, and plasma proteins.

Body protein turnover in both healthy individuals and critically ill patients may be determined by several different methods (Table 6-4). They range from simple noninvasive measurements that can easily be performed in a clinical setting, such as nitrogen balance (NB), to expensive and more

complicated tests, such as tracer methodology, arteriovenous differences across tissue beds, and the use of molecular biology techniques.[10] All methods have limitations.

Nitrogen Balance

NB is calculated in clinical settings to help assess protein requirements and adequacy. This technique is used to determine minimum levels of human protein and amino acid requirements. Determining NB using urinary urea is an approximation based on certain assumptions, such as urea accounting for about 80% of the total urinary nitrogen losses. The urinary urea nitrogen concentration is affected by stress and increased urinary excretion of non–urea nitrogen. NB determined with total urinary nitrogen (Kjeldahl method) is consistently more reliable than the urine urea nitrogen measurement but is typically not available for routine clinical measurements. Stool and skin losses of nitrogen are usually estimated to be about 2 g/d, unless there is excessive diarrhea or ostomy/fistula losses. In such cases, the effluent should also be collected and measured for total nitrogen, if possible. There are also negligible losses that are not accounted for clinically, such as menstrual losses and nasal secretion.

The NB equation used clinically is as follows:

$$NB = Nitrogen\ Intake - Nitrogen\ Output$$

TABLE 6-4 Measurement of Protein Metabolism

Method	Characteristics
Nitrogen balance	• Measure of nitrogen input minus nitrogen output. • Can be used in clinical setting. • Decreased accuracy in certain clinical conditions (renal dysfunction, high-output fistula, and ostomy).
Arteriovenous amino acid differences across organs	• Invasive method. • A tracer amino acid should be infused. • Samples of blood are obtained from both the arterial and venous catheter. • The measurements are made across muscle beds.
Tracer methodology	• Constant infusion method used in human studies. • No requirement for a steady state. • Ideal for measuring acute changes in patients. • Important research tool.
Urinary creatinine excreted over 24 hours	• Indirect measurement of muscle mass. • Has high variation.
Urinary 3-methyl histidine excretion	• Can be used as a measure of muscle protein degradation. • Compromised accuracy with organ dysfunction.

where nitrogen intake is the total nitrogen intake, including enteral tube feeding and/or oral intake and parenteral nutrition (PN), and nitrogen output is the sum of nitrogen losses from urine, stool, skin, and body fluids:[26]

Nitrogen Output (g/d) = [Urinary Urea Nitrogen (mg/100 mL) × Urinary Volume (L/d)/100] + 20% of Urinary Urea Losses + 2 g

In clinical settings, a 24-hour urine collection is necessary for accurate urea nitrogen measurements. Adjustments need to be made in certain patients. Many other factors affect the accuracy of NB measurement. In addition to renal dysfunction, errors in estimating intake, or incomplete collections of urine, stool, fistula, or ostomy losses may affect balance results. NB, which may also be affected by changes in the muscle glutamine pool, has been reported to be significantly decreased in critical illness.[27]

Because NB measures the net difference between nitrogen intake and output, it is a useful value to measure the gross utilization of administered protein; however, it does not provide information about how the administered protein is used within the body (eg, for protein synthesis, formation of nonessential amino acids, oxidation, or gluconeogenesis). NB is a poor indicator for characterizing interorgan amino acid flux and changes in protein turnover. More sensitive tools such as isotopically labeled tracers can be used to determine substrate balance across an organ and amino acid circulation. Practice Scenario 6-1 discusses the use of NB in a critical care setting.

Practice Scenario 6-1

Question: What are the best ways to evaluate protein adequacy after traumatic injury?

Scenario: A 36-year-old man was admitted to the trauma center after a collision with a tree while riding a motorcycle. He sustained major abdominal injuries, including a ruptured spleen, severe liver contusions, and small bowel lacerations, as well as 3 fractured ribs, a fractured pelvis, and a right femur fracture. He required multiple blood transfusions (10 units) during the first 24 hours in the hospital. After resuscitation and stabilization, he was taken to the operating room for intra-abdominal exploration, splenectomy, and repair of small bowel lacerations, which required 2 small bowel resections. Also noted was a large right retroperitoneal hematoma, which appeared stable. He also underwent an open reduction internal fixation of his femur fracture and stabilization of his pelvic fracture. His previous medical history was notable for alcohol abuse. His pertinent objective data include the following:
- Height: 73 inches
- Weight: 95 kg
- Ideal body weight: 84 kg
- Estimated energy needs (25 to 30 kcal/kg): 2375 to 2850 kcal/d
- Estimated protein needs (1.5 g/kg): 142 g/d

He was initially started on nasogastric feedings on postoperative Day 3 with a standard high-calorie, high-protein tube feeding, which was discontinued after 24 hours because of very high gastric residuals (>250 mL). Parenteral nutrition (PN) was started as a total nutrient admixture to meet the patient's needs until a nasojejunal tube was placed.

Intervention: On Day 3 of PN, the nutrition support team was consulted because the patient was experiencing worsening azotemia, with his blood urea nitrogen (BUN) rising to 63 mg/dL and a creatinine level of 1.9 mg/dL. His urine output and creatinine clearance were within normal limits. His liver function tests were also elevated, with the transaminases 5 times normal, total bilirubin 2.9 mg/dL, and direct bilirubin 1.8 mg/dL.

The primary team requested an evaluation of the protein dose provided by the feeding regimen for potential overfeeding.

Answer: A clinically useful and practical tool for assessing protein requirements in hospitalized patients is nitrogen balance (NB). When PN or tube feeding is the sole source of nutrition intake, accurate determination of nitrogen intake is easier. Collection of output is usually where errors in calculating NB occur. Gastrointestinal (GI) losses need to be accounted for, but they are often difficult to collect and analyze in a clinical setting. If there is significant fluctuation in daily plasma BUN levels (>10 mg/dL), the change in plasma urea nitrogen generation over the 24-hour collection period should also be included in the output calculations.

Rationale: Although clinical guidelines help define protein requirements in critical illness, it is often necessary to adjust protein goals depending on the clinical condition of the patient (eg, worsening renal function, where protein may need to be decreased) or results of NB data used in clinical monitoring.[26]

The NB equation was determined as follows: A 24-hour urine collection was started on Day 4 of PN. The patient's BUN was stable, and there were no additional excess GI losses via drains, tubes, and so on. The PN solution provided 2450 kcal and 130 g protein over the same 24-hour period as the urine collection. The patient was on nothing by mouth status.

The PN provided 20.8 g nitrogen; urine output was 2870 mL; and urine urea nitrogen was 16 g. Therefore, the NB was calculated as follows:

20.8 g Nitrogen In − [16 g Urea Nitrogen + (20% for Other Urine Nitrogen, or 3.2 g) + (Estimated Other Nitrogen from Skin and GI Losses, or 2 g)] = −0.4 g, or Nitrogen Equilibrium

This NB equation suggests that the feeding regimen is adequate.

Arteriovenous Amino Acid Differences Across Organs

A more invasive tool for measuring amino acid flux across tissues and organs is arteriovenous differences. Catheters placed in an artery and vein are used to measure the amino acids in blood delivered to the tissue and the amino acids from the blood leaving the tissue. Most commonly, these measurements are made across muscle beds, such as the leg or arm. By combined measurements of arteriovenous differences of both amino acid concentrations and the isotopically labeled amino acid tracer in and out of the organs, this method can provide quantitative information on the rates of protein synthesis and degradation, namely protein turnover in the organ or tissue. The tracer amino acid is usually given by primed continuous infusion, and replicate samples of blood are obtained from both the arterial and venous catheters at steady-state conditions. Typically, net fluxes of 13C-, 15N-, and 2H-labeled amino acids (and sometime their metabolites) across tissues are used to investigate changes in protein turnover. Muscle biopsies have also been used along with arteriovenous difference measurements to obtain information on the dynamics of intramuscular pool of amino acids. This method allows assessment of intracellular amino acid recycling and trans-membrane transport.[28]

Tracer Methodology to Measure Protein Turnover

Nonradioactive stable isotope tracer amino acids to measure whole body protein turnover were first used in the 1950s, but the accuracy was limited by because the technology lacked the necessary sensitivity to detect the stable isotope enrichment of ^{15}N-glycine in biological samples. It was not until 1969 that a simpler tracer model using ^{15}N-glycine was developed by Picou and Taylor-Roberts. The tracer was originally administered orally with the metabolite being measured in the urine. Current investigations in human subjects are commonly using the method of primed constant intravenous (IV) or intragastric infusion of amino acid tracers to achieve a steady state, in which the isotope abundance in the metabolic pool reaches a plateau level. The labeled tracers are identical to the endogenous metabolites in the body except for the substituted atom that is labeled by a heavy isotope. The major assumption of the mathematical model is that the amino acid tracer is well mixed with the metabolic pool of the free amino acids within the body; then the ratio of the labeled/natural amino acids in the metabolic pool is used to calculate the metabolic rates of this amino acid along the major pathways of its metabolism, including the rates of protein synthesis and breakdown.

Another approach of measuring tissue protein metabolism is the tracer incorporation method. The advancement of mass spectrometry technology has enabled the enrichment of free and protein-bound amino acids to be measured in very small samples of plasma or tissue. The protein synthesis rate of a special tissue is calculated based on the incorporation rate of the labeled amino acid into the proteins. A limitation of the tracer incorporation method is the time required to reach a steady state in isotope infusions; additionally, it is not useful in those critically ill patients who cannot be in a pathophysiological steady state during the period of isotope infusion. An alternative approach to measure protein synthesis rates in isolated tissues and cell cultures is the flooding-dose technique. This technique minimizes the intra- and extracellular amino acid enrichment differences. It does not require a long period of stable isotope infusion, and the measurement can be completed in less than 30 minutes. This technique is ideal for measuring acute changes of protein synthesis rate in specific tissues of interest in patients.[29] More recent methodology is being developed using pulse tracer injections, coupled with muscle biopsies, to mea-

sure fractional protein breakdown as well as synthetic rates of muscle proteins. Tracer methodology is an important research tool for gaining further insight into protein and amino acid flux in health and disease in living subjects in vivo.

Other Measures of Protein Breakdown

Other methods have been used to specifically evaluate muscle protein breakdown, such as 3-methyl histidine excretion and creatinine excretion to measure creatinine height index. The amount of urinary creatinine excreted over 24 hours is an indirect measure of muscle mass; however, significant day-to-day variation in creatinine excretion occurs in both healthy individuals and hospitalized patients with acute illness and renal dysfunction.[25] Three-methyl histidine is an amino acid residue formed only by the myofibrillar proteins actin and myosin. It is not reused for protein synthesis; therefore, its excretion rate from the urine can be used as a measure of myofibrillar protein degradation. However, its accuracy is affected in patients with compromised renal function; also, muscle myofibrillar contents in the diet interfere the measurements. In addition, there are no available objective standards for comparison.[25] However, urinary 3-methyl histidine can serve as one of the parameters, combined with NB and/or protein turnover measurements, to assess the protein metabolism status of critically ill patients.

Role of Proteins in Organs and Body Systems

Gastrointestinal Tract

Because the GI tract is a metabolically active organ, it plays an important role in amino acid homeostasis. The GI tract actively regulates amino acid flow from the diet by extracting those amino acids it needs for maintenance and function. Reed and Burrin[30] estimate that a minimum of 25% of protein intake is used within the splanchnic bed, largely by the GI tract. In the presence of a low-protein diet, GI tract growth is preserved over growth of other peripheral tissues or muscle.[30,31] A large proportion of the amino acids used by the GI tract, especially the small intestine, are involved in secretory protein synthesis. Within the intestinal cell, amino acids may also be used for synthesis of nucleic acids, the antioxidant glutathione, apoproteins as components of lipoproteins, or other nitrogen-containing compounds.[30] In addition, amino acids provide an important energy source to the GI tract. Dietary glutamate and aspartate account for a significant proportion of the energy source for the small intestine.[30] Glutamine released by the lung and skeletal muscle is used as a primary source of energy for the enterocyte, and it may have trophic effects on the mucosal cells of the GI tract. Glutamine is also used by the immune system—which is abundant within the GI tract as gut-associated lymphoid tissue—as a precursor to nucleotide synthesis, especially for the quick-turnover proteins.[32]

Liver

The liver is a key organ for protein metabolism because of its high capacity for uptake and metabolism of amino acids. It also plays an essential role in regulating the flow of dietary amino acids and other nitrogenous compounds derived from tissue degradation into the systemic circulation.[33] Approximately 57% of the amino acids extracted by the liver are either oxidized or used to synthesize plasma proteins.[34] Some of these essential plasma proteins made by the liver play important roles such as maintenance of oncotic pressure in the blood (albumin), transport functions (albumin, prealbumin, transferrin, lipoproteins, some globulins), clotting functions (fibrinogen, prothrombin), and enzymatic reactions (alanine aminotransferase, aspartate aminotransferase). Amino acids are transported across the basolateral membrane of the enterocyte to the portal vein circulation (Figure 6-1). Carrier systems also exist for amino acid transport into the hepatocyte as the only site for oxidation of the essential (indispensable) amino acids, excluding the BCAAs.[8,10]

Another important function of the liver is the metabolism of toxic nitrogenous wastes that have accumulated from exogenous protein intake or from protein breakdown during catabolic states such as trauma or sepsis.[35] The accumulation and elimination of nitrogenous wastes such as ammonia from protein degradation is accomplished by hepatic ureagenesis. Urea is subsequently excreted in the urine by the kidneys. Carbon skeletons from the degradation of the gluconeogenic amino acids (alanine, glycine, cysteine, serine, threonine, asparagine, arginine, aspartic acid, histidine, glutamic acid, glutamine, isoleucine, methionine, proline, valine, and phenylalanine) can be metabolized by the liver to glucose. Gluconeogenesis, another major homeostatic role of the liver, provides glucose when glucose supply is limited in the fasting state. Also, in critically ill patients, hepatic glucose production is increased, which can contribute to hyperglycemia in these patients.

Musculoskeletal System

BCAAs are minimally extracted by the liver; instead, they mostly enter the systemic circulation for metabolism largely by muscles. Musculoskeletal uptake of amino acids following a protein-containing meal leads to a net protein synthesis within muscle.[8] The fed state supplies amino acids from dietary protein as a source of energy and helps replenish the amino acid stores. Muscle mass is maintained in a relative steady state with a fraction of the muscle protein broken down and resynthesized daily (protein turnover).[34] Most amino acids are released from the muscle in proportion to their concentrations within the muscle.[36] The release of BCAA is more conservative than that of other amino acids. However, alanine and glutamine release from muscle is higher than their concentrations within muscle. Alanine and glutamine have a key role in muscle BCAA metabolism by participating in the process to remove the nitrogen wastes that are produced during BCAA oxidation.[10,36]

The glucose-alanine cycle is another means for the musculoskeletal system to eliminate nitrogen waste while replenishing its energy supply. Glycolysis is the process of glucose oxidation within the muscle that produces alanine via the action of alanine transaminase (ie, alanine aminotransferase). Alanine is then transported through the bloodstream to the liver where its carbon atoms are used in gluconeogenesis to produce glucose, which is delivered back to the muscle. The amino group from alanine degradation within the liver is converted to urea and eventually excreted by the kidneys.[37]

Leucine is the only amino acid that undergoes a complete oxidation pathway via the formation of acetyl coenzyme A in muscle, although some of its intermediates, such as alpha-ketoisocaproate, after transamination may leave muscle and be further oxidized in other tissues or organs. In the fasting state, leucine levels rise both in the bloodstream and within the muscle. In the muscle, it is oxidized to acetyl coenzyme A, an energy source for that muscle. This process simultaneously spares pyruvate oxidation in the tricarboxylic acid cycle. Pyruvate could be reduced to lactate in the absence of oxygen (anaerobic respiration) by the action of lactate dehydrogenase and released by the muscle. The carbon skeleton of pyruvate is also transferred to liver in the form of either lactate or alanine (by transamination) as the precursor for gluconeogenesis. Therefore, leucine oxidation by the skeletal muscle may have some effect in sparing some essential amino acids as gluconeogenic precursors.[8]

Kidney

The kidney plays an important role in the interorgan exchange and synthesis of a variety of amino acids.[38] The kidney, preferentially, extracts specific amino acids, such as glycine, alanine, glutamine, glutamate, phenylalanine, and aspartate. The kidney is also a major site for arginine, histidine, and serine production,[8] and it is involved in the conversions of phenylalanine to tyrosine, and glycine to serine.[38] Aside from the liver, the kidney is the only organ with the necessary enzymes for conversion of the gluconeogenic amino acids to glucose during the process of gluconeogenesis.

Kidneys also remove nitrogenous waste from the body. Enzymes within the kidney catalyze the removal of ammonia from glutamate and glutamine, promoting the excretion of nitrogenous wastes in the urine. Urea, the hepatic metabolite of ammonia, is excreted by the kidneys, and, under normal circumstances, 80% of the body's nitrogenous wastes are excreted as urinary urea nitrogen.[8]

Specialized parenteral glutamine-dipeptides are thought to require the kidney as a metabolic mediator. The kidney uses some of the glutamine, whereas the remainder is released into the bloodstream.[38] The kidney is also the site of conversion of enterally supplemented glutamine into arginine. Glutamine is first metabolized by the gut, and its nitrogen contributes to the formation of the nonproteinogenic amino acid citrulline, which is subsequently converted by the kidneys to arginine (see "Conditionally Essential Amino Acids in Clinical Practice" section, later in this chapter).[35,38]

Brain and Central Nervous System

Essential amino acids are actively transported into the neurons and are present in higher concentrations in neurons than within the plasma. These amino acids perform a variety of important functions as neurotransmitters, evoking signals between neurons and other cells. Tryptophan acts as a precursor to the sleep-regulating hormone melatonin and the excitatory neurotransmitter serotonin.[8]

Many nonessential amino acids are required for neurotransmitter synthesis and themselves act as neurotransmitters. Tyrosine is used to synthesize the catecholamines (dopamine, norepinephrine, and epinephrine). Catecholamine levels rise within the blood during stress, causing an increase in heart rate, blood pressure, and blood glucose. Both glycine and taurine act as inhibitory neurotransmitters. In a vitamin B_6–dependent reaction, glutamate is converted to gamma-aminobutyric acid, which acts as an inhibitory neurotransmitter within the central nervous system. Glutamate may also act as an excitatory neurotransmitter or combine with ammonia through the action of glutamine synthetase to form glutamine. Glutamine then diffuses freely into the blood or cerebrospinal fluid, helping to rid the brain of ammonia.[8]

Neuropeptides also act as potent neurotransmitters, primarily in the hypothalamus, and consist of more than 100 different peptides. These complex molecules are more potent than other neurotransmitters, thus requiring only small amounts to produce profound effects on hormone release, endocrine function, and modulation of mood and behavior. Neuropeptides are responsible for mediating sensory and emotional responses including hunger, thirst, sex drive, pleasure, and pain. The enkephalins and endorphins are similar to opiates, affecting pain sensation, body temperature, and blood pressure regulation. CCK is one of the most abundant neuropeptides in the central nervous system (see Chapter 1). Although the function of CCK within the brain is not fully understood, it may play a role in the control of food intake or in the pathogenesis of certain types of anxiety and/or schizophrenia. Vasopressin also performs a variety of functions within the body, including specific hormonal actions in the brain with respect to memory formation, blood pressure and temperature regulation, and pair bonding.[8,39]

Other Organs and Body Systems

In addition, amino acids are precursors for at least 2 important compounds that widely exist in almost all tissues and organs and exert important regulatory roles in metabolism—namely, (1) glutathione formed from glycine, cysteine, and glutamate via the gamma glutamyl cycle, and (2) nitric oxide formed from arginine via nitric oxide synthase. Glutathione exists in all tissues and plays important roles against oxidative damage to the tissues. Nitric oxide plays multiple roles in modulating hemodynamics, immune function, and neurotransmission. These functions are important in disease conditions, especially in critical illness. The availability of their precursor amino acids in nutrition support is a factor related to the quantity and function of these important mediators.

Food and Protein

Adaptation to Fasting and Starvation

Protein is the primary substrate for gluconeogenesis during starvation metabolism. The fasting state occurs as blood glucose levels return to a baseline level before the start of the next meal with a decrease in insulin levels and rise in glucagon levels.[40] Tissues such as the brain and red blood cells require a constant supply of glucose, even when there is no exogenous supply (as during fasting). The breakdown of hepatic glycogen stores (glycogenolysis) for glucose production begins within 2 to 3 hours of fasting, and stores could be depleted in approximately 24 hours.[10]

Gluconeogenesis from amino acids and other noncarbohydrate sources, such as glycerol and lactic acid, occurs in both the liver and the kidney and begins within 4 to 6 hours of the last meal.[41] After approximately 2 days of starvation, the brain switches its fuel source from glucose to ketone bodies; however, blood cells and the adrenal medulla continue to rely on glucose as the primary source of energy substrate. This adaptation to starvation involves the conversion in the liver of free fatty acids to ketone bodies. As the metabolically active lean mass is diminished with starvation, metabolic processes occurring within these tissues are also reduced, accounting for a reduction in resting energy expenditure. Within approximately 1 week, adaptation to starvation with a ketone-based fuel system minimizes gluconeogenesis and further protein breakdown.[42,43]

Determining Protein Quality

Protein quality is evaluated by calculating the protein digestibility-corrected amino acid score (PDCAAS). PDCAAS was proposed in 1991 by the Food and Agriculture Organization/World Health Organization (FAO/WHO) and has been adopted by the Food and Nutrition Board of the Health and Medicine Division (formerly Institute of Medicine) of the National Academies of Science.[44] The PDCAAS indicates the overall quality of a protein because it represents the relative adequacy of its most limiting amino acid. The PDCAAS is estimated as follows:

PDCAAS (%) = [(mg of limiting amino acid in 1 g of test protein)/(mg of same amino acid in 1 g of reference protein)] × fecal true digestibility percentage

For example, if a protein has a PDCAAS of 40% and the lowest amino acid content is for lysine, then 40% of that protein can be used for protein synthesis. The highest PDCAAS is 100%, which would mean that 100% of the amino acids of that protein after digestion can be used for protein synthesis, or that the protein contains all essential amino acids in adequate proportions. Given that typical diets contain many sources of dietary protein, foods could function as "complementary proteins" if they are higher in the amino acid that is limiting in other protein.[45]

An important benefit to using the PDCAAS is that this approach uses human amino acid requirements whereas animal bioassays were used in the past.[35] An additional step is added to this method: the lowest amino acid ratio is then multiplied by its true protein digestibility. This ensures that the appropriate levels of essential amino acids are provided in the diet.

Determining Protein Content in Food

Historically, the protein content of foods was determined by multiplying total nitrogen, as measured by the Kjeldahl method, by a conversion factor. This approach is based on 2 assumptions: first, that carbohydrates and fats do not contain nitrogen, and, second, that almost all nitrogen in the diet is present as amino acids in proteins. Based on early estimates, the average nitrogen content of proteins was estimated to be 16%, which led to the use of the following calculation to convert nitrogen to protein:[46]

Protein = Nitrogen × 6.25

where the conversion factor 6.25 was calculated by dividing 1 by 16%.

However, estimating nitrogen content of dietary protein with the use of a single factor may not accurately reflect true nitrogen content. Not all nitrogen in foods is protein-based. For example, nitrogen may be part of amino acids, nucleotides, creatine, and choline, where it is referred to as *nonprotein nitrogen*. Only a small percentage of nonprotein nitrogen is available to synthesize nonessential amino acids. Moreover, the nitrogen content of specific amino acids varies with the molecular weight of the amino acid and the number of nitrogen atoms it contains (1 to 4, depending on the amino acid in question). Based on this information, we know that the nitrogen content of proteins varies from 13% to 19%, and nitrogen conversion factors range from 5.26 to 7.69.

Other factors that have been used to determine dietary protein content include "Jones" factors, which are nitrogen conversion factors for specific foods.[47] For example, Jones factors for animal protein such as meat, milk, and eggs are between 6.25 and 6.38, whereas those for vegetable proteins are in the range of 5.7 to 6.25. The difference between the conventional 6.25 conversion factor and the Jones factor is only about 1% for mixed diets. The protein content for enteral and parenteral formulations is also determined by amino acid analysis. The protein content of the enteral or parenteral formula can be calculated from its amino acid concentrations. It is important to realize, however, that the total amount of protein provided from an IV amino acid mixture is about 17% less than what would be assumed. When a peptide bond is made, a molecule of water is released; thus, the weight of a peptide bond is 18 mass units less than its molecular weight.[48] In essence, to provide 1.0 to 1.5 g of protein per kg of body weight via PN, one needs to administer 1.2 to 1.8 g of a mixed amino acid solution.[48]

Protein in Clinical Practice

Optimizing Nitrogen-Energy Relationships

Loss of significant body protein is associated with disability and death. This process is accelerated in critical illness due to increased protein catabolism and prolonged bed rest and can be further hastened by an inadequate nutrient intake. However, providing energy from nonprotein sources in amounts to meet energy demands has important effects on NB. Calloway and Spector reported nitrogen sparing in early experiments with healthy active men when energy was supplied without protein.[49] Maximum protein sparing occurred at approximately 700 nonprotein kcal. Additional increases in calories

energy intake did not improve NB. However, addition of protein in dietary intake further improved nitrogen sparing. The researchers concluded that, with fixed but adequate protein intake, the energy level is a determinant factor in nitrogen equilibrium, and, with fixed and adequate energy intake, protein intake determines nitrogen equilibrium.

The Recommended Dietary Allowance for protein is set at 0.8 g/kg/d for healthy adults, based on NB studies performed in men and women who were receiving their full energy requirements. Adding 25%, or 2 standard deviations, to the balance data meets the needs of 97.5% of a normally distributed population.[44]

Critical illness is associated with increased protein turnover, protein catabolism, and negative NB, usually associated with hypermetabolism. The increased metabolic rate and accelerated net protein loss demand greater energy and protein intake. In fact, protein requirements double in critical illness, to approximately 15% to 20% of total energy; this increment could be much higher in very severe injury such as a large-area burn. For example, the estimated protein requirement for a patient with multiple traumas who requires 2600 kcal/d for maintenance would be at least 98 to 120 g/d. With regard to critically ill patients, there is controversy regarding whether full energy provision in the first week of intensive care is beneficial.[50] Many of the permissive underfeeding studies have some methodological limitations. However, outcomes seem to be similar when comparing full energy feeds with underfeeding in the first week of intensive care, keeping in mind that it is unusual to provide full energy needs in the first week if relying on enteral feedings alone.

Clearly, the goals for a patient who is at nutrition risk or malnourished should be to meet full energy and protein needs as early as possible.[51] Current practice dictates that energy goals should meet energy demands—which, ideally, are determined by indirect calorimetry, or, alternatively, are calculated with energy equations—and protein intake should be at least 1.5 g/kg/d. However, recommendations in trauma and burns suggest protein requirements as high as 2.5 g/kg/d.[52,53] NB is difficult to attain in critically ill patients and may not be a realistic goal. Exogenous protein will improve nitrogen retention by increasing synthesis, but it has little effect on protein catabolic rates.

Protein Requirements in Critical Illness

Nutrient requirements of critically ill patients are remarkably different than in normal individuals because of profound alterations in carbohydrate, lipid, and protein metabolism. The primary goal of nutrition therapy in critical illness is to preserve lean body mass and support metabolic functions. Lean-tissue loss inevitably occurs because of the rapid rates of protein breakdown, mobilization of amino acids from the periphery to the liver for gluconeogenesis, and production of acute-phase proteins, to support the immune system in host defense, to the wound to promote healing, and to the kidney for acid-base balance. Immobilization after critical illness and, in some cases, starvation and prolonged bed rest also contribute to lean-tissue wasting. A generalized hypoaminoacidemia occurs in critical illness due to the increased uptake of amino acids to meet the needs of the rapidly turning over central proteins (liver, kidney, immune cells). Therefore, providing adequate exogenous amino acids could potentially improve clinical outcomes by increasing protein synthesis to ameliorate the inflammatory response and by mitigating the loss of muscle protein observed in the first week of critical illness and beyond when critical illness is prolonged.[52,54–57]

After injury, sepsis, or critical illness, protein turnover rates, synthesis, breakdown, and oxidation of protein are increased. The degree of increase is determined by the severity of the illness and metabolic response. The negative NB seen after minor elective surgery is due primarily to a decrease in protein synthesis. However, with severe sepsis and injury, both synthesis and catabolism are elevated and feeding further increases turnover. An older (1987) protein turnover study by Shaw and associates suggested that feeding protein in patients with sepsis at 1.1 g/kg/d decreases net protein-loss catabolism. When protein intake was increased to 1.6 g/kg/d, catabolism was decreased further; however, catabolism increased again when protein intake was greater than 1.6 g/kg/d.[58] Studies such as the one by Shaw et al[58] from 30-plus years ago could be criticized for their low numbers of patient enrollment and for possibly overfeeding critically ill patients; however, numerous other studies using different methods and clinical observations mostly serve as a basis for the current protein recommendations of 1.2 to 1.5 g/kg/d. Several recently published comprehensive reviews of protein requirements in critical illness suggest that most critically ill patients may require much more than 1.5 g/kg/d,[52,54,55] and this recommendation is corroborated by recently published research suggesting the same.[59–61] Further support can be lent from the report that the oxidation rates of the most essential amino acids measured by their ^{13}C-labeled tracers were about 50% higher in critically ill patients than in the healthy subjects.[61] Therefore, considering the protein requirement for healthy individuals is 0.8 to 1.0 g/kg/d, the protein requirement of critically ill patients could be at the level of 1.5g/kg/d. Using data from the 2013 International Nutrition Survey, Nicolo and colleagues evaluated the energy and protein intakes of 2828 patients who were in the intensive care unit (ICU) for 4 days or longer.[61] Patients who received at least 80% of their protein requirements had shorter times to discharge alive (TDA) and reduced mortality. Receiving more than 80% of energy requirements did not have any effect on TDA or survival.

The risks of feeding too much protein include prerenal azotemia, with the excess protein increasing the burden to the kidneys to work to excrete excess urea nitrogen. Excess protein feeding over the long term can result in kidney stones and increased risk for osteoporosis. Nevertheless, adequately fed, underweight patients may require protein up to 25% more than their normal weight counterparts, or more than 1.9 g/kg/d.[62,63]

To determine the adequate protein supply to support a specific patient, the clinician must take into consideration the nutrition status of that patient on admission and the underlying disease. Clinical studies of underweight critically ill patients have not been performed; however, as weight decreases, there is a loss of both fat and muscle and the more rapidly turning over or metabolically active central protein compartments

(liver, heart, lungs, brain) make up a greater proportion of the total body weight; therefore, metabolic rate and protein requirements may be higher per kilogram of body weight in an underweight versus normal or overweight individual.[64–67]

Conditionally Essential Amino Acids in Clinical Practice

Some amino acids may exert pharmacological action during critical illness when administered at higher doses than normally consumed in food or standard nutrition support. For example, glutamine metabolism during critical illness has been extensively investigated during the past 20 years. Glutamine is the most abundant amino acid in the body, accounting for more than 50% of the intracellular free amino acid pool in muscle. It is the vital fuel for rapidly dividing cells such as fibroblasts, reticuloendothelial cells, malignant cells, and gut epithelial cells. Glutamine carries 2 nitrogen moieties per molecule, and, along with alanine, it serves as the body's primary nitrogen shuttle between muscle and visceral organs. In some clinical conditions, such as exercise, trauma, and sepsis, the body's glutamine requirement exceeds the mammalian's ability to synthesize glutamine; this imbalance leads to a fall in plasma and intracellular glutamine levels. This fall in glutamine concentration is associated with atrophy of intestinal mucosa, impairment of immune function, decreased protein synthesis, and even "second-hit" sepsis due to the impaired gut barrier function against bacterial translocation. Low plasma and muscle concentrations of glutamine in critical illness are correlated with increased mortality, leading to the hypothesis that replenishment of glutamine levels has a therapeutic value in certain clinical conditions. However, the REDOX trial, which included 40 ICUs and randomly assigned 1223 ventilated ICU patients to receive glutamine (IV and enteral), antioxidants, both glutamine and antioxidants, or placebo, suggested a trend toward an increased 28-day mortality and significant hospital and 6-month mortality in those patients that received glutamine.[68] However, the amount of glutamine (approximately 60 g) administered in this trial was much higher than that administered in previous trials. Some smaller recent trials suggest glutamine supplementation may be beneficial in selected burn and surgical patient populations, but larger randomized controlled trials need to be performed before glutamine supplementation can be routinely recommended.[69–71]

Arginine and cysteine, the former having an important role in immunomodulation, may also have pharmacological properties. Arginine has demonstrated importance in immune function and wound healing. It is essential for young mammals, but adults can synthesize it de novo. Plasma arginine levels are usually dependent on dietary intake because the rate of endogenous synthesis cannot increase in response to an inadequate supply. Arginine is a urea-cycle intermediate. It is deaminated to citrulline and used to synthesize polyamines and nitric oxide, which affects respiratory, cardiovascular, renal, and immunological function. Arginine and cysteine also enhance lymphocyte function and may prove useful in treating inflammatory diseases and AIDS.[62] Arginine is a key component of some immune-enhancing enteral nutrition formulas.[72] It also plays a role in promoting wound healing, partially because of its relationship to the metabolic pathway of arginine-ornithine-proline. See Chapters 23 and 24 for more on this topic.

Additional proteins with pharmacological potential include carnitine and choline. Carnitine is a trimethylated amino acid similar in structure to choline, which is required as a cofactor for transformation of free long-chain fatty acids into acylcarnitines and their transport into the mitochondria. Although a primary deficiency in carnitine is rare, it has been documented in preterm infants and in chronic renal failure. Carnitine is discussed in greater detail in Chapter 5.

Choline is also an essential nutrient necessary for proper membrane structure, which is not part of PN formulations. It can be manufactured in the liver from methionine, but synthesis may be impaired in patients on long-term PN or in premature infants. IV methionine is metabolized differently than orally or enterally consumed methionine, which may be partially responsible for the choline deficiency that develops with PN.[73] Small amounts of choline are available in the form of lecithin present in lipid injectable emulsions, but, despite this, low choline levels have been documented in patients receiving PN.[74] There is some evidence that choline deficiency is partially responsible for the hepatic abnormalities prevalent in patients on long-term PN, specifically hepatic steatosis. There are no available IV forms of choline. Repletion, if necessary, needs to be via the oral or enteral route.

Finally, creatine and beta-hydroxy beta-methylbutyrate (HMB) have been marketed as ergogenic aids in the sports medicine literature. They have both been extensively studied and have consistently been shown to increase lean body mass and improve strength when combined with resistance training.[75] Creatine has also been studied in diseases associated with muscle wasting (amyotrophic lateral sclerosis and muscular dystrophy).[76] HMB is a metabolite of leucine, but its mechanism of action remains elusive. It has been used as a supplement with glutamine in wasting associated with AIDS.[77] The ingestion of 3 g of HMB per day in the elderly promotes an increase in strength and lean body mass when combined with resistance exercise.[78,79] Its role in the treatment of the sarcopenia of aging is currently under investigation.[80]

References

1. Murray RK, Granner DK, Mayes PA, et al. *Harpers Illustrated Biochemistry*. 26th ed. New York: McGraw-Hill; 2003:14–20.
2. Young VR, Pellett PL. Plant proteins in relation to human protein and amino acid nutrition. *Am J Clin Nutr*. 1994;59(5 Suppl): 1203S–1212S.
3. Reeds PJ. Dispensable and indispensable amino acids for humans. *J Nutr*. 2000;30(suppl):S1835–S1840.
4. Nelson DL, Cox MM. *Lehninger Principles of Biochemistry*. 4th ed. New York: W.H. Freeman; 2005:85–89.
5. Walsh JH, Dochray GJ. *Gut Peptides*. New York: Raven Press; 1994:305–340.
6. Solcia E, Fiocca R, Rindi G, et al. The pathology of the gastrointestinal endocrine system. *Endocrinol Metab Clin North Am*. 1993;22:795–821.
7. Whitney EN, Cataldo CB, Rolfes SR. Protein: amino acids. In: Rolfes SR, Pinna, K, Whitney E, eds. *Understanding Normal and Clinical Nutrition*. 7th ed. Pacific Grove, CA: Brooks/Cole; 2005: 180–211.
8. Gropper SS, Smith JL, Groff JL. Protein. In: Gropper SS, Smith JL, eds. *Advanced Nutrition and Human Metabolism*. 5th ed. Belmont, CA: Wadsworth Learning; 2009:179–249.
9. Anderson CE. Energy and metabolism. In: Schneider HA, Anderson CE, Coursin DB. eds. *Nutrition Support of Medical Practice*. 2nd ed. Philadelphia, PA; Harper & Row; 1983:10–22.
10. Matthews DE. Proteins and amino acids. In: Shils ME, Olson JA, Rose AC, eds. *Modern Nutrition in Health and Disease*. 10th ed. Baltimore, MD: Williams & Wilkins; 2006:23–61.
11. Trier JS. Intestinal absorption: alimentary tract, liver, biliary tree and pancreas. In: Stein JH, ed. *Internal Medicine*. Vol I. Boston, MA: Little, Brown; 1983:11–16.
12. Beyer PL. Digestion, absorption, transport, and excretion of nutrients. In: Mahan LK, Escott-Stumps S, eds. *Krause's Food, Nutrition, and Diet Therapy*. 10th ed. Philadelphia, PA: WB Saunders; 2000:3–18.
13. Gardner ML. Absorption of intact proteins and peptides. In: Johnson LR, Alpers DH, Christensen J, et al., eds. *Physiology of the Gastrointestinal Tract*. 3rd ed. New York: Raven Press; 1994:1795–1820.
14. Ganapathy V, Brandsch M, Leibach FH. Intestinal transport of amino acids and peptides. In: Johnson LR, Alpers DH, Christensen J, et al., eds. *Physiology of the Gastrointestinal Tract*. 3rd ed. New York: Raven Press; 1994:1773–1794.
15. Adibi SA, Gray S, Menden E. The kinetics of amino acid absorption and alteration of plasma composition of free amino acids after intestinal perfusion of amino acid mixtures. *Am J Clin Nutr*. 1967;20:24–33.
16. Fairclough PD, Hegarty JE, Silk DBA, Clark ML. A comparison of the absorption of two protein hydrolysates and their effects on water and electrolyte movements in the human jejunum. *Gut*. 1980;21:829–834.
17. Silk DBA, Fairclough PD, Clark ML, et al. Use of peptide rather than a free amino acid nitrogen source in chemically defined elemental diets. *JPEN J Parenter Enteral Nutr*. 1980;4:548–553.
18. Zaloga GP. Physiological effects of peptide-based enteral formulas. *Nutr Clin Pract*. 1990;5:231–237.
19. Alpers DH. Uptake and fate of absorbed amino acids and peptides in the mammalian intestine. *Fed Proc*. 1986;45:2261–2267.
20. Grimble GK. The significance of peptides in clinical nutrition. *Annu Rev Nutr*. 1994;14:419–447.
21. DiMagno EP, Go VLW, Summerskill WHJ. Relations between pancreatic enzyme outputs and malabsorption in severe pancreatic insufficiency. *New Engl J Med*. 1973;288:813–815.
22. Zachos M, Tandeur M, Griffiths AM. A meta-analysis of enteral nutrition as primary therapy of active Crohn's disease: does formula composition influence efficacy? *Cochrane Database Syst Rev*. 2001;3:1–24.
23. Griffiths AM. Enteral nutrition in management of Crohn's disease. *JPEN J Parent Enter Nutr*. 2005;29(suppl):S108–S117.
24. Nelson DL, Cox MM. *Lehninger Principles of Biochemistry*. 4th ed. New York: Freeman; 2004:1044–1045.
25. Young LS, Stoll S. Protein in nutrition support. In Matarese LE, Gottschlich MM, eds. *Contemporary Nutrition Support Practice: A Clinical Guide*. 2nd ed. Philadelphia, PA: Saunders; 1998:97–109.
26. Wilmore DW. *Metabolic Management of the Critically Ill*. New York: Plenum Publishing; 1977:193.
27. Walser M. Misinterpretation of nitrogen balances when glutamine stores fall or are replenished. *Am J Clin Nutr*. 1993;5:414–416.
28. Wagenmakers AJM. Tracers to investigate protein and amino acid metabolism in human subjects. *Proc Nutr Soc*. 1999;58:987–1000.
29. Garlick PJ, Wernerman J, McNurlan MA, Heys SD. Organ-specific measurements of protein turnover in man. *Proc Nutr Soc*. 1991;50:217–225.
30. Reeds PJ, Burrin DG. The gut and amino acid homeostasis. *Nutrition*. 2000;16:666–668.

31. Ebner S, Schoknecht P, Reeds PJ, Burrin DG. Growth and metabolism of gastrointestinal and skeletal muscle tissues in protein malnourished neonatal pigs. *Am J Physiol.* 1994;266:R1736–R1741.

32. Scheppach W, Loges C, Bartram P, et al. Effects of free glutamine and alanyl-glutamine dipeptide on mucosal proliferation of the human ileum and colon. *Gastroenterology.* 1994;107:429–434.

33. Van de Poll MCG, Siroen MPC, Van Leeuwen PAM, et al. Interorgan amino acid exchange in humans: consequences for arginine and citrulline metabolism. *Am J Clin Nutr.* 2007;85(1):167–172.

34. Ettinger S. Macronutrients: carbohydrates, proteins, and lipids. In: Mahan LK, Escott-Stumps S, eds. *Krause's Food, Nutrition, and Diet Therapy.* 10th ed. Philadelphia, PA: WB Saunders; 2000:31–66.

35. Fukagawa NK, Yu Y-M. Nutrition and metabolism of proteins and amino acids. In: Gibney MJ, Lanham-New SA, Cassidy A, Vorster HH, eds. *Introduction to Human Nutrition.* 2nd ed. Oxford, UK: Wiley-Blackwell; 2009:49–73.

36. Young VR, Meredith C, Hoerr R, et al. Amino acid kinetics in relation to protein and amino acid requirements: the primary importance of amino acid oxidation. In: Garrow JS, Halliday D, eds. *Substrate and Energy Metabolism in Man.* London: John Libbey; 1985:119–134.

37. King MW. Medical biochemistry: glucose-alanine cycle 1996. www.dentistry.leeds.ac.uk/biochem/theme/glucose-alaninecycle.html. Accessed April 22, 2006.

38. Van de Poll MCG, Soeters PB, Deutz NE, et al. Renal metabolism of amino acids: its role in interorgan amino acid exchange. *Am J Clin Nutr.* 2004;79:185–197.

39. Cooper PE. Neuroendocrinology. In: Bradley WG, Daroff RB, Fenichel GM, Jankovic J, eds. *Neurology in Clinical Practice.* Vol 1: *Principles of Diagnosis and Management.* 4th ed. Philadelphia, PA: Elsevier; 2004:849–868.

40. Champe PC, Harvey RA. Metabolism in starvation, diabetes mellitus, and injury. In: Champe PC, Harvey RA, eds. *Lippincott's Illustrated Reviews: Biochemistry.* 2nd ed. Philadelphia, PA: JB Lippincott Co.; 1994:291–302.

41. Marks DB, Marks AD, Smith CM. Fasting. In: Smith C, Marks A, Lieberman M, eds. *Basic Medical Biochemistry—A Clinical Approach.* Baltimore, MD: Williams & Wilkins; 1996:27–34.

42. Cahill GF Jr, Aoki TT. Partial and total starvation. In: Kinney JM, ed. *Assessment of Energy Metabolism in Health and Disease: Report of the First Ross Conference on Medical Research.* Columbus, OH: Ross Laboratory; 1980:129–134.

43. Borum PR. Nutrient metabolism. In: Gottschlich MM, ed. *The Science and Practice of Nutrition Support: A Case-Based Core Curriculum.* Dubuque, IA: Kendall Hunt; 2001:17–29.

44. World Health Organization. *Energy and Protein Requirements. Report of a Joint FAO/WHO/UNO Expert Consultation.* Geneva, Switzerland: World Health Organization; 1985.

45. Castellanos VH, Litchford MD, Campbell WW. Modular protein supplements and their applications to long-term care. *Nutr Clin Pract.* 2006;21:485–504.

46. Food and Agriculture Organization of the United Nations. Food Energy—Methods of Analysis and Conversion Factors. Special Report of a Technical Workshop. Rome, 3–6 December 2002. 2003. http://www.fao.org/docrep/006/Y5022E/Y5022E00.HTM. Accessed December 19, 2016.

47. Jones DB. *Factors for Converting Percentages of Nitrogen in Foods and Feeds into Percentages of Proteins.* Washington, DC: US Department of Agriculture; 1942.

48. Hoffer LJ. How much protein do parenteral amino acid mixtures provide? *Am J Clin Nutr.* 2011;94:1396–1398.

49. Calloway DH, Spector H. Nitrogen balance as related to calorie and protein intake in active young men. *Am J Clin Nutr.* 1954;2:405–412.

50. Arabi YM, Aldawood AS, Haddad SH, et al. Permissive underfeeding on standard enteral feeding in critically ill adults. *N Engl J Med.* 2015;372:2398–408.

51. McClave SA, Codner P, Patel J, et. al. Should we aim for full enteral feeding in the first week of illness? *Nutr Clin Pract.* 2016;31:425–431.

52. Hoffer LJ, Bistrian BR. Appropriate protein provision in critical illness: a systematic and narrative review. *Am J Clin Nutr.* 2012;96:591–600.

53. Jacobs DG, Jacobs DO, Kudsk KA, et al. Practice management guidelines for nutrition support of the trauma patient. *J Trauma.* 2004;57:660–679.

54. Hoffer LJ, Bistrian BR. Why critically ill patients are protein deprived. *JPEN J Parenter Enteral Nutr.* 2013;37:300–309.

55. Hoffer JL. Human protein and amino acid requirements. *JPEN J Parenter Enteral Nutr.* 2016;40:460–474.

56. Burke PA, Young LS, Bistrian BR. Metabolic vs nutrition support: a hypothesis. *JPEN J Parenter Enteral Nutr.* 2010;34:546–548.

57. Reid CL, Campbell IT, Little RA. Muscle wasting and energy balance in critical illness. *Clin Nutr.* 2004;23:273–280.

58. Shaw JH, Wildbore M, Wolf RR. Whole body protein kinetics in severely septic patients: the response to glucose infusion and total parenteral nutrition. *Ann Surg.* 1987;205:288–294.

59. Clifton GL, Robertson CS, Constant CF. Enteral hyperalimentation in head injury. *J Neurosurg.* 1985;62:186–193.

60. Dickerson RN, Pitts SL, Maish GO III, et. al. A reappraisal of nitrogen requirements for patients with critical illness and trauma. *J Trauma Acute Care Surg.* 2012;73:549–557.

61. Nicolo M, Heyland DK, Chittams J, et. al. Clinical outcomes related to protein delivery in a critically ill population: a multicenter, multinational observation study. *JPEN J Parenter Enteral Nutr.* 2016;40:45–51.

62. Stehle P. Nutrition support in critical illness: amino acids. In: Cynober L, Moore FA, eds. *Nutrition in Critical Care.* Nestlé Nutrition Workshop Series Clinical and Performance Program. Basel, Switzerland: Nestlé Ltd; 2003:57–73.

63. Campbell IT. Limitations of nutrient intake. the effect of stressors: trauma, sepsis and multiple organ failure. *Eur J Clin Nutr.* 1999;53(Suppl 1):S143–S147.

64. Hoffer LJ. Protein and energy provision in critical illness. *Am J Clin Nutr.* 2003;78:906–911.

65. Ahmad A, Duerksen DR, Munroe S, Bistrian BR. An evaluation of resting energy expenditure in hospitalized, severely underweight patients. *Nutrition.* 1999;15:384–388.

66. Kurpad AV, Regan MM, Raj T, et al. Lysine requirements of chronically undernourished adult Indian men, measured by a 24-h indicator amino acid oxidation and balance technique. *Am J Clin Nutr.* 2003;77:101–108.

67. Winter TA, O'Keefe SJ, Callahan M, Dip, N, Marks T. The effect of severe undernutrition and subsequent refeeding on whole-body metabolism and protein synthesis in human subjects. *JPEN J Parenter Enteral Nutr.* 2005;29:221–228.

68. Heyland D, Musceder J, Wischmeyer PE, et al. A randomized trial of glutamine and antioxidants in critically ill patients. *N Engl J Med.* 2013;368:1489-1497.

69. McClave SA, Taylor BE, Martindale RG, et al. Guidelines for the provision and assessment of nutrition support therapy in the adult critically ill patient: Society of Critical Care Medicine (SCCM) and American Society for Parenteral and Enteral Nutrition (ASPEN). *JPEN J Parenter Enteral Nutr.* 2016;40:159–211.

70. Griffiths RD, Allen KD, Andrews FJ, Jones C. Infection, multiple organ failure, and survival in the intensive care unit: influence of glutamine-supplemented parenteral nutrition on acquired infections. *Nutrition.* 2002;18:546–552.

71. Alpers DH. Glutamine: do the data support the cause for glutamine supplementation in humans? *Gastroenterology.* 2006;130:S106–S116.

72. McCowen KC, Bistrian BR. Immunonutrition: problematic or problem solving? *Am J Clin Nutr.* 2003;77:764–770.

73. Buchman AL. Choline deficiency during parenteral nutrition in humans. *Nutr Clin Pract.* 2003;18:353–358.

74. Chawla RK, Berry CJ, Kutner MH, et al. Plasma concentrations of transulfuration pathway products during nasoenteral and intravenous hyperalimentation of malnourished patients. *Am J Clin Nutr.* 1985;42:577–584.

75. Wandrag L, Brett SJ, Frost G, Hickson M. Impact of supplementation with amino acids or their metabolites on muscle wasting in patients with critical illness or other muscle wasting illness: a systemic review *J Hum Nutr Diet.* 2015; 28(4):313–330.

76. Sakkas GK, Schambelan M, Mulligan K. Can the use of creatine supplementation attenuate muscle loss in cachexia and wasting? *Curr Opin Clin Nutr Metab Care.* 2009;12(6):623–627.

77. Clark RH, Feleke G, Din M, et al. Nutritional treatment for acquired immunodeficiency virus-associated wasting using beta-hydroxy beta methyl butyrate, glutamine, and arginine: a randomized, double-blind, placebo-controlled study. *JPEN J Parenter Enteral Nutr.* 2000;24(3):133–139.

78. Flakoll P, Sharp R, Baier S, et al. Effect of beta-hydroxy-beta-methylbutyrate, arginine, and lysine supplementation on strength, functionality, body composition, and protein metabolism in elderly women. *Nutrition.* 2004;20:445–451.

79. Vukovich MD, Stubbs NB, Bohlken RM, et al. Body composition in 70-year-old adults responds to dietary beta-hydroxy-beta-methylbutyrate (HMB) similarly to that of young adults. *J Nutr.* 2001;131:2049–2052.

80. Phillips SM. Nutritional supplements in support of resistance exercise to counter age-related sarcopenia. *Adv Nutr.* 2015; 6(4):452–460.

7 Fluids, Electrolytes, and Acid-Base Disorders

Todd W. Canada, PharmD, BCNSP, BCCCP, FASHP, FTSHP, and Linda M. Lord, NP, CNSC, ACNP-BC

CONTENTS

Acknowledgments: Ginger Langley, PharmD, BCNSP, BCPS, CPHQ, and Sharla Tajchman, PharmD, BCNSP, BCPS, were coauthors of this chapter for the second edition.

Objectives

1. Describe factors that influence fluid movement between the intracellular fluid (ICF) and extracellular fluid (ECF) compartments.
2. Calculate replacement and maintenance fluid requirements for various patient populations.
3. Recommend appropriate treatment for common electrolyte abnormalities.
4. Evaluate and treat acid-base disorders based on the clinical presentation and accompanying laboratory data.

Test Your Knowledge Questions

1. The administration of 1 liter 0.9% sodium chloride (NaCl) to a normonatremic patient will increase the intravascular and interstitial fluid compartments by:
   A. 1000 mL and 0 mL, respectively
   B. 0 mL and 1000 mL, respectively
   C. 750 mL and 250 mL, respectively
   D. 250 mL and 750 mL, respectively
2. Assuming the same weight and serum sodium concentration, which of the following patients has the greatest free water deficit?
   A. A 35-year-old man
   B. A 75-year-old man
   C. A 35-year-old woman
   D. A 75-year-old woman
3. A patient with severe intractable nausea and vomiting is at risk for which of the following acid-base disorders?
   A. Hyperchloremic metabolic alkalosis
   B. Hyperchloremic metabolic acidosis
   C. Hypochloremic metabolic alkalosis
   D. Hypochloremic metabolic acidosis

Test Your Knowledge Answers

1. The correct answer is **D**. A solution of 0.9% NaCl (154 mEq/L) is isotonic and, therefore, does not contribute to an osmotic gradient. Isotonic saline enters and remains in the ECF. Thus, administering 1 liter 0.9% NaCl expands the ECF by 1 liter. The intravascular volume accounts for 25% of the ECF and will expand by 250 mL. The remaining 750 mL will be distributed to the interstitial fluid compartment.
2. The correct answer is **A**. Free water deficit is calculated as follows:

Free Water Deficit = TBW × [1 − (140/Serum Sodium)]

where free water deficit and total body water (TBW) are measured in liters and serum sodium is measured in mEq/L. Given the same body weight and serum sodium concentration, the only variable is the percentage of TBW. The percentage of TBW increases as the proportion of lean body mass (LBM) to adipose tissue increases. In general, the percentage of TBW decreases with age and is lower in females than in males. Younger men would be expected to have the highest proportion of LBM and the highest percentage of TBW and would therefore have the largest free water deficit.

3. The correct answer is **C**. Gastric fluids contain approximately 130 mEq chloride (Cl^-) per liter and are very acidic (pH 1 to 2). Losing large amounts of gastric fluids via vomiting, especially for a prolonged period of time, can result in a hypochloremic metabolic alkalosis as the loss of acid from the stomach leaves the body with a relative excess of alkali.

Background

Body fluids differ with regard to their distribution and the substances dissolved within them. These substances include electrolytes and nonelectrolytes, such as glucose and proteins. Even with variations in daily intake, fluid and electrolyte balance is achieved through a complex system of regulatory mechanisms that maintain an environment conducive to normal cell function. Because nearly all biochemical reactions are influenced by hydrogen ion concentration, cell function also depends on acid-base homeostasis. In practice, disruptions of fluid, electrolyte, and acid-base homeostasis are common, and the results can profoundly affect organ systems. This chapter discusses normal body requirements, the distribution and homeostasis of water and electrolytes, as well as the evaluation and treatment of common fluid, electrolyte, and acid-base disorders.

Fluid Compartments

Water, the most abundant substance in the body, constitutes approximately 50% to 60% of body weight. TBW is a function of weight, age, sex, and the relative amount of body fat. Of all body tissues, adipose tissue is the least hydrated. Thus, individuals with more body fat have proportionally less TBW content.[1]

TBW is distributed among the ICF, ECF, and transcellular fluid (TCF) compartments. Approximately two-thirds of TBW is contained in ICF and the remaining one-third is in ECF. The TCF compartment accounts for about 3% of TBW and includes specialized fluids such as cerebrospinal fluid, the aqueous humor of the eye, and secretions of the gastrointestinal (GI) tract. The ECF is the most clinically important fluid compartment because it contains the intravascular and interstitial spaces.[2]

Osmotic pressure, the pressure required to maintain equilibrium with no net movement of solvent, is of prime importance in determining the distribution of water between the extracellular and intracellular spaces. Each compartment contains a major osmotically active solute that ultimately determines its osmotic pressure. Sodium is the dominant extracellular osmole holding water in the extracellular space, whereas potassium is the primary intracellular osmole holding water within the cells. Activity of cellular sodium-potassium-adenosine triphosphatase (Na^+-K^+-ATPase) pumps allows for the maintenance of these unique solute compositions of the ECF and ICF and plays a key role in the regulation of cell volume.[1]

To better illustrate the dynamics of water distribution between the ICF and ECF, consider the exogenous administration of intravenous (IV) fluids. If 1 liter 5% dextrose in water (solute-free water) is infused, the dextrose is metabolized and the resulting water distributes proportionately to all fluid compartments. In other words, two-thirds (667 mL) of the fluid distributes into the ICF and one-third (333 mL) distributes into the ECF. Of the one-third distributed into the ECF, 25% (85 mL) remains in the intravascular space. In contrast, IV administration of 1 liter 0.9% NaCl (isotonic saline) is distributed completely to the ECF where one-quarter (250 mL) remains in the intravascular space. Thus, when choosing IV fluids. isotonic saline is approximately 3 times more efficient than 5% dextrose in water at expanding the intravascular space. Alternatively, the addition of hypertonic fluid (eg, 3% NaCl) to the ECF increases its tonicity, establishing an osmotic gradient that results in the movement of water out of cells and into the ECF until osmotic equilibrium is attained. The osmolalities of both compartments increases—that of the ECF because of the addition of NaCl and that of the ICF from water loss. The volume change is proportional to the degree of increase in ECF osmolality (Figure 7-1).[3]

Although osmotic forces determine the distribution of water between the ICF and ECF spaces, the plasma oncotic and hydrostatic pressures govern the movement of fluid between the plasma and interstitial fluid. These forces are generally balanced, and compartment sizes are therefore maintained in a steady state despite large fluid exchanges between compartments. Disruption in oncotic and/or hydrostatic pressure results in a net flow of fluid from one compartment to another. When these disruptions favor a plasma-to-interstitial fluid shift,

third spacing, the accumulation of excess fluid in the interstitial space (edema) or in the potential fluid spaces (effusion),[4] occurs. Although the fluid will be absorbed back into the extracellular compartment over a period of days to weeks, the acute reduction in blood volume, if not replaced, can lead to severe volume depletion. This phenomenon is common during critical illness when capillary permeability increases, resulting in the leakage of albumin from the intravascular to the interstitial space and reduced plasma oncotic pressure, which favors the movement of fluid from the intravascular to the interstitial space. Third spacing can occur with intestinal obstruction, severe acute pancreatitis, crush injuries, bleeding, peritonitis, obstruction of a major venous system, and other conditions.

Fluid Balance

After taking into account insensible losses, fluid gains (input) should be in balance with fluid losses (output) over a period of several days. On average, a healthy adult requires 30 to 40 mL of fluid per kg of body weight per day to maintain this balance.[5,6] However, weight-based estimates tend to overestimate fluid requirements for large individuals and underestimate them for small people. Water intake is derived primarily from the diet (including water generated from the oxidation of carbohydrates, proteins, and fats), whereas various sources of water loss contribute to total fluid output. In most cases, sensible (easily measurable) losses from the GI tract and kidneys account for most fluid loss, although insensible (not easily measurable) losses from the lungs and skin can contribute up to 1 L/d.[1]

FIGURE 7-1 Water Distribution to the Extracellular Fluid and Intracellular Fluid and Composition of Commonly Used Intravenous Fluids

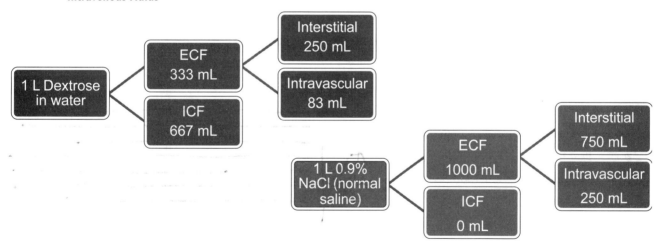

Solution	Dextrose, g/L	Sodium, mEq/L	Chloride, mEq/L	Tonicity	Free Water, mL/L[a]
D5W (5% dextrose)	50	0	0	Hypotonic	1000
0.45% NaCl (½ normal saline)	0	77	77	Hypotonic	500
0.9% NaCl (normal saline)	0	154	154	Isotonic	0
3% NaCl (hypertonic saline)	0	513	513	Hypertonic	−2331
Lactated Ringer's	0	130	109	Isotonic	0

ECF, extracellular fluid; ICF, intracellular fluid; NaCl, sodium chloride.
[a]Amount of water available to correct a free water deficit associated with hypernatremia.

Calculating Fluid Requirements

Various approaches are used to estimate fluid requirements in adults. Formulas used to calculate daily fluid requirements should account for the patient's weight, age, and clinical status. Water is needed to support an individual's LBM, which fluctuates with weight and decreases with age. Some formulas are energy based (1 mL per kcal consumed[7] or 1 mL per kcal required[8]), and others are weight based, such as the simple calculation of 25 to 35 mL/kg.[9] Some weight-based calculations set a minimum of 1500 mL/d.[10] For example, the Holliday-Segar formula[11] is 1500 mL for the first 20 kg body weight plus 20 mL/kg for the remaining kg of body weight.

Weight-based formulas may lead to fluid overload in patients with severe cardiac issues or kidney distress.[8] Fluid-restricted patients whose physical activity is limited may benefit from use of the energy-based formulas to prevent fluid overload.[8]

To prevent dehydration, some experts discourage the use of energy-based formulas in individuals age 65 years or older and recommend the use of one of the following formulas for the older adult: (1) an adjusted Holliday-Segar formula (1500 mL for the first 20 kg body weight plus 15 mL/kg for remaining body weight) or (2) 30 mL/kg with a minimum of 1500 mL; or (3) 1500 to 2000 mL/d.[10,12-14]

Nutrition support clinicians must ensure that sufficient fluid is given to individuals who are vulnerable to dehydration, cannot express thirst, or are in a setting where the signs of dehydration are not closely monitored. When patients discharged home or to an alternate care facility receive nutrition support with inadequate fluid, they can become rapidly dehydrated and suffer symptoms such as hypotension, confusion, extreme thirst, and constipation that may not initially be attributed to dehydration.

Some practitioners have found clinical success by calculating fluid needs (mL/d) with the following 2 formulas and then using the average of the results.

Equation 1 (based on body weight and age):[9]

Ages 18–55 years: 35 mL × Body Weight (kg)

Ages 56–75 years: 30 mL × Body Weight (kg)

Ages >75 years: 25 mL × Body Weight (kg)

Fluid-restricted adults (eg, those with kidney disease, cardiac disease, or fluid overload states):
≤25 mL × Body Weight (kg)

Equation 2 (Holliday-Segar formula adjusted for age):[12-14]

Ages ≤50 years: 1500 mL for first 20 kg Body Weight + [20 mL × Remaining Body Weight (kg)]

Ages >50 years: 1500 mL for first 20 kg Body Weight + [15 mL × Remaining Body Weight (kg)]

Very muscular, active individuals likely require more water than in the volume estimated by these equations because they have an increased percentage of LBM. Conversely, the use of an obesity-adjusted weight should be used to calculate the fluid needs of obese individuals to account for their increased percentage of body fat. When an individual gains excess weight, about 75% is typically fat tissue and 25% is lean (although the proportions can vary widely among individuals).[15] An obesity-adjusted weight is often used when an individual's weight is equal to or greater than 125% ideal body weight (IBW), unless the excess weight is due to muscle mass. For this method, which has not been validated but is in common use, IBW is calculated as follows:

Women: IBW (lb) =
100 lb for 5 ft in height + 5 lb for each inch over 5 ft
Men: IBW (lb) =
106 lb for 5 ft in height + 6 lb for each inch over 5 ft

Then, the obesity-adjusted weight is obtained by subtracting the IBW (± 10%) from the actual weight and adding back one-quarter (25%) of the difference to the IBW:

Obesity-Adjusted Body Weight (lb) =
[(Actual Weight − IBW) × 0.25] + IBW

The adjusted weight is then converted to kilograms to perform the fluid calculations. For example, to estimate the fluid requirements for a 61-year-old woman who is 5 feet, 4 inches tall and weighs 160 pounds, the clinician would proceed as follows:

1. Calculate IBW: 100 lb + (5 × 4 lb) = 120 lb
2. Calculate obesity-adjusted weight:
[(160 lb − 120 lb) × 0.25] + 120 lb = 130 lb (59 kg)
3. Calculate fluid requirements using Equation 1:
30 mL × 59 kg = 1770 mL/d
4. Calculate fluid requirements using Equation 2:
1500 mL + [15 × (59 kg −20 kg)] = 2085 mL/d
5. Calculate the mean of the results from steps 3 and 4:
(1770 mL/d + 2085 mL/d)/2 = ~1900 mL/d

For obese, chronically inactive individuals, an additional approach is to calculate both energy and fluid requirements using IBW instead of an obesity-adjusted weight.

Additional fluid must be provided for patients with severe diarrhea or emesis; large draining wounds; excessive diaphoresis; constant drooling; paracentesis losses; drains; high gastric, fistula, and ostomy outputs; or persistent fevers. Fluid needs increase by 7% for each °F above normal (13% for each °C above normal). Women who are lactating also have increased fluid requirements.

Fluid losses should be measured when possible, but outputs are not always collectable. Weighing wound dressings before and after placement may help determine the fluid loss from open wounds. Excessive diaphoresis that soaks bed linens is usually equal to at least 1 liter of fluid.[16]

Fluids in the Nutrition Support Prescription

Parenteral nutrition (PN) formulas can usually meet a patient's calculated fluid needs. For patients receiving enteral tube feedings, the tube feeding formula provides a portion of the fluid needs, but additional water is usually required. Enteral tube feeding formulas are 67% to 87% water (approximately 160 to 210 mL water per 8-oz container). The remainder is solids consisting of macro- and micronutrients (see Chapter 11). The more energy-dense a formula is, the lower the percentage of water volume is. Manufacturers do not usually list water content on the formula label, although the information is available elsewhere in product documentation. After accounting for the water in the parenteral or enteral formula, the patient's remaining fluid needs are provided with water flushes (if enteral nutrition support), oral fluid (if allowed), or additional IV fluids. When parenteral or enteral formulas are held, it is important to continue to provide the fluids needed by some other means to prevent dehydration.

Regardless of the method used to determine the initial fluid prescription, the fluid volume must be adjusted regularly based on fluctuations in intake and output as well as patient clinical status (eg, organ/system function). Fluid imbalances can occur quickly; therefore, patients receiving nutrition support and their caregivers must be educated on the signs and symptoms of under- and overhydration. See Practice Scenario 7-1 for a discussion of maintenance fluids in a common clinical condition.[1,17-20]

Practice Scenario 7-1

Question: How would you manage maintenance fluids for a patient with heart failure?

Scenario: RA is a 65-year-old man weighing 75 kg with an ideal body weight of 66 kg. His past medical history is significant for heart failure and diabetes, and he was admitted to your hospital for heart failure exacerbation. Physical examination revealed jugular venous distention, rales, and 3+ pitting edema in bilateral lower extremities. On admission, RA was receiving oxygen therapy at 8 L/min via a nasal cannula and was unable to tolerate an oral diet. An intravenous (IV) solution with 0.9% sodium chloride was initiated at 125 mL/h. On hospital Day 3, RA's oxygen requirements increased, necessitating noninvasive positive pressure ventilation and transfer to the intensive care unit (ICU).

Intervention: Upon transfer to the ICU, the intensivist started a continuous IV furosemide infusion and changed IV fluids to 0.45% sodium chloride at 10 mL/h to maintain IV access.

Answer: Maintenance fluid requirements for a healthy 75-kg man would be 25 to 35 mL/kg/d (1875 to 2625 mL/d). However, patients who present with fluid overload secondary to heart failure exacerbations cannot tolerate normal maintenance fluid requirements. For patients with heart failure, daily fluid intake should be approximately 20 to 25 mL per kg of estimated dry weight, and calculated fluid requirements should take into account clinical symptoms (ie, edema, fatigue, shortness of breath). Additionally, sodium should be restricted to less than 2000 mg (87 mEq) per day.[19,18] Because RA has a history of heart failure and was admitted with fluid overload and shortness of breath, 3 liters of maintenance IV fluids per day contributed to further respiratory

decompensation, requiring aggressive diuresis and ICU transfer. The restriction of IV fluids and sodium along with diuresis resulted in decreased oxygen requirements and improvement in other clinical symptoms associated with fluid overload.

Rationale: Heart failure patients with evidence of significant fluid overload should initially be treated with loop diuretics and sodium and fluid restriction. Therapy for hospitalized patients with decompensated heart failure should begin as soon as possible because early interventions have been associated with better outcomes.[19,20] After admission to the hospital, patients should be carefully monitored in accordance with the severity of their symptoms and the results of initial findings on the physical examination and laboratory assessment.

Serum osmolality (water balance) is maintained within the normal range of 280 to 295 mOsm/kg. This point is essential because imbalances of only 1% to 2% initiate mechanisms to return the serum osmolality to normal.[1] Two mechanisms regulate water balance: (1) the thirst sensation, and (2) control of renal water excretion by antidiuretic hormone (ADH). The body responds to a water load by suppressing ADH secretion, resulting in decreased collecting tubule water reabsorption and excretion of excess water. The correction of a water deficit requires the intake and retention of exogenous water achieved by increases in thirst and ADH release. Efficiency of this regulatory system is incomplete if the patient has any renal impairment or abnormality in the thirst mechanism (eg, lack of access to water for a mechanically ventilated patient).

Fluid and Electrolyte Disorders

Terminology

Disorders of fluid balance can be classified as disturbances of volume, concentration, or composition. These disturbances often occur simultaneously in clinical practice. Excessive gain of fluid (ie, water and solute such as sodium) is referred to as *volume overload* or *hypervolemia*. Conversely, excessive fluid loss is known as *volume depletion* or *hypovolemia*. Volume depletion often follows GI hemorrhage, vomiting, diarrhea, and diuresis.[21] *Overhydration* refers to the gain of water alone, whereas *dehydration* is the loss of water only. These 2 conditions are recognized by a change in serum sodium concentration and plasma osmolality.[2] A *disturbance of composition* refers to a gain or loss of potassium, magnesium, calcium, phosphate, chloride, bicarbonate, or hydrogen ions.

General Management Principles

Some fluid losses contain significant amounts of electrolytes, minerals, or proteins that require replacement along with water. Knowledge of the composition of specific body fluids is therefore useful. Table 7-1 shows the volume of fluid secreted and its electrolyte content throughout the GI tract.[5] Abnormalities in renal excretion and excessive losses from the GI tract (eg, vomiting, nasogastric suctioning, diarrhea) are often primary contributors to electrolyte imbalances. Identifying the etiology of the electrolyte imbalance is essential to providing safe and effective treatment.

TABLE 7-1 Volume and Average Electrolyte Content of Gastrointestinal Secretions

Source/Type of Secretion	Volume, L/d	Na⁺	K⁺	Cl⁻	HCO₃⁻
Saliva	1.5	10	26	10	30
Stomach	1.5	60	10	130	0
Duodenum	Variable	140	5	80	0
Ileum	3	140	5	104	30
Colon	Variable	60	30	40	0
Pancreas	Variable	140	5	75	115
Bile	Variable	145	5	100	35

Electrolyte Concentration, mEq/L

Cl⁻, chloride; HCO₃⁻, bicarbonate; K⁺, potassium; Na⁺, sodium.
Source: Adapted with permission from reference 5: Whitmire SJ. Fluids and electrolytes. In: Matarese LE, Gottschlich MM, eds. *Contemporary Nutrition Support Practice: A Clinical Guide*. Philadelphia, PA: Saunders: 1998:130. Copyright © Laura E. Matarese and Michele M. Gottschlich.

The therapeutic approach to fluid and electrolyte disorders requires clinicians to determine the time frame in which the abnormality occurred. Generally, the development of an acute abnormality (less than 48 hours) is associated with symptoms that require immediate treatment (eg, altered mental status with acute hyponatremia). The development of a chronic electrolyte disorder is often asymptomatic, and the patient may be harmed if the disorder is corrected too rapidly, as in the case of chronic hyponatremia. In the absence of symptoms, the chronologic trends in electrolyte values are generally more important than the absolute value on any given day.[2] Clinicians should review all available electrolyte values because patients often have multiple electrolyte abnormalities.

Figure 7-2 illustrates several key principles that warrant consideration when evaluating and treating electrolyte disorders in clinical practice. Upon initial review of laboratory data, clinicians should first determine whether the reported electrolyte levels are consistent with the patient's clinical condition. If laboratory results are inconsistent, the accuracy of the specimen collection should be validated before further treatment is considered. This step is crucial to prevent inappropriately treating electrolyte values that may be caused by errors in sample collection or handling. If a collection error or specimen mishandling is confirmed, a new specimen should be collected and further analyzed. If the laboratory result is valid, clinicians should then develop a treatment regimen based on the aberrant electrolyte level.

If an electrolyte level is above the normal range, therapy should be directed toward the removal of exogenous sources of the electrolyte or facilitating its elimination. The most appropriate treatment regimen often depends on the severity of the electrolyte disorder and the presence or absence of symptoms. Potential treatments to consider include removing electrolyte supplementation from IV fluids or PN, changing an enteral nutrition formulation that contains the electrolyte(s) to another product, discontinuing medications that could be contributing to the electrolyte disorder, management of acid-base abnormalities (eg, metabolic acidosis), and/or inducing renal or GI elimination of the electrolyte.

Electrolyte replacement is the treatment for electrolyte levels below the normal range. To determine whether oral or IV electrolyte replacement is appropriate, patient-specific factors should be considered. IV electrolyte replacement is preferred for patients with impaired GI tract function (eg, diarrhea, malabsorption), those with difficulty swallowing, those who are *nil per os* status, and those who have critically low electrolyte levels. Conservative electrolyte replacement is often indicated for patients with impaired renal function unless they are actively receiving renal replacement therapy. Patients with volume overload should receive volume-restricted electrolyte replacement or oral therapy whenever possible. When considering IV electrolyte replacement, the options for IV access (peripheral vs central) should be identified. Peripheral administration has limits for volume and the rate of administration, especially for potassium and calcium, and exceeding these limits can result in tissue damage and potential patient harm.

To optimize and minimize electrolyte replacement, clinicians should assess the presence of concurrent electrolyte abnormalities. For example, to optimize replacement in a patient with hypomagnesemia and hypokalemia, magnesium should be repleted before potassium because potassium levels are rarely corrected unless the magnesium deficit is corrected first. The use of potassium phosphate to correct concurrent hypokalemia and hypophosphatemia is an example of minimizing electrolyte replacement.

Sodium

At its normal serum concentration of 135 to 145 mEq/L, sodium (Na⁺) is the principal cation in the ECF. Sodium functions as the major osmotic determinant in regulating ECF volume and water distribution in the body. Other functions of sodium include determining the membrane potential of cells and the active transport of molecules across cell membranes.

Hyponatremia

Hyponatremia (serum sodium concentration less than 135 mEq/L) occurs in 25% of hospitalized patients.[22] Symptoms include headache, nausea, vomiting, muscle cramps, lethargy, restlessness, disorientation, depressed reflexes, seizures, and coma. Clinical manifestations related to central nervous system (CNS) dysfunction are more likely when the serum sodium concentration drops rapidly and when it falls below 125 mEq/L.[2] Mortality rates are increased significantly when serum sodium drops below 120 mEq/L.[23]

The hyponatremic patient requires a systematic assessment. Upon recognition of clinically relevant hyponatremia (serum sodium less than 130 mEq/L), clinicians should determine the patient's serum sodium concentration and volume status to identify the etiology of the hyponatremia and appropriate treatment options.

FIGURE 7-2 Algorithm for the Management of Electrolyte Disorders

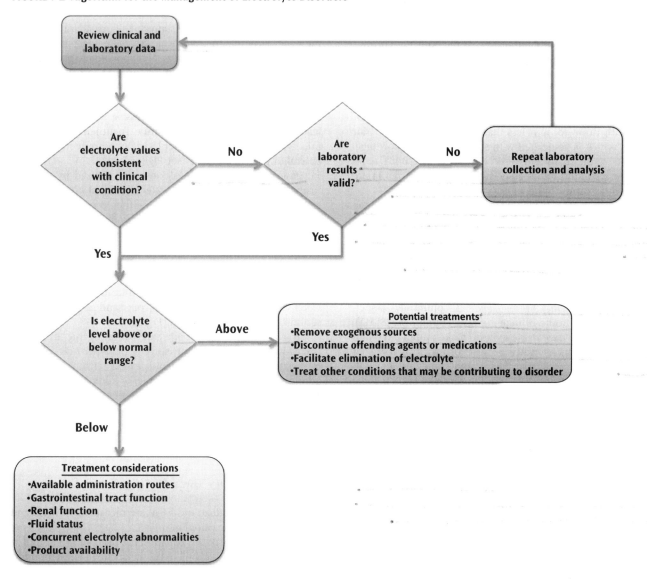

Serum osmolality can be directly measured, or it can be calculated with the following equation:

Serum Osmolality =
$$2 \times \{[(\text{Serum Na}^+) + (\text{Serum Glucose})/18] + [\text{BUN}/2.8]\}$$

where serum osmolality is measured in mOsm/kg, serum sodium is measured in mEq/L, and serum glucose and blood urea nitrogen (BUN) are measured in mg/dL.

Serum and calculated osmolalities should be relatively close in value. If there is a difference between the 2 values, the patient should be assessed for possible ingestion of toxic substances (ethylene glycol, propylene glycol) that can cause a gap between serum and calculated osmolality. Such a gap is referred to as an *osmolar gap* when the difference is more than 10 mOsm/kg.

Hypertonic hyponatremia (serum osmolality greater than 290 mOsm/L) is caused by the presence of osmotically active substances other than sodium in the ECF. Common causes include hyperglycemia and mannitol administration. The correction of serum sodium related to hyperglycemia can be estimated with the following equation:

Corrected Na⁺ =
$$\text{Serum Na}^+ + [0.016 \times (\text{Serum Glucose}) - 100]$$

where sodium is measured in mEq/L and serum glucose is measured in mg/dL.

Isotonic hyponatremia (serum osmolarity within the normal range, approximately 275 to 300 mOsm/L) occurs when the fraction of serum that is composed of water is reduced (indicating an excess of plasma proteins or lipids). With recent advances in laboratory analysis, isotonic hyponatremia is rarely observed.

Hypotonic hyponatremia (serum osmolarity less than 275 mOsm/L) warrants a detailed assessment of volume status and urine sodium osmolality. In *hypovolemic hypotonic hyponatremia*, patients lose more sodium in relation to water. Therefore, it is critical to determine the source of fluid loss. Urine osmolality in these patients is always greater than serum osmolality, which indicates concentrated urine and the body's attempt to retain fluid. Renal losses are usually caused by diuretic use and identified by urine sodium more than 20 mEq/L. Extrarenal losses can be caused by diarrhea, GI fistula output, excessive sweating, burns, open wounds, and fluid drains (eg, peritoneal, pleural, biliary, or pancreatic drains) and may be associated with urine sodium less than 20 mEq/L. Cerebral salt wasting, which is associated with subarachnoid hemorrhage, may also result in hypovolemic hyponatremia. Both renal and extrarenal fluid losses associated with hyponatremia are treated with isotonic fluids to expand the ECF volume.

Patients with *hypervolemic hypotonic hyponatremia* have some element of end-organ damage (renal failure, hepatic failure with ascites, heart failure), resulting in fluid retention or third spacing. These patients retain more water than sodium, and treatment involves both fluid and sodium restriction. Sodium restriction may seem counterintuitive for hyponatremia; however, increased sodium intake increases fluid retention.

Euvolemic hypotonic hyponatremia is commonly associated with the syndrome of inappropriate antidiuresis (SIAD). Patients with SIAD have stable sodium intake/output but retain additional amounts of water because of excessive levels of ADH (which is released from the pituitary gland and, in small amounts, from lung alveoli). Common causes of SIAD include brain or CNS malignancies, head trauma, lung malignancies, and pneumonia. With euvolemic hypotonic hyponatremia, urine osmolality is always greater than serum osmolality and urine sodium is greater than 20 mEq/L, indicating that the kidneys are inappropriately concentrating urine and volume status is adequate, thus differentiating this condition from hypovolemic hypotonic hyponatremia. The mainstay of treatment for SIAD is to restrict fluids to 500 to 1000 mL/d; if the patient is symptomatic, exogenous salt is also administered. SIAD refractory to conventional treatment may require pharmacologic therapy with loop diuretics and/or vasopressin-2 receptor antagonists such as conivaptan or tolvaptan. Other causes of euvolemic hypotonic hyponatremia are psychogenic polydipsia (the ingestion of large amounts of free water), hypothyroidism, and reset osmostat. Treatment revolves around correcting the underlying disorder and fluid restriction.

Figure 7-3 presents an algorithm for the evaluation, etiology, and treatment of hyponatremia.[5] To prevent osmotic demyelination, the targeted rate of sodium correction for hyponatremia should not exceed 10 to 12 mEq/L/d if the condition is acute or 6 to 8 mEq/L/d if the condition is chronic or of unknown duration.[24]

Hypernatremia

Hypernatremia (serum sodium greater than 145 mEq/L) occurs in approximately 2% of hospitalized patients, and serum sodium levels greater than 160 mEq/L are associated with a significant increase in mortality.[25,26] Clinical manifestations of hypernatremia are associated with neurologic sequelae that range from mild (headache, dizziness, confusion) to severe (seizures, coma, and death). The approach to determine the etiology of hypernatremia is similar to the method used to identify causes of hyponatremia.

An assessment of volume status is the first step in diagnosing hypernatremia. In *hypovolemic hypernatremia*, patients have above-normal serum osmolality. In hypovolemic patients, it is important to determine the source of fluid loss. Renal losses are commonly caused by diuretic use, solute diuresis associated with hyperglycemia or azotemia, or acute tubular necrosis. Extrarenal losses (diarrhea, excessive sweating) can also lead to hypovolemic hypernatremia. Treatment of hypovolemic hypernatremia involves replacing hypotonic fluids via an enteral or parenteral route (see Figure 7-4).[5]

Euvolemic hypernatremia is commonly caused by diabetes insipidus. These patients have water losses that exceed sodium losses. Diabetes insipidus can be either central or nephrogenic in etiology (Table 7-2). Central diabetes insipidus is an impairment of ADH secretion, whereas the nephrogenic condition occurs when the kidneys cannot respond to ADH circulating in the serum. Both types of diabetes insipidus lead to excessive water losses via urine. Treatment differs for the 2 disorders, but both conditions require the replacement of water via the enteral or parenteral route and normalization of serum calcium and potassium (Figure 7-4).[5]

Hypervolemic hypernatremia can be iatrogenic in nature (excessive administration of isotonic or hypertonic sodium) or related to mineralocorticoid excess (from exogenous administration, Cushing's syndrome, or adrenal malignancy). Treatment involves correcting the underlying disorder, administering diuretics, and replacing water (Figure 7-4).[5]

When treating hypernatremia, the following equation may be used to calculate the free water deficit for the initial replacement volume:

$$\text{Free Water Deficit} = \text{TBW} \times [1 - (140/\text{Serum Na}^+)]$$

where free water deficit and TBW are measured in liters and serum sodium is measured in mEq/L.

However, the use of this equation has been shown to underestimate free water losses by 1 to 2.5 liters; thus, clinical monitoring is required to normalize the serum sodium concentration.[27] Because of the risk for cerebral edema and neurologic impairment, sodium correction should not exceed 10 mEq/L/d when hypernatremia is chronic or of an unknown duration.[24] Acute hypernatremia may be corrected at a rate of 2 mEq sodium per liter per hour until the serum sodium reaches 145 mEq/L.[24]

Potassium

At its normal serum concentration of 3.5 to 5 mEq/L, potassium (K^+) is the major intracellular cation. In contrast to sodium, which is restricted primarily to the ECF, 98% of total body potassium is located within cells. Potassium plays a critical role in cell metabolism, including protein and glycogen synthesis. Additionally, the ratio of potassium concentrations in the cell and the ECF is vital to maintaining resting membrane potential and therefore crucial for normal neural and muscular function. Normal daily potassium requirements range from 0.5 to 2 mEq/kg.[6]

FIGURE 7-3 Evaluation of Hyponatremia

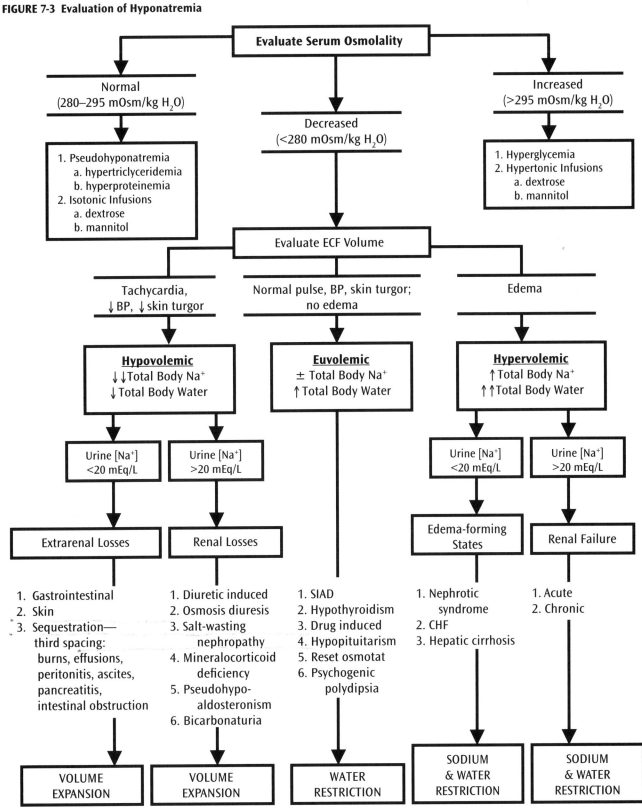

BP, blood pressure; CHF, congestive heart failure; ECF, extracellular fluid; H₂0, water; Na⁺, sodium; SIAD, syndrome of inappropriate antidiuresis.
Source: Adapted with permission from reference 5: Whitmire SJ. Fluids and electrolytes. In: Matarese LE, Gottschlich MM, eds. *Contemporary Nutrition Support Practice: A Clinical Guide.* Philadelphia, PA: Saunders: 1998:129. Copyright © Laura E. Matarese and Michele M. Gottschlich.

FIGURE 7-4 Evaluation of Hypernatremia

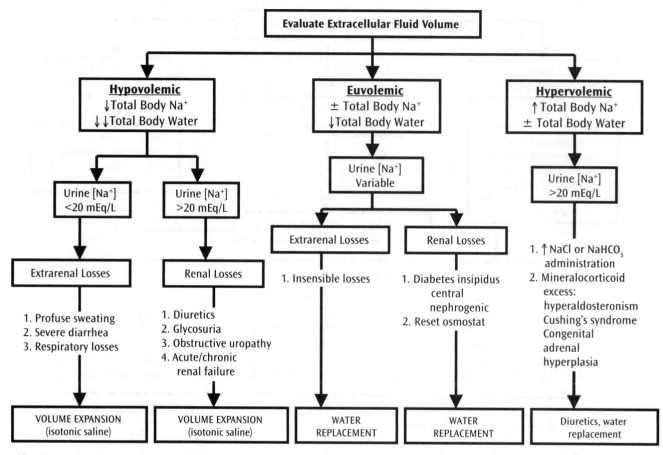

Na⁺, sodium; NaCl, sodium chloride; NaHCO₃, sodium bicarbonate.
Source: Adapted with permission from reference 5: Whitmire SJ. Fluids and electrolytes. In: Matarese LE, Gottschlich MM, eds. *Contemporary Nutrition Support Practice: A Clinical Guide*. Philadelphia, PA: Saunders: 1998:130. Copyright © Laura E. Matarese and Michele M. Gottschlich.

TABLE 7-2 Causes of Diabetes Insipidus

Nephrogenic causes
- Hypokalemia
- Hypercalcemia
- Lithium toxicity
- Polycystic kidney disease
- Advanced renal disease
- Drugs:
  - Amphotericin B
  - Cidofovir
  - Foscarnet
  - Osmotic diuretics
  - Demeclocycline

Central causes
- Cerebral hemorrhage
- Head trauma
- Neurosurgery (pituitary)
- CNS infection
- CNS malignancy

CNS, central nervous system.

Regulation of the internal distribution of potassium seems to be extremely efficient, as the movement of only 1.5% to 2% of cellular potassium to the ECF can result in a potentially fatal increase in the plasma potassium concentration to levels as high as 8 mEq/L or more.[1] Of all the factors that influence this distribution, the Na⁺-K⁺-ATPase pump and the plasma potassium concentration are the most important in the daily regulation of potassium balance.[28] Other factors affecting potassium distribution include those regulating the activity of the Na⁺-K⁺-ATPase pump—specifically insulin and catecholamines—as well as exercise, extracellular pH, and cellular breakdown.

Hypokalemia

Hypokalemia is a common electrolyte abnormality. When defined as a serum potassium concentration less than 3.6 mEq/L, it is found in over 20% of hospitalized patients.[29] Clinical manifestations vary among individuals and are influenced by the rapidity of onset and the degree of hypokalemia. Patients are typically asymptomatic when the disorder is mild (serum potassium 3.0 to 3.5 mEq/L); with lower serum potassium concentrations, nonspecific symptoms such as generalized weakness, lethargy, and constipation are more likely. More severe consequences of hypokalemia can include muscle necrosis, ascending paralysis, arrhythmias, and death.[30]

Hypokalemia is often the result of abnormal potassium losses via the urine or stool. It can also develop from a transcellular shift of potassium from the ECF into cells or inadequate dietary intake. Metabolic alkalosis and increases in insulin and catecholamines (ie, epinephrine or norepinephrine) are potential causes of transcellular shifts of potassium into the cells. As shown in Table 7-3, many medications can also cause hypokalemia. The table lists drugs associated with magnesium depletion because hypokalemia is often refractory to treatment in the setting of hypomagnesemia.

Goals of therapy for hypokalemia include avoidance or resolution of symptoms, restoring the serum potassium concentration to normal, and preventing hyperkalemia. Hypokalemia

is treated by administration of oral or IV potassium supplements. Commonly used oral and enteral potassium supplements are listed in Table 7-4. IV potassium supplements are available as chloride, acetate, and phosphate salts. Potassium acetate is used as an alternative to potassium chloride in the presence of a metabolic acidosis because acetate is converted to bicarbonate by a normally functioning liver. Potassium phosphate is used to correct coexisting hypokalemia and hypophosphatemia.

Potassium supplements are best administered orally in a moderate dosage over a period of several days to 1 week to achieve complete potassium repletion. An oral potassium dosage of 10 to 30 mEq/d is generally sufficient to prevent hypokalemia, whereas dosages of 40 to 100 mEq/d may be required for treatment.

Oral correction of hypokalemia is generally safer and reduces the risk of overcorrection and rebound hyperkalemia. Potassium chloride can be given in a capsule, tablet, or liquid formulation. Although several liquid preparations are available and less expensive than capsules and tablets, they often have an unpleasant taste and are poorly tolerated. The slow-release tablets are well tolerated but have been associated with ulceration and bleeding of the GI tract.[31] Oral potassium dosages of 40 to 100 mEq/d divided into 2 to 4 doses are usually sufficient to correct hypokalemia.[32,33]

IV potassium supplementation is reserved for the treatment of severe hypokalemia or when the condition of the GI tract precludes the use of oral agents. Recommendations for IV potassium replacement doses vary according to the severity of hypokalemia and the presence of renal insufficiency (Table 7-5).[32-36] Infusion rates should generally not exceed 10 to 20 mEq/h; however, infusion rates as high as 40 mEq/h have been used for emergent cases or severely symptomatic patients. If an infusion rate exceeding 10 mEq/h is required, continuous cardiac monitoring is recommended to detect any signs of hyperkalemia. Administration via a central venous catheter is recommended to minimize phlebitis and burning. Total daily potassium supplementation, in most cases, should not exceed 40 to 100 mEq/d (or 0.5 to 1.2 mEq/kg/d). However, some patients with severe potassium wasting may require doses of 200 mEq/d (1.5 mEq/kg/d) or higher with additional cardiac monitoring.

Additional caveats to consider when replacing a potassium deficit include the diluent (dextrose vs saline) and the presence of hypomagnesemia. When possible, dextrose solutions should be avoided because they may worsen the hypokalemia by stimulating insulin release that promotes an intracellular shift of potassium.[37] A magnesium deficit should be corrected because hypomagnesemia may result in refractory hypokalemia related to accelerated renal potassium loss or the impairment of Na^+-K^+-ATPase pump activity.[38]

Hyperkalemia

Because of the body's effective regulatory mechanisms, hyperkalemia (serum potassium greater than 5.0 mEq/L) rarely occurs in healthy individuals. In contrast to the relatively large decrease in total body potassium needed to cause a slight decrease in serum potassium, even a small excess of total body

TABLE 7-3 Causes of Drug-Induced Hypokalemia

Mechanism	Examples

Increased renal potassium loss	• Diuretics:
	  – Acetazolamide
	  – Thiazides
	  – Indapamide
	  – Metolazone
	  – Bumetanide
	  – Furosemide
	  – Torsemide
	• Fludrocortisone
	• Hydrocortisone
	• Drugs associated with magnesium depletion:
	  – Aminoglycosides
	  – Cisplatin
	  – Foscarnet
	  – Amphotericin B
	  – Posaconazole

Excess potassium loss in stool	• Patiromer • Phenolphthalein • Sodium polystyrene sulfonate • Sorbitol

Potassium shift from ECF to ICF	• B$_2$-adrenergic agonists:
	  – Epinephrine
	  – Albuterol
	  – Terbutaline
	  – Pirbuterol
	  – Salmeterol
	  – Isoproterenol
	  – Ephedrine
	  – Pseudoephedrine
	• Theophylline
	• Caffeine
	• Verapamil intoxication
	• Insulin (all types)

ECF, extracellular fluid; ICF, intracellular fluid.

TABLE 7-4 Commonly Used Oral Potassium Replacement Products

Dosage Form	Brand Names	Strength	Clinical Considerations
Enteral or oral administration			
Potassium bicarbonate: effervescent tablet for solution	Klor-Con/EF, K-Lyte	25 mEq/tablet	Dissolve in 90 mL water; orange flavor
Potassium chloride:			
• Effervescent tablet for solution	K-Lor, Klor-Con	20 mEq/tablet	Dissolve in 120 mL water; fruit flavor
• Powder for solution	Klor-Con/25	25 mEq/packet	Dilute in 120 mL cold water or juice for administration; contains sorbitol, which may cause diarrhea
• Solution		20 mEq/15 mL 40 mEq/15 mL	
Potassium phosphate:			
• Tablet for solution	K-Phos	500 mg (3.7 mEq potassium)	Dissolve in 90 mL water
• Powder for solution	Phos-NaK	250 mg (7.1 mEq potassium, 8 mmol phosphorus) per packet	Dilute in 75 mL water; fruit flavor
• Tablet	K-Phos No. 2	2.3 mEq potassium, 8 mmol phosphorus per tablet	
Oral administration only			
Potassium chloride:			
• Capsule, extended-release, microencapsulated	Micro K	8 mEq/600 mg 10 mEq/750 mg	Swallow whole; capsules may be opened and contents sprinkled on applesauce and swallowed immediately without chewing
• Tablet, extended-release	Micro K	8 mEq/600 mg 10 mEq/750 mg 20 mEq/1500 mg	Swallow whole; do not crush or chew; larger tablet size with higher doses; difficult to swallow; potential noncompliance issues
• Tablet, extended-release, microencapsulated	Klor-Con M10 Klor-Con M15 Klor-Con M20	10 mEq/750 mg 15 mEq/1125 mg 20 mEq/1500 mg	Tablet may be broken in half; whole tablet may be dissolved in 120 mL water or ½ tablet in 60 mL water
• Tablet, extended-release, wax matrix	Klor-Con	8 mEq/600 mg 10 mEq/750 mg	Do not crush or chew; swallow whole

TABLE 7-5 Empirical Treatment of Hypokalemia

Serum Potassium Concentration, mEq/L	Intravenous Potassium Dose, mEq[a]
3–3.4	20–40
2.5–2.9	40–80
<2.5	80–120

[a]These dosing guidelines are recommended for patients with normal renal function. Patients with renal impairment should receive 50% of the initial empirical dose. Rate of infusion: 10 to 20 mEq potassium per hour; maximum infusion rate: 40 mEq/h. Continuous cardiac monitoring and infusion via a central venous catheter are recommended for infusion rates >10 mEq potassium per hour.

potassium will elicit a sharp increase in the serum concentration.[39] Clinical manifestations of hyperkalemia are related to changes in neuromuscular and cardiac function. Patients are often asymptomatic until the serum potassium concentration exceeds 5.5 mEq/L.[32] Signs and symptoms of hyperkalemia include muscle twitching, cramping, weakness, ascending paralysis, electrocardiogram changes (eg, tall, peaked T-waves; prolonged PR-interval; widened QRS complex; shortened QT interval), and arrhythmias (eg, bradyarrhythmias, ventricular fibrillation, asystole).

Although hyperkalemia can be caused by extracellular shifts of potassium and increased potassium ingestion, it most often occurs in the setting of chronic kidney disease (CKD). Increased potassium intake alone rarely causes hyperkalemia.

Extracellular shifts of potassium are relatively common and are often a result of metabolic acidosis, tissue catabolism, and pseudohyperkalemia. Metabolic acidosis results in an extracellular potassium shift to maintain electroneutrality because some of the excess hydrogen ions are buffered intracellularly.[40] In general, for every 0.1 decrease in pH, potassium will increase by an average of 0.6 mEq/L but the increase can range from 0.3 to 1.3 mEq/L. Tissue destruction or breakdown causes the release of intracellular potassium into the ECF. Pseudohyperkalemia signifies an artifactual increase in serum potassium related to the release of intracellular potassium during or after blood sampling. This finding is most commonly associated with trauma during venipuncture, but it can also occur with the measurement of serum potassium in patients with marked leukocytosis (100,000/mm^3) or thrombocytosis (400,000/mm^3) or when the blood sample is contaminated with infused potassium or hydrolyzed. Therefore, if a serum potassium level is inappropriately elevated for the clinical situation, a repeat potassium level should be obtained to confirm the diagnosis and avoid unwarranted treatment. Drug-induced causes of hyperkalemia are listed in Table 7-6.[41]

Table 7-7 lists therapies for the treatment of hyperkalemia.[42-44] The choice of treatment depends on the degree of hyperkalemia and the severity of symptoms. Goals of therapy include antagonizing the cardiac effects of potassium, reversing symptoms (if present), and returning the serum potassium

TABLE 7-6 Causes of Drug-Induced Hyperkalemia

Mechanism	Examples
Impaired renal potassium excretion	• Potassium-sparing diuretics (spironolactone, eplerenone, triamterene, amiloride) • Nonsteroidal anti-inflammatory agents • ACE-inhibitors • Angiotensin-II receptor blockers • Aliskiren • Trimethoprim • Pentamidine • Cyclosporine • Tacrolimus • Everolimus • Heparin • Aripiprazole • Canagliflozin
Increased potassium input	• Potassium supplements • Salt substitutes • Stored packed red blood cells • Penicillin G potassium
Potassium shift from ICF to ECF	• Beta blockers • Succinylcholine • Digoxin intoxication

ACE, angiotensin-converting-enzyme; ECF, extracellular fluid; ICF, intracellular fluid.

concentration to normal. If feasible, all sources of exogenous potassium and other medications that can cause hyperkalemia should be discontinued or dosages should be decreased. IV calcium gluconate should be given to symptomatic patients and those with electrocardiogram changes to restore membrane excitability to normal. Insulin and dextrose, sodium bicarbonate, and beta$_2$-adrenergic agonists cause potassium to move intracellularly. Loop and thiazide diuretics, cation-exchange resins (eg, sodium polystyrene sulfonate), and dialysis facilitate potassium removal. Serum potassium should be monitored frequently during the treatment of symptomatic patients because many of the therapies employed for acute hyperkalemia redistribute potassium and do not remove it from the body. Upon symptom resolution, continued potassium monitoring is recommended every 4 to 12 hours after therapeutic interventions until potassium levels return to normal.

Magnesium

At its normal serum concentration of 1.8 to 2.8 mg/dL, magnesium (Mg^{2+}) is mostly found in the ICF.[45] Total body magnesium content is approximately 25 g (2000 mEq), of which 50% to 60% is in bone.[46] The rest is located in cardiac muscle, skeletal muscle, and the liver, with about 2% in the ECF. Magnesium is essential in the activation of more than 300 enzymatic reactions, including those involved in glucose metabolism, fatty acid synthesis and breakdown, and DNA and protein metabolism.[47] Magnesium is also required for the maintenance of the Na$^+$-K$^+$-ATPase pump and, hence, cell membrane action potential. It is a structural component of bone and a factor in parathyroid hormone (PTH) secretion, neuromuscular transmission, cardiovascular excitability, vasomotor tone, and muscle contraction.

Cellular and extracellular magnesium concentrations are carefully regulated by the GI tract, kidney, and bone. Healthy people absorb approximately 30% to 40% of ingested magnesium. Magnesium absorption occurs primarily in the distal jejunum and ileum and varies inversely with intake. Renal elimination normally accounts for approximately one-third of absorbed magnesium. However, with increased magnesium intake, renal magnesium excretion increases to maintain normal serum concentrations.[48]

Hypomagnesemia

Hypomagnesemia (serum magnesium less than 1.8 mg/dL), has been reported in 6.9% to 47% of hospitalized patients,[49-52] and in as many as 65% of patients in ICUs.[53] Neuromuscular hyperexcitability is the primary symptom of magnesium deficiency.[54] Latent tetany, as elicited by positive Chvostek and Trousseau signs, may be present. Frank, generalized seizures may also occur in severe cases. Concomitant electrolyte abnormalities in the setting of magnesium deficiency include hypokalemia and hypocalcemia. Both are refractory to treatment until the magnesium deficit is corrected. Hypomagnesemia occurs in approximately 38% to 61% of patients with hypokalemia and 22% to 28% of patients with hypocalcemia.[52,55,56] Magnesium depletion is also associated with

TABLE 7-7 Treatment of Hyperkalemia

Treatment	Dose	Onset	Duration	Action
Calcium gluconate[a,b]	1–2 g (4.65–9.3 mEq) intravenously over 10 min	1–2 min	10–30 min	Antagonizes cardiac conduction abnormalities
Sodium bicarbonate[a]	50–100 mEq intravenously over 2–5 min	30 min	2–6 h	Shifts potassium intracellularly
Regular insulin with dextrose	5–20 units intravenously with 50–120 mL of 50% dextrose injection	15–45 min	2–4 h	Shifts potassium intracellularly
Albuterol	10–20 mg nebulized	30 min	1–2 h	Shifts potassium intracellularly
Furosemide	20–80 mg intravenous push	5–15 min	4–6 h	Promotes renal potassium loss
Patiromer sorbitex calcium	8.4 g/d; may adjust in increments of 8.4 g at weekly intervals up to 25.2 g/d	4-7 h	≥24 h	Nonabsorbable cation-exchange polymer that increases fecal potassium excretion
Sodium polystyrene sulfonate	15–60 g orally or rectally	1 h	4–6 h	Increases fecal potassium elimination
Hemodialysis	Variable	Immediate	Variable	Removes potassium from plasma

[a]First-line therapies in hyperkalemic emergencies.
[b]Repeat dose in 5 minutes if abnormal electrocardiogram persists. Calcium chloride may be used, but calcium gluconate is preferred for peripheral administration (less venous irritation). Calcium chloride (1 g = 13.6 mEq) provides 3 times more calcium than calcium gluconate (1 g = 4.65 mEq).

cardiac complications, including electrocardiogram changes, arrhythmias, and increased sensitivity to cardiac glycosides (digoxin).[57] Additionally, hypomagnesemia may reduce insulin sensitivity and glucose cellular uptake, impair insulin secretion, and reduce lipoprotein lipase.[58]

Hypomagnesemia can occur with decreased intake or absorption, excessive losses, or redistribution into the ICF. Common causes of reduced magnesium intake or absorption include protein-energy malnutrition, prolonged administration of magnesium-free IV fluids or PN, alcoholism, presence of an ileostomy or colostomy, malabsorption syndromes, short bowel syndrome, and intestinal bypass operations. Magnesium losses can occur via the GI tract or the kidneys. Renal losses may be caused by acute tubular necrosis, renal tubular acidosis, Bartter syndrome, hyperaldosteronism, or they may be induced by drugs such as thiazide and loop diuretics, cisplatin, cyclosporine, amphotericin B, aminoglycosides, and foscarnet.[59] Intracellular shifts of magnesium may be seen during refeeding, diabetic ketoacidosis, hyperthyroidism, and myocardial infarction.

Because only about 1% to 2% of total body magnesium is located in the ECF, serum levels may not correlate with intracellular concentrations or total body magnesium levels. Therefore, treatment of hypomagnesemia is largely empirical. Both oral and IV formulations of magnesium are available to replace estimated deficits. Table 7-8 lists commonly used oral and enteral magnesium supplements. The IV route of administration is often preferred because issues with administration, slow onset of action, and GI intolerance limit the use of oral supplements. Table 7-9 provides recommended dosing regimens for the treatment of hypomagnesemia according to severity.[60–63] Maximal magnesium sulfate infusion rates should not exceed 1 g/h (8 mEq/h) in asymptomatic patients because more than 50% of the dose may be lost in the urine as renal magnesium

reabsorption is exceeded.[61,63] Similarly, recommended empirical doses should be reduced by approximately 50% or more when administered to patients with renal impairment to reduce the risk of hypermagnesemia. IV treatment of hypomagnesemia can be generally expected to produce a serum magnesium change of 0.1 mg/dL for each gram (8 mEq) administered, although the plasma concentration typically takes up to 48 hours after the bolus to equilibrate.[64,65] Additionally, replacing magnesium concurrently with potassium reduces renal potassium excretion and cardiac dysrhythmias observed clinically.[66]

Hypermagnesemia

Hypermagnesemia (serum magnesium greater than 2.8 mg/dL) occurs primarily in the setting of CKD in combination with magnesium intake. Hypermagnesemia is generally well tolerated, but it can affect neurologic, neuromuscular, and cardiac function when magnesium levels exceed 4.8 mg/dL.[50] Physical findings include nausea, vomiting, diaphoresis, flushing, sensation of heat, depressed mental functioning, drowsiness, muscular weakness, loss of deep tendon reflexes, hypotension, and bradycardia.

IV calcium (chloride or gluconate) should be administered to patients with symptomatic severe hypermagnesemia to reverse the cardiac and neuromuscular effects.[46,67] Therapy for patients with asymptomatic hypermagnesemia includes the removal of exogenous sources of magnesium (eg, PN, IV fluids), magnesium restriction, and loop diuretics.

Calcium

Normal total serum calcium (Ca^{2+}) concentrations range from 8.6 to 10.2 mg/dL. Calcium is one of the most abundant

TABLE 7-8 Commonly Used Oral Magnesium Replacement Products

Dosage Form	Brand Names	Strength	Clinical Considerations
Enteral or oral administration			
Magnesium gluconate: solution	Magonate	4.8 mEq/5 mL (1000 mg/5 mL)	
Magnesium sulfate: solution		4 mEq/mL (500 mg/mL)	
Oral administration only			
Magnesium chloride:			
• Tablet, enteric-coated	Slow-Mag	5 mEq	Do not crush or chew; swallow whole; contains 106 mg elemental calcium
• Tablet, delayed-release	Mag 64	5 mEq	Do not crush or chew; swallow whole; contains 110 mg elemental calcium
Magnesium gluconate tablet	Mag G / Magtrate	2.4 mEq/500 mg / 2.4 mEq/500 mg	
Magnesium lactate: caplet, sustained-release	Mag-Tab SR	7 mEq	Do not crush or chew; swallow whole
Magnesium oxide:			
• Capsule	Mag-Caps / Uro-Mag	7 mEq / 7 mEq/140 mg	
• Capsule, soft gel	MagGel	28.6 mEq/600 mg	
• Tablet	Mag-Ox 400 / MG Plus Protein	20 mEq/500 mg / 11 mEq	Large tablet size; potential noncompliance issues Chelated to soy protein; reduced gastrointestinal side effects

TABLE 7-9 Empirical Treatment of Hypomagnesemia

Severity	Serum Magnesium Concentration, mg/dL	Intravenous Magnesium Dose[a]
Mild to moderate	1–1.5	16–32 mEq (2–4 g) magnesium sulfate; ≤1 mEq/kg
Severe	<1	32–80 mEq (4–10 g) magnesium sulfate; ≤1.5 mEq/kg

[a]These dosing guidelines are recommended for patients with normal renal function. Patients with renal impairment should receive 50% of the initial empirical dose. If hypomagnesemia is asymptomatic, the maximum rate of infusion is 8 mEq (1 g) magnesium sulfate per hour, ≤96 mEq (12 g) magnesium sulfate over 12 hours. Up to 32 mEq (4 g) magnesium sulfate may be infused over 4 to 5 minutes in severe symptomatic hypomagnesemia.

cations in the body and accounts for 1% to 2% of adult human body weight.[46] It is essential to many physiological functions, including the preservation of cell membrane integrity, neuromuscular activity, regulation of endocrine secretory activities, blood coagulation, activation of the complement system, and bone metabolism.[68] Serum calcium concentrations are under hormonal control primarily mediated by PTH, vitamin D, and calcitonin.[1] Low serum calcium concentrations stimulate the release of PTH, which increases bone resorption, augments renal conservation of calcium, and activates vitamin D, which in turn increases intestinal calcium absorption. Calcitonin is released by the thyroid gland in response to elevated serum calcium concentrations and acts to inhibit bone resorption and increase urinary calcium excretion. In healthy individuals, any excess calcium is excreted in the urine, whereas any decrease in total serum calcium is met by an increase in calcium mobilization from bone to restore the serum calcium concentration to normal.

About 99% of total body calcium is found in teeth and bones, with less than 1% in the serum.[69] Serum calcium exists in 3 forms: complexed, protein bound, and ionized. The ionized fraction of calcium, with a normal range of 1.12 to 1.3 mmol/L, is the metabolically active form and is of greatest physiological importance.[68] Serum pH, phosphorus, and albumin levels affect the percentage of ionized calcium. A metabolic alkalosis decreases the percentage of ionized calcium, as does an increase in serum phosphorus. Hypoalbuminemia decreases total serum calcium but does not affect ionized calcium levels. For each 1 g/dL decrease in albumin below 4 g/dL, total serum calcium decreases by approximately 0.8 mg/dL.[70] Total calcium can be adjusted for hypoalbuminemia, as follows:

$$\text{Corrected Total Serum Ca}^{2+} = \text{Measured Total Serum Ca}^{2+} + [0.8 \times (4 - \text{Serum Albumin})]$$

where serum calcium is measured in mg/dL and serum albumin is measured in g/dL.

However, direct measurement of ionized calcium is the most accurate method to assess calcium abnormalities. Direct measurement is especially important in critically ill patients because this equation often overestimates the corrected calcium concentration.[71]

Hypocalcemia

Hypocalcemia (total serum calcium less than 8.6 mg/dL or ionized calcium less than 1.12 mmol/L) frequently occurs secondary to hypoalbuminemia; however, this hypocalcemia is usually not clinically significant as long as the ionized calcium concentration remains normal.[26] Causes of hypocalcemia include decreased vitamin D activity (vitamin D deficiency, hyperphosphatemia, pseudohypoparathyroidism), decreased PTH activity (acute pancreatitis, hypomagnesemia, hypoparathyroidism), citrate anticoagulation during continuous renal replacement therapy, and hungry bone syndrome (which can occur after total parathyroidectomy or thyroidectomy). Hypocalcemia is common in critically ill patients and is also associated with sepsis, rhabdomyolysis, and massive blood transfusions (secondary to citrate preservative in the blood bank binding with serum calcium).[71,72] Drugs implicated in the etiology of hypocalcemia include bisphosphonates, calcitonin, furosemide, foscarnet, and long-term therapy with phenobarbital and phenytoin.[73] Clinical manifestations may be cardiovascular (ie, hypotension, decreased myocardial contractility, or prolonged QT interval) or neuromuscular (ie, distal extremity paresthesias, Chvostek sign, Trousseau sign, muscle cramps, tetany, or seizures).

Acute symptomatic hypocalcemia (total serum calcium less than 7.5 mg/dL or ionized calcium less than 0.9 mmol/L) requires prompt correction with IV calcium gluconate or calcium chloride.[74] Although calcium chloride (10 mL 10% solution = 272 mg [13.6 mEq] elemental calcium) contains 3 times more elemental calcium than an equivalent amount of calcium gluconate (10 mL 10% solution = 92 mg [4.65 mEq] elemental calcium), it may cause tissue necrosis if extravasation occurs.[75,76] Initially, 1 g of calcium chloride (13.6 mEq calcium) or 3 g calcium gluconate (14 mEq calcium) may be given over 10 minutes to control hypocalcemia symptoms. Continuous infusions of IV calcium may be required for severe acute hypocalcemia refractory to intermittent bolus doses.[74] Guidelines for the acute treatment of hypocalcemia are provided in Table 7-10.[77,78] If concomitant hypomagnesemia is present, magnesium supplements should be provided to facilitate the correction of hypocalcemia.[79,80] In cases of hypocalcemia related to elevated serum phosphorus levels, treatment with phosphate binders is warranted prior to calcium replacement to reduce the risk of soft tissue calcification. Chronic or asymptomatic hypocalcemia can be treated with

TABLE 7-10 Empirical Treatment of Acute Hypocalcemia

Serum Ionized Calcium Concentration, mmol/L	Intravenous Calcium Dose
1–1.12	1–2 g (4.65–9.3 mEq) calcium gluconate over 1–2 hours
<1	2–4 g (9.3–18.6 mEq) calcium gluconate over 2–4 hours

TABLE 7-11 Common Calcium Supplements

Calcium Salt	Available Dosage Forms	Elemental Calcium, %
Calcium acetate	Tablet	25
Calcium carbonate	Powder for solution Suspension Chewable tablet Soft chew tablet Tablet	40
Calcium citrate	Granules for solution Capsule Tablet	21
Calcium glubionate	Powder for solution Capsule Tablet	9
Calcium lactate	Tablet	13

oral calcium supplements and vitamin D.[32] Common calcium supplements are listed in Table 7-11. Recent evidence suggests that dose-dependent calcium administration with PN for critically ill patients who are not on mechanical ventilation or vasopressor support is associated with an increased mortality, acute respiratory failure, and new-onset shock; therefore, the risk vs benefit should be assessed in these patients prior to IV calcium use.[81]

Hypercalcemia

Hypercalcemia (total serum calcium greater than 10.2 mg/dL or ionized calcium greater than 1.3 mmol/L) most often occurs in hyperparathyroidism and cancer with bone metastases (primarily breast cancer, lung cancer, and multiple myeloma). It can also occur with toxic levels of vitamin A or vitamin D, chronic ingestion of milk and/or calcium carbonate–containing antacids in the setting of renal insufficiency (milk-alkali syndrome), adrenal insufficiency, immobilization, tuberculosis, and use of various medications (eg, thiazide diuretics and lithium).[68] Early clinical manifestations are nonspecific and include fatigue, nausea, vomiting, constipation, anorexia, and confusion. In more severe causes, cardiac arrhythmias (bradycardia) may be present.

Mild hypercalcemia (total serum calcium 10.3 to 11.9 mg/dL) usually responds well to hydration and ambulation. Severe hypercalcemia (total serum calcium equal to or greater than 14 mg/dL) requires immediate treatment because it can lead to acute renal failure, obtundation, ventricular arrhythmias, coma, and death.[69,82,83] IV hydration using 0.9% NaCl should be started promptly at 200 to 300 mL/h to reverse the volume depletion caused by hypercalcemia. After adequate hydration is achieved, 40 to 80 mg IV furosemide may be used to enhance renal calcium excretion if the patient is vigilantly monitored to avoid further volume depletion, although diuretic use remains controversial in the treatment of hypercalcemia. Saline hydration can reduce serum calcium levels by 2 to 3 mg/dL within the first 48 hours of treatment. Calcitonin can also be used to treat acute hypercalcemia, but tachyphylaxis often limits its usefulness after 48 hours. Hemodialysis may be necessary in life-threatening hypercalcemia or in patients with CKD. Although bisphosphonates have a primary role in the treatment of hypercalcemia of malignancy, their delayed onset of action of 4 to 10 days renders these agents useful only as maintenance therapy.

Phosphorus

The normal serum phosphorus concentration of 2.7 to 4.5 mg/dL reflects less than 1% of total body phosphorus, with most phosphorus found in bones and soft tissues.[68] Phosphorus is the main intracellular anion (which exists primarily as phosphate in the serum) and has many important functions, including bone and cell membrane composition and maintenance of normal pH. It provides energy-rich bonds in the form of adenosine triphosphate and is required in all cellular functions that require energy.[84–86] Adequate total body phosphorus is necessary for carbohydrate use, glycolysis, maintenance of normal pH, 2,3-diphosphoglycerate synthesis and function (which are necessary for oxygen release from hemoglobin and, ultimately, tissue oxygenation), neurologic function, and muscular function (especially the myocardium and diaphragm).[84–90]

Serum phosphorus concentrations are determined by intake, intestinal absorption, renal excretion, hormonal regulation of bone resorption and deposition, and distribution between intracellular and extracellular compartments. Carbohydrate and insulin administration, catecholamines, and alkalosis are causes of intracellular shifts of phosphorus. Alternatively, cellular destruction and acidosis result in the release of phosphorus from the cell to the ECF.[68]

Hypophosphatemia

Hypophosphatemia (serum phosphorus concentration less than 2.7 mg/dL) can cause a variety of adverse effects. Manifestations may be neurologic (ataxia, confusion, paresthesias), neuromuscular (weakness, myalgia, rhabdomyolysis), cardiopulmonary (cardiac and ventilatory failure), or hematologic (reduced 2,3-diphosphoglycerate concentration, hemolysis).[2] Hypophosphatemia is common in chronic alcoholism, critical illness, respiratory and metabolic alkalosis, following the treatment of diabetic ketoacidosis, and in patients receiving phosphate-binding medications.[84–86] The administration of carbohydrate loads or PN is likely to cause hypophosphatemia if an inadequate amount of phosphate is provided, especially in malnourished patients at risk for developing severe hypophosphatemia and refeeding syndrome.[87,88,91,92] See Practice Scenario 7-2 for a discussion of prevention of refeeding syndrome.[92]

Practice Scenario 7-2

Question: How can complications be prevented when providing nutrition support therapy to a malnourished esophageal cancer patient?

Scenario: JR is a 37-year-old man (weight, 68 kg; height, 6 feet; usual body weight, 78 kg) with esophageal cancer status post esophagectomy and chemoradiation. He is admitted to the hospital for progressive weight loss (10-kg weight loss in the previous 2 months) and failure to thrive. On hospital Day 2, a percutaneous jejunostomy tube is placed and a 1.5 kcal/mL high-protein enteral formula is started and advanced to 70 mL/h within 24 hours. On hospital Day 4, JR falls while attempting to get out of bed and attributes this event to new-onset muscle weakness and pain. His laboratory test values are as follows:

Day	Na+, mEq/L	K+, mEq/L	Cl-, mEq/L	HCO3-, mEq/L	BUN, mg/dL	Creatinine, mg/dL	Glucose, mg/dL	Mg, mg/dL	Phos, mg/dL
1	133	3.6	99	27	3	0.3	89	1.8	2.8
2	132	3.6	98	28	4	0.3	97	1.7	2.6
4	138	2.6	102	21	8	0.4	105	1.2	1.4

Intervention: The rate of enteral feeds is reduced to 20 mL/h. Intravenous electrolyte replacement is ordered to correct electrolyte abnormalities, and serum chemistry monitoring is ordered every 12 hours. The nutrition support team initiates daily administration of thiamin 100 mg via the feeding tube.

Answer: Nutrition support therapy should be advanced cautiously for patients at risk for refeeding. In this case, JR received 2520 kcal/d (35 kcal/kg/d) with no enteral feeding titration. This aggressive feeding rate and energy provision resulted in a massive intracellular shift of potassium, magnesium, and phosphorus that caused symptomatic hypokalemia, hypomagnesemia, and hypophosphatemia. Electrolyte abnormalities should be corrected as soon as they are identified, and nutrition support therapy should be decreased to a safe rate of 500 kcal/d before the rate is further advanced. Thiamin supplementation is also indicated to facilitate efficient carbohydrate metabolism, correct existing thiamin deficiency, and prevent potential lactic acidosis and Wernicke encephalopathy. The energy prescription should be advanced to meet estimated nutrition needs as permitted by the resolution of symptoms and normalization of serum electrolyte values (eg, 480 kcal/d for 2 days, then 960 kcal/d for 1 day, then 1440 kcal/d for 1 day, then 100% of energy goal).[92]

Rationale: JR was at significant risk for refeeding complications secondary to significant weight loss prior to the initiation of enteral feeds. Severely malnourished patients such as those undergoing anticancer treatment, especially radiation to the gastrointestinal tract, are at an increased risk for electrolyte abnormalities and fluid shifts upon the initiation of nutrition support. Electrolyte abnormalities should be corrected prior to nutrition support therapy, and electrolyte concentrations should be closely monitored as the amount of energy administered is carefully increased to meet estimated needs.

Treatment of hypophosphatemia varies according to the degree of severity and the presence of symptoms. Asymptomatic mild hypophosphatemia may be treated with oral phosphate supplements if the GI tract is functional. Table 7-12

TABLE 7-12 Common Oral Phosphate Replacement Products

Dosage Form	Brand Names	Strength	Clinical Considerations
Enteral or oral administration			
Potassium phosphate:			
• Tablet for solution	K-Phos	500 mg (3.7 mEq potassium, 3.7 mmol phosphate per tablet)	Dissolve in 90 mL water
• Powder for solution	Phos-NaK	250 mg/packet (7.1 mEq potassium, 8 mmol phosphate per packet)	Dilute in 75 mL of water; fruit flavor
Sodium phosphate	OsmoPrep	1.5 g sodium phosphate per tablet (10.8 mmol phosphate, 13.6 mEq sodium per tablet)	Dilute in 240 mL water. Saline laxative; concern for renal failure when used for bowel cleansing in high-risk patients (age >55 years, dehydration, baseline kidney disease, bowel obstruction, active colitis, medications that affect renal perfusion)

lists the most commonly used oral and enteral phosphate supplements.[93] Limitations of oral phosphate supplementation include diarrhea and unreliable absorption. Patients with symptomatic, moderate, or severe hypophosphatemia as well as patients who cannot tolerate oral phosphate formulations should receive IV potassium or sodium phosphate to correct serum phosphorus levels.[31] Phosphate boluses should always be ordered as millimoles of phosphate. Phosphate is present in 2 different valence states at physiological pH. Phosphorus supplements combine both monobasic and dibasic salts, with the ratio of the 2 being dependent on pH. Thus, milliequivalents of phosphate are not exactly known. IV potassium phosphate is preferred unless the potassium concentration is greater than 4 mEq/L (3 mmol potassium phosphate = 4.4 mEq potassium) or renal insufficiency exists. Dosing recommendations (Table 7-13) are largely empirical because serum phosphorus concentrations may not accurately reflect total body stores.[94-96] Reduced phosphate dosages (approximately 50%) are recommended for patients with renal impairment to prevent the development of hyperphosphatemia. Infusion rates should not exceed 7 mmol/h because faster infusion rates can often cause thrombophlebitis and soft tissue calcium-phosphate deposition.[97,98] If potassium phosphate is

being used to replete phosphate, the rate of infusion of potassium may also be rate-limited.

Hyperphosphatemia

Hyperphosphatemia (serum phosphorus greater than 4.5 mg/dL) most often occurs in the setting of CKD. Hyperphosphatemia can also be caused by the endogenous release of phosphorus into the ECF from cellular destruction, such as with massive trauma, cytotoxic agents (especially in the treatment of lymphomas and leukemias with large tumor burden), hypercatabolism, hemolysis, rhabdomyolysis, and malignant hyperthermia. Transcellular shifts of phosphorus from the ICF to the ECF caused by a respiratory or metabolic acidosis may also result in hyperphosphatemia. The administration of large quantities of phosphate-containing laxatives or enemas, especially in the elderly, has been reported to contribute to severe hyperphosphatemia and end-organ damage (renal failure).[99]

The most serious complication of hyperphosphatemia is soft tissue and vascular calcification.[39] Calcification occurs when the calcium-phosphorus product (ie, total serum calcium × serum phosphorus) exceeds 55 mg^2/dL^2.[2,100,101] Additional consequences of hyperphosphatemia include secondary hyperparathyroidism and renal osteodystrophy. Other signs and symptoms are secondary to the development of hypocalcemia and manifest as anorexia, nausea, vomiting, dehydration, and neuromuscular irritability.

Exogenous sources of phosphorus (eg, dietary sources, PN, and phosphate-containing enemas or laxatives) should be decreased or eliminated in the setting of hyperphosphatemia. Conventional aluminum- and calcium-based phosphate binders can be used to reduce intestinal absorption of phosphorus. However, calcium-free binders (ie, lanthanum carbonate, sevelamer hydrochloride or carbonate) are at least as effective and without the untoward risks of anemia and osteomalacia seen with use of aluminum-based agents.[102] Dialysis may be required to treat severe hyperphosphatemia associated with

TABLE 7-13 Empirical Treatment of Hypophosphatemia

Severity	Serum Phosphorus Concentration, mg/dL	Intravenous Phosphate Dose, mmol/kg[a]
Mild	2.3–2.7	0.08–0.16
Moderate	1.5–2.2	0.16–0.32
Severe	<1.5	0.32–1

[a]These guidelines are recommended for patients with normal renal function. Patients with renal impairment should receive 50% of the initial empirical dose. Maximum infusion rate is 7 mmol phosphate per hour. Potassium phosphate is preferred over sodium phosphate when the serum potassium concentration is <4 mEq/L.

CKD. In patients with normal renal function, volume repletion is usually sufficient.

Acid-Base Disorders

Nearly all biochemical reactions are influenced by the pH of their fluid environment. Accordingly, the acid-base balance of body fluids is critical and tightly regulated. Alterations in acid-base balance can have adverse consequences and, when severe, can be life-threatening.

Terminology

An understanding of acid-base terminology is critical to accurately diagnose and manage acid-base disorders. An *acid* is a substance that can donate hydrogen ions (H^+). A *base* is a substance that can accept or combine with hydrogen ions.[1] The free H^+ concentration determines the acidity of body fluids and is represented by the *pH*. Because the pH varies inversely with the H^+ concentration, an increase in the H^+ concentration reduces the pH and a decrease in the H^+ concentration elevates the pH. The pH of arterial blood is normally maintained within the narrow range of 7.35 to 7.45. A pH below 7.35 is called *acidemia*; a pH greater than 7.45 is called *alkalemia*.[1] Processes that tend to raise or lower the H^+ concentration are called *acidosis* and *alkalosis*, respectively. Recognizing the distinction between these terms is necessary to evaluate acid-base disorders in patients in whom both acidotic and alkalotic processes may coexist (mixed acid-base disorders).

Acid-Base Physiology

Although small amounts of acidic substances enter the body via ingested foods, most hydrogen ions originate as byproducts or end products of cellular metabolism. Metabolism of carbohydrates and fats alone results in the daily production of approximately 15,000 mmol carbon dioxide (CO_2), which combines with water to form carbonic acid (H_2CO_3). Protein metabolism accounts for another 50 to 100 mEq of daily acid (noncarbonic acid) production.[103] A progressive accumulation of acid would occur if these substances were not excreted from the body.

The concentration of H^+ in body fluids must be tightly regulated to maintain a pH compatible with life (6.80 to 7.80).[1] The process of H^+ regulation involves 3 sequential steps: (1) chemical buffering by extracellular and intracellular mechanisms; (2) control of the partial pressure of CO_2 in the blood by alterations in the rate of alveolar ventilation; and (3) control of the plasma bicarbonate concentration by changes in renal H^+ excretion.

Buffering prevents large changes in the H^+ concentration in the body. This process is the body's first line of defense and occurs immediately to resist changes in pH. Buffer systems are primarily weak acids and base pairs that can take up or release H^+ so that changes in the free H^+ concentration are minimized. The principal buffer system is the carbonic acid/bicarbonate (H_2CO_3/HCO_3^-) system. Other buffer systems, including proteins, phosphate, and hemoglobin, also contribute to the maintenance of normal pH.

The principal role of the lungs in maintaining acid-base balance is to regulate the pressure exerted by dissolved CO_2 gas in the blood (PCO_2). Of all the chemicals influencing respiration, CO_2 is the most powerful respiratory stimulant. Both the rate and depth of ventilation can be altered to allow for the excretion of CO_2 generated by diet and cellular metabolism. Adjustments in the rate and depth of ventilation begin to compensate for acid-base disturbances within minutes. Conditions that impair respiratory system functioning (eg, opiate overdose) have the potential to cause acid-base imbalances.

The final and slowest mechanism by which the body maintains acid-base balance is via alterations in renal H^+ excretion. Two processes achieve this: (1) reabsorption of filtered HCO_3^- and (2) excretion of the H^+ produced daily as a result of protein metabolism. Of all the regulatory mechanisms involved in acid-base homeostasis, only the kidneys have the ability to regulate levels of alkaline substances in the blood and eliminate metabolic acids (organic acids other than carbonic acid) from the body.

Assessment

Blood gases are used to assess a patient's oxygenation and acid-base status. Arterial blood gases (ABGs) reflect the ability of the lungs to oxygenate blood, whereas venous blood gases (VBGs) reflect tissue oxygenation. Blood gas measurements consist of the pH, PCO_2, partial pressure of oxygen in the blood (PO_2), oxygen saturation (SaO_2), calculated HCO_3^-, and the base excess. Table 7-14 lists normal values for ABGs and VBGs.

As previously described, the pH reflects the degree of blood acidity. The PCO_2 provides information on the lung's ability to excrete CO_2, and changes in PCO_2 are associated with respiratory processes that can lead to acid-base disorders. Increases in PCO_2 represent an acidosis, and decreases in PCO_2 represent an alkalosis. PO_2 reflects the ability of hemoglobin to carry oxygen. The higher the PO_2 value, the more saturated hemoglobin is with oxygen. The PO_2 value is directly related to the SaO_2 (eg, when PO_2 is high, the SaO_2 of the blood is high).

Either the calculated HCO_3^- reported in a blood gas or the measured serum HCO_3^- can be used to evaluate acid-base

TABLE 7-14 Normal Blood Gas Values

pH	7.40 (7.35–7.45)	7.36 (7.33–7.43)
	Arterial Blood Gas	**Mixed Venous Blood Gas**
PCO_2, mm Hg	35–45	41–51
PO_2, mm Hg	80–100	35–40
O_2 saturation, %	95	70–75
HCO_3^-, mEq/L	22–26	24–28
Base excess	−2 to +2	0 to +4

HCO_3^-, bicarbonate; O_2, oxygen; PCO_2, partial pressure of carbon dioxide in the blood; PO_2, partial pressure of oxygen in the blood.

status. Changes in HCO_3^- are associated with metabolic processes that can lead to acid-base disorders. HCO_3^- is the base component of the carbonic acid/bicarbonate buffer system. Increases in serum or calculated HCO_3^- represent an alkalosis, and decreases represent an acidosis. HCO_3^- can also be reported by clinical laboratories as total CO_2 content, which is the sum of measured serum HCO_3^- plus dissolved CO_2 in blood plus carbonic acid. Thus, the values for total CO_2 content are slightly higher than measured serum HCO_3^- alone.

Base excess is a calculated value that estimates the metabolic component of an acid-base disorder. An elevated base excess indicates metabolic alkalosis, whereas a base deficit occurs in metabolic acidosis.

An analysis of acid-base disorders requires a systematic approach to avoid misdiagnosis and inappropriate treatment. The following stepwise approach is useful in evaluating even the most complex cases:

- Step 1: Assess the pH of blood to determine whether the patient is acidemic (pH less than 7.4) or alkalemic (pH greater than 7.4). If the pH is 7.4, an acid-base disorder cannot be ruled out. A mixed acid-base disorder or compensation may be present.
- Step 2: Assess the PCO_2 to determine whether a respiratory process may be contributing to an acid-base disorder. If the PCO_2 is elevated, the patient has a respiratory acidosis. If the PCO_2 is low, the patient has a respiratory alkalosis (Table 7-15).
- Step 3: Assess the serum HCO_3^- to determine whether a metabolic process may be contributing to an acid-base disorder. If the HCO_3^- is elevated, the patient has a metabolic alkalosis (Table 7-16). If the HCO_3^- is low, the patient has a metabolic acidosis (Table 7-17).
- Step 4: Calculate the anion gap (refer to the "Metabolic Acidosis" section later in the chapter for the equation) to determine whether metabolic acidosis is present. This calculation is critical to determine the etiology of the acid-base disorder and select the appropriate treatment.
- Step 5: Determine whether the acid-base disorder is acute or chronic, and use the recommended formulas in Table 7-18 to determine whether the acid-base disorders are appropriately compensated. If compensation is not appropriate, the patient has a mixed acid-base disorder.

Respiratory Acidosis

Respiratory acidosis is a clinical disorder characterized by a reduced pH, an elevation in the PCO_2, and a variable increase in the serum HCO_3^- concentration (Table 7-19).[1] Respiratory acidosis almost always results from decreased effective alveolar ventilation, not an increase in CO_2 production. Hypoventilation can occur when any step in the ventilatory process is compromised. Table 7-15 includes common causes of respiratory acidosis.

Respiratory Alkalosis

Respiratory alkalosis is a clinical disturbance characterized by an elevated pH, a decrease in PCO_2, and a variable

TABLE 7-15 Causes of Respiratory Acid-Base Disorders

Respiratory acidosis
- Central depression of respiration
- Drugs (opioids, anesthetics, sedatives)
- Stroke
- Head injury
- Sleep apnea
- Perfusion abnormalities
- Massive pulmonary embolism
- Cardiac arrest
- Airway or pulmonary abnormalities:
  - Hypoxemia or tissue abnormalities
  - Airway obstruction
  - Asthma
  - Chronic obstructive pulmonary disorder
  - Severe pulmonary edema
  - Severe pneumonia
  - Acute respiratory distress syndrome
  - Smoke inhalation
  - Pneumothorax
- Neuromuscular abnormalities:
  - Brainstem or cervical cord injury
  - Guillain-Barré syndrome
  - Myasthenia gravis
  - Multiple sclerosis
- Obesity hypoventilation (Pickwickian syndrome)
- Mechanical ventilator hypoventilation
- Parenteral or enteral nutrition overfeeding

Respiratory alkalosis
- Central stimulation of respiration
- Anxiety
- Pain
- Fever
- Brain tumors
- Vascular accidents
- Head trauma
- Pregnancy
- Catecholamines
- Salicylate toxicity
- Peripheral stimulation
- Pulmonary embolus
- Asthma
- High altitudes
- Pneumonia
- Pulmonary edema
- Severe anemia
- Mechanical ventilator hyperventilation
- Hepatic encephalopathy

reduction in serum HCO_3^- concentration (Table 7-19).[1] Respiratory alkalosis occurs when effective alveolar ventilation is increased beyond the level necessary to eliminate metabolically produced CO_2. Table 7-15 includes common causes of hyperventilation that can result in respiratory alkalosis.

TABLE 7-16 Causes of Metabolic Alkalosis

Saline responsive (urine chloride <20 mEq/L)
- Gastrointestinal loss
- Vomiting
- Nasogastric suction
- Renal loss
- Diuretic therapy
- Excessive bicarbonate administration
- Rapid correction of hypocapnia

Saline-resistant (urine chloride >20 mEq/L)
- Excess mineralocorticoids
- Cushing's syndrome
- Hyperaldosteronism
- Profound hypokalemia (serum potassium <2 mEq/L)
- Excessive licorice ingestion (eg, from chewing tobacco)

TABLE 7-17 Causes of Metabolic Acidosis

Normal anion gap
- Gastrointestinal loss of HCO_3^-:
  - Diarrhea
  - Pancreatic or small bowel fistula
  - Obstructed ileal loop conduit
  - Ketoacidosis
  - Ureterosigmoidostomy
  - Anion-exchange resins
- Renal loss of HCO_3^-:
  - Type 2 renal tubular acidosis
  - Carbonic anhydrase inhibitors
  - Hyperparathyroidism
  - Hypoaldosteronism
- Ingestion of ammonium chloride or parenteral nutrition containing chloride salts

Increased anion gap
- Increased production of endogenous acid:
  - Lactic acidosis
  - Ketoacidosis (diabetic, starvation, alcoholic)
  - Inborn errors of metabolism
- Failure to excrete acids:
  - Renal failure
- Ingestion of exogenous acid:
  - Salicylates, methanol, ethanol

HCO_3^-, bicarbonate

Metabolic Acidosis

Metabolic acidosis is a clinical disturbance characterized by a reduced pH, reduced serum HCO_3^- concentration, and compensatory hyperventilation resulting in a decrease in PCO_2 (Table 7-19).[1] Metabolic acidosis can be induced by 2 fundamental mechanisms: (1) an inability of the kidneys to excrete the dietary H^+ load or (2) an increase in the generation of H^+ either by the addition of H^+ or the loss of HCO_3^-.

TABLE 7-18 Renal and Respiratory Compensation to Primary Acid-Base Disorders

Disorder	Primary Disturbance	Compensatory Response
Metabolic acidosis	HCO_3^-	1.2 mm Hg decrease in PCO_2 for every 1 mEq/L decrease in HCO_3^-
Metabolic alkalosis	HCO_3^-	0.7 mm Hg increase in PCO_2 for every 1 mEq/L increase in HCO_3^-
Acute respiratory acidosis	PCO_2	1 mEq/L increase in HCO_3^- for every 10 mm Hg increase in PCO_2
Chronic respiratory acidosis	PCO_2	3.5 mEq/L increase in HCO_3^- for every 10 mm Hg increase in PCO_2
Acute respiratory alkalosis	PCO_2	2 mEq/L decrease in HCO_3^- for every 10 mm Hg decrease in PCO_2
Chronic respiratory alkalosis	PCO_2	4 mEq/L decrease in HCO_3^- for every 10 mm Hg decrease in PCO_2

HCO_3^-, bicarbonate; PCO_2, partial pressure of carbon dioxide in the blood.

TABLE 7-19 Characteristics of the Primary Acid-Base Disorders

Disorder	pH	Primary Disturbance	Compensatory Response
Metabolic acidosis	↓	↓ HCO_3^-	↓ PCO_2
Metabolic alkalosis	↑	↑ HCO_3^-	↑ PCO_2
Respiratory acidosis	↓	↑ PCO_2	↑ HCO_3^-
Respiratory alkalosis	↑	↓ PCO_2	↓ HCO_3^-

HCO_3^-, bicarbonate; PCO_2, partial pressure of carbon dioxide in the blood.

The anion gap represents unmeasured serum anions (proteins, phosphate, sulfate, and organic ions) and unmeasured serum cations (potassium, calcium, and magnesium).[104] Therefore, calculating the anion gap is often useful in the differential diagnosis of metabolic acidosis. It is equal to the difference between the serum concentrations of the major measured cation and the major measured anions:[1]

Anion Gap = [Serum Na^+] – ([Serum Cl^-] + [Serum HCO_3^-])

where all values are measured in mEq/L.

Normal anion gap is 9 mEq/L (range 3 to 11 mEq/L). Albumin accounts for a significant portion of the unmeasured serum anions. For every 1 g/dL decrease in serum albumin, 2.5 mEq/L must be added to the anion gap.

The anion gap is used to differentiate between the 2 main types of metabolic acidosis: normal anion gap acidosis (hyperchloremic acidosis) and elevated anion gap acidosis. In the setting of normal anion gap acidosis, there is a milliequivalent-for-milliequivalent replacement of extracellular HCO_3^- by Cl^-; thus, the anion gap does not change because the sum of the major measured anions remains constant. Increased GI or renal bicarbonate losses cause this disorder, also known as *hyperchloremic metabolic acidosis*. Elevated anion gap acidosis is associated with an accumulation of unmeasured anions, which leads to an elevation in the anion gap. Metabolic acidosis with an elevated anion gap commonly results from increased endogenous organic acid production. Table 7-17 lists common causes of metabolic acidosis with an increased or normal anion gap. Practice Scenario 7-3 discusses the management of metabolic acidosis.

Practice Scenario 7-3

Question: How would you alter the electrolyte composition of a parenteral nutrition (PN) formulation for a patient with an elevated end ileostomy output?

Scenario: BB was a 54-year-old woman with a 30-year history of Crohn's disease. Her disease course had included small bowel strictures resulting in multiple small bowel resections, ultimately requiring the creation of an end ileostomy. She was admitted to the hospital for progressive weight loss and fatigue, elevated ileostomy output (3 to 4.5 L/d), and acute renal failure secondary to volume depletion. Albumin and prealbumin on admission were 2.1 g/dL and 18.6 mg/dL, respectively. Intravenous fluids with 0.9% sodium chloride (NaCl) were started at 125 mL/h in addition to a regular diet. By Day 3, BB developed a severe metabolic acidosis and continued to experience ileostomy output greater than 3 L/d. The dietitian reported BB primarily consumed high-fat, fried foods and milkshakes. The patient's laboratory test results for the first 3 days included the following results:

Day	Na+, mEq/L	K+, mEq/L	Cl−, mEq/L	HCO3−, mEq/L	BUN, mg/dL	Creatinine, mg/dL
1	131	3.3	97	18	69	1.4
2	137	4.1	112	14	30	1.2
3	137	4.1	114	12	23	1.1

Intervention: PN formulated to correct the metabolic acidosis was started on Day 3. The patient was counseled to restrict her diet to small, frequent meals.

Answer: The PN formulation for a high-output ileostomy patient should contain maximum amounts of acetate salts to prevent and/or correct a hyperchloremic metabolic acidosis. In this patient, PN was started at 50% of estimated energy needs to reduce the risk for refeeding syndrome and acetate salts were maximized. Common acetate additives for PN include sodium acetate and potassium acetate. Based on patient laboratory parameters, the amounts of sodium and potassium acetate should be tailored for individual needs/tolerance. In addition, the sodium concentration

in the PN should be equal to that of 0.9% NaCl (normal saline) to approximate the sodium concentration of ileostomy fluid.

Rationale: Patients with high-output ileostomies are at risk for acid-base disturbances secondary to anatomical changes. The management of high-output ileostomies (greater than 1 L/d) should include fluid replacement that approximates the electrolyte composition of ileal fluid (Table 7-1).

Metabolic Alkalosis

Metabolic alkalosis is characterized by an elevation in the pH, an increase in the serum HCO_3^- concentration, and compensatory hypoventilation, resulting in a rise in the PCO_2 (Table 7-19).[1] Loss of gastric acid (HCl) as a result of vomiting or nasogastric suction and loss of intravascular volume and chloride as a result of diuretic use are common causes of metabolic alkalosis. This disorder is observed in approximately 33% to 55% of hospitalized patients with acid-base disturbances.[105] Metabolic alkalosis in this setting is often caused by the overzealous treatment of metabolic acidosis with bicarbonate or an excess of acetate in PN solutions, which is metabolized to bicarbonate with a normally functioning liver. In addition, the transcellular shift of H^+ that typically occurs with severe hypokalemia may contribute to the development of a metabolic alkalosis.

Under normal circumstances, the kidneys are able to correct a metabolic alkalosis by excreting the excess HCO_3^- in the urine. Therefore, some degree of impairment in renal HCO_3^- excretion must be present for maintenance of metabolic alkalosis.[1] In general, the mechanisms that sustain metabolic alkalosis can be classified into volume-mediated processes (saline responsive) and volume-independent processes (saline unresponsive). The urine chloride concentration is useful in the differential diagnosis of metabolic alkalosis and predicts those patients likely to respond to volume replacement.

Saline-responsive metabolic alkalosis (urine chloride less than 20 mEq/L) is by far the more prevalent disorder. Common causes are listed in Table 7-16. In these disorders, the increase in HCO_3^- reabsorption that maintains the alkalosis can be reversed by the administration of half-isotonic or isotonic saline. Although adequate NaCl repletion will usually normalize the plasma HCO_3^- concentration, it will not reverse metabolic alkalosis associated with moderate to severe hypokalemia. Only the administration of potassium chloride will correct this disorder.

Saline-resistant disorders (urine chloride greater than 20 mEq/L) are commonly associated with hyperaldosteronism and are characterized by a high urinary chloride concentration. Management of these disorders typically consists of the treatment of the underlying cause of the mineralocorticoid excess. Aggressive potassium repletion should also be employed when hypokalemia is present with metabolic alkalosis in primary hyperaldosteronism.

Mixed Acid-Base Disorders

Patients may simultaneously have more than one acid-base disturbance (ie, a mixed acid-base disorder). The diagnosis of a mixed disorder requires an understanding of the extent of the renal and respiratory compensations for each of the simple acid-base disturbances (Table 7-18). If a given set of blood gases does not fall within the range of expected responses for a simple acid-base disturbance, a mixed disorder should be suspected. Common examples include (1) mixed respiratory acidosis and metabolic acidosis, (2) mixed respiratory alkalosis and metabolic alkalosis, (3) mixed metabolic acidosis and respiratory alkalosis, and (4) mixed metabolic alkalosis and respiratory acidosis.

References

1. Rose BD, Post TW. *Clinical Physiology of Acid-Base and Electrolyte Disorders*, 5th ed. New York: McGraw-Hill; 2001.
2. Canada TW, Boullata JI. Fluid and electrolytes. In: Rolandelli RH, Bankhead R, Boullata JI, Compher CW, eds. *Enteral and Tube Feeding*. 4th ed. Philadelphia, PA: Elsevier Saunders; 2005: 95–109.
3. Moukarzel A. Understanding and managing fluid and electrolyte abnormalities. In: *A.S.P.E.N. 22nd Clinical Congress Course Syllabus*. Orlando, FL:1999:247–254.
4. Hansen M. Fluid balance. In: Hansen M, ed. *Pathophysiology: Foundations of Disease and Clinical Intervention*. Philadelphia, PA: Saunders; 1998:160–175.
5. Whitmire SJ. Fluids and electrolytes. In: Matarese LE, Gottschlich MM, eds. *Contemporary Nutrition Support Practice: A Clinical Guide*. Philadelphia, PA: Saunders; 1998.
6. Mirtallo J, Canada T, Johnson D, et al. Safe practices for parenteral nutrition. *JPEN J Parenter Enteral Nutr*. 2004;28(Suppl):S39–S70.
7. Adolph EF. The metabolism and distribution of water in body and tissues. *Physiol Rev*. 1933;13(3):336–371.
8. Tannenbaum SL, Castellanos VH, George V, Arheart KL. Current formulas for water requirements produce different estimates. *JPEN J Parenter Enteral Nutr*. 2012;36(3):299–305.
9. Clinical nutrition: fluid requirements in adults. Nutrition 411. January 11, 2017. http://www.consultant360.com/n411/content/fluid-requirements-adults. Accessed August 17, 2017.
10. Chernoff R. Meeting the nutritional needs of the elderly in the institutional setting. *Nutr Rev*. 1994;52(4):132–136.
11. Holliday MA, Segar WE. The maintenance need for water in parenteral fluid therapy. *Pediatrics*. 1957;19:823–832.
12. Chidester JC, Splanger AA. Fluid intake in the institutionalized elderly. *J Am Diet Assoc*. 1997;97(1):23–28.
13. Kayser-Jones J, Schell ES, Porter C, et al. Factors contributing to dehydration in nursing homes: inadequate staffing and lack of professional supervision. *J Am Geriatr Soc*. 1999;47(10):1187–1194.
14. Holben DH, Hassell JT, Williams JL, Helle B. Fluid intake compared with establishes standards and symptoms of dehydration among elderly residents of a long-term-care facility. *J Acad Nutr Diet*. 1999;99(11):1447–1450.
15. Forbes GB. Lean body mass-body fat interrelationships in in humans. *Nutr Rev*. 1987;45:225–231.
16. Metheny NM. Nursing assessment. In: Metheny NM. *Fluid and Electrolyte Balance: Nursing Considerations*. Philadelphia, PA: Lippincott; 1987:1135.
17. Alvelos M, Ferreira A, Bettencourt P, et al. The effect of dietary sodium restriction on neurohumoral activity and renal dopaminergic response in patients with heart failure. *Eur J Heart Fail*. 2004;6(5):593–599.
18. Damgaard M, Norsk P, Gustafsson F, et al. Hemodynamic and neuroendocrine responses to changes in sodium intake in compensated heart failure. *Am J Physiol Regul Integr Comp Physiol*. 2006;209:R1294–R1301.
19. Peacock WF, Fonarow GC, Emerman CL, et al. Impact of early initiation of intravenous therapy for acute decompensated heart failure on outcomes in ADHERE. *Cardiology*. 2007;107:44–51.
20. Maisel AS, Peacock WF, McMullin N, et al. Timing of immunoreactive B-type natriuretic peptide levels and treatment delay in acute decompensated heart failure: an ADHERE (Acute Decompensated Heart Failure National Registry) analysis. *J Am Coll Cardiol*. 2008;52:534–540.
21. Mange K, Matsuura D, Cizman B, et al. Language guiding therapy: the case of dehydration versus volume depletion. *Ann Intern Med*. 1997;127:848–853.
22. Hawkins RC. Age and gender as risk factors for hyponatremia and hypernatremia. *Clin Chim Acta*. 2003;337:169–172.
23. Anderson RJ, Chung, HM, Kluge R, et al. Hyponatremia: a prospective analysis of its epidemiology and the pathogenic role of vasopressin. *Ann Intern Med*. 1985;102:164–168.
24. Sterns RH. Disorders of plasma sodium-causes, consequences, and correction. *N Engl J Med*. 2015;372:55–65.
25. Kumar S, Berl T. Sodium. *Lancet*. 1998;352:220–228.
26. Snyder NA, Feigal DW, Arieff A. Hypernatremia in elderly patients. A heterogeneous, morbid, and iatrogenic entity. *Ann Intern Med*. 1987;107:309–319.
27. Cheuvront SN, Kenefick RW, Sollanek KJ, Ely BR, Sawka MN. Water-deficit equation: systematic analysis and improvement. *Am J Clin Nutr*. 2013;97:79–85.
28. Clausen T, Everts ME. Regulation of the Na,K-pump in skeletal muscle. *Kidney Int*. 1989;35:1–13.
29. Paice BJ, Paterson KR, Onyanga-Omara F, et al. Record linkage study of hypokalaemia in hospitalized patients. *Postgrad Med J*. 1986;62:187–191.
30. Gennari FJ. Hypokalemia. *N Engl J Med*. 1998;339:451–458.
31. Strom BL, Carson JL, Schinnar R, et al. Upper gastrointestinal tract bleeding from oral potassium chloride. Comparative risk from microencapsulated vs. wax matrix formulations. *Arch Intern Med*. 1987;147:954–957.
32. Kraft MD, Btaiche IF, Sacks GS, Kudsk KA. Treatment of electrolyte disorders in adult patients in the intensive care unit. *Am J Health Syst Pharm*. 2005;62:1663–1682.
33. Cohn JN, Kowey PR, Whelton PK, Prisant LM. New guidelines for potassium replacement in clinical practice: a contemporary review by the National Council on Potassium in Clinical Practice. *Arch Intern Med*. 2000;160:2429–2436.
34. Kruse JA, Carlson RW. Rapid correction of hypokalemia using concentrated intravenous potassium chloride infusions. *Arch Intern Med*. 1990;150:613–617.
35. Kruse JA, Clark VL, Carlson RW, Geheb MA. Concentrated potassium chloride infusions in critically ill patients with hypokalemia. *J Clin Pharmacol*. 1994;34:1077–1082.
36. Hamill RJ, Robinson LM, Wexler HR, Moote C. Efficacy and safety of potassium infusion therapy in hypokalemic critically ill patients. *Crit Care Med*. 1991;19:694–699.
37. Agarwal A, Wingo CS. Treatment of hypokalemia. *N Engl J Med*. 1999;340:154–155.
38. Whang R, Whang DD, Ryan MP. Refractory potassium repletion. A consequence of magnesium deficiency. *Arch Intern Med*. 1992;152:40–45.
39. Lutarewych MA, Batlle DC. Disorders of potassium balance. In: Androgue HJ, ed. *Contemporary Management in Critical Care: Acid-Base and Electrolyte Disorders*. Vol. 1. New York: Churchill Livingstone; 1991:193–232.
40. Adrogue HJ, Madias NE. Changes in plasma potassium concentration during acute acid-base disturbances. *Am J Med*. 1981;71:456–467.
41. Perazella MA. Drug-induced hyperkalemia: old culprits and new offenders. *Am J Med*. 2000;109:307–314.

42. Kunau RT, Stein JH. Disorders of hypo and hyperkalemia. *Clin Nephrol*. 1977;7:173–190.

43. Mandal AK. Hypokalemia and hyperkalemia. *Med Clin North Am*. 1997;81:611–639.

44. Williams ME. Endocrine crises. Hyperkalemia. *Crit Care Clin*. 1991;7:155–174.

45. Connolly E, Worthley L. Intravenous magnesium. *Crit Care Resusc*. 1999;1:162–172.

46. Reinhart RA. Magnesium metabolism. A review with special reference to the relationship between intracellular content and serum levels. *Arch Intern Med*. 1988;148:2415–2420.

47. Zaloga GP, Roberts PR. Calcium, phosphorus, and magnesium disorders. In: Ayres SM, Grenvik NA, Holbrook PR, Shoemaker WC, eds. *Textbook of Critical Care*. 4th ed. Philadelphia, PA: Saunders; 2000:905–928.

48. Institute of Medicine. *Dietary Reference Intakes for Calcium, Phosphorus, Magnesium, Vitamin D, and Fluoride*. Washington, DC: National Academies Press; 1997.

49. Whang R. Magnesium deficiency: pathogenesis, prevalence, and clinical implications. *Am J Med*. 1987;82:24–29.

50. Wong ET, Rude RK, Singer FR, Shaw ST. A high prevalence of hypomagnesemia and hypermagnesemia in hospitalized patients. *Am J Clin Pathol*. 1983;79:348–352.

51. Rubeiz GJ, Thill-Baharozian M, Hardie D, Carlson RW. Association of hypomagnesemia and mortality in acutely ill medical patients. *Crit Care Med*. 1993;21:203–209.

52. Whang R, Oei TO, Aikawa JK, et al. Predictors of clinical hypomagnesemia. Hypokalemia, hypophosphatemia, hyponatremia, and hypocalcemia. *Arch Intern Med*. 1984;144:1794–1796.

53. Ryzen E, Wagers PW, Singer FR, Rude RK. Magnesium deficiency in a medical ICU population. *Crit Care Med*. 1985;13:19–21.

54. Rude RK, Singer FR. Magnesium deficiency and excess. *Annu Rev Med*. 1981;32:245–259.

55. Desai TK, Carlson RW, Geheb MA. Prevalence and clinical implications of hypocalcemia in acutely ill patients in a medical intensive care setting. *Am J Med*. 1988;84:209–214.

56. Boyd JC, Bruns DE, Wills MR. Frequency of hypomagnesemia in hypokalemic states. *Clin Chem*. 1983;2:178–179.

57. Rude RK. Magnesium metabolism and deficiency. *Endocrinol Metab Clin North Am*. 1993;22:377–395.

58. Das UN. Beneficial actions of magnesium in metabolic syndrome: why and how? *Nutrition*. 2016;32:1308–1310.

59. Dacey MJ. Hypomagnesemic disorders. *Crit Care Clin*. 2001;17:155–173.

60. Dickerson RN, Brown RO. Hypomagnesemia in hospitalized patients receiving nutritional support. *Heart Lung*. 1985;14:561–569.

61. Oster JR, Epstein M. Management of magnesium depletion. *Am J Nephrol*. 1988;8:349–354.

62. Sacks GS, Brown RO, Dickerson RN, et al. Mononuclear blood cell magnesium content and serum magnesium concentration in critically ill hypomagnesemic patients after replacement therapy. *Nutrition*. 1997;13:303–308.

63. Hebert P, Mehta N, Wang J, et al. Functional magnesium deficiency in critically ill patients identified using a magnesium loading test. *Crit Care Med*. 1997;25:749–755.

64. Shechter M, Hod H, Chouraqui P, Kaplinsky E, Rabinowitz B. Magnesium therapy in acute myocardial infarction when patients are not candidates for thrombolytic therapy. *Am J Cardiol*. 1995;75:321–323.

65. Raghu C, Peddeswara Rao P, Seshagiri Rao D. Protective effect of intravenous magnesium in acute myocardial infarction following thrombolytic therapy. *Int J Cardiol*. 1999;71:209–215.

66. Hamill-Ruth RJ, McGory R. Magnesium repletion and its effect on potassium homeostasis in critically ill adults: results of a double-blind, randomized, controlled trial. *Crit Care Med*. 1996;24:38–45.

67. Van Hook JW. Endocrine crises. Hypermagnesemia. *Crit Care Clin*. 1991;7:215–223.

68. Popovtzer MM. Disorders of calcium, phosphorus, vitamin D, and parathyroid hormone activity. In: Schrier RW, ed. *Renal and Electrolyte Disorders*. 6th ed. Philadelphia, PA: Lippincott Williams & Wilkins; 2003:216–277.

69. Bushinsky DA, Monk RD. Electrolyte quintet: calcium. *Lancet*. 1998;352:306–311.

70. Singer FR, Bethune JE, Massry SG. Hypercalcemia and hypocalcemia. *Clin Nephrol*. 1977;7:154–162.

71. Dickerson RN, Alexander KH, Minard G, Croce MA, Brown RO. Accuracy of methods to estimate ionized and "corrected" serum calcium concentrations in critically ill multiple trauma patients receiving specialized nutrition support. *JPEN J Parenter Enteral Nutr*. 2004;28:133–141.

72. Zivin JR, Gooley T, Zager RA, Ryan MJ. Hypocalcemia: a pervasive metabolic abnormality in the critically ill. *Am J Kidney Dis*. 2001;37:689–698.

73. Guise TA, Mundy GR. Clinical review 69: evaluation of hypocalcemia in children and adults. *J Clin Endocrinol Metab*. 1995;80:1473–1478.

74. Olinger ML. Disorders of calcium and magnesium metabolism. *Emerg Med Clin North Am*. 1989;7:795–822.

75. Jucgla A, Sais G, Curco N, et al. Calcinosis cutis following liver transplantation: a complication of intravenous calcium administration. *Br J Dermatol*. 1995;132:275–278.

76. Semple P, Booth C. Calcium chloride; a reminder. *Anaesthesia*. 1996;51:93.

77. Dickerson RN, Morgan LM, Cauthen AD, et al. Treatment of acute hypocalcemia in critically ill multiple-trauma patients. *JPEN J Parenter Enteral Nutr*. 2005;29:436–441.

78. Dickerson RN, Morgan LM, Croce MA, Minard G, Brown RO. Treatment of moderate to severe acute hypocalcemia in critically ill trauma patients. *JPEN J Parenter Enteral Nutr*. 2007;31:228–233.

79. Anast CS, Winnacker JL, Forte LR, Burns TW. Impaired release of parathyroid hormone in magnesium deficiency. *J Clin Endocrinol Metab*. 1976;42:707–717.

80. Fatemi S, Rzyen E, Flores J, et al. Effect of experimental human magnesium depletion on parathyroid hormone secretion and 1,25–dihydroxyvitamin D metabolism. *J Clin Endocrinol Metab*. 1991;73:1067–1072.

81. Dotson B, Larabell P, Patel JU, et al. Calcium administration is associated with adverse outcomes in critically ill patients receiving parenteral nutrition: results from a natural experiment created by a calcium gluconate shortage. *Pharmacotherapy*. 2016;36:1185–1190.

82. Davis KD, Attie MF. Management of severe hypercalcemia. *Crit Care Clin*. 1991;7:175–190.

83. Minisola S, Pepe J, Piemonte S, Cipriani C. The diagnosis and management of hypercalcemia. *BMJ*. 2015;350:h2723. doi:10.1136/bmj.h2723.

84. Peppers MP, Geheb M, Desai T. Endocrine crises. Hypophosphatemia and hyperphosphatemia. *Crit Care Clin*. 1991;7:201–214.

85. Knochel JP. The pathophysiology and clinical characteristics of severe hypophosphatemia. *Arch Intern Med*. 1977;137:203–220.

86. Stoff JS. Phosphate homeostasis and hypophosphatemia. *Arch Intern Med*. 1982;72:489–495.

87. Sheldon GF, Grzyb S. Phosphate depletion and repletion: relation to parenteral nutrition and oxygen transport. *Ann Surg*. 1975;182:683–689.

88. Travis SF, Sugerman HJ, Ruberg RL, et al. Alterations of red-cell glycolytic intermediates and oxygen transport as a consequence

of hypophosphatemia in patients receiving intravenous hyperalimentation. *N Engl J Med*. 1971;285:763–768.

89. Newman JH, Neff TA, Ziporin P. Acute respiratory failure associated with hypophosphatemia. *N Engl J Med*. 1977;296:1101–1103.

90. Aubier M, Murciano D, Lecocguic Y, et al. Effect of hypophosphatemia on diaphragmatic contractility in patients with acute respiratory failure. *N Engl J Med*. 1985;313:420–424.

91. Brooks MJ, Melnik G. The refeeding syndrome: an approach to understanding its complications and preventing its occurrence. *Pharmacotherapy*. 1995;15:713–726.

92. Doig GS, Simpson F, Heighes PT, et al. Restricted versus continued standard caloric intake during the management of refeeding syndrome in critically ill adults: a randomised, parallel-group, multicentre, single-blind controlled trial. *Lancet Respir Med*. 2015;3:943–952.

93. US Food and Drug Administration. Information for healthcare professionals: oral sodium phosphate (OSP) products for bowel cleansing (marketed as Visicol and OsmoPrep, and oral sodium phosphate products available without a prescription). FDA Alert 12/11/2008. https://www.fda.gov/Drugs/DrugSafety/PostmarketDrugSafetyInformationforPatientsandProviders/ucm126084.htm. Accessed August 12, 2017.

94. Lentz RD, Brown DM, Kjellstrand CM. Treatment of severe hypophosphatemia. *Ann Intern Med*. 1978;89:941–944.

95. Vannatta JB, Whang R, Papper S. Efficacy of intravenous phosphorus therapy in the severely hypophosphatemic patient. *Arch Intern Med*. 1981;141:885–887.

96. Andress DL, Vannatta JB, Whang R. Treatment of refractory hypophosphatemia. *South Med J*. 1982;75:766–767.

97. Rosen GH, Boullata JI, O'Rangers EA, et al. Intravenous phosphate repletion regimen for critically ill patients with moderate hypophosphatemia. *Crit Care Med*. 1995;23:1204–1210.

98. Clark CL, Sacks GS, Dickerson RN, et al. Treatment of hypophosphatemia in patients receiving specialized nutrition support using a graduated dosing scheme: results from a prospective clinical trial. *Crit Care Med*. 1995;23:1504–1511.

99. Brunelli SM, Lewis JD, Gupta M, et al. Risk of kidney injury following oral phosphosoda bowel preparations. *J Am Soc Nephrol*. 2007;18:3199–3205.

100. Block GA, Port FK. Re-evaluation of risks associated with hyperphosphatemia and hyperparathyroidism in dialysis patients: recommendations for a change in management. *Am J Kidney Dis*. 2000;35:1226–1237.

101. Goodman WG, Goldin J, Kuizon BD, et al. Coronary artery calcification in young adults with end-stage renal disease who are undergoing dialysis. *N Engl J Med*. 2000;342:1478–1483.

102. Ritz E. The clinical management of hyperphosphatemia. *J Nephrol*. 2005;18:221–228.

103. Kurtz I, Maher T, Hulter HN, et al. Effect of diet on plasma acid base composition in normal humans. *Kidney Int*. 1983;24:670–680.

104. Winter SD, Pearson JR, Gabow PA, et al. The fall of the serum anion gap. *Arch Intern Med*. 1990;150:311–313.

105. Hodgkin JE, Soeprono FF, Chan DM. Incidence of metabolic alkalemia in hospitalized patients. *Crit Care Med*. 1980;8:725–728.

8 Vitamins and Trace Elements

Liam McKeever, MS, PhD, RDN

CONTENTS

Acknowledgments: Susan F. Clark, RDN, PhD, was the author of this chapter for the second edition. The author also thanks Sarah Peterson, RDN, PhD, CNSC, Kelly Roehl MS, RDN, CNSC, and Carol Braunschweig, RD, PhD, for their support and advice in this process, as well as Kelly Hagemes, RN, for his assistance editing the Practice Scenarios..

Objectives

1. Describe the known metabolism, functions, and requirements for essential vitamins and minerals in human nutrition.
2. Assess signs and symptoms of vitamin and mineral deficiency and toxicity.
3. Detect how various disease conditions can influence micronutrient metabolism.
4. Demonstrate clinical examples of potential vitamin and mineral interactions, deficiencies, and toxicities.

Test Your Knowledge Questions

1. What amount of retinol is equivalent to 24 mcg of beta-carotene from food?
   A. 2 mcg
   B. 4 mcg
   C. 2 mcg
   D. 1 mg
2. Which of the following nutrients does *not* engage in conversion of homocysteine to methionine?
   A. Choline
   B. Vitamin D
   C. Vitamin B_{12}
   D. Folate
3. The first B vitamin deficiency to manifest in people with alcoholism is usually:
   A. Niacin
   B. Pantothenic acid
   C. Vitamin B_6
   D. Thiamin
4. Which of the following trace elements is regulated at the level of absorption but not excretion?
   A. Zinc
   B. Copper
   C. Manganese
   D. Iron

Test Your Knowledge Answers

1. The correct answer is **A**. One mcg retinol has the vitamin A activity of 12 mcg beta-carotene. Therefore, 24 mcg beta-carotene is equivalent to 2 mcg retinol.
2. The correct answer is **B**. Vitamin B_{12} and folate are needed to convert the cardiac risk factor homocysteine back into methionine. Alternatively, choline may be used for this conversion.
3. The correct answer is **D**. Very small amounts of thiamin are stored in the liver. Therefore, this B vitamin tends to be the first to become deficient in malabsorptive or inadequate intake situations.
4. The correct answer is **D**. The control mechanisms that keep iron levels stable in the body occur at the absorption phase. It is very difficult to eliminate iron except in conditions of blood loss (eg, blood donation or menstruation).

Background

Micronutrients are essential to macronutrient metabolism as well as countless other processes in the body. This chapter examines 14 vitamins and 9 trace elements, and the review of each micronutrient is broadly separated into 2 sections. The first section covers background information regarding absorption, digestion, biochemical functions, and excretion. The second section presents information of direct clinical relevance to nutrition support clinicians, including recommended intakes, at-risk populations, nutrient half-life, diagnostic laboratory tests, clinical signs and symptoms of deficiency/toxicity, nutrient-nutrient interactions, nutrient-medication interactions, and treatment considerations. Ultratrace elements are also briefly discussed.

Assessment of Micronutrient Status

Evaluation of vitamin and trace element status relies on a variety of biochemical measurements. Deficiencies of vitamins and trace elements generally occur in several phases, and alterations in metabolism can occur at biochemical, clinical, morphological, and functional levels. Generally, the biochemical alterations occur before other changes are evident. In fact, by the time clinical, morphological, or functional alterations occur, the concentration of that nutrient in biological fluids will already be greatly reduced. Therefore, early identification of biochemical changes is essential.

A person's age, lifestyle, or disease state can alter both the intake and requirements for specific micronutrients. The ability to identify at-risk populations for specific nutrient deficiencies increases the likelihood of detection.

Understanding of the biological half-lives of the various nutrients gives us a method to at least vaguely assess the impact of the duration of a patient's inadequate intake on the likelihood of deficiency. In this context, *half-life* is defined as the time it takes for half the amount of an ingested nutrient to be eliminated from the body. Assuming the half-life of a nutrient is the same at all levels of physiological concentration, we expect the nutrient to be approximately 97% eliminated from the system within 5 half-lives. However, the half-lives for most nutrients increase as the concentration of the nutrient decreases due to the activation of nutrient retention mechanisms.

Dietary Reference Intakes

The Dietary Reference Intakes (DRIs) are designed to reflect the latest understanding of nutrient requirements based on optimizing health in individuals and groups. The primary goal of DRI values is to prevent nutrient deficiencies and reduce nutrition-related disease. The following are definitions and descriptions of the 4 DRI categories for micronutrients:

- *Estimated Average Requirement (EAR)*—the intake that meets the estimated nutrient needs of 50% of the individuals in a group. The EAR must be derived from scientific studies, and it serves as the basis for developing the Recommended Dietary Allowance (RDA). It can also be used for evaluating the adequacy of group intakes and planning recommendations for group intakes.
- *Recommended Dietary Allowance (RDA)*—the intake that meets the nutrient needs of almost all (97% to 98%) individuals in that group. The RDA may be 2 standard deviations (SD) above the EAR if the variation in requirement for a micronutrient is well defined (RDA = EAR + 2 SD of EAR), or it may be 1.2 times the EAR if the variation is inconsistent or unavailable (RDA = 1.2 × EAR, which assumes a coefficient of variation of 10%).
- *Adequate Intake (AI)*—the average observed or experimentally derived intake by a defined population or subgroup that seems to sustain a defined nutrition-related state, such as normal circulating nutrient values, growth, or other

functional indicators of health. If the EAR cannot be determined for a micronutrient, the RDA cannot be set. In these cases, the AI serves as a goal for intake.

- *Tolerable Upper Intake Level (UL)*—the maximum intake by an individual that is unlikely to pose risks of adverse health effects in almost all individuals. There is no established benefit of consuming nutrients at levels above the RDA or AI. Therefore, the UL is *not* intended to be a recommended level of intake. For most nutrients, the UL refers to total intakes from food, fortified food, and nutrient supplements.

The Food and Nutrition Board of the Health and Medicine Division (formerly Institute of Medicine) of the National Academies of Science has published DRI reports for the following nutrient groups:

- Calcium, phosphorus, magnesium, vitamin D, and fluoride
- Folate, vitamin B_{12}, other B vitamins, and choline
- Vitamin C, vitamin E, selenium, and carotenoids
- Vitamin A, vitamin K, and trace elements
- Energy and macronutrients
- Electrolytes and water

The DRIs are periodically updated by the Health and Medicine Division, with the most recent updates being calcium and vitamin D in 2011.[1] As new bioavailability information is gained about micronutrients, DRIs are debated and may be changed in the future.[2]

Vitamins

Vitamins are essential organic substances needed in small amounts in the diet to maintain fundamental functions of the body such as growth, metabolism, and cellular integrity. Vitamins contribute to energy metabolism through their supportive role in macronutrient metabolism. In humans, 13 vitamins plus the dietary component choline are considered essential. These include 8 B vitamins (thiamin, niacin, riboflavin, folate, vitamin B_6, vitamin B_{12}, biotin, and pantothenic acid); vitamin C (ascorbic acid); and the fat-soluble vitamins A, D, E, and K. Most vitamins are not related chemically and thus differ in their biochemical and physiological roles.

Malabsorption, medications, certain disease states, or excesses of dietary substances such as alcohol can influence nutrient intake as well as the digestion, absorption, and transport of vitamins, which consequently alter vitamin requirements and nutrition status. Clinicians must use a nutrition-focused physical assessment to identify nutrient deficiencies in tandem with the appropriate biochemical assays to determine the adequacy of a patient's vitamin status. A consultation with multidisciplinary nutrition support teams also improves the nutrition status of patients and the overall safety and efficacy of care.[3]

Fat-Soluble vs Water-Soluble Vitamins

Vitamins are broadly grouped into those that are fat-soluble (vitamins A, D, E, and K) vs those that are water-soluble (vitamin C, the 8 B vitamins, and choline) to account for differences in absorption, transportation, and excretion in the body. In the duodenum, fat-soluble vitamins are incorpo-

FIGURE 8-1 Absorption of Fat-Soluble Vitamins

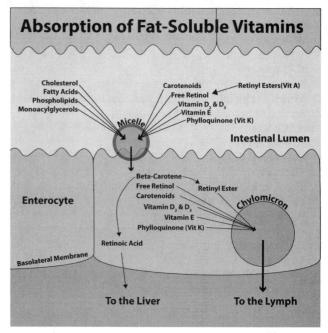

Fat-soluble vitamins are absorbed into the enterocyte via the micelle. Here all fat-soluble vitamins except for retinoic acid are repacked into a chylomicron to enter the lymph system.

rated into micelles for absorption into the enterocyte. From there, they are repackaged into chylomicrons for distribution to the extrahepatic tissues. Some are even repackaged into very low-density lipoproteins for redistribution (Figure 8-1). Ultimately, they are stored in adipocytes or excreted through the feces (predominantly) or the urine. In general, fat-soluble vitamins tend to be absorbed better when taken with dietary fat because they are processed similarly to fat. Patients with fat-malabsorptive disorders, either through decreased pancreatic sufficiency, decreased bile acid release or production, or decreased intestinal surface area, are at risk for fat-soluble vitamin deficiencies.

Vitamin A

Vitamin A represents a subgroup of compounds known as *retinoids* that have biological activity of retinol. Several plant-derived carotenoids, once metabolized, also possess vitamin A activity. Vitamin A exists in 3 forms: retinol, retinaldehyde (retinal), and retinoic acid. Beta-carotene, the primary provitamin A carotenoid, can be split into 2 molecules of retinal and is a dietary precursor of retinol. Retinol can be oxidized reversibly to retinal, or it can be further oxidized to retinoic acid, each having unique biochemical functions. The intracellular metabolism of retinol involves 4 major processes: it may (1) be esterified and stored, (2) be converted to active metabolites such as retinoic acid or retinal, (3) form covalent bonds with cell proteins, or (4) be catabolized to an excretory form.

Generally, dietary vitamin A exists as retinoids in animal tissues and carotenoids in plants; however, there are carotenes in butterfat, and some plant-based foods such as breakfast cereals and margarines may be fortified with retinyl ester, the most stable form of vitamin A. Typically, vitamin A is ingested as retinyl ester and must be freed by acidic digestion, the emulsifying action of bile salts, and the subsequent integration of retinol into micelles. The micelles are transported to the intestinal cell, where the retinol is then reesterified by intracellular binding proteins and packaged into chylomicrons. The chylomicrons enter the mesenteric lymphatic system and pass into systemic circulation where retinol is removed primarily by the liver.[4] Once in the liver, the vitamin enters the hepatocyte for storage. Although the liver is the primary storage site of vitamin A, extrahepatic locations (eg, adipose tissue, kidneys, bone marrow, lungs, eyes) also contain significant amounts of vitamin A.[4]

Approximately 90% of dietary vitamin A is absorbed. In contrast, dietary carotenoids are absorbed primarily in the upper small intestine at a lower efficiency of approximately 8%.[4] Overall, vitamin A absorption depends on the amount of dietary fat intake as well as disease states that influence fat absorption. Retinol-binding protein (RBP) is a liver-synthesized protein that is required to transport retinol from the liver to the target tissues. Synthesis of this protein is tightly regulated by the availability of retinol and, therefore, is sensitive to the nutrition status of the individual.[4] In the plasma, RBP is bound to the protein transthyretin (TTR), also called *prealbumin*. The protein complex TTR-RBP is responsible for the plasma transport of retinol. Measurement of these binding proteins is used to assess vitamin A status.

Functions of Vitamin A

Vision

Proper vision relies upon impulses sent through the optic nerve to vision centers in the brain. Rods and cones send these impulses. Cones are necessary for vision in bright-light conditions whereas rods are needed for dim-light conditions. The rods of the eye contain a vitamin A–dependent pigment complex called *rhodopsin* (formerly called *visual purple*), which is a combination of opsin and cis-retinal. In dim conditions, when light enters the eyes, it converts the cis-retinal to trans-retinal, effectively cleaving rhodopsin, which releases the nerve impulse to the vision centers of the brain. The trans-retinal is regenerated to cis-retinal, rejoins with opsin, and repeats the cycle. When vitamin A is in short supply, the formation of rhodopsin is impeded, leading to night blindness.[5]

Epithelial Cell Regulations

Vitamin A as retinoic acid regulates epithelial cell differentiation. For example, retinoic acid is necessary for the transformation of keratinocytes into mature skin cells. In the absence of vitamin A, keratinocytes grow uncontrolled, causing hyperkeratosis of the skin, and they grow in nondermal areas such as the conjunctiva of the eyes. When keratinocytes replace mucus-secreting cells and cells of the conjunctiva, they cause dryness (xeropthalmia) and rough corneal keratin deposition (Bitot's spots).[5]

Wound Healing

Vitamin A as retinoic acid is also needed for epithelial cell growth. During the inflammatory phase, vitamin A increases the number of macrophages and monocytes in the wound, stimulates epithelialization, and increases collagen deposition by fibroblasts.[6] Vitamin A can also reverse the inhibitory effects of corticosteroids on wound healing.[7]

Bone and Cellular Health

Toxic amounts of vitamin A are known to have negative skeletal effects. In a prospective cohort comparing postmenopausal women who consumed 2000 mcg retinol per day vs those who consumed 500 mcg/d, the risk of hip fractures was almost double in the women who consumed 2000 mcg/d, an amount less than the UL for vitamin A of 3000 mcg/d.[8] Thus, chronic intake of retinol may contribute to the development of osteoporotic hip fractures.

Elevated serum levels of vitamin A occur in both chronic and acute renal failure because the binding capacity of RBP is exceeded, which allows more of the vitamin to circulate unbound with the potential to damage cell membranes.[9] It is prudent to supplement vitamin A with caution in renal failure and in accordance with standard practice guidelines.[10]

Clinical Applications

Recommended Intakes for Adults

The RDA for vitamin A is as follows:
- 900 RAE for men
- 700 RAE for women
- 770 RAE for pregnant women
- 1300 RAE for lactating women

RAE refers to *retinoic acid equivalent*, which equals any of the following: 1 mcg retinol, 3.33 IU retinol, 12 mcg food-based beta-carotene, 24 mcg alpha-carotene, or 24 mcg beta-cryptoxanthin. Note that oil-based oral beta-carotene supplements are highly absorbable, yielding 1 RAE for every 2 mcg beta-carotene.[4]

The UL for retinol is 3000 RAE (3000 mcg). Retinol consumption greater than 3000 mcg/d during the periconceptional period places women at risk for delivering neonates with birth malformations, and this finding was an influencing factor on determining the UL. However, more than 50 possible signs of vitamin A toxicity[4,11] have been observed at intakes as low as 1800 mcg/d. Long-term intake of preformed vitamin A in amounts as 3 or 4 times the RDA can lead to toxicity symptoms, but toxicity is more common at intake levels 10 times the RDA.[5]

Sources

Food sources of vitamin A include liver, fortified milk, eggs, and dark-green and yellow-orange vegetables.[12]

Populations at Risk for Deficiency

Patients with fat-malabsorptive disorders and pregnant women with low vitamin A intake may be at risk for vitamin A deficiency.

Half-Life of the Nutrient in the Body

The half-life of retinol is approximately 140 days.[13]

Assessment of Vitamin A Status

Table 8-1 lists clinical signs and symptoms of vitamin A deficiency and toxicity.[11,14] Serum retinol results from laboratory testing are interpreted as follows:[5]
- ≤0.35 mcmol/L (10 mcg/dL): low/depleted
- ≥1.05 mcmol/L (30 mcg/dL) to 3.5 mcmol/L (100 mcg/dL): adequate
- ≥3.5 mcmol/L (100 mcg/dL): toxic

Nutrient-Nutrient Interactions

Because retinol circulates attached to RBP and TTR as a complex, the presence of either protein-energy malnutrition and/or zinc deficiency may compromise circulating serum vitamin A levels. Decreased circulating serum retinol levels may reflect an impaired RBP synthesis and mobilization secondary to inflammatory processes or disease and do not require correction by vitamin A supplementation.[15]

Medication-Nutrient Interactions

Cholestyramine (bile acid sequestrant), lomitapide (lipid-lowering agent), octreotide (antidiarrheal), orlistat (weight control medication), and mineral oil (laxative) decrease absorption of vitamin A through fat malabsorption. In general, corticosteroids (anti-inflammatories) also may cause decreased serum vitamin A.[7]

Treatment Considerations

If patients have a vitamin A deficiency, daily supplementation with 606 to 60,600 RAE (2000 to 200,000 IU) of vitamin A may be warranted.[5]

Vitamin A administration is commonly used to enhance wound healing in patients with comorbidities (diabetes, tumors, and radiation).[6] A wide dosage range of 3000 to 15,000 RAE/d orally for 7 days, or 3000 RAE/d intramuscularly for 7 days, has been recommended to counteract the inhibitory effects that steroids have on collagen synthesis and connective tissue repair, although results have been inconsistent.[16] The application of topical vitamin A can minimize delayed wound healing in patients requiring long-term corticosteroid treatment.[16] Oral administration of 3000 to 4500 RAE/d is recommended to enhance wound healing with concurrent corticosteroid therapy.[16]

Vitamin D

Vitamin D refers to both ergocalciferol (vitamin D_2) and cholecalciferol (vitamin D_3), which are either consumed in the diet or synthesized in the skin from the compound 7-dehydrocholesterol postexposure to solar or artificial ultraviolet (UVB) light (D_3). Sun exposure lasting 5 to 15 minutes in the spring, summer, and fall between the hours of 10 AM and 3 PM may be enough to achieve adequate vitamin D levels.[17] About 80% of dietary vitamin D intake is incorporated into a micelle, primarily in the distal small intestine, although uptake is more rapid in the duodenum.[14] Vitamin D absorption occurs in tandem with fat and bile salts via passive diffusion into the intestinal cell where it is packaged as chylomicrons for entrance into the lymphatic system and then into the blood. Approximately 40% of the cholecalciferol is transported via chylomicrons (Figure 8-1), although some is transferred from the chylomicron to a vitamin D–binding protein (DBP) for export to extrahepatic tissues. The chylomicron remnant delivers the remaining vitamin D to the liver. Cholecalciferol synthesized from the skin is transported to the liver bound to DBP; however, some is deposited in muscle and adipose before its liver uptake. These different mechanisms for vitamin D transport influence the distribution in the body.

Once vitamin D is transported to the liver, it undergoes the first of 2 hydroxylation steps at carbon 25 via the enzyme 25-hydroxylase to form 25-hydroxy-D (calcidiol), its major circulating form that has no biological activity.[14] Although this enzyme is not tightly regulated, its efficiency is dependent

TABLE 8-1 Selected Clinical Signs and Symptoms of Vitamin A Deficiency or Toxicity

System	Deficiency	Toxicity
Skin	Follicular hyperkeratosis	Pruritus
Hair	None	Alopecia
Eyes	Roughened conjunctiva, Bitot's spots, xeropthalmia, night blindness	Vision disorders, conjunctivitis
Mouth	None	Cheilitis
Nervous system	None	Ataxia
Bones	Excessive bone deposition	Bone loss, bone pain, hip fractures
Other	Impaired wound healing	Hyperlipidemia, renal osteodystrophy, membrane dryness, muscle pain, hepatotoxicity, birth defects

Source: Data are from references 11 and 14.

on vitamin D status. Enzymatic conversion is more efficient during vitamin D deprivation. When 25-hydroxy-D is transported to the kidneys, it may undergo a second hydroxylation at carbon 1 to form the active form of the vitamin 1,25-dihydroxyvitamin D (calcitriol).[18] Other tissues are also capable of this reaction and thus may make calcitriol for their own (ie, autocrine) uses. (Technically, the terms *calcidiol* and *calcitriol* refer only to the D_3 versions of these molecules. It has become common convention, however, to conflate the D_2 versions of these molecules into these terms and this approach has been taken here.)

Calcitriol made by the kidneys is released into the circulation, where it is necessary for bone mineralization and intestinal calcium uptake, among other actions. The activity of the enzyme is highly controlled via the vitamin D receptor and is affected by several factors that influence calcium homeostasis. Vitamin D can be stored in adipose tissue for later use or converted to calcidiol in the liver. Excretion is primarily via bile, with minimal amounts lost via urine.

Functions of Vitamin D

Calcium Homeostasis

When describing vitamin D functions, it is important to note that calcitriol is the active form. The principal function of vitamin D is to maintain serum calcium and phosphorus levels to support neuromuscular function, bone calcification, and other cellular processes. In its active form, calcitriol functions to maintain circulating serum levels of calcium and phosphorus within normal ranges.

When blood calcium levels are low, the parathyroid glands respond by secreting parathyroid hormone (PTH). PTH increases blood calcium levels as follows:[5]

- PTH in the kidneys stimulates increased renal calcium retention and the conversion of calcidiol (inactive vitamin D) to the active form, calcitriol.
- Both calcitriol and PTH act on the bone, stimulating osteoclast activity for the resorption of calcium into the bloodstream.
- Calcitriol travels to the intestines to increase exogenous calcium absorption. Once serum calcium has normalized, PTH secretion decreases, effectively halting the cycle.

Pleiotropic Effects of Vitamin D

Recent literature suggests that vitamin D may be important in the management of multiple other medical conditions, such as musculoskeletal disorders, falls, immunity, autoimmunity, infections, cancer, diabetes or glucose intolerance, and cardiovascular disease.[19-21] The potential effects of vitamin D on the cardiometabolic system are thought to be mediated by a variety of mechanisms related to the inflammatory response and have been associated with therapeutic doses greater than the current DRI. Although some experts now recommend up to 800 to 1000 IU vitamin D per day to prevent deficiency in select populations, such as older adults, the most recent RDAs are 600 IU for healthy adults younger than 70 years and 800 IU for those age 70 years or older.

Vitamin D and Nosocomial Infection

Vitamin D receptors are expressed throughout the innate and adaptive immune system and may play a role in fighting infection. Macrophages are activated by calcitriol,[22,23] increasing their capacity for oxidative bursts of cytokines, acid phosphatases, and hydrogen peroxide in response to pathogens.[24] Furthermore, vitamin D enhances the motility and phagocytic activity of neutrophils.[24] These aspects of vitamin D have profound implications for hospital-acquired infections, such as *Clostridium difficile*. Low calcidiol levels have been associated with increased incidence of *C. difficile*[22] infection as well as increased severity of infection in those who are positive for *C. difficile*.[23] Low calcidiol levels decrease the body's ability to make calcitriol within the macrophages, thereby diminishing this aspect of immune function. Prospective randomized controlled trials are needed to determine whether supplementing vitamin D affects rates of *C. difficile* infection.

Clinical Applications

Recommended Intakes for Adults

The vitamin D RDA for adults younger than 70 years is 600 IU (15 mcg), and the RDA for adults age 70 years or older is 800 IU (20 mcg). The UL for individuals age 9 years and older is 4000 IU (100 mcg). These DRIs assume minimal sun exposure.

Sources

Sources of vitamin D include sunlight as well as fish liver oils, fatty fish, fortified milk, and breakfast cereals.

Populations at Risk for Deficiency

Individuals with inadequate sun exposure are at risk for vitamin D deficiency; populations at risk include older adults, nursing home residents, dark-skinned individuals, people who wear clothing or veils that expose very little skin, people who are indoors much of the time or use sunscreen daily, and exclusively breastfed infants.[19-21] Patients with extensive skin damage (eg, burns), fat-malabsorptive disorders, or renal disease (insufficient renal calcitriol production), and those on long-term parenteral nutrition (PN) are also at risk. One study suggests that patients on home PN had a high prevalence of vitamin D deficiency despite oral vitamin D supplementation.[25]

Half-Life of the Nutrient in the Body

The half-life of calcitriol is 4 to 6 hours.[26] The half-life for calcidiol can be 2 to 3 weeks but may be as high as 2 to 3 months in patients with high adiposity.[26]

Assessment of Vitamin D Status

Calcitriol is not a good marker of vitamin D status. When calcidiol levels fall, both serum calcium and phosphorus levels

TABLE 8-2 Interpretation of Serum Calcidiol Levels

Status	Calcidiol Level, ng/mL
Sufficient	>30
Insufficient	>20 to ≤30
Deficient	≤20

Source: Data are from reference 5.

TABLE 8-3 Clinical Signs and Symptoms of Vitamin D Deficiency or Toxicity

System	Deficiency	Toxicity
Bones	Osteomalacia	Calcification of soft tissues (cardiovasculature, lungs)
Nervous system	Tetany	Confusion, psychosis, tremor
Other	Hypocalcemia	Hypercalcemia, hypercalciuria

Source: Data are from reference 5.

decrease, which stimulates PTH secretion to increase renal production of vitamin D's active form, calcitriol.[21] Consequently, circulating levels of the calcitriol are often normal or elevated in vitamin D deficiency, making it a less-sensitive indicator of vitamin D status.

The measurement of serum calcidiol is a reasonable assay to evaluate vitamin D status.[27,28] (See Table 8-2.[5]) However, vitamin D adequacy is more clearly defined using surrogate markers such as PTH and calcium. Normal circulating calcidiol levels vary with the degree of sun exposure and range from 54 to 90 ng/mL.[29]

Vitamin D deficiency and toxicity may affect bones, the nervous system, and calcium levels in the blood or urine. See Table 8-3 for clinical signs and symptoms.[5]

Nutrient-Nutrient Interactions

Excess vitamin D stimulates hepatic oxidation, and excretion of vitamin K.[5]

Medication-Nutrient Interactions

Cholestyramine (bile acid sequestrant), lomitapide (lipid-lowering agent), orlistat (weight control medication), octreotide (antidiarrheal), and mineral oil (laxative) decrease absorption of vitamin D through fat malabsorption. Phenobarbital (anticonvulsant), phenytoin (antiepileptic), valproic acid (antiepileptic), and rifampin (antibiotic) increase the metabolism of vitamin D and may decrease serum levels. Corticosteroids (anti-inflammatories), carbamazepine (antiepileptic), and isoniazid (antitubercular) also may cause decreased serum vitamin D levels. Vitamin D may increase the drug effects of digoxin (antiarrhythmic).[7]

Treatment Considerations

Serum calcidiol (25-hydroxy) concentrations are expected to increase by 1 ng/mL for every 100 IU vitamin D ingested per day. Vitamin D deficiency is typically treated with 50,000 IU Vitamin D once per week for 8 weeks; the dose is then lowered to approximately 1000 IU/d for several months.[5] Maintaining 25-hydroxyvitamin D concentrations between 78 and 100 nmol/L is associated with maximum bone health and the prevention of chronic diseases.[21,27,28] Patients receiving long-term PN patients are prone to hypovitaminosis D and must be monitored to ensure optimal levels of calcidiol, calcitriol, PTH, and calcium.

Vitamin E

Vitamin E activity has been found in 8 naturally occurring compounds: 4 tocopherols (α, β, γ, and δ) and 4 tocotrienols (α, β, γ, and δ), each with varying degrees of biological activity.[14] Evidence indicates that these 8 forms of vitamin E are functionally unique. The most active and naturally occurring form is the RRR isomer of α-tocopherol, which exhibits antioxidant activity and inhibits cell proliferation, platelet aggregation, and monocyte adhesion.[14] γ-Tocopherol represents the predominant form of vitamin E in a typical American diet; it has anti-inflammatory, antineoplastic, and natriuretic properties.[30]

In 2000, the Food and Nutrition Board of the Institute of Medicine determined that only α-tocopherol should be considered sufficient to meet the vitamin E recommendations because evidence for the activity of other forms of the vitamin were insufficient. α-Tocopherol has 8 different isomers, all of which provide some vitamin E activity. The RRR isomer of α-tocopherol is special in that it is selectively recognized by receptors in the liver and incorporated into very low-density lipoproteins (VLDL) for distribution to the tissues. This capacity for VLDL incorporation greatly increases its half-life compared with other forms of vitamin E and other isomers of α-tocopherol, which are only distributed in the chylomicron phase of lipid circulation.

Since the recommendations of the Food and Nutrition Board were issued, the evidence for the vitamin E activity of the tocotrienols and γ-tocopherol has grown. Tocotrienols have neuroprotective, antioxidant, anticancer, and cholesterol-lowering effects that are different from the properties of tocopherols.[30] Some vitamin E molecules, such as γ-tocopherols, δ-tocopherols, and α-tocotrienols, have emerged with roles in health and disease that are distinct from the function of α-tocopherols.[5]

Vitamin E absorption depends on dietary fat absorption and occurs primarily in the jejunum via nonsaturable, passive diffusion. Absorption varies from about 20% to 50%, decreasing as intake increases.[14,30,31] At pharmacological doses (200 mg), absorption drops to less than 10%.[14] Tocopherols are found free in foods; however, the tocotrienols are esterified and must be hydrolyzed before they are absorbed via pancreatic and duodenal esterases located in the lumen. Vitamin E is incorporated into micelles within the lumen of the small intestine (Figure 8-1). Once taken up by the enterocytes, vitamin E is transported as part of a lipoprotein complex through the lymph into circulation. Adipose tissue, muscle, and the liver serve as the major storage sites. Excretion occurs primarily via the urine and bile, but significant amounts are found in the feces because of the body's limited absorption of vitamin E.

Functions of Vitamin E

The principal biochemical function of vitamin E is the maintenance of membrane integrity in body cells via its action as an antioxidant. By inhibiting lipid peroxidation, vitamin E protects the integrity of all biological membranes.[14] It also acts as an antioxidant by trapping peroxyl free radicals in cell membranes to protect against oxidation. Thus, sufficient vitamin E is critical in the oxidative stress states (chronic inflammation, sepsis, systemic inflammatory response syndrome [SIRS], and organ failure).[31]

Clinical Applications

Recommended Intakes for Adults

The RDA for vitamin E for all adults is 15 mg. The UL is 1000 mg. Values for vitamin E are often expressed in international units (IU). IU conversions are substance-specific and vary by the type of vitamin E ingested: 1 mg vitamin E can equal anywhere from 1 to 1.5 IU depending on the form. For example, 15 mg of naturally occurring d-α-tocopherol is 22.5 IU. In synthetic supplements, α-tocopherol is often a mixture of *D* and *L* forms in which 15 mg vitamin E equals 16.5 IU.

Sources

Food sources of vitamin E include vegetable oils, wheat germ, asparagus, and peanuts.

Populations at Risk for Deficiency

Patients at risk for vitamin E deficiency include those with fat-malabsorptive disorders such as prolonged steatorrhea, Crohn's disease, cystic fibrosis, compromised biliary function, or resection of the ileum or small intestine. Patients receiving long-term PN without vitamin E supplementation are also at risk.

Half-Life of the Nutrient in the Body

The half-life of RRR-α-tocopherol is 44 to 60 hours. The half-lives of other isomers of α-tocopherol are much shorter. For example, the half-life of SRR-α-tocopherol is 15 hours.[32]

Assessment of Vitamin E Status

Relevant diagnostic laboratory tests for vitamin E levels include plasma or serum Vitamin E (α-tocopherol), which may be interpreted as follows:[33]
- <0.5 mg/dL: deficient
- 0.5 to 2.0 mg/dL: normal
- >2.0 mg/dL: toxicity

In addition, a ratio of plasma α-tocopherol (mcmol/L) to plasma cholesterol (mmol/L) below 2.2 indicates a risk for vitamin E deficiency.[33] Table 8-4 lists clinical signs of vitamin E deficiency or toxicity.[11,30–34]

Nutrient-Nutrient Interactions

An intake of more than 1200 mg vitamin E per day interferes with absorption and metabolism of vitamin K and may be problematic for patients receiving warfarin therapy. Daily intake of 800 to 1200 mg vitamin E may decrease platelet adhesion.[14,30,31]

Medication-Nutrient Interactions

Cholestyramine (bile acid sequestrant), lomitapide (lipid-lowering agent), orlistat (weight control medication), octreotide (antidiarrheal), and mineral oil (laxative) decrease absorption of vitamin E through fat malabsorption. A form of vitamin E that has been altered to be soluble in water increases the absorption of cyclosporine (immunosuppressant).[7]

TABLE 8-4 Clinical Signs and Symptoms of Vitamin E Deficiency or Toxicity

System	Deficiency	Toxicity
Skin	Ceroid pigmentation (age spots)	Bruising from decreased vitamin K absorption
Eyes	Vision changes	None
Bone	None	Inclusion bodies in bone marrow
Nervous system	Ophthalmoplegia, ptosis, vision loss, dysarthria, ataxia, neuronal degeneration	None
Other	Hemolytic anemia, increased platelet aggregation, urinary creatinine wasting	Thrombocytopenia, cerebral hemorrhage, impaired neutrophil function, abrogated granulocytopenic response to antigen, impaired coagulation. Prolonged depletion: skeletal muscle lesions with ceroid deposits in smooth muscle

Source: Data are from references 11 and 30–34.

Treatment Considerations

Vitamin E deficiency is rare, but it usually requires treatment with oral vitamin E intakes of 200 to 2000 mg/d.[35] Thrombocytopenia and cerebral hemorrhages resulting in death have been reported at pharmacological doses below the UL (50 mg/d and 1000 mg/d).[34,36] Consistent intake of excessive amounts of vitamin E is contraindicated in patients with a coagulation defect.[30]An intake of more than 1200 mg vitamin E per day interferes with vitamin K and may be problematic for patients receiving warfarin therapy (see previous "Nutrient-Nutrient Interactions" discussion).

Vitamin K

Vitamin K is a generic name for a family of compounds that are synthesized by gut microflora in the distal small intestine and colon; these compounds include phylloquinones (K_1), which are found in plants, and menaquinones (K_2), which are found in fish oils and meats. Menadione (K_3) is a common synthetic form that is converted to K_2 by intestinal flora. Some of the menaquinones may be synthesized in vivo from vitamin K_1. Phylloquinone absorption occurs primarily in the jejunum by a saturable, energy-dependent process. Like the absorption of other fat-soluble nutrients, vitamin K absorption depends on the presence of lipids, which stimulate the bile salt and pancreatic enzyme release necessary for its incorporation into chylomicrons for transport (Figure 8-1). Absorption of vitamin K normally varies from 40% to 80%. With any impairment in the lipid absorption process, such as in the case of a biliary obstruction or a significant small bowel resection, absorption decreases to 20% to 30%.[14,37] The absorption and usefulness of the menaquinone synthesized by bacteria are still unknown. Mineral oil and other nonabsorbable lipids interfere with vitamin K absorption. There is no storage mechanism for vitamin K in the body.[14,37]

Functions of Vitamin K

Clotting

Vitamin K is involved in a variety of enzymatic reactions within the body that affect blood coagulation. The primary biochemical function of vitamin K is as a cosubstrate in the posttranslational carboxylation of proteins at designated glutamic acid residues. As part of a membrane-bound carboxylase system, vitamin K functions in the posttranslational gamma-carboxylation of clotting factors (II, VII, IX, and X), and normally occurring anticoagulant proteins C and S.[14] Clotting is often measured in terms of prothrombin time (PT). Variations in methods for determining PT cause variance in test results. To account for this variance, a standardized measure of PT, the international normalized ratio (INR), is used.

Patients on anticoagulation therapy (warfarin therapy) may find that ingestion of excess vitamin K decreases the ability to achieve a therapeutic INR.[38] Warfarin and vitamin K have an antagonistic relationship with each other regarding their effect on INR. Warfarin increases the INR, whereas vitamin K decreases the INR. Achieving a therapeutic INR (typi-

cally between 2 and 3) requires a balance between warfarin administration and vitamin K ingestion. One study in healthy patients anticoagulated with a low warfarin dose found that every 100 mcg increase in vitamin K beyond an initial amount of 150 mcg causes a 0.2 decrease in INR. Therefore, assessment of vitamin K intake is an essential part of warfarin therapy.[39] The amount of vitamin K from sources of nutrition support can quickly add up. These sources include obvious ones, such as parenteral multivitamin infusions, but also less obvious sources such as lipid emulsions and propofol administration.

Bone Health

Vitamin K may be involved in bone health through its role in converting protein-bound glutamate to gamma-carboxy-glutamate (Gla). Osteocalcin is a bone Gla-protein that facilitates calcium binding to the hydroxyapatite matrix of bone.[40] Emerging evidence in human intervention studies suggests that vitamin K may benefit bone health, particularly when coadministered with vitamin D.[37]

Several mechanisms have been proposed to explain vitamin K modulation of bone metabolism.[35] One relates to the Gla content of osteocalcin, which accounts for up to 80% of the total Gla content of mature bone. Undercarboxylation of osteocalcin secondary to inadequate vitamin K can impair the ability of osteocalcin to bind to the bone mineral matrix and thus regulate bone mineralization. There is also increasing evidence that vitamin K positively affects calcium balance, a key mineral in bone metabolism.[37,40] Some researchers contend that the DRI for vitamin K should be increased given its role in bone health.[37,40]

Clinical Applications

Recommended Intakes for Adults

The AI for vitamin K for men is 120 mcg, and AI for women is 90 mcg. A UL has not been established for vitamin K.

Sources

Food sources of vitamin K include liver, green leafy vegetables, broccoli, peas, and green beans.[41] Other sources of vitamin K are propofol and lipid injectable emulsions (ILEs). The amount of vitamin K in ILE varies depending on the composition of the ILE and the manufacturing process.[42]

Populations at Risk for Deficiency or Adverse Effects

The following conditions and therapies increase a patient's risk for vitamin K deficiency:
- Fat malabsorption
- Inflammatory bowel disease
- Antibiotic therapy
- Long-term PN without lipid emulsion
- *Nil per os* status

Patients on anticoagulant therapy may require closer monitoring of vitamin K. Some adverse effects have been reported when large doses of this vitamin were given to individuals who had severely compromised liver function.[43] In addition, menadione, a water-soluble synthetic vitamin K analog, has produced fatal anemia, hyperbilirubinemia, severe jaundice,[5] and anaphylactoid reaction.[44]

Half-Life of the Nutrient in the Body

The first half-life of phylloquinone is 15 minutes. The half-life then slows down to about 2.5 hours.[4]

Body pool turnover has been reported to be 1.5 days;[45] however, another study found liver pool of phylloquinone to decrease by two-thirds in 3 days.[4]

Assessment of Vitamin K Status

The INR is the most common laboratory procedure used to monitor warfarin therapy and detect potential bleeding problems. A more sensitive indicator of vitamin K status is the measurement of plasma phylloquinone, the major circulating form. Fasting phylloquinone reference values in healthy adults are 0.15 to 1.0 mcg/L and reflect both dietary depletion and repletion.[46] Refer to Table 8-5 for clinical signs and symptoms of vitamin K deficiency.[14,26,37,47]

Nutrient-Nutrient Interactions

Excess vitamin A or vitamin E can diminish absorption of vitamin K. Excess serum/plasma vitamin D levels stimulate hepatic oxidation and excretion of vitamin K.[5]

Medication-Nutrient Interactions

Cholestyramine (bile acid sequestrant), lomitapide (lipid-lowering agent), orlistat (weight control medication), octreotide (antidiarrheal), and mineral oil (laxative) decrease absorption of vitamin K through fat malabsorption. Vitamin K negates the effects of warfarin and must be carefully titrated to optimize anticoagulation therapy. Vitamin K metabolism is increased by phenobarbital (sedative) and phenytoin (antiepileptic).[7]

Treatment Considerations

Guidelines for treating vitamin K deficiency do not exist. However, oral or injected supplementation of 2.5 to 10 mg vitamin K twice weekly to daily is common.

TABLE 8-5 Clinical Signs and Symptoms of Vitamin K Deficiency

System	Deficiency
Skin	Bruising, prolonged bleeding
Bones	Decreased bone density
Other	Increased prothrombin time

Source: Data are from references 14, 26, 37, and 47.

The literature continues to support recommendations for increased vitamin K intake to reduce bone loss and fracture risk, especially among older adults.[48]

As noted, warfarin and vitamin K counter each other in the goal of achieving a therapeutic INR. Therefore, once the goal INR is met, daily vitamin K intake should remain consistent. Increased vitamin K intake without adjustment of warfarin leads to an increased risk of clotting whereas decreased vitamin K intake could increase the risk of bleeding.

Administration of warfarin with continuous enteral nutrition leads to decreased warfarin absorption. Currently, the evidence suggests that warfarin binds irreversibly with plastic tubing. More rapid administration of warfarin through the tubing results in less warfarin binding and more warfarin administered to the patient.[49]

If a patient on anticoagulation therapy has difficulty achieving a therapeutic INR, consider all sources of vitamin K, including from lipid emulsions and fat-based medicines (propofol).[42] See Practice Scenario 8-1.[50]

Practice Scenario 8-1

Question: What considerations should be made when a patient on warfarin therapy is receiving parenteral nutrition (PN)?

Scenario: A 52-year-old man with a diagnosis of stage IV colon cancer status post chemotherapy presents to the emergency department with severe nausea, vomiting, abdominal pain, and distention. The patient reports that his last bowel movement was 5 days ago and he has had nothing but sips of fluid since that time. He also reports "cramping" pain in his left calf and edema is noted in that extremity. A computed tomography scan of the abdomen is positive for ileus. Doppler ultrasound of the left lower extremity reveals deep vein thrombosis (DVT). A nasogastric tube is inserted and connected to low-intermittent suction for abdominal decompression, and intravenous fluids are started for dehydration. A heparin drip is initiated per the hospital's DVT protocol, and the patient is transferred to the intensive care unit for further management. Within 48 hours of admission, patient is still unable to tolerate oral feedings, and PN is initiated. As the patient's condition improves, he is advanced to a liquid diet with supplemental PN and transitioned to warfarin therapy with a target international normalized ratio (INR) of 2 to 3. During the course of the warfarin therapy, his INR remains subtherapeutic despite frequent increases in the warfarin dose until it reaches abnormally high levels.

Intervention: The nutrition support clinician assesses the patient's vitamin K intake from PN sources and its impact on warfarin dosage. PN is adjusted to decrease vitamin K intake to achieve therapeutic INR at a stable warfarin dose. If possible, the patient is switched to a multivitamin product that does not contain vitamin K, such as M.V.I.-12 (Hospira). If the lipid emulsion provides a high dose of vitamin K, it may also be adjusted.

Answer: All sources of vitamin K must be accounted for in the management of a patient on warfarin. PN provides a significant amount of vitamin K. Parenteral multivitamins such as Infuvite contain 150 mcg vitamin K per unit dose (10 mL). Depending upon their fat source, lipid emulsions provide anywhere from 0 to 1000 mcg vitamin K per liter.

Rationale: Vitamin K is necessary for the formation of key clotting factors. Warfarin acts as a vitamin K antagonist and is thus an anticoagulant. Proper dosing of warfarin requires that vitamin K intake be (1) known and (2) consistent. The variable vitamin K content in lipid emulsions along with the periodic nature of their administration adds an extra challenge to the provision of nutrition support to patients receiving warfarin therapy. For example, a 250-mL bag of the 20% lipid emulsion Intralipid has 132.5 mcg vitamin K. If this product is given in addition to a daily multivitamin infusion of 150 mcg vitamin K, the daily intake of vitamin K will be 2 to 3 times the Adequate Intake without a commensurate adjustment in warfarin, making achievement of the target INR difficult. Another considerable source of vitamin K may be the sedative lipid propofol, which is 10% soybean oil. Soybean oil has approximately 1.7 mcg vitamin K per mL. If a patient were receiving both warfarin and propofol, the propofol might need to be discontinued to achieve a therapeutic INR; however, it would be unusual for patients to be receiving both of these medications concomitantly.[50]

Vitamin C

The total amount of naturally occurring and biologically active vitamin C is available as ascorbic acid (reduced form) and dehydroascorbic acid (oxidized form). Vitamin C absorption occurs predominately in the ileum, with some absorption in the jejunum via the sodium/energy-dependent active transport system. The transport systems for vitamin C are both saturable and dose dependent—that is, absorption efficiency decreases as intake increases. At pharmacological doses (12 g/d), vitamin C absorption falls to about 16%, whereas at low intakes (less than 20 mg/d), absorption can reach 98%. At normal intakes (20 to 120 mg/d), absorption is 80% to 90%.[51] Serum ascorbic acid levels rise with dietary intakes of 70 to 140 mg vitamin C per day, and then saturation is reached (at 80 to 90 mcmol/L). Once serum ascorbic acid levels reach 80 mcmol/L, renal clearance sharply increases,[14] which explains why few toxic effects are associated with high vitamin C intake.

Functions of Vitamin C

Ascorbic acid serves as an antioxidant, reacting directly with superoxide, hydroxyl radicals, and singlet oxygen.[52] Vitamin C also provides reducing equivalents for a variety of reactions and acts as a cofactor for reactions that require a reduced metal. As a result, vitamin C has very complex functional roles, such as the synthesis of collagen, carnitine, and neurotransmitters; the enhancement of intestinal absorption of nonheme iron; cholesterol hydroxylation into bile acids; the reduction of toxic transition (variable positive oxidative states) metals; the reductive protection of folic acid and vitamin E; and the immune-mediated and antibacterial functions of white blood cells.[14]

Clinical Applications

Recommended Intakes for Adults

The following RDAs have been set for vitamin C:
- Men: 90 mg
- Women: 75 mg
- Pregnant women: 100 mg
- Lactating women: 120 mg

The UL for vitamin C is 2000 mg.

Sources

Food sources of vitamin C include citrus fruits and other fruits and vegetables.[41]

Populations at Risk for Deficiency

Older adults and patients with malabsorptive disorders or poor diets combined with alcoholism are at increased risk of vitamin C deficiency. Type 2 diabetes mellitus and certain types of cancer may increase vitamin C turnover. People who smoke tobacco need more vitamin C because of tobacco use increases free radical production.

Half-Life of the Nutrient in the Body

The half-life of vitamin C varies according to serum status. In replete states, vitamin C half-life is approximately 30 minutes. When plasma levels of vitamin C are less than approximately 70 mcmol/L, the half-life is 8 to 40 days because of renal reabsorption.[53] Studies report daily intake of less than 10 mg vitamin C causes frank signs of scurvy within approximately 30 days.[5]

Assessment of Vitamin C Status

Plasma ascorbic acid analysis is the most feasible procedure for evaluating the status of vitamin C in individuals as well as in population groups. (See Table 8-6.[14]) Although the concentration of ascorbic acid in leukocytes reflects body stores, this measurement is technically difficult to perform. Table 8-7 presents clinical signs and symptoms of vitamin C deficiency and toxicity.[14,54]

Nutrient-Nutrient Interactions

Vitamin C assists in the absorption of iron (Fe) by reducing Fe^{3+} to Fe^{2+}. For this reason, patients taking oral iron supple-

TABLE 8-6 Interpretation of Plasma/Serum Ascorbic Acid Levels

Status	Plasma/Serum Ascorbic Acid Level, mcmol/L (mg/dL)
Sufficient	>23 (0.4)
Low	12–23 (0.2–0.4)
Deficient	≤11 (0.2)

Source: Data are from reference 14.

TABLE 8-7 Clinical Signs and Symptoms of Deficiency or Toxicity

System	Deficiency	Toxicity
Skin	Capillary rupture, delayed wound healing, petechiae, perifollicular hemorrhage, hyperkeratotic papules	None
Hair	Corkscrew hairs	None
Mouth	Bleeding gums (from weakened collagen)	None
Joints	Joint effusions	None
Other	Hypochondriasis, increased susceptibility to infection	Nausea, vomiting, diarrhea, kidney stones

Source: Data are from references 14 and 54.

ments should consume them with a source of vitamin C. However, this absorptive benefit plateaus at 75 mg vitamin C.[5] This same iron-reductive mechanism has been theorized to increase oxidative stress if vitamin C is taken in excess because the resulting Fe^{2+} is capable of reacting with hydrogen peroxide to form the highly deleterious hydroxyl radical.[55]

Medication-Nutrient Interactions

One study found that vitamin C in amounts of 3g/d or more decreased acetaminophen excretion by 75%. Patients taking allopurinol (xanthine oxidase inhibitor) should refrain from ingesting large amounts of vitamin C because they increase the potential for renal calculi. Tetracycline (antibiotic), aspirin, and corticosteroids increase urinary vitamin C wasting.[7]

Treatment Considerations

Oral supplementation of 100 mg vitamin C 3 times per day is recommended to treat vitamin C deficiency. An initial intravenous (IV) dose of 60 to 100 mg may also be given.[5] Vitamin C intake less than 10 mg/d over a prolonged period can result in classic deficiency signs and symptoms.[14,54] Scurvy is rare today because it is preventable with as little as 10 mg vitamin C per day.[41]

Supplementation of vitamin C (100 to 200 mg/d) is now common in patients who have wounds, including stage I and II pressure ulcers.[6,11,14] Surgical and burn patients are frequently reported to have ascorbate deficiency.[6] Reports indicate that vitamin C status deteriorates during hospitalization and from medical or surgical stress, which can negatively impact wound healing.[15,56] Hyperglycemia is common in acute stress states and prevents vitamin C transport, which is needed for normal leukocyte function.[56] Vitamin C supplementation improves leukocyte function, but the extent to which it influences immune response is unclear.

Reports of vitamin C toxicity are uncommon. People given 5 to 15 g/d, which is well above the UL, have reported nausea and vomiting. The hypothesis that rebound scurvy occurs fol-lowing the cessation of large vitamin C doses is controversial. Individuals with renal failure, kidney stones, or iron overload disease, and patients receiving heparin or warfarin therapy should avoid large vitamin C doses. Vitamin C intake increases both oxalate formation and absorption.[57] Furthermore, vitamin C competitively inhibits renal reabsorption of uric acid. Health benefits for vitamin C intakes beyond 500 mg/d are unsubstantiated. Therefore, patients prone to oxalate- or uric acid–based kidney stones should not exceed 500 mg vitamin C intake per day. The relationship between excess vitamin C and oxalate formation is even more pronounced in renal failure. Vitamin C doses greater than 100 mg/d to 500 mg/d can precipitate oxalate crystals in soft tissues of patients with renal failure, increasing the risk of kidney stones and further compromising renal function.[10]

Thiamin Vit B₁

Thiamin (vitamin B_1) consists of a central carbon to which a nitrogen-containing ring and a sulfur-containing ring are attached. Thiamin is readily inactivated by prolonged exposure to heat or alkaline solutions. There are 3 forms of thiamin: thiamin monophosphate (TMP), thiamin triphosphate (TTP), and thiamin pyrophosphate (TPP). TPP is the biologically active coenzyme and is also known as thiamin diphosphate (TDP).

Before absorption, intestinal phosphatases hydrolyze the phosphates, leaving free thiamin. Absorption of thiamin can occur by either active or passive diffusion, depending on the concentration of intestinal thiamin.[14] At low physiological concentrations, thiamin is absorbed via a specific energy-dependent, saturable active transport mechanism. It is mainly absorbed in the proximal small intestine, especially the jejunum, via a carrier-mediated process. Thiamin absorption is passive during high intake. Approximately 30 mg of thiamin is stored in the body as either TPP or TMP, with most found in the skeletal muscle (50%).[14] Alcohol abuse is the most common cause of impaired thiamin absorption. In the blood, thiamin is bound to albumin, with most thiamin present in the red blood cells as TPP. Following absorption, most free thiamin is taken up by the liver and is phosphorylated into its coenzyme form, TPP. Whether excess intake is given orally or intravenously, most unused thiamin is rapidly excreted in the urine. A UL has not been set because suitable data are lacking.[58]

Functions of Thiamin

Key biochemical functions that require thiamin include energy transformation, synthesis of pentoses and reduced nicotinamide adenine dinucleotide phosphate (NADPH), as well as membrane and nerve conduction. TPP plays a major role in carbohydrate metabolism, serving as a magnesium-coordinated coenzyme for the oxidative decarboxylation of α-ketoacids (pyruvate and α-ketoglutarate), and for the activity of transketolase in the pentose phosphate pathway. As a structural component of nerve membranes, TTP may also function in nerve conduction.[14]

Thiamin deficiency affects the central nervous system. Patients at risk for a deficiency include those with recurrent vomiting or alcoholism, gastric surgery patients, and those who have an increased demand with marginal nutrition status.[11]

The classic thiamin deficiency neurologic diseases are beriberi and Wernicke encephalopathy, which can develop into Wernicke-Korsakoff syndrome. Beriberi is usually characterized by muscle weakness in the lower extremities coupled with impaired nerve conduction. It is caused primarily by inadequate thiamin intake with adequate carbohydrate intake. Acute post–gastric reduction surgery neuropathy, also called *bariatric beriberi*, has become more prevalent as the numbers of bariatric surgeries has increased. Although the neuropathy is multifactorial in origin, thiamin deficiencies along with vitamin B12 deficiencies have been implicated in 40% of the cases.[59] Wernicke encephalopathy is generally precipitated by ethanol abuse. The classic triad of symptoms encompasses ocular abnormalities, gait ataxia, and mental status changes.[11,14] Approximately 80% of patients with Wernicke encephalopathy develop Wernicke-Korsakoff syndrome, resulting in psychosis and memory disturbances. In the absence of thiamin, the resultant inhibition of pyruvate dehydrogenase drives carbohydrate metabolism toward lactic acid fermentation, resulting in a build-up of lactic acid. Untreated thiamin deficiency can result in fatal lactic acidosis.[60]

Clinical Applications

Recommended Intakes for Adults

The following RDAs for thiamin have been set:
- Men 1.2 mg
- Women: 1.1 mg
- Pregnant women: 1.4 mg
- Lactating women: 1.5 mg
As noted previously, a UL has not been established for thiamin.

Sources

Food sources of thiamin include enriched or fortified whole grain products, pork products, sunflower seeds, and wheat germ.

Populations at Risk for Deficiency

Populations at risk for thiamin deficiency include individuals with chronic alcoholism, patients receiving long-term PN or dialysis, patients with refeeding syndrome or malabsorption, women with hyperemesis gravidarum, patients experiencing protracted vomiting or decreased intake after bariatric surgery, and patients who receive insufficient thiamin supplementation during shortages of injectable multivitamin solutions.[11,55]

Half-Life of the Nutrient in the Body

The biological half-life of thiamin is 9 to 18 days,[14] and thiamin deficit occurs with 14 to 20 days of inadequate intake.[61,62] Because of its short biological half-life, thiamin deficiency is often the first nutrient deficiency noted when food intake is limited or when absorption is impaired by alcohol abuse.

Assessment of Thiamin Status

The preferred method for differentiating normal thiamin status from subclinical thiamin deficiency is the measurement of erythrocyte transketolase activity, with and without the in vivo addition of TDP.[14] Transketolase is a TPP-dependent enzyme. This enzyme is measured in hemolyzed blood before and after the addition of TPP, and its resulting increased activity is quantified. This test provides a sensitive, specific biochemical functional measurement of thiamin status. A normal value, which indicates an acceptable thiamin status, is 0% to 15% increase in enzyme activity with the addition of TPP. A low value (or marginally deficient status) is an increase of 16% to 24%, whereas a deficient status (or a high risk of deficiency) is an increase greater than 25%. Adequacy of thiamin can also be assessed by the measurement of thiamin in whole blood; values less than 1.7 mcg/dL denote deficiency. Table 8-8 presents clinical signs and symptoms of thiamin deficiency.[63,64]

Thiamin is remarkably nontoxic. Toxic effects of thiamin have been reported with an excess of 3 g/d (ie, 50 mg per kg body weight); otherwise, it is generally recognized as safe.

Nutrient-Nutrient Interactions

Magnesium is necessary for the conversion of thiamin to its active form, thiamin diphosphate. Thus, a magnesium deficiency effectively renders thiamin unusable.[61]

Medication-Nutrient Interactions

Furosemide (diuretic) therapy has been shown to cause thiamin deficiency secondary to the drug's diuretic effect, which results in increased urinary thiamin excretion. Theophylline (bronchodilator) decreases serum thiamin.[62]

Treatment Considerations

Some experts recommend prophylactic thiamin dosing when a deficiency is probable, especially in patients with a history of alcohol abuse who are receiving PN.[62,65] The standard recommendation is 5 to 20 mg parenteral thiamin per day; however,

TABLE 8-8 Clinical Signs and Symptoms of Thiamin Deficiency

System	Deficiency
Eyes	Nystagmus
Nervous system	Dry beriberi: paresthesia, weakness in lower extremities Wernicke-Korsakoff syndrome and Wernicke encephalopathy: mental status changes, global confusion, nystagmus, polyneuritis, gait ataxia, and stupor
Other	Wet beriberi: high-output cardiac failure, dyspnea, hepatomegaly, tachycardia, oliguria, sodium and water retention, elevated lactic acid

Source: Data are from references 63 and 64.

wider ranges between 50 to 300 mg/d (IV, intramuscular, or oral) have been suggested.[11,62,65] In cases of Wernicke encephalopathy or Wernicke-Korsakoff syndrome, recommendations vary greatly. For patients with suspected Wernicke encephalopathy or Wernicke-Korsakoff syndrome, a recent compilation of the evidence suggests 100 to 200 mg IV or intramuscular thiamin 3 times daily before high-carbohydrate meals for 3 to 5 days followed by 100 mg oral thiamin supplementation 3 times daily for 1 to 2 weeks and then once daily thereafter.[66] For confirmed Wernicke encephalopathy or Wernicke-Korsakoff syndrome, increasing the initial dosing period to 200 to 500 mg thiamin 3 times daily and sustaining this regimen for 5 to 7 days before switching to the oral regimen is recommended.[66]

The clinician should be aware that hypersensitivity and anaphylactic reactions are possible, especially if thiamin is given repeatedly via the parenteral route.[11,14] It is also important to note that thiamin supplementation is only effective if magnesium is replete. For this reason, it may be advisable to give patients an initial dose of 1000 mg magnesium sulfate (approximately 200 mg elemental magnesium) unless repletion status is known.[61] See Practice Scenario 8-2.

Practice Scenario 8-2

Question: How does thiamin deficiency affect nutrient metabolism?

Scenario: A patient presents to the emergency department with shortness of breath, restlessness, and mild confusion. Severe edema in the lower extremities and abdominal ascites secondary to alcoholic liver cirrhosis are noted. The patient's spouse states that the patient's oral food intake has been inadequate for the past month because of "binge drinking." The physician orders furosemide 40 mg. By Day 2, the patient's restlessness progresses to combative behavior, increased confusion, nystagmus, and leg tremor. Arterial blood gas is indicative of metabolic lactic acidosis, which is unresponsive to treatment. Wernicke encephalopathy secondary to inadequate thiamin deficiency is suspected. The patient's serum magnesium is 1.5 mg/dL, which is slightly below normal.

Intervention: Furosemide is discontinued and replaced with oral spironolactone. A multivitamin is administered along with thiamin (200 mg 3 times daily) for 5 days. The initial dose is given with 1 g magnesium sulfate. The confusion and agitation, as well as the metabolic lactic acidosis, resolve within 6 hours of initial treatment. The patient is sent home on an oral thiamin supplement of 100 mg 3 times daily. Two weeks later, this dose is decreased to 100 mg/d.

Answer: Thiamin is necessary for the conversion of pyruvate to acetyl coenzyme A (acetyl-CoA), a major step in the transformation of glucose to **adenosine triphosphate**. In the absence of thiamin, energy metabolism is impaired. As pyruvate builds up, it is driven toward lactic acid fermentation, which causes the spike in lactate and contributes to metabolic acidosis. Furthermore, thiamin is necessary for the Krebs cycle enzyme α-ketoglutarate

dehydrogenase. Together, these conditions decrease the acetyl-CoA entering the Krebs cycle from carbohydrate metabolism and limit the energy substrates produced in the Krebs cycle from fatty acid–derived acetyl-CoA.

Rationale: Wernicke's encephalopathy is a thiamin deficiency–induced neurologic disorder. Its main symptoms include ataxia, ophthalmoplegia, and mental confusion. Severe alcoholism frequently causes thiamin deficiency through the following mechanisms:

- People with alcoholism often replace nutrient-dense energy sources with energy from alcohol intake, which can lead to malnutrition.
- Ethanol inhibits intestinal thiamin absorption.
- The active form of thiamin, thiamin pyrophosphate, is synthesized in the liver, making liver cirrhosis a possible contributing factor in thiamin deficiency.

The placement of this patient on furosemide may have compounded thiamin deficiency. Furosemide is a diuretic that promotes urinary thiamin wasting. Once furosemide is discontinued, the patient's diuretic is switched to spironolactone. The treatment protocol includes supplementation of both thiamin and magnesium sulfate. Magnesium is a necessary cofactor in the conversion of thiamin to its active form in the liver. If magnesium is depleted, administered thiamin cannot be utilized. Therefore, unless magnesium adequacy is a certainty, supplementation with magnesium is advisable. This patient is given 1 g magnesium sulfate (approximately 200 mg elemental magnesium by weight). These doses are followed by a high-carbohydrate meal, which is thought to enhance thiamin absorption.

Riboflavin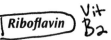

Riboflavin (vitamin B_2) chemically contains 3 linked 6-membered rings, with a sugar alcohol attached to the middle ring. It is a precursor to 2 major coenzyme derivatives, flavin mononucleotide (FMN) and flavin adenine dinucleotide (FAD), which are involved in a wide variety of enzymatic reactions in intermediary metabolism. Dietary sources of riboflavin are primarily in the coenzyme forms, whereas the free form is found in milk and enriched grain products. All these forms can be used to meet the requirement for riboflavin.

Before absorption, riboflavin dissociates from the coenzyme derivatives in the stomach via the action of hydrochloric acid (HCl). The extent of absorption is proportionate to the dose and occurs predominately in the proximal portion of the small intestine via a saturable, sodium-dependent carrier mechanism. Riboflavin deficiency results in an increased intestinal uptake, whereas high riboflavin intake results in decreased absorption efficiency. The upper limit of absorption is estimated to be approximately 66.4 mcmol/d (25 mg/d).[14] Several factors can enhance or impair riboflavin absorption. Evidence indicates that the presence of food increases riboflavin absorption, most likely by delaying the intestinal transit time.[14] Bile salts also increase the absorption of riboflavin. In contrast, several metals and drugs can impede riboflavin. For example, many of the divalent metals, such as copper, zinc, iron, and manganese, form chelates with riboflavin and prevent its absorption.[14] The clinical significance of this binding may become relevant when deciding the amount of supplementation of these trace elements. Alcohol ingestion can also impair both the digestion and absorption of riboflavin. Once absorbed into the mucosal cells, riboflavin then enters the portal circulation destined for the liver, where it undergoes phosphorylation into FMN and FAD. The synthesis of these coenzymes is under hormonal control; adrenocorticotropic hormone, aldosterone, and the thyroid hormones stimulate synthesis.[14] Riboflavin undergoes little metabolism before it is excreted in the urine. Intake that exceeds plasma saturation levels is lost via the urine primarily as free riboflavin.

Functions of Riboflavin

The major biochemical function of riboflavin is to serve as a component of FMN and FAD as an electron transport intermediary for oxidation-reduction reactions. As a component of FMN and FAD, riboflavin participates in pyridine- and non-pyridine-dependent dehydrogenases, oxygen and monooxygen reductases, disulfide reductases, and one-electron transfers. FAD is a key player in macronutrient metabolism because of its ability to receive electrons from the breakdown of fatty acid oxidation and Krebs cycle intermediates and donate them to the electron transport chain for the production of adenosine triphosphate (ATP). Although seldom recognized, riboflavin also has antioxidant activity because the coenzyme FAD is required for the enzyme glutathione reductase, a pivotal enzyme protecting against lipid peroxides. Riboflavin deficiency has been associated with increased lipid peroxidation, especially in association with excessive ethanol intake.[14] Other micronutrient pathways that require riboflavin include the conversion of vitamin B_6 to its active form, the synthesis of the active form of folate, and the catabolism of choline. Riboflavin deficiency rarely occurs alone and is most often accompanied by multiple nutrient abnormalities, such as deficits of the other B-complex vitamins.

Clinical Applications

Recommended Intakes for Adults

The RDA for riboflavin is 1.3 mg for men and 1.1 mg for women. A UL for riboflavin has not been established because suitable data are lacking.[58] Riboflavin toxicity from food or supplements is rare.[58,67]

Sources

Food sources of riboflavin include organ meats, milk, bread products, and fortified cereals.[58]

Populations at Risk for Deficiency

Individuals with alcoholism are at risk for riboflavin deficiency because intake and absorption are limited. Patients with thyroid disorders may have riboflavin deficiencies as a result of altered riboflavin metabolism. Patients with type 2 diabetes, trauma, or extreme stress may excrete more riboflavin than

normal. Patients with chronic malabsorptive disorders are also at risk for riboflavin deficiency.

Half-Life of the Nutrient in the Body

The half-life of riboflavin is 66 to 84 minutes.[68]

Assessment of Riboflavin Status

The erythrocyte glutathione reductase activity coefficient (EGR-AC) assay is a sensitive, functional indicator of riboflavin status and the method of choice for its analysis.[69] An EGR-AC value less than 1.2 (ie, less than 20% stimulation of activity upon addition of FAD) indicates an acceptable riboflavin status. A value between 1.2 and 1.4 indicates marginal status, and a value greater than 1.4 indicates a riboflavin deficiency.[14] This assay is invalid in individuals with a glucose 6-phosphate dehydrogenase deficiency.[14,58]

Although riboflavin is not associated with a specific deficiency disease, characteristic symptoms of overt deficiency are known (see Table 8-9).[14]

Nutrient-Nutrient Interactions

Alcohol as well as divalent metals such as copper, zinc, iron, and manganese form chelates with riboflavin and prevent riboflavin absorption.[14]

Medication-Nutrient Interactions

Tricyclic antidepressant medications and tetracycline (antibiotic) inhibit riboflavin absorption.[7]

Treatment Considerations

Riboflavin deficiency is rare in the general US population. However, suboptimal riboflavin status can be found in critically ill patients.[70] If a patient has riboflavin deficiency, supplement 10 to 20 mg riboflavin daily until the deficiency is resolved.[5]

TABLE 8-9   Clinical Signs and Symptoms of Riboflavin Deficiency

System	Deficiency
Skin	Seborrheic dermatitis of face and scrotum
Eyes	Visual impairment, corneal vascularization, photophobia
Mouth	Cheilosis, angular stomatitis, glossitis, edema, and hyperemia of oral and pharyngeal mucosa, sore throat
Nervous system	Peripheral nerve dysfunction
Other	Normochromic normocytic anemia

Source: Data are from reference 14.

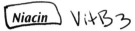 Vit B3

The term *niacin* (vitamin B_3) is a generic descriptor for the vitamin's water-soluble active forms, nicotinic acid and nicotinamide. Nicotinamide serves as a component of 2 coenzymes: nicotinamide adenine dinucleotide (NAD) and NADP. In dietary sources of animal origin, niacin occurs mainly in these 2 forms. In addition to dietary sources, NAD can be synthesized from the essential amino acid tryptophan: 60 mg tryptophan produces 1 mg niacin.

Absorption and Metabolism

Both nicotinic acid and nicotinamide are absorbed rapidly and efficiently from the stomach and intestine by active transport (at low concentrations) or passive diffusion (at high concentrations).[14] Both NAD and NADP are enzymatically hydrolyzed in the intestinal mucosa to release nicotinamide, the major form in the blood. The amount of niacin excreted in the urine is related to the form of niacin ingested and niacin status of the individual. Very little nicotinamide and nicotinic acid is excreted because they both are actively reabsorbed from the glomerular filtrate. Excess niacin is methylated in the liver to form methylnicotinamide, one of the primary urinary metabolites.

Functions of Niacin

The nicotinamide portion of NAD and NADP serves as a hydrogen donor or an electron acceptor for more than 200 enzymes involved in intermediary metabolism.[14] In this role, niacin functions in the metabolism of amino acids, fatty acids, and carbohydrates, accepting electrons from key macronutrient intermediates to form reduced nicotinamide adenine dinucleotide (NADH) and later donating those electrons to the electron transport chain for the production of ATP. Following hydrolysis, hepatic NAD releases adenosine diphosphate ribose, which, in turn, may be transferred to acceptor proteins and functions in the repair of DNA, as well as calcium mobilization.[14,58] Niacin, as NADPH, is also involved with reducing the antioxidants dehydroascorbate (oxidized vitamin C) and glutathione, thus serving as a general regenerator of the body's antioxidant systems. In addition, NADPH is required for activation of folate.

Pellagra

The classic niacin deficiency disease is pellagra, which is rare in developed nations. It can affect the gastrointestinal (GI) tract, the skin, and the nervous system, and presents as "three Ds": dermatitis, diarrhea, and dementia. In the United States, dietary deficiency of niacin is rare because many food products are fortified with niacin.[14]

Niacin as Treatment for Hyperlipidemia

Pharmacological doses of nicotinic acid are used to treat hyperlipidemia but may cause vasodilatation as a result of prostaglandin release. Most individuals taking 3 g/d will experience this phenomenon and other effects.[14,58] Low-dose aspirin, ibu-

profen, or naproxen therapy taken 30 minutes before nicotinic acid helps mitigate these adverse effects. Pharmacological doses of niacin have been shown in some studies to inhibit adipocyte lipolysis as well as very low-density and low-density lipoprotein synthesis,[71] while raising high-density lipoprotein cholesterol. However, these changes have not translated into decreased cardiovascular risk.[72]

Clinical Applications

Recommended Intakes for Adults

The RDAs for niacin are as follows:
- Men: 16 mg
- Women: 14 mg
- Pregnant women: 18 mg
- Lactating women: 17 mg

The UL for niacin is 35 mg.

Sources

Food sources of niacin include meat, fish, poultry, enriched and fortified breads, and fortified cereals.[56]

Populations at Risk for Deficiency

Patients with malabsorptive disorders, individuals with alcoholism, older adults, and patients on the antitubercular medication isoniazid or mercaptopurine are at risk for niacin deficiency.[5]

Half-Life of the Nutrient in the Body

The biological half-life of niacin is 20 to 45 minutes. One study found that approximately 70% of administered niacin was excreted in urine within 96 hours.[73]

Assessment of Niacin Status

Tests to measure the urinary excretion of 2 major niacin-methylated metabolites, N-methylnicotinamide (NMN) and 2-pyridone, are the most common methods to determine niacin status. A niacin deficiency is defined as urinary levels of NMN less than 5.8 mcmol/d and urinary excretion of 2-pyridone less than 2 mg/g of creatinine.[14,58] The measurement of plasma levels of 2-pyridone or NMN may also be used to assess niacin status.[58] A decreased concentration of NAD in red blood cells, coupled with a low plasma tryptophan concentration, may also suggest niacin deficiency.[14] Clinical signs and symptoms of niacin deficiency and toxicity are listed in Table 8-10.[5,14,58]

Nutrient-Nutrient Interactions

Nutrient interactions with niacin have not been identified.

Medication-Nutrient Interactions

Isoniazid (tuberculosis treatment) may decrease niacin levels by inhibiting niacin production from tryptophan.

TABLE 8-10 Clinical Signs and Symptoms of Niacin Deficiency or Toxicity

System	Deficiency	Toxicity
Skin	Dermatitis, sun sensitivity causing symmetrical pigmented rash	Flushing, heat, vasodilation, itching
Mouth	Glossitis	None
Nervous system	Dementia, apathy, fatigue, memory loss, peripheral neuritis, and extremity paralysis	None
Other	Diarrhea, vomiting	Gastrointestinal irritation, severe hepatitis, glucose intolerance, myopathy

Source: Data are from references 5, 14, and 58.

Mercaptopurine (cancer/autoimmune treatment) may cause niacin deficiency by interfering with the conversion of niacin to NAD.[7]

Treatment Considerations

Advanced stages of pellagra are treated via intramuscular injections of nicotinic acid (50 to 100 mg) 3 times daily for 3 to 4 days, followed by oral therapy of nicotinic acid.[11]

Vitamin B6

There are 3 forms of vitamin B_6: pyridoxine, pyridoxal, and pyridoxamine. These 3 forms are metabolically, chemically, and functionally related and can be converted to the active coenzymes pyridoxal phosphate (PLP) and pyridoxamine phosphate (PMP). Plant foods contain the more stable pyridoxine, whereas animal products have more pyridoxal and PLP. Ingested phosphorylated forms must undergo hydrolysis to remove the phosphate group via intestinal phosphatases prior to absorption.[14]

Absorption and Metabolism

Uptake of pyridoxine, pyridoxal, and pyridoxamine by intestinal epithelial cells occurs via a carrier-mediated, pH-dependent mechanism before entry into the portal vein. Absorption rates range from 71% to 82%.[11,14] After uptake by the liver, the hepatocyte converts the dephosphorylated pyridoxine, pyridoxal, and pyridoxamine into the metabolically active PLP form. Both PLP and pyridoxal are released for transport to the extrahepatic tissues, with muscle containing most of the PLP (75% to 80%).[14] Approximately 60% to 90% of the vitamin B_6 in the plasma is in the form of PLP, and most of this is bound to albumin for transport. The major excretory metabolite is urinary 4-pyridoxic acid, the oxidation product of pyridoxal.

Functions of Vitamin B6

The coenzyme forms of vitamin B_6 participate in more than 100 enzymatic reactions. These reactions include, but are not limited to, protein, amino acid, and lipid metabolism; gluconeogenesis; steroid receptor binding; central nervous system development; neurotransmitter synthesis; heme biosynthesis; and normal immune function.[14] Vitamin B_6 as PLP and PMP plays a key coenzyme role in the interconversion of amino acids by facilitating transamination and deamination reactions. Vitamin B_6 also provides a pathway for decreasing levels of homocysteine, facilitating its conversion to cysteine.[5]

Routes of Toxicity

Adverse effects due to high food intakes of vitamin B_6 have been reported,[11,14] and large oral supplemental doses (greater than 500 mg/d) have resulted in a variety of adverse effects. Doses as low as 100 mg/d have been associated with Lhermitte's sign, which suggests an effect on the spinal cord.[11,14] Adverse effects have also been related to prolonged intakes of 300 mg/d. Patients undergoing intestinal transplantation given 50 mg/d more than the UL of 100 mg had an accumulation of PLP within the red cells 30 times the upper limit of normal.[74] Patients with intakes greater than 2000 mg/d have impaired motor control and paresthesia. Animal research suggests this nervous system impairment is caused by degeneration of the gasserian and dorsal root ganglia.[75] Clinicians should adopt a cautious approach to vitamin B_6 supplementation.

Clinical Applications

Recommended Intakes for Adults

RDAs for vitamin B_6 are as follows:
- Men and women ages 50 years or younger: 1.3 mg
- Men older than 50 years: 1.7 mg
- Women older than 50 years: 1.9 mg
- Pregnant women: 1.9 mg
- Lactating women: 2.0 mg

The UL for vitamin B_6 is 100 mg.

Sources

Food sources of vitamin B_6 include fortified cereals, organ meats, and whole grains.[11,58]

Populations at Risk for Deficiency

Individuals with alcoholism, renal patients maintained on dialysis, older adults, and people receiving medication therapies that inhibit vitamin activity (ie, isoniazid, penicillamine, corticosteroids, and/or anticonvulsants) are at risk for vitamin B_6 deficiency.

Half-Life of the Nutrient in the Body

The half-life of vitamin B_6 is approximately 25 days.[58]

Assessment of Vitamin B₆ Status

A combination of the following 3 tests is recommended to assess vitamin B₆ status because each individual test has limitations:[14,58]

- Direct plasma PLP levels, which respond to intake, reflect liver stores, and plateau in 6 to 10 days.
- 24-hour urinary excretion of 4-pyridoxic acid, a hepatic B₆ metabolite. Excretion of greater than 3 mcmol/d suggests adequate status.
- The activation of erythrocyte aspartate aminotransferase (EAST) and erythrocyte alanine aminotransferase (EALT) by PLP, which is used to evaluate long-term vitamin B₆ status. An EAST index value less than 1.6 and an EALT index value less than 1.25 reflect adequate B₆ status.

In critically ill intestinal transplant patients, intracellular (red cell) PLP concentrations are a more reliable measure of status than are plasma measurements.[74]

Table 8-11 presents clinical signs and symptoms of vitamin B₆ deficiency and toxicity.[5,11,14,76]

Nutrient-Nutrient Interactions

Because vitamin B₆ is needed for the interconversion of one amino acid to another, B₆ deficiency may lead to alterations in the amino acid pool.

Medication-Nutrient Interactions

Isoniazid (tuberculosis medication), oral contraceptives, corticosteroids (anti-inflammatories), and penicillamine (chelating agent) all have potential to diminish vitamin B₆ levels or activity.[5,7]

Treatment Considerations

Vitamin B₆ deficiency may be treated with 100 mg vitamin B₆ per day.[5] Patients receiving isoniazid may be given 25 to 50 mg/d as prophylactic against deficiency.[7]

Recently, patients with a neuromyopathic disorder associated with progressive muscle weakness and gait disturbances

TABLE 8-11 Clinical Signs and Symptoms of Vitamin B₆ Deficiency or Toxicity

System	Deficiency	Toxicity
Skin	Seborrheic dermatitis	Dermatologic lesions
Mouth	Angular stomatitis, cheilosis, glossitis	—
Nervous System	Epileptiform convulsions, confusion, depression	Sensory neuropathy, ataxia, areflexia, impaired cutaneous and deep sensations
Other	Microcytic anemia	—

Source: Data are from references 5, 11, 14, and 76.

2-years post–intestinal transplantation were found to have PLP deficiency. Patients who undergo intestinal transplantation should have their preoperative PLP status assessed, and serial long-term monitoring is warranted postoperatively in intestinal transplantation patients receiving PN. In these patients, preemptive replacement of vitamin B₆ should be done when indicated.[76]

Vitamin B₁₂

Naturally occurring vitamin B₁₂ is found exclusively in foods of animal origin. These foods provide vitamin B₁₂ in the coenzyme forms methylcobalamin, hydroxylcobalamin, and deoxyadenosylcobalamin. The complex structure of cobalamin contains a corrin ring with cobalt incorporated into the center. The only reliable sources of vitamin B₁₂ come from animal products or synthetic non-animal-based B₁₂ supplementation. Cyanocobalamin is the form primarily used in supplements and fortified foods. Oral vitamin B₁₂ is relatively nontoxic in its naturally occurring forms. A rare allergic reaction to crystalline cyanocobalamin, which is the form used in many oral formulations, has been reported.[14] Because suitable data are unavailable, a UL for vitamin B₁₂ could not be set.[58] All forms are readily converted into the biologically active forms, methylcobalamin and deoxyadenosylcobalamin.

Absorption and Metabolism

The digestion and absorption process for vitamin B₁₂ is complex and dependent on normal GI function. Vitamin B₁₂ is released from ingested proteins via the action of HCl and pepsin in the gastric secretions. The free B₁₂ binds to the glycoprotein haptocorrin (also called *R-protein* or *transcobalamin I*), which is secreted by the salivary glands and swallowed with food. This complex travels into the small intestine, where pancreatic proteases hydrolyze haptocorrin and free B₁₂ is released.[14] In the duodenum, free B₁₂ encounters another glycoprotein, intrinsic factor (IF), which is produced by the gastric parietal cells. The IF-B₁₂ complex moves into the ileum, where it attaches to a specific IF receptor, cubilin, on the GI epithelial cells for absorption into the enterocyte.[77] Three to four hours after intestinal absorption, the vitamin is transferred to a specific transport protein, transcobalamin II. This carrier protein enters the portal circulation. It is first taken up by the liver and then by bone marrow and erythrocytes. Unlike other water-soluble vitamins, vitamin B₁₂ can be stored in the liver.[14,78]

Adults with normal gastric function absorb approximately 50% of dietary vitamin B₁₂. Because B₁₂ is secreted into the bile, most is reabsorbed via enterohepatic circulation. Failure of any of these processes can decrease B₁₂ absorption. For example, pancreatic insufficiency could interfere with the release of free B₁₂ from haptocorrin, preventing its attachment to IF and reducing the amount of B₁₂ absorbed. Individuals with impaired HCl production, such as older adults, patients with *Helicobacter pylori* infections, and those taking histamine-2 (H₂) antagonists or proton pump inhibitors have reduced absorption.[14,77] Patients who have had a portion or all of the ileum or stomach removed and patients with chronic malabsorption syndromes also have reduced absorption.

Functions of Vitamin B_{12}

The Methyl-Folate Trap

Vitamin B_{12} is needed for the conversion of homocysteine to the benign amino acid methionine. Elevated homocysteine levels have been associated with increased risk for cardiovascular disease, stroke, dementia, Alzheimer's disease, and osteoporosis.[79–81] Vitamin B_{12} must be converted to 1 of its 2 coenzyme forms, methylcobalamin or 5'-deoxyadenosylcobalamin, to be metabolically active. Methylcobalamin is a cofactor for methionine synthetase, the enzyme that converts homocysteine to methionine. Simultaneously, this conversion of homocysteine to methionine involves the demethylation of 5-methyltetrahydrofolate into its active form, tetrahydrofolate (THF) (Figure 8-2).[5] When vitamin B_{12} is lacking, folate becomes "trapped" in its methyl, or inactive, form. For this reason, vitamin B_{12} deficiency often presents as folate deficiency and is, therefore, commonly misdiagnosed. A second major known reaction requiring B_{12} (as deoxyadenosylcobalamin) is the conversion of methylmalonyl coenzyme A (CoA) to succinyl-CoA and for the degradation of certain amino acids and odd chain fatty acids. Between these 2 reactions, B_{12} prevents a host of deficiency symptoms.

Stages of Vitamin B_{12} Deficiency

There are 4 stages of vitamin B_{12} status: stage I, low serum B_{12}; stage II, low cell stores of B_{12}; stage III, a biochemical deficiency; and stage IV, a clinically apparent deficiency.[82] The first manifestations of marginal or inadequate vitamin B_{12} status are usually neurologic and are possibly followed by hematologic and GI abnormalities. Other common age-related problems associated with vitamin B_{12} deficiency include cognitive decline, cardiovascular disease, and bone fractures.[14,81–83] Clinical vitamin B_{12} deficiency has been associated with malabsorption syndromes that may occur in patients after gastrectomy, gastric bypass, or ileal resection, or those with Crohn's disease.[84] Vitamin B_{12} deficiency has also been reported in some vegetarian/vegan populations.[85]

FIGURE 8-2 Conversion of Homocysteine to Methionine

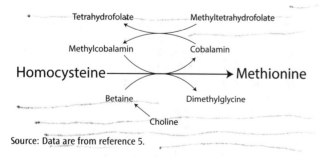

Source: Data are from reference 5.

Clinical Applications

Recommended Intakes for Adults

RDAs for vitamin B_{12} are as follows:
- Men and women: 2.4 mcg
- Pregnant women: 2.6 mcg
- Lactating women: 2.8 mcg

As noted previously, a UL for vitamin B_{12} has not been established.

Sources

Food sources of vitamin B_{12} include fortified cereals, meat, fish, poultry, and eggs.[58]

Populations at Risk for Deficiency

Patients with malabsorption syndromes, vegetarian and vegan populations, and patients with low HCl secretion are at risk for vitamin B_{12} deficiency.

Half-Life of the Nutrient in the Body

The serum half-life of vitamin B_{12} is approximately 6 days. The half-life of B_{12} in the liver is approximately 12 months.[86]

Assessment of Vitamin B_{12} Status

The earliest indicator compromised vitamin B_{12} status is a low serum level of holotranscobalamin II, the primary delivery protein for vitamin B_{12}. However, this laboratory test is not routinely available in hospital settings. The decrease in serum vitamin B_{12} levels occurs later than the decrease in holotranscobalamin II and suggests a decline in cellular stores. In fact, serum vitamin B_{12} levels may even be maintained at the expense of its stores.[58] The serum levels of methylmalonic acid (MMA) and homocysteine are elevated in more than 90% of individuals with a vitamin B_{12} deficiency.[82] Homocysteine serum concentrations may also be elevated in folic acid deficiency and, therefore, are not a specific indicator of B_{12} deficiency. Measuring the serum concentration of vitamin B_{12} is the procedure of choice for determining B_{12} status. According to the World Health Organization, serum values of B_{12} less than 150 pg/mL (110 pmol/L) denote a deficiency for all ages.[87] Other sources suggest that levels less than either 300 or 350 pg/mL should be considered B_{12} deficient.[4]

Because of the close interrelationships between vitamin B_{12} and folic acid, especially in the presence of megaloblastic anemia, the status of both vitamins should be determined simultaneously. Megaloblastic anemia is recognizable as a mean corpuscular volume (MCV) >100 fL/cell. However, the absence of megaloblastic anemia should not be taken as lack of B_{12} deficiency because folate can mask B_{12} deficiency. Serum homocysteine and MMA are increased in B_{12} deficiency; measurements of both are useful when diagnosing vitamin B_{12} deficiency.[71,72] Normal serum MMA levels are 0.08 to 0.56 mcmol/L. Homocysteine levels between 5 and 15 mcmol/L

TABLE 8-12 Clinical Signs and Symptoms of Vitamin B$_{12}$ Deficiency

System	Deficiency
Bone	Bone marrow changes, bone fractures
Mouth	Glossitis
Nervous system	Diminution of vibration and/or position sense, hand/feet paresthesia, unsteadiness, cognitive decline, confusion, depression, mental slowness, poor memory, delusions, or overt psychosis
Other	Megaloblastic anemia, leukopenia, thrombocytopenia, cardiovascular disease, neutrophil nuclei hypersegmentation

Source: Data are from references 81 through 83.

are considered normal. Homocysteine and MMA values greater than normal ranges do support vitamin B$_{12}$ deficiency.

Patients with vitamin B$_{12}$ deficiency may exhibit a variety of clinical signs and symptoms. See Table 8-12 for details.[81-83]

Nutrient-Nutrient Interactions

An excess intake of vitamin C (500 mg) in a single dose may temporarily impair the vitamin B$_{12}$ bioavailability from foods and destroy the vitamin.[14]

Medication-Nutrient Interactions

Metformin (insulin sensitizer), proton pump inhibitors (PPIs) (gastroesophageal reflux disease medications), and colchicine (anti-gout agent) decrease vitamin B$_{12}$ absorption. Tetracycline (antibiotic), oral contraceptives, and octreotide (antidiarrheal) decrease serum B$_{12}$. Methyldopa (antihypertensive) increases the need for B$_{12}$ supplementation, and rifampin (antitubercular) confounds B$_{12}$ assay measurements.[7]

Treatment Considerations

Vitamin B$_{12}$ supplementation may be done by intramuscular injection or via a sublingual, nasal spray, oral, or gel B$_{12}$ preparation. The common doses for treating B$_{12}$ deficiency are intramuscular injections of either 100 mcg or 1000 mcg at 1-month intervals until corrected. If patients have symptomatic B$_{12}$ deficiency, injections may initially be done more frequently than monthly.

Adult vegans and strict vegetarians with normal vitamin B$_{12}$ absorption may safely take a standard multivitamin supplement to avoid a B$_{12}$ deficiency.

Folic Acid

Folic acid (folate, folacin) is also called *pteroylglutamate* or *pteroylmonoglutamate*. The metabolically active forms of folate have reduced (tetrahydro-) pteridine rings with up to 11 glutamic

acids (polyglutamates) attached. Pteroylpolyglutamate is the form of folate in foods and often contains up to 9 glutamate residues. Prior to absorption, polyglutamates are converted to the monoglutamate form by hydrolytic zinc-dependent enzymes (conjugases) located in the jejunal brush border.[14] The monoglutamates produced are actively transported via a pH-dependent, carrier-mediated mechanism.[14] Within the intestinal cell and before entry into the portal circulation, the monoglutamate form of folate undergoes a reduction to THF, which is then converted to either N^5-methyltetrahydrofolate (N^5-MTHF) or N^{10}-formyltetrahydrofolate. These 2 forms are secreted into the bile and recirculate via enterohepatic circulation. They may account for as much as 50% of the folate that reaches the peripheral tissues.[14] The predominant form found in the plasma is N^5-MTHF, which is loosely bound to albumin and folate-binding proteins (also called *folate carriers* or *folate receptors*). Folate transport across membranes into cells of various tissues occurs via a carrier-mediated process. Folate-binding proteins are found within the intestinal brush border and facilitate cellular folate uptake. Intracellularly, N^5-MTHF is demethylated via a vitamin B$_{12}$–dependent enzyme and converted back into a tetrahydrofolate form to become the active coenzyme capable of transferring 1-carbon units. Excretion of folate metabolites is minimal, due to reabsorption via enterohepatic bile circulation.

Both zinc deficiency and chronic alcohol consumption can impair the conjugase activity and, thus, the absorption of folate. Any change in luminal jejunal pH secondary to drug therapy or disease can also limit folate absorption. Conditions or diseases that impair bile secretion may also limit folate recirculation.

Functions of Folate

The primary biochemical role of folic acid is as a coenzyme in the transfer of single carbon fragments from one compound to another for amino acid metabolism and nucleic acid synthesis.[14,58] Folate (THF) functions as a coenzyme to accept 1-carbon groups generated from amino acid metabolism. These THF derivatives serve as donors of 1-carbon units for the synthesis of amino acids, purines, and pyrimidines. THF donates a methyl group to cobalamin (B$_{12}$) for the regeneration of methionine from homocysteine (Figure 8-2).

Dietary folate equivalents (DFEs) are used to express folate requirements and to reflect differences in absorption of food vs synthetic folate (1 DFE = 1 mcg food folate, 0.6 mcg fortified/supplemental folic acid taken with food, or 0.5 mcg supplemental folic acid taken without food).

Pregnant women are at greater risk of developing a folate deficiency secondary to the increased demand for DNA synthesis for embryonic development. Folate deficiency causes the DNA misincorporation of uracil in place of thymine, leading to DNA fragility and strand breakage that cause neural tube defects (NTDs) during fetal development.[5] Since the US Food and Drug Administration (FDA) mandated folate fortification of cereal and grain products in January 1998, the number of reported cases of NTDs has declined.[88] Low serum folate levels during pregnancy have also been associated with poor pregnancy outcomes.[89]

Clinical Applications

Recommended Intakes for Adults

The RDAs for folate are as follows:
- Men and women: 400 DFE
- Pregnant women: 600 DFE
- Lactating women: 500 DFE

The UL for folic acid is 1000 mcg.

Women of childbearing age should take a synthetic daily supplement with 400 mcg folic acid to prevent NTDs in offspring. Women who have a history of delivering neonates with NTDs should take 4000 mcg synthetic folic acid per day beginning 1 month prior to attempting conception through the first 3 months of pregnancy.[90]

Sources

Food sources of folate include enriched grain foods, dark-green leafy vegetables, and fortified cereals.[58]

Populations at Risk for Deficiency

People with alcoholism are at risk for folate deficiency because of decreased folate intake and absorption. As noted earlier, folate deficiency is a risk for pregnant women because of the increased demand for the nutrient for DNA synthesis in embryonic development. Other populations at risk for folate deficiency include periconceptual and premenopausal women and patients taking phenytoin, cholestyramine, or sulfasalazine.

Half-Life of the Nutrient in the Body

The half-life of folate is approximately 90 days.[91] With deficient intake, plasma folate levels decrease within 1 month. If this deficiency is not corrected, red blood cells can become folate deficient within 3 to 4 months and megaloblastic anemia can occur within 4 to 5 months.[5]

Assessment of Folate Status

There are 4 stages of folate deficiency:[14]
- Stage 1 is early negative balance with serum folate levels less than 3 ng/mL (6.8 nmol/mL).
- Stage 2 is tissue depletion when red blood cell folate levels are less than 160 ng/mL (362.67 nmol/mL).
- Stage 3 is folate-deficient erythropoiesis, indicated by neutrophil hypersegmentation and an abnormal deoxyuridine suppression test (correctable by folate in vitro).
- Stage 4 is a clinical folate deficiency, manifested by megaloblastic or macrocytic anemia.

The goal is early detection and correction of deficiency. As has been discussed, vitamin B$_{12}$ status and homocysteine concentrations should be determined in tandem with folate status. New methodologies to accurately assess folate status via folate derivatives are under development and hold promise for the future.[14]

TABLE 8-13 Clinical Signs and Symptoms of Folate Deficiency

System	Deficiency
Mouth	Cheilosis
Nervous system	Nervous instability, dementia
Other	Megaloblastic or macrocytic anemia, neutrophil hypersegmentation (early indicator of deficiency), diarrhea, weight loss, depression of cell-mediated immunity, cardiovascular disease

Source: Data are from references 14 and 58.

Patients with folate deficiency may exhibit a variety of clinical signs and symptoms. See Table 8-13 for details.[14,58]

Nutrient-Nutrient Interactions

Zinc deficiency can impair the absorption rate of folate.

Medication-Nutrient Interactions

Carbamazepine (antiepileptic), estrogen therapy, oral contraceptives, phenobarbital (sedative), phenytoin (antiepileptic), and triamterene (diuretic) cause decreased folate in the serum. Cholestyramine (bile acid sequestrant), metformin (insulin sensitizer), sulfasalazine (anti-inflammatory), and pancrelipase (pancreatic enzyme) decrease folate absorption. Trimethoprim (antibiotic) interferes with folate metabolism. Rifampin (antitubercular agent) confounds folate assay measurements.[7]

Treatment Considerations

Treatment for folate deficiency is 1 to 5 mg folate daily.[5] Excessive amounts of folic acid (100 times the RDA) may result in seizures in individuals on phenytoin therapy. Some evidence supports folate treatment of 10 mg/d to improve hyperhomocysteinemia as well as endothelial dysfunction via improvements in coagulation and free radical scavenger activity.[92] No signs of toxicity were observed when women were given 10 mg folic acid daily for 4 months.[14] Allergic reactions to oral and parenteral folic acid products have been observed.[14,58] As mentioned earlier in this chapter, the metabolism and functions of folate and vitamin B$_{12}$ are interrelated. Consumption of large folate amounts can mask a B$_{12}$ deficiency.

Biotin

Biotin (vitamin B$_7$) is ubiquitous in the diet and exists in the free biotin and the protein-bound coenzyme form biocytin, which is biotin bound to the amino acid lysine. Free biotin is absorbed via facilitated diffusion. Biocytin requires the enzyme biotinidase in the small intestine to cleave the protein portion from biocytin, releasing the free vitamin for jejunal absorption.[14] Evidence suggests that biotinidase may also function as a biotin carrier protein.[93]

Functions of Biotin

Biotin is necessary for the genetic expression of more than 2000 enzymes. Additionally, biotin functions as a cofactor for 4 carboxylase enzymes in mammalian systems, which transport carbon dioxide (carboxyl units) to various substrates. These biotin-dependent carboxylases catalyze vital reactions in important metabolic pathways: acetyl-coA carboxylase for fatty acid synthesis, pyruvate carboxylase for gluconeogenesis, propionyl-CoA carboxylase for propionate metabolism, and 3-methylcrotonyl-CoA carboxylase for branched-chain amino acid catabolism.

Overall, biotin deficiency is rare because biotin is synthesized by colonic microflora.[5] However, approximate 1 person in 60,000 has biotinidase deficiency, an inherited autosomal recessive trait.[93] These individuals improve clinically when they are given pharmacological doses of biotin (5 to 20 mg/d).

Clinical Applications

Recommended Intakes for Adults

The AIs for biotin are: 30 mcg for men and nonpregnant women and 35 mcg during pregnancy. A UL for biotin has not been established because there are no reports of biotin toxicity.[58]

Sources

Food sources of biotin include liver; smaller amounts are also found in other cuts of meat and in fruits.[58,93]

Populations at Risk for Deficiency

Biotin deficiencies have been reported in association with long-term PN, in people with alcoholism, and in patients with partial gastrectomy.

Half-Life of the Nutrient in the Body

The half-life of biotin is 1.8 hours. Inadequate biotin intake manifests as deficiency within 2 to 4 weeks.[94]

Assessment of Biotin Status

Commonly used methods for determining biotin status include measurements of serum biotin concentrations and 24-hour urinary excretion of biotin. The most valid indicators of biotin status are an abnormally decreased urinary excretion of biotin and an abnormally increased urinary excretion of 3-hydroxyisovaleric acid.[93] Whole blood or serum biotin concentrations of less than 200 pg/mL indicate biotin deficiency but are not as reliable as urinary analysis. A urinary concentration of biotin less than 6 mcg/d is a better indicator of deficiency.[5]

TABLE 8-14 Clinical Signs and Symptoms of Biotin Deficiency

System	Deficiency
Skin	Pallor, erythematous seborrheic dermatitis
Hair	Alopecia
Eyes	Vision problems
Mouth	Glossitis, cheilosis
Nervous system	Nervous instability, dementia, hallucinations, paresthesia in extremities, depression
Other	Hypotonia, anorexia, nausea, vomiting, lethargy, muscle pain, ketolactic acidosis, elevated cholesterol

Source: Data are from references 14 and 93.

Patients with biotin deficiency may exhibit a variety of clinical signs and symptoms. See Table 8-14 for details.[14,93]

Nutrient-Nutrient Interactions

No nutrient interactions with biotin have been identified.

Medication-Nutrient Interactions

Carbamazepine (antiepileptic) decreases serum biotin.[7]

Treatment Considerations

Patients with biotin deficiency who are given 3 to 20 mg/d usually improve. Even at high intakes of biotin, no evidence of toxicity was observed when patients with biotin-responsive, inborn errors of metabolism or acquired biotin deficiency were treated with daily doses of either 200 mg of biotin orally or 20 mg intravenously.[14,58]

Pantothenic Acid

Pantothenic acid (vitamin B5) is a component of the CoA molecule and the acyl carrier protein of fatty acid synthetase complex.[14] Dietary CoA is hydrolyzed to pantothenic acid in the intestinal lumen. Absorption is either by passive diffusion or via a saturable, sodium-dependent active transport. Absorbed pantothenic acid is transported via the erythrocytes throughout the body.[14] Most of the pantothenic acid in the body tissues is in the form of CoA, which is hydrolyzed to pantothenic acid before excretion in the urine.[14]

Functions of Pantothenic Acid

As a component of CoA, pantothenic acid is involved in energy released from fat, carbohydrate, and ketogenic amino acids. In this form, pantothenic acid is also involved in gluconeogenesis, heme and sterol synthesis, and most acetylation reactions. As CoA, pantothenic acid is required for the synthesis of bile salts, cholesterol, steroid hormones, and fatty acids. It is also

---

responsible for the transport of long-chain fatty acids into the mitochondria for catabolism through beta-oxidation. Signs and symptoms of a pantothenic acid deficiency have only been observed after the administration of metabolic antagonists (ie, omega methylpantothenate) or feeding a synthetic diet free of this vitamin.

Clinical Applications

Recommended Intakes for Adults

AIs for pantothenic acid are as follows:
- Men and women: 5 mg
- Pregnant women: 6 mg
- Lactating women: 7 mg

The UL for pantothenic acid has not been established because the available data were insufficient.[14,58] Toxicity due to pantothenic acid is rare.[58]

Sources

Food sources of pantothenic acid include sunflower seeds, beef liver, mushrooms, peanuts, eggs, broccoli, and milk.

Populations at Risk for Deficiency

Pantothenic acid deficiency often occurs in conjunction with multiple other nutrient deficiencies or with conditions such as diabetes mellitus, inflammatory bowel disease, and alcoholism. Absorption of pantothenic acid is likely impaired with both inflammatory bowel disease and alcoholism.[14] Individuals who ingest large amounts of ethanol may have an increased requirement for this vitamin.[58]

Half-Life of the Nutrient in the Body

The half-life of pantothenic acid is unknown.

Assessment of Pantothenic Acid Status

Pantothenic acid status is reflected by both whole blood assays and urinary excretion determined by a 24-hour urine collection. A blood value less than 1 mcmol pantothenic acid per liter is considered low.[14] Urinary pantothenic acid excretion is a more reliable indicator of status because it is closely related to dietary intake and is likely the easiest test to conduct and interpret. A urinary pantothenic acid concentration less than 1 mg/d (in adults) indicates a poor status or nutriture of the vitamin.[5]

Table 8-15 presents the clinical signs and symptoms of pantothenic acid deficiency and toxicity.[5,14]

Nutrient-Nutrient Interactions

Nutrient interactions with pantothenic acid have not been identified.

Medication-Nutrient Interactions

Tetracycline (antibiotic) may cause decreased serum pantothenic acid.[7]

TABLE 8-15 Clinical Signs and Symptoms of Pantothenic Acid Deficiency or Toxicity

System	Deficiency	Toxicity
Skin	Poor wound healing	None
Nervous system	Neuromuscular disturbances, numbness, parethesias, staggering gait, mental depression, listlessness, irritability, restlessness, malaise, sleep disturbances	None
Other	Muscle cramps, fatigue, nausea, abdominal cramps, vomiting, diarrhea, hypoglycemia, increased insulin sensitivity, compromised immune function, diminished engraftment	Rare mild gastrointestinal distress

Source: Data are from references 5 and 14.

Treatment Considerations

Although no UL has been set for pantothenic acid, diarrhea has been reported with supplementation more than 10 g/d. Supplementation less than 10 g/d seems to be nontoxic.[58]

Choline

Choline is found in a wide variety of foods. Nearly all dietary choline is in the form of choline phosphatides such as lecithin and sphingomyelin. Betaine, the oxidized form of choline, is also present in the diet, but it cannot be directly converted to choline.[14] Dietary choline is absorbed by the small intestine, and uptake occurs via choline transporter proteins before it is delivered to the liver via the portal vein. Choline is primarily converted to the major phospholipid phosphatidylcholine (lecithin). When the body's choline supply is low, choline is recycled in the liver and redistributed from the kidneys, lungs, and the intestines to the liver and brain.[96] Very small amounts of choline are excreted in the urine; excess choline is converted to betaine, a methyl donor providing methyl groups to compounds such as homocysteine (Figure 8-2).[14]

Functions of Choline

Choline is needed for neurotransmitter synthesis (acetylcholine), cell membrane signaling (phospholipids), and lipid transport (lipoproteins). Its by-product, betaine, is a methyl group donor and may act as a substitute for vitamin B$_{12}$ in the regeneration of methionine from homocysteine.[14,96,97] As such, choline is essential for cell membrane integrity, methyl metabolism, cholinergic neurotransmission, transmembrane signaling, and the transport and metabolism of lipid cholesterol.[58] Endogenous de novo synthesis of choline occurs via the sequential methylation of phosphatidylethanolamine with S-adenosylmethionine as the methyl donor.[14] However, this de novo synthesis of choline alone is insufficient to meet human needs. In sum, the demand for choline is influenced by methionine, folic acid, vitamin B_{12}, and betaine, all of which are involved in metabolic methyl-exchange reactions.[14]

Observational research has linked choline deficiency with long-term PN support. Evidence indicates that choline deficiency may contribute to PN-induced liver dysfunction, causing hepatic steatosis and eventual hepatic failure. Humans who were given PN formulations without choline developed fatty livers and liver damage, which were corrected in part by giving choline.[58,98] Reductions in plasma choline concentrations observed in long-term PN also correlate with abnormal hepatic aminotransferase levels.[98] Individuals receiving PN secondary to short bowel syndrome who develop a choline deficiency are more susceptible to these hepatic consequences. Impairment of verbal and visual memory in choline-deficient PN patients may be related to insufficient acetylcholine synthesis. IV choline supplementation is needed for optimal long-term PN support to minimize fatty liver infiltration.[98] The UL for choline is set to avoid the adverse effects of excessive intakes.[14,58]

Significant evidence demonstrates a relationship between choline deficiency and the development of diseases such as liver disease, atherosclerosis, cancer, and possibly neurologic disorders (eg, NTDs, Alzheimer's disease, and memory problems).[96] The current literature suggests that the AI set for choline may be too low because some people develop organ dysfunction even at levels that meet the AI.[99]

Clinical Applications

Recommended Intakes for Adults

The AIs for choline are 550 mg for men and 425 mg for women. The UL for choline is 3.5 g.

Sources

Food sources of choline include milk, liver, eggs, and peanuts.

Populations at Risk for Deficiency

Whenever the demand for choline is high (during pregnancy, lactation, hypermetabolic states), sufficient choline intake becomes a critical concern. Postmenopausal women may be at risk for choline deficiency because de novo synthesis of phosphotidyl-choline diminishes with diminished estrogen.[99] Patients on long-term PN support without choline are also at risk.

Half-Life of the Nutrient in the Body

The half-life of choline is unknown.

Assessment of Choline Status

Plasma choline levels reflect dietary intake, but they do not decline below 50% of normal levels, even following a short fast. Maintaining a plasma choline concentration of 10 mcmol/L is desirable in adults for optimal health through-

TABLE 8-16 Clinical Signs and Symptoms of Choline Deficiency or Toxicity

System	Deficiency	Toxicity
Skin	None	Sweating
Mouth	None	Excessive salivation
Nervous system	Impairment of verbal and visual memory	None
Other	Hepatic steatosis	Hypotension, anorexia, fishy body odor, hepatotoxicity

Source: Data are from reference 14.

out life.[100] Table 8-16 notes signs and symptoms of choline deficiency and toxicity.[14]

Nutrient-Nutrient Interactions

Choline in the form of its metabolite betaine can replace vitamin B_{12} to replenish methionine from homocysteine through methyl group donation.

Medication-Nutrient Interactions

Interactions between choline and medications have not been identified.

Treatment Considerations

Currently, there are no parenteral supplements for choline. The dextrose and protein components of PN formulations contain no choline. However, choline is part of lipid emulsions in the form of phosphatidylcholine. A 20% emulsion contains 13.2 mcmol choline per mL.[101]

Trace Elements

Minerals are required for virtually all aspects of metabolism. *Trace elements* are defined as minerals required by humans in amounts less than 100 mg/d. The minerals discussed in this chapter include iron, zinc, copper, manganese, selenium, iodine, chromium, fluoride, and molybdenum. Absorption, transport, excretion, function, deficiency and toxicity characteristics, and requirements are reviewed, with emphasis placed on alterations in metabolism, transport, and excretion that occur with chronic and acute illnesses. The physiological changes sometimes associated with trace element deficiencies can be subtle, which often makes diagnosis difficult. In addition, trace minerals interact with each other and compete for receptor sites, and these activities may influence or interfere with the absorption of select minerals.

Iron

Iron (Fe) is a component of every living cell and has long been recognized to be essential for the maintenance of health. The amount of iron present in an individual varies based on age, sex, weight, and nutrition status. Total body stores contain about 2 to 4 g, with differences between the sexes. On average, menstruating women have 40 mg iron per kg of body weight, whereas the average for men is 50 mg/kg.[14]

Normal iron balance is regulated via alterations in absorption. Iron in food occurs in a heme or nonheme form. Approximately 18.5% of iron in the typical diet is from heme iron derived from hemoglobin and myoglobin molecules found in animal flesh. Heme iron is more efficiently absorbed than nonheme iron, which is found primarily in plant foods. About 15% to 35% of ingested heme iron is absorbed.[4] The amount of nonheme iron absorbed varies depending on other dietary constituents and is estimated at 2% to 20%.[4] Factors that enhance nonheme iron absorption include the presence of organic compounds that increase acidity, such as vitamin C, HCl, lactic acid, and the acidic amino acids aspartic and glutamic acid. These components maintain iron in the ferrous form (Fe^{2+}), which is better absorbed compared to ferric iron (Fe^{3+}). Iron deficiency is another key factor that enhances absorption.

Absorption and Metabolism

Absorption mechanisms differ for heme iron vs nonheme iron. Heme iron is absorbed intact into the enterocyte after the globin fraction is removed, and it is then hydrolyzed to ferrous iron by the intestinal cell. In the stomach, nonheme iron is released from food components, usually in the ferric form, and is then converted to ferrous iron via the action of gastric acid. This ferrous iron can traverse the intestinal cell's glycocalyx and brush border by binding to receptors. The primary sites of iron absorption are in the duodenum and jejunum.

Following absorption into the enterocyte and depending on the body's requirements, iron is transported out of the enterocyte by ferroportin into the bloodstream, where it is bound to transferrin, or it is stored in the intestinal cell, where it binds to apoferritin to form ferritin. Ferritin is a short-term form of iron storage. The iron incorporated into transferrin binds to transferrin receptors on the cell's surface. The number of transferrin receptors depends on the cell's iron requirement. An elevated need for iron increases the number of receptors on the cell's surface. Hence, the extent of iron stores in the body determines how much iron will be absorbed.[14,102] When iron stores are adequate, all the iron-binding sites for transferrin are saturated and transport into the blood is inhibited. In contrast, when iron stores are low, transferrin receptors increase to allow for more iron binding, thus shifting iron directly from the intestinal cells into the blood. When the amount of iron in the body exceeds the storage capacity of ferritin, some of the ferritin is degraded to the insoluble iron-protein compound hemosiderin, which also acts as a long-term iron storage site. These mechanisms allow the body to control iron absorption. In addition, the body limits the amount of iron excreted per day. Because most iron is conserved and recycled, tight regulation of iron absorption is a necessity.

Hepcidin and Iron Regulation

Iron homeostasis is partially maintained by the peptide hormone hepcidin, which is synthesized in the liver. Hepcidin is a key homeostatic regulator of iron metabolism that senses iron status and is also involved in pathological regulation of iron in response to infection, inflammation, hypoxia, and anemia.[102,103] During iron deficiency states, serum hepcidin concentrations are low, whereas concentrations are elevated in the anemia associated with the inflammation of chronic disease. Hepcidin enhances the degradation of the protein ferroportin, effectively blocking iron from exiting the cell for systemic circulation (Figure 8-3).[5] Hepcidin regulates both plasma iron concentrations and tissue distribution via the inhibition of dietary iron absorption, iron recycling by macrophages, and the mobilization of iron from hepatic stores.[103]

Iron and the Acute-Phase Response

The acute-phase response to injury and infection suppresses iron transport, at least partly due to the upregulation of hepcidin production.[104] Clinically, serum iron levels are depressed, while serum ferritin levels are increased.[105] Sequestration of iron into a storage form following injury and infection is thought to be physiologically protective to the host on several fronts. It reduces the availability of iron for iron-dependent microorganism proliferation.[106] It may also reduce potential for free radical production and oxidative damage to membranes and DNA.[14,103] Iron is an essential component of hemoglobin, which is necessary for oxygen transport, and

FIGURE 8-3 Iron Regulation by Hepcidin

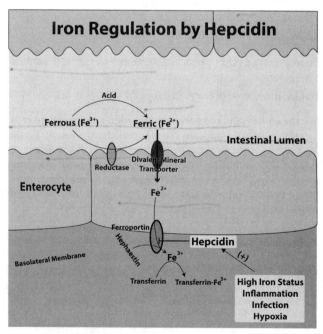

High hepcidin levels block the exit of iron from the enterocyte.
Source: Data are from reference 5.

myoglobin, which is necessary for muscle iron storage. Iron is also an important component of cytochromes, which are necessary for the oxidative production of cellular energy as ATP.

Iron Deficiency

The diagnosis of iron deficiency and iron deficiency anemia is challenging. Iron deficiency is an anemia that is usually microcytic and hypochromic. Iron depletion and the development of iron deficiency occur in stages. An assessment includes several hematological indices: hemoglobin, plasma iron, iron-binding capacity, ferritin, transferrin, erythrocyte protoporphyrin, transferrin receptor, and MCV.[14,107,108] These indices are examined in context with the nutrition-related and medical history. Early stages of iron depletion result in decreased transferrin saturation and are characterized by reduced plasma iron and elevated plasma transferrin. If depletion continues, serum ferritin, which reflects iron body stores, decreases to levels of less than 10 ng/mL in women and less than 20 ng/mL in men.

Ferritin is a positive acute-phase protein. Therefore, calculation of plasma ferritin concentrations must be adjusted to remove the effects of inflammation associated with chronic disease. It is recommended that ferritin and C-reactive protein are measured together to discern a more accurate ferritin concentration.[14,105,107–110] Another sensitive indicator of early iron deficiency is elevated levels of erythrocyte protoporphyrin. This iron measure has limitations because it is altered when hemoglobin synthesis is blunted, during situations of hemodilution, or in the presence of inflammation. Given these hematological changes, iron deficiency anemia is subsequently confirmed by a decreased MCV and a decreased hemoglobin concentration.[107,108] The currently used indicators of iron status have limitations, some of which are related to the inflammation of chronic disease. However, serum hepcidin is emerging as a more useful indicator of deficient iron stores.[111] This measure could significantly aid in the differential diagnosis of anemia of inflammation and iron deficiency anemia.

Clinical Applications

Recommended Intakes for Adults

The RDAs for iron are as follows:
- Men: 8 mg
- Premenopausal women: 18 mg
- Postmenopausal women: 8 mg
- Pregnant women: 27 mg
- Lactating women: 9 mg

The UL for iron is 45 mg.

Sources

Food sources of iron include meats, seafood, beans, dark leafy greens, broccoli, peas, bran, and enriched grain foods.

Populations at Risk for Deficiency

Individuals at risk for developing iron deficiency include women of childbearing age, patients hospitalized with excess blood sampling or blood loss, and individuals with decreased gastric acid production, including some older adults (gastric acid production diminishes with aging). The concomitant use of medications that reduce stomach acidity such as antacids, H_2 antagonists, or PPIs can impair iron absorption. Ineffective iron absorption also occurs in malabsorptive states such as celiac disease, Crohn's disease, or pernicious anemia and during frank achlorhydria. In addition, reduced iron absorption occurs after Roux-en-Y gastric bypass or other GI surgery, after injury, or during inflammation.[15,103,108,112]

Half-Life of the Nutrient in the Body

Iron metabolism is a somewhat closed system. Unlike most nutrients, iron is regulated at the level of absorption, not excretion. Therefore, once iron successfully enters the body, it is very difficult to eliminate. Men and women lose approximately 1 mg iron per day by sloughed epithelial cells from intestines and skin. Premenopausal women lose an additional 0.3 to 0.4 mg/d on average from losses accrued during menstruation. There are very few other mechanisms of iron elimination in place, making iron potentially very toxic if it is consumed in excess.[5]

Assessment of Iron Status

To determine whether iron malabsorption is present, serum iron levels should be measured before and 2 to 4 hours after the patient is given 325 mg of oral ferrous sulfate. If the iron level does not rise above the pretreatment value, the result indicates poor iron absorption.[14]

The stages of iron depletion and deficiency are as indicated as follows:[5]
- Stage 1: depleted iron stores—serum ferritin level 20 mcg/L or less
- Stage 2: non-anemia iron deficiency—transferrin saturation 15% or less and red blood cell protoporphyrin equal to or greater than 100 mcg/dL
- Stage 3: iron deficiency anemia—microcytic/hypochromic red blood cells (MCV equal to or less than 80 fL)

Iron toxicity or overload results from exposure to iron that exceeds the body's physiological protection mechanisms. A serum ferritin value great than 150 ng/mL in women and greater than 200 ng/mL in men suggests iron overload; values above 700 ng/mL are usually associated with symptomatic hemochromatosis.[106] Hemochromatosis is a genetic disorder that increases the amount of iron absorbed from the diet. This increased iron is stored in the organs, especially the liver, and may cause organ damage over time. Iron therapy in patients with preexisting hemochromatosis is contraindicated.

Patients with iron deficiency exhibit a variety of clinical signs and symptoms. Signs of iron toxicity may occur in the skin or organs. See Table 8-17 for details.[14,105–108]

Nutrient-Nutrient Interactions

Certain dietary factors reduce nonheme iron absorption by forming insoluble iron complexes. These factors include phytic acid in grain fibers; oxalic acid in spinach, chard, tea, and

TABLE 8-17 Clinical Signs and Symptoms of Iron Deficiency or Toxicity

System	Deficiency	Toxicity
Skin	Pallor	Skin pigmentation
Nails	Koilonychia	None
Eyes	Conjunctival pallor	None
Mouth	Glossitis	None
Nervous system	Impaired behavioral and intellectual performance	None
Other	Microcytic, hypochromic anemia; tachycardia; poor capillary refilling; fatigue; sleepiness; headache; anorexia; nausea; reduced work performance, impaired ability to maintain body temperature in cold environments; decreased resistance to infections; increased lead absorption; and adverse outcomes during pregnancy	Organ damage (ie, liver cirrhosis, heart enlargement, pancreatic damage)

Source: Data are from references 14 and 105–108.

chocolate; polyphenols in coffee, tea, and cocoa; and other nutrients such as calcium, zinc, and manganese.[14] Nutrient-nutrient interactions such as these have clinical significance, especially because increased doses of zinc and manganese are often standard recommendations in critical illness.[107,108] Iron absorption may be competitively impaired when zinc or manganese supplements are provided via the GI tract; these can contribute to compromised iron status.[107,108] Chromium toxicity can contribute to iron deficiency anemia because of chromium's receptor site competition with iron.[5]

Medication-Nutrient Interactions

Medications that decrease iron absorption include oral bisphosphonates (osteoporosis treatment), caffeine, phosphate binders, calcium polycarbophil (bulk-forming fiber therapy [Fibercon]), cholestyramine (bile acid sequestrant), magnesium hydroxide, miglitol (diabetes medication), oral contraceptives, PPIs, sodium bicarbonate (antacid), tetracyclines (antibiotic), and levothyroxine (thyroid hormone).[7]

Eltrombopag (thrombocytopenia medication) and vorapaxar (antithrombotic) decrease serum iron levels. Carbamazepine (antiepileptic) may decrease iron levels if taken long term.[7]

Epoetin alfa (erythropoietin) uses iron. Therefore, patients using this drug may require iron supplementation.[7]

Iron decreases the absorption of cefdinir (antibiotic), ciprofloxacin (antibiotic), levofloxacin (antibiotic), and dolutegravir sodium (HIV antiviral). Iron increases the absorption of methyldopa (antihypertensive).[7]

Treatment Considerations

The recommended treatment for iron deficiency is 150 to 200 mg elemental iron per day.[113] Common oral preparations include ferrous sulfate, gluconate, and fumarate. Although the fumarate form has the highest absorption rate, the preferred forms remain ferrous sulfate and gluconate. These forms are relatively inexpensive and possess good bioavailability. Because oral iron is better absorbed in an acidic environment, it is recommended that iron supplements be taken with a source of ascorbic acid (eg, orange juice). Foods that reduce iron absorption (eg, tea tannins or phytates) or medications that increase the gastric pH (eg, antacids, PPIs, or H_2 blockers) should be avoided.

Adverse effects of oral iron preparations include nausea, epigastric discomfort, and constipation. Enteric-coated, delayed release ferric compounds (eg, ferric bisglycinate) are often better tolerated but may be released in the GI tract distal to the site of optimal absorption.

Standard parenteral trace element products do not include iron, in part to avoid iron's potential contribution to microbial growth and damaging oxidative reactions. Parenteral iron preparations should be considered only when a patient cannot take anything by mouth or does not respond adequately to oral supplementation.[107,109] Currently, 6 parenteral iron preparations are available: low–molecular weight iron dextran, high–molecular weight iron dextran, sodium ferric gluconate, iron sucrose, ferumoxytol, and soluble ferric pyrophosphate. Iron sucrose and ferumoxytol have been associated with lower rates of adverse effects.

Soluble ferric pyrophosphate (Triferic), a more recently introduced source of IV iron, has been shown effective in hemodialysis patients with end-stage renal failure whose iron needs are increased due to erythropoietin administration. Soluble ferric pyrophosphate is unique in that it is deliverable through the dialysate. Furthermore, it bypasses physiologic mechanisms of iron sequestration, making it more readily transported to the marrow to facilitate erythropoiesis.[114]

According to package insert information, no test dose is required by for iron sucrose (Venofer), ferric gluconate (Ferrlecit), ferumoxytol (Feraheme), or soluble ferric pyrophosphate (Triferic). A test dose of 0.5 mL is required for iron dextran to evaluate tolerance and avoid anaphylactic reactions.

The dextran formulation, or bound Fe, is the preferable form to add to PN.[106] Iron dextran may be added to dextrose-amino acid solutions, but it should not be added to total nutrient admixtures because it can destabilize these emulsions. It seems to be safe, is devoid of lipid peroxide formation, and is preferred over free iron as a form of parenteral addition.

A parenteral administration of iron may contribute to oxidative reactions that exacerbate tissue damage. In addition, excessive amounts of circulating iron may also stimulate bacterial proliferation; therefore, parenteral use of iron is not recommended during acute illness or sepsis. During the recovery phase of stress, iron can be administered parenterally or otherwise with or without erythropoietin. For similar reasons, additional enteral iron is also not recommended during the acute-phase response to an infection.[106]

Zinc

Zinc (Zn) is involved in numerous aspects of cellular metabolism. It is hydrolyzed from amino acids and nucleic acids via the action of gastric HCl and other enzymes in the small intestine before absorption. A reduced gastric acidity can decrease zinc availability for absorption. Zinc is found bound to cellular proteins in virtually all cells in the body. More than 95% of the body's zinc content is intracellular.

Approximately 20% to 40% of ingested zinc is absorbed from the small intestine, primarily in the duodenum and jejunum and, to a lesser extent, in the ileum. Absorption occurs by a carrier-mediated (saturable) process and a nonmediated diffusion process.[14] The transcellular movement of zinc into the mucosal cell is modulated by metallothionein, a protein responsible for the regulation of zinc absorption. If zinc is not transferred to the blood or zinc intake is high, metallothionein synthesis increases.

After the transfer from the intestine, zinc binds to albumin for transport to the liver. The liver releases zinc into the circulation bound to albumin (70%) or α-macroglobulins (approximately 30%).[4] Diseases or physiological conditions characterized by hypoalbuminemia can impair hepatic release of zinc. Plasma zinc levels are also subject to a variety of stimuli including dietary zinc intake, fasting, and acute infections. During fasting, plasma zinc concentrations increase. However, during infections, zinc is redistributed, resulting in hypozincemia. Within hours after an injury, plasma zinc levels decrease by 10% to 69%; the extent and type of injury determine the duration and magnitude of this reduction.[56] The stress of acute infection precipitates the secretion of cytokines such as interleukin-1 and interleukin-6, which act to increase the hepatic zinc uptake. These acute-phase responses are protective to the host and need to be considered when evaluating zinc status.

Various inhibitors of zinc absorption may deplete the zinc status. These include other minerals, vitamins, proteins, phytic acid, alcohol, physiological factors, and disease processes.[14] Phytic acid and calcium supplements decrease zinc absorption by as much as 50%. Certain milk proteins may have a negative effect on absorption as well. In addition, the long-term ingestion of large amounts of zinc can compete with copper and iron for absorption. Key excretion routes include the GI tract, the kidneys, and the skin.

Functions of Zinc

The overall biochemical functions of zinc can be categorized as catalytic, structural, and regulatory in nature. Zinc is important as a catalyst for enzymes in all 6 enzyme classes, which include more than 200 enzymes.[14] Examples of these enzymes include alkaline phosphatase, carbonic anhydrase, alcohol dehydrogenase, and the RNA polymerases I, II, and III. The structural role of zinc includes its function in metalloenzymes and in the zinc-finger motif in proteins (ie, zinc-finger proteins), through which zinc exerts a regulatory role in gene expression.[14] Zinc is necessary for other physiological processes, such as lipid peroxidation, apoptosis, neuromodulation, cellular proliferation and differentiation, wound healing, insulin synthesis and glucose control, and immune function.[14,115] Zinc may also have mild antimicrobial and anti-inflammatory properties.

The diagnosis of zinc deficiency is difficult, in part because of zinc redistribution during the acute-phase response to infection, inadequate biomarkers of zinc status, and the diversity of clinical symptoms. Zinc deficiency affects both the innate and adaptive immune systems and thus affects the immune response, resulting in lymphopenia, impaired phagocytic function, and natural killer cells coupled with an altered secretion of cytokines.[115] Furthermore, zinc deficiency affects vitamin A metabolism via the following 2 mechanisms:[14]

- Decreasing retinol mobilization from the liver
- Decreasing zinc-dependent enzyme conversion of retinol to retinal, which is critical to the vision cycle

A zinc deficiency could therefore precipitate a secondary vitamin A deficiency. Zinc deficiency also decreases the work capacity of muscles, which can have detrimental effects on respiratory muscle function, worsen hepatic dysfunction, and cause glucose intolerance. The underlying mechanisms for this problem have not been identified.[115,116] Zinc deficiency may occur secondary to acrodermatitis enteropathica, a heritable disorder of zinc metabolism.

Clinical Applications

Recommended Intakes for Adults

The RDAs for zinc are as follows:
- Men: 11 mg
- Women: 8 mg
- Pregnant women: 11
- Lactating women: 12 mg

The UL for zinc is 40 mg. This UL was set because observed copper deficiency is induced by excess zinc (see nutrient-nutrient interactions later in this section). Acute zinc toxicity was reported when 150 mg of zinc was administered daily. Death occurred when large IV doses (1.5 g zinc over 3 days) were given. Other toxicities have been associated with chronic oral intakes of 300 mg/d.[14]

Sources

Food sources of zinc include seafood, meats, greens, and whole grains.

Populations at Risk for Deficiency

Zinc deprivation has been reported in a variety of populations including older adults, people with alcoholism, postoperative patients, burn patients, patients with malabsorptive diseases or conditions (eg, intestinal bypass or resection), and patients with renal disease. Patients with liver disease may be at risk for deficiency.[117] Zinc deficiency has also been known to occur in patients with sickle cell anemia, acrodermatitis enteropathica, or malignancy, and it may contribute to macular degeneration.[14,51] Wound drainage or any clinical condition causing GI zinc losses can further contribute to a declining zinc status.

Half-Life of the Nutrient in the Body

The half-life of zinc is approximately 180 days.[118]

Assessment of Zinc Status

In healthy populations, plasma and urinary zinc have been confirmed as the most reliable biomarkers to assess zinc status.[119] In a clinical setting, the measurement of serum or plasma zinc concentration presents a conundrum. During SIRS, serum zinc will fall to about half the normal level and remain depressed until resolved. This decline is secondary to zinc sequestration, which represents a host mechanism to control leukocyte cytokine production.[56] Table 8-18 explains how to interpret plasma zinc levels.

In situations where SIRS is suspected, evaluating serum C-reactive protein, an acute-phase protein, may help differentiate between a declining serum or plasma zinc level related to an acute-phase response and a declining level associated with increased requirements.[15,120] An elevated C-reactive protein level is consistent with the acute-phase reaction. Although an analysis of leukocyte zinc and lymphocyte 5'-nucleotidase activities provides more specific and sensitive indicators of zinc status, the current laboratory procedures are too tedious to perform. Table 8-19 lists clinical signs and symptoms of

TABLE 8-18 Interpretation of Plasma Zinc Levels

Status	Plasma Zinc Level, mcg/dL
Sufficient	>85
Marginal	>70 to ≤85
Low	≤70

TABLE 8-19 Clinical Signs and Symptoms of Zinc Deficiency or Toxicity

System	Deficiency	Toxicity
Skin	Rash (periorificial, perianal, buttocks), impaired wound healing and epithelization	None
Hair	Alopecia	None
Eyes	Impaired night vision	None
Nervous system	Alterations in taste and smell	None
Other	Impaired immune function, hypogonadism, anorexia, diarrhea	Gastric distress, nausea, and dizziness; decreased immune function; decreased levels of high-density lipoprotein cholesterol

Source: Data are from reference 14.

zinc deficiency and toxicity.[14] Clinical manifestations of deficiency are noted at serum or plasma zinc levels less than 33 mcg/dL. These values should be interpreted cautiously with hypoalbuminemia because zinc transport depends on adequate albumin levels.

Nutrient-Nutrient Interactions

Zinc deficiency can cause a secondary vitamin A deficiency. High levels of calcium or iron compete with zinc for binding to ligands and chelators necessary for zinc absorption. High levels of zinc (greater than 40 mg/d) may cause copper deficiency due to increased metallothionein production. Copper binds strongly to metallothionein and is effectively trapped in the enterocyte. See Practice Scenario 8-3 for further discussion of zinc-copper interactions.

Practice Scenario 8-3

Question: Besides inadequate iron intake, what other mineral deficiencies or excesses may create hematological indices consistent with iron deficiency anemia and why?

Scenario: A 28-year-old school teacher presents to the emergency department with toxic inhalation injury from smoke and heat exposure during a fire at her high school. Her medical history indicates that iron deficiency anemia was diagnosed 1 month ago and is being treated with oral iron supplementation. The patient's husband states that "she is constantly sucking zinc lozenges, 5 to 10 per day, to avoid getting sick." Because of her history of anemia, complete blood count and comprehensive metabolic panel are ordered along with serum ferritin. Laboratory test data reveal hemoglobin of 9 g/dL and serum ferritin of 10 mcg/L. Serum copper and ceruloplasmin tests are ordered to rule out copper deficiency anemia secondary to her potentially excessive zinc consumption. Both values are below normal: serum copper 0.8 mcmol/L; ceruloplasmin 28 mg/L. Within 2 hours of admission, the patient develops respiratory stridor, indicative of impending airway compromise. She is intubated and placed on mechanical ventilation.

Intervention: Within 1 week on enteral nutrition, patient's hemoglobin levels improve remarkably. Upon release, patient is instructed to continue her iron supplementation and stop consuming zinc lozenges until the anemia has resolved, at which point she should not use more than 2 lozenges per day.

Answer: Copper deficiency interferes with iron absorption and metabolism and thus effectively creates copper deficiency anemia (iron deficiency anemia in patients with iron replete status). Zinc toxicity creates a copper deficiency, initiating the same anemic mechanisms. Also, chromium toxicity can contribute to iron deficiency anemia due to its receptor site competition with iron.

Rationale: Zinc lozenges have been found effective in reducing the symptoms and duration of the common cold. These popular products are sold over the counter. One lozenge of the Cold-Eeze brand contains 13.3 mg of elemental zinc, and product labeling suggests that 1 lozenge can be taken every 2 to 4 hours until cold symptoms subside. Other zinc lozenge products contain up to 27 mg zinc. Considering the Tolerable Upper Intake Level (UL) of zinc consumption is 40 mg, patients taking zinc lozenges prophylactically may exceed the UL for zinc consumption for prolonged periods of time. High levels of zinc stimulate the increased expression of metallothionein, a protein that binds copper strongly, trapping it in the enterocyte. In this way, zinc toxicity leads to copper deficiency. Copper is necessary for the transport of iron out of cells. Iron is prepared for transport out of the enterocyte through oxidation by the copper-dependent enzyme hephaestin and out of other cells by ceruloplasmin. In copper deficiency, iron is trapped inside the cell and iron absorption via the enterocyte ceases. The patient in this case study caused an iron deficiency status despite iron repletion by inducing a copper deficiency through excessive zinc consumption.

Medication-Nutrient Interactions

Tetracycline (antibiotic), ciprofloxacin (antibiotic), levofloxacin (antibiotic), phosphate binders, calcium polycarbophil (bulk-forming fiber therapy [Fibercon]), eltrombopag (thrombocytopenia medication), and ferrous salts decrease zinc absorption. Corticosteroids, (anti-inflammatory), hydrochlorothiazide (antihypertensive), and propofol (sedative) increase urinary zinc wasting. Oral contraceptives may decrease serum zinc levels. Zinc decreases absorption of dolutegravir sodium (HIV antiviral).[7]

Treatment Considerations

Zinc supplementation, although often indicated, can alter the status of other nutrients.[116] Supplementation with 50 mg zinc per day increased urinary zinc excretion. Parenteral zinc doses of 30 mg/d induced an exaggerated acute-phase response.[56] Zinc doses of 25 to 150 mg/d can induce a copper deficiency through the upregulation of metallothionein, which binds copper and prevents its ability to leave the cell.[14] Additional zinc is recommended in patients with losses from thermal injury or hypermetabolic states such as traumatic brain injury, and in patients with excessive GI losses such as diarrhea, decubitus ulcers, and high fistula outputs.[121] Doses of 80 mg zinc per day in combination with other antioxidant nutrients can reduce the development of age-related macular degeneration.[120] Typical recommendations for wound healing are up to 40 mg zinc (176 mg zinc sulfate) for 10 days.[14] The standard oral adult replacement dose is 220 mg twice daily (50 mg elemental zinc).[122]

Copper

Copper (Cu) homeostasis is maintained primarily by excretion rather than by absorption. Most of the copper in food is in the Cu^{2+} ionic state bound to organic compounds such as amino acids. Hence, digestion is necessary to free the copper before absorption. Gastric secretions, HCl, and pepsin assist in the release of bound copper in the stomach, which has some degree of copper absorption capacity. Most absorption, however, occurs

throughout the small intestine, especially in the duodenum. Two mechanisms involved in copper absorption include a saturable, active transport system and a nonsaturable, passive diffusion.[14] Like other transport systems, the active transport system for copper operates during low dietary copper intakes, whereas passive diffusion is activated during high dietary intakes. Typically, the intestinal absorption of copper ranges from about 12% to 75%, with higher intakes associated with low absorptive capacity. The reverse is true at low intakes. Hence, the amount of copper absorbed depends on dietary copper availability and the body's current copper status. The efficiency of copper absorption changes to regulate copper status, with changes in fecal excretion mediating the process. For example, as copper stores increase, biliary copper excretion increases. Dietary factors that negatively influence copper absorption include phytates, dietary fiber, zinc, iron, large doses of calcium gluconate, molybdenum, and large doses of vitamin C. Protein carriers, albumin, and specific copper transporters (CTR1, ATP7A) transport copper from the intestinal cell into the hepatocytes and Kupffer cells within the liver.[14,123] Following hepatic uptake, copper is either incorporated into liver enzymes (cytochrome c oxidase, superoxide dismutase) or the acute-phase protein ceruloplasmin, which is then either secreted into the blood for transport to extrahepatic tissues or excreted in bile.

Aside from transporting copper to cells via the specific ceruloplasmin cell surface receptor, ceruloplasmin acts as a scavenger of free radicals. It also catalyzes the oxidation of ferrous ion. Both serum ceruloplasmin and copper levels increase proportionally to the severity of the acute-phase reaction. Serum ceruloplasmin levels may rise during an infection to increase copper transport to stimulate cuproenzyme synthesis and inactivate inflammation-induced free radicals. These responses are considered a nonspecific host defense mechanism. Postprandially, 60% to 95% of circulating copper exists as a constituent of ceruloplasmin.[14]

Functions of Copper

Copper is involved in a myriad of biological processes. It primarily functions in oxidation-reduction and electron-transfer reactions involving oxygen (eg, cytochrome c oxidase).[14] The 3 copper enzymes that have a role in antioxidant defense are superoxide dismutases, ceruloplasmin, and copper thioneins. Ceruloplasmin is also responsible for manganese (Mn^{2+}) oxidation and oxidation of ferrous iron (Fe^{2+}) to ferric (Fe^{3+}) iron. Select copper-dependent enzymes and their roles include lysyl oxidase, necessary for the formation of cross-linkages found in collagen and elastin; dopamine monooxygenase, necessary for the conversion of dopamine to norepinephrine; peptidylglycine α-amidating monooxygenase, necessary for the activation and deactivation of various peptide hormones; and other copper-containing enzymes, which are used for the formation and maintenance of myelin. In addition, copper is necessary for cholesterol metabolism, glucose metabolism, and the formation of melatonin pigment.[14,123]

Copper deficiency can lead to impaired absorption of iron. Iron must be in its ferric state to leave the enterocyte and bind to transferrin. Hephaestin, a copper-dependent protein catalyzes the oxidation of ferrous iron to ferric iron as iron leaves the enterocyte on the vehicle of ferroportin. In copper deficiency, iron cannot exit the enterocyte, causing a microcytic, hypochromic copper deficiency anemia.[5]

Clinical Applications

Recommended Intakes for Adults

The RDAs for copper are as follows:
- Men and women: 900 mcg
- Pregnant women: 1000 mcg
- Lactating women: 1300 mcg

The UL for copper is 10 mg.

Sources

Food sources of copper include liver, cocoa, beans, nuts, whole grains, and dried fruits.

Populations at Risk for Deficiency

Individuals at greatest risk for developing copper deficiency include patients with malabsorptive disorders such as celiac disease, patients recovering from undernutrition associated with chronic diarrhea, patients recovering from intestinal surgery, and those receiving hemodialysis where copper losses can be excessive. Individuals who have had bariatric surgery may also be at increased risk of deficiency. Copper deficiency can be a complication of celiac disease with hematological alterations and debilitating, often irreversible neurologic deficits.[124]

Copper toxicity is uncommon because the body regulates copper storage via biliary excretion. As a result, impaired biliary excretion or cholestasis may cause copper retention in the hepatocyte, leading to oxidative damage.[14] Chronic ingestion of excessive copper amounts can result in liver cirrhosis in those with a genetic predisposition (eg, Wilson disease) with an accumulation of copper in the liver and other organs.[14,125]

Half-Life of the Nutrient in the Body

The half-life of copper is 13 to 33 days.[126]

Assessment of Copper Status

The preferred biomarker to assess copper status is serum copper concentration because it reflects changes in both depleted and repleted patients.[127] Values less than approximately 0.7 mcg/dL represent the early stages of copper depletion. Serum ceruloplasmin levels are also useful data but may not reflect hepatic copper stores.[127] A serum ceruloplasmin value less than 20 mg/dL is considered early copper deficiency.[5] Serum ceruloplasmin levels, and subsequently serum copper levels, increase in response to SIRS; therefore, the identification of SIRS by the measurement of serum C-reactive protein concentration may assist in the interpretation of findings from laboratory tests of copper levels.[127]

Patients with copper deficiency or toxicity may exhibit an array of clinical signs and symptoms of the condition. See Table 8-20 for details.[11,14,123,125]

TABLE 8-20 Clinical Signs and Symptoms of Copper Deficiency or Toxicity

System	Deficiency	Toxicity
Skin	Hypopigmentation	None
Hair	Hypopigmentation	None
Eyes	None	Kayser-Fleischer rings[a]
Mouth	None	Metallic taste
Nervous system	Sensory ataxia, lower extremity spasticity, paresthesia in extremities, myeloneuropathy	None
Other	Hypochromic microcytic anemia, leukopenia, neutropenia, hypercholesterolemia, increased erythrocyte turnover, abnormal electrocardiographic patterns	Blood in urine, liver damage

[a]copper-colored ring around the iris.
Source: Data are from references 11, 14, 123, and 125.

Nutrient-Nutrient Interactions

Overzealous zinc supplementation can hamper copper absorption. Copper deficiency causes iron deficiency by decreasing release of iron from the enterocyte. (See Practice Scenario 8-3.) Excess molybdenum increases urinary copper wasting.

Medication-Nutrient Interactions

H_2 antagonist or PPI medications decrease copper absorption. Oral contraceptives increase serum copper.[7]

Treatment Considerations

Prophylactic copper supplementation is recommended for individuals with celiac disease when anemia or neutropenia is present.[14] No clinically significant deleterious effects of copper ingestion have been observed with copper intakes equal to 0.5 mg/kg/d. Doses between 10 to 15 mg can cause a metallic taste, diarrhea, and vomiting. Because copper is excreted via the liver, it should not be administered, or should be administered with caution, in patients with hepatic dysfunction. There is a risk of iatrogenic hepatic copper overload in patients receiving PN, which has the potential to do irreparable harm to the liver.[128] Autopsy reports for adult patients who received long-term PN have revealed alarming results concerning copper accumulation. Major elevations in copper (and manganese) were found, which suggests the current parenteral copper recommendations may need to be modified.[129] Molybdenum, in the form of tetrathiomolybdate, is used in the treatment of copper toxicity because molybdenum induces urinary copper wasting.[5]

Manganese

Manganese (Mn) is a ubiquitous mineral found in a wide range of oxidative states; however, in humans, it occurs only in the divalent state. Although the specific mechanism for manganese absorption is unclear, it seems to resemble the mechanism for iron absorption. Manganese is absorbed in the Mn^{2+} state throughout the small intestine.[14] Approximately 1% to 5% of dietary manganese is absorbed. The absorption process is quickly saturated, such that absorption decreases when manganese intake is high, thus protecting the body against toxicity. Absorption of manganese can be influenced by iron because iron competes for common binding sites with manganese.[130]

Manganese enters the liver via the portal circulation. In the liver, it is oxidized by ceruloplasmin to Mn^{3+}, possibly complexes with transferrin, and is delivered to extrahepatic tissues.[130] Nearly 100% of manganese is excreted via the hepatobiliary system into the feces. Dietary excess is quickly excreted by the liver into bile to maintain manganese homeostasis and to prevent toxicity. Manganese toxicity can result in severe abnormalities of the central nervous system.[14,131]

Functions of Manganese

Manganese functions as a constituent of various metalloenzymes and as an activator of certain enzymes. (See Figure 8-4.[55]) The manganese-containing metalloenzymes include arginase, which is necessary for urea formation; pyruvate carboxylase, which is necessary for carbohydrate synthesis from pyruvate; and manganese superoxide dismutase, which provides the essential preparatory step in the neutralization of free radicals, produced from the electron transport chain, to water.[55] Manganese also activates numerous enzymes such as glycosyltransferases, phosphoenolpyruvate carboxylase, and glutamine synthetase.[14]

Clinical Applications

Recommended Intakes for Adults

The AIs for manganese are as follows:
- Men: 2.3 mg
- Women: 1.8 mg
- Pregnant women: 2 mg
- Lactating women: 2.6 mg

The UL for manganese is 11 mg.

Sources

Food sources of manganese include nuts, oats, and other whole grains.

Populations at Risk for Deficiency or Toxicity

Manganese deficiency is rare unless the mineral is totally absent from the diet. Because manganese is almost exclusively eliminated via the hepatobiliary system, any patient with hepatobiliary disease, such as cholestatic liver disease, may be predisposed to manganese toxicity.[132] Populations at risk for developing manganese toxicity include those receiving long-term PN (greater than 30 days) who develop obstruction of the biliary duct and are unable to excrete manganese.[131,133] More than 50% of home PN patients have exhibited manganese toxicity coupled with clinically significant cerebral and hepatic complications.[132]

Half-Life of the Nutrient in the Body

The half-life of manganese is approximately 40 days.[134]

FIGURE 8-4 Management of Reactive Species by Manganese- and Selenium-Dependent Enzymes in the Mitochondria

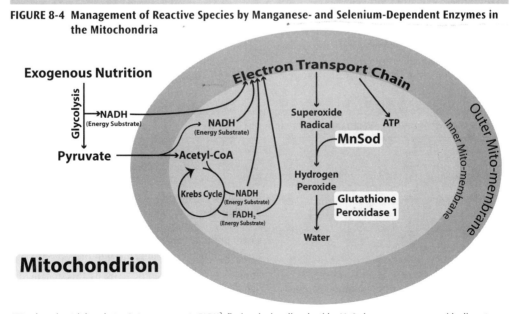

ATP, adenosine triphosphate; CoA, coenzyme A; $FADH_2$, flavin adenine dinucleotide; MnSod, manganese superoxide dismutase; NADH, nicotinamide adenine dinucleotide.
Source: Data are from reference 55.

Assessment of Manganese Status

Reliable biomarkers for determining manganese status have not been identified. Consistent changes in blood or plasma manganese have not been seen in manganese-depleted and manganese-repleted human subjects.[14] Magnetic resonance imaging (MRI) can detect toxicity; however, the procedure is expensive.[14] Monitoring whole blood manganese levels is best to monitor trace element status because levels correlate well with MRI abnormalities. Normal blood levels for manganese range from 4.7 to 18.3 ng/mL.

Patients with manganese deficiency or toxicity may exhibit an array of clinical signs and symptoms of the condition. See Table 8-21 for details.[14,67]

Nutrient-Nutrient Interactions

Iron competes for similar bindings sites with Mn^{2+} and may impair manganese absorption.[130]

Medication-Nutrient Interactions

Tetracycline (antibiotic) may chelate with manganese, decreasing manganese absorption.[7]

Treatment Considerations

As previously mentioned, both manganese and copper levels were elevated in the autopsies of home PN patients.[129] Reports of manganese brain deposition have occurred with IV manganese administration of 1.1 mg/d. An oral manganese intake less than 10 mg/d is considered safe.[1]

Selenium

The nonmetal selenium (Se) exists in ionic states as Se^{2-}, Se^{4+}, and Se^{6+}. Selenium content in food depends on soil concentration, which varies widely throughout the world. Most selenium in foods is complexed with derivatives of the amino acids methionine and cysteine. Selenomethionine, the primary dietary form, is derived from plant sources, and sele-

nocysteine is derived from animal sources of food; both are called *selenoproteins*. The bioavailability of ingested selenium is approximately 50% to 100%.[14]

Functions of Selenium

Following absorption, selenium is bound to the major plasma protein selenoprotein P. The role of selenoprotein P in selenium transport remains unclear, but it is thought to act as an antioxidant, particularly in the neutralization of the strongly oxidizing reactive species peroxynitrite.[5] Selenium homeostasis is maintained almost equally through urinary and fecal excretion. The best understood biochemical function of selenium is as a required cofactor in glutathione, iodine, and thyroid metabolism.[14,135] Some selenium-dependent enzymes include glutathione peroxidase and the iodothyronine deiodinases.

Glutathione peroxidase catalyzes reactions to eliminate hydrogen peroxide, a by-product of nutrient substrate processing at the electron transport chain (Figure 8-4). Iodothyronine deiodinase catalyzes the deiodination of iodine, triiodothyronine, and reverse triiodothyronine, thus playing a key role in the regulation of metabolism. Selenoprotein P is associated with oxidative defense properties.[14,135,136] Approximately 50% of plasma selenium is found as selenoprotein P and 30% is found as glutathione peroxidase.

Available selenium is distributed to selenoproteins in a hierarchical fashion. Therefore, in deficient states, some selenium-dependent processes will continue to function while others are impeded.[137] For example, glutathione peroxidase, which converts hydrogen peroxide to water, sits low on the selenium hierarchy and is likely affected early in selenium deficiency.

Clinical Applications

Recommended Intakes for Adults

The RDAs for selenium are as follows:
- Men and women: 55 mcg
- Pregnant women: 60 mcg
- Lactating women: 70 mcg

The UL for selenium is 400 mcg.

TABLE 8-21 Clinical Signs and Symptoms of Manganese Deficiency or Toxicity

System	Deficiency	Toxicity
Bones/joints	Abnormal bone and cartilage formation	None
Nervous system	Ataxia	Hyperirritability, violent tendencies, hallucinations, disturbances of libido, ataxia, manganese deposition in the basal ganglia secondary to perioperative parenteral nutrition support following gastrointestinal surgery, Parkinson-like motor dysfunction (ie, tremors, difficulty walking, facial muscle spasms)
Other	Poor reproductive performance, congenital abnormalities in offspring, abnormal bone/cartilage formation, growth retardation, and defects in lipid/carbohydrate metabolism	Immune system and reproductive dysfunction, nephritis, pancreatitis, hepatic damage, testicular damage

Source: Data are from references 14 and 67.

Sources

Food sources of selenium include fish, organ meats, eggs, milk, and shellfish.

Populations at Risk for Deficiency

Cardiomyopathy and skeletal muscle weakness have been reported in patients who received long-term PN without selenium supplementation and patients with thermal injury.[14,114,136] Medications in the statin class of cholesterol-lowering agents inhibit the enzyme 3-hydroxy-3-methylglutaryl CoA reductase and can induce myopathy by interfering with the synthesis of selenoproteins.[138] Depressed serum selenium levels in trauma patients postinjury have resulted in decreased thyroxine deiodination, which might explain the posttrauma changes observed in thyroid metabolism.[139]

Half-Life of the Nutrient in the Body

The half-life of selenium is approximately 100 days.[140]

Assessment of Selenium Status

The plasma or serum selenium concentration reflects the recent intake of selenium, whereas the erythrocyte concentration indicates long-term selenium status. The measurement of plasma glutathione peroxidase reflects the functional status of selenium; erythrocyte values less than 10.5 U/mL denote deficiency. As a general guideline, plasma or serum concentrations of selenium greater than 100 mcg/L represent adequate selenium status,[42] whereas 70 mcg/L tends to be the cut-off for deficiency.[5] The plasma or serum selenium concentration can be assessed using a variety of methodologies.[141] Table 8-22 lists clinical signs and symptoms of selenium deficiency and toxicity.[14,135]

TABLE 8-22 Clinical Signs and Symptoms of Selenium Deficiency or Toxicity

System	Deficiency	Toxicity
Skin	None	Skin lesions
Hair	None	Hair loss
Nails	None	Nail loss
Bone	None	Tooth decay
Nervous system	None	Peripheral neuropathy
Other	Increased susceptibility to mercury exposure, altered thyroid hormone metabolism, congestive cardiomyopathy secondary to Keshan disease, nausea, vomiting	Fatigue, irritability

Source: Data are from references 14 and 135.

Nutrient-Nutrient Interactions

The iodine-dependent selenoprotein deiodinases are necessary for the interconversion between the various forms of iodothyronine. Selenium deficiency decreases production of these deiodinases limiting this important role of iodine.[5]

Medication-Nutrient Interactions

Eltrombopag (thrombocytopenia medication) decreases selenium absorption.[7]

Treatment Considerations

Clear recommendations for the treatment of selenium deficiency are lacking. However, studies performed in populations where selenium deficiency was prevalent found that participants needed approximately 75 mcg/d.[4]

Selenium toxicity is known as *selenosis*. Due to the potential for selenosis, the consumption of less than 200 mcg of selenium per day or no more than 5 mcg per kg body weight per day has been recommended.[14]

Iodine

Iodine (I) can refer to the element in any ionic form but generally refers to iodide (I_2), the molecular form. The iodide content in foods varies depending on the soil concentration and the amount of fertilizer used in plant cultivation. The predominant source of dietary iodide comes from iodized salt; other dietary sources are either bound to amino acids or are found free as iodate (IO_3), which is reduced by glutathione to iodide during digestion. Iodide is rapidly absorbed in the stomach and the upper small intestine.[14,142] Absorbed iodide appears in the portal blood, where most is rapidly taken up by the thyroid (70% to 80%) for the synthesis of thyroid hormones. Lesser amounts of iodide are found in the kidneys, salivary glands, and other tissues. The kidneys are the principal route of excretion.

Functions of Iodine

Iodine functions as an integral component of the thyroid hormones thyroxine (T_4) and triiodothyronine (T_3).[14] The metabolically active form of T_3 regulates the rate of cell metabolism, as well as the activity and growth in multiple tissues, including fetal and neuronal tissues, and those in the periphery.[14]

When iodine is deficient, insufficient T_4 is produced, thereby eliminating its negative feedback on thyroid-stimulating hormone (TSH). This lack of negative feedback results in a constant release of TSH from the pituitary gland, which causes hyperplasia of the thyroid gland (goiter) as an adaptation designed to more effectively capture iodide from the blood.

Iodine is generally well tolerated when thyroid function is normal. If iodine deficiency is present and iodine intake is increased too rapidly, normal control mechanisms are ineffective and thyrotoxicosis can occur. Clinical signs of this so-called Jod-Basedow phenomenon are described in later in this section in the discussion of assessment of iodine status. This phenomenon is especially problematic for older adults.[14,142]

Clinical Applications

Recommended Intakes for Adults

The RDAs for iodine are as follows:
- Men and women: 150 mcg
- Pregnant women: 220 mcg
- Lactating women: 290 mcg

The UL for iodine is 1100 mcg.

Sources

Food sources of iodine include saltwater fish, seafood, and iodized salt.[1]

Populations at Risk for Deficiency

Iodine deficiency is a risk for individuals on low-salt diets, individuals who take salt from unfortified sources (eg, sea salt), and people from areas where the iodine level in the soil is low.

Half-Life of the Nutrient in the Body

The half-life of iodine is 66 to 80 days.[143]

Assessment of Iodine Status

Assessment of iodine status focuses on both the physical examination and biomarkers (Table 8-23).[142] Urinary iodine, measured in repeated 24-hour samples or in random samples, is a useful and reliable indicator of iodine status, and values correlate well with thyroglobulin concentrations, a biomarker for thyroid function.[142] Data from field studies note that a mean urinary iodine value less than 5 mcg/L suggests a risk for iodine deficiency; also, in pregnant women, a value less than 2 mcg/L implies a serious risk that their infants will be born with cretinism.[14,142] Iodine deficiency may also be indicated by elevated serum levels of total T_4 (ie, greater than 24 ng/dL in adults ages 20 to 49 years; greater than 181 ng/dL in adults ages 50 to 90 years).

TABLE 8-23 Clinical Signs and Symptoms of Iodine Deficiency or Toxicity

System	Deficiency	Toxicity
Biochemical markers	Elevated TSH	Elevated TSH
Other	Jod-Basedow phenomenon: nodular goiter, weight loss, tachycardia, muscle weakness, skin warmth	Depressed thyroid activity

TSH, thyroid-stimulating hormone.
Source: Data are from reference 142.

Nutrient-Nutrient Interactions

The iodine-dependent thyroid hormones T_3 and T_4 depend on selenoprotein deiodinases to interconvert between active and inactive forms of thyroid hormone. Therefore, this major role of iodine is altered in the presence of a selenium deficiency. Furthermore, cruciferous vegetables contain compounds that compete with iodide for entry into the thyroid gland. Such foods are termed *goitrogens*. In animal studies, diets exclusively high in goitrogenic foods caused goiter.[5]

Medication-Nutrient Interactions

Lithium (antimanic agent) inhibits thyroid hormone release from the thyroid.[5]

Treatment Considerations

In adults, iodine intakes between 50 and 1000 mcg/d are generally considered safe.[67] Iodine requirements in adult patients receiving EN or PN range between 70 and 150 mcg/d.[142] Parenteral micronutrient formulations currently available in the United States do not contain iodine. Hospitalized patients receive iodine primarily from iodine-containing antiseptic preparations absorbed via the skin.

Chromium

Chromium (Cr) is an essential trace metal required for glucose and lipid metabolism. It is ubiquitous within nature and in the food supply and can exist in several oxidation states from Cr^{2+} to Cr^{6+}. The trivalent form seems to be the biologically relevant form. Most chromium in the food supply is in the trivalent form, which is the most stable. The Cr^{6+} compounds are strong oxidizing agents that are readily reduced to Cr^{3+} in an acidic environment.

Absorption and Transport

Absorption of dietary chromium within the intestines is rapid, yet poor, ranging from 0.4% to 3%, whereas the remainder is excreted in the feces.[14] A dose-dependent relationship exists; as intake increases, absorption efficiency decreases. Absorption averages 2% at intakes of 10 mcg, whereas it decreases to 0.5% at doses of 40 mcg. Cr^{6+} is absorbed more readily than Cr^{3+}.[14,144] Some Cr^{3+} is soluble in the stomach and may form complexes with ligands in the acid environment. The remaining chromium is absorbed via nonmediated passive diffusion throughout the intestine, primarily in the jejunum.

Although little is known about the mechanism for Cr^{3+} absorption, the transport modality in the blood is more clearly understood. Trivalent chromium binds competitively with transferrin and is then transported into the blood along with iron. Consequently, chromium uses the iron transport system for movement from the blood into cells, where a rapid transfer from transferrin to the oligopeptide chromodulin occurs.[14,144] Chromodulin, formerly called *glucose tolerance factor*, binds 4 Cr^{3+} molecules. Interestingly, increases in serum glucose are accompanied by increases in chromium excretion, which suggests that chromium stored or maintained in the blood is mobilized in response to increases in insulin concentrations and is ultimately excreted in the urine as chromodulin.

Functions of Chromium

Chromium potentiates the action of insulin; therefore, it has a role in glucose, protein, and lipid metabolism and, as such, is required for growth. The biologically active form of chromium is chromodulin, which serves some role in insulin signaling, amplifying the tyrosine kinase activity of the insulin receptor.[14,144] Conditions that lead to increased urinary excretion of chromium include type 2 diabetes and pregnancy.[14] Individuals with these conditions may benefit from chromium supplementation.

Evidence for chromium deficiency in humans is sparse. Chromium deficiency can result in impaired glucose and amino acid use, increased plasma low-density lipoprotein cholesterol levels, and peripheral neuropathy.[14,120] Chromium deficiency has been reported in adult patients who underwent massive bowel surgery and subsequently received PN.[144] To date, the only cases of chromium deficiency reported in humans have been in patients receiving PN without an adequate chromium replacement.

Clinical Applications

Recommended Intakes for Adults

The AIs for chromium are as follows:
- Men younger than 50 years: 35 mcg
- Men age 50 years or older: 30 mcg
- Women younger than 50 years: 25 mcg
- Women age 50 years or older: 20 mcg
- Pregnant women: 30 mcg
- Lactating women: 45 mcg

The UL for chromium has not be set.

Sources

Food sources of chromium include whole grain products, egg yolks, beer, processed meats, mushrooms, and legumes.[1]

Populations at Risk for Deficiency

Patients receiving PN without chromium supplementation are at risk for chromium deficiency.

Half-Life of the Nutrient in the Body

Estimates regarding the half-life of chromium range from a few days to more than 1 month.[145]

Assessment of Chromium Status

Chromium status is difficult to determine because the mineral is present in the blood in extremely low concentrations, which

TABLE 8-24 Clinical Signs and Symptoms of Chromium Deficiency or Toxicity

System	Deficiency	Toxicity
Nervous system	Peripheral neuropathy	None
Other	Weight loss, hyperglycemia refractory to insulin, glycosuria, elevated plasma free fatty acids	Muscle rhabdomyolysis,[a] liver dysfunction,[b] renal failure[b]

[a]Observed in patients taking 1200 mcg Cr^{3+} per day.
[b]Observed in patients taking 600–1200 mcg Cr^{3+} per day.
Source: Data are from reference 144.

approach detection limits.[144] Normal serum, erythrocyte, and urine chromium values are less than 0.05 to 0.5 mcg/L, less than 20 to 36 mcg/L, and 0.1 to 2 mcg/L, respectively.[146] Refer to Table 8-24 for signs and symptoms of chromium deficiency and toxicity.[144]

Nutrient-Nutrient Interactions

Iron status can be compromised with chromium supplementation because chromium and iron compete for binding sites on transferrin. Serum ferritin levels decrease at chromium intakes of 200 mcg/d.

Medication-Nutrient Interactions

Corticosteroids (anti-inflammatories) cause increased urinary chromium wasting.[7]

Treatment Considerations

The use of chromium supplements is probably unnecessary for the general population, and the use of certain chromium forms—such as Cr^{3+} picolinate ($Cr[pic]_3$), the most common product—is potentially harmful.[128] $Cr[pic]_3$ causes liver dysfunction as well as renal and chromosomal damage at levels as low as 600 mcg/d.[5,144] Intakes of 1200 mcg/d may cause muscle rhabdomyolysis.[144]

Glucose control improved in patients with type 2 diabetes taking 200 mcg $Cr(pic)_3$ per day.[147] Based on this evidence, individuals with altered glucose metabolism might benefit from pharmacological doses of chromium. However, safety issues related to $Cr(pic)_3$ supplementation remain a concern.

Fluoride

Fluoride (F) is almost completely absorbed (50% to 100%) from the GI tract, and most is absorbed from the stomach.[5] Absorption generally occurs via passive diffusion and is inversely related to pH. Therefore, factors that promote gastric acid secretion increase the absorption rate of fluoride. In contrast, factors that inhibit gastric acid secretion decrease absorption. Fluoride appears in the plasma promptly after absorption, primarily in the ionic form. Removal of fluoride from the circulation occurs via kidney excretion (50%) or by deposition in the calcified tissue (bone and developing teeth).

Functions of Fluoride

Although fluoride has not been proven to be an essential trace element in humans, it plays a role in bone mineralization and the hardening of tooth enamel.[148] The major biochemical function of fluoride is to protect calcified tissues against pathological demineralization by forming fluorapatite crystals rather than the usual hydroxyapatite crystals. Fluoride helps inhibit and reverse the initiation and progression of dental caries; for this reason, it is considered to be a "beneficial element for humans."[148] Fluoride also stimulates new bone formation by stimulating osteoblasts, and it may reduce the risk for osteoporosis.[12] Some studies suggest that it may inhibit the calcification of aorta and soft tissues.[149]

Unequivocal or specific signs and symptoms of fluoride deficiency in humans do not exist. When an individual is deficient in fluoride, he or she has an increased risk for developing dental caries.[12]

Acute fluoride toxicity may result in a variety of symptoms.[149] Chronic excessive fluoride intake (eg, more than 5 mg/d) may result in enamel and skeletal fluorosis. Skeletal fluorosis has several stages. The preclinical stage (stage 1) is characterized by slight increases in bone mass and higher fluoride concentrations in the bone.[148] Signs and symptoms of stage 1 include stiffness, joint pain, and some osteosclerosis of the pelvis and vertebra.[148] Stages 2 and 3 involve the calcification of ligaments, osteosclerosis, exostoses, long bone osteoporosis, muscle wasting, and neurologic defects.[148]

The swallowing of fluoridated toothpaste represents a major source of fluoride toxicity. The American Dental Association recommends that children ages 2 through 6 years use only a pea-sized amount of fluoridated toothpaste when brushing the teeth and not swallowing.[150] There are no recommendations for adults.

Clinical Applications

Recommended Intakes for Adults

The AIs for fluoride are 4 mg for men and 3 mg for women, including during pregnancy and lactation. The UL for fluoride is 10 mg.

Sources

Sources of fluoride include fluoridated water, toothpaste, and dental treatments; tea; and seaweed.

Populations at Risk for Lower Fluoride Intake

Populations with nonfluoridated water as their primary water source may have lower serum fluoride levels.

Half-Life of the Nutrient in the Body

Fluoride leaves the bloodstream for excretion or deposition in bone with a half-life of several hours. Due to its deposition in bone, its true half-life may be up to 2 decades.[151]

Assessment of Fluoride Status

Plasma and urinary fluoride levels may be monitored to detect toxicity. Normal ranges for ionic fluoride are 0.01 to 0.2 mcg/mL in the plasma and 0.2 to 1.1 mg per liter of urine. Serum fluoride concentrations greater than 190 ng/mL have been associated with skeletal fluorosis.[5] Refer to Table 8-25 for clinical signs and symptoms of fluoride deficiency and toxicity.[149]

Nutrient-Nutrient Interactions

Calcium and magnesium form insoluble complexes when combined with fluoride.

Medication-Nutrient Interactions

Phosphate binders and calcium polycarbophil (bulk-forming fiber therapy [Fibercon]) interfere with fluoride supplement absorption.[7]

Treatment Considerations

Fluoride treatment is not a part of nutrition care. For cases of toxicity, identifying and removing the source of fluoride intake (toothpaste, supplements) is key.

Molybdenum

Molybdenum (Mo) is an ultratrace element because the estimated dietary requirement is less than 100 mg/d. Other ultratrace elements are discussed later in this chapter.

TABLE 8-25 Clinical Signs and Symptoms of Fluoride Deficiency or Toxicity

System	Deficiency	Toxicity
Eyes	None	Lacrimation
Mouth	None	Excessive salivation
Bone	Increased risk of dental caries	Enamel and skeletal fluorosis (mottled teeth)
Nervous system	None	Convulsions, sensory disturbances, paralysis, coma
Other	None	Nausea, vomiting, diarrhea, abdominal pain, pulmonary disturbances, cardiac insufficiency, arrhythmias, weakness

Source: Data are from reference 149.

Molybdenum exists as the ionic states Mo^{4+} and Mo^{6+} and is generally bound to either sulfur or oxygen. Human absorption ranges from 85% to 93%. The absorption rate is highest in the proximal small intestine. The transport of molybdenum occurs by an active carrier-mediated process when molybdenum blood concentrations are low and via passive diffusion when blood concentrations are high. Molybdenum is transported as molybdate, which is loosely attached to erythrocytes, and tends to bind albumin and α-macroglobulin.[152] After absorption, molybdenum elimination occurs as molybdate via the kidneys. High dietary intakes of molybdenum increase excretion. Hence, molybdenum regulation is controlled through excretion rather than absorption.

Functions of Molybdenum

Biochemically, molybdenum functions as a cofactor for the metalloenzymes aldehyde oxidase, xanthine oxidase, and sulfite oxidase, and it catalyzes the hydroxylation of various substrates.

Molybdenum deficiency is rarely caused by inadequate dietary intake alone. However, in at least one case, a patient with short bowel syndrome who received prolonged PN developed a syndrome of hypermethioninemia, hypouricemia, hyperoxypurinemia, hypouricosuria, and low urinary sulfate excretion, along with mental disturbances that progressed to a coma.[14] Contributing factors included the loss of the molybdenum -dependent enzyme, sulfite oxidase activity, and inadequate molybdenum intake.[14]

Excessive dietary intake (10 to 15 mg molybdenum per day) or exposure to an environmental molybdenum contamination may result in a gout-like syndrome with elevated blood levels of molybdenum, uric acid, and xanthine oxidase.[14]

Clinical Applications

Recommended Intakes for Adults

The AIs for molybdenum are 45 mcg for men and women; AIs increase to 50 mcg for women who are pregnant or lactating. The UL for molybdenum is 2 mg.

Sources

Food sources of molybdenum include beans, grains, and nuts.[1]

Populations at Risk for Deficiency

Molybdenum deficiency is unlikely, but it has occurred in patients receiving long-term PN.

Half-Life of the Nutrient in the Body

The half-life of molybdenum is not documented. The *half-time* (time to clear 50% of molybdenum from the blood) is reportedly a few hours to a few days for small animals.[153]

Assessment of Molybdenum Status

There is no standardized laboratory method for molybdenum analysis. Values in the literature on molybdenum blood levels

TABLE 8-26 Clinical Signs and Symptoms of Molybdenum Deficiency or Toxicity

System	Deficiency	Toxicity
Eyes	Dislocation of ocular lens, altered vision	None
Nervous system	Altered mental status, attenuated brain growth, neurologic damage	None
Other	Tachycardia, tachypnea, elevated methionine, headache, lethargy, nausea, vomiting	Rare: hyperuricemia, gout-like symptoms

Source: Data are from references 5 and 14.

vary widely, with normal molybdenum serum/plasma levels reported from 0.58 ± 0.21 to 0.8 ± 0.2 mcg/L.[154] For the clinical signs and symptoms of molybdenum deficiency and toxicity, refer to Table 8-26.[5,14]

Nutrient-Nutrient Interactions

Moderate doses of molybdenum (ie, 0.54 mg/d) are associated with copper wasting in the urine.[14,154] The compound responsible, tetrathiomolybdate, is therefore used to treat copper toxicity (Wilson disease).[5]

Medication-Nutrient Interactions

No medication interactions with molybdenum are known.

Treatment Considerations

In one case study, a patient with molybdenum deficiency secondary to 18 months of PN was successfully treated with 300 mcg ammonium molybdate (equivalent to 163 mcg molybdenum).[5]

Ultratrace Elements

Ultratrace elements are defined as those elements with estimated dietary requirements less than 100 mg/d.[5] The ultratrace elements include aluminum, arsenic, boron, bromine, cadmium, chromium, fluorine, germanium, lead, lithium, molybdenum, nickel, rubidium, selenium, silicon, tin, and vanadium. Research findings regarding the essentiality of these elements vary depending on the quality of the experimental evidence and should be interpreted with caution.[8,154] However, research on boron suggests a relationship between adequate boron intake and health, perhaps making it a more relevant nutrition concern than previously thought.[155] There is also substantial circumstantial evidence for the essentiality of arsenic, nickel, silicon, and vanadium.[1] With the exceptions of chromium, fluoride, molybdenum, and selenium, RDAs or AIs are not assigned to the ultratrace elements.

Parenteral Vitamins

In 2000, the FDA issued new parenteral multivitamin drug dosing requirements (Table 8-27).[65,156,157] Dosages for thiamin, vitamin B_6, vitamin C, and folic acid increased, and vitamin K was added to the multivitamin formulation. The addition of vitamin K raises some concern for patients who receive long-term parenteral multivitamin products and use oral anticoagulant therapy to maintain patency of their IV access devices. In these patients, regular monitoring of the INR is needed, and warfarin doses may need to be adjusted because of the vitamin K content in the multivitamin product. Two parenteral multivitamin products are currently available for adult patients, one with vitamin K and one without vitamin K, but both meet the FDA mandate. Other sources of IV vitamin K are found in ILE, but the amount varies from 0 to 290 mcg/L.[44] Weekly IV supply of 250 to 500 mcg phytonadione, a synthetic form of phylloquinone, is adequate to preserve coagulation in PN patients.[44] Clinicians should carefully consider the impact of the administration of parenteral vitamins outside of these FDA dosing requirements as well as what impact additional amounts have on other micronutrients.

The parenteral multivitamin supplementation of certain other nutrients, such as vitamin D, can present clinical challenges. Vitamin D preparations for PN are challenging because high-dose parenteral formulas of vitamin D are unavailable or not recommended in the United States. Currently, US patients receiving PN receive a daily multivitamin infusion that contains 200 to 400 IU (5 to 10 mcg) of vitamin D. An intramuscular form of high-dose vitamin D is available outside of the United States, but it is not currently recommended in the United States because of solubility and absorption inconsistencies, unpredictable clinical response, and significant pain upon administration. Sun exposure and UVB radiation therapy from tanning beds are alternative and effective methods to ensure vitamin D status for long-term PN patients;[158] however, these methods may increase the risk of skin cancer. For issues related to other parenteral vitamins, see the relevant sections earlier in this chapter.

Parenteral Trace Elements

The American Medical Association (AMA) and the American Society for Parenteral and Enteral Nutrition (ASPEN) have published recommendations for daily parenteral intake of the trace elements zinc, copper, manganese, and chromium (Table 8-28).[65,156,159] Selenium supplementation of 20 to 60 mcg/d is also now recommended for patients receiving PN therapy.[65] Other information about parenteral dosing is found in sections on the various trace elements.

In 2009, ASPEN performed a review of commercially available parenteral products and found them to contain potentially toxic levels of manganese, copper, and chromium. Since the 1980s, studies have shown manganese toxicity, excess hepatic copper, and potentially nephrotoxic chromium levels in adults on long-term PN. The FDA has yet to issue recommendations for product reformulation despite these well-documented issues. Currently, ASPEN is working with the FDA to resolve this problem to improve the safety and effectiveness of PN support formulations.[160]

Enteral Vitamin and Mineral Adequacy

Data on the clinical implications regarding micronutrient stability in enteral formulations are limited. Variability in enteral

---

TABLE 8-27 Parenteral Multivitamin Dosing Requirements

Vitamin	Amount Per Day
Fat-soluble vitamins	
Vitamin A (retinol)	1 mg
Vitamin D (ergocalciferol or cholecalciferol)	5 mcg
Vitamin E (α-tocopherol)	10 mg
Vitamin K (phylloquinone)	150 mcg
Water-soluble vitamins	
B_1 (thiamin)	6 mg
B_2 (riboflavin)	3.6 mg
B_6 (pyridoxine)	6 mg
B_{12} (cyanocobalamin)	5 mcg
Niacin	40 mg
Folic acid	600 mcg
Pantothenic acid	5 mg
Biotin	60 mcg
Vitamin C (ascorbic acid)	200 mg

Source: Data are from references 65, 156, and 157.

TABLE 8-28 Parenteral Trace Element Supplementation for Adults

Trace Element	Dose per Day		GI Losses
	Previous Recommendations (AMA, 1979)[14]	Current Recommendations (ASPEN, 2012)[159]	
Zinc	2.5–4.0 mg	2.5–5 mg[a]	Varies[b]
Copper	0.5–1.5 mg	0.3–0.5 mg	500 mcg/d
Chromium	10–15 mcg	10–15 mcg	20 mcg/d[c]
Iron	None	None	Not applicable
Manganese	150–800 mcg	60–100 mcg	Unknown
Selenium	None	20–60 mcg	Unknown

AMA, American Medical Association; ASPEN, American Society for Parenteral and Enteral Nutrition; GI, gastrointestinal.

[a]In hypermetabolic patients, increase dose by 2 mg zinc per day until 6–12 mg/d is achieved.

[b]An additional 12 mg zinc per liter of small bowel losses or 17 mg zinc per liter of stool or ileostomy losses may be needed.

[c]Check glycated hemoglobin (A1C) every 6 months.

Source: Data are from references 14, 65, 156, and 159.

feeding containers, light exposure, hang times, storage temperatures, and shelf life beyond 1 year can diminish micronutrient value.[161,162] Specific nutrient losses of thiamin, riboflavin, and vitamins A and E have been reported at storage temperatures between 20°C and 30°C compared with 4°C. Storing EN for more than 9 months also results in a loss of these nutrients.[163] Requirements that manufacturers include stability information in product information for EN formulas would help clinicians in product selection and administration. Adherence to the EN practice standards mitigates most of the stability issues.[162]

Best Practice: The Clinician's Role in Micronutrient Management in Times of Shortages

During shortages of parenteral vitamins or trace elements, a professional practice consultation is critical. Clinicians involved in the delivery of specialized nutrition therapy should seek the recommendations on usage from ASPEN, the American Society of Health-System Pharmacists Drug Shortages Resource Center, or the FDA's Drug Shortage Program, and Current Drug Shortages bulletins. Some strategies recommended include reassessing the indication of micronutrient supplementation, providing oral doses, and prioritizing the most vulnerable populations. To avoid micronutrient deficiencies in patients receiving EN or PN, clinicians collectively need to continually monitor and reassess the need for micronutrient supplementation.[164]

References

1. Ross AC, Manson JE, Abrams SA, et al. The 2011 Dietary Reference Intakes for calcium and vitamin D: what dietetics practitioners need to know. *J Am Diet Assoc.* 2011;111(4):524–527.

2. Hambidge KM. Micronutrient bioavailability: Dietary Reference Intakes and a future perspective. *Am J Clin Nutr.* 2010;91(5):1430S–1432S.

3. Institute of Medicine. *Dietary Reference Intakes for Vitamin A, Vitamin K, Arsenic, Boron, Chromium, Copper, Iodine, Iron, Manganese, Molybdenum, Nickel, Silicon, Vanadium, and Zinc.* Washington, DC: National Academies Press; 2002. doi:10.17226/10026.

4. Ross AC. *Modern Nutrition in Health and Disease.* 11th ed. Philadelphia, PA: Wolters Kluwer Health; 2014.

5. Gropper SA, Smith JL, Groff JL. *Advanced Nutrition and Human Metabolism.* 6th ed. Belmont, CA: Wadsworth Cengage Learning; 2012.

6. Arnold M, Barbul A. Nutrition and wound healing. *Plast Reconstr Surg.* 2006;117(7 Suppl):42S–58S.

7. Pronsky ZM. *Food Medication Interactions.* 18th ed. Birchrunville, PA: Food-Medication Interactions; 2015.

8. Feskanich D, Singh V, Willett WC, Colditz GA. Vitamin A intake and hip fractures among postmenopausal women. *JAMA.* 2002;287(1):47–54.

9. Cabral PC, Diniz Ada S, de Arruda IK. Vitamin A and zinc status in patients on maintenance haemodialysis. *Nephrology (Carlton).* 2005;10(5):459–463.

10. Brown RO, Compher C. A.S.P.E.N. clinical guidelines: nutrition support in adult acute and chronic renal failure. *JPEN J Parenter Enteral Nutr.* 2010;34(4):366–377.

11. Kumar N. Neurologic presentations of nutritional deficiencies. *Neurol Clin.* 2010;28(1):107–170.

12. Institute of Medicine. *Dietary Reference Intakes for Calcium, Phosphorus, Magnesium, Vitamin D, and Fluoride.* Washington, DC: National Academies Press; 1997. doi:10.17226/5776.

13. Gannon BM, Tanumihardjo SA. Comparisons among equations used for retinol isotope dilution in the assessment of total body stores and total liver reserves. *J Nutr.* 2015;145(5):847–854.

14. Shils ME, Shike M. *Modern Nutrition in Health and Disease.* 10th ed. Philadelphia, PA: Lippincott Williams & Wilkins; 2006.

15. McClave SA, Taylor BE, Martindale RG, et al. Guidelines for the provision and assessment of nutrition support therapy in the adult critically ill patient: Society of Critical Care Medicine (SCCM) and American Society for Parenteral and Enteral Nutrition (A.S.P.E.N.). *JPEN J Parenter Enteral Nutr.* 2016;40(2):159–211.

16. Stechmiller JK. Understanding the role of nutrition and wound healing. *Nutr Clin Pract.* 2010;25(1):61–68.

17. Holick MF. The vitamin D epidemic and its health consequences. *J Nutr.* 2005;135(11 Suppl):2739S–2748S.

18. Seifert M, Tilgen W, Reichrath J. Expression of 25-hydroxyvitamin D-1alpha-hydroxylase (1alphaOHase, CYP27B1) splice variants in HaCaT keratinocytes and other skin cells: modulation by culture conditions and UV-B treatment in vitro. *Anticancer Res.* 2009;29(9):3659–3667.

19. Holick MF. Vitamin D: evolutionary, physiological and health perspectives. *Curr Drug Targets.* 2011;12(1):4–18.

20. Norman AW. From vitamin D to hormone D: fundamentals of the vitamin D endocrine system essential for good health. *Am J Clin Nutr.* 2008;88(2):491S–499S.

21. Pittas AG, Laskowski U, Kos L, Saltzman E. Role of vitamin D in adults requiring nutrition support. *JPEN J Parenter Enteral Nutr.* 2010;34(1):70–78.

22. Quraishi SA, Litonjua AA, Moromizato T, et al. Association between prehospital vitamin D status and hospital-acquired *Clostridium difficile* infections. *JPEN J Parenter Enteral Nutr.* 2015;39(1):47–55.

23. van der Wilden GM, Fagenholz PJ, Velmahos GC, et al. Vitamin D status and severity of *Clostridium difficile* infections: a prospective cohort study in hospitalized adults. *JPEN J Parenter Enteral Nutr.* 2015;39(4):465–470.

24. Youssef DA, Miller CW, El-Abbassi AM, et al. Antimicrobial implications of vitamin D. *Dermatoendocrinol.* 2011;3(4):220–229.

25. Kumar PR, Fenton TR, Shaheen AA, Raman M. Prevalence of vitamin D deficiency and response to oral vitamin D supplementation in patients receiving home parenteral nutrition. *JPEN J Parenter Enteral Nutr.* 2012;36(4):463–469.

26. Basson A. Vitamin D and Crohn's disease in the adult patient: a review. *JPEN J Parenter Enteral Nutr.* 2014;38(4):438–458.

27. Heaney RP. Vitamin D in health and disease. *Clin J Am Soc Nephrol.* 2008;3(5):1535–1541.

28. Seamans KM, Cashman KD. Existing and potentially novel functional markers of vitamin D status: a systematic review. *Am J Clin Nutr.* 2009;89(6):1997S–2008S.

29. Hollis BW. Circulating 25-hydroxyvitamin D levels indicative of vitamin D sufficiency: implications for establishing a new effective dietary intake recommendation for vitamin D. *J Nutr.* 2005;135(2):317–322.

30. Zingg JM. Vitamin E: an overview of major research directions. *Mol Aspects Med.* 2007;28(5–6):400–422.

31. Biesalski HK. Vitamin E requirements in parenteral nutrition. *Gastroenterology.* 2009;137(5 Suppl):S92–S104.

32. Traber MG. Vitamin E regulatory mechanisms. *Annu Rev Nutr.* 2007;27:347–362.

33. Ahuja JK, Goldman JD, Moshfegh AJ. Current status of vitamin E nutriture. *Ann N Y Acad Sci.* 2004;1031:387–390.

34. Bell SJ, Grochoski GT. How safe is vitamin E supplementation? *Crit Rev Food Sci Nutr.* 2008;48(8):760–774.

35. Morgan SL, Weinsier RL. *Fundamentals of Clinical Nutrition.* 2nd ed. St. Louis, MO: Mosby; 1998.

36. Steiner M. Vitamin E, a modifier of platelet function: rationale and use in cardiovascular and cerebrovascular disease. *Nutr Rev.* 1999;57(10):306–309.

37. Bugel S. Vitamin K and bone health in adult humans. *Vitam Horm.* 2008;78:393–416.

38. Dickerson RN, Garmon WM, Kuhl DA, Minard G, Brown RO. Vitamin K-independent warfarin resistance after concurrent administration of warfarin and continuous enteral nutrition. *Pharmacotherapy.* 2008;28(3):308–313.

39. Schurgers LJ, Shearer MJ, Hamulyak K, Stocklin E, Vermeer C. Effect of vitamin K intake on the stability of oral anticoagulant treatment: dose-response relationships in healthy subjects. *Blood.* 2004;104(9):2682–2689.

40. Cockayne S, Adamson J, Lanham-New S, et al. Vitamin K and the prevention of fractures: systematic review and meta-analysis of randomized controlled trials. *Arch Intern Med.* 2006;166(12): 1256–1261.

41. Institute of Medicine. *Dietary Reference Intakes for Vitamin C, Vitamin E, Selenium, and Carotenoids.* Washington, DC: National Academies Press; 2000. doi:10.17226/9810.

42. Cheung LK, Agi R, Hyman DJ. Warfarin resistance associated with parenteral nutrition. *Am J Med Sci.* 2012;343(3):255–258.

43. Shearer MJ. Vitamin K in parenteral nutrition. *Gastroenterology.* 2009;137(5 Suppl):S105–S118.

44. Edmunds MW, Mayhew MS, Setter SM. *Pharmacology for the Primary Care Provider.* 4th ed. St. Louis, MO: Elsevier; 2013.

45. Olson RE, Chao J, Graham D, Bates MW, Lewis JH. Total body phylloquinone and its turnover in human subjects at two levels of vitamin K intake. *Br J Nutr.* 2002;87(6):543–553.

46. Booth SL, Al Rajabi A. Determinants of vitamin K status in humans. *Vitam Horm.* 2008;78:1–22.

47. Nakano T, Tsugawa N, Kuwabara A, et al. High prevalence of hypovitaminosis D and K in patients with hip fracture. *Asia Pac J Clin Nutr.* 2011;20(1):56–61.

48. Booth SL. Vitamin K status in the elderly. *Curr Opin Clin Nutr Metab Care.* 2007;10(1):20–23.

49. Klang M, Graham D, McLymont V. Warfarin bioavailability with feeding tubes and enteral formula. *JPEN J Parenter Enteral Nutr.* 2010;34(3):300–304.

50. MacLaren R, Wachsman BA, Swift DK, Kuhl DA. Warfarin resistance associated with intravenous lipid administration: discussion of propofol and review of the literature. *Pharmacotherapy.* 1997;17(6):1331–1337.

51. Marian M, Sacks G. Micronutrients and older adults. *Nutr Clin Pract.* 2009;24(2):179–195.

52. Mandl J, Szarka A, Banhegyi G. Vitamin C: update on physiology and pharmacology. *Br J Pharmacol.* 2009;157(7):1097–1110.

53. Hickey SR, Roberts HJ, Miller NJ. Pharmacokinetics of oral vitamin C. *J Nutr Environ Med.* 2008;17(3):169–177.

54. Schleicher RL, Carroll MD, Ford ES, Lacher DA. Serum vitamin C and the prevalence of vitamin C deficiency in the United States: 2003–2004 National Health and Nutrition Examination Survey (NHANES). *Am J Clin Nutr.* 2009;90(5):1252–1263.

55. Halliwell B, Gutteridge JMC. *Free Radicals in Biology and Medicine.* 5th ed. ed. Oxford, UK: Oxford University Press; 2015.

56. McClave SA, Martindale RG, Vanek VW, et al. Guidelines for the provision and assessment of nutrition support therapy in the adult critically ill patient: Society of Critical Care Medicine (SCCM) and American Society for Parenteral and Enteral Nutrition (A.S.P.E.N.). *JPEN J Parenter Enteral Nutr.* 2009;33(3):277–316.

57. Massey LK, Liebman M, Kynast-Gales SA. Ascorbate increases human oxaluria and kidney stone risk. *J Nutr.* 2005;135(7):1673–1677.

58. Institute of Medicine. *Dietary Reference Intakes for Thiamin, Riboflavin, Niacin, Vitamin B6, Folate, Vitamin B12, Pantothenic Acid, Biotin, and Choline.* Washington, DC: National Academies Press; 1998. doi:10.17226/6015.

59. Kazemi A, Frazier T, Cave M. Micronutrient-related neurologic complications following bariatric surgery. *Curr Gastroenterol Rep.* 2010;12(4):288–295.

60. Cho YP, Kim K, Han MS, et al. Severe lactic acidosis and thiamine deficiency during total parenteral nutrition: case report. *Hepatogastroenterology.* 2004;51(55):253–255.

61. Giacalone M, Martinelli R, Abramo A, et al. Rapid reversal of severe lactic acidosis after thiamine administration in critically ill adults: a report of 3 cases. *Nutr Clin Pract.* 2015;30(1):104–110.

62. Sica DA. Loop diuretic therapy, thiamine balance, and heart failure. *Congest Heart Fail.* 2007;13(4):244–247.

63. Hanninen SA, Darling PB, Sole MJ, Barr A, Keith ME. The prevalence of thiamin deficiency in hospitalized patients with congestive heart failure. *J Am Coll Cardiol.* 2006;47(2):354–361.

64. Keith ME, Walsh NA, Darling PB, et al. B-vitamin deficiency in hospitalized patients with heart failure. *J Am Diet Assoc.* 2009; 109(8):1406–1410.

65. Mirtallo J, Canada T, Johnson D, et al. Safe practices for parenteral nutrition. *JPEN J Parenter Enteral Nutr.* 2004;28(6):S39–S70.

66. Latt N, Dore G. Thiamine in the treatment of Wernicke encephalopathy in patients with alcohol use disorders. *Intern Med J.* 2014;44(9):911–915.

67. National Research Council. *Recommended Dietary Allowances.* 10th ed. Washington, DC: National Academies Press; 1989.

68. Litt JZ. *Litt's Drug Eruption Reference Manual: Including Drug Interactions.* 11th ed. London, UK: Taylor & Francis; 2005.

69. Hoey L, McNulty H, Strain JJ. Studies of biomarker responses to intervention with riboflavin: a systematic review. *Am J Clin Nutr.* 2009;89(6):1960S–1980S.

70. Gariballa S, Forster S, Powers H. Riboflavin status in acutely ill patients and response to dietary supplements. *JPEN J Parenter Enteral Nutr.* 2009;33(6):656–661.

71. Al-Mohaissen MA, Pun SC, Frohlich JJ. Niacin: from mechanisms of action to therapeutic uses. *Mini Rev Med Chem.* 2010;10(3): 204–217.

72. Digby JE, Ruparelia N, Choudhury RP. Niacin in cardiovascular disease: recent preclinical and clinical developments. *Arterioscler Thromb Vasc Biol.* 2012;32(3):582–588.

73. Menon RM, Adams MH, Gonzalez MA, et al. Plasma and urine pharmacokinetics of niacin and its metabolites from an extended-release niacin formulation. *Int J Clin Pharmacol Ther.* 2007;45(8):448–454.

74. Vasilaki AT, McMillan DC, Kinsella J, et al. Relation between pyridoxal and pyridoxal phosphate concentrations in plasma, red cells, and white cells in patients with critical illness. *Am J Clin Nutr.* 2008;88(1):140–146.

75. Schaumburg H, Kaplan J, Windebank A, et al. Sensory neuropathy from pyridoxine abuse. A new megavitamin syndrome. *N Engl J Med.* 1983;309(8):445–448.

76. Matarese LE, Dvorchik I, Costa G, et al. Pyridoxal-5'-phosphate deficiency after intestinal and multivisceral transplantation. *Am J Clin Nutr.* 2009;89(1):204–209.

77. Moestrup SK. New insights into carrier binding and epithelial uptake of the erythropoietic nutrients cobalamin and folate. *Curr Opin Hematol.* 2006;13(3):119–123.

78. Laine L, Ahnen D, McClain C, Solcia E, Walsh JH. Review article: potential gastrointestinal effects of long-term acid suppression with proton pump inhibitors. *Aliment Pharmacol Ther.* 2000;14(6):651–668.

79. de Bree A, Verschuren WM, Blom HJ, et al. Coronary heart disease mortality, plasma homocysteine, and B-vitamins: a prospective study. *Atherosclerosis.* 2003;166(2):369–377.

80. Herrmann M, Kraenzlin M, Pape G, Sand-Hill M, Herrmann W. Relation between homocysteine and biochemical bone turnover markers and bone mineral density in peri- and post-menopausal women. *Clin Chem Lab Med.* 2005;43(10):1118–1123.

81. McCracken C. Challenges of long-term nutrition intervention studies on cognition: discordance between observational and intervention studies of vitamin B12 and cognition. *Nutr Rev.* 2010;68(Suppl 1):S11–S15.

82. Hankey GJ, Eikelboom JW, Baker RI, et al; VITATOPS Trial Study Group. B vitamins in patients with recent transient ischaemic attack or stroke in the VITAmins TO Prevent Stroke (VITATOPS) trial: a randomised, double-blind, parallel, placebo-controlled trial. *Lancet Neurol.* 2010;9(9):855–865.

83. McLean RR, Jacques PF, Selhub J, et al. Plasma B vitamins, homocysteine, and their relation with bone loss and hip fracture in elderly men and women. *J Clin Endocrinol Metab.* 2008;93(6): 2206–2212.

84. Handzlik-Orlik G, Holecki M, Orlik B, Wylezol M, Dulawa J. Nutrition management of the post-bariatric surgery patient. *Nutr Clin Pract.* 2015;30(3):383–392.

85. Rizzo G, Lagana AS, Rapisarda AM, et al. Vitamin B_{12} among vegetarians: status, assessment and supplementation. *Nutrients.* 2016;8(12).

86. Adams JF. Biological half-life of vitamin B12 in plasma. *Nature.* 1963;198:200.

87. de Benoist B. Conclusions of a WHO Technical Consultation on folate and vitamin B_{12} deficiencies. *Food Nutr Bull.* 2008;29(2 Suppl):S238–S244.

88. Stevenson RE, Allen WP, Pai GS, et al. Decline in prevalence of neural tube defects in a high-risk region of the United States. *Pediatrics.* 2000;106(4):677–683.

89. Tamura T, Picciano MF. Folate and human reproduction. *Am J Clin Nutr.* 2006;83(5):993–1016.

90. Centers for Disease Control and Prevention. Recommendations for the use of folic acid to reduce the number of cases of spina bifida and other neural tube defects. *MMWR* 1992;41:RR-14.

91. Nijhout HF, Reed MC, Budu P, Ulrich CM. A mathematical model of the folate cycle: new insights into folate homeostasis. *J Biol Chem.* 2004;279(53):55008–55016.

92. Mayer O, Simon J, Rosolova H, et al. The effects of folate supplementation on some coagulation parameters and oxidative status surrogates. *Eur J Clin Pharmacol.* 2002;58(1):1–5.

93. Wolf B. Clinical issues and frequent questions about biotinidase deficiency. *Mol Genet Metab.* 2010;100(1):6–13.

94. Bitsch R, Salz I, Hotzel D. Studies on bioavailability of oral biotin doses for humans. *Int J Vitam Nutr Res.* 1989;59(1):65–71.

95. Mock NI, Malik MI, Stumbo PJ, Bishop WP, Mock DM. Increased urinary excretion of 3-hydroxyisovaleric acid and decreased urinary excretion of biotin are sensitive early indicators of decreased biotin status in experimental biotin deficiency. *Am J Clin Nutr.* 1997;65(4):951–958.

96. Zeisel SH, da Costa KA. Choline: an essential nutrient for public health. *Nutr Rev.* 2009;67(11):615–623.

97. Perez C, Koshy C, Ressl S, Nicklisch S, Kramer R, Ziegler C. Substrate specificity and ion coupling in the Na+/betaine symporter BetP. *EMBO J.* 2011;30(7):1221–1229.

98. Buchman AL. Choline deficiency during parenteral nutrition in humans. *Nutr Clin Pract.* 2003;18(5):353–358.

99. Fischer LM, daCosta KA, Kwock L, et al. Sex and menopausal status influence human dietary requirements for the nutrient choline. *Am J Clin Nutr.* 2007;85(5):1275–1285.

100. Zeisel SH, Char D, Sheard NF. Choline, phosphatidylcholine and sphingomyelin in human and bovine milk and infant formulas. *J Nutr.* 1986;116(1):50–58.

101. Marriott BM, ed. Food Components to Enhance Performance: An Evaluation of Potential Performance-Enhancing Food Components for Operational Rations. Washington, DC: National Academies Press; 1994. doi:10.17226/4563.

102. Young MF, Glahn RP, Ariza-Nieto M, et al. Serum hepcidin is significantly associated with iron absorption from food and supplemental sources in healthy young women. *Am J Clin Nutr.* 2009;89(2):533–538.

103. Munoz M, Garcia-Erce JA, Remacha AF. Disorders of iron metabolism. Part 1: molecular basis of iron homoeostasis. *J Clin Pathol.* 2011;64(4):281–286.

104. D'Angelo G. Role of hepcidin in the pathophysiology and diagnosis of anemia. *Blood Res.* 2013;48(1):10–15.

105. Thurnham DI, McCabe LD, Haldar S, et al. Adjusting plasma ferritin concentrations to remove the effects of subclinical inflammation in the assessment of iron deficiency: a meta-analysis. *Am J Clin Nutr.* 2010;92(3):546–555.

106. Forbes A. Iron and parenteral nutrition. *Gastroenterology.* 2009; 137(5 Suppl):S47–S54.

107. Clark SF. Iron deficiency anemia. *Nutr Clin Pract.* 2008;23(2): 128–141.

108. Munoz M, Garcia-Erce JA, Remacha AF. Disorders of iron metabolism. Part II: iron deficiency and iron overload. *J Clin Pathol.* 2011;64(4):287–296.

109. Clark SF. Iron deficiency anemia: diagnosis and management. *Curr Opin Gastroenterol.* 2009;25(2):122–128.

110. Thurnham DI, Northrop-Clewes CA, Knowles J. The use of adjustment factors to address the impact of inflammation on vitamin A and iron status in humans. *J Nutr.* 2015;145(5):1137S–1143S.

111. Pasricha SR, McQuilten Z, Westerman M, et al. Serum hepcidin as a diagnostic test of iron deficiency in premenopausal female blood donors. *Haematologica.* 2011;96(8):1099–1105.

112. Ruz M, Carrasco F, Rojas P, et al. Iron absorption and iron status are reduced after Roux-en-Y gastric bypass. *Am J Clin Nutr.* 2009;90(3):527–532.

113. Alleyne M, Horne MK, Miller JL. Individualized treatment for iron-deficiency anemia in adults. *Am J Med.* 2008;121(11): 943–948.

114. Albright T, Al-Makki A, Kalakeche R, Shepler B. A review of ferric pyrophosphate citrate (triferic) use in hemodialysis patients. *Clin Ther.* 2016;38(10):2318–2323.

115. Heyland DK, Jones N, Cvijanovich NZ, Wong H. Zinc supplementation in critically ill patients: a key pharmaconutrient? *JPEN J Parenter Enteral Nutr.* 2008;32(5):509–519.

116. Wiernsperger N, Rapin J. Trace elements in glucometabolic disorders: an update. *Diabetol Metab Syndr.* 2010;2:70.

117. Mohammad MK, Zhou Z, Cave M, Barve A, McClain CJ. Zinc and liver disease. *Nutr Clin Pract.* 2012;27(1):8–20.

118. Muirhead N, Kertesz A, Flanagan PR, et al. Zinc metabolism in patients on maintenance hemodialysis. *Am J Nephrol.* 1986;6(6): 422–426.

119. Lowe NM, Fekete K, Decsi T. Methods of assessment of zinc status in humans: a systematic review. *Am J Clin Nutr.* 2009;89(6): 2040S–2051S.

120. Fuhrman MP. Micronutrient assessment in long-term home parenteral nutrition patients. *Nutr Clin Pract.* 2006;21(6): 566–575.

121. McClave SA, Codner P, Patel J, et al. Should we aim for full enteral feeding in the first week of critical illness? *Nutr Clin Pract.* 2016;31(4):425–431.

122. Stechmiller JK CL, Logan KM. Nutrition support for wound healing. *Support Line.* 2009(31):2–7.

123. Uauy R, Maass A, Araya M. Estimating risk from copper excess in human populations. *Am J Clin Nutr.* 2008;88(3):867S–871S.

124. Halfdanarson TR, Kumar N, Hogan WJ, Murray JA. Copper deficiency in celiac disease. *J Clin Gastroenterol.* 2009;43(2): 162–164.

125. Shike M. Copper in parenteral nutrition. *Gastroenterology.* 2009;137(5 Suppl):S13–S17.

126. Barceloux DG. Copper. *J Toxicol Clin Toxicol.* 1999;37(2): 217–230.

127. Harvey LJ, Ashton K, Hooper L, Casgrain A, Fairweather-Tait SJ. Methods of assessment of copper status in humans: a systematic review. *Am J Clin Nutr.* 2009;89(6):2009S–2024S.

128. Blaszyk H, Wild PJ, Oliveira A, Kelly DG, Burgart LJ. Hepatic copper in patients receiving long-term total parenteral nutrition. *J Clin Gastroenterol.* 2005;39(4):318–320.

129. Howard L, Ashley C, Lyon D, Shenkin A. Autopsy tissue trace elements in 8 long-term parenteral nutrition patients who received the current U.S. Food and Drug Administration formulation. *JPEN J Parenter Enteral Nutr.* 2007;31(5):388–396.

130. Aschner JL, Aschner M. Nutritional aspects of manganese homeostasis. *Mol Aspects Med.* 2005;26(4–5):353–362.

131. Dobson AW, Erikson KM, Aschner M. Manganese neurotoxicity. *Ann N Y Acad Sci.* 2004;1012:115–128.

132. Dickerson RN. Manganese intoxication and parenteral nutrition. *Nutrition.* 2001;17(7–8):689–693.

133. Hardy G. Manganese in parenteral nutrition: who, when, and why should we supplement? *Gastroenterology.* 2009;137(5 Suppl): S29–S35.

134. Stellman JM, International Labour Office. *Encyclopaedia of Occupational Health and Safety.* 4th ed. Geneva, Switzerland: International Labor Office; 1998.

135. Boosalis MG. The role of selenium in chronic disease. *Nutr Clin Pract.* 2008;23(2):152–160.

136. Shenkin A. Selenium in intravenous nutrition. *Gastroenterology.* 2009;137(5 Suppl):S61–S69.

137. Meplan C. Selenium and chronic diseases: a nutritional genomics perspective. *Nutrients.* 2015;7(5):3621–3651.

138. Moosmann B, Behl C. Selenoproteins, cholesterol-lowering drugs, and the consequences: revisiting of the mevalonate pathway. *Trends Cardiovasc Med.* 2004;14(7):273–281.

139. Andrews PJ. Selenium and glutamine supplements: where are we heading? A critical care perspective. *Curr Opin Clin Nutr Metab Care.* 2010;13(2):192–197.

140. Griffiths NM, Stewart RD, Robinson MF. The metabolism of [75Se]selenomethionine in four women. *Br J Nutr.* 1976;35(3): 373–382.

141. Ashton K, Hooper L, Harvey LJ, et al. Methods of assessment of selenium status in humans: a systematic review. *Am J Clin Nutr.* 2009;89(6):2025S–2039S.

142. Zimmermann MB, Crill CM. Iodine in enteral and parenteral nutrition. *Best Pract Res Clin Endocrinol Metab.* 2010;24(1): 143–158.

143. Kramer GH, Hauck BM, Chamberlain MJ. Biological half-life of iodine in adults with intact thyroid function and in athyreotic persons. *Radiat Prot Dosimetry.* 2002;102(2):129–135.

144. Moukarzel A. Chromium in parenteral nutrition: too little or too much? *Gastroenterology.* 2009;137(5 Suppl):S18–S28.

145. O'Flaherty EJ, Kerger BD, Hays SM, Paustenbach DJ. A physiologically based model for the ingestion of chromium(III) and chromium(VI) by humans. *Toxicol Sci.* 2001;60(2):196–213.

146. Tietz NW, Finley PR, Pruden E, Amerson AB. *Clinical Guide to Laboratory Tests.* 2nd ed. Philadelphia, PA: Saunders; 1990.

147. Broadhurst CL, Domenico P. Clinical studies on chromium picolinate supplementation in diabetes mellitus—a review. *Diabetes Technol Ther.* 2006;8(6):677–687.

148. Warren JJ, Levy SM. Current and future role of fluoride in nutrition. *Dent Clin North Am.* 2003;47(2):225–243.

149. Eren E, Ozturk M, Mumcu EF, Canatan D. Fluorosis and its hematological effects. *Toxicol Ind Health.* 2005;21(10):255–258.

150. Fluoride toothpaste use for young children. *J Am Dent Assoc.* 2014;145(2):190–191.

151. National Research Council. *Fluoride in Drinking Water: A Scientific Review of EPA's standards.* Washington, DC: National Academies Press; 2006. doi:10.17226/11571.

152. Schwarz G, Mendel RR. Molybdenum cofactor biosynthesis and molybdenum enzymes. *Annu Rev Plant Biol.* 2006;57:623–647.

153. Vyskocil A, Viau C. Assessment of molybdenum toxicity in humans. *J Appl Toxicol.* 1999;19(3):185–192.

154. Brown Bowman BA, Russell RM, International Life Sciences Institute–Nutrition Foundation. *Present Knowledge in Nutrition.* 9th ed. Washington, DC: ILSI Press; 2006.

155. Nielsen FH. Is boron nutritionally relevant? *Nutr Rev.* 2008;66(4): 183–191.

156. American Medical Association Department of Foods and Nutrition. Multivitamin preparations for parenteral use. A statement by the Nutrition Advisory Group. American Medical Association Department of Foods and Nutrition, 1975. *JPEN J Parenter Enteral Nutr.* 1979;3(4):258–262.

157. US Food and Drug Administration. Parenteral multivitamin products (notices). *Federal Register.* 2000;65(77):21200–21201.

158. Koutkia P, Lu Z, Chen TC, Holick MF. Treatment of vitamin D deficiency due to Crohn's disease with tanning bed ultraviolet B radiation. *Gastroenterology.* 2001;121(6):1485–1488.

159. Vanek VW, Borum P, Buchman A, et al. A.S.P.E.N. position paper: recommendations for changes in commercially available parenteral multivitamin and multi-trace element products. *Nutr Clin Pract.* 2012;27(4):440–491.

160. Vanek VW, Borum P, Buchman A, et al. A call to action to bring safer parenteral micronutrient products to the U.S. market. *Nutr Clin Pract.* 2015;30(4):559–569.

161. American Society for Parenteral and Enteral Nutrition Board of Directors. Clinical guidelines for the use of parenteral and enteral nutrition in adult and pediatric patients, 2009. *JPEN J Parenter Enteral Nutr.* 2009;33(3):255–259.

162. Bankhead R, Boullata J, Brantley S, et al. Enteral nutrition practice recommendations. *JPEN J Parenter Enteral Nutr.* 2009;33(2): 122–167.

163. Frias J, Vidal-Valverde C. Stability of thiamine and vitamins E and A during storage of enteral feeding formula. *J Agric Food Chem.* 2001;49(5):2313–2317.

164. Guenter P. Safe practices for enteral nutrition in critically ill patients. *Crit Care Nurs Clin North Am.* 2010;22(2):197–208.

CLINICAL FOUNDATIONS OF NUTRITION SUPPORT

9 Malnutrition Screening and Assessment

Andrea K. JeVenn, MEd, RD, LD, CNSC, Marianne Galang, RD, LD, CSO,
Peggy Hipskind, MA, RD, LD, and Christan Bury, MS, RD, LD, CNSC

CONTENTS

Acknowledgments: Gordon L. Jensen, MD, PhD, Pao Ying Hsiao, MS, RD, and Dara Wheeler, RD, were the authors of this chapter in the second edition.

Objectives

1. Review definitions of malnutrition, including those that recognize the impact of inflammation.
2. Describe the rationale for a comprehensive nutrition assessment.
3. Describe practical nutrition screening and assessment techniques suitable for routine clinical applications.
4. Demonstrate an approach to nutrition assessment that uses information from the patient's anthropometrics, medical and surgical history, family and social history, medication review, clinical presentation, biochemical data, nutrient intake data, and nutrition-focused physical examination.

Test Your Knowledge Questions

1. Which of the following is an example of a patient condition anticipated to manifest with a severe systemic inflammatory response?
   A. Anorexia nervosa with body mass index (BMI) of 15
   B. Major depression with compromised dietary intake and 5% loss of body weight
   C. Homebound older adult with restricted access to food and 10% loss of body weight
   D. Thermal burn injury of second and third degrees covering 15% body surface area

2. A physician informs you that a patient has a serum albumin of 2.8 g/dL and prealbumin of 14 mg/dL and asks whether these laboratory findings mean the patient is malnourished. What is the most appropriate response?
   A. The patient's protein intake is inadequate, and the patient should receive prompt nutrition support.
   B. Together, these markers indicate that the patient has moderate protein-energy malnutrition.
   C. Consideration of medical history, clinical diagnosis, and laboratory signs of the inflammatory response would help you interpret these findings.
   D. For most hospitalized patients, albumin and prealbumin have excellent sensitivity and specificity to identify malnutrition.

3. Which of the following is one of the best validated screening indicators for malnutrition risk?
   A. Patient reports a nonvolitional weight loss.
   B. Patient reports following a low-carbohydrate, weight loss diet.
   C. Patient is 2 days status post laparoscopic cholecystectomy.
   D. Patient reports a recent flu-like febrile illness.

Test Your Knowledge Answers

1. The correct answer is **D**. The burn injury is significant and will be associated with severe systemic inflammatory response. The diagnosis, clinical signs, physical examination data, and laboratory indicators for such a patient will support this conclusion. The other answers describe states of starvation that are not likely to be associated with severe systemic inflammatory response.

2. The correct answer is **C**. By themselves, these proteins should be interpreted with caution because they lack specificity and sensitivity as indicators of nutrition status. Both albumin and prealbumin may be reduced by the systemic response to injury, disease, or inflammation. Patients with low albumin or prealbumin levels may or may not be malnourished. The patient's medical history, clinical diagnosis, and laboratory signs of the inflammatory response can help clarify whether inflammation is present and whether the patient is malnourished.

3. The correct answer **A**. Of the options provided, the only well-validated indicator to screen for malnutrition risk is a nonvolitional weight loss. The other options might be noted in screening and assessment but are not themselves validated measures of malnutrition risk.

Introduction

Nutrition screening and assessment are integral tools used to direct the nutrition care of a patient. Each has the ability to detect malnutrition, but they are distinct from each other.[1] Nutrition screening is used "to identify an individual who may be malnourished or at risk for malnutrition and to determine if a comprehensive nutrition assessment is indicated."[2] Results from the screen may indicate the need for a complete nutrition assessment (for patients deemed at risk for malnutrition) or the need to rescreen at a future date (if the screen is negative).[1,3,4] A nutrition assessment is "a comprehensive approach to defining the nutrition state that uses a combination of the following: medical, nutrition, and medication histories; physical examination; anthropometric measurements; and laboratory data."[2] Comparatively, screening is a simpler and quicker means to identify individuals at nutrition risk, whereas assessment is a more rigorous evaluation to detect a variety of nutrition abnormalities, including malnutrition, and is the basis to guide therapeutic interventions, enhance nutrition status, and improve outcomes.[1] In the United States, both Centers for Medicare and Medicaid Services and the Joint Commission recognize the importance of screening and assessing patients for nutrition abnormalities.[3,4] US hospital policy makers are required to develop and implement strategies using a collaborative and interdisciplinary approach to determine individual patient needs through routine screening and assessment protocols.[4] Such activities can be accomplished by healthcare team members who have appropriate training, education, and scope of practice as defined by state laws.[4,5] Nutrition screening is usually performed by nursing staff on admission.[6,7] Screening and assessment practices are part of a continuous process that involves reevaluation and monitoring to ensure delivery of suitable nutrition interventions throughout the continuum of care.[1]

Malnutrition—or, more specifically, undernutrition—in hospitalized patients has been a documented concern for decades.[8,9] It has been associated with increased complications, such as poor wound healing, compromised immune status, impairment of organ functions, and increased mortality. Malnutrition is also associated with increased use of healthcare resources.

The prevalence of malnutrition is difficult to isolate and ranges from 30% to 50%, depending on the setting and criteria used to define it.[10,11] In 2010, only 3.2% of US hospital patients had a documented diagnosis of malnutrition at discharge.[11] Lack of practitioner awareness and confusion generated by various conflicting definitions and criteria of malnutrition have led to poor detection and treatment of undernutrition.[10,12,13] However, practitioners can increase identification of malnutrition through appropriate screening and assessment methods. To this end, this chapter describes notable approaches to adult malnutrition, including Subjective Global Assessment (SGA), the set of clinical characteristics proposed by the American Society for Parenteral and Enteral Nutrition (ASPEN) and the Academy of Nutrition and Dietetics (AND) as a means to define and improve reporting of malnutrition,[14] and the European Society for Clinical Nutrition and Metabolism (ESPEN)

2015 consensus statement that established criteria to diagnose malnutrition.[15] Practical nutrition screening and assessment techniques suitable for routine clinical applications are also reviewed.

Defining Malnutrition

Malnutrition (undernutrition) has been defined in many ways. All definitions include an inadequacy of nutrients to maintain a person's health that is caused by one or more of the following factors: insufficient intake, impaired absorption, increased nutrient requirements, and altered nutrient transport and utilization.[14] Beyond this broad conceptualization of malnutrition, definitions vary in their terminology and the criteria used to define this condition.[14,15] Clinicians have historically used SGA to diagnose malnutrition because it has been validated for use in many populations.[1,16,17] It is commonly used today; and the Canadian Nutrition Society has adopted it for diagnosing malnutrition.[18] Other nutrition societies have initiated alternate processes to consistently characterize elements of malnutrition.[14,15,18] In the United States, concerns brought forth by the Centers for Medicare and Medicaid Services, and a desire to promote a national standard for consistent diagnosis[19] prompted ASPEN and AND to develop an etiology-based methodology that incorporates the inflammatory process into the characterization of malnutrition in adults in clinical settings.[14] Subsequently, in 2015, ESPEN proposed a minimal set of straightforward, well-defined, and generally accepted parameters, independent from etiological factors, to identify malnutrition across a broad spectrum of patients.[15] These national and international efforts to find a unifying set of malnutrition characteristics aim to enhance clinical patient care, augment the legitimacy of nutrition practice, and, ultimately, expand the scientific field of nutrition.[15,19]

Role of Inflammation in Malnutrition

For many years, investigators and clinicians have recognized that infection is consistent with critical deterioration of lean body mass,[20,21] and such observations have led to the postulate that the identification of acute and chronic inflammation is integral to determine the etiology of malnutrition.[10] Therefore, SGA and the ASPEN/AND method attempt to evaluate the presence and severity of the inflammatory process and how inflammation contributes to a patient's malnutrition.[14,18,22] For example, SGA uses metabolic stress from disease as a proxy for inflammation.[18,22]

The onset of an inflammatory process begins with an insult to the body from pathogens, trauma, or other disease-causing agents. The ensuing inflammatory response increases cytokine production. Cytokines subsequently signal hepatocytes to suppress the production of negative acute-phase proteins in favor of freeing amino acids for production of positive acute-phase proteins.[23] Anorexia often accompanies inflammation, further compromising nutrition status. Some disorders and interventions may precipitate malnutrition because they adversely affect the body's ability to ingest or absorb nutrients, or because they impose diet restrictions or other limitations.

The presence of inflammation may reduce the effectiveness of nutrition interventions, and the associated malnutrition may, in turn, blunt the effectiveness of medical therapies.[24] During proinflammatory states, hepatic transport proteins, such as albumin and prealbumin, are poor indicators of nutrition status. The down regulation of negative acute-phase proteins allows for more amino acids to be used for producing positive acute-phase proteins, which help mitigate consequences of infection and modify the immune response.

Approaches to Diagnosing Malnutrition

Although this chapter focuses on 3 internationally recognized malnutrition assessment tools (SGA, the ASPEN/AND malnutrition characteristics, and the ESPEN diagnostic criteria), an abundance of other malnutrition assessment tools have been developed (see Table 9-1 for examples).[14,15,22,25-27] Historically, clinicians have also determined the severity of malnutrition by a variety of nonstandardized methods, such as depleted serum proteins, poor oral intake, and low BMI.

Subjective Global Assessment

SGA is a prominently used, validated, and reliable assessment tool for diagnosing nutrition status, which relies on the patient's medical history and physical assessment (see Figure 9-1).[16,17,22,28] SGA is comprised of 5 components that consider medical history (weight changes, dietary intake, gastrointestinal [GI] symptoms, functional capacity, and metabolic stress from disease) and 3 components focusing on physical examination (muscle wasting, fat depletion, and nutrition-related edema). The clinician subjectively tallies information obtained during the physical examination, and results are used to classify an individual as well nourished, moderately malnourished, or severely malnourished.[22] The SGA is not a specific grading system, but rather a weighted system where weight loss, oral intake, and physical assessment are most important for making clinical decisions. The remaining components of SGA (GI symptoms, functional capacity, and metabolic demand) are used to confirm clinician findings and are less influential for making a malnutrition diagnosis.[22] SGA attempts to account for inflammation by accounting for metabolic stress from disease as a proxy.[18,22] For patients who are critically ill, where SGA may have limited use, ASPEN and the Society of Critical Care Medicine recommend that clinicians use the Nutrition Risk Score (NRS-2003) or Nutrition Risk in Critically Ill (NUTRIC) tool to determine nutrition risk and plan appropriate interventions.[29] Practice Scenario 9-1 illustrates the clinical use of SGA.[22,30-32]

ASPEN/AND Classification

The etiology-based classification system developed by ASPEN/AND has elements similar to those of SGA (see Table 9-1), but the ASPEN/AND method includes a modern understanding of how proinflammatory states affect malnutrition and seeks to identify an etiology on a case-by-case basis as a framework for determining malnutrition. This approach recognizes

TABLE 9-1 Comparison of Nutrition Assessment Instruments

	SGA[22]	ASPEN/AND Malnutrition Clinical Characteristics[14]	ESPEN Consensus Statement[15]	MNA[25,26]	PG-SGA[27]
Nutrition history[a]	X	X	X	X	X
Biochemical data		X[b]		X	
Anthropometrics					
Weight change	X	X	X	X	X
BMI			X	X	
Other				X	
Physical examination					
Muscle mass	X	X	X		X
Fat stores	X	X			X
Fluid status	X	X			X
Functional capacity	X	X		X	X
Medical history					
GI symptoms	X				X
Medical conditions	X	X[b]			X
Neurologic issues				X	

AND, Academy of Nutrition and Dietetics; ASPEN, American Society for Parenteral and Enteral Nutrition; BMI, body mass index; ESPEN, European Society for Clinical Nutrition and Metabolism; GI, gastrointestinal; MNA, Mini Nutritional Assessment; PG-SGA, Scored Patient-Generated Subjective Global Assessment; SGA, Subjective Global Assessment.
[a]Intake and diet histories.
[b]Laboratory test data and medical history are used indirectly to assess level of inflammation.
Source: Data are from references 14, 15, 22, and 25–27.

3 underlying etiologies for malnutrition. The first etiology, social/environmental/behavioral circumstances, describes an absence of inflammation, such as pure starvation. The other etiologies, chronic illness and acute illness or injury, incorporate different degrees of inflammation. Chronic illness describes inflammation of a longer-term condition with a mild to moderate intensity. Acute illness or injury recognizes inflammation of a much greater intensity that is associated with a short-lived process.[14,33] Table 9-2 presents examples of medical conditions and their associated malnutrition etiology.[33,34] The table is not all-inclusive, and the determination of malnutrition etiology is subject to clinician judgment. The patient's medical diagnosis alone should not be used to determine the malnutrition etiology; consider all parameters for evidence of inflammation. Table 9-3 lists inflammatory markers that can assist in evaluating patients for the presence and severity of inflammation.[34] This table is also not all-inclusive; inflammatory markers should be considered within the larger scope of the patient's medical situation. For example, an acute exacerbation, infection, or other complication can be superimposed onto an existing chronic condition or disease.[14,33] Etiologies associated with a patient's malnutrition can also change over time because of the fluid nature of illness.[14]

Identifying the etiology of malnutrition is only part of the ASPEN/AND assessment process. Once the malnutrition etiology has been identified, the severity of malnutrition can be elucidated as moderate or severe (see Figure 9-2).[10,14,35] Two characteristics must be present to diagnosis malnutrition,

and the gravity of these factors establishes the severity of malnutrition.

Characteristics used in the ASPEN/AND classification can sometimes be ambiguous; for instance, a characteristic may not be related to nutrition (eg, edema during heart failure) or may not be present in individuals who are at high nutrition risk (eg, a previously healthy patient who is experiencing a trauma event).[14] For the severity of malnutrition to have a useful meaning to healthcare professionals and in research, the diagnosis requires a standardized methodology. In an attempt to improve objectivity and uniformity, ASPEN and AND developed 6 malnutrition clinical characteristics as part of their classification, which is built on the foundational principles of SGA. However, the ASPEN/AND approach has been criticized for its complexity, subjective interpretations of inflammation and disease burden, requirement of physical assessment skills, lack of recognition for body composition measures other than a physical examination, limitations of functional assessment, and the use of edema as a characteristic of malnutrition for this population.[18] This method of diagnosing malnutrition has yet to be validated, but studies of this nature are on the horizon. Practice Scenarios 9-2 and 9-3 illustrate the clinical application of ASPEN/AND recommendations for malnutrition assessment.[14,36–40]

ESPEN Criteria

The initial ESPEN consensus statement aimed to characterize malnutrition clearly and simply, without regard for

FIGURE 9-1 Decision Tree for Determining Severity of Malnutrition Using Subjective Global Assessment

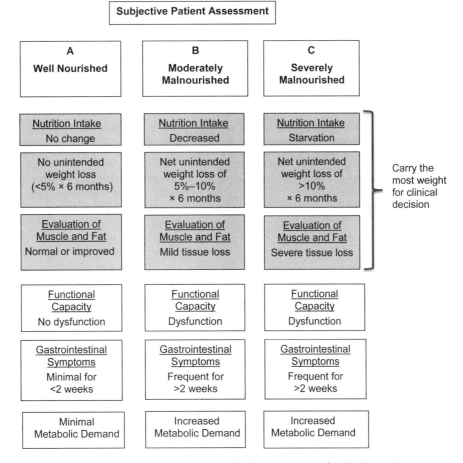

Select an option from each characteristic (intake, weight, physical assessment, functional capacity, gastrointestinal symptoms and metabolic demand), and then select the Subjective Global Assessment rank (A, B, C) based on subjective weight of the categories.
Source: Data are from reference 22.

inflammation as an etiology, so that the characterization could be generally applied to all patients independent of setting.[15] The ESPEN consensus established that (1) all criteria should be objective; (2) visceral proteins are not good prognostic indicators; (3) functional measures are not specific enough to assess nutrition; and (4) the final criteria would be few in number.[15] The 3 criteria chosen for evaluating malnutrition are unintentional weight loss, low BMI (as established by the World Health Organization, with allowances for age-specific variations), and decreased fat-free mass index (FFMI)[33] based on gender (see Figure 9-3 and Table 9-4).[14,15,18,22] Specific cutoff points were proposed for each characteristic, with clinicians analyzing the variables if a validated screening tool indicated the patient was at nutrition risk.[15] Further delineation for malnutrition severity was not described,[15] but a grading system has been proposed for future use.[18] The ESPEN consensus has been criticized as being overly restrictive, using parameters that are difficult to apply when assessing obese populations, and relying on body composition measures that are

not universally available in all settings.[18] Like the ASPEN/AND methodology, ESPEN's process has not yet been validated. Practice Scenario 9-4 illustrates the use of the ESPEN malnutrition assessment criteria in clinical practice.[15,31,41–43]

Nutrition Screening

The Joint Commission requires nutrition screening programs for most US healthcare facilities (ie, acute and long-term care) for the purpose of systematically identifying individuals at nutrition risk.[4] Many screening tools share similar elements, despite the lack of standards establishing the essential components or the qualifications of the person using the screen.[6] The screening process typically involves use of an instrument, such as the Malnutrition Screening Tool (MST) or NUTRIC score[29] or a set of standardized criteria that aids in quickly determining whether additional information is required to warrant a nutrition intervention. During the nutrition screen, the individual is assigned a level of nutrition risk based on a

Practice Scenario 9-1

Question: According to Subjective Global Assessment (SGA) criteria,[22] what severity of malnutrition best describes a patient who presents with cirrhosis complicated by portal hypertension, ascites, and edema?

Scenario: A 52-year-old man presented with an established history of cirrhosis and portal hypertension in the setting of long-term ethanol abuse. He had gained 10 pounds (4.5 kg) over the prior 2 weeks and exhibited massive ascites. Additional findings included mild encephalopathy (grade 1) with poor concentration, asterixis, and scleral icterus.

Upon admission, his clinical and laboratory criteria included the following: temperature, 36.7°C (normal: 36.1–37.2°C); albumin, 1.7 g/dL (normal: 3.9–4.9 g/dL); prealbumin, 6.8 mg/dL (normal: 17–36 mg/dL); white blood cell count, 3900/mcL (normal: 3700–11,000/mcL); total bilirubin, 3.8 mg/dL (normal: 0.2–1.3 mg/dL); aspartate aminotransferase, 96 IU/L (normal: 6–40 IU/L); alanine aminotransferase, 111 IU/L (normal: 20–60 IU/L); alkaline phosphatase, 162 IU/L (normal: 44–147 IU/L); and prothrombin time, 18 seconds (normal: 11–14 seconds).

A family member reported that the patient's food intake had been severely compromised for at least 1 month. Upon further probing, the family member reported intakes less than 50% of the patient's usual intakes. The patient complained of chronic early satiety, loss of appetite, and diarrhea due to lactulose. At presentation, the patient was 68 inches (172.7 cm) in height and weighed 161 pounds (73 kg). Family reported his usual weight as approximately 150 pounds (68 kg).

Physical findings were notable for ascites as well as grade 3–4+ lower extremity edema. The physical examination was limited because of fluid retention but revealed severe subcutaneous fat loss in the triceps and chest and severe muscle wasting in the deltoids. Muscle wasting in the quadriceps could not be assessed because of edema. The patient had physical limitations and spent most of his time lying in bed or sitting in a chair.

Intervention: Promote adequate energy intake with balanced macronutrients, sodium-restricted diet, and replacement of appropriate micronutrients (refer to Chapter 27). The patient may benefit from protein-energy supplements and vitamin/mineral replacement.

Answer: The patient's SGA ranking is C: Severely Malnourished. Malnutrition is identified by his poor nutrition intake, muscle wasting, and loss of subcutaneous fat, and supported by data showing his decreased functional capacity, persistent gastrointestinal symptoms for greater than 2 weeks, and increased metabolic demand (see Figure 9-1).

Rationale: Cirrhosis is a condition with an increased metabolic demand that is consistent with characteristics of moderately or severely malnourished (SGA rankings B and C, respectively).[22] Abnormal liver function tests (total bilirubin, aspartate aminotransferase, alanine aminotransferase, alkaline phosphatase, albumin, prothrombin time, and prealbumin) are consistent with a diagnosis

of liver failure and cannot be reliably interpreted to support malnutrition.[30] The presence of gastrointestinal symptoms for more than 2 weeks (SGA rankings B and C) is considered significant and has prevented adequate intake.[22]

The patient's family reported food intakes to be less than 50% of usual intake for 1 month (SGA ranking C). This finding is consistent with severe, prolonged, restricted energy intake and helps support a diagnosis of malnutrition.[22]

In this case, ascites and severe edema are the major contributors to the patient's weight change, masking any true losses that may be occurring. It is not feasible to use weight change as reliable evidence supporting a diagnosis of malnutrition for this patient.

Muscle in the lower extremities was difficult to evaluate because of fluid accumulation but the physical examination identified severe muscle loss of the deltoids (SGA ranking C) and subcutaneous fat loss of the triceps and chest (SGA ranking C). These findings are concerning in a patient who has not been eating well for a prolonged period of time and are suggestive of improper nutrition when all other causes have been ruled out.[22] If available, other body composition measures, such as dual-energy x-ray absorptiometry, computed tomography, and magnetic resonance imaging, may be used to demonstrate and confirm loss of muscle and subcutaneous fat.[31,32]

Ascites and lower extremity edema are indicative of cirrhosis and are not a direct result of malnutrition in this patient. In this situation, edema and ascites interfere with the clinician's accurate evaluation of weight loss.

A notable indication of physical decline is seen by the increased time he spends in a bed or chair (SGA rankings B and C). His functional decline may be related to malnutrition, but it is not the sole, definitive cause.

set of standardized guidelines. Risk levels guide how quickly the individual must be rescreened or assessed. According to a 2014 survey,[6] most facilities screen patients on admission or within 24 hours of admission. Nurses perform screens most frequently, but it is not uncommon for dietitians to screen patients also. In this survey, 38% of respondents indicated that a validated screening tool was used, and the most frequently reported tools were MST, Nutrition Risk Classification, Simple Screening Tool, and SGA.[6] Refer to Table 9-5 for a list of commonly used screening tools that have been assessed and validated.[25,26,29,44–53]

Nutrition Assessment

Nutrition assessment is an in-depth, systematic process that aims to integrate and interpret various forms of data about a patient to identify nutrition-related problems.[54] The elements of a nutrition assessment include anthropometrics, client history (medical and surgical history, family and social history, and medication review), current clinical presentation, biochemical data, nutrient intake data, nutrition-focused physical examination findings, and functional status. These considerations are all important when thoroughly evaluating the nutrition status of a patient.[55]

TABLE 9-2 Inflammatory States Associated with Various Medical/Surgical Diagnoses

Malnutrition Etiology	Associated Inflammatory Condition	Common Medical/Surgical Diagnosis
Acute illness/injury (short duration)	Heightened, intense inflammatory response	Critical illness; major infection/sepsis; adult respiratory distress syndrome; systemic inflammatory response syndrome; severe burns; major abdominal surgery; multitrauma; closed head injury; severe acute pancreatitis; postoperative ileus
Chronic illness (≥3-month duration)	Mild to moderate inflammatory response	Cardiovascular disease; congestive heart failure; cystic fibrosis; inflammatory bowel disease; celiac disease; chronic pancreatitis; rheumatoid arthritis; solid tumors; hematologic malignancies; sarcopenic obesity; diabetes mellitus; metabolic syndrome; cerebrovascular accident; neuromuscular disease; dementia; organ failure/transplant of the kidney, liver, heart, lung, or gut; periodontal disease; pressure wounds; chronic obstructive pulmonary disease; HIV; lupus; small bowel obstruction; prolonged ileus
Social/behavioral/environmental circumstances	No inflammatory response	Starvation; anorexia nervosa; compromised food intake in the setting of financial disparity; dementia; alcohol/drug abuse; pain; small bowel obstruction

Source: Data are from references 33 and 34.

TABLE 9-3 Suggested Parameters to Assess for the Presence of Inflammation

Biochemical data:
- Depleted albumin, prealbumin, transferrin
- Elevated CRP, ferritin
- Hyperglycemia
- Leukocytosis, leukopenia
- Thrombocytopenia

Microbiological data:
- Urine cultures (urinary tract infection)
- Blood cultures (bloodstream infections)
- Fecal cultures (gastrointestinal infections)
- Bodily fluid cultures (infected abscess, pleural fluid, sputum, ascites)

Imaging:
- Chest x-ray (pneumonia, infiltrations, inflammation)
- CT, MRI, PET scan; abdominal/pelvic x-ray (abscess, pancreatitis, cancer, inflammatory process, bowel obstruction)
- Gastric emptying study/small bowel follow-through (gastroparesis, dysmotility)
- EGD/colonoscopy (IBD, radiation enteritis, GVHD, gastritis, ulcers, fistula, strictures)
- ECHO (vegetation, endocarditis)

Clinical manifestations:
- Fever, hypothermia, chills, night sweats
- Tachycardia, low blood pressure
- Rashes; skin redness, swelling, tenderness
- Discharge from eyes or nose
- Swelling or redness of mouth and gums
- Pain with urination, productive cough, burns

CRP, C-reactive protein; CT, computed tomography; ECHO: echocardiogram; EGD: esophagogastroduodenoscopy; GVHD: graft-versus-host disease; IBD: inflammatory bowel disease; MRI, magnetic resonance imaging; PET, positron emission tomography.
Source: Data are from reference 34.

FIGURE 9-2 Practical Application Process to Determine Etiology and Severity of Malnutrition Using the ASPEN/AND Clinical Characteristics

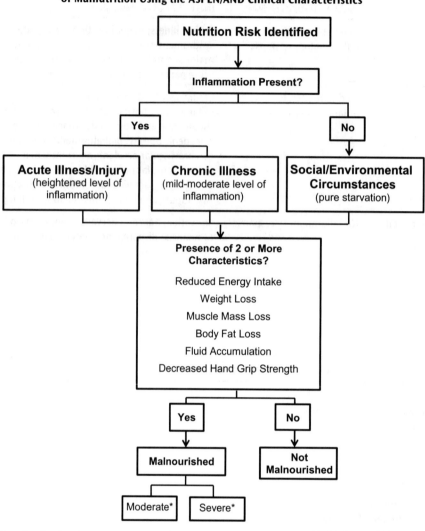

*Severity of malnutrition determined by seriousness of characteristics, as defined by ASPEN and AND malnutrition criteria. AND, Academy of Nutrition and Dietetics; ASPEN; American Society for Parenteral and Enteral Nutrition.
Source: Data are from references 10, 14, and 35.

Practice Scenario 9-2

Question: According to the American Society for Parenteral and Enteral Nutrition and Academy of Nutrition and Dietetics criteria for malnutrition,[14] what etiology and severity of malnutrition best describes a patient who presents with anorexia nervosa?

Scenario: A 36-year-old woman was admitted to the hospital with a diagnosis of anorexia nervosa and a long-standing history of restrictive eating behavior without purging. Her typical intakes were described as being less than 500 kcal/d for at least the past year. She reported a highly active lifestyle and exercises in excess of 2 h/d. Upon admission, her clinical and laboratory criteria included the following: temperature, 37°C (normal: 36.1°C–37.2°C); resting heart rate, 50 bpm (normal:

60–100 bpm); albumin, 4.0 g/dL (normal: 3.9–4.9 g/dL); prealbumin, 25 mg/dL (normal: 17–36 mg/dL); C-reactive protein, 0.7 mg/dL (normal: <1.0 mg/dL); white blood cell count, 6200/mcL (normal: 3700–11,000/mcL); and fasting glucose, 75 mg/dL (normal: 65–100 mg/dL).

Upon admission, the patient was 66 inches (167.6 cm) in height and weighed 92.6 pounds (42 kg), with a body mass index (BMI) of 15. Four weeks prior, she weighed 97.9 pounds (44.5 kg), and 6 months ago, she weighed 123.6 pounds (56.2 kg). The nutrition-focused physical examination findings were as follows:

- Subcutaneous fat loss: severe orbital, triceps, and midaxillary line losses.
- Muscle loss: severe wasting in temporalis, pectoralis, deltoid, interosseous, latissimus dorsi, quadricep, and gastrocnemius muscles.

- Lanugo and dry mucus membranes.
- Marked underweight status was evident, and weight loss of 41.6 pounds (18.9 kg) had occurred over 6 months.

Intervention: The clinicians resuscitated the patient cautiously to avoid refeeding syndrome while continually reassessing her nutrition status. Establishing a baseline for serum markers and intake and ouput records is recommended to help with monitoring and managing refeeding syndrome (see Chapters 13 and 17). Suggested daily assessment includes, but is not limited to, orthostatic vital signs, daily weight, fluid retention and shifts, intakes and outputs, and laboratory indicators (sodium, potassium, phosphorus, and magnesium). The initial energy goal may be set at 1500 kcal/d for women or 1750 kcal/d for men. Providing this amount of energy, in conjunction with potassium and phosphorus supplementation, can help with stabilize electrolyte levels during refeeding.[36]

Answer: The etiology of this patient's malnutrition is social/behavioral/environmental circumstances. Based on her energy intake, muscle and fat wasting, and significant weight loss, her malnutrition is characterized as severe protein-energy malnutrition.

Rationale: History, clinical diagnosis, and laboratory markers determine the etiological framework of the patient's malnutrition. Anorexia nervosa is consistent with starvation without an inflammatory component. Restrictive eating behaviors and weight loss support this diagnosis. Review of the patient's laboratory test data finds no signs of active inflammation. In the absence of inflammation, albumin and prealbumin and most other laboratory results typically remain within normal ranges.[37]

The patient's compromised energy and protein intake over the past year provided less than 50% of her needs for at least 1 month. Her weight loss is categorized as a severe loss because she lost 5.6% of her body weight over 1 month and 25% of her body weight over 6 months.[14] Additionally, her BMI indicates underweight status. No edema was noted at the time of assessment. Orthostatic vital signs are indicative of malnutrition and dehydration. Dehydration is also suggested by her noticeably dry, cracked lips and mucus membranes, but dehydration alone cannot account for the patient's drastic weight decline over 6 months. The nutrition-focused physical examination of muscle and fat revealed severe muscle and fat wasting, which is consistent with anorexia nervosa.[37] Furthermore, lanugo development is typically a result of loss of adipose stores.[38]

Handgrip dynamometry is recommended to assess handgrip strength, which has been correlated to nutrition status,[39] but it was not performed in this scenario because the patient had an active lifestyle and her functional status did not seem to be a relevant characteristic of her state of malnourishment.

Practice Scenario 9-3

Question: According to American Society for Parenteral and Enteral Nutrition (ASPEN) and Academy of Nutrition and Dietetics (AND) criteria for malnutrition,[14] what etiology and severity of malnutrition best describes a multiple trauma victim early in his course of recovery?

Scenario: A previously healthy 38-year-old man experienced multitrauma secondary to a motor vehicle accident. A computed tomography (CT) scan revealed a ruptured spleen, grade III liver laceration, left femur fracture, and bilateral pulmonary contusions. He underwent damage control celiotomy, splenectomy, and packing of the liver and then was transferred on a ventilator to the trauma intensive care unit, where he continued to be resuscitated. Upon admission, his clinical and laboratory criteria for systemic inflammatory response syndrome included the following: temperature, 39.2°C (normal: >38°C or <36°C); heart rate, 112 bpm (normal: >90 bpm); respiratory rate, 26 breaths/min (normal: >20 breaths/min); white blood cell count, 2100/mcL (normal: >12,000/mcL); and partial pressure of carbon dioxide (PCO_2), 30 mm Hg (normal: less than 32 mm Hg).

His family reported that the patient's usual body weight was 190 pounds (86.4 kg), and they said that he had not experienced any weight or diet changes prior to the injury. He was also fairly active in recreational sports when he was not at work.

He was markedly edematous, weighing 15 pounds (6.8 kg) more than his usual body weight with the bed scale reading 205 pounds. He was 73 inches (185.4 cm) in height, and his BMI was 25.1 (based on his family's report of a usual weight of prior to hospitalization). His open abdomen was dressed. The physical examination was limited because of hemodynamic instability (severe edema in the quadriceps and moderate edema in the gastrocnemius and interosseous muscles), body positioning, and the use of restraints. Muscle mass evaluation could only be performed in the temporal region and the upper chest and shoulder areas (muscles in these areas appeared normal). No subcutaneous fat loss was noted in the orbital area, and muscle loss was not seen in the temporalis, pectoralis, or deltoid muscles.

Indirect calorimetry showed that he had an increased metabolic rate with a resting energy expenditure of 2750 kcal/d. The family reported that the last time he ate was the evening before the injury. Because the medical team anticipated that oral nutrition intake would be compromised for a week or longer, enteral nutrition (EN) was started within 24 hours of admission. A complete nutrition assessment was unable to classify this patient's severity of malnutrition on hospital Day 2, but his Nutrition Risk in Critically Ill (NUTRIC) score was calculated to be 5, and a plan was initiated to provide EN via orogastric access.

Over the next 7 days, the patient underwent various surgeries, procedures, and tests to address his complex medical issues. During that time, a CT scan found intra-abdominal fluid collection, which required drainage, and also showed diminished muscle mass at the lumbar 3 region. Enteral feeds, while tolerated, had been frequently turned on and off and provided an average of 65% to 70% of his estimated needs.

At a subsequent nutrition assessment, his clinical laboratory data were as follows: temperature, 38.9°C (normal: 36.1–37.2°C); heart rate, 98 bpm (normal: 60–100 bpm); respiratory rate, 26 breaths/min (normal: 12–20 breaths/min); white blood cell count, 16,500/mcL (normal: 3700–11,000/mcL); C-reactive protein, 11.6 mg/dL (normal: less than 1.0 mg/dL); albumin, 2.6 g/dL (normal: 3.9–4.9 g/dL); prealbumin, 11.0 mg/dL (normal: 17–36 mg/dL); fasting glucose, 180 mg/dL (normal: 65–100 mg/dL).

His physical examination found no subcutaneous fat loss in the orbital area, triceps, or midaxillary line. There was mild wasting in the temporalis and pectoralis muscles but none in the deltoids. Muscle loss elsewhere could not be assessed because of moderate or severe edema (interosseous, quadricep, gastrocnemius muscles) or body position (latissimus dorsi).

Intervention: Enteral feedings (an immune-modulating formula) were initiated within 24 hours of admission (see Chapters 10, 13, and 24).

Answer: Using the ASPEN/AND criteria, the etiology of this patient's malnutrition was acute illness/injury and indicated by inadequate nutrition intake and muscle loss. The malnutrition was of moderate severity.

Rationale: Multiple trauma requiring urgent surgical interventions and procedures is consistent with acute systemic inflammatory response. Further evidence of this heightened inflammatory response is seen in laboratory markers: leukocytosis, elevated C-reactive protein with depressed albumin and prealbumin levels, and hyperglycemia without a history of diabetes. Signs of severe acute systemic inflammatory response are caused by hormonal, metabolic, and immunological mediators that include cytokines. Nutrition intervention is intended to support vital immune system, wound healing, and organ system functions to help the patient through this phase of acute inflammatory response. Trauma victims are often not malnourished at baseline, but they are at risk of becoming severely malnourished due to acute metabolic dysregulation and associated catabolism.

Prior to his injury, the patient was eating normally. After injury, he was at risk for an extended duration of compromised nutrient intake during a time of significant catabolism, and clinicians therefore decided to initiate EN promptly. Despite this proactive decision, medical interventions took priority, and tube feeds were not consistently infused, so he was only able to receive an average of 65% to 70% of his estimated needs over the prior week. Even with aggressive nutrition support during this acute phase, trauma patients will likely remain in negative nitrogen balance and have low albumin and prealbumin due to the marked proinflammatory state.[40] Provision of less than adequate EN contributes to a picture of malnutrition in this situation.

Determining accurate body mass changes over a specific time period was not feasible for this patient. Because of the appreciable edema, observed weight changes would not help the clinician to further support a diagnosis of malnutrition.

The patient's BMI before the injury was normal and may provide a generalized idea of his baseline physique. The patient did not appear wasted in the first examination, but it was difficult to fully assess muscle and fat stores. Further into his hospitalization, some signs of muscle wasting started to emerge at the clavicle and temporalis. This loss was confirmed by reviewing CT scans focusing on musculature at the L3 region. No decline in adipose tissue was obvious. It has been demonstrated that significant amounts of muscle mass can be lost during the first week in an intensive care setting.[40]

The initial physical examination revealed anasarca and pitting edema of the dependent areas and lower extremities, making muscle and fat store evaluation, as well as weight loss, quite difficult. At follow-up, the severity of upper body edema abated, while persisting in the lower extremities. Fluid accumulation of this

magnitude and immediacy are indicative of the patient's medical problems and treatment course, not nutrition status.

Handgrip dynamometry is recommended to assess handgrip strength, which has been correlated to nutrition status,[39] but grip strength and physical performance testing are not feasible in an acutely injured and sedated patient.

The amount and type of information obtained will be influenced by the health status of the patient, clinical setting, use of evolving evidence-based practices, and whether the evaluation is an initial assessment or a reassessment.[54] Multi-item assessment instruments (Table 9-5) have been developed to assist in identifying indicators of nutrition status.

Anthropometric Data

The anthropometric measures used in nutrition assessment are relatively simple physical measurements that provide information about body size and composition. Findings are compared with standards (for the same gender and age) and/or with previous measurements of the same individual. Trends can be particularly useful in assessment.

Height

Accurate measurement of height is indicated because a variety of anthropometric measures are standardized for height. When individuals are able to stand without assistance, height should be measured in a standing position, without shoes, using a wall-mounted stadiometer. For adults who are unable to stand, height can be estimated by doubling the arm span measurement (from the patient's sternal notch to the end of the longest finger). Stature in older persons can also be estimated from knee height measured with a caliper device, as follows:[56]

Men: Stature (cm) = [2.02 × Knee Height (cm)] – [0.04 × Age (y)] + 64.19

Women: Stature (cm) = [1.83 × Knee Height (cm)] – [0.24 × Age (y)] + 84.8

Body Weight

Actual measured body weight and weight change trends are particularly important components of nutrition assessment. Weight should be measured on admission to a clinical area, then re-evaluated frequently throughout the duration of the stay.[14] To improve accuracy and reliability of body weight measures, individuals who can stand should be weighed in a consistent manner, without shoes or overgarments. Chair and bed scales are available for those who cannot stand. These instruments should be used according to manufacturers' guidelines for the most accurate results.

Clinicians need to interpret weights as part of the larger clinical presentation. For example, among individuals with substantial disease burden, measures of weight can be erroneously skewed by factors such as dehydration, excessive fluid accumulation, or presence of tumors.[34,57]

FIGURE 9-3 Decision Tree to Determine Presence of Malnutrition Using the ESPEN Criteria

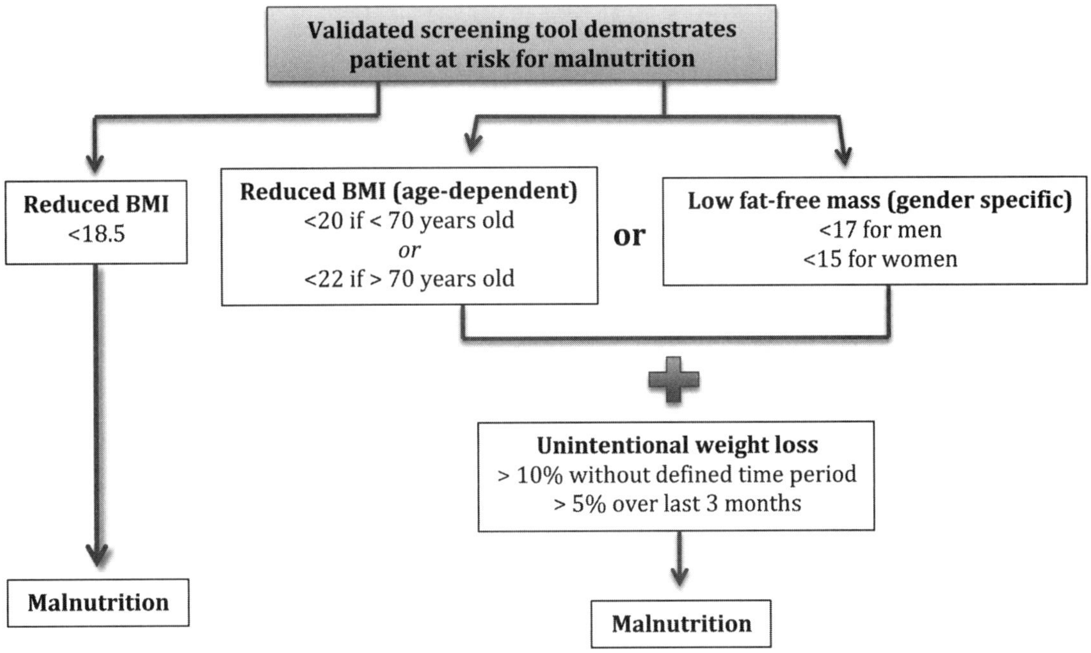

BMI, body mass index; ESPEN, European Society for Clinical Nutrition and Metabolism.
Source: Data are from reference 18.

TABLE 9-4 Comparison of SGA, ASPEN/AND, and ESPEN Nutrition Assessment Methods

	SGA[22]	ASPEN/AND[14]	ESPEN[15]
Laboratory markers	• Not used	• Used to determine presence of inflammation	• Not recommended

Physical examination	• Muscle wasting:
	  – Quadriceps
	  – Deltoids
	• Fat depletion:
	  – Triceps
	  – Chest
	• Nutrition-related edema:
	  – Ankle
	  – Sacral area
	  – Ascites
		• Muscle wasting:
		  – Temporalis
		  – Pectoralis
		  – Deltoids
		  – Scapular
		  – Interosseous
		  – Quadriceps
		  – Gastrocnemius
		• Fat depletion:
		  – Orbital
		  – Triceps
		  – Midaxillary at the iliac crest
		• Fluid accumulation:
		  – Nutrition-related edema
		  – Effect on weight
			• FFMI:
			  – Men: <17
			  – Women: <15
			• BMI:
			  – <18.5 or
			  – <20 for persons age <70 y
			  – <22 for persons age ≥70 y

Medical history	• Weight changes • Nutrition intake • GI symptoms • Functional capacity • Metabolic stress from disease	• Unintentional weight loss • Nutrition intake • Functional capacity • Chronic illness, acute illness, or social/behavioral/environmental circumstances	• Unintentional weight loss (also inclusive of decreased food intake, appetite loss, nutrient requirement/intake imbalances)

AND, Academy of Nutrition and Dietetics; ASPEN, American Society for Parenteral and Enteral Nutrition; BMI, body mass index; ESPEN, European Society for Clinical Nutrition and Metabolism; FFMI, fat-free mass index; GI, gastrointestinal; SGA, Subjective Global Assessment.
Source: Data are from references 14, 15, and 22.

Practice Scenario 9-4

Question: According to the European Society for Clinical Nutrition and Metabolism (ESPEN) consensus,[15] would an elderly patient who presents to clinic with obesity and frailty be considered malnourished?

Scenario: A 70-year-old woman presented for a follow-up clinic appointment with long-standing obesity, osteoarthritis, type 2 diabetes, hypercholesterolemia, and metabolic syndrome. Her medications included a statin, a diabetes oral agent, and a nonsteroidal anti-inflammatory. Her chief complaint was worsening knee pain and swelling that interfered with her mobility. She lived in her own home but was generally house-bound. An adult daughter accompanied the patient and reported that her mother had been running a low-grade fever intermittently at home over the past week.

Vital sign and laboratory tests revealed the following: temperature, 37.9°C (normal: 36.1–37.2°C); resting heart rate, 96 bpm (normal: 60–100 bpm); blood pressure, 135/85 mm Hg (normal: <120/<80 mm Hg); albumin, 3.2 g/dL (normal: 3.9–4.9 g/dL); C-reactive protein: 3.1 mg/dL (normal: <1.0 mg/dL); white blood cell count, 14,100/mcL (normal: 3700–11,000/mcL); fasting glucose, 142 mg/dL (normal: 65–100 mg/dL); glycated hemoglobin A1C, 7.0% (normal: 4%–5.6%); cholesterol, 180 mg/dL (normal: <200 mg/dL); high-density lipoprotein cholesterol, 45 mg/dL (normal: 40–59 mg/dL); and triglycerides, 125 mg/dL (normal: <150 mg/dL).

The daughter checked on her mother once a week and brought meals during those visits. The patient described feeling disinterested in food, getting full quickly, and experiencing occasional nausea for the past 3 to 4 weeks. She estimated food consumption of one-half to two-thirds of her usual meal intake during that time. She indicated that she might have lost 10 to 20 pounds (4.5 to 9 kg) over the past 6 months without trying and said her pants fit more loosely than usual.

Upon evaluation, her height was 62 inches (157.5 cm), weight was 180 pounds (81.8 kg), and body mass index (BMI) was 33. A review of her medical records confirmed a 20-pound (9-kg) weight loss since her last visit 6 months ago and documented a usual weight of 200 pounds. The patient had difficulty pulling herself from a seated position in the chair and ambulating. Furthermore, she reported feeling less energetic for the past 2 months, which she associated with worsening knee discomfort. An intake nurse used the Mini Nutritional Assessment–Short Form (MNA-SF) to screen this patient, which resulted in a low score.

Physical examination revealed truncal adiposity with a waist circumference of 90 cm (35.4 inches). The physical examination elicited limited information about muscle and fat stores; although the patient insisted she was thinner than usual, only mild muscle loss could be observed in the temporalis and along her clavicle bone. Her fat-free mass index (FFMI) was calculated to be 12 based on results from a recent bioelectric impedance analysis (BIA).

Intervention: Clinicians encouraged the patient to follow a consistent carbohydrate diet regimen with regular, high-quality meals and snacks (see Chapter 34) and supplement with a daily multivitamin with minerals. In view of her lipid profile on statin therapy, additional restriction of cholesterol or fat did not seem warranted while addressing her other nutrition problems. Family engagement was encouraged, and social services were consulted about participation with Meals on Wheels and a diabetes management team.

Answer: According to the ESPEN consensus statement, this patient is malnourished (see Figure 9-3) due to weight loss and a low FFMI.

Rationale: The patient's decreased food intake over the past month, occasional nausea, early satiety, and disinterest in food contributed to the patient's low MNA-SF score during the nutrition screen. These issues could further be compounded by her homebound status and limited resources. Her reports of lower-than-usual food intakes, in the context of weight loss and physical symptoms of muscle loss, are concerning.

Although the patient unintentionally lost 10% of her usual body weight over the last 6 months, her BMI and waist circumference at presentation were consistent with obesity. Individuals who are obese may be at risk for malnutrition or malnourished (see Chapter 35).[41,42] In this case, the patient's BMI did not reflect a diagnosis of malnutrition according to the ESPEN consensus criteria; however, her unexpected weight loss, which occurred as a result of diminished nutrition intake, did.[15]

Based solely on physical examination, it is difficult to subjectively quantify changes in total adiposity in individuals with obesity; however, the patient stated that her pants were looser, which likely indicated losses along the midaxillary line. Loss of muscle mass can also be difficult to observe and palpate in obese patients, but information provided by BIA allowed for better quantification of FFMI deficits than BMI alone would have provided.[43] While FFMI attempts to distinguish whether tissue is muscle or adipose, it is important to note that fat-free mass includes organs, connective tissue, and bone, along with skeletal and nonskeletal muscle.[31] According to ESPEN consensus, women whose FFMI is below 15 can be considered malnourished if accompanied by a significant amount of weight loss (5% in the last 3 months or 10% over an undefined period of time).[15] Other body composition measures, such as computed tomography, dual-energy x-ray absorptiometry, or magnetic resonance imaging, may be used to demonstrate loss of muscle and to confirm sarcopenic obesity.[15]

Reference tables of standards for ideal body weight relative to height, such as the Metropolitan Height and Weight Tables,[58] are not routinely recommended for use because they suffer notable limitations, including subjective interpretation of frame size and inadequate availability of reference data for many population groups. Ideal body weight may be of use for specific disease states and conditions as a means to determine energy and protein needs for certain patients, but there is no agreement on the consistent use of this parameter for nutrition assessment. For patients who are ill, usual body weight is a more suitable parameter than ideal body weight.[54]

Body Mass Index

BMI is a ratio of body weight to height:

$$BMI = \text{Weight (kg)/Height (m)}^2$$

TABLE 9-5 Selected Nutrition Screening Instruments and Their Characteristics

Instrument	Nutrition-Related Indicators	Severity of Illness Indicators	Intended Population, Validity, and Reliability

MNA-SF[25,26,44,46]	• Unintentional weight loss
	• Appetite
	• Food intake problem
		• Disease severity
		• Homebound
		• Dementia/depression
			• Ambulatory and subacute patients:
			  – 98%–100% sensitivity
			  – 70%–100% specificity
			  – Reliability: no data
			• Hospitalized, elderly patients:[a]
			  – 100% sensitivity
			  – 52.8% specificity
			  – AUC: 0.95

MST[44–46]	• Appetite
	• Unintentional weight loss
		• Not applicable	• Oncology patients:
			  – 100% sensitivity
			  – 81%–92% specificity
			  – Reliability: $\kappa = 0.83$–0.88
			• Acute, hospitalized patients:
			  – 74%–93% sensitivity
			  – 76%–93% specificity
			  – Reliability: $\kappa = 0.84$–0.93
			• Hospitalized, elderly patients:[a]
			  – 90.3% sensitivity
			  – 84.7% specificity
			  – AUC: 0.92

MUST[44,45,47]	• BMI
	• Unintentional weight loss
	• Problems with food intake
		• Disease severity	• Hospitalized, medical-surgical patients:
			  – 61% sensitivity
			  – 76% specificity
			  – Agreement between MUST and SGA: $\kappa = 0.26$
			• Hospitalized, elderly patients:[a]
			  – 87.1% sensitivity
			  – 86.1% specificity
			  – AUC: 0.89

Simple, 2-Part[44]	• Unintentional weight loss
	• Subcutaneous fat loss
		• Not applicable	• Acute, hospitalized patients:
			  – 63% sensitivity
			  – 97% specificity
			  – Reliability: no data

NST/BAPEN[44]	• Unintentional weight loss
	• Appetite
	• Weight
	• Height
	• Food intake problem
		• Not applicable	• Acute, hospitalized patients:
			  – 86% sensitivity
			  – 95% specificity
			  – Reliability: $\kappa = 0.66$

NRS-2002[44,45,48]	• Unintentional weight loss
	• BMI
		• Disease severity
		• Impaired general condition
		• Age >70 years
			• Acute, hospitalized patients:
			  – 39%–70% sensitivity
			  – 83%–85% specificity
			  – Agreement with SGA: 79.2%
			  – Agreement with MNA: 84.6%
			• Hospitalized medical-surgical patients:
			  – 62% sensitivity
			  – 93% specificity
			  – Agreement with SGA: $\kappa = 0.48$
			• Hospitalized, elderly patients:[a]
			  – 90.3% sensitivity
			  – 83.3% specificity
			  – AUC: 0.89

(continued)

TABLE 9-5 Selected Nutrition Screening Instruments and Their Characteristics *(continued)*

Instrument	Nutrition-Related Indicators	Severity of Illness Indicators	Intended Population, Validity, and Reliability

SNAQ[45,49–51]	• Unintentional weight loss
	• Decreased appetite
	• Use of supplemental drinks/tube feeds
		• Not applicable	• Hospitalized, medical-surgical patients:
			  – 76%–88% sensitivity
			  – 83%–91% specificity
			  – AUC: 0.85
			  – Reliability: κ = 0.69
			• Hospitalized, medical-surgical patients:
			  – 81.5% sensitivity
			  – 76.4% specificity
			• Hospitalized, elderly patients:[a]
			  – 79% sensitivity
			  – 90.3% specificity
			  – AUC: 0.93

NUTRIC Score[29,52,53]	• Not applicable	• APACHE II
		• SOFA (with or without IL-6)
		• Number of comorbidities
		• Days from hospital to ICU admission
			• Critically ill patients:
			  – Predictive of 28-day mortality (C-index 0.783)
			  – Among 28-day survivors, strongly associated with days observed on mechanical ventilation (P <0.0001)
			  – Recommended to assist with identification of critically ill patients most likely to gain from aggressive nutrition interventions

APACHE, Acute Physiology and Chronic Health Evaluation; AUC, area under the curve; BMI, body mass index; C-index, concordance index; ICU, intensive care unit; IL-6, interleukin 6; MNA-SF, Mini Nutrition Assessment–Short Form; MST, Malnutrition Screening Tool; MUST, Malnutrition Universal Screening Tool; NRS-2002, Nutritional Risk Screening 2002; NST/BAPEN, Nutrition Screening Tool/British Association of Parenteral and Enteral Nutrition; NUTRIC, Nutrition Risk in Critically Ill; SGA, Subjective Global Assessment; SNAQ, Short Nutrition Assessment Questionnaire; SOFA, sequential organ failure assessment.
[a]Compared with SGA.
Source: Data are from references 25, 26, 29, and 44–53.

It is a practical measure of body size and an indirect measure of body adiposity,[59] but it does not account for sex, age, race, fitness levels, or variations in abdominal adiposity and therefore should be interpreted cautiously.[60] Flegal and colleagues have shown that mortality rate sharply increased when BMI was less than 18.5 or greater than 35.[61] Persons categorized into the highest or lowest BMI ranges may also be at heightened risk for malnutrition. The ESPEN consensus statement included low BMI as a defining characteristic of malnutrition,[15] but ASPEN and AND did not include BMI as a malnutrition clinical characteristic because malnutrition can occur at any BMI.[41,57,62,63]

The National Institutes of Health guidelines[64] for interpretation of BMI in adults are as follows:
• BMI less than 18.5: underweight
• BMI 18.5 to 24.9: normal weight
• BMI 25 to 29.9: overweight
• BMI 30 to 34.9: class I obesity
• BMI 35 to 39.9: class II obesity
• BMI equal to or greater than 40: extreme (class III) obesity

Weight History

One of the most important historical elements in a nutrition assessment is prior weight loss (specifically, nonvolitional weight reduction). This information can be obtained from the medical record, the patient, a caregiver, or family member. Weight loss should be interpreted through an evaluation of other confounding factors—such as whether the loss was intentional, the presence of edema or dehydration, and the length of time in which change occurred—and in comparison with the individual's typical or usual body weight.[14,45] The clinical relevance of weight loss varies according to its degree and duration. Significant, unintentional weight loss is a highly substantiated marker of malnutrition.[41,57,62,63] Both SGA and the ESPEN consensus consider weight loss when defining malnutrition.[15,22] As described by the ASPEN/AND characteristics, severity of malnutrition is influenced by the percentage of weight lost compared with an individual's usual weight during a defined length of time.[14] Table 9-6 outlines the time frames and percentages of meaningful weight lost for each malnutrition etiology in the ASPEN/AND classification.[14]

Client History

Medical, surgical, family, and psychosocial histories, along with the current clinical status of a patient, are known to affect an array of nutrition abnormalities.[54,55] Clinicians who conduct nutrition assessments must understand how diseases, medical conditions, and surgical interventions can alter

TABLE 9-6 Weight Loss Characteristics That Support a Diagnosis of Malnutrition Using the ASPEN/AND Methodology

Malnutrition Etiology	Weight Loss Over Time	
	Nonsevere/Moderate Malnutrition	Severe Malnutrition
Acute illness/injury	• 1%–2% in 1 week • 5% in 1 month • 7.5% in 3 months	• >2% in 1 week • >5% in 1 month • >7.5% in 3 months
Chronic illness	• 5% in 1 month • 7.5% in 3 months • 10% in 6 months • 20% in 1 year	• >5% in 1 month • >7.5% in 3 months • >10% in 6 months • >20% in 1 year
Social/environmental circumstance	• 5% in 1 month • 7.5% in 3 months • 10% in 6 months • 20% in 1 year	• >5% in 1 month • >7.5% in 3 months • >10% in 6 months • >20% in 1 year

AND, Academy of Nutrition and Dietetics; ASPEN, American Society for Parenteral and Enteral Nutrition.

Source: Data are from reference 14.

digestion, absorption, ingestion, and metabolism of micro- and macronutrients. Likewise, an understanding of how nutrients affect disease processes is essential.[55]

A review of medications is part of a comprehensive nutrition assessment. Practitioners should be familiar with the potential nutrient interactions of drugs that are commonly used to treat their patients. A pharmacy consult can be helpful. Nutrition status may be adversely affected by medications that interfere with food intake (eg, by causing anorexia or taste changes) or with the absorption, metabolism, and excretion of nutrients. Drug levels may also be altered by foods and nutrients that modify drug absorption, metabolism, and excretion. During the assessment, clinicians should also investigate the patient's use of herbal supplements and complementary medicine products.[55] See Chapters 18 and 19 for further discussion of drug-nutrient interactions and dietary supplements, respectively.

Biochemical Data

Laboratory assays can be used as supportive evidence regarding nutrition status, particularly organ/system function and the magnitude of inflammation. Indeed, the principle purpose of laboratory assays is to help evaluate physiological and metabolic abnormalities related to disease and trauma. Traditional use of nutrition laboratory biomarkers, such as the negative phase proteins, are notably more useful for their role as indicators of inflammatory conditions than as primary predictors of nutrition status (see Tables 9-7 and 9-8).[10,14,29,65–84] Clinical history and physical examination data provide more accurate information than serum laboratory markers for assessing nutrition status.[85] Laboratory findings are useful as supportive data for nutrition deficiencies, but they should be interpreted with caution because they lack specificity and sensitivity as direct indicators of nutrition status.[10,66] As previously noted, although laboratory markers are beneficial for evaluating inflammation, they must be used in conjunction with other assessment data, such as clinical history, physical examination, and functional

assessment, to diagnose malnutrition.[10,14] Indicators such as leukocytosis, C-reactive protein elevation, cytokines, and hyperglycemia may suggest inflammatory response.[10] Refer to the disease-specific chapters in Part III of this book for further information on interpreting laboratory test data.

Nutrient Intake Data

Assessment of nutrient intake can be used to detect imbalanced nutrition consumption, which can help identify nutrient deficiencies or excesses. Inadequate energy intake, impaired digestion, and impaired absorption play key roles in the development of malnutrition.[86] Therefore, clinicians should thoroughly assess a patient's nutrient intake, including oral food and beverage consumption, enteral feedings, and parenteral infusions. Then, the intakes can be compared with estimated energy, protein, fluid, and micronutrient requirements for that individual. Detailed discussion of energy and protein needs for patients can be found in Chapters 2 and 4, respectively, as well as in the disease- and condition-specific chapters in Part III.

The SGA, ESPEN, and ASPEN/AND criteria for malnutrition all include nutrient intake data, albeit nonuniformly.[14,15,22] For example, the ASPEN/AND characteristics focus on energy provision and suggest reporting intakes as a percentage of estimated energy requirements over time (see Table 9-9).[14]

Clinicians should consider several elements when attempting to obtain an accurate representation of nutrition intake. They should be cognizant of natural, random variations in daily nutrient and energy intake of humans.[87] Determining specific food quantities is appropriate but can be complicated because clinicians and patients may not share a mutual understanding about portion sizes.[88] Certain populations are also prone to underreport food intake.[88–90] Clinicians should also pose questions about therapeutics, weight reduction, vegetarian or macrobiotic diets, cultural/religious practices, fad diets, food intolerances and allergies, and other dietary restrictions.

TABLE 9-7 Laboratory Tests Traditionally Used to Detect Malnutrition

Test	Description	Interpretation	Recommendations for Use as an Indicator of Nutrition Status
Albumin[10,14,29,66–71]	• Maintain colloidal osmotic pressure of plasma; binds to many other sources • Negative acute-phase reactant • Half-life: 14–20 days	• Indicator of inflammatory condition; proxy measure for underlying injury, disease, or inflammation • A predictor for morbidity and mortality • Reflection of acute-phase response • Lack of consistent change with loss of weight, reduced energy intakes, or nitrogen balance • Lacks sensitivity and specificity for malnutrition • Affected by hydration, infection, disease, and other inflammatory conditions	• Does not accurately represent nutrition status in ICU setting • Should not be used as marker of nutrition status
Prealbumin[29,67,69–75]	• Major plasma protein; binds thyroxin • Plays a role in metabolism of vitamin A • Carrier of retinol-binding protein • Negative acute-phase reactant • Half-life: 2–3 days	• Sensitive to short-term changes in inflammation • Affected by hydration, infection, disease, and other inflammatory conditions	• Should not be used as marker of nutrition status • Reflection of acute-phase response; does not accurately represent nutrition status in ICU setting
Transferrin[29,67,70–78]	• Iron transport • Indirectly assessed as TIBC • Negative acute-phase reactant • Half-life: 8–10 days	• Sensitive to short-term changes in inflammation • Lacks sensitivity and specificity for malnutrition • Affected by hydration, infection, disease, and other inflammatory conditions • Altered by perturbation in iron status	• Should not be used as marker of nutrition status • Reflection of acute-phase response; does not accurately represent nutrition status in ICU setting
Retinol-binding protein[29,69,71,79,80]	• Binds to prealbumin • Vitamin A transport • Negative acute-phase reactant • Half-life: 12 hours	• Also affected by vitamin A and zinc deficiency and renal disease	• Should not be used as marker of nutrition status • Reflection of acute-phase response; does not accurately represent nutrition status in ICU setting

ICU, intensive care unit; TIBC, total iron-binding capacity.
Source: Data are from references 10, 14, 29, and 66–80.

Thorough evaluation of nutrition intake also considers types and quantities of supplements, including vitamins, minerals, protein supplements, probiotics, and nutrition drinks and shakes. Alternate sources of nutrition should also be reviewed, including enteral and parenteral nutrition, intravenous fluids, calorically emulsified medications, beverages, and alcohol. Furthermore, it is prudent to discuss the availability and financial affordability of food, the individual's ability to prepare foods, and any other social/behavioral practices that may influence the individual's nutrient intake.[55] In some cases, caregivers can be used as a proxy to report dietary intake.

Multiple nutrient intake assessment methods are available, and the appropriate method to choose depends on the population of interest, availability of resources, skills of the

TABLE 9-8 Laboratory Tests Used to Detect Inflammation

Test	Description	Interpretation	Recommendations for Use
C-reactive protein[29,68,69,81,82]	• Has proinflammatory and anti-inflammatory roles • Positive acute-phase reactant	• Assists in evaluation of inflammatory conditions along with negative acute-phase reactants • Has proinflammatory and anti-inflammatory roles	• Still investigational; should not be used as surrogate marker of nutrition status
White blood cell count[83]	• Found in the lymphatic system • Some diseases and conditions may elicit elevated laboratory values as a response to inflammation • Suppressed levels may indicate a condition that suppresses the immune system	• Assists in evaluation of inflammatory conditions along with negative acute-phase reactants • Intense exercise or severe emotional or physical stress can increase a white blood cell count; test is not used to evaluate these conditions	• Inflammatory marker
Cytokines (interleukins, interferons, tumor necrosis factor α)[29,83,84]	• One of a group of proteins that assist in regulation and/or promotion of an immune response	• Prognostic use of cytokine measurements as indicators of inflammatory status is being investigated • Can be impaired (along with insulin signaling) by muscle atrophy	• Still investigational; should not be used as surrogate marker of nutrition status

Source: Data are from references 29, 68, 69, and 81–84.

TABLE 9-9 Energy Intake Characteristics That Support a Diagnosis of Malnutrition Using the ASPEN/AND Methodology

Malnutrition Etiology	Nonsevere/Moderate Malnutrition	Severe Malnutrition
Acute illness/injury	<75% of estimated energy requirement for >7 days	≤50% of estimated energy requirement for ≥5 days
Chronic illness	≤75% of estimated energy requirement for ≥1 month	≤75% of estimated energy requirement for ≥1 month
Social/environmental circumstance	<75% of estimated energy requirement for ≥3 months	≤50% of estimated energy requirement for ≥1 month

AND, Academy of Nutrition and Dietetics; ASPEN, American Society for Parenteral and Enteral Nutrition.
Source: Data are from 14.

healthcare professional, feasibility, and purpose. Table 9-10 describes common methods.[5,91]

Both the 24-hour recall method and a modified version of the diet history are commonly used in clinical settings to evaluate a specific individual's intake. Originally developed by Burke and Stuart,[91] the diet history obtains information about an individual's past diet and can include queries of information about the types and frequency of intake of various foods. The original Burke diet history method included a detailed interview about usual food intake, a food frequency checklist, and a 3-day diet record, but this level of detail is often omitted in the clinical setting, where a modified diet history is obtained. Querying patients for a history of nutrition intake practices is a fundamental part of any nutrition assessment.

Once dietary intake data has been collected, it can be entered into a nutrition software program that provides an analysis of the energy and nutrients of the diet. It is important that the food database software contains data on foods and preparation methods relevant to the target population. The analysis is typically based on information from a database with values for food ingredients derived from the US Department of Agriculture National Nutrient Database for Standard Reference. Among the more widely used programs are Nutritionist Pro (Axxya Systems, Stafford, TX), Nutrition Data System for Research (University of Minnesota, Nutrition Coordinating Center, Minneapolis, MN), and Food Processor (ESHA Research, Salem, OR). Selection of diet analysis software will depend on cost, system requirements, usability, and available features.

Reports of nutrient intake generated by the diet analysis software can then be compared with recommendations and calculated estimations. The Dietary Reference Intakes (DRIs)[92] are a set of nutrient recommendations established by the Health and Medicine Division (formerly Institute of

TABLE 9-10 Nutrition Intake Assessment Methods

Method	Procedure	Characteristics	Limitations
Prospective			
Diet record/food diary	• Self-recorded food and beverage intake, usually for a brief time (3–7 days).	• Food portions may be weighed or estimated using household measurements. • Can be used to record compliance to a diet regimen or to self-monitor food intake. • Does not rely on self-recall. • Provides information on food preparation and meal timing. • Usually used in outpatient settings.	• Captures recent intake which may or may not reflect usual intake. • High participant burden. • Act of recording can influence food intake. • Analysis can be cumbersome. • Data collection influenced by literacy skills and participants' ability to judge/record portion sizes. • Quality declines as duration lengthens.
Nutrient intake analysis	• Direct observation; clinician does a visual analysis of meal before and after being served to estimate food intake. Nutrients from enteral and parenteral sources are also documented. • Recommended duration is ≥72 hours.	• Typically used with hospitalized patients or those in residential facilities. • Includes a "calorie count" to assess whether subject is likely meeting nutrient needs. • Cost-effective; quick.	• If meal tray is removed/discarded before clinician can observe, food intake cannot be estimated. • Relies on clinician ability to estimate portion size. • 1 or 2 meal evaluations may not provide realistic portrayal of usual intakes. • Inaccurate/incomplete records are commonplace.
Retrospective			
24-hour recall	• Self-recall of exact food and beverage consumption for previous 24 hours.	• Low participant burden. • Trained interviewer using prompts can collect more detailed information. • Can be administered via telephone or in-person. • Can be inexpensive and quick. • Does not influence food intake.	• Accuracy depends on participant's ability to recall and estimate portion size. • Multiple recalls may need to be conducted to capture usual food intake. • Influenced by language barriers. • Tendency to exaggerate low intakes.
Food frequency questionnaire	• Self-reported frequency of consumption from selected list of foods.	• Provides assessment of long-term (6–12 months) diet intake patterns. • May or may not query portion size. • Low subject burden. • Is easily self-administered. • Commonly used with large-scale populations. • Easily standardized. • Focuses on consumptions of food groups. • Must be culture-specific.	• Use with special populations should be validated. • Intake is often misreported. • Language barriers affect results. • Food intake during times of illness is usually significantly different from usual intakes, and recorded data may not be representative of current situation. • No meal pattern data. • Accuracy depends on knowledge of portion sizes. • Not designed for current intake assessment.
Prospective and retrospective			
Diet history	• Original approach included 3 elements: detailed interview about food intake, checklist of foods, and 3-day diet record.	• Often modified in clinical settings. • The 3 elements can be used to cross-check reported intake.	• High interviewer burden/time-consuming. • Relies on participant recall and portion size estimation.

Source: Data are from references 54 and 90.

Medicine) of the National Academies of Sciences, Engineering and Medicine. The DRIs include Adequate Intakes, Recommended Dietary Allowances, Tolerable Upper Intake Levels, and Estimated Average Requirements. DRI values are intended to define amounts that support most healthy individuals. Therefore, clinicians should exercise caution when using them to evaluate nutrient intakes of individuals with diseases.

Nutrient intake data can be highly subjective and may provide limited insight into a patient's overall consumption of nutrients.[89] The data should be used in combination with other components of a nutrition assessment to evaluate the patient's nutrition status. Measurement of nutrient intake is complex, and each approach to nutrient intake assessment is subject to both systematic errors (eg, the subject's ability to recall intake or accurately estimate portion size) and random errors (eg, misreporting of true intake by certain population groups). Because potential sources of error cannot be eliminated entirely, practitioners must understand the nature of the errors and how they may affect analysis and interpretation of the data.[88,89,93]

Nutrition-Focused Physical Examination

Compared with other techniques or the use of laboratory indexes, clinical history and physical examination can provide more accurate information about the nutrition status of patients.[85] Malnutrition and micronutrient abnormalities can broadly affect organs and tissues resulting in physical sequela that may be readily detected by the trained practitioner with the use of a nutrition-focused physical examination (NFPE).[34]

NFPE is an easy-to-learn, economical, and efficient way to confirm the presence of malnutrition or another nutrition problem.[35] Unlike physical examinations conducted by nurses or physicians, an NFPE focuses primarily on changes to muscle, fat stores, fluid retention, and/or other physical signs that can result from micronutrient deficiencies or excesses.[35] Tables 9-11 and 9-12 provide guidelines for evaluating muscle and subcutaneous fat with this technique.[35] Although not part of the ASPEN/AND clinical characteristics to diagnose malnutrition, an NFPE should also evaluate the various parts of the body where high cell turnover occurs (eg, hair, skin, mouth, tongue) because they are among the most likely to rapidly show signs

TABLE 9-11 Characteristics of Muscle Status Used in Nutrition Assessment

Muscle Status	Upper Body	Lower Body[a]
Normal	• Temporalis muscle is well defined; easy to see and palpate. • Pectoralis major protrudes or is flat; clavicle is visible but not sharply defined in women; not typically seen in men. • Deltoid muscle, around the shoulders and upper arms, looks curved. • Trapezius, supraspinatus, and infraspinatus muscles, around the neck base and above the scapula, show no signs of hollowing; scapular bones are not prominent. • Interosseous and dorsal side of thumb muscles bulge or look flat.	• Muscles around knee are visible/palpable and well-rounded; patella is not prominent. • Quadriceps and gastrocnemius muscles (posterior calf) are developed and rounded; may appear less developed if person is not very active.
Mild to moderate loss	• Temporalis muscle is slightly depressed. • Pectoralis major is diminished; clavicle is moderately prominent in women; visible in men. • Shoulder blades and acromion process become more evident as deltoid diminishes. • Trapezius starting to look hollow; scapular bones and upper spine are somewhat prominent. • Interosseous muscles are slightly depressed; may also be characteristic of aging.	• Patella is slightly prominent, yet rounded. • Inner thigh starts to appear concave; may see gap between thighs when knees pressed together. • Gastrocnemius muscles look less developed than normal.
Severe loss	• Temporalis muscle is depressed, hollow-looking; facial bones prominent. • Clavicle sharply protrudes, minimal pectoralis muscle palpable. • Deltoid muscle not readily palpable around shoulders, upper arms; scapula and acromion process edges are sharply angular. • Trapezius has deeply hollowed appearance; scapular bones are well defined with sharp angles; upper spine is clearly visible. • Dorsal muscle between forefinger and thumb is deeply concave; bones between interosseous muscles are prominent.	• Patella is sharply prominent with little sign of surrounding muscle. • Quadriceps with prominent concave shape between thighs; lack definition. • Posterior calves are thin and lack muscle definition.

[a]Area is less sensitive to change than upper body muscle.

Source: Data are from reference 35.

TABLE 9-12 Characteristics of Subcutaneous Fat Status Used in Nutrition Assessment

| Subcutaneous Fat Status | Body Region | | |
	Orbital Area[a]	Upper Arm	Thoracic and Lumbar Region/Midaxillary Line
Normal	• Fat pads protrude slightly or are flat.	• Gentle pinch of skinfold underneath triceps with fingers yields ample fat tissue.	• Iliac crest does not protrude. • Ribs are not visible.
Mild to moderate loss	• Faintly dark circles are visible around eyes. • Area surrounding the eye is moderately concave.	• Gentle pinch of skinfold underneath triceps with fingers yields some fat tissue; finger tips closer together.	• Iliac crest is visible. • Ribs are visible but without marked depressions between them.
Severe loss	• Dark circles are visible around eyes. • Eye socket is extremely concave. • Skin is loose.	• Gentle pinch of skinfold underneath triceps results in fingers touching; little to no fat tissue.	• Iliac crest and ribs are protruding. • Sharp depressions seen between ribs.

[a]Loss may be obscured by fluid retention.
Source: Data are from reference 35.

TABLE 9-13 Muscle and Fat Characteristics That Support a Diagnosis of Malnutrition Using the ASPEN/AND Methodology

| Malnutrition Etiology | Fat or Muscle Loss Severity | |
	Nonsevere/Moderate Malnutrition	Severe Malnutrition
Acute illness/injury	Mild	Moderate
Chronic illness	Mild	Severe
Social/environmental circumstance	Mild	Severe

AND, Academy of Nutrition and Dietetics; ASPEN, American Society for Parenteral and Enteral Nutrition.
Source: Data are from reference 14.

of possible nutrient deficiencies (refer to Chapter 8 for further information about micronutrient deficiencies).[94] Symptoms of nutrition abnormalities tend to be nonspecific; therefore, other possible causes must be considered.[35] For example, peripheral edema is often associated with reduced albumin in the setting of inflammatory response, but this issue may or may not be related to nutrition adequacy.[95] Table 9-13 identifies how information from an NFPE is interpreted according to the ASPEN/AND methodology.[14] Figure 9-1 details its use in SGA.[22]

Pathophysiological Changes of Muscle and Fat

Lean muscle mass and adipose stores play a defining role in the nutrition status of individuals. Both the stress response and starvation affect nutrient utilization and the breakdown of body components, but stress-related inflammation and starvation affect fat stores and muscle mass at different rates and to varying degrees of severity.[96] Therefore, clinicians performing an NFPE to assess muscle mass and fat stores must recognize the differences between these 2 metabolic pathways (starvation vs inflammation) and understand their implications for patients' rates of recovery and nutrition status.[14]

During starvation, preservation of lean body mass is the ultimate goal. Initially, glycogen is used as the primary energy source, but these reserves are quickly depleted, forcing the body to use amino acids to make glucose and support energy requirements.[97] Eventually, further adaptation occurs and resting energy expenditure decreases as fat becomes the main energy source, providing ketones as fuel as a means to preserve muscle mass.[35,97]

In contrast, the metabolic pathway of the stress response is characterized by extreme catabolism and negative nitrogen balance, driven by a storm of hormones and cell mediators to mount an immune defense and repair tissues during injury and illness.[10,97] All of these reactions accelerate muscle breakdown to generate energy.[97] Amino acids are displaced from muscles and used for gluconeogenesis.[10] Additionally, cytokines act to inhibit repair and synthesis of new muscle tissue, promote muscle breakdown, and affect muscle function. Muscle degradation continues unabated while the condition persists, creating a much faster rate of skeletal and lean muscle loss than seen in starvation.[97] The stress response mechanisms also work against nutrition interventions aimed at preservation.[10]

Evaluation of Muscle Mass and Adipose Tissue

Losses of lean mass and adipose tissue have long been recognized as a means to identify malnutrition, although evaluation of such losses is not universally part of routine nutrition assessment. Loss of lean mass is strongly correlated with functionality, increased hospital length of stay, and mortality in patients with chronic and acute illness, regardless of their weight or BMI.[28,31,98] Individuals who present to the hospital with preexisting diminished muscle mass and minimal fat stores are also noted to have slower recovery and rehabilitation after hospitalization.[14,40]

Muscle atrophy is a loss of bulk and tone that is detectable by palpation.[14,99] The upper body is more often used than the lower body to help identify fat and muscle loss because the upper body is typically less affected by edema, is more accessible to the clinician, and has been identified as a good reflection of overall muscle mass.[35,63] Tables 9-11 and 9-12 describe how to assess muscle and fat during a physical examination.[35] Routine monitoring of these body components during hospitalization helps detect potentially related changes in nutrition status.[10]

Sarcopenia is defined as the age-related loss of muscle mass and has been associated with a decline in function.[100] The etiology of sarcopenia can be related to various factors, including inflammatory and cytokine-driven oxidative stress[10] as well as protein synthesis and neuromuscular integrity.[101] Sarcopenic obesity refers to reduced muscle mass, and perhaps muscle quality, that is disproportionate to fat mass.[102] Sarcopenic obesity may further aggravate the catabolic process of cachexia and muscle loss.[103,104] From the ages of 20 years to 80 years, muscle mass declines by approximately 30%. These changes in muscle size do not always correlate with changes in strength, but it is suggested that the quality of muscle may also change.[102] The European Workgroup on Sarcopenia in Older People recommends defining sarcopenia using the inclusion of low muscle mass and either low strength and/or low muscle function and performance.[101] Conditions affecting sarcopenia include but are not limited to lack of muscle use, chronic disease, insulin resistance, and poor nutrition.

Cachexia is defined as loss of muscle mass, irrespective of adipose tissue changes, which accompanies underlying illnesses and is often associated with inflammation, insulin resistance, decreased appetite and intake, and protein catabolism. Because of its multifaceted and profound inflammatory state, cachexia is not responsive to nutrition support; however, symptom management (eg, psychological, oral, GI, pharmacological, and metabolic interventions) is imperative.[105] An individual found to be cachectic will also meet the criteria for sarcopenia, but the sarcopenic individual is not always cachectic.[101]

In obese and overweight individuals, weight changes may not identify individuals with underlying cachexia, particularly in cancer-related cachexia. These individuals have been noted to have lean muscle changes and associated comorbidities, comparable with those of their underweight counterparts.[104] See Chapter 35 for additional information on overweight and obesity.

Body Composition Assessment Tools

Body composition can be measured in several ways. Anthropometric measurements such as skinfolds and body part circumferences are easy to obtain, noninvasive, and inexpensive, but they have had limited practical applications in inpatient care settings.[31] These methods tend to be insensitive and presume that subcutaneous adipose tissue thickness has a constant compressibility.[31,32] Additionally, comparative standards for these measurements are based on states of balanced hydration, and measurements may not correlate well with whole lean body mass or muscle loss in critically ill patients.[99]

Several body composition assessment instruments that are used in research require specialized equipment or are not widely available or practical for routine clinical applications at the bedside.[31] Examples of these instruments include labeled water–isotope dilution techniques, 3-dimensional body surface imaging, air displacement plethysmography, total body count of naturally occurring potassium isotope, and water displacement (or hydrodensitometry).[102] Tools used more routinely in clinical practice to differentiate lean soft tissue and fat mass include bioelectrical impedance analysis, dual-energy x-ray absorptiometry, magnetic resonance imaging, computed tomography (CT), and ultrasound.[31,32]

Long-standing staples in diagnostics, CT and bedside ultrasound have emerged over the last several years as body composition assessment tools used in the clinical setting by physicians and registered dietitians. Analyzing CT images at the third lumbar vertebrae (L3) region is a precise and valid means to quantify and distinguish between lean and adipose tissue.[106,107] In certain clinical scenarios, such as cancer treatment or intensive care of the critically ill, serial CT scans can demonstrate changes in lean tissue over time.[31] However, CT scans are not available for all patients, emit high doses of radiation, and are costly.[31,32] Analyzing and interpreting the CT results can be achieved by specialized software packages[108] or by collaborating with a radiologist.

Investigators have studied the use of bedside ultrasound to quantify muscle layer thickness in mid–upper arm, forearm, and quadriceps muscles of hospitalized and critically ill patients.[109–112] The quadriceps muscle has been shown to be indicative of overall lean body mass,[22,113] and it is relatively accessible for ultrasound examination in most hospitalized and ICU patients. Bedside ultrasound is not as accurate as CT scans, and the measurement can be subject to errors related to the selection of reliable site, repeatability among different clinicians, patient edema, and force of compressibility.[114] Clinicians should therefore exercise caution when considering whether ultrasound results indicate malnutrition; however, given the ease, accessibility, and safety of bedside ultrasound in critically ill patients, its use shows promise as a quantifiable tool to assess lean body mass in an ICU setting.[31,109,115] Refer to Table 9-14 for more information about body composition tools.[31,32,40,102,111,115–126]

Fluid Accumulation/Edema

Fluid accumulation affects changes in weight, and ASPEN/ AND consider it to be a characteristic that can be used to

TABLE 9-14 Body Composition Tools Commonly Used in Hospital and Ambulatory Settings

Test	Description	Advantages	Disadvantages
Skinfold and circumference measurements[32,116,117]	• Body composition measurements. • Skinfold calipers measure the percentage of subcutaneous fat. • A tape measure is used to measure waist, hip, and neck circumferences.	• Typical coefficient of variation is ≥10%. • Accessible, noninvasive.	• Clinicians require training to reliably measure skinfolds and circumferences. • Low degree of precision. • Reliability and validity of estimations of overall body fat are questionable because of comorbidities associated with centralized obesity.
Bioelectrical impedance[31,32,118–120]	• Based on differential resistance of body tissues. • Measures conductivity of water, with results used to estimate fat-free mass and lean mass.	• Can be accurate in healthy, nonobese individuals. • Easily accessible, benign technique available to clinicians. • Equipment is portable. • Accurately measures body water. • Requires population-specific validation of regression equations.	• Subject to error in a clinical setting. • Most formulas underestimate fat. • Affected by hydration status.
Dual-energy x-ray absorptiometry[121–124]	• Often used to evaluate bone density, but can be used for soft tissue measurements with appropriate x-ray absorptiometry software. • Can compare truncal and appendicular components.	• Precise differentiation between tissues. • Content-specific to measured areas. • Noninvasive, repeatable. • Can be used in outpatient/ambulatory setting for long-term follow-up.	• Modest radiation exposure. • Measurements affected by hydration status. • Impractical in most clinical settings.
Magnetic resonance imaging[31]	• Whole body, cross-sectional images are developed via the alignment of protons generated by a strong magnetic field.	• Most accurate method for visualizing all body compartments. • Safe, does not use radiation.	• Highly specialized. • Costly. • Requires patient participation.
Computed tomography[31,32,40,102,125]	• Imaging technique that uses high-dose radiation to differentiate adipose tissue, skeletal muscle, visceral organs, and bone.	• At the L3 vertebrae, can precisely provide qualitative and quantitative evaluation of skeletal muscle and adipose tissue.	• High radiation exposure. • Expensive. • Requires specialized training to accurately identify muscle/fat stores at L3 region. • Specific software needed.
Ultrasound[31,32,111,115,126]	• High-frequency sound waves travel from a transducer through the skin and bounce back at different frequencies to differentiate among tissues (muscle, adipose, bone).	• Due to ease, availability, low cost, and noninvasiveness, an emerging bedside tool to measure muscle mass. • Can be used serially to determine changes in muscle mass.	• Subject to technical errors. • Accuracy of image can be affected by edema.

Source: Data are from references 31, 32, 40, 102, 111, and 115–126.

support a diagnosis of malnutrition.[14] Edema, an excess of interstitial fluid accumulation, can be caused by a variety of diseases, conditions, and medications,[127] but it is rarely the direct result of malnutrition.[14] Therefore, clinicians should exercise caution when using this characteristic to justify the presence of malnutrition in a patient. Ordinarily, the human body is a very capable fluid and electrolyte regulator.[128] Abrupt changes in fluid and sodium intake from the diet do not disrupt biological functionality and cause edema, as long as the heart and kidneys are relatively healthy.[129] Edema may be present during cases of volume depletion where interstitial and intravascular fluids shift into the surrounding tissues because of oncotic pressure changes and capillary leak syndrome. Prolonged periods of time with frank deficiencies in protein consumption, as well as the physiological response to refeeding syndrome, can also result in edema.[127] When assessing edema, clinicians should seek to identify the underlying cause.[14,130] Table 9-15 shows the severity of edema and how it correlates with the ASPEN/AND malnutrition criteria.[14]

Routine observation of signs and symptoms with a physical examination is as important as monitoring weight fluctuations to evaluate for the presence of, or changes in, edema.[131] Table 9-16 illustrates a technique to evaluate the severity of edema in the lower extremities, such as over the tibia bone or ankle.[132] Clinical manifestations of fluid retention may not be noticeable until it accounts for at least 10% of body weight[129] or when interstitial fluid volume increases by 2.5 to 3 liters.[130] In many situations, fluid accumulation diminishes the accuracy of weight changes[14,22] and can impede physical examination of muscle and fat stores.[133] Additionally, extra fluid in the lungs or around the heart,[131] or small pockets of ascites, might only be visible on imaging studies. Therefore, fluid retention can be present without being appreciable on a physical examination.[127] Alternate indications of the presence of edema include distended neck veins, increased blood pressure, ill-fitting rings or shoes, declining serum sodium levels, and rapid weight increase.[127,131,134,135]

Micronutrient Abnormalities

Physical signs associated with micronutrient deficiencies or excesses must be interpreted carefully because they might be caused by environmental factors, diseases, or infections and do not necessarily indicate a micronutrient problem. Oral intake

data, assessment by dermatologic examination, or laboratory findings can help confirm or rule out possible abnormalities identified in the NFPE. Micronutrient irregularities are covered more extensively in Chapter 8.

Functional Status

Measures of strength and functional status have been recognized as an important component of the nutrition assessment, but they are widely underused.[136] Functional status is a measurement of the capacity of an individual to perform usual activities. Muscle function and strength can be affected by inflammatory conditions, acute and chronic diseases, atrophy from lack of use, and sensory-loss from neuromuscular damage. Muscle function, as assessed by handgrip, shows a direct relationship with measures of functional status and physical components of quality of life.[137] Anthropometry, measurements that focus on size and proportions of bodily muscle and fat, has limitations as it does not reflect muscle function and strength. The development of useful and practical techniques for assessing functional status is a current topic of interest and research.[136]

The use of a handgrip dynamometer to gauge muscle strength is a validated tool for determining functional status of an individual[94,138] and can be useful in nutrition assessment.[136] The handgrip dynamometer may not be available or practical in all clinical settings because the patient must be correctly positioned and able to use bilateral, upper-extremity strength.[138] Alternatively, manual muscle testing has shown some reliability as a strength and muscle function assessment tool.[139] Other measures of physical performance that are being investigated for use and practicality include the 30-second chair stand; stair climb test; 4- × 10-meter, fast-paced walk; timed up-and-go test; and 6-minute walk test.[136]

Self-evaluation of physical performance and functioning has been part of validated nutrition assessment tools and quality-of-life measures. Obtaining a patient's perspective regarding his/her functional status may be useful if a handgrip dynamometer is not available.[27,136] Validated nutrition assessment tools that include self-evaluation of functional status include the SGA,[22] the Dialysis Malnutrition Score,[27,140] and the Patient-Generated Subjective Global Assessment.[27] The ASPEN/AND malnutrition clinical characteristics also incorporate functional status into the assessment of malnutrition

TABLE 9-15 Fluid Accumulation Characteristics That Support a Diagnosis of Malnutrition Using the ASPEN/AND Methodology

Malnutrition Etiology	Degree of Fluid Accumulation	
	Nonsevere/Moderate Malnutrition	Severe Malnutrition
Acute illness/injury	Mild	Moderate to severe
Chronic illness	Mild	Severe
Social/environmental circumstance	Mild	Severe

AND, Academy of Nutrition and Dietetics; ASPEN, American Society for Parenteral and Enteral Nutrition.
Source: Data are from reference 14.

TABLE 9-16 Assessing the Degree of Edema

	Edema Classification	Depth and Rebound Time	Severity of Edema
(illustration)	0	No distortion occurs after pressure applied; bone structure is readily identifiable.	None
(illustration) 2 mm or less	1+	Depression is barely noticeable; rebound occurs immediately.	Mild
(illustration) 2–4 mm	2+	Applied pressure causes deeper pit; rebound occurs after a few seconds.	Moderate
(illustration) 4–6 mm	3+	Pitting is even more pronounced; rebound occurs after about 10–12 seconds.	Severe
(illustration) 6–8 mm	4+	Pressure causes very deep pit; rebound generally takes longer than 20 seconds.	Severe

Source: Data are from reference 132. Artwork reprinted with permission, Cleveland Clinic Center for Medical Art & Photography © 2014–2016. All Rights Reserved.

(see Table 9-17).[14] Quality-of-life measures that evaluate functional ability include the Katz Index of Independence in Activities of Daily Living, Lawton Instrumental Activities of Daily Living, Karnofsky Performance Scale Index, and Eastern Cooperative Oncology Group Performance status tool.

Conclusion

This chapter has introduced various approaches to understanding adult malnutrition that highlight the importance of the inflammatory process along with some practical nutrition

TABLE 9-17 Functional Status Characteristics That Support a Diagnosis of Malnutrition Using the ASPEN/AND Methodology

Malnutrition Etiology	Nonsevere/Moderate Malnutrition	Severe Malnutrition
Acute illness/injury	N/A	Measurably reduced functional status
Chronic illness	N/A	Measurably reduced functional status
Social/environmental circumstances	N/A	Measurably reduced functional status

AND, Academy of Nutrition and Dietetics; ASPEN, American Society for Parenteral and Enteral Nutrition.
N/A, not applicable.
Source: Data are from reference 14.

screening and assessment methods suitable for routine clinical applications. Initiatives to globally refine and validate a means to diagnose and define malnutrition are ongoing and will likely be updated as new information emerges.[14,18] Currently, no single clinical or laboratory measure provides a comprehensive assessment of nutrition status. Therefore, a complete assessment of nutrition status should include a review of the client's anthropometrics, medical and surgical history, family and social history, medication use, clinical presentation, and biochemical data; additionally, the clinician should obtain nutrient intake data and perform an NFPE (including a functional status assessment). All of these components are integral to confirm the presence of malnutrition and generate an appropriate care plan.

References

1. Mueller C, Compher C, Ellen DM, American Society for Parenteral and Enteral Nutrition Board of Directors. A.S.P.E.N. clinical guidelines: nutrition screening, assessment, and intervention in adults. *JPEN J Parenter Enteral Nutr.* 2011;35(1):16–24.
2. American Society for Parenteral and Enteral Nutrition (A.S.P.E.N.) Board of Directors and Clinical Practice Committee. Definition of terms, style, and conventions used in A.S.P.E.N. Board of Directors–approved documents. American Society for Parenteral and Enteral Nutrition. May 2015. http://www.nutritioncare.org/Guidelines_and_Clinical_Resources/Clinical_Practice_Library/Special_Reports. Accessed July 22, 2016.
3. Centers for Medicare and Medicaid Services. CMS State Operations Manual. Appendix A: Survey Protocol, Regulations, and Interpretive Guidelines for Hospitals. Revised October 17, 2008. https://www.cms.gov/Regulations-and-Guidance/Guidance/Transmittals/downloads/R37SOMA.pdf. Accessed June 15, 2017.
4. The Joint Commission. The Joint Commission Comprehensive Accreditation and Certification Manual. https://e-dition.jcrinc.com/MainContent.aspx. Accessed July 14, 2016.
5. The Joint Commission. Standards FAQ Details. Nutritional screen—who may document. https://www.jointcommission.org/standards_information/jcfaqdetails.aspx?StandardsFaqId=933&ProgramId=46. Accessed May 30, 2017.
6. Patel V, Romano M, Corkins MR, et al. Nutrition screening and assessment in hospitalized patients: a survey of current practice in the United States. *Nutr Clin Pract.* 2014;29(4):483–490.
7. Chima CS, Dietz-Seher C, Kushner-Benson S. Nutrition risk screening in acute care: a survey of practice. *Nutr Clin Pract.* 2008;23(4):417–423.
8. Bistrian BR, Blackburn GL, Hallowell E, Heddle R. Protein status of general surgical patients. *JAMA.* 1974;230(6):858–860.
9. Bistrian BR, Blackburn GL, Sherman M, Scrimshaw NS. Therapeutic index of nutritional depletion in hospitalized patients. *Surg Gynecol Obstet.* 1975;141(4):512–516.
10. Jensen GL, Bistrian B, Roubenoff R, Heimburger DC. Malnutrition syndromes: a conundrum vs continuum. *JPEN J Parenter Enteral Nutr.* 2009;33(6):710–716.
11. Corkins MR, Guenter P, DiMaria-Ghalili RA, et al. A.S.P.E.N. data brief 2014: use of enteral and parenteral nutrition in hospitalized patients with a diagnosis of malnutrition: United States, 2010. *Nutr Clin Pract.* 2014;29(5):698–700.
12. Singh H, Watt K, Veitch R, Cantor M, Duerksen DR. Malnutrition is prevalent in hospitalized medical patients: are housestaff identifying the malnourished patient? *Nutrition.* 2006;22(4):350–354.
13. Volkert D, Saeglitz C, Gueldenzoph H, Sieber CC, Stehle P. Undiagnosed malnutrition and nutrition-related problems in geriatric patients. *J Nutr Health Aging.* 2010;14(5):387–392.
14. White JV, Guenter P, Jensen G, et al. Consensus statement: Academy of Nutrition and Dietetics and American Society for Parenteral and Enteral Nutrition: characteristics recommended for the identification and documentation of adult malnutrition (undernutrition). *JPEN J Parenter Enteral Nutr.* 2012;36(3):275–283.
15. Cederholm T, Bosaeus I, Barazzoni R, et al. Diagnostic criteria for malnutrition: an ESPEN consensus statement. *Clin Nutr.* 2015;34(3):335–340.
16. Sheean PM, Peterson SJ, Gurka DP, Braunschweig CA. Nutrition assessment: the reproducibility of Subjective Global Assessment in patients requiring mechanical ventilation. *Eur J Clin Nutr.* 2010;64(11):1358–1364.
17. de Mutsert R, Grootendorst DC, Boeschoten EW, et al. Subjective Global Assessment of nutritional status is strongly associated with mortality in chronic dialysis patients. *Am J Clin Nutr.* 2009;89(3):787–793.
18. Cederholm T, Barazzoni R, Austin P, et al. ESPEN guidelines on definitions and terminology of clinical nutrition. *Clin Nutr.* 2017;36(1):49–64.
19. Guenter P, Jensen G, Patel V, et al. Addressing disease-related malnutrition in hospitalized patients: a call for a national goal. *Jt Comm J Qual Patient Saf.* 2015;41(10):469–473.
20. Scrimshaw NS, Taylor CE, Gordon JE. Interactions of nutrition and infection. *Am J Med Sci.* 1959;237(3):367–403.
21. Keusch GT. The history of nutrition: malnutrition, infection and immunity. *J Nutr.* 2003;133(1 Suppl):336S–340S.
22. Detsky AS, McLaughlin JR, Baker JP, et al. What is Subjective Global Assessment of nutritional status? *JPEN J Parenter Enteral Nutr.* 1987;11(1):8–13.
23. Gabay C, Kushner I. Acute-phase proteins and other systemic responses to inflammation. *N Engl J Med.* 1999;340(6):448–454.
24. Norman K, Pichard C, Lochs H, Pirlich M. Prognostic impact of disease-related malnutrition. *Clin Nutr.* 2008;27(1):5–15.

25. Guigoz Y. The Mini Nutritional Assessment (MNA) review of the literature: what does it tell us? *J Nutr Health Aging*. 2006; 10(6):466–487.

26. Kaiser MJ, Bauer JM, Ramsch C, et al. Frequency of malnutrition in older adults: a multinational perspective using the Mini Nutritional Assessment. *J Am Geriatr Soc*. 2010;58(9):1734–1738.

27. Bauer J, Capra S, Ferguson M. Use of the scored Patient-Generated Subjective Global Assessment (PG-SGA) as a nutrition assessment tool in patients with cancer. *Eur J Clin Nutr*. 2002;56(8):779–785.

28. Pirlich M, Schutz T, Norman K, et al. The German hospital malnutrition study. *Clin Nutr*. 2006;25(4):563–572.

29. Taylor BE, McClave SA, Martindale RG, et al. Guidelines for the provision and assessment of nutrition support therapy in the adult critically ill patient: Society of Critical Care Medicine (SCCM) and American Society for Parenteral and Enteral Nutrition (A.S.P.E.N.). *Crit Care Med*. 2016;44(2):390–438.

30. American Gastroenterological Association. American Gastroenterological Association medical position statement: evaluation of liver chemistry tests. *Gastroenterology*. 2002;123(4):1364–1366.

31. Prado CM, Heymsfield SB. Lean tissue imaging: a new era for nutritional assessment and intervention. *JPEN J Parenter Enteral Nutr*. 2014;38(8):940–953.

32. Earthman CP. Body Composition tools for assessment of adult malnutrition at the bedside: a tutorial on research considerations and clinical applications. *JPEN J Parenter Enteral Nutr*. 2015; 39(7):787–822.

33. Jensen GL, Mirtallo J, Compher C, et al. Adult starvation and disease-related malnutrition: a proposal for etiology-based diagnosis in the clinical practice setting from the International Consensus Guideline Committee. *JPEN J Parenter Enteral Nutr*. 2010; 34(2):156–159.

34. Malone A, Hamilton C. The Academy of Nutrition and Dietetics/ the American Society for Parenteral and Enteral Nutrition consensus malnutrition characteristics: application in practice. *Nutr Clin Pract*. 2013;28(6):639–650.

35. Fischer M, JeVenn A, Hipskind P. Evaluation of muscle and fat loss as diagnostic criteria for malnutrition. *Nutr Clin Pract*. 2015; 30(2):239–248.

36. Moises A, Rome E. Anorexia nervosa and bulimia nervosa. *ACP Hospitalist*. September 2011. www.acphospitalist.org/archives/2011 /09/focus.htm. Accessed June 15, 2017.

37. Rome ES, Strandjord SE. Eating disorders. *Pediatr Rev*. 2016; 37(8):323–336.

38. Mehler PS, Brown C. Anorexia nervosa: medical complications. *J Eat Disord*. 2015;3:11.

39. Norman K, Stobaus N, Gonzalez MC, Schulzke JD, Pirlich M. Hand grip strength: outcome predictor and marker of nutritional status. *Clin Nutr*. 2011;30(2):135–142.

40. Puthucheary ZA, Rawal J, McPhail M, et al. Acute skeletal muscle wasting in critical illness. *JAMA*. 2013;310(15):1591–1600.

41. Rosenbaum K, Wang J, Pierson RN, Kotler DP. Time-dependent variation in weight and body composition in healthy adults. *JPEN J Parenter Enteral Nutr*. 2000;24(2):52–55.

42. Han TS, Tajar A, Lean ME. Obesity and weight management in the elderly. *Br Med Bull*. 2011;97:169–196.

43. Schutz Y, Kyle UU, Pichard C. Fat-free mass index and fat mass index percentiles in Caucasians aged 18–98 y. *Int J Obes Relat Metab Disord*. 2002;26(7):953–960.

44. Skipper A, Ferguson M, Thompson K, Castellanos VH, Porcari J. Nutrition screening tools: an analysis of the evidence. *JPEN J Parenter Enteral Nutr*. 2012;36(3):292–298.

45. Young AM, Kidston S, Banks MD, Mudge AM, Isenring EA. Malnutrition screening tools: comparison against two validated nutrition assessment methods in older medical inpatients. *Nutrition*. 2013;29(1):101–106.

46. Ferguson M, Capra S, Bauer J, Banks M. Development of a valid and reliable malnutrition screening tool for adult acute hospital patients. *Nutrition*. 1999;15(6):458–464.

47. Elia M. The "MUST" report, nutritional screening of adults: a multidisciplinary responsibility. British Association for Parenteral and Enteral Nutrition; 2003. www.bapen.org.uk/pdfs/must /must_exec_sum.pdf. Accessed June 15, 2017.

48. Kondrup J, Rasmussen HH, Hamberg O, et al. Nutritional risk screening (NRS 2002): a new method based on an analysis of controlled clinical trials. *Clin Nutr*. 2003;22(3):321–336.

49. Kruizenga HM, Van Tulder MW, Seidell JC, et al. Effectiveness and cost-effectiveness of early screening and treatment of malnourished patients. *Am J Clin Nutr*. 2005;82(5):1082–1089.

50. Kruizenga HM, Seidell JC, de Vet HC, Wierdsma NJ, van Bokhorst-de van der Schueren MA. Development and validation of a hospital screening tool for malnutrition: the Short Nutritional Assessment Questionnaire (SNAQ). *Clin Nutr*. 2005;24(1):75–82.

51. Rolland Y, Perrin A, Gardette V, Filhol N, Vellas B. Screening older people at risk of malnutrition or malnourished using the Simplified Nutritional Appetite Questionnaire (SNAQ): a comparison with the Mini-Nutritional Assessment (MNA) tool. *J Am Med Dir Assoc*. 2012;13(1):31–34.

52. Heyland DK, Dhaliwal R, Jiang X, Day AG. Identifying critically ill patients who benefit the most from nutrition therapy: the development and initial validation of a novel risk assessment tool. *Crit Care*. 2011;15(6):R268.

53. Rahman A, Hasan RM, Agarwala R, Martin C, Day AG, Heyland DK. Identifying critically-ill patients who will benefit most from nutritional therapy: further validation of the "modified NUTRIC" nutritional risk assessment tool. *Clin Nutr*. 2016;35(1):158–162.

54. Hammond K. *Assessment: Dietary and Clinical Data*. 12th ed. St Louis, MO: Saunders Elsevier; 2008.

55. Brantley SL, Russell MK, Mogensen KM, et al. American Society for Parenteral and Enteral Nutrition and Academy of Nutrition and Dietetics: revised 2014 standards of practice and standards of professional performance for registered dietitian nutritionists (competent, proficient, and expert) in nutrition support. *J Acad Nutr Diet*. 2014;114(12):2001–2008.

56. Chumlea WC, Roche AF, Steinbaugh ML. Estimating stature from knee height for persons 60 to 90 years of age. *J Am Geriatr Soc*. 1985;33(2):116–120.

57. Klein S, Kinney J, Jeejeebhoy K, et al. Nutrition support in clinical practice: review of published data and recommendations for future research directions. National Institutes of Health, American Society for Parenteral and Enteral Nutrition, and American Society for Clinical Nutrition. *JPEN J Parenter Enteral Nutr*. 1997;21(3):133–156.

58. Society of Actuaries and Association of Life Insurance Medical Directors. 1979 Build Study. Chicago, IL: Metropolitan Life Insurance Company; 1980.

59. Heymsfield SB, Cefalu WT. Does body mass index adequately convey a patient's mortality risk? *JAMA*. 2013;309(1):87–88.

60. Primeau V, Coderre L, Karelis AD, et al. Characterizing the profile of obese patients who are metabolically healthy. *Int J Obes (Lond)*. 2011;35(7):971–981.

61. Flegal KM, Kit BK, Orpana H, Graubard BI. Association of all-cause mortality with overweight and obesity using standard body mass index categories. *JAMA*. 2012;309(1):71–82.

62. Blackburn GL, Bistrian BR, Maini BS, Schlamm HT, Smith MF. Nutritional and metabolic assessment of the hospitalized patient. *JPEN J Parenter Enteral Nutr*. 1977;1(1):11–22.

63. Keys A. Caloric undernutrition and starvation, with notes on protein deficiency. *J Am Med Assoc*. 1948;138(7):500–511.

64. National Heart, Lung, and Blood Institute. Classification of overweight and obesity by BMI, waist circumference, and associated

disease risks. https://www.nhlbi.nih.gov/health/educational/lose_wt/BMI/bmi_dis.htm. Accessed May 30, 2017.

65. Bharadwaj S, Ginoya S, Tandon P, et al. Malnutrition: laboratory markers vs nutritional assessment. *Gastroenterol Rep (Oxf)*. 2016;4(4):272–280.

66. Jensen GL. Inflammation as the key interface of the medical and nutrition universes: a provocative examination of the future of clinical nutrition and medicine. *JPEN J Parenter Enteral Nutr.* 2006; 30(5):453–463.

67. Lexicomp Online. Albumin. Updated June 3, 2016. Accessed June 27, 2017.

68. Rall LC, Roubenoff R, Harris TB. *Albumin as a Marker of Nutritional and Health Status.* New York: Raven; 1995.

69. Banh L. Serum proteins as markers of nutrition: what are we treating? *Pract Gastroenterol.* 2006;43:46–63. https://med.virginia.edu/ginutrition/articles-from-practical-gastroenterology. Accessed May 30, 2017.

70. Pagana KD, Pagana TJ, Pagana TN. *Mosby's Diagnostic and Laboratory Test Reference.* 12th ed. St. Louis, MO: Elsevier; 2015.

71. Davis CJ, Sowa D, Keim KS, Kinnare K, Peterson S. The use of prealbumin and C-reactive protein for monitoring nutrition support in adult patients receiving enteral nutrition in an urban medical center. *JPEN J Parenter Enteral Nutr.* 2012;36(2):197–204.

72. Ingenbleek Y, Young V. Transthyretin (prealbumin) in health and disease: nutritional implications. *Annu Rev Nutr.* 1994;14:495–533.

73. Carpentier YA, Barthel J, Bruyns J. Plasma protein concentration in nutritional assessment. *Proc Nutr Soc.* 1982;41(3):405–417.

74. Boles JM, Garre MA, Youinou PY, et al. Nutritional status in intensive care patients: evaluation in 84 unselected patients. *Crit Care Med.* 1983;11(2):87–90.

75. Goldberg DM, Brown D. Advances in the application of biochemical tests to diseases of the liver and biliary tract: their role in diagnosis, prognosis, and the elucidation of pathogenetic mechanisms. *Clin Biochem.* 1987;20(2):127–148.

76. Roza AM, Tuitt D, Shizgal HM. Transferrin: a poor measure of nutritional status. *JPEN J Parenter Enteral Nutr.* 1984;8(5): 523–528.

77. Fletcher JP, Little JM, Guest PK. A comparison of serum transferrin and serum prealbumin as nutritional parameters. *JPEN J Parenter Enteral Nutr.* 1987;11(2):144–147.

78. Spiekerman AM. Proteins used in nutritional assessment. *Clin Lab Med.* 1993;13(2):353–369.

79. Sachs E, Bernstein LH. Protein markers of nutrition status as related to sex and age. *Clin Chem.* 1986;32(2):339–341.

80. Smith FR, Goodman DS. The effects of diseases of the liver, thyroid, and kidneys on the transport of vitamin A in human plasma. *J Clin Invest.* 1971;50(11):2426–2436.

81. Pepys MB. C-reactive protein fifty years on. *Lancet.* 1981;1(8221): 653–657.

82. Deodhar SD. C-reactive protein: the best laboratory indicator available for monitoring disease activity. *Cleve Clin J Med.* 1989;56(2):126–130.

83. American Association of Clinical Chemistry. Lab Tests Online. https://labtestsonline.org. Accessed July 14, 2016.

84. Brandt C, Pedersen BK. The role of exercise-induced myokines in muscle homeostasis and the defense against chronic diseases. *J Biomed Biotechnol.* 2010;2010:520258.

85. Baker JP, Detsky AS, Wesson DE, et al. Nutritional assessment: a comparison of clinical judgment and objective measurements. *N Engl J Med.* 1982;306(16):969–972.

86. Kondrup J. Can food intake in hospitals be improved? *Clin Nutr.* 2001;20(1):153–160.

87. Tarasuk V, Beaton GH. Day-to-day variation in energy and nutrient intake: evidence of individuality in eating behaviour? *Appetite.* 1992;18(1):43–54.

88. Schoeller DA. Limitations in the assessment of dietary energy intake by self-report. *Metabolism.* 1995;44(2 Suppl 2):S18–S22.

89. Subar AF, Freedman LS, Tooze JA, et al. Addressing current criticism regarding the value of self-report dietary data. *J Nutr.* 2015;145(12):2639–2645.

90. Johnson RK. Dietary intake: how do we measure what people are really eating? *Obes Res.* 2002;10(Suppl 1):63S–68S.

91. Burke BS, Stuart HC. A method of diet analysis: application in research and pediatric practice. *J Pediatrics.* 1938;12(4):493–503.

92. Institute of Medicine. Dietary Reference Intakes Tables and Application. https://www.nal.usda.gov/fnic/dri-tables-and-application-reports. Accessed May 30, 2017.

93. Smiciklas-Wright H, Mitchell DC, Lindiwe JH. Dietary intake assessment: methods for adults. In: Berdanier CD, ed. *Handbook of Nutrition and Food.* 2nd ed. Boca Raton, FL: CRC Press; 2007.

94. Jensen GL, Hsiao PY, Wheeler D. Adult nutrition assessment tutorial. *JPEN J Parenter Enteral Nutr.* 2012;36(3):267–274.

95. Sterns RH. Pathophysiology and etiology of edema in adults. In: Post TW, ed. *UpToDate.* Waltham, MA: UpToDate; 2014. www.uptodate.com. Accessed August 24, 2016.

96. Jensen GL. Malnutrition and inflammation—"burning down the house": inflammation as an adaptive physiologic response versus self-destruction? *JPEN J Parenter Enteral Nutr.* 2015;39(1):56–62.

97. Winkler MF, Malone AM. Medical nutrition therapy for metabolic stress: sepsis, trauma, burns, and surgery. In: Mahan LK, Escott-Stump S, eds. St Louis, MO: Saunders; 2008:1021–1041.

98. Thibault R, Pichard C. The evaluation of body composition: a useful tool for clinical practice. *Ann Nutr Metab.* 2012;60(1):6–16.

99. Puthucheary Z, Montgomery H, Moxham J, Harridge S, Hart N. Structure to function: muscle failure in critically ill patients. *J Physiol.* 2010;588(23):4641–4648.

100. Mitchell WK, Williams J, Atherton P, et al. Sarcopenia, dynapenia, and the impact of advancing age on human skeletal muscle size and strength; a quantitative review. *Front Physiol.* 2012;3:260.

101. Cruz-Jentoft AJ, Baeyens JP, Bauer JM, et al. Sarcopenia: European consensus on definition and diagnosis: report of the European Working Group on Sarcopenia in Older People. *Age Ageing.* 2010;39(4):412–423.

102. Fielding RA, Vellas B, Evans WJ, et al. Sarcopenia: an undiagnosed condition in older adults. Current consensus definition: prevalence, etiology, and consequences. International working group on sarcopenia. *J Am Med Dir Assoc.* 2011;12(4):249–256.

103. Martin L, Birdsell L, Macdonald N, et al. Cancer cachexia in the age of obesity: skeletal muscle depletion is a powerful prognostic factor, independent of body mass index. *J Clin Oncol.* 2013; 31(12):1539–1547.

104. Prado CM, Lieffers JR, McCargar LJ, et al. Prevalence and clinical implications of sarcopenic obesity in patients with solid tumours of the respiratory and gastrointestinal tracts: a population-based study. *Lancet Oncol.* 2008;9(7):629–635.

105. Peterson SJ, Mozer M. Differentiating sarcopenia and cachexia among patients with cancer. *Nutr Clin Pract.* 2017;32(1):30–39.

106. Sheean PM, Peterson SJ, Gomez Perez S, et al. The prevalence of sarcopenia in patients with respiratory failure classified as normally nourished using computed tomography and Subjective Global Assessment. *JPEN J Parenter Enteral Nutr.* 2014;38(7): 873–879.

107. Shen W, Punyanitya M, Wang Z, et al. Total body skeletal muscle and adipose tissue volumes: estimation from a single abdominal cross-sectional image. *J Appl Physiol.* 2004;97(6):2333–2338.

108. Gomez-Perez SL, Haus JM, Sheean P, et al. Measuring abdominal circumference and skeletal muscle from a single cross-sectional computed tomography image: a step-by-step guide for clinicians using National Institutes of Health ImageJ. *JPEN J Parenter Enteral Nutr.* 2016;40(3):308–318.

109. Gruther W, Benesch T, Zorn C, et al. Muscle wasting in intensive care patients: ultrasound observation of the M. quadriceps femoris muscle layer. *J Rehabil Med.* 2008;40(3):185–189.

110. Campbell IT, Watt T, Withers D, et al. Muscle thickness, measured with ultrasound, may be an indicator of lean tissue wasting in multiple organ failure in the presence of edema. *Am J Clin Nutr.* 1995;62(3):533–539.

111. Mourtzakis M, Wischmeyer P. Bedside ultrasound measurement of skeletal muscle. *Curr Opin Clin Nutr Metab Care.* 2014;17(5):389–395.

112. Reid CL, Campbell IT, Little RA. Muscle wasting and energy balance in critical illness. *Clin Nutr.* 2004;23(2):273–280.

113. Arbeille P, Kerbeci P, Capri A, et al. Quantification of muscle volume by echography: comparison with MRI data on subjects in long-term bed rest. *Ultrasound Med Biol.* 2009;35(7):1092–1097.

114. Teigen L, Kuchnia AJ, Mourtzakis M, Earthman CP. The use of technology for estimating body composition: strengths and weaknesses of common modalities in a clinical setting. *Nutr Clin Pract.* 2017;31(1):20–29.

115. Tillquist M, Kutsogiannis DJ, Wischmeyer PE, et al. Bedside ultrasound is a practical and reliable measurement tool for assessing quadriceps muscle layer thickness. *JPEN J Parenter Enteral Nutr.* 2014;38(7):886–890.

116. Lean ME, Han TS, Deurenberg P. Predicting body composition by densitometry from simple anthropometric measurements. *Am J Clin Nutr.* 1996;63(1):4–14.

117. Hall JC, O'Quigley J, Giles GR, Appleton N, Stocks H. Upper limb anthropometry: the value of measurement variance studies. *Am J Clin Nutr.* 1980;33(8):1846–1851.

118. Elia M. The bioimpedance "craze." *Eur J Clin Nutr.* 1993;47(12):825–827.

119. Jebb SA, Elia M. Techniques for the measurement of body composition: a practical guide. *Int J Obes Relat Metab Disord.* 1993;17(11):611–621.

120. Roubenoff R, Baumgartner RN, Harris TB, et al. Application of bioelectrical impedance analysis to elderly populations. *J Gerontol A Biol Sci Med Sci.* 1997;52(3):M129–M136.

121. Pietrobelli A, Formica C, Wang Z, Heymsfield SB. Dual-energy X-ray absorptiometry body composition model: review of physical concepts. *Am J Physiol.* 1996;271(6):E941–E951.

122. Rubiano F, Nunez C, Heymsfield SB. A comparison of body composition techniques. *Ann N Y Acad Sci.* 2000;904:335–338.

123. Heymsfield SB, Wang Z, Baumgartner RN, Ross R. Human body composition: advances in models and methods. *Annu Rev Nutr.* 1997;17:527–558.

124. Siervo M, Jebb SA. Body composition assessment: theory into practice: introduction of multicompartment models. *IEEE Eng Med Biol Mag.* 2010;29(1):48–59.

125. Baracos V, Kazemi-Bajestani SM. Clinical outcomes related to muscle mass in humans with cancer and catabolic illnesses. *Int J Biochem Cell Biol.* 2013;45(10):2302–2308.

126. Barber L, Barrett R, Lichtwark G. Validity and reliability of a simple ultrasound approach to measure medial gastrocnemius muscle length. *J Anat.* 2011;218(6):637–642.

127. Braunwald E, Loscalzo J. Edema. In: Longo DL, Fauci AS, Kasper DL, et al, eds. *Harrison's Principles of Internal Medicine.* 18th ed. New York: McGraw Medical; 2012.

128. Sterns RH. Etiology, clinical manifestations, and diagnosis of volume depletion in adults. In: Post TW, ed. *UpToDate.* Waltham, MA: UpToDate; 2014. www.uptodate.com. Accessed February 2, 2016.

129. Rosenthal LD, Cumbler E. Evaluation of peripheral edema. Epocrates. 2016. https://online.epocrates.com/noFrame/showPage?method=diseases&MonographId=609&ActiveSectionId=11. Accessed June 15, 2017.

130. Edema. In: Stern SDC, Cifu AS, Altkorn D, eds. *Symptom to Diagnosis: An Evidence-Based Guide.* 2nd ed. New York: McGraw Medical; 2009:248–265.

131. Sterns RH. Clinical manifestations and diagnosis of edema in adults. In: Post TW, ed. *UpToDate.* Waltham, MA: UpToDate; 2014. www.uptodate.com. Accessed January 30, 2016.

132. Med-Health.net. Edema grading. http://www.med-health.net/edema-grading.html. Accessed July 18, 2017.

133. Lawson CM, Daley BJ, Sams VG, Martindale R, Kudsk KA, Miller KR. Factors that impact patient outcome: nutrition assessment. *JPEN J Parenter Enteral Nutr.* 2013;37(5 Suppl):30S–38S.

134. Phelps KR. Edema. In: Walker HK, Hall WD, Hurst JW, ed. *Clinical Methods: The History, Physical, and Laboratory Examinations.* 3rd ed. Boston, MA: Butterworths; 1990.

135. Hogan M. *Medical-Surgical Nursing.* 2nd ed. Salt Lake City, UT: Prentice Hall; 2007.

136. Russell MK. Functional assessment of nutrition status. *Nutr Clin Pract.* 2015;30(2):211–218.

137. Norman K, Stobaus N, Smoliner C, et al. Determinants of hand grip strength, knee extension strength, and functional status in cancer patients. *Clin Nutr.* 2010;29(5):586–591.

138. Dowhan L, DeChicco R, Welsh R, et al. Comparison between handgrip dynamometry and manual muscle testing performed by registered dietitians in measuring muscle strength and function of hospitalized patients. *JPEN J Parenter Enteral Nutr.* 2016;40(7):951–958.

139. Heymsfield SB, McManus C, Stevens V, Smith J. Muscle mass: reliable indicator of protein-energy malnutrition severity and outcome. *Am J Clin Nutr.* 1982;35(5 Suppl):S1192–S1199.

140. Kalantar-Zadeh K, Kleiner M, Dunne E, Lee GH, Luft FC. A modified quantitative Subjective Global Assessment of nutrition for dialysis patients. *Nephrol Dial Transplant.* 1999;14(7):1732–1738.

10 Overview of Enteral Nutrition

Jennifer Doley, MBA, RD, CNSC, FAND, and Wendy Phillips, MS, RD, CNSC, CLE, FAND

CONTENTS

Acknowledgments: Susan L. Brantley, MS, RD, LDN, CNSC, and Mary E. (Beth) Mills, MS, RD, LDN, CNSC, were the authors of this chapter for the second edition.

Objectives

1. Identify indications and contraindications for enteral nutrition (EN) in specific patient populations.
2. Describe factors to consider when developing appropriate EN feeding regimens.
3. Identify and describe methods used to assess the tolerance, efficacy, and safety of EN delivery.

Test Your Knowledge Questions

1. Which of the following is a benefit of EN compared with parenteral nutrition (PN) or no nutrition?
   A. Maintenance of normal gallbladder function
   B. Reduced gastrointestinal (GI) bacterial translocation
   C. More efficient nutrient metabolism
   D. All of the above

2. High-protein hypocaloric EN feeding providing 65% to 70% of energy needs, as determined by indirect calorimetry (IC), is recommended for intensive care unit (ICU) patients with which of the following conditions?
   A. Malnutrition
   B. Obesity
   C. Liver failure
   D. Acute respiratory distress syndrome (ARDS)
3. Risk factors for aspiration include all of the following *except:*
   A. Malnutrition
   B. Use of naso-/oro-feeding tube
   C. Bolus EN feeding
   D. Supine position

Test Your Knowledge Answers

1. The correct answer is **D**. EN provides nutrients to the small intestine, stimulating the release of cholecystokinin, which helps maintain normal gallbladder function and reduce the risk of cholecystitis. Luminal nutrients provide GI structural support and help maintain the gut-associated and mucosa-associated lymphoid tissues vital to immune function. Immunoglobulin A (IgA), which is secreted within the GI tract in response to intraluminal nutrients, can prevent bacterial adherence and translocation. Nutrients from EN more closely mimic normal oral feeding, and undergo first-pass metabolism, promoting more efficient nutrient utilization.[1]

2. The correct answer is **B**. Patients with malnutrition should receive more than 80% of their estimated nutrient needs within 48 to 72 hours of intubation. Delays in initiating and advancing EN result in greater energy and protein deficits, which may contribute to higher infection and mortality rates. Studies indicate obese patients benefit from low-calorie, high-protein feedings to minimize the metabolic complications of feeding, preserve lean body mass (LBM), and mobilize fat stores. In patients with ARDS, studies indicate no difference in outcomes between those receiving eucaloric feedings and those receiving trophic feedings.[2]

3. The correct answer is **A**. Although malnutrition may result in generalized weakness and contribute to swallow dysfunction, malnutrition by itself is not recognized as a risk factor for aspiration. Conditions that manipulate or affect the function of the lower esophageal sphincter, such as the presence of a feeding tube in the esophagus, increase the risk of reflux and thus aspiration. Bolus feedings, which increase the volume of contents in the stomach, and the supine position also increase the risk of reflux.

Introduction

Enteral nutrition is defined as "nutrition provided through the gastrointestinal tract via a tube, catheter, or stoma that delivers nutrients distal to the oral cavity."[3] The history of EN, including the first rectal feedings;[4] the early "formula" mixtures of wine, eggs, milk, and other food substances;[5] and the growth and use of EN as a routine

intervention in modern-day critical care units can be found elsewhere.[5,6] Common indications for EN include stroke and other neurologic disorders that impair swallowing ability, oral intubation for mechanical ventilation preventing oral nutrition intake, or the need to feed the gut distal to an obstruction or high-output fistula.[7] A functional GI tract, with sufficient length and absorptive capacity, is necessary for effective nutrient delivery using EN.[1,8] EN can be tailored to the care setting, such as critical care and acute care units, long-term care facilities, or the home.

Enteral formulas are composed of a variety of sources of macronutrients, micronutrients, and water in different quantities to meet the individual goals of nutrition therapy. Because the formula itself may not be sufficient to meet the need for specific nutrients, additional amino acids, probiotics, vitamins, trace minerals, and fiber components may be added to EN regimens to provide specific therapeutic benefits.

The safety and efficacy of EN use has been demonstrated in several patient populations, including those with head injuries, trauma, burns, major surgery, and pancreatitis.[2]

Before initiating EN, clinicians should consider ethical issues, including the patient and/or family's wishes, quality of life, goals of care, and risks and benefits of nutrition therapy in the context of the patient's diagnosis, prognosis, and long-term care goals.[9] See Chapter 39 for more information on ethical issues.

Benefits

When comparing alternative feeding methods for patients who cannot ingest food and fluids by mouth, EN is preferred over PN.[2] Using the GI tract as much as possible for digestion and absorption of nutrients helps maintain the functional integrity of the gut. Nutrients provided via the enteral route undergo first-pass metabolism, promoting efficient nutrient utilization. The presence of nutrients in the small intestine maintains normal gallbladder function by stimulating the release of cholecystokinin, reducing the risk of cholecystitis that may occur if patients are kept *nil per os* (NPO [nothing by mouth]) or fed solely with PN.[1]

In addition to the benefit of maintaining normal digestive and absorptive capabilities, luminal nutrients provide GI structural support and help maintain the gut-associated and mucosa-associated lymphoid tissues vital to immune function. IgA, which is secreted within the GI tract in response to intraluminal nutrients, can prevent bacterial adherence and translocation. Additionally, in several prospective randomized clinical trials, EN has been shown to reduce infectious complications associated with pneumonia, sepsis, intravenous (IV) line sepsis, and intra-abdominal abscess. Finally, the provision of EN is, overall, less expensive than PN.[1,10,11] Therefore, whenever feasible, EN is a superior choice to PN.

Contraindications

While EN remains the preferred route of nutrition support when feasible, there are times when use of the GI tract is contraindicated. Patients with the conditions listed in Table 10-1 may require PN instead of EN.[1,8,12]

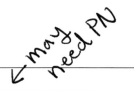
← may need PN

TABLE 10-1 Contraindications for Enteral Nutrition

- Severe short bowel syndrome (<100–150 cm remaining small bowel in the absence of the colon or 50–70 cm remaining small bowel in the presence of the colon)
- Other severe malabsorptive conditions
- Severe GI bleed
- Distal high-output GI fistula
- Paralytic ileus
- Intractable vomiting and/or diarrhea that does not improve with medical management
- Inoperable mechanical obstruction
- When the GI tract cannot be accessed—for example, when upper GI obstructions prevent feeding tube placement

GI, gastrointestinal.
Source: Data are from references 1, 8, and 12.

Assessment

After determining whether the patient is an appropriate candidate for EN, several factors need to be assessed to make necessary decisions regarding EN initiation. Expected duration of EN therapy, feeding modality, aspiration and refeeding risk, primary diagnosis, and comorbidities will all drive decisions regarding feeding tubes, formulas and administration schedules.

Access

When choosing a feeding tube, several factors should be considered, including—but not limited to—expected duration of therapy, desired feeding location (such as stomach or small intestine), administration mode (such as continuous or bolus), and the expertise of clinicians available for feeding tube placement.

Options for short-term EN therapy include tubes inserted through the nose or mouth into the stomach, past the pylorus into the duodenum, or distal to the ligament of Treitz into the jejunum. Long-term options include gastrostomy, jejunostomy, and gastrojejunostomy tubes for patients who will require nutrition therapy for longer than 4 to 6 weeks. These tubes can be placed using percutaneous endoscopic methods; radiological methods using fluoroscopy, ultrasound, or computed tomography (CT) are also available. When possible, the least-invasive placement method should be used; however, open or laparoscopic surgical placement may be necessary or convenient if another abdominal surgery is already being performed.

Clinical factors may influence the choice of feeding tube. Patients who are awake and alert often prefer small-bore, flexible tubes to limit discomfort. These tubes may reduce the risk of upper GI bleeding and therefore may be appropriate for patients who are overly anticoagulated or have esophageal varices.[13] Patients with significant ascites, unusual GI anatomy, or hiatal hernias may require surgically placed tubes if the gastroenterologist determines that endoscopic placement is not possible or may cause complications. See Chapter 12 for more information about enteral access and devices.

Formula Selection

Several commercially prepared enteral formulas are available to meet the needs of a variety of patients, and these products are generally categorized as standard or disease-specific. Standard formulas provide macronutrients and micronutrients in sufficient proportions to meet normal requirements for most patients. They have an energy density of 1 to 2 kcal/mL, and some contain fiber while others do not.[14] Most formulas, whether standard or disease-specific, do not provide sufficient fluid to meet hydration needs, thus necessitating the provision of additional water.

Disease-specific formulas include those designed for patients with renal or hepatic disease, diabetes, pulmonary disease (chronic obstructive pulmonary disease and ARDS), and immunocompromised patients. For patients with malabsorption, elemental or semi-elemental formulas may be beneficial as they are easily digested and absorbed.[15] Evidence supporting the use of disease-specific formulas is limited, and guidelines support the use of standard EN formulas in most patient populations.[1,2]

Manufacturers frequently develop new products with differing amounts or the addition of specific micronutrients, as well as altered macronutrient components and profiles, based on data from recent controlled studies, clinical practice guidelines, and expert recommendations.[6] Although homemade blenderized formulas can be used, they are more susceptible than commercial formulas to microbial contamination and are generally not used in the hospital setting.[14]

Modular components can be coadministered via the feeding tube to further individualize EN provision to meet specific nutrition goals. Increased energy content can be achieved by the addition of hydrolyzed cornstarch and maltodextrin as a carbohydrate component, and fat content can be increased through the addition of oils such as fish oils, medium-chain triglycerides, and safflower oils. Additionally, protein content can be increased through the addition of powdered calcium caseinates and whey protein concentrates. Individual amino acids such as glutamine and arginine are available and can be added via the enteral route if needed in quantities beyond what the EN formula provides.[16–19] Modulars typically are not mixed directly with EN formulas because they may clog the feeding tube. See Chapter 11 for more information on EN formulations.

Refeeding Risk

Although no standard definition or diagnostic criteria for refeeding syndrome exists, it is generally characterized by fluid and electrolyte shifts resulting from sodium and carbohydrate provision to malnourished patients. Although refeeding can occur with oral intake, it is more commonly associated with enteral, and especially parenteral, nutrition. Symptoms are generally seen in adults within 2 to 5 days of starting nutrition.[20]

Hypophosphatemia is present in almost all cases of refeeding;[21] other biochemical abnormalities may include hypokalemia, hypomagnesemia, hypocalcemia, hyperglycemia, and thiamin deficiency. These abnormalities are generally caused

TABLE 10-2 Potential Signs and Symptoms of Refeeding

- Electrolyte abnormalities
  - Hypophosphatemia
  - Hypokalemia
  - Hypomagnesemia
  - Hypocalcemia
  - Hyponatremia
- Cardiovascular conditions
  - Arrhythmias
  - Hypotension
  - Heart failure
  - Cardiac arrest
- Thiamin deficiency
- Fluid retention
- Hyperglycemia
- Neurologic conditions
  - Weakness
  - Numbness
  - Paresthesia
  - Myalgia
  - Vertigo
- Respiratory conditions
  - Shortness of breath
  - Pulmonary edema
  - Respiratory failure

Source: Data are from reference 21.

by increased use of these nutrients for carbohydrate metabolism. Refeeding can manifest as asymptomatic depletion of serum phosphorus, but, in severe cases, it can result in cardiopulmonary compromise.[20,21] See Table 10-2 for potential signs and symptoms of refeeding syndrome.[21]

Ideally, refeeding should be prevented; therefore, it is important to recognize risk factors, which include severe malnutrition, prolonged NPO status, and GI or renal conditions resulting in electrolyte losses (see Practice Scenario 10-1).[20,21] The use of medications that can result in electrolyte depletion, such as diuretics, is also a risk factor. Before starting nutrition support in at-risk patients, serum electrolytes should be checked and repleted if needed. Although EN formulas generally provide more than 100% of the Recommended Dietary Allowance for thiamin, additional thiamin supplementation may be beneficial, especially for patients at risk for deficiency, such as those with malnutrition or alcohol dependency.[20] The typical dose for repletion is 100 mg of thiamin daily for 5 to 7 days.

Practice Scenario 10-1

Questions: How do you assess the risk for refeeding in a patient requiring enteral nutrition (EN) therapy? How can you reduce the risk for refeeding in the enterally fed patient?

Scenario: A 62-year-old homeless man with alcohol dependency is admitted to the intensive care unit (ICU) with altered mental status. He is unable to provide a medical, diet, or weight history;

however, medical records indicate the patient has cirrhosis and has been admitted frequently for delirium tremens. The patient is underweight, with a body mass index of 17 and significant fat and muscle wasting. He is *nil per os* (NPO) on admission. On hospital Day 2, the patient is intubated to protect his airway due to worsening confusion and agitation. Serum laboratory results from the day of admission indicate potassium level of 3.1 mmol/L, phosphorus level of 2.2 mmol/L, and magnesium level of 1.6 mmol/L. Medications include multivitamin, thiamin, and folate administered via intravenous infusion. Enteral nutrition (EN) is started within 24 hours of intubation. On the morning following EN initiation, serum laboratory results indicate potassium level of 2.9 mmol/L, phosphorus level of 1.4 mmol/L and magnesium level of 1.5 mmol/L.

Intervention: Electrolyte replacement protocols are followed to replenish potassium, phosphorus, and magnesium levels on the day of admission. Electrolytes are rechecked prior to the initiation of EN and are within normal ranges. A standard EN formula is started at a rate of 20 mL/h and advanced slowly, by 10 mL every 12 hours, to a goal rate of 60 mL/h, which provides 25 kcal/kg. Electrolyte replacement protocols are again used to replete electrolyte levels, and the levels are rechecked per protocol until they are within normal range. The patient is monitored closely for other signs of refeeding, including cardiac arrhythmia.

Answer: Risk factors for refeeding include malnutrition, poor nutrition intake, and increased GI losses from ileostomies, diarrhea, or fistulas. The dietitian diagnoses the patient with severe malnutrition. Although the patient cannot provide a diet history, one can presume that, because of current alcohol dependency, homelessness, and altered mental status, the patient's nutrition intake prior to admission was limited. In recognition of these factors, EN was initiated at a low rate and advanced slowly to reduce the risk for refeeding. Depleted electrolyte levels were replaced prior to the start of EN, and again after EN initiation, and were rechecked frequently until normal levels were achieved. Thiamin was also provided as part of the standard regimen for treatment of active alcohol dependency; if not already provided, thiamin supplementation should have been initiated because of the risk for deficiency and refeeding.

Rationale: Biochemical abnormalities of refeeding syndrome may include hypophosphatemia, hypokalemia, hypomagnesemia, hypocalcemia, hyperglycemia, and thiamin deficiency, which are generally caused by increased use of these nutrients for carbohydrate metabolism. Severe cases of refeeding can result in cardiopulmonary compromise.[20,21]

Slowly advancing EN to goal rate in high-risk patients is recommended. Bankhead and colleagues[8] suggest initiating EN at 25% of goal rate and advancing to goal over 3 to 5 days. However, nutrition support providers should use clinical judgment to develop an individualized plan for advancement, considering the presence and severity of malnutrition, electrolyte levels prior to the start of EN, and assessment of refeeding risks compared with the benefits of early EN feeding.[8] In some cases, if electrolytes—especially phosphorus and potassium—

are severely depleted, it is prudent to delay advancement of EN to the goal rate.

Rapid identification of the signs and symptoms of refeeding is important to minimize complications; for this reason, serum electrolytes should be monitored daily once nutrition is initiated. Once electrolytes are repleted and electrolyte levels are stabilized, daily laboratory monitoring may no longer be required. Treatment of refeeding syndrome depends on the symptoms, but, in most cases, it can generally be managed by electrolyte replacement.[20] Electrolyte replacement protocols or guidelines may be beneficial.[22] See Chapter 13 for more information on EN complications.

Aspiration Risk

Aspiration, or the inhalation of GI or oropharyngeal contents into the lungs, can result in pneumonia and its consequences, including death. Dysfunctional swallowing can lead to aspiration of oral secretions and orally ingested foods and beverages, whereas regurgitation or reflux results in aspiration of stomach contents, the latter being relevant to EN administration. It should also be noted that aspiration of gastric contents is less likely to result in bacterial colonization of the respiratory tract than oral secretions.[23] As with refeeding, prevention is ideal, and risk factors should therefore be assessed when choosing a feeding tube and developing an EN regimen. See Table 10-3.[24]

Traditionally, a key strategy to decrease the incidence of aspiration in patients receiving EN has been postpyloric feeding tube placement, which reduces the volume of stomach contents. In a 2015 Cochrane review, the authors concluded that there was moderate-quality evidence to suggest that postpyloric feeding resulted in a 30% lower rate of aspiration than gastric feeding.[25]

Although experts have concluded that postpyloric feeding reduces aspiration, evidence that it reduces risk of pneumonia

TABLE 10-3 Risk Factors for Aspiration

- Inability to protect the airway related to
  - Reduced level of consciousness
  - Neurologic deficit
- Delayed gastric emptying related to
  - Gastroparesis
  - Medications (eg, opiods)
  - Hyperglycemia
  - Electrolyte abnormalities
- Presence of naso- or oroenteric feeding tube
- Gastroesophageal reflux disease
- Supine position
- Vomiting
- Bolus enteral feedings
- Mechanical ventilation
- Age >70 years
- Transport outside the intensive care unit
- Inadequate nurse-to-patient ratio
- Poor oral care

Source: Data are from reference 24.

is less clear; some studies have concluded that small bowel feeding did reduce incidence of pneumonia,[26,27] but other studies have not.[28,29] Most research suggests that although the incidence of pneumonia may be higher in gastric feeding, there is no difference in length of stay or mortality in gastric vs small bowel feeding; therefore, gastric feeding is considered safe for most patients.[2] Gastric feeding is preferable if waiting for migration of a feeding tube tip past the pylorus will delay the early initiation of EN; evidence indicates that gastric feeding increases nutrient provision.[30,31] However, postpyloric feeding is still recommended for patients at high risk for aspiration.[2] See Chapter 13 for more information on EN complications.

Intervention

Administration

After assessment of the patient has helped establish the route of feeding and formula to be used, decisions regarding EN initiation need to be made, including timing, modality, administration regimen, and energy, protein, and fluid goals.

Timing

In the hospital setting, the ideal time to start EN can vary depending on degree of illness and nutrition status on admission. Little has been published regarding the initiation of EN for noncritically ill patients; however, the American Society for Parenteral and Enteral Nutrition (ASPEN) *Enteral Nutrition Handbook* suggests that EN does not need to be initiated for a well-nourished patient until no or inadequate intake reaches 7 to 14 days.[1] Other sources suggest initiating EN within 5 to 7 days for well-nourished patients, and even sooner in malnourished patients.[32]

Early EN initiation is recommended in high-risk critically ill patients. Although definitions vary by study or protocol, "early" is usually defined as EN that is initiated within 24 to 48 hours of the initial insult, such as surgery, mechanical ventilation, or neurologic injury. Early initiation has been shown to significantly reduce mortality and infectious morbidity; for this reason, it is recommended that EN begin within 24 to 48 hours in this population.[2]

Early EN is recommended for specific subsets of the critically ill population, including patients with moderate to severe acute pancreatitis. Comparing early EN to late EN, and early EN to no nutrition provision, research has demonstrated positive outcomes, such as reduced infection rates, with early EN.[33-35] (See Chapter 28 for information on pancreatitis.) Similar research on post–liver transplant patients has also found significant improvements in infection rates, length of stay and survival.[36-38] (See Chapter 27 for information on liver disease and Chapter 31 for a discussion of solid organ transplantation.) Other critically ill populations, including trauma, traumatic brain injury, open abdomen in the absence of bowel injury, burns, and sepsis all seem to benefit when EN is initiated within 48 hours, if the patient is hemodynamically stable.[2] Burn patients in particular may benefit from even earlier EN initiation, within 4 to 6 hours of injury, if possible.[2,39,40]

(See Chapter 23 for more information on critical care and sepsis and Chapter 24 for coverage of trauma, surgery, and burns).

Modality

Enteral feeding may be administered by a continuous, intermittent drip, or bolus method. Factors such as the patient's preexisting and current medical conditions, location of the feeding tube tip, and the patient's expected tolerance to EN should be considered when selecting the delivery method.[41] The choice of feeding modality is also affected by the level of care, and the modality may change as the patient transitions across the continuum of care, from the ICU, to a lower acuity hospital unit, to a long-term care facility or the home. Patients may be fed with one method, or a combination of methods may be used to improve EN tolerance and quality of life. Some patients transition from one method of feeding administration to another as their clinical status evolves.

Continuous Feeding

Pump-assisted continuous drip infusions are the preferred method for feeding patients who are critically ill, are mechanically ventilated using an oro-tracheal method, are at risk for refeeding syndrome, have poor glycemic control, are being fed via jejunostomy tube, or have demonstrated intolerance to intermittent gravity drip or bolus feedings.[41] A variety of enteral feeding pumps are available on the market, ranging from lightweight portable pumps for home use to more durable pumps for use at home and in healthcare facilities.

The gravity drip method (without the use of a pump) may be used to provide continuous drip feedings to the noncritically ill patient living at home or outside the hospital setting. To determine the EN infusion rate, divide the total daily formula volume desired by the number of hours per day the formula will be administered. Table 10-4 shows a sample calculation of a continuous EN prescription. It is helpful to describe the volume of feeding in terms with which the patient and family are familiar, such as 60 mL/h equals ¼ cup (or 4 tablespoons) of formula infused over an entire hour, or 1 mL per minute.[42]

Cyclic Feeding

Cyclic feeding provides EN by pump or gravity drip over a time period that is less than 24 hours. Depending on the patient's volume tolerance, infusion times may be decreased from 24 hours per day down to as little as 8 hours.[43] As a patient recovers from critical illness, this method may be used to transition from 24-hour continuous feedings to 12-hour or shorter nocturnal feedings; it may increase the patient's volitional intake during the day and increase mobility by providing time in which the patient is free from tubing and pump connections.[43]

Intermittent Feeding

Intermittent feedings can be delivered by infusion pump or by the gravity drip method. This feeding regimen is usually selected for patients with feeding tubes that terminate in the stomach to accommodate the larger volumes administered in

TABLE 10-4 | Sample Calculations for a Continuous Feeding Regimen

1. Calculate daily nutrient needs:
   - 1900 kcal
   - 80 g protein
   - 2100 mL water
2. Choose EN formula:
   - Standard formula
   - 1.2 kcal/mL, 55 g protein per liter, 810 mL free water per liter
3. Calculate total volume of formula needed:
   - 1900 kcal ÷ 1.2 kcal/mL = 1583 mL/d
4. Divide by desired hours of infusion:
   - 1583 mL ÷ 24 hours = 65.9 mL/h
5. Round to nearest 5 mL, and calculate final volume:
   - 65 mL/h × 24 hours = 1560 mL/d
6. Calculate protein and water provision:
   - Protein: 1.56 liters × 55 g/L = 85.8 g/d
   - Water: 1.56 liters × 810 mL/L = 1264 mL/d
7. Determine additional protein and fluid needs:
   - Protein: No protein modular necessary
   - Water: 2100 mL – 1264 mL = 836 mL/d
8. Calculate water flushes (if not receiving fluid from other sources):
   - 836 mL ÷ 4 flushes/d = ~200 mL 4 times per day
9. Final EN regimen provides:
   - 1560 mL/d × 1.2 = 1872 kcal
   - 1.56 L/d × 55 = 86 g protein
   - (1.56 L/d × 810) + (200 mL × 4) = 2063 mL water

a shorter time period. Volumes can range from 240 to 720 mL (1 to 3 cups), be administered in a time period ranging from 20 to 60 minutes, and be provided anywhere from 4 to 6 times per day depending on the volume of formula required to meet the patient's specific needs.[41]

Patients receiving EN at home may try to mimic the feeding regimen used in the hospital by setting alarms to awaken and administer feeds every 4 to 6 hours, even during the night. Therefore, the patient and family should be instructed that intermittent feeding can occur entirely during waking hours, which improves quality of life and more closely matches their pre-illness or family meal schedule. This schedule adjustment can be accomplished by increasing the feeding volume, if tolerated, so as to decrease the total number of feeds. (See Chapter 38 for more information on home nutrition support.)

Bolus Feeding

Bolus feedings are accomplished by providing a set volume of formula at specified time intervals over a very short period of time, usually with a feeding syringe. A typical feeding regimen might provide 240 mL of formula over a 4- to 10-minute timeframe, with infusions 3 to 6 times per day and at least 3 hours between feedings.[43] Bolus feeds can also be administered using a gravity drip method. The rate of formula infusion using a gravity drip bag is regulated by adjusting a roller clamp. When using a syringe without a plunger as a funnel, the rate of delivery of formula is controlled by raising or lowering a formula-filled syringe or adjusting the rate of pressure applied when using the syringe plunger.[43] Bolus feedings mimic normal meals, provide freedom of movement, can be administered in more convenient settings (even outside the home), and are usually the least expensive delivery option.[43] (See Practice Scenario 10-2 for further discussion of the use of bolus feedings vs continuous enteral administration and Chapter 12 for more information on enteral access and devices.)

Practice Scenario 10-2

Question: When would a continuous enteral infusion be preferred over a bolus administration schedule?

Scenario: A 76-year-old man suffered a stroke with subsequent dysphagia and had a gastrostomy tube placed 7 days ago. After tolerating continuous enteral nutrition (EN) for 5 days, yesterday he was switched to a trial run of bolus feeds to prepare for discharge. Having been administered the volume of bolus feeds required to meet his nutrition needs using a feeding schedule that would work best for his caregivers, he exhibited nausea and distension, despite regular bowel movements. Gut motility medications were tried, with little improvement. The dietitian was asked to provide an alternative feeding plan to facilitate discharge.

Intervention: Bolus feeds of half the previously ordered volume were tried, and the patient tolerated these well. The dietitian documented intolerance of high-volume bolus feedings and worked with case management staff to obtain a feeding pump to administer continuous feeding during night-time hours to reduce the volume required during the day. Caregivers were instructed on the volume of EN to provide for the 4 boluses received during the day, and to administer them slowly, over 30 to 60 minutes, whenever possible. The patient was given this enteral feeding regimen in the hospital and then discharged home after demonstrating tolerance. The patient was instructed to follow up with a dietitian after discharge, as tolerance of the new feeding schedule improved, to assess the feasibility of transitioning to full-volume bolus feedings, thus eliminating the need for a feeding pump at home.

Answer: Patients who do not tolerate bolus feedings are good candidates for home continuous or intermittent feeds using a feeding pump, but adequate documentation must be provided to the insurance company for payment of needed supplies. Smaller, portable pumps are available for home use. For instances when it is preferable not to use the pump, such as social settings, a large-volume syringe can be used, with the rate of delivery of formula controlled by raising or lowering the formula-filled syringe or adjusting the rate of pressure applied when using the syringe plunger.

Rationale: Patients with dysphagia, such as this stroke patient, may require EN because they are at risk to aspirate oral secretions and orally ingested foods and beverages. Reflux can result in aspiration of stomach contents, including the enteral formula. This patient with abdominal distension and nausea is at high risk for reflux that could lead to aspiration due to his inability to

swallow safely, increasing his risk for aspiration, pneumonia, and further complications. Therefore, it is appropriate to change the feeding schedule to include continuous feeding to reduce the risk of aspiration.[41-43]

Initiation and Advancement

While assessment of GI function is necessary, initiation of EN should not be delayed in the absence of overt signs of GI contractility, such as bowel sounds or bowel movements, even in the critically ill population, because delayed EN will increase the risk of compromising the GI mucosal barrier and immune function.[2] Initial rate and advancement regimens should be individualized and based on the patient's clinical status, including acuity of illness, risk for refeeding, and expected tolerance of EN.

Stable noncritically ill patients generally tolerate EN initiated at the goal rate. If EN is not started at the goal rate, it should be rapidly advanced to the goal within 24 to 48 hours to maximize nutrient delivery.[1] Standard EN protocols for noncritically ill patients often include starting full strength feeds at 50 mL per hour and advancing by 15 mL per hour every 4 hours until the goal rate is met.[44] Bolus feedings can be advanced by volumes of 60 to 120 mL every 8 to 12 hours until goal volume is reached; more rapid advancement may be well tolerated by some patients at low risk for refeeding.[1]

In critically ill patients, EN is commonly started at a volume of 10 to 40 mL per hour and advanced to the goal rate by 10 to 20 mL per hour every 8 to 12 hours.[1] However, initiation at lower rates and slow advancement to the goal has been shown to be a major contributor to energy and protein deficits in this population.[45,46] Many critically ill patients can tolerate rapid advancement of EN to the goal rate within 24 to 48 hours, which results in smaller energy and protein deficits.[2,46] In fact, several studies have reported no difference in tolerance between critically ill patients who were started at the goal rate vs those whose EN was advanced more slowly.[46-48]

Volume-based feeding, in which EN is prescribed in terms of the goal volume per day rather than the goal volume per hour, is a more recent feeding method used in the critically ill population. Parameters vary by protocol, but they generally include starting EN at the goal rate, or rapidly advancing to the goal. The use of EN protocols, including those that are volume-based, such as FEED ME (*Feed Early Enteral Diet Adequately for Maximum Effect*) and PEP uP (*Enhanced Protein-Energy Provision via the Enteral Route Feeding Protocol*), have been shown to significantly improve nutrient delivery.[49-52]

EN initiation should be delayed in those critically ill patients who are considered hemodynamically unstable, generally defined as those with a mean arterial blood pressure of less than 50 mmHg, or those who are starting vasopressor medications or require increasing doses to maintain blood pressure. Although a rare complication in patients receiving EN, ischemic bowel may occur as a result of reduced blood flow to the gut, a potential consequence of low blood pressure. EN may be initiated in patients on low-dose stable vasopressors, but these patients should be monitored closely for signs of intolerance.[2] (See Chapter 23.)

Goal

EN should be advanced to the goal rate, as tolerated, within 24 to 48 hours in those patients who are determined to be at high nutrition risk or malnourished, with the goal of providing more than 80% of estimated energy and protein needs within 48 to 72 hours. In this high-risk population, rapid advancement to the goal reduces mortality and infection rates.[2] However, meeting 80% to 100% of estimated energy needs as soon as possible may not benefit all patients. Critically ill obese patients, regardless of diagnosis, may benefit from high-protein hypocaloric EN to minimize the metabolic complications of feeding, preserve LBM and mobilize fat stores. Hypocaloric feeding is defined as 65% to 70% of energy needs as estimated by IC; if IC is not available, calculations should be used to determine an appropriate hypocaloric regimen for the obese population.[2] (See Chapter 35 for more information on obesity.)

In patients with sepsis, guidelines[2] suggest that 60% to 70% of energy needs be provided in the first week of EN; EN should then be advanced to provide more than 80% of needs after the first week. It should be noted, however, that sufficient protein should be provided for all patients, if possible, as adequacy of protein provision is more closely correlated with positive outcomes than is adequate energy provision.[2]

Patients with ARDS or acute lung injury who are expected to be ventilated for more than 72 hours, and who are not at high nutrition risk or malnourished may receive either trophic EN (defined as 10 to 20 mL/h or up to 500 kcal/d) or full EN; no difference in outcomes has been demonstrated between these feeding regimens.[2] (See Chapter 23.)

Other Considerations

In the administration of EN, it is important to address numerous factors, including water provision, medication administration, and issues affecting the safety of EN.

Water Flushes

Flushing the enteral feeding tube with water helps prevent tube obstruction. Factors that increase the risk for clogging the feeding tube include the use of a fiber-containing formulas, use of small-diameter tubes, use of silicone rather than polyurethane tubes, checking gastric residual volumes (GRVs), and improper medication administration via the tube.[5] In addition to the minimum water flushes needed to maintain tube patency, water flushes should be provided to meet hydration needs, especially if the patient is not receiving IV hydration or drinking fluids.

The most frequently studied flush solutions to maintain tube patency are water, carbonated beverages, and cranberry juice. Water is the superior choice because it maintains patency the best and helps keep the patient adequately hydrated.[8] Sterile water is often used in the hospital, but tap water is generally used by patients at home. The 2009 ASPEN EN practice guidelines recommend flushing feeding tubes with at least 30 mL of water every 4 hours during continuous feeding or before and after intermittent or bolus feedings in adult patients.[8] The feeding tube should also be flushed with 30 mL of water after GRV checks.

Medication Administration

Many patients who depend on EN for nutrient delivery must also use the same access device for medication administration. The coadministration of formula and medications must be carefully managed to avoid tube obstruction and ensure medication safety and efficacy. When possible, a pharmacist should be consulted before the medication regimen or EN modality is changed. See Table 10-5 for helpful tips for administering medications via the enteral feeding tube,[53] and refer to Chapter 18 for information on drug-nutrient interactions.

TABLE 10-5 Tips for Administering Medications via the Enteral Feeding Tube

- Medication form:
  - Use liquid or suspension forms whenever possible. However, liquid medications may contain sorbitol or be hyperosmotic, which can lead to diarrhea. If diarrhea does occur, an alternate medication regimen may be needed.
  - If a tablet form must be used, consult with the pharmacist to ensure it can be safely crushed and dispersed in water prior to administration. Enteric-coated, sublingual, or sustained-release tablets generally should not be crushed.
  - Confirm appropriate medication delivery route with the pharmacist. Medications that depend on gastric acid for breakdown or absorption may need to be substituted or given by an alternate method if feeding tube placement is in the duodenum or jejunum.
- Medication administration:
  - Stop EN prior to the administration of medications; restart as soon as possible to ensure adequate nutrient delivery. Only delay restarting EN when it is necessary to avoid altered drug bioavailability.
  - Flush the tube with at least 30 mL of water before and after giving medications through the tube.
  - Give each medication separately and flush the tube with 5 mL of warm water between medications.
  - Do not mix medications or dosage forms, as this can affect drug stability and efficacy.
  - If the tube is smaller than 12 French, avoid using it to give crushed medications, if possible.
  - Do not add medications to the EN formula, as this can increase the incidence of tube occlusions, interfere with medication and nutrient bioavailability, affect GI function, and increase the risk of microbial contamination.

EN, enteral nutrition; GI, gastrointestinal.
Source: Data are from reference 53.

Safety Considerations

Safety of EN delivery can be compromised by microbial contamination or tubing misconnections, both of which can have potentially fatal consequences.

Open vs Closed Feeding Systems

Ready-to-use EN formulas come in either closed or open systems. A closed system consists of a sterile container of prefilled formula that is ready to administer to the patient and is spiked with an administration set. Open systems involve cans, bottles, or tetra-paks of formula that must be poured into an EN feeding bag or syringe before delivery to the patient. Patient safety and ease of use should be evaluated when determining which system to use. The EN delivery system least likely to contribute to infection through bacterial contamination is the safest, whereas the system with the fewest required administration steps is generally the easiest to use.

The risk of microbial contamination increases as manipulation and handling of the formula and administration set increase.[54-58] Contamination can occur during preparation if additional modular components must be added to the formula, when the feeding is transferred to the administration container, during assembly of the feeding system, and during administration to the patient.[17,59,60] To reduce the risk of bacterial contamination of a closed or open system, individuals who prepare and deliver formula must use clean preparation techniques and properly wash their hands.[16] Improper hand washing is one of the major causes of contamination of EN.[17-19]

Many studies support the use of closed over open systems because a closed system involves less manipulation of and human/environmental contact with the EN formula and feeding administration sets.[59,61-65] However, some studies imply that as long as proper administration procedures and hygiene rules are followed, an open system formula can be safely used,[66-68] and there is no benefit of using one system over another.[17,69,70] In addition to a decreased risk of bacterial contamination with a closed system, administration of formulas using a closed system requires fewer steps than administration of formulas using an open system,[71] thus saving time and healthcare resources.[17,72]

The administration of bacteria-contaminated formulas can cause complications including abdominal distension,[73] diarrhea,[60,74,75] and bacteremia.[76,77] Other rare but serious complications may include sepsis, pneumonia, and infectious enterocolitis, all of which ultimately lead to increased patient burden, longer hospital stays, and higher healthcare costs.[16,17,60,63,64,75,78-81] (See Chapter 13 for additional information on EN complications.)

Tubing Misconnections

Hospitalized patients receive nutrition, medication, and fluids through a variety of tubes and catheters that are often connected using small-bore connectors such as Luer connectors. Enteral misconnections can occur when an enteral feeding system is inadvertently connected to another system, such as an IV catheter or a peritoneal dialysis catheter, and formula is delivered outside of the GI tract to the lungs, bloodstream, or abdominal cavity. Historically, connectors were often compatible between different delivery systems, leading to patient injury and death when medicines, enteral formulas, or air were accidentally delivered through the wrong tubing.

The International Organization for Standardization provided safety requirements for new EN connectors, and a workgroup including manufacturers, clinicians, and governmental agencies developed a new design, now referred to as the ENfit connector.[82] In February 2015, the US Food and Drug Administration published final guidance for manufacturers of small-bore EN connectors to reduce the risks of misconnections. Enteral tubing misconnections will be much less likely to occur once manufacturers have fully implemented these recommendations.[83] (See Chapter 12 for more about enteral access and devices.)

Monitoring

The hospitalized patient receiving EN must be monitored to quickly identify and treat complications such as refeeding, aspiration, and GI intolerance, as well as to assess whether nutrients and fluids are adequately provided. Monitoring should include physical assessment, laboratory data, anthropometrics, vital signs, and measurement of intake and output.[1]

Tolerance

Traditionally, GRVs have been regularly used to assess EN tolerance; however, the most recent Society of Critical Care Medicine/American Society for Parenteral and Enteral Nutrition (SCCM/ASPEN) guidelines for nutrition support in critical illness do not recommend checking GRV.[2] A number of factors can compromise the accuracy of GRV checks, including feeding tube type, diameter, and position; viscosity of GRVs; technique, including size of the syringe and time and effort spent; and the position of the patient.[84,85]

GRVs have not been found to correlate with incidence of pneumonia[86,87] or aspiration; furthermore, checking GRVs can increase episodes of feeding tube occlusion, reduce the total volume of EN delivered, and take up valuable nursing time.[24] High GRVs have been identified as one of the primary reasons EN is held; holding EN repeatedly or for prolonged periods can increase the risk for development of an ileus.[2]

Some experts assert that checking GRVs may still be of value in some patient populations, namely those that are at high risk for GI dysfunction, such as patients in the surgical ICU and the most severely ill patients.[84] However, to provide adequate nutrient intake, EN should not be routinely held for high GRVs, and other methods of assessing GI function should be used. These indicators include passage of flatus and stool, stool frequency and consistency, physical examination to assess bowel sounds and abdominal girth, and abdominal radiographs. If GRVs are checked, the SCCM/ASPEN guidelines suggest that, in the absence of other signs of intolerance such as vomiting or abdominal distention, EN should not be held for GRVs of less than 500 mL.[2]

For most individuals on long-term stable EN, no formal assessment of GI tolerance is necessary. This is especially true for patients in the home setting, and for individuals who can effectively communicate any GI issues they may experience, such as nausea, bloating, or abdominal discomfort. (See Chapter 13 for information on EN complications and Chapter 38 for a discussion of home nutrition support.)

Hydration

Fluid is an important component of any EN regimen, especially in patients who are not receiving fluids intravenously or by mouth. Patients at high risk for dehydration include those with increased fluid losses. In addition to urine, excessive losses may occur in patients with high-volume GI output from diarrhea, colostomies, ileostomies, or fistulas; also, patients with high fevers, burns, or extensive wounds may lose higher than normal amounts of fluid from the skin. Although most risk factors for dehydration are related to medical issues, EN may contribute to dehydration if the formula provided is highly osmolar, which may result in osmotic diuresis related to an increased renal solute load.

Patients receiving EN should be assessed for signs of dehydration, including poor skin turgor, dry mucous membranes, and elevated serum blood urea nitrogen, creatinine, and sodium.

Excessive fluid intake may also be an issue, especially in patients with heart failure or renal dysfunction. In these populations, input, output, and weight should be monitored daily; additionally, regular physical assessment should be conducted to examine extremities for edema. Fluid management should be coordinated with the primary care provider, as fluid restrictions or diuretic medications may be necessary. (See Chapter 7 for discussion of fluid requirements and Chapter 29 for information about renal disease.)

Glycemic Control

Hyperglycemia is common in hospitalized patients, even in those without diabetes, particularly in the ICU setting. Causes are multifactorial and include increased release of counterregulatory hormones that stimulate gluconeogenesis, proinflammatory cytokines that result in insulin resistance, provision of steroid and adrenergic medications, and excess dextrose administration via IV fluid solutions and medications. Hyperglycemia negatively affects patient outcomes, resulting in higher infection rates, longer hospital stays, and increased mortality.[88]

Although earlier studies indicated improved outcomes with tight blood glucose (BG) control, more recent research has shown the opposite effect, presumably because higher incidences of hypoglycemia are associated with tight BG control. Therefore, according to the SCCM/ASPEN Guidelines, a target BG range of 140 to 180 mg/dL is recommended for hospitalized patients.[2] BG levels in patients with diabetes should be monitored regularly, generally every 4 to 6 hours; in the critically ill population, even for patients without diabetes, the same monitoring schedule should be followed if BG levels are greater than 180 mg/dL.[88] Sliding-scale insulin regimens and the use of oral hypoglycemia medications should not be used because they can delay the achievement of BG control and are associated with a higher incidence of renal dysfunction in hospitalized patients.

Several professional groups, such as the American Academy of Physicians and SCCM, have published specific guidelines on the use of insulin protocols to manage hyperglycemia in hospitalized patients.[88]

BG control can be achieved via continuous insulin drips; therefore, EN initiation and advancement to the goal rate should not be postponed because a critically ill patient has elevated BG levels. Although high-fat, low-carbohydrate formulas with fiber have been developed for patients with hyperglycemia, their efficacy has not been established.[2] Use of these products is generally not recommended because the higher fat content may delay gastric emptying, affecting tolerance and thereby limiting the ability to achieve goal volumes. (See Chapter 34 for more information about diabetes and glycemic control.)

Adequacy

The assessment of whether nutrition provision is adequate can be challenging in the acute care setting. Albumin and prealbumin, traditionally used as markers of nutrition status, are now known to be indicative of inflammatory status and not nutrition intake. No serum laboratory values effectively indicate nutrition status or adequacy of nutrition provision.

Especially in the ICU, body weight measurements are often unreliable if bed scales are not properly calibrated; furthermore, linens, dressings, tubing and other equipment on the bed can contribute to unreliable measurements. Weight should still be monitored; however, in the short term, weight changes are more likely to indicate changes in fluid status rather than adequacy of nutrition provision. In patients receiving long-term EN, weight should be monitored regularly because weight trends generally reflect adequacy of EN provision. However, it is important to consider the effects of inflammation and immobility in patients who are chronically critically ill, as both factors are associated with loss of LBM and are not completely attenuated by adequate nutrition provision.[2]

Radiographic imaging techniques, such as CT, magnetic resonance imaging (MRI), and ultrasound, are emerging as instruments to measure LBM. These tools are most beneficial in a hospital setting, where scans are already performed for the purpose of medical diagnosis. There are drawbacks to each type of radiographic imaging, including high radiation exposure with CTs, cost of CTs and MRIs, and the need for skilled ultrasound technicians.[89] Although radiographic imaging may be useful in assessment of LBM, and thus perhaps in estimation of nutrient needs, using these methods to monitor changes in LBM as a measure of nutrition support adequacy has not been studied. Changes in LBM in the setting of acute illness, especially in the critically ill population, are more likely a result of immobility and increased protein losses caused by the inflammatory process.

Nitrogen balance (NB) can be used as a tool to assess adequacy of protein provision. Measurement of urinary urea is used to estimate nitrogen losses, and 24-hour urine collection is required for accurate measurement, although some practitioners have collected urine for shorter time periods and extrapolated results to 24 hours. Research suggests, however, that collections of less than 12 hours may be less reliable.[90]

Measurement of protein intake during the same time period is also required; for this reason, estimations are most accurate for patients receiving EN or PN as the sole source of nutrition. A positive NB suggests adequate protein provision. Accuracy of NB can be limited by multiple factors, including impaired renal function; also, incomplete collection of GI losses from fistulas, stool, or ostomies can affect NB results. (See Chapter 6 for a discussion of how to calculate and interpret NB.)

Conclusion

Current evidence indicates that EN is a safe and effective mode of nutrient delivery in patients who cannot meet nutrition needs via oral intake. Benefits of EN include maintenance of gut integrity and immune function, reduced incidence of infectious complications, and attenuation of some negative metabolic consequences of illness. Many factors must be considered when developing an EN regimen, including indications for EN, as well as the individual patient's nutrition status, risk for complications, severity of illness, and comorbidities. Decisions regarding EN regimens, including when to initiate, formula selection, and enteral access, modality, advancement, and goals, will affect the efficacy and safety of feeding. Patients receiving EN feedings should be monitored for signs of complications such as refeeding, GI intolerance, and hyperglycemia.

References

1. Boullata J, Nieman Carney L, Guenter P, eds. *The A.S.P.E.N. Enteral Nutrition Handbook.* Silver Spring, MD: American Society for Parenteral and Enteral Nutrition; 2010.
2. McClave SA, Taylor BE, Martindale RG, et al. Guidelines for the provision and assessment of nutrition support therapy in the adult critically ill patient: Society of Critical Care Medicine (SCCM) and American Society for Parenteral and Enteral Nutrition (A.S.P.E.N.). *JPEN J Parenter Enteral Nutr.* 2016;40(2):159–211.
3. American Society for Parenteral and Enteral Nutrition. A.S.P.E.N definition of terms, style, and conventions used in A.S.P.E.N. Board of Directors–approved documents. 2015. http://www .nutritioncare.org/Guidelines_and_Clinical_Resources/Clinical _Practice_Library/Special_Reports. Accessed December 20, 2016.
4. McCamish MA, Bounous G, Geraghty ME. History of enteral feedings: past and present perspectives. In: Rombeau JL, Rolandelli RH, Kersey R, eds. *Clinical Nutrition Enteral and Tube Feeding.* 3rd ed. Philadelphia, PA: WB Saunders; 1997:1–11.
5. Bartlett RH. Nutrition in critical care. *Surg Clin N Am.* 2011; 91:595–607.
6. Skipper A. Enteral nutrition. In: Skipper A, ed. *Dietitian's Handbook of Enteral and Parenteral Nutrition.* 3rd ed. Sudbury, MA: Jones & Bartlett Learning; 2012:259–280.
7. A.S.P.E.N. Board of Directors and the Clinical Guidelines Task Force. Guidelines for the use of parenteral and enteral nutrition in adult and pediatric patients. *JPEN J Parenter Enteral Nutr.* 2002;26(Suppl):1SA-138SA (errata 2002;26:144).
8. Bankhead R, Boullata J, Brantley S, Corkins M, et al. Enteral nutrition practice recommendations. *JPEN J Parenter Enteral Nutr.* 2009;33(2):122–167.
9. Schwartz DB, Olfson K, Goldman B, Barrocas A, Wesley JR. Incorporating palliative care concepts into nutrition practice: across the age spectrum. *Nutr Clin Pract.* 2016;31(3):305–315.
10. Reddy P, Malone M. Cost and outcome analysis of home parenteral and enteral nutrition. *JPEN J Parenter Enteral Nutr.* 1998;22(5):302–310.
11. Academy of Nutrition and Dietetics Evidence Analysis Library. Critical illness: enteral and parenteral nutrition. What is the effect of enteral nutrition versus parenteral nutrition on the cost of medical care in critically ill patients? 2006. http://www.andeal .org/topic.cfm?cat=1032. Accessed June 26, 2016.
12. DiBaise J, Parrish CR. Short bowel syndrome in adults—part 5: trophic agents in the treatment of short bowel syndrome. *Pract Gastroenterol.* 2015;141:10–18.
13. Osman D, Djibre M, Da Silva D, Gouenok C. Management by the intensivist of gastrointestinal bleeding in adults and children. *Ann Intensive Care.* 2012;2(1):46.
14. Malone A. Enteral formula selection. In: Charney P, Malone A, eds. *ADA Pocket Guide to Enteral Nutrition.* Chicago, IL: American Dietetic Association; 2006:63–122.
15. Chen Y, Peterson S. Enteral nutrition formulas: which formula is right for your adult patient? *Nutr Clin Pract.* 2009;24(3):344–355.
16. Marion ND, Rupp ME. Infection control issues of enteral feeding systems. *Curr Opin Clin Nutr Metab Care.* 2000;3(5):363–366.
17. Herlick SJ, Vogt C, Pangman V, Fallis W. Clinical research: comparison of open versus closed systems of intermittent enteral feeding in two long term care facilities. *Nutr Clin Pract.* 2000;15(6):287–298.
18. Williams TA, Leslie GD. A review of the nursing care of enteral feeding tubes in critically ill adults: part II. *Intensive Crit Care Nurs.* 2005;21(1):5–15.
19. McKinlay J, Wildgoose A, Wood W, Gould IM, Anderton A. The effect of system design on bacterial contamination of enteral tube feeds. *J Hosp Infect.* 2001;47(2):138–142.
20. Miller SJ. Death resulting from overzealous total parenteral nutrition: the refeeding syndrome revisited. *Nutr Clin Pract.* 2008;23(2):166–171.
21. Skipper A. Refeeding syndrome or refeeding hypophosphatemia: a systematic review of cases. *Nutr Clin Pract.* 2012;27(1):34–40.
22. Flesher ME, Archer KA, Leslie BD, McCollom RA, Martinka GP. Assessing the metabolic and clinical consequences of early enteral feeding in the malnourished patient. *JPEN J Parenter Enteral Nutr.* 2005;29(2):108–117.
23. Bonten MJ, Gaillard CA, van Tiel FH, Smeets HG, van der Geest S, Stobberingh EE. The stomach is not a source for colonization of the upper respiratory tract and pneumonia in ICU patients. *Chest.* 1994;105(3):878–884.
24. McClave SA, DeMeo MT, DeLegge MH, et al. North American summit on aspiration in the critically ill patient: consensus statement. *JPEN J Parenter Enteral Nutr.* 2002;26(6 Suppl):S80–S85.
25. Alkhawaja S, Martin C, Butler RJ, Gwadry-Sridhar F. Post-pyloric versus gastric tube feeding for preventing pneumonia and improving nutritional outcomes in critically ill adults. *Cochrane Database Syst Rev.* 2015;CD008875. doi:10.1002/14651858.CD008875.pub2.
26. Heyland DK, Drover JW, Dhaliwal R, Greenwood J. Optimizing the benefits and minimizing the risks of enteral nutrition in the critically ill: role of small bowel feeding. *JPEN J Parenter Enteral Nutr.* 2003;26(6 Suppl):S51–S57.
27. Metheny NA, Stewart BJ, McClave SA. Relationship between feeding tube site and respiratory outcomes. *JPEN J Parenter Enteral Nutr.* 2011;35(3):346–355.
28. Ho KM, Dobb GJ, Webb SA. A comparison of early gastric and post-pyloric feeding in critically ill patients: a meta-analysis. *Intensive Care Med.* 2006;32(5):639–649.
29. Marik PE, Zaloga GP. Gastric versus post-pyloric feeding: a systematic review. *Crit Care.* 2003;7(3):R46–R51.
30. Zhang Z, Xu X, Ding J, Ni H. Comparison of postpyloric tube feeding and gastric tube feeding in intensive care unit patients: a meta-analysis. *Nutr Clin Pract.* 2013;28(3):371–380.

31. Saran D, Brody RA, Stankorb SM, Parrott SJ, Heyland DK. Gastric vs small bowel feeding in critically ill neurologically injured patients: results of a multicenter observational study. *JPEN J Parenter Enteral Nutr*. 2015;39(8):910–916.

32. Stroud M, Duncan H, Nightingale J. Guidelines for enteral feeding in adult hospital patients. *Gut*. 2003;52(Suppl 7):vii1–vii12.

33. Sun JK, Li WQ, Ke L, et al. Early enteral nutrition prevents intra-abdominal hypertension and reduces the severity of severe acute pancreatitis compared with delayed enteral nutrition: a prospective pilot study. *World J Surg*. 2013;37(9):2053–2060.

34. Wereszczynska-Siemiatkowska U, Swidnicka-Siergiejko A, Siemiatkowski A, Dabrowski A. Early enteral nutrition is superior to delayed enteral nutrition for the prevention of infected necrosis and mortality in acute pancreatitis. *Pancreas*. 2013;42(4):640–646.

35. Wu XM, Liao YW, Wang HY, Ji KQ, Li GF, Zang B. When to initialize enteral nutrition in patients with severe acute pancreatitis? A retrospective review in a single institution experience (2003–2013). *Pancreas*. 2015;44(3):507–511.

36. Ei S, Shinoda M, Itano O, Obara H, et al. Effects of addition of early enteral nutritional support during the postoperative phase in patients after living-donor liver transplantation. *Ann Transplant*. 2015;20:357–365.

37. Mehta PL, Alaka KJ, Filo RS, Leaman SB, Milgrom ML, Pescovitz MD. Nutrition support following liver transplantation: comparison of jejunal versus parenteral routes. *Clin Transplant*. 1995;9(5):364–369.

38. Ikegami T, Shirabe K, Yoshiya S, et al. Bacterial sepsis after living donor liver transplantation: the impact of early enteral nutrition. *J Am Coll Surg*. 2012;214(3):288–295.

39. Chiarelli A, Enzi G, Casadei A, Baggio B, Valerio A, Mazzoleni F. Very early nutrition supplementation in burned patients. *Am J Clin Nutr*. 1990;51(6):1035–1039.

40. Vicic VK, Radman M, Kovacic V. Early initiation of enteral nutrition improves outcomes in burn disease. *Asia Pac J Clin Nutr*. 2013;22(4):543–547.

41. Clohessy SRJ. Administration of enteral nutrition: initiation, progression, and transition. In: Rolandelli RH, Bankhead R, Boullata J, Compher CW, ed. *Clinical Nutrition Enteral and Tube Feeding*. 4th ed. Philadelphia, PA: WB Saunders; 2005:243–247.

42. Parrish CR. Enteral feeding: the art and science. *Nutr Clin Pract*. 2003;18(1):76–85.

43. Lord LM, Harrington M. Enteral nutrition implementation and management. In: Merritt R, De Legge MH, Holcombe B, ed. *The ASPEN Nutrition Support Practice Manual*. Silver Spring, MD: American Society for Parenteral and Enteral Nutrition; 2005:76–89.

44. Abad-Jorge A, Banh L, Cumming C. *Adult Enteral and Parenteral Nutrition Handbook*. 5th ed. Charlottesville: University of Virginia Health System; 2011.

45. Kozeniecki M, McAndrew N, Patel JJ. Process-related barriers to optimizing enteral nutrition in a tertiary medical intensive care unit. *Nutr Clin Pract*. 2016;31(1):80–85.

46. Dijkink S, Fuentes E, Quraishi SA, et al. Nutrition in the surgical intensive care unit: the cost of starting low and ramping up rates. *Nutr Clin Pract*. 2016;31(1):86–90.

47. Adam S, Batson S. A study of problems associated with the delivery of enteral feed in critically ill patients in five ICUs in the UK. *Intensive Care Med*. 1997;23(3):261–266.

48. Taylor SJ, Fettes SB, Jewkes C, Nelson RJ. Prospective, randomized, controlled trial to determine the effect of early enhanced enteral nutrition on clinical outcome in mechanically ventilated patients suffering head injury. *Crit Care Med*. 1999;27(11):2525–2531.

49. Heyland DK, Dhaliwal R, Lemieux M, Wang M, Day AG. Implementing the PEPuP protocol in critical care units in Canada: results of a multicenter, quality improvement study. *JPEN J Parenter Enteral Nutr*. 2015;39(6):698–706.

50. Taylor B, Brody R, Denmark R, Southard R, Byham-Gray L. Improving enteral delivery through the adoption of the "Feed Early Enteral Diet Adequately for Maximum Effect (FEED ME)" protocol in a surgical trauma ICU: a quality improvement review. *Nutr Clin Pract*. 2014;29(5):639–648.

51. Ventura AMC, Waitzberg DL. Enteral nutrition protocols for critically ill patients: are they necessary? *Nutr Clin Pract*. 2015;30(3):351–362.

52. Lee ZY, Barakatun-Nisak MY, Airini IN, Heyland DK. Enhanced protein-energy provision via the enteral route in critically ill patients (PEP uP Protocol): a review of evidence. *Nutr Clin Pract*. 2016;31(1):68–79.

53. Boullata J. Drug administration through an enteral feeding tube: the rationale behind the guidelines. *Am J Nurs*. 2009;109(10):34–42.

54. Beattie TK, Anderton A. Microbiological evaluation of four enteral feeding systems which have been deliberately subjected to faulty handling procedures. *J Hosp Infect*. 1999;42(1):11–20.

55. Anderton A, Aidoo KE. Decanting—a source of contamination of enteral feeds? *Clin Nutr*. 1990;9(3):157–162.

56. Weenk GH, Kemen M, Werner HP. Risks of microbiological contamination of enteral feeds during the set up of enteral feeding systems. *J Human Nutr Diet*. 1993;6:307–316.

57. Chan L, Yasmin AH, Ngeow YF, Ong GSY. Evaluation of the bacteriological contamination of a closed feeding system for enteral nutrition. *Med J Malaysia*. 1994;49(1):62–67.

58. Patchell CJ, Anderton A, MacDonald A, George RH, Booth IW. Bacterial contamination of enteral feeds. *Arch Dis Child*. 1994;70(4):327–330.

59. Moffitt SK, Gohman SM, Sass KM, Faucher KJ. Clinical and laboratory evaluation of a closed enteral feeding system under cyclic feeding conditions: a microbial and cost evaluation. *Nutrition*. 1997;13(7):622–628.

60. Fernandez-Crehuet Navajas M, Jurado Chacon D, Guillen Solvas JF, Galvez Vargas R. Bacterial contamination of enteral feeds as a possible risk of nosocomial infection. *J Hosp Infect*. 1992;21(2):111–120.

61. Beattie TK, Anderton A. Decanting versus sterile prefilled nutrient containers—the microbiological risks in enteral feeding. *Int J Environ Health Res*. 2001;11(1):81–93.

62. Marlon ND, Rupp ME. Infection control issues of enteral feeding systems. *Curr Opin Clin Nutr Metab Care*. 2000;3(5):363–366.

63. Bott L, Husson MO, Guimber D, et al. Contamination of gastrostomy feeding systems in children in a home-based enteral nutrition program. *J Pediatr Gastroenterol Nutr*. 2001;33(3):266–270.

64. Vanek VW. Closed versus open enteral delivery systems: a quality improvement study. *Nutr Clin Pract*. 2000;15(5):234–243.

65. Wagner DR, Elmore MF, Knoll DM. Evaluation of "closed" vs "open" systems for the delivery of peptide-based enteral diets. *JPEN J Parenter Enteral Nutr*. 1994;18(5):453–457.

66. Lyman B, Gebhards S, Hensley C, Roberts C, San Pablo W. Safety of decanted enteral formula hung for 12 hours in a pediatric setting. *Nutr Clin Pract*. 2011;26(4):451–456.

67. Schroeder P, Fisher D, Volz M, Paloucek J. Microbial contamination of enteral feeding solutions in a community hospital. *JPEN J Parenter Enteral Nutr*. 1983;7(4):364–368.

68. Fagerman KE. Limiting bacterial contamination of enteral nutrient solutions: 6-year history with reduction of contamination at two institutions. *Nutr Clin Pract*. 1992;7(1):31–36.

69. Donius MA. Contamination of a prefilled ready-to-use enteral feeding system compared with a refillable bag. *JPEN J Parenter Enteral Nutr*. 1993;17(5):461–464.

70. Lee CH, Hodgkiss IJ. The effect of poor handling procedures on enteral feeding systems in Hong Kong. *J Hosp Infect*. 1999;42(2):119–123.

71. Foster M, Phillips W, Parrish C. Transition to ready to hang enteral feeding system: one institution's experience. *Pract Gastroenterol.* 2015;147:28–38.

72. Luther H, Barco K, Chima C, Yowler CJ. Comparative study of two systems of delivering supplemental protein with standardized tube feedings. *J Burn Care Rehabil.* 2003;24(3):167–172.

73. Freedland CP, Roller RD, Wolfe BM, Flynn NM. Microbial contamination of continuous drip feedings. *JPEN J Parenter Enteral Nutr.* 1989;13(1):18–22.

74. Anderson KR, Norris DJ, Godfrey LB, Avent CK, Butterworth CE. Bacterial contamination of tube-feeding formulas. *JPEN J Parenter Enteral Nutr.* 1984;8(6):673–678.

75. Okuma T, Nakamura M, Totake H, Fukunaga Y. Microbial contamination of enteral feeding formulas and diarrhea. *Nutrition.* 2000;16(9):719–722.

76. Levy J, Van Laethem Y, Verhaegen G, Perpete C, Butzlet JP, Wenzel RP. Contaminated enteral nutrition solutions as a cause of nosocomial bloodstream infection: a study using plasmid fingerprinting. *JPEN J Parenter Enteral Nutr.* 1989;13(3):228–234.

77. Baldwin BA, Zagoren AJ, Rose N. Bacterial contamination of continuously infused enteral alimentation with needle catheter jejunostomy—clinical implications. *JPEN J Parenter Enteral Nutr.* 1984;8(1):30–33.

78. Chan L, Yasmin AH, Ngeow YF, Ong GS. Evaluation of the bacteriological contamination of a closed feeding system for enteral nutrition. *Med J Malaysia.* 1994;49(1):62–67.

79. Anderton A. Bacterial contamination of enteral feeds and feeding systems. *Clin Nutr.* 1993;12(Suppl. 1):16–32.

80. Desport JC, Mounier M, Preux PM, et al. Evaluation of the microbial safety of a new 1.5 l enteral feeding diet reservoir system. *Clin Nutr.* 2004;23(5):983–988.

81. Lafourcade P, Boulestrau H, Arnaud-Battandier F, et al. Is a 24-h cyclic closed enteral feeding system microbiologically safe in geriatric patients? *Clin Nutr.* 2002;21(4):315–320.

82. American National Standards Institute and Association for the Advancement of Medical Instrumentation. Small-bore connectors for liquids and gases in healthcare applications—part 1: general requirements. Updated December 30, 2010. http://my.aami.org/aamiresources/previewfiles/8036901_1012_preview.pdf. Accessed August 4, 2016.

83. US Food and Drug Administration. Center for Devices and Radiological Health. Safety considerations to mitigate the risks of misconnections with small-bore connectors intended for enteral applications. Updated February 11, 2015. http://www.fda.gov/downloads/MedicalDevices/DeviceRegulationandGuidance/GuidanceDocuments/UCM313385.pdf. Accessed August 4, 2016.

84. Elke G, Felbinger TW, Heyland DK. Gastric residual volume in critically ill patients: a dead marker or still alive? *Nutr Clin Pract.* 2015;30(1):59–71.

85. Ellis RJB, Fuehne J. Examination of accuracy in the assessment of gastric residual volumes: a simulated controlled study. *JPEN J Parenter Enteral Nutr.* 2015;39(4):434–440.

86. Montejo JC, Minambres E, Bordeje L, et al. Gastric residual volume during enteral nutrition in ICU patients: the REGANE study. *Intensive Care Med.* 2010;36(8):1386–1393.

87. Pinilla JC, Samphire J, Arnold C, Liu L, Thiessen B. Comparison of gastrointestinal tolerance to two enteral feeding protocols in critically ill patients: a prospective, randomized controlled trial. *JPEN J Parenter Enteral Nutr.* 2001;25(2):81–86.

88. Davidson P, Kwiatkowski CA, Wien M. Management of hyperglycemia and enteral nutrition in the hospitalized patient. *Nutr Clin Pract.* 2015;30(5):652–659.

89. Prado CM, Heymsfield SB. Lean tissue imaging: a new era for nutritional assessment and intervention. *JPEN J Parenter Enteral Nutr.* 2014;38(8):940–953.

90. Candio JA, Hoffman MJ, Lucke JF. Estimation of nitrogen excretion based on abbreviated urinary collections in patients on continuous parenteral nutrition. *JPEN J Parenter Enteral Nutr.* 1991;15(2):148–151.

11 Enteral Nutrition Formulations

Susan Roberts, MS, RDN, LD, CNSC, and Rachelle Kirsch, RDN, LD, CNSC

CONTENTS

Acknowledgments: Gail Cresci, PhD, RD, LD, CNSC, Jennifer Lefton, MS, RD, CNSC, and Dema Halasa Esper, MS, RD, LD, were the authors of this chapter for the second edition.

Objectives

1. Identify and evaluate enteral formulas for nutrition support of the general patient on tube feeding.
2. Recognize enteral product attributes of importance for the patient with food allergies or intolerances.
3. Analyze and appraise evidence associated with the selection of enteral products marketed for specific diseases or conditions.
4. Design an enteral formulary based upon patient populations.

Test Your Knowledge Questions

1. A 55-year-old man presented to the hospital after a traumatic fall from a ladder while working at home. A computed tomography (CT) scan of the head showed significant subdural hematoma with midline shift. After admission to the intensive care unit (ICU), the patient was intubated and sedated, with an orogastric tube to suction and removal of 200 mL gastric content. The patient's abdomen was soft and nondistended. Nephrology was consulted, and the patient was started on continuous venovenous hemodialysis. What type of enteral formula would best meet his needs?
   A. A formula restricted in fluid, protein, and electrolytes
   B. A formula not restricted in protein but restricted in fluid and electrolytes
   C. A formula restricted in fluid but not restricted in protein or electrolytes
   D. A formula not restricted in fluid or protein but restricted in electrolytes

2. A 60-year-old, critically ill patient has been tolerating a standard 1 kcal/mL enteral feeding formula well for the past week. She begins having frequent bouts of loose stools, requiring placement of a rectal tube. What should be the clinician's next suggestion?
   A. Change to a peptide-based formula.
   B. Determine the cause of diarrhea.
   C. Add pre- and probiotics to the feeding regimen.
   D. Change to a fiber-supplemented formula.

3. What should a clinician do when considering the use of enteral formulas marketed for specific disease conditions?
   A. Use formulas as indicated by the product manufacturer to meet patient's needs.
   B. Use standard polymeric formulas for all patients.
   C. Use specialty formulas only when patients exhibit signs and symptoms of intolerance to standard polymeric formulations.
   D. Evaluate the studies used to support the use of specialty formulas and apply clinical judgment to select the appropriate enteral product for the individual patient.

Test Your Knowledge Answers

1 The correct answer is C. Not all patients with acute renal failure require fluid restrictions, but, of the answers provided, a formula restricted in fluid but not protein or electrolytes is the best option. There is no need to restrict protein in patients that are dialyzed. Additionally, electrolytes such as potassium and phosphorus need only be restricted when serum levels are chronically high.

2. The correct answer is B. Determining the cause of acute diarrhea is the correct answer. The feeding formula that she had been tolerating well during the past week is the least likely cause of the diarrhea. Assessment to identify newly ordered medications that can cause diarrhea or possible infections such as *Clostridium difficile* may help to determine the cause of diarrhea. If no obvious cause of diarrhea can be found, then a different feeding formula may be tried.

3. The correct answer is D. Standard polymeric formulas are indicated for most patients requiring enteral nutrition (EN) support. When considering the use of specialty products, the clinician must use clinical judgment regarding the efficacy, tolerance, and benefit of these formulas and specifically evaluate the studies used to support these formulas, paying close attention to the quality, patient population, and clinical outcomes of the studies that are used to support their use.

Introduction

Clinicians must make many decisions when initiating EN, including identifying an appropriate enteral formulation that will meet the patient's needs. Currently, more than 100 enteral formulas are available for use in the United States, and they vary greatly with respect to concentration and composition.[1,2] This chapter reviews the composition of enteral formulations that are currently available and their indications for use.

Enteral formulations are considered "medical foods" by the US Food and Drug Administration (FDA).[3] The FDA defines medical foods as "a food which is formulated to be consumed or administered enterally under the supervision of a physician and which is intended for the specific dietary management of a disease or condition for which distinctive nutrition requirements, based on recognized scientific principles, are established by medical evaluation."[3] Therefore, their labels can make structure and function claims without the approval of the FDA. A *structure and function claim* is a claim that a specific nutrient is intended to affect the normal structure or function in humans. The mere quantity of enteral formula options and the lack of clinical research to support structure and function claims pose challenges for clinicians when selecting an optimal enteral formula. EN practice recommendations from the American Society for Parenteral and Enteral Nutrition (ASPEN) include the following statements regarding enteral formulation selection:[1]

- The veracity (accuracy, credibility) of adult enteral formula labeling and product claims is dependent on formula vendors.
- Nutrition support clinicians and consumers are responsible for determining the veracity of information about adult enteral formulations.
- Interpret enteral formulation content/labeling and health claims with caution until such time as more specific regulations are in place.

These practice recommendations were based on expert opinion and editorial consensus.[4] The provision of EN has long been the standard of care for patients who are unable to meet their energy and protein needs orally.[5] EN not only provides both macro- and micronutrients but also supports the structural integrity of the gastrointestinal (GI) tract.[5]

Formula Composition

Carbohydrate

Carbohydrate (see Chapter 3) is the primary macronutrient and principal energy source in most enteral formulations. Enteral formulations typically offer 40% to 70% of their energy as carbohydrate.[6] Carbohydrates contribute to osmolality, digestibility, and sweetness of enteral formulations.[7]

Most formulations contain oligosaccharides or polysaccharides.[7,8] Polymeric formulas use primarily corn syrup solids as their source of carbohydrate; hydrolyzed formulas use maltodextrin or hydrolyzed cornstarch (Tables 11-1 and 11-2).[1,7-9]

Oral products contain simpler or less-complex carbohydrates, such as sucrose, to increase the palatability of the product. Due to the prevalence of lactose intolerance, most formulations do not contain lactose.[7,8]

Fiber

Fiber, a polysaccharide found in plant foods that is not digested by humans, is added to some enteral formulations.

Common fiber sources in enteral formulations are guar gum and soy fiber.[1] Most enteral formulations with fiber contain a combination of both soluble and insoluble fiber. Soluble-fermentable fiber is fermented by the gut microbiota in the distal intestine to produce short-chain fatty acids (SCFAs). The SCFAs are a source of energy for colonocytes, and they help to increase intestinal mucosal growth and promote water and sodium absorption (see Chapter 4).[8] Soluble fiber may help control diarrhea due to its ability to increase sodium and water absorption via its fermentation byproducts, the SCFAs. Some studies of enteral formulations supplemented with soluble fiber have been shown to reduce the incidence of diarrhea.[2,10] Insoluble fiber is not effectively fermented by the gut microbiota, but it may help to decrease transit time by increasing fecal weight.[8] Current ASPEN and Society of Critical Care

TABLE 11-1 Classification of Enteral Formulation: Common Terms and Definitions

Term	Definition
Standard, polymeric	Formula containing macronutrients as nonhydrolyzed protein, fat, and carbohydrate
Elemental and semi-elemental	Contains partially or completely hydrolyzed nutrients (protein) and altered fats to maximize absorption
Blenderized	Formulated with a mixture of blenderized whole foods, with or without the addition of standard formula; best suited for patients with a healed feeding site and for those who adhere to safe food practices and tube maintenance
Disease-specific	Targeted for organ dysfunction or specific metabolic conditions
Modular	Used for supplementation to create a formula or enhance nutrient content of a formula or diet

Source: Data are from reference 1.

TABLE 11-2 Macronutrient Sources in Enteral Formulations

Enteral Formulation	Carbohydrate	Fat	Protein
Polymeric	Corn syrup solids Hydrolyzed cornstarch Maltodextrin Sucrose Fructose Sugar alcohols	Borage oil Canola oil Corn oil Fish oil High-oleic sunflower oil MCT Menhaden oil Mono- and diglycerides Palm kernel oil Safflower oil Soybean oil Soy lecithin	Casein Sodium, calcium, magnesium, and potassium caseinates Soy protein isolate Whey protein concentrate Lactalbumin Milk protein concentrate
Elemental	Cornstarch Hydrolyzed cornstarch Maltodextrin Fructose	Fatty acid esters Fish oil MCT Safflower oil Sardine oil Soybean oil Soy lecithin Structured lipids	Hydrolyzed casein Hydrolyzed whey protein Crystalline L-amino acids Hydrolyzed lactalbumin Soy protein isolate

MCT, medium-chain triglycerides.

Medicine (SCCM) guidelines suggest that clinicians consider fiber-containing formulation if patients have persistent diarrhea, and they suggest that both insoluble and soluble fiber be avoided if patients are at a high risk for bowel ischemia and have severe dysmotility.[11]

The tolerance of fiber-supplemented enteral formulations should be monitored closely, particularly in critically ill patients. Cases of bowel obstruction from the use of these formulations have been reported.[12,13] It may be safer to use a fiber-free formulation for critically ill patients who are at risk for gut dysmotility or bowel ischemia.[14]

The prebiotic fibers in fiber-containing formulas may provide benefits to some patients.[1] For example, some enteral formulations contain fructooligosaccharides (FOS), prebiotics that help promote growth of beneficial bacteria (lactobacilli and *Bifidobacterium*) in the distal bowel and are fermented to produce SCFAs.[15] Although FOS add sweetness to products, they provide less direct energy because they are not fully absorbed, and they indirectly may increase energy harvest by the microbiota, due to SCFA yield (see Chapter 4 for further information on prebiotics).

A systematic review compared the use of fiber-containing enteral formulas to formulas that did not contain fiber and concluded that fiber-containing formulas reduced bowel frequency when baseline bowel frequency was high and increased bowel frequency when baseline bowel frequency was low.[16] The same review found that fiber may also speed up transit time, increase fecal bulk, reduce constipation, and improve gut barrier function through the stimulation of colonic bacteria.[16]

Fat

Fat (see Chapter 5) added to enteral formulations serves as a concentrated energy source and provides essential fatty acids (EFAs; ie, linoleic and linolenic acid). A mixture of long-chain triglycerides (LCTs) and medium-chain triglycerides (MCTs) are often used in enteral formulations. Corn and soybean oil are the most common sources of LCTs used; however, safflower, canola, and fish oils are also used.

Palm kernel and coconut oil may be added to enteral formulations as a source of MCTs, which offer several advantages. They are absorbed directly into the portal circulation and do not require chylomicron formation for absorption. They also do not require pancreatic enzymes or bile salts for digestion and absorption. MCTs are cleared from the bloodstream rapidly and cross the mitochondrial membrane without the need for carnitine, where they are oxidized to carbon dioxide (CO_2) and water and therefore not stored.[7] However, because MCTs do not provide EFAs, most enteral formulations contain a mixture of LCTs and MCTs.

Some enteral formulations contain structured lipids as their fat source. Structured lipids are a chemical re-esterification of LCTs and MCTs on the same glycerol backbone, offering advantages of MCTs while including enough LCTs to meet EFA needs. Considerable attention has been devoted in recent years to ω-3 fatty acids because of their health benefits. Although both ω-6 and ω-3 fatty acids share the same enzyme systems as they are desaturated and elongated, their end products are different. ω-3 fatty acids are metabolized to prostaglandins of the 3 series and leukotrienes of the 5 series, which are associated with anti-inflammatory effects, slowing of platelet aggregation, immune enhancement, and antiarrhythmic properties. ω-6 fatty acids are metabolized to prostaglandins of the 2 series and leukotrienes of the 4 series, which are involved in inflammation, platelet aggregation, and immunosuppression. Some enteral formulations have altered the ratio of ω-6 to ω-3 fatty acids to include more ω-3 fatty acids for their anti-inflammatory effects. Research on enteral formulations supplemented with ω-3 fatty acids is discussed in the sections of this chapter on immune-modulating formulations and formulations for pulmonary conditions.

Protein

Protein (see Chapter 6) is a source of nitrogen and energy in enteral formulations. Enteral formulations may have intact proteins, hydrolyzed proteins, or free amino acids.[3] *Intact protein* refers to whole protein or protein isolates. Casein and soy protein isolates are the most commonly used types of intact protein. Lactalbumin, whey, and egg albumin are also sources of intact protein. Formulations with intact proteins require normal levels of pancreatic enzymes for digestion and absorption.

Formulations with hydrolyzed protein, small peptides (more than 3 amino acid residues), dipeptides and tripeptides, and free amino acids are referred to as *semi-elemental* or *elemental formulations*. The intestine expresses both free amino acid and peptide transport systems so it is able to absorb both free amino acids and di- and tripeptides. Any peptide greater than 3 amino acid residues requires further hydrolyzation prior to absorption.[17] Some research has suggested nitrogen absorption is greater with peptide-based formulations than with those containing only free amino acids.[16,18] Semi-elemental or elemental formulations are intended for patients with GI dysfunctions such as short bowel syndrome, malabsorption, or pancreatic exocrine insufficiency (see the section on formulations for GI disorders and malabsorption later in chapter).

Some enteral formulations add specific amino acids (eg, glutamine and arginine) at pharmacological levels to function in wound and muscle repair. See Chapter 6 for additional information on glutamine and arginine.

Vitamins and Minerals

Most enteral formulations provide adequate amounts of vitamins and minerals to meet Dietary Reference Intakes (DRIs) when provided in volumes of 1000 to 1500 mL/d.[17] Supplementation should be considered for patients when the enteral formulation does not meet their vitamin and mineral needs, or if the volume of feeding provided is inadequate to meet DRIs for vitamins and minerals.

Some disease-specific enteral formulations, such as those intended for patients with renal disease, may have low or high amounts of specific vitamins and minerals.[7] Practitioners should pay close attention to the vitamin and mineral content of the enteral formulations used to avoid adverse clinical outcomes associated with inadequate or excessive micronutrient intakes. Specialty formulas for renal disease are discussed later in this chapter.

Electrolytes

Standard enteral formulations contain modest amounts of electrolytes, typically enough to meet daily needs in most patients when the formula is provided in adequate amounts to meet DRIs. The amounts of electrolytes in disease-specific formulations may be altered because of the disease process targeted (eg, renal failure). When recommending an enteral formulation, attention should be made to the disease or medical condition of the patient and the medical therapy provided.

Water

Enteral formulas contain roughly 70% to 85% water by volume.[7,19] In general, the more energy dense the formula, the less free water it contains. Enteral formulations are not intended to meet the patient's total fluid needs. The percentage of water from enteral formulations should be included in the patient's total fluid intake. Adequate hydration is important in maintaining tissue perfusion and electrolyte balance.[5] Metabolic changes such as fever and hyperparathyroidism, and medical therapies such as diuretics and dialysis affect a patient's fluid needs.[5] Most patients receiving EN require an additional source of water to meet their fluid needs. Water is often provided through the feeding tube for hydration and as flushes to maintain feeding tube patency. When EN is implemented, intravenous (IV) fluids must be accounted for and adjusted as required to meet the patient's needs.

Osmolality

Osmolality of an enteral formulation is the concentration of free particles, molecules, or ions in a given solution, and it is expressed as milliosmoles per kilogram of water (mOsm/kg).[7] The osmolality of enteral formulations ranges from 280 to 875 mOsm/kg. As the content of free particles, ions, or molecules increases in the product, so does the osmolality. For instance, formulas containing sucrose have a higher osmolality than those with cornstarch or maltodextrin, and formulas with single amino acids or high amounts of di- and tripeptides have a higher osmolality than those with intact proteins.

Hypertonic enteral formulations (osmolality greater than 320 mOsm/kg) have frequently been blamed for formula intolerance (eg, diarrhea). When hyperosmolar formulas containing sucrose are delivered directly into the small intestine, dumping syndrome can occur, but this problem is unlikely to occur when peptide or single amino acids are provided in a similar manner. However, other than simple sugar–related hyperosmolality, the osmolality of an enteral formulation has little to do with formula tolerance. Formula tolerance or diarrhea is most often related to the severity of illness, comorbid conditions, enteric pathogens, or the concomitant use of medications administered through the enteral access device.[20] Additionally, the average gastric tube–fed patient will dilute

the enteral formula with 1 to 2 liters of saliva and gastric juices. The osmolality of several items on a clear liquid diet and many medications given via the enteral route is much higher than the osmolality of enteral formulations. Further information on enteral feeding complications and tolerance is covered in Chapter 13.

Food Allergies and Intolerances

Researchers estimate that up to 15 million Americans have food allergies.[21] It is important that the clinician complete a diet history including any food intolerances or allergies as part of the nutrition assessment. This evaluation can be helpful in determining whether a reported allergy is a food intolerance or a true food allergy. For example, some patients report a milk allergy but actually have lactose intolerance.

Enteral formulations may contain milk, soy, corn, or egg products, all of which are common allergens. However, most enteral formulations are lactose free and gluten free. Clinicians must be knowledgeable about the ingredients in enteral formulations that may not be suitable for those with food allergies. Product manufacturers can provide ingredients lists and guidance about the suitability of products for patients with common allergies.

Oral Products

Enteral formulations used as oral supplements are available in either liquid form or as powders that must be reconstituted as liquids. These products are used for individuals who are unable to ingest adequate nutrients in the form of a standard oral diet.[22] Additional oral products are available in the form of juices and nutrient-dense bars, cookies, puddings, and soups. These products provide approximately 40% to 60% of total energy from carbohydrates, 15% to 25% from protein, and 15% to 35% from fat. DRIs for vitamins and minerals can often be met by ingesting a portion of these oral supplements daily. These products may contain a blend of soluble and insoluble dietary fiber.

The efficacy of oral supplements has been studied mostly in older adults. Nutritional supplements containing protein and energy are often prescribed in this population because older adults are vulnerable to malnutrition and deterioration of nutrition status due to acute and chronic illnesses. Two reviews have assessed the effectiveness of oral supplements on anthropometric indexes, muscular skeletal strength, and functional status. Milne and colleagues reported that supplementation produces a small but consistent weight gain in older adults and that mortality may be reduced in older adults who are undernourished.[23] Reduction of length of hospital stay and improved functional status was not found in this review, which concluded that further clinical trials are needed to determine additional benefits from oral nutrition supplementation.[23] In an earlier review, Stratton and Elia indicated community-dwelling individuals with chronic obstructive pulmonary disease (COPD) or a body mass index (BMI) less than 20 seemed to show the greatest weight gain with the use of oral supplementation.[24]

Patients with muscle wasting diseases (eg, cancer, acquired immunodeficiency syndrome [AIDS], or sarcopenia) may also benefit from oral nutrition supplements containing added amino acids and anti-inflammatory agents to attenuate lean muscle loss and improve immune function.[25] However, early intervention with an oral nutrition supplement seems to be imperative to gain the benefit.

Varieties of oral supplements are available in different flavors, textures, and consistencies. When they are used, they should be used on a daily schedule that is suitable for the specific individual. However, supplementation should not replace the benefits of eating a balanced diet; the goal is to augment the energy and nutrients that can be received from whole foods.

Formulations Indicated for Specific Diseases or Conditions

In addition to standard EN formulations, numerous disease-specific EN formulations are on the market. As noted earlier, enteral formulations are classified as medical foods and are not regulated by the FDA as medications are; therefore, they do not require rigorous premarket research to determine whether they are indicated for various clinical conditions. Many specialty EN formulas contain hydrolyzed proteins and free amino acids and are marketed as being more easily digested than standard formulations; however, the superiority of these specialty products over polymeric formulas has not been clearly demonstrated and there is limited research in this area.[5] Research that has been conducted with these formulations is typically performed by private investigators, and the funding may or may not be supported by the formula company. Therefore, the evaluation of the efficacy of disease-specific formulations is mostly left up to the clinician. When evaluating research on the efficacy of a disease-specific enteral formula, clinicians should consider several factors (Table 11-3). It is important to note the quality of the research study and the patient populations included in the study to determine the value of the research results and whether the study endpoints are applicable to clinical practice. Standard, or polymeric, formulas are commonly used for patients requiring EN support, and they generally meet the needs for most noncritically ill patients who have normal digestion function. However, some patients may require a specialized formula to better meet their nutrition needs. Multiple practice guidelines are available to help guide the clinician with use of disease-specific enteral formulas.

TABLE 11-3 Considerations When Evaluating Research on Specialized Enteral Formulas

- In vitro (animal) vs in vivo (human) study
- Quality of study design:
  - Prospective randomized controlled trial
  - Retrospective review
  - Case reports
- Similarity of patient population studied to patients being cared for (demographic factors, clinical status, clinical environment, etc)
- Generalizability of results

Diabetes and Glucose Intolerance

Hyperglycemia is common in hospitalized patients and may be due to many factors, including preexisting and undiagnosed diabetes mellitus, interventions such as nutrition support and medications, insulin resistance, and the stress response.[26] One study, which included more than 3 million patients in US hospitals, reported the incidence of hyperglycemia (defined as blood glucose greater than 180 mg/dL) as approximately 32% in both ICU and non-ICU patients.[27] Glycemic control in hospitalized patients is important because hyperglycemia, hypoglycemia, and glycemic variability have each been associated with morbidity and mortality.[28-31] Guidelines recommend maintaining blood glucose between 140 and 180 mg/dL in the hospital setting.[11,32,33]

Provision of EN that contains glucose from carbohydrate sources can contribute to hyperglycemia.[26] Therefore, several diabetes-specific formulas have been developed and are marketed for use in patients with diabetes and hyperglycemia (see Table 11-4). Refer to Chapter 34 for additional information on EN for patients with diabetes.

In general, diabetes-specific formulas are lower in carbohydrate (33% to 40% of total energy), higher in monounsaturated fat and total fat (42% to 54% of total energy), and provide more fiber (14 to 16 g/L) than standard polymeric EN formulas.[32] The rationale is that this mixture of macronutrients (lower carbohydrate and higher fat content) and fiber will slow gastric emptying and lead to better glycemic control.[1] However, current recommendations from the American Diabetes Association (ADA) for individuals with diabetes do not endorse a specific dietary macronutrient distribution. Instead, their guidelines state "evidence suggests that there is not an ideal percentage of calories from carbohydrate, protein, and fat for all patients with diabetes"[34(p3823)] and "macronutrient distribution should be based on individualized assessment of current eating patterns, preferences, and metabolic goals."[34(p3823)] According to the ADA, the ideal quantity of carbohydrate intake as well as insulin therapy should be individualized for each patient.[34] The ADA guidelines do not provide fiber recommendations for individuals with diabetes,[34] but fiber may not be appropriate in all patients, especially those who are critically ill.[11] Additionally, patients with diabetes who also have gastroparesis may have difficulty tolerating diabetes-specific formulas because of their higher fat and fiber content.[35] Although the particular ADA guidelines cited here were not developed specifically for hospitalized patients on EN, the recommendation for individualized care applies to patients in the hospital setting. Hospitalized patients have complex nutrition needs, and clinicians must consider many factors—such as elevated energy and protein needs in the ICU, presence of or risk for malnutrition, wounds or risk for wound development, and gastric emptying—in addition to glucose control when determining the optimal nutrition intervention for a specific patient. Furthermore, factors other than nutrition that influence glucose control (see Chapter 34). Therefore, strategies for achieving glycemic targets, including selection of the optimal EN formula, must be individualized in the context of the patient's overall needs.[1] Both overfeeding and underfeeding are risks with EN support; underfeeding is more common than overfeeding with

TABLE 11-4 Select Enteral Formulations Promoted for Use in Patients with Diabetes or Glucose Intolerance

Product (Company)	Energy, kcal/mL	Protein g/L (% kcal)	Sources	Carbohydrate g/L (% kcal)	Sources	Fat g/L (% kcal)	Sources
Diabetisource AC (Nestlé)	1.2	60 (20)	Soy protein isolate, L-arginine	100 (36)	Corn syrup, fructose, tapioca dextrin, vegetables, fruits, guar gum, soy fiber, FOS	58.8 (44)	Canola oil, refined fish oil (anchovy, sardine)
Glucerna 1.0 Cal (Abbott)	1.0	41.8 (16.7)	Sodium caseinate, calcium caseinate	95.6 (34.3)	Corn maltodextrin, soy fiber, fructose	54.4 (49)	High-oleic safflower oil, high-oleic canola oil, soy lecithin
Glucerna 1.2 Cal (Abbott)	1.2	60 (20)	Sodium caseinate, soy protein isolate milk protein concentrate	114.5 (35)	Corn maltodextrin, isomaltulose, fructose, sucromalt, glycerin, FOS, oat and soy fiber	60 (45)	High-oleic safflower oil, high-oleic canola oil, soy lecithin
Glucerna 1.5 Cal (Abbott)	1.5	82.5 (22)	Sodium caseinate, calcium caseinate, soy protein isolate	133.1 (33)	Corn maltodextrin, isomaltulose, fructose, sucromalt, glycerin, FOS, oat and soy fiber	75 (45)	High-oleic safflower oil, high-oleic canola oil, soy lecithin
Nutren Glytrol (Nestlé)	1.0	45.2 (18)	Calcium caseinate, potassium caseinate	100 (40)	Maltodextrin, modified cornstarch, pea fiber, gum acacia, FOS, inulin	47.6 (42)	Canola oil, high-oleic safflower oil, MCT, soy lecithin

Product (Company)	Osmolality, mOsm/kg	Volume to Provide 100% RDI, mL	% H$_2$O	Fiber, g/L	Additional Information
Diabetisource AC (Nestlé)	450	1250	82	15.2	Arginine: 4 g/L Vitamin E: 32 mg/L Vitamin C: 240 mg/L Chromium: 160 mcg/L
Glucerna 1.0 Cal (Abbott)	355	1420	85.3	14.4	Vitamin A: 6300 IU/L Vitamin C: 215 mg/L Chromium: 85 mcg/L
Glucerna 1.2 Cal (Abbott)	720	1250	80.5	16.1	Vitamin A: 7730 IU/L Vitamin E: 39 IU/L Vitamin C: 260 mg/L Chromium: 160 mcg/L
Glucerna 1.5 Cal (Abbott)	875	1000	75.9	16.1	Vitamin A: 8660 IU/L Vitamin E: 48 IU/L Vitamin C: 325 mg/L Chromium: 200 mcg/L
Nutren Glytrol (Nestlé)	280	1500	84	15.2	Vitamin A: 5080 IU/L Vitamin E: 30 IU/L Vitamin C: 140 mg/L Chromium: 124 mcg/L

FOS, fructooligosaccharides; MCT, medium-chain triglycerides; RDI, Reference Daily Intake.
Manufacturers may change product ingredients or nutritional content. Always check current product information.
Source: Data are from the manufacturers, Abbott Nutrition (https://abbottnutrition.com) and Nestlé Health Science (https://www.nestlehealthscience.us).

EN, especially in the ICU setting. Clinicians should closely monitor actual intake of energy and protein along with blood glucose levels because iatrogenic underfeeding of both energy and protein, particularly in patients at high nutrition risk, have been associated with poor patient outcomes.[36,37]

Research evaluating diabetes-specific formulas has been done for several decades. Many studies have included small sample sizes, short-term follow-up of 24 hours or less,[38–42] subjects who were healthy volunteers or patients outside of the hospital environment,[38–42] and oral consumption of diabetes-specific formulas.[39–41,43] Therefore, the ability to extrapolate their results to patients who require enteral feeding in a hospital setting is restricted.[37–46] However, a few studies have evaluated glycemic parameters and outcomes in hospitalized patients receiving a diabetes-specific formula via a feeding tube.[47–49]

Pohl and colleagues[47] conducted a randomized controlled trial in 4 rehabilitation units and 1 nursing home to evaluate the use of a diabetes-specific formula vs a standard formula. Patients with dysphagia due to a neurologic insult (N = 105) who had preexisting hyperglycemia and/or elevated hemoglobin A1c (A1C) levels were included in the study. They were prescribed 27 kcal/kg/d and followed for up to 84 days. Outcome parameters included changes from baseline to Day 84 in total insulin requirements, fasting blood glucose levels, and A1C levels. Of the 55 patients that were in the study at Day 84, those who received the diabetes-specific formula had, compared to baseline, decreased total daily insulin requirements (–8 vs 2 units/d; P <0.0001) and decreased fasting glucose (–39 vs –12 mg/dL; P <0.0001). The diabetes-specific formula group also experienced fewer hypoglycemic events compared to the group receiving the standard formula (5 vs 1). There was no difference in the change in A1C levels from baseline to Day 84 for the 2 groups (–1.3 vs –1.2, P = 0.56), which suggests that the statistical difference seen in fasting glucose levels was not necessarily clinically significant. Additionally, no data were reported on the actual amount of EN infused, which also could have affected the results. However, the authors concluded that the diabetes-specific formulas resulted in improved glycemic control compared with the standard formula.[47]

León-Sanz et al compared glycemic control in tube-fed patients with type 2 diabetes admitted to the hospital due to neurologic disorders or head and neck cancer surgery.[48] Patients were randomly assigned in a nonblinded fashion to a diabetes-specific formula or a formula classified as high in carbohydrate and followed for up to 14 days in the hospital. Of the 108 patients initially enrolled, 63 were included in the final analysis; the others withdrew or did not meet the study criteria, including energy intake less than 75% of the target energy goal. There was no difference in the amount of energy delivered, daily insulin dose, daily insulin dose/kg, daily kcal per unit of insulin, or A1C. The mean glucose level on study Day 8 in the group receiving the high-carbohydrate formula was 21% higher than at baseline (198 vs 229 mg/dL, P = 0.006) whereas the mean blood glucose in the group receiving the diabetes-specific formula was 215 mg/dL at baseline and 229 mg/dL at study Day 8. However, there was no difference in the blood glucose levels of the 2 groups at study Day 15, and there was no statistical difference between the 2 groups at any point in time. The clinical significance of this difference from baseline to Day 8 is questionable, and both group's glucose levels increased during that time period. It is unclear from the data provided whether other factors, such as medications, could have influenced the glucose levels at Day 8. Overall, the results of this study do not provide support for the use of diabetes-specific formulas, although the study conclusion statement promotes the diabetes-specific formula over the high-carbohydrate formula for improved glycemic control.[48]

Mesejo et al evaluated the impact of 3 enteral formulas on glycemic parameters and clinical outcomes in critically ill hyperglycemic patients (N = 157) on mechanical ventilation in a prospective, open-label, randomized multicenter trial.[49] Inclusion criteria included an ICU stay of 48 hours or longer following random assignment and use of EN expected for at least 5 days. Patients were excluded if they had insulin-dependent diabetes, an Acute Physiology and Chronic Health Evaluation score equal to or less than 10, renal or hepatic failure, life expectancy of 48 hours or less, or BMI equal to or greater than 40, or if they required parenteral nutrition. The primary outcome measured was the amount of insulin therapy needed to maintain the blood glucose level between 110 and 150 mg/dL, and blood glucose was managed using an insulin infusion. Secondary outcomes were glycemic control through measurement of plasma blood glucose and glycemic variability, ICU-acquired infection, days on mechanical ventilation, ICU length of stay, and mortality at Day 28 and 6 months. The 3 formulas studied were a standard high-protein EN formula (n = 53), a commonly used diabetes-specific formula (n = 52), and a "new-generation" diabetes-specific formula (n = 52). The new-generation formula contained more protein than the other 2 formulas as well as slowly digested carbohydrates and ω-3 fatty acids. EN was prescribed at 25 kcal/kg, started within 48 hours of ICU admission via a nasogastric tube, and infused continuously over 24 hours with interruption for 8 hours on study Days 3, 7, 14, 21 and 28 to obtain blood tests. The energy and protein intakes of all 3 groups were similar. However, grams of carbohydrate intake per day was lower in the new-generation formula group compared to the high-protein formula group (110.6 vs 151.3 g/d; P <0.001). The insulin requirements (19.1 vs 23.7 units; P <0.05) and plasma glucose levels (138.6 vs 146.1 mg/dL; P <0.01) were lower in the new-generation formula group compared with the high-protein formula group, but they were not different from the group receiving the other diabetes-specific formula. The glycemic variability was also more pronounced in the high-protein formula group in comparison to the new-generation formula group. However, other glycemic measures—such as peak glucose level and percentage of patients with a blood glucose level maintained between 80 and 150 mg/dL—and the number of infections were not different among the 3 groups. The rate of tracheobronchitis per 1000 ventilator days was higher in the high-protein formula group than in the 2 groups receiving the diabetes-specific formulas (10 vs 7; P <0.01). However, the overall rate of infection, days on mechanical ventilation, ICU length of stay, and mortality rate at all time points were not different for the 3 groups. The authors concluded that the new-generation diabetes-specific formula, in comparison to a high-protein formula, improves glucose homeostasis and may reduce risk of ICU-acquired infections. They attributed the lack of difference in important clinical outcomes, such as time on mechanical ventilation, length of stay in the ICU, and mortality, to a small sample size and lack of power to detect a difference in these outcomes.[49] While some statistical differences were achieved in glycemic measures in this study, they may not be clinically important, and the results do not provide a clear indication for the use of diabetes-specific formulas in the study population.

Currently, standard enteral formulas used in conjunction with appropriate energy provision and insulin therapy are promoted for patients with diabetes or stress-induced hyperglycemia. North American nutrition support guidelines for critically ill patients do not recommend the use of diabetes-specific formulas based on the evidence available.[11,50,51] Diabetes-specific formulas may be an option if glucose control cannot be achieved despite an optimal insulin regimen.[51] More well-designed, adequately powered, prospective, randomized controlled trials are needed to evaluate the impact of diabetes-specific formulas on glycemic control and important clinical outcomes, including mortality, quality of life and functional status postdischarge, in patients with diabetes or stress-induced hyperglycemia. See Practice Scenario 11-1 for a discussion of the best approach to enteral formula selection and glycemic control in a critical care setting.[11,32,33,50-52]

Practice Scenario 11-1

Question: What is the best approach to enteral nutrition (EN) management in a postoperative patient with type 2 diabetes?

Scenario: A 56-year-old man with a past medical history of type 2 diabetes and hypertension was admitted to the surgical intensive care unit (ICU) following an aortic valve replacement. On postoperative Day 1, the patient was intubated and sedated, and received intravenous (IV) fluids at 100 mL/h using 5% dextrose with half-normal saline. The patient was 5 feet, 10 inches (178 cm) tall and weighed 80 kg, which was 5 kg less than what he weighed 2 months prior to admission. A review of laboratory values found that they were all insignificant, except for blood glucose levels, which were consistently higher than 180 mg/dL since the patient was admitted to the ICU. Elevated blood glucose levels were treated with regular insulin subcutaneously every 4 hours following a standard glucose monitoring schedule. The patient's energy requirements were estimated to be 2000 kcal/d, and protein requirements were estimated to be 96 to 120 g/d (1.2 to 1.5 g/kg/d). Enteral feedings were initiated on ICU Day 1 using a diabetes-specific formula at 30 mL/h, and insulin management was unchanged. After initiation of enteral feedings, blood glucose levels continued to be higher than 180 mg/dL.

Intervention: On ICU Day 2, the EN order was changed to a standard high-protein, 1.0 kcal/mL polymeric enteral formula. The infusion rate was increased to goal rate of 80 mL/h to provide 1920 kcal and 119 g protein. The IV fluids were decreased to 50 mL/h and changed to ½ normal saline. A continuous IV insulin infusion was also started to maintain blood glucose levels within the range of 140 to 180 mg/dL.

Answer: A diabetes-specific enteral formula is not necessary in ICU patients with diabetes and hyperglycemia. In this case, the patient was experiencing hyperglycemia prior to initiation of EN because of his type 2 diabetes, postsurgical stress, and IV fluids, which were providing approximately 400 kcal from dextrose. A standard formula is indicated because evidence supporting use of a diabetes-specific formula in critically ill patients to control blood glucose levels is limited. Providing regular insulin on an "as

needed" basis is not effective in controlling blood glucose within the recommended range of 140 to 180 mg/dL, which practice guidelines indicate is beneficial to minimize complications and improve patient outcomes;[11,32,33] therefore, a continuous insulin infusion was needed to improve blood glucose control.

Rationale: Hyperglycemia is common in the ICU setting in patients with and without diabetes. Based on the evidence to date, diabetes-specific formulas are not the first-line intervention for managing hyperglycemia in the ICU.[11,50,51] Instead, blood glucose control should be optimized by appropriate energy provision and insulin therapy, frequently through continuous IV insulin infusion in the critical care setting.[52] (See Chapter 34 for more information on nutrition support in patients with diabetes mellitus.)

Gastrointestinal Disorders and Malabsorption

GI disorders, particularly those affecting the lower GI tract, can impair nutrient utilization and absorption. Additionally, exocrine pancreatic function may be reduced in various clinical conditions, which can lead to altered digestion and absorption of intact proteins and long-chain lipids. Persistent feeding intolerance or malabsorption can compromise nutrition status, warranting specialized nutrition support. Elemental and semi-elemental formulas are often used for patients who have known GI disorders or for those who exhibit signs and symptoms of intolerance to polymeric formulations.[1] Historically, patients were kept on nothing by mouth (NPO) orders when they experienced malabsorption; however, current research indicates it is important to enterally feed patients to maintain gut integrity and immunity.[11]

As knowledge of the immunologic and barrier functions of the intestine has increased, enteral formulations specifically for GI disorders have emerged (Table 11-5). These products contain hydrolyzed proteins (peptides and amino acids) and MCTs to aid in nutrient digestion and absorption. A few of these products contain ω-3 fatty acids, which affect inflammatory metabolism (see Chapters 5 and 24). Prebiotics, such as synthetic FOS and inulin, have been added to some of the formulations to support growth of beneficial colonic bacteria (eg, lactobacilli and bifidobacteria) along with increased production of SCFAs, which have been shown to enhance fluid and electrolyte absorption.[53] Further review of prebiotics can be found in Chapter 4.

The use of peptide-based formulas has not been extensively evaluated, and the results of the available studies have been contradictory.[54-57] Two studies found that the incidence or frequency of diarrhea was reduced by using a peptide-based formula,[54,55] but other studies found that the frequency of diarrhea increased or stayed the same following the change to a peptide-based formula.[56,57] The European Society for Clinical Nutrition and Metabolism (ESPEN) does not recommend the routine use of elemental formulas with Crohn's disease, ulcerative colitis, or short bowel syndrome.[58] ASPEN also recommends that routine elemental and disease-specific formulas be avoided in critically ill patients because no clear benefit to patient outcome has been shown in the literature.[11] Clinicians should thoroughly investigate the etiology of a patient's

TABLE 11-5 Select Enteral Formulations Marketed for Use in Patients with Gastrointestinal Disorders and Malabsorption

Product (Company)	Energy, kcal/mL	Protein			Carbohydrate			Fat		
		g/L (% kcal)	Source		g/L (% kcal)	Source		g/L (% kcal)	Source	
Peptamen (Nestlé)	1.0	40 (16)	Enzymatically hydrolyzed whey protein		128 (51)	Maltodextrin, cornstarch		40 (33)	MCT, soybean oil	
Peptamen 1.5 (Nestlé)	1.5	68 (18)	Enzymatically hydrolyzed whey protein		188 (49)	Maltodextrin, cornstarch		56 (33)	MCT, soybean oil	
Peptamen AF (Nestlé)	1.2	76 (25)	Enzymatically hydrolyzed whey protein		112 (35)	Maltodextrin, cornstarch, FOS, inulin		54 (40)	MCT, fish oil, soybean oil (EPA/DHA 2.4 g/L)	
Peptamen with Prebio (Nestlé)	1.5	68 (18)	Enzymatically hydrolyzed whey protein		184 (48)	Maltodextrin, cornstarch, FOS, inulin		56 (34)	MCT, soybean oil	
Peptamen Intense VHP (Nestlé)	1.0	92 (37)	Partially hydrolyzed whey protein concentrate		76 (29)	Maltodextrin, cornstarch, FOS, inulin, guar gum		38 (34)	MCT, fish oil, high-linoleic safflower oil	
Tolerex (Nestlé)	1.0	20.5 (8.0)	100% free amino acids (L-glutamine, 3.5g/L; L-arginine, 2.4 g/L)		226 (90)	Maltodextrin, modified food starch		2 (2.0)	Safflower oil	
Vital 1.0 Cal (Abbott)	1.0	40 (16)	Whey protein hydrolysate, partially hydrolyzed sodium caseinate		130 (51)	Maltodextrin, sucrose, short-chain FOS		38.1 (33)	Structured lipids (canola oil, MCT)	
Vital 1.5 Cal (Abbott)	1.5	67.5 (18)	Whey protein hydrolysate, partially hydrolyzed sodium caseinate		187 (49)	Maltodextrin, sucrose, short-chain FOS		57.1 (33)	Structured lipids (canola oil, MCT)	
Vital AF 1.2 Cal (Abbott)	1.2	75 (25)	Whey protein hydrolysate, hydrolyzed sodium caseinate		110.6 (36)	Corn maltodextrin, short-chain FOS		53.9 (39)	Structured lipids (canola oil/MCT); EPA and DHA from fish oil; soy oil	
Vital High Protein (Abbott)	1.0	87.5 (35)	Whey protein hydrolysate, hydrolyzed sodium caseinate		112 (45)	Corn maltodextrin, sucrose, cellulose		23.2 (20)	Marine oil, MCT	
Vivonex T.E.N. (Nestlé)	1.0	38.3 (14)	100% free amino acids (L-glutamine, 4.8 g/L; L-arginine, 3.9 g/L)		206 (83)	Maltodextrin, modified food starch		3 (3)	Safflower oil	
Vivonex RTF (Nestlé)	1.0	50 (20)	100% free amino acids (L-arginine, 5.3 g/L)		176 (70)	Maltodextrin, modified food starch		11.6 (10)	Soybean oil, MCT	
Vivonex Plus (Nestlé)	1.0	45 (17)	100% free amino acids (L-glutamine, 9.5 g/L; L-arginine, 6.3 g/L)		190 (77)	Maltodextrin, modified food starch		6.7 (6)	Soybean oil	

DHA, docosahexaenoic acid; EPA, eicosapentaenoic acid; FOS, fructooligosaccharides; MCT, medium-chain triglycerides.
Manufacturers may change product ingredients or nutritional content. Always check current product information.
Source: Data are from the manufacturers, Abbott Nutrition (https://abbottnutrition.com) and Nestlé Health Science (https://www.nestlehealthscience.us).

diarrhea or malabsorption, rather than assuming the enteral formula is the cause—for example, other potential causes might be medication use, the rate of formula or fluid infusion into the small intestine is too rapid, or small intestinal bacterial overgrowth (eg, *C. difficile* infection).[11] However, updated specialized formulations for GI disorders containing added components such as prebiotics and ω-3 fatty acids warrant further investigation.

Hepatic Failure

Malnutrition is prevalent in patients with liver failure.[59–61] Multiple factors contribute to malnutrition in this patient population, including inadequate intake, malabsorption, decreased protein synthesis, altered metabolism of nutrient substrates, and hypermetabolism.[60,62] (See Chapter 27 for more information on liver disease.)

Hepatic encephalopathy is a complication of liver failure, and elevated blood ammonia has been implicated in this condition, although the mechanism is still not completely understood.[63] The branched-chain amino acids (BCAAs) leucine, valine, and isoleucine have been promoted for use in hepatic encephalopathy because they clear ammonia in the skeletal muscles, decreasing cerebral ammonia levels and reducing the uptake of aromatic amino acids (AAAs) across the blood-brain barrier.[64] Due to impaired hepatic deamination, patients with liver failure may have alterations in amino acid levels, namely higher levels of AAAs (tyrosine, tryptophan, and phenylalanine) compared to BCAAs. This altered ratio of AAAs to BCAAs allows more AAAs to enter the brain and contribute to production of false neurotransmitters, which contribute to symptoms seen in hepatic encephalopathy.[65] Therefore, formulations with a lower amount of total protein, increased amounts of BCAAs, and decreased amounts of AAAs compared with standard EN formulas, were developed for use in this patient population.

However, there is no evidence that use of high-BCAA formulations alter patient outcomes compared to provision of a standard enteral formula.[10] Historically, protein restriction was used in patients with liver failure, but this approach is no longer recommended because it leads to a further decline in nutrition status and lean body mass (LBM) and may result in higher ammonia levels.[11,62] A systematic review and meta-analysis including 16 randomized clinical trials and 827 patients was conducted to evaluate outcomes associated with BCAA supplementation in patients with hepatic encephalopathy.[66] Of these trials, 8 studies supplemented BCAA orally, 7 provided IV BCAA, and 1 included both. BCAA supplementation was found to have a beneficial effect on hepatic encephalopathy, but it did not lead to improvements in mortality, quality of life, or nutrition-related outcomes. Additionally, BCAA supplementation was associated with an increased risk of nausea and vomiting.[66]

Immunonutrition

Over the last 2 decades, the enteral administration of arginine, glutamine, ω-3 polyunsaturated fatty acids, nucleotides, and antioxidants has been studied for an effect on immune-related responses to injury and illness.[1] Enteral formulas that contain these nutrients are called *immune-modulating formulations* (IMFs). The specific nutrients in IMFs (Table 11-6) are thought to have the potential to modulate the metabolic response to surgery or stress.

Metabolism of arginine differs in surgical versus nonsurgical patients. Therefore, the effects of IMFs are likely to differ between these 2 groups.[67] Some immunonutrition studies have included supplemental parenteral nutrition, and data analysis techniques vary among the studies. Most of the literature on immunonutrition has focused on patients elective GI surgeries in the pre- and perioperative states, and the findings demonstrate favorable outcomes in hospital length of stay.[1] A recent systematic review and meta-analysis assessed the effect of arginine-enriched enteral formulations on patients undergoing surgery for head and neck cancers, and the use of arginine-containing formulations was associated with reduction in fistulas and hospital length of stay.[68]

Numerous published meta-analysis and systematic reviews[46–54,69] have evaluated outcomes of IMFs in predominantly surgical and critical care populations. Patients who received an IMF had decreased risk for infections/infectious complications,[67,69–76] reduced length of stay,[67,69–74] and reduced mortality.[67] The 2016 SCCM/ASPEN guidelines for the critically ill do not recommend the routine use of IMFs with severe sepsis. They also recommend that IMF use be reserved for the postoperative patients in the surgical ICU.[11] The Canadian Practice Guidelines recommend that IMFs not be used for critically ill patients, and they note that this recommendation does not apply to elective surgical patients, where IMFs are associated with significant reduction in infections.[77] ESPEN guidelines cite no general recommendation for use of IMFs in patients with severe illness and sepsis.[58] The most recent Surviving Sepsis Campaign guidelines recommend against the use of immunonutrition in patients with severe sepsis.[78]

Pulmonary Failure and Acute Respiratory Distress Syndrome

Respiratory failure is associated with poor compensation in the presence of elevated CO_2 levels. When oxidized, macronutrients yield different amounts of CO_2; therefore, the respiratory quotient (RQ), a value that describes CO_2 production in relation to oxygen consumption, varies for carbohydrate (1.0), protein (0.8), and lipid (0.7); RQ for lipogenesis is 1.0 to 1.3.[79] In the 1980s, it was found that parenteral nutrition formulations containing high amounts of carbohydrates were associated with CO_2 retention, and when the carbohydrate content was decreased, respiration improved.[80–82] These studies led to the development of pulmonary failure–specific enteral formulas, which were designed for patients with chronic lung disease and acute pulmonary failure to help with weaning from mechanical ventilation. However, subsequent research showed that total energy provision or overfeeding was more important than the composition (high carbohydrate vs high fat) of the formula in respiratory status of mechanically ventilated patients.[83]

Pulmonary failure can be classified as chronic or acute lung disease, although some patients have both conditions—

TABLE 11-6 Select Enteral Formulations Marketed as Immune Modulating (Feeding Tube Use)

Product (Company)	Energy, kcal/mL	Protein g/L (% kcal)	Protein Source	Carbohydrate g/L (% kcal)	Carbohydrate Source	Fat g/L (% kcal)	Fat Source
Impact (Nestlé)	1.0	56 (22)	Sodium caseinate, calcium caseinate, L-arginine	132 (53)	Maltodextrin, hydrolyzed cornstarch	28 (25)	Palm kernel oil, refined fish oils, high-oleic sunflower oil, high-linoleic safflower oil
Impact Peptide 1.5 (Nestlé)	1.5	94 (25)	Hydrolyzed casein, L-arginine	140 (37)	Maltodextrin, cornstarch	63.6 (38)	MCT, fish, refined fish oil, soybean oil
Perative (Abbott)	1.3	66.7 (20.5)	Partially hydrolyzed sodium caseinate, whey hydrolysate, L-arginine	180.3 (54.5)	Corn maltodextrin, FOS	37.3 (25)	Canola oil, MCT, corn oils, soy lecithin
Pivot 1.5 (Abbott)	1.5	93.8 (25)	Partially hydrolyzed sodium caseinate, whey hydrolysate, L-arginine	172.4 (45)	Corn syrup solids, FOS	50.8 (30)	MCT, structured lipids, canola oil, soy oil

FOS, fructooligosaccharides; MCT, medium-chain triglycerides.
Manufacturers may change product ingredients or nutritional content. Always check current product information.
Source: Data are from the manufacturers, Abbott Nutrition (https://abbottnutrition.com) and Nestlé Health Science (https://www.nestlehealthscience.us).

for example, a patient with COPD could have pneumonia. Specialized enteral formulations are available for 2 different patient populations with pulmonary failure: ambulatory, noncritically ill patients vs critically ill patients with acute respiratory distress syndrome (ARDS) or acute lung injury (ALI) (Tables 11-7 and 11-8). In general, these specialized formulas are energy dense because these patients typically require fluid restriction or need a concentrated source of nutrition because of their altered respiratory function and elevated nutrition requirements. The formulations are low in carbohydrate (27% of kcal) and high in lipid (55% of kcal), and contain moderate amounts of protein. The formulations for ambulatory and critically ill patients vary by the type of lipid they contain. The product marketed for ambulatory patients contains corn and safflower oils (ω-6 fatty acids), and the formulation marketed for the ARDS/ALI population contains fish oil and borage oil (with a ratio of ω-6 to ω-3 fatty acids of 1.8:1) in addition to added antioxidants. High doses of ω-6 fatty acids are not recommended in critically ill patients because of their potential to exacerbate the inflammatory state already present. ω-3 fatty acids from fish and borage oil have been investigated as a means to reduce inflammation and improve pulmonary function and outcome in patients with ARDS and ALI.[84]

A Cochrane systematic review evaluated the impact of nutritional supplementation in randomized controlled trials on a variety of parameters in patients with stable COPD.[85] The review included 17 studies and 632 patients who received nutritional supplementation for at least 2 weeks. Nutritional supplementation led to significant weight gain, especially in malnourished patients. The review also reported a significant change from baseline in fat-free mass index/fat-free mass,

fat mass/fat mass index, midarm muscle circumference, and 6-minute walk test, as well as a significant improvement in skinfold thickness for all patients. In addition, there were significant improvements in respiratory muscle strength and measurements of quality of life in malnourished patients with COPD. Although some of the studies included in the review used a pulmonary-specific formula, most used a standard formula or some other means to improve nutrition intake. A comparison between pulmonary-specific supplements and standard EN formulas was not carried out in this review. Therefore, the findings cannot be attributed to specifically to pulmonary-specific formulas, but it seems that nutritional supplementation is beneficial in stable COPD patients.[85]

Research findings are inconsistent regarding outcomes in critically ill patients with ARDS/ALI receiving specialized EN formulations containing fish oils, borage oil, or gamma-linolenic acid, as well as antioxidants. Early research studies demonstrated positive clinical outcomes with the use of this type of formula compared to a pulmonary formula with high ω-6 content or a standard EN formula. Positive outcomes reported include improved oxygenation, fewer new organ failures, more ventilator-free and ICU-free days, and lower mortality.[86–89] However, subsequent research has not replicated these findings.[90–95] Based on the evidence to date, the 2016 SCCM/ASPEN guidelines for critically ill patients do not recommend the use of this specialized formula for ARDS/ALI.[11] Additionally, the guidelines do not recommend the use of a high-fat/low-carbohydrate formula containing high levels of ω-6 fatty acids.[11] In contrast, the Canadian Clinical Practice Guidelines recommend that clinicians consider this specialized formula with fish and borage oil and supplemental antioxidants for patients with ARDS/ALI.[96] The disparity between the 2 guide-

CHAPTER 11: ENTERAL NUTRITION FORMULATIONS **239**

TABLE 11-7 Select Enteral Formulations Marketed for Use in Patients with Pulmonary Failure (Feeding Tube or Oral Use)

Product (Company)	Energy, kcal/mL	Protein g/L (% kcal)	Protein Source	Carbohydrate g/L (% kcal)	Carbohydrate Source	Fat g/L (% kcal)	Fat Source
Nutren Pulmonary (Nestlé)	1.5	68 (18)	Calcium-potassium caseinate	100 (27)	Maltodextrin	94.8 (55)	Canola oil, corn oil, MCT
Pulmocare (Abbott)	1.5	62.6 (16.7)	Sodium caseinate, calcium caseinate	105.7 (28.2)	Sucrose, maltodextrin	93.3 (55.1)	Canola oil, corn oil, safflower oil, MCT

Product (Company)	Osmolality, mOsm/kg	Volume Providing 100% RDI, mL	% H_2O	Fiber, g/L
Nutren Pulmonary (Nestlé)	330 (450 vanilla flavor)	1000	78	0
Pulmocare (Abbott)	475	947	78.5	0

MCT, medium-chain triglycerides; RDI, Reference Daily Intake.
Manufacturers may change product ingredients or nutritional content. Always check current product information.
Source: Data are from the manufacturers, Abbott Nutrition (https://abbottnutrition.com) and Nestlé Health Science (https://www.nestlehealthscience.us).

TABLE 11-8 Select Enteral Formulation Marketed for Use in Patients with Acute Respiratory Distress Syndrome or Acute Lung Injury (Feeding Tube Use)

Product (Company)	Energy, kcal/mL	Protein g/L (% kcal)	Protein Source	Carbohydrate g/L (% kcal)	Carbohydrate Source	Fat g/L (% kcal)	Fat Source
Oxepa (Abbott)	1.5	62.7 (16.7)	Sodium caseinate, calcium caseinate	105.3 (28.1)	Sugar, maltodextrin	93.8 (55.2)	Canola oil, MCT, fish oil, borage oil

Product (Company)	Osmolality, mOsm/kg	Volume Providing 100% RDI, mL	% H_2O	Fiber, g/L	Additional Information
Oxepa (Abbott)	535	946	78.5	0	Vitamin A: 11,910 IU/L Vitamin E: 320 IU/L Vitamin C: 850 mg/L Selenium: 74 mcg/L

MCT, medium-chain triglyceride; RDI, Reference Daily Intake.
Manufacturers may change product ingredients or nutritional content. Always check current product information.
Source Data are from the manufacturer, Abbott Nutrition (https://abbottnutrition.com).

lines is likely related to differences in the studies included and methods for analyzing data used to develop recommendations. Until further evidence is available on outcomes associated with this specialized EN formula, clinicians should use their judgment to decide whether to use a pulmonary-specific or a standard EN formula.

Renal Failure

Both acute and chronic renal failure is associated with malnutrition risk.[97,98] Patients with chronic kidney disease (CKD) on dialysis have increased protein needs and may require fluid and electrolyte restrictions.[99] Patients with CKD who are not yet on dialysis may slow progression of the CKD by limiting dietary protein intake.[100] In addition to considering the patient's comorbidities and metabolic state, the clinician should take into account the nutrition-related implications of the medical therapy used to treat renal dysfunction (eg, continuous renal replacement therapy vs hemodialysis vs predialysis treatment) to determine the appropriate nutrition prescription. Patients with acute kidney injury (AKI) are usually critically ill, hypermetabolic, and hypercatabolic, and they often have other organ dysfunctions.[101,102] Optimal nutrition management in AKI includes providing adequate macronutrient support to correct underlying conditions and prevent ongoing loss of organ function, supplementing micronutrients and

© 2017 ASPEN, www.nutritioncare.org

vitamins during renal replacement therapy, and adjusting electrolyte replacement based on the degree and extent of renal dysfunction.[98,101,102] (See Chapter 29 for additional discussion of renal disease.)

Functionally, the kidneys excrete nitrogenous waste and help maintain fluid, electrolyte, and vitamin and mineral homeostasis. EN formulations intended for patients with renal insufficiency and CKD are altered compared to standard formulas in the amounts of fluid (water), protein, electrolytes, vitamins, and minerals they provide (see Table 11-9). Protein content varies depending on the intended patient population. Formulas intended for patients with kidney dysfunction not yet on dialysis are protein restricted, whereas those intended for patients on dialysis have higher protein content because dialysis causes catabolism and protein wasting, increasing the protein requirement. Patients on continuous renal replacement therapies also have higher protein needs related to the

loss of protein to exchange fluids. However, routine use of a renal-specific EN formula is not necessary in patients with CKD or AKI.[11,103]

A systematic review published in 2005 included 18 studies and 541 patients on maintenance dialysis who were receiving EN, mostly as an oral supplement.[103] Of the 18 studies, 2 compared outcomes with oral intake of a renal-specific formula vs a standard formula. No differences were seen between the groups in serum albumin levels, protein and energy intake, performance status, or GI complaints. Additionally, the researchers noted electrolyte status was not adversely affected when oral supplements with low levels of electrolytes were used along with a standard diet. However, when a low-electrolyte supplement was used as the sole source of nutrition, hypophosphatemia, hypokalemia, and hyponatremia occurred occasionally. Overall, in maintenance dialysis patients, nutritional supplementation, whether standard or

TABLE 11-9 Select Enteral Formulations Marketed for Use in Patients with Renal Failure (Feeding Tube or Oral Use)

Product (Company)	Energy, kcal/mL	Protein g/L (% kcal)	Source	Carbohydrate g/L (% kcal)	Source	Fat g/L (% kcal)	Source
Nepro with Carb Steady (Abbott)	1.8	81 (18)	Sodium caseinate, calcium caseinate, magnesium caseinate, milk protein isolate	161 (34)	Corn syrup solids, sucrose, corn maltodextrin, glycerin, FOS	96 (48)	Safflower oil, canola oil
Novosource Renal (Nestlé)	2.0	90.7 (18)	Sodium caseinate, calcium caseinate, soy protein isolate	183 (37)	Corn syrup, sugar	100 (45)	Canola oil, corn oil
RenalCal (Nestlé)[a]	2.0	34.4 (7)	Whey protein concentrate, amino acid blend	290.4 (57)	Maltodextrin, cornstarch	82.4 (36)	MCT, corn oil, canola oils
Suplena with Carb Steady (Abbott)[b]	1.8	45 (10)	Milk protein isolate, sodium caseinate	196 (42)	Corn maltodextrin, isomaltulose, sucrose, glycerin, FOS	96 (48)	Safflower oil, canola oil

Product (Company)	Osmolality, mOsm/kg	Volume Providing 100% RDI, mL	% H₂O	Fiber, g/L	Sodium, mg/L	Potassium, mg/L	Magnesium, mg/L	Phosphorus, mg/L
Nepro with Carb Steady (Abbott)	745	944	72.7	12.6	1060	1060	210	720
Novosource Renal (Nestlé)	800	1000	72	0	945	945	197	819
RenalCal (Nestlé)[a]	600	1000	70	0	60	80	20	100
Suplena with Carb Steady (Abbott)[b]	780	944	73.8	12.7	802	1139	211	717

FOS, fructooligosaccharides; MCT, medium-chain triglycerides; RDI, Reference Daily Intake.
Manufacturers may change product ingredients or nutritional content. Always check current product information.
[a]Per manufacturer's product handbook, RenalCal is intended for oral supplementation and short-term tube feeding. It is not intended for use via oral or enteral route as a sole source of nutrition, and use of the product requires careful monitoring because of the negligible electrolyte content.
[b]Suplena is marketed for individuals with renal failure who are not receiving dialysis.
Source: Data are from the manufacturers, Abbott Nutrition (https://abbottnutrition.com) and Nestlé Health Science (https://www.nestlehealthscience.us).

renal-specific, seems to improve energy and protein intake and raise serum albumin levels; however, most studies did not report clinical outcomes.[103] The decision to use a renal-specific oral supplement in patients with CKD should be based on the individual patient's nutrition, fluid, and electrolyte status. The SCCM/ASPEN guidelines for critically ill patients recommend the use of standard high-protein EN formulas for patients with AKI. Patients with hyperkalemia or hyperphosphatemia may require a renal-specific formula.[11]

Conditions Requiring Fluid Restriction

Table 11-10 lists standard, energy-concentrated (up to 2 kcal/mL) enteral formulas that can be used instead of disease-specific formulas when the patient's clinical condition calls for restricted volume. For example, these formulas may be appropriate in patients with renal failure who require fluid restriction but do not require electrolyte restriction. The SCCM/ASPEN guidelines recommend the use of concentrated formulas in patients with acute respiratory failure because the presence of concomitant fluid overload, pulmonary edema, and renal failure are associated with worse clinical outcomes.[11] These formulas may also be used in other disease states or conditions, such as liver and heart failure, that result in fluid overload, hypervolemic hyponatremia, decreased urine output, early satiety, and elevated nutrition needs.[60] These formulations are available for use as oral supplements or via feeding tubes.

Wasting Conditions

Chronic wasting diseases, such as AIDS and cancer, contribute to patient morbidity and mortality. (See Chapter 32 for discussion of HIV/AIDS and Chapter 33 for information on cancer.) Tumor-induced and host-derived products facilitate wasting (eg, proinflammatory cytokines cause metabolic and neuro-

endocrine disturbances in the host).[104] Proteolysis-inducing factor has been identified as a cause of protein catabolism, which contributes to the skeletal muscle mass depletion seen in cancer cachexia.[105-107] In addition to the disease process, many factors—including anorexia, pain, malabsorption, early satiety due to ascites, bowel or gastric outlet obstruction, and GI toxicities related to chemotherapy and medication side effects—contribute to loss of LBM and malnutrition, and the specific factors vary depending on the type of cancer.[108] Preservation of muscle mass is crucial for patient rehabilitation, but the exact mechanisms involved with muscle wasting are still disputed and optimal nutrition support in the ICU has yet to be defined.[109]

Muscle loss is associated with an imbalance between protein synthesis to protein degradation, with the latter being greater. The conditionally essential amino acids glutamine and arginine are associated with improving immune function and wound complications when supplemented at pharmacological levels.[73,74] Beta-hydroxy beta-methylbutyrate (HMB), a metabolite of the BCAA leucine, is a dietary supplement that results in positive patient outcomes when provided with or without arginine and glutamine. HMB promotes anabolism by increasing protein synthesis and inhibiting the ubiquitin-proteasome pathway controlling protein degradation, thereby conserving and even promoting accretion of LBM.[110] Trauma patients receiving only HMB supplementation had improved (less negative) nitrogen balance compared with patients receiving an isonitrogenous placebo and an isonitrogenous combination of HMB, arginine, and glutamine.[111] HMB helps preserve LBM in patients with sarcopenia,[112,113] cancer cachexia,[114] and AIDS.[115] Additionally, HMB supplementation is associated with improved immune status with surrogate markers cluster of differentiation 3 and cluster of differentiation 8 levels as well as decreased viral load in patients with AIDS.[115]

Enteral formulations have evolved to include these amino acids and are marketed to enhance muscle mass and improve

TABLE 11-10 Select Enteral Formulations Marketed for Use in Patients Requiring Fluid Restriction (Feeding Tube or Oral Use)

Product (Company)	Energy, kcal/mL	Protein g/L (% kcal)	Protein Source	Carbohydrate g/L (% kcal)	Carbohydrate Source	Fat g/L (% kcal)	Fat Source
Nutren 2.0 (Nestlé)	2.0	84 (16)	Soy protein isolate, sodium caseinate	216 (43)	Corn syrup, maltodextrin	92 (41)	MCT, canola oil
TwoCal HN (Abbott)	2.0	83.5 (16.7)	Sodium caseinate, calcium caseinate	218.5 (43.2)	Corn syrup solids, corn maltodextrin, sucrose, FOS	90.5 (40.1)	Safflower oil, canola oil, MCT

Product (Company)	Osmolality, mOsm/kg	Volume Providing 100% RDI, mL	% H2O	Fiber, g/L	Sodium, mg/L	Potassium, mg/L	Phosphorus, mg/L	Magnesium, mg/L
Nutren 2.0 (Nestlé)	780	750	69	0	1500	2100	1480	560
TwoCal HN (Abbott)	725	948	70	5	1450	2440	1050	425

FOS, fructooligosaccharides; MCT, medium-chain triglycerides; RDI, Reference Daily Intake.
Manufacturers may change product ingredients or nutritional content. Always check current product information.
Data are from reference 4 and the manufacturers, Abbott Nutrition (https://abbottnutrition.com) and Nestlé Health Science (https://www.nestlehealthscience.us).

wound healing (Table 11-11). There are limited supportive data for the routine use and effectiveness of these supplements in patients with wasting syndrome. May and colleagues evaluated a combined supplement of HMB, arginine, and glutamine vs a control supplement in patients with stage 4 cancer (N = 24). After 4 weeks of supplementation, the intervention group gained 0.95 ± 0.66 kg body mass (1.12 ± 0.68 kg fat-free mass) whereas the controls lost 0.26 ± 0.78 kg body mass (1.34 ± 0.78 kg fat-free mass), and the weight changes were maintained over 24 weeks of evaluation.[114]

Wound Healing

Compared with patients who are not malnourished, those with malnutrition are likely to have worse outcomes, including poor wound healing or accelerated development of wounds (see Chapters 9 and 21). Nutrients, beyond energy and protein, that have been linked with improving patient outcomes include glutamine, arginine, ω-3 fatty acids, zinc, selenium, and vitamins A, C, and E (see Chapter 21).[116]

Pharmacological dosing of various nutrients is linked with improved wound healing.[117] EN formulations and supplements targeted for wound healing are available (Tables 11-6,

11-11, and 11-12). These formulations may or may not provide complete nutrition in addition to these wound-healing nutrients.

As discussed previously, provision of the IMFs, which contain arginine, ω-3 fatty acids, antioxidants, and sometimes glutamine, decreases the incidence of patient complications including anastomotic dehiscence. These effects have been demonstrated in GI surgery and trauma populations.[67,74,75] A systematic review and meta-analysis examined the impact of enteral tube feeding or oral nutritional supplements on pressure ulcer incidence and healing.[118] The review examined 5 randomized controlled trials to compare nutrition support to routine care (usual diet and pressure ulcer care) and concluded that the use of high-protein oral nutritional supplements reduced the risk of developing pressure ulcers by 25% in high-risk patients (eg, elderly, postsurgical, and chronically hospitalized patients). This review[118] and others[117] have suggested a high-protein diet, along with adequate serum levels of vitamin A and zinc, can assist patients at risk for pressure ulcers (eg, nursing home residents, spinal cord patients, those with wounds) as long as other protective behaviors such as weight control, exercise, and healthy lifestyle are involved (see Chapter 21).

TABLE 11-11 Oral Products Marketed for Use in Patients with Wound Healing and Muscle Repair

Product (Company)	Energy, kcal[a]	Protein g[a] (% kcal)	Protein Source	Carbohydrate g[a] (% kcal)	Carbohydrate Source	Fat g[a] (% kcal)	Fat Source
Ensure Enlive (Abbott)	350	20 (23)	Sodium caseinate, calcium caseinate, milk protein concentrate	44 (49)	Corn maltodextrin, sucrose, short-chain FOS	11 (28)	Canola oil, corn oil
Juven (Unflavored) (Abbott)	70/pkt	14/pkt (85)	L-arginine, L-glutamine	4/pkt (15)	Sucrose	0	None
Arginaid (Nestlé)	25	4.5 (72)	L-arginine	2 (28)	Citric acid, malic acid	0	None
Arginaid Extra (Nestlé)	250	10.5 (17)	Whey protein isolate, L-arginine	52 (83)	Sucrose, corn syrup solids	0	None

Product (Company)	Osmolality, mOsm/kg	% H₂O	Fiber, g[a]	Vitamin A, IU[a]	Vitamin C, mg[a]	Zinc, mg[a]	Additional Information
Ensure Enlive (Abbott)	780	75	3.0	1250	36	3.8	
Juven (Abbott)	451	0	0	0	0	0	
Arginaid (Nestlé)	170	0	0	0	260	0	Mix with 237 mL water. 4.5 g L-arginine per pkt
Arginaid Extra (Nestlé)	1340	83	0	1000	250	15	4.5 g L-arginine per 237 mL

FOS, fructooligosaccharides; pkt, packet.
Manufacturers may change product ingredients or nutritional content. Always check current product information.
[a]Data are per 237 mL unless otherwise indicated.
Source: Data are from the manufacturers, Abbott Nutrition (https://abbottnutrition.com) and Nestlé Health Science (https://www.nestlehealthscience.us).

TABLE 11-12 Select High-Protein Enteral Formulations (Feeding Tube Use)

Product (Company)	Energy, kcal/mL	Protein g/L (% kcal)	Protein Source	Carbohydrate g/L (% kcal)	Carbohydrate Source	Fat g/L (% kcal)	Fat Source
Replete (Nestlé)	1.0	64 (25)	Sodium caseinate, calcium caseinate	112 (45)	Maltodextrin	34 (30)	Canola oil, MCT
Replete Fiber (Nestlé)	1.0	64 (25)	Sodium caseinate, calcium caseinate, soy protein isolate	124 (45)	Maltodextrin, corn syrup, pea fiber, gum acacia, FOS, inulin	35 (30)	MCT
Perative (Abbott)	1.3	66.7 (20.5)	Partially hydrolyzed sodium caseinate, whey hydrolysate, L-arginine	180.3 (54.5)	Corn maltodextrin, FOS	37.3 (25)	Canola oil, MCT, corn oil, soy lecithin
Promote (Abbott)	1.0	62.5 (25)	Sodium caseinate, soy protein isolate	130 (52)	Corn maltodextrin, sucrose	26 (23)	Soy oil, MCT, safflower oil
Promote with Fiber (Abbott)	1.0	62.5 (25)	Sodium caseinate, calcium caseinate, soy protein isolate	138 (50)	Corn maltodextrin, oat fiber	28 (25)	Safflower oil, soy oil, MCT

Product (Company)	Osmolality, mOsm/kg	Volume Providing 100% RDI, mL	% H_2O	Fiber, g/L	Vitamin A, IU/L	Vitamin C, mg/L	Zinc, mg/L
Replete (Nestlé)	300	1500	84	0	3466	200	16
Replete Fiber (Nestlé)	330	1500	84	15.2	3466	340	24
Perative (Abbott)	460	1155	79	6.5	8675	260	20
Promote (Abbott)	340	1000	83.9	0	7250	345	24
Promote with Fiber (Abbott)	380	1000	83.1	14.4	7250	340	24

FOS, fructooligosaccharides; MCT, medium-chain triglycerides; RDI, Reference Daily Intake.
Manufacturers may change product ingredients or nutritional content. Always check current product information.
Source: Data are from the manufacturers, Abbott Nutrition (https://abbottnutrition.com) and Nestlé Health Science (https://www.nestlehealthscience.us).

Obesity

The 2016 SCCM/ASPEN critical care guidelines state that the critically ill obese patient should receive high-protein, hypocaloric feedings to preserve LBM and mobilize adipose stores.[11] In this population, weight loss may increase insulin sensitivity, facilitate nursing care, and reduce the risk of comorbidities.[11] The rationale is that severe obesity increases risks of insulin resistance, sepsis, infections, organ failure, and deep venous thrombosis. The goal for energy provision for obese patients should not exceed 65% to 70% of energy requirements as calculated by indirect calorimetry (IC).[11] If IC is unavailable, clinicians can use weight-based equations that estimate 11 to 14 kcal per kg of *actual* body weight for patients with BMI between 30 and 50, and 22 to 25 kcal per kg of *ideal* body weight for patients with BMI greater than 50.[11] Studies have found that daily provision of more than 2 g of protein per kg with hypocaloric feeding is adequate to achieve nitrogen balance, preserve LBM, and allow for adequate wound healing in the morbidly obese patient.[11]

Most enteral formulations have a high nonprotein calorie–to–nitrogen ratio (NPC:N), which requires clinicians to add a large amount of protein modular to meet the protein needs of the obese patient.[11] Enteral formulations that provide 1 kcal/mL have a lower NPC:N and also provide additional fluid, which is often needed for obese critically ill patients.[11] There may be some benefit in the use of immune-modulating formulas in this population, as low-grade systematic inflammatory response syndrome, insulin resistance, and metabolic syndrome may predispose obese, critically ill patients to a heightened immune-response with acute illness.[11] This area of focus requires additional research because there is currently a lack of outcome data. See Chapter 35 for further discussion of nutrition care for patients with obesity.

Modular Products

Sometimes, the ideal formula may not exist, perhaps because a facility's enteral formulary is limited or because products are unavailable. In these situations, clinicians must use modular products to meet a patient's specific needs. Modular products are typically single-nutrient products and are available for use in addition to the selected enteral formulations. Protein powders are the most common modular components (Table 11-13). Modular protein products have been evaluated based on their amino acid profile and the protein digestibility corrected amino acid score (PDCAAS). The PDCAAS assesses the bioavailability of essential amino acids of a protein module.[120] Manufacturers have used these scores to suggest that one modular protein product is superior to another. Modular products are also available for carbohydrate powders, MCT oil, and amino acids (eg, glutamine or arginine). Modular products are commonly used to fortify tube feedings or meals served on food trays. Liquid variations of modular products are available, but they often are hyperosmolar and caution should therefore be taken when administering them into a feeding tube. Powder and liquid protein modulars can be mixed into beverages and oral supplements. They also can be administered to patients receiving tube feedings but should not be mixed with the formula. Instead, they should be given as a separate flush via the feeding tube.

Developing an Enteral Product Formulary

Many healthcare facilities choose to develop an enteral formulary. The benefits of a formulary are inventory control and cost savings. Additionally, a formulary simplifies product-selection competency by professional staff.[4]

To develop a product formulary, one should evaluate the facility's patient population, current use of products, and contractual requirements. Clinicians should use the best available evidence to select appropriate products for an enteral formulary. Simply matching a medical diagnosis to a formula that is specifically marketed for that diagnosis could lead to inappropriate nutrition support provision as well as significantly increased costs to the facility.[4] The following factors should be considered when developing an enteral formulary:[120]

- Patient acuity
- Digestive and absorptive capacity, organ dysfunction, and metabolic requirements of most patients
- Formulation components that may be contraindicated
- Need for fluid restriction
- Need for added formulation components

Enteral formulary contracts should include a clause that allows the facility to purchase a noncompeting product if it better meets the nutrition needs of patients.[4] Healthcare facilities must complete a cost-benefit analysis when developing a formulary to choose appropriate products and limit expenditure.

Open vs Closed Systems

Enteral formulations are available as ready-to-feed liquids, ready-to-hang liquids, or powders that must be reconstituted. Each of these systems has advantages and disadvantages. With ready-to-feed products, enteral formulations must be transferred from a can, bottle, or brick pack to a refillable administration set or bag before delivery. In theory, this "open system" method increases the risk of formula contamination. In addition, more nursing time is required to administer an open system. Open systems are limited to a hang time of 8 to 12 hours to decrease risk of contamination.[5] Any nonsterile formula, such as powder formula, that needs to be reconstituted with sterile water should not hang for more than 4 hours; if the reconstituted formula is not used immediately, it can be refrigerated for 24 hours after preparation.[5] Compared to liquid formulations, powdered formulas are more susceptible to contamination because they require more manipulation during preparation.

Ready-to-hang (closed-system) enteral formulations are packaged in sealed bags or rigid containers that hold volumes of 1000, 1500, or 2000 mL. Administration tubing (eg, "spike sets") must be attached to the container before use; however, because no further manipulation of the formulation should occur, opportunities for contamination should be reduced. Hang times for closed systems for enteral formulations range from 24 to 48 hours. In addition to reducing the potential for contamination, these systems offer greater convenience

TABLE 11-13 Select Protein Modulars

Product (Company)	Energy, kcal/mL	Protein g/serving	Protein Source	Carbohydrate g/serving	Carbohydrate Source	Fat g/serving	Fat Source
ProMod (Abbott)	100/1-oz serving	10	Hydrolyzed collagen	14	Glycerin	0	None
Beneprotein (Nestlé)	25/scoop	6	Whey protein isolate	0	None	0	None

Manufacturers may change product ingredients or nutritional content. Always check current product information.
Data are from the manufacturers, Abbott Nutrition (https://abbottnutrition.com) and Nestlé Health Science (https://www.nestlehealthscience.us).

to both nurses and patients. Less nursing time is required to administer enteral formulations through a closed system than an open one. Despite their obvious advantages, closed-system containers have some drawbacks. Greater amounts of formulas may be wasted with closed systems in situations where feeding intolerance is common or in unstable patients where changes in the formula occur frequently. A more serious concern with closed systems is the potential for misconnection errors. Container design may allow the insertion of an IV spike set and inadvertent IV administration of enteral formulation, a life-threatening medical error.[121] A sentinel event alert from the Joint Commission in 2006 has raised awareness of this potentially deadly error and emphasized the importance of appropriate staff education concerning proper use of these products. Since the alter was issued, several innovations have been made to the previous enteral tubing design. A cross-spike unique "nutrition source connector" and ENFit, a "patient access connector" have been developed; the ENFit connector will not allow connectivity with other therapeutic devices and provides a locking feature that prevents disconnections.[5] In 2015, the ENFit female connector and ENFit Transition Con-

nector were introduced, and in 2016, the release of the ENFit male connector was released completed the transition.[5] (See Chapter 12 for further information.)

Formula Safety

As mentioned previously, the 4-phase process to gain FDA approval required for pharmaceutical agents is not required for enteral formulations. Safety concerns about enteral formulations focus on the potential for contamination. *C. difficile* colonization has been reported in tube-fed patients.[122] Approximately 30% to 75% of formulations prepared in the hospital have been found to be contaminated with bacteria, and at least half of those had bacterial counts in excess of federal limits (greater than 10^4 colony-forming units/mL).[4] Although the literature has not established a strong link between formula contamination and formula tolerance, best practice is to employ methods to reduce formula contamination.[4] Storage, preparation, handling, administration, and hang time of formulations should all be considered when evaluating the potential for contamination. Table 11-14 presents ASPEN's

TABLE 11-14 ASPEN Practice Recommendations for Adult Enteral Formula Safety

1. Each institution should define an ongoing quality control process for EN formula preparation, distribution, storage, handling, and administration. (B)
2. Institutions should maintain written policies and procedures for safe EN formula preparation and handling, as well as maintain an ongoing surveillance program for contamination. These should be based on HACCP and the USP good compounding practices. (B)
3. EN formulas should be prepared for patient use in a clean environment using aseptic technique by specially trained personnel. Strict aseptic technique (done under sterile conditions) should be used in the preparation and administration of enteral formulas. (A)
4. All personnel involved in preparing, storing, and administering EN formulas should be capable and qualified for the tasks and follow accepted best practices. (C)
5. Sterile, liquid EN formulas should be used in preference to powdered, reconstituted formulas whenever possible. (A)
6. Store unopened commercially available liquid EN formulas under controlled (dark, dry, cool) conditions. (B)
7. Maintain a rapid enteral feeding formula inventory turnover well within the product's expiration date. (C)
8. Formulas reconstituted in advance should be immediately refrigerated, and discarded within 24 hours of preparation if not used; formulas should be exposed to room temperature for no longer than 4 hours, after which they should be discarded. (B)
9. Use purified water or sterile water for irrigation supply, formula reconstitution, and medication dilution. Consider purified water for enteral access device flushes in at-risk patients. (B)
10. Strict adherence to manufacturer's recommendations for product use results in less contamination of EN. (A)
11. Use of disposable gloves is recommended in the administration of EN. (A)
12. Formula decanted from a screw cap is preferable instead of a flip top because formula poured from a screw cap was associated with less microbial growth. (A)
13. A recessed spike on a closed-system container is preferable. (B)
14. A feeding pump with a drip chamber prevents retrograde contamination of the EN formula from the feeding tube. (A)
15. Sterile, decanted formula should have an 8-hour hang time. (B)
16. Administration sets for open system enteral feedings should be changed at least every 24 hours. (B)
17. Powdered, reconstituted formula, and EN formula with additives should have a 4-hour hang time. (C)
18. Closed-system EN formulas can hang for 24 to 48 hours per manufacturer's guidelines. (A)
19. Administration sets for closed-system EN formulas should be changed per manufacturer guidelines. (A)

ASPEN, American Society for Parenteral and Enteral Nutrition; EN, enteral nutrition; HACCP, hazard analysis and critical control points; USP, US Pharmacopeia Convention.
Source: Adapted with permission from reference 4: Bankhead R, Boullata J, Brantley S, et al. A.S.P.E.N. enteral nutrition practice recommendations. *JPEN J Parenter Enteral Nutr.* 2009;33(2):122–167.

current practice recommendations to reduce the risk of enteral formulation contamination.[4]

References

1. Brown B, Roehl K, Betz M. Enteral nutrition formula selection: current evidence and implications for practice. *Nutr Clin Pract.* 2015;30(1):72–85.

2. Spapen H, Diltoer M, Van Malderen C, et al. Soluble fiber reduces the incidence of diarrhea in septic patients receiving total enteral nutrition: a prospective, double-blind, randomized, and controlled trial. *Clin Nutr.* 2001;20(4):301–305.

3. US Food and Drug Administration. Frequently asked questions about medical foods. 2016(May). http://www.fda.gov/downloads /Food/GuidanceRegulation/GuidanceDocumentsRegulatory Information/UCM500094.pdf. Accessed January 16, 2017.

4. Bankhead R, Boullata J, Brantley S, et al. Enteral nutrition practice recommendations. *JPEN J Parenter Enteral Nutr.* 2009;33(2): 122–167.

5. Kozeniecki M, Fritzshall R. Enteral nutrition for adults in the hospital setting. *Nutr Clin Pract.* 2015;30(5):634–651.

6. Charney P. Enteral nutrition: indications, options, and formulations. In: Gottschlich MM, ed. *The Science and Practice of Nutrition Support: A Core-Based Care Curriculum.* Dubuque, IA: Kendall/ Hunt Publishing; 2001:141–166.

7. Trujillo EB. Enteral nutrition: a comprehensive overview. In Matarese LE, Gottschlich MM, eds. *Contemporary Nutrition Support Practice: A Clinical Guide.* Philadelphia, PA: Saunders; 1998:192–201.

8. Malone AM. Enteral formulations. In Cresci GA, ed. *Nutrition Support for the Critically Ill Patient: A Guide to Practice.* Boca Raton, FL: CRC Press; 2005:253–277.

9. Malone A. Enteral formula section: a review of selected product categories. *Pract Gastroenterol.* 2005;24:44–74.

10. Rushdi TA, Pichard C, Khater YH. Control of diarrhea by fiber-enriched diet in ICU patients on enteral nutrition: a prospective randomized controlled trial. *Clin Nutr.* 2004;23(6):1344–1352.

11. McClave SA, Taylor BE, Martindale RG, et al. Guidelines for the provision and assessment of nutrition support therapy in the adult critically ill patient: Society of Critical Care Medicine (SCCM) and American Society for Parenteral and Enteral Nutrition (ASPEN). *JPEN J Parenter Enteral Nutr.* 2016;40(2):159–211.

12. Scaife CL, Saffle JR, Morris SE. Intestinal obstruction secondary to enteral feedings in burn trauma patients. *J Trauma.* 1999;47(5): 859–863.

13. McIvor AC, Meguid MM, Curtas S, Warren J, Kaplan DS. Intestinal obstruction from cecal bezoar, a complication of fiber-containing tube feedings. *Nutrition.* 1990;6(1):115–117.

14. McClave SA, Chang WK. Feeding the hypotensive patient: does enteral feeding precipitate or protect against ischemic bowel? *Nutr Clin Pract.* 2003;18(4):279–284.

15. Ettinger S. Macronutrients: carbohydrates, proteins, and lipids. In: Mahan K, Escott-Stump S, eds. *Krause's Food, Nutrition, and Diet Therapy.* 11th ed. Philadelphia, PA: Saunders; 2004:37–74.

16. Elia M, Engfer MB, Green CJ, Silk DBA. Systematic review and meta-analysis: the clinical and physiological effects of fibre-containing enteral formulae. *Aliment Pharmacol Ther.* 2008;27(2):120–145.

17. Silk DB, Fairclough PD, Clark ML, et al. Use of a peptide rather than free amino acid nitrogen source in chemically defined "elemental" diets. *JPEN J Parenter Enteral Nutr.* 1980;4(6):548–553.

18. Craft IL, Geddes D, Hyde CW, Wise IJ, Matthews DM. Absorption and malabsorption of glycine and glycine peptides in man. *Gut.* 1968;9(4):425–437.

19. Lord LM, Lipp J, Stull S. Adult tube feeding formulas. *Medsurg Nurs.* 1996;5(6):407–419; quiz 420–421.

20. Eisenberg PG. Causes of diarrhea in tube-fed patients: a comprehensive approach to diagnosis and management. *Nutr Clin Pract.* 1993;8(3):119–123.

21. Food Allergy Research and Education. http://www.foodallergy .org. Accessed January 16, 2017.

22. American Society for Parenteral and Enteral Nutrition Board of Directors. Guidelines for the use of parenteral and enteral nutrition in adult and pediatric patients. *JPEN J Parenter Enteral Nutr.* 2002;26(1 Suppl):1SA–138SA.

23. Milne AC, Potter J, Vivanti A, Avenell A. Protein and energy supplementation in elderly people at risk from malnutrition. *Cochrane Database Syst Rev.* 2009(2):CD003288.

24. Stratton RJ, Elia M. Are oral nutritional supplements of benefit to patients in the community? Findings from a systematic review. *Curr Opin Clin Nutr Metab Care.* 2000;3(4):311–315.

25. Lynch GS, Schertzer JD, Ryall JG. Therapeutic approaches for muscle wasting disorders. *Pharmacol Ther.* 2007;113(3): 461–487.

26. Davidson P, Kwiatkowski CA, Wien M. Management of hyperglycemia and enteral nutrition in the hospitalized patient. *Nutr Clin Pract.* 2015;30(5):652–659.

27. Swanson CM, Potter DJ, Kongable GL, Cook CB. Update on inpatient glycemic control in hospitals in the United States. *Endocr Pract.* 2011;17(6):853–861.

28. Signal M, Le Compte A, Shaw GM, Chase JG. Glycemic levels in critically ill patients: are normoglycemia and low variability associated with improved outcomes? *J Diabetes SciTech.* 2012;6(5): 1030–1037.

29. van Hooijdonk RT, Mesotten D, Krinsley JS, Schultz MJ. Sweet spot: glucose control in the intensive care unit. *Semin Respir Crit Care Med.* 2016;37(1):57–67.

30. Krinsley JS, Preiser JC. Time in blood glucose range 70 to 140 mg/dl >80% is strongly associated with increased survival in non-diabetic critically ill adults. *Crit Care.* 2015;19:179.

31. Penning S, Pretty C, Preiser JC, et al. Glucose control positively influences patient outcome: a retrospective study. *J Crit Care.* 2015;30(3):455–459.

32. McMahon MM, Nystrom E, Braunschweig C, Miles J, Compher C. A.S.P.E.N. clinical guidelines: nutrition support of adult patients with hyperglycemia. *JPEN J Parenter Enteral Nutr.* 2013;37(1):23–36.

33. Moghissi ES, Korytkowski MT, DiNardo M, et al. American Association of Clinical Endocrinologists and American Diabetes Association consensus statement on inpatient glycemic control. *Diabetes Care.* 2009;32(6):1119–1131.

34. Evert AB, Boucher JL, Cypress M, et al. Nutrition therapy recommendations for the management of adults with diabetes. *Diabetes Care.* 2013;36(11):3821–3842.

35. Sadiya A. Nutritional therapy for the management of diabetic gastroparesis: clinical review. *Diabetes Metab Syndr Obes.* 2012;5:329–335.

36. Heyland DK, Dhaliwal R, Wang M, Day AG. The prevalence of iatrogenic underfeeding in the nutritionally "at-risk" critically ill patient: Results of an international, multicenter, prospective study. *Clin Nutr.* 2015;34(4):659–666.

37. Nicolo M, Heyland DK, Chittams J, Sammarco T, Compher C. Clinical outcomes related to protein delivery in a critically ill population: a multicenter, multinational observation study. *JPEN J Parenter Enteral Nutr.* 2016;40(1):45–51.

38. Ceriello A, Lansink M, Rouws CH, van Laere KM, Frost GS. Administration of a new diabetes-specific enteral formula results in an improved 24h glucose profile in type 2 diabetic patients. *Diabetes Res Clin Pract.* 2009;84(3):259–266.

39. Vanschoonbeek K, Lansink M, van Laere KM, et al. Slowly digestible carbohydrate sources can be used to attenuate the post-

prandial glycemic response to the ingestion of diabetes-specific enteral formulas. *Diabetes Educ.* 2009;35(4):631–640.

40. Voss AC, Maki KC, Garvey WT, et al. Effect of two carbohydrate-modified tube-feeding formulas on metabolic responses in patients with type 2 diabetes. *Nutrition.* 2008;24(10):990–997.

41. Garcia-Rodriguez CE, Mesa MD, Olza J, et al. Postprandial glucose, insulin and gastrointestinal hormones in healthy and diabetic subjects fed a fructose-free and resistant starch type IV-enriched enteral formula. *Eur J Nutr.* 2013;52(6):1569–1578.

42. Lansink M, Hofman Z, Genovese S, Rouws CH, Ceriello A. Improved glucose profile in patients with type 2 diabetes with a new, high-protein, diabetes-specific tube feed during 4 hours of continuous feeding. *JPEN J Parenter Enteral Nutr.* 2016(Jan). Epub ahead of print.

43. de Luis DA, Izaola O, de la Fuente B, et al. A randomized clinical trial with two doses of an enteral diabetes-specific supplements in elderly patients with diabetes mellitus type 2. *Eur Rev Med Pharmacol Sci.* 2013;17(12):1626–1630.

44. Elia M, Ceriello A, Laube H, et al. Enteral nutritional support and use of diabetes-specific formulas for patients with diabetes: a systematic review and meta-analysis. *Diabetes Care.* 2005;28(9):2267–2279.

45. Peters AL, Davidson MB. Effects of various enteral feeding products on postprandial blood glucose response in patients with type I diabetes. *JPEN J Parenter Enteral Nutr.* 1992;16(1):69–74.

46. Peters AL, Davidson MB, Isaac RM. Lack of glucose elevation after simulated tube feeding with a low-carbohydrate, high-fat enteral formula in patients with type I diabetes. *Am J Med.* 1989;87(2):178–182.

47. Pohl M, Mayr P, Mertl-Roetzer M, et al. Glycemic control in patients with type 2 diabetes mellitus with a disease-specific enteral formula: stage II of a randomized, controlled multicenter trial. *JPEN J Parenter Enteral Nutr.* 2009;33(1):37–49.

48. Leon-Sanz M, Garcia-Luna PP, Sanz-Paris A, et al. Glycemic and lipid control in hospitalized type 2 diabetic patients: evaluation of 2 enteral nutrition formulas (low carbohydrate-high monounsaturated fat vs high carbohydrate). *JPEN J Parenter Enteral Nutr.* 2005;29(1):21–29.

49. Mesejo A, Montejo-Gonzalez JC, Vaquerizo-Alonso C, et al. Diabetes-specific enteral nutrition formula in hyperglycemic, mechanically ventilated, critically ill patients: a prospective, open-label, blind-randomized, multicenter study. *Crit Care.* 2015;19:390.

50. Critical Care Nutrition. Canadian clinical practice guidelines: composition of enteral nutrition: (carbohydrate/fat): high fat/low CHO. 2015. http://www.criticalcarenutrition.com/docs/CPGs%202015/4.2a%202015.pdf. Accessed September 30, 2016.

51. Academy of Nutrition and Dietetics Evidence Analysis Library. Critical illness guideline. 2012. http://www.andeal.org/topic.cfm?menu=5302&cat=4800. Accessed September 30, 2016.

52. American Diabetes Association. Position statement 13. Diabetes care in the hospital. *Diabetes Care.* 2016;39(Suppl 1):S99–S104.

53. Guarner F, Malagelada JR. Gut flora in health and disease. *Lancet.* 2003;361(9356):512–519.

54. Mowatt-Larssen CA, Brown RO, Wojtysiak SL, Kudsk KA. Comparison of tolerance and nutritional outcome between a peptide and a standard enteral formula in critically ill, hypoalbuminemic patients. *JPEN J Parenter Enteral Nutr.* 1992;16(1):20–24.

55. Brinson RR, Kolts BE. Diarrhea associated with severe hypoalbuminemia: a comparison of a peptide-based chemically defined diet and standard enteral alimentation. *Crit Care Med.* 1988;16(2):130–136.

56. Heimburger DC, Geels VJ, Bilbrey J, Redden DT, Keeney C. Effects of small-peptide and whole-protein enteral feedings on serum proteins and diarrhea in critically ill patients: a randomized trial. *JPEN J Parenter Enteral Nutr.* 1997;21(3):162–167.

57. Meredith JW, Ditesheim JA, Zaloga GP. Visceral protein levels in trauma patients are greater with peptide diet than with intact protein diet. *J Trauma.* 1990;30(7):825–828; discussion 828–829.

58. Kreymann KG, Berger MM, Deutz NE, et al. ESPEN guidelines on enteral nutrition: intensive care. *Clin Nutr.* 2006;25(2):210–223.

59. Dasarathy S. Cause and management of muscle wasting in chronic liver disease. *Curr Opin Gastroenterol.* 2016;32(3):159–165.

60. Hasse JM, DiCecco SR. Enteral Nutrition in chronic liver disease: translating evidence into practice. *Nutr Clin Pract.* 2015;30(4):474–487.

61. Nishikawa H, Yoh K, Enomoto H, et al. Factors associated with protein-energy malnutrition in chronic liver disease: analysis using indirect calorimetry. *Medicine (Baltimore).* 2016;95(2):e2442.

62. Abdelsayed GG. Diets in encephalopathy. *Clin Liver Dis.* 2015;19(3):497–505.

63. Parekh PJ, Balart LA. Ammonia and its role in the pathogenesis of hepatic encephalopathy. *Clin Liver Dis.* 2015;19(3):529–537.

64. Kawaguchi T, Taniguchi E, Sata M. Effects of oral branched-chain amino acids on hepatic encephalopathy and outcome in patients with liver cirrhosis. *Nutr Clin Pract.* 2013;28(5):580–588.

65. Holecek M. Three targets of branched-chain amino acid supplementation in the treatment of liver disease. *Nutrition.* 2010;26(5):482–490.

66. Gluud LL, Dam G, Les I, et al. Branched-chain amino acids for people with hepatic encephalopathy. *Cochrane Database Syst Rev.* 2015(9):CD001939.

67. Marik PE, Zaloga GP. Immunonutrition in high-risk surgical patients: a systematic review and analysis of the literature. *JPEN J Parenter Enteral Nutr.* 2010;34(4):378–386.

68. Vidal-Casariego A, Calleja-Fernández A, Villar-Taibo R, Kyriakos G, Ballesteros-Pomar MD. Efficacy of arginine-enriched enteral formulas in the reduction of surgical complications in head and neck cancer: a systematic review and meta-analysis. *Clin Nutr.* 2014;33(6):951–957.

69. Osland E, Hossain MB, Khan S, Memon MA. Effect of timing of pharmaconutrition (immunonutrition) administration on outcomes of elective surgery for gastrointestinal malignancies: a systematic review and meta-analysis. *JPEN J Parenter Enteral Nutr.* 2014;38(1):53–69.

70. Heys SD, Walker LG, Smith I, Eremin O. Enteral nutritional supplementation with key nutrients in patients with critical illness and cancer: a meta-analysis of randomized controlled clinical trials. *Ann Surg.* 1999;229(4):467–477.

71. Beale RJ, Bryg DJ, Bihari DJ. Immunonutrition in the critically ill: a systematic review of clinical outcome. *Crit Care Med.* 1999;27(12):2799–2805.

72. Heyland DK, Novak F, Drover JW, et al. Should immunonutrition become routine in critically ill patients? A systematic review of the evidence. *JAMA.* 2001;286(8):944–953.

73. Montejo JC, Zarazaga A, López-Martínez J, et al. Immunonutrition in the intensive care unit. A systematic review and consensus statement. *Clin Nutr.* 2003;22(3):221–233.

74. Waitzberg DL, Saito H, Plank LD, et al. Postsurgical infections are reduced with specialized nutrition support. *World J Surg.* 2006;30(8):1592–1604.

75. Cerantola Y, Hübner M, Grass F, Demartines N, Schäfer M. Immunonutrition in gastrointestinal surgery. *Br J Surg.* 2011;98(1):37–48.

76. Drover JW, Dhaliwal R, Weitzel L, et al. Perioperative use of arginine-supplemented diets: a systematic review of the evidence. *J Am Coll Surg.* 2011;212(3):385–399, 399.e381.

77. Dhaliwal R, Cahill N, Lemieux M, Heyland DK. The Canadian Critical Care Nutrition Guidelines in 2013: an update on current recommendations and implementation strategies. *Nutr Clin Pract.* 2014;29(1):29–43.

78. Levy MM, Artigas A, Phillips GS, et al. Outcomes of the Surviving Sepsis Campaign in intensive care units in the USA and Europe: a prospective cohort study. *Lancet Infect Dis.* 2012; 12(12):919–924.

79. Stapel SN, de Grooth HJ, Alimohamad H, et al. Ventilator-derived carbon dioxide production to assess energy expenditure in critically ill patients: proof of concept. *Crit Care.* 2015; 19:370.

80. Askanazi J, Elwyn DH, Silverberg PA, Rosenbaum SH, Kinney JM. Respiratory distress secondary to a high carbohydrate load: a case report. *Surgery.* 1980;87(5):596–598.

81. Covelli HD, Black JW, Olsen MS, Beekman JF. Respiratory failure precipitated by high carbohydrate loads. *Ann Intern Med.* 1981;95(5):579–581.

82. Dark DS, Pingleton SK, Kerby GR. Hypercapnia during weaning. A complication of nutritional support. *Chest.* 1985;88(1):141–143.

83. Talpers SS, Romberger DJ, Bunce SB, Pingleton SK. Nutritionally associated increased carbon dioxide production. Excess total calories vs high proportion of carbohydrate calories. *Chest.* 1992;102(2):551–555.

84. DeMichele SJ, Wood SM, Wennberg AK. A nutritional strategy to improve oxygenation and decrease morbidity in patients who have acute respiratory distress syndrome. *Respir Care Clin N Am.* 2006;12(4):547–566, vi.

85. Ferreira IM, Brooks D, White J, Goldstein R. Nutritional supplementation for stable chronic obstructive pulmonary disease. *Cochrane Database Syst Rev.* 2012;12:CD000998.

86. Gadek JE, DeMichele SJ, Karlstad MD, et al. Effect of enteral feeding with eicosapentaenoic acid, gamma-linolenic acid, and antioxidants in patients with acute respiratory distress syndrome. Enteral Nutrition in ARDS Study Group. *Crit Care Med.* 1999;27(8):1409–1420.

87. Pontes-Arruda A, Aragao AM, Albuquerque JD. Effects of enteral feeding with eicosapentaenoic acid, gamma-linolenic acid, and antioxidants in mechanically ventilated patients with severe sepsis and septic shock. *Crit Care Med.* 2006;34(9):2325–2333.

88. Pontes-Arruda A, Demichele S, Seth A, Singer P. The use of an inflammation-modulating diet in patients with acute lung injury or acute respiratory distress syndrome: a meta-analysis of outcome data. *JPEN J Parenter Enteral Nutr.* 2008;32(6):596–605.

89. Singer P, Theilla M, Fisher H, et al. Benefit of an enteral diet enriched with eicosapentaenoic acid and gamma-linolenic acid in ventilated patients with acute lung injury. *Crit Care Med.* 2006;34(4):1033–1038.

90. Grau-Carmona T, Moran-Garcia V, Garcia-de-Lorenzo A, et al. Effect of an enteral diet enriched with eicosapentaenoic acid, gamma-linolenic acid and anti-oxidants on the outcome of mechanically ventilated, critically ill, septic patients. *Clin Nutr.* 2011;30(5):578–584.

91. Santacruz CA, Orbegozo D, Vincent JL, Preiser JC. Modulation of dietary lipid composition during acute respiratory distress syndrome: systematic review and meta-analysis. *JPEN J Parenter Enteral Nutr.* 2015;39(7):837–846.

92. Li C, Bo L, Liu W, Lu X, Jin F. Enteral immunomodulatory diet (omega-3 fatty acid, gamma-linolenic acid and antioxidant supplementation) for acute lung injury and acute respiratory distress syndrome: an updated systematic review and meta-analysis. *Nutrients.* 2015;7(7):5572–5585.

93. Garcia de Acilu M, Leal S, Caralt B, et al. The role of omega-3 polyunsaturated fatty acids in the treatment of patients with acute respiratory distress syndrome: a clinical review. *Biomed Res Int.* 2015;2015:653750.

94. Rice TW, Wheeler AP, Thompson BT, et al. Enteral omega-3 fatty acid, gamma-linolenic acid, and antioxidant supplementation in acute lung injury. *JAMA.* 2011;306(14):1574–1581.

95. Kagan I, Cohen J, Stein M, et al. Preemptive enteral nutrition enriched with eicosapentaenoic acid, gamma-linolenic acid and antioxidants in severe multiple trauma: a prospective, randomized, double-blind study. *Intensive Care Med.* 2015;41(3):460–469.

96. Critical Care Nutrition. Canadian clinical practice guidelines: composition of enteral nutrition: fish oils, borage oils and antioxidants. 2015. http://www.criticalcarenutrition.com/docs/CPGs %202015/4.1b(i)%202015.pdf. Accessed September 30, 2016.

97. Knap B, Arnol M, Romozi K, et al. Malnutrition in renal failure: pleiotropic diagnostic approaches, inefficient therapy and bad prognosis. *Ther Apher Dial.* 2016;20(3):272–276.

98. Oh WC, Gardner DS, Devonald MA. Micronutrient and amino acid losses in acute renal replacement therapy. *Curr Opin Clin Nutr Metab Care.* 2015;18(6):593–598.

99. Campbell KL, Ash S, Zabel R, et al. Implementation of standardized nutrition guidelines by renal dietitians is associated with improved nutrition status. *J Ren Nutr.* 2009;19(2):136–144.

100. Banerjee T, Liu Y, Crews DC. Dietary patterns and CKD progression. *Blood Purif.* 2016;41(1-3):117–122.

101. Gervasio JM, Garmon WP, Holowatyj M. Nutrition support in acute kidney injury. *Nutr Clin Pract.* 2011;26(4):374–381.

102. McCarthy MS, Phipps SC. Special nutrition challenges: current approach to acute kidney injury. *Nutr Clin Pract.* 2014;29(1): 56–62.

103. Stratton RJ, Bircher G, Fouque D, et al. Multinutrient oral supplements and tube feeding in maintenance dialysis: a systematic review and meta-analysis. *Am J Kidney Dis.* 2005;46(3):387–405.

104. Tisdale MJ. Inhibition of lipolysis and muscle protein degradation by EPA in cancer cachexia. *Nutrition.* 1996;12(1 Suppl): S31–S33.

105. Smith HJ, Lorite MJ, Tisdale MJ. Effect of a cancer cachectic factor on protein synthesis/degradation in murine C2C12 myoblasts: modulation by eicosapentaenoic acid. *Cancer Res.* 1999;59(21):5507–5513.

106. Smith KL, Tisdale MJ. Mechanism of muscle protein degradation in cancer cachexia. *Br J Cancer.* 1993;68(2):314–318.

107. Lorite MJ, Smith HJ, Arnold JA, et al. Activation of ATP-ubiquitin-dependent proteolysis in skeletal muscle in vivo and murine myoblasts in vitro by a proteolysis-inducing factor (PIF). *Br J Cancer.* 2001;85(2):297–302.

108. Falconer JS, Fearon KC, Plester CE, Ross JA, Carter DC. Cytokines, the acute-phase response, and resting energy expenditure in cachectic patients with pancreatic cancer. *Ann Surg.* 1994;219(4): 325–331.

109. Wandrag L, Brett SJ, Frost G, Hickson M. Impact of supplementation with amino acids or their metabolites on muscle wasting in patients with critical illness or other muscle wasting illness: a systematic review. *J Hum Nutr Diet.* 2015;28(4):313–330.

110. Siddiqui R, Pandya D, Harvey K, Zaloga GP. Nutrition modulation of cachexia/proteolysis. *Nutr Clin Pract.* 2006;21(2):155–167.

111. Kuhls DA, Rathmacher JA, Musngi MD, et al. Beta-hydroxy-beta-methylbutyrate supplementation in critically ill trauma patients. *J Trauma.* 2007;62(1):125–131; discussion 131–132.

112. Flakoll P, Sharp R, Baier S, et al. Effect of beta-hydroxy-beta-methylbutyrate, arginine, and lysine supplementation on strength, functionality, body composition, and protein metabolism in elderly women. *Nutrition.* 2004;20(5):445–451.

113. Baier S, Johannsen D, Abumrad N, et al. Year-long changes in protein metabolism in elderly men and women supplemented

with a nutrition cocktail of beta-hydroxy-beta-methylbutyrate (HMB), L-arginine, and L-lysine. *JPEN J Parenter Enteral Nutr.* 2009;33(1):71–82.

114. May PE, Barber A, D'Olimpio JT, Hourihane A, Abumrad NN. Reversal of cancer-related wasting using oral supplementation with a combination of beta-hydroxy-beta-methylbutyrate, arginine, and glutamine. *Am J Surg.* 2002;183(4):471–479.

115. Clark RH, Feleke G, Din M, et al. Nutritional treatment for acquired immunodeficiency virus-associated wasting using beta-hydroxy beta-methylbutyrate, glutamine, and arginine: a randomized, double-blind, placebo-controlled study. *JPEN J Parenter Enteral Nutr.* 2000;24(3):133–139.

116. Scholl D, Langkamp-Henken B. Nutrient recommendations for wound healing. *J Intraven Nurs.* 2001;24(2):124–132.

117. Hayes GL, McKinzie BP, Bullington WM, Cooper TB, Pilch NA. Nutritional supplements in critical illness. *AACN Adv Crit Care.* 2011;22(4):301–316; quiz 317–318.

118. Stratton RJ, Ek AC, Engfer M, et al. Enteral nutritional support in prevention and treatment of pressure ulcers: a systematic review and meta-analysis. *Ageing Res Rev.* 2005;4(3):422–450.

119. Choban PS, Dickerson RN. Morbid obesity and nutrition support: is bigger different? *Nutr Clin Pract.* 2005;20(4):480–487.

120. Castellanos VH, Litchford MD, Campbell WW. Modular protein supplements and their application to long-term care. *Nutr Clin Pract.* 2006;21(5):485–504.

121. Neven A, Wilson R, Kochevar M, McMahon MM. Compatibility of IV administration sets with closed enteral nutrition containers. *JPEN J Parenter Enteral Nutr.* 2000;24(6):369.

122. Bliss DZ, Johnson S, Savik K, Clabots CR, Willard K, Gerding DN. Acquisition of *Clostridium difficile* and *Clostridium difficile*-associated diarrhea in hospitalized patients receiving tube feeding. *Ann Intern Med.* 1998;129(12):1012–1019.

12 Enteral Access Devices

John C. Fang, MD, and Merin Kinikini, DNP, FNP, RD, CNSC

CONTENTS

Objectives

1. Define the patient and tube selection criteria for various enteral access devices.
2. Understand the insertion techniques for the different types of enteral access devices.
3. Describe proper care and maintenance of enteral access devices.
4. Know the complications of enteral access devices.

Test Your Knowledge Questions

1. If a nasoenteric feeding tube cannot be unclogged using water flushes, what is the next most reliable method for unclogging the tube before it is replaced?
   - A. Administer cola through the tube, and let it sit for a few hours.
   - B. Administer Clog Zapper (CORPAK MedSystems, Buffalo Grove, IL), and flush within 30 to 60 minutes.
   - C. Wait a few hours to see whether the clog dissolves spontaneously.
   - D. Administer a mixture of pancreatic enzymes and bicarbonate solution, allow it to sit for 1 to 2 hours (or longer), and then flush with warm water.

2. You perform a telephone evaluation of a patient who relates increased redness, pain, and swelling around his existing low-profile gastrostomy tube (G-tube). He has not been seen in the clinic for more than 6 months and, when asked, states that he has been doing quite well on his enteral tube feeds. In fact, the patient states he has gained over 20 pounds. You would proceed as follows:
   A. Congratulate him on gaining the weight and tell him to continue his present tube feeding plan.
   B. If possible, have him come to the clinic or call the clinician managing the tube to rule out buried bumper syndrome.
   C. Direct him to put some triple antibiotic around the site and call back in a couple of weeks if the discomfort continues.
   D. Tell him to put hot packs on it, take acetaminophen, and rest for a few days.

3. An 18-year-old female patient with cystic fibrosis had a standard-profile, solid internal bolster, 20-Fr percutaneous endoscopic gastrostomy (PEG) tube placed 1 year ago because of her inability to take in enough energy orally and weight loss. She has done very well, with her weight stabilizing and no complications of the PEG. The original tube is now getting stiff and cracking, and the patient wants a replacement tube. The patient has a very supportive family environment, is very active, and is concerned about the cosmetic appearance of the tube itself. What type of replacement tube would you recommend?
   A. Standard-profile, 20-Fr percutaneous G-tube with solid internal bolster
   B. Standard-profile, 20-Fr percutaneous G-tube with balloon internal bolster
   C. Low-profile, 20-Fr percutaneous G-tube with solid internal bolster
   D. Low-profile, 20-Fr percutaneous G-tube with balloon internal bolster

Test Your Knowledge Answers

1. The correct answer is **D**. Pancreatic enzyme solutions have been studied, and, in one report, this method of unclogging tubes had a 90% success rate when the tube was allowed to sit for 2 hours. The mixture of 1 tablet of a pancreatic enzyme (pancrelipase [Viokase] 6000 units, protease 19,000 units, amylase 30,000 units) and 325 mg sodium bicarbonate (half of a 650-mg tablet) is crushed and mixed with 5 mL of warm water and instilled into the feeding tube for 30 minutes to 2 hours. This method can be tried an additional time (for up to 24 hours), if the shorter waiting period is ineffective. However, if the clog is from a medication and does not clear the first time, the tube should be replaced. Answer A is a common misconception. Administering an acidic solution can actually worsen formula and many medication clogs. Clog Zapper is a commercial mixture of papain, α-amylase, and citric acid solution. It has a lower success rate than pancreatic enzyme solutions. Waiting longer will not help a tube become unclogged.

2. The correct answer is **B**. Whenever a patient with a low-profile feeding tube gains or loses a significant amount of weight, there is a risk that the tube is no longer sized correctly. This risk is greatest with weight gain, because that can cause abnormal internal pressure from the bolster or balloon (one that has deflated enough to be pulled into the abdominal wall), which can erode the gastric mucosa. If this process continues, buried bumper syndrome may develop. It results from growth of the gastric mucosa partially or completely over the internal bumper, or excess pressure on the tissues in-between the abdominal wall and gastric mucosa, usually because of excessive tension between the internal and external bumpers or a partially deflated balloon. Poor wound healing, significant weight gain without adjusting the external bumper or changing to a longer, low-profile feeding tube, or lack of routine changes with a balloon tube can contribute as well. Patients are often unaware of this problem until the tube site becomes extremely painful. As the skin becomes irritated and swells, it magnifies the problem. This patient needs to be evaluated soon and have the feeding tube exchanged for either a longer, low-profile tube or a standard tube. If the process has progressed too far, infection may also occur and more intensive treatment with antibiotics and tube removal may be required.

3. The correct answer is **D**. A low-profile, 20-Fr percutaneous G-tube with balloon internal bolster is appropriate for this patient. Because she is very active, standard-profile tubes are less appealing than low-profile, skin-level tubes. Because the patient is concerned about her appearance, a low-profile tube is also a better option. Solid internal bolsters last longer, but they cause significant discomfort when removed and therefore require a clinic or hospital visit to be replaced. Therefore, a low-profile, balloon internal bolster, percutaneous G-tube is the best replacement option. Because the patient and her family are so involved in her care and supportive, they can likely be trained to exchange a low-profile, balloon-type replacement PEG on their own, thus further minimizing future office visits to exchange the feeding tube.

Introduction

Enteral nutrition (EN) is the preferred method of feeding in the presence of a functional gastrointestinal (GI) tract when the patient cannot take in enough nutrition orally (see Chapter 10). Delivery of EN to the patient will require an enteral access device. To determine the type of enteral access device that is best for the patient, many factors must be evaluated. The underlying disease, gastric and small bowel function, short- and long-term goals, anticipated length of therapy, risk factors related to the method of tube placement, and ethical considerations are all considered when determining the type of enteral access device. To choose the appropriate feeding tube and location in the GI tract, nutrition support clinicians should involve the patient and family in the decision-making process and understand their own institution's specific resources and expertise. These factors are essential for the successful delivery of enteral feedings in the hospital or nonhospital setting. Nutrition support clinicians should also provide the appropriate postplacement care of feeding tubes to prevent and manage complications of enteral access devices.

Enteral Access Device Selection

Several factors help the clinician determine the optimal type of enteral access device to place. A clear rationale for enteral feedings, the potential length of EN therapy, and a plan for enteral access placement must be determined. Both a thorough history, including the patient's current and past medical and surgical conditions, and a focused physical assessment, including the anatomy and function of the upper airway, esophagus, and digestive tract, are imperative to select the appropriate enteral access device.

The estimated duration of EN therapy, or the desire for an enteral feeding trial to assess for tube feeding tolerance before an invasive procedure, are the main factors in determining nasal tube placement vs percutaneous enterostomy. Generally, tubes used for short-term therapy (less than 4 to 6 weeks) are placed nasally (or, in some cases, orally) at the bedside. Placement may be done blindly, with the aid of an electromagnetic tracking device (CORPAK MedSystems, Buffalo Grove, IL), endoscopically, or fluoroscopically in interventional radiology.[1] These tubes include nasogastric, nasoduodenal, nasojejunal, and nasogastric-jejunal tubes. For long-term placement, (longer than 4 to 6 weeks), percutaneous enterostomy tubes can be placed into the stomach or small bowel using endoscopic, fluoroscopic, laparoscopic, and open laparotomy techniques (see Practice Scenario 12-1).[2-8]

When long-term access is needed, percutaneous feeding tubes are indicated and the condition of the external abdominal wall, ability to correct coagulopathies (including use of anticoagulant medications), and patient tolerance to anesthesia must be assessed. Percutaneous access devices can be placed with local anesthesia of the abdominal wall and minimal or moderate intravenous (IV) sedation; therefore, these devices may be a better option than those placed under general anesthesia, especially in the patient who may not tolerate general anesthesia. Available expertise in endoscopy and radiology for placement of gastrojejunal and direct jejunal tubes may vary significantly per institution. In some clinical settings, direct jejunal tubes must be placed surgically. Previous surgical scars in the abdominal wall, existing surgical wounds and fistulas, the presence of or future requirements for ostomies, percutaneous or intra-abdominal infusion devices, ascites, and peritoneal dialysis catheters must be assessed as part of the decision-making process.

Practice Scenario 12-1

Question: Is a patient with head and neck cancer a candidate to receive an enteral feeding device? If so, what type of enteral feeding tube should be used?

Scenario: A 72-year-old man was diagnosed with metastatic squamous cell carcinoma of the tongue. He is scheduled to receive a 6-week course of a combination of chemotherapy and radiation therapy followed by reassessment of tumor response. Physical examination reveals a thin man who weighs 80 kg and has lost approximately 11 kg in the past 3 months, which represents a weight loss of 14% of his previous body weight. His electrolytes, complete blood count, liver function tests, and albumin are within normal limits.

Intervention: The patient received a percutaneous gastrostomy tube (G-tube) using the introducer method technique performed by an interventional radiologist.

Answer: This patient could benefit from an enteral feeding tube to address both his existing malnutrition as well as likely further decreases in oral intake related to mucositis, nausea, and vomiting from chemoradiation. As the expected duration of therapy will be more than 6 weeks, the preference would be to place a percutaneous G-tube over a nasoenteric feeding tube. A percutaneous G-tube would also be more convenient for the patient, as bolus feeding is much easier through a larger-bore gastric tube than a smaller-bore nasoenteric tube.

Rationale: During radiation and chemotherapy treatment for head and neck cancer, patients almost always experience dysphagia, odynophagia, and mucositis. In fact, these problems are so prevalent that some clinicians advocate placing "prophylactic" G-tubes before treatment starts.[2,3] This type of therapy can help the patient maintain hydration and meet energy and protein goals while dysphagia is severe. One study showed that patients who had a prophylactic G-tube placed before treatment lost 5% less weight than the control group.[3] In addition to the timing of gastrostomy placement, controversy also surrounds the type of feeding tube to place in patients with head and neck cancer. Some centers contend that keeping a nasogastric tube (vs percutaneous G-tube) will preserve the muscles of swallowing and allow the patient to independently feed more quickly after therapy is completed.[4,5] The general consensus is that patients have less dysphagia and a shorter duration of therapy with the nasoenteric tube, but they lose less weight with the percutaneous G-tube.[6] Clearly, more research is warranted. In this case, a percutaneous G-tube is chosen because of the preexisting malnutrition, the expected development of further nutrition impairment with chemoradiotherapy, and the estimated length of time that a feeding tube will be required. To help minimize the risk of prolonged dysphagia, a patient with head and neck cancer needs to be seen by a speech therapist during the time a nasoenteric tube or percutaneous G-tube tube is used. With either type of tube, the patient can continue to practice swallowing food and liquids as tolerated and do the recommended swallowing exercises.

Using the pull technique for percutaneous G-tube placement may carry a risk for tumor implantation because the G-tube is dragged through the cancer field, potentially seeding the gastrostomy tract with tumor cells.[7] To minimize this risk, the "introducer" method can be used by interventional radiologists, surgeons, or endoscopists to place a percutaneous G-tube. In this technique, the stomach is insufflated and anchored to the anterior abdominal wall with T-fasteners. Serial dilators are then used to enlarge the tract, and the G-tube is introduced percutaneously. In this manner, the tube is not pulled through the region with active cancer and risk for tumor seeding is decreased.[8]

The decision to place an enteral access device for gastric or small bowel feedings is based on gastric motility, gastric aspiration risk, alterations in GI anatomy (eg, postsurgical), and coexisting medical conditions. Gastric feeding is generally reserved for the patients with normal gastric emptying and a low risk of gastric aspiration, although more and more institutions are using gastric feeds as a first-line approach, even in the intensive care setting. Small bowel feedings are preferred in the presence of gastric outlet obstruction, gastroparesis, severely increased risk of aspiration, and pancreatitis. The use of gastrojejunal tube systems, which allow for simultaneous gastric decompression and small bowel feedings, may be indicated for gastric outlet obstruction, severe gastroesophageal reflux, gastroparesis, and early (postoperative) feeding.[9,10] The use of small bowel feeding to reduce risk for aspiration pneumonia is controversial, although recent data and meta-analysis suggest this feeding approach may be of benefit (see Practice Scenario 12-2).[11-15]

Practice Scenario 12-2

Question: What type of long-term tube (stomach or small bowel) should patients receive if they have the preexisting condition of gastroesophageal reflux disease (GERD)? Does the answer change if the patient is in the intensive care unit (ICU)?

Scenario: A 35-year-old man sustained a closed head injury in a car crash. He is expected to have oral dysphagia for many weeks, and the intensivist asks which type of feeding tube would be the best option. Previous history includes long-standing GERD for which the patient was taking an over-the-counter acid-suppression medication.

Intervention: The patient receives a bedside percutaneous gastrostomy tube with a solid internal bolster.

Answer: This patient can benefit from a tube that most closely mimics the physiological state of the body. He will likely be undergoing extensive rehabilitation with many different therapy sessions. He may also be confused for a period of time, and the fewer tubes and lines that are visible for the patient to grab, the safer he will be. The least-expensive option is to bolus feed, thus eliminating the need for bags, tubing, and a feeding pump. The goal of a tube in the stomach is to work toward 3 or 4 bolus feeds per day, which mimics breakfast, lunch, dinner, and an evening snack.

Rationale: The question often arises as to whether a tube placed in the stomach leads to increased risk for aspiration pneumonia, especially in the setting of GERD, ICU, or dementia. To minimize this risk, many hospital physicians will order a gastrostomy-jejunostomy tube, instead of a gastric tube, to safely feed the patient below the pylorus. Numerous studies have been done comparing the risk for aspiration pneumonia with feeding in the stomach vs small bowel, and the results are conflicting. Guidelines from the American Society for Parenteral and Enteral Nutrition (ASPEN) suggest that gastric residual volumes do not need to be checked in the ICU setting, as they do not correlate with increased risk of aspiration, and the ASPEN guidelines continue to recommend feeding into the stomach as the first-line option.[15]

Whenever possible, we should feed our patients into the stomach. This route is the most physiologically normal for the body, ensuring appropriate mixing of nutrients with gastric acid. It also allows for flexibility of schedules, is the safest with regards to formula contamination secondary to no formula hang time, allows for blenderized diets, and is the most cost-effective. If the patient does not tolerate gastric feeding or has an aspiration event, the feeding can be diverted to the small intestine.

Enteral Feeding Tube Devices

Physical Characteristics

Patient comfort and tube performance are the key criteria in choosing a brand of feeding tube. Commercially manufactured feeding tubes are usually made of polyurethane or silicone, and each material has specific advantages and disadvantages (Table 12-1). Most nasogastric or nasoenteric tubes are constructed of polyurethane because it allows for a relatively larger inner tube diameter for a given outer diameter size. Most percutaneous tubes are constructed from silicone because of its inherent material longevity and comfort. Rubber tubes, used in Foley catheters and red rubber surgical jejunostomy tubes, are inferior because they degrade rapidly and lack internal (red rubber) or external (Foley catheter) retaining devices. With the new mandate to have ENFit connectors (new connectors engineered to not allow connectivity with connectors for any other clinical use) on all enteral feeding devices by 2017, the use of Foley catheters or red rubber catheters for enteral feeding will no longer be possible.[16-18]

Tube Types

Nasoenteric feeding tubes come in a wide array of diameters and lengths, with an equally wide array of internal stylets, feeding and medication ports, and weighted or unweighted tip configurations (Table 12-2). All feeding tube sizes are reported by the tube's external diameter measurement. However, flow through the tubes and susceptibility to clogging depend on a tube's inner diameter. The inner diameter may vary depending on the specific material used to construct the tube. In general,

TABLE 12-1 Comparison of Polyurethane and Silicone Tube Characteristics

	Polyurethane	Silicone
Comfort	Lower	Higher
Stiffness	Higher	Lower
Wall width	Thinner	Thicker
Fungal degradation	More resistant	Less resistant
Common use	Nasoenteric feeding tubes	Percutaneous (abdominal) feeding tubes

TABLE 12-2 Nasoenteric and Percutaneous Enterostomy Tube Sizes

Tube Type	Size, Fr	Length, cm
Nasogastric	8–16	38–91
Nasoenteric	8–12	91–240
Gastrostomy	12–30	Not applicable
Gastrojejunal	6–14	Not applicable
Jejunal extension through existing gastrostomy	8-12	15–95
Dual-lumen (gastric and jejunal)	16–30	Not applicable
Single-lumen (jejunal only)	12–24	15–58
Low-profile gastrostomy (replacement)	12–24	0.8–6.5
Low-profile gastrojejunostomy	14–22	15–45

FIGURE 12-1 Nasoenteric Feeding Tube Ports

Y Port　　　　　　**Single Port**

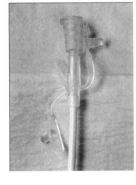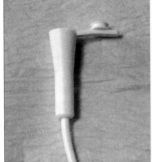

polyurethane tubes with the same outer diameter as a silicone tube will have a larger internal diameter that may be less likely to clog.

Stylets or guidewires are provided with most nasoenteric feeding tubes to provide tube structure and/or guidance while passing these relatively floppy tubes. They are designed to be shorter than the length of the tube and to have a flexible distal tip to avoid perforation of the GI wall. A water-activated lubricant may be used to coat the tube's internal lumen to allow easier removal of these stylets or guidewires after the tube is in place. Commercially available nasoenteric feeding tubes have either 1 port for feeding or 2 in a "Y" configuration: one for feeding and the other for medication and/or irrigation (Figure 12-1). These ports can accommodate either a feeding set or a syringe, or both. Dual ports allow concomitant feeding and medication administration and/or irrigation. However, to prevent clogging, medications should be administered through the tube only after enteral feedings are held and the feeding tube is flushed with water.

The US Food and Drug Administration has recognized that serious errors can occur when enteral feeding tubes are inadvertently connected to nonenteral feeding connectors (eg, IV lines, peritoneal catheters, tracheostomy tubes). Such errors have resulted in patient injury and deaths, and they are widely recognized as underreported. The Global Enteral Device Supplier Association is a nonprofit trade association formed to introduce the new international standards for enteral feeding connectors that are designed to increase patient safety and optimal delivery of EN by reducing the risk of tubing misconnections. These ENFit connectors will make it nearly impossible to connect non–enteral feeding catheters to enteral access devices including pumps, connectors, and feeding tubes (Figure 12-2).[16,17]

Feeding tube tips come in a wide variety of sizes, number of distal feeding delivery holes, and end vs side feeding holes. There are no specific data to favor any particular design. Therefore, the choice is determined by the preference of the individual clinician, institutional availability and mode of placement. Initially, weighted tube tips were thought to facilitate transpyloric passage. However, critical analysis of the literature does not demonstrate a clear advantage with the use of either weighted or unweighted tips.[19]

Percutaneous enterostomy feeding tubes are also available in a wide array of diameters and lengths (Table 12-2). The internal retention bolsters of percutaneous tubes are constructed of either solid material (silicone or polyurethane) or silicone balloons (Figure 12-3). Solid internal bolsters are more common with initial percutaneous enterostomy tube placement because they have greater longevity. Balloon-type internal bolsters are inserted more commonly with radiologic and surgical tube placement, and they are used as replacement devices in the office setting because of their ease in placement. If placed in the small bowel, the balloon is typically filled to a volume of 3 to 4 mL so it will not obstruct the lumen. These balloons generally only have a lifespan of about 4 to 6 months.[20] If possible, use of a nonballoon tube is preferred for direct jejunal tube placement to avoid occluding the narrower jejunal lumen.

An enteral feeding tube is available with a solid internal bolster constrained in a dissolvable capsule that can be placed in the same manner as a balloon tube. This tube may be used for laparoscopic initial gastric or direct jejunal tube placement, as well as for replacement tubes. It combines the longevity of a solid internal bolster with the ease of placement of a balloon-type internal bolster tube.

Percutaneous enterostomy feeding tubes may also have multiple ports. Typically, separate ports are included for feeding and medication and/or irrigation. If the internal bolster is of the balloon type, an additional third port is present for balloon inflation or deflation.

Percutaneous gastrojejunal feeding tubes are inserted into the stomach with a smaller-bore extension tube that passes through the pylorus into the jejunum. Some gastrojejunal tubes are specifically designed with separate gastric and jejunal lumens and have ports that allow for both jejunal feeding and gastric decompression (Figure 12-4). Direct percutaneous jejunostomy tubes are placed directly into the jejunum without passage through the stomach. Low-profile tubes are

FIGURE 12-2 ENFit Connectors for All Feeding Tubes

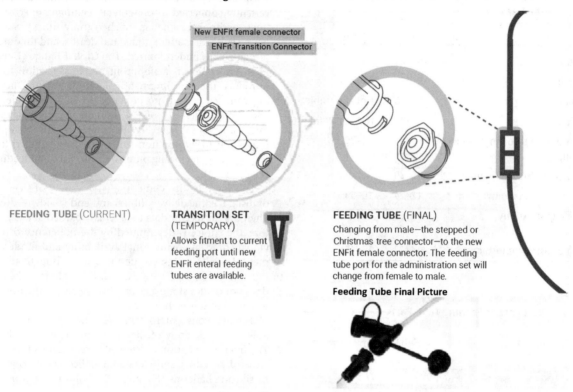

FEEDING TUBE (CURRENT)

TRANSITION SET
(TEMPORARY)

Allows fitment to current feeding port until new ENFit enteral feeding tubes are available.

FEEDING TUBE (FINAL)

Changing from male—the stepped or Christmas tree connector—to the new ENFit female connector. The feeding tube port for the administration set will change from female to male.

Feeding Tube Final Picture

Source: Used with permission from the Global Enteral Device Supplier Association (GEDSA).

FIGURE 12-3 Percutaneous Endoscopic Gastrostomy Tube Internal Bolsters

Solid Type   Balloon Type

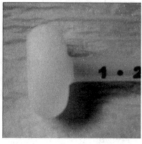 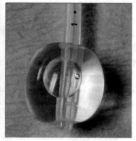

FIGURE 12-4 Percutaneous Endoscopic Gastrojejunostomy Feeding Ports

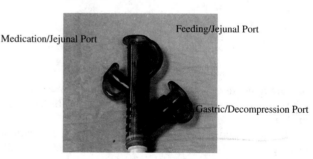

skin-level devices that are used as initial placement or, more commonly, for replacement devices for gastrostomies, gastrojejunostomies, and jejunostomies (Figure 12-5). They are an excellent option for the patients who are concerned about the cosmetic appearance of a feeding tube. This device can also be more comfortable for patients who are active, sleep in the prone position, or need only intermittent therapy. To attach a feeding connector to the skin-level device, the patient will need adequate manual dexterity or caregiver assistance.

Enteral Access Insertion Methods

Nasal Tubes

Nasogastric and nasoenteric feeding tubes are inserted when short-term access is indicated. They can also provide an opportunity to assess tolerance of enteral feedings before placement of a percutaneous enterostomy if longer-term access is required. They may be passed transorally or transnasally, although the nasal approach will be better tolerated in conscious patients. Nasogastric or nasoenteric feeding tube

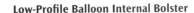

FIGURE 12-5 Replacement Percutaneous Endoscopic Gastrostomy Tubes

Low-Profile Solid Internal Bolster   **Low-Profile Balloon Internal Bolster**

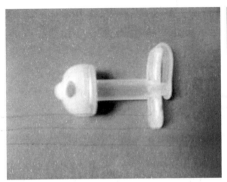 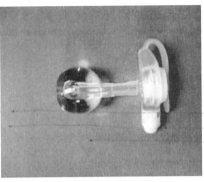

Standard-Profile Solid Internal Bolster

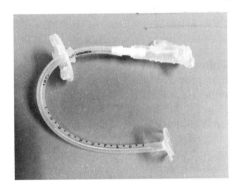

placement is contraindicated if the patient has an obstructing head, neck, and esophageal pathology or injury that prevents safe insertion. Nasogastric or nasoenteric feeding tubes should not be used for feeding until confirmation of proper position is obtained. Plain abdominal or chest radiography is the gold standard for confirmation of placement. However, recent studies suggest that radiographic confirmation may not be required when electromagnetic imaging technology is used for placement by an experienced tube team with demonstrated success.[21,22] Other methods, including auscultation, pH set up, and capnography are unreliable and still require radiographic confirmation.[23–26]

Nasogastric tubes are the easiest feeding tubes to insert. Placement may be performed by a variety of clinicians (physicians, dietitians, nurses) as long as they have been appropriately trained. If possible, larger, stiffer tubes used for gastric decompression should be converted to a smaller-bore feeding tubes (ie, 6 to 12 Fr) for patient comfort and to decrease the risk of associated complications. The most reliable method for measuring the length of the tube necessary for gastric placement is termed *NEMU* (which stands for "direct distance from nose to earlobe to midumbilicus"), although many clinicians continue to use the NEX ("nose-earlobe-xiphoid") process.[27] Placement of a nasogastric tube requires passage through a patent nare and may be facilitated by concurrent

patient swallowing. Aspiration of gastric contents, auscultation of insufflated air over the stomach, and absence of patient coughing or choking suggest, but cannot confirm, correct tube placement. As noted previously, correct position within the GI tract lumen should be confirmed radiographically.

Nasoenteric feeding tubes are placed anywhere distal to the pylorus, whereas nasojejunal tubes are placed distal to the ligament of Treitz. Placing a tube in either of these positions requires more skill than placing a nasogastric tube. Nasoenteric tubes can be placed at the bedside, endoscopically, or fluoroscopically. Bedside placement usually requires experienced personnel with specialized training. An older method that is still practiced in many centers uses the technique described by Zaloga.[28] This technique requires the patient to lie on the right side; the feeding tube tip is bent and advanced slowly with a combination of air insufflation, tube rotation, and auscultation. Prokinetics (erythromycin or metoclopramide) are often added to bedside techniques and may increase success rates.[29,30] A systemic review by Booth showed that IV erythromycin (in doses of 200 to 500 mg) had the highest success rate.[29]

Recently, devices have been developed to assist with nasoenteric tube placement including a bedside magnet and electromagnetic imaging system. Success rates greater than 90% have been reported when these systems, especially the electromagnetic one, are used.[31–33] Nasojejunal placement is most reliably achieved with endoscopic or fluoroscopic techniques, but these methods are costly, require advanced training, and have particular risks (radiation exposure with regards to radiology and sedation with endoscopy). The reported success rate for bedside nasoenteric tube placement ranges from 56% to 92%, with better than 90% success rates reported for endoscopic and fluoroscopic placement. However, success rates are lower for placement distal to the ligament of Treitz.[34]

Percutaneous Enterostomy Tubes

Enterostomy tubes are placed when long-term access (longer than 4 to 6 weeks) is required. These tubes may be placed by endoscopic, fluoroscopic, or surgical methods. These methods have similar success rates, although there is less morbidity and cost with endoscopic or fluoroscopic techniques.[35–39]

Routine preprocedural testing of coagulation parameters and platelets is no longer recommended for patients undergoing enterostomy tube placement, but these tests should be considered if there is concern for abnormal coagulation due to anticoagulant medication, medical history of excessive bleeding, or recent antibiotic use. American Society of Gastrointestinal Endoscopy guidelines consider placement of a percutaneous feeding tube to be a high-bleeding-risk procedure.[40] Patients are then stratified into high and low risk for thromboembolic complications. Thienopyridines (eg, clopidogrel) should be held, whenever possible, for 5 to 7 days before PEG placement. If holding the thienopyridine is not possible, some institutions will add epinephrine to the lidocaine for local anesthesia (vasoconstriction), watch out for vessels on the skin and mucosa, and make sure the bolsters are relatively firm (not tight) for 3 to 4 days before loosening them. Aspirin regimens should be continued in patients with high thromboembolic risk.[40] Warfarin should be held 5 days before PEG placement and high-risk patients should be bridged with short-acting heparin. The new, direct-acting oral anticoagulants should be held for at least 48 hours before high-risk procedures and restarted up to 48 hours after the procedure.[41] Consultation with relevant cardiology, neurology, and anticoagulation services is suggested. Prophylactic antibiotics are administered when enterostomy tubes are placed, as they have been shown to decrease peristomal infection rates when using endoscopic methods for initial placement.[42,43]

Gastrostomy Tubes

PEG is the most common technique for obtaining long-term enteral access, and it is generally performed under moderate sedation.[44] Specific contraindications for endoscopic placement include obstruction of the GI tract proximal to the stomach and the inability to transilluminate the abdominal wall for identification of a safe abdominal access site.[45] Additional relative contraindications include ascites, coagulopathy, gastric varices, active head and neck cancers, morbid obesity, and neoplastic, infiltrative, or inflammatory disease of the gastric or abdominal wall.[46]

The most common method of PEG tube insertion is the Ponsky (pull) technique.[47] Air is insufflated into the stomach via an endoscope. The optimal site for PEG tube placement is determined through simultaneous endoscopic transillumination of the abdominal wall and endoscopically visualized finger indentation at the site. A small incision is made at this site, and a needle/trocar is inserted through the abdominal wall and into the stomach. A guidewire is passed through the needle/trocar and grasped with a snare passed through the endoscope; then, the guidewire, snare, and endoscope are withdrawn through the mouth. A G-tube is affixed to the guidewire and pulled through the esophagus into the stomach and out the abdominal wall. The G-tube is held in place by a solid, mushroom-type internal retention device and an external bumper. Advantages of PEG placement include performance at bedside, lack of radiation, and ability to perform diagnostic and therapeutic endoscopic procedures simultaneously.

Percutaneous G-tubes can also be placed using fluoroscopic guidance. There are 2 general fluoroscopic placement techniques. In the first, a nasogastric tube is placed to insufflate the stomach, a safe window is identified under fluoroscopy, and 1 to 4 T-fasteners are used to perform a gastropexy to secure the stomach wall to the abdominal wall. A needle is used to obtain gastric access, the guidewire is advanced through the needle, and the tract is dilated sequentially until there is a large enough hole for the tube to go through. Lastly, the G-tube is placed through the tract using a peel-away sheath.[48,49] The second, less commonly performed fluoroscopic method uses a slightly curved 18-gauge needle or vascular sheath; it is advanced into the stomach and pointed toward the gastroesophageal junction after gastric insufflation. The guidewire is then advanced with or without help of an angiographic catheter into the esophagus and oropharynx and out of the mouth. A G-tube is then threaded over the wire, advanced until it emerges from the abdominal wall, and then pulled into the desired position.[37,50] Advantages of fluoroscopic gastrostomy placement include lack of need for conscious sedation in some patients, ability to perform in patients with severe stenosis/trauma of the upper GI tract, and potentially decreased risk of tumor seeding from upper aerodigestive tract cancers (Practice Scenario 12-1). Reported success rates for either fluoroscopic or endoscopic gastrostomies are greater than 95%.[51]

A G-tube inserted using the laparoscopic or open (laparotomy) method is performed in the operating room using general anesthesia. Surgical placement of feeding tubes is used when patients are undergoing another abdominal operation, when endoscopic and radiologic attempts fail, and/or in the presence of an aerodigestive tract obstruction or facial trauma. Direct laparoscopic gastric tube placement is also done when endoscopic or radiologic placement fails or is not available.

Laparoscopic technique accesses the peritoneal cavity by way of small ports that enter through the abdominal wall.[47] A pneumoperitoneum is created through a port inserted just below the umbilicus through which a camera is passed. The stomach is accessed and manipulated through a second port entering in the left lower quadrant and a third port (if required) entering through the right upper quadrant. T-fasteners or laparoscopic sutures are placed to affix the stomach to the abdominal wall. The procedure then proceeds in a manner similar to fluoroscopic gastrostomy, with a hollow needle advanced percutaneously into the stomach lumen followed by wire, dilators, peel-away sheath, and finally the G-tube.[52–55]

The Stamm technique is the most commonly used surgical placement of an open G-tube.[9,45] It requires a small laparotomy in the upper midline of the abdomen. The G-tube is brought into the stomach through a small stab wound in the upper abdominal wall. A small incision is made into the stomach through which the feeding tube enters and around which purse-string sutures are placed to secure the stomach around the G-tube. The stomach is then sutured to the anterior abdominal wall. This tube may be held in place with an inflated balloon or sutured to the abdominal wall to prevent tube migration.

Gastrojejunal Tubes

In the situation of impaired gastric motility, pancreatitis, or pancreatic surgery, or any time that enteral feeding into the small bowel with simultaneous stomach decompression is required, a gastrojejunal tube should be placed.[56,57] Percutaneous endoscopic gastrojejunostomy may be performed immediately or any time after G-tube placement. Most commonly, a guidewire is placed through the existing gastrostomy, grasped endoscopically, and carried into the jejunum. The endoscope is then withdrawn, leaving the guidewire in place. The jejunal extension tube is threaded over the guidewire into the small bowel.[45,58] A more recently described technique uses reclosable clips. The jejunal feeding tube with a suture on its tip is inserted through the PEG or stoma into the stomach lumen. A clip is passed through the working channel of an endoscope and used to grasp the suture and drag the tube into the jejunum as the endoscope is advanced. The suture is then clipped to the jejunal mucosa, securing the feeding tube to the small bowel.[59]

Fluoroscopic gastrojejunal access is becoming much more common. Initial steps are similar to fluoroscopic gastrostomy placement, as previously described. In addition, to facilitate placement of the gastrojejunostomy, puncture of the stomach is performed in the direction of the pylorus. A guidewire is advanced through the stomach to the ligament of Treitz, and the jejunal extension tube is advanced over the wire into the jejunum.[60,61] Fluoroscopic techniques can be used when the patient cannot undergo endoscopy; however, fluoroscopic placement does require transport of the patient to the radiology suite.

Gastrojejunal tubes can be placed during laparotomy or with laparoscopy methods, using any of the previously discussed methods. Using manual and/or endoscopic methods, the jejunal tube is positioned into the small bowel. The gastric component of the tube is left in the stomach. The patient benefits from gastric decompression while receiving enteral feeds into the small bowel, but there is greater risk of the jejunal tube piece migrating back into the stomach on a regular basis.

Jejunostomy Tubes

Direct percutaneous endoscopic jejunostomy is a modification of the pull PEG technique. A pediatric colonoscope or enteroscope is advanced into the small bowel. Transillumination and finger palpation are performed over the jejunum instead of the stomach. A sounding needle and/or trocar is passed through the anterior abdominal wall into the jejunum.

An insertion wire is advanced through the trocar and grasped. The procedure is then completed as per the pull-type PEG.[61,62]

Direct jejunostomy tube placement is performed in a variety of fluoroscopic ways. In general, identification of the target bowel loop is performed by advancing an angiographic catheter into the proximal jejunum and insufflating it with air and contrast,[63] or by placing an angioplasty balloon[64] or snare loop[65] in the desired location to serve as a target. The jejunal loop is accessed with a needle, and a T-fastener device is then delivered to secure the jejunal loop against the abdominal wall. A guidewire is then advanced through the needle, the tract is dilated, and the jejunostomy tube is placed.

Direct percutaneous jejunostomy using either endoscopic or fluoroscopic guidance is not available in all institutions. It is considerably more difficult technically than percutaneous gastrostomy, even though the methods are similar. Success rates range from 68% to 100% for endoscopic jejunostomy and from 87% to 100% for fluoroscopic jejunostomy.[66] Higher rates of successful endoscopic placement have been reported when balloon enteroscopes are used.[67,68] Endoscopic jejunostomy tubes are more stable than fluoroscopic tubes because the endoscopic tubes have solid, mushroom-type internal bolsters and larger tube diameters (18 to 20 Fr vs 10 to 14 Fr).

The technique of laparoscopic jejunostomy is similar to laparoscopic gastrostomy. Ports are placed in the left upper quadrant and lower abdominal midline. The jejunum is manipulated to affix it to the abdominal wall with T-fasteners. Then a guidewire is placed into the lumen of the jejunum, and a jejunostomy tube is advanced into the small bowel through a peel-away sheath.[47,53] An advantage with this approach is that a larger-diameter tube (18 to 20 Fr) with a solid bolster can be placed. An open jejunostomy is placed using a Witzel technique. In this procedure, a submucosal tunnel is created in the small bowel through which the jejunostomy tube is threaded; this method prevents leakage of small bowel contents onto the abdominal wall.[10] Less commonly, a needle-catheter jejunostomy may be placed by laparotomy or laparoscopy.[10,69] In this procedure, a needle is threaded into the small bowel. A guidewire is passed into the jejunum. A small jejunostomy catheter (5 to 8 Fr) is passed over this guidewire into the jejunum. The small-bore size of needle-catheter jejunostomies make them prone to occlusion. Because endoscopic and radiologic methods for jejunostomies are complex, surgical jejunostomies are common.

Removal and Replacement of Percutaneous Enterostomy Tubes

Enterostomy tubes can be safely removed or replaced after the stoma tract has matured. Although maturation usually occurs 1 to 2 weeks after initial placement, many clinicians prefer to wait 4 to 6 weeks prior to removal to ensure that the stoma tract is mature. This longer waiting period is especially valid in patients who are on steroids, immunosuppressed, obese, or otherwise suspected of poor wound healing. Removal of G-tubes before stoma tract maturation may result in the stomach or small bowel falling away from the abdominal wall, allowing bowel contents to leak into the peritoneum. If this problem occurs, tube replacement with the assistance of endoscopy, interventional radiology, or even surgery is required.

A standard-profile or low-profile replacement G-tube can be exchanged at the bedside without endoscopy or fluoroscopy. However, gastrojejunostomy and some direct jejunostomy tubes require endoscopy or fluoroscopic guidance for replacement. A percutaneous feeding tube with a solid internal bolster can be removed at the bedside using the traction method. The patient is placed in the supine position with knees bent to relax the abdominal muscles. The exposed gastric tubing is firmly grasped and pulled forcefully. Removal for solid internal bolster devices may be painful, and some clinicians advocate mild sedation for the procedure. For devices held in place with an inflated balloon, the balloon is deflated and the tube is gently removed; sedation is not required for this procedure.

If the tube is exchanged with a low-profile device, the length of the existing stoma tract is measured before choosing and placing the correctly sized replacement device. The replacement device is then lubricated and advanced through the stoma tract into place. Replacement feeding tubes are held in place with an inflated internal balloon or a solid silicone internal retention bolster (Figure 12-5). When using a balloon replacement tube, follow the manufacturer's recommendations regarding balloon volume. Generally, 5 to 20 mL of sterile water should be used for gastric tubes and 3 to 4 mL sterile water for small bowel tubes. Correct tube position can be checked after replacement by aspiration of gastric contents or auscultation of insufflated air. However, these methods are not completely reliable. If there is any concern for misplacement, the tube position should be assessed with fluoroscopic or endoscopic imaging (Practice Scenario 12-3).[70]

Practice Scenario 12-3

Question: What is the complication in a patient with percutaneous gastrostomy tube (G-tube) who develops abdominal pain after tube exchange?

Scenario: The patient is a 24-year-old woman with a history of severe gastric and small bowel dysmotility. She has a 24-Fr gastric balloon decompression tube that was initially placed several years ago and is regularly changed by the patient at home. She most recently uneventfully changed her gastric tube the day before she presented to the emergency department with severe abdominal pain. The patient awoke in the middle of the night with gastric leakage and intense pain around her feeding tube. She was unable to aspirate any gastric fluid from the feeding tube or move the tube within the tract. Her skin was very reddened and ulcerated from the leakage of gastric fluid.

Intervention: The patient had a radiologic evaluation of her feeding tube, and the tip was located within the gastric wall with leakage of the Gastrografin dye into the subcutaneous tissue. No peritoneal leakage was noted. The percutaneous G-tube was removed and a new G-tube placed through the same tract. Proper position was confirmed by instillation of contrast through the tube with filling of the stomach with contrast noted.

Answer: Dislodgement of her abdominal feeding tube occurred after replacement. Healthcare providers should have an extremely

low threshold for confirming tube position if there is any concern for tube malposition after replacement.

Rationale: If a patient develops abdominal pain after percutaneous feeding tube replacement, the concern is that the tube was potentially placed within the stoma tract instead of correctly into the gastric lumen or perforated into the peritoneal space. This problem most often occurs when there has been difficulty with tube replacement, but it can also occur when replacement is reported to go smoothly. When a malpositioned tube is suspected, the tube position should be evaluated fluoroscopically or endoscopically. Treatment depends on how severe the problem is and if there has been contamination of enteral feeds into the peritoneal cavity. If significant peritoneal contamination has not occurred, the malpositioned tube can be removed and another tube placed using the same tract. If there is no further leakage into the peritoneal cavity, the tube is safe to use. If more significant disruption of the tract occurs and a new tube cannot be placed at the existing site, the patient can be supported through a nasoenteric feeding tube while the stoma tract closes and any infection is treated.[70] If significant leakage has occurred and abdominal sepsis develops, the patient is supported with intravenous fluids and antibiotics, and a surgical consultation is obtained. Necrotizing fasciitis has been reported in severe cases of untreated, uncontrolled infection. This condition is a surgical emergency with high morbidity and mortality. Emergency consultation for wide surgical debridement is indicated.

Postinsertion Care

Oral Hygiene and Skin Care

Regardless of the tube type or insertion technique, all patients require appropriate oral hygiene. It is often important for preventing aspiration pneumonia in ventilator-dependent patients or those with a depressed level of consciousness.

Patients with nasal tubes benefit from skin care to the nasal area to address prolonged exposure to tape and adhesive products. Repositioning the nasal tube and avoiding pressure to the nares is important to prevent pressure necrosis.

Patients and caregivers may use mild soap and water to cleanse the stoma site for percutaneous tubes. The area should be rinsed and dried thoroughly.

Routine use of antibiotic ointments or hydrogen peroxide at the tube site is not recommended. Dressings can be applied if there is drainage from the stoma site; however, they should not be placed with excessive tension, which can promote infection and buried bumper syndrome.

Prevention of Clogging

All feeding tubes are prone to clogging. Usual causes include suboptimal flushing, not flushing prior to and after each medication administration, accumulation of pill fragments, frequent checking of residuals, and administration of high-protein or high-fiber formulas.[45,58] Compliance with intermittent flushing protocols is essential to prevent clogging. Water should be used as the flush fluid of choice. Two reports have demonstrated superiority of prophylactic use of pancreatic enzymes to prevent tube occlusion compared with standard water flushes.[71,72]

Medications in liquid form may contain higher amounts of sorbitol/sugar, have a higher osmolality and/or a higher viscosity, and may be costlier than tablet forms. Giving a crushed and diluted medication could therefore be preferable; however, crushed pills can be more likely to clog a small-bore tube than medication in a liquid form. Clearly, each patient should be evaluated individually, and in conjunction with a pharmacist, to determine the best way to deliver a medication to a tube feeding patient. Whether a medication is in pill or liquid form, each medication should be given separately with a water flush before and after each medication administration.[30] See Chapter 18 for further discussion of enteral administration of drugs.

Enteral Access Device Complications

Nasal Tubes

Complications of nasogastric and nasoenteric feeding tubes can be divided into those occurring during the insertion procedure or those occurring in the postprocedure period. The overall rate for procedure-related complications—including epistaxis, aspiration, and circulatory or respiratory compromise—is approximately 10%. The most-dreaded procedural complication is initial misplacement of the nasoenteric tube into the bronchopulmonary tree. This complication occurs in 2% to 4% of nasoenteric tube placements. Notably, it is unsuspected in 80% of occurrences, and it results in pneumothorax in up to 50% of cases.[23,73–75] Radiography is the gold standard for ensuring correct placement and should be performed before the feeding tube is used. Published data demonstrate that adopting radiographic confirmation protocols decreases inadvertent use of incorrectly placed feeding tubes.[24] As stated previously, use of a bedside electromagnetic imaging system by experienced clinicians may obviate the need for radiographic confirmation.[21,22]

Postprocedural complications include inadvertent tube dislodgement, tube malfunction, sinusitis, tube occlusion, tube feeding aspiration, and intestinal ischemia. Dislodgement occurs in 25% to 41% of cases.[76–78] The use of a nasal bridle decreases tube dislodgment rates dramatically.[79] Gunn and colleagues reported that the incidence of accidental dislodgement decreased from 36% to 10% when a magnet-based system was used to place the nasal bridle.[80] Malfunction of the tube, including breaking, cracking, or kinking of the tube, occurs 11% to 20% of the time.[77,78]

When accurately diagnosed by sinus needle puncture and aspiration, sinusitis occurs about 12% of the time.[81] This problem is believed secondary to obstruction of physiological sinus drainage by the nasoenteric tube.

Tube occlusion is a frequent problem (20% to 45%) and often requires tube replacement.[78,82,83] Risk factors for tube occlusion include increasing tube length, decreasing tube caliber, inadequate water flushing, frequent medication delivery, and use of the tube to measure residual volumes.[83] When feeding tubes become clogged, simple flushing with water can relieve the obstruction in one-third of patients.[84] If this method fails, the installation of pancreatic enzymes can reopen an additional 50% of the occluded tubes.[84,85] Mechanical

dislodgement may also be achieved using a cytology brush, an endoscopic retrograde cholangiopancreatography catheter, or a commercial corkscrew device.[86] Finally, replacing the nasal feeding tube is the last resort.

Rarely, the provision of EN to a hypotensive, critically ill patient may be associated with intestinal ischemia, which is usually evidenced by increasing GI intolerance (increased tube output, abdominal pain and distension, ileus). This complication is best avoided by cessation of enteral feeding pending further evaluation in hypotensive patients. These patients typically require increasing doses of vasopressor agents with progressive GI intolerance.[34,87]

Enterostomy Tubes

Complications of percutaneous enterostomy tubes can be divided into procedural and postprocedural events. Incidence of procedure-related complications (eg, intraprocedural aspiration, hemorrhage, perforation of the GI lumen, and prolonged ileus) is 1.5% to 4%, and procedure-related mortality is rare, occurring in 0% to 2% of cases.[70] Risk factors for aspiration include the supine position, advanced age, need for sedation, and neurologic impairment.[88] Pneumoperitoneum as a result of the percutaneous procedure is common and in the absence of peritoneal signs is of no clinical consequence.[89] Infusion of water-soluble contrast with fluoroscopic or computed tomography imaging is the test of choice if peritonitis is suspected. The procedural and long-term mortality rate directly related to PEG placement is very low despite the up to 50% annual mortality in patients receiving G-tubes.[88] This very high rate of mortality is a function of the significant comorbidities of the patients rather than the procedure or the feeding tube itself.

The overall postprocedure complication rate for enterostomy tubes ranges from 4.8% to 10.8%.[72] Minor postprocedural complications are 2 to 3 times more common than major ones (Table 12-3). Peristomal infection is the most

TABLE 12-3 Major and Minor Complications of Enterostomy Tube Placement

Complication	Reported Frequency, %
Major complications	
Aspiration	0.3–1.0
Hemorrhage	0–2.5
Peritonitis/necrotizing fasciitis	0.5–1.3
Death[a]	0–2.1
Minor complications	
Peristomal infection	5.4–30
Peristomal leakage	1–2
Buried bumper syndrome	0.3–2.4
Inadvertent removal	1.6–4.4
Fistulous tracts	0.3–6.7

[a]Data are for percutaneous endoscopic gastrostomy placement.

common complication of gastrostomy placement.[44,90] Most of these infections are mild. In rare cases, necrotizing fasciitis with high morbidity and mortality can develop. Prophylactic antibiotics before tube placement, early recognition of wound infections, treatment with antibiotics, local wound care, and debridement, if necessary, are the keys to successful management.[44,46,91]

Leakage around the gastrostomy site is a common and underrecognized problem in nutrition support.[92] Risk factors include infection, excessive cleansing with irritant solutions (eg, hydrogen peroxide, povidone-iodine), and excessive tension and side torsion on the external portion of the feeding tube. Prompt treatment of infection, good ostomy skin care, loosening of the outer bumper, and stabilizing the G-tube to prevent tension torsion on the tube will address these issues.[86]

Buried bumper syndrome results from growth of the gastric mucosa over the internal bumper (see Practice Scenario 12-3). Risk factors include excessive tension between the internal and external bumpers, poor wound healing, and significant weight gain.[93-95] Treatment is based on maintaining the stoma tract while restoring the internal bumper entirely within the stomach lumen.[96,97]

As noted previously, accidental G-tube removal should be addressed urgently. If a standard tube is not promptly available, a suitably sized Foley or red rubber catheter can be used to keep the tract open until a standard replacement tube can be placed. In patients prone to pulling tubes, the use of an abdominal binder, placing mittens on the patient's hands, cutting down the external tube length to 6 to 8 cm, or switching to a low-profile device can reduce the risk of future removal.[70]

Gastrojejunal and Jejunal Tubes

Complications of gastrojejunal tubes and jejunal tubes are similar to those described previously for G-tubes. Gastrojejunal feeding tubes are also complicated by frequent (up to 70%) malfunction, migration, and/or occlusion of the smaller jejunal extension tube.[98,99] Additional complications of direct jejunostomy tubes include jejunal volvulus and/or small bowel perforation.[100] Although more distal feeding with jejunal tubes is often recommended by expert opinion, there is no clear evidence that it markedly decreases a patient's aspiration risk. ASPEN guidelines recommend feeding into the stomach as a first choice. However, as stated previously, recent data and meta-analysis suggest that jejunal feeding may be associated with decreased risk of aspiration pneumonia.[11-14] Clearly, this issue needs more quality research before a definitive recommendation can be suggested.

Conclusion

Enteral feeding remains the feeding route of choice in the presence of a functional GI tract. Success depends on using the best insertion method available to place the appropriate access device in the appropriate location of the GI tract. Proper care and maintenance of enteral access devices are critical to successful EN therapy. Clinicians should also focus on the prevention and early recognition and management of device-related complications.

References

1. Vanek V. Ins and outs of enteral access: part 1—short-term enteral access. *Nutr Clin Pract*. 2002;17:275–283.
2. Nguyen N, North D, Smith H, et al. Safety and effectiveness of prophylactic gastrostomy tubes for head and neck cancer patients undergoing chemoradiation. *Surg Oncol*. 2006;15(4):199–203.
3. Chang J, Gosling T, Larsen J, et al. Prophylactic gastrostomy tubes for patients receiving radical radiotherapy for head and neck cancers: a retrospective review. *J Med Imaging Radiat Oncol*. 2009; 53(5):431–432.
4. Paleri V, Patterson J. Use of gastrostomy in head and neck cancer: a systematic review to identify areas for future research. *Clin Otolaryngol*. 2010;35:177–189.
5. Corry J. Feeding tubes and dysphagia: cause or effect in head and neck cancer patients. *J Med Imaging Radiat Oncol*. 2009;53(5): 431–432.
6. Bossola M. Nutritional interventions in head and neck cancer patients undergoing chemoradiotherapy: a narrative review. *Nutrients*. 2015;7(1):265–276.
7. Tsai J, Schattner M. Percutaneous endoscopic gastrostomy site metastasis. *Gastrointest Endosc Clin N Am*. 2007;17(4):777.
8. Foster J, Filocamo P, Nava H, et al. The introducer technique is the optimal method for placing percutaneous endoscopic gastrostomy tubes in head and neck cancer patients. *Surg Endosc*. 2007;21(6):897–901.
9. Vanek V. Ins and outs of enteral access: part 2—long-term access—esophagostomy and gastrostomy. *Nutr Clin Pract*. 2003; 18(1):50–74.
10. Vanek V. Ins and outs of enteral access; part 3—long-term access—jejunostomy. *Nutr Clin Pract*. 2003;18(3):201–220.
11. Metheny N, Stewart B, McClave S. Relationship between feeding tube site and respiratory outcomes. *JPEN J Parenter Enteral Nutr*. 2011;35(3):346–355.
12. Hsu C, Sun S, Lin S, et al. Duodenal versus gastric feeding in medical intensive care unit patients: a prospective, randomized, clinical study. *Crit Care Med*. 2009;37(6):1866–1872.
13. Panagiotakis P, DiSario J, Hilden K, et al. DPEJ prevents aspiration in high-risk patients. *Nutr Clin Pract*. 2008;23(2):172–175.
14. Dhaliwal R, Cahill N, Lemieux M et al. The Canadian Critical Care Nutrition Guidelines in 2013: an update on current recommendations and implementation strategies. *Nutr Clin Pract*. 2014;29(1):29–43.
15. McClave SA, Taylor BE, Martindale RG, et al. Guidelines for the provision and assessment of nutrition support therapy in the adult critically ill patient: Society of Critical Care Medicine (SCCM) and American Society for Parenteral and Enteral Nutrition (A.S.P.E.N.). *JPEN J Parenter Enteral Nutr*. 2016;40(2): 159–211.
16. US Food and Drug Administration. Safety considerations to mitigate risks of misconnections with small bore connectors intended for enteral applications. February 11, 2015. https://www.fda .gov/downloads/medicaldevices/deviceregulationandguidance /guidancedocuments/ucm313385.pdf. Accessed May 10, 2017.
17. Global Enteral Device Supplier Association (GEDSA) website. gedsa.org. Accessed August 15, 2016.
18. Stay Connected website. stayconnected.org. Accessed August 15, 2016.
19. Levy H. Nasogastric and nasoenteric feeding tubes. *Gastrointest Endosc Clin N Am*. 1998;8:529–549.
20. Heiser M, Malaty H. Balloon-type versus non-balloon-type replacement percutaneous endoscopic gastrostomy: which is better? *Gastroenterol Nurs*. 2001;24(2):58–63.
21. Powers J, Luebbehusen M, Spitzer T, et al. Verification of an electromagnetic placement device compared with abdominal

radiograph to predict accuracy of feeding tube placement. *JPEN J Parenter Enteral Nutr.* 2011;35(4):535–539.

22. Koopman M, Kudsk K, Szotkowski M, et al. A team-based protocol and electromagnetic technology eliminate feeding tube placement complications. *Ann Surg.* 2011;253(2):287–302.

23. Rassias A, Ball P, Corwin H. A prospective study of tracheopulmonary complications associated with the placement of narrow-bore enteral feeding tubes. *Crit Care.* 2009;2(1):25–28.

24. Marderstein E, Simmons R, Ochoa J. Patient safety: effect of institutional protocols on adverse events related to feeding tube placement in the critically ill. *J Am Coll Surg.* 2004;199(1):39–47.

25. Gray R, Tynan C, Reed L, et al. Bedside electromagnetic-guided feeding tube placement: an improvement over traditional placement technique? *Nutr Clin Pract.* 2007;22(4):436–444.

26. Stark S, Sharpe J, Larson G. Endoscopically placed nasoenteral feeding tubes. Indications and techniques. *Am Surg.* 1991;57(4):203–205.

27. Ellett MLC, Beckstrand J, Flueckiger J, Perkins SM, Johnson CS. Predicting the insertion distance for placing gastric tubes. *Clin Nurs Res.* 2005;14(1):11–27.

28. Zaloga G. Bedside method for placing small bowel feeding tubes in critically ill patients. A prospective study. *Chest.* 1991;100(6):1643–1646.

29. Booth C, Heyland D, Paterson W. Gastrointestinal promotility drugs in the critical care setting: a systematic review of the evidence. *Crit Care Med.* 2002;30(7):1429–1435.

30. Lord L, Weiser-Maimone A, Pulhamus M, et al. Comparison of weighted versus unweighted feeding tubes for efficacy of transpyloric intubation. *JPEN J Parenter Enteral Nutr.* 1993;7(3):271–273.

31. Akers AS, Pinsky M. Placement of a magnetic small bowel feeding tube at the bedside: the syncro-bluetube. *JPEN J Parenter Enteral Nutr.* 2017;41(3):496–499. doi:10.1177/0148607115594235.

32. Smithard D, Barrett NA, Hargroves D, Elliot S. Electromagnetic sensor-guided enteral access systems: a literature review. *Dysphagia.* 2015;30(3):275–285.

33. Gerritsen A, can der Poel MJ, de Rooig T, et al. Systematic review on bedside electromagnetic-guided, endoscopic, and fluoroscopic placement of nasoenteral feeding tubes. *Gastrointest Endosc.* 2015;81(4):836–847.

34. McClave S, Chang W. Complications of enteral access. *Gastrointest Endosc.* 2003;58(5):739–751.

35. Cosentini E, Sauntner T, Gnant M, et al. Outcomes of surgical, percutaneous endoscopic, and percutaneous radiologic gastrostomies. *Arch Surg.* 1998;133(10):1076–1083.

36. Moller P, Lindberg C, Zilling T. Gastrostomy by various techniques: evaluation of indications, outcome, and complications. *Scand J Gastroenterol.* 1999;34(10):1050–1054.

37. Laasch H, Wilbraham L, Bullen K, et al. Gastrostomy insertion: comparing the options—PEG, RIG, or PIG? *Clin Radiol.* 2003;58(5):398–405.

38. Stiegmann G, Goff J, Silas D, et al. Endoscopic versus operative gastrostomy: final results of a prospective randomized trial. *Gastrointest Endosc.* 1990;36(1):1–5.

39. Scott J, de la Torre RA, Unger S. Comparison of operative versus percutaneous endoscopic gastrostomy tube placement in the elderly. *Am Surg.* 1991;57(5):338–340.

40. American Society of Gastrointestinal Endoscopy Standards of Practice Committee. The management of antithrombotic agents for patients undergoing GI endoscopy. *Gastrointest Endosc.* 2016; 83(1):3–16.

41. Veitch AM, Vanbiervliet G, Gerschlick AH, et al. Endoscopy in patients on antiplatelet or anticoagulant therapy, including direct oral anticoagulants: British society of gastroenterology (BSG) and European Society of Gastrointestinal Endoscopy (ESGE) guidelines. *Endoscopy.* 2016;48(4):385–402.

42. Banerjee S, Shen B, Baron T, et al. Antibiotic prophylaxis for GI endoscopy. *Gastrointest Endosc.* 2008;67(6):791–798.

43. Lipp A, Lusardi G. Systemic antimicrobial prophylaxis for percutaneous endoscopic gastrostomy. *Cochrane Data Syst Rev.* 2013; 14(11):CD005571.

44. Gossner L, Keymling J, Hahn E, et al. Antibiotic prophylaxis in percutaneous endoscopic gastrostomy (PEG): a prospective randomized clinical trial. *Endoscopy.* 1999;31(2):119–124.

45. DiSario J, Baskin W, Brown R, et al. Endoscopic approaches to enteral nutritional support. *Gastrointest Endosc.* 2002;55:901–908.

46. Jain N, Larson D, Schroeder K, et al. Antibiotic prophylaxis for percutaneous endoscopic gastrostomy: a prospective, randomized, double-blind clinical trial. *Ann Intern Med.* 1987; 107(6):824–828.

47. Ponsky J, Gauderer M. Percutaneous endoscopic gastrostomy: a non-operative technique for feeding gastrostomy. *Gastrointest Endosc.* 1981;27(1):9–11.

48. Cope C. Suture anchor for visceral drainage. *Am J Roentgenol.* 1986;146:160–162.

49. Coleman C, Coons H, Cope C, et al. Percutaneous enterostomy with the Cope suture anchor. *Radiology.* 1990;174(3 Pt 1):889–891.

50. Funaki B, Zaleski G, Lorenz J, et al. Radiologic gastrostomy placement: pigtail-placement versus mushroom-retained catheters. *Am J Roentgenol.* 2000;175(2):375–379.

51. Duszak R, Mabry M. National trends in gastrointestinal access procedures: an analysis of Medicare services provided by radiologists and other specialists. *J Vasc Interv Radiol.* 2003;14(8):1031–1036.

52. Lorentzen T, Skjoldbye B, Nolsoe C, et al. Percutaneous gastrostomy guided by ultrasound and fluoroscopy. *Acta Radiol.* 1995;36(2):159–162.

53. Grant J. Comparison of percutaneous endoscopic gastrostomy with Stamm gastrostomy. *Ann Surg.* 1988;207(5):598–603.

54. Duh Q, Senokozlieff-Englehart A, Choe Y, et al. Laparoscopic gastrostomy and jejunostomy: safety and cost with local vs. general anesthesia. *Arch Surg.* 1999;134(2):151–156.

55. Lydiatt D, Murayama K, Hollins R, et al. Laparoscopic gastrostomy versus open gastrostomy in head and neck cancer patients. *Laryngoscope.* 1996;106:407–410.

56. Ho C. Radiologic placement of gastrostomy/jejunostomy tubes in high-risk patients. *Nutr Clin Pract.* 1997;12(suppl):S17–S19.

57. Ho C, Yeung E. Percutaneous gastrostomy and transgastric jejunostomy. *Am J Roentgenol.* 1992;158:251–257.

58. DeLegge M, Patrick P, Gibbs R. Percutaneous endoscopic gastrojejunostomy with a tapered tip, nonweighted jejunal feeding tube: improved placement success. *Am J Gastroenterol.* 1996; 91(6):1130–1134.

59. Udorah MO, Fleischman MW, Bala V, Cai Q. Endoscopic clips prevent displacement of intestinal feeding tubes: a long-term follow-up study. *Dig Dis Sci.* 2010;55(2):371–374.

60. Peitgen K, Walz M, Krause U, et al. First results of laparoscopic gastroscopy. *Surg Endosc.* 1997;11(6):658–662.

61. Varadarajulu S, DeLegge M. Use of a 19-gauge injection needle as a guide for direct percutaneous endoscopic jejunostomy tube placement. *Gastrointest Endosc.* 2003;57(7):942–945.

62. Shike M, Latkany L, Gerdes H, et al. Direct percutaneous endoscopic jejunostomies for enteral feeding. *Gastrointest Endosc.* 1996;44(5):536–540.

63. Yang Z, Shin J, Song H, et al. Fluoroscopically guided percutaneous jejunostomy: outcomes in 25 consecutive patients. *Clin Radiol.* 2007;62:1061–1065.

64. Szymski G, Albazzaz A, Funaki B, et al. Radiologically guided placement of pull-type gastrostomy tubes. *Radiology.* 1997;205(3):669–673.

65. Richard H, Widlus D, Malloy P. Percutaneous fluoroscopically guided jejunostomy placement. *J Trauma.* 2008;65(5):1072–1077.

66. Itkin N, DeLegge M, Fang J, et al. Multidisciplinary practical guidelines for gastrointestinal access for enteral nutrition and decompression from the Society of Interventional Radiology and American Gastroenterological Association (AGA) Institute, with endorsement by Canadian Interventional Radiological Association (CIRA) and Cardiovascular and Interventional Radiological Society of Europe (CIRSE). *Gastroenterology.* 2011;141(2):742–765.

67. Al-Bawardy B, Gorospe EC, Alexander JA, et al. Outcomes of double-balloon enteroscopy-assisted direct percutaneous endoscopic jejunostomy tube placement. *Endoscopy.* 2016;48(6):552–556.

68. Velazquez-Avina J, Beyer R, Diaz-Tobar CP, et al. New method of direct percutaneous endoscopic jejunostomy tube placement using balloon-assisted enteroscopy with fluoroscopy. *Dig Endosc.* 2015;27(3):317–322.

69. Hicks M, Surratt R, Picus D, et al. Fluoroscopically guided percutaneous gastrostomy and gastroenterostomy: analysis of 158 consecutive cases. *Am J Roentgenol.* 1990;154:725–728.

70. Lynch C, Fang J. Prevention and management of complications of PEG tubes. *Pract Gastroenterol.* 2004;22:66–76.

71. Sriram K, Jayanthi V, Lakshmi R, et al. Prophylactic locking of enteral feeding tubes with pancreatic enzymes. *JPEN J Parenter Enteral Nutr.* 1997;21(6):353–356.

72. Bourgault A, Heyland D, Drover J, et al. Prophylactic pancreatic enzymes to reduce feeding tube occlusions. *Nutr Clin Pract.* 2003;18(5):398–401.

73. McWey R, Curry N, Schabel S, et al. Complications of nasoenteric feeding tubes. *Am J Surg.* 1988;155(2):253–257.

74. Odocha O, Lowery R, Mezghebe H, et al. Tracheopleuropulmonary injuries following enteral tube insertion. *J Natl Med Assoc.* 1989;81(3):275–281.

75. Roubenoff R, Ravich W. Pneumothorax due to nasogastric feeding tubes: report of four cases, review of the literature, and recommendations for prevention. *Arch Intern Med.* 1989;149(1):184–188.

76. Damore LJ, Andrus C, Herrmann V, et al. Prospective evaluation of a new through-the-scope nasoduodenal enteral feeding tube. *Surg Endosc.* 2002;11:460–463.

77. Lee S, Mathiasen R, Lipkin C, et al. Endoscopically placed nasogastrojejunal feeding tubes: a safe route for enteral nutrition in patients with hepatic encephalopathy. *Am Surg.* 2002;68:196–200.

78. McClave S, Sexton L, Spain D, et al. Enteral tube feeding in the intensive care unit: factors impeding adequate delivery. *Crit Care Med.* 1999;27(7):1252–1256.

79. Bechtold ML, Nguyen DL, Palmer LB et al. Nasal bridles for securing nasoenteric tubes: a meta-analysis. *Nutr Clin Pract.* 2014;29(5):667–671.

80. Gunn S, Early B, Zenati M, et al. Use of a nasal bridle prevents accidental nasoenteral feeding tube removal. *JPEN J Parenter Enteral Nutr.* 2009;33(1):50–54.

81. Brandt C, Mittendorf E, Rassias A, et al. Endoscopic placement of nasojejunal feeding tubes in ICU patients. *Surg Endosc.* 1999;13(12):1211–1214.

82. Patrick P, Marulendra S, Kirby D, et al. Endoscopic nasogastricjejunal feeding tube placement in critically ill patients. *Gastrointest Endosc.* 1997;45(1):72–76.

83. Bosco J, Gordon F, Zelig M, et al. A reliable method for the endoscopic placement of a nasoenteric feeding tube. *Gastrointest Endosc.* 1994;40(6):740–743.

84. Marcuard S, Stegall K, Trogdon S. Clearing obstructed feeding tubes. *JPEN J Parenter Enteral Nutr.* 1989;13(1):81–83.

85. Stahlfeld K, Hiltner L. Clogged feeding tube management now that Viokase is unavailable. *JPEN J Parenter Enteral Nutr.* 2011;35:11.

86. McClave S. Managing complications of percutaneous and nasoenteric feeding tubes. *Tech Gastrointest Endosc.* 2001;3:62–68.

87. Smith-Choban P, Max M. Feeding jejunostomy: a small bowel stress test? *Am J Surg.* 1988;155(1):112–117.

88. Safadi B, Marks J, Ponsky J. Percutaneous endoscopic gastrostomy. *Gastrointest Endosc Clin N Am.* 1998;8:551–568.

89. Wojtowycz M, Arata JA Jr, Micklos T, et al. CT findings after uncomplicated percutaneous gastrostomy. *Am J Roentgenol.* 1988;151:307–309.

90. James A, Kapur K, Hawthorne A. Long-term outcome of percutaneous endoscopic gastrostomy feeding in patients with dysphagic stroke. *Age Ageing.* 1998;27:671–676.

91. Akkersdijk W, van Bergeijk JD, van Egmond T, et al. Percutaneous endoscopic gastrostomy (PEG): comparison of push and pull methods and evaluation of antibiotic prophylaxis. *Endoscopy.* 1995;27:313–316.

92. Lin H, Ibrahim H, Kheng J, et al. Percutaneous endoscopic gastrostomy: strategies for prevention and management of complications. *Laryngoscope.* 2001;111(10):1847–1852.

93. Ségal D, Michaud L, Guimber D, et al. Late-onset complications of percutaneous endoscopic gastrostomy in children. *Pediatr Gastroenterol Nutr.* 2001;33:495–500.

94. Venu R, Brown R, Pastika B, et al. The buried bumper syndrome: a simple management approach in two patients. *Gastrointest Endosc.* 2002;56:582–584.

95. Walton G. Complications of percutaneous endoscopic gastrostomy in patients with head and neck cancer—an analysis of 42 consecutive patients. *Ann R Coll Surg Engl.* 1999;81(4):272–276.

96. Ma M, Semlacher E, Fedorak R, et al. The buried gastrostomy bumper syndrome: prevention and endoscopic approaches to removal. *Gastrointest Endosc.* 1995;4:505–508.

97. Boyd J, DeLegge M, Shamburek R, et al. The buried bumper syndrome: a new technique for safe, endoscopic PEG removal. *Gastrointest Endosc.* 1995;41:508–511.

98. DiSario J, Foutch P, Sanowski R. Poor results with percutaneous endoscopic gastrojejunostomy. *Gastrointest Endosc.* 1990;36(3):257–260.

99. DeLegge M, Duckworth PF Jr, McHenry L, et al. Percutaneous endoscopic jejunostomy: a dual center safety and efficacy trial. *JPEN Parenter Enteral Nutr.* 1995;19(3):239–243.

100. Maple J, Baron T, Petersen B. The frequency, severity, and spectrum of adverse events associated with direct percutaneous endoscopic jejunostomy (DPEJ). *Gastrointest Endosc.* 2005;61(5):AB80.

13 Complications of Enteral Nutrition

Ainsley M. Malone, MS, RD, LD, CNSC, FAND, FASPEN, David S. Seres, MD, FASPEN, PNS, and Linda M. Lord, NP, CNSC, ACNP-BC

CONTENTS

Objectives

1. Understand the risk factors, signs and symptoms, and management of gastrointestinal (GI) complications, including nausea and vomiting, abdominal distention, malabsorption, diarrhea, and constipation.
2. Consider the risk for complications related to pulmonary aspiration of enteral formulations and the methods to detect and prevent aspiration-related problems.
3. Compare the metabolic complications associated with enteral nutrition (EN) vs parenteral nutrition (PN).
4. Review strategies to identify and prevent dehydration in patients receiving EN.

Test Your Knowledge Questions

1. Which of the following actions is most appropriate for enhancing gastric emptying during the administration EN?
   A. Keep the bed in Trendelenburg position.
   B. Decrease the rate of a continuous feeding infusion, or change from bolus to continuous feeding.
   C. Switch to an enteral formulation with a higher fat content.
   D. Switch to an enteral formulation with a higher protein content.
2. Which of the following is the most appropriate initial action for the management of tube feeding–associated diarrhea?
   A. Change to an enteral formulation with fiber.
   B. Review the patient's medication administration record to determine whether hyperosmolar agents are being administered.
   C. Change to a peptide-based enteral formulation.
   D. Use an antimotility agent.
3. Which of the following methods is not recommended to minimize contamination of enteral feeding formula?
   A. Washing hands and donning clean gloves before preparing enteral formula.
   B. Immediate use of enteral formula from a newly opened container.
   C. Infusing reconstituted powdered formulas or formulas with added modular components in 1 bag for up to 8 hours.
   D. Changing an "open" feeding container every 24 hours.

Test Your Knowledge Answers

1. The correct answer is **B**. Factors that delay gastric emptying include large boluses of fluid given at one time, increased rate of formula infusion, increased fat content of the solution, and infusion of solutions colder than room temperature. Elevation of the head of the bed (HOB) and turning of the patient slightly to the right side allows gravity to help drain the stomach; however, such positions are often difficult to achieve in the hospital environment.
2. The correct answer is **B**. If clinically significant diarrhea develops during EN, the most appropriate initial action is to evaluate whether hyperosmolar medications that could result in liquid stooling are being administered. If none are in use, testing for the presence of *Clostridium difficile*; if those results are negative, the addition of fiber from a formulation that contains fiber or supplemental fiber may be beneficial. Adding an antimotility agent or changing to a peptide-based formula should be considered if diarrhea continues despite these initial interventions. PN should be initiated only if the other treatment modalities fail.
3. The correct answer is **C**. A formula prepared from reconstituted powder or with added modular components should be infused for no more than 4 hours. Infusion times greater than 4 hours are associated with formula contamination. The use of good handwashing technique and clean gloves and immediately using a newly opened formula container will minimize contamination. Changing an "open" feeding container every 24 hours will minimize bacterial growth that can contaminate formula.

Background

Enteral tube feeding is the preferred feeding modality when the GI tract is functional and the patient is unable or unwilling to consume an adequate oral diet. The enteral route is promoted as an efficacious and cost-effective method of providing nutrients to patients (see Chapter 10). However, enteral tube feeding is not without its challenges. The administration of EN may be complicated by disease, illness, or trauma; treatment side effects; and iatrogenic conditions. Distinguishing the potential causes of a complication is essential to preventing or managing it. GI, pulmonary aspiration, and metabolic complications that can contribute to a patient's morbidity and mortality are reviewed in this chapter. Chapter 12 reviews complications specific to enteral feeding devices, and Chapter 18 discusses drug-nutrient interactions.

Clinicians must thoroughly evaluate patients before EN is initiated to identify and, when feasible, avoid or minimize potential problems. Ongoing monitoring and reassessment should be a standard component of follow-up care.

Gastrointestinal Complications

Nausea and Vomiting

Nausea and/or vomiting occur in 7% to 26% of critically ill patients who receive EN support.[1-3] Vomiting, especially in minimally responsive patients, is believed to increase the risk of pulmonary aspiration, pneumonia, and sepsis. Multiple etiologies exist for nausea and vomiting with EN. Delayed gastric emptying is the most commonly identified problem.[4-6] Potential causes of slowed emptying include the following:[7-13]

- Diabetic gastropathy
- Hypotension
- Sepsis
- Stress
- Anesthesia and surgery
- Infiltrative gastric neoplasms
- Various autoimmune diseases
- Surgical vagotomy
- Pancreaticoduodenectomy
- Opiate analgesic medications (morphine sulfate, codeine, fentanyl)
- Anticholinergics (chlordiazepoxide hydrochloride and clidinium bromide)
- Excessively rapid infusion of formula
- Infusion of a very cold solution or one containing a large amount of fat or fiber

If delayed gastric emptying is suspected, appropriate interventions include reducing or discontinuing all narcotic medications, switching to a low-fiber, low-fat, and/or isotonic formula, administering the feeding solution at room temperature, temporarily reducing the rate of infusion by 20 to 25 mL/h, changing the infusion method from bolus to continuous, and/or administering a prokinetic agent such as metoclopramide or erythromycin.[5,6,10-12] Once tolerance is achieved, the rate or volume will typically be gradually increased every 6 to 24 hours until nutrition goals are met.[5,6] If nausea or vomiting occurs as the rate of administration or bolus volume of the EN increases, the rate or volume should be reduced to the greatest tolerated amount, with an attempt to increase the rate again after symptoms abate. If these efforts to increase the rate/volume of EN fail, small bowel access (eg, nasojejunal tube or transgastric jejunostomy tube) should be considered.

Abdominal distention in a patient with nausea indicates a need to monitor the abdomen closely—before the next bolus tube feeding or every 4 hours for continuous feeding. As discussed in greater detail later in the chapter, gastric residual volume (GRV) is often used to assess EN tolerance. However, elevated GRVs alone do not correlate with intolerance.[14] Furthermore, in a prospective, randomized trial, checking GRVs did not decrease the incidence of ventilator-associated pneumonia (VAP) in critically ill patients,[15] and the Society of Critical Care Medicine (SCCM) and American Society for Parenteral and Enteral Nutrition (ASPEN) do not recommend routine checks of GRVs in critically ill patients.[14]

If GRVs are low but nausea persists, patients may benefit from antiemetic medications. Clinicians should also monitor stool frequency in patients who complain of nausea. Obstipation or fecal impaction may lead to distention and nausea, particularly in institutionalized patients or those with chronic critical illness. Distention and vomiting may be caused by diarrheal illness such as *Clostridium difficile* colitis.

Abdominal Distention

Abdominal and gastric distention are common reasons why EN is interrupted.[1,2] Distention and its associated symptoms of bloating and cramping may be caused by GI ileus, obstruction, obstipation, ascites, or diarrheal illness. Additionally, excessively rapid formula administration or infusion of very cold formula may contribute to abdominal distention. Use of fiber-containing formulas can cause abdominal distention because fiber ferments and produces gas in the gut. Theoretically, the role of fiber in slowing gastric emptying may also be a factor.

Abdominal distention is diagnosed by visual inspection and palpation as well as from patient reports. Attempts have been made to define distention objectively (eg, an increase of abdominal girth of more than 8 to 10 cm),[16] but careful clinical evaluation remains the most practical means of assessment. If an ileus or bowel obstruction is suspected based on physical examination and symptoms, it may be confirmed by a flat and upright abdominal x-ray. However, upright films are often impractical in hospitalized patients and these "plain" films may be nondiagnostic. Therefore, cross-sectional imaging (eg, computed tomography) may be needed to confirm the diagnosis. Nevertheless, plain radiology remains the appropriate screening method if ileus or obstruction are suspected.

Another simple method of assessing distention, particularly when the position of the feeding tube is in question, is to inject a small amount of contrast material through the feeding tube and observe intestinal anatomy and motility on a follow-up, single x-ray or under fluoroscopy. This technique can often provide a clear picture of the clinical situation. If intestinal appearance and function are normal, EN may be continued

despite the distention. Feedings may need to be discontinued, however, if motility is poor, the bowel is markedly dilated, or the patient's discomfort too severe.

Maldigestion/Malabsorption

Maldigestion refers to impaired breakdown of nutrients into absorbable forms (eg, lactose intolerance). Clinical manifestations of maldigestion include bloating, abdominal distention, and diarrhea.

Maldigestion may result in significant *malabsorption*, defined as defective mucosal uptake and transport of nutrients (fat, carbohydrate, protein, vitamins, electrolytes, minerals, or water) from the small intestine. Clinical manifestations of malabsorption include unexplained weight loss; steatorrhea; diarrhea; and signs of vitamin, mineral, or essential macronutrient deficiency, such as anemia, tetany, bone pain, pathologic fractures, bleeding, dermatitis, neuropathy, and glossitis.

Methods used to screen for malabsorption include the following (listed in order of complexity):[17]

- Gross and microscopic examination of the stool
- Qualitative determination of fat and protein content of a random stool collection
- Measurement of serum carotene concentration
- Measurement of serum citrulline levels
- Measurement of d-xylose absorption
- Radiologic examination of intestinal transit time and motility

When laboratory data, history, and/or radiologic examination suggest maldigestion or malabsorption, diagnosis can involve the following:[17]

- Intake-output balance (stool collections for quantitative fecal fat assessment)
- Tests for the maldigestion/malabsorption of specific nutrients, such as lactose tolerance test, Schilling test to screen for abnormal absorption of vitamin B_{12}, essential fatty acid profile for lipid malabsorption, and various radioisotopic tests to identify iron, calcium, amino acid, folic acid, pyridoxine, and vitamin D malabsorption
- Endoscopic small bowel biopsy, which is helpful in diagnosing mucosal disorders such as celiac disease, tropical sprue, and Whipple disease (see Chapter 26 for additional information on the diagnosis of celiac disease)

Causes of maldigestion/malabsorption include gluten-sensitive enteropathy, Crohn's disease, diverticular disease, radiation enteritis, enteric fistulas, human immunodeficiency virus, pancreatic insufficiency, short-gut syndrome, small intestinal bacterial overgrowth (SIBO), and numerous other syndromes. Although it is common practice to use predigested enteral products when malabsorption is suspected, only weak data support their use to prevent intolerance[18] or overcome malabsorption/maldigestion during enteral feeding (see Chapter 11). Selected patients with severe malabsorption that is unresponsive to medical therapy or supplementation may require PN.[6,17,19]

Diarrhea

Diarrhea is the most commonly reported GI side effect in patients receiving EN.[20] No definition of diarrhea is universally accepted.[21] However, a clinically useful definition is any abnormal volume or consistency of stool. Normal stool water content is 250 to 500 mL/d. Diarrhea has also been defined as greater than 500 mL stool output every 24 hours or more than 3 stools per day for at least 2 consecutive days.[22,23] Stool volume can be measured by placing a collection device in the toilet or by using a bedpan; in incontinent patients, it can be measured via a fecal management system or by placing a pad under the patient and weighing it after each stool (assuming 1 g equals 1 mL of stool).

Etiologies

Common causes of diarrhea in patients receiving EN include medications, primary GI disease, and bacterial infection. Characteristics of the formula (osmolality, fat content) and specific components in the formula (eg, lactose) are less likely to cause diarrhea.[24,25]

Drug-Induced Diarrhea

The hypertonicity of some drugs—such as electrolyte supplements (potassium, phosphorus, magnesium) and medications delivered in liquid form that contain magnesium or sorbitol in the vehicle—may cause diarrhea. As little as 10 to 20 g of sorbitol can lead to GI side effects, including diarrhea.[6,26–29] Table 13-1 outlines the sorbitol content of selected liquid medications.[25]

Drugs with direct effects on the gut, such as antibiotics, proton pump inhibitors, and prokinetic medications, can also cause diarrhea (see Table 13-2).[30] Antibiotic-associated diarrhea (AAD) is a

TABLE 13-1 Sorbitol Content of Selected Medications

Generic Name	Trade Name	% Sorbitol[a]
Acetaminophen elixir	Tylenol	35.0
Amantadine	Symmetrel	72.0
Cimetidine	Tagamet	46.1
Doxycycline	Vibramycin	70.0
Furosemide	Lasix	35.0
Guaifenesin and codeine	Robitussin AC	35.0
Hydroxyzine	Vistaril	116.0
Indomethacin	Indocin	35.0
Isoniazid[b]	—	70.0
Metoclopramide	Reglan	28.0–42.0
Nortriptyline	Aventyl	64.0
Pseudoephedrine and triprolidine	Actifed	49.0

[a]Weight per volume.
[b]Generic version.
Adapted with permission from reference 25: McCarthy MS, Fabling JC, Bell DE. Drug-nutrient interactions. In: Shikora SA, Martindale RG, Schwaitzberg SD, eds. *Nutrition Considerations in the Intensive Care Unit: Science, Rationale and Practice.* Dubuque, IA: Kendall-Hunt; 2002:153. Copyright 2002 American Society for Parenteral and Enteral Nutrition.

TABLE 13-2 Medications Associated with Increased Incidence of Diarrhea

- Ampicillin
- Bisacodyl
- Caffeine
- Clindamycin
- Colchicine
- Digoxin
- Erythromycin
- Hydralazine
- Lactulose
- Magnesium-containing preparations
- Metoclopramide
- Methotrexate
- Neomycin
- Penicillamine
- Procainamide
- Quinidine
- Theophylline

Reprinted from reference 30: Ratnaike RN, Jones TE. Mechanisms of drug-induced diarrhea in the elderly. *Drugs Aging.* 1998;13(3):245–253. Reprinted with permission of Springer.

common medication effect, occurring in up to 25% of patients treated with antibiotics, and *C. difficile* colitis affects 10% to 20% of all patients who develop AAD.[31]

The osmotic load of some medications may make diarrhea inevitable. Any drug in a liquid vehicle given via a small bowel feeding tube should be diluted to avoid a hypertonic-induced, dumping-like syndrome. Most drugs and electrolytes (eg, potassium) should be mixed with a minimum of 30 to 60 mL of water per 10-mEq dose to avoid direct irritation of the gut.

Gastrointestinal Diseases

Many primary diseases of the intestine, including inflammatory bowel disease, short bowel syndrome, gluten-sensitive enteropathy, and acquired immunodeficiency syndrome, may result in malabsorption or secretory diarrhea (see Table 13-3).[32] Recognition and treatment of these diseases can minimize diarrhea. In some disease states, PN may be required. In others, use of specialized enteral products are proposed to facilitate absorption.

Infusion of Hyperosmolar Feeding Solutions

Hyperosmolar EN products rarely cause clinically significant diarrhea unless they are infused at a very high rate or administered by bolus into the small bowel. The highest osmolality of a tube feed is around 750 mOsm/L, which is about 2.5 times greater than normal serum. In contrast, electrolyte supplements have osmolalities in the range of 5000 to 7500 mOsm/L and are far more likely to cause osmotic diarrhea. If the clinician suspects that the hyperosmolality of an enteral formula is causing diarrhea, changing to an isotonic formula may be beneficial. Diluting the formula with water, a measure

TABLE 13-3 Conditions Associated with Secretory Diarrhea

- Infection with enterotoxic organisms such as *Clostridium difficile*
- Abuse of stimulant laxatives
- Intestinal resection
- Inflammatory bowel disease
- Bile acid malabsorption
- Fatty acid malabsorption
- Chronic infections
- Celiac sprue
- Small intestinal lymphoma
- Villous adenoma of the rectum
- Zollinger–Ellison syndrome
- Collagen vascular diseases
- Congenital defects
- Malignant carcinoid syndrome

Source: Reprinted with permission from reference 32: Fine KD, Krejs GJ, Fordtran JS. Diarrhea. In: Sleisenger MH, Fordtran JS, eds. *Gastrointestinal Disease: Pathophysiology, Diagnosis, Management.* 5th ed. Philadelphia, PA: Saunders; 1995:1043. Copyright Elsevier.

that was once common for patients with diarrhea, may result in suboptimal nutrient provision, and formula dilution has not been shown to improve tolerance.[33,34] In addition, this practice is discouraged because it contaminates formula.

Specific Components of Enteral Formulas

Polymeric enteral formulas with intact protein are recommended for initial use in most individuals starting EN (see Chapter 11).[35] Older studies comparing intact protein with peptide-based formulas did not find the latter to be better tolerated.[36,37] In a recent, randomized pilot trial comparing a peptide-based formula with a polymeric formula in critically ill patients, the number of days of adverse GI events, including diarrhea, was significantly reduced with the peptide-based formula, but the incidence of diarrhea itself was not significantly different between the 2 groups.[18]

Most formulas are lactose free, but diarrhea related to lactose intolerance may be observed during the transition from EN to an oral diet. Some patients are lactase deficient prior to the onset of illness, and others develop a transient lactase deficiency during their illness. A lactose-restricted diet may help reduce diarrhea in patients with lactase deficiency.

Management Strategies

A systematic approach can be effective in the management of diarrhea (Practice Scenario 13-1).[14,38–40] A 2007 observational study confirmed improvement in diarrhea incidence following the use of a defined diarrhea protocol.[23] Figure 13-1 provides an algorithm for treatment of diarrhea in tube-fed patients.[41] If clinically significant diarrhea develops during EN, clinicians should consider the following options:

- Medical assessment of the patient to rule out infectious or inflammatory causes, fecal impaction, diarrheagenic medications, and so on

- Use of an antidiarrheal agent (loperamide, diphenoxylate, paregoric, or octreotide) once *C. difficile* infection has been ruled out or is being treated
- Changing the formula type (eg, from an intact protein product to a peptide-based formula)
- Addition of soluble fiber or insoluble fiber to the medication regimen and/or changing to an enteral formula with added fiber, except in unstable critically ill patients[14]
- Continuation of EN as tolerated and initiation of PN to complete delivery of macro- and micronutrients if intolerance or malabsorption is severe and prolonged

Practice Scenario 13-1

Question: How does a nutrition support clinician select an enteral formula for a tube-fed patient who experiences diarrhea?

Scenario: Isotonic, fiber-free, nasogastric enteral feeding was initiated in a 78-year-old man following surgical intervention for a perforated duodenal ulcer, for which he was receiving a proton pump inhibitor. His postoperative course was complicated by hospital-acquired pneumonia requiring ventilator support and the use of antibiotic therapy. Enteral nutrition (EN) was initiated and advanced over a 72-hour period. At first, the patient demonstrated good tolerance to the EN with a slightly distended abdomen; hypoactive to active bowel sounds were heard; and he had 1 to 2 semiloose stools per day. However, after 5 days of feeding, he developed 4 to 5 watery stools per day and a fecal management system was required.

Intervention: The nutrition support clinician reviewed the patient's medication profile and determined that he was not receiving hypertonic or sorbitol-based medications and a prokinetic agent was not in use. The clinician recommended obtaining a stool culture to assess for the presence of *Clostridium difficile* and the use of an enteral formula high in soluble fiber to assist in controlling the patient's diarrhea.

Answer: The inclusion of a gelatinous soluble fiber (eg, psyllium) in the EN regimen is one approach to manage diarrhea.

Rationale: Diarrhea in patients receiving EN can have many causes. A review of this patient's medication record does not identify any motility agents, sorbitol-based drugs, or hypertonic medications, but antibiotics and/or the proton pump inhibitor may be contributing factors.

Several management strategies can be employed to help control the patient's diarrhea. One is to add fiber to his EN regimen. Multiple small studies have demonstrated that the addition of soluble fiber to EN improves diarrhea,[38,39] and adding fiber to EN is the recommended standard of care.[14] However, the beneficial effect has been small, and a meta-analysis that aggregated data from 400 subjects found no difference in diarrhea in patients receiving EN with fiber vs EN without fiber.[40] Interestingly, hospital length of stay was reduced in supplemented patients in this analysis, but no difference in mortality was seen.[40] The addition of fiber can be achieved by using a fiber-containing enteral formula or by using a fiber modular supplement. A fiber-containing formula is usually preferable because modular fiber supplements can clog feeding tubes.

Testing for the presence of *C. difficile* in the stool is recommended in any patient deemed at risk for *C. difficile* infection. If the *C. difficile* results are negative, and offending medications cannot be stopped, the initiation of antidiarrheal agents is appropriate. Changing the enteral formula to a peptide-based formulation may be an option if other interventions are ineffective, but these formulas are costlier than intact-nutrient formulas. The addition of fiber to the EN regimen or changing the formulation should never be the primary intervention or the end of the evaluation or intervention for diarrhea.

Small Intestinal Bacterial Overgrowth

Bacterial overgrowth in the GI tract can cause severe enteritis with marked diarrhea, abdominal cramps and pain, hypoalbuminemia, protein catabolism, cachexia, fever, and even sepsis. Increasingly, SIBO is seen in patients after Roux-en-Y gastric bypass surgery.[42] SIBO is difficult to diagnose definitively, especially in patients with blind intestinal limbs, such as those who have undergone Roux-en-Y bypass. Techniques such as hydrogen breath testing may provide false-negative results in these patients, necessitating empiric treatment. In patients who have altered GI anatomy or have been treated

with prolonged antibiotic therapy, SIBO should be considered in the differential diagnosis if they present with bloating, abdominal pain, and/or otherwise unexplained catabolism/hypoalbuminemia. Prolonged use of broad-spectrum antibiotics increases the incidence of SIBO.[43,44] Treatment is often empiric and includes antibiotics. Nonabsorbable antibiotics are the treatment of choice, but systemic antibiotics are often necessary when the overgrowth is suspected to be in a nonalimentary bowel limb because the oral medication will not pass through the effected segment of bowel. Refer to Chapter 26 for additional discussion of SIBO.

Complications Related to Formula Contamination

Whenever enterally fed patients have diarrhea, abdominal upset, or fever, the contamination of enteral formula and the enteral delivery system should be considered as a potential cause of the problem. Contamination of enteral formulas can lead to diarrhea, abdominal distention, pneumonia, infectious enterocolitis, bacteremia, septicemia, and death.[45–47] Neonates, critically ill and immune-suppressed patients, and those with a compromised gastric acid microbial barrier may be at greater risk for morbidity and mortality related to formula contamination.

Enteral feeding formula can become contaminated with microorganisms during formula storage, preparation, or

FIGURE 13-1 Algorithm for Management of Diarrhea

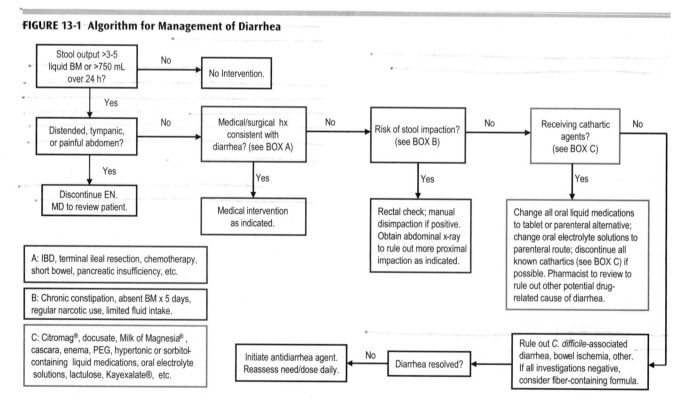

BM, bowel movements; *C. difficile*, *Clostridium difficile*; EN, enteral nutrition; hx, history; IBD, inflammatory bowel disease; MD, Doctor of Medicine; PEG, percutaneous endoscopic gastrostomy.
Source: Adapted from reference 41: Greenwood J. Critical Care Nutrition at the Clinical Evaluation Research Unit. Study tools: management of diarrhea algorithm. 2010. www.criticalcarenutrition.com/docs/tools/Diarrhea.pdf. Accessed June 4, 2017. Reproduced with permission from Critical Care Nutrition: www.criticalcarenutrition.com.

administration. Enteral formulas that require minimal handling with sterile technique, such as those supplied in "closed-system" containers or sterile formulas that are carefully transferred to a feeding receptacle, have a lower incidence of microbial contamination compared with those that require reconstitution, mixing, or dilution (see Chapter 11). This difference translates to a small reduction in the incidence of diarrhea with formulas that require minimal handling, but no other clinical benefit has been demonstrated.[48]

Enteral "open" delivery systems provide liquid formula delivered via syringe or poured into a bag and delivered to the patient by gravity drip or pump. Formulas poured into feeding bags directly from cans, screw-top plastic bottles, and Brik Paks, have hang times from 4 to 12 hours; specific hang times depend on the feeding protocol at the facility and the manufacturer's recommendations. Reconstituted powdered formulas or formulas with added modular components delivered by gravity drip or pump should hang no more than 4 hours at room temperature. Enteral "closed" delivery systems use prefilled, sterile bottles or non-air-dependent containers that are accessed with a spike or screw-top tubing. These are administered by pump infusion and allow for longer hang times of 24 to 48 hours.

Formulas provided in liquid form undergo heat sterilization, whereas powdered formulas are not required to be sterile and may contain contaminants. To minimize the risk for contamination, powdered formulas should ideally be reconstituted with sterile water.[49] Preparation and administration of any type of formula must always involve trained personnel using good handwashing, clean gloves, and aseptic technique in a clean environment.

Formulas should be used immediately after being opened, or after reconstitution with sterile water, with strict adherence to the manufacturer-recommended hang times for room-temperature formula. If formula is leftover after the intended volume is poured into the feeding system, the excess should be refrigerated immediately and stored according to the manufacturer's recommendations, typically a maximum of 24 to 48 hours.

For example, if the formula rate is 25 mL/h and the formula hang time is 8 hours, a maximum of 200 mL of formula can be poured into the feeding bag and administered at room temperature during that 8-hour period; any formula leftover after the feeding bag is filled should be immediately refrigerated for future use.

Use of a blender to add carbohydrate and protein modular additives to formula carries a high risk for contamination during the mixing process and should be avoided.[50] The lids of cans should be cleansed with isopropyl alcohol and allowed to dry before pouring the formula into the delivery receptacle.[51] Feeding bags do not need to be rinsed with water before additional formula is added, but formula should not be added until the previous formula has infused. The feeding bag itself should be changed every 24 hours.[52]

Lyman and colleagues investigated the risk for formula contamination and associated complications in pediatric patients who received sterile, undiluted formula provided from cans into enteral feeding bags over 12-hour hang times.[53] Aseptic technique and clean gloves were used; the cans and the hub of the tubing were cleansed with alcohol wipes; and touch contamination was avoided. No bacterial contamination was found in 90% of formula cultures, and acceptable, very low-level bacterial contamination was identified in 5% of cultures. The 5% of patients who were exposed to unacceptable bacterial contamination of formula did not show any clinical signs of bacterial gastroenteritis (increased stool output, fever, or clinical deterioration).

The risk of contamination is reduced with the "closed" delivery system because the formula is less exposed to contact with anything nonsterile.[54,55] However, prefilled containers require the attachment of tubing, so touch contamination is still a risk. Contamination is reduced with delivery systems that have recessed spike sets and recessed nutrient container seals.[56,57] These features prevent inadvertent touching of the parts of the closed delivery system that come into contact with the formula. Tubing used with "closed" delivery systems, such as spike sets, should be replaced every 24 hours to lower the incidence of diarrhea.[48]

Enteral formulas may also become contaminated in a retrograde manner if the patient's endogenous microorganisms (from stomach, throat, lungs) reproduce within the feeding tube and then migrate into the enteral delivery system.[58] These microorganisms may then proliferate within the feeding formula and be reinfused to the patient in greater numbers. Most enteral delivery tubing systems contain a drip chamber that minimizes the occurrence of this problem during formula delivery.[59,60] However, if formula infusions are interrupted, the stagnant period could allow microorganisms to proliferate.

The procedure of checking for GRV pulls potentially pathogenic microorganisms up the feeding tube and can lead to a contaminated feeding tube hub and contaminated gloves.[61] The exposure of a patient's body fluids in this manner is labeled a "dirty" procedure. In a "clean" procedure, the individual checking GRV will remove gloves, thoroughly wash hands (or use a hand sanitizer), and put on clean gloves before administering the enteral formula. Research on the benefits and risks of GRV assessment is discussed in greater detail later in this chapter.

The Y-ports of enteral delivery systems are used to deliver medications and water flushes to minimize disconnection of the enteral formula. Mathus-Vliegen and colleagues took cultures in enteral feeding systems and identified bacterial contamination of more than 100 CFU/mL in 48.1% of the "closed" delivery systems at the Y-port vs a 2.4% contamination rate in the formula containers.[58] The investigators determined that the contamination was caused by either administration of medications through the Y-port or retrograde movement of microorganisms from the feeding tube to the delivery system. Although this study looked at the results of cultures and not clinical outcomes of patients, Mathus-Vliegen et al recommended that tube feedings not be allowed to remain within the delivery system without the infusion process occurring and that delivery sets be changed frequently.

Lopez valves are 3-way stopcocks that are frequently attached to enteral feeding tubes that do not contain a clamp, such as nasogastric, balloon gastrostomy, balloon gastrojejunostomy, and jejunostomy tubes. These 3-way valves swivel to block or allow fluid passage. An in vitro investigation showed the development of a bacterial biofilm in Lopez valves within 3 days when the valves were attached to enteral bags delivering a continuous drip, polymeric formula inoculated with *Pseudomonas aeruginosa* on Day 1.[62] The bag and tubing were changed every 24 hours, and sterile formula was used on Days 2 and 3. Biofilms are resistant to antibiotics and the patient's own immune response and can cause acute or chronic infections. The authors of this study suggest changing Lopez valves at intervals of 3 days or less and perhaps at each tubing change.

An investigation of hospitalized patients showed that the incidences *C. difficile* infection and *C. difficile*–associated diarrhea were significantly higher in tube-fed patients compared with non-tube-fed patients, and risk was greatest for those receiving postpyloric tube feeding. The investigators recommended testing for *C. difficile* while investigating other etiologies for diarrhea in tube-fed patients.[45] Alterations in the fecal microbiota were found to occur in patients receiving enteral tube feedings who developed diarrhea.[63] The patients who developed diarrhea had significantly higher concentrations of clostridia and lower concentrations and proportions of bifidobacteria, which may be involved in the pathogenesis of the diarrhea.

The implementation of enteral quality control programs and institutional protocols can reduce enteral formula contamination to acceptable levels.[49,64] An enteral quality control program should define the process for receiving, distributing, storing, preparing, handling, and administering enteral formula, and identify who is responsible for each task. The formula container should be visually inspected for damage, and the expiration date should be noted. Proper handwashing or application of a hand sanitizer should be performed before the feeding administration set and formula are handled. If clinicians wear gloves to perform other patient care needs, they must put on clean gloves before handling formula and enteral devices. A clean area, such as a clean towel or underpad, should be set up beneath the feeding tube connection. Flip-top cans should be wiped with isopropyl alcohol and allowed to dry. Once opened, the formula should be inspected for altered formula characteristics such as formula separation, thickening, clumping, or curdling. If a powdered formula or modular component requires reconstitution or dilution, sterile water should be used. Aseptic technique should be used in preparing the formula, when pouring formula into a receptacle or spiking the formula container, and when connecting the administration set or syringe to the feeding tube. Recommendations for formula hang times at room temperature, refrigeration times, and timing for feeding set changes should be followed. "Closed" EN delivery systems should be used whenever feasible. If an "open" delivery system is used, new formula should not be added to remaining formula in the feeding bag. The addition of a 3-way stopcock increases contamination risk; therefore, the manufacturer's recommendations should be followed for cleaning and routine replacement schedules should be established. Disconnections within the enteral delivery system should be minimized. When they are necessary, the distal end of the delivery system should be covered with a clean cap, and long periods of formula stagnation should be avoided. All related equipment, such as flush syringes and their containers, must be kept as clean and dry as

possible, and enteral equipment should be stored away from potential sources of contamination, such as dirty wounds, fistula, or ostomy dressings and supplies. It is also important to educate patients and their caregivers on the ways to minimize contamination risk with tube feeding delivery.

Constipation, Impaction, and Intestinal Bezoar

Constipation is difficult to define because normal defecation patterns range from 4 stools each day to 1 stool every 4 or 5 days. With EN, the variation in defecation patterns increases depending on the residue and extent of absorption of an enteral feeding product. The best clinical definition of constipation is the accumulation of excess waste in the colon, often up to the transverse colon or even the cecum. A rectal examination and plain abdominal x-ray are often effective for diagnosis and can differentiate constipation from small bowel obstruction or ileus. With uncomplicated constipation, small bowel dilatation is rarely found.

Common causes of constipation include dehydration and either inadequate or excessive fiber in the diet.[7,28,65] To avoid dehydration, patients receiving EN require adequate fluid (see discussion of dehydration later in this chapter). Hydration may be problematic when a concentrated formula is needed for fluid restriction. If a patient has constipation and the usual hydration volume is contraindicated, the addition of a stool softener (docusate sodium or docusate calcium, or various emollients) and a laxative or cleansing enema may be considered. Chronic use of stimulants (eg, senna) often results in tachyphylaxis and is not indicated. Frequent rectal exams and abdominal radiographs may be required in patients with serious constipation.

Fiber helps propel waste through the colon, and inadequate fiber intake can result in infrequent bowel movements with significant buildup of waste in the colon. If fiber is added to the enteral regimen, administering a minimum of 1 mL of fluid per kcal enterally may help prevent solidification of waste in the colon and constipation. Patients often need additional fluid to facilitate regular stool output and minimize the chance of impaction. Inadequate physical activity can also contribute to constipation. Patients should ambulate whenever possible. Shorter-chain fibers are recommended for prevention of constipation in hemodynamically stable patients.[14]

A variant of constipation is *impaction*, a firm collection of stool in the distal colon (sigmoid colon or rectum). Liquid stool will seep around an impaction, occasionally at high volume. If impaction is near to the rectum, it can be diagnosed and may be treated by rectal examination. Impaction higher up in the sigmoid colon cannot be easily detected by examination, and a high level of clinical suspicion should be maintained in patients at risk. Impaction should be considered in patients, particularly older adults and patients who are bedbound, when stool volumes have been small and then become liquid. Impaction may be the cause of confusion and agitation in older adults.[66] Enemas, cathartics (sorbitol, lactulose), and even endoscopy may be required to treat severe impaction.

Finally, case reports[67] have described rare but life-threatening complications caused by intestinal bezoar associated with tube feeds that contain fiber. These bezoars may present insidiously as obstruction or bowel perforation, have been reported most often in severely ill patients for whom hypomotility is more likely, and can be, in the experience of one of the authors, fatal. SCCM/ASPEN guidelines recommend that fiber be avoided in patients who are not hemodynamically stable,[14] but the risk factors are not well understood.

Intestinal Ischemia

Intestinal ischemia has several etiologies and is rarely nutrition related; however, in case reports of ischemia in conjunction with EN,[68] nonocclusive bowel necrosis (NOBN) has been associated with a high degree of morbidity and possibly with death. Neonates, critically ill and immune-suppressed patients, and patients with a compromised gastric acid microbial barrier may be at greater risk for NOBN. Underlying factors possibly associated with NOBN include the use of jejunal feedings, hyperosmolar formulas, and feeding in the presence of hypotension, as well as disordered peristalsis. Typical signs of enteral feeding intolerance, including abdominal distention and nausea and vomiting, are common with NOBN, but the symptoms are nonspecific and may be observed in enterally fed patients in the intensive care unit (ICU) without NOBN. NOBN may present later in the patient's clinical course rather than shortly after enteral feeding initiation. In a review of NOBN among surgical patients, the mean day of diagnosis after EN initiation was Day 6 with a range from Day 4 to Day 18.[69]

Although it is difficult to predict who may develop NOBN in conjunction with enteral feedings, precautionary measures may be preventive. Delaying EN until the patient is fluid-resuscitated is likely of greatest importance. According to a review of case series reports of patients who developed NOBN, all reports cited the presence of hypotension and/or hypovolemia as precipitating factors.[68] Other considerations may include the initial use of an isotonic and fiber-free enteral formula. Ongoing monitoring of EN is essential because acute changes in abdominal assessment can prompt early recognition and treatment of NOBN. A patient who previously demonstrated enteral feeding tolerance and then develops abdominal distention, abdominal pain, and an acute change in nasogastric tube output should be fully evaluated.

Pulmonary Aspiration Complications

Pulmonary aspiration is defined as the inhalation of material into the airway. This problem is of concern in all patients, and its occurrence in those receiving EN has received considerable attention. The assumption is that patients could develop pneumonia if they inhale gastric contents and/or the tube feeding formula into the airway. However, while there is a strong association between tube feeding and pneumonia, and a stronger association between tube feeding and aspiration, causal relationships have not been established. In fact, pulmonary aspiration can be asymptomatic (silent aspiration), and aspiration of saliva is a normal phenomenon during sleep. In a 2-day study of 10 normal volunteers, half aspirated overnight.[70] In contrast, the incidence of pneumonia is low. In a report on US veterans, for example, the incidence of

community-acquired pneumonia was 4.4 cases of pneumonia per 1000 patient years.[71] Thus, aspiration seems to be a poor surrogate for pneumonia risk, given the disparity between the apparent incidence of aspiration and low incidence of pneumonia. On the other hand, it is incontrovertible that inhalation of significant volumes of vomitus is highly likely to be deleterious.

Chemical pneumonitis and/or pneumonia can result from pulmonary aspiration of significant volumes of enteral formula; however, aspiration of very small amounts of fluid alone is likely insufficient to cause pneumonia. The progression from aspiration to aspiration pneumonia is hard to predict and may depend on the quantity and acidity of the formula in addition to the particulates and contaminants in the formula. Age, immune status, and comorbidities also are likely to strongly influence the development of aspiration pneumonia.

When the quantity and acidity of the formula overwhelm either the patient's natural defense mechanisms or the patient's altered pulmonary defense mechanisms, pneumonia is more likely to occur. Acute symptoms of clinically significant aspiration include dyspnea, wheezing, frothy or purulent sputum, hypoxia, cyanosis, anxiety, and agitation. Patients can also have a fever, tachycardia, tachypnea, rhonchi and rales, leukocytosis, leukopenia, and a new or progressing infiltrate on chest film. When pneumonia develops in ventilated patients, it is labeled VAP. Aspiration and VAP are also discussed in Chapter 25.

Incidence and Risk Factors

Pulmonary aspiration of tube feeding formula is one of the most feared complications of EN support because it can lead to acute pulmonary pathology. Aspiration pneumonia may account for 5% to 15% of pneumonia in hospitalized patients,[72] but diagnostic criteria vary, and proving that aspiration was the cause of pneumonia is nearly impossible. In addition to pneumonia, potential complications of aspiration include pneumonitis, atelectasis, empyema, bronchitis, acute lung injury, and acute respiratory distress syndrome. However, relating pathologic respiratory developments to the aspiration of tube feeding formula is difficult because pulmonary aspiration can also occur when a patient inhales oropharyngeal and gastric secretions.

Reported incidence of aspiration in tube-fed patients varies and depends on the patient population studied and the technique and criteria used to identify aspiration. Investigations using advanced aspiration detection techniques have reported the presence of gastric contents in the tracheal secretions of 22% to 31% of critically ill, tube-fed patients.[73,74] These studies identified aspiration of gastric contents by detecting either pepsin (a major enzyme in gastric fluid) or yellow microscopic beads (added to tube feeding formula) in tracheal aspirates. When pepsin-positive secretions were used, Metheny et al identified low HOB elevation, vomiting, gastric tube feedings (as opposed to small bowel feedings), low Glasgow coma score, and GI reflux disease as risk factors for aspiration.[74] Patients with a higher number of pepsin-positive secretions and those with paralytic agents and high sedation levels were at higher risk for pneumonia, but a causal relationship was not proven.

Additional risk factors associated with an increased incidence of aspiration include a malpositioned feeding tube, transportation within the hospital, and inadequate nursing staff.[75,76]

Detection

No reliable method to detect pulmonary aspiration of tube feeding formula is currently available for routine clinical use. Radiographic findings are generally nonspecific and insensitive. However, after an episode of emesis and regurgitation of tube feeding formula, aspiration of feeding formula or vomitus can be presumed if a patient develops dyspnea, cyanosis, and agitation and there is evidence of a new infiltrate on chest film. Patients with dysphagia may aspirate saliva and develop aspiration pneumonia independent of the presence of gastric contents. Regardless of the underlying cause, aspiration is a medical urgency. Emergency measures may include sitting the patient upright, orotracheal suctioning, oxygen, and antibiotics.

Methods historically used to detect pulmonary aspiration of formula include tinting enteral formula with blue dye or checking tracheal secretions with glucose oxidase strips. These methods are unsatisfactory because they are neither sensitive nor specific.[74] Numerous problems surround the practice of tinting formulas. The dose of food coloring has never been standardized, and concerns about bacterial contamination, allergic reactions, and false-positive guaiac testing have been raised. More importantly, a Public Health Advisory issued by the US Food and Drug Administration on September 29, 2003, reported blue discoloration of body parts and fluids followed by refractory hypotension, metabolic acidosis, and death in patients receiving tube feedings containing Food Drug and Cosmetic Blue No. 1 dye.[77] Based on this report and the method's lack of sensitivity, specificity, or standardization, the practice of tinting enteral formulas should be abandoned.

Glucose oxidase strips can be used to detect a high glucose level in tracheal aspirates, which might indicate that the aspirates contain feeding formula. However, high tracheal concentrations of glucose can also be found in aspirates of nonfed patients and those with elevated blood glucose levels, as well as in aspirates that contain some blood.[78,79] A study using an animal model demonstrated a correlation between pepsin levels in tracheal aspirates and aspiration pneumonia, with a sensitivity of 90% and a specificity of 100%; however, this assay is not available for routine clinical use.[80]

Risk Assessment

Gastric Residual Volume

Because elevated GRVs can predict vomiting or reflux, clinicians have used GRV to determine the risk for aspiration. To measure GRV, the clinician withdraws or suctions fluid intermittently from enteral access devices with a syringe or by gravity drainage. Then, in the hope of preventing aspiration, tube feedings may be held when the GRV is determined to be too high. However, interpretation of GRVs is highly subjective and the accuracy of GRV measurements can be influenced by many factors, including the diameter and position of the tube tip,

the number and location of the tube's openings, the patient's position altering the level of stomach fluid, and the skill of the clinician.

Studies of the value of GRV measurement have reached conflicting conclusions. For example, Metheny and colleagues reported that frequent aspirators (ie, patients with greater than 40% pepsin-positive secretions) had a significantly higher incidence of GRVs of at least 200 mL times 2 or 250 mL times 1.[81] These investigators noted that aspiration can occur without high GRVs, but that it occurs more frequently when GRVs are high. Based on her research findings, Metheny encourages facilities to keep GRV checks in nursing protocols.[82] Conversely, McClave and associates found no correlation between GRVs greater than 200 mL or greater than 400 mL and aspiration in critically ill, mechanically ventilated patients receiving gastric tube feedings by either a nasogastric feeding tube or gastrostomy tube.[83] These investigators identified aspiration by the addition of yellow microscopic beads to the tube feeding formula and use of calorimetric fluoroscopy for detection in the tracheal aspirate, and they noted less aspiration with the gastrostomy tube feedings compared with the nasogastric tube feedings.

Other investigations have evaluated not obtaining GRV at all, holding gastric tube feedings for varying levels of GRV, re-instilling vs discarding of GRV and the frequency of GRV checks in relation to the incidence of VAP and non–ventilator pneumonia, rates of emesis/regurgitation, and the achievement of tube feeding volume goals in critically ill patients. Selected findings from such studies are reviewed here.

A "before and after" study at 1 hospital compared the effects of obtaining vs not obtaining GRVs in 205 critically ill, ventilated, medical patients who had an aggressive, nasogastric, continuous tube feeding schedule initiated within 48 hours of admission with the intent to reach goal feedings within 24 hours.[1] In the "before" group, GRVs were obtained every 6 hours and re-instilled if they were 250 mL or less. If the GRV were greater than 250 mL or emesis occurred, the tube feeding was decreased to the previous rate and intravenous (IV) erythromycin was initiated. In the "after" group, no GRVs were obtained and the protocol to lower the tube feeding rate and initiate IV erythromycin was used for emesis only. All patients had the HOB elevated 45°. The median daily volume of enteral feeding was significantly higher in the "after" group (1489 kcal/d vs 1381 kcal/d), and there were no differences in incidence of emesis (approximately 25% in each group) or VAP rates (19.6% in "before" group vs 18.4% in "after" group).

A more recent, prospective multicenter study also compared the effects of obtaining vs not obtaining GRVs. In this trial, 449 critically ill, ventilator-dependent patients (over 90% in the medical ICU) receiving nasogastric tube feedings were randomly assigned to GRV checks every 6 hours (control group) and no GRV checks (intervention group).[15] Tube feedings were initiated at goal rates within 36 hours after intubation. HOB was elevated 30° to 45°, and oral care with chlorhexidine was given every 6 to 8 hours. Up to 250 mL GRV was re-instilled in the control group. Intolerance was defined as GRV greater than 250 mL and/or vomiting in the control group and vomiting alone in the intervention group. There was significantly more vomiting in the intervention group (41.8% vs 26.5% of patients over the study period), perhaps because the control group received more erythromycin. Notably, VAP occurrence was similar in both groups (15.8% in control group vs 16.7% in intervention group). The proportion of patients that received 100% of their energy goal was reportedly higher in the intervention group, but the amounts of enteral formula lost through vomiting or residual discard were not measured and it is likely that energy intake was overestimated.

The prospective REGANE study investigated the consequences of using a higher GRV as the point at which tube feeding is held. The investigators randomly assigned 329 critically ill, ventilated patients (80% medical patients) receiving nasogastric tube feedings in multiple ICUs to holding feedings for 6 hours after a GRV equal to or greater than 200 mL (control group) vs a GRV equal to or greater than 500 mL (study group).[84] It was not reported whether any of the GRV was re-instilled. All patients had the HOB elevated 30° to 45° and received metoclopramide every 8 hours for the first 3 days of feedings. VAP rates were similar for both groups (27.3% in control group vs 28% in study group). The percentage of prescribed formula received was significantly higher in the study group but only for the first week (88.20% vs 84.48%). Some patients received PN to help meet nutrient needs.

A single-institution investigation of 122 surgical and medical ICU patients receiving nasogastric tube feedings studied the effects of re-instilling GRV vs discarding it. Participants were randomly assigned to the "return" or "discard" (control) group.[85] GRV checks were obtained every 6 hours, and the "return" group had up to 250 mL GRV re-instilled with the remaining volume discarded. GRV was completely discarded in the control group. All patients had the HOB elevated 30° to 45°, were on continuous tube feeding schedules, and received 40 mg omeprazole daily; some patients also received PN. Feedings were held if patients had GRV greater than 500 mL, experienced vomiting, had diarrhea for more than 48 hours, and underwent radiologic or surgical procedures. The "return" group had a significantly lower incidence of subsequent high GRV. The authors suggested that the re-instilling of the GRV may have an impact on gastric function by maintaining GRV at "closer physiological levels."[85] (The stomach empties intermittently, and a certain volume of fluid needs to be reached to promote gastric contractions and emptying.[86] The volume required to facilitate this process varies among individuals and is unknown.) The frequency of hyperglycemia in the "return" group was significantly higher.[85] No differences were found in obstruction of the nasally placed feeding tubes, intolerance episodes (nausea, vomiting, diarrhea and abdominal distention), discomfort episodes, or hypokalemic episodes. The authors reported no difference in enteral feeding delays (defined as >20% difference between feeding prescribed and amount administered per day), with the administered feeding averaging 89% of prescribed in the control group and 93% of prescribed in the intervention group, but the study did not account for feeding lost via discarded GRV. The authors stated that there was no difference in pulmonary aspiration between groups based on blood glucose levels in tracheal aspirates;[85] however, this method does not measure formula content, and it is therefore not useful for detection of tube feeding formula

aspiration.[87] This study suggests that re-instilling up to 250 mL GRV poses no additional risk for increased accumulation of gastric fluid levels or GI intolerance, but it did not address the incidence of pulmonary aspiration between groups.[85]

A single-institution, randomized controlled trial studied the frequency of GRV checks in 357 medical and surgical critically ill patients (98% on mechanical ventilation) receiving tube feedings by a nasogastric tube or a nasoenteric tube (with a concurrent nasogastric tube).[88] Tube feedings were administered by a continuous drip, and target feeding goals were to be achieved within Day 1 of ICU admission; some patients in the study received PN. All participants had GRV checks every 4 hours initially. The intervention group progressed to GRV checks every 8 hours once they tolerated the goal feeding volume for at least 4 hours (ie, GRV was less than the volume of the previous 2 hours' feeding). GRV checks continued every 4 hours in the control group. Up to 300 mL of GRV was re-instilled, and the remaining volume was discarded as per the facility's usual practice. If the GRV were greater than the volume of the previous 2 hours' feeding, prokinetics were considered and, in the intervention group, the frequency of GRV checks reverted, at least temporarily, to every 4 hours. Despite the aggressive early EN protocol, the percentage of subjects who received at least 80% of prescribed feeding volume was only 48% in the control group and 50% in the intervention group. The mean number of daily GRV checks was 5.4 for the control group and 3.4 for the intervention group. Incidence of regurgitation was significantly higher in the intervention group (3.6% vs 2.1%), but the incidence of pneumonia did not significantly differ between groups (14.1% in control group vs 13.2% in intervention group). Because regurgitation was increased in the intervention group, the investigators did not advocate decreasing the frequency of GRV checks.[88]

One review of GRV monitoring has addressed the evidence for and against monitoring.[89] It noted, with some important caveats, that recent prospective, randomized trials of critically ill, ventilator patients showed no benefit from adjusting EN based on GRV checks. Surgical and trauma patients, who are at higher risk for aspiration pneumonia, have not been fully evaluated. The authors also noted that in trials where enteral feedings continued despite elevated GRVs, strict protocols were employed to prevent gastric reflux and aspiration of contaminated oral secretions, including HOB elevation, regular oral decontamination, and use of prokinetic agents. They also pointed out that with the recent introduction of more aggressive, volume-based or top-down feeding protocols, GRV checks should be considered at least during the initial days of feeding and in patients at risk for enteral feeding intolerance. The review stressed the overall importance of viewing patient characteristics and the EN delivery strategy when designing protocols for the use or abolishment of GRV checks.

Alternate Techniques to Detect Delayed Gastric Emptying

Alternate techniques for detecting gastric emptying delays during enteral feedings are either experimental or of unproven value. Methods such as scintigraphy, the paracetamol absorption test, the carbon-isotope breath test, refractometry, ultrasound, and gastric impedance tend to be time-consuming, are difficult to perform at the bedside, and require standardization and validation in critically ill patients.[89,89a]

Minimizing Aspiration Risk

Since there is no reliable and standardized bedside method to determine gastric emptying, identifying patients at high risk for aspiration is difficult. However, preventive measures and protocols aimed at risk reduction have been tested with some benefits. For example, raising the HOB 30° to 45° during gastric feedings has been associated with decreased esophageal and pharyngeal reflux of gastric contents and a lowered incidence of aspiration pneumonia.[90] A written physician's order set for HOB elevation and the hourly recording of the bed angle on bedside flowsheets have been recommended to improve compliance.[91]

A protocol including HOB elevation of 30°, GRV checks every 4 hours, and prokinetics for those with elevated GRVs was studied in critically ill, mechanically ventilated patients being fed through nasally inserted feeding tubes.[92] The protocol used a decision tree to direct actions depending on amount of GRV obtained. When the GRV was greater than 200 mL, a prokinetic agent was to be given once and then repeated if GRV remained higher than 200 mL. If the GRV was equal to or greater than 200 mL after the prokinetic intervention, the EN delivery method was changed to a small bowel feeding tube. With this protocol in place, the practice of HOB elevation increased from 38% to 88% and the shift of patients to small bowel feeding tubes increased from 39% to 68%. Aspiration incidence decreased from 88% to 39%, and the occurrence of pneumonia decreased from 48% to 19%.

Juve-Udina and colleagues studied the effects of EN protocol use in medical and surgical ICU patients. The protocols included HOB elevation 30° to 45°, continuous tube feeding schedules, use of omeprazole, and the re-instillation of GRVs (up to 250 mL). The protocols also called for holding EN for GRVs greater than 500 mL, vomiting, or diarrhea for more than 48 hours. With these protocols, patients received 93% of prescribed EN, 93% of the GRVs were less than 150 mL, and 2.3% of patients had GRV greater than 250 mL. However, the study did not adequately address the incidence of pulmonary aspiration.[85]

Guidelines

SCCM/ASPEN 2016 guidelines suggest that GRVs should not be used as part of routine care to monitor ICU patients receiving EN. If ICUs still use GRVs, SCCM/ASPEN further recommend that clinicians avoid holding EN for GRVs less than 500 mL in the absence of other signs of feeding intolerance (quality of evidence: low).[14]

Guidelines recently published in other nations have not concurred with the SCCM/ASPEN recommendations. The 2013 Canadian critical care nutrition guidelines deem that abandoning GRV checks or using a 500-mL threshold is premature, question the external validity of the current trials, and suggest a GRV threshold of 250 to 500 mL.[93] The German Society for Nutritional Medicine (2013) proposes the omission of GRV checks in medical ICU patients as long as the medical team adjusts the enteral infusion as needed, such as when vomiting occurs. It recommends obtaining GRV checks in surgical ICU patients and adjusting the EN delivery rate when GRV reaches 200 mL.[94]

It may be advisable to follow different protocols for gastrostomy tubes, as opposed to nasal tubes. Gastrostomy tubes are positioned in the anterior abdomen and are unlikely to allow full withdrawal of stomach contents during GRV checks. A GRV of 100 mL or greater with a gastrostomy tube has been suggested as a prudent trigger for careful evaluation of the patient for GI symptoms.[83]

Prevention Methods

Tube-fed patients should be assessed for signs of tube feeding intolerance (eg, abdominal distention, feeling of fullness, discomfort, nausea, or emesis) at 4-hour intervals,[35] and measures should be implemented to reduce aspiration risk. These measures include HOB elevation of at least 30° to 45° or positioning the patient upright in a chair (if such positioning is contraindicated, consider the reverse Trendelenburg position), good oral care twice daily (with chlorhexidine in critically ill patients), continuous tube feeding schedules, use of minimal sedation techniques, and appropriate and timely oropharyngeal suctioning (eg, prior to lowering the HOB, deflating the cuff of endotracheal tubes, or extubation).

The American Academy of Critical-Care Nurses (AACN) advocates that clinicians check GRV every 4 hours to help determine tolerance to gastric tube feedings while also assessing patients for other signs of GI intolerance, such as nausea, emesis and abdominal distention and discomfort. AACN also recommends residual checks with both gastric or small bowel feeding tubes every 4 hours to help determine changes in tube placement.[95] Changes in the volume (and pH, if measurable) of aspirate can indicate movement of a feeding tube between the small bowel, stomach, and esophagus. Tube placement should also be checked by noting any change in the visible tube length or marking at nares/stoma every 4 hours,[95] as well as after emesis, coughing episodes, or events during which the tube was tugged. If tube placement is questionable, a radiograph should be obtained. Feeding tube position should be assessed with routine chest and abdominal radiographs. See Chapter 12 for additional discussion of the assessment of enteral tube placement.

Unless the patient is vomiting, GRVs up to 250 mL should be re-instilled to replace fluid, electrolytes, and feeding formula. Prokinetic agents and small bowel feedings should be considered for patients determined to be at high aspiration risk.[14] Continued study is required to delineate methods to assess risk of aspiration during tube feeding and to develop strategies to prevent this complication.

Metabolic Complications

EN, by itself, is unlikely to cause metabolic derangements, other than refeeding syndrome, or specific nutritional deficiencies. However, patients receiving EN are likely to have underlying conditions that predispose them to metabolic derangements (see Table 13-4).[16,96] The nutrition support

TABLE 13-4 Metabolic Complications of Enteral Nutrition

Problem	Possible Causes	Prevention or Therapy
Hypertonic dehydration	• Excessive fluid loss • Inadequate fluid intake • Concentrated (energy, protein) formula administered to a patient who cannot express thirst	• Monitor daily fluid I/O. • Monitor body weight daily.[a] • Estimate fluid losses.[b] • Monitor serum electrolytes, urine-specific gravity, BUN, and Cr daily.[c] • Provide enteral or IV fluid as indicated.
Overhydration	• Excessive fluid intake • Rapid refeeding • Catabolism of lean body mass with potassium loss • Refeeding syndrome • Renal, hepatic, or cardiac insufficiency	• Monitor I/O daily. • Assess fluid status daily. • Monitor body weight daily.[a] • Check aldosterone levels, which will be elevated with sodium retention. • Consider use of less-concentrated formula. • Diuretic therapy.
Hypokalemia	• Refeeding syndrome • Catabolic stress • Depleted body cell mass • Effect of ADH and aldosterone • Diuretic therapy • Excessive losses (diarrhea, NGT) • Metabolic alkalosis • Insulin therapy • Dilution	• Supplement potassium to normal before initiation of TF. • Monitor serum potassium daily until stable with patient at goal TF rate. • Supplement potassium and chloride. • Consider supplementation protocol.
Hyperkalemia	• Metabolic acidosis • Poor perfusion (eg, congestive heart failure) • Renal failure • Excessive potassium intake from TF, IV fluid, oral diet	• Correct acidosis, if possible; recheck serum potassium. • Correct serum potassium before initiation of TF, if possible. • Monitor serum potassium daily. • Treat cause of poor perfusion. • Potassium-binding resin, glucose, and/or insulin therapy. • Eliminate potassium from IV fluids; reduce potassium in TF and oral diet.
Hyponatremia	• Dilution, from elevated ADH levels • Hepatic, cardiac, or renal insufficiency • Reduced sodium intake relative to output • Depletion of total body sodium, extracellular mass, ECF, SIADH	• Consider addition of table salt to TF. • Monitor sodium level daily. • Assess fluid status. • Diuretic therapy, if indicated. • Fluid and/or sodium restriction.
Hypernatremia	• Inadequate fluid intake with increased fluid loss (sweating, osmotic diuresis) • Increased sodium intake (IV fluid)	• Monitor daily I/O. • Monitor electrolytes and BUN:Cr daily.[c] • Monitor body weight daily.[a] • Estimate fluid loss.[b] • Replace fluid loss via enteral or parenteral route to replete ECF.
Hypophosphatemia	• Refeeding syndrome • Excessive energy intake • Binding by epinephrine • Sucralfate, antacids • Insulin therapy	• Supplement phosphorus to achieve normal level before initiation of TF. • Monitor serum phosphorus daily and replete as necessary as clinical course changes. • Supplement phosphorus as sodium or potassium form, as clinically indicated, via enteral or parenteral route.

(continued)

TABLE 13-4 Metabolic Complications of Enteral Nutrition *(continued)*

Problem	Possible Causes	Prevention or Therapy
Hyperphosphatemia	• Renal insufficiency	• Phosphate-binder therapy.
Hypercapnia	• Overfeeding energy • Excessive carbohydrate provision in patient with respiratory dysfunction	• Choose TF product with lower phosphorus content. • Measure energy requirement via IC, if possible. • If IC is unavailable, provide maintenance energy needs only until hypercapnia resolves. • Provide appropriate balance of carbohydrate, protein, and fat; consider providing 30%–50% of total energy as fat.
Hypozincemia	• Excessive losses (NGT, protein-losing enteropathy, ostomy, wound)	• Supplement zinc via enteral or parenteral route.
Vitamin K deficiency	• Inadequate vitamin K intake • Prolonged use of low-fat or low–vitamin K formula • Antibiotic use, cirrhosis, malabsorption, pancreatic insufficiency	• Supplement vitamin K. • Consider probiotic agents. • Measure PT and PTT or INR daily until stable.
Thiamin deficiency	• Chronic alcoholism • Advanced age • Long-term malnutrition • Malabsorption • Antacid therapy • Dialysis	• Supplement thiamin for 3–7 days. • Consider addition of folate and multivitamin in cases of alcoholism or chronic disease.
Essential fatty acid deficiency	• Inadequate linoleic acid intake	• Provide ≥4% of energy needs as linoleic acid. • Add modular fat component to TF if needed. • Provide 5 mL safflower oil per day via enteral route.
Hyperglycemia	• Refeeding syndrome • Diabetes mellitus, sepsis, catabolism, trauma, or other disease states or conditions • Insulin resistance • Glucocorticoids • Excessive carbohydrate	• Correct serum glucose levels before initiation of TF, if possible. • Monitor serum glucose every 6 hours, or per protocol. • Treat underlying disease. • Maintain appropriate intervascular volume and hydration. • Provide OHA or insulin therapy as needed to maintain serum glucose as low as possible. • Consider providing 30%–50% of total energy as fat. • Consider use of a product with fiber.
Hypoglycemia	• Abrupt cessation of EN in a patient receiving OHA or insulin	• Monitor serum glucose every 6 hours, or per protocol. • Treat with glucose (IV or via tube) to increase serum level to >100 mg/dL. • Taper TF gradually.

ADH, antidiuretic hormone; BUN, blood urea nitrogen; Cr, creatinine; ECF, extracellular fluid; IC, indirect calorimetry; INR, international normalized ratio; I/O, intake/output; IV, intravenous; NGT, nasogastric tube; OHA, oral hypoglycemic agent; PT, prothrombin time; PTT, partial thromboplastin time; SIADH, syndrome of inappropriate antidiuretic hormone secretion; TF, tube feeding.
[a]Weight change >0.2 kg/d reflects change in ECF volume.
[b]Mild fluid loss = 3% weight decrease; moderate loss = 6% weight decrease; severe loss = 10% weight decrease.
[c]BUN:Cr is usually 1:10 in state of normal hydration.
Source: Data are from references 16 and 96.

regimen may be the sole source of nutrients, fluids, and electrolytes for the patient. Therefore, the nutrition support clinician must be well schooled in the underlying medical issues that may affect formula selection, the fluid and electrolyte prescription, and the response to feeding in previously starved or electrolyte-depleted patients. Nutrition support clinicians must work closely and as part of a team with the primary healthcare providers to set therapeutic goals and monitor the patient's progress.

Many people assume that patients receiving EN are at less risk for metabolic complications than those receiving PN (see Chapter 17). Certainly, PN carries greater potential for metabolic alterations because the content of individual nutrients can be manipulated in PN solutions and the formulation is administered intravenously. However, with the exception of hyperglycemia studies, few randomized controlled trials have compared the metabolic effects of EN vs PN or EN vs no intervention.[97] Therefore, it is unclear whether enteral feedings may cause metabolic alterations or if EN provides any advantage over PN with regard to metabolic complications.

Refeeding Syndrome

The potential for the serious electrolyte deficiencies associated with refeeding syndrome should be anticipated in all malnourished patients, especially those with large electrolyte losses. Patients at increased risk for refeeding syndrome include those with diarrhea, high-output fistulas, or vomiting (Table 13-5).[98] The frequency of refeeding syndrome with EN therapy has not been reported, but the syndrome may be life-threatening if it is uncorrected.

Refeeding syndrome, which has been reviewed extensively elsewhere,[99-101] occurs after nutrition formulas are started, but it may also arise in malnourished patients who are resuscitated with standard IV solutions containing dextrose. With refeeding syndrome, decrements in electrolyte levels may occur in a matter of hours and may lead to arrhythmias, respiratory and cardiac failure, aspiration, and death (see Chapter 17). Although refeeding syndrome is typically associated with the use of PN, its incidence in patients receiving EN has been well documented.[98,101,102] The nutrition support clinician should examine the patient's chart for previous episodes

TABLE 13-5 Risk Factors for Refeeding Syndrome

- Malnutrition
- Inadequate nutrition intake for >2 weeks
- Poorly controlled diabetes
- Cancer, both before and during treatment
- Anorexia nervosa
- Short bowel syndrome
- Inflammatory bowel disease
- Being an older adult living alone
- Low birth weight and premature birth
- Chronic infections (eg, HIV)

Source: Data are from reference 98.

of hypophosphatemia, hypomagnesemia, or hypokalemia because these abnormalities may suggest multiple, unrecognized electrolyte deficiencies.

Electrolyte deficiencies may occur in the presence of normal serum levels. For potassium, a total body deficit of approximately 80 mEq is required before serum levels drop below normal. All patients should be evaluated for refeeding risk prior to EN initiation, with the assessment including the factors outlined in Table 13-5,[49,98] and any electrolyte abnormalities should be corrected.[49] ASPEN recommends that EN for patients at risk for refeeding syndrome should provide only 25% of the energy goal on Day 1, with attention to the energy contribution from IV fluids, and then cautiously advanced toward the energy goal over the next 3 to 5 days as dictated by clinical status and/or stable electrolyte levels.[49]

Hyperglycemia

Hyperglycemia is more commonly associated with PN than EN. The enteral products developed to improve glycemic control are typically higher in fat and contain fiber, both to slow gastric emptying and decrease the glycemic index. These effects may not be desirable in acutely ill patients in whom antropyloric dysfunction (poor gastric emptying, gastroparesis) commonly complicates gastric feeding. Furthermore, absorption of glucose from continuous feeds is more affected by the rate of carbohydrate delivery than the glycemic index, because glycemic index refers to the rate of glucose increase after a bolus. Slow advancement of EN and close collaboration with the medical team should allow for adequate glucose control with standard feeding products. Glycemic control should be considered a primarily medical issue in the acutely ill patient. Diabetes-specific enteral products may help improve the ease of glycemic control in chronic care, but they have yet to be consistently proven to be of benefit in the acutely ill.[103-105] See Chapters 15 and 34 for further discussion of formula selection and glycemic control.

Dehydration

Dehydration is an excessive fluid volume deficit, which may be accompanied by sodium imbalance. It is caused by insufficient fluid intake (orally, by tube, or intravenously) and/or excessive fluid losses, such as from fever, diarrhea, vomiting, significant blood volume loss, chronic illness (eg, diabetes, kidney disease), overuse of diuretics, drainage tube or paracentesis losses, wound seepage, or high nasogastric, fistula, or ostomy outputs.

Dehydration is associated with an increased risk for falls, pressure ulcers, constipation, urinary tract infections, respiratory infections, and medication toxicities. Persistent dehydration can lead to delirium, renal failure, coma, and death.

Hospital-Acquired Dehydration

Hospital patients are at risk for dehydration and its complications. A retrospective investigation compared hospitalized US veterans between 1997 and 2000.[106] The overall development of dehydration in this group of patients was 3.5%. Mortality rates at 30 days and 6 months postdischarge were significantly higher (about double) for those patients who developed dehydration during their hospital stay compared with those who did not. For the patients who had volume-depleted dehydration, the mortality rate was 13.8% (vs 6.0% for controls) at 30 days and 29.3% (vs 14.7% for controls) at 6 months.

Risk Factors

Patients who are tube fed are at risk for dehydration. Enteral formulas alone typically do not meet total fluid needs; therefore, patients require additional water flushes. The risk for dehydration is greater in older adults. They have lower water reserves because of the decrease in lean body mass that occurs with aging. Other age-related changes that increase dehydration risk include altered sense of thirst, diminished cognition, dysphagia, dysgeusia, hyposmia, reduced kidney function, impairment of hormonal modulators of sodium and water balance (lowered aldosterone secretion, vasopressin release, and renin activity), and limitations in function.[107–109] Younger tube-fed patients with characteristics similar to those described for older adults, patients with chronic disease, and those at risk for adverse drug reactions are also at higher risk for dehydration.

Detection

Clinicians need to assess for multiple signs and symptoms to determine whether a patient is dehydrated. Early signs include dry mouth and eyes, thirst, light-headedness (especially when standing), headache, fatigue, loss of appetite, flushed skin, heat intolerance, and dark urine with a strong odor. Tongue dryness can be a simple, quick, reliable, cost-effective way to identify dehydration in the older adults, provided that other etiologies of dry mouth, such as diuretic and anticholinergic use, are ruled out.[110] Alternatively, moist mucous membranes without tongue furrows can help rule out dehydration.[110] Dehydrated patients usually develop orthostatic hypotension (a drop in systolic blood pressure of 20 mm Hg or more on standing) and a rise in pulse rate by at least 10 beats per minute. Signs of progressive dehydration include dysphagia, clumsiness, poor skin turgor (sternum: more than 2 seconds), sunken eyes with dim vision, painful urination, muscle cramps, and delirium.

Laboratory results for dehydrated patients usually show an elevation, relative to predehydration levels, in blood urea nitrogen (BUN), plasma osmolality, and hematocrit, whereas serum sodium levels can be elevated, low, or normal, depending on the etiology of the dehydration. In dehydration, the BUN level usually rises out of proportion to the usual BUN-to-creatinine ratio of 20:1. The BUN:creatinine ratio should be evaluated in the context of the patient's nutrition state and underlying renal function. Patients with low muscle mass have low creatinine concentrations. A rise in creatinine from 0.2 mg/dL to 0.4 mg/dL in a patient with severe loss of muscle mass signals a drop by 50% in glomerular filtration rate. BUN reflects protein intake as well as hydration and renal function. A patient with renal failure and no protein intake may have a normal or even low BUN concentration. A severely cachectic patient with renal failure with a creatinine level significantly lower than 1 mg/dL, a BUN level greater than 100 mg/dL, and a BUN:creatinine ratio greater than 100:1 might still be adequately hydrated.

An elevated urine-specific gravity (greater than 1.028) paired with low urine output usually reflects dehydration. Typical urine-specific gravity measurements are 1.010 to 1.025.[111] One report showed that assessment of hydration status by comparing urine color to a standardized color reference chart was comparable to urine-specific gravity and osmolality results.[112] When greater precision and accuracy in assessment are not required, clinicians may infer that tube-fed patients who achieve and maintain urine that is pale yellow or straw-colored are not dehydrated.

In hospitalized patients at risk for dehydration, fluid status can be tracked by strict intake and output measurements (including ostomy, fistula, liquid stool, drains, nasogastric tube, paracentesis outputs) and daily weights. The minimum urine output required to remove waste is 30 mL/h or about 700 mL/d. The urine output range for adults is typically 0.5 to 2.0 mL/kg/h,[113] and an output of at least 1 mL/kg/h is useful as a guideline for adequate urine output. When evaluating daily weight changes and intake and output volumes, clinicians can assume that 1 kg of weight change equals 1 liter of fluid. If a patient loses weight while total fluid output exceeds total fluid intake by more than 800 to 1000 mL/d (the volume equal to insensible losses from lungs, feces, and skin), dehydration may develop. However, higher urine outputs with concurrent weight loss are expected when fluid overload is resolving.

Prevention

Clinicians need to be attuned to the fluid needs of their tube-fed patients to be sure they are providing maintenance fluid needs and replacing any additional losses. Ongoing assessments are required, and fluid intake should be increased if a patient has a fever, emesis, diarrhea, high fistula and ostomy outputs, or hyperglycemia. For patients with fever, increase fluid intake by 12% per degree Celsius above 37.8°C.[113] If a patient misses a feeding, then the fluid content of that feeding should be replaced. At times, the replacement of large fluid losses cannot be accomplished via the GI tract. The clinician may then need to consider IV fluid therapy.

When a patient is being diuresed, the clinician must be watchful and determine when the patient achieves a euvolemic state and then initiate adequate fluids to prevent dehydration. The presence of edema, indicating total body fluid and salt overload, does not guarantee intravascular volume adequacy. Aggressive diuresis of an acutely ill patient may lead to low vascular volume, which may be difficult to detect but can lead to renal, cardiac, or other organ failure as well as hypoperfusion, and hypotension. Useful signs of intravascular volume depletion in acutely ill patients include an increased heart rate, decreased or more concentrated urine, and an increase in oxygen extraction (an increase in the difference between arterial and venous oxygen concentration). Chapter 7 discusses methods for estimating fluid requirements for patients receiving EN.

Conclusion

All interventions, including EN, involve risks. The potential complications of EN range from uncomfortable GI symptoms to life-threatening problems. Fortunately, careful assessment, use of evidence-based nutrition support protocols, and ongoing monitoring of patients receiving EN can help prevent many complications and spur prompt intervention when complications do occur.

References

1. Poulard F, Dimet J, Martin-Lefevre L, et al. Impact of not measuring residual gastric volume in mechanically ventilated patients receiving early enteral feeding: a prospective before-after study. *JPEN J Parenter Enteral Nutr.* 2010;34:125–130.

2. Montejo JC, Grau T, Acosta J, et al. Multicenter, prospective, randomized, single-blind study comparing the efficacy and gastrointestinal complications of early jejunal feeding with early gastric feeding in critically ill patients. *Crit Care Med.* 2002;30:796–800.

3. Heyland DK, Cahill NE, Dahliwal R, et al. Enhanced protein-energy provision via the enteral route in critically ill patients: a single center feasibility trial of the PEPuP protocol. *Crit Care.* 2010;14:R78.

4. Beyer PL. Complications of enteral nutrition. In: Matarese LE, Gottschlich MM, eds. *Contemporary Nutrition Support Practice: A Clinical Guide.* 2nd ed. Philadelphia, PA: Saunders; 1998:215–216.

5. Kozar RA, McQuiggan MM, Moore FA. Trauma. In: Merritt RM, ed. *The A.S.P.E.N. Nutrition Support Practice Manual.* Silver Spring, MD: American Society for Parenteral and Enteral Nutrition; 2005:271–276.

6. Malone AM, Brewer CK. Monitoring for efficacy, complications and toxicity. In: Rolandelli RH, ed. *Clinical Nutrition: Enteral and Tube Feeding.* 4th ed. Philadelphia, PA: Saunders; 2005:276–290.

7. Vickery G. Basics of constipation. *Gastroenterol Nurs.* 1997;20:125–128.

8. Davies A, Prentice W. Fentanyl, morphine, and constipation. *J Pain Sympt Manage.* 1998;16:141–144.

9. Ukleja A. Altered GI motility in critically Ill patients: current understanding of pathophysiology, clinical impact, and diagnostic approach. *Nutr Clin Pract.* 2010;25:16–25.

10. Ali T, Hasan M, Hamadani M, et al. Gastroparesis. *South Med J.* 2007;100:281–286.

11. Taylor SJ, Manara AR, Brown J. Treating delayed gastric emptying in critical illness: metoclopramide, erythromycin, and bedside (cortrak) nasointestinal tube placement. *JPEN J Parenter Enteral Nutr.* 2010; 34:289–294.

12. Rhoney DH, Parker D, Formea CM, et al. Tolerability of bolus versus continuous gastric feeding in brain-injured patients. *Neurol Res.* 2002;24:613–620.

13. Sidery MB, Macdonald IA, Blackshaw PE. Superior mesenteric artery blood flow and gastric emptying in humans and the differential effects of high fat and high carbohydrate meals. *Gut.* 1994;35:186–190.

14. McClave SA, Taylor BE, Martindale RG, et al. Guidelines for the provision and assessment of nutrition support therapy in the adult critically ill patient: Society of Critical Care Medicine (SCCM) and American Society for Parenteral and Enteral Nutrition (A.S.P.E.N.). *JPEN Parenter Enteral Nutr.* 2016;40(2):159–211.

15. Reignier J, Mercier E, Le Gouge A, et al; Clinical Research in Intensive Care and Sepsis (CRICS) Group. Effect of not monitoring residual gastric volume on risk of ventilator-associated pneumonia in adults receiving mechanical ventilation and early enteral feeding. *JAMA.* 2013;309(3):249–256.

16. Ideno KT. Enteral nutrition. In: Gottschlich MM, Matarese LM, Shronts EP, eds. *Nutrition Support Dietetics Core Curriculum.* 2nd ed. Silver Spring, MD: American Society for Parenteral and Enteral Nutrition; 1993:98–99.

17. Wall-Alonso E, Sullivan MM, Byrne TA. Gastrointestinal and pancreatic disease. In: Matarese LE, Gottschlich MM, eds. *Contemporary Nutrition Support Practice: A Clinical Guide.* 2nd ed. Philadelphia, PA: Saunders; 2003:412–444.

18. Seres DS, Ippolito PR Pilot study evaluating the efficacy, tolerance and safety of a peptide-based enteral formula versus a high protein enteral formula in multiple ICU settings (medical, surgical, cardiothoracic). *Clin Nutr.* 2016;36(3):706–709. doi:10.1016/j.clnu.2016.04.016.

19. Russell MK. Monitoring and complications. In: Charney P, Malone A, eds. *ADA Pocket Guide to Enteral Nutrition.* Chicago, IL: American Dietetic Association, 2005:189–209.

20. Wiesen P, Van Gossum A, Preiser JC. Diarrhoea in the critically ill. *Curr Opin Crit Care.* 2006;12:149–154.

21. Brito-Ashurst I, Preiser JC. Diarrhea in critically ill patients: the role of enteral feeding. *JPEN J Parenter Enteral Nutr.* 2016;40:913–923.

22. Williams MS, Harper R, Magnuson B, et al. Diarrhea management in enterally fed patients. *Nutr Clin Pract.* 1998;13:225–229.

23. Ferrie S, East V. Managing diarrhea in intensive care. *Aust Crit Care.* 2007;20:7–13.

24. deBrito-Ashurst I, Preiser JC. Diarrhea in critically ill patients: the role of enteral nutrition. *JPEN J Parenter Enteral Nutr.* 2016;40(7):913–923.

25. McCarthy MS, Fabling JC, Bell DE. Drug–nutrient interactions. In: Shikora SA, Martindale RG, Schwaitzberg SD, eds. *Nutrition Considerations in the Intensive Care Unit: Science, Rationale and Practice.* Dubuque, IA: Kendall-Hunt; 2002:153–171.

26. Reese JL, Means ME, Hanrahan K, et al. Diarrhea associated with nasogastric feedings. *Oncol Nurs Forum.* 1996;23:59–68.

27. Kely TW, Patrick MR, Kely TW, Patrick MR, Hillman KM. Study of diarrhea in critically ill patients. *Crit Care Med.* 1983;11:7–9.

28. Edes TE, Walk BE, Austin JL. Diarrhea in tube-fed patients: feeding formula is not necessarily the cause. *Am J Med.* 1990;88:91–93.

29. Monturo CA. Diarrhea in patients receiving enteral nutrition. *Oncol Nurs Forum.* 1995;22:1288.

30. Ratnaike RN, Jones TE. Mechanisms of drug-induced diarrhea in the elderly. *Drugs Aging.* 1998;13(3):245–253.

31. Bartlett JG. Antibiotic-associated diarrhea. *N Engl J Med.* 2002; 346:334–339.

32. Fine KD, Krejs GJ, Fordtran JS. Diarrhea. In: Sleisenger MH, Fordtran JS, eds. *Gastrointestinal Disease: Pathophysiology, Diagnosis, Management.* 5th ed. Philadelphia, PA: Saunders; 1995:1043.

33. Keohane PP, Attrill H, Love M, et al. Relationship between osmolality of diet and gastrointestinal side effects in enteral nutrition. *BMJ.* 1984;288:678–680.

34. Gottschlich MM, Warden GD, Michel M, et al. Diarrhea in tube fed burn patients: incidence, etiology, nutritional impact, and prevention. *JPEN J Parenter Enteral Nutr.* 1988;12:338–345.

35. Escuro AA, Hummell AC. Enteral formulas in nutrition support practice: is there a better choice for your patient? *Nutr Clin Pract.* 2016;31:709–722. doi:10.1177/0884533616668492.

36. Ford EG, Hull SF, Jennings LM, Andrassy RJ. Clinical comparison of tolerance to elemental or polymeric enteral feedings in the postoperative patient. *J Am Coll Surg.* 1992;11:11–16.

37. Heimburger DC, Geels VJ, Bilbrey J, Redden DT, Keeney G. Effects of small-peptide and whole-protein enteral feedings on

serum proteins and diarrhea in critically ill patients: a randomized trial. *JPEN J Parenter Enteral Nutr.* 1997;21:162–167.

38. Spapen H, Diltoer M, Van Malderen C, et al. Soluble fiber reduces the incidence of diarrhea in septic patients receiving total enteral nutrition: a prospective, double-blind, randomized, and controlled trial. *Clin Nutr.* 2001;20(4):301–305.

39. Rushdi TA, Pichard C, Khater YH. Control of diarrhea by fiber-enriched diet in ICU patients on enteral nutrition: a prospective randomized controlled trial. *Clin Nutr.* 2004;23(6):1344–1352.

40. Yang G, Wu XT, Zhou Y, Wang YL. Application of dietary fiber in clinical enteral nutrition: a meta-analysis of randomized controlled trials. *World J Gastroenterol.* 2005;11:3935–3938.

41. Greenwood J. Critical Care Nutrition at the Clinical Evaluation Research Unit. Study tools: management of diarrhea algorithm. 2010. www.criticalcarenutrition.com/docs/tools/Diarrhea.pdf. Accessed June 4, 2017.

42. Sabate JM, Coupaye M, Castel B, et al. Consequences of small intestinal bacterial overgrowth in obese patients before and after bariatric surgery. *Obes Surg.* 2017;27(3):599–605. doi:10.1007/s11695-016-2343-5.

43. Schiller LR, Sellin JH. Diarrhea. In: Feldman M, Friedman LS, Brandt LJ, eds. *Gastrointestinal and Liver Disease.* 10th ed. Philadelphia, PA: Saunders; 2016:221–241.

44. Hecht GA, Gaspar J, Malespin M. Approach to the patient with diarrhea. In: Podolsky DK, Camilleri M, Fitz JG, et al, eds. *Yamada's Textbook of Gastroenterology.* Oxford, UK: Wiley; 2015:735–757.

45. Bliss DZ, Johnson S, Savik K, et al. Acquisition of *Clostridium difficile* and *Clostridium difficile*-associated diarrhea in hospitalized patients receiving tube feeding. *Ann Intern Med.* 1998;129:1012–1019.

46. Anderton A. Bacterial contamination of enteral feeds and feeding systems. *Clin Nutr.* 1993;12(Suppl 1):16–32.

47. Okuma T, Nakamura M, Totake H, et al. Microbial contamination of enteral feeding formulas and diarrhea. *Nutrition.* 2000;16:719–722.

48. Anderton A, Nwoguh CE, McKune I, et al. A comparative study of the numbers of bacteria present in enteral feeds prepared and administered in hospital and the home. *J Hosp Infect.* 1993;23:43–49.

49. Boullata J, Carrera AL, Harvey L, et al. ASPEN safe practices for enteral nutrition therapy. *JPEN J Parenter Enteral Nutr.* 2017;41:15–103.

50. Perry J, Stankorb SM, Salgueiro M. Microbial contamination of enteral feeding products in thermoneutral and hyperthermal ICU environments. *Nutr Clin Pract.* 2015;30(1):128–133.

51. Fagerman KE. Limiting bacterial contamination of enteral nutrient solutions: 6-year history with reduction of contamination at two institutions. *Nutr Clin Pract.* 1992;7:31–36.

52. Kohn CL. The relationship between enteral formula contamination and length of enteral delivery set usage. *JPEN J Parenter Enteral Nutr.* 1991;15:567–571.

53. Lyman B, Gebhards S, Hensley C, Roberts C, San Pablo W. Safety of decanted enteral formula hung for 12 hours in a pediatric setting. *Nutr Clin Pract.* 2011;26(4):451–456.

54. Vanek V. Closed versus open enteral delivery systems: a quality improvement study. *Nutr Clin Pract.* 2000;15:234–243.

55. Wagner DR, Elmore MF, Knoll DM. Evaluation of "closed" versus "open" systems for the delivery of peptide-based enteral diets. *JPEN J Parenter Enteral Nutr.* 1994;18:453–457.

56. Beattie TK, Anderton A. Microbiological evaluation of four enteral feeding systems which have been deliberately subjected to faulty handling procedures. *J Hosp Infect.* 1999;42:11–20.

57. McKinlay J, Wildgoose A, Wood W, Gould IM, Anderton A. The effect of system design on bacterial contamination of enteral tube feeds. *J Hosp Infect.* 2001;47(2):138–142.

58. Mathus-Vliegen EMH, Bredius WJ, Binnekade JM. Analysis of sites of bacterial contamination in an enteral feeding system. *JPEN J Parenter Enteral Nutr.* 2006;30(6):519–525.

59. Moffitt SK, Gohman SM, Sass KM, et al. Clinical and laboratory evaluation of a closed enteral feeding system under cyclic feeding conditions: a microbial and cost evaluation. *Appl Nutr Invest.* 1997;13:622–628.

60. Payne-James JJ, Rana SK, Bray MJ, et al. Retrograde (ascending) bacterial contamination of enteral diet administration systems. *JPEN J Parenter Enteral Nutr.* 1992;16(4):369–373.

61. Matlow A, Jacobson M, Wray R, et al. Enteral tube hub as a reservoir for transmissible enteric bacteria. *Am J Infect Control.* 2006;34:131–133.

62. Solseng T, Vinson H, Gibbs P, Greenwald B. Biofilm growth on the Lopez enteral feeding valve cultured in enteral nutrition: potential implications for medical-surgical patients, nursing care and research. *Med Surg Nurs.* 2009;18(4):225–233.

63. Whelan K, Judd PA, Tuohy KM, et al. Fecal microbiota in patients receiving enteral feeding are highly variable and may be altered in those who develop diarrhea. *Am J Clin Nutr.* 2009;89(1):240–247.

64. Ho SS, Tse MM, Boost MV. Effect of an infection control program on bacterial contamination of enteral feed in nursing homes. *J Hosp Infect.* 2012;82(1):49–55.

65. Wong K. The role of fiber in diarrhea management. *Support Line.* 1998;20:16–20.

66. Obokhare I. Fecal impaction: a cause for concern? *Clin Colon Rectal Surg.* 2012;25:53–58.

67. McIvor AC, Meguid MM, Curtas S, Warren J, Kaplan DS. Intestinal obstruction from cecal bezoar: a complication of fiber-containing tube feedings. *Nutrition.* 1990;6(1):115–117.

68. Marvin RG, McKinley BA, McQuiggan M, et al., Nonocclusive bowel necrosis occurring in critically ill trauma patients receiving enteral nutrition manifests no reliable clinical signs for early detection. *Am J Surg.* 2000;179:7–12.

69. Spalding DR, Behranwala KA, Straker P, et al. Non-occlusive small bowel necrosis in association with feeding jejunostomy after elective upper gastrointestinal surgery. *Ann R Coll Surg Engl.* 2009;91: 477–482.

70. Gleeson K, Eggli DF, Maxwell SL. Quantitative aspiration during sleep in normal subjects. *Chest.* 1997;111(5):1266–1272.

71. McLaughlin JM, Johnson MH, Kagan SA, Baer SL, Clinical and economic burden of community-acquired pneumonia in the Veterans Health Administration, 2011: a retrospective cohort study. *Infection.* 2015;43(6):671–680. doi:10.1007/s15010-015-0789-3.

72. DiBardino DM, Wunderink RG. Aspiration pneumonia: a review of modern trends. *J Crit Care.* 2015;30(1)40-48.

73. McClave SA, Lukan JK, Stefater JA, et al. Poor validity of residual volumes as a marker for risk of aspiration in critically ill patients. *Crit Care Med.* 2005;33(2):324–330.

74. Metheny N, Clouse RE, Chang YH, et al. Tracheobronchial aspiration of gastric contents in critically ill tube-fed patients: frequency, outcomes and risk factors. *CCM.* 2006;34(4):1007–1015.

75. Kollef MH, Von Harz B, Prentice D, et al. Patient transport from intensive care increases the risk of developing ventilator-associated pneumonia. *Chest.* 1997;112:765–773.

76. Amaravadi RK, Dimick JB, Pronovost PJ, et al. IC nurse-to-patient ratio is associated with complications and resource use after esophagectomy. *Intensive Care Med.* 2000;26:1857–1862.

77. US Food and Drug Administration. FDA Public Health Advisory: subject: reports of blue discoloration and death in patients receiving enteral feedings tinted with the dye, FD&C Blue No. 1. September 29, 2003. https://www.fda.gov/forindustry/coloradditives/coloradditivesinspecificproducts/inmedicaldevices/ucm142395.htm. Accessed June 30, 2017.

78. Kinsey GC, Murray MJ, Swensen SJ, et al. Glucose content of tracheal aspirates: implications for the detection of tube feeding aspiration. *Crit Care Med.* 1994;22(10):1557–1562.

79. Metheny N, Dahms T, Stewart B, et al. Verification of inefficacy of the glucose method in detecting aspiration associated with tube feedings. *Med Surg Nurs.* 2005;14:112–121.

80. Metheny NA, Dahms TE, Chang YH, et al. Detection of pepsin intratracheal secretions after forced small-volume aspirations of gastric juice. *JPEN J Parenter Enteral Nutr.* 2004;28:79–84.

81. Metheny NA, Schallom L, Oliver DA, et al. Gastric residual volume and aspiration in critically ill patients receiving gastric feedings. *Am J Crit Care.* 2008;17(6):512–519.

82. Metheny NA. Residual volume measurement should be retained in enteral feeding protocols. *Am J Crit Care.* 2009;17(1):62–64.

83. McClave SA, Lukan JK, Stefater JA, et al. Poor validity of residual volumes as a marker for risk of aspiration in critically ill patients. *Crit Care Med* 2005;33:324–330.

84. Montejo JC, Minambres E, Bordeje L, et al. Gastric residual volume during enteral nutrition in ICU patients: the REGANE study. *Intensive Care Med.* 2010;36:1386–1393.

85. Juve-Udina ME, Valls-Miro C, Carreno-Granero A, et al. To return or to discard? Randomized trial on gastric residual volume management. *Intensive Crit Care Nurs.* 2009;25:258–267.

86. Williams TA, Leslie G, Mills L, et al. Frequency of aspirating gastric tubes for patients receiving enteral nutrition in the ICU: a randomized controlled trial. *JPEN J Parenter Enteral Nutr.* 2014;38(7):809–816.

87. Rice TW. Gastric residual volume: end of an era. *JAMA.* 2013;309(3):283–284.

88. Williams TA, Leslie GD. Should gastric aspirate be discarded or retained when gastric residual volume is removed from gastric tubes? *Austral Critical Care.* 2010;23(4):215–217.

89. Elke G, Felbinger, TW, Heyland, DK. Gastric residual volume in critically ill patients: a dead marker or still alive? *Nutr Clin Pract.* 2015;30(1):59–71.

89a. Moreira TV, McQuiggan M. Methods for the assessment of gastric emptying in critically ill, enterally fed adults. *Nutr Clin Pract.* 2009;24(2):261–273.

90. Metheny NA, Frantz RA. Head-of-bed elevation in critically ill patients: a review. *Crit Care Nurs.* 2013;33:53–65.

91. Metheny NA. Effectiveness of an aspiration risk-reduction protocol. *Nurs Res.* 2010;59(1):18–25.

92. Drakulovic MB, Torres A, Bauer TT, et al. Supine body position as a risk factor for nosocomial pneumonia in mechanically ventilated patients: a randomized trial. *Lancet.* 1999;354(9193):1851–1858.

93. Dhaliwal R, Cahill N, Lemieux M, Heyland DK. The Canadian critical care nutrition guidelines in 2013: an update on current recommendations and implementation strategies. *Nutr Clin Pract.* 2014;29:29–43.

94. Hartl WH, Parhofer KG, Kuppinger D, Rittler P; German Society for Nutritional Medicine (DGEM) Steering Committee. S3-guideline of the German Society for Nutritional Medicine (DGEM) in cooperation with the GESKES and the AKE monitoring of artificial nutrition: specific aspects. *Aktuel Ernahrungsmed.* 2013;38:e90–e100.

95. AACN Clinical Resources Task Force. AACN practice alert. Prevention of aspiration in adults. *Crit Care Nurs.* 2016;36(1):e20–e24.

96. Lord L, Trumbore L, Zaloga G. Enteral nutrition implementation and management. In: Merritt RM, Souba WW, Kohn-Keeth C, et al, eds. *The A.S.P.E.N. Nutrition Support Practice Manual.* Silver Spring, MD: American Society for Parenteral and Enteral Nutrition; 1998:5.10–5.14.

97. Braunschweig CL, Levy P, Sheean PM, Wang X. Enteral compared with parenteral nutrition: a meta-analysis. *Am J Clin Nutr.* 2001;74:534–542.

98. Patel U, Sriram K. Acute respiratory failure due to refeeding syndrome and hypophosphatemia induced by hypocaloric enteral nutrition. *Nutrition.* 2009;25:364–367.

99. Crook MA, Hally V, Panteli JV, et al. The importance of the refeeding syndrome. *Nutrition.* 2001;17:632–637.

100. Brooks MJ, Melnik G. The refeeding syndrome: an approach to understanding its complications and preventing its occurrence. *Pharmacotherapy.* 1995;15:713–726.

101. Khan LU, Ahmed J, Khan S, Macfie J. Refeeding syndrome: a literature review. *Gastroenterol Res Pract.* 2011;(2011):410971. doi:10.1155/2011/410971.

102. Lubart E, Leibovitz A, Dror Y, et al., Mortality after nasogastric tube feeding initiation in long-term care elderly with oropharyngeal dysphagia—the contribution of refeeding syndrome. *Gerontology.* 2009;55:393–397.

103. Academy of Nutrition and Dietetics Evidence Analysis Library. Enteral Nutrition and Diabetes. https://www.andeal.org/topic.cfm?menu=5302&cat=1491 Accessed June 29, 2017.

104. Elia M, Ceriello A, Laube H, et al. Enteral nutritional support and use of diabetes-specific formulas for patients with diabetes: a systematic review and meta-analysis. *Diabetes Care.* 2005;28:2267–2279.

105. Mesejo A, Montejo-Gonzalez JC, Vaquerizo-Alonso C, et.al. Diabetes-specific enteral nutrition formula in hyperglycemic, mechanically ventilated, critically ill patients: a prospective, open-label, blind-randomized, multicenter study. *Crit Care.* 2015;19:390–403.

106. Wakefield BJ, Mentes J, Holman JE, et al. Postadmission dehydration: risk factors, indicators, and outcomes. *Rehabil Nurs.* 2009;34(5):209–216.

107. Feinsod F, Levenson M, Rapp SA, et al. Dehydration in frail, older residents in long-term care facilities. *J Am Med Dir Assoc.* 2004;5(Suppl 2):S35–S41.

108. Xiao H, Barber J, Campbell ES. Economic burden of dehydration among hospitalized elderly patients. *Am J Health-Syst Pharm.* 2004;61:2534–2540.

109. Vivanti A, Harvey K, Ash S. Developing a quick and practical screen to improve the identification of poor hydration in geriatric and rehabilitative care. *Arch Gerontol Geriatr.* 2010;50:156–164.

110. McGee S, Abernethy WB, Simel DL. The rational clinical examination: is this patient hypovolemic? *JAMA.* 1999;281:1022–1029.

111. Armstrong LE, Maresh CM, Castellani JW, et al. Urinary indices of hydration status. *Int J Sport Nutr.* 1994;4:265–279.

112. Wakefield B, Mentes J, Diggelmann L, et al. Monitoring hydration status in elderly veterans. *West J Nurs Res.* 2002;24(2):132–142.

113. The Merck Manual. Dehydration in children. www.merckmanuals.com/professional/print/sec20/ch293/ch293b.html. Accessed July 4, 2011.

14 Overview of Parenteral Nutrition

Jay M. Mirtallo, MSc, RPh, BCNSP, FASHP, FASPEN

CONTENTS

Acknowledgments: Meera Patel, PharmD, BCPS, was a coauthor of this chapter for the second edition.

Objectives

1. Determine the appropriate indications for parenteral nutrition (PN).
2. Decide the best PN route based on the patient's nutrition, metabolic, and clinical status.
3. Initiate and manage PN therapy.
4. Describe the effects of PN on patient outcomes.

Test Your Knowledge Questions

1. What is the optimal nutrition support for a malnourished patient when enteral nutrition (EN) is not feasible for a prolonged period?
   A. Central parenteral nutrition (CPN)
   B. Nasogastric enteral tube feedings
   C. Postpyloric enteral tube feedings
   D. Peripheral parenteral nutrition (PPN)
2. In which patient condition or treatment could PN elicit an improved patient outcome?
   A. Cancer chemotherapy
   B. Preoperative care of surgery patients with upper gastrointestinal (GI) cancer
   C. Allogeneic bone marrow transplantation
   D. Critical illness

3. CPN is contraindicated in which of the following conditions?
   A. Do not resuscitate (DNR) status
   B. Peritonitis
   C. Intestinal hemorrhage
   D. High-output fistulas
4. PN should be discontinued when which of the following criteria are met?
   A. A clear liquid diet is ordered.
   B. Tube feeding is initiated at 10% of goal rate.
   C. Solid food is well tolerated by mouth.
   D. Advancement to a regular diet is poorly tolerated.

Test Your Knowledge Answers

1. The correct answer is **A**. The benefits of CPN are more closely associated with patients with malnutrition, although those benefits have not been consistently shown.[1] Newer studies of the impact of PN on malnourished cancer patients' body composition (2010)[2] and performance scores (2011)[3] provide a perspective of PN on outcomes not currently considered in American Society for Parenteral and Enteral Nutrition (ASPEN) guidelines (2009)[4] that may expand the role of CPN in clinical practice.

2. The correct answer is **B**. A review of PN literature has reported improved outcomes in patients with upper GI tract malignancies when PN is initiated 7 days before surgery.[5] An early report of a decrease in length of stay and infectious complications in allogeneic bone marrow transplant patients receiving PN has not been confirmed.[6] A review of published data on the use of PN in cancer chemotherapy, in the perioperative period, and during critical illness reports no positive effect of PN on clinical outcomes and a significant increase in infectious complications in patients randomly assigned to PN therapy as compared with those receiving no nutrition support.[5]

3. The correct answer is **A**. Trujillo and colleagues[7] abstracted indications for PN from the 1993 ASPEN guidelines as peritonitis, intestinal hemorrhage, intestinal obstruction, intractable vomiting, paralytic ileus, severe pancreatitis, stool output greater than 1 L/d, high-output fistulas, short bowel syndrome, and bone marrow recipients. PN therapy was contraindicated for patients who were classified as well nourished and had inadequate EN for less than 7 days; patients who had a DNR status and were deemed to warrant comfort measures only or were terminally ill; and those receiving adequate EN.

4. The correct answer is **C**. The goal of PN therapy is to maintain the nutrition status of the patient until some form of EN is tolerated. Critically ill patients whose therapy is withdrawn during the terminal stages of their disease process are the exception to this goal. In most other situations, GI function returns or appropriate enteral access is obtained, and PN is tapered as the amount of reliable enteral intake increases. PN support may be discontinued when patients can tolerate solid food by mouth, unless advanced age, debilitation, malignancy, or cultural food practices complicate the transition to oral intake. In those circumstances, a detailed transitional feeding plan should be established.[8]

Background

A successful infusion of hypertonic parenteral nutrients by Dudrick and colleagues[9] in the late 1960s was a major advancement in providing nutrition to patients with a nonfunctioning GI tract. Although intravenous (IV) nutrition has been of interest since the 17th century,[10,11] Dudrick et al were interested in "patients seriously depleted of protein and in whom it was known that operation would carry an increased risk of various complications, both infectious and non-infectious."[11] Initially, challenges to providing PN therapy included selecting sources of safe IV nutrients and establishing adequate venous access for hypertonic nutrient administration. Venous access problems were resolved by subclavian vein catheterization use, which minimized thrombotic complications associated with peripheral PN infusions (see Chapter 16). Early PN formulations consisted of dextrose and protein hydrolysates of either casein or fibrin. Protein hydrolysates were replaced by newer, crystalline amino acids, which are better utilized and lack preformed ammonia. Lipid injectable emulsions (ILEs) were not available in the United States until the 1970s and were used primarily as a source of essential fatty acids. It was not until the 1980s that ILEs were routinely used as an energy source. This development coincided with approval by the US Food and Drug Administration for fat emulsions to be compounded in the same container as other IV nutrients. Such a formulation is commonly referred to as a *3-in-1 admixture* or *total nutrient admixture* (TNA).

PN has been used in several clinical situations. When PN was first used, it was shown to provide a significant benefit to patients with GI fistulas who were unable to ingest nutrients by mouth.[11] Home PN has become a lifeline for patients with short bowel syndrome, allowing them to resume a nearly normal lifestyle (see Chapter 30). New knowledge and technology have improved patient selection for PN, whereas individualized therapies and improved PN techniques have improved the safety of this therapy. The refinement of PN will continue to make it a useful therapy for patients with complex diseases whose GI tracts are nonfunctional.

The parenteral feeding formulation is a complex mixture containing up to 40 different chemical (nutrient) components that may cause problems with stability and compatibility (see Chapter 15). Serious harm and death have resulted from improperly compounded parenteral feeding formulations. Two deaths were attributed to the infusion of calcium phosphate precipitates, resulting from an improper admixture process.[12] Other complications, such as venous catheter infections, hepatobiliary disease, and glucose disorders, have contributed to patient morbidity (see Chapters 16 and 17).[13,14] The risks of complications can be minimized through careful patient selection and by having knowledgeable clinicians oversee the specialized nutrition support program. Nehme[15] reports that patients whose PN was managed by an interdisciplinary team had significantly reduced metabolic, fluid, and electrolyte complications as compared with patients managed by individual clinicians. In Nehme's report, 8 of 11 patients with hyperglycemic, nonketotic dehydration and 2 of 7 patients with rebound hypoglycemia died in the group managed by individual clinicians, whereas no deaths occurred in the group managed by the interdisciplinary team.

Interdisciplinary teams are also more likely to follow ASPEN guidelines regarding the use of PN.[7]

The benefit of PN in various conditions continues to be debated. Its use warrants a thorough evaluation of risks and benefits. The benefits can be difficult to determine because the patient's underlying disease process often affects measurable outcomes more than PN does.

Routes of Infusion

The components of a parenteral feeding formulation determine its osmolarity and infusion route. PN may be prepared for peripheral venous infusion or infusion through a central venous access device. PN may also be prepared as a TNA or a 2-in-1 solution. The latter contains all necessary IV macronutrients and micronutrients in the same container except ILE, which may be infused separately (see Chapter 15).

Parenteral feeding formulations are hypertonic to body fluids and, if administered inappropriately, may result in venous thrombosis, suppurative thrombophlebitis, or extravasation. Specifically, the osmolarity of a parenteral feeding formulation is primarily dependent on the dextrose, amino acid, and electrolyte content. Dextrose contributes approximately 5 mOsm/g; amino acids yield approximately 10 mOsm/g; and electrolytes provide approximately 1 mOsm per mEq of individual electrolyte additive. For example, the estimated osmolarity of a 1-liter total volume parenteral feeding formulation providing 150 g of dextrose, 50 g of amino acids, and 150 mEq of electrolyte additives is 1400 mOsm/L. Central venous administration is necessary for this PN feeding formulation because the maximum osmolarity tolerated by a peripheral vein is 900 mOsm/L.[16]

Central Parenteral Nutrition

CPN is often referred to as *total parenteral nutrition* because the entire nutrient needs of the patient may be delivered by this route. A complete, balanced formulation includes dextrose; amino acids; ILEs; electrolytes such as potassium, magnesium, and phosphorus; vitamins; and multiple trace elements, such as zinc, copper, manganese, chromium, and selenium. The glucose content (usually 150 to 600 g/d), along with amino acids and electrolytes, provides a hyperosmolar (1300 to 1800 mOsm/L) formulation that must be delivered into a large-diameter vein, such as the superior vena cava adjacent to the right atrium. The rate of blood flow in these large vessels rapidly dilutes the hypertonic parenteral feeding formulation to that of body fluids, minimizing the risk of complications associated with an IV infusion of hypertonic solutions. CPN provides complete nutrition in a reasonable fluid volume and may be concentrated to provide adequate energy and protein for those patients requiring fluid restriction. Because central venous access can be maintained for prolonged periods (weeks to years), CPN is preferred for use in patients who will require PN support for longer than 7 to 14 days, including those patients receiving care at home or other extended healthcare environments, such as assisted living or extended care facilities and nursing homes (see Chapters 36 and 38).

Peripheral Parenteral Nutrition

PPN is similar in composition to CPN, but it has lower concentrations of nutrient components to allow for peripheral venous administration. The dextrose dose in PPN is 150 to 300 g/d (5% to 10% of final concentration), and the amino acid content is 50 to 100 g/d (3% of final concentration). Large fluid volumes must be administered with PPN to provide energy and protein doses comparable to those of CPN. PPN is usually an undesirable option for patients with fluid restriction because concentrating the solution to meet their fluid requirements frequently results in a hyperosmolar solution that is not suitable for peripheral administration. PPN may be used in patients to provide partial or total nutrition support when they are not able to ingest adequate energy orally or enterally, or when CPN is not feasible. However, this therapy is typically used for short periods (up to 2 weeks) because patients' tolerance is limited and because there are few suitable peripheral veins. PPN is generally not indicated in malnourished patients requiring longer periods of nutrition support.

Patients considered for PPN must meet 2 criteria: (1) they must have good peripheral venous access, and (2) they should be able to tolerate large volumes of fluid (2.5 to 3 L/d). They should require at least 5 days but no more than 2 weeks of partial or total PN. Contraindications to PPN are listed in Table 14-1.[17] The use of PPN is controversial, with many believing that the risk of complications outweighs any potential benefit because candidates for this therapy have only minor, if any, nutrition deficits. When using PPN in critically ill patients, it is difficult to provide adequate doses of energy, protein, and micronutrients in a limited fluid volume. PPN formulations are hyperosmolar (600 to 900 mOsm/L) and may cause phlebitis and may require frequent peripheral IV site rotations (at least every 48 to 72 hours). ILE may be used to increase the energy density of the peripheral parenteral feeding formulation without increasing the osmolarity, and it has been reported to improve peripheral vein tolerance of PPN.[17] The use of midline catheters is recommended in patients needing PPN for more than 6 days due to the catheters' length and lower probability of dislodging compared with other peripheral cannulas; however, midline catheters do not eliminate the risk of thrombophlebitis.[18] Liu and colleagues recently found a favorable response when colorectal

---

TABLE 14-1 Contraindications to Peripheral Parenteral Nutrition

- Significant malnutrition
- Severe metabolic stress
- Large nutrient or electrolyte needs (potassium is a strong vascular irritant)
- Fluid restriction
- Need for prolonged parenteral nutrition (>2 weeks)
- Renal or liver compromise

Source: Data are from reference 17.

cancer patients at nutrition risk received a preoperative PPN formula that included multivitamins and trace elements and was infused at a volume of 1500 mL/d. Micronutrient inclusion resulted in lower C-reactive protein and higher albumin levels as well as a reduced anastomotic leak rate and shorter length of hospital stay.[19]

Approaches to Parenteral Nutrition

As practice has evolved, new concepts and approaches to PN related to specific patient conditions have surfaced, including permissive underfeeding, hypocaloric feeding, and supplemental PN to avoid energy deficits. *Permissive underfeeding* is a concept relevant to critically ill patients who do not tolerate nutrition, especially PN, well. This approach is intended to minimize complications of PN delivery by providing only 80% of estimated energy requirements until the patient's condition improves.[20] *Hypocaloric feeding* is used in both EN and PN therapy for obese patients to meet protein requirements but provide less energy than the estimated requirement.[21] This approach is also designed to minimize the metabolic complications of PN while improving nitrogen balance. It is used for patients with a body mass index greater than 30, unless weight loss is not intended. It may be used in critically ill and other hospitalized patients. Very little data are available for long-term (greater than 30 days) use of this approach. (See Chapter 35 for more information on nutrition support and obesity.) Lastly, *supplemental PN* is an approach designed to minimize the energy deficit that accumulates during periods of no nutrition or undernutrition. It is used in those circumstances where EN is insufficient to meet energy needs.[20,22]

Indications for Parenteral Nutrition

General Guidelines

Malnutrition is associated with increased patient complications and mortality.[23] Although PN has been shown to improve several markers of nutrition status, prospective, randomized trials have rarely shown PN to improve patient outcomes.[5,24] However, many of these trials have been criticized for inadequate study designs, including inconsistent control for nutrition status, extent or type of underlying disease, or consistency in nutrient type and dose.[24] PN has been shown to benefit patients with moderate-to-severe malnutrition who have no or inadequate oral or EN for prolonged periods. This finding is particularly relevant to the following populations: patients receiving perioperative support; patients with acute exacerbations of Crohn's disease, GI fistulas, or extreme short bowel syndrome; and critical care and cancer patients.[5,25]

PN is costly, and it may result in serious complications when used inappropriately.[26] The costs of PN include not only the admixture but also expenses related to placing venous access, laboratory monitoring, and treatment of complications.[26] As such, the use of PN is scrutinized by patients, providers, and payers.[5] The therapy should only be used in those patients who will demonstrably benefit from it.[27] Iden-

tifying these patients is not an easy task because the effects of the nutrition components of care may be confounded by the underlying disease process and its treatment. Specific guidelines for the implementation of PN have been developed by ASPEN,[28] and Table 14-2 outlines criteria that may be used to determine the appropriate application of PN.[29] These criteria can be easily adapted to a nutrition consultation form designed to educate the clinician requesting PN on the pertinent patient variables that identify a candidate for PN (Figure 14-1). By completing the nutrition consultation request section, the individual requesting PN addresses the previously mentioned criteria. Considerations include the patient's nutrition status, GI function, and the extent and severity of the underlying disease. See Practice Scenario 14-1 for a discussion of indications for PN.

TABLE14-2 Indications for Parenteral Nutrition

Considerations for PN use:
- PN may be appropriate for patients who are unable to meet nutrition requirements with EN. These patients are already or have the potential of becoming malnourished.
- PPN may be used in selected patients to provide partial or total nutrition support for up to 2 weeks when those patients cannot ingest or absorb oral or enteral tube–delivered nutrients, or when CPN is not feasible.
- CPN support is necessary when PN is indicated for longer than 2 weeks, peripheral venous access is limited, nutrient needs are large, or fluid restriction is required, and the benefits of PN outweigh the risks.

Use CPN when:
- The patient has failed the EN trial with appropriate tube placement (postpyloric).
- EN is contraindicated or the GI tract has a severely diminished function because of the underlying disease or treatment. Specific applicable conditions are as follows:
  - Paralytic ileus
  - Mesenteric ischemia
  - Small bowel obstruction
  - GI fistula, except when enteral access may be placed posterior to the fistula or volume of output (less than 200 mL/d) supports a trial of EN
- The exact duration of starvation that can be tolerated without increased morbidity is unknown, as can occur in postoperative nutrition support. Expert opinion suggests that wound healing will be impaired if PN is not started within 5 to 10 days postoperatively for patients who cannot eat or tolerate enteral feeding.[29]
- The patient's clinical condition is considered in the decision to withhold or withdraw therapy. Conditions where nutrition support is poorly tolerated and should be withheld until the condition improves are severe hyperglycemia; azotemia; encephalopathy and hyperosmolality; and severe fluid and electrolyte disturbances.

CPN, central parenteral nutrition; EN, enteral nutrition; GI, gastrointestinal; PN, parenteral nutrition; PPN, peripheral parenteral nutrition.
Source: Data are from reference 29.

FIGURE 14-1 Nutrition Assessment and Recommendation Form

Date: Time:	Consulting Service:		
IBW (Kg)	Actual Weight (Kg)	Dosing Weight (Kg)	Recent wt loss (Kg)

Indication
☐ Acute Pancreatitis ☐ SBO ☐ Ileus ☐ Fistula ☐ Short Bowel Syndrome ☐ Intractable Vomiting/Diarrhea
Other: _____

PMH
☐ DM1 ☐ DM2 ☐ CHF ☐ CRI ☐ ESRD- HD ☐ Liver Disease Other: _____

Current Medical Problems
☐ Hyperglycemia ☐ Sepsis ☐ Pregnancy ☐ Hyper TG ☐ ARF Other: _____

Current Medications

Glucose Control ☐ Insulin drip: _____ ☐ ICU- SSI every: _____ ☐ SSI ( ) every: _____ ☐ Oral Hypoglycemics: _____ ☐ Octreotide: _____ ☐ Steroids: _____	Sedation ☐ Propofol drip: _____	GI Meds ☐ PPI (IV, po, tube) _____ ☐ H2 blocker: _____

Nutrient Access ☐ PICC ☐ Central Line ☐ NG/OG-Tube	Estimated Daily Needs Calories: _____ Kcals / day Protein: _____ Grams / day

Baseline nutritional status
☐ Acute Malnutrition (acute injury/illness) ☐ Chronic disease related malnutrition
☐ Chronic Malnutrition (starvation) ☐ Well Nourished at baseline
☐ NPO for 24-72 hours ☐ NPO > 72 hours
☐ Currently receiving enteral nutrition meeting _____% goals

Refeeding risk	☐ Low ☐ Moderate ☐ High

Baseline Labs:

Na	K+	Cl	Bicarb	BUN	Crea	Gluc	Ca	Alb	Corr Ca

Mg	Phos	Chol	Trig	WBC	PLT	Hgb	HCT	PAB	ICa

CrCl: _____ ml/min   CBGs: _____

Impression	
Recommendation/ Formula	☐ Modified/Special Diet ☐ Enteral/Tube Feeding ☐ Parenteral Nutrition
Goals of Therapy	☐ _____ ☐ _____ ☐ _____
Consult Completed By	

Sample/simulated form that may facilitate nutrition assessment by including key components required to diagnose malnutrition, determine the indications for enteral or parenteral nutrition, and establish a nutrition care plan that is documented for the patient. Alb, albumin; ARF, acute renal failure; Bicarb, bicarbonate; BUN, blood urea nitrogen; Ca, calcium; CBGs, complete blood gases; CHF, congestive heart failure; Chol, cholesterol; Cl, chloride; Corr Ca; corrected calcium; Crea, creatinine; CrCl, creatinine clearance; CRI, chronic renal insufficiency; DM1, type 1 diabetes; DM2, type 2 diabetes; ESRD-HD, end-stage renal disease on hemodialysis; GI, gastrointestinal; Gluc, glucose; H$_2$ blocker, H-2 receptor antagonist; HCT, hematocrit; Hgb, hemoglobin; Hyper TG, hypertriglyceridemia; IBW, ideal body weight; ICa, ionized calcium; ICU, intensive care unit; IV, intravenous; K+, potassium; Mg, magnesium; Na, sodium; NG/OG, nasogastric/orogastric; NPO, *nil per os*; PAB, prealbumin; Phos, phosphorus; PICC, peripherally inserted central catheter; PLT, platelets; PMH, patient medical history; PO, *per os*; PPI, proton-pump inhibitor; SBO, small bowel obstruction; SSI, sliding-scale insulin; Trig, triglycerides; WBC, white blood cell count.

Practice Scenario 14-1

Question: When is parenteral nutrition (PN) indicated?

Scenario: A 47-year-old woman was admitted with recurring gastrointestinal (GI) problems. Her nutrition parameters were listed as follows:

1. Weight loss: 8.4 kg
2. Weight change: 11%
3. Period of weight change: 35 days
4. Intake history: <25% estimated nutrition needs
5. Prealbumin: 8 mg/dL

Abdominal scan findings demonstrated a bowel obstruction with pockets of fluid collections consistent with an intra-abdominal abscess.

Intervention: At surgery, the patient was found to have a complete bowel obstruction, multiple adhesions, recurrence of Crohn's disease, and a large suprapubic abscess. The surgical procedure consisted of an exploratory laparotomy, lysis of adhesions, small bowel resection to remove the disease-affected bowel, and drainage of the abdominal abscess. A nasogastric tube was placed, which drained 1500 to 2000 mL on postoperative Day 1.

Answer: The patient was at a high risk of developing postoperative complications such as wound dehiscence, wound infection, pneumonia, and renal failure. Because the problem with the GI tract was not expected to be resolved in 7 to 10 days, PN was indicated.[25]

Rationale: Whether PN is indicated is dependent on the severity of the patient's malnutrition, the length of time the patient will not be able to use the enteral route for nourishment, and the influence of the underlying clinical condition on the safety and efficacy of therapy. When a nutrition consult form (Figure 14-1) was completed, the patient met 2 criteria for severe malnutrition: (1) more than 10% weight loss over a 2- to 3-month period, and (2) inadequate oral intake for more than 7 days before her surgery. Because of the severity of malnutrition in this patient, some form of nutrition support was indicated. The problem with the GI tract precluded the use of EN and was not expected to be resolved within 7 to 10 days; therefore, PN was indicated.[25]

Gastrointestinal Function

Symptoms such as nausea, vomiting, diarrhea, and abdominal distention or cramps may preclude the use of the GI tract for prolonged periods. We do not know how long patients can endure inadequate oral nutrition and semi- or complete starvation before there is an impact on clinical outcomes. Generally, treatment toxicities in cancer patients that preclude an adequate oral intake for more than a week are an indication for PN.[6] In critically ill patients at high nutrition risk or severely malnourished, PN is indicated if EN is not feasible.[20] For critically ill patients with normal nutrition risk or no malnutrition, PN should be avoided for up to 7 days.[20]

For the severely malnourished patient, PN is indicated when an impairment of the GI tract occurs. PN is indicated in other conditions that preclude the use of the GI tract for more than 7 to 10 days.[22] PN is often used when enteral tube feedings are unsuccessful as evidenced by GI intolerance or pulmonary aspiration. In some cases, enteral access is contraindicated or attempts at achieving enteral access may have failed. Finally, in certain conditions, the GI tract should not be used until the underlying problem is treated (Table 14-2).

Clinical Status

PN should only be initiated in patients who are hemodynamically stable and who can tolerate the fluid volume and protein, carbohydrate, and ILE doses necessary to provide adequate nutrient substrate. Table 14-3 lists examples of situations where the administration of PN warrants caution. Table 14-4 describes laboratory tests to use when assessing and monitoring patients receiving PN.[8,30]

Specific Guidelines

Gastrointestinal Disorders

PN has not been shown to improve patient outcomes as the primary management of acute exacerbations of Crohn's disease or ulcerative colitis.[5,31] A retrospective analysis of data for PN use in patients with small bowel fistulas suggests an improvement in mortality rates and spontaneous and surgical closures, except when the fistula arises from the bowel with active Crohn's disease.[5] Data suggest that bowel rest is not necessary to achieve remission in Crohn's disease.[31] (See Chapter 26 for more information on GI disorders.)

TABLE 14-3 Clinical Conditions Warranting Cautious Use of Parenteral Nutrition

Condition	Suggested Criteria[a]
Hyperglycemia	Glucose >300 mg/dL
Azotemia	BUN >100 mg/dL
Hyperosmolality	Serum osmolality >350 mOsm/kg
Hypernatremia	Na >150 mEq/L
Hypokalemia	K <3 mEq/L
Hyperchloremic metabolic acidosis	Cl >115 mEq/L
Hypophosphatemia	Phosphorus <2 mg/dL
Hypochloremic metabolic alkalosis	Cl <85 mEq/L

BUN, blood urea nitrogen; Cl, chloride; K, potassium; Na, sodium.
[a]There is no published evidence to support the specific criteria noted in this column. These values are suggestions by the author and should be modified based on clinical judgment about the specific patient in question or the environment in which parenteral nutrition is being administered, such as intensive care unit, general medical ward, long-term care facility, or the home.

TABLE 14-4 Suggested Monitoring for Parenteral Nutrition

Parameter	Baseline	Initiation	Critically Ill Patients	Stable Patients
CBC with differential	Yes		Weekly	Weekly
INR, PT, PTT	Yes		Weekly	Weekly
Electrolytes: Na, K, Cl, CO_2, Mg, Ca, phosphorus, BUN, Cr	Yes	Daily × 3	Daily	1–2 × per week
Serum triglycerides	Yes	Day 1	Weekly	Weekly
Serum glucose	Yes	Daily × 3	Daily	1–2 × per week
Capillary glucose		As needed	≥3 × day until consistently <150 mg/dL	As needed
Weight	Yes	Daily	Daily	2–3 × per week
Intake and output	Yes	Daily	Daily	Daily unless fluid status is assessed by physical exam
ALT, AST, ALP, total bilirubin	Yes	Day 1	Weekly	Monthly
Nitrogen balance	As needed		As needed	As needed

ALP, alkaline phosphatase; ALT, alanine aminotransferase; AST, aspartate aminotransferase; BUN, blood urea nitrogen; Ca, calcium; CBC, complete blood cell count; Cl, chloride; CO_2, bicarbonate; Cr, serum creatinine; INR, international normalized ratio; K, potassium; Mg, magnesium; Na, sodium; PT, prothrombin time; PTT, partial thromboplastin time.
Source: Data are from references 8 and 30.

Pancreatitis

The role of PN in treating pancreatitis has evolved substantially since PN was first used. GI or bowel rest and PN no longer have a role in pancreatitis. Recent reviews highlight the importance of maintaining GI integrity with EN as a means to avoid complications from pancreatitis and improve outcomes from the disease.[32] PN is unlikely to benefit patients with mild, acute, or chronic relapsing pancreatitis when the conditions last for less than 1 week.[33] PN should be avoided unless EN is not feasible because of GI ileus, small bowel obstruction, or the inability to properly place an enteral feeding tube. Despite improvements in delivery and tolerance of EN in pancreatitis patients, 5% to 10% of patients will have GI intolerance and require PN.[34] When PN is needed, it is recommended that PN energy administration not exceed 25 to 35 kcal/kg/d and glucose be adequately controlled.[33] It is also recommended to consider glutamine (0.3 g alanyl-glutamine [Ala-Gln] dipeptide per kg) to minimize the effect of being *nil per os* (nothing by mouth) on GI integrity.[35] (See Chapter 28 for more information on pancreatitis.)

Perioperative Malnutrition

The stress of surgical procedures produces an abundance of proinflammatory cytokines, which increase metabolic rate and cause catabolism, resulting in a depletion of lean body mass and aberrations in glycemic control. Studies have shown that patients at the highest risk of adverse postsurgical outcomes are those with low visceral protein stores (specifically, albumin) at baseline.[20] The ratio of prealbumin to C-reactive protein may predict diminishing inflammation and, therefore, a patient's return to normal anabolic metabolism facilitated by feeding (PN) and subsequent repletion.[36] Well-designed and appropriately timed nutrition support in this population may help attenuate metabolic and oxidative stress and, as a result, improve postsurgical recovery. Early nutrition support in both the pre- and postoperative phases is associated with better patient outcomes. EN is the preferred form, mainly due to its protective effect on the GI mucosal barrier. Perioperative PN is reserved for patients with severe malnutrition at baseline, in whom the risk of surgery would outweigh any benefit because of the high risk of postoperative complications; maximal benefit is derived in severely malnourished patients who receive PN for more than 7 to 10 days.[36] However, recent (2011) evidence has found that PN using contemporary doses of energy and protein has effects comparable to EN in malnourished cancer patients undergoing surgery.[1] Therefore, PN in the perioperative patient may be useful in treating malnutrition when other nutrition options are not feasible. (See Chapters 24 and 33 for more information on surgery and cancer, respectively.)

Critical Illness

Critical illness is characterized by a catabolic state that is generally the result of systemic inflammatory response to infectious or traumatic insult. In this state, gut failure is common because of preferential blood supply to vital organs. Additionally, mesenteric ischemia resulting from hemodynamic compromise and the use of vasopressors is a potential problem in critical illness not usually seen in other conditions. These facts notwithstanding, the ASPEN/Society of Critical Care Medicine guidelines recommend the enteral route as the preferred means of nutrition support in this population, with the greatest benefit derived in patients started on enteral feedings within 24 to 48 hours of intensive care unit admission.[20] The benefit of EN is largely due to (1) its positive impact on the immune barrier and decreasing the permeability of the GI tract to enteric organisms, which can contribute to the overall detrimental systemic inflammatory response, and (2) the low risk of mesenteric ischemia when introducing EN.[20] Expert recommendations[20] place PN as a last resort in this patient group; in patients whose baseline nutrition status was normal, it is reserved for those cases when EN cannot be initiated for more than 7 days. Critically ill patients requiring PN usually meet all the following criteria: (1) are malnourished at baseline; (2) will not reliably ingest or absorb significant amounts of EN for a period of greater than 7 to 10 days; and (3) have been adequately resuscitated from any hemodynamic compromise. PN is also indicated for patients who are hemodynamically stable and have a paralytic ileus, acute GI bleeding, or complete bowel obstruction (see Chapters 23 and 24). Recent guidelines suggest a role for supplemental PN as described previously.[20] These guidelines also provide methods to minimize the complications of PN, such as the use of hypocaloric feeding and maintaining target glucose of 140 or 150 to 180 mg/dL.[20]

Cancer

Routine PN use in patients receiving chemotherapy or radiation is associated with increased infectious complications and no improvement in clinical response, survival, or toxicity to chemotherapy.[4] ASPEN guidelines for the provision of nutrition support in adult patients receiving anticancer therapy recommend a thorough assessment of the patient's nutrition status and the use of PN only in those who are malnourished and likely to be unable to ingest and absorb adequate nutrients for a period of 7 to 14 days.[4] EN is preferred in cancer patients with functional GI tracts. EN is also preferred in patients undergoing a hematopoietic cell transplant because glycemic control is better during EN than PN.[4] Data suggest favorable outcomes in both of these patient groups with the use of immune-enhancing EN.[37] Until more specific data are available, indications for these patients are similar to those for other conditions (see Chapter 33). Recent research has found PN to have some beneficial results in cancer patients, which may lead to a broader use of PN in the future. As discussed previously, Klek et al found the effects of PN and EN in malnourished cancer patients undergoing surgery to be comparable.[1] Pelzer and colleagues used bioelectrical impedance analysis to demonstrate improvements in body composition in pancreatic cancer patients who had lost weight while receiving EN.[2]

Home Parenteral Nutrition

In general, indications for home PN are the same as those for hospitalized patients, but careful consideration must be given to the capabilities of the patient and caregivers as well as the safety of the home environment for PN. For home PN candidates, the duration of PN is prolonged (more than 2 weeks), and hospitalization is no longer needed for medical reasons. However, federal (Medicare) and state (Medicaid) healthcare programs have developed criteria that must be met before home PN–associated costs are reimbursed. Medicare requires documentation that the patient's GI tract is nonfunctional ("artificial gut"), and this condition is permanent (at least 90 days of therapy is needed). The patient must also have documented evidence of inability to tolerate enteral feeding (malabsorption, obstruction).

Outcomes in home PN patients vary depending on the underlying disease causing their nonfunctional GI tract. Cancer patients have more frequent PN complications, which are more likely to result in readmission to the hospital.[3,38] Also, the extent of the disease or its responsiveness to treatment is likely to influence the success of home PN in cancer patients with extensive disease. However, performance status (Karnofsky performance status score [KPF] greater than 50) has been associated with longer survival in incurable cancer patients receiving home PN.[3] Improvements in quality of life, KPF, and nutrition status in advanced cancer patients have also been observed.[39]

Whether PN can be initiated in the home is controversial. Table 14-5 lists circumstances where the clinical risk warrants caution when considering the initiation of PN in the home. (See Chapter 38 for additional information on home nutrition support.)

The Parenteral Nutrition System

Outcomes from PN are dependent on the system by which it is managed within the healthcare system. ASPEN guidelines provide practical advice for PN[40] use as well as safe practices.[41] As noted, successful use of PN depends on an adequate system to order, transcribe, prepare (compound), dispense, and administer.[16] PN is a complex therapy requiring trained professionals to initiate and manage it.[42,43] Outcomes are optimized when interdisciplinary care or nutrition support teams manage PN.[44,45] Although the system is generally safe, PN is likely to cause patient harm when the system fails.[46,47]

Pace and colleagues[48] used ASPEN guidelines to assess the overuse of PN, the underuse of EN, and the need to update hospital policies and procedures to reflect recent advances and changes in nutrition support practice. A performance model was used to revise policies and procedures and to educate staff. This process resulted in a 52% decrease in PN use during a 4-year period, an increase in appropriate PN use from 74% to 95%, and an elimination of PPN use.

In a tertiary care teaching hospital, PN use was evaluated in 209 patients managed by either individual medical or surgical

TABLE 14-5 Conditions Warranting Caution When Initiating Parenteral Nutrition in the Home

Medical conditions:	Electrolyte disorders:
• Diabetes mellitus	• Hypernatremia
• Congestive heart failure	• Hypokalemia
• Pulmonary disease	• Hyperchloremic metabolic acidosis
• Severe malnutrition	• Hypophosphatemia
• Hyperemesis gravidarum	• Hypochloremic metabolic alkalosis

services or a metabolic support service.[3] Indications for PN were derived from ASPEN guidelines.[28] PN therapy was considered preventable if the patient had a functional small bowel but there was no suitable enteral access. PN was contraindicated if the patients were classified as well nourished and had inadequate EN for fewer than 7 days; had DNR status and were deemed to warrant comfort measures only or were terminally ill; or were receiving adequate EN. Of the PN regimens initiated, 62% were indicated, 23% were preventable, and 15% were not indicated. Compliance to established guidelines was improved when patients were managed by the metabolic support service.[3]

PN should be reserved for use in patients who are unable to tolerate enteral nutrients for prolonged periods of time because of physical or physiological impediments. PN has been associated with complications and patient harm including infections related to the introduction of IV catheters and their manipulations[49] or the administration of a viable growth medium;[50] metabolic complications from overfeeding or refeeding; and problems caused by other errors during prescription, transcription, or preparation.[16,51] In response to these errors, guidelines and expert recommendations have been developed to curb harm resulting from PN use.[52] Although the overall error rates may have decreased with the use of these recommendations, errors still occur and occasionally result in patient harm. In a prospective observational study, Sacks and colleagues[47] found 74 errors in a cohort of 4730 prescriptions for PN (ie, an overall error rate of 1.56%). Of these errors, 67 (91%) were classified as nonharmful, whereas 6 (8%) resulted in temporary harm to a patient. Most errors occurred during the transcription and administration phase in this study. As suggested by the work of Sacks and colleagues, the incorporation of nutrition guidelines may help decrease error rates. In addition, the use of a multistep, double-check process that requires the verification of an electronically transcribed order against the actual written order may significantly decrease error rates.[47]

In addition to incorporating systematic procedures for electronically transcribing and compounding PN accurately, the use of multidisciplinary teams in the ordering phase has been shown to help ensure the appropriate use of PN.[3] See Practice Scenarios 14-2 through 14-5 for discussions of proper initiation, advancement, monitoring, and discontinuation of PN.[3,6,14,53] A 2011 study querying PN practices in statewide hospitals[54] indicates that nutrition support teams and certified nutrition support clinicians can help reduce the inappropriate use of PN and, as a result, substantially lower costs. In this study, of the 278 PN cases reviewed by registered dietitians, PN was inappropriately prescribed in 32% of cases, resulting in 552 days and $138,000 in preventable hospital costs.[54]

Practice Scenario 14-2

Question: How should parenteral nutrition (PN) be initiated?

Scenario: PN is to be initiated in a 53-year-old man who has chronic disease–related malnutrition and a complete bowel obstruction. Nutrition-related and metabolic parameters in the patient are as follows:

- White blood cell (WBC) count: 9.6×10^9/L
- Sodium (Na): 135 mEq/L
- Potassium (K): 4.1 mEq/L
- Chloride (Cl): 103 mEq/L
- Bicarbonate (CO_2): 24 mmol/L
- Blood urea nitrogen (BUN): 6 mg/dL
- Creatinine (Cr): 1.1 mg/dL
- Glucose: 234 mg/dL
- Magnesium (Mg): 1.8 mEq/L
- Calcium (Ca): 9.8 mg/dL
- Phosphorus: 1.5 mg/dL
- Prealbumin: 2 mg/dL
- Weight loss: 20 kg
- % weight loss: 14%
- Time of weight change: 45 days

Intervention: PN is initiated at a low rate (100 g dextrose per day) with a supplemental dose of phosphorus prior to the start of PN and an increased dose of phosphorus in PN.

Answer: A favorable clinical response to PN may be delayed by the patient's catabolic state. Glucose and phosphorus problems should be corrected before PN is initiated. Then, PN should be initiated slowly, beginning with a low energy dose.

Rationale: The metabolic response to stress or injury influences the efficiency by which nutrients are incorporated into the body (see Chapters 23 and 24). Also, tolerance to nutrition support is influenced by abnormalities in carbohydrate, protein, and fat metabolism that are characterized in the stressed patient as hyperglycemia, insulin resistance, uremia, encephalopathy, hyperosmolality, and hypertriglyceridemia. Severe deficits in electrolytes may be present and exacerbated by the initiation of a parenteral feeding formulation (see Chapter 7). In some conditions, caution in initiating PN is warranted (Table 14-3). The patient's laboratory data demonstrate elevated serum glucose and hypophosphatemia. Both conditions should be corrected before PN is initiated and should be addressed in the PN formula. Use of a nutrition consultation form (eg, Figure 14-1) not only assists with determining the appropriate indication for PN but also establishes a framework by which PN may be safely initiated. This patient is severely malnourished and, as such, at significant risk of developing refeeding syndrome.[53] PN should be initiated slowly, beginning at a low energy dose. Electrolyte abnormalities should be corrected before initiating PN.

Practice Scenario 14-3

Question: When can parenteral nutrition (PN) be advanced to the goal infusion rate?

Scenario: PN is initiated in a 61-year-old woman who has a history of type 2 diabetes.

Intervention: PN is initiated at a low energy dose. The following morning, the patient's blood glucose concentration is in the range of 210 to 240 mg/dL. The patient's blood pressure and other vital signs are within acceptable parameters.

Answer: PN should be advanced only when the following criteria are met: stable blood pressure, pulse, and respiration rates; and normal serum phosphorus, potassium, and glucose concentrations. The best practice is to control the patient's blood glucose before advancing the rate of PN to its goal rate. A reasonable goal for blood glucose is 140 to 180 mg/dL.[53]

Rationale: Because PN contributes significantly to the fluid intake of the patient, patients with limited cardiac function may not tolerate the PN infusion. Therefore, patients should be assessed for signs and symptoms of congestive heart failure and pulmonary edema. In addition, vital signs such as blood pressure and pulse may be adversely affected by PN. It is prudent to not advance the parenteral feeding formulation rate until the following criteria are met: stable blood pressure, pulse, and respiration rates; and normal serum phosphorus, potassium, and glucose concentrations. Hyperglycemia is frequently encountered in patients receiving PN (see Chapter 17).[14] The dextrose content of intravenous fluids and medications may contribute to excessive glucose administration in patients receiving PN.[14] The best practice is to control the patient's blood glucose before advancing the rate of PN to its goal rate.

Practice Scenario 14-4

Question: Once parenteral nutrition (PN) is infusing at its goal rate, what approach to monitoring should be taken?

Scenario: PN is advanced to the goal rate in a patient with normal renal function but a gastrointestinal fistula draining 800 mL/d. Laboratory values are normal after the acute replacement of potassium and magnesium and a correction of a metabolic acidosis.

Intervention: Follow-up laboratory tests are done on a daily/as-needed basis, and capillary blood glucose checks continue 4 times a day with sliding-scale insulin coverage.

Answer: Initially, fluid, electrolyte, and renal status should be monitored daily. Routine blood glucose monitoring should also be conducted daily. Metabolic parameters (triglycerides and liver function tests) should be obtained periodically. The effectiveness of PN may be further assessed by measuring serum visceral proteins on a weekly basis and determining nitrogen balance in patients with functioning kidneys and adequate urine output.

Rationale: Because PN may be a large source of fluid and electrolytes as well as other nutrients, serum levels of electrolytes, blood urea nitrogen, creatinine, and glucose should be assessed daily during the initial period of PN therapy. Patients receiving PN may be predisposed to fluid and electrolyte disturbances because of fluid losses from the gastrointestinal tract, drug therapy such as diuretics, or electrolyte losses during periods of semi- or complete starvation. Other parameters of fluid and electrolyte status to monitor are fluid intakes and outputs, as well as daily weights in combination with physical assessment for signs and symptoms of dehydration or edema.

Patients receiving PN often experience metabolic disturbances. In addition to serum electrolytes and blood glucose monitoring, the periodic assessment of serum triglycerides is necessary if lipid injectable emulsions are administered. Abnormal hepatic function has also been associated with PN. Hepatic function should be assessed before initiating PN and then weekly.[53] See Table 14-4 for more on laboratory tests used in assessment and monitoring of PN.[3]

Practice Scenario 14-5

Question: When and how should parenteral nutrition (PN) therapy be discontinued?

Intervention: Following a surgical procedure for a bowel obstruction and the drainage of intra-abdominal abscess, PN is initiated in a 65-year-old woman. On postoperative Day 8, nasogastric tube output dramatically declines, the patient is noted to have bowel sounds, and she has a bowel movement. At this time, the nasogastric tube is removed and orogastric tube feedings are initiated.

Answer: PN may be discontinued when the patient can meet and tolerate an adequate percentage of their estimated energy and protein needs via the enteral route.

Rationale: The goal of PN therapy is to maintain the nutrition status of the patient until some form of enteral nutrition is tolerated. The exception is the critically ill patient in whom therapy is withdrawn during the terminal stages of the disease process. In most other situations, the problem with the gastrointestinal tract resolves or the appropriate enteral access is obtained. PN is tapered as the amount of reliable enteral intake increases. It may be discontinued when the patient can consume solid food or when he or she tolerates an adequate percentage of the estimated energy and protein needs.[6] In this patient, enteral tube feedings are initiated 8 days after the operation and advanced to the goal infusion rate within 72 hours of initiation. PN therapy is decreased by 50% on postoperative Day 9 and discontinued on postoperative Day 10.

To prevent rebound hypoglycemia, PN may be tapered over 1 to 2 hours. If PN needs to be stopped emergently, a 10% dextrose in water solution should be infused at either the same rate as the PN or at a rate of at least 50 mL/h. When cyclic PN infusion is used in the home, some form of tapering is usually required during the last 2 hours of the cycle. Finally, PN may be rapidly discontinued if the patient is tolerating tube feeding in amounts adequate to maintain normal blood glucose levels.

A review by Taylor and colleagues also suggests that the incorporation of a dietitian in the care of critically ill patients leads to a higher quality assessment of these patients' nutrition needs.[55] Dietitians are vital in thoroughly assessing patients' nutrition needs, including their fluid and electrolyte requirements, as well as suggesting the appropriate route and timing of nutrition provision. Additionally, research led by dietitians has provided insight into the achievement of optimal blood glucose control and the use of specialized nutrition. Dietitians and other qualified nutrition support clinicians help adjust patients' nutrition plans according to changes in physiological status.[54]

Conclusion

ASPEN guidelines are useful in identifying patients who are likely to benefit from PN. CPN provides adequate nutrients to maintain and replete the patient's nutrition stores. PPN may be useful for limited periods in maintaining nutrition status until the GI tract is functional. Recent evidence strongly supports EN to be the preferred mode of nutrition support in critical illness and pancreatitis because of its ability to maintain the integrity of the GI tract and properly support the systemic inflammatory response. PN should be reserved for those patients who are malnourished or at significant nutrition risk and have a contraindication to EN or in whom GI intolerance persists beyond 7 days. Current experience with PN in malnourished patients has demonstrated improvements in body composition with PN; PN outcomes comparable with those of EN when contemporary doses of energy and protein are used; improved quality, safety, and utilization when PN is managed by nutrition support teams; positive PN outcomes in long-term patients; improved PN performance measures; and better quality of life for some patients. Even though PN can cause several complications, these may be minimized when managed well by trained individuals, allowing for beneficial effects to be achieved.

References

1. Klek S, Sierzega M, Szybinski P, et al. Perioperative nutrition in malnourished surgical cancer patients—a prospective, randomized, controlled clinical trial. *Clin Nutr.* 2011;30:708–713.

2. Pelzer U, Arnold D, Govercin M, et al. Parenteral nutrition support for patients with pancreatic cancer. Results of a phase II study. *BMC Cancer.* 2010;10:86–91.

3. Chermesh I, Mashiach T, Amit A, et al. Home parenteral nutrition (HTPN) for incurable patients with cancer with gastrointestinal obstruction: do the benefits outweigh the risks? *Med Oncol.* 2011;28:83–88.

4. August DA, Huhmann MB. A.S.P.E.N. clinical guidelines: nutrition support therapy during adult anticancer treatment and in hematopoietic cell transplantation. *JPEN J Parenter Enteral Nutr.* 2009;33(5):472–500.

5. Klein S, Kinney J, Jeejeebhoy K, et al. Nutrition support in clinical practice: review of published data and recommendations for future research directions. Summary of a conference sponsored by the National Institutes of Health, American Society for Parenteral and Enteral Nutrition, and American Society for Clinical Nutrition. *JPEN J Parenter Enteral Nutr.* 1997;2:133–156.

6. Weisdorf SA, Lysne J, Wind D, et al. Positive effect of prophylactic total parenteral nutrition on long-term outcome of bone marrow transplantation. *Transplantation.* 1987;43(6):833–838.

7. Trujillo EB, Young LS, Chertow GM, et al. Metabolic and monetary costs of avoidable parenteral nutrition use. *JPEN J Parenter Enteral Nutr.* 1999;23(2):109–113.

8. Sacks GS, Mayhew S, Johnson D. Parenteral nutrition implementation and management. In: Merritt R, ed. *The A.S.P.E.N. Nutrition Support Practice Manual.* 2nd ed. Silver Spring, MD: American Society for Parenteral and Enteral Nutrition; 2005:108–117.

9. Dudrick SJ, Wilmore DW, Vars HM, Rhoads JE. Long-term total parenteral nutrition with growth, development, and positive nitrogen balance. *Surgery.* 1968;64(1):134–142.

10. Dudrick SJ. Early developments and clinical applications of total parenteral nutrition. *JPEN J Parenter Enteral Nutr.* 2003;27(4):291–299.

11. Rhoads JE, Dudrick SJ. History of intravenous nutrition. In: Rombeau JL, Caldwell MD, eds. *Clinical Nutrition, Parenteral Nutrition.* 2nd ed. Philadelphia, PA: Saunders; 1993:1–10.

12. Lumpkin MM. Safety alert: hazards of precipitation associated with parenteral nutrition. *Am J Hosp Pharm.* 1994;51(11):1427–1428.

13. Btaiche IF, Khalidi N. Metabolic complications of parenteral nutrition in adults, Part 2. *Am J Health Syst Pharm.* 2004;61(19): 2050–2059.

14. Pleva M, Mirtallo JM, Steinberg SM. Hyperglycemic events in nonintensive care unit patients receiving parenteral nutrition. *Nutr Clin Pract.* 2009;24(5):626–634.

15. Nehme AE. Nutritional support of the hospitalized patient. *JAMA.* 1980;283(19):1906–1908.

16. Mirtallo J, Canada T, Johnson D, et al. Safe practices for parenteral nutrition. *JPEN J Parenter Enteral Nutr.* 2004;28(6 Suppl):S39–S70.

17. Anderson ADG, Palmer D, MacFie J. Peripheral parenteral nutrition. *Br J Surg.* 2003;90(9):1048–1054.

18. Pittiruti M, Hamilton H, Biffi R, et al. ESPEN guidelines on parenteral nutrition: central venous catheters (access, care, diagnosis and therapy of complications). *Clin Nutr.* 2009;28(4):365–377.

19. Liu MY, Tang HC, Hu SH, Yang HL, Chang SJ. Influence of preoperative peripheral parenteral nutrition with micronutrients after colorectal cancer patients. *Biomed Res Int.* 2015;2015:535431. Epub 2015(Apr 27). doi:10.1155/2015/535431.

20. McClave SA, Taylor BE, Martindale RG, et al. Guidelines for the provision and assessment of nutrition support therapy in the adult critically ill patient. Society of Critical Care Medicine (SCCM) and American Society for Parenteral and Enteral Nutrition (A.S.P.E.N.). *JPEN J Parenter Enteral Nutr.* 2016;40(2):159–211.

21. Choban PS, Dickerson RN. Morbid obesity and nutrition support: is bigger different? *Nutr Clin Pract.* 2005;20(4):480–487.

22. Oshima T, Heidegger C-P, Pichard C. Supplemental parenteral nutrition is the key to prevent energy deficits in critically ill patients. *Nutr Clin Pract.* 2016;31(3):431–437.

23. Dempsey DT, Mullen JL, Buzby GP. The link between nutritional status and clinical outcome. Can nutritional intervention modify it? *Am J Clin Nutr.* 1988;47(2 Suppl):352–356.

24. Mirtallo JM. Parenteral nutrition: can outcomes be improved? *JPEN J Parenter Enteral Nutr.* 2013;37(2):181–189.

25. McClave SA, Martindale RG, Taylor B, Gramlich L. Appropriate use of parenteral nutrition through the perioperative period. *JPEN J Parenter Enteral Nutr.* 2013;37(suppl):73S–82S.

26. Twomey PL, Patching SC. Cost effectiveness of nutritional support. *JPEN J Parenter Enteral Nutr.* 1985;9(1):3–10.

27. Mullen JL, Buzby GP, Matthews DC, Smale BF, Rosato EF. Reduction of operative morbidity and mortality by combined preoperative and postoperative nutrition support. *Ann Surg.* 1980;192(5):604–613.

28. A.S.P.E.N. Board of Directors and the Clinical Guidelines Task Force. Guidelines for the use of parenteral and enteral nutrition in adult and pediatric patients. *JPEN J Parenter Enteral Nutr.* 2002:26(1 Suppl):1SA–138SA.

29. A.S.P.E.N. Board of Directors. Guidelines for the use of parenteral and enteral nutrition in adult and pediatric patients. *JPEN J Parenter Enteral Nutr.* 1993;17(4 Suppl):1SA–52SA.

30. A.S.P.E.N. Board of Directors. *A.S.P.E.N.'s Adult Parenteral Nutrition (PN) Support Pathway.* Silver Spring, MD: American Society for Parenteral and Enteral Nutrition; 1998.

31. Koretz RL, Lipman TO, Klein S. AGA technical review: parenteral nutrition. *Gastroenterology.* 2001;121(4):970–1001.

32. Italian Association for the Study of the Pancreas (AISP); Pezzilli R, Zerbi A, Campra D, et al. Consensus guidelines on severe acute pancreatitis. *Dig Liver Dis.* 2015;47(7):532–543. Epub 2015(Apr 2). doi:10.1016/j.dld.2015.03.022.

33. Mirtallo JM, Forbes A, McClave SA, et al. International consensus guidelines for nutrition therapy in pancreatitis. *JPEN J Parenter Enteral Nutr.* 2012;36(3):284–291. doi:10.1177/0148607112440823.

34. Bakker OJ, van Brunschot S, van Santvoort HC, et al; Dutch Pancreatitis Study Group. Early versus on-demand nasoenteric tube feeding in acute pancreatitis. *N Engl J Med.* 2014; 371(21):1983–1993. doi:10.1056/NEJMoa1404393.

35. Yong L, Lu QP, Liu SH, et al. Efficacy of glutamine-enriched nutrition support for patients with severe acute pancreatitis: a meta-analysis. *JPEN J Parenter Enteral Nutr.* 2016; 40(1):83–94. Epub 2015(Feb 5). doi:10.1177/0148607115570391.

36. Kudsk KA, Tolley EA, DeWitt RC, et al. Preoperative albumin and surgical site identify surgical risk for major postoperative complications. *JPEN J Parenter Enteral Nutr.* 2003;27(1):1–9.

37. Braga M, Gianotti L, Vignali A, Carlo VD. Preoperative oral arginine and n-3 fatty acid supplementation improves the immunometabolic host response and outcome after colorectal resection for cancer. *Surgery.* 2002;132(5):805–814.

38. Hurley RS, Campbell SM, Mirtallo JM, Wade VR, Murphy C. Outcomes of cancer and non-cancer patients on HPN. *Nutr Clin Pract.* 1990;5(2):59–62.

39. Vashi PG, Dahik S, Popiel B, et al. A longitudinal study investigating quality of life and nutritional outcomes in advanced cancer patients receiving home parenteral nutrition. *BMC Cancer.* 2014;14:593–602.

40. Boullata JI, Gilbert K, Sacks G, et al. A.S.P.E.N. guidelines: parenteral nutrition ordering, order review, compounding, labeling, and dispensing. *JPEN J Parenter Enteral Nutr.* 2014;38:334–377.

41. Ayers P, Adams S, Boullata J, et al. A.S.P.E.N. parenteral nutrition safety consensus recommendations. *JPEN J Parenter Enter Nutr.* 2014;38:296–333.

42. Guenter P, Boullata JI, Ayers P, et al. Standardized competencies for parenteral nutrition prescribing. The American Society for Parenteral and Enteral Nutrition model. *Nutr Clin Pract.* 2015;30(4):570–576.

43. Boullata JI, Holcombe B, Sacks G, et al. Standardized competencies for parenteral nutrition order review and parenteral nutrition preparation including compounding. The ASPEN model. *Nutr Clin Pract.* 2016;31(4):548–555.

44. A.S.P.E.N. Practice Management Task Force; DeLegge M, Wooley JA, Guenter P, et al. The state of nutrition support teams and update on current models for providing nutrition support therapy to patients. *Nutr Clin Pract.* 2010;25(1):76–84.

45. Hvas CL, Farrer K, Donaldson E, et al. Quality and safety impact on the provision of parenteral nutrition through introduction of a nutrition support team. *Euro J Clin Nutr.* 2014;68:1294–1299. doi:10.1038/ejcn.2014.186.

46. Seres D, Sacks GS, Pedersen CA, et al. Parenteral nutrition safe practices: results of the 2003 American Society for Parenteral and Enteral Nutrition survey. *JPEN J Parenter Enteral Nutr.* 2006;30(3):259–265.

47. Sacks GS, Rough S, Kudsk KA. Frequency and severity of harm of medication errors related to the parenteral nutrition process in a large university teaching hospital. *Pharmacotherapy.* 2009;29(8): 966–974.

48. Pace NM, Long JB, Elerding S, et al. Performance model anchors successful nutrition support protocol. *Nutr Clin Pract.* 1997; 12(6):274–279.

49. Dimick JB, Swoboda S, Talamini MA, et al. Risk of colonization of central venous catheters: catheters for total parenteral nutrition vs catheters for other purposes. *Am J Crit Care.* 2003;12(4):328–335.

50. Gupta N, Hocevar SN, Moulton-Meissner HA, et al. Outbreak of *Serratia marcescens* bloodstream infections in patients receiving parenteral nutrition prepared by a compounding pharmacy. *Clin Infect Dis.* 2014;59(1):1–8. Epub 2014(Apr 11). doi:10.1093/cid/ciu218.

51. Storey MA, Weber RJ, Besco K, et al. Evaluation of parenteral nutrition errors in an era of drug shortages. *Nutr Clin Pract.* 2016;31:211–217.

52. American Society for Parenteral and Enteral Nutrition. Parenteral nutrition safety toolkit. https://www.nutritioncare.org/Guidelines_and_Clinical_Resources/Toolkits/Parenteral_Nutrition_Safety_Toolkit. Accessed September 5, 2016.

53. Mundi MS, Nystrom EM, Hurley DL, McMahon M. Management of parenteral nutrition in hospitalized adult patients. *JPEN J Parenter Enteral Nutr.* 2016. Epub ahead of print 2016(Sept 28). doi:10.1177/0148607116667060.

54. Martin K, DeLegge M, Nichols M, et al. Assessing appropriate nutrition ordering practices in tertiary care medical centers. *JPEN J Parenter Enteral Nutr.* 2011;35(1):122–130.

55. Taylor B, Renfro A, Mehringer L. The role of the dietitian in the intensive care unit. *Curr Opin Clin Nutr Metab Care.* 2005; 8(2): 211–216.

15 Parenteral Nutrition Formulations

Rina Patel, PharmD, BCNSP

CONTENTS

Acknowledgments: Jacqueline R. Barber, PharmD, BCNSP, FASHP, and Gordon S. Sacks, PharmD, BCNSP, FCCP, were authors of this chapter for the second edition.

Objectives

1. List 12 components typically incorporated into a parenteral nutrition (PN) formulation.
2. Summarize the major differences in commercially available crystalline amino acid formulations.
3. Compare the dextrose–amino acid (2-in-1) system for PN vs the total nutrient admixture (TNA) system in terms of convenience, stability, compatibility, and potential to support microbial growth if contaminated.
4. Describe the factors that influence the stability of PN formulations.

5. Explain the benefits of in-line filtration for PN formulations.
6. List guidelines for hang times of various PN components.
7. Perform calculations to construct a practical PN regimen given a patient's specific macronutrient needs.

Test Your Knowledge Questions

1. Which of the following may increase the risk of phlebitis with peripherally administered parenteral nutrition (PPN)?
   A. Osmolarity equal to or less than 900 mOsm/L
   B. Potassium 100 mEq/L
   C. Calcium less than 5 mEq/L
   D. Addition of heparin to the PPN
2. What is the smallest pore size filter that recommended for TNA?
   A. 0.22 μm
   B. 0.5 μm
   C. 1.2 μm
   D. 5 μm
3. Which of the following will increase the solubility of calcium and phosphate in a PN formulation?
   A. Use of calcium as the chloride salt
   B. Use of phosphate as the sodium salt
   C. Increased amino acid concentration
   D. Increased temperature
4. According to recommendations by the National Advisory Group on Standards and Practice guidelines for parenteral nutrition formulations and the American Society for Parenteral and Enteral Nutrition (ASPEN) parenteral nutrition safety consensus,[1] the amount of dextrose used in preparation of a PN formulation is required to appear on the label as:
   A. The percentage of original concentration and volume (eg, dextrose 50% water, 500 mL)
   B. The percentage of final concentration after admixture (eg, dextrose 25%)
   C. Grams per liter of PN admixed (eg, dextrose 250 g/L)
   D. Grams per day (eg, dextrose 250 g/d)

Test Your Knowledge Answers

1. The correct answer is **B**. Potassium can be quite irritating to peripheral veins. Potassium in concentrations less than 60 mEq/L and preferably less than 40 mEq/L is generally suggested for fluids administered via the peripheral vein. All the other choices may actually *decrease* the risk of phlebitis.[2-5]
2. The correct answer is **C**. The 1.2-μm filter is not a sterilizing filter, but it will remove large microorganisms such as *Candida albicans* and large particles that might otherwise lodge in pulmonary capillaries if allowed to pass through. A 0.22-μm filter is used for the 2-in-1 dextrose and amino acid type of PN, and it does qualify as a sterilizing filter. Because fat particles are generally between 0.1 μm and 1 μm in size, lipid injectable emulsion (ILE) could occlude 0.22-μm and 0.5-μm filters, or the emulsion could be destabilized if used with these filters. The 5-μm filter removes particulate matter, but it would allow many types of microbial contaminants to pass through.[1]

3. The correct answer is **C**. The higher the concentration of amino acids in the formulation, the less likely precipitation is to occur. Amino acids can form soluble complexes with calcium, which reduce the effective concentrations of free calcium available to form insoluble precipitates with phosphorus ions. Calcium chloride is more dissociated than calcium gluconate, making the risk of precipitation with phosphate higher. The salt form of phosphate does not affect calcium solubility if the phosphate amount remains constant; that is, 1 mmol of phosphate as the sodium salt has the same potential to precipitate with calcium as 1 mmol of phosphate as the potassium salt. Precipitation is more likely to occur at warmer temperatures because the dissociation of calcium salts increases as the temperature rises, promoting the availability of ions to form insoluble complexes with phosphate.[6]
4. The correct answer is **D**. Grams of dextrose per day is the information most consistent with that found on a nutrient label, supports the use of the 24-hour nutrient infusion system, and requires the least number of calculations to determine the daily energy amount. The quantity per liter may appear on the label in a second column in parentheses.[1]

Formulation Components

Components used in formulating PN typically include energy substrates such as carbohydrate, protein (as amino acids), and fat, as well as electrolytes, vitamins, and trace elements. Sterile water for injection may be added to provide necessary volume to the PN formulation. Various combinations of these components are incorporated into the PN regimen for intravenous (IV) administration based on the patient's individual requirements.

Carbohydrate Energy Substrates

The most commonly used carbohydrate energy substrate is dextrose, which, in its hydrated form, provides 3.4 kcal/g. Dextrose is commercially available in multiple concentrations ranging from 2.5% to 70% as well as in combinations with other components of the PN formulation. According to the United States Pharmacopeia (USP), dextrose solutions are acidic, with a pH ranging from 3.5 to 6.5, and vary in osmolarity depending on their concentration. Higher dextrose concentrations (greater than 10%) are generally reserved for central venous administration because of their propensity to cause thrombophlebitis in peripheral veins.[7]

Glycerol (glycerin), a sugar alcohol that provides 4.3 kcal/g is another, less frequently used carbohydrate energy substrate. It is contained in 1 standardized commercially available PN (SCAPN) formulation marketed for peripheral administration. This formulation has been shown to be protein-sparing,[8,9] and it has been reported to induce less insulin response than dextrose-based regimens,[8,10] although another study found higher serum insulin levels with glycerol use.[9] A brief discussion of rationales for the clinical use of this product is included in the section on SCAPN.

Protein

Crystalline amino acids are used in PN formulations to provide protein and yield 4 kcal/g when oxidized for energy. Nitrogen content varies depending on the concentration of the amino acid formulation and the mixture of individual amino acids; however, for nitrogen balance calculations, amino acid products are generally assumed to be 16% nitrogen (6.25 g amino acids = 1 g nitrogen). Standard or balanced amino acid products are mixtures of essential and nonessential amino acids. They are available from different manufacturers in stock solutions with concentrations ranging from 3.5% to 20%, although 8.5%, 10%, and 15% are most frequently used for PN compounding. Modified or specialty amino acid products are specifically formulated for certain disease states or special conditions (Table 15-1).[7] Commercially available amino acid formulations may also contain various concentrations and combinations of electrolytes and/or buffers, in addition to the inherent or endogenous electrolyte content (eg, acetate) of the individual amino acids. Clinicians should be cognizant that the electrolyte content of certain amino acid formulations may affect the amounts of electrolytes that need to or can be added to the PN formulation. For example, FreAmine III and HepatAmine both contribute an additional 10 mEq/L sodium

TABLE 15-1 Commercially Available Crystalline Amino Acid Solutions

Brand Name (Manufacturer)	Type	Stock Concentrations	Electrolytes (Excluding Chloride and Acetate)
Travasol (Baxter IV Systems)	Standard	10%	• None
FreAmine III (B. Braun Medical)	Standard	10%	• Sodium, 10 mEq/L; phosphate, 10 mmol/L
Aminosyn (Hospira)	Standard	8.5%, 10%	• None
Aminosyn II (Hospira)	Standard	8.5%, 10%, 15%	• 8.5% concentration: sodium, 32 mEq/L • 10% concentration: sodium, 38 mEq/L • 15% concentration: sodium, 50 mEq/L
Aminosyn with electrolytes (Hospira)	Standard with electrolytes	3.5%M, 7%, and 8.5% with electrolytes[a]	• Aminosyn 3.5%M: sodium, 40 mEq/L; potassium, 13 mEq/L; magnesium, 3 mEq/L; phosphate, 3.5 mmol/L • Aminosyn 7% and 8.5% with electrolytes: sodium, 65 mEq/L; potassium, 65 mEq/L; magnesium, 10 mEq/L; phosphate, 30 mmol/L
Clinisol (Baxter IV Systems)	Standard/concentrated	15%	• None
Plenamine (B. Braun Medical)	Standard/concentrated	15%	• None
ProSol (Baxter IV Systems)	Standard/concentrated	20%	• None
HepatAmine[a] (B. Braun Medical)	BCAA-enriched	8%	• Sodium, 10 mEq/L; phosphate, 10 mmol/L
FreAmine HBC[b] (B. Braun Medical)	BCAA-enriched	6.9%	• Sodium, 10 mEq/L
Aminosyn HBC[b] (Hospira)	BCAA-enriched	7%	• None
NephrAmine[c,d] (B. Braun Medical)	EAA	5.4%	• Sodium, 5 mEq/L
Aminosyn RF[c,e] (Hospira)	EAA	5.2%	• None

BCAA, branched-chain amino acids; EAA, essential amino acids; HBC, high–branched chain.
[a]Contains 36% BCAA; formulated for hepatic failure.
[b]Contains 45% BCAA; formulated for metabolic stress
[c]Formulated for renal failure
[d]Contains essential amino acids only, including histidine.
[e]Contains essential amino acids, including histidine, plus arginine.

and 10 mmol/L phosphate, and Aminosyn II contributes a varying amount of sodium depending on the concentration of the formulation.

Modified Amino Acid Formulations

Specialty amino acid formulations are available for use in certain disease states or conditions (Table 15-1). These products are generally more expensive than standard formulations and should be reserved for patients meeting the intended indications who are expected to benefit clinically from their use. ASPEN has published guidelines for the use of these products in clinical practice.[11,12]

The modified amino acid formulation designed for use in hepatic encephalopathy contains increased amounts of branched-chain amino acids (BCAA) and decreased amounts of aromatic amino acids (AAA) compared to standard parenteral amino acid formulations (eg, Hepatamine contains 36% BCAA and 2.1% AAA, whereas Travasol contains 19% BCAA and 7.8% AAA).[13] An altered metabolism in patients with hepatic failure can result in a high serum ratio of AAA to BCAA. This imbalance is thought to increase transport of AAA into the brain, where they serve as precursors to neurotransmitters that may be responsible for altered mental status. Indications for this modified amino acid formulation are very limited. See Chapter 27 for a discussion of nutrition in liver disease, including the appropriate use and cost-effectiveness of specialized amino acid formulations.

The modified amino acid formulations marketed for use in renal failure are composed primarily of essential amino acids. This preference for essential amino acids is based on the theory that nonessential amino acids can be physiologically recycled from urea, whereas essential amino acids must be provided from the diet. Despite the need for fluid restriction in many renal failure patients, these formulations are more dilute (5.2% to 5.4%) than commonly used standard amino acid formulations (8.5% and 10%). Essential amino acid formulas offer no significant advantage over the standard formulations and may result in metabolic complications; therefore, indications for these formulations are very limited.[12,13] Standard formulations are recommended and usually prescribed for patients with renal failure. See Chapter 29 for further discussion of nutrition in renal failure.

Modified amino acid formulations are also available for use in metabolic stress, trauma, thermal injury, and/or hypercatabolic states. These products are formulated based on the theory that increased amounts of BCAA are beneficial during severe metabolic stress because of increased skeletal muscle catabolism; therefore, these products provide increased amounts of leucine, isoleucine, and valine. Although the use of BCAA-enriched formulations slightly improves nitrogen balance in certain patient groups, clinical evidence does not support improved outcomes.[11] Refer to Chapters 23 and 24 for more information on specialized nutrition support in critical care, trauma, and burns.

Concentrated amino acid formulations are available for use when patients require fluid restriction. These formulations are highly concentrated (15% or 20%), but they are otherwise similar in composition to the standard amino acid formulations. The amounts of certain electrolytes, such as chloride and acetate, may be different in concentrated formulations than in the standard formulations. Generally, the acetate content is higher in the more concentrated products than in standard stock concentrations. However, chloride salts may be used to balance the chloride:acetate ratio in the final PN formulation to avoid iatrogenic acid-base disturbances.

Lipid Injectable Emulsions

ILEs are used to provide energy as well as essential fatty acids for PN formulations. Until recently, 3 ILE products were available in the United States: 2 formulations composed solely of long-chain triglycerides (LCTs; carbon chain length equal to or greater than 14), which are 100% soybean oil–based formulations and a 50:50 blend of safflower oil and soybean oil.[14,15] However, because of a lack of supply of safflower oil and manufacturing limitations, the product with a 50:50 blend of safflower oil and soybean oil has been out of stock with no expected release date.

ILE formulations are commercially available in concentrations of 20% (2 kcal/mL) and 30% (2.9 to 3 kcal/mL, depending on the manufacturer). The ILE 30% formulation is approved only for the compounding of a 3-in-1 admixture (ie, TNA), not for direct IV administration. Previously, ILEs were available in 10% (1.1 kcal/mL) concentration, but 10% ILE formulations are currently marketed only in premixed products and products with a lipid emulsion such as propofol. The higher phospholipid:triglyceride ratio in the 10% ILE, compared to the 20% ILE, increases the presence of free phospholipids, which interfere with lipoprotein lipase activity, thereby decreasing the lipid clearance rate.

The major component fatty acids in the 100% soybean oil–based ILE include linoleic acid (44% to 62%), oleic acid (19% to 30%), palmitic acid (7% to 10%), α-linolenic acid (4% to 11%), and stearic acid (1.4% to 5.5%). Safflower oil contains only a trace of α-linolenic acid; thus, the ILE product using a 50:50 mix of soybean oil and safflower oil contains half as much ω-3 fatty acid (ie, α-linolenic acid) as ILE using 100% soybean oil.

Concerns about the high content of proinflammatory ω-6 polyunsaturated fatty acids (PUFA) in traditional ILE led to the development of alternative ILE formulations made from various oil sources.[16] Some of these ILEs have been available worldwide for many years. However, it was not until July 2016 that the US Food and Drug Administration (FDA) approved a combination ILE product marketed as Smoflipid (Fresenius Kabi AG, Bad Homburg VDH, Germany) for use in the United States.[17] "Smof" refers to the types of oils in Smoflipid: soybean oil; medium-chain triglycerides (MCTs; saturated fatty acids with a carbon length of 6 to 12); olive oil; and fish oil. This ILE contains a mixture of 30% soybean oil (LCTs), 30% MCTs, 25% olive oil, and 15% fish oil, and it is available as a 20% solution (ie, 6% soybean, 6% MCTs, 5% olive oil, and 3% fish oil).[17,18] It is contraindicated in patients with a known hypersensitivity to soybean, fish, egg, or peanut protein. The major component fatty acids in Smoflipid are oleic acid (23% to 35%), linoleic acid (14% to 25%), caprylic acid (13% to 24%), palmitic acid (7% to 12%), capric acid (5% to 15%), steric acid (1.5% to 4%), α-linolenic acid (1.5% to 3.5%), eicosapentaenoic acid (EPA; 1% to 3.5%), and docosahexae-noic acid (DHA; 1% to 3.5%). The mean essential fatty acid concentrations of Smoflipid are 35 mg/mL (range 28 to 50 mg/mL) for linoleic acid and 4.5 mg/mL (range 3 to 7 mg/mL) for α-linolenic acid. Smoflipid's essential acid concentration is thus lower than the concentration in the traditionally available soybean oil–based ILE. Because their compositions vary, Smoflipid and soybean oil–based ILE are not generically interchangeable products.

Smoflipid capitalizes on the beneficial attributes of oils from non–soybean oil sources while reducing the amounts and detrimental effects of ω-6 fatty acids. It may be useful in patients who do not tolerate soybean oil–based ILE during critical illness or metabolic stress, and also in patients with carnitine deficiency because the transport of MCTs into mitochondria is carnitine-independent.[19] Compared with soybean oil–based ILE, Smoflipid has been associated in clinical use with reduced liver changes and the preservation of antioxidant capacity in pediatric home PN patients, adult intestinal failure long-term PN patients, and critically ill patients.[20-22] PN-associated liver disease (PNALD) is thought to be multifactorial in nature. ω-6 PUFA in soybean oil–based ILE can lead to the development of proinflammatory cytokines derived from linoleic and arachidonic acids.[16] Furthermore, intravenously administered phytosterols (ie, plant sterols contained in plant-derived lipid formulations such as soybean oil) have been associated with the development of PNALD. Another proposed mechanism of hepatic injury from ILE is oxidative stress; therefore, antioxidants, such as vitamin E, in ILE may provide a protective effect, although this effect has not been established in humans. Clinicians should keep in mind that long-term safety data for Smoflipid, such as the risk of essential fatty acid deficiency (EFAD), are limited.

Other components of ILE formulations include an egg phospholipid emulsifier, which contributes 15 mmol phosphate per liter; glycerin to render the formulation isotonic; and sodium hydroxide to adjust the final pH to a range of 6 to 9.[23]

Each gram of fat provides 9 kcal. Furthermore, the glycerol in ILE adds energy such that 10% ILE supplies 1.1 kcal/mL, 20% ILE supplies 2 kcal/mL, and 30% ILE supplies 2.9 to 3 kcal/mL.

Whether infused separately from amino acids and dextrose or as a TNA, the ILE infusion rate should not exceed 0.11 g/kg/h.[24] Greater infusion rates are associated with increased risk of adverse effects such as hypertriglyceridemia, infectious complications, and fat overload syndrome, which is characterized by headaches, seizures, fever, jaundice, hepatosplenomegaly, abdominal pain, respiratory distress, pancytopenia, and shock.

The daily dose of ILE should not exceed 60% of total energy requirements or 2.5 g/kg/d.[11] Many clinicians limit soybean oil–based ILE to 1 g/kg/d because of the higher ω-6 fatty acid provision. This concern about ω-6 fatty acids is especially relevant in critically ill patients; for this patient population, the ASPEN/Society of Critical Care Medicine (SCCM) guidelines suggest that clinicians either withhold soybean oil–based ILE or limit it to a maximum of 100 g (often divided into 2 doses) during the first week following initiation of PN if the patient is at risk for EFAD.[25]

Table 15-2 lists soybean oil–, MCT-, olive oil–, and fish oil–based ILE formulations currently available worldwide and in the United States.[16,26]

Structured Lipids and Fish Oil– and Olive Oil–Based Fat Emulsions

Structured lipids containing laboratory-developed, chemically altered triglyceride molecules with specific fatty acids at the 3 binding sites of the glycerol backbone have been investigated in various patient populations.[27,28] Specific fatty acids in structured lipids may include linoleic acid, a medium-chain fatty acid, and a very long–chain ω-3 fatty acid, or various combinations of these or other fatty acids not found in nature. Because fatty acids at the 1 and 3 position of the glycerol backbone may be hydrolyzed more rapidly than those at the 2 position, the metabolism of structured lipids may be significantly different than that of typical LCT or MCT-LCT mixtures. Although currently under investigational study, structured lipid products are not commercially available for IV use in the United States.[29,30]

Fish oil–based ILE incorporate ω-3 fatty acids into ILE in an effort to produce less-inflammatory and nonthrombogenic prostaglandins by the metabolic pathways responsible for lipoprotein breakdown. Studies indicating this effect have been performed in patients with sepsis,[31] atopic dermatitis,[32] and severe ulcerative colitis,[33] and those undergoing elective surgery.[34] Omegaven (Fresenius Kabi AG, Bad Homburg VDH, Germany) is an ILE that contains 100% fish oils with no oils from plant or vegetable sources. The most dramatic impact of ILE rich in ω-3 fatty acids has been seen in the treatment of pediatric intestinal failure associated liver disease, with more rapid and frequent cholestasis reversal with fish oil–based ILE compared to soybean oil–based ILE.[26,35,36] Of note, the low arachidonic acid and linoleic acid content of fish oil–based ILE raises concerns for the development of EFAD when used as monotherapy, especially in the pediatric population or those on long-term PN, although in 1 study this problem was not demonstrated for up to 18.4 weeks (median; interquartile range [IQR], 8.7–36.4 weeks).[37]

Olive oil has also been substituted for a portion of LCT in ILE to reduce the risks of conventional LCT ILE products in critically ill patients. Olive oil–based fat emulsions, such as Clinolipid, offer advantages over the current polyunsaturated LCT ILE, including decreased peroxidation[38] and a lack of in vitro lymphocyte function inhibition.[39] The FDA approved Clinolipid (Baxter Healthcare, Deerfield, IL) in 2013, but it is not currently available on the US market. Data from clinical trials with olive oil–based ILE reveal these products to be clinically safe and well tolerated with a tendency to preserve hepatic function. Because olive oil contains approximately 20% ω-6 fatty acids, the supply of linoleic acid is enough to avoid the risk of EFAD.

In an observational, prospective multicenter study of the effects of different ILE formulations on clinical outcomes in 451 critically ill patients, the use of olive oil– and fish oil–based ILE was associated with faster termination of mechanical ventilation and less time to intensive care unit discharge alive compared with soybean oil–based ILE.[40]

TABLE 15-2 Comparison of Lipid Injectable Emulsion Products

	Intralipid	Liposyn III	Smoflipid	Lipofundin MCT/LCT	Clinolipid	Omegaven
Manufacturer/distributor	Fresenius Kabi	Hospira	Fresenius Kabi	B. Braun	Baxter	Fresenius Kabi
Availability in the United States	Available	Unavailable	Available	Unavailable	FDA-approved but unavailable	Available for compassionate use only
Oil source, %						
Soybean	100	50	30	50	20	0
Safflower	0	50	0	0	0	0
Coconut (MCT)	0	0	30	50	0	0
Olive	0	0	25	0	80	0
Fish	0	0	15	0	0	100
Fat composition						
Palmitic, g/100 mL	1	0.88	0.9	0.55	0.75–1.9	0.25–1
Stearic, g/100 mL	0.4	0.32	0.33	0.2	0.07–0.5	0.05–0.2
Oleic,[a] g/100 mL	2.6	1.82	2.8	1.16	4.4–8	0.6–1.3
Linoleic,[b] g/100 mL	5	6.54	2.85	2.66	1.4–2.2	0.1–0.7
α-Linolenic,[c] g/100 mL	0.9	0.39	0.275	0.1	0.05–0.4	< 0.2
EPA,[c] g/100 mL	0	0	0.25	0	0	1.28–2.82
Arachidonic,[b] g/100 mL	0	0	0.05	0	0.025	0.1–0.4
DHA,[c] g/100 mL	0	0	0.05	0	0	1.44–3.09
Phytosterols, mg/L	348 ± 33	383	47.6	NP	327 ± 8	0
α-Tocopherol, mg/L	38	NP	163–225	100	32	150–296
ω-6:ω-3 ratio	7:1	7:1	2.5:1	7:1	9:1	1:8

DHA, docosahexaenoic acid; EPA, eicosapentaenoic acid; FDA, US Food and Drug Administration; LCT, long-chain triglyceride; MCT, medium-chain triglyceride; NP, not provided.
[a] ω-9 fatty acid.
[b] ω-6 fatty acid.
[c] ω-3 fatty acid.
Source: Data are from manufacturers and references 16 and 26.

Electrolytes

Maintenance or therapeutic amounts of various electrolytes are added to PN formulations in amounts that depend on the patient's requirements. Standard daily ranges for adults are listed in Table 15-3.[1] Acetate and chloride do not have specific ranges for intake; rather, they are adjusted as needed to maintain acid-base balance.[1] Electrolytes are available in various parenteral salt forms, but not all electrolytes are not intended to be added to PN (Table 15-4). Calcium gluconate and magnesium sulfate are the preferred forms of these cations for use in PN formulations because they are less likely to produce physicochemical incompatibilities compared to calcium chloride, calcium gluceptate, and magnesium chloride. Electrolytes are available commercially as individual salts and as "cocktails" (or combination products) for ease in admixing. They are also pre-added in specified amounts to certain stock amino acid formulations or SCAPN. Clinicians should carefully evaluate the composition of electrolyte combination products for compatibility (eg, calcium chloride may be incompatible with some combination products).

Vitamins

Commercially available vitamin products for PN supplementation include single vitamin products and multivitamin products that include both fat-soluble and water-soluble vitamins. Injectable multivitamin products for use in adults include ascorbic acid, retinol, ergocalciferol or cholecalciferol, thiamin, riboflavin, pyridoxine, niacinamide, dexpanthenol, dl-α tocopheryl acetate, folic acid, cyanocobalamin, biotin, and phytonadione. Parenteral formulations for single vitamins are not commercially available for biotin, pantothenic acid, riboflavin, vitamin A, vitamin D, or vitamin E. Table 15-5 lists the composition of adult parenteral multivitamin products available in the United States.[41,42] Micronutrient requirements and

TABLE 15-3 Daily Electrolyte Requirements

Electrolyte	Parenteral Requirement
Sodium	1–2 mEq/kg
Potassium	1–2 mEq/kg
Chloride	As needed to maintain acid-base balance
Acetate	As needed to maintain acid-base balance
Calcium	10–15 mEq
Magnesium	8–20 mEq
Phosphate	20–40 mmol

Source: Data are from reference 1.

TABLE 15-4 Commercially Available Parenteral Electrolyte Salts

Electrolyte	Salt Form
Sodium	Acetate, chloride, phosphate, bicarbonate,[a] lactate[a]
Potassium	Acetate, chloride, phosphate
Chloride	Sodium, potassium
Acetate	Sodium, potassium
Calcium	Gluconate,[b] gluceptate, chloride[c]
Magnesium	Sulfate,[b] chloride
Phosphate	Sodium, potassium

Note: 1 mmol of sodium phosphate contains 1.33 mEq of sodium; 1 mmol of potassium phosphate contains 1.47 mEq of potassium.
[a]Avoid adding in parenteral nutrition (PN) mixtures; not intended to be added to PN mixtures.
[b]Preferred salt form for use in PN formulations.
[c]Avoid adding to PN mixtures; there is a very high risk of precipitation, and compatibility data are limited. Calcium chloride is not interchangeable with calcium gluconate.

clinical indications of deficiencies and toxicities are reviewed in Chapter 8.

Trace Elements

Commonly used trace elements in PN formulations include zinc, copper, chromium, manganese, and selenium. These nutrients are commercially available as single-entity products and in various multi–trace element combinations and concentrations for adults, pediatrics, and neonates.[43] Table 15-6 lists the composition ranges of adult parenteral multi–trace element products available in the United States.

In 2012, ASPEN recommended that commercially available multi–trace element products should undergo significant modifications. Furthermore, ASPEN also stated that, when the multiple-element products are inappropriate, single-element products should be used to meet individual patient needs.[44] ASPEN's recommendations for adult trace element products

TABLE 15-5 Composition of Adult Parenteral Multivitamin Products Available in the United States[a]

Component	Dose (10 mL)
Fat-soluble vitamins	
Vitamin A (retinol)	1 mg (3300 USP units)
Vitamin D (ergocalciferol or cholecalciferol)	5 mcg (200 USP units)
Vitamin E (dl-α tocopheryl acetate)	10 mg (10 USP units)
Vitamin K (phytonadione)[a]	150 mcg
Water-soluble vitamins	
Vitamin B$_1$ (thiamin)	6 mg
Vitamin B$_2$ (riboflavin 5-phosphate sodium)	3.6 mg
Vitamin B$_6$ (pyridoxine HCl)	6 mg
Niacinamide	40 mg
Dexpanthenol (d-pantothenyl alcohol)	15 mg
Biotin	60 mcg
Folic acid	600 mcg
Vitamin B$_{12}$ (cyanocobalamin)	5 mcg
Ascorbic acid	200 mg

HCl, hydrogen chloride; USP, United States Pharmacopeia.
[a]One manufacturer provides a product that is phytonadione free.

TABLE 15-6 Composition of Adult Parenteral Multi–Trace Element Products Available in the United States

Component	Dose Provided from Daily Dose of Multi–Trace Element Product
Copper (cuprous chloride or cupric sulfate)	1–1.3 mg
Chromium (chromic chloride)	10–12 mcg
Manganese (manganese chloride or sulfate)	270–500 mcg
Selenium (sodium selenite or selenious acid)[a]	0–60 mcg
Zinc (zinc chloride or sulfate)	3–6.5 mg
Iron (ferric chloride)[b]	1.1 mg
Iodine (potassium iodide)[b]	130 mcg
Molybdate (sodium molybdate dihydrate)[b]	19 mcg
Fluoride (sodium fluoride)[b]	950 mcg

[a]MTE-4 products do not contain selenium.
[b]Addamel N contains additional elements as noted.

included decreasing copper to 0.3 to 0.5 mg/d, decreasing manganese to 55 mcg/d, manufacturing a product with no chromium (or a maximum of 1 mcg/d), and including selenium in all products at a higher dose of 60 to 100 mcg/d. ASPEN also recommended that trace element contamination in PN formulations be limited to less than 0.1 mg/d and 40 mcg/d of copper and manganese, respectively. These recommendations were based on the discrepancy between adult parenteral trace element requirements and the doses provided by multi–trace element products, findings of organ accumulation of copper, manganese, and chromium in long-term PN patients,[45] and reports of PN contaminant levels of copper, manganese, and chromium that met between 63% and 100% of a patient's daily requirements.[46]

Iron

Other elements that may be supplemented in PN include molybdenum, iodine, and iron. Five injectable iron products are available, all as single-entity products. Only iron dextran is approved for addition to PN, but this supplement should only be considered for dextrose–amino acid formulations, because ILE formulations are disrupted by iron.[47]

Other Specific Nutrients

Glutamine

Glutamine, an amino acid found in the human body, is described as having a role in intestinal integrity, immune function, and protein synthesis during stress states. Crystalline amino acid formulations do not contain glutamine, and there has been interest in adding glutamine to PN, either as a separate entity or as part of the amino acid stock formulations. However, no FDA-approved IV form of glutamine is commercially available in the United States for admixture in PN solutions, because of poor solubility and stability and compatibility limitations. Studies of glutamine-supplemented PN have used extemporaneous preparations of powdered L-glutamine sterilized by filtration as well as commercially available products not available in the United States. Parenteral glutamine supplementation is no longer recommended for adult critically ill patients because recent literature indicates either a lack of infectious and mortality benefit or even higher mortality rates when IV glutamine is compared with placebo.[25,48,49]

Carnitine

Carnitine is a quaternary amine necessary for proper transport and metabolism of long-chain fatty acids into the matrix of the mitochondria for beta-oxidation. Carnitine deficiency itself can lead to impaired fatty acid oxidation, which is thought to increase the possibility of other consequences such as hepatic steatosis. Carnitine is not present in any commercially available PN formulation component, but an IV form of L-carnitine is commercially available to be added to PN formulations for the treatment of carnitine deficiency and for selected patients who have a documented deficiency or are susceptible to a deficiency, such as neonates and infants. Limited stability data exist for the addition of carnitine to PN.[50]

Parenteral Nutrition Product Shortages

PN product shortages have occurred in the United States because of a variety of factors, including acquisition issues with raw materials, manufacturing/production interruptions, and consolidation of the market. ASPEN assembled a group of experts to establish guidelines for managing shortages of ILE formulations, amino acids, multivitamins, electrolyte/mineral injections, and trace element products (Tables 15-7 through 15-11).[51-56] Recommendations should only be used in the event of a national shortage of these products and should not be employed during routine (ie, nonshortage) clinical practice. Although there are no substitutions for these products, dose conservation and alternate measures can be used during the shortage period. See Practice Scenario 15-1 for an example of PN product shortage and its implications.[57,58]

TABLE 15-7 Considerations for Use of Lipid Injectable Emulsion in Adults During a National Shortage

- ILE should not be administered to adult, mild to moderately undernourished hospitalized patients receiving PN for less than 2 weeks.
- Adult, hospitalized patients receiving PN longer than 2 weeks should receive a total of 100 g of soybean oil–based ILE per week to avoid EFAD.
- No additional ILE is necessary in adult, hospitalized critically ill patients receiving propofol.
- Home or long-term care adult patients should receive a minimum of 100 g of soybean oil–based ILE per week to avoid EFAD.
- ILE should be included as a component of PN on a daily basis for special patient populations requiring PN (eg, patients with glucose intolerance, severely malnourished patients, patients at risk for refeeding syndrome, pregnant patients).
- Consider using a more recently available ILE formulation (eg, Smoflipid) during a soybean oil–based ILE shortage, although the dose and frequency of administration to prevent EFAD may be different than soybean oil–based ILE.[a]
- Monitor patients for signs and symptoms of EFAD.
- Consider compounding PN in a single, central location to decrease inventory waste.

ASPEN, American Society for Parenteral and Enteral Nutrition; EFAD, essential fatty acid deficiency; ILE, lipid injectable emulsion; PN, parenteral nutrition.
[a]Not part of the ASPEN Clinical Practice Committee Shortage Subcommittee's 2013 considerations (the US Food and Drug Administration approved Smoflipid in 2016).
Source: Adapted with permission from reference 51: Clinical Practice Committee Shortage Subcommittee. A.S.P.E.N. parenteral nutrition intravenous fat emulsion product shortage considerations. *Nutr Clin Pract.* 2013;28:4:528–529. Information on use of Smoflipid is from reference 52.

TABLE 15-8 Considerations for Use of Intravenous Amino Acids in Adults During a National Shortage

- Review all amino acid products currently available in the United States. Although supply in one concentration may be limited, a different concentration may be available.
- Reserve high-concentration amino acid products (eg, >10%) for use in fluid-restricted PN patients.
- Only use neonatal/pediatric-specific amino acids or disease-specific amino acids for the indicated patient populations.
- Evaluate PN patient population to determine if a SCAPN is appropriate for use.
- Be aware that different brands of amino acids vary with respect to pH, electrolyte composition (eg, phosphate), and calcium phosphate solubility. Therefore, compatibility and stability issues must be considered when substituting amino acid products.
- Consider compounding PN in a single, central location to decrease inventory waste.

PN, parenteral nutrition; SCAPN, standardized commercially available PN formulation.
Source: Adapted with permission from reference 53: Plogsted S, Adams SC, Allen K, et al. Clinical Practice Committee's Nutrition Product Shortage Subcommittee. Parenteral nutrition amino acids product shortage considerations. *Nutr Clin Pract*. 2016;31:4:560–561.

TABLE 15-9 Considerations for Use of Intravenous Multivitamins in Adults During a National Shortage

- Reserve IV multivitamins for patients receiving solely PN or those with therapeutic medical need for IV multivitamins.
- Consider using oral or enterally administered multivitamin preparations when oral/enteral intake is initiated (excluding patients with malabsorption syndromes). Note: Many oral liquid medications contain sorbitol, which may cause diarrhea and gastrointestinal intolerance.
- When supplies of adult multivitamins are no longer available, ration IV multivitamins in PN (eg, reduce the daily dose by 50% or provide multivitamin doses 3 times a week).
- If a 13-vitamin product cannot be obtained, a 12-vitamin product (without vitamin K) may be used with vitamin K supplementation of 150 mcg/d or 5–10 mg/wk.
- If supplies of adult IV multivitamins are exhausted, administer the following individual parenteral vitamins on a daily basis: thiamin, 6 mg; ascorbic acid, 200 mg; pyridoxine, 6 mg; and folate, 0.6 mg. 100 mcg cyanocobalamin should be administered at least once per month.
- Substituting pediatric IV multivitamins for use in adults is not recommended because it may contribute to a shortage of pediatric products. The vitamin composition of pediatric products differs from adult products and may be inappropriate for use.
- Adult IV multivitamins should not be administered to neonates because these products contain propylene glycol, polysorbate, and aluminum, which may create toxic side effects.
- Observe patients for an increase in deficiencies with ongoing shortages. Increase awareness and assessment for signs and symptoms of vitamin deficiencies. Monitor serum vitamin concentrations or other appropriate serum biochemical markers to evaluate vitamin status.
- Consider compounding PN in a single, central location to decrease inventory waste.

IV, intravenous; PN, parenteral nutrition.
Source: Adapted with permission from reference 54: Plogsted S, Adams SC, Allen K, et al. Clinical Practice Committee's Nutrition Product Shortage Subcommittee. Parenteral nutrition multivitamin product shortage considerations. *Nutr Clin Pract*. 2016;31:4:556–559.

TABLE 15-10 Considerations for Use of Parenteral Electrolyte/Mineral Products in Adults During a National Shortage

- Reserve IV electrolyte and mineral products for patients receiving solely PN or those with a therapeutic medical need for IV electrolyte and mineral products.
- Consider using oral or enterally administered electrolyte and mineral products when oral/enteral intake is initiated (excluding patients with malabsorption syndromes or nonfunctioning gastrointestinal tract).
- Minimize the use of electrolyte/mineral additives to IV fluids and enteral nutrition products.
- If appropriate for your PN patient population, consider using a standardized, commercially available multi-electrolyte/mineral product or SCAPN with standard electrolytes.
- Consider decreasing the daily amount of electrolytes added to PN and monitor serum electrolyte concentrations closely.
- Consider using a different concentration or salt form if one is available and there are no issues with compatability.
- Observe patients for an increase in deficiencies with ongoing shortages. Increase awareness and assessment for signs and symptoms of electrolyte and mineral deficiencies. Monitor serum vitamin concentrations or other appropriate serum biochemical markers to evaluate vitamin status.
- Consider compounding PN in a single, central location to decrease inventory waste.

IV, intravenous; PN, parenteral nutrition; SCAPN, standardized commercially available PN formulation.
Source: Adapted with permission from reference 55: Plogsted S, Adams SC, Allen K, et al. Clinical Practice Committee's Nutrition Product Shortage Subcommittee. Parenteral nutrition electrolyte and mineral shortage considerations. *Nutr Clin Pract*. 2016;31:4:132–134.

TABLE 15-11 Considerations for Use of Parenteral Trace Element Products in Adults During a National Shortage

- Reserve IV trace elements for patients receiving solely PN or those with therapeutic medical need for IV trace elements.
- Consider using oral or enterally administered multivitamin/multimineral/multi–trace element supplement products when oral/enteral intake is initiated (excluding patients with malabsorption syndromes). Supplements may not have a full spectrum of trace elements nor contain a daily enteral maintenance dose and generally have a lower bioavailability than IV formulations.
- If IV multi–trace element products are no longer available, administer individual parenteral trace element entities.
- When supplies of adult multi–trace element products are no longer available, ration IV multi–trace element products in PN (eg, reduce the daily dose by 50% or provide multi–trace elements 3 times a week).
- Consider withholding IV adult multi–trace element products for the first month of therapy to newly initiated adult PN patients who are not critically ill and do not have preexisting deficits.
- Substituting pediatric/neonatal IV multi–trace elements for use in adults is not recommended because it may contribute to a shortage of pediatric products. The composition of pediatric multi–trace element products differs from adult products and may be inappropriate for use.
- Observe patients for an increase in deficiencies with ongoing shortages. Increase awareness and assessment for signs and symptoms of trace element deficiencies. Monitor serum trace element concentrations or other appropriate serum biochemical markers to evaluate trace element status.
- Consider compounding PN in a single, central location to decrease inventory waste.

IV, intravenous; PN, parenteral nutrition.
Source: Adapted with permission from reference 56: Clinical Practice Committee Shortage Subcommittee. A.S.P.E.N. parenteral nutrition trace element product shortage considerations. *Nutr Clin Pract*. 2014;29:2:249–251.

Practice Scenario 15-1

Question: What is the most appropriate strategy to provide calcium to a patient receiving parenteral nutrition (PN) in the event of an intravenous (IV) calcium gluconate shortage?

Scenario: AC, a surgical patient requiring central PN, has a single-lumen peripherally inserted central catheter. Pertinent anthropometric and laboratory data are as follows: weight, 40 kg; height, 170 cm; sodium, 145 mmol/L (normal, 135 to 145 mmol/L); potassium, 3.5 mmol/L (normal, 3.5 to 5 mmol/L); chloride, 105 mmol/L (normal, 98 to 107 mmol/L); bicarbonate, 21 mmol/L (normal, 22 to 30 mmol/L); blood urea nitrogen, 37 mg/dL (normal, 7 to 20 mg/dL); creatinine, 0.8 mg/dL (normal, 0.6 to 1.2 mg/dL); calcium, 7.1 mg/dL (normal, 8.5 to 10.2 mg/dL); magnesium, 1.4 mEq/L (normal, 1.6 to 2.2 mEq/L); phosphate, 1.3 mg/dL (normal, 2.5 to 4.5 mg/dL); albumin, 2.6 g/dL (normal, 3.5 to 5 g/dL); and ionized calcium, 2.25 mEq/L (normal, 2 to 2.5 mEq/L).

The patient's energy and protein requirements are estimated to be 25 to 30 kcal/kg/d and 1.5 g/kg/d, respectively. A total nutrient admixture formulation containing dextrose, 175 g/d; amino acids, 60 g/d; and lipid injectable emulsion, 37 g/d in a volume of 1200 mL/d to infuse at 50 mL/h is prescribed to meet the patient's nutrition and fluid requirements. Additionally, IV fluids via a peripheral site are added to this regimen to correct dehydration. Because of a national shortage of IV concentrated calcium gluconate, the only salt form available for use is calcium chloride. The daily additives ordered for this 1200 mL/d PN formulation are as follows:
- Sodium acetate, 40 mEq
- Potassium chloride, 80 mEq
- Sodium phosphate, 45 mmol
- Calcium chloride, 15 mEq
- Magnesium sulfate, 24 mEq
- Multivitamins, 10 mL
- Multiple trace elements, 5 mL

Intervention: Calcium is removed from the PN formulation and ionized calcium concentrations are monitored for evidence of calcium deficiency.

Answer: The patient is evaluated for signs related to low serum calcium concentrations, such as tetany and other central nervous system or cardiovascular symptoms. If calcium supplementation is necessary, administer calcium chloride separately from the PN formulation, taking care not to infuse IV calcium through the same catheter as the PN formulation.

Rationale: After correcting the total calcium level for a decreased albumin concentration of 2.6 g/dL, AC's estimated total serum calcium concentration of 8.2 mg/dL is below normal (normal, 8.5 to 10 mg/dL); however, the ionized calcium concentration is within the normal range. In this case, the dose of calcium in the PN can be removed to avoid precipitation from the addition of calcium chloride, a form of calcium that is less soluble than calcium gluconate, the preferred form of calcium for use in PN solutions. One of the most-feared PN incompatibilities is the formation and infusion of calcium phosphate precipitates into the patient. The infusion of particulate matter, such as insoluble complexes of calcium phosphate, may block capillaries and have deleterious effects on vital organs such as the brain, lungs, kidneys, and liver. Case reports of pulmonary emboli and diffuse granulomatous interstitial pneumonitis have been attributed to calcium phosphate precipitates infused via PN formulations.[57,58]

Parenteral Nutrition Preparation

Admixtures: Dextrose–Amino Acid Formulations vs Total Nutrient Admixtures

PN admixtures may be prepared for the administration in either of 2 formats—the traditional dextrose–amino acid (2-in-1) formulation, or the TNA system, which is also referred to as a *3-in-1 admixture* or *all-in-1 admixture*. The dextrose–amino acid format incorporates the dextrose and amino acid–base solutions along with the prescribed electrolytes, minerals, vitamins, and trace elements in either a single container or multiple containers each day. ILE is administered separately as a piggyback infusion. In contrast, the TNA system incorporates dextrose, amino acids, ILE, and the prescribed micronutrients together in the same container for final administration.

Specific advantages and disadvantages are associated with the use of each PN formulation system.[59] Many institutions and home care providers have embraced the TNA system for its overall convenience and cost advantages. Although these advantages are significant, especially in the home care setting, they must be weighed against the disadvantages, along with

the circumstances of each situation.[60–62] A brief discussion of the major points follows.

Historically, the dextrose–amino acid format evolved as PN substrates were developed and refined, and standards of practice for specialized nutrition support matured. Concerns for the potential of ILE to support bacterial and fungal growth (if contaminated) led to the Centers for Disease Control and Prevention (CDC) guidelines limiting the hang times of ILE given in the piggyback fashion to a maximum of 12 hours.[63] At times, and with shorter infusion durations (4 to 6 hours), the faster infusion rates predisposed susceptible patients to hypertriglyceridemia that could have been lessened by infusing ILE at a slower rate. Under these circumstances and to simplify administration procedures, prescribers began adding ILE directly to the PN admixture to provide the total daily infusion in a single container. This innovation resulted in increased convenience for administration and a potential decreased risk of microbial contamination because TNA required fewer manipulations or entries into the IV line. Initial concerns that an ILE hang time greater than 12 hours would increase the risk for infection were not realized when the individuals preparing and administering PN adhered to proper sterile technique at all points in the process.[64] Table 15-12

TABLE 15-12 Advantages and Disadvantages of the Total Nutrient Admixture System

Advantages:

- All components are aseptically compounded by the pharmacy.
- Preparation is more efficient for pharmacy personnel, especially when it is automated.
- Administering TNA involves less manipulation than administering 2-in-1 formulations plus separate ILE, and there is therefore less risk of contamination of the system during administration.
- If contamination does occur, the bacterial growth is more inhibited or slower with TNA than with separate ILE, although there is no clinical difference in infectious complications between 2-in-1 vs 3-in-1 formulations.[66]
- TNA may be more cost-effective overall in certain settings:
  - It requires less nursing time because it is administered via a single container per day and there is no piggyback ILE to administer.
  - The supply and equipment expenses are lower with TNA because only 1 infusion pump and IV tubing are needed.
- In home care settings, TNA is more convenient to store, involves fewer supplies, and is easier to administer.
- In some situations, dextrose and venous access tolerance may be better with TNA than with 2-in-1 formulations.
- TNA may have possible applications in fluid-restricted patients because ILE 30% is restricted to use in TNA.
- Fat clearance may be better when ILE is administered over more than 12 hours.

Disadvantages:

- Larger particle size of admixed ILE precludes use of 0.22-µm (bacteria-eliminating) filter and requires the larger pore size filter of 1.2 µm.
- Admixed ILE is less stable and more prone to separation of lipid components.
- TNA formulations are more sensitive to destabilization with greater divalent and monovalent electrolyte concentrations.
- TNA formulations are more sensitive to destabilization with low concentrations of dextrose and amino acids.
- TNA formulation may be unstable when the final concentration of ILE is low.
- Compatibility and solubility of calcium gluconate and sodium/potassium phosphate are less in TNA formulations than in 2-in-1 formulations.
- Lower pH amino acid formulations may destabilize the ILE portion of admixture.
- It is difficult to visualize precipitate or particulate material in the opaque admixture.
- Certain medications are incompatible with the ILE portion of TNA.
- The risk for catheter occlusion is greater and the catheter lifespan is shorter with daily ILE.[66]
- TNA is less stable over time than dextrose–amino acid PN formulations with separate ILE.

ILE, lipid injectable emulsion; IV, intravenous; PN, parenteral nutrition; TNA, total nutrient admixture.
Source: Data are from references 61–66.

presents the major advantages and disadvantages of the TNA system for PN.[61-66.]

Either system may be infused via a central venous access device. If PN is to be administered via a true peripheral line, as opposed to a peripherally inserted central catheter, certain criteria are important to decrease risk of thrombophlebitis and damage to peripheral vein(s). Osmolarity should be kept below 900 mOsm/L;[66] calcium and potassium concentrations should be kept low (for some institutions, this may translate to calcium equal to or less than 5 mEq/L and potassium equal to or less than 40 mEq/L whenever possible), and ILEs are usually given daily to provide adequate energy and decrease osmolarity.[1,2] In TNA, the desired concentration of dextrose and amino acids (greater than 10% and greater than 4%, respectively) to help prevent lipid destabilization from divalent cations may limit the ability to adhere to the osmolarity restrictions of PPN (see Practice Scenario 15-2, later in this chapter). In a dextrose–amino acid system for PPN, the ILE is usually piggybacked into the same line and infused over 24 hours, with the ILE bag replaced at 12 hours to adhere to the 12-hour limit on hang time. Some investigators have hypothesized that this technique of using daily ILE along with the dextrose–amino acid formulation may confer a protective effect on venous tolerance by the dilution of the PPN formulation and/or by some buffering action in the vein.[5] However, this co-infusion of ILE has not been shown to reduce thrombophlebitis.[66] There has also been success in reducing or preventing thrombophlebitis through the addition of heparin and/or small amounts of hydrocortisone to PPN.[67] Another technique to minimize thrombophlebitis includes the use of a nitroglycerin patch at the venous insertion site.[67] These strategies have been reported in the literature but are not commonly seen in current practice.

National Standards for Compounded Sterile Preparations

A primary responsibility of pharmacists is to ensure that PN is prepared safely. Compounding an accurate formulation free of microbial and particulate matter is an essential component of this process. Organizations such as the USP and the American Society of Health-System Pharmacists (ASHP) have developed multiple procedures to assist pharmacists in complying with sterile product admixture guidelines.

The USP is a private, nonprofit organization recognized by the federal government as the official group responsible for setting national standards for drug purity and safety and issues standards on the pharmaceutical compounding of sterile products. On January 1, 2004, the USP formally adopted Chapter {797},[68] the first official monograph enforceable by regulatory agencies concerning the procedures and requirements for compounded sterile preparations (CSPs). Much of the same information was previously published as recommendations in nonenforceable materials, including USP Chapter {1206}, which focused on dispensing for home care and guidelines related to sterile product preparation published by ASHP.[69] Although Chapter {797} discusses the standards that apply to all sterile dosage forms that are compounded, this chapter reviews only information pertinent to PN and its implications.

Chapter {797} defined 3 different risk levels (low, medium, and high) for each CSP based on the potential for microbial contamination. The low-risk level typically involves a simple, closed-system aseptic transfer. A medium-risk level involves reconstitution of several sterile commercial products for transfer into several small-volume minibags or a large-volume parenteral preparation, such as PN. A high-risk compounding activity involves the preparation from bulk, nonsterile ingredients or the preparation from sterile ingredients that are exposed to less than the International Organization for Standardization (ISO) Class 5 standards. ISO Class 5 standards do not allow circulating particles 0.5 µm or larger to exceed 100 particles per cubic foot. A low- or medium-risk product becomes high risk when any added component is high risk; thus, a PN formulation with L-glutamine compounded from nonsterile powder becomes a high-risk product.

Of note, Chapter {797} underwent review from 2010 to 2015 with expected publication of revisions in the summer of 2017, after this book goes to press. It is anticipated that major revisions will include (1) possible introduction of the terminology *in-use time* to refer to the time before which a conventionally manufactured product used to make a CSP must be used once it has been opened or punctured, or the time before which a CSP must be used after it has been opened or punctured, and (2) consolidation of the 3 microbial risk categories for CSPs (ie, low, medium, and high risk) into 2 categories (ie, Category 1 and 2), which are distinguished primarily by the conditions under which they are made and the time within which they are used.

The in-use time will depend on the type of product/CSP and the environment where the manipulation occurs (eg, the environment meets or does not meet ISO Class 5 standards). It is proposed that Category 1 CSPs are those assigned a maximum beyond-use-date (BUD) equal to or less than 12 hours at controlled room temperature or equal to or less than 24 hours when refrigerated, if they are made in accordance with all applicable standards for Category 1 CSPs. Category 2 CSPs are those that may be assigned a BUD greater than 12 hours at room temperature or greater than 24 hours when refrigerated, if they are made in accordance with all the applicable standards for Category 2 CSPs. These minimum requirements may include personnel qualifications, media fill testing, and environmental monitoring. Some criteria that distinguish the proposed standards for Category 1 and Category 2 CSPs include the location of primary engineering control, release testing, and, as mentioned, BUD assignment. These BUDs for CSPs are based on the risk of microbial contamination, not physical or chemical stability. The BUD for Category 2 CSPs is based on the method of achieving sterility, starting components (ie, sterile vs nonsterile), sterility testing with results known before dispensing, the presence of a preservative, and storage conditions (ie, room temperature 20°C to 25°C; refrigerator 2°C to 8°C; or freezer –25°C to –10°C). BUD is the date or time after which a CSP should not be stored, transported, or administered and is determined from the date and time the preparation was compounded. For example, the BUD for unspiked ILE in the original packing is determined by the manufacturer's expiration date.

Automated Compounding Devices

Automated compounding devices (ACDs) were originally developed to help streamline the manufacturing sequence for multiple-ingredient preparations, such as PN formulations, by automatically delivering individual components in a predetermined sequence under computerized control. The main advantage ACDs offer is enhanced accuracy of the dosage form. Instead of trying to compound easily measured volumes (eg, 250- or 500-mL increments for amino acids or dextrose), pharmacies can program ACDs to pump any volume of a formulation from large stock containers. When ACDs are used, PN formulations can be more easily tailored to meet patient-specific needs, and the process is more efficient. Also, ACDs should improve enforcement of proper compounding sequence and reduce the likelihood of touch contamination. For institutions compounding more than a few PN formulations per day, ACDs are associated with decreased pharmacy labor and supply costs. This advancement in technology also reduces the risk of extrinsic contaminants that might be introduced with manually prepared formulations, such as "coring" of rubber vial tops and fibers from alcohol swabs. Ultimately, ACDs enable clinicians to provide more precise and safe preparations to patients.

ACDs are also available for the addition of the micronutrient components to PN formulations. These types of ACDs may reduce labor and supply costs if an institution compounds many PN formulations daily. Some of these devices interface with barcode readers, which may help minimize compounding errors. However, ACDs may not be cost-effective for institutions that make only a few PN formulations per day. The ACD uses a cassette with tubing that must be changed daily, and this equipment represents a significant cost that may or may not be offset by any savings in labor or supply costs. Furthermore, pharmacies with limited space may simply not have enough space available for the ACD.

Pharmacy personnel should assess the volume and weight accuracy of ACDs each day that they are used to compound CSPs to ensure the correct quantities of ingredients are delivered into the final PN container. Also, prior to PN compounding, an independent double-check of the initial daily ACD set-up should be done using a printed checklist. In facilities that care for adults, pediatric, and neonatal patients, PN preparation for each population should take place at a separate allocated location or time.

To reduce the risk of transcription errors, institutions that use computerized-physician order entry for PN ordering and ACDs for PN compounding should ideally have a system that is fully integrated, wherein the entered PN order is electronically transmitted to the ACD without requiring re-entry of any data.[70] In addition, organizations should implement soft and hard (or catastrophic) limits for PN ingredients that are employed during prescribing, order review, and compounding. These warning limits should be weight-based and determined by pharmacists' review to ensure consistency with the needs of the specific patient population.

Quality Control for the Preparation of Parenteral Nutrition Admixtures

USP Chapter {797} describes the procedures for ensuring accuracy and precision of the compounding process.[68] For conventional manual compounding of PN formulations, the additive vials and syringes must be inspected prior to dispensing the final product. A pharmacist other than the compounding personnel is preferred for confirming that the measured volumes in syringes correspond with the PN order. The major methods used for verifying the accuracy of the compounding process by ACDs are volumetric and gravimetric analysis. Each ACD has its own set of internal surveillance checks that assist the compounding pharmacist. These devices have the capability to measure each nutrient volume added to the final PN container. If the weight of the final PN container is different than the theoretical weight calculated by the automated system (the sum of the volume of each ingredient multiplied by its specific gravity), the ACD alerts the pharmacist to a possible error in the admixture process. Gravimetric analysis may also be used to assess the precision of the final PN admixture. Gravimetric analysis can be used as a quality control measure for manual or automated compounded systems, and is a method of quality assurance that can be applied independent of the ACD. Pharmacists can use an analytic balance to determine the weight of individual additive containers that have a narrow margin of safety. For example, if overfill for a final PN formulation were supplied solely from a potassium chloride container, the consequences of this error could be fatal. Thus, pharmacists can employ gravimetric techniques to assess the accuracy of individual additives delivered to the final PN formulation.

Refractometry is also used to determine whether PN formulations have been compounded properly. The refractive index of dextrose and amino acids can be measured with a refractometer and compared to values established for known concentrations of dextrose and amino acids in PN base formulations. If the measured refractive indices differ substantially from predicted values, the base formulation may have been improperly admixed. Refractometers cannot be used with ILE; therefore, alternative methods must be used to assess the integrity of TNA systems. Factors other than incorrect preparations can result in refractive indices deviating from predicted values. For example, Kitzen and colleagues[71] found that revised equations for predicting refractive indices may be needed when final dextrose concentrations exceed 15%. Instead of indirectly measuring final dextrose concentrations with refractometric analysis, certain instruments use chemical analysis to directly measure final dextrose concentrations. Although dextrose concentrations of PN formulations administered in clinical practice may exceed the range of detection, samples can be diluted and compared against control solutions to determine whether the formulation is within an acceptable margin of error.

Chapter {797} also states that the pharmacist should visually inspect each CSP for physical defects (eg, check TNA for phase separation) and package integrity (eg, check for leakage or improper seals). The pharmacist is also responsible for monitoring the quality of all CSPs after they leave the pharmacy for distribution.[68] This responsibility involves oversight of the processes for packaging, handling, and transport of the PN formulation to the patient or caregiver. For example, written procedures must be developed to ensure that the PN formulation is not exposed to extremes in temperature or light. The use of seals on all ports of PN containers can enhance product integrity during handling and transport. Close attention to quality and control after dispensing is required for home care products because significant time and handling usually occur between the PN production in the pharmacy and delivery to the patient or caregiver.

Standardized Commercially Available Parenteral Nutrition Formulations

As noted earlier, SCAPN products are available for central and peripheral vein administration as dextrose–amino acid (2-in-1) formulations with and without electrolytes and 3-in-1 formulations with electrolytes. To prevent a chemical reaction that alters the integrity of the dextrose and amino acids (ie, the Maillard reaction), an internal membrane separates the macronutrients into different chambers of the product and is broken so the components can be mixed just before administration. SCAPN formulations require the addition of the multivitamin injection shortly before administration because vitamins are essential components of PN that are not stable when added more than 24 hours in advance of use.

ProcalAmine (B. Braun Medical, Bethlehem, PA) is a glycerol-based product that can be used for short-term PPN administration; it contains a final concentration of amino acids of 3%, a final concentration of glycerol of 3%, and electrolytes.[72,73] Because glycerol is a sugar alcohol, this product can be premixed and sterilized in a single bottle without undergoing the Maillard reaction that precludes the heat sterilization of mixed dextrose and amino acid solutions. This product must be protected from light until administration. Compatibility data are unavailable for the addition of multivitamin products to ProcalAmine.

The 2-in-1 products for central vein infusion generally contain final concentrations of dextrose of 10%, 15%, 20%, or 25% and final concentrations of amino acids of 2.75%, 4.25%, or 5%; may or may not include a standard package of electrolytes; and have an osmolarity greater than 900 mOsm/L. The 2-in-1 products for peripheral vein infusion have a final concentration of dextrose of 5% and final concentrations of amino acids of 2.75%, 3.5%, or 4.25%; may or may not include electrolytes; and have an osmolarity less than 900 mOsm/L. The 3-in-1 products with electrolytes are available for (1) central vein infusion as dextrose 9.7%, amino acids 3.3%, and lipids 3.8%, with an osmolarity of 1060 mOsm/L; or (2) peripheral vein infusion as dextrose 6.7%, amino acids 2.4%, and lipids 3.5%, with an osmolarity of 750 mOsm/L.

Specific advantages and disadvantages are associated with the use of SCAPN products. Potential advantages include a reduction in costs, decreased compounding time, less risk for ordering and compounding errors, and fewer bloodstream infections.[74] Furthermore, these products are shelf stable and heat sterilized, allowing for more time before expiration than compounded PN. For these reasons, SCAPN products may be preferred in settings where PN is used infrequently or irregularly, such as in rural hospitals or long-term care facilities. SCAPN products may also be used for first-dose or starter PN, as a backup system, and during after-hour and weekend shifts. The use of SCAPN products has increased in the setting of shortages of amino acid products for PN compounding.

However, SCAPN products may not be appropriate for all patients, such as those with increased protein requirements or labile fluid status (eg, obese or critically ill patients), because these products provide standardized concentrations of amino acids, dextrose, and fluid; generally, the concentrations of amino acid and dextrose are lower than customized PN. In addition, because the electrolyte composition is standardized in SCAPN products, these formulations may not be appropriate for patients with conditions that cause significant electrolyte wasting (eg, high-output ostomy) or conditions that decrease electrolyte clearance (eg, renal insufficiency).

Stability and Compatibility of Parenteral Nutrition Formulations

Although the terms *stability* and *compatibility* have been used interchangeably in the medical literature, the terms have distinct meanings in reference to parenteral admixtures. The *stability* of PN formulations refers to the degradation of nutritional components that changes their original characteristics. A classic example is the Maillard reaction, mentioned previously, that occurs between IV dextrose and certain amino acids such as lysine, resulting in a brownish discoloration of the final formulation. Stability may also refer to the ability of PN additives, including medications, to maintain their chemical integrity and pharmacological activity. Photodegradation from light exposure, particularly fluorescent light, results in a loss of some vitamins, including cyanocobalamin, folic acid, phytonadione, pyridoxine, riboflavin, thiamin, and retinol.[75] In contrast, *compatibility* issues with PN formulations generally involve the formation of precipitates. These precipitates may be solid, such as crystalline matter, or liquid, such as phase separation of oil and water in a TNA. The distinction between stability and compatibility with ILEs can be difficult to discern, because all emulsions are inherently unstable systems that will return to their oil and water components over time. However, ILEs clearly have compatibility issues—for example, the addition of trivalent cations such as iron dextran to an ILE results in phase separation of the ILE components. Most studies evaluating additive and Y-site compatibility with PN formulations evaluate only physical compatibility; a few include stability. For example, octreotide is listed as physically compatible when admixed in tested PN formulations, but a study including stability data found highly variable drug activity.[76] Manufacturer information warns that the glycosylation of octreotide and the subsequent loss of activity may occur when the drug is added to PN formulations.[77] Unstable substances should not be added to PN regardless of physical compatibility.

When discussing medication incompatibilities, a distinction should be made between the use of dextrose–amino acid and TNA formulations. The presence of the ILE in the same container and its chemical properties explain why some drugs are compatible in dextrose–amino acid formulations but not in a TNA formulation. A few medications, usually fat-soluble drugs, are compatible with TNA but not dextrose–amino acid formulations (Table 15-13).[76,78]

Ultimately, medications should not be added to PN formulations unless there is clear evidence from the literature

TABLE 15-13 Physical Compatibility[a] of Parenteral Nutrition with Selected Medications via Y-Site Administration

Medication	Dextrose–Amino Acids	TNA
Acyclovir 7 mg/mL D5W	I	I
Amikacin 5 mg/mL D5W	C	C
Amphotericin B 0.6 mg/mL D5W	I	I
Ampicillin 20 mg/mL 0.9% NaCl	C	C
Butorphanol 0.04 mg/mL D5W	C	C
Cefazolin 20 mg/mL D5W	I	C
Ceftazidime 40 mg/mL D5W	C	C
Cimetidine 12 mg/mL D5W	C	C
Ciprofloxacin 1 mg/mL D5W	I	C
Cyclosporine 5 mg/mL D5W	I	I
Dopamine 3200 mcg/mL D5W	C	I
Dobutamine 4 mg/mL D5W	C	C
Famotidine 2 mg/mL D5W	C	C
Fentanyl 12.5 mcg/mL D5W	C	C
Fentanyl 50 mcg/mL undiluted	C	C
Ganciclovir 20 mg/mL D5W	I	I
Gentamicin 5 mg/mL D5W	C	C
Haloperidol 0.2 mg/mL D5W	C	I
Heparin 100 unit/mL undiluted	C	I
Hydromorphone 0.5 mg/mL D5W	C	I
Insulin 1 unit/mL D5W	C	C
Lorazepam 0.1 mg/mL D5W	C	I
Midazolam 2 mg/mL D5W	I	I
Morphine 1 mg/mL D5W	C	C
Morphine 15 mg/mL undiluted	NA	I
Ofloxacin 4 mg/mL D5W	C	C
Ondansetron 1 mg/mL D5W	C	I
Potassium phosphate 3 mmol/mL undiluted	I	I
Ranitidine 2 mg/mL D5W	C	C
Sodium bicarbonate 1 mEq/mL undiluted	I	C
Tacrolimus 1 mg/mL D5W	C	C
Ticarcillin/clavulanate 30/0.1 mg/mL D5W	C	C
Tobramycin 5 mg/mL D5W	C	C
Trimethoprim/sulfamethoxazole 0.8/4 mg/mL D5W	C	C
Vancomycin 10 mg/mL D5W	C	C
Zidovudine 4 mg/mL D5W	C	C

C, compatible; D5W, 5% dextrose in water; I, incompatible; NA, not available; NaCl, sodium chloride; TNA, total nutrient admixture.

[a]Certain medications that are physically compatible when coadministered with PN may not be suitable for coadministration because of loss of activity or inactivation of the medication.

Source: Data are from references 76 and 78.

or standard references to support stability, compatibility, and maintenance of pharmacological and therapeutic efficacy that is specific to the nutrient composition in the PN to be dispensed.

Stability of Intravenous Fat Emulsion and Total Nutrient Admixture Formulations

ILE consists of an interior oil phase dispersed in an external water phase. Polar and nonpolar regions on the same fat droplet are responsible for maintaining stability. The polar regions create a negative charge, or zeta potential, on the surface of the fat droplet that promotes repulsion between neighboring lipid particles of the same charge.[57,62] When the surface charge becomes less negative, fat droplets begin to aggregate into larger fat globules (greater than 1 μm in diameter), and the emulsion becomes unstable. Clinically, the ILE becomes unsafe for administration at this point, and fat globules may lodge in the pulmonary vasculature, compromising respiratory function. Standards for globule size distribution in ILE are provided in USP {729}.

Factors that may alter the electrical charge on the fat droplet surface include reductions in pH and the addition of electrolyte salts. A pH in the range of 6 to 9 (ie, the manufactured pH) is most favorable for ILE stability, whereas additives lowering the pH below 5 or increasing the pH above 10 may irreversibly destabilize or "crack" the emulsion.[62] When a cracked ILE occurs, the oil phase separates from the water phase. Initially, subtle changes in the uniformly white appearance of the emulsion occur, but the oil-water separation may progress to show yellow oil streaks throughout the bag or an amber oil layer at the top of the admixture bag. A TNA with these changes is unsafe for use. Low pH is especially damaging because, in addition to effects on the electrical charge, the egg phospholipid emulsifier begins to degrade.

MCTs, which are usually derived from coconut or palm kernel oils, improve ILE stability by displacing LCTs at the droplet surface and by reducing stress on the emulsifier because of the shorter hydrocarbon chain.[79]

The final pH of a PN formulation is generally very near that of the amino acid solution unless the buffering capacity of the amino acids has been overwhelmed by other PN components. Therefore, the most critical factor influencing the pH of a PN formulation is the crystalline amino acid solution used for compounding. The pH of crystalline amino acid solutions varies by brand and ranges from about 5.2 to 7. Those with a pH of 5.3 or less, such as Aminosyn, Aminosyn HBC, and Aminosyn RF, are not appropriate for use in a TNA preparation. Amino acid solutions with a pH in the range of 5.8 to 7, including Aminosyn II, FreAmine, HepatAmine, Travasol, Prosol, and Clinisol products, are generally acceptable for use in TNA compounding. Certain crystalline amino acid solutions used for pediatric patients and some concentrated solutions (15% and 20%), such as Plenamine, may be marginal for use in TNA formulations because the pH (5.4 to 5.7) is borderline for ILE stability. Use of these amino acid formulations can be particularly problematic in home care where PN is made several days in advance of use and when other factors influencing TNA stability are marginal for ILE stability.

The addition of cysteine hydrochloride, as is routine with neonatal PN formulations and some pediatric PN formulations, renders the pH of the final admixture to be less than 5, promoting ILE destabilization. However, some prescribers may request the use of pediatric amino acid products in adult PN patients because the pediatric amino acid formulations are the only products with taurine, and L-cysteine hydrochloride may be added to an adult PN formulation to increase calcium phosphate solubility (eg, when a patient is eliminating high amounts of calcium in response to foscarnet therapy).

Because a concentrated dextrose solution has an acidic pH, it should not be added directly to ILE; rather, dextrose should be combined first with the amino acid solution during the compounding process. The amino acid solution serves as a buffer, and low final concentrations of amino acids (less than 4%) may not provide adequate buffer capacity to prevent destabilization of a TNA. Low ILE concentrations, especially below 2% or 2.5%, may also result in an unstable TNA.[80,81] When compounding PN for 3 to 7 days in advance of use, final ILE concentrations may need to be higher for a stable TNA formulation, especially if other components contribute to destabilization. Stability studies should be reviewed carefully to ensure that the assigned BUD is reasonable for the final concentrations of base components and the combination of additives in the PN formulation. Manufacturers' data often list a range of dextrose, amino acids, and ILE concentrations that have been evaluated for TNA stability, but they seldom include the specific combinations of base components, electrolytes, vitamins, and trace elements present in the PN formulations reported. Although this information from the manufacturer provides some guidance to stability limits, it does not provide adequate data to fully inform practice. For instance, a range of final concentrations for each base component (dextrose, amino acids, and ILE) is typically listed. Dextrose 10%, amino acids 1%, and ILE 1% might each be listed as within the range tested, but that does not mean this particular combination was tested. Although a final concentration of ILE 1% may be stable with amino acids 5% or higher, this ILE concentration is not likely to be compatible with the final concentration of amino acids 1%; however, this possible incompatibility is not stated. Clinicians involved in home PN must be particularly vigilant in assessing appropriate combinations of final concentrations and the BUD assigned. A PN formulation may be stable when used within 30 hours of compounding in the hospital, but it may begin to destabilize before use when assigned a longer BUD. Practice Scenario 15-2 further explores the topic of TNA stability.[62,81–85]

Practice Scenario 15-2

Question: What are the limitations in compounding (ie, 3-in-1 vs 2-in-1) when compounding a peripheral parenteral nutrition (PPN) formulation?

Scenario: SG is an 83-year-old man who fell from a stepladder at home and was admitted for repair of a hip fracture and mandibular fracture, and for observation due to altered mental status. He has been *nil per os* for 5 days because of the mandibular fracture and impending surgery. On hospital Day 7 (postoperative Day 2), SG is advanced to full liquids but experiences abdominal pain and distention. A partial small bowel obstruction is confirmed with abdominal x-ray. The nutrition support team is consulted for the initiation of PPN because long-term (greater than 10 days) parenteral nutrition (PN) is not anticipated, and SG's primary physician does not want him to have a central venous line placed because of the risk for a central line infection.

Intervention: A 2-in-1 PN formulation with a separate infusion of lipid injectable emulsion (ILE) is prepared for SG.

Answer: Total nutrient admixtures (TNAs) should be used with extreme caution or not at all as PPN formulations.

Rationale: Although published data are scarce, if final concentrations are less than 4% for amino acids, less than 10% for dextrose, or less than 2% for ILE, TNA stability is compromised, and coalescence of submicrometer droplets into large fat globules often occurs before the 30-hour beyond-use date assignment.[81] As a result, use of TNA for PPN formulations often does not meet stability requirements, and ILE should be infused separately to preserve a stable and safe formulation.

When reduced final concentrations of amino acids and dextrose are used for compounding PN solutions, a lack of data makes it difficult to accurately predict solubility limits between calcium (as the organic gluconate salt) and inorganic phosphate (as sodium or potassium salts). Low-osmolarity PN formulations, such as PPNs, seem to pose a high threat for calcium phosphate precipitation.[82] The forms of calcium phosphate that may arise from the interaction between these 2 ions are monobasic calcium phosphate ($Ca[H_2PO_4]_2$), dibasic calcium phosphate ($CaHPO_4$), and tribasic calcium phosphate ($Ca_3[PO_4]_2$). Dibasic calcium phosphate (which is virtually insoluble in water) poses the greatest potential threat for lethal precipitants in the PN admixture and is commonly implicated in reports of significant morbidity and mortality among patients receiving incompatible mixtures. Comparatively, monobasic calcium phosphate is roughly 60 times more soluble.[83]

Excess cation amounts, especially divalent cations such as calcium (Ca^{2+}) or magnesium (Mg^{2+}), can reduce or neutralize the negative surface charge exerted by the emulsifier, thereby removing the repulsive force and allowing fat particles to combine.[62] To prevent lipid destabilization with divalent cation concentrations between 16 and 20 mEq/L, the final concentration of monohydrated dextrose must be greater than 10% and the final concentration of amino acid must be greater than 4%.[81] Trivalent cations (ie, Fe^{3+}) have even greater destabilizing effects. Because of instability issues, no dosage of iron dextran can be added to any TNA; furthermore, other parenteral iron products are also not safe, even if they were to be approved for addition to PN. As with base components, clinicians involved in home PN must be especially alert for inappropriate concentrations of electrolytes because the process of coalescence is not immediate, and formulations that are stable for 30 hours may not be stable for longer periods of time. Coalescence indicates that a fusion of fat droplets has occurred, and the individual droplet size has increased. Formulations should no longer be infused after coalescence occurs because increased droplet sizes have produced organ damage in experimental animal models.[84,85]

Calcium and Phosphate

Microprecipitates can develop within PN formulations as a result of incompatible combinations. In 1994, the FDA released a safety alert in response to reports of 2 deaths and at least 2 cases of respiratory distress associated with the administration of PN formulations thought to contain an insoluble or unstable intermediate (ie, calcium phosphate crystals).[58,86] Diffuse microvascular pulmonary emboli containing calcium phosphate were confirmed in patient autopsies.

Calcium phosphate solubility is a substantial compatibility concern with PN formulations. For patient safety, all healthcare professionals who prescribe PN formulations that deviate from pre-established standards should be familiar with limitations for the addition of calcium and phosphate. Ideally, the compounding pharmacist serves as a secondary check for calcium phosphate solubility rather than as a single evaluator.

Several factors can influence the calcium and phosphate solubility in a PN formulation (Table 15-14).[6] The pH of the final PN formulation plays a major role in dictating the solubility of calcium and phosphate. A low pH favors the presence of monobasic calcium phosphate, a relatively soluble salt form of calcium. Increasing the pH results in a greater availability of dibasic phosphate to bind with free calcium ions and increases the chance of precipitation. Thus, lowering the pH of the PN admixture reduces the likelihood that calcium and phosphate will precipitate. This concept has been applied extensively in compounding pediatric PN formulations.[87] For example, relatively large doses of calcium

TABLE 15-14 Factors That Influence Calcium and Phosphorus Compatibility in Parenteral Nutrition Formulations

Increased risk of calcium phosphate precipitation:

- Increased calcium concentration
- Increased phosphate concentration (including amino acids with phosphorus content)
- Calcium chloride salt use (vs calcium gluconate)
- Increased temperature of PN admixture

Increased calcium phosphate solubility:

- Increased amino acid concentration
- Increased dextrose concentration
- Lower pH of the PN admixture

PN, parenteral nutrition.
Source: Data are from reference 6: Trissel LA. *Trissel's Calcium and Phosphate Compatibility in Parenteral Nutrition*. Houston, TX: TriPharma Communications; 2001.

and phosphorus are routinely required in neonatal PN formulations to optimize bone formation. Although pediatric amino acid products are formulated at a lower pH, L-cysteine hydrochloride can be added to further decrease pH and thereby increase calcium and phosphate solubility.[88] Because L-cysteine is considered a semiessential amino acid in premature infants, its addition to pediatric formulations serves a dual purpose. However, an acidic pH creates an unfavorable environment for ILE, which may destabilize the final emulsion. For this reason, clinicians are discouraged from using TNA admixtures in the neonatal and pediatric populations, where lowering the pH is an effective technique for increasing calcium phosphate solubility.

The concentration or amounts of calcium and phosphate ions are directly related to the risk of precipitation.[6] As the concentration of either micronutrient rises, precipitation is more likely to occur. A variety of resources are available to assist clinicians in determining appropriate calcium and phosphate concentrations to avoid precipitation. Product-specific solubility curves have been published that depict solubility limits for calcium and phosphate salts.[6,89] Unfortunately, most of these curves were developed using fixed concentrations of amino acids, dextrose, calcium, and phosphate and often omitted other components that might influence calcium phosphate solubility. Furthermore, stability studies beyond 48 hours are lacking. These factors make use of such curves for determining solubility characteristics of patient-specific formulations difficult; nevertheless, these solubility curves likely provide the best guidance in determining calcium phosphate solubility. When ACDs are used in the admixture process, the manufacturer's software may be helpful in predicting calcium and phosphate solubility for a given formulation.

Pharmacists can help minimize the risk of precipitation by verifying the need for large calcium doses (greater than 2 times the Recommended Dietary Allowance with the prescriber. Low total serum calcium concentrations may arise from hypoalbuminemia, fluid retention, or acid-base disturbances, and supplemental calcium may be unnecessary. One practitioner has reported that reducing daily calcium doses from 13.5 mEq to 4.5 mEq in PN for stability reasons did not influence serum calcium concentrations.[89] However, the risk of metabolic bone disease must be considered when calcium provision is below the recommended 10 to 15 mEq/d for adults because serum calcium is maintained at the expense of bone calcium during inadequate intake.[1] If a patient has hypoalbuminemia, ionized calcium concentrations can be measured to assess whether additional calcium is needed.

The salt form of calcium added to the PN formulation can have a dramatic impact on the risk of precipitation. Calcium gluconate and calcium glucepate are generally less dissociated salt forms of calcium than the chloride salts.[90] As a result, the amount of free calcium available to form insoluble complexes with phosphate is reduced. Solubility curves for calcium phosphate are specific for calcium salt and cannot be interchanged; most solubility curves are for calcium gluconate. High localized phosphate or calcium concentrations can occur if the final container is not sufficiently agitated or the contents are not adequately dispersed during the compounding process.

Medication Additives

Precipitates from medication incompatibilities or emulsion disruption from medication additives have also been reported. Studies of medications with dextrose–amino acid and TNA formulations during simulated Y-site administration have been performed, and incompatibilities ranged from the formation of precipitates to haziness, discoloration, and emulsion disruption with frank separation of oil and water phases. Table 15-13 summarizes the Y-site compatibility of selected medications with dextrose–amino acid and TNA formulations.[76,78] Compatibility by Y-site infusion (co-infusion) is not synonymous with admixture into the PN formulation because the time of exposure of the medication to PN components is greatly increased with admixture. In addition, pharmacokinetic variables must be considered with admixture of a medication into PN because the medication must be safe and effective when administered as a continuous infusion or over the cycle time of a PN formulation.

Aluminum Contamination

Trace element contamination is found in most parenteral formulation components that are expected to be free of minerals. These trace elements include, but are not limited to, arsenic, aluminum, chromium, zinc, manganese, and copper.[66] The amount of contamination varies among manufacturers and even among lots, vial sizes, and concentrations from the same manufacturer. (Further information regarding trace element contamination can be found earlier the chapter, in the Trace Elements section.)

On July 26, 2004, federal regulations regarding the labeling of aluminum content in large-volume parenteral formulations (LVPs), pharmacy bulk packaging (PBP), and small-volume parenteral formulations (SVPs) became effective.[91] Despite significant aluminum content in albumin, blood products, and certain medications, only products regulated by the Endocrine and Metabolic Products Division of the FDA, including products used in compounding PN formulations, are governed by the regulation.

The maximum aluminum load permitted in LVPs, including dextrose solutions, amino acid solutions with and without electrolytes, and SCAPN, is 25 mcg/L. Labels on PBPs and SVPs must include the statement "not more than 25 mcg per liter of aluminum" or provide the aluminum content in micrograms per liter at product expiration. Thus, the label must contain the potential maximum aluminum content but not necessarily the actual amount of aluminum at the time of use. Aluminum content increases over time and is influenced by the container material and closures. Products with an affinity for aluminum can leach aluminum from glass containers and elastomeric closures, causing a significant rise in aluminum contamination over the shelf life of the product. Specific amino acids, calcium salts, and phosphate salts have a high affinity for aluminum; therefore, storage of these products in plastic containers typically results in significantly less aluminum content at expiration than storage in glass containers.[92,93] Raw product contamination with aluminum also contributes to the aluminum load and may be responsible for some of the significant variability in aluminum content among different salt forms of products, such as calcium gluconate and calcium chloride.

Aluminum is widespread in the environment; however, under normal circumstances, less than 1% of ingested aluminum is absorbed from the gastrointestinal tract.[93,94] The lungs also serve as an effective barrier. Unfortunately, the body has no effective barriers to aluminum contaminants in parenteral products and must rely on excretion to prevent toxicity. The kidneys are the primary route for the elimination of aluminum and remove unbound aluminum from the blood. The 95% of aluminum bound to protein, primarily transferrin, cannot be excreted; thus, elimination occurs slowly as equilibrium between bound and unbound aluminum maintains about 5% of the aluminum available for filtration via the kidneys.[94,95] Eventually, about 60% of infused aluminum is eliminated in patients with adequate renal function.[93] The remaining aluminum is deposited in tissues, including the brain, bones, liver, and lungs.

Adult patients at risk for aluminum toxicity include those with (1) significant renal dysfunction, (2) a high intake of parenteral products such as PN, or (3) iron deficiency.[91,94] These patients have impaired excretion or excessive exposure such that aluminum accumulation is likely to occur. Progressive encephalopathy, patchy osteomalacia, reduced parathyroid hormone secretion, and erythropoietin-resistant microcytic anemia have been associated with aluminum toxicity. The final FDA ruling regarding the labeling of aluminum content selected 4 to 5 mcg/kg/d as the upper limit of acceptable aluminum exposure and requires a warning statement in the manufacturer's product information to this effect.[91] There is no mandate for the calculation of potential aluminum load or for the inclusion of this information on compounded PN in the FDA ruling; however, minimizing aluminum exposure is an important clinical consideration for patients at risk for toxicity, such as pediatric patients and patients requiring long-term PN.

Administration

Use of Filters

The 1994 FDA safety alert on calcium phosphate precipitation highlighted the need for filtration of PN at the bedside. Relatively large-pore filters (5 μm) are adequate for the removal of precipitates (eg, calcium phosphate) and particulate matter (eg, plastic fragments from the bag) from a PN formulation. Filters, however, are not a substitute for good compounding practices intended to prevent precipitate formation.

The risk of infection associated with the preparation and administration of PN formulations further emphasizes the need for proper filtration techniques. In vitro studies have demonstrated that 0.22-μm filters can remove pathogenic microorganisms, such as *Staphylococcus epidermidis*, *Escherichia coli*, and *Candida albicans*, from a PN administration line.[96]

The limitations of filters must also be recognized. Because fat particle sizes, even in the most stable formulations (including undiluted ILE from the manufacturer), contain fat droplets in excess of 5 μm, 0.22-μm filters are inappropriate for use with ILE.[97] Current recommendations include using 1.2-μm filters with ILE-containing PN formulations (ie, 3-in-1 formulations/TNAs and separately infused ILE) to avoid particle shearing and instability that may occur with filters of smaller pore size. Despite the inability to remove bacterial contaminants such as *S. epidermidis* and *E. coli*, a 1.2-μm filter does trap larger organisms including *C. albicans*.

A 0.22-μm filter should be used for dextrose–amino acid PN admixtures (ie, 2-in-1 formulations). Therefore, if a 2-in-1 dextrose–amino acid admixture is administered with a separate infusion of ILE, 2 filters would be required: (1) a 0.22-μm in-line filter for the dextrose–amino acid admixture and (2) a 1.2-μm filter for the ILE, which can be either infused via a separate vascular access or infused via a Y-connector with the filter placed closer to the patient than the 0.22-μm filter. In-line filters should be changed with each new administration of PN (ie, every 24 hours for TNA and dextrose–amino acid formulations and every 10 to 12 hours for ILE infused separately).

In-line filters can increase the incidence of occlusion alarms during PN administration. Nursing interventions for frequent infusion pump alarms are often needed because of decreased flow rates or occlusions associated with filter use. However, these alarms should be recognized as a potential sign of a precipitate and should be investigated by a qualified clinician. An occluded filter should never be removed to allow a PN formulation to infuse freely without the use of any device to reduce the infusion of particulates and microprecipitates. Although filters may reduce the potential for patients to become infected by contaminated PN formulations, they do not completely eliminate this risk. As such, the CDC does not endorse the use of in-line filters solely for the purpose of infection control.

Administration Tubing and Containers

PN formulations are provided in a single bag, unless the ILE is administered separately. PN should be refrigerated and protected from light exposure from the time it is compounded until it is administered. Administration tubing should be attached to the PN container, using sterile technique, immediately prior to administration. Because fat-containing fluids extract di-2-ethylhexyl phthalate (DEHP) from containers that use DEHP as a plasticizer (eg, polyvinyl chloride containers), PN administration sets should be free of DEHP to prevent DEHP contamination of the PN formulation. Administration sets, like in-line filters, should be changed with every new infusion container (ie, every 24 hours for TNA and dextrose–amino acid formulations and every 10 to 12 hours for ILE infused separately).[70]

Lipid Injectable Emulsion Hang Time

Due to enhanced microbial growth potential with the infusion of ILE separate from formulations that contain dextrose and amino acids, the CDC recommends a 12-hour limit on the hang time for ILE.[63] The CDC states that ILE incorporated into a TNA can hang for up to 24 hours.[63] The USP has also endorsed using ILE products within 12 hours of opening the original manufacturer's container if the ILEs are infused as separate preparations from dextrose and amino acids.[68] However, TNA/3-in-1 formulations may be administered over 24 hours. The administration and hang time of 3-in-1 formulations is extended because bacterial growth is inhibited by the reduced pH (pH approximately 5.6 to 6) and the increased total osmolarity with the combination of all 3 substrates in 1 container.

The manufacturer may or may not specify a maximum hang time in the product information; however, since the release of USP Chapter {797}, which includes the CDC recommended times, abiding by maximum hang time is considered the standard of practice. It is generally preferable to infuse an entire container of lipids over 12 hours to prevent wastage, although this rate of infusion must be balanced with adequate clearance of fats from the blood.

Calculation of Parenteral Nutrition Formulations

Common stock solutions of dextrose for use in manual PN compounding include 30%, 50%, and 70% concentrations. These are frequently supplied from the manufacturer in 500-mL partial-fill bags or bottles; that is, the bags or bottles in which they are supplied have a potential capacity of slightly more than 1 liter, allowing for the addition of amino acids and other additives to the formulation. Common stock solutions of amino acids for use in manual PN compounding include 8.5% and 10% concentrations. Manufacturers are transitioning from glass bottles to flexible plastic containers for ILE. These containers are made from nonphthalate plastics (plastics that do not contain DEHP), typically polypropylene or a copolymer of propylene, with an overwrap system that protects the ILE from oxygen exposure.

A variety of regimens can be constructed that will approximate the patient's predicted needs. If the PN formulation is going to be compounded manually, the pharmacy should be consulted before an order for a nonstandard formulation (ie, a formulation with unusual volumes of dextrose vs amino acids) is prescribed to determine the feasibility of mixing such a formulation and perhaps to explore alternative formulations that would be easier to compound.

Figure 15-1 illustrates a method of calculating the appropriate amounts of dextrose, amino acids, and ILE for the manual preparation of a PN formulation (ie, in an institution that does not use an ACD and does not prepare TNA formulations). Figure 15-2 (examples 1 and 2) provides the calculations for a fluid-restricted PN formulation (ie, 1.5 liter) with the same provision of energy and protein. The calculations are based on the use of commercially available products.

FIGURE 15-1 Calculation of Parenteral Nutrition Formulation for Manual Preparation

Clinical presentation: LT is a 45-year-old man hospitalized after a motor vehicle collision in which he suffered multiple injuries, including a liver laceration and several bone fractures. A feeding jejunostomy tube was placed during an emergent laparotomy. However, the patient develops abdominal distention following initiation of enteral tube feedings; therefore, the feedings are discontinued and PN is initiated on Day 2 of hospitalization. The patient is 72 inches tall, with a precollision weight estimated at 74 kg. The nutrition support team determines that the patient should receive 1.5 g protein/kg/d and between 25 and 30 total kcal/kg/d. The hospital pharmacy compounds PN formulations manually (ie, no ACD) and does not prepare TNA formulations.

Calculations:

1. Calculate fluid and energy requirements.

    Fluid Requirements = 30 mL/kg/d × 74 kg = 2220 mL/d
    Energy Requirements = 25–30 kcal/kg/d × 74 kg = 1850–2220 total kcal/d

2. *Calculate amounts of dextrose and protein.* Usually, dextrose is administered at a maximum rate of 3 mg/kg/min to not exceed the maximum amount of dextrose the liver can oxidize (ie, 5 mg/kg/min). The protein requirement is 1.5 g/kg/d.

    Amount of Dextrose = 74 kg × 3 mg/kg/min × 1440 min/d ÷ 1000 g/kg = 320 g dextrose
    Amount of Protein = 1.5 g/kg/d × 74 kg = 111 g/d

3. *Calculate energy from dextrose and protein.* Round off the grams of dextrose and protein to amounts amenable to manual compounding. Then, multiply these amounts by the energy per gram.

    Energy Supplied by Dextrose = 300 g/d × 3.4 kcal/g = 1020 kcal/d
    Energy Supplied by Protein (Amino Acids) = 100 g/d × 4 kcal/g = 400 kcal/d

4. Calculate energy to be supplied by ILE.

    Energy from ILE to Meet *Maximum* Energy Goal = 2220 kcal/d – 1020 kcal/d (from dextrose) – 400 kcal (from protein) = 800 kcal
    Energy from ILE to Meet *Minimum* Energy Goal = 1850 kcal/d – 1020 kcal/d (from dextrose) – 400 kcal/d (from protein) = 430 kcal

5. *Choose a standard amount of ILE that approximates the energy goal calculated in step 4.* ILE 20% has 2 kcal/mL. Therefore, 250 mL ILE will provide 500 kcal.

The final prescription for the PN formulation:
*   Dextrose: 300 g/d. Choosing dextrose 30% for compounding, 30 g/100 mL = 300 g/*x* mL; solving for *x* yields 1000 mL dextrose 30%.
*   Amino acids: 100 g/d. Choosing amino acids 10% for compounding, 10 g/100 mL = 100 g/*x* mL; solving for *x* yields 1000 mL amino acids 10%.
*   ILE: 250 mL/d of 20% ILE infused for 12 hours = 21 mL/h.
*   Estimate 30 mL/L for additives (electrolytes, multivitamins, and trace elements): 30 mL/L × 2 L/d = 60 mL/d.
*   The sum of the volumes of dextrose, amino acids, ILE, and additives is 2310 mL, which is close to the estimated fluid requirement of 2220 mL/d.
*   The dextrose, amino acids and additives will be supplied over 24 hours (2060 mL ÷ 24 hours = 86 mL/h for 2-in-1 PN infused continuously). The ILE is administered separately, typically piggybacked over 12 hours onto the primary PN administration set at a port distal to the 0.22-μm filter.

ACD, automated compounding device; ILE, lipid injectable emulsion; PN, parenteral nutrition; TNA, total nutrient admixture.

FIGURE 15-2 Calculation for Fluid-Restricted Parenteral Nutrition Formulation

Clinical presentation: A patient weighing 80 kg has estimated requirements of 30 kcal/kg/d and 1.5 g protein per kg per day. Between 20% and 30% of total energy will be provided as ILE. The volume of PN formulation is restricted to 1.5 L/d.

Estimated requirements calculations:

Total Energy = 30 kcal/kg/d × 80 kg = 2400 kcal/d
Protein = 1.5 g/kg/d × 80 kg = 120 g/d
Minimum Energy from ILE = 2400 kcal/d × 0.2 = 480 kcal/d
Maximum Energy from ILE = 2400 kcal/d × 0.3 = 720 kcal/d

Example 1:
Stock solutions used by the pharmacy for compounding PN are amino acids 10%, dextrose 70%, and ILE 20%. PN formulations are manually compounded without an ACD as dextrose–amino acids formulations.

Calculations:
Using amounts amenable to manual compounding:
- Amino acids 10%: 1000 mL yields 100 g; 100 g × 4 kcal/g yields 400 kcal/d
- 70% dextrose: 250 mL yields 175 g; 175 g × 3.4 kcal/g yields 595 kcal/d
- 20% ILE: 250 mL × 2 kcal/mL yields 500 kcal/d; the ILE will be piggyback infused
- Therefore, 400 + 500 + 595 = 1495 kcal/d in 1500 mL/d

Discussion:
Meeting the energy and protein needs of the fluid-restricted patient can be challenging or, in some cases, impossible. Amino acid stock solutions in 15% and 20% concentrations are available commercially. They are more expensive on a gram of protein basis than amino acids 8.5% or 10% formulations, especially if the pharmacy is purchasing 500 mL containers for manual compounding as opposed to larger stock bottles of amino acids 15% or 20% formulations for automated compounding. The 20% amino acid solution is available only as a 2-liter volume unit for automated compounding. Dextrose 50% or 70% should be used for compounding PN in situations of fluid restriction.

If the pharmacy does not routinely use higher concentrated macronutrient stock solutions, the best plan would be to use amino acids 10%, dextrose 70%, and ILE 20%, as outlined previously. Compounding this solution would require a special mix by the pharmacy because the volumes of dextrose and amino acids are not equal. The protein and energy provided by this regimen are significantly less than the patient's estimated requirements.

Example 2:
Stock solutions used by the pharmacy for compounding PN are amino acids 20%, dextrose 70%, and ILE 30%. The pharmacy compounds TNA solutions with an ACD.

Calculations:
- Protein: 20 g/100 mL = 120 g/x mL; solving for x yields 600 mL of amino acids 20%; 120 g amino acids × 4 kcal/g = 480 kcal/d from amino acids.
- ILE: Because the PN formulation volume is restricted to 1.5 L/d, provide 30% of energy (720 kcal/d) with ILE 30%, which has a greater energy density (3 kcal/mL) than dextrose 70% (2.38 kcal/mL). 720 kcal/d ÷ 3 kcal/mL = 240 mL ILE.
- Dextrose: Energy needed from dextrose = 2400 kcal/d – 480 kcal/d (from amino acids) – 720 kcal/d (from ILE) = 1200 kcal/d. 1200 kcal ÷ 3.4 kcal/g = 353 g dextrose. Dextrose 70% provides 70 g/100 mL = 353 g/x mL. Solving for x = 504 mL.

Thus, the volume for the macronutrients is 600 mL amino acids 20% + 240 mL ILE 30% + 504 mL dextrose 70% = 1344 mL/d. Additives, including electrolytes, parenteral multiple vitamins, and trace minerals, will provide an additional 100 to 120 mL/d. A final volume of 1500 mL/d or less can be achieved.

Discussion:
If the pharmacy prepares TNA formulations and stocks amino acids 20% formulation and ILE 30%, then the second scenario could be recommended. The daily goal of 120 g protein and 2400 kcal with 20% to 30% of kcal provided as ILE could be supplied in a volume slightly less than 1500 mL.

ACD, automated compounding device; ILE, lipid injectable emulsion; PN, parenteral nutrition; TNA, total nutrient admixture.

References

1. Mirtallo JM, Canada TW, Johnson D, et al. Safe practices for parenteral nutrition. *JPEN J Parenter Enteral Nutr.* 2004;28(Suppl):S39–S70.

2. Isaacs JW, Millikan WJ, Stackhouse J, et al. Parenteral nutrition of adults with a 900 milliosmolar solution via peripheral veins. *Am J Clin Nutr.* 1977;30:552–559.

3. Hatton J, Cohen JL. Potassium. In: Baumgartner TG, ed. *Clinical Guide to Parenteral Micronutrition.* 3rd ed. Chicago, IL: Fujisawa USA; 1997:239–254.

4. Gazitua R, Wilson K, Bistrian BR, et al. Factors determining peripheral vein tolerance to amino acid infusions. *Arch Surg.* 1979;114:897–900.

5. Fujiwara T, Kawarasaki H, Fonkalsrud E. Reduction of post-infusion venous endothelial injury with Intralipid. *Surg Gynecol Obstet.* 1984;158:57–65.

6. Trissel LA. *Trissel's Calcium and Phosphate Compatibility in Parenteral Nutrition.* Houston, TX: TriPharma Communications; 2001.

7. Mirtallo JM. Parenteral formulas. In: Rombeau JL, Rolandelli RH, eds. *Parenteral Nutrition.* 3rd ed. Philadelphia, PA: WB Saunders; 2001:118–139.

8. Singer P, Bursztein S, Kirvela O, et al. Hypercaloric glycerol in injured patients. *Surgery.* 1992;112:509–514.

9. Fairfull-Smith RJ, Stoski D, Freeman JB. Use of glycerol in peripheral parenteral nutrition. *Surgery.* 1982;92:728–732.

10. Lev-Ran A, Johnson M, Hwang DL, et al. Double-blind study of glycerol vs. glucose in parenteral nutrition of post-surgical insulin-treated diabetic patients. *JPEN J Parenter Enteral Nutr.* 1987;11:271–274.

11. A.S.P.E.N. Board of Directors and The Clinical Guidelines Task Force. Guidelines for the use of parenteral and enteral nutrition in adult and pediatric patients. *JPEN J Parenter Enteral Nutr.* 2002;26(Suppl):1SA–138SA.

12. Brown RO, Compher C; A.S.P.E.N. Board of Directors. Clinical guidelines: nutrition support in adult acute and chronic renal failure. *JPEN J Parenter Enteral Nutr.* 2010;34;4:366–377.

13. Melnick G. Value of specialty intravenous amino acid solutions. *Am J Health Syst Pharm.* 1996;53:671–674.

14. Drugs.com. Liposyn II. https://www.drugs.com/pro/liposyn-ii.html. Accessed February 17, 2017.

15. Intralipid [package insert]. Baxter Healthcare Corporation: Deerfield, IL. Revised May 2016.

16. Vanek VW, Seidner DL, Bistrian B, et al. A.S.P.E.N. position paper: clinical role for alternative fat emulsions. *Nutr Clin Pract.* 2012;27:150–192.

17. Smoflipid [package insert]. Fresenius Kabi: Austria GmbH. Revised April 2015.

18. Waitzberg DL, Torrinhas RS, Jacintho TM. New parenteral emulsions for clinical use. *JPEN J Parenter Enteral Nutr.* 2006;30:351–367.

19. Ulrich H, Pastores SM, Katz DP, et al. Parenteral use of medium-chain triglycerides: a reappraisal. *Nutrition.* 1996;2:231–238.

20. Antebi H, Mansoor O, Ferrier C, et al. Liver function and plasma antioxidant status in intensive care unit patients requiring total parenteral nutrition: comparison of 2 fat emulsions. *JPEN J Parenter Enteral Nutr.* 2004;28:142–148.

21. Goulet O, Antebi H, Wolf C. A new intravenous fat emulsion containing soybean oil, medium-chain triglycerides, olive oil, and fish oil: a single-center, double-blind, randomized study on efficacy and safety in pediatric patients receiving home parenteral nutrition. *JPEN J Parenter Enteral Nutr.* 2010;34:485–495.

22. Klek S, Chambrier C, Singer P, et al. Four-week parenteral nutrition using a third generation lipid emulsion (SMOFlipid)—a double-blind, randomized, multicenter study in adults. *Clinical Nutrition.* 2013;32:224–231.

23. Sacks GS, Driscoll DF. Does lipid hang time make a difference? Time is of the essence. *Nutr Clin Pract.* 2002;17:283–290.

24. Klein S, Miles JM. Metabolic effects of long-chain and medium-chain triglycerides in humans. *JPEN J Parenter Enteral Nutr.* 1994;18:396–397.

25. McClave SA, Taylor BE, Martindale RG, et al. Guidelines for the provision and assessment of nutrition support therapy in the adult critically ill patient: Society of Critical Care Medicine (SCCM) and American Society for Parenteral and Enteral Nutrition (A.S.P.E.N.). *JPEN J Parenter Enteral Nutr.* 2016;40:159–211.

26. De Meijer VE, Gura KM, Le HD, Meisel JA, Puder M. Fish oil-based lipid emulsions prevent and reverse parenteral nutrition-associated liver disease: the Boston experience. *JPEN J Parenter Enteral Nutr.* 2009;33:541–547.

27. Bellantone R, Bossola M, Carriero C, et al. Structured versus long-chain triglycerides: a safety, tolerance, and efficacy randomized study in colorectal surgical patients. *JPEN J Parenter Enteral Nutr.* 1999;23:123–127.

28. Nijveldt RJ, Tan AM, Prins HA, et al. Use of a mixture of medium-chain triglycerides and long chain triglycerides versus long-chain triglycerides in critically ill surgical patients: A randomized prospective double-blind study. *Clin Nutr.* 1998;17:23–29.

29. Gottschlich MM. Selection of optimal lipid sources in enteral and parenteral nutrition. *Nutr Clin Pract.* 1992;7:152–165.

30. Merritt RJ, ed. *The A.S.P.E.N. Nutrition Support Practice Manual.* 2nd ed. Silver Spring, MD: American Society for Parenteral and Enteral Nutrition; 2006.

31. Mayer K, Gokorsch S, Fegbeutel C, et al. Parenteral nutrition with fish oil modulates cytokine response in patients with sepsis. *Am J Respir Crit Care Med.* 2003;167:1321–1328.

32. Mayser P, Mayer K, Mahloudjian M, et al. A double-blind, randomized, placebo-controlled trial of n-3 vs. n-6 fatty acid based lipid infusion in atopic dermatitis. *JPEN J Parenter Enteral Nutr.* 2002;26:151–158.

33. Grimminger F, Führer D, Papavassilis C, et al. Influence of intravenous n-3 lipid supplementation on fatty acid profiles and lipid mediator generation in a patient with severe ulcerative colitis. *Eur J Clin Invest.* 1993;23:706–715.

34. Weiss G, Meyer F, Matthies B, et al. Immunomodulation by perioperative administration of n-3 fatty acids. *Br J Nutr.* 2002;87(Suppl):S89–S94.

35. Soden JS, Lovell MA, Brown K, et al. Failure of resolution of portal fibrosis during omega-3 fatty acid lipid emulsion therapy in two patients with irreversible intestinal failure. *J Pediatr.* 2010;156:327–331.

36. Puder M, Valim C, Meisel JA, et al. Parenteral fish oil improves outcomes in patients with parenteral nutrition-associated liver injury. *Ann Surg.* 2009;250:395–402.

37. Gura KM, Lee S, Valim C, et al. Safety and efficacy of a fish-oil based fat emulsion in the treatment of parenteral nutrition-associated liver disease. *Pediatrics.* 2008;121:e678–e686.

38. Goulet O, de Potter S, Antebi H, et al. Long-term efficacy and safety of a new olive-oil based intravenous fat emulsion in pediatric patients: a double-blind randomized study. *Am J Clin Nutr.* 1999;70:338–345.

39. Granot D, Blum S, Zbinden I, et al. Effect of ClinOleic®, an olive-oil based parenteral lipid emulsion on lymphocyte function in vitro. *Clin Nutr.* 1996;15:9(Suppl 1):3.

40. Edmunds CE, Brody RA, Parrot S, et al. The effects of different IV fat emulsion on clinical outcomes in critically ill patients. *Crit Care Med.* 2014;42:1168–1177.

41. US Food and Drug Administration. Notices/parenteral multivitamin products. *Fed Regist.* 2000;65:21200–21201.

42. American Medical Association Department of Foods and Nutrition. Multivitamin preparations for parenteral use: a statement

by the Nutrition Advisory Group. *JPEN J Parenter Enteral Nutr.* 1979;3:258–262.

43. American Medical Association Department of Foods and Nutrition. Guidelines for essential trace element preparations for parenteral use. A statement by an expert panel. *JAMA.* 1979;241:2051–2054.

44. Vanek VW, Borum P, Buchman A, et al. A.S.P.E.N. position paper: recommendations for changes in commercially available parenteral multivitamin and multi-trace element products. *Nutr Clin Pract.* 2012;27:440–491.

45. Howard L, Ashley C, Lyon D, Shenkin A. Autopsy tissue trace elements in 8 long-term parenteral nutrition patients who received the current U.S. Food and Drug Administration formulation. *JPEN J Parenter Enteral Nutr.* 2007;31:388–396.

46. Pluhator-Murton MM, Fedorak RN, Audette RJ, et al. Trace element contamination of total parenteral nutrition, 1: contribution of component solutions. *JPEN J Parenter Enteral Nutr.* 1999;23:222–227.

47. Kumpf VJ. Update on parenteral iron therapy. *Nutr Clin Pract.* 2003;18:318–326.

48. Heyland D, Muscedere J, Wischmeyer PE, et al. Canadian Critical Care Trials Group: a randomized trial of glutamine and antioxidants in critically ill patients. *N Engl J Med.* 2013;368:1489–1497.

49. Andrews PJ, Avenell A, Noble DW, et al. Scottish Intensive care Glutamine or seleNium Evaluative Trial Trials Group: randomised trial of glutamine, selenium, or both, to supplement parenteral nutrition for critically ill patients. *BMJ.* 2011;342:d1542.

50. Borum PR. Is L-carnitine stable in parenteral nutrition solutions prepared for preterm neonates? *Neonatal Intensive Care.* 1993;6:30–32.

51. Clinical Practice Committee Shortage Subcommittee. A.S.P.E.N. parenteral nutrition intravenous fat emulsion product shortage considerations. *Nutr Clin Pract.* 2013;28:4:528–529.

52. American Society for Parenteral and Enteral Nutrition. 2017 parenteral nutrition lipid injectable emulsion product shortage considerations. http://www.nutritioncare.org/News/General _News/2017_Parenteral_Nutrition_Lipid_Injectable_Emulsion _Product_Shortage_Considerations. Accessed March 15, 2017.

53. Plogsted S, Adams SC, Allen K, et al. Clinical Practice Committee's Nutrition Product Shortage Subcommittee. Parenteral nutrition amino acids product shortage considerations. *Nutr Clin Pract.* 2016;31:4:560–561.

54. Plogsted S, Adams SC, Allen K, et al. Clinical Practice Committee's Nutrition Product Shortage Subcommittee. Parenteral nutrition multivitamin product shortage considerations. *Nutr Clin Pract.* 2016;31:4:556–559.

55. Plogsted S, Adams SC, Allen K, et al. Clinical Practice Committee's Nutrition Product Shortage Subcommittee. Parenteral nutrition electrolyte and mineral shortage considerations. *Nutr Clin Pract.* 2016;31:4:132–134.

56. Clinical Practice Committee Shortage Subcommittee. A.S.P.E.N. parenteral nutrition trace element product shortage considerations. *Nutr Clin Pract.* 2014;29:2:249–251.

57. Barnett MI. Physical stability of all-in-one admixtures: factors affecting fat droplets. *Nutrition.* 1989;5:348–349.

58. US Food and Drug Administration. Safety alert: hazards of precipitation associated with parenteral nutrition. *Am J Hosp Pharm.* 1994;51:1427–1428.

59. Mattox TW, Crill C. Parenteral nutrition. In: DiPiro JT, Talbert RL, Yee GC, et al, eds. *Pharmacotherapy.* 9th ed. New York: McGraw-Hill; 2014:2405–2426.

60. Mirtallo JM. Should the use of total nutrient admixtures be limited? *Am J Hosp Pharm.* 1994;51:2831–2834.

61. Driscoll DF. Use of total nutrient admixtures should not be limited. *Am J Health Syst Pharm.* 1995;52:893–895.

62. Driscoll DF. Total nutrient admixtures: theory and practice. *Nutr Clin Pract.* 1995;10:114–119.

63. Centers for Disease Control and Prevention. Guidelines for the prevention of intravascular catheter-related infections. *MMWR.* 2002;51:1–28.

64. D'Angio RG, Reichers KC, Gilsdorf RB, Costantino JM. Effect of the mode of lipid administration on parenteral nutrition-related infections. *Ann Pharmacother.* 1992;26:14–17.

65. Gervasio J. Total nutrient admixtures (3-in-1): pros vs cons in adults. *Nutr Clin Pract.* 2015;30:3:331–335.

66. Boullata JI, Gilbert K, Sacks G, et al. A.S.P.E.N. clinical guidelines: parenteral nutrition ordering, order review, compounding, labeling, and dispensing. *JPEN J Parenter Enteral Nutr.* 2014;38:334–377.

67. Tighe MJ, Wong C, Martin IG, et al. Do heparin, hydrocortisone, and glyceryl trinitrate influence thrombophlebitis during full intravenous nutrition via peripheral vein? *JPEN J Parenter Enteral Nutr.* 1995;19:507–509.

68. Chapter {797}. Pharmaceutical compounding—sterile preparations. Physical tests. In: *United States Pharmacopeia 28/National Formulary 23.* Rockville, MD: US Pharmacopeial Convention; 2005:2461–2477.

69. American Society of Health-System Pharmacists. ASHP guidelines on quality assurance for pharmacy-prepared sterile products. *Am J Health Syst Pharm.* 2000;57:1150–1169.

70. Ayers P, Adams S, Boullata J, et a. A.S.P.E.N. parenteral nutrition safety consensus recommendations. *JPEN J Parenter Enteral Nutr.* 2014;38:296–333.

71. Kitzen JM, Halberstadt DJ, Nguyen H, et al. The effect of dextrose and amino acid composition on the refractive indices of parenteral nutrition solutions. *Hosp Pharm.* 1996;31:817–822.

72. Waxman K, Day AT, Stellin GP, et al. Safety and efficacy of glycerol and amino acids in combination with lipid emulsion for peripheral parenteral nutrition support. *JPEN J Parenter Enteral Nutr.* 1992;16:374–378.

73. Freeman JB, Fairfull-Smith R, Rodman GH, et al. Safety and efficacy of a new peripheral intravenously administered amino acid solution containing glycerol and electrolytes. *Surg Gynecol Obstet.* 1983;156:625–631.

74. Hall JW. Safety, cost and clinical considerations for the use of premixed parenteral nutrition. *Nutr Clin Pract.* 2015;30:3:325–330.

75. Smith JL, Canham JE, Wells PA. Effect of phototherapy light, sodium bisulfite, and pH on vitamin stability in total parenteral nutrition admixtures. *JPEN J Parenter Enteral Nutr.* 1988;12:394–402.

76. Trissel LA, Gilbert DL, Martinez JF, et al. Compatibility of medications with 3-in-1 parenteral nutrition admixtures. *JPEN J Parenter Enteral Nutr.* 1999;23:67–74.

77. Octreotide acetate (Sandostatin) [package insert]. East Hanover, NJ: Novartis Pharmaceuticals Corporation; 2002.

78. Trissel LA, Gilbert DL, Martinez JF, et al. Compatibility of parenteral nutrient solutions with selected drugs during simulated Y-site administration. *Am J Health Syst Pharm.* 1997;54:1295–1300.

79. Wanten GJ. Parenteral lipid tolerance and adverse effects: fat chance for trouble. *JPEN J Parenter Enteral Nutr.* 2015;39:33S-38S.

80. Driscoll DF. Physicochemical stability assessments of lipid emulsions of varying oil composition. *Clin Nutr.* 2001;20:8–10.

81. Driscoll DF. Lipid injectable emulsions 2006. *Nutr Clin Pract.* 2006;21:381–386.

82. Joy J, Silvestri AP, Franke R, et al. Calcium and phosphate compatibility in low-osmolarity parenteral nutrition admixtures intended for peripheral vein administration. *JPEN J Parenter Enteral Nutr.* 2010;34:46–54.

83. Newton DW, Driscoll DF. Calcium and phosphate compatibility: revisited again. *Am J Health Syst Pharm.* 2008;65:73–80.

84. Brown R, Quercia RA, Sigman R. Total nutrient admixtures: a review. *JPEN J Parenter Enteral Nutr.* 1986;10:650–658.

85. Driscoll DF. Lipid injectable emulsions: pharmacopeial and safety issues. *Pharm Res.* 2006;23:1959–1969.

86. Knowles JB, Cusson G, Smith M, et al. Pulmonary deposition of calcium phosphate crystals as a complication of home parenteral nutrition. *JPEN J Parenter Enteral Nutr.* 1989;13:209–213.

87. Eggert LD, Rusho WJ, MacKay MW, et al. Calcium and phosphorus compatibility in parenteral nutrition solutions for neonates. *Am J Hosp Pharm.* 1982;39:49–53.

88. Schmidt GL, Baumgartner TG, Fischlschweiger W, et al. Cost containment using cysteine HCL acidification to increase calcium/phosphate solubility in hyperalimentation solutions. *JPEN J Parenter Enteral Nutr.* 1986;10:203–207.

89. Mirtallo JM. The complexity of mixing calcium and phosphate. *Am J Hosp Pharm.* 1994;51:1535–1536.

90. Driscoll DF, Newton DW, Bistrian BR. Precipitation of calcium phosphate from parenteral nutrition fluids. *Am J Hosp Pharm.* 1994;51:2834–2836.

91. US Food and Drug Administration. Aluminum in large and small volume parenterals used in total parenteral nutrition. *Fed Regist.* 2000;65:4103–4111.

92. Bohrer D, do Nascimento PC, Binotto R, Carlesso R. Influence of the glass packing on the contamination of pharmaceutical products by aluminum. Part II: amino acids for parenteral nutrition. *J Trace Elem Med Biol.* 2001;15:103–108.

93. Bohrer D, do Nascimento PC, Binotto R, et al. Contribution of raw material to the aluminum contamination in parenterals. *JPEN J Parenter Enteral Nutr.* 2002;26:383–388.

94. Klein GL. Aluminum in parenteral solutions revisited—again. *Am J Clin Nutr.* 1995;61:449–456.

95. Yokel RA, McNamara PJ. Aluminum toxicokinetics: an updated mini-review. *Pharmacol Toxicol.* 2001;88:159–167.

96. Mershon J, Nogami W, Williams JM, et al. Bacterial/fungal growth in a combined parenteral nutrient solution. *JPEN J Parenter Enteral Nutr.* 1986;10:498–502.

97. McKinnon BT. FDA safety alert: hazards of precipitation associated with parenteral nutrition. *Nutr Clin Pract.* 1996;11:59–65.

16 Parenteral Access Devices

Antoinette M. Neal, BSN, RN, CRNI, VA-BC, CNSC, and Kathryn Drogan, MS, NP, ANP-BC

CONTENTS

Acknowledgments: Elizabeth A. Krzywda, APNP, MSN, Deborah A. Andris, APNP, MSN, and Charles E. Edmiston, Jr., PhD, coauthored this chapter for the second edition.

Objectives

1. Identify the vascular anatomy pertinent to the placement of peripheral and central venous catheters (CVCs).
2. Describe aspects of device selection for parenteral nutrition (PN).
3. Differentiate characteristics of various venous access devices (VADs).
4. Discuss the maintenance of VADs.
5. Identify patient risk factors for and etiology, pathogenesis, and management of device-related infectious and noninfectious complications.

Test Your Knowledge Questions

1. Which of the following is the most appropriate VAD strategy for a patient requiring long-term PN therapy?
   A. Use a midclavicular catheter as a cost-effective measure.
   B. Place a percutaneous nontunneled catheter to initiate PN and then replace it with an implanted port.
   C. Place a single-lumen, tunneled cuffed catheter.
   D. Place a triple-lumen, antibiotic-coated catheter to ensure adequate access for future needs.
2. Thrombotic occlusions are most commonly treated with which of the following?
   A. Thrombolytics
   B. Anticoagulants
   C. 10% hydrochloric acid
   D. Sodium bicarbonate
3. Which of the following practices has been shown to reduce the risk for catheter-related bloodstream infections (CRBSIs)?
   A. Systemic use of antimicrobial prophylaxis at the time of insertion or access
   B. Routine replacement of central venous access devices (CVADs)
   C. Use of the "Central Line Bundle" of insertion and maintenance practices
   D. Selection of an internal jugular site as opposed to subclavian site

Test Your Knowledge Answers

1. The correct answer is **C**. A single-lumen tunneled catheter is the preferred device. The tunneled catheter was originally developed for patients with long-term PN.[1] Tunneled catheters have been demonstrated to be safe and effective in long-term therapies ranging from months to years.[2] A midclavicular catheter does not provide central access and, therefore, would not be an appropriate catheter choice. Percutaneous nontunneled catheters with additional features of multiple lumens and an antibiotic/antimicrobial coating provide PN access in the acute care setting for a shorter duration of time. It would be best to start with selection of the optimal device for the current therapy rather than a planned replacement. Ports are an alternative to external-lumen catheters, and patients need to understand that repeated needle sticks will be required for daily therapy.

2. The correct answer is **A**. Catheter occlusions are often secondary to a thrombotic problem, such as an intraluminal thrombus, an extraluminal fibrin sleeve, or vessel thrombosis.[3] The successful use of thrombolytics (eg, streptokinase, urokinase, alteplase) to treat catheters occluded with a thrombus is well documented. Nonthrombogenic factors in catheter occlusion include intraluminal drug and lipid precipitates. Pharmacological agents that change the pH within the lumen increase the solubility of the precipitate.[3]

3. The correct answer is **C**. The Central Line Bundle for insertion and maintenance includes (1) hand hygiene, (2) maximal barrier precautions, (3) skin antisepsis with chlorhexidine gluconate (CHG), (4) optimal catheter site selection, and (5) daily review of line necessity, with the prompt removal of unnecessary lines.[4] The use of this bundle has been documented to decrease the incidence of catheter-related infections. The systemic use of antimicrobial prophylaxis at the time of insertion or access is not recommended and may actually promote the resistance of microbial populations associated with catheter infections. The routine replacement of CVADs is not recommended, and catheters should only be removed when clinically indicated. Studies have shown a lower rate of catheter-related infections in line placements via the subclavian site.[5]

Introduction to Vascular Access

Vascular access is the means by which intravenous (IV) fluids, medications, and nutrition support are provided to patients across the continuum of healthcare. Ever since the circulation of blood was discovered centuries ago, humans have developed and improved on ways to access vascular circulation. As vascular access continues to evolve, clinicians following evidence-based practices can improve patients' outcomes and quality of life and reduce risks for complications,[6] particularly when they are part of a specialty vascular access team trained to select the proper site, standardize vascular access insertions, maintain vascular access, reassess the patient's need for a VAD, and promptly remove unneeded devices.[7] The Healthcare Infection Control Practices Advisory Committee of the Centers for Disease Control and Prevention (CDC) has published guidelines to help clinicians create specialized vascular access teams that can reduce and eliminate bloodstream infections (BSIs) in patients with vascular access. The guidelines state that "the goal of an effective program should be elimination of CRBSI from all patient care areas."[8] Additionally, the guidelines note that specialized IV teams "have shown unequivocal effectiveness in reducing the incidence of CRBSI, associated complications, and costs."[8]

Physiological Principles

Venous blood flow returns blood from the body to the heart and lungs. It involves negative thoracic pressure during inspiration as well as muscle contractions and valves with peripheral veins.[9] In the upper and lower extremities, the system of paired valves prevents retrograde blood flow against gravity. In the large central veins, such as the inferior vena cava (IVC) and superior vena cava (SVC), blood flow relies on negative intrathoracic pressure and abdominal and diaphragmatic muscle movement, not valves. Unlike arteries, veins can compensate for occlusions via a rich collateral circulation.

Vascular Anatomy

The superficial veins of the upper extremity are visible and palpable because they lie in the superficial fascia. These vessels include the basilic, cephalic, and median antecubital veins. The median antebrachial vein drains the venous plexus on the palmar surface of the hand. It travels up the ulnar side of the front of the forearm and ends in the basilic vein or in the median antecubital; in a small proportion of cases, it divides into a branch that joins the basilic vein and a branch that joins the cephalic vein, below the elbow.

The SVC is the main vessel for venous return from the upper trunk emptying into the right atrium.[2] The subclavian vessels receive the external jugular veins and join with the internal jugular vein to form the brachiocephalic vein. The right brachiocephalic vein is directed vertically downward in the thorax. The left brachiocephalic vein crosses over to the right chest. The right and left brachiocephalic veins join to form the SVC. The SVC is approximately 7 cm long and 20 to 30 mm in diameter. The estimated blood flow in the SVC is 2000 mL/min, making it the preferred vessel for central access and the infusion of PN solutions. The rate of blood flow in the central vein rapidly dilutes PN, which is hypertonic with an osmolarity greater than 900 mOsm/L. Along with PN, concentrated antibiotics, and vesicants can be infused into central venous blood flow without causing damage to veins Figure 16.1).[10]

Veins in the lower body include the iliac veins, which are the major leg veins. They join at the fifth lumbar vertebra to form the IVC, the large vein that carries deoxygenated blood from the lower body, legs, and torso to the right atrium of the heart. This vein runs posterior to the abdominal cavity alongside the right vertebral column of the spine. If the SVC becomes thrombosed or occluded, catheter placement in the IVC may be warranted. Although this approach is not routine, it may be the only central venous option available. Long-term access to the IVC is feasible without undue concern when access to the SVC is prohibited.[11]

Catheter Technology

Catheter Measurements

Catheter size is expressed as diameter, French size, and gauge. Diameter can refer to the internal or external diameter and is measured in millimeters. Depending on the catheter material, the internal diameter may vary between catheters with the same external diameter. French size is a measure of the outer diameter (1 mm = 3 Fr). Gauge is a unit of measure that is inversely proportional to the catheter's outer diameter. The total catheter length depends on the site of insertion and any catheter trimming that is done at the time of insertion.

Central Venous Catheter Features

Most CVCs are available in multilumen versions. This option provides for simultaneous infusion of multiple solutions or

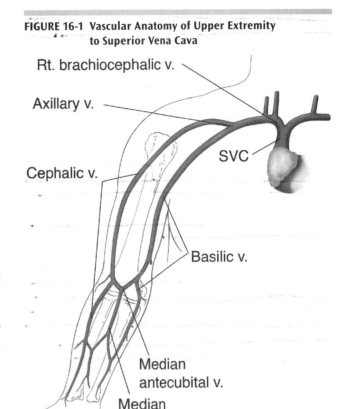

FIGURE 16-1 Vascular Anatomy of Upper Extremity to Superior Vena Cava

Rt., right; SVC, superior vena cava; v., vein.
Source: Reprinted with permission from reference 10: Bennett JD, Papadouris D, Rankin RN, et al. Percutaneous inferior vena caval approach for long-term central venous access. *J Vasc Interv Radiol.* 1997;8(5):851–855.

incompatible drugs. Design may vary among manufacturers in terms of both lumen size and distal tip configurations.

Cuffs attached to CVCs are designed to serve as subcutaneous anchors and mechanical barriers. Dacron cuffs are most often attached to tunneled catheters. These cuffs are positioned in the subcutaneous tissue and serve to anchor the catheter by facilitating fibrous ingrowth. Collagen cuffs impregnated with silver ions can be attached to the catheter at insertion or are available preattached. The gradual release of the silver ion exerts short-term antimicrobial activity.[12] Specialized valves have been developed to help prevent retrograde blood flow, catheter occlusions, and air embolisms. A Groshong catheter is a VAD with a pressure sensitive 3-way slit valve on the tunneled catheter. This valve eliminates the need for daily heparinized flushes and catheter clamping before disconnection at the catheter hub.

Catheter Materials

Many inert biomaterials are available for catheter construction. However, upon insertion into the patient, some materials may produce a variety of adverse effects. The ideal biomaterial is nontoxic, nonpyrogenic, easily sterilized, biocompatible with host tissues, and durable. The compounds that most closely achieve these ideals include polyvinylchloride (PVC), polyethylene, polyurethane, silicone elastomer, and hydrogels. PVC is a long-chain polymer that has many applications in the biomedical device field. Although this material is relatively inert, it is also quite rigid and demonstrates a high surface energy that is attractive to serum proteins. PVC catheters have been associated with an increase in thrombus formation and phlebitis compared with other polymeric catheters. Some reports suggest that plasticizing substances added during manufacturing to confer catheter flexibility may leach out following placement and provoke an acute inflammatory reaction.[13]

Catheters are most often made of polyurethane or silicone. Polyurethane catheters are characterized by a smooth surface, which demonstrates resistance to hydrolytic enzymes. Polyurethane offers greater tensile strength than silicone and lower degrees of microbial colonization.[14] The material's properties of biocompatibility and versatility hold promise for future catheter technology.[15]

Catheters constructed of silicone demonstrate excellent elasticity and softness and cause less damage to the vessel intima. In addition, silicone elastomer has a low inflammatory-provoking potential in the tissues, and the surface is less attractive for adherence of microbial populations when compared with other biomaterials used in catheter construction. The material tends to be chemically inert to blood, with reduced platelet adherence; however, serum protein will adsorb to the surface. Therefore, fibrin sleeve formation is seen as a common complication of silicone devices.[16]

A unique class of hydrophilic polymers has a cross-linked, 3-dimensional structure, which allows water absorption—in some cases, up to 90% of the catheter's dry weight. This polymer has been bonded to catheter surfaces. The polymer's negatively charged surface mimics the electrical characteristics of the host vessel wall, resulting in enhanced biocompatibility with a reduction in thrombogenicity. These catheters are stiffer on insertion and subsequently soften after placement in the vessel. Unfortunately, the hydrogels as a group lack the tensile strength and durability of other catheter materials, such as silicone elastomer. Acute hypersensitivity reactions have been associated with midline catheters composed of an elastomeric hydrogel material.[17]

Types of Access

Central and peripheral access are not defined by the initial point of entry into the vascular system but rather by the position of the distal catheter tip. In a peripheral catheter, the tip position is located outside of the central vessels (the SVC or IVC). A CVC is a catheter with the tip in the distal SVC, IVC, or right atrium.[18] Table 16-1 summarizes options for parenteral access,[8,11,19-22] and specific types are further discussed in the sections that follow.

Short-Term Venous Access

Peripheral Venous Access

Venous access into a peripheral vein is a simple, inexpensive means of providing infusion therapy with proven short-term

results. Peripheral veins in the upper extremities in the hands and arms can be accessed with peripheral catheters. Steel-winged and sheath-over needles are 2 types of short peripheral catheters. The catheters discussed in this chapter are sheath-over needles. Steel-winged devices are for single-dose administration only, and the device is not to be left in place.[23]

The short peripherally placed catheter is a widely used tool. Up to 80% of hospital patients require at least 1 peripheral venous catheter; their use is the most frequent invasive procedure in hospitals.[24] However, peripheral venous access has limitations; therefore, the clinical team should collaboratively decide whether to place a short peripheral catheter based on the projected treatment plan. Peripheral vein preservation should also be considered when planning for vascular access. A short peripheral catheter is appropriate for nonirritant, nonvesicant, and nonhyperosmolar infusion therapy with relatively short duration (eg, less than 1 week). Catheter tips located in a peripheral vessel are not appropriate for the infusion of PN that has a final concentration exceeding 10% dextrose or other additives that result in an osmolarity of greater than 900 mOsm/L.[18,25] Peripheral sites are reserved for short-term therapies and times when fluid restriction is not necessary.[25]

Peripheral devices are considered to have the lowest risk of complications and are the most commonly used VADs; however, documented rates of infections are rarely reported and well-designed prospective studies are lacking to adequately support this commonly held belief.[26]

The leading complication associated with peripheral access is peripheral venous thrombophlebitis. The hallmark signs and symptoms of infusion phlebitis (an inflammation of the cannulated vein) are pain, erythema, tenderness, or a palpable cord.[27] This phenomenon has been related to multiple risk factors, including catheter material, catheter diameter, operator skill, infusates, and duration of cannulation. The duration of catheter cannulation was once believed to be the most common risk factor; therefore, it previously was recommended that standard peripheral cannula be rotated to a new site every 48 to 72 hours. This concept has been challenged, and a recent review found no conclusive benefit to routinely changing catheters.[28] Rather, peripheral catheters should be changed when clinically indicated (refer to Table 16-1). CDC guidelines recommend close monitoring of peripheral access, with the peripheral IV line removed no more frequently than every 72 to 96 hours, unless clinically indicated.[8]

Peripheral catheters include standard peripheral cannulas and midline catheters. Midline catheters were initially introduced in 1950, temporarily removed from the market in the 1990s, and are now available in redesigned forms. Recently introduced midline catheters with short midlines of 8 to 10 cm are all-in-one devices with the needle, wire, and introducer combined for ease and speed of access; they are inserted using the accelerated Seldinger technique (described in next section).[29] When longer midline catheters (20 cm in length) are used, the tip location is advanced no further than the axillary vein, which maintains the tip into the peripheral vasculature.[28] Midline catheters have lower phlebitis rates than standard, short peripheral catheters and lower rates of infection than CVADS.[29] These catheters are suitable for peripherally

TABLE 16-1 Vascular Access Devices

Catheter Type	Placement	Advantages	Disadvantages
Peripheral access			
Peripheral catheters	• Percutaneous peripheral insertion. • Enter and terminate in peripheral veins in the hand and lower arm. • Placed with ultrasonography or other vein-locating devices. • Can use visible light devices that provide transillumination to visualize and locate difficult vessels. • Consider the use of near-infrared light technology to aid in locating viable venous access while decreasing procedure time.	• Least expensive. • Least risk for catheter-related infections. • Do not require a special placement room. • Clinicians are easily trained in placement.	• Must be immediately removed when infiltration is suspected or when the following complications are clinically indicated: discoloration, redness, or blanching; disruption of sensation, pain, tenderness, numbness; localized swelling; exudate; increased skin temperature; induration. • Site must be visualized frequently (eg, every 4 hours). • Not appropriate for infusates >900 mOsm/L or dextrose concentrations >10%.
Midline catheters	• Percutaneous peripheral insertion. • Typically inserted in veins above the antecubital fossa. • The catheter tip resides in the basilic or cephalic vein, with the tip at or before the axilla, distal to the shoulder.	• Used for therapies lasting 2–4 weeks.	• Not appropriate for infusions requiring central access. • Not appropriate for infusates >900 mOsm/L or dextrose concentrations >10%.
Midclavicular catheters	• Percutaneous peripheral insertion.	• None identified. Literature does not support use of these catheters.	• Not appropriate for infusions requiring central access. • Risk of mural thrombosis. • Increased risk of penetrating the veins intima, causing rupture to the innominate or subclavian vein, which can easily go unnoticed.
Central access			
Percutaneous central catheters, nontunneled	• Placed via direct puncture and cannulation of the internal jugular, subclavian, or femoral vein. • Typically 15–25 cm long.	• Useful in acute or short-term care (often inserted for 7–14 days). • Economical, easily removable.	• Catheter breakage cannot be repaired. • Patient is self-care difficult; not recommended for home care. • Requires sutures to prevent dislodgment. • High risk for catheter-related infections.
PICC, nontunneled	• Percutaneous placement via a peripheral vein.	• Can be used in acute and home care for therapies ranging from several weeks to months. • Low risk of placement complications. • Can be placed in radiology suite or at patient bedside.	• Self-care is impractical and unsafe because the catheter must be secured during dressing change and because aseptic technique requires 2 sterile gloved hands to perform dressing and cap change. • Because of the placement location, dressings can easily become wet, soiled, and loose. • Can interfere with daily activities.

(continued)

TABLE 16-1 Vascular Access Devices *(continued)*

Catheter Type	Placement	Advantages	Disadvantages
Internal jugular catheters, cuffed or noncuffed; tunneled or nontunneled	• Internal jugular insertion.	• Can preserve the subclavian site in patients with renal disease (eg, hemodialysis patients with advanced kidney disease) by avoiding or preventing subclavian vein stenosis.	• May be easily dislodged if not tunneled and if the catheter does not have a cuff. • Removal requires small procedure.
Tunneled, cuffed catheters	• Percutaneous insertion into subclavian or jugular vessels, with distal tip located the lower third of the SVC.	• Can be placed for long-term usage. • Placement location can be determined collaboratively with clinician and patient (usually placed on chest wall). • Can be covered with clothing. • An integrated cuff on the device anchors the catheter within the subcutaneous tissue and limits entry of bacteria along the extraluminal surface of the device. • Dressings and sutures can be removed after 1 month. • Self-care is easy. • Repair kits are available.	• Must be placed in operating room or other specialized room. • Removal requires small procedure.
TIVADs	• Percutaneous venous placement via subclavian, jugular, or peripheral vessels.	• Can be used for long-term therapies. • Options for placement location are available. • Site care is required only when device is accessed. • Maintenance frequency varies from monthly to 90 days, depending on type of port. • Cosmetically more desirable. • No external catheter for breakage.	• Must be placed in operating room or other specialized room. • Surgical procedure required for insertion and removal. • Most expensive CVADs to place and remove. • Require needle access; needle dislodgment can result in infiltration. • When accessed continuously, infection risk is not reduced and tissue area over port may start to break down from dressings and needle in port.
Translumbar, transhepatic, transcollateral central catheters	• Translumbar, transhepatic, transcollateral insertion.	• Viable option when all other vascular access options are unavailable.	• Placement requires skilled, trained interventional radiology unit clinicians. • CT-guided puncture is associated with higher radiation doses, although newer versions of CT fluoroscopy have lower radiation doses. • Self-care maybe challenging, depending on the catheter exit site.

CT, computed tomography; CVAD, central venous access device; PICC, peripherally inserted central catheter; SVC, superior vena cava; TIVAD, totally implanted vascular access device.

Source: Data are from references 8, 10, and 19–22.

compatible solutions where treatment is considered for 2 to 6 weeks. Because of the extended dwell time, frequent venous site changes are not needed with midline catheters.

Percutaneous Nontunneled Catheters

Nontunneled, noncuffed CVADs are most commonly used in the acute care setting for therapies of short duration. Most often, access is obtained with a percutaneous venipuncture using a subclavian, jugular, or femoral approach. Percutaneous insertion techniques include the Seldinger approach, which involves accessing a vein or artery with a small needle, introducing a flexible guidewire, removing the needle, and advancing the catheter over the wire and into the vessel. The modified Seldinger technique involves accessing a vein with a small needle (21 or 22 gauge) into which a guidewire is threaded, removing the needle, and inserting an introducer/dilator unit over the guidewire to help dilate the tissue to allow for larger-diameter catheters. The wire and dilator can be removed separately or as one unit, leaving the introducer in the vein. The catheter is inserted through the introducer; the introducer can then be removed or peeled away. To prevent dislodgment of the catheter, sutures or securement devices are placed at the exit site, and a sterile dressing is used.

The dwell time of this temporary catheter is limited to 5 to 7 days; the device has the option of up to 5 lumens, allowing for separate access and concurrent infusion of multiple treatments.[2] Advantages to nontunneled catheters include lower placement costs, ease of removal, and the ability to exchange catheters over a guidewire. A guidewire exchange can be used to replace a malfunctioning nontunneled catheter when no evidence of infection is present. However, routinely scheduled catheter exchanges over a guidewire are no longer recommended as an effective means of preventing catheter-related infections.[5] Prospective studies have demonstrated a higher rate of infection when catheters are routinely exchanged over a guidewire.[30,31] The potential drawback associated with catheter guidewire exchanges is contamination of the new catheter.

Percutaneous nontunneled catheters are not appropriate for the home care setting. In that setting, they should be exchanged for a long-term catheter.

Central Venous Access Devices

The most common sites of venipuncture for central access include the cephalic, basilic, subclavian, jugular, and femoral veins (see Figure 16-2). Repeated use of the subclavian vein is associated with risk of stenosis, which can have serious consequences in patients with renal concerns who require arteriovenous fistulas or shunts for hemodialysis. The right internal jugular vein is the most direct approach to the SVC for patients with chronic kidney disease who may require dialysis.[32,33] According to the Michigan Appropriateness Guide for Intravenous Catheters (MAGIC) expert panel, clinicians should consult a nephrologist before peripherally inserted central catheter (PICC) insertion if any questions or ambiguity exist regarding the severity of underlying kidney disease.[21] These authors also stress the imperative to preserve peripheral and

central veins for possible hemodialysis or creation of arteriovenous fistula and grafts.[21]

In the United States alone, more than 7 million CVADs are placed annually, accounting for over 15 million CVAD days.[34] CVAD access has become the foundation for short- and long-term medication administration. Placement is required in patients receiving life-sustaining PN. Despite the routine use, these devices carry risk for complications—which can be related to insertion technique—causing vascular injury, infection, and misplacement. Morbidity and mortality risks create significant healthcare burdens in hospital cost, length of stay, and patient quality of life.[34]

Advances in technology with ultrasound-guided imaging, tip-placement location devices, and antibiotic-impregnated catheters play an important part in ensuring that CVAD insertion technique is safe. The CDC has developed guidelines for healthcare personnel who insert catheters as well as for those responsible for surveillance and control of infections across the healthcare continuum.[8]

CVADs provide access blood aspiration required for laboratory monitoring as well as increased options for medications and infusions. These devices are not limited by drug pH, osmolarity, or volume, and they reduce the risk for extravasation of vesicant drugs.

Conceptually, CVADs can be grouped into 3 broad categories: nontunneled, tunneled, and implanted.[2,18] This general classification provides a basis for catheter selection. No catheter is ideal for all situations; therefore, catheter choice is guided by the advantages and disadvantages associated with various options (see Table 16-1).

Long-Term Venous Access

Peripherally Inserted Central Catheters

A PICC is a catheter inserted via a peripheral vein with the tip in the SVC. These catheters are classified as nontunneled CVADs. Although they are nontunneled, PICCs are a common means for securing central vascular access in acute care and home settings. Median cubital, cephalic, basilic, and brachial veins with sufficient diameter for PICC cannulation can be used (Figure 16-2).

In adults, a venous site where the catheter-to-vein ratio is equal to or less than 45% should be selected to minimize the risk of venous thrombosis.[11,21,35] The peripheral approach decreases the risks associated with a thoracic approach to catheter placement. Licensed clinicians (mainly nurses and physicians with specialized training) place these catheters. PICC line placement can occur in the patient's home, at the bedside, or in an interventional radiology suite.

PICCs offer several advantages, including safer insertion in the arm, cost-effectiveness, and the convenience of placement by vascular access teams,[21] and the use of PICCs has grown worldwide. Despite the advantages of PICCs, their use may lead to significant complications, such as luminal occlusions, malpositioning, and dislodgement. Additionally, superficial thrombophlebitis and infection at PICC insertion site may occur even when the insertion was uneventful.

FIGURE 16-2 Long-Term Vascular Access for Parenteral Nutrition

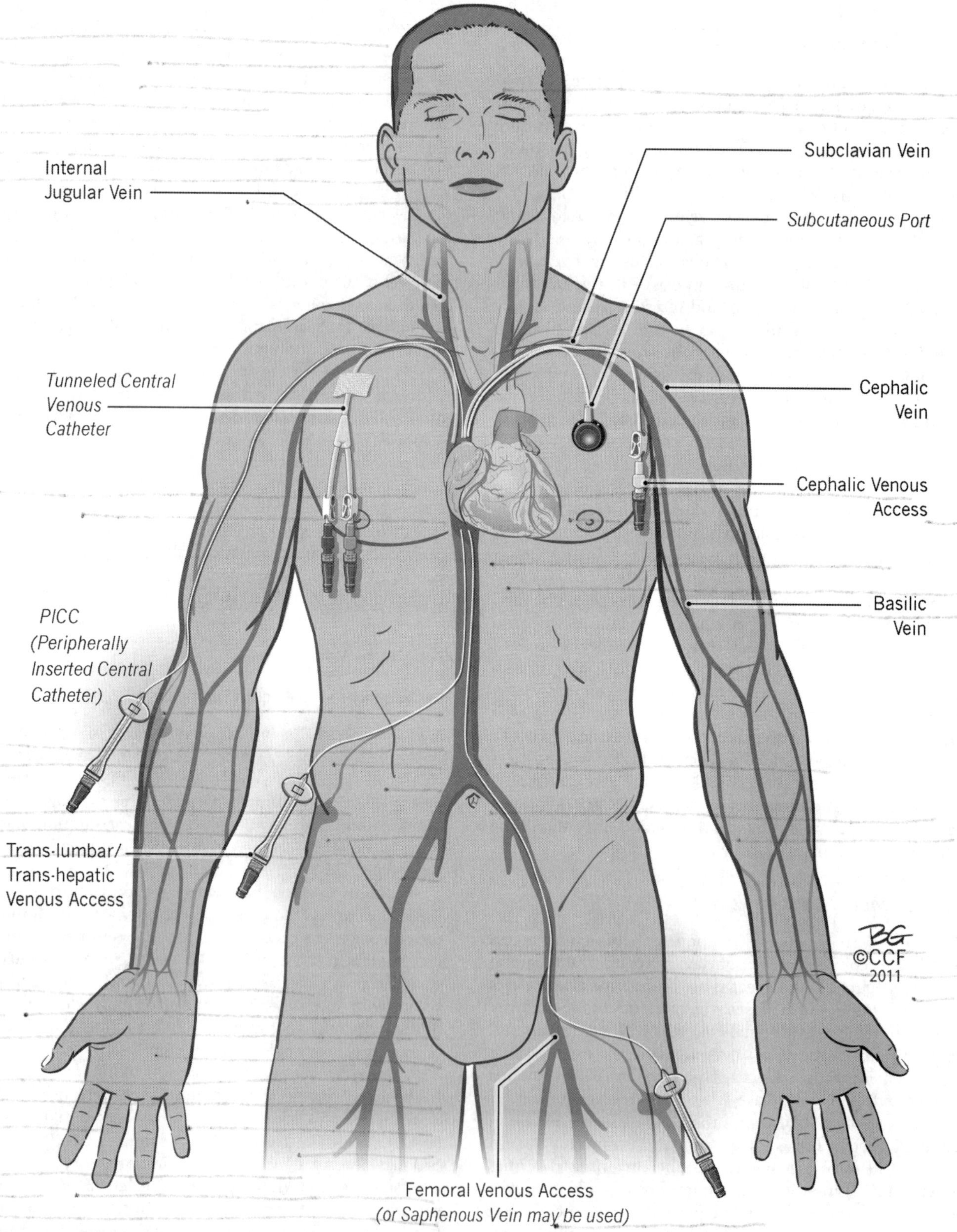
Internal Jugular Vein
Subclavian Vein
Subcutaneous Port
Tunneled Central Venous Catheter
Cephalic Vein
Cephalic Venous Access
Basilic Vein
PICC (Peripherally Inserted Central Catheter)
Trans-lumbar/ Trans-hepatic Venous Access
©CCF 2011
Femoral Venous Access
(or Saphenous Vein may be used)

Source: Reprinted with permission, Cleveland Clinic Center for Medical Art & Photography ©2011–2017. All Rights Reserved.

CRBSI
└ Catheter-related bloodstream infection

Morbid complications include venous thromboembolism and CRBSI.[11,21] PICCs should therefore be used with caution in patients who have cancer or are critically ill.[11,21,36,37]

Stabilization devices are necessary to maintain PICC placement and avoid malposition. However, even with appropriate devices, PICCs may migrate. The MAGIC expert panel concluded that advancements of migrated PICCs are inappropriate regardless of how far a PICC is dislodged, and the panel rated guidewire exchange as appropriate if there are no signs of local or systemic infection.[21] Guidewire exchanges are also rated as appropriate when changes to existing PICC characteristics (such as the number of lumens or power-injection compatibility) are needed.[21] As with the selection of all CVCs, the collaboration of an interdisciplinary team is needed to determine the most appropriate device for the therapy and the patient. The MAGIC panel rated PICCs as appropriate for infusions of irritants and vesicants, such as PN and chemotherapy, for any length of duration, with PICC lines dwelling for months.[21] The Sustain Registry, a research database established in the United Sates to track and monitor patient outcomes on PN, documented 292 patients with PICC lines and noted that these lines remained in place for months to years.[38]

The availability of a skilled caregiver is an important factor when considering PICC placement. A patient or unskilled clinician cannot adequately dress or maintain the PICC site because aseptic technique is required. Sterile technique must be maintained throughout the dressing change procedure.[11] Use of an extension set allows patients and caregivers to independently flush lines and infuse PN. Long-term care of the PICC by skilled clinicians may create an additional financial burden for the patients already receiving an expensive therapy.[39]

Tunneled Central Venous Catheters

The development of PN support served as an impetus for the technological development of long-term CVADs. Initially, central venous access was accomplished using surgically created arteriovenous fistulas. In an attempt to improve vascular access, a silicone elastomer catheter was inserted by subclavian venipuncture, with the distal tip placed into the midatrium.[1] The Broviac catheter served as a model for the original tunneled catheter using an extravascular segment with an attached cuff that was brought through a subcutaneous tunnel on the anterior chest (Figure 16-2).

Theoretically, catheter tunneling decreases the risk of catheter infection by separating the exit and venipuncture sites.[40,41] Catheter tunneling has, in general, been correlated with lower rates of infection. In one prospective study, catheter-related sepsis was confirmed in 28% of patients with nontunneled catheters and 11.5% of those with tunneled catheters.[41] However, the benefit and cost-effectiveness of catheter tunneling has been debated.[42] When members of an infusion therapy team cared meticulously for nontunneled catheters in a cohort study of cancer patients, the catheter-related infection rate for the less-expensive nontunneled devices was comparable to the infection rate for tunneled catheters (0.13 vs 0.14 per 100 catheter days).[43]

Tunneled catheters have been demonstrated to be safe and effective in long-term therapies ranging from months to years.

Advantages to these catheters include ease of self-care by the patient, placement on chest wall so they are covered by clothing, decreased risk of dislodgment, and the ability to repair the external lumen in the event of catheter breakage.

Translumbar, Transhepatic, and Transcollateral Venous Access

Long-term administration of PN hinges on the maintenance of patent venous access. Central venous occlusions caused by thrombi from hypercoagulation and septic incidents put patients in jeopardy of losing their life-sustaining therapy.[44] When repeated catheterizations to common vein sites affect the continued likelihood of the vein's preservation, alternative access sites may become the patient's only viable option. Although unusual, insertion of a CVAD into the translumbar, transhepatic, and transcollateral venous circulation may be the only way to provide access for PN and medications.[2,20] These alternate routes for permanent venous access use the IVC, with the catheter tip above the level of the diaphragm.[23] Proper anatomical, radiologic, and technical knowledge will influence the success of the procedures, which are best performed by a trained interventional radiology unit (Figure 16-2).[20]

Totally Implanted Venous Access Devices (Subcutaneous Ports)

Totally implanted venous access devices (TIVADs) were first developed in 1982 as an alternative to external-lumen tunneled catheters.[45] These devices consist of a silicone or polyurethane catheter attached to a portal reservoir made of stainless steel, polysulfone, or titanium with a self-sealing silicone elastomer septum.[46] TIVADs can be implanted into a subcutaneous pocket in the upper chest, upper arm, or forearm. Variations of the initial port design have included larger septums, double-lumen ports, side-entry ports, and power ports designed to be used for computed tomography (CT) contrast injection. A lower-profile port, the peripheral access system port, is half the length and one-third the height of an implanted chest port. It is placed in the inner surface of the upper arm, which may be cosmetically appealing to patients. Multiple TIVAD options are available to accommodate a patient's anatomy, clinical needs, and preferences. Obtaining access involves locating and palpating the port and then inserting a noncoring needle into the silicone septum. Ports can be accessed up to 1000 to 2000 times. TIVADs have evolved to include a valve in the proximal tip of the catheter, and these closed-ended port catheters offer an extended maintenance interval (Figure 16-2).

Device Selection and Patient Assessment

Device Selection

Few prospective randomized studies are available to compare the complications and outcomes associated with various CVADs.[47] Overall, existing data support the safety of indwelling devices. Early studies demonstrated that implanted ports have the lowest rates of CRBSI. These studies included a large prospective study, which demonstrated significantly lower rates of infection in cancer patients with implanted ports as compared with tunneled catheters.[48] When studying outcomes, the type of catheter is not the sole variable; instead, multiple factors influence the potential for catheter complications and successful outcomes. Selection of the VAD should therefore address all these factors, including the patient's characteristics, preferences, medical history, comorbidities, and infusion needs, as well as available device options.[2]

Patient Assessment

Device selection should align the patient and his or her therapy with the appropriate catheter. The goal is to choose a device that is safe, meets the patient's access needs, and is cost-effective. Many factors play a role in the decision-making process, including the type of medication or solution to be delivered, the overall therapeutic regimen, the anticipated duration of therapy, the patient's lifestyle, the potential impact of the device on the patient's body image, and his or her activity level.

In the home care setting, the patient's cognitive ability and willingness to perform necessary tasks also need to be assessed because these factors will influence the degree of care and maintenance the patient will be able to provide. If the patient is unable to participate on a certain level, a device requiring less maintenance may be indicated. The need for and availability of an additional caregiver will affect the cost as well as the need for long-term home nursing assistance. The "ideal" goal of home therapy of a lifelong nature is to restore the patient to his or her prior level of function. When choosing a device, one must allow for an increasing level of activity as the patient condition improves and even considers an eventual return to work. See Chapter 38 for further discussion of home nutrition support.

Collaboration between the patient and the clinical team offers the patient autonomy to make informed decisions regarding care. The likelihood of optimal outcomes is greater when the right device is chosen for the right therapy in the right location for the patient. Clinicians must assess the education needs of the patient and caregivers to ensure the success of discussions regarding ongoing care, maintenance of the VAD, and potential complications.[2]

A vascular access history and a focused physical examination are components of the selection/preoperative assessment process. A comprehensive preoperative assessment may decrease the rate of insertion-related complications. In a randomized prospective study, 3 factors were associated with the failure of placement of a CVC in the subclavian vein: prior surgery or radiation in the region, body mass index greater than 30 or less than 20, and previous catheterization.[49] A vascular access history identifies any previous devices, their location, and the length of time they were in place. Prior device-associated complications, such as thrombosis, infection, withdrawal occlusion, or difficult placement, should be noted. Previous chest, neck, or breast surgery or clavicular fracture may alter normal anatomical landmarks used during insertion. The physical examination should focus on identifying any lesions, tumors, previous surgical procedures, venous abnormalities, or breaks in skin integrity near the intended placement site. The medication history screens for the use of drugs that could affect coagulation status, such as aspirin, nonsteroidal anti-inflammatory agents, warfarin, or heparin. If the patient is receiving anticoagulants or antiplatelet medications, these medications should be held with a possible transition to low–molecular weight heparin based on the individual's risk of thromboembolism.[50]

Venous duplex ultrasonography or venous angiography can be obtained when clinicians have concerns regarding venous patency. Studies support the use of the subclavian approach except in chronic kidney patients; in those patients, the National Kidney Foundation Kidney Disease Outcomes Quality Initiative guidelines should be followed.[33,51] The MAGIC expert panel has acknowledged the imperative in patients with renal disease to preserve peripheral and central veins for possible hemodialysis or creation of arteriovenous fistulae and grafts; therefore, regardless of the vascular indication, the panel rated insertion of devices (PICCs, midline catheters) into the arm veins as inappropriate for such patients.[21] If venous access is needed for 5 days or fewer, the panel recommended a peripheral IV in the dorsum of the hand (avoiding the forearm veins) for peripheral-compatible infusates such as peripheral PN. If longer-duration venous access is needed for a nonperipherally compatible drug or solution, the use of a tunneled, 4-Fr single-lumen or 5-Fr double-lumen inserted into the jugular vein and tunneled into the distal SVC was rated appropriate.[21] When selecting a CVAD, clinicians should choose the device with the least number of lumens or ports appropriate for the patient. Unnecessary lumens require more manipulation and access of the catheter, thereby increasing the risk for CVAD-related infection and complications.[5,52]

Contraindications to elective placement of a long-term CVAD include sudden clinical deterioration with a change in the treatment plan; a new, unexplained fever; or absolute neutropenia (less than 1000 white blood cells per mL). When platelet counts are less than 50,000, platelet administration within 2 hours of catheter insertion should be considered.

Catheter Insertion and Maintenance

Catheter placement is not without risks. Arterial, venous, and other organ injuries can occur along with bleeding and hematomas.[34] Complications can be immediate or delayed. Subsequent morbidity and mortality increase healthcare costs and decrease patient satisfaction and quality of life.[34] CDC guidelines[8] recommend that healthcare providers implement an effective strategy to educate clinicians regarding the indications for catheter use, proper procedures for insertion and maintenance, and appropriate infection control measures to prevent intravascular catheter-related infections and possible insertion complications.

Catheter Insertion

Depending on the type, catheters may be inserted at the bedside or in the home, procedure room, operating room, or interventional radiology suite. With regard to infection risk, the setting may be less critical than the use of maximal barrier precautions such as cap, mask, disposable gown, gloves, and large drape. Two landmark studies demonstrated a decrease in catheter colonization at the time of catheter insertion with use of these measures, thereby lowering the catheter-related sepsis risk.[53,54]

Insertion of a CVAD requires the application of care bundle guidelines (discussed in detail later in the chapter),[4] hand hygiene, skin antisepsis using 0.5% chlorhexidine in alcohol solution, maximal sterile barrier precautions, and selection of appropriate venous access. Along with the care bundle, proper technique is advanced through the use of a standardized checklist, proper education of staff, and empowerment of staff to stop the procedure if a break in protocol is noted.[23] Long-term CVADs are usually placed after the patient has received a local anesthetic with or without additional IV sedation. Catheter insertion is commonly performed by 1 of 2 techniques: the percutaneous approach (Seldinger or modified Seldinger) or venous cutdown.[55-57] Tunneled catheters are passed subcutaneously to a site 3 to 10 cm distal to the venotomy with the cuff 2 to 3 cm from the exit site. The percutaneous approach is associated with a risk of pneumothorax, arterial puncture, and catheter pinch-off.

Immediate complications of CVAD insertion may include pneumothorax, air embolism, arterial puncture, arrhythmia, and bleeding. Pneumothorax is the most common immediate complication, with an incidence of 1% to 3%. Symptoms of pneumothorax include dyspnea, cough, hypoxia, chest pain, and tachycardia.[58] A cutdown approach virtually eliminates the risk of a pneumothorax. A venous cutdown is performed using the cephalic, external jugular, or internal jugular vein. In this technique, the vein is dissected and a venotomy allows the clinician to directly visualize the vessel while inserting the catheter.

Arrhythmias can occur when the guidewire or catheter is advanced too far and enters the right atrium of the heart.[59] Large-volume blood loss during CVAD insertion is uncommon, but anticoagulants may need to be held prior to the procedure to prevent bleeding issues.

Cardiac tamponade is a very rare, but often fatal complication of CVAD insertion.[60] It can occur immediately or several months after placement of the CVAD. The guidewire or tip of the catheter may puncture the wall of the heart initially, or it may later migrate into the heart.[61] Symptoms include chest pain, dyspnea, tachycardia, nausea, hypotension, and enlarged neck veins.[60] If cardiac tamponade is suspected, any infusions should immediately be stopped and the catheter not used until it is evaluated. The use of imaging to guide insertion and confirm correct catheter tip placement in the SVC helps prevent cardiac tamponade.[43,60,61]

The long-standing mandate to verify catheter placement and check for pneumothorax with a postprocedure chest x-ray has recently been challenged.[62,63] In a retrospective review of 205 patients that underwent elective subclavian venous port placement, complications included pneumothorax (2%) and catheter malposition (2.4%).[62] Pneumothorax was not identified on the postprocedure chest x-ray but found on a repeat chest x-ray when the patient was symptomatic. The catheter malpositions were recognized with intraoperative fluoroscopy and corrected.

The use of ultrasound guidance technology has improved placement of CVADs by increasing successful placement rates, reducing the number of needle punctures, and lowering the incidence of needle-stick complications. When ultrasound guidance is available, well-trained clinicians should therefore use it to place CVADs.[23] In one of the largest published studies,

Cavanna and colleagues prospectively monitored the safety of ultrasound-guided CVAD placement. A total of 1978 procedures were done, with a single needle puncture in achieved 98% of all procedures and no occurrence of pneumothorax.[63]

Confirmation of correct tip location is mandatory before the PICC can be used. Historically, the gold standard for confirming accurate tip placement of a PICC line into the lower third of the SVC or the cavoatrial junction has been a chest x-ray. Confirmation of tip location by postprocedural chest radiography remains an acceptable practice.[11] However, methods for identifying PICC placement during the insertion procedure are more accurate, allow for more rapid initiate of infusion therapy, and reduce costs. Electrocardiography (ECG)–guided CVAD placement provides real-time tip confirmation during the insertion procedure. The ECG-guided method for tip location relies on the identification of the patient's P wave and monitoring changes in it by using the catheter as an intravascular electrode. As the catheter moves in relation to the right atrium, the amplitude of the P wave increases or decreases. An exaggerated, positive P wave deflection is the target that determines optimum tip location.[64] Anomalies in the cardiac dysrhythmias and the presence of a P wave on ECG may prohibit the use of this technology,[23] and only trained clinicians should attempt to use it.

Catheter Site Maintenance

Care of the catheter exit site and hub play a pivotal role in decreasing the risk for catheter-related sepsis.[65,66] General care principles prevail regardless of the type of catheter. Site care and management techniques are aimed at maintaining vascular access and reducing the risk of complications (Table 16-2).[23] Assessment of the catheter skin junction and surrounding area for redness, tenderness, swelling, and drainage is done by visual inspection and palpation through the intact dressing, as well as through patient reports.[23] CVADs and midline catheters should be assessed daily, and short peripheral catheters should be checked at least every 4 hours.[23] Home care patients and those receiving outpatient therapy should be instructed to check the site at least once a day and report any signs or symptoms of complications.[23]

The catheter exit site should be cleansed with an appropriate antiseptic agent—chlorhexidine gluconate (CHG), 70% alcohol, or 10% povidone-iodine. Maki and colleagues[67] pioneered research in this area by comparing these agents, and they found 2% aqueous chlorhexidine to be significantly more effective than the other 2 agents in decreasing both local infection and catheter-related sepsis. Acetone has not been found to decrease infection risk and is no longer recommended as a component of the site care regimen.[68] In a 2005 review of evidence, Hibbard noted significantly improved immediate, persistent, and cumulative antimicrobial activity with products that combine 2% CHG and 70% isopropyl alcohol.[69] The CDC guidelines recommend that the skin should be prepped with a greater than 0.5% CHG preparation containing alcohol.[8] In the event that CHG is contraindicated, tincture of iodine, iodophor, or 70% alcohol can be used as an alternative.[5]

Whichever skin antisepsis agent is used, guidelines for appropriate dry times must be followed and skin must be allowed to dry completely before the dressing is applied.

Alcohol/chlorhexidine solutions must dry at least 30 seconds, and iodophors need at least 1.5 to 2 minutes to dry.[11] Risk of medical adhesive–related injury associated with engineered stabilization devices (ESDs) must be addressed; frequent monitoring of sites and use of skin barriers along with adhesive removers can assist in maintaining insertion sites. Refer to Table 16-2 for further information on the care and maintenance of each vascular access site.[11,46]

Routine use of antibiotic ointments at the catheter insertion site is not recommended because they may change normal bacterial flora and contribute to the emergence of resistant bacteria or fungi.[12] However, recent studies have reexamined the application of antibiotic and antiseptic ointments to the catheter site in high-risk patients, such as those who are critically ill or on hemodialysis.[5,70,71] In these studies, use of either povidone-iodine or mupirocin ointments was associated

TABLE 16-2 Central Venous Catheter Maintenance

	Site Care	Flushing[a]
Nontunneled CVC	• Perform skin antisepsis as a sterile procedure.[b] • Change dressing at established intervals,[c] when integrity of the dressing is compromised, and when moisture, blood, or drainage is present.[d]	• Internal volume is 0.1–0.53 mL. • Minimum flushing is equal to twice the internal volume of the VAD system plus 20%. • Flush before and after each use or daily if not in use.
Tunneled cuffed CVC: internal jugular; translumbar, transhepatic, and transcollateral	• Perform skin antisepsis as a sterile procedure.[b] • Change dressing at established intervals,[c] when integrity of the dressing is compromised, and when moisture, blood, or drainage is present.[d] • When subcutaneous tunnel is well healed, consideration may be given to no dressing.	• Internal volume is 0.15–1.8 mL. • Minimum flushing is equal to twice the internal volume of the VAD system plus 20%. • Flush before and after each use, or daily if not in use.
PICC	• Perform skin antisepsis as a sterile procedure.[b] • Change dressing at established intervals (changing TSM with ESD),[c] when integrity of the dressing is compromised, and when moisture, blood, or drainage is present.[d] • Avoid use of tape or sutures because they are not effective alternatives to ESD. • Do not use rolled bandages with or without elastic properties to secure as they do not adequately secure the device.	• Internal volume is 0.04–1.2 mL. • Minimum flushing is equal to twice the internal volume of the VAD system plus 20%. • Flush before and after each use, or daily if not in use.
Ports	• Perform skin antisepsis as a sterile procedure.[b] • Replace noncoring needle every 7 days when port is being used. • Maintain a sterile dressing over the site when the port remains accessed. • Change dressing at established intervals,[c] when integrity of the dressing is compromised, and when moisture, blood, or drainage is present.[d] • If gauze is used to support the wings of a noncoring needle in an implanted port and does not obscure the insertion site, it is not considered a gauze dressing.	• Internal volume is 0.5–1.5 mL. • Minimum flushing is equal to twice the internal volume of the VAD system plus 20%. • Flush before and after each use, or daily if port is not in use but remains accessed. • Flush every 4–6 weeks when not in use with 0.9% NaCl followed by 3–5 mL heparin 10–100 units/mL. • Flush Groshong port every 90 days when not in use with 10 mL 0.9% NaCl.

CHG, chlorhexidine gluconate; CLABSI, central line–associated bloodstream infection; CVAD, central venous access device; CVC, central venous catheter; ESD, engineered stabilization device; NaCl, sodium chloride; PICC, peripherally inserted central venous catheter; TSM, transparent semipermeable membrane; VAD, venous access device.

[a]Flushing CVADs with 10 mL 0.9% NaCl may remove fibrin deposits, drug precipitate, and other debris from the lumen; parenteral nutrition may require larger flush volumes. Split-valve needleless connectors and certain other needleless connectors do not require a heparin flush secondary to their design.

[b]Skin antisepsis guidelines: The preferred skin antiseptic agent is 0.5% chlorhexidine in alcohol solution. If chlorhexidine alcoholic solution is contraindicated, alternative antisepsis solutions include iodine, iodophor (povidone-iodine), and 70% alcohol. Allow skin antisepsis to fully dry prior to dressing placement: Chlorhexidine alcoholic solutions must dry for at least 30 seconds; iodophors need to dry for at least 1.5 to 2 minutes. Dressing should be changed at established intervals, when the integrity of the dressing is compromised, or if moisture, blood, or drainage is present.

[c]Change TSM every 5–7 days. Change gauze dressing every 2 days. Gauze dressing under a TSM is considered a gauze dressing and should be changed at least every 2 days.

[d]Use chlorhexidine-impregnated dressings over CVADs to reduce infection risk when the extraluminal route is the primary source of infection. Even when organizations show a low baseline CLABSI rate, the use of CHG dressings further reduces the CLABSI rate. The efficacy of CHG dressings in long-term (>14 days) CVAD use has not been shown when intraluminal sources of infection are the primary source of infection.

Source: Data are from references 10 and 46.

with a decrease in colonization (primarily in nasal carriers of *Staphylococcus aureus*) and lower rates of BSIs. Despite these findings, concern for the emergence of resistant organisms remains a prime consideration.[5]

Either sterile gauze or transparent dressings should be used to cover the catheter exit site. Studies comparing these 2 types of dressing have yielded no difference in catheter-site colonization rates.[5] Once the Dacron cuff has been incorporated into the subcutaneous tissue, some clinicians advocate cleansing the exit site with mild soap and water and using no dressing.

Hub Care

A hub is the end of the VAD that connects to the medication tubing or caps.[72] CRBSIs arising from the hub or the intraluminal source indicate a lapse in aseptic technique, which may occur during manipulation of the VAD hubs or needleless catheter connectors or with the addition of stopcocks. Mermel[73] reports that 31% of nurses in one study did not properly disinfect the needleless catheter connectors before accessing the catheter, and 17% of the discarded blood drawn through these needleless connectors had microbial growth, which increased the risk of CRBSI. The design of some needleless connectors can lead to suboptimal cleaning and thereby increase the risk for contamination. Protocols focusing on care of the catheter hub are as critical as those emphasizing care of the exit site.[73]

In most cases, a needleless connector is attached to the hub, which allows direct access to the catheter and obviates the use of needles. The primary purpose of needleless connectors is to protect healthcare personnel by eliminating the use of needles and subsequent needle sticks.[11] Originally, these devices consisted of a simple split-septum design with no internal mechanism, but connectors have become more sophisticated.[70] Connectors with a mechanical valve designed to control the flow within the system, as well as devices that affect fluid displacement within the device, have been developed. Needleless connectors are potential sites for intraluminal contamination if infection prevention practices are not implemented.[11] Microbial barriers that incorporate the use of either silver or CHG are a new feature of some needleless connectors. This technology was developed after studies found that the use of 70% alcohol to cleanse the connector did not reliably prevent entry of microorganisms into the catheter.[74] Under in vitro conditions, an innovative silver nanohub technology demonstrated a resistance to microbial contamination and biofilm formation involving selective microbial pathogens such as methicillin-resistant *Staphylococcus aureus* (MRSA), vancomycin-resistant enterococci (VRE), *Pseudomonas aeruginosa*, coagulase-negative staphylococci, and *Enterobacter cloacae*.[75,76]

Although disinfection of the hub is seen as an important step in preventing infection, there is a lack of consensus on the optimal agent. Available data suggest that vigorous scrubbing with an antiseptic such as CHG for 15 seconds may be preferable. The Infusion Nurses Society recommends that clinicians "Perform a vigorous mechanical scrub for manual disinfection of the needless connector prior to each VAD access and allow to air dry. Length of contact time for scrubbing and drying depends on the design of the needleless connector and the properties of the disinfecting agent."[18] Acceptable disinfecting

agents include 70% isopropyl alcohol, iodophors, or greater than 0.5% chlorohexidine in alcohol solution.[5] There is no demonstrated benefit to changing connectors more frequently than every 96 hours.[11]

Catheter Patency

VADs should be assessed for blood return prior to each infusion and flushed with normal saline after each infusion to clear all infused medication or solutions. These steps help ensure catheter patency by reducing the risk of incompatible medications causing precipitation, and decreasing the risk of intraluminal occlusion by the reflux of blood into or remaining in the catheter. Single-use flushing and locking solutions should be utilized. A VAD should never be forcibly flushed, and the use of a 10-mL syringe when flushing reduces the risk of catheter damage.

The role of routine anticoagulant flush solutions such as heparin to maintain catheter patency has been debated.[66] A 2010 study found that routine use of a heparin flush (10 units/mL) decreased thrombotic occlusions.[77] However, case studies raise the possibility that patients can develop heparin-induced thrombocytopenia with minimal heparin exposure when a heparin flush is used to maintain the patency of VADs.[78] Institutions have revised their use of heparin in response to these findings. Although institutions continue to use heparin, recommendations suggest using the smallest amount necessary to maintain patency. All flush solutions should be single-use products. The flushing volume of the solution should be twice the volume of the catheter and should not interfere with coagulation factors. Alternate anticoagulants such as ethylenediaminetetraacetate (EDTA) may be beneficial not only in maintaining patency but also providing anti-infective properties.[66] Split-valve needleless connectors and certain other needleless connectors do not require a heparin flush secondary to their design (see Table 16-2).

Vascular Access Locks

Locking a VAD is defined as the instillation of a limited amount of antimicrobial or antiseptic solution, with sufficient volume to fill the internal priming volume of the catheter, following routine catheter flush.[23] Locking solutions usually dwell for the period of time when the catheter is not in use, to prevent intraluminal clot formation and/or catheter colonization.[79] These solutions may be used for therapeutic and prophylactic purposes to prevent CRBSIs in patients who have a history of multiple infections despite other methods of CRBSI reduction as well other patients at high risk for CRBSI. The use of locking solutions may help decrease morbidity and mortality associated with CRBSI, shorten hospital length of stays, reduce rates of premature loss of CVADs and lower healthcare costs.[80] There is no clear evidence regarding the dwell time or concentration needed for locking solutions to be effective,[23] and some types of catheter materials are incompatible with the safe administration of antimicrobial locks.

Antibiotic lock therapy solutions contain higher concentrations of antibiotics, which are chosen based on the infecting organism.[23] The emergence of antimicrobial-resistant bacterial strains is a concern with the use of antibiotic lock therapy. Because biofilm that forms naturally can be difficult to penetrate with antibiotic lock therapy, even higher concentrations of ongoing antibiotics are needed.[80] Infusion Nurses Society guidelines recommend aspirating all antimicrobial locking solutions from the CVAD at the end of the locking period because flushing the lock solution into the patient's bloodstream could increase the development of antibiotic resistance.[11]

Although the use of antibiotic or antimicrobial locks can be an effective strategy for the treatment of CRBSIs and catheter salvage, the prophylactic use of antimicrobial locks to prevent CRBSI is controversial. The CDC guidelines recommend that the practice should be limited to patients with long-term catheters who have a history of multiple CRBSIs,[8] and a systematic review of clinical trials supported this recommendation.[81]

Antiseptic lock solutions include ethanol, taurolidine, citrate, 26% sodium chloride, and EDTA. Ethanol locking solutions exhibit bactericidal and fungicidal properties and have been shown to eradicate organisms in biofilm to prophylactically prevent and treat CRBSI.[80,82] In high-risk patients, use of ethanol locking solutions has reduced the risk for CRBSI. Hypothetically, prophylactic use of such solutions could be beneficial for all PN patients, although results from a 2017 study by Salonen and colleagues did not support this theory.[83] Ongoing studies continue to evaluate the safety and effectiveness of antiseptic lock and ethanol locking solutions. In a small study of home PN patients (59 participants), Davidson and associates found that antiseptic lock and ethanol locking solutions (used in 51 and 8 patients, respectively) reduced the overall rate of infections per 1000 catheter days.[80] These investigators support continued clinical trials on the use of such solutions to prevent or treat CRBSI in high-risk PN populations.[80]

Ethanol locking solution concentrations have been trialed as high as 98%, but no specific ethanol dilution has been determined to be most effective. Concentrations of ethanol locking solutions from 7% to 70% have been studied. In vitro studies demonstrated precipitates of plasma proteins in CVADs with ethanol concentrations greater than 28%.[11,82,84] Because ethanol locking solution was associated with CVAD lumen occlusion, the authors of these studies recommend that concentration of ethanol not exceed 28%.[11,82,84] The risks and benefits for the patient should be weighed before higher concentrations of ethanol locking solutions are used.[82] Heparin and ethanol lock therapy has been documented to cause precipitation leading to catheter occlusions and complications.[85] Observational studies have noted that some practices withdraw ethanol locking solution prior to use of the catheter, whereas other practices continue to flush the ethanol locking solution through with 0.9% sodium chloride and proceed with the daily therapy.[85] CVADs made of polyurethane material have ruptured and split when ethanol lock solutions were used for intraluminal locking. However, ethanol can be safely instilled into a silicone catheter.[23] Clinicians should follow catheter manufacturers' guidelines regarding the safe use of ethanol and locking solutions.

Taurolidine, a product that is not readily available in the United States, has been studied in Europe as an agent in the prevention of CRBSI, especially in the high-risk PN population. In a 10-year retrospective study with 22 home PN

patients, Saunders and colleagues found that CRBSI rates decreased from 5.71 infections per 1000 patient PN days before taurolidine to 0.99 infections per 1000 PN days after taurolidine; these preliminary data suggest the benefit of its use as primary prophylaxis.[86] Other studies continue to investigate this theory.[83,86]

Device Stabilization

The VAD must be anchored to prevent migration of the catheter and loss of access. Effective catheter stabilization helps prevent subtle movement of the catheter tip against the wall of the blood vessel, which can create irritation and promote thrombosis formation. Evidence suggests that the appropriate use of stabilization devices also reduces the incidence of CRBSI.[87] In recognition of these benefits, the Infusion Nurses Society and CDC guidelines recommend the use of manufactured securement devices to stabilize intravascular catheters whenever feasible.[5,11] Methods commonly used to stabilize catheters include steristrips and ESDs. A device or system designed and engineered to control the movement at the catheter hub should not interfere with the assessment and monitoring of access or impede vascular circulation or delivery of the prescribed therapy.[23] Sutures should be avoided as a permanent method to secure catheters because they increase the risk for catheter-site infections. Subcutaneous ESDs currently on the market meet the Infusion Nurses Society standards with favorable patient outcomes and patient inserter satisfaction.[23]

The use of adhesive-based ESDs is associated with a risk for medical adhesive–related skin injury. An alternative securement system consists of a securement device and a bordered transparent dressing. A gentle silicone adhesive is used to integrate the molded plastic device with a breathable base, allowing ease of removal and decreased risk of skin injury.[88]

Device-Related Complications

VADs have been associated with infectious and noninfectious complications. Infectious complications are the most common. Noninfectious or mechanical complications include catheter occlusion, thrombosis, and breakage. Catheter occlusion is the most common noninfectious complication observed with the long-term use of VADs.

Catheter-Related Infections

Definitions

The CDC has published standardized definitions for types of catheter-related infections. The use of consistent definitions will improve accuracy when comparing infection rates and treatments (Table 16-3).[89] Another important terminology distinction concerns the terms *catheter-related bloodstream infection* (CRBSI) and *central line–associated bloodstream infection* (CLABSI). CRBSI is a clinical term used for diagnosis and treatment of a BSI.[8] CLABSI is a surveillance term used by the CDC's National Healthcare Safety Network to determine a causal relationship between the catheter and BSI.[8] CLABSI is a laboratory-confirmed BSI in which the central line or

TABLE 16-3 Types of Catheter-Related Infections

Infection Type	CDC Definition
Exit site	Erythema or induration within 2 cm of the catheter exit site, in the absence of concomitant BSI and without concomitant purulence.
Tunnel	Tenderness, erythema, or site induration >2 cm from the catheter site along the subcutaneous tract of a tunneled (eg, Hickman or Broviac) catheter, in the absence of concomitant BSI.
Pocket	Purulent fluid in the subcutaneous pocket of a totally implanted intravascular catheter that might or might not be associated with spontaneous rupture and drainage or necrosis of the overlaying skin, in the absence of concomitant BSI.
Bloodstream	Bacteremia/fungemia in a patient with an intravascular catheter with at least 1 positive blood culture obtained from a peripheral vein, clinical manifestations of infections (ie, fever, chills, and/or hypotension), and no apparent source for the BSI except the catheter. One of the following should be present: a positive semiquantitative (>15 CFU/catheter segment) or quantitative (>10^3 CFU/catheter segment catheter) culture whereby the same organism (species and antibiogram) is isolated from the catheter segment and peripheral blood; simultaneous quantitative blood cultures with a ≥5:1 ratio CVC vs peripheral; differential period of CVC culture vs peripheral blood culture positivity of >2 hours.

BSI, bloodstream infection; CDC, Centers for Disease Control and Prevention; CFU, colony-forming unit; CVC, central vein catheter.

Source: Definitions are reprinted from reference 89: O'Grady NP, Alexander M, Dellinger EP, et al; Centers for Disease Control and Prevention. Guidelines for the prevention of intravascular catheter-related infections. Appendix A: examples of clinical definitions for catheter-related infections. *MMWR.* 2002;51(RR10);27–28. https://www.cdc.gov/mmwr/preview/mmwrhtml/rr5110a2.htm. Accessed August 18, 2017.

umbilical catheter was in place for more than 2 calendar days on the date of event, with day of device placement being Day 1, *and* the line was also in place on the date of event or the day before. If a central line or umbilical catheter were in place for more than 2 calendar days and then removed, the date of event of the laboratory-confirmed BSI must be the day of discontinuation or the next day to be a CLABSI. If the patient is admitted or transferred to a facility with an implanted central line (port) in place, and that is the patient's only central line, the day of first access (ie, line placement, insertion of needle into the port, infusion or withdrawal through the line) in an inpatient location is considered Day 1. Such lines continue to be eligible for a CLABSI once they are accessed until they are either discontinued (removed from body) or the day after patient discharge (as per the Transfer Rule). Simply "de-accessing" a port (eg, removal of port needle but port remains in body) does not result in the patient's removal from CLABSI surveillance or from including the central line in central line day counts.[90] Although these definitions are distinct, they can be confusing and are often used interchangeably.

Signs and Symptoms

Signs and symptoms of CRBSI include elevated white blood cell count (greater than 10,500/mcL), fever, chills, malaise, nausea, vomiting, hypotension, tachycardia, headache, and backache. Symptoms at the insertion site include tenderness, erythema, swelling, purulent exudate. Of note, fever may be masked by medications such as acetaminophen, ibuprofen, aspirin, and oral steroids.[91]

Microbial Etiology and Pathogenesis

CVC-related infections can originate from 1 of 4 recognized sources: endogenous skin flora at the insertion site,

contamination of the catheter hub by hands or devices, hematogenous seeding from a distant infection source, and contamination of infusate.[5] The 2 primary portals for the contamination of CVCs have been identified as the skin insertion site and the hub.[73] Hub contamination is the most frequent cause of intraluminal contamination in the long-term use of VADs.[92] However, migration of endogenous skin flora from the insertion site, which results in extraluminal colonization of the catheter, is a more prevalent source of infection in patients with short-term catheters. Hematogenous seeding is an elusive mechanism that requires documentation of a primary infection at a distant site. Infusate contamination is rarely associated with catheter infection.

Gram-positive, coagulase-negative staphylococci have emerged as a major nosocomial isolate and are the predominant pathogens associated with infections from biomedical devices.[5] The coagulase-negative staphylococci are frequently capable of producing a biofilm composed of an exopolysaccharide (glycocalyx) matrix. The exopolysaccharide allows the staphylococcal cells to cling tenaciously to the surface of a catheter or biomedical device (Figure 16-3).[93] Biofilms can form on CVAD surfaces as soon as 24 hours after device insertion.[94] The extracellular matrix stabilizes the biofilm and protects the embedded bacteria cells from antibiotics and host phagocytes.[95] Once a biofilm matures, it becomes increasingly resistant to antibiotic therapy and more difficult to eliminate.[94] In addition, selected strains of *Staphylococcus epidermidis* that produce a biofilm often express phenotypic resistance to traditional antimicrobial agents.[96] The presence of a biofilm associated with a catheter-related infection increases the difficulty of successfully treating the infection without removing the catheter.[97]

Bacterial cells from the biofilm can slough off and travel in the bloodstream, causing other infections such as sepsis and urinary tract infections.[95] Removal of the CVAD and initiation of systemic antibiotic therapy is the usual treatment.[94] Treating

FIGURE 16-3 The Role of Biofilm to Protect Bacteria on a Medical Device

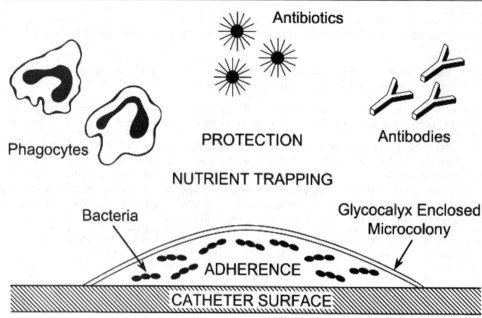

The exopolysaccharide (glycocalyx) substance elaborated by selected bacterial populations (staphylococci) facilitates microbial persistence and provides a protective environment on the catheter surface, preventing normal host defense mechanisms, such as opsonizing antibodies and phagocytic cells, from effectively dealing with the microbial pathogens. In addition, microbial populations enmeshed in the glycocalyx matrix are sequestered from the therapeutic activity of systemic antimicrobial agents.

Source: Reprinted with permission from the American Society for Parenteral and Enteral Nutrition from reference 93: Krzywda EA, Andris DA, Edmiston CE, Wallace JR. Parenteral access devices. In: Gottschlich M, ed. *The A.S.P.E.N. Nutrition Support Core Curriculum: A Case-Based Approach: The Adult Patient.* Silver Spring, MD: American Society for Parenteral and Enteral Nutrition; 2007:300–322.

a CRBSI becomes increasingly challenging when the microbes form a biofilm. However, a promising treatment for biofilms are antimicrobial catheter locks, which are discussed earlier in the chapter.

S. aureus was at one time the most frequently reported pathogen associated with CRBSI.[98] Adherence of *S. aureus* to a catheter surface is mediated by surface receptors that involve specific host protein interactions. The importance of this microorganism has been compounded by the emergence of MRSA, which accounts for more than 50% of all *S. aureus*.[99] This resistance has contributed to an increase in the use of vancomycin to treat nosocomial BSIs. Hand contamination is the primary means of nosocomial acquisition of BSIs. However, microbial aerosols produced during periods of rhinorrhea may also contribute to the distribution of these organisms, emphasizing the importance of maximal barrier precautions, including masks, while inserting central lines.

Enterococci account for 9% of nosocomial BSIs.[8] *Enterococcus faecalis* causes 90% of clinical enterococcal infections, whereas 5% to 10% are associated with *E. faecium*. The emergence of VRE is associated with several sentinel risk factors, including (1) previous antibiotic therapy involving third-generation cephalosporins and vancomycin use; (2) gastrointestinal colonization with VRE; (3) the severity of the underlying disease; (4) a prolonged hospital stay; and (5) the use of indwelling VADs. Enterococcal BSIs may arise from

the patient's own endogenous flora or through nosocomial transmission involving the hands of healthcare workers and exposure to contaminated surfaces.[100] The increasing use of IV prophylactic vancomycin, especially in the neutropenic or high-risk population, has contributed to the emergence of VRE in the vascular access population.[18]

In general, Candida (yeast) is associated with a 9% catheter-related sepsis rate.[98] The pathogenesis of these infections suggest that endogenous colonization is the principal mechanism of nosocomial acquisition.

Enterobacter spp., *Escherichia coli*, *Klebsiella pneumoniae*, and *Pseudomonas aeruginosa* are infrequent causes of CRBSI. However, in the past, clusters of catheter infections associated with specific isolates such as Enterobacter or Acinetobacter spp. may suggest the contamination of infusate solutions.[99] Infections involving Pseudomonas spp. and *Stenotrophomonas maltophilia* often require catheter removal with a positive tip culture, because contamination with these specific pathogens is associated with a high rate of treatment failures.

Within the long-term PN patient population, many of the common microbial pathogens are the same as those seen in acute care patients. Specifically, coagulase-negative staphylococci occur in approximately 60% of CVC infections followed by *Klebsiella pneumoniae*, *S. aureus*, and Enterococcus spp. Additionally, Candida species, including *C. parapsilosis*, *C. glabrata*, and *C. albicans*, are often recovered from long-term

CVCs used for PN.[100] Recurrent gram-negative infections of central lines have been observed in patients with short-bowel syndrome receiving PN.[101]

Central Line Bundles and Other Risk Reduction Strategies

CVCs pose the greatest risk for the development of a CRBSI,[102] and nosocomial BSIs associated with CVCs have an attributed mortality of 12% to 25%.[55] Prevention is the key to decreasing CRBSIs and is the main focus of the CDC's 2011 guidelines.[8] In 2003, Harbarth and associates[56] published a systematic review of the literature on potentially preventable nosocomial infections in healthcare and estimated that preventive measures could reduce the incidence of CRBSI in CVCs by about 56% (from 8.7 episodes to 3.8 episodes per 1000 catheter days).

The current focus on patient safety has brought the problem of CRBSIs under closer scrutiny by regulatory agencies and consumer groups. Several states have enacted laws mandating public disclosure of hospital-acquired infections, including central line infection rates. In response to this heightened awareness of the problem of CRBSIs, the Institute for Healthcare Improvement (IHI) has proposed a set of evidence-based practices as a "Central Line Bundle," which has been designed to reduce the incidence of infections associated with central lines.[4]

Based on CDC guidelines, the IHI Central Line Bundle has 5 components: (1) hand hygiene, (2) maximal barrier precautions, (3) CHG skin antisepsis, (4) optimal catheter site selection, and (5) daily review of line necessity, with the prompt removal of unnecessary lines.[4] Maximal barrier precautions (use of a cap, mask, sterile gown, sterile gloves, as well as a sterile full body drape) should be observed during the insertion of CVCs, PICCs, or guidewire exchange.[5] Recent published studies have documented that the use of a catheter line care bundle incorporating maximal barrier precautions and CHG skin antisepsis is effective in reducing the incidence of CRBSIs.[103–107] According to the bundle concept, these measures are considered as a single intervention rather than as a set of individual processes. Failure to complete any aspect of the bundle is regarded as noncompliance with the entire protocol. Prospective clinical trials in which central line bundles have been rigorously implemented have yielded impressive reductions in the incidence of CRBSIs. Some centers have virtually eliminated central line infections in intensive care units (ICUs) that employed the IHI bundle.[108,109]

Implementation of the Central Line Bundle has resulted in a significant reduction in the global rate of CRBSIs, and the adjunctive addition of selective evidence-based interventions has allowed many institutions to essentially eliminate line-associated infections within selective critical care patient populations.[110] These results underscore the importance of evidence-based practice and how strict adherence to standards of care can improve patient outcomes (Practice Scenario 16-1).[5,111,112]

Practice Scenario 16-1

Question: What is the appropriate treatment of catheter-related bloodstream infection (CRBSI) in a patient with a tunneled cuffed vascular access catheter?

Scenario: A 55-year-old woman on long-term home parenteral nutrition (PN) presents to the clinic with a fever and shaking chills that started 2 hours after beginning her PN infusion. The patient had been receiving home PN for 8 months after a complicated surgical history that had resulted in stenosis of the superior mesenteric and celiac arteries, bowel ischemia, small bowel resection, and short-bowel syndrome. A single-lumen, tunneled, cuffed silicone elastomer catheter is in place.

The patient's vital signs are as follows: temperature, 101.8°F; blood pressure, 130/80 mm Hg; pulse, 100 beats/min; respiratory rate, 18 breaths/min. Her skin is warm and dry, and the catheter site is clean, nontender, with no erythema. Laboratory testing is significant for a white blood cell count of 15,000/mcL (normal: 5,000 to 10,000/mcL) and an elevated blood glucose level of 160 mg/dL (normal: 70 to 120 mg/dL). CRBSI is suspected, and blood cultures are obtained both through the catheter and a peripheral venipuncture. Results show *Staphylococcus epidermidis* growth from the catheter specimen within 4 hours, and the same organism is identified in the peripheral sample in 10 hours.

Intervention: Treatment includes both systemic antibiotic therapy as well as a 70% ethanol catheter lock of 2 mL daily with a 6-hour dwell time. The patient is discharged home with treatment planned for 7 days, and home PN is continued.

Answer: The gold standard for the diagnosis of a CRBSI requires catheter removal; however, in patients that require long-term intravenous therapies, catheter salvage rather than removal is desirable. Blood cultures are obtained using a method of "differential time to positivity." Central venous catheter blood cultures that become positive more than 2 hours sooner than the peripheral culture are considered predictive for CRBSIs, with 85% sensitivity and 81% specificity. In this patient, blood cultures confirmed a CRBSI. Catheter salvage using both a 70% ethanol lock as well as systemic antibiotic therapy will often successfully treat a CRBSI.

Rationale: The decision to remove an infected CVC depends, in part, on the virulence of the microorganism.[111] Removal of the catheter is recommended for documented fungal infections and *S. aureus*. Ethanol 70% is an antiseptic that provides bactericidal activity against a broad range of organisms and is less likely to promote resistance.[112] A growing number of studies have documented the efficacy of locking catheters as both a treatment option as well as a method of prevention in patients with recurrent CRBSIs.[5]

In initial trials, antiseptic- or antibiotic-impregnated catheters were found to reduce the risk of microbial colonization and CRBSI for short-term access.[113,114] The CDC guidelines[8] recommend that clinicians "use a chlorhexidine/silver sulfadiazine or minocycline/rifampin-impregnated CVC in patients whose catheter is expected to remain in place >5 days if, after successful implementation of a comprehensive strategy to reduce rates of CLABSI, the CLABSI rate is not decreasing." This technology alters the polymeric catheter surface to achieve increased resistance to microbial colonization. Its use should be part of a comprehensive strategy to prevent infection, including education of those inserting and managing catheters, verifying the use of maximal barrier precautions, and using a greater than

0.5% chlorhexidine preparation with alcohol for skin antisepsis during CVAD insertion.[8] In a prospective randomized trial, significantly decreased rates for both catheter colonization and CRBSI were demonstrated with the use of a CHG and silver sulfadiazine coating on the external lumen of CVCs.[114] However, a more recent investigation comparing a chlorhexidine/silver sulfadiazine-impregnated double-lumen CVC to a standard CVC found no difference in the colonization rate between both devices in ICU patients.[115] An economic analysis employing a Markov decision model has suggested that the cost-effectiveness of using an antimicrobial-impregnated CVC within the ICU patient population is "highly uncertain."[116] Despite the CDC recommendation, infection control personnel are sometimes reluctant to universally adopt this technology as a risk-reducing strategy. However, clinical investigations suggest that the fear that the use of selective antimicrobial-impregnated catheters will promote antimicrobial resistance among hospital-acquired pathogens seems unfounded.[117,118] Limited reports in the literature address CHG hypersensitivities, especially with the use of CHG-impregnated CVC.[5] An Australian case report noted an anaphylactic event following insertion of a CHG-impregnated CVC.[119]

Several investigations have concluded that the use of 70% ethanol–impregnated caps can effectively reduce the incidence of CRBSIs by more than 40%, decrease the length of stay, and lower hospital costs.[120,121] Many institutions have recently incorporated ethanol caps for CVCs in their standard of care, and Sweet and associates demonstrated a significant reduction of CVC infections from 2.5% to 0.2% using this technology.[121]

An adjunctive intervention strategy that is supported by strong evidence-based data is the use of a CHG-impregnated sponge, which is affixed at the catheter exit site following line insertion. In a multicenter, randomized clinical study involving over 1600 ICU patients and more than 28,000 catheter days, the use of the CHG-impregnated sponges significantly reduced the rate of CRBSI from 1.1 per 1000 catheter days to 0.6 per 1000 catheter days ($P < 0.03$).[110] In the same study, the use of this technology reduced the risk of catheter-related infections by 60% among patients with a low background rate of CRBSIs.[110]

To reduce the risk of CRBSI, the CVAD should not be used for blood sampling when PN is administered.[11,18,122] The use of a designated single-lumen catheter to administer PN and other, lipid-based solutions may be appropriate. A pharmacist should be consulted about IV administration of medications to patients receiving PN; co-infusing medications with PN may lead to incompatibility and instability of the infusion, thus increasing risk of intraluminal contamination.[11,18,122,123]

Noninfectious Complications

Noninfectious complications of CVADs include air embolism, pulmonary embolism, catheter migration, cardiac tamponade, and nerve injury.[59,60] Air embolism is a rare but often fatal complication; its severity is related to the amount of air entering the bloodstream. Symptoms of air embolism include sudden chest pain, dyspnea, headache, and confusion. If air embolism is suspected, catheter lumens should be clamped and the patient immediately placed in Trendelenburg with a left lateral decubitus position.[124] To prevent air embolism, occlusion of catheter lumens should be maintained at all times when not in use.

Pulmonary embolism is a blood clot that usually breaks off from another thrombus in the body, travels to the lungs, and occludes a pulmonary blood vessel.[125] Risk factors for developing a pulmonary embolism include a diagnosis of cancer, immobility for long periods of time, recent surgery or trauma, deep vein thrombosis (DVT), and other thrombus elsewhere in the body.[125,126] Symptoms include sudden onset dyspnea, chest pain, back pain, decreased oxygen saturation, and tachycardia. Diagnosis of a pulmonary embolism is obtained with a CT scan or ventilation-perfusion (VQ) scan, and the most common treatment is anticoagulation therapy.[126]

Migration of the catheter can cause the tip to enter the heart chambers. Puncture of the pericardium can result in cardiac tamponade, as described earlier in this chapter.[61]

Phrenic nerve injury is a rare complication of tunneled CVAD insertions. It can occur initially or several months after insertion and can lead to paralysis of the diaphragm.[127] Symptoms include respiratory distress, decreased air flow in the lung on the affected side, decreased oxygen saturation, and elevated respiratory rate.[127] Findings on chest x-ray show a one-sided elevation of the diaphragm.[127] Delayed phrenic nerve injury is most likely caused by inflammation from the CVAD or a blood clot. Delayed nerve injury to the diaphragm is usually not reversible.[127]

Device Occlusion

Catheter occlusion is the most common noninfectious catheter-related complication and has historically occurred in up to 50% of CVCs.[128] Occlusion can be secondary to thrombotic or nonthrombotic causes. Catheter patency is defined by 2 criteria: the ability to infuse without resistance and the ability to aspirate blood without resistance. When either of these criteria is not met, the catheter is occluded (Table 16-4).

Thrombotic Occlusion

Thrombotic causes are the primary source of catheter dysfunction.[128] In the early 19th century, Virchow proposed a triad of key factors resulting in the development of vessel thrombosis: (1) vessel wall damage, (2) blood flow changes, and (3) a systemic alteration in coagulation.[104] Today, these factors continue to form a physiological explanation for catheter-related thrombosis. Vessel wall injury occurs with catheter placement. Venous thrombi are composed of fibrin, and trauma induced by the catheter tip against the vessel wall binds platelets and blood cells. In response to this injury, coagulation factors are activated. Fibrin becomes cross-linked and erythrocytes interweave with platelets and leukocytes. In addition, blood flow dynamics are altered by the presence of a catheter in a vessel. Evidence suggests that as catheter size increases venous blood flow decreases.[35] The MAGIC expert panel has recommended that a 1:3 catheter-to-vein ratio be used to reduce the risk for catheter-related DVT.[21] Malignancy and certain other diseases can produce procoagulants that alter the physiological equilibrium and predispose the patient to thrombotic phenomena.

TABLE 16-4 Types of Catheter Occlusions

Etiology	Signs	Treatment
Intraluminal occlusion	Resistance to infusion/aspiration	• Blood clotting: use thrombolytic in volume to fill catheter lumen. • Drug/lipid precipitate: use appropriate pharmacologic agent: (0.1 N hydrochloric acid, sodium bicarbonate, ethyl alcohol).
Fibrin sheath—distal catheter tip	Inability to aspirate blood sample	• Thrombolytic agents given as catheter infusion or via overfill method. • Endovascular catheter stripping.
Vessel or pericatheter thrombosis	Resistance to infusion and aspiration	• Thrombolytic agents given as systemic infusion and/or catheter directed. • Endovascular stenting.
Mechanical occlusion	Resistance to infusion and aspiration	• Rectify closed clamp, tight suture, or catheter malposition. • Pinch-off syndrome: remove catheter.

The initiation of a thrombotic process on a catheter surface occurs minutes after vascular catheter insertion. In a landmark study, Horshal and colleagues[129] described the presence of fibrin sheaths surrounding subclavian CVCs. Upon autopsy inspection, all catheters were noted to have circumferential fibrin sheaths. The origin of these collections seemed to occur at 2 points. The most common point was where the catheter entered the vessel. The second point identified was at the intima adjacent to the distal catheter tip.

Risk factors for thrombus formation include catheter tip position, catheter material, type of infusate, and length of catheter duration. A prospective study of 444 patients with indwelling CVCs identified 3 significant baseline factors associated with the incidence of catheter-related thrombosis: multiple insertion attempts, ovarian cancer, and previous CVC insertion.[130] The incidence of symptomatic catheter-related thrombosis varies from 0.3% to 28.3%; when assessed by venography, catheter-related thrombosis is reported to range from 27% to 66%.[131] Rates of thrombotic complications associated with PICCs range from 1% to 4% (based on symptoms alone) to 23% (based on radiographic findings).[132,133]

Catheter-related thrombosis can be differentiated according to the location and extent of the thrombus.[3] Distinct thrombotic occlusions include an intraluminal clot, a fibrin sheath formation, a mural thrombus, or thrombosis of the vessel.

Intraluminal clotting related to inadequate flushing or blood reflux can result in sluggish catheter function as well as catheter occlusion. When a saline flush following blood aspiration and the administration of blood products is inadequate, intraluminal clotting may occur. The volume of flush solution is recommended to be at least twice the volume of the catheter (eg, 5 to 10 mL normal saline).[66] Fibrin sheaths can encase the catheter and distal catheter tip. *Venous thrombosis* refers to a thrombus in the vessel that may partially or totally occlude the vessel. This mural thrombus may initially present as a venous obstruction.

The primary finding that suggests a catheter-related thrombosis is loss of catheter patency. Fibrin sheath formation at the distal catheter tips often presents as an occlusion when attempting to withdraw blood or solution from the catheter lumen with a syringe. Catheters remain fully functional for infusion; however, blood cannot be aspirated from the lumen. Physiologically, the fibrin sheath acts as a one-way valve. As negative pressure is applied, the sheath is pulled over the open catheter tip and prevents blood aspiration. Catheter phlebography has demonstrated the presence of presumed fibrin collections encasing the distal catheter tips. In some cases, the sheath may extend to the venous entry site and result in extravasation of infusate into the surrounding tissues.

Catheter-related venous thrombosis may present as a catheter occlusion, with clinical symptoms of vascular obstruction, such as neck vein distension, edema, tingling or pain over the ipsilateral arm and neck, a tight feeling in the throat, and a prominent venous pattern over the anterior chest.[134] SVC thrombosis can result in a permanent vascular obstruction, chronic venous insufficiency, and loss of future access.[130]

Treatment depends on the extent of the thrombus, the severity of symptoms, the need to reestablish access, and available alternatives. Treatment is most successful when the cause of the catheter occlusion is correctly identified. The effectiveness and safety of the use of thrombolytics in the treatment of intraluminal clot and fibrin sheath formation has been documented.[3,135] Historically, streptokinase and urokinase have been used as thrombolytics. These agents lyse thrombus by activating and converting plasminogen to plasmin, which degrades fibrin clots. Alteplase, a tissue plasminogen activator, is an approved thrombolytic agent for CVAD occlusions.[23] Alteplase 2 mg in a 2-mL volume is injected into the catheter and allowed to dwell for 30 minutes to 4 hours, then aspiration of solution with a syringe is attempted. If patency is not reestablished, the dose may be repeated.

In patients with catheter-associated mural or venous thrombosis, catheter removal is not recommended as the first treatment.[134] In a pilot study,[134] the use of standard dalteparin/warfarin in patients with upper extremity DVT secondary to a CVC maintained access without the risk of recurrence or extension of the DVT. Catheter-directed thrombolysis has typically been used in patients with a recent onset of symptoms, extensive edema, and an impairment of function.

Early evidence suggested low-dose anticoagulation therapy might have a prophylactic benefit in patients at risk for catheter-related thrombosis. However, this practice is no longer supported; an analysis of randomized studies found no significant effect for either vitamin K antagonists or heparin on symptomatic DVT.[136] Catheter tip placement has been identified as a prognostic factor for thrombosis. Catheter tips that are positioned during placement in the lower vena cava have a decreased rate of thrombosis than those with tips more proximal in the vena cava.[133]

Thrombosis has been linked to an increased risk of infection.[137] Fibrin sheaths, rich in fibrin and fibronectin, promote bacterial adherence. In a study of 72 postmortem examinations, catheter-related septicemia was demonstrated only in patients with underlying mural thrombosis.[137] In a prospective study, van Rooden and colleagues evaluated 105 patients for catheter-related infections and thrombosis.[138] In patients with 2 or more positive cultures, 71.4% developed thrombosis; the incidence of thrombosis was 3.3% in patients with a negative or single positive culture. These results highlight the potential benefit of using thrombolytics in the treatment and prevention of CRBSIs.

Nonthrombotic Occlusion

The leading causes of intraluminal occlusions are drug-heparin interactions, PN formulations with inappropriate calcium-to-phosphate ratios, and lipid residue.[3] Lipid occlusions may slowly accumulate within the catheter lumen, resulting in sluggish catheter flow before a complete occlusion. The compounding of total nutrient admixtures requires close attention to prevent the precipitation of components. The use of a 0.9% normal saline flush between all IV medications, infusions, and heparin is the key to prevention. Various factors can lead to a nonthrombotic or mechanical catheter occlusion, including external clamps, kinking of the catheter, occluded port needles, and constricting sutures (see Practice Scenario 16-2).[133,139,140]

Practice Scenario 16-2

Question: How do you successfully establish catheter patency in an occluded central catheter?

Scenario: A 70-year-old man with a pseudo-obstruction has a single-lumen tunneled catheter for administration of parenteral nutrition (PN). After his hospital discharge, he was transferred to an intermediate skilled nursing facility. Within the first week at this facility, the nurse began the nightly PN infusion; 3 hours after PN infusion, the pump alarms signaled occlusion. The clinician assessed the situation and reported the following findings: (1) no extrinsic compression from clamps, sutures, or kinked catheter

tubing was noted; (2) postural changes, such as raising the ipsilateral arm and shrugging the shoulders forward, relieved the occlusion; (3) recent infusion history included only PN with no recent blood draws or medications; and (4) there were no physical signs of edema, redness, pain, or dilated vessels.

Intervention: In view of the assessment of an occlusion that resolves with postural changes, catheter pinch-off syndrome is suspected. The physician is contacted and arrangements are made for a chest x-ray and possible catheter replacement.

Answer: Catheter pinch-off syndrome is an often-unrecognized cause of catheter occlusion. A pinch-off presents as an intermittent mechanical obstruction related to postural changes caused by catheter compression between the clavicle and the first rib.[133] In some patients, a narrow anatomical triangle exists at the junction of the axillary vein and the subclavian vein. This junction is in the lateral aspect of the clavicle, and pinch-off may occur with medial placement of a percutaneous central venous catheter (CVC) in this area. Changing the patient's position by raising the ipsilateral arm, which opens this angle, relieves the occlusion. In a prospective study of 1457 CVC placements, pinch-off syndrome was identified in 1.1% of the catheters.[139] Chest x-rays will demonstrate a luminal narrowing of the catheter.

Rationale: Pinch-off syndrome can lead to catheter transection and embolus; therefore, removal is recommended.[140]

Infusion Delivery Devices

Infusion delivery devices, or pumps, are an integral component of PN therapy. These devices add a level of safety by ensuring accuracy of rate and volume delivery of IV infusions, as well as issuing alerts about problems such as air in the line or occlusion. Significant advances in device design have led to the availability of a variety of infusion pumps on the market. Ease of operation, mobility, and acquisition cost have been major incentives for technological advances. This new technology has allowed ambulatory electronic infusion devices to be widely used in home settings. Patients can manage these devices easily, allowing them to have more independence, as well as increased acceptance of IV treatments. The US Food and Drug Administration provides information about these devices, including safety issues, in the Medical Devices section of its website.[141]

References

1. Broviac JW, Cole JJ, Scribner BH. A silicone rubber atrial catheter for prolonged parenteral alimentation. *Surg Gynecol Obstet.* 1973;136(4):602–606.
2. Sansivero GE. Features and selection of vascular access devices. *Semin Oncol Nurs.* 2010;26(2):88–101.
3. Baskin JL, Pui CH, Reiss U, et al. Management of occlusion and thrombosis associated with long-term indwelling central venous catheters. *Lancet.* 2009;374(9684):159–169.
4. Institute for Healthcare Improvement. *How-to Guide: Prevent Central Line-Associated Bloodstream Infections.* Cambridge, MA: Institute for Healthcare Improvement; 2012.

5. O'Grady NP, Alexander M, Burns LA, et al. Guidelines for the prevention of intravascular catheter-related infections. *Am J Infect Control.* 2011;39(4 Suppl 1):S1–S34.

6. Harpel J. Best practices for vascular access resource teams. *J Infus Nurs.* 2013;36(1):46–50. doi:10.1097/NAN.0b013e3182798862.

7. Johnson D, Snyder T, Strader D, Zamora A. Positive influence of a dedicated vascular access team in an acute care hospital. *J Assoc Vasc Access.* 2017;22(1):35–37.

8. Centers for Disease Control and Prevention. Guidelines for the Prevention of Intravascular Catheter-Related Infections, 2011. https://www.cdc.gov/hai/pdfs/bsi-guidelines-2011.pdf. Accessed July 17, 2017.

9. Sansivero GE. Venous anatomy and physiology. Considerations for vascular access device placement and function. *J Intraven Nurs.* 1998;21(5 Suppl):S107–S114.

10. Bennett JD, Papadouris D, Rankin RN, et al. Percutaneous inferior vena caval approach for long-term central venous access. *J Vasc Interv Radiol.* 1997;8(5):851–855.

11. Gorski L, Hadaway L, Hagle M. Infusion therapy standards of practice. *J Infus Nurs.* 2016;39(1 Suppl):S1–S156.

12. Crnich CJ, Maki DG. The promise of novel technology for the prevention of intravascular device-related bloodstream infection. II. Long-term devices. *Clin Infect Dis.* 2002;34(10):1362–1368.

13. Kim SW, Petersen RV, Lee ES. Effect of phthalate plasticizer on blood compatibility of polyvinyl chloride. *J Pharm Sci.* 1976; 65(5):670–673.

14. Zdrahala RJ, Zdrahala IJ. Biomedical applications of polyurethanes: a review of past promises, present realities, and a vibrant future. *J Biomater Appl.* 1999;14(1):67–90.

15. Brown JM. Polyurethane and silicone: myths and misconceptions. *J Intraven Nurs.* 1995;18(3):120–122.

16. Larsson N, Stenberg K, Linder LE, Curelaru I. Cannula thrombophlebitis: a study in volunteers comparing polytetrafluoroethylene, polyurethane, and polyamide-ether-elastomer cannulae. *Acta Anaesthesiol Scand.* 1989;33(3):223–231.

17. Centers for Disease Control and Prevention. Adverse reactions associated with midline catheters—United States, 1992–1995. *JAMA.* 1996;275(10):749–750.

18. Ayers P, Adams S, Boullata J, et al. A.S.P.E.N. parenteral safety consensus recommendations. *JPEN J Parenter Enteral Nutr.* 2014; 38(3):296–333. doi:10,1177/0148607113511992.

19. Cook LS. Continuing controversy of midclavicular catheters. *J Infus Nurs.* 2007;30(5):267–273.

20. Yaacob Y, Zakaria R, Mohammad Z, Ralib ARM, Muda AS. The vanishing veins: difficult venous access in a patient requiring translumbar, transhepatic, and transcollateral central catheter insertion. *Malays J Med Sci.* 2011;18(4):98–102.

21. Chopra V, Flanders S, Saint S, et al. The Michigan Appropriateness Guide for Intravenous Catheters (MAGIC): results from a multispecialty panel using the RAND/UCLA appropriateness method. *Ann Intern Med.* 2015;163(6 Suppl):S1–S40. doi:10.7326/M15-0744.

22. Richardson D. Vascular access nursing: standards of care and strategies in the prevention of infection. A primer on central venous catheters (part 2 of a 3-part series). J Assoc Vasc Access. 2007;12(1):19–27.

23. Gorski L, Hadaway L, Hagle M, et al. *Policies and Procedures for Infusion Therapy.* 5th ed. Norwood, MA: Infusion Nurses Society; 2016.

24. Marsh N, Webster J, Mihala G, Rickard CM. Devices and dressings to secure peripheral venous catheters to prevent complications. *Cochrane Database System Rev.* 2015;(6):CD011070. doi:10.1002/14651858.CD011070.pub2.

25. Gura KM. Is there still a role for peripheral parenteral nutrition? *Nutr Clin Pract.* 2009;24(6):709–717.

26. Zingg W, Pittet D. Peripheral venous catheters: an under-evaluated problem. *Int J Antimicrob Agents.* 2009;34(Suppl 4): S38–S42.

27. Uslusoy E, Mete S. Predisposing factors to phlebitis in patients with peripheral intravenous catheters: a descriptive study. *J Am Acad Nurse Pract.* 2008;20(4):172–180.

28. Adams D, Little A, Vinsant C, Khandelwal S. The midline catheter: a clinical review. *J Emergency Med.* 2016;51(3):252–258.

29. Moureau N, Chopra V. Indications for peripheral, midline and central catheters: summary of the MAGIC recommendations. *Br J Nurs.* 2016;25(8 Suppl):S15–S24. doi:10.12968/bjon.2016.25.8S15.

30. Cobb DK, High KP, Sawyer RG, et al. A controlled trial of scheduled replacement of central venous and pulmonary-artery catheters. *N Engl J Med.* 1992;327(15):1062–1068.

31. Marschall J, Mermel LA, Fakih M, et al. Strategies to prevent central line-associated bloodstream infections in acute care hospitals. *Infect Control Hosp Epidemiol.* 2014;35:753–77118.

32. Gordon AC, Salkien JC, Johns D, Owen R, Gray RR. US-guided puncture of the internal jugular vein: complications and anatomic considerations *J Vasc Interv Radiol.* 1998;9(2):333–338.

33. Hoggard J, Saad T, Schon D, et al. Guidelines for venous access in patients with chronic kidney disease. A position statement from the American Society of Diagnostic and Interventional Nephrology, Clinical Practice Committee and the Association for Vascular Access. *Semin Dial.* 2008;21(2):186–191.

34. Kombau C, Lee KC, Hughes GD, Firstenberg MS. Central line complications. *Int J Crit Illn Inj Sci.* 2015;5:170–178.

35. Nifong T, McDevitt T. The effect of catheter to vein ratio on blood flow rates in a simulated model of peripherally inserted central venous catheters. *Chest.* 2011;140(1):48–53. doi:10.1378/chest.10-2637.

36. Chopra V, Anand S, Hickner A, et al. Risk of venous thromboembolism associated with peripherally inserted central catheters: a systemic review and meta-analysis. *Lancet.* 2013;382(9889): 311–325.

37. Chopra V, Ohoro J, Rogers M, et al. The risk of bloodstream infection associated with peripherally inserted central catheters compared with central venous catheters in adults : a systemic review and meta-analysis. *Infect Control Hosp Epidemiol.* 2013;34(9):908–918.

38. Winkler MF, DiMaria-Ghalili RA, Guenter P, et al. Characteristics of a cohort of home parenteral nutrition patients at the time of enrollment in the sustain registry. *JPEN J Parenter Enteral Nutr.* 2016;40(8):1140–1149.

39. Opilla M. Peripherally inserted central catheter experience in long term home parenteral nutrition patients. *J Assoc Vasc Access.* 2017;22(1):42–45.

40. de Cicco M, Panarello G, Chiaradia V, et al. Source and route of microbial colonisation of parenteral nutrition catheters. *Lancet.* 1989;2(8674):1258–1261.

41. Keohane PP, Jones BJ, Attrill H, et al. Effect of catheter tunnelling and a nutrition nurse on catheter sepsis during parenteral nutrition. A controlled trial. *Lancet.* 1983;2(8364):1388–1390.

42. Darouiche RO, Berger DH, Khardori N, et al. Comparison of antimicrobial impregnation with tunneling of long-term central venous catheters: a randomized controlled trial. *Ann Surg.* 2005;242(2):193–200.

43. Raad I, Davis S, Becker M, et al. Low infection rate and long durability of nontunneled silastic catheters. A safe and cost-effective alternative for long-term venous access. *Arch Intern Med.* 1993; 153(15):1791–1796.

44. Borroughs SG, Farmer DG. Intestinal transplantation. In: DiBaise JK, Rees Parrish C, Thompson JS, eds. *Short Bowel Syndrome: Practical Approach to Management.* Boca Raton, FL: CRC Press; 2016: 301–320.

45. Gullo SM. Implanted ports. Technologic advances and nursing care issues. *Nurs Clin North Am.* 1993;28(4):859–871.

46. Bard Access Systems. Resources: implantable port devices product literature. http://www.bardaccess.com/resources/literature/ports. Accessed August 17, 2017.

47. Bouza E, Guembe M, Munoz P. Selection of the vascular catheter: can it minimise the risk of infection? *Int J Antimicrob Agents.* 2010;36(Suppl 2):S22–S25.

48. Groeger JS, Lucas AB, Thaler HT, et al. Infectious morbidity associated with long-term use of venous access devices in patients with cancer. *Ann Intern Med.* 1993;119(12):1168–1174.

49. Mansfield PF, Hohn DC, Fornage BD, Gregurich MA, Ota DM. Complications and failures of subclavian-vein catheterization. *N Engl J Med.* 1994;331(26):1735–1738.

50. Nagelhout J, Elisha S, Waters E. Should I continue or discontinue that medication? *AANA J.* 2009;77(1):59–73.

51. National Kidney Foundation Kidney Disease Quality Outcomes Initiative. Clinical Practice Guidelines and Clinical Practice Recommendations 2006 Updates: Vascular Access. https://www2.kidney.org/professionals/KDOQI/guideline_upHD_PD_VA/va_guide1.htm. Accessed August 19, 2017.

52. Kirby D, Corrigan M, Speerhas R, Emery D. Home parenteral nutrition tutorial. *JPEN J Parenter Enteral Nutr.* 2012;36(6):632–644.

53. Mermel LA, McCormick RD, Springman SR, Maki DG. The pathogenesis and epidemiology of catheter-related infection with pulmonary artery Swan-Ganz catheters: a prospective study utilizing molecular subtyping. *Am J Med.* 1991;91(3B):197S–205S.

54. Raad II, Hohn DC, Gilbreath BJ, et al. Prevention of central venous catheter-related infections by using maximal sterile barrier precautions during insertion. *Infect Control Hosp Epidemiol.* 1994;15(4):231–238.

55. Safdar N, Fine JP, Maki DG. Meta-analysis: methods for diagnosing intravascular device-related bloodstream infection. *Ann Intern Med.* 2005;142(6):451–466.

56. Harbarth S, Sax H, Gastmeier P. The preventable proportion of nosocomial infections: an overview of published reports. *J Hosp Infect.* 2003;54(4):258–266.

57. O'Grady NP, Alexander M, Dellinger EP, et al. Guidelines for the prevention of intravascular catheter-related infections. *Am J Infect Control.* 2002;30(8):476–489.

58. Thompson EC, Calver LE. Safe subclavian vein cannulation. *Am Surg.* 2005;71(2):180–183.

59. McGee DC, Gould MK. Preventing complications of central venous catheterization. The *N Engl J Med.* 2003;348(12):1123–1133.

60. Azevedo AC, deLima IF, Brito V, Centeno MJ, Fernandes A. Cardiac tamponade: a rare complication of central venous catheter—a clinical report. *Brazil J Anesthesiol.* 2016(Sep 18). Epub ahead of press. doi:10.1016/j.bjane.2015.04.005.

61. Collier PE, Goodman GB. Cardiac tamponade caused by central venous catheter perforation of the heart: a preventable complication. J Am Coll Surg. 1995;181(5):459–463.

62. Brown JR, Slomski C, Saxe AW. Is routine postoperative chest x-ray necessary after fluoroscopic-guided subclavian central venous port placement? *J Am Coll Surg.* 2009;208(4):517–519.

63. Cavanna L, Civardi G, Vallisa D, et al. Ultrasound-guided central venous catheterization in cancer patients improves the success rate of cannulation and reduces mechanical complications: a prospective observational study of 1,978 consecutive catheterizations. *World J Surg Oncol.* 2010;8:91.

64. Mifflin N, Vanno S, Evan A, Stewart A, Catt J. Paradoxical electrocardiographic rhythm during peripherally inserted central catheter insertion from persistent left superior vena cava. *J Assoc Vasc Access.* 2017;22(1):15–18.

65. Krzywda EA, Andris DA. Twenty-five years of advances in vascular access: bridging research to clinical practice. *Nutr Clin Pract.* 2005;20(6):597–606.

66. Ryder M. Evidence-based practice in the management of vascular access devices for home parenteral nutrition therapy. *JPEN J Parenter Enteral Nutr.* 2006;30(1 Suppl):S82–S93.

67. Maki DG, Ringer M, Alvarado CJ. Prospective randomised trial of povidone-iodine, alcohol, and chlorhexidine for prevention of infection associated with central venous and arterial catheters. *Lancet.* 1991;338(8763):339–343.

68. Maki DG, McCormack KN. Defatting catheter insertion sites in total parenteral nutrition is of no value as an infection control measure. Controlled clinical trial. *Am J Med.* 1987;83(5):833–840.

69. Hibbard JS. Analyses comparing the antimicrobial activity and safety of current antiseptic agents: a review. *J Infus Nurs.* 2005;28(3):194–207.

70. Fukunaga A, Naritaka H, Fukaya R, Tabuse M, Nakamura T. Povidone-iodine ointment and gauze dressings associated with reduced catheter-related infection in seriously ill neurosurgical patients. *Infect Control Hosp Epidemiol.* 2004;25(8):696–698.

71. Johnson DW, MacGinley R, Kay TD, et al. A randomized controlled trial of topical exit site mupirocin application in patients with tunnelled, cuffed haemodialysis catheters. *Nephrol Dial Transplant.* 2002;17(10):1802–1807.

72. Centers for Disease Control and Prevention. Central venous catheter hub cleaning prior to accessing. Centers for Disease Control and Prevention (CDC) Dialysis Bloodstream Infection (BSI) Prevention Collaborative protocol. https://www.cdc.gov/dialysis/pdfs/collaborative/protocol-hub-cleaning-final-3-12.pdf. Accessed August 17, 2017.

73. Mermel LA. What is the predominant source of intravascular catheter infections? *Clin Infect Dis.* 2011;52(2):211–212.

74. Menyhay SZ, Maki DG. Disinfection of needleless catheter connectors and access ports with alcohol may not prevent microbial entry: the promise of a novel antiseptic-barrier cap. *Infect Control Hosp Epidemiol.* 2006;27(1):23–27.

75. Maki DG. In vitro studies of a novel antimicrobial luer-activated needleless connector for prevention of catheter-related bloodstream infection. *Clin Infect Dis.* 2010;50(12):1580–1587.

76. Edmiston CE, Markina V. Reducing the risk of infection in vascular access patients: an in vitro evaluation of an antimicrobial silver nanotechnology luer activated device. *Am J Infect Control.* 2010;38(6):421–423.

77. Jonker MA, Osterby KR, Vermeulen LC, Kleppin SM, Kudsk KA. Does low-dose heparin maintain central venous access device patency? A comparison of heparin versus saline during a period of heparin shortage. *JPEN J Parenter Enteral Nutr.* 2010;34(4):444–449.

78. Sancar E, May S. Heparin-induced thrombocytopenia. Medscape: 2015. http://emedicine.medscape.com/article/1357846-overview#a5. Accessed September 23, 2016.

79. Goossens GA. Flushing and locking of venous catheters: available evidence and evidence deficit. *Nurs Res Pract.* 2015;2015:985686. doi:10.1155/2015/985686.

80. Davidson JB, Edakkanambeth Varayil J, Okano A, et al. Prevention of subsequent catheter-related bloodstream infection using catheter locks in high-risk patients receiving home parenteral nutrition. *JPEN J Parenter Enteral Nutr.* 2017;41(4):685–690. doi:10.1177/0148607115604118.

81. Snaterse M, Ruger W, Scholte OP, Reimer WJ, Lucas C. Antibiotic-based catheter lock solutions for prevention of catheter-related bloodstream infection: a systematic review of randomised controlled trials. *J Hosp Infect.* 2010;75(1):1–11.

82. Schilcher G, Schlagenhauf A, Schneditz D, et al. Ethanol causes protein precipitation—new safety issues for catheter locking

techniques. *PLOS One*. 2013;8(12):e84869. doi:10.1371/journal.pone.0084869.

83. Salonen B, Bonnes S, Vallumseta N, et al. A prospective double blind randomized controlled study on the use of ethanol locks in HPN patients. *Clin Nutr*. 2017(May 17). Epub ahead of print. doi:10.1016/j.clnu.2017.05.009.

84. Mermel L, Alang N. Adverse effects associated with ethanol catheter lock solutions a systematic review. *J Antimicrob Chemother*. 2014;(69):2611–2619. doi:10.1093/jac/dku182.

85. Mezoff E, Fei L, Troutt M, et al. Ethanol lock efficacy and associated complications in children with intestinal failure. *JPEN J Parent Enteral Nutr*. 2016;40(6):815–819. doi:10.1177/0148607115574745.

86. Saunders J, Naghibi M, Leach Z, et al. Taurolidine locks significantly reduce the incidence of catheter-related blood stream infections in high-risk patients on home parenteral nutrition. *Eur J Clin Nutr*. 2014;69(2):282–284. doi:10.1038/ejcn.2014.32.

87. Yamamoto AJ, Solomon JA, Soulen MC, et al. Sutureless securement device reduces complications of peripherally inserted central venous catheters. *J Vasc Interv Radiol*. 2002;13(1):77–81.

88. Krenik KM, Smith GE, Bernatchez SF. Catheter securement systems for peripherally inserted and nontunneled central vascular access devices: clinical evaluation of a novel sutureless device. *J Infus Nurs*. 2016;39(4):210–217. doi:10.1097/NAN.0000000000000174.

89. O'Grady NP, Alexander M, Dellinger EP, et al; Centers for Disease Control and Prevention. Guidelines for the Prevention of Intravascular Catheter-Related Infections. Appendix A: Examples of Clinical Definitions for Catheter-Related Infections. *MMWR*. 2002;51(RR10);27–28. https://www.cdc.gov/mmwr/preview/mmwrhtml/rr5110a2.htm. Accessed August 18, 2017.

90. Centers for Disease Control and Prevention. Device associated module: bloodstream infection event (central line-associated bloodstream infection and non-central line-associated bloodstream infection). January 2017. https://www.cdc.gov/nhsn/pdfs/pscmanual/4psc_clabscurrent.pdf. Accessed July 17, 2017.

91. Gorski L, Hadaway L, Hagle M, et al. Infusion-related complications: identification and intervention. In: *Policies and Procedures for Infusion Therapy*. 5th ed. Norwood, MA: Infusion Nurses Society; 2016:170–173.

92. Gaynes R, Edwards JR. Overview of nosocomial infections caused by gram-negative bacilli. *Clin Infect Dis*. 2005;41(6):848–854.

93. Krzywda EA, Andris DA, Edmiston CE, Wallace JR. Parenteral access devices. In: Gottschlich M, ed. *The A.S.P.E.N. Nutrition Support Core Curriculum: A Case-Based Approach: The Adult Patient*. Silver Spring, MD: American Society for Parenteral and Enteral Nutrition; 2007: 300–322.

94. Gominet M, Compain F, Beloin C, Lebeaux D. Central venous catheters and biofilms: where do we stand in 2017? *APMIS*. 2017;125(4):365–375. doi:10.1111/apm.12665.

95. Donlan R. Biofilms: microbial life on surfaces. *Emerg Infect Dis*. 2002;8(9):881–890.

96. Mehall JR, Saltzman DA, Jackson RJ, Smith SD. Fibrin sheath enhances central venous catheter infection. *Crit Care Med*. 2002;30(4):908–912.

97. Costerton W, Veeh R, Shirtliff M, et al. The application of biofilm science to the study and control of chronic bacterial infections. *J Clin Invest*. 2003;112(10):1466–1477.

98. Schaberg DR, Culver DH, Gaynes RP. Major trends in the microbial etiology of nosocomial infection. *Am J Med*. 1991;91(3B):72S–75S.

99. Klevens RM, Edwards JR, Tenover FC, et al. Changes in the epidemiology of methicillin-resistant *Staphylococcus aureus* in intensive care units in US hospitals, 1992-2003. *Clin Infect Dis*. 2006;42(3):389–391.

100. Boyce JM, Opal SM, Chow JW, et al. Outbreak of multidrug-resistant *Enterococcus faecium* with transferable vanB class vancomycin resistance. *J Clin Microbiol*. 1994;32(5):1148–1153.

101. Ena J, Dick RW, Jones RN, Wenzel RP. The epidemiology of intravenous vancomycin usage in a university hospital. A 10-year study. *JAMA*. 1993;269(5):598–602.

102. Trautner BW, Darouiche RO. Catheter-associated infections: pathogenesis affects prevention. *Arch Intern Med*. 2004;164(8):842–850.

103. Schulman J, Stricof R, Stevens TP, et al. Statewide NICU central-line-associated bloodstream infection rates decline after bundles and checklists. *Pediatrics*. 2011;127(3):436–444.

104. Koll BS, Straub TA, Jalon HS, et al. The CLABs collaborative: a regionwide effort to improve the quality of care in hospitals. *Jt Comm J Qual Patient Saf*. 2008;34(12):713–723.

105. Galpern D, Guerrero A, Tu A, Fahoum B, Wise L. Effectiveness of a central line bundle campaign on line-associated infections in the intensive care unit. *Surgery*. 2008;144(4):492–495.

106. Marra AR, Cal RG, Durao MS, et al. Impact of a program to prevent central line-associated bloodstream infection in the zero tolerance era. *Am J Infect Control*. 2010;38(6):434–439.

107. Furuya EY, Dick A, Perencevich EN, et al. Central line bundle implementation in US intensive care units and impact on bloodstream infections. *PLoS One*. 2011;6(1):e15452.

108. Reduction in central line-associated bloodstream infections among patients in intensive care units—Pennsylvania, April 2001–March 2005. *MMWR Morb Mortal Wkly Rep*. 2005;54(40):1013–1016.

109. Berenholtz SM, Pronovost PJ, Lipsett PA, et al. Eliminating catheter-related bloodstream infections in the intensive care unit. *Crit Care Med*. 2004;32(10):2014–2020.

110. Timsit JF, Schwebel C, Bouadma L, et al. Chlorhexidine-impregnated sponges and less frequent dressing changes for prevention of catheter-related infections in critically ill adults: a randomized controlled trial. *JAMA*. 2009;301(12):1231–1241.

111. Raad II, Hanna HA. Intravascular catheter-related infections: new horizons and recent advances. *Arch Intern Med*. 2002;162(8):871–878.

112. Maiefski M, Rupp ME, Hersman ED. Ethanol lock technique: review of the literature. *Infect Control Hosp Epidemiol*. 2009;30(11):1096–1108.

113. Darouiche RO, Raad II, Heard SO, et al. A comparison of two antimicrobial-impregnated central venous catheters. Catheter Study Group. *N Engl J Med*. 1999;340(1):1–8.

114. Maki DG, Stolz SM, Wheeler S, Mermel LA. Prevention of central venous catheter-related bloodstream infection by use of an antiseptic-impregnated catheter. A randomized, controlled trial. *Ann Intern Med*. 1997;127(4):257–266.

115. Camargo LF, Marra AR, Buchele GL, et al. Double-lumen central venous catheters impregnated with chlorhexidine and silver sulfadiazine to prevent catheter colonisation in the intensive care unit setting: a prospective randomised study. *J Hosp Infect*. 2009;72(3):227–233.

116. Halton KA, Cook DA, Whitby M, Paterson DL, Graves N. Cost effectiveness of antimicrobial catheters in the intensive care unit: addressing uncertainty in the decision. *Crit Care*. 2009;13(2):R35.

117. Aslam S, Darouiche RO. Prolonged bacterial exposure to minocycline/rifampicin-impregnated vascular catheters does not affect antimicrobial activity of catheters. *J Antimicrob Chemother*. 2007;60(1):148–151.

118. Ramos ER, Reitzel R, Jiang Y, et al. Clinical effectiveness and risk of emerging resistance associated with prolonged use of antibiotic-impregnated catheters: more than 0.5 million catheter days and 7 years of clinical experience. *Crit Care Med*. 2011;39(2):245–251.

119. Kluger M. Anaphylaxis to chlorhexidine-impregnated central venous catheter. *Anaesth Intens Care.* 2003;31(6):697–698.

120. Wright MO, Tropp J, Schlora DM, et al. Continuous passive disinfection of catheter hubs prevents contamination and bloodstream infection. *Am J Infect Control.* 2013;41:33–38.

121. Sweet MA, Cumpston A, Briggs F, Craig M, Hamadani M. Impact of alcohol-impregnated port protectors and needleless neutral pressure connectors on central line-associated bloodstream infections and contamination of blood cultures in an inpatient oncology unit. *Am J Infect Control.* 2012;40:931–934.

122. Buchman A, Opilla M, Kwasny M, Diamantidis T, Okamoto R. Risk factors for the development of catheter related blood stream infections in patients receiving home parenteral nutrition. *JPEN J Parenter Enteral Nutr.* 2014; 38(6):744–749. doi:10.1177/0148607113491783.

123. Loveday J, Wilson JR, Pratt R, et al. epic3: national evidence-based guidelines for preventing healthcare-associated infections in NHS hospitals in England. *J Hosp Infect.* 2014;86(Suppl 1): S1–S70. doi:10.1016/S0195-6701(13)60012-2.

124. Gordy S, Rowell S. Vascular air embolism. *Int J Crit Illn Inj Sci.* 2013;3(1):73–76.

125. Konstantinides SV, Barco S, Lankeit M, Meyer G. Management of pulmonary embolism. *J Am Coll Cardiol.* 2016;76(8):976–990.

126. Burns KE, McLaren A. Catheter-related right atrial thrombus and pulmonary embolism: a case report and systematic review of the literature. *Can Respir J.* 2009;6(5):163–165.

127. Shawyer A, Chippington S, Quyam S, Schulze-Neick I, Roebuck D. Phrenic nerve injury after image-guided insertion of a tunnelled right internal jugular central venous catheter. *Pediatr Radiol.* 2012;42:875–877.

128. Moureau N, Poole S, Murdock MA, Gray SM, Semba CP. Central venous catheters in home infusion care: outcomes analysis in 50,470 patients. *J Vasc Interv Radiol.* 2002;13(10):1009–1016.

129. Hoshal VL, Ause RG, Hoskins PA. Fibrin sleeve formation on indwelling subclavian central venous catheters. *Arch Surg.* 1971; 102(4):353–358.

130. Lee AY, Levine MN, Butler G, et al. Incidence, risk factors, and outcomes of catheter-related thrombosis in adult patients with cancer. *J Clin Oncol.* 2006;24(9):1404–1408.

131. Verso M, Agnelli G. Venous thromboembolism associated with long-term use of central venous catheters in cancer patients. *J Clin Oncol.* 2003;21(19):3665–3675.

132. Kovacs MJ, Kahn SR, Rodger M, et al. A pilot study of central venous catheter survival in cancer patients using low-molecular-weight heparin (dalteparin) and warfarin without catheter removal for the treatment of upper extremity deep vein thrombosis (The Catheter Study). *J Thromb Haemost.* 2007;5(8):1650–1653.

133. Cadman A, Lawrence JA, Fitzsimmons L, Spencer-Shaw A, Swindell R. To clot or not to clot? That is the question in central venous catheters. *Clin Radiol.* 2004;59(4):349–355.

134. Kucher N. Clinical practice. Deep-vein thrombosis of the upper extremities. *N Engl J Med.* 2011;364(9):861–869.

135. Ponec D, Irwin D, Haire WD, et al. Recombinant tissue plasminogen activator (alteplase) for restoration of flow in occluded central venous access devices: a double-blind placebo-controlled trial—the Cardiovascular Thrombolytic to Open Occluded Lines (COOL) efficacy trial. *J Vasc Interv Radiol.* 2001;12(8):951–955.

136. Akl EA, Vasireddi SR, Gunukula S, et al. Anticoagulation for patients with cancer and central venous catheters. *Cochrane Database Syst Rev.* 2011;(4):CD006468.

137. Raad II, Luna M, Khalil SA, et al. The relationship between the thrombotic and infectious complications of central venous catheters. *JAMA.* 1994;271(13):1014–1016.

138. van Rooden CJ, Schippers EF, Barge RM, et al. Infectious complications of central venous catheters increase the risk of catheter related thrombosis in hematology patients: a prospective study. *J Clin Oncol.* 2005;23(12):2655–2660.

139. Andris DA, Krzywda EA, Schulte W, Ausman R, Quebbeman EJ. Pinch-off syndrome: a rare etiology for central venous catheter occlusion. *JPEN J Parenter Enteral Nutr.* 1994;18(6):531–533.

140. Mirza B, Vanek VW, Kupensky DT. Pinch-off syndrome: case report and collective review of the literature. *Am Surg.* 2004; 70(7): 635–644.

141. US Food and Drug Administration. Medical Devices: Infusion Pumps. https://www.fda.gov/MedicalDevices/Productsand MedicalProcedures/GeneralHospitalDevicesandSupplies /InfusionPumps. Accessed August 19, 2017.

17 Complications of Parenteral Nutrition

Vanessa J. Kumpf, PharmD, BCNSP, and Jane Gervasio, PharmD, BCNSP, FCCP

CONTENTS

Objectives

1. Identify potential acute and long-term metabolic complications associated with parenteral nutrition (PN).
2. Describe the laboratory and clinical monitoring parameters required to identify metabolic complications associated with PN.
3. List clinically relevant metabolic complications that develop from administration of inadequate or excessive nutrients.
4. Develop strategies to avoid and treat metabolic complications associated with PN.

Test Your Knowledge Questions

1. Which of the following is the most common metabolic complication associated with PN?
   A. Hyperglycemia
   B. Essential fatty acid deficiency (EFAD)
   C. Azotemia
   D. Hyperammonemia
2. One day after initiating PN in a critically ill adult patient, the patient's laboratory values are as follows: serum potassium, 3.1 mEq/L (normal: 3.4–4.8 mEq/L); serum phosphorus 1.6 mg/dL (normal: 2.5–4.8 mg/dL); and serum magnesium, normal. The PN regimen is providing protein 90 g, dextrose 150 g, no lipid, minimum volume, potassium 80 mEq, phosphate 40 mmol, and standard doses of sodium, magnesium, calcium, vitamins, and trace elements. The patient weighs 60 kg and has a body mass index (BMI) of 18. The most appropriate response to these laboratory data is:
   A. Increase potassium and phosphate in the PN, and decrease macronutrient doses with tonight's PN bag.
   B. Provide supplemental intravenous (IV) doses of potassium and phosphate today, but do not change the macronutrient doses with tonight's PN bag.
   C. Increase potassium and phosphate in the PN, and advance dextrose to 225 g with tonight's PN bag.
   D. Provide supplemental IV doses of potassium and phosphate today, and advance dextrose to 225 g with tonight's PN bag.
3. Which of the following measures would be considered most beneficial in a patient who develops cholestasis while receiving long-term PN that is infused over 12 hours nightly?
   A. Stop all oral and enteral intake.
   B. Switch from a cyclic to continuous method of PN administration.
   C. Decrease lipid injectable emulsion (ILE) dose from 1.5 g/kg/d to 1 g/kg twice weekly.
   D. Increase protein dose from 1 g/kg/d to 2 g/kg/d.
4. Which of the following PN modifications is recommended to help prevent and/or treat osteoporosis in a long-term PN patient?
   A. Maintain protein intake of at least 2 g/kg/d.
   B. Provide more than 20 mEq calcium per day.
   C. Add injectable vitamin D to the PN formulation.
   D. Provide 20 to 40 mmol phosphorus per day.

Test Your Knowledge Answers

1. The correct answer is A. Hyperglycemia is the most common metabolic complication that occurs with PN. Hyperglycemia is associated with overfeeding but is also common in appropriately fed patients, where it is attributed to insulin suppression and resistance as well as gluconeogenesis from stress and infection. Nondiabetic hospitalized patients receiving IV dextrose infusions at rates greater than 4 mg/kg/min have a 50% chance of developing hyperglycemia.[1] EFAD is associated with fat-free PN and can be avoided by administering minimal amounts of ILE. Azotemia is usually associated with renal or hepatic dysfunction or protein overfeeding. Hyperammonemia rarely occurs now that crystalline amino acids are used in PN.
2. The correct answer is B. Management and prevention of refeeding syndrome and refeeding hypophosphatemia involve (1) identifying patients at risk, (2) serum electrolyte monitoring with aggressive replacement, and (3) slowly increasing energy intake.[2-5] In this critically ill patient who experiences hypophosphatemia and hypokalemia after the initiation of PN, the electrolyte abnormalities should be treated quickly with supplemental, IV replacement doses. Energy intake from PN should not be advanced until the electrolyte deficiencies are corrected.
3. The correct answer is C. Cholestasis has been associated with ILE doses greater than 1 g/kg/d in adult patients receiving long-term PN,[6] and the patient may therefore benefit from a trial of lowering the ILE dose. Cyclic infusion has been shown to reduce serum liver enzyme and conjugated bilirubin concentrations when compared with continuous infusion.[7] Enteral feeding should be attempted to promote enterohepatic circulation of bile acids. The protein dose does not seem to play a role in the development of cholestasis in adults.
4. The correct answer is D. An inadequate phosphorus dose may increase urinary calcium excretion; therefore, the American Society for Parenteral and Enteral Nutrition (ASPEN) recommends that phosphorus doses of 20 to 40 mmol/d be added to the PN formulation.[8] Although patients receiving PN are vulnerable to a negative calcium balance, calcium supplementation in the PN formulation is limited by calcium's physical compatibility with phosphorus, and higher calcium doses are offset by higher urinary losses. ASPEN recommends that calcium gluconate 10 to 15 mEq/d be added to the PN formulation.[8] High protein doses (2 g/kg/d vs 1 g/kg/d) in PN formulations have been associated with increased urinary calcium excretion in adult patients. Excessive vitamin D doses can be detrimental to the bone because they can suppress parathyroid hormone (PTH) and promote bone resorption, and individual forms of parenteral ergocalciferol or cholecalciferol are not available.

Background

Parenteral nutrition–associated complications can be categorized as mechanical, metabolic, and infectious. Metabolic complications are more commonly associated with PN rather than enteral nutrition. Therefore, patients receiving PN

TABLE 17-1 Monitoring to Identify/Prevent Metabolic Complications in Patients Receiving Parenteral Nutrition

Parameter	Frequency of Monitoring	
	Initiation of Therapy (Acute Care)	Long-Term Therapy
Capillary glucose	Every 6 hours until patient is advanced to PN goal and as needed to maintain glucose level of 140–180 mg/dL	Not routine; done on as-needed basis to coordinate with PN infusion cycle
Basic metabolic panel, phosphorus, magnesium	Daily, until patient is advanced to PN goal and stable; then 1–2 times/wk	Weekly; then decrease frequency in stable patients
CBC (with differential)	Baseline; then 1–2 times/week	Monthly; then decrease frequency in stable patients
Liver function: ALT, AST, ALP, total bilirubin, INR	Baseline; then weekly	Monthly; then decrease frequency in stable patients
Serum triglycerides	Baseline if patient is at risk for hypertriglyceridemia; then as needed	Not routine; done on as-needed basis
Iron studies, 25-hydroxyvitamin D	Not routine	Baseline; then every 3–6 months
Zinc, copper, selenium, manganese	Not routine	Baseline; then every 6 months
Weight	Daily	Daily
Total fluid intake/output	Daily until stable; then as needed	As-needed basis

ALP, alkaline phosphatase; ALT, alanine aminotransferase; AST, aspartate aminotransferase; CBC, complete blood count; INR, international normalized ratio; PN, parenteral nutrition.

require close monitoring for prevention and early detection of complications. Mechanical complications related to the venous access device and infectious complications are discussed in Chapter 16. This chapter focuses on the recognition, prevention, and treatment of metabolic complications associated with PN in the adult patient. Refer to Table 17-1 for an overview of monitoring recommendations to identify or prevent such complications.

Macronutrient-Related Complications

Hyperglycemia

Hyperglycemia is the most common complication associated with PN administration and can be caused by various factors. Stress-associated hyperglycemia in acutely ill and septic patients often develops as a result of insulin resistance, increased gluconeogenesis and glycogenolysis, and suppressed insulin secretion.[1] Excess carbohydrate administration has been associated with hyperglycemia, hepatic steatosis, and increased carbon dioxide production. ASPEN recommends target blood glucose concentrations between 140 to 180 mg/dL in adult hospitalized patients receiving nutrition support.[9] Similarly, the Society of Critical Care Medicine (SCCM) recommends blood glucose concentrations be maintained between 150 to 180 mg/dL for the general intensive care unit (ICU) population.[10] PN should be initiated at half of the estimated energy needs, or approximately 150 to 200 g dextrose, for the first 24 hours. Delivery of less dextrose (approximately 100 g) may be warranted if the patient has a low BMI or poor glucose control. Carbohydrate

administration should not exceed a rate of 4 to 5 mg/kg/min or 20 to 25 kcal/kg/d in acutely ill patients.[11]

Blood glucose concentrations can be controlled with insulin therapy, which may be administered subcutaneously, intravenously via an insulin infusion, or directly in the PN solution. Capillary blood glucose concentrations should be monitored every 6 to 8 hours in patients receiving short-acting subcutaneous insulin and more frequently in critically ill patients receiving insulin infusion therapy. An initial insulin regimen of 0.05 to 0.1 units per gram of dextrose in the PN solution is common, or 0.15 to 0.2 units per gram of dextrose may be used in patients who are already hyperglycemic. Supplemental short-acting or rapid-acting insulin may be administered subcutaneously if needed, using a sliding scale regimen. Two-thirds of the total amount of sliding scale insulin required over 24 hours may then be added to the next day's PN formulation. Only regular insulin should be added to the PN formulation. When administering repeat doses of insulin, clinicians must take into account the duration of action of the insulin formulation previously provided before administering the next dose. Giving the subsequent dose too soon is referred to as "stacking" insulin and can result in hypoglycemia.

The dextrose dose in the PN formulation should not be advanced until the patient's blood glucose concentrations are controlled. The insulin dose should be proportionally increased and decreased with respect to the PN dextrose dose. Alternatively, an insulin infusion may be instituted to provide consistent and safe glucose control. A proportional increase in fat content or frequency may be necessary to increase energy from PN.

Rarely, hyperglycemia may be related to chromium deficiency. Insulin is less effective in patients with chromium deficiency. Increasing the chromium dose in the PN formulation beyond the standard amount in commercially prepared multiple trace element injections may be necessary.[12,13]

Hyperglycemia is associated with worsened clinical outcomes, such as increased risk of infection, poor wound healing, and inability to gain weight. Uncontrolled hyperglycemia may result in hyperosmolar hyperglycemia, nonketotic dehydration, coma, and death secondary to osmotic diuresis.[14] Refer to Chapter 34 for additional information on hyperglycemia and the administration of insulin.

Hypoglycemia

PN-associated hypoglycemia can occur from excess insulin administration via the PN solution, IV infusion, or subcutaneous injection. Excessive or erroneous administration of insulin is a severe medication error, and resulting hypoglycemia may be life-threatening. Treatment includes initiation of a 10% dextrose infusion, administration of an ampule of 50% dextrose, and/or stopping any source of insulin administration. Treatment with oral carbohydrate, such as glucose gel or chewable tablets, can be considered for management of mild hypoglycemia in suitable patients who are likely to tolerate it.

Abrupt discontinuation of PN solutions has been associated with rebound hypoglycemia.[15] Studies have not reported symptomatic hypoglycemia after abruptly stopping PN infusions given over 16 to 24 hours.[16,17] However, some patients had asymptomatic hypoglycemia.

Patients requiring large doses of insulin have a greater propensity for rebound hypoglycemia, but predicting which patients will experience rebound hypoglycemia is difficult. Therefore, to reduce the risk of rebound hypoglycemia in susceptible patients, a 1- to 2-hour taper down of the infusion, or half the infusion rate, may be necessary. If a PN solution must be discontinued quickly, a dextrose-containing fluid should be infused for 1 or 2 hours following PN discontinuation to avoid a possible rebound hypoglycemia. Obtaining a capillary blood glucose concentration 30 minutes to 1 hour after the PN solution is discontinued will help identify rebound hypoglycemia. See Chapter 34 for additional discussion of this topic.

Essential Fatty Acid Deficiency

ILE is generally provided as a source of essential fatty acids and as a nonprotein energy source (see Chapters 5 and 15). Depending on the length of the PN therapy and the nutrition status of the patient, ILE-free PN may result in EFAD. Two polyunsaturated fatty acids, linoleic and α-linolenic, cannot be synthesized by the body and are considered essential. Clinical manifestations of EFAD include scaly dermatitis, alopecia, hepatomegaly, thrombocytopenia, fatty liver, and anemia.[18] A triene:tetraene ratio of more than 0.2 indicates EFAD and can occur within 1 to 3 weeks in adults receiving ILE-free PN.[19] The adult requirements for linoleic acid are met through exogenous sources or endogenously through the lipolysis of adipose tissue. However, when hypertonic dextrose is infused, insulin

is secreted and lipolysis is reduced. Thus, an exogenous source of fat must be provided.

To prevent EFAD, 1% to 2% of daily energy requirements should be derived from linoleic acid and about 0.5% of energy from linolenic acid.[8] This goal translates to approximately 250 mL of 20% or 500 mL of 10% soy-based ILE administered over 8 to 10 hours, twice a week. Alternatively, 500 mL of a 20% soy-based ILE can be given once a week. When using an alternative oil–based ILE, such as those containing medium-chain triglycerides, olive oil, and fish oil, a greater amount of ILE is required to meet essential fatty acid requirements because these non-soy-based products contain lower quantities of linoleic and linolenic acid. In patients who do not tolerate ILE, a trial of topical skin application or oral ingestion of oils may be given to alleviate biochemical EFAD.[20,21]

Immunosuppression

Soy-based ILEs have been associated with immunosuppressive effects, reticuloendothelial system dysfunction, and exaggerated systemic inflammatory response. The 18-carbon ω-6 fatty acid preparation (ie, linoleic acid) has been postulated to suppress the immune response by activating the arachidonic pathway. Evidence suggest that certain long-chain fatty acids may impair immune function by interfering with phagocytosis and chemotaxis and may increase the patient's risk of infection. The alternative oil–based ILEs now available in the United States have demonstrated fewer proinflammatory and immunosuppressive properties compared with soy-based ILEs (see Chapter 5). Although alternative oil–based products are safe and effective, further research is necessary to determine which patient populations and medical conditions will benefit from them.[22]

Withholding or limiting soy-based ILE in critically ill patients for the first week of PN has been suggested as a strategy to reduce immunosuppression complications. The 2016 ASPEN and SCCM guidelines for nutrition support therapy in the adult critically ill patient support this recommendation; however, ASPEN and SCCM gave the quality of evidence a very low rating.[23] The recommendation is primarily based on research from one study involving trauma patients receiving fat-free PN over the first 10 days of hospitalization.[24] The study reported that the elimination of ILE from the PN improved clinical outcomes (eg, decreased infectious morbidity, decreased hospitalization, shortened ICU length of stay, and shortened duration of mechanical ventilation). However, the study is more than 20 years old and has not been duplicated. Also, it has been criticized, in part because the goals for energy delivery in the study were based on nonprotein calories (not total calories). Consequently, the total amount of energy delivered was greater than reported, and overfeeding may have contributed to the complications associated with the PN with ILE.[23,24]

Hypertriglyceridemia

Hypertriglyceridemia can occur with dextrose overfeeding or with rapid administration rates of ILE (greater than 0.11 g/kg/h).[8] Hyperlipidemia may impair immune response, alter pulmonary hemodynamics, and increase the risk of pancreatitis.[25,26] Reducing the dose and/or lengthening the infusion time of ILE will help minimize these effects. ILE intake should be restricted to less than 30% of total energy, or 1 g/kg/d; also, if ILE is administered separately, it should be provided slowly over at least 8 to 10 hours.[25] Serum triglyceride concentrations should be checked prior to ILE administration in any patient with a known history of hyperlipidemia or risk of hypertriglyceridemia. ASPEN recommends that serum triglyceride concentrations greater than 400 mg/dL be avoided when infusing ILE, and clinicians should reduce the ILE dose or discontinue ILE if this level of hypertriglyceridemia occurs.[8] The dose of ILE should also be reduced or discontinued in mechanically ventilated patients receiving propofol for sedation because propofol is supplied as a 10% ILE.

Pancreatitis due to ILE-induced hyperlipidemia is rare unless serum triglyceride concentrations exceed 1000 mg/dL. ILE is considered safe for use in patients with pancreatitis without hypertriglyceridemia.[27] See Chapter 28 for further discussion of pancreatitis.

Adverse Reactions to Lipid Injectable Emulsions

Although the incidence of complications associated with ILE use is low, potential complications include allergic or infusion-related adverse reactions. Allergic reactions to ILE are rare, but they can occur, especially in patients with history of egg allergy. The allergic reaction is most likely a result of the egg phospholipid that is used as an emulsifier. Other acute, infusion-related adverse reactions associated with ILE include dyspnea, cyanosis, flushing, sweating, dizziness, headache, back or chest pain, nausea, and vomiting.

Azotemia

When protein administration is excessive, the metabolic demand of disposing of the byproducts of protein metabolism increases. Prerenal azotemia can result from dehydration, excess protein, and/or inadequate energy from nonprotein sources (eg, in patients with anorexia nervosa). Intolerance to the protein load is exhibited by an increase in blood urea nitrogen. Patients with hepatic or renal disease are prone to developing azotemia because their ability to metabolize and eliminate urea is impaired. When urea clearance is impaired, patients may require dialysis to help eliminate urea and allow for the adequate intake of protein.

Hyperammonemia was a greater risk when protein hydrolysates contained excessive amounts of ammonia and insufficient arginine for urea cycle metabolism. This complication has become a rare occurrence since the advent of crystalline amino acid solutions, although it has been observed with the new crystalline amino acid solutions in patients with urea cycle defects, such as ornithine transcarbamylase deficiency.[28,29]

Patients who develop prerenal azotemia may benefit from a reduction in the amount of amino acids provided. Protein restriction in patients in liver failure with hyperammonemia and encephalopathy has not been demonstrated to improve outcomes and thus is discouraged. In patients with hepatic failure and hepatic encephalopathy, the use of high branched-chain, low aromatic amino acid formulations has provided inconsistent results and is not recommended (see Chapter 27 for discussion of the appropriate use of specialized amino acid formulations in liver disease). Protein should *not* be restricted in critically ill patients with acute kidney injury receiving continuous renal replacement therapy or hemodialysis, especially in the setting of malnutrition (see Chapter 29 for more information on acute kidney injury).

Micronutrient-Related Complications

Fluid and Electrolytes

Once macronutrient tolerance has been established, the routine management of the patient receiving PN centers on fluid and electrolytes (see Chapter 7). The requirements vary depending on the patient's renal, fluid, and electrolyte status when starting PN, as well as the underlying disease process and any losses he or she may incur.[30,31] To identify necessary adjustments in the PN solution composition and volume, clinicians must routinely monitor patients for fluid and electrolyte shifts between the intracellular and extracellular space or changes in total body water or electrolyte status.

When determining the patient's fluid and electrolyte status, clinicians also need to evaluate concurrent IV fluids and medications provided during PN therapy. All fluids being infused should be considered when the PN formulation is prescribed. If the patient has excessive losses, fluid and electrolyte replacement with separate IV fluids outside of the PN formulation may be necessary. Treatment involves replacing the lost fluids with IV fluid of similar electrolyte composition. Accurate intake and output records are necessary to show the amount of loss from various body fluids. See Chapter 7 for a complete review of fluid and electrolytes and Practice Scenario 17-1 for a discussion of metabolic monitoring during PN.

Practice Scenario 17-1

Question: What parameters should be monitored, and with what frequency, to help identify and prevent metabolic complications in a patient initiating parenteral nutrition (PN)?

Scenario: A 52-year-old woman, postoperative Day 7, presents with a small bowel obstruction. She has elevated gastric residual volumes, abdominal distention, and hypoactive bowel sounds. She is 165 cm in height and weighs 63 kg, with no muscle or adipose tissue wasting or signs of edema noted. Serum laboratory values include the following: albumin, 3.7 g/dL; prealbumin, 16 mg/dL; sodium, 139 mmol/L; potassium, 3.9 mmol/L; chlorine, 101 mmol/L; carbon dioxide, 25 mmol/L; blood urea nitrogen, 10 mg/dL; creatinine, 0.7 mg/dL; glucose, 112 mg/dL; ionized calcium, 4.7 mg/dL; phosphate, 3.3 mg/dL; and magnesium, 1.9 mg/dL. Vital signs include heart rate, 74 bpm; blood pressure, 118/70 mm Hg; input, 2400 mL/d; and output, 2370 mL/d.

Intervention: The patient's maintenance intravenous fluid is discontinued, and PN is initiated.

Answer: Before PN is initiated, the nutrition support team should evaluate the patient's vital signs, intake/output, and physical examination data to determine her fluid status, and a complete metabolic panel as well as phosphate, and magnesium levels should be obtained and assessed. If electrolytes, specifically potassium, phosphate, and magnesium, are depleted, they should be repleted before PN is administered. After PN is initiated, electrolytes should be evaluated daily until levels are stable, in part to assess for potential refeeding syndrome. PN may be administered slowly and titrated to goal over a period of days to prevent hyperglycemia. Glucose levels should be monitored at least every 6 hours until the patient is euglycemic. If insulin is administered, more frequent glucose monitoring may be necessary because the patient is at increased risk for hypoglycemia. Prealbumin can be evaluated initially and serially during PN administration. Below-normal prealbumin can be a useful indicator of inflammatory metabolism, and normal levels can indicate that normal postprandial metabolism and anabolism are possible (see Chapter 9 for further discussion).

Rationale: Initial presentation of the patient does not suggest any additional concerns beyond the standard considerations of fluid status, electrolytes, and glucose levels. Her electrolytes are within normal values, her vital signs and fluid status are appropriate, and she has no signs of wasting. The complication of hyperglycemia must be considered when PN is initiated. Additionally, until she is stable, daily electrolyte monitoring is necessary.

Vitamins

Vitamins are essential for effective nutrient utilization, and a sustained exogenous intake of vitamins is essential to avoid deficiency (see Chapter 8). However, excessive amounts of lipid-soluble vitamins A, D, E, and K can be toxic. Provision of adequate vitamin intake in the PN patient may be complicated by conditions that increase requirements, such as sepsis, trauma, or recovery following surgery. Identifying vitamin deficiency or toxicity can be difficult because serum vitamin concentrations do not always directly correlate with body stores and clinical symptoms are often nonspecific. Therefore, adult patients receiving PN should receive a standard daily dose of parenteral multivitamins.[32] Clinicians should not delay IV multivitamin therapy until a patient develops clinical signs of vitamin deficiency and must take measures to address product shortages.

Certain clinical situations warrant special attention. Patients receiving both PN and warfarin therapy require close monitoring because the vitamin K (150 mcg) included in the 13-vitamin preparation interacts with warfarin and can result in therapeutic failure. Patients with a history of prolonged poor dietary intake or alcohol abuse are at risk for developing thiamin deficiency, especially with initiation of carbohydrate. Acute thiamin deficiency can result in alterations in mental status and peripheral nervous system dysfunction (ie, Wernicke's encephalopathy). Several cases of lactic acidosis due to thiamin deficiency, including 3 deaths, were reported in patients receiving PN without thiamin during a period of parenteral multivitamin shortage.[33] Supplemental thiamin (50 to 100 mg/d) and folic acid (1 mg/d) beyond what is provided in the parenteral multivitamin preparation for the initial 5 to 7 days of PN therapy has been recommended in patients with a history of prolonged poor dietary intake.[34]

Vitamin toxicity, particularly of the fat-soluble vitamins, is a potential complication of PN. Vitamin A toxicity has been reported in patients with chronic renal failure receiving PN, and some clinicians have recommended reducing the frequency of fat-soluble vitamin administration to twice per week in these patients. However, because there are no injectable multivitamin preparations available without fat-soluble vitamins, water-soluble vitamin deficiency is a risk with restricted dosing. Furthermore, because some water-soluble vitamins may be lost with hemodialysis, provision of water-soluble vitamins to patients receiving dialysis has been recommended.[35] An oral vitamin B complex supplement or individual parenteral vitamin B supplementation, as available, can be used to address this recommendation.

Several vitamins are known to undergo substantial degradation after addition to the PN formulation. This issue is not considered a significant problem in the acute care setting because of the relatively short time period between compounding and administration. However, because PN formulations are compounded in a batch fashion for patients in the home setting, degradation is a risk with these solutions. Vitamin A degradation was clearly demonstrated in a home PN patient who developed night blindness within 6 months of receiving PN that was prepared on a weekly basis with the vitamins added to the PN formulation by the pharmacy before delivery.[36] Although the patient's night blindness resolved after a therapeutic dose of vitamin A, the source of the problem was not identified until symptoms returned 6 months later. Substantial amounts of vitamin A were likely lost to degradation and adsorption to the plastic matrix of the bag because the vitamins were added to the PN formulation up to a week before administration. To avoid this problem, the patient or caregiver must perform the task of adding vitamins to the PN formulation prior to administration in the home setting.[8] Home nutrition support is further discussed in Chapter 38.

Interruptions in parenteral multivitamin product supply have been an ongoing issue in the United States and could possibly harm patients if not appropriately managed (see Chapter 15). ASPEN offers the following advice to help clinicians cope with parenteral multivitamin product shortages:[37]

- Reserve a supply of IV multivitamins for those patients receiving solely PN.
- Use oral or enterally administered multivitamins whenever possible.
- To ensure fair allocation of products nationwide, do not stockpile parenteral multivitamins.
- Do not use pediatric IV multivitamins for adult patients.
- When all options to obtain IV multivitamins have been exhausted, ration use by reducing the dose by 50% or giving 1 dose 3 times a week.
- If IV multivitamins are no longer available, administer individual thiamin, ascorbic acid, pyridoxine, and folic acid daily.

Trace Elements

Trace element deficiencies are relatively uncommon in patients receiving PN, but they can occur when intake is insufficient or utilization or excretion is increased over a prolonged period. For example, a patient with high intestinal losses may become zinc deficient. Cardiomyopathy caused by selenium deficiency has been reported in patients receiving long-term PN without selenium supplementation.[38,39] Trace element toxicity is also a potential complication in patients receiving long-term PN and those with hepatobiliary disease. Available parenteral multi–trace element preparations may exceed actual requirements in many patients receiving PN.[40] In addition, many of the components of the PN formulation may be contaminated with trace elements such as zinc, copper, manganese, chromium, selenium, and aluminum.[41] Tissue elevations of copper, manganese, and chromium have been noted on autopsy in patients receiving long-term PN.[42] Although serum trace element monitoring is recommended at baseline and routine follow-up in patients receiving long-term PN, serum levels are unreliable measures of total body balance.[43] Empiric adjustments in trace element intake may be warranted. Clinicians should consider reducing manganese and copper dosing in patients with hepatobiliary disease because the disease impairs excretion. Removal of supplemental manganese from the PN formulation and reduction in the copper dose are often necessary in long-term PN patients to minimize the risk for toxicity.

Interruptions in the supply of IV multi–trace element and individual trace element products have resulted in shortage situations in the United States. To address parenteral multi–trace element shortages, ASPEN suggests rationing the supply by reducing doses by half, limiting the frequency of administration to 3 times a week, and using the oral/enteral route when feasible. Withholding multi–trace element products for the first month of PN therapy from newly initiated adult patients who are not critically ill and do not have preexisting deficits could also be considered. If a multi–trace element supply is no longer available, individual trace element components should be given parenterally, as available, or otherwise provided by the oral/enteral route.[44]

Iron is not a component of the PN formulation, primarily because of compatibility limitations. Parenteral iron supplementation at repletion doses is warranted in conditions of iron deficiency when the oral route is ineffective or not tolerated and can be provided as an infusion separate from the PN formulation. Delivery of parenteral iron to replete iron stores to patients receiving PN may be provided on an as-needed basis as determined by routine monitoring of iron status.[45,46] See Chapters 8 and 15 for more information about trace elements in PN.

Refeeding Syndrome

Refeeding syndrome refers to the adverse effects of metabolic and physiological shifts of fluid, electrolytes, vitamins, and minerals (eg, phosphorus, magnesium, potassium, thiamin) that can occur as a result of aggressive nutrition support or nutrition repletion of a malnourished patient; it is a risk during the first 2 to 5 days after the start of nutrition support.[47] In periods of prolonged starvation, the body adapts by deriving energy from fat (ketone production), reducing energy expenditure, decreasing insulin secretion, and utilizing intracellular minerals and electrolytes. With the reintroduction of carbohydrate during nutrition repletion, glucose again becomes the primary fuel source. Insulin release is stimulated and results in enhanced update of glucose, electrolytes, minerals, and water into cells. The carbohydrate administration increases the demand for intracellular phosphorus to synthesize adenosine triphosphate, resulting in a further depletion of phosphorus. Additionally, carbohydrate administration results in an increased need for thiamin, potassium, and magnesium. These resulting electrolyte and vitamin deficits cause symptoms of neuromuscular, cardiovascular, and respiratory compromise. Moreover, fluid and sodium from the nutrition delivery further burdens the compromised organs, resulting in fluid overload and edema. Because these deleterious effects are the result of aggressively feeding a malnourished or starved patient, energy and fluid should be initiated and advanced slowly and electrolytes and vitamins administered as aggressively as necessary in at-risk patients (see Practice Scenario 17-2).[47-50]

Practice Scenario 17-2

Question: How can the complications of refeeding syndrome be minimized when providing parenteral nutrition (PN) to a nutritionally depleted patient?

Scenario: A 54-year-old man with a history of gastric cancer is status post partial gastrectomy and small bowel resection. His nasogastric output is 1250 mL/d with absent bowel sounds. A kidney, ureter, and bladder x-ray is consistent with a small bowel ileus. The patient's height is 180 cm and he weighs 66 kg (body mass index: 20). His usual body weight was 75 kg, and he shows signs of moderate wasting of lean muscle and adipose stores as well as slight edema postsurgery. His prealbumin is 10 mg/dL and his albumin is 3.1 g/dL.

Intervention: Intravenous fluids are tapered as PN is initiated on postoperative Day 8.

Answer: The nutrition support team should start nutrition slowly by providing half of the goal energy requirements, or approximately 15 kcal/kg/d, on the first day of PN. The first bag should contain about 1000 kcal. Recommendations differ with regard to initial protein dosing. Since the effect of protein on glycolysis is not as concerning as dextrose, starting at the goal protein dose (1.2 to 1.5 g/kg/d) is recommended.[47] Dextrose and fat should comprise the rest of the formulation, although dextrose should not exceed approximately 200 g/d. Nutrition should be slowly increased to the full nutrition goal over the next 2 to 5 days, based on the patient's tolerance. Clinicians should monitor electrolytes daily, paying close attention to sodium, potassium, phosphorous, and magnesium. Daily intake and output, as well as the patient's weight, must be assessed. Vitamins and trace elements should be administered daily.

Rationale: The patient is at risk for refeeding syndrome complications because he is severely malnourished; his lean muscle and adipose stores are moderately wasted, and he has experienced significant weight loss. He should be monitored closely for electrolyte abnormalities and volume overload. The monitoring parameters suggested in Table 17-1 can help identify and prevent metabolic complications when initiating PN therapy.

The term *refeeding hypophosphatemia* has been used to describe decreased serum phosphorus concentrations after the initiation of nutrition in patients who do not have the other metabolic abnormalities associated with refeeding syndrome.[50] Hypophosphatemia may also result from other causes, including cellular phosphate redistribution, poor phosphate intake, or renal tubular phosphate loss. Even without the other complications associated with refeeding syndrome, hypophosphatemia is concerning, and phosphorus should be replaced as needed; however, labeling the complication *refeeding syndrome* is arguably not necessary.[48–51]

Hepatobiliary Complications

Disorders of the liver and biliary system are commonly reported in patients receiving PN. These complications may be life-threatening and are particularly concerning in patients who depend on long-term PN support. We do not yet fully understand how PN influences the development of liver disease. Historically, it was thought that some existing component of the PN formulation or a nutrient not provided by the PN formulation caused the liver disease. However, that simplistic concept has been replaced. Today, we recognize that liver dysfunction can result from a complex set of risk factors that affect patients receiving PN, such as the primary risk factor of intestinal failure. The term *PN-induced liver disease* has therefore been replaced with the interchangeable terms *PN-associated liver disease* (PNALD)[52] and *intestinal failure–associated liver disease*[53] to refer to hepatic dysfunction secondary to intestinal failure that occurs in the setting of PN.

Types of Hepatobiliary Disorders

The types of hepatobiliary disorders associated with PN in adult patients are usually different from those seen in pediatric patients, although age-related distinctions become less evident in patients receiving long-term PN. The 3 types of hepatobiliary disorders associated with PN therapy are steatosis, cholestasis, and gallbladder sludge/stones; these disorders may coexist.[54] Steatosis (hepatic fat accumulation) is more common in adults than in pediatric patients and is generally benign. It typically presents as modest elevations of serum aminotransferase concentrations that occur within 2 weeks of PN therapy, and concentrations may return to normal even when PN is continued. Most patients are asymptomatic. Steatosis seems to be a complication of overfeeding and has probably decreased in prevalence over the years as estimates of PN energy requirements have been lowered. Although steatosis is generally thought to be a nonprogressive lesion, it may progress to fibrosis or cirrhosis in patients receiving long-term PN.[6]

PN-associated cholestasis (PNAC) is a condition of impaired secretion of bile or frank biliary obstruction that occurs predominantly in children, but it may also occur in adult patients receiving long-term PN. PNAC typically presents as elevated alkaline phosphatase, γ-glutamyl transpeptidase, and conjugated (direct) bilirubin concentrations with or without jaundice. Although both γ-glutamyl transpeptidase and alkaline phosphatase are sensitive markers for hepatobiliary disease, they lack specificity because levels may be elevated in other diseases as well. An elevated serum conjugated bilirubin (eg, greater than 2 mg/dL) is considered the prime indicator for cholestasis. PNAC is a serious complication because it may progress to cirrhosis and liver failure.

Gallbladder stasis during PN therapy may lead to the development of gallstones or gallbladder sludge with subsequent cholecystitis. This complication is related more to the lack of enteral stimulation than the PN infusion itself. The lack of oral intake results in decreased cholecystokinin (CCK) release and impaired bile flow and gallbladder contractility. The duration of PN therapy seems to correlate with the development of biliary sludge.[55] Biliary sludge may progress to acute cholecystitis in the absence of gallstones. This condition is also referred to as *acalculous cholecystitis*.

Prevalence

Prevalence rates of PNALD vary greatly. In adult patients receiving PN, the reported incidence of abnormal enzyme elevations ranges from 25% to 100%.[54] However, few studies have correlated enzyme changes to permanent hepatic function or histological damage. The risk for and severity of liver disease seem to increase as the duration of PN usage lengthens. The prevalence of chronic cholestasis in a group of 90 patients receiving home PN for permanent intestinal failure was 55% at 2 years, 64% at 4 years, and 72% at 6 years.[6]

Many studies evaluating the prevalence of PNALD have also attempted to identify risk factors unrelated to the PN therapy. Bacterial and fungal infections are associated with cholestasis. Sepsis likely causes liver inflammation because of the release of proinflammatory cytokines that are activated by endotoxins. This point is especially relevant in the long-term PN patient, who may experience recurrent central line–associated bloodstream infections. Many patients receiving PN have disorders that predispose them to small intestinal bacterial overgrowth (SIBO), which is another risk factor for liver disease. SIBO occurs when large amounts of bacteria normally confined to the colon and lower small bowel populate the upper small intestine (see Chapter 26). It has been postulated that these anaerobic bacteria in the small intestine may produce hepatotoxins. Massive intestinal resection has also been identified as a risk factor for PNALD.[6,56] A small bowel remnant less than 50 cm in length has been significantly associated with chronic cholestasis.[6]

Parenteral Nutrition–Related Risk Factors

Although supporting data are limited, various factors related to the nutrient composition of the PN formulation could contribute to the development of liver complications. Therefore, it is important to evaluate the merits of these potential risk factors to design a PN formulation that minimizes risk of PNALD.

Energy

Clinical studies suggest that the development of steatosis during PN administration is primarily related to excessive energy intake.[42] Overfeeding in general or an excess of individual energy substrates (carbohydrate, fat, protein) can contribute to liver complications. The administration of excessive energy is thought to promote hepatic fat deposition by stimulating insulin release, which, in turn, promotes lipogenesis and inhibits fatty acid oxidation.[54]

Carbohydrate

Dextrose-based PN regimens that contain little or no fat have been implicated in the development of steatosis. Excess carbohydrates deposit in the liver as fat, and a dextrose-based PN regimen may result in EFAD, which may lead to impaired lipoprotein formation and triglyceride secretion, resulting in steatosis. Providing balanced amounts of energy from dextrose and fat seems to decrease the incidence of steatosis, possibly by decreasing hepatic triglyceride uptake and promoting fatty acid oxidation.[54] A balanced PN formulation should provide 70% to 85% of nonprotein energy as carbohydrate and 15% to 30% as fat.[8] In addition, the carbohydrate content of PN should not exceed 7 g/kg/d in adults.[8]

Protein

Early sources of amino acids for parenteral use included protein hydrolysates contaminated with significant amounts of aluminum. Animal studies suggest that high levels of aluminum exposure may lead to the development of cholestasis. The replacement of protein hydrolysates with crystalline amino acids has significantly reduced the overall aluminum contamination in PN formulations. Amino acid–associated aluminum toxicity is no longer considered a risk factor for the development of liver complications.[57] Although the role that amino acids play in the development of cholestasis in adults is unclear, it does not seem to be as significant as the role they play in cholestasis in infants.

Lipid Injectable Emulsion

The role of ILE in the development of liver complications may involve the fat source, the phytosterol content, or the dose. The most commonly used ILE in the United States is soybean oil–based and contains high concentrations of ω-6 fatty acids and significant amounts of phytosterols. Phytosterols are inefficiently metabolized to bile acids by the liver, and it has been postulated that they may impair bile flow and cause biliary sludge and stones. Adult patients with short bowel syndrome (SBS) receiving ILE-containing PN have been shown to have much higher serum phytosterol levels than other patients with SBS or healthy controls.[58] Case reports of children with PN-related cholestasis have documented high serum phytosterol

levels.[59] In addition, the high ω-6 fatty acid content of soybean-based ILE may potentially initiate or worsen inflammatory states and can have immunosuppressive effects.[60] The presence of phytosterols and proinflammatory ω-6 fatty acids may contribute to the hepatotoxic effects seen in patients receiving long-term PN with a soybean oil–based ILE. The use of a fish oil–based ILE, primarily composed of ω-3 fatty acids and containing no phytosterols, has shown promising results in reversing PNALD in pediatric patients when used in place of soybean oil–based ILE.[61,62] Further study evaluating the safety and efficacy of fish oil–based ILE for the prevention and treatment of PNALD is needed before its use can be recommended.[22,63,64] A newer-generation ILE product containing a combination of soybean, medium-chain triglyceride, olive, and fish oils has recently become available (see Chapters 5 and 15). Compared with soybean oil alone, it offers a shift in the ω-6:ω-3 ratio toward an anti-inflammatory effect, which, theoretically, may reduce the risk for PNALD or provide a treatment option for patients with PNALD. However, further study is required to investigate these hypotheses.[64,65]

The ILE dose is another concern when evaluating PN options. Although liver complications have been associated with EFAD, they can also occur when the ILE dose is excessive. Steatosis can occur when the ILE infusion rate exceeds the liver's ability to clear the phospholipids and fatty acids, leading to direct deposition in the liver. Cholestasis may also be associated with high ILE doses, especially with long-term use. Multivariate analysis demonstrated that chronic cholestasis and severe PNALD were strongly associated with ILE intake greater than 1 g/kg/d in patients receiving long-term PN.[6] The results demonstrated no association between dextrose intake or nonprotein energy intake and PNALD.

Carnitine

Carnitine plays an important role in fat metabolism (see Chapters 5 and 15). Primary carnitine deficiency has been associated with the development of steatosis. Because carnitine is not routinely added to PN, a patient's plasma carnitine concentrations may decrease below the reference range within a few weeks of starting PN therapy. Carnitine supplementation has been shown to help mobilize hepatic fat stores and prevent steatosis in neonates receiving PN.[59] However, low serum carnitine concentrations do not necessarily correlate with hepatic dysfunction in adults. Bowyer and colleagues studied carnitine supplementation in adult patients receiving home PN who had abnormal serum liver enzymes and low serum carnitine concentrations. The investigators found no improvement in liver enzymes after carnitine was supplemented for 1 month, despite normalization of serum carnitine concentrations.[66] The role of carnitine in the prevention and treatment of PN-associated liver complications in adults remains to be established.

Choline

Choline is essential for normal function of all cells and required for lipid transport and metabolism. This nutrient is found in many foods, but it is not a component of PN formulations because it is assumed that endogenous synthesis is possible from methionine contained in the crystalline amino acid solution. However, the conversion of methionine to choline may be less efficient when methionine is given parenterally than when given orally.[67] Low plasma-free choline concentrations have been reported in patients receiving long-term PN and have been associated with elevated serum hepatic aminotransferase concentrations.[68] Steatosis resolved following choline supplementation in a small group of adult patients receiving long-term PN but did not resolve in a control group.[69]

At present, an injectable choline preparation is not commercially available. ASPEN recommends that a commercially available parenteral choline product be developed for routine addition to adult and PN formulas, either as an individual product or incorporated into a multivitamin product.[40]

Strategies to Manage Parenteral Nutrition–Associated Hepatobiliary Complications

When a patient receiving PN develops liver complications, clinicians should review all aspects of care to identify and eliminate or treat the various contributing factors. Table 17-1 provides monitoring parameters, and Table 17-2 outlines strategies to consider when a patient receiving PN develops liver complications. See Practice Scenario 17-3 for a discussion of management of cholestasis in an adult patient on long-term PN.

TABLE 17-2 Strategies to Manage Parenteral Nutrition–Associated Liver Complications

---

- Rule out non-PN etiologies for liver problems, such as hepatotoxic medications, herbal supplements, biliary obstruction, hepatitis, and sepsis.

- Consider PN modifications:
  - Decreasing dextrose.
  - Decreasing ILE (<1g/kg/d).
  - Providing a balance of dextrose and ILE.
  - Cyclic PN infusion.

- Maximize enteral intake:
  - Encourage oral diet.
  - Tube feeding, even at slow rate.

- Prevent/treat bacterial overgrowth:
  - Use enteral antibiotics, such as metronidazole, neomycin, doxycycline, ciprofloxacin, or rifaximin.
  - In CIPO patients, consider agents to enhance motility, such as metoclopramide or erythromycin.

- Pharmacotherapy:
  - Aggressively treat infection.
  - Prescribe ursodeoxycholic acid (ursodiol).
  - Treat pruritus with cholestyramine, rifampin, or phenobarbital.

- Consider intestinal transplantation for patients with PN failure.

CIPO, chronic intestinal pseudo-obstruction; ILE, lipid injectable emulsion; PN, parenteral nutrition.

Practice Scenario 17-3

Question: How can a parenteral nutrition (PN) formulation be modified to minimize and manage the development of cholestasis in an adult patient requiring long-term PN?

Scenario: A 72-year-old woman with a history of ovarian cancer and short bowel syndrome due to intestinal ischemia presents to the intestinal failure clinic for home-PN management after receiving home PN for the past year. She has approximately 120 cm of small bowel remaining with an end jejunostomy. A recent liver biopsy shows cholestasis and steatosis, and laboratory studies show elevated levels of serum transaminase, alkaline phosphatase, and conjugated/direct bilirubin (8 mg/dL). The patient is eating a regular diet and empties the ostomy appliance 10 times daily. Her weight is 50 kg and has been stable; her body mass index is 18.9. The home PN regimen provides protein 60 g, dextrose 250 g, and lipid 50 g; standard amounts of electrolytes, vitamins, and trace elements; and a volume of 2500 mL cycled over 15 hours nightly through a single-lumen tunneled catheter.

Intervention: The frequency of lipid injectable emulsion (ILE) is reduced from daily to twice weekly, and the amount of dextrose is increased proportionally to account for the decrease in energy from lipid. A trial of stopping ILE for 1 to 2 weeks could also be considered. The infusion cycle is shortened from 15 to 12 hours. Trace element levels are obtained, and supplemental copper and manganese are removed from the PN formulation.

Answer: Because the patient's weight is stable and the PN formulation provides 32 kcal/kg/d, neither the amount of dextrose nor the overall energy dose from PN seems excessive. Although the dose of ILE does not exceed 1 g/kg/d, a trial to decrease the dose/frequency may be beneficial. Infusing PN over a cyclic period rather than a continuous, 24-hour infusion rate may reduce risk for PN-associated liver disease (PNALD). The impact of changing the PN cycle from 15 to 12 hours may be minimal, but all efforts to minimize risk are warranted as long as the patient tolerates the changes. Finally, the dose of copper and manganese should be reduced or eliminated and levels monitored in this patient because her excretion of these elements is impaired.

Rationale: The PN formulation should be reviewed whenever liver complications develop. Although the PN therapy may not be implicated as the cause of the complication, it may contribute to or exacerbate the problem. Overfeeding should be avoided, and a trial of a lower-energy regimen may be warranted. Infection has been identified as a risk factor for development of PNALD; therefore, efforts to minimize the risk of infection are especially crucial. In the long-term patient who develops cholestasis, limiting the ILE dose may be beneficial.

Oral and Enteral Nutrition

Oral and enteral nutrition should be optimized whenever feasible in the patient on long-term PN because even small amounts of dietary or enteral intake may promote enterohepatic circulation of bile acids. Oral nutrition is generally preferable to tube feeding, for obvious reasons, but tube feeding may offer certain advantages in select patients. For example, patients with chronic intestinal pseudo-obstruction who depend on PN and require gastric decompression may tolerate jejunal feeding at a slow rate during a portion of the day or night. These patients may need medications to enhance motility, and multiple trials may be required before they achieve feeding tolerance. During periods of acute illness, enteral tolerance may be more difficult to achieve, and setbacks can be expected; however, clinicians should attempt to restart enteral feeding as soon as possible once the patient's condition has stabilized.

Patients with SBS should be encouraged to maximize oral intake because at least some of their intake will be absorbed. Depending on the severity of the SBS, a reduction in energy from PN may be necessary to prevent unwanted weight gain. However, the patient's fluid requirements generally remain high because stool output tends to increase when oral intake increases. See Chapter 30 for further discussion of nutrition support for patients with SBS.

Cyclic Infusion

Cyclic PN infusion refers to the infusion of a PN formulation over a period of less than 24 hours (generally 8 to 12 hours). This type of regimen gives the patient time off PN. Continuous PN infusion can result in hyperinsulinemia and fat deposition in the liver, thereby potentially increasing the risk of liver complications. Cyclic PN infusion has been shown to reduce serum liver enzyme and conjugated bilirubin concentrations when compared with continuous PN infusion.[7] Allowing time off PN each day may reduce the risk of PNALD, especially in patients who depend on long-term PN.

Pharmacotherapeutic Options

In addition to enteral intake, medications can be used to help stimulate bile flow and maintain gallbladder contractility. Ursodiol (ursodeoxycholic acid) is a form of bile acid widely used to treat various chronic cholestatic liver diseases, and it has been shown to improve biochemical markers of cholestasis. When given orally at therapeutic doses, it becomes the predominant biliary bile acid and is thought to displace potentially hepatotoxic bile salts. Data about using ursodiol to treat PNAC are limited. The medication may improve biochemical markers and symptoms of pruritis,[70] but there is no evidence that the progression of disease is delayed. No IV form of ursodiol is available; therefore, the use of ursodiol is limited to patients who can absorb oral medications.

CCK-octapeptide is a synthetic fragment of CCK that produces the biologic activities of CCK. It is available in an injectable form, but there is not enough evidence to support its use in the prevention or treatment of PNAC.

Phenobarbital has been used to relieve pruritus in patients with cholestasis and treat other types of cholestatic liver disease. However, evidence supporting its use to treat PNAC is lacking.

Transplantation

In the long-term PN patient with significant or progressive liver disease, an isolated intestinal or combined liver/intestinal transplant may be the only treatment option.[71,72] The Centers for Medicare and Medicaid Services (CMS) have approved reimbursement of intestinal transplantation for patients with intestinal failure who fail PN therapy. One of the CMS criteria to define PN failure is the development of impending or overt liver failure. The choice of an isolated small bowel transplantation vs a combined small bowel and liver transplantation depends on the extent of liver disease. Although many patients can stop PN after an intestinal transplantation, other life-threatening complications and quality-of-life issues must be considered before deciding on this intervention (see Chapter 31).

Metabolic Bone Disease

Osteoporosis and osteomalacia are associated with long-term PN use. Osteoporosis is the most common form of metabolic bone disease and is characterized by low bone mass, compromised bone strength, and deterioration of bone tissue and architecture.[73] It is a silent disease until it is complicated by fractures. According to World Health Organization criteria, the diagnosis of osteoporosis is based on a bone mineral density measurement that is more than 2.5 standard deviations below the mean score for young-adult, ethnicity- and sex-matched controls. It is reported as a T-score below –2.5. A T-score that ranges between –1 and –2.5 is considered low bone mass (osteopenia).

Osteomalacia is characterized as softening and bending of the bones that occurs because the bones contain osteoid tissue that has failed to calcify. This problem is generally caused by vitamin D deficiency. The diagnosis of osteomalacia requires a bone biopsy for histologic examination of bone tissue. Therefore, this condition is difficult to identify. Some patients may have a combination of osteoporosis and osteomalacia.

Prevalence

The prevalence of PN-associated metabolic bone disease is unknown, but compromised bone health is of concern in all patients requiring long-term PN. Pironi and colleagues reported osteoporosis in 41% of patients after at least 6 months of home PN,[74] and Cohen-Solal and associates identified osteoporosis in 67% of patients on long-term PN because of intestinal failure.[75] Many diseases, conditions, and medications increase the risk for bone loss (Table 17-3). Because almost all patients receiving long-term PN manifest at least 1 of these risk factors, it is unclear whether PN itself contributes to accelerated bone loss. In a follow-up study in a relatively large patient group receiving long-term PN according to more current protocols, participants had moderate bone loss that was not statistically different from bone loss in age- and sex-matched, healthy subjects.[76]

Parenteral Nutrition–Related Factors

Various factors related to the nutrient composition of the PN formulation could potentially interfere with bone

TABLE 17-3 Risk factors for Bone Loss

Postmenopausal osteoporosis
Long-term parenteral nutrition

Endocrine disease:
- Cushing's syndrome
- Hypogonadism
- Amenorrhea
- Hyperthyroidism
- Hyperparathyroidism

Gastrointestinal disease:
- Crohn's disease
- Short bowel syndrome
- Malabsorption

Malignancy:
- Multiple myeloma
- Leukemia

Medications:
- Corticosteroids
- Heparin
- Warfarin
- Levothyroxine overreplacement
- Phenytoin
- Phenobarbital
- Leuprolide
- Methotrexate

Genetic disease:
- Osteogenesis imperfecta

Immobilization:
- Spinal cord injury
- Prolonged bed rest

Other:
- Alcohol abuse
- Anorexia nervosa
- Roux-en-Y gastric bypass

metabolism.[77,78] Therefore, the PN formulation should be designed to minimize the risk for bone problems.

Calcium

Calcium plays a vital role in maintaining bone integrity by decreasing bone turnover and slowing bone loss. Patients receiving PN are at risk for negative calcium balance because of limited intake and increased urinary calcium loss. Calcium supplementation in the PN formulation is limited by the mineral's physical compatibility with phosphorus, and there seems to be a threshold for calcium uptake when given parenterally. Higher calcium doses provided in the PN formulation are offset by higher urinary calcium losses. Therefore, ASPEN recommends daily intake of 10 to 15 mEq calcium gluconate from the PN formulation.[8]

An inadequate phosphorus dose may increase urinary calcium excretion. Phosphorus seems to enhance calcium reabsorption by the renal tubules and thereby promote a positive calcium balance. The ASPEN recommendation for intake of phosphorus from the PN formulation is 20 to 40 mmol/d.[8]

Higher protein doses (2 g/kg/d vs 1 g/kg/d) in PN formulations have been associated with increased urinary calcium excretion. For this reason, reducing protein intake to maintenance doses whenever possible has been recommended.[77,79]

Chronic metabolic acidosis is associated with hypercalciuria and metabolic bone disease.[80] Correction of the acidosis with acetate in the PN formulation can reduce urinary calcium excretion; therefore, adequate acetate amounts should be added to the PN formulation to avoid metabolic acidosis.[77]

Finally, cyclic PN infusion results in higher urinary calcium losses when compared with continuous infusion.[81] However, this potential disadvantage associated with cyclic infusion should be weighed against its potential benefits to the liver and quality of life in long-term PN patients.

Vitamin D

Data regarding vitamin D requirements in patients receiving PN are controversial. Both vitamin D deficiency and vitamin D toxicity can result in bone disease. The adult multivitamin preparation used for PN formulations contains 200 IU of vitamin D (ergocalciferol or cholecalciferol). Vitamin D can be detrimental to the bone when excessive doses are given because it can suppress PTH secretion and directly promote bone resorption. There are reports that short-term removal of vitamin D from the PN formulation resulted in decreased hypercalciuria and an improvement in osteomalacia, although the results may have been influenced by the presence of significant aluminum contamination. In 9 patients receiving long-term PN who had low serum PTH and low 1,25-hydroxyvitamin D, long-term (average of 4.5 years) removal of vitamin D resulted in normal PTH and 1,25-hydroxyvitamin D concentrations and improved bone mineral density of the spine.[82] Although vitamin D removal may benefit certain patients, such as those with a low serum PTH concentration, it is impractical because there are no commercially available injectable multivitamin preparations without vitamin D. Certainly, excessive supplementation of vitamin D should be avoided.

Vitamin D status should be monitored to identify deficiency states, which can result in bone disease and poor mineralization. The prevalence of vitamin D deficiency is higher in patients with intestinal malabsorption syndromes than in the general population.[83,84] It is reasonable to provide PN patients with the maintenance vitamin D dose contained in the injectable multivitamin preparation. However, when supplemental doses of vitamin D are required to treat deficiency, the oral route is required because individual parenteral ergocalciferol or cholecalciferol products are not commercially available.

Aluminum

Osteomalacia was associated with PN formulations that contained significant aluminum contamination from protein hydrolysates. A low-turnover bone disease and decreased bone formation were described in patients with elevated plasma, urine, and bone aluminum concentrations. Aluminum contamination of PN formulations is significantly lower now that crystalline amino acids have replaced protein hydrolysates. However, aluminum contamination is still a concern and has prompted the US Food and Drug Administration (FDA) to establish labeling requirements. Manufacturers of large-volume parenteral products, small-volume parenteral products, and pharmacy bulk packages used in PN compounding are required to measure the aluminum content of the product and disclose the concentration on the label.[85] Large-volume parenteral products, including amino acid and concentrated dextrose solutions, ILE, and sterile water for injection, are required to contain no more than 25 mcg aluminum per liter. The FDA does not limit the aluminum content in small-volume parenteral products (ie, electrolyte salts) and pharmacy bulk packages (ie, parenteral multivitamins and trace element solutions), but manufacturers are required to state the maximum aluminum level at expiry in the product labeling.

Magnesium

Hypocalcemia is a prominent manifestation of magnesium deficiency. Magnesium deficiency results in decreased mobilization of calcium from bone through several mechanisms. Hypomagnesemia causes an increased release of magnesium ions at the bone surface in exchange for increased bone uptake of calcium ions from the serum. In addition, chronic severe hypomagnesemia inhibits PTH release, resulting in inappropriately low PTH levels for the degree of hypocalcemia. The response of bone to PTH can also be diminished, resulting in functional hypoparathyroidism. Hypomagnesemic hypocalcemia should be treated with magnesium supplementation because it is often refractory to calcium therapy alone. Magnesium deficiency can also lead to hypophosphatemia because of increased phosphorus excretion.

Copper

Copper deficiency impairs bone formation and can cause osteoporosis (see Chapter 8). Bone disease has been reported in infants receiving a copper-free PN formulation.[78]

Prevention and Management

Because most patients with osteoporosis are asymptomatic, a screening process is important to identify patients at risk. Clinicians should perform a thorough history, physical examination, and laboratory assessment to identify risk factors. Patients receiving long-term PN may lose height because of compression fractures of the vertebral bodies. A baseline dual-energy x-ray absorptiometry scan is recommended for all patients who require long-term PN therapy. In addition to routine laboratory monitoring, patients with low bone mineral density may require further diagnostic testing, including measurement of thyroid-stimulating hormone, intact PTH, 25-hydoxyvitamin D, 24-hour urine calcium and magnesium, urine markers of bone turnover (such as N-telopeptide collagen), and serum markers of bone turnover (such as osteocalcin and C-telopeptide collagen).

Strategies to prevent and treat osteoporosis should be considered in all patients who require long-term PN therapy, as outlined in Table 17-4. The PN formulation should be designed to minimize hypercalciuria; provide adequate magnesium, calcium, and phosphorus; avoid metabolic acidosis; provide vitamins and trace elements; and minimize aluminum contamination.[71] Individual products with the lowest-reported maximal aluminum content should be used in PN compounding whenever possible; for example, sodium phosphate is preferable to potassium phosphate.[86] Patients with osteoporosis should be educated on lifestyle modifications, low-intensity exercises, and fall prevention measures to minimize risk. Medications that improve bone mineral density and decrease fracture risk in patients with osteoporosis may also be used to prevent or treat osteoporosis. Medications that decrease bone resorption include bisphosphonates, raloxifene (a selective estrogen-receptor modulator), calcitonin,

TABLE 17-4 Strategies to Prevent and Treat Osteoporosis in Patients Receiving Long-Term Parenteral Nutrition

Strategy	Considerations
PN modifications	• Avoid high doses of protein. • Avoid excessive doses of sodium. • Calcium: 10 to 15 mEq/d. • Phosphorus: 20 to 40 mmol/d. • Treat metabolic acidosis. • Maintain adequate magnesium intake. • Maintain adequate copper intake. • Minimize aluminum contamination. • Avoid adding heparin.
Lifestyle modifications	• Weight-bearing exercises. • Stop smoking. • Reduce caffeine intake. • Reduce alcohol intake.
Fall prevention measures	• Increase safety of home. • Discontinue medications that may increase risk of falls, if possible.
Calcium	• Consider oral supplementation.
Vitamin D	• Consider oral supplementation, if patient has vitamin D deficiency.
Pharmacological treatment	• Perform a comprehensive risk assessment after the initial treatment period. • Do not consider any pharmacotherapy to be indefinite in duration. • Individualize treatment decisions. • Avoid oral route for bisphosphonate therapy due to malabsorption and tolerance issues in PN patients. • Consider endocrinology referral for management.

PN, parenteral nutrition.

estrogen, and the monoclonal antibody denosumab. Teripa-ratide is the only FDA-approved medication that stimulates bone formation.[74]

Summary

A thorough monitoring plan is required to identify and prevent short- and long-term metabolic complications in all patients receiving PN. Refeeding syndrome and hyperglycemia are significant risks in patients receiving PN in the acute care setting. In patients receiving long-term PN, potential complications include micronutrient abnormalities, hepatobiliary problems, and metabolic bone disease. Even though the PN itself may not be the sole cause of these complications, efforts to minimize contributing risk factors from the PN formula should be taken.

References

1. Lewis KS, Kane-Gill SL, Bobek MB, et al. Intensive insulin therapy for critically ill patients. *Ann Pharmacother.* 2004;38:1243–1251.
2. Mehanna HM, Moledina J, Travis J. Refeeding syndrome: what it is, and how to prevent and treat it. *BMJ.* 2008;336:1495–1498.
3. Byrnes MC, Stangenes J. Refeeding in the ICU: an adult and pediatric problem. *Curr Opin Clin Nutr Metab Care.* 2011;14:186–192.
4. Weinsier RL, Krumdieck CL. Death resulting from overzealous total parenteral nutrition: the refeeding syndrome revisited. *Am J Clin Nutr.* 1981;34:393–399.
5. Brown KA, Dickerson RN, Morgan LM, et al. A new graduated dosing regimen for phosphorus replacement in patients receiving nutrition support. *JPEN J Parenter Enteral Nutr.* 2006;30:209–214.
6. Cavicchi M, Beau P, Crenn P, et al. Prevalence of liver disease and contributing factors in patients receiving home parenteral nutrition for permanent intestinal failure. *Ann Intern Med.* 2000;132:525–532.
7. Hwang TL, Lue MC, Chen LL. Early use of cyclic TPN prevents further deterioration of liver functions for the TPN patients with impaired liver function. *Hepatogastroenterology.* 2000;47:1347–1350.
8. Task Force for the Revision of Safe Practices for Parenteral Nutrition. Safe practices for parenteral nutrition. *JPEN J Parenter Enteral Nutr.* 2004;28(6 Suppl):S39–S70.
9. McMahon MM, Nystrom E, Braunschweig C, Miles J, Compher C. A.S.P.E.N clinical guidelines: nutrition support of adult patients with hyperglycemia. *JPEN J Parenter Enteral Nutr.* 2013;37:23–36.
10. Jacobi J, Bircher N, Krinsley J, et al. Guidelines for the use of an insulin infusion for management of hyperglycemia in critically ill patients. *Crit Care Med.* 2012;40:3251–3276.
11. McMahon MM. Management of parenteral nutrition in acutely ill patients with hyperglycemia. *Nutr Clin Pract.* 2004;19:120–128.
12. Hopkins LL Jr, Ransome-Kuti O, Majaj AS. Improvement of impaired carbohydrate metabolism by chromium (III) in malnourished infants. *Am J Clin Nutr.* 1968;21:203–211.
13. Jeejeebhoy KN, Chu RC, Marliss EB, et al. Chromium deficiency, glucose intolerance, and neuropathy reversed by chromium supplementation in a patient receiving long-term total parenteral nutrition. *Am J Clin Nutr.* 1977;30:531–538.
14. McCurdy DK. Hyperosmolar hyperglycemia nonketotic diabetic coma. *Med Clin North Am.* 1970;54:683–699.
15. Stout SM, Cober MP. Metabolic effects of cyclic parenteral nutrition infusion in adults and children. *Nutr Clin Pract.* 2010;25:277–281.

16. Krzywda EA, Andris DA, Whipple JK, et al. Glucose response to abrupt initiation and discontinuation of total parenteral nutrition. *JPEN J Parenter Enteral Nutr.* 1993;17:64–67.
17. Eisenberg PG, Gianino S, Clutter WE, et al. Abrupt discontinuation of cycled parenteral nutrition is safe. *Dis Colon Rectum.* 1995;38:933–939.
18. Hamilton C, Austin T, Seidner DL. Essential fatty acid deficiency in human adults during parenteral nutrition. *Nutr Clin Pract.* 2006;21:387–394.
19. Holman RT, Smythe L, Johnson S. Effect of sex and age on fatty acid composition of human serum lipids. *Am J Clin Nutr.* 1979;32:2390–2399.
20. Miller DG, Williams SK, Palombo JD, et al. Cutaneous application of safflower oil in preventing essential fatty acid deficiency in patients on home parenteral nutrition. *Am J Clin Nutr.* 1987;46:419–423.
21. Friedman Z, Shochat SJ, Maisels MJ, et al. Correction of essential fatty acid deficiency in newborn infants by cutaneous application of sunflower-seed oil. *Pediatrics.* 1976;58:650–654.
22. Vanek VW, Seidner DL, Allen P, et al. A.S.P.E.N. position paper: clinical role for alternative intravenous fat emulsions. *JPEN J Parenter Enteral Nutr.* 2012;27:150–192.
23. McClave SA, Taylor BE, Martindale RG, et al. Guidelines for the provision and assessment of nutrition support therapy in the adult critically ill patient: Society of Critical Care Medicine (SCCM) and American Society for Parenteral and Enteral Nutrition (A.S.P.E.N.). *JPEN J Parenter Enteral Nutr.* 2016;40:159–211.
24. Battistella FD, Widergren JT, Anderson JT, et al. A prospective, randomized trial of intravenous fat emulsion administration in trauma victims requiring total parenteral nutrition. *J Trauma.* 1997;43:52–58.
25. Seidner DL, Mascioli EA, Istfan NW, et al. Effects of long-chain triglyceride emulsions on reticuloendothelial system function in humans. *JPEN J Parenter Enteral Nutr.* 1989;13:614–619.
26. Carpentier YA, Kinney JM, Sidebrova VS, et al. Hypertriglyceridemia clamp: a new model for studying lipid metabolism. *Clin Nutr.* 1990;9(Suppl 1):1–9.
27. Adamkin DH, Gelke KN, Andrews BF. Fat emulsions and hypertriglyceridemia. *JPEN J Parenter Enteral Nutr.* 1984;8:563–567.
28. Kapila S, Saba M, Lin CH, Bawle EV. Arginine deficiency-induced hyperammonemia in a home total parenteral nutrition-dependent patient: a case report. *JPEN J Parenter Enteral Nutr.* 2001;25:286–288.
29. Felig DM, Brusilow SW, Boyer JL. Hyperammonemic coma due to parenteral nutrition in a woman with heterozygous ornithine transcarbamylase deficiency. *Gastroenterology.* 1995;109:282–284.
30. Sacks GS, Mayhew S, Johnson D. Parenteral nutrition implementation and management. In: Merritt RM, ed. *The A.S.P.E.N. Nutrition Support Practice Manual.* 2nd ed. Silver Spring, MD: American Society for Parenteral and Enteral Nutrition; 2005:108–117.
31. Kraft MD, Btaiche IF, Sacks GS, et al. Treatment of electrolyte disorders in adult patients in the intensive care unit. *Am J Health Syst Pharm.* 2005;62:1663–1682.
32. Ayers P, Adams S, Boullata J, et al. A.S.P.E.N. parenteral nutrition safety consensus recommendations. *JPEN J Parenter Enteral Nutr.* 2014;38:296–333.
33. Centers for Disease Control and Prevention. Lactic acidosis traced to thiamin deficiency related to nationwide shortage of multivitamins for total parenteral nutrition—United States, 1997. *JAMA.* 1997;278:109–111.
34. Kraft MD, Btaiche IF, Sacks GS. Review of the refeeding syndrome. *Nutr Clin Pract.* 2005;20:625–633.

35. American Society for Parenteral and Enteral Nutrition Board of Directors and the Clinical Guidelines Task Force. Guidelines for the use of parenteral and enteral nutrition in adult and pediatric patients. *JPEN J Parenter Enteral Nutr.* 2002;26(1 Suppl): 1SA–138SA.

36. Howard L, Chu R, Feman S, et al. Vitamin A deficiency from long-term parenteral nutrition. *Ann Intern Med.* 1980;93:576–577.

37. Plogsted S, Adams SC, Allen K, et al. Parenteral nutrition multivitamin product shortage considerations. *Nutr Clin Pract.* 2016; 31:556–559.

38. Fleming CR, Lie JT, McCall JT, et al. Selenium deficiency and fatal cardiomyopathy in a patient on home parenteral nutrition. *Gastroenterology.* 1982;83:689–693.

39. Yusef SW, Rehman Q, Casscells W. Cardiomyopathy in association with selenium deficiency: a case report. *JPEN J Parenter Enteral Nutr.* 2002;26:63–66.

40. Vanek VW, Borum P, Buchman A, et al. A.S.P.E.N. position paper: recommendations for changes in commercially available parenteral multivitamin and multi-trace element products. *Nutr Clin Pract.* 2012;27:440–491.

41. Pluhator-Murton MM, Fedorak RN, Audette RJ, et al. Trace element contamination of total parenteral nutrition: 1. Contribution of component solutions. *JPEN J Parenter Enteral Nutr.* 1999; 23:222–227.

42. Howard L, Ashley C, Lyon D, et al. Autopsy tissue trace elements in 8 long-term parenteral nutrition patients who received the current U.S. Food and Drug Administration formulation. *JPEN J Parenter Enteral Nutr.* 2007;31:388–396.

43. Fessler TA. Trace elements in parenteral nutrition: a practical guide for dosage and monitoring for adult patients. *Nutr Clin Pract.* 2013;28:722–729.

44. Plogsted S, Adams SC, Allen K, et al. Parenteral nutrition trace element product shortage considerations. *Nutr Clin Pract.* 2016;31(6):843–847. doi:10.1177/0884533616670374.

45. Koruru P, Abraham BP. The role of ferric carboxymaltose in the treatment of iron deficiency anemia in patients with gastrointestinal disease. *Ther Adv Gastroenterol.* 2016;9:76–85.

46. Kumpf VJ. Update on parenteral iron therapy. *Nutr Clin Pract.* 2003;18:318–326.

47. Solomon SM, Kirby DF. The refeeding syndrome: a review. *JPEN J Parenter Enteral Nutr.* 1990;14:90–97.

48. Walmsley RS. Refeeding syndrome: screening, incidence, and treatment during parenteral nutrition. *J Gastroenterol Hepatol.* 2013;28:113–117.

49. O'Connor G, Nicholis D. Refeeding hypophosphatemia in adolescents with anorexia nervosa: a symptomatic review. *Nutr Clin Pract.* 2013;298:358–364.

50. Skipper A. Refeeding syndrome or refeeding hypophosphatemia: a systematic review of cases. *Nutr Clin Pract.* 2012;27:34–40.

51. Crook MA. Refeeding syndrome: problems with definition and management. *Nutrition.* 2014;30:1448–1455.

52. Kumpf VJ. Parenteral nutrition-associated liver disease in adult and pediatric patients. *Nutr Clin Pract.* 2006;21:279–290.

53. Beath SV, Kelly DA. Total parenteral nutrition-induced cholestasis: prevention and management. *Clin Liver Dis.* 2016;20:159–176.

54. Quigley EMM, Marsh MN, Shaffer JL, et al. Hepatobiliary complications of total parenteral nutrition. *Gastroenterology.* 1993;104: 286–301.

55. Messing B, Bories C, Kunstlinger F, et al. Does total parenteral nutrition induce gallbladder sludge formation and lithiasis? *Gastroenterology.* 1983;84:1012–1019.

56. Luman W, Shaffer JL. Prevalence, outcome and associated factors of deranged liver function tests in patients on home parenteral nutrition. *Clin Nutr.* 2002;21:337–343.

57. Buchman A. Total parenteral nutrition-associated liver disease. *JPEN J Parenter Enteral Nutr.* 2002;26(5 Suppl):S43–S48.

58. Ellegard L, Sunesson A, Bosaeus I. High serum phytosterol levels in short bowel patients on parenteral nutrition support. *Clin Nutr.* 2005;24:415–420.

59. Btaiche IF, Khalidi N. Parenteral nutrition-associated liver complications in children. *Pharmacotherapy.* 2002;22:188–211.

60. Calder PC. Hot topics in parenteral nutrition: rationale for using new lipid emulsions in parenteral nutrition and a review of the trials performed in adults. *Proc Nutr Soc.* 2009;68:252–260.

61. Bharadwaj S, Gohel T, Deen OJ, DeChicco R, Shatnawei A. Fish-oil based lipid emulsion: current updates on a promising novel therapy for the management of parenteral nutrition-associated liver disease. *Gastroenterol Rep.* 2015;3:110–114.

62. de Meijer VE, Gura KM, Meisel JA, et al. Parenteral fish oil monotherapy in the management of patients with parenteral nutrition-associated liver disease. *Arch Surg.* 2010;145:547–551.

63. Wales PW, Allen N, Worthington P, et al. A.S.P.E.N. clinical guidelines: support of pediatric patients with intestinal failure at risk of parenteral nutrition-associated liver disease. *JPEN J Parenteral Enteral Nutr.* 2014;38:538–557.

64. Biesboer AN, Stoehr NA. A product review of alternative oil-based intravenous fat emulsions. *Nutr Clin Pract.* 2016;31:610–618.

65. Mundi MS, Salonen BR, Bonnes S. Home parenteral nutrition: fat emulsions and potential complications. *Nutr Clin Pract.* 2016; 31:629–641.

66. Bowyer BA, Miles JM, Haymond MW, et al. L-carnitine therapy in home parenteral nutrition patients with abnormal liver tests and low plasma carnitine concentrations. *Gastroenterology.* 1988;94:434–438.

67. Chawla RK, Berry CJ, Kutner MH, et al. Plasma concentrations of transsulfuration pathway products during nasoenteral and intravenous hyperalimentation of malnourished patients. *Am J Clin Nutr.* 1985;42:577–584.

68. Buchman AL, Moukarzel AA, Jenden DJ, et al. Low plasma free choline is prevalent in patients receiving long-term parenteral nutrition and is associated with hepatic aminotransferase abnormalities. *Clin Nutr.* 1993;12:33–37.

69. Buchman AL, Ament ME, Sohel M, et al. Choline deficiency causes reversible hepatic abnormalities in patients receiving parenteral nutrition: proof of a human choline requirement: a placebo-controlled trial. *JPEN J Parenteral Enteral Nutr.* 2001;25:260–268.

70. San Luis VA, Btaiche IF. Ursodiol in patients with parenteral nutrition-associated cholestasis. *Ann Pharmacother.* 2007;41:1867–1872.

71. Pironi L, Arends J, Bozzetti F, et al. ESPEN guidelines on chronic intestinal failure in adults. *Clin Nutr.* 2016;35:247–307.

72. Iyer KR. Surgical management of short bowel syndrome. *JPEN J Parenter Enteral Nutr.* 2014;38(Suppl 1):53S–59S.

73. Cosman F, deBeur SJ, LeBoff MS, et al. Clinician's guide to prevention and treatment of osteoporosis. *Osteoporos Int.* 2014;25: 2359–2381.

74. Pironi L, Labate AM, Pertkiewicz M, et al. Prevalence of bone disease in patients on home parenteral nutrition. *Clin Nutr.* 2002; 21:289–296.

75. Cohen-Solal M, Baudoin C, Joly F, et al. Osteoporosis in patients on long-term home parenteral nutrition: a longitudinal study. *J Bone Miner Res.* 2003;18:1989–1994.

76. Haderslev KV, Tjellesen L, Haderslev PH, et al. Assessment of the longitudinal changes in bone mineral density in patients receiving home parenteral nutrition. *JPEN J Parenter Enteral Nutr.* 2004;28:289–294.

77. Seidner DL. Parenteral nutrition-associated metabolic bone disease. *JPEN J Parenter Enteral Nutr.* 2002;26(5 Suppl):S37–S42.

78. Buchman AL, Moukarzel A. Metabolic bone disease associated with total parenteral nutrition. *Clin Nutr.* 2000;19:217–231.

79. Bengoa JM, Sitrin DM, Wood RJ, et al. Amino acid–induced hypercalciuria in patients on total parenteral nutrition. *Am J Clin Nutr*. 1983;83:264–269.

80. Cunningham J, Fraher LJ, Clemens TL, et al. Chronic acidosis in metabolic bone disease: effect of alkali on bone density and vitamin D metabolism. *Am J Med*. 1982;73:199–204.

81. Wood RJ, Bengoa JM, Sitrin MD, et al. Calciuretic effect of cyclic versus continuous total parenteral nutrition. *Am J Clin Nutr*. 1985;41:614–619.

82. Verhage AH, Cheong WK, Allard JP, et al. Increase in lumbar spine bone mineral content in patients on long-term parenteral nutrition without vitamin D supplementation. *JPEN J Parenter Enteral Nutr*. 1995;19:431–436.

83. Margulies SL, Kurian D, Elliott MS, Han Z. Vitamin D deficiency in patients with intestinal malabsorption syndromes—think in and outside the gut. *J Dig Dis*. 2015;16:617–633.

84. Fan S, Ni X, Wang J, et al. High prevalence of suboptimal vitamin D status and bone loss in adult short bowel syndrome even after weaning off parenteral nutrition. *Nutr Clin Pract*. 2017; 32:258–265.

85. US Food and Drug Administration. Amendment of regulations on parenteral nutrition; delay of effective date. *Fed Register*. 2003; 68:32979–32981.

86. Smith BS, Kothari H, Hayes BD, et al. Effect of additive selection on calculated aluminum content of parenteral nutrient solutions. *Am J Health Syst Pharm*. 2007;64:730–739.

18 Drug-Nutrient Interactions

Amber Verdell, PharmD, BCPS, BCNSP,
and Carol J. Rollins, MS, RD, CNSC, PharmD, BCNSP, FASPEN

CONTENTS

Objectives

1. Describe 3 different types of drug-nutrient interactions (DNIs) related to parenteral nutrition (PN) or enteral nutrition (EN), and give an example of each.
2. List 2 drug- or formula-related factors that may contribute to DNIs with PN formulations and EN formulations.
3. Determine when intermittently stopping enteral feeding or changing the EN formulation is more likely to result in successful management or prevention of a DNI.
4. List the usual steps for administering a drug via the feeding tube or when PN is also being administered, and explain why these steps are more appropriate than other methods including admixture of a drug with parenteral or enteral feeding formulations.

Test Your Knowledge Questions

1. An alert and oriented adult patient is receiving a continuous infusion of a standard, fiber-containing EN formulation through an 8-Fr nasogastric (NG) tube. Drugs administered by bolus administration through the side port of the tube are phenytoin suspension 400 mg daily and nizatidine 150 mg every 12 hours. The feeding tube becomes occluded and must be removed. A new tube is placed because a long-term tube will not be considered until after a swallow study is completed 2½ weeks from now. Which of the following measures is most appropriate for preventing occlusion of the new tube?
   A. Replace the 8-Fr tube with an 18-Fr NG tube.
   B. Flush the feeding tube with 15 mL of water before and after administering each medication.
   C. Discontinue the fiber-containing enteral feeding formulation, and initiate feeding with a fiber-free formulation.
   D. Hold the feeding infusion for 2 hours before and after administering phenytoin.

2. The EN formulation for a home patient receiving EN through a percutaneous gastrostomy was recently changed from a high-protein, fiber-containing, 1 kcal/mL formulation to the only 1.5 kcal/mL formulation available in the local store. The new product is marketed for use in patients with compromised pulmonary function and contains low amounts of carbohydrate, 55% of energy from fat, about 15% less protein per day than the 1 kcal/mL formulation, and no fiber. What component of the new formulation is most likely to contribute to interactions resulting from slow gastric emptying?
   A. Lower fiber content
   B. Lower protein content
   C. Higher fat content
   D. Higher energy density

3. Which of the following is the preferred method of administering a hospitalized patient's antihypertensive medication when tube feeding is started due to poor oral intake?
   A. By the oral route
   B. As an oral liquid via the feeding tube
   C. As a crushed tablet via the feeding tube
   D. By the intravenous (IV) route

4. A medication that is ordered as a liquid to be administered via the feeding tube is available in the pharmacy in the IV form, as a capsule (powdered drug in a hard gelatin capsule), and as a film-coated tablet. What is the most appropriate and cost-effective choice for administration of this medication?
   A. Administer the IV form via the IV route.
   B. Administer the IV form via the feeding tube.
   C. Make a slurry of the capsule's powder and administer via the feeding tube.
   D. Crush the tablet to a fine powder and administer via the feeding tube.

Test Your Knowledge Answers

1. The correct answer is **B**. The most likely cause of the feeding tube occlusion is improper flushing technique (see Chapters 12 and 13). The tube should be flushed with a minimum of 15 mL of water before and after each medication, but 30 mL is commonly recommended and may be required to properly flush longer or larger tubes.[1,2] Although the risk of occlusion is potentially greater with an 8-Fr small-bore tube than with an 18-Fr tube, the discomfort associated with such a large-bore tube would make it a poor choice for nasoenteral access in an alert patient, especially when needed for more than 2 weeks. Switching from a fiber-containing to a fiber-free EN formulation would have little influence on risk of tube occlusion. The fiber used in EN formulations has been processed to a degree that makes its viscosity similar to that of polymeric, fiber-free formulations.[3] Holding the feeding infusion for 2 hours before and after phenytoin administration has been recommended as a method to enhance drug absorption; it would not be expected to influence tube occlusion.

2. The correct answer is **C**. High fat intake slows gastric emptying. High protein intake and high energy density can also slow gastric emptying but have less effect than high fat. In addition, protein intake will be lower with the new formulation. Low fiber intake has been associated with slow colonic transit and constipation rather than altered gastric emptying.

3. The correct answer is **A**. The oral route is preferred whenever possible because it is the route by which oral medications are designed to be administered. If the patient is allowed to take adequate water to swallow the medication, the oral route should be considered. For medications to be taken with food, the patient should have either food from oral ingestion or enteral formulation in the stomach before medication administration by mouth. Medications that are not administered via the feeding tube will not cause tube occlusion, making oral administration a very effective method of preventing tube occlusion caused by medications.

4. The correct answer is **C**. IV administration is generally the most expensive method and requires IV access. Use of IV dosage forms via the gastrointestinal (GI) tract is not usually recommended because these dosage forms are not designed to withstand the environment of the GI tract (gastric acid), and adequate amounts may not reach the bloodstream after presystemic metabolism in the GI tract mucosa (eg, cytochrome P450 [CYP450] metabolism) and first-pass metabolism in the liver. Crushing a film-coated tablet can be difficult because the film coating tends to remain intact and can become sticky when wetted with water. That makes administration via a feeding tube challenging. Most hard gelatin capsules can be opened and the powder inside combined with water to make a slurry for administration via a feeding tube.

Background

Interactions between medications (ie, drugs) and PN or EN have the potential to adversely affect patient outcomes because of loss of feeding access, loss of access for drug administration, or inappropriate response to drugs and/or altered absorption of nutrients. Numerous factors must be considered to prevent or mitigate DNIs, including the route and method of drug administration, the dosage form, and the medication's pharmacokinetic properties (primarily absorption and metabolism), as well as its stability and compatibility characteristics. Factors related to nutrition support that may influence DNIs include the type and site of access, method of administration, and content of the PN or EN formulation.

Unfortunately, the US Food and Drug Administration does not require manufacturers to evaluate drugs for altered pharmacokinetic parameters or potential DNIs when administered via tube into the stomach, duodenum, or jejunum. Few DNIs are well studied in patients receiving PN or EN therapy, and studies that do exist often focus on in vitro physical interactions or use small numbers of healthy volunteers with simulated feeding access (eg, ingesting an EN formulation by mouth rather than by feeding tube). Studies in patients are typically not blinded, lack placebo control, and are retrospective in nature. Observational studies and case reports from very small numbers of patients are often the only data available. Thus, understanding of the mechanism of interaction is often poor, and the strength of evidence supporting methods to prevent or mitigate DNIs in patients receiving PN or EN therapy is seldom strong. Even the limited data available in the literature are sometimes conflicting, leading to multiple approaches to manage a DNI. Despite these limited and conflicting data, it is often possible to identify general principles that apply to management of DNIs. This chapter presents general principles to consider with DNIs and discusses specific issues related to the concurrent administration of drugs with PN or EN therapy. The chapter is not intended to be inclusive of all potential DNIs that the clinician may encounter; rather, it is intended to illustrate certain common clinical dilemmas.

Types of Interactions

The American Society for Parenteral and Enteral Nutrition has defined a DNI as "an event that occurs when nutrient availability is altered by a medication, or when a drug effect is altered or an adverse reaction is caused by the intake of nutrients."[4] This is a broad definition that encompasses many types and potential mechanisms of interaction between drugs and nutrients. Table 18-1 illustrates one system for classifying DNIs; other systems using somewhat different categories and terminology are also in use.[5] The focus of this chapter is primarily on the physical, pharmaceutical, and pharmacokinetic interactions because these are the types most likely to present problems specific to PN or EN therapy, although they can occur in patients receiving an oral diet as well. Other types of interactions, such as electrolyte alterations related to specific medications, also occur in patients receiving nutrition support, but they tend to be independent of the route of nutrition and will occur whether the patient receives PN, EN, or an oral diet.

Physical Interactions

Interactions that result in altered physical characteristics of the nutrition formulation or the drug occur with both PN and EN therapy. Occlusion of the feeding access device is frequently the outcome of physical interactions. Other outcomes can include reduced bioavailability of the drug or nutrients, although studies seldom address effects of DNIs on nutrients. Physical interactions typically occur in the delivery device before the drug or nutrients reach the patient; therefore, this type of interaction can be referred to as an ex vivo interaction.[5] Variables to consider when assessing the

TABLE 18-1 Classification of Drug-Nutrient Interactions

Type of Interaction	Effects of Interaction	Associated Factors
Physical	• Precipitation in PN or EN formulations • Disruption of emulsion for ILEs or EN formulation • Altered viscosity, change in consistency, clumping, or curdling of EN formulation	• Drug and formulation pH • Reactive chemical moieties • Protein complexity • Time • Temperature • Duration of exposure
Pharmaceutical	• Loss of drug activity • Toxicity	• Alteration of a specialized dosage form or administration by a different route than that for which it was designed
Pharmacokinetic	• Loss of drug activity • Toxicity	• Occurs before the drug or nutrient reaches the site of action • Altered absorption, presystemic metabolism, hepatic metabolism
Pharmacodynamic	• Loss of drug activity • Toxicity	• Occurs at the site of action • Binding sites or receptors usually involved
Pharmacological	• Inability to provide PN or EN therapy because of adverse effects	• Extension of a drug's normal pharmacological actions

EN, enteral nutrition; ILE, lipid injectable emulsion; PN, parenteral nutrition.

risk of physical interactions include the pH at which the drug and the PN or EN formulation is most stable; presence of cations and anions known to react chemically; concentration and chemical complexity of nutrients; and time, temperature, and duration of exposure to one another. This latter factor is one reason that admixture of drugs with a PN or EN formulation is very different than y-site administration or coadministration.

Parenteral Nutrition

Many studies evaluating compatibility between drugs and PN rely on visual inspection, measured turbidity, or increased particle count. Visually evident physical changes, such as turbidity, haziness, cloudiness, color changes, or precipitate formation in PN formulations, indicate incompatibility, as does emulsion disruption in lipid-containing PN. Drugs that show no evidence of physical interaction with PN are generally classified as compatible. However, some interactions result in a loss of drug or nutrient activity that requires chemical or molecular analysis for detection; no visible changes occur in the product(s). Admixture of octreotide acetate to PN formulations results in no visible changes (visibly compatible); nevertheless, incompatibility occurs due to development of a glycosyl octreotide conjugate and loss of drug activity (chemically incompatible).[6,7] In addition, injectable multivitamin preparations are compatible with PN formulations, although some vitamins, such as thiamin, have limited stability and begin to very quickly lose their activity once added to the PN formulation because of hydrolysis, photodegradation, or other forms of chemical degradation (see Chapter 15) that may not be visible. Visual compatibility does not ensure chemical stability and drug or nutrient activity.

Safety guidelines that address the stability and compatibility of PN formulations have been developed.[8-10] When drugs are administered with PN, either by admixture or co-infusion, the method of administration should ensure that both the drug and the PN formulation are stable and free from incompatibility. General principles for evaluating compatibility of drugs with a PN formulation include obtaining data for both physical compatibility and chemical stability of the drug and PN components whenever possible.

Both physical compatibility and chemical stability are influenced by pH. Because most PN formulations have a slightly acidic pH (5 to 6.5), drugs requiring a high pH or low pH for best solubility are typically incompatible with PN (see Practice Scenario 18-1 for a discussion of drug compatibility with PN). Increasing time of exposure between the PN and drug increases the risk of interactions; therefore, admixture of a drug into a PN formulation poses greater risk of interaction than co-infusion. Factors to consider include (1) details related to the specific drug formulation (eg, with or without preservative, salt form) and drug concentrations evaluated, (2) specific components in the PN formulation, and (3) environmental conditions during evaluation (temperature[s] in particular). Dextrose and amino acid concentration, specific brand of amino acids used for compounding, inclusion of lipid injectable emulsion (ILE), the specific type of ILE, electrolyte concentrations and specific electrolytes added, and addition of

trace elements, heparin, insulin, and other components can all influence compatibility and stability of PN formulations. When admixing a drug with PN, efficacy and toxicity profiles must be acceptable with administration by continuous infusion rather than intermittent infusion. Clinical application of principles of drug compatibility and PN formulations is discussed in Chapter 15.

Practice Scenario 18-1

Question: What factor(s) is most likely to result in occlusion of the vascular access device (VAD) when a patient is receiving several drugs and parenteral nutrition (PN) through the VAD?

Scenario: A 44-year-old man who underwent hematopoietic cell transplant 6 weeks ago is currently receiving PN with separate lipid injectable emulsion and patient-controlled analgesia with morphine sulfate (1 mg/mL concentration) through his tunneled VAD. Ceftazidime, fluconazole, and foscarnet are also administered through the VAD. Calcium chloride, 1 g every 8 hours, is ordered for adding to PN to address the patient's increased calcium requirements. This form of calcium is chosen because of a shortage of calcium gluconate and because the patient requires high phosphate content in the PN, which would limit addition of calcium gluconate. Medications are ordered for "minimum fluid" to limit fluid administration because he receives platelet and red blood cell transfusions 3 or 4 times weekly. The VAD is double lumen; however, the patient's nurse states that 1 lumen is occluded. Two attempts to clear the catheter with a thrombolytic agent failed. The morphine has continued through the patent line. Foscarnet, ceftazidime, fluconazole, and PN are on hold until access can be obtained.

Intervention: A 0.1-N hydrochloric acid solution is ordered. After confirming acceptability of hydrochloric acid use with the patient's silicone catheter, the nurse instilled the ordered dose in the occluded lumen and allowed it to dwell for 30 minutes before attempting to withdraw the solution. The procedure is repeated once because the catheter was still "sluggish" after the first attempt.

Answer: Several factors, including pH, time, administration method, and PN composition can contribute to physical interactions that occlude the VAD. When the pH of PN and the pH at which a drug is most soluble differ significantly, there is a high risk of the drug precipitating when co-infused with PN. The administration regimen should be reviewed. In addition, the composition of the PN and the co-infused drug should be reviewed. A high concentration of a potentially incompatible component of PN (eg, phosphate) and/or a high concentration of a potentially incompatible product to be co-infused (eg, calcium chloride) will increase precipitation risk. Electrolyte concentrations are typically several times higher in a supplemental dose than in PN; thus, the rationale that an electrolyte such as calcium is usually in PN and therefore can be co-infused is erroneous. Precipitation of calcium phosphate is the most likely cause of VAD occlusion if calcium is co-infused with PN, particularly when the co-infusion occurs below the PN filter.

Rationale: Evidence supports most antibiotics in the cephalosporin class, including ceftazidime, as compatible with PN; therefore, ceftazidime is unlikely to have caused the occlusion.[7] Data also support fluconazole compatibility with PN. Limited evidence suggests foscarnet is compatible for co-infusion with PN; however, other data indicate its incompatibility with calcium-containing solutions. Given this mixed picture of compatibility, foscarnet may cause problems if co-infused with PN containing calcium. In this case, the patient is receiving calcium chloride outside the PN. Calcium is known to precipitate with phosphate when the solubility product of calcium phosphate is exceeded, which is likely to occur if calcium chloride is co-infused with PN containing phosphate. Thrombolytic agents are not effective in clearing drug precipitate. Altering the pH within the VAD lumen to make the drug more soluble can often clear the occlusion. However, the risk vs benefit of attempting line salvage should be considered. Generally, salvage is more likely to be attempted with a long-term tunneled or implanted VAD. However, the compatibility between catheter materials and the recommended clearance solution should be confirmed prior to attempting salvage. Many peripherally inserted central catheters are made from polyurethane whereas tunneled catheters are often composed of silicone. With calcium phosphate precipitate, decreasing the pH by instilling 0.1 N hydrochloric acid will increase calcium phosphate solubility and may be effective in clearing the occlusion. Discussion with the nurse reveals the infusion arrangement changed last evening. The patient was receiving a blood transfusion when his calcium dose was due, and he was to receive platelets once the red cell transfusion was completed. Therefore, the nurse co-infused calcium chloride with the PN, which contained above-standard amounts of potassium phosphate due to effects of foscarnet. A 0.22-micron filter was on the PN lumen of a bifurcation device connected to the catheter lumen; however, there was no filter after the calcium mixed with the PN solution.

Enteral Nutrition

Use of enteral feeding tubes as a drug delivery device increases the risk of various interactions between the drug, the EN formulation, and the feeding tube. Physical interactions can be a significant problem when drugs are allowed to mix with EN formulations. Several studies have evaluated physical compatibility between various drugs in liquid form (elixirs, solutions, suspensions) and EN formulations. Almost all of these studies were performed more than 25 years ago and tested relatively few drugs and even fewer EN formulations.[11-16] Direct application of these results to current clinical practice is difficult because drug and EN formulations may have been altered by the manufacturer while maintaining the same product name. Nevertheless, principles of compatibility can be gleaned from these studies.

Both the drug and the EN formulation affect the risk of physical interactions. The presence of complex protein (ie, intact or whole protein, not hydrolyzed protein or free amino acids) seems to be a critical property for determining risk of developing a physical interaction. Protein source (caseinates, soy, whey) may have some effect on interactions; however, fiber content, nitrogen content, and dilution of the EN formulation

have not been shown to affect the risk of physical interactions with drugs in studies reported in the literature.[11-15,17] Theoretically, dilution of the EN formula is expected to improve drug dissolution and reduce interactions; however, formula dilution is not recommended because it increases risk of microbial contamination.[2] Two factors are of particular importance with drugs in liquid form: (1) acidic pH, and (2) base components, especially sugar-water syrups, alcohol-containing elixirs, or oil-based products.[11-13,17,18] These factors are probably more important than the drug per se in most cases; however, it is important to recognize that pH and base components are selected to optimize solubility of a particular drug.

Overall, approximately one-third of drugs in liquid dosage forms evaluated for physical interactions with EN formulations have demonstrated undesirable effects (precipitation, curdling, clumping) with at least 1 EN formulation.[11-14,17,18] Of 25 drugs reported to be incompatible with intact protein formulations in these studies, only 3 (1 potassium chloride liquid and 2 oil-based products—medium chain triglyceride oil and methenamine suspension) were incompatible with a hydrolyzed EN formulation. Of the 12 drugs tested with both fiber-free and fiber-containing EN formulations, 1 drug (Reglan syrup, Baxter Healthcare Corporation, Deerfield, IL) was reported as incompatible with fiber and compatible without fiber. The formulation tested contained soy polysaccharide as the fiber source. There are no data for EN formulations containing soluble fiber (guar gum, acacia, gum arabic, pectin) or fructooligosaccharides. Soluble fibers have a propensity to form gels. Therefore, the risk of undesirable interactions between drugs and EN formulations containing these fiber sources may be greater than with soy polysaccharide, although the relatively low amounts of soluble fiber in current EN formulations may mitigate the risk. An acidic pH was reported for all but 2 of the incompatible drugs, the exceptions being antacids (Mylanta II, McNeil Consumer Pharmaceuticals Co., Fort Washington, PA; Riopan, Takeda Pharmaceuticals International, Inc., Deerfield, IL), both with pH 7.5. Characteristics of the antacids other than pH, such as their composition of divalent and trivalent cations and formulation as suspensions, likely contributed to the incompatibility.

The protein source for all of the intact protein EN formulations in these studies included caseinates.[11-14] There is limited evidence that soy protein results in finer precipitate than caseinates, and whey-based formulations are unlikely to curdle and clump when mixed with acidic drug products because of the acid-stable characteristics of whey protein.[17] However, these are primarily observations that should be confirmed in scientifically rigorous studies with current EN and drug formulations. The data suggest protein denaturation, especially for caseinates, may be responsible for much of the physical incompatibility when drugs in liquid dosage form and EN formulations interact.

Preventing or Mitigating Physical Interactions

Physical interactions are best avoided by not allowing drugs to mix with either PN or EN formulations. Ideally, drugs should be administered via a route other than the feeding administration device (vascular access device [VAD] or feeding tube), although that is not always possible. There are a few exceptions where products are added directly to the PN or EN formulation, including drugs such as insulin and histamine-2 receptor antagonists in PN. For patients who are allowed oral intake, the best route for administration of oral drugs is by mouth (see Practice Scenario 18-2 for a discussion of oral vs tube administration of medications). Routes such as rectal, transdermal, sublingual, intramuscular, and subcutaneous can be considered when drugs are available in these forms.

Practice Scenario 18-2

Question: What is the most effective method for preventing feeding tube occlusion related to medication administration in a patient receiving jejunal feedings to supplement inadequate oral intake associated with gastroparesis?

Scenario: A 63-year-old woman is admitted to the hospital because of nausea and weight loss. The gastrointestinal workup, including small bowel follow-through, indicates gastroparesis, likely secondary to type 2 diabetes mellitus. Thin liquids empty from the stomach with only slight delay; however, progression of thick liquids and solids into the duodenum is severely delayed. A percutaneous gastrojejunostomy tube is placed by interventional radiology, and the patient is started on tube feeding in addition to a modified consistency (thin liquid) diet. Although the patient's chart from another hospital indicates poor response to prokinetic agents, metoclopramide is ordered and home medications are restarted, including levothyroxine, lovastatin, amlodipine, calcium citrate, and fluoxetine.

Intervention: Medications are ordered for administration through the feeding tube. After reviewing the chart, the nutrition support clinician recommends changing the order to oral administration of medications.

Answer and Rationale: Medication administration through a feeding tube is a contributing factor to tube occlusion. Medications administered by mouth do not cause tube occlusion. In this case, the patient is allowed an oral diet with thin liquids to reduce gastric stasis. Medications taken with water should have minimal effect on gastric emptying compared with water alone, and thin liquids empty with only slight delay per the gastrointestinal evaluation.

When a drug must be administered through the same device as the PN or EN formulation, feeding should be stopped, and the access device should be flushed with fluid that is compatible with the PN or EN formulation as well as the drug. The access device should be flushed before and after drug administration and between drugs if multiple drugs are administered. The "flush" volume must be adequate to clear the administration device of the feeding formulation or the drug. Sodium chloride 0.9% is the usual fluid of choice for flushing VADs, but 5% dextrose solution is sometimes required. Minimum flush volume for VADs is typically specified by the manufacturer based on catheter size and type. Water is the fluid of choice for flushing enteral feeding tubes.[19] Other fluids should

generally be avoided to reduce the risk of interactions with the EN formulation. Acidic products, such as carbonated beverages and cranberry juice, may be particularly problematic.[20,21] The minimum recommended volume used to flush enteral feeding tubes in adults is 15 mL, although larger volumes are often used.[2]

Other potential methods of preventing physical interactions with PN and EN formulations include altering the infusion time, the nutrition formulation, or the drug. For PN, a cyclic regimen might allow an incompatible drug to infuse during the off time, although this approach is rarely effective for drugs administered more than once daily. Ideally, a therapeutically equivalent drug with evidence of compatibility for coadministration with the PN formulation could be used if changing the administration schedules is not possible. Altering the PN formulation to omit the interacting component may be possible in limited circumstances and for a limited duration. For example, it may be possible to omit the ILE for a few days while other vascular access is obtained when the emulsion is known to be the incompatible component and the patient's clinical condition is acceptable for this approach.

Changing to a hydrolyzed or free amino acid EN formulation rather than an intact protein source could be considered, although these formulas tend to be considerably more expensive and this approach is not typically a preferred way to prevent interactions. Viable options in some cases include alternative dosage forms (eg, powder from a capsule can be made into a slurry rather than using an elixir) or drugs that are therapeutic equivalents (different drug with the same therapeutic effect) but with different potential to interact.

Pharmaceutical Interactions

Dosage Forms

Interactions that occur because a drug dosage form is altered are more likely to occur with EN therapy and are seldom necessary for consideration with PN therapy. Drug dosage forms include the drug itself and other nonmedicinal components (excipients) necessary to make a stable and efficacious product that has suitable administration characteristics (eg, palatable for oral administration, nonirritating for dermal administration). Some dosage forms are designed for specific applications, such as enteric-coated tablets to protect drugs from gastric acid or the stomach from an irritating drug, long-acting products to reduce the number of daily doses, and sublingual or rectal products that avoid first-pass metabolism in the liver. Altering certain dosage forms can dramatically increase or decrease drug bioavailability and trigger adverse effects or, conversely, destroy the active ingredient. Thus, pharmaceutical interactions can also be classified as pharmacokinetic interactions.

The most common method of altering a dosage form is to crush or dissolve solid dosage forms to create a liquid for administration via the feeding tube. When a solid dosage form is to be administered via a feeding tube, it must first be determined that crushing or dissolving will not disrupt the drug's pharmaceutical activity. Solid dosage forms that are appropriate to crush should be prepared as a very fine powder and mixed with warm water before administering through the tube. In addition, many capsules may be opened and the contents administered after forming a slurry with water from the powder or finely crushed solids. Consult manufacturers' product information and the medical literature for information regarding crushing tablets or capsules. A frequently updated list of dosage forms that should not be crushed is available.[22]

As a general rule, special dosage forms such as long-acting, sustained-release, slow-release, or delayed-release forms containing several doses in 1 tablet or capsule should not be crushed or dissolved. These dosage forms are designed to slowly release the drug in the GI tract, often over 12 to 24 hours. Crushing may cause immediate release of the total drug dose, increasing the risk of toxicity and reducing efficacy. A 200-mg, extended-release morphine capsule is designed to gradually release drug over 24 hours; when crushed or dissolved before administration, the full 200-mg dose is immediately released, resulting in increased risk of respiratory depression and, potentially, respiratory arrest. However, conventional (non-extended-release) morphine is usually dosed every 4 to 6 hours so the patient is likely to experience pain, and potentially withdrawal symptoms if the conventional dosage form is given according to the schedule intended for the extended-release formulation. Figure 18-1 provides a graphic representation of expected effects on serum concentrations of a drug from crushing a once-daily, slow-release formulation compared with an every-6-hour, immediate-release formulation or oral administration of the once-daily formulation without crushing. The risk of toxicity from crushing an extended-release formulation is exacerbated when bioavailability is increased disproportionately as the drug dose increases, as it does with diltiazem.[23] The metabolic effects of the immediate release of large drug doses intended for extended delivery, such as nifedipine from crushing an extended-release tablet,

can be life-threatening.[24] Drugs whose names are followed by initials such as CD, CR, ER, LA, SA, SR, TR, XL, or XR generally need to be taken intact and should not be crushed or dissolved for administration.

Enteric-coated products, often denoted by EC after the name, are another special dosage form that generally should not be altered for administration. The coating is intended to protect a drug from destruction by gastric acid or to protect the stomach from irritation caused by the drug. When the coating is disrupted by crushing or dissolving the tablet, adverse effects are likely to occur if the medication is administered into the stomach. In one case, the drug is destroyed by exposure to gastric acid, and the patient receives less than the desired dose, thereby placing the patient at risk for treatment failure. Gastric irritation from removal of a protective tablet coating may also result in treatment failure if the patient experiences emesis from the drug. Administration into the jejunum negates the need for an enteric coating since the jejunum is where the coating is designed to dissolve. Therefore, dissolving the coating in bicarbonate solution, then crushing the tablet is acceptable for jejunal administration, although the process can be slow (30 to 45 minutes) and caution is still required to avoid tube occlusion.[25,26]

Enteric coatings should be distinguished from film coatings on tablets. Film coatings are used to make tablets easier to swallow or to mask unpleasant taste, but they do not impart special characteristics such as those associated with enteric coatings. Crushed film-coated tablets should not result in altered drug activity or increased risk of adverse effects. However, as with enteric coatings, film coatings can be problematic because they often remain as undissolved pieces that become sticky in water and can occlude the feeding tube. Sublingual dosage forms are designed to dissolve under the tongue for absorption via oral mucosa. Enteric mucosal and

FIGURE 18-1 Expected Blood Concentration Effects of Crushing a Once-Daily, Slow-Release Product

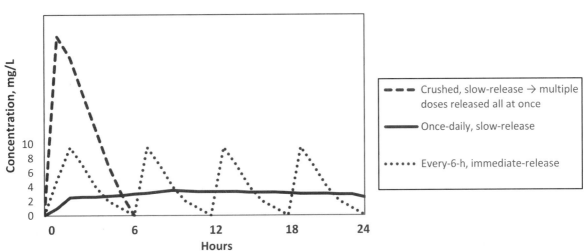

The graph depicts expected blood concentration effects of crushing a once-daily, slow-release product (high peak followed by near zero concentration by 6 hours) compared with an immediate-release product dosed every 6 hours (4 moderate size peaks between 9 and 10 mg/L evenly spaced across 24 hours) or the normal oral administration of the once-daily, slow-release product (concentration consistently between 2 and 4 mg/L over 24 hours).
Source: Reprinted by permission of Carol J. Rollins.

endoplasmic reticulum enzymes (eg, CYP450) and transporters (eg, P-glycoprotein and anion-transporting polypeptides) are bypassed with this route, thereby eliminating presystemic metabolism. In addition, blood flow is not routed to the liver, so first-pass effects from hepatic enzymes, including hepatic CYP450 enzymes, are eliminated. Sublingual doses are typically small compared with oral doses, and sublingual doses administered via a feeding tube are unlikely to provide an appropriate treatment dose of the drug. Buccal doses are similar to sublingual doses in this respect.

Dosage forms designed to disintegrate rapidly in the mouth before swallowing (solutabs) avoid the need for crushing and administering through the feeding tube when the patient is able to take such products by mouth. Pellets contained inside microencapsulated dosage forms should generally not be crushed because they are either enteric coated and/or time-released. Intact pellets may be administered through the feeding tube, provided the pellets are small enough to completely pass through the tube. Usually, a larger tube (minimum 16-Fr gastrostomy tube) is necessary for successful administration of these dosage forms. Suggestions for administering the microencapsulated beads or pellets include pouring them down the tube or suspending them in an acidic juice before administering through the tube.[27] Using an acidic juice as the vehicle for microencapsulated pieces should reduce the risk of the beads or pellets sticking to the tube. However, water should be used to clear the tube of the EN formulation before and after administration of the acidic juice–drug mixture to avoid physical DNIs between the EN formulation and an acidic product (see Practice Scenario 18-3 for an example of such a drug administration situation).[25,28–30] If the feeding tube diameter is too small to administer intact beads or pellets, a therapeutic option with better characteristics for tube administration is highly recommended. For a few drugs with no viable options, such as pancreatic enzymes, it may be necessary to dissolve an enteric coating on the beads or pellets in a sodium bicarbonate solution, then crush and administer the drug with a small volume of sodium bicarbonate solution.

Practice Scenario 18-3

Question: Which of the available dosage forms of lansoprazole should be ordered, and how should it be administered through a nasal-jejunal feeding tube?

Scenario: A 49-year-old man is receiving lansoprazole due to a gastrointestinal bleed. He is being fed via a small-bore nasal-jejunal tube because of poor nutrition status, inability to take an oral diet, and aspiration risk while on mechanical ventilation. He was taken off mechanical ventilation yesterday and is transferring from the intensive care unit (ICU) to a medicine unit today. His continuous intravenous infusion of lansoprazole was stopped today and administration via the feeding tube is ordered.

Intervention: The ICU pharmacist discusses the options for acid suppression with the physician and obtains an order to change lansoprazole to famotidine.

Answer: Lansoprazole is problematic for administration through a small-bore feeding tube using commercially available dosage forms. Either an extemporaneously prepared oral suspension or therapeutic alternatives should be considered to avoid occlusion of the feeding tube. In addition, the continued need for acid suppression once the patient is off mechanical ventilation, especially after he leaves the ICU, should be addressed. If acid suppression is to continue, the histamine-2 receptor antagonist on the hospital's formulary may be adequate. Otherwise, extemporaneous preparation of a suspension will be required or specific manufacturer's directions for an orally disintegrating tablet (ODT) followed.

Rationale: Lansoprazole is available as a delayed-release capsule and as a delayed-release ODT. These dosage forms should not be crushed because of the delayed-release characteristics. The capsule can be opened and intact granules administered with apple juice (40 mL recommended) via feeding tube.[28] However, the tube must be of adequate size (equal to or greater than 16 Fr) to allow intact granules to pass through the tube without causing occlusion. Because of the risk of tube occlusion, caution must be used with any ODT administered through a small-bore feeding tube.[28] Specific directions for administration of the lansoprazole ODT are provided by the manufacturer and should be followed to minimize the risk of occlusion.[29] A histamine-2 receptor antagonist available in a liquid dosage form or crushable tablet, such as famotidine, can be considered if acid suppression is still necessary once the patient leaves the ICU. Recipes are available for preparation of an oral lansoprazole liquid dosage form; however, this approach requires preparation from the available delayed-release capsule.[25,30]

Administration of IV dosage forms via the GI tract is similar to altering a dosage form. In general, IV dosage forms are poorly suited to withstand gastric acidity and enzyme activity within the GI tract. Substantial drug loss can occur, resulting in poor drug absorption and delivery to the site of activity. IV electrolyte preparations are an exception and seem to be effective when administered via the GI tract. However, the osmolality of such preparations can be very high and potentially result in GI intolerance, including osmotic diarrhea. Oral liquid dosage forms can also have a high osmolality and result in diarrhea or cramping. The osmolality of oral liquids and IV drugs often exceeds 1000 mOsm/kg and may be several thousand mOsm/kg.[18,31,32] The effect of high osmolality is most pronounced when a large volume is needed for each dose of drug. Diluting hyperosmolar products with water before administration reduces the osmolality and may reduce the risk of GI intolerance.

Sweetening agents such as mannitol, sucrose, and sorbitol are used in many oral liquid dosage forms and contribute to increased osmolality. Sorbitol is particularly troublesome because the cumulative daily dose from oral liquid drugs can reach 20 to 50 g, an amount commonly used as an osmotic laxative.[33,34] With only 5 to 10 g of sorbitol daily, a considerable portion of people experience bloating and flatulence.[35] An important factor in promoting EN tolerance is identification, prevention, and management of diarrhea due to the sorbitol content or hypertonicity of concurrent liquid medications. See

Chapter 13 for additional discussion of diarrhea as a complication of EN.

Preventing or Mitigating Pharmaceutical Interactions

Methods of preventing or mitigating pharmaceutical interactions include using immediate-release dosage forms rather than long-acting forms and avoiding special dosage forms, such as enteric-coated or sublingual, when they must be crushed or dissolved for administration through the feeding tube. Proper tube flushing cannot prevent pharmaceutical interactions. However, flushing with adequate quantities of water remains an important technique to prevent concomitant physical interactions. Pharmaceutical interactions may also be minimized by using alternate routes of administration or by using a therapeutic alternative that is available in a form conducive to administration via the feeding tube. Exposure to sorbitol may be controlled by use of alternate administration routes or by use of therapeutic alternatives. Unfortunately, current information on the sorbitol content of a drug is often unavailable, so selecting a therapeutic alternative with less sorbitol may not be easy. The drug manufacturer is generally the best source of information for current sorbitol content. Published information may not reflect current content, and a wide variation in sorbitol content can be found in versions of a given product from different manufacturers. Many pediatric drugs in liquid form, such as antibiotics, are now formulated without sorbitol.[25,29]

Pharmacokinetic Interactions

Definition

The term *pharmacokinetics* refers to studies of the time course for drug absorption, distribution, metabolism, and excretion.[36] However, the term can also be applied to nutrients because these same processes occur with nutrients. Pharmacokinetic DNIs are characterized by alterations in one or more pharmacokinetic parameters of a drug or nutrient due to an interaction between them. Changes in drug absorption and metabolism are most often reported. The effects of drugs on nutrient pharmacokinetics are rarely evaluated. Pharmacokinetic DNIs occur as the result of multiple factors, including those related to administration of EN or PN, the drug, and the PN or EN formulation. The disease process resulting in a requirement for EN or PN can also contribute to pharmacokinetic DNIs, especially as it affects protein status, organ perfusion, and GI motility.

Apparent Absorption and Metabolism

Bioavailability describes the amount of drug that reaches systemic circulation after administration. Drug or nutrient loss during administration, adverse pH effects, complex formation between nutrient(s) and drug, presystemic metabolism in the gut mucosa (eg, CYP450 metabolism), and hepatic first-pass metabolism can cause product losses that decrease bioavailability. Product loss during administration may reflect a chemical interaction that results in deterioration of the drug or nutrient without causing a change in the physical appearance of the PN or EN formulation or the drug product. A change in product color without precipitate formation or changes in viscosity may also indicate an interaction. Photodegradation, oxidation, and hydrolysis are typical chemical reactions resulting in stability problems. These chemical reactions tend to be exacerbated by pH changes, increased time of exposure (eg, admixture in a PN formulation rather than co-infusion), and increased temperature. Photodegradation requires light exposure and tends to be limited by opaque formulations, including ILEs and most EN formulations.

Amino acids are frequently associated with chemical reactions in PN and EN formulations. The Maillard reaction occurs between the amine group of amino acids, including those in proteins, and the carbonyl moiety of certain carbohydrates, resulting in a browning reaction that alters taste, appearance, and, potentially, nutritional value. The carbohydrates involved are reducing sugars (eg, glucose, lactose). Sucrose and complex carbohydrates commonly found in EN formulations do not react unless hydrolyzed to monosaccharides. Heat (eg, heat sterilization) and water accelerate the reaction.

The potential for chemical reactions and stability issues exists whenever a solid dosage form of drug is made into a liquid form. Water tends to accelerate chemical reactions that result in loss of drug activity. Solid dosage forms (tablets, capsules) may not contain protective additives or stabilizers needed for liquid dosage forms of the same drug. Aspirin illustrates the effect of water on stability; an aspirin tablet dissolved in water quickly loses most of its pharmacological activity. Therefore, solid drug dosage forms should be prepared as a slurry with water just before administration through the feeding tube. Occasionally, extended stability data for extemporaneous liquid preparations are available, and the pharmacist can make the liquid product a few days in advance.[7,25,30]

Administration-Related Factors

Tubing and Bag Characteristics

Adsorption of a drug or nutrient into a container or administration tubing results in product loss without changes in the physical appearance of the products and is difficult to separate from chemical instability without sophisticated analysis. Specific chemical characteristics of the container or administration set must be considered before extrapolating data from a study to the practice site. Results of studies conducted in foreign markets relative to the clinician's practice may be especially problematic for extrapolation because differences in container and tubing characteristics, as well as medication formulation, may influence results.

Products with high fat solubility are more likely to undergo adsorption with plastics, but other drugs (eg, insulin) can also be adsorbed. The classic example of nutrient loss to the container is vitamin A loss into diethylhexylphthalate (DEHP)-containing plastics.[37] ILEs actually leach DEHP from the bags into the emulsion, as does the castor oil emulsion used in formulating certain fat-soluble drugs, such as cyclosporine A. Although not DNIs in the usual sense, these interactions are concerning because the solubilized DEHP may pose a health risk.[38]

Loss of certain drugs into feeding tubes has been suggested.[39–41] A small in vitro study to determine the extent of warfarin binding to polyurethane feeding tube material evaluated warfarin recovery from a mixture of simulated gastric fluid and a crushed warfarin tablet, and the investigators found significantly less recovery when pieces of feeding tube were added to the container vs no feeding tube.[39] In contrast, it is likely that most, if not all, of the drug losses during in vitro studies with phenytoin and carbamazepine suspensions were caused by adherence to the intraluminal surface of the tube; diluting the suspensions before administration reduced drug losses.[40,41] Irrigating the feeding tubes after drug administration also reduced drug loss. Thus, suspensions, especially viscous suspensions, are best diluted to a relatively thin consistency before administration through a feeding tube. Slurries made from a powdered or crushed drug should also be a thin consistency to avoid drug loss in the feeding tube. In addition, the tube must be adequately flushed to remove any residual drug. Failure to properly flush the tube may result in physical DNIs between the drug retained in the feeding tube and the EN formulation, resulting in a high likelihood of feeding tube occlusion.

Site of Delivery

The site of drug delivery has minimal effect on PN-associated DNIs but can be a major administration-related factor for EN therapy. For PN therapy, the delivery sites are peripheral vein or central venous circulation, and the primary difference in PN formulations is the lower osmolarity of peripheral PN. On the other hand, efficacy and bioavailability of EN therapy may be greatly altered by site of delivery. Drugs with a "local" effect must be delivered to that locale. Antacids and sucralfate are examples of drugs with a local effect; they have no therapeutic effect with postpyloric delivery because they act locally in the stomach. Drug or nutrient absorption from the GI tract requires that the product be in a ready state for absorption. Nutrients must be released from the food matrix and specific complexes (eg, vitamin B_{12} and intrinsic factor) or valences (eg, ferric vs ferrous iron) may be needed. Drugs generally must be dissolved and have some portion in the nonionized (noncharged) state. The site of feeding and drug delivery determines the environment to which a product is exposed, thereby affecting readiness for absorption. The location of the tube's distal tip determines the delivery environment for products administered through a feeding tube.

Delivery Environment

Feeding tubes can deliver drugs and nutrients to the stomach, duodenum, or jejunum (see Chapter 12). The environment changes from highly acidic to moderate acidity to near neutrality as the tip of the feeding tube moves deeper into the GI tract. These environmental changes in pH influence the degree of absorption. Feeding and drug delivery into the stomach allow most of the normal physiological functions associated with digestion to be utilized. The stomach serves as a mixing chamber, helping release nutrients from the food matrix and mixing foods and drugs with gastric acid. Drugs soluble in acid generally complete the dissolution process in the stomach. Drugs that are not soluble in acid dissolve once they reach the small bowel.

Little absorption actually occurs in the stomach; rather, the vast majority of absorption occurs in the small bowel because of the enormous surface area. Thus, gastric emptying is a rate-controlling step for absorption, and any nutrient or drug that alters the gastric emptying rate will affect pharmacokinetic parameters. Table 18-2 lists several EN formulation characteristics and drug examples that may be associated with altered gastric emptying.[42–44] The rate of nutrient and drug absorption typically follows the direction of change in gastric emptying. Slow gastric emptying slows absorption, and rapid gastric emptying increases the absorption rate.

Effects of altered gastric emptying on bioavailability, or extent of absorption, can be difficult to predict and are dependent on the chemical characteristics and mechanisms of absorption for a particular drug or nutrient. Rapid gastric emptying accompanied by rapid GI transit can result in poor absorption because there is insufficient contact time between the drug or nutrient and the absorptive surface of the small bowel. Rapid gastric emptying in the presence of normal small bowel motility is expected to reduce the extent of absorption for nutrients and drugs that require an acidic environment to create readiness for absorption. Slow gastric emptying allows increased release of nutrients from the food matrix, increased exposure to acid, and slower presentation of chyme to the small bowel. Thus, slow gastric emptying increases the extent of absorption for nutrients such as iron, calcium, and magnesium that benefit from acid exposure and for nutrients such as riboflavin that undergo active absorption by a saturable mechanism in the upper small bowel. Dissolution of acid-soluble (eg, tetracycline) and poorly soluble (eg, carbamazepine, digoxin) drugs is improved with slow gastric emptying; however, bioavailability depends on stability in an acid environment. For example, bioavailability increases for carbamazepine, an acid-stable drug, but decreases for digoxin, which is hydrolyzed in the presence of acid.

Delivery of the EN formulation and drugs into the small bowel bypasses problems with gastric emptying. Experience with use of short- and long-term jejunal feeding using both hydrolyzed and intact protein formulations suggests that delivery beyond the duodenum has negligible effects on overall nutrient absorption. The effect of delivery into the small bowel on drugs largely depends on their solubility and need for acid exposure for absorption. Poorly soluble drugs that benefit from an increased time for dissolution and drugs that require exposure to acid are expected to exhibit reduced bioavailability with administration into the small bowel. Thus, drugs such as carbamazepine, itraconazole, and tetracycline are likely to have reduced bioavailability with postpyloric administration. Limited data support poor itraconazole absorption with jejunal administration.[45]

The balance between reduced dissolution and less acid destruction with postpyloric administration of poorly soluble but acid-labile drugs, such as digoxin, is difficult to predict. Reduced hydrolytic products (0.6% vs 2.9%) and greater nonmetabolized digoxin recovery (96.3% vs 90.8%) were reported with jejunal administration compared with oral intake in a small study, suggesting that the balance may be in favor of

TABLE 18-2 Factors Associated with Delayed Gastric Emptying

Factors	Amount/Characteristics	Concomitant Effect on Gastrointestinal Motility
Formulation-related:		
• Long-chain fats[a]	• High concentration	• Decrease (gastric)
• Protein	• High concentration	• Decrease (gastric)
• pH	• Low	• Decrease (gastric)
		• Increase (small bowel)
Osmolarity, mOsm/L	• <250 and >800	• Decrease (gastric)
		• Increase (small bowel)
Viscosity	• High	• Decrease (gastric)
Volume	• Large	• Decrease (gastric)
		• Increase (small bowel)
Drug particle size	• Large or tablets	• Decrease (gastric)
Drugs:[b]		
• Anticholinergic agents		• Decrease (gastric and small bowel)
• Narcotic agents		• Decrease (gastric and small bowel)
• Octreotide		• Decrease (gastric and small bowel)

[a]Greatest effect of formulation-related factors.
[b]This list of drugs is not all-inclusive.
Sources: Data are from references 42, 43, and 44.

reduced destruction.[46] Because serum digoxin levels were not reported in this study, it is unclear if more nonmetabolized digoxin in the jejunum results in greater drug absorption. Published data, including the manufacturers' package inserts, rarely provide information on the proportion of a drug absorbed in specific segments of the small bowel. Fortunately, most drugs have a wide therapeutic range and seem to be efficacious and nontoxic, despite potential changes in bioavailability related to the delivery site and environment. For drugs with a narrow therapeutic index, it is advisable to monitor for changes in the serum drug level whenever administration occurs through a feeding tube.

Administration Regimen

Food is known to interact with many drugs and alter pharmacokinetic profiles, particularly absorption and metabolism.[44] Recommendations for oral administration of many drugs commonly include directions for taking the drug with or without food. Logic suggests that an EN formulation is equivalent to oral food ingestion; however, limited data indicate that the method of EN administration influences GI tract response. Particular patterns of GI motility and secretions are associated with the "fed" state, including slowed gastric emptying and increased release of digestive enzymes and GI tract secretions. The "nonfed" state is associated with more rapid gastric emptying and fewer digestive enzymes and secretions.

A study of hydralazine pharmacokinetics in 8 healthy volunteers receiving an EN formulation via NG tube reported similar results with fasting and continuous infusion of the EN formulation.[47] Hydralazine parameters with bolus administration of the EN formulation were similar to those with a standard breakfast (controlled for effects of nutrient content, such as fat) and differed from fasted parameters. These results suggest that holding continuous EN administration for drugs to be taken on an empty stomach (1 hour before or 2 hours after a meal) is not necessary. However, extrapolating results from a single investigation of a particular drug in healthy subjects to other patient populations and other medications is difficult. There is little evidence of therapeutic failure in most cases when continuous EN administration is stopped only during the short time needed to properly flush the tube and administer the drug (a few notable exceptions are discussed later in the chapter). Clinical experience does, however, suggest that holding EN administration for approximately 1 to 2 hours every 6 to 8 hours for drug administration is likely to result in inadequate nutrition support and deterioration in nutrition status unless a volume-based feeding protocol is used.

Drug-Related Factors

Factors associated with the drug itself can result in pharmacokinetic DNIs. These factors include the dosage form, chemical characteristics, and susceptibility to presystemic enzymatic degradation, cellular transport, and hepatic metabolism. For PN formulations, drug-related factors are largely associated with stability of the IV dosage form and the potential for loss of drug activity due to chemical reactions (photodegradation, oxidation, hydrolysis). As discussed previously in this chapter, alteration of dosage forms and chemical characteristics relative to the delivery environment are important drug-related factors pertinent to EN therapy. Susceptibility of drugs to presystemic enzymatic degradation, cellular transport, and hepatic metabolism can play a major role in apparent absorption for drugs administered into the GI tract; however, these processes are not specific to EN therapy and are reviewed only briefly here.

Presystemic Metabolism

Metabolism that occurs before reaching systemic circulation is known as *presystemic metabolism* and occurs in both the gut mucosa and liver. The CYP450 enzyme system includes many isoenzymes involved in drug metabolism and is a major component of presystemic metabolism. It is estimated that about 60% of drugs currently available are metabolized by CYP450 isoenzymes, specifically CYP3A4.[48] Drug interactions with grapefruit juice are the classic example of CYP450-mediated DNIs. Grapefruit juice inhibits the isoenzyme CYP3A4, thereby increasing serum levels of drugs normally metabolized by this isoenzyme.[49] Considerable research has been devoted to understanding effects of the CYP450 system on drug metabolism and DNIs because these enzymes can dramatically alter bioavailability, and, in some cases, this can result in life-threatening DNIs. In addition, drug transporters have increasingly been recognized for their importance in drug metabolism and disposition.

The best-known transporter is P-glycoprotein, which serves as an efflux mechanism to pump xenobiotics (drugs and other chemicals or substances not normally present in the body), out of cells and prevent entry to the compartment that the cells protect. P-glycoprotein is located on the luminal surface of cells lining the small bowel and prevents systemic absorption of certain drugs. The bile canalicular membrane in the liver and cells in the renal proximal tubule also contain P-glycoprotein. Organic anion-transporting polypeptides serve as uptake transporters in the intestine, opposing the efflux effect of P-glycoprotein.[50] The net effect of inhibition, induction, and interaction between CYP450 enzymes, uptake transporters, and efflux transporters can be complex and requires continued research to understand. To date, there are no data to suggest that any component of EN formulations significantly inhibits or induces these enzymes and transporters.

Therapeutic Index

Drugs with a narrow therapeutic index require serum drug concentrations within a small range to avoid therapeutic failure or toxicity. Any alteration in absorption of these drugs can be problematic; thus, routine monitoring of serum drug levels or surrogate markers (eg, prothrombin time [PT]/international normalized ratio [INR] for warfarin) is generally conducted. Monitoring of narrow therapeutic index drugs is also advised with initiation and changes in an EN regimen.

Formula-Related Factors

Macronutrients

The association of complex proteins and fiber with physical DNIs was discussed previously in this chapter. Protein may also influence drug metabolism through effects on enzymes of the mixed-function oxidase system in the liver.[44,51] Activity of the mixed-function oxidase system seems to be stimulated with high protein intake and with riboflavin, niacin, and large ascorbic acid doses, thereby increasing clearance of drugs metabolized by these enzymes. Protein intake may also influence blood flow, with low intake reducing flow to the kidney and lowering renal elimination of some drugs. However, most data on protein effects come from animal studies, and more research is required before any definitive statement or recommendations can be made regarding the effect of protein on DNIs in the clinical setting. Nutrients that alter gastric emptying and GI motility can alter the rate and extent of drug absorption, thereby contributing to DNIs. The effects of macronutrients on gastric emptying and GI motility are included in Table 18-2.

Micronutrients

Micronutrients in EN formulations have the potential to cause DNIs. Divalent and trivalent minerals (calcium, magnesium, and iron) are known to form complexes with certain drugs, such as tetracycline and ciprofloxacin, which results in poor absorption of the drugs. Degradation products from micronutrients have also been reported to cause physical interactions. For example, oxalate from ascorbic acid degradation has been reported to interact with calcium in PN formulations, forming an insoluble precipitate.[52]

The vitamin K content of EN formulations is a concern because of potential DNIs with warfarin. Formation of vitamin K–dependent blood clotting factors in the liver (Factors II, VII, IX, X) is inhibited by warfarin, resulting in an anticoagulation effect. Significant vitamin K intake from an EN formulation can antagonize this anticoagulant effect and result in treatment failure. Most EN formulations marketed today contain modest amounts of vitamin K and provide daily vitamin K intake similar to average dietary intake from foods (90 to 120 mcg/d in adults).[53] Consistent intake of an EN formulation containing less than 100 mcg vitamin K per 1000 kcal is not expected to cause warfarin resistance. Nonetheless, warfarin resistance has been reported in EN patients with relatively low vitamin K intake and seems to respond to changes in the warfarin administration schedule.[54,55] This evidence suggests a mechanism other than vitamin K antagonism of warfarin activity, because the duration of warfarin antagonism is several days, not hours. This interaction is discussed further in the "Specific Drug–Enteral Nutrition Interactions" section later in this chapter.

Disease-Related Factors

The alterations in body composition associated with malnutrition may affect the risk of pharmacokinetic DNIs. Pharmacokinetic parameters can be affected by decreased serum concentrations of visceral proteins, especially albumin, which binds many drugs (eg, phenytoin, valproic acid, warfarin). Edema, increased body water, and decreased lean muscle mass may also affect pharmacokinetic parameters. Other disease-related factors include alterations in organ function and perfusion, as well as effects on GI motility. A full discussion of disease-related factors is beyond the scope of this chapter.

Specific Drug–Enteral Nutrition Interactions

There are many potential DNIs involving EN therapy; however, a few drugs are particularly troublesome and have generated more discussion than most. Four of these drugs are discussed in this section.

Phenytoin

Phenytoin is a notorious drug for interaction with EN therapy. Many studies and case reports have been published, but few are prospective, randomized, controlled trials. There are multiple theories regarding the interaction and many proposed solutions. Four prospective, randomized, controlled trials of phenytoin and EN in healthy volunteers have been reviewed.[56,57] Only 1 study investigated the effect of the EN formulation delivered through a feeding tube while the others investigated the effect of oral EN on serum phenytoin concentrations. None of these studies found an interaction between phenytoin and EN formulations. Countering these results were 25 reports and studies with less rigorous designs (no randomization or placebo control) that supported an interaction in patients.[56] Theories regarding the mechanism of interaction focus on issues related to pH[58-61] and phenytoin binding, either to tubing[40] or to an EN component.[62] Dosage form issues (eg, suspension, chewable tablets, capsule, IV formulation), chemical form (phenytoin acid vs phenytoin sodium), and solubility are encompassed in the discussion of pH.

Of the various methods proposed to manage the phenytoin-EN interaction, none is completely reliable, and monitoring of serum phenytoin concentrations is highly recommended. Holding administration of the EN formulation for at least 1 hour, and possibly 2 hours, before and after phenytoin administration seems to produce the most consistent results.[62,63] However, some practitioners choose to continue adjusting the phenytoin dose to achieve therapeutic serum concentrations because adjustment of the EN infusion schedule can create problems related to inadequate EN delivery. Relatively high phenytoin doses are typically required to achieve therapeutic levels with this approach, and close monitoring of serum concentrations is required when the EN is discontinued. Dilution of phenytoin suspension is also recommended when the suspension is administered through a feeding tube.[40] Regardless of the method used, consistency of administration is important to control one of the variables influencing the phenytoin concentration.

Carbamazepine

Carbamazepine is a relatively insoluble drug and is acid stable; thus, slow gastric emptying improves bioavailability. Limited data suggest that EN therapy reduces bioavailability, possibly by altering solubility. Relative bioavailability of 90% was reported in a randomized, crossover study comparing administration of carbamazepine suspension via NG tube with continuous EN and oral intake after an overnight fast in 7 healthy males.[64] Serum carbamazepine concentrations with tube feeding were significantly lower at 8 hours, and the lower maximum concentration approached statistical significance,

although the small study size limited the ability to show significance. In vitro recovery of carbamazepine also seemed to be reduced after it was mixed with an intact protein EN formulation (58% recovery) compared with recovery after mixture with a simulated gastric juice (79% recovery).[65] Recovery was similar for the EN formulation and simulated intestinal juice (59% recovery). These data suggest that postpyloric administration of carbamazepine may result in poor bioavailability.

Binding of carbamazepine to a component of EN formulations has not been demonstrated; thus, it is unclear if holding administration of the EN formulation for 2 hours before and after the drug dose, as has been recommended, is the best method of mitigating this potential interaction.[66,67] Adequate dilution of the suspension (or slurry from a crushed tablet) prior to administration and adequate flushing after the dose should be the first choice of methods to mitigate the EN-carbamazepine interaction because this approach does not affect delivery of adequate nutrition. When adequate dilution and flushing fail in patients with postpyloric administration, it would be reasonable to hold feedings before and after drug administration in this population. Gastric administration may be cautiously monitored without routinely holding the EN formulation, unless there is evidence of an interaction. Carbamazepine suspension should be diluted at least 1:1, preferably 3:1, with water if administered via a feeding tube because drug loss in the feeding tube seems to be reduced with dilution.[41]

Fluoroquinolones

Bioavailability of some fluoroquinolone antibiotics seems to be reduced by EN formulations. Studies in healthy volunteers have reported a 25% to 28% decrease in ciprofloxacin bioavailability when it is administered with an EN formulation, and decreases of 27% to 67% have been reported in hospitalized patients.[68-70] Reduced bioavailability is also reported with repeated doses of ciprofloxacin via NG tube in critically ill patients receiving continuous infusion of an EN formulation.[71,72] Jejunal feeding has the greatest potential of reducing ciprofloxacin bioavailability because significant absorption normally occurs in the duodenum; however, the limited data available do not provide clear evidence of clinically significant differences in absorption based on the site of administration.[47,68,73-75] It is unclear whether reduced bioavailability with gastric or jejunal feeding is clinically significant because serum drug concentrations above the minimum inhibitory concentration have been reported for many pathogenic microorganisms with either administration route.[73,76]

Complex formation of ciprofloxacin with divalent cations in the EN formulation was initially thought to be responsible for reduced bioavailability of ciprofloxacin with EN therapy. Fluoroquinolones are known to bind with divalent cations, and manufacturers' instructions advise separating drug administration from intake of foods, dietary supplements, or other drugs containing calcium, magnesium (eg, antacids), or iron. However, an in vitro study failed to find a correlation between cation content of the EN formulation and loss of different fluoroquinolones mixed directly into the formulation.[77] Ciprofloxacin loss was greatest (82.5%), followed by levofloxacin (61%) and ofloxacin (46%). The amount of loss seemed to increase with the degree of hydrophilicity of the individual drug. Limited in vivo data support this finding. Better bioavailability of ofloxacin (90%) compared with ciprofloxacin (72%) has been reported in healthy volunteers receiving the antibiotics with an EN formulation.[76] Currently, many facilities follow a policy of holding administration of the EN formulation for at least 1 hour before a fluoroquinolone dose and 2 hours after the dose, as recommended previously.[67] This approach seems to minimize effects of the DNI on ciprofloxacin and norfloxacin; however, data supporting the holding of EN are very limited, especially in patients actually receiving tube feedings. Evidence from studies of 16 critically ill patients and 12 healthy volunteers does not support holding gatifloxacin or moxifloxacin, respectively.[78,79] The studies were small; however, when the drug was crushed and administered via a feeding tube with or without an EN formula, there were no clinically relevant effects on serum concentrations.

For each of the fluoroquinolones, well-designed studies of adequate size comparing proper drug dilution and adequate flush volumes with holding of EN therapy are necessary to confirm the validity of holding or not holding feedings. Nonetheless, in the absence of such a study, holding feedings remains a potential method of mitigating EN interactions with ciprofloxacin or norfloxacin; however, holding feedings with other fluoroquinolones should not be done routinely.

Warfarin

One proposed mechanism for warfarin resistance with low vitamin K intake is binding of warfarin to a component of the EN formulation, most likely protein.[80] Warfarin resistance due to protein binding has not been adequately studied to confirm whether protein binding is an in vivo mechanism of DNI. The study used to promote protein binding as a mechanism of interaction was conducted in vitro at a pH outside the physiological range.[80] Use of a free amino acid (elemental) EN formulation is expected to prevent the interaction if protein binding actually causes the DNI; however, this premise has not been tested. Given the higher cost of elemental formulas, the potential for the high osmolality to cause GI intolerance, and the greater difficulty in justifying use of these formulas, practitioners may elect to manage the interaction by other methods (ie, increase the warfarin dose or change to an alternative anticoagulant therapy). Many questions remain relative to the theory of warfarin-EN protein binding, including the reversibility of such binding during or after absorption, and potential for release of warfarin from protein during protein metabolism. Binding of warfarin to the protein component of EN remains a theory with limited data to support this mechanism of interaction.

A recent in vitro study presents data supporting another potential mechanism for the warfarin-EN interaction.[39] Loss of warfarin was demonstrated when drug was infused through a polyurethane feeding tube under defined laboratory conditions and when weighed amounts of sliced feeding tube were added to beakers containing 3 different concentrations of warfarin. Binding of warfarin to the polyurethane feeding tube material did not seem to be a saturable process in this study. The authors concluded that holding EN around administration

of warfarin through a feeding tube should not affect bioavailability of warfarin, and they did not recommend holding feedings to mitigate the warfarin-EN interaction. This study only evaluated warfarin binding to polyurethane feeding tube material under simulated gastric conditions. Further studies are needed to determine whether other feeding tube materials or small bowel conditions would produce the same effects.

The mechanism of interaction between warfarin and EN has not been clearly delineated, and no definitive recommendation can be provided for mitigating warfarin resistance associated with relatively low vitamin K intake. Nonetheless, interactions involving warfarin can be life-threatening. Response to warfarin therapy must be closely monitored when EN therapy is started, stopped, or altered (see Practice Scenario 18-4).[80,81]

Practice Scenario 18-4

Question: Should tube feeding be held when a therapeutic international normalized ratio (INR) is not achieved with the home dose of warfarin after tube feeding starts?

Scenario: A 68-year-old man was admitted to the hospital with suspected sepsis and required mechanical ventilation. His past medical history included hypertension, recurrent deep vein thrombosis, and osteoarthritis with left knee replacement 2 months ago. Medications before admission included lisinopril, 20 mg tablet daily; acetaminophen/hydrocodone, 500/5 mg, 1 tablet every 6 hours and up to 2 additional tablets daily as needed for pain; paroxetine, 20 mg tablet daily; and warfarin, 5 mg tablet daily.

Broad-spectrum antibiotic coverage was initiated immediately after admission. Antibiotics were changed to high-dose intravenous (IV) nafcillin on hospital Day 3, based on blood culture results. Tube feeding was started on hospital Day 5 through a small-bore nasogastric (NG) tube and reached goal rate within 48 hours. Mechanical ventilation was stopped on Day 10, and the patient was transferred to a medical floor. Tube feeding was continued due to possible esophageal damage, as was IV nafcillin and a heparin infusion. Lisinopril and warfarin were initiated through the feeding tube at home dosages. Morphine liquid was ordered via NG tube, with 1 mg IV morphine allowed every 4 hours, as needed for pain. After 2 weeks of gradually increasing the daily warfarin dose from 5 mg (home dose) to 12 mg, the INR remained subtherapeutic at 1.4.

Answer: The pharmacist recommends restarting paroxetine and changing to acetaminophen/hydrocodone (home medication) for pain management, rather than holding tube feedings around warfarin administration.

Rationale: Assessing drug interactions with warfarin before altering the tube feeding regimen is important. Paroxetine increases INR. The patient received paroxetine at home and will likely be discharged on this medication. Acetaminophen interrupts the vitamin K cycle through effects of the N-acetyl (p)-benzoquinone imine metabolite on vitamin K–dependent carboxylase, an enzyme in the vitamin K cycle.[81] Standard doses of acetaminophen increase INR significantly in some patients. Nafcillin decreases INR and could contribute to warfarin resistance. Keeping the warfarin concentration relatively high in the slurry prepared for administration through the feeding tube and administering it rapidly would be an appropriate administration technique. Holding tube feedings for 1 to 2 hours on each side of the warfarin dose, and adjusting the feeding rate to provide full daily volume, may be reasonable if the INR does not increase within a few days of restarting acetaminophen/hydrocodone and paroxetine at the home doses; however, data supporting this action are limited. Binding of warfarin with a component of the EN formulation has been proposed to explain warfarin resistance with modest vitamin K intake.[80] Use of a free amino acid (elemental) EN formulation should prevent the interaction if protein binding actually causes the drug-nutrient interaction; however, no studies support this approach. A low-molecular-weight heparin or one of the new oral anticoagulants could also be used for anticoagulation, but the risks and benefits must be carefully considered for each patient.

Potential methods of mitigating the warfarin-EN interaction include rapidly administering a concentrated form of the drug to minimize contact with the feeding tube, separating warfarin administration from EN administration, increasing the warfarin dose until a therapeutic PT/INR is achieved, or changing to an alternative anticoagulation therapy that does not interact with EN therapy. Minimizing contact with the feeding tube has a low potential to cause unintended consequences and is a reasonable first approach. If this option fails to resolve warfarin resistance, separating the warfarin dose from EN by holding EN for at least 1 hour before and after the warfarin dose can be tried; however, if the interaction is actually with the feeding tube material, avoiding contact between the drug and EN formulation is unlikely to improve warfarin response. If the warfarin resistance does improve, any increases in PT/INR should be evident within a few days. Increasing the warfarin dose periodically until a therapeutic INR is achieved can result in high drug doses that may place the patient at risk for bleeding should EN administration be reduced for any reason. In addition to routine monitoring, the PT/INR should be re-evaluated with any change in the EN regimen.

Summary

DNIs are an important consideration with both PN and EN therapy. The consequences of such interactions range from relatively benign to life-threatening. Pharmacists typically have the most specific training regarding drug interactions and should be involved in decisions related to DNIs; however, all nutrition support clinicians should be involved in establishing safe practices that minimize the risk of various types of DNIs occurring and limit adverse effects associated with such interactions. Few DNIs that occur with nutrition support, especially EN, are well studied or well understood and further research is needed to better mitigate such interactions.

References

1. Rollins CJ. General pharmacologic issues. In: Matarese LE, Gottschlich MM, eds. *Contemporary Nutrition Support Practice*. 2nd ed. Philadelphia, PA: Saunders; 2003:315–335.
2. Bankhead R, Boullata J, Brantley S, et al. A.S.P.E.N. enteral nutrition practice recommendations. *JPEN J Parenter Enteral Nutr*. 2009;33:122–167.
3. Scheppach W, Burghardt W, Bartram P, et al. Addition of dietary fiber to liquid formula diets: the pros and cons. *JPEN J Parenter Enteral Nutr*. 1990;14:204–209.
4. American Society for Parenteral and Enteral Nutrition. Definition of terms, style, and conventions used in A.S.P.E.N. guidelines and standards. *Nutr Clin Pract*. 2005;20:281–285.
5. Chan LN. Drug-nutrient interaction in clinical nutrition. *Curr Opin Clin Nutr Metab Care*. 2002;5:327–332.
6. Sandostatin (octreotide acetate) injection, Novartis Pharma Stein AG, Stein, Switzerland. https://www.pharma.us.novartis.com/sites/www.pharma.us.novartis.com/files/sandostatin_inj.pdf. Accessed October 2, 2016.
7. *Handbook on Injectable Drugs*. 18th ed. Bethesda, MD: American Society of Health-System Pharmacists; 2015.
8. Task Force for the Revision of Safe Practices for Parenteral Nutrition. Safe practice for parenteral nutrition formulations. *JPEN J Parenter Enteral Nutr*. 2004;28(6 Suppl):S39–S70.
9. Ayers P, Adams S, Boullata J, et al. A.S.P.E.N. parenteral nutrition safety consensus recommendations. *JPEN J Parenter Enteral Nutr*. 2014;38(3):296–333.
10. Boullata JI, Gilbert K, Sacks G, et al. A.S.P.E.N. clinical guidelines: parenteral nutrition ordering, order review, compounding, labeling, and dispensing. *JPEN J Parenter Enteral Nutr*. 2014;38(3):334–377.
11. Fagerman KE, Ballou AE. Drug compatibilities with enteral feeding solutions co-administered by tube. *Nutr Support Serv*. 1988;8:31–32.
12. Altman E, Cutie AJ. Compatibility of enteral products with commonly employed drug additives. *Nutr Support Serv*. 1984;4:8–17.
13. Cutie AJ, Altman E, Lenkel L. Compatibility of enteral products with commonly employed drug additives. *JPEN J Parenter Enteral Nutr*. 1983;7:186–191.
14. Burns PE, McCall L, Wirsching R. Physical compatibility of enteral formulas with various common medications. *J Am Diet Assoc*. 1988;88:1094–1096.
15. Holtz L, Milton J, Sturek JK. Compatibility of medications with enteral feedings. *JPEN J Parenter Enteral Nutr*. 1987;11:183–186.
16. Strom JG, Miller SW. Stability of drugs with enteral nutrient formulas. *Drug Intell Clin Pharm*. 1990;24:130–134.
17. Rollins CJ. Tube feeding formula and medication characteristics contributing to undesirable interactions (abstract). *JPEN J Parenter Enteral Nutr*. 1999;23:S13.
18. Klang M, McLymont V, Ng N. Osmolality, pH, and compatibility of selected oral liquid medications with an enteral nutrition product. *JPEN J Parenter Enteral Nutr*. 2013;37(5):689–694.
19. Boullata JI, Carrera AL, Harvey L, et al. A.S.P.E.N. safe practices for enteral nutrition therapy. *JPEN J Parenter Enteral Nutr*. 2016;41:15–103.
20. Nicolau DP, Davis SK. Carbonated beverages as irrigants for feeding tubes. *Ann Pharmacother*. 1990;24:840.
21. Metheny N, Eisenberg P, McSweeney M. Effect of feeding tube properties and three irrigants on clogging rates. *Nurs Res*. 1988;37:165–169.
22. Mitchell JF. Oral dosage forms that should not be crushed. Do not crush list. www.ismp.org/Tools/DoNotCrush.pdf. Accessed September 22, 2016.
23. Höglund P, Nilsson LG. Pharmacokinetics of diltiazem and its metabolites after repeated multiple-dose treatments in healthy volunteers. *Ther Drug Monitor*. 1989;11:551–557.
24. Schier JG, Howland MA, Hoffman RS, et al. Fatality from administration of labetalol and crushed extended-release nifedipine. *Ann Pharmacother*. 2003;37:1420–1423.

25. Jew R, Soo-Hoo W, Erush S, Amiri E. *Extemporaneous Formulations for Pediatric, Geriatric and Special Needs Patients.* Bethesda, MD: American Society of Health-System Pharmacists; 2016.

26. Rollins, CJ, Baggs JH. Adult enteral nutrition. In: *Koda-Kimble and Young's Applied Therapeutics: The Clinical Use of Drugs.* 10th ed. Philadelphia, PA: Lippincott Williams Wilkins; 2013:904.

27. Beckwith MC, Barton RG, Graves C. A guide to drug therapy in patients with enteral feeding tubes: dosage form selection and administration methods. *Hosp Pharm.* 1997;32:57–64.

28. Wensel TM. Administration of proton pump inhibitors in patients requiring enteral nutrition. *P&T.* March 2009;34:143–160.

29. Drugs.com. Lansoprazole orally disintegrating tablets. https://www.drugs.com/pro/lansoprazole-orally-disintegrating-tablets.html. Accessed October 2, 2016.

30. Rollins CJ, Thomson CA, Crane T. Pharmacotherapeutic issues. In: Rolandelli RH, Bankhead R, Boullata JI, et al, eds. *Clinical Nutrition: Enteral and Tube Feeding.* 4th ed. Philadelphia, PA: Elsevier Saunders; 2005:291–305.

31. Niemiec PW, Vanderveen TW, Morrison JI, et al. Gastrointestinal disorders caused by medication and electrolyte solution osmolality during enteral nutrition. *JPEN J Parenter Enteral Nutr.* 1983; 7:387–389.

32. Dickerson RN, Melnik G. Osmolality of oral drug solutions and suspensions. *Am J Hosp Pharm.* 1988;45:832–834.

33. Lutomski DM, Gora ML, Wright SM, et al. Sorbitol content of selected oral liquids. *Ann Pharmacother.* 1993;27:269–274.

34. Johnston KR, Govel LA, Andritz MH. Gastrointestinal effects of sorbitol as an additive in liquid medications. *Am J Med.* 1994;97: 185–191.

35. Hyams JS. Sorbitol intolerance: an unappreciated cause of functional gastrointestinal complaints. *Gastroenterology.* 1983;84: 30–33.

36. Introduction to pharmacokinetics and pharmacodynamics. In: Spruill WJ, Blouin RA, DiPiro JT et al, eds. *Concepts in Clinical Pharmacokinetics.* 6th ed. Bethesda, MD: American Society of Health-System Pharmacists; 2014:1–20.

37. Howard L, Chu R, Feman S, et al. Vitamin A deficiency from long-term parenteral nutrition. *Ann Intern Med.* 1980;93:576–577.

38. Feigal DW. FDA public health notification: PVC devices containing the plasticizer DEHP. http://www.fda.gov/MedicalDevices/Safety/AlertsandNotices/PublicHealthNotifications/UCM062182. Accessed August 15, 2016.

39. Klang M, Graham D, McLymont V. Warfarin bioavailability with feeding tubes and enteral formula. *JPEN J Parenter Enteral Nutr.* 2010;34:300–304.

40. Cacek AT, DeVito JM, Koonce JR. In vitro evaluation of nasogastric administration methods for phenytoin. *Am J Hosp Pharm.* 1986;43:689–692.

41. Clark-Schmidt AL, Garnett WR, Lowe DR, et al. Loss of carbamazepine suspension through nasogastric feeding tubes. *Am J Hosp Pharm.* 1990;47:2034–2037.

42. Cullen J, Kelly K. Gastric motor physiology and pathophysiology. *Surg Clin North Am.* 1993;73:1145–1160.

43. Fleischer D, Li C, Zhou Y. Drug, meal and formulation interactions influencing drug absorption after oral administration. *Clin Pharmacokinet.*1999;36:233–254.

44. Singh BN. Effects of food on clinical pharmacokinetics. *Clin Pharmacokinet.* 1999;37:213–255.

45. Kintzel PE, Rollins CJ, Yee WJ, et al. Low itraconazole serum levels following administration of itraconazole suspension to critically ill allogeneic bone marrow transplant recipients. *Ann Pharmacother.* 1995;29:140–143.

46. Magnusson JO. Metabolism of digoxin after oral and jejunal administration. *Br J Clin Pharmacol.* 1983;16:741–742.

47. Semple HA, Koo W, Tam YK, et al. Interactions between hydralazine and oral nutrients in humans. *Ther Drug Monit.* 1991;13: 304–308.

48. Zhou S, Chan SY, Goh BC, et al. Mechanism-based inhibition of cytochrome P450 3A4 by therapeutic drugs. *Clin Pharmacokinet.* 2005;44:279–304.

49. Dresser GK, Bailey DG. The effects of fruit juices on drug disposition: a new model for drug interactions. *Eur J Clin Invest.* 2003; 33(Suppl 2):10–16.

50. Cvetkovic M, Leake B, Fromm MF, et al. OATP and P-glycoprotein transporters mediate the cellular uptake and excretion of fexofenadine. *Drug Metab Dispos.* 1999;27:866–871.

51. Williams L, Davis JA, Lowenthal DT. The influence of food on the absorption and metabolism of drugs. *Med Clin North Am.* 1993;77:815–829.

52. Gupta DV. Stability of vitamins in total parenteral nutrient solutions. *Am J Hosp Pharm.* 1986;43:2132.

53. Institute of Medicine. Vitamin K. In: *Dietary Reference Intakes for Vitamin A, Vitamin K, Arsenic, Boron, Chromium, Copper, Iodine, Iron, Manganese, Molybdenum, Nickel, Silicon, Vanadium, and Zinc.* Washington, DC: National Academies Press; 2001:162–196. http://www.nap.edu/openbook.php?record_id=10026&page=162#. Accessed October 4, 2016.

54. Petretich DA. Reversal of osmolite-warfarin interaction by changing warfarin administration time [letter]. *Clin Pharm.* 1990;9:93.

55. Dickerson RN, Garman WM, Kuhl DA, et al. Vitamin K–independent warfarin resistance after concurrent administration of warfarin and continuous enteral nutrition. *Pharmacotherapy.* 2008;28:308–313.

56. Au Yeung SC, Ensom MHH. Phenytoin and enteral feedings: does evidence support an interaction? *Ann Pharmacother.* 2000;34: 896–905.

57. Doak KK, Curtis EH, Dunnigan KJ, et al. Bioavailability of phenytoin acid and phenytoin sodium with enteral feedings. *Pharmacotherapy.* 1998;18:637–645.

58. Splinter MY, Seifert CF, Bradberry JC, et al. Recovery of phenytoin suspension after in vitro administration through percutaneous endoscopic gastrostomy Pezzer catheters. *Am J Hosp Pharm.* 1990;47:373–377.

59. Fleisher D, Sheth N, Kou JH. Phenytoin interaction with enteral feedings administered through nasogastric tubes. *JPEN J Parenter Enteral Nutr.* 1990;14:513–516.

60. Hooks MA, Longe RL, Taylor AT, Francisco GE. Recovery of phenytoin from an enteral nutrient formula. *Am J Hosp Pharm.* 1986;43:685–688.

61. Guidry JR, Eastwood TF, Curry SC. Phenytoin absorption on volunteers receiving selected enteral feedings. *West J Med.* 1989; 150:659–661.

62. Gilbert S, Hatton J, Magnuson B. How to minimize interaction between phenytoin and enteral feedings: two approaches—therapeutic options. *Nutr Clin Pract.* 1996;11:28–31.

63. Bauer LA. Interference of oral phenytoin absorption by continuous nasogastric feedings. *Neurology.* 1982;32:570–572.

64. Bass J, Miles MV, Tennison MB, et al. Effects of enteral tube feeding on the absorption and pharmacokinetic profile of carbamazepine. *Epilepsia.* 1989;30:364–369.

65. Kassam RM, Friesen E, Locock RA. In vitro recovery of carbamazepine from Ensure. *JPEN J Parenter Enteral Nutr.* 1989;13:272–276.

66. Estoup M. Approaches and limitations of medication delivery in patients with enteral feeding tubes. *Crit Care Nurse.* 1994;14: 68–79.

67. Engle KK, Hannawa TE. Techniques for administering oral medications to critical care patients receiving continuous enteral nutrition. *Am Society Health-Syst Pharm.* 1999;56:1441–1444.

68. Healy DP, Brodbeck MC, Clendening CE. Ciprofloxacin absorption is impaired in patients given enteral feedings orally and via gastrostomy and jejunal tubes. *Antimicrob Agents Chemother.* 1996;40:6–10.

69. Mueller BA, Brierton DG, Abel SR, et al. Effect of enteral feeding with Ensure on oral bioavailabilities of ofloxacin and ciprofloxacin. *Antimicrob Agents Chemother.* 1994;38:2101–2105.

70. Piccolo ML, Toossi Z, Goldman M. Effect of coadministration of a nutritional supplement on ciprofloxacin absorption. *Am J Hosp Pharm.* 1994;51:2697–2699.

71. Mimoz O, Binter V, Jacolot A, et al. Pharmacokinetics and absolute bioavailability of ciprofloxacin administered through a nasogastric tube with continuous enteral feeding to critically ill patients. *Intensive Care Med.* 1998;24:1047–1051.

72. de Marie S, VandenBergh MF, Buijk SL, et al. Bioavailability of ciprofloxacin after multiple enteral and intravenous doses in ICU patients with severe gram-negative intra-abdominal infections. *Intensive Care Med.* 1998;24:343–346.

73. Sahai J, Memish Z, Conway B. Ciprofloxacin pharmacokinetics after administration via a jejunostomy tube. *J Antimicrob Chemother.* 1991;28:936–937.

74. Yuk JH, Nightingale CH, Quintiliani R, et al. Absorption of ciprofloxacin administered through a nasogastric or a nasoduodenal tube in volunteers and patients receiving enteral nutrition. *Diag Microbiol Infect Dis.* 1990;13:99–102.

75. Staib AH, Beerman D, Harder S, et al. Absorption differences of ciprofloxacin along the human gastrointestinal tract determined using remote-control drug delivery device. *Am J Med.* 1989;97(Suppl 5A):66S–69S.

76. Cohn SM, Sawyer MD, Burns GA, et al. Enteric absorption of ciprofloxacin during tube feeding in the critically ill. *J Antimicrob Chemother.* 1996;38:871–876.

77. Wright DH, Pietz SL, Konstantinides FN, et al. Decreased in vitro fluoroquinolone concentrations after admixture with an enteral feeding formulation. *JPEN J Parenter Enteral Nutr.* 2000;24: 42–48.

78. Kanji S, McKinnon PS, Barletta JF, et al. Bioavailability of gatifloxacin by gastric tube administration with and without concomitant enteral feeding in critically ill patients. *Crit Care Med.* 2003;31(5):1347–1352.

79. Burkhardt O, Stass H, Thuss U, et al. Effects of enteral feeding on the oral bioavailability of moxifloxacin in healthy volunteers. *Clin Pharmacokinet.* 2005;44(9):969–976.

80. Penrod LE, Allen JB, Cabacungan LR. Warfarin resistance and enteral feedings: two case reports and a supporting in vitro study. *Arch Phys Med Rehabil.* 2001;82:1270–1273.

81. Thijssen HH, Soute BA, Vervoort LM, et al. Paracetamol (acetaminophen) warfarin interaction: NAPQI, the toxic metabolite of paracetamol, is an inhibitor of enzymes in the vitamin K cycle. *Thromb Haemost.* 2004;92:797–802.

19 Dietary Supplements

Gerard E. Mullin, MD

CONTENTS

Acknowledgments: Joseph L. Boullata, PharmD, RPh, BCNSP, Michele Nicolo, MS, RD, CDE, CNSC, LDN, and Kathleen W. Stratton, JD, MA, RD, LDN, were the authors of this chapter for the second edition.

Objectives

1. Understand the current terminology defined by the National Center for Complementary and Alternative Medicine (NCAAM) in relation to dietary supplements and complementary and alternative medicine (CAM).
2. Describe current regulatory issues and trends relating to dietary supplements, including labeling requirements, advertising, product quality, legal actions, and adverse event reporting.
3. Identify potential safety problems with dietary supplements including adverse effects, interactions with prescription medications, and issues involving either intrinsic or extrinsic ingredients.

Test Your Knowledge Questions

1. Which of the following claims for a dietary supplement would most likely cause the US Food and Drug Administration (FDA) to consider that the supplement should be regulated as a drug rather than as a dietary supplement?
   A. Supports strong bones and teeth
   B. Treats influenza
   C. Promotes urinary health
   D. Improves immune function

2. Which of the following best describes dietary supplement use in the United States?

   A. Only a minority of the population uses dietary supplements.

   B. Most patients report their dietary supplement use to their primary care providers.

   C. Most patients think that their health care providers are knowledgeable about dietary supplements.

   D. Many patients using prescription medicines concomitantly use dietary supplements.

3. Even if Current Good Manufacturing Practices (CGMPs) promulgated by the Dietary Supplement Health and Education Act of 1994 (DSHEA) are properly implemented, which of the following is still likely to occur?

   A. A dietary supplement product adulterated with a prescription drug such as sibutramine is being marketed and sold.

   B. A dietary supplement product is analyzed and found to have much less of the active ingredient than what is indicated on the label.

   C. A dietary supplement product is analyzed and found to have much more of the active ingredient than what is indicated on the label.

   D. A dietary supplement product is marketed and sold, but there are no studies to confirm its efficacy for any condition.

Test Your Knowledge Answers

1. The correct answer is **B**. Under the DSHEA, manufacturers of dietary supplements may make statements regarding product ability to affect structure or function of the body. Manufacturers refer to these as "structure-function claims," which are regulated by the FDA for labeling and the US Federal Trade Commission (FTC) for merchandizing and marketing. Any claim regarding diagnosis, treatment, cure, or prevention of a disease is disallowed and subject to fines and prosecution. Therefore, a claim to support strong bones and teeth would be allowed as a structure claim, if true. The claims to promote urinary health and support the immune system would be function claims. The claim that a product treats influenza is an obvious claim regarding treatment of disease and would thus be disallowed.

2. The correct answer is **D**. Surveys have shown varying percentages of the US population using dietary supplements. Data from a large nationwide survey published in 2016 indicated that the use of dietary supplements remained stable between 1999 and 2012, with 52% of US adults reporting use of any supplements in 2011–2012.[1] Many persons using dietary supplements do not report this use to their allopathic health providers. Patients may not disclose supplement use because they do not think of supplements as products that may interact with their medications or because they believe that the health provider will be judgmental about their use. Abundant data indicate that the latter belief is overwhelmingly the most common reason why patients do not disclose the supplements they use, and there is strong evidence to validate patients' fear of reprisal. Although most patients think that their healthcare provider should be knowledgeable regarding dietary supplements, only about half of patients in a recent survey reported that providers actually were knowledgeable. In contrast, surveys of healthcare providers indicate that they are often reluctant to recommend CAM modalities even though they report having good to excellent awareness of the potential benefit of these modalities. Many patients using dietary supplements also use prescription medications; this concomitant use could result in supplement interactions with medication or increased incidence of adverse events.

3. The correct answer is **D**. The DSHEA mandates that CGMPs be set up for the dietary supplement industry. Under these CGMPs, process controls are supposed to be in place at each step of manufacturing. Thus, the dietary supplements arriving on the shelf should contain the correct ingredients in the correct amounts and should be free of adulterants. There should be consistency between lots in terms of content. Unfortunately, the FDA does not have sufficient resources to inspect all manufacturing plants and final products. However, examples of random testing of the authenticity of dietary supplements sold in large national retail chains by New York State agencies caught national attention in 2015 and led to legal action against the retailers, which ultimately paid large settlements.[2] The CGMPs do not address whether there are any data supporting the efficacy of dietary supplements.

Introduction

Dietary supplements are widely used by consumers and are probably used by some patients receiving nutrition support. Nutrition support clinicians are in an important position to not only identify patient use but also provide information to patients and other healthcare providers about dietary supplement indications, efficacy, safety, and legal regulation. This chapter provides an overview of the subject. More complete information on specific dietary supplement ingredients is available from specialized resources (Table 19-1). A relatively small number of ingredients account for a large portion of the most popular dietary supplement products.

Current Use in Adults

In the United States, annual sales of dietary supplement products exceed $36 billion.[3] The reported prevalence of dietary supplement use varies by the population evaluated and the products included in the survey. As noted earlier, US survey data indicates that the use of dietary supplements remained stable between 1999 and 2012, with 52% of US adults reporting use of any supplements in 2011–2012.[1] National Health and Nutrition Examination Survey data published in 2011 suggests that approximately 53% of adults use dietary supplements.[4] Other surveys confirm similar rates of dietary supplement use among older adults.[5]

However, clinicians may be unaware of their patients' use of dietary supplements. The results of a 2002 study in a community hospital indicate that, of the patients taking dietary supplements, less than half reported their supplement use to their primary providers. Documentation of dietary supple-

---

TABLE 19-1 Select Resources on Dietary Supplements

Reference books:

- Barnes J, Anderson LA, Phillipson JD, eds. *Herbal Medicines*. 3rd ed. London, UK: Pharmaceutical Press; 2007.
- Coates PM, Betz JM, Blackman MR, et al, eds. *Encyclopedia of Dietary Supplements*. 2nd ed. London, UK: Informa Healthcare; 2010.
- Cupp MJ, Tracy TS, eds. *Dietary Supplements: Toxicology and Clinical Pharmacology*. 2nd ed. Totowa, NJ: Humana Press; 2007.
- Dasgupta A, Hammett-Stabler C, eds. *Herbal Supplements*. Hoboken, NJ: Wiley; 2011.
- Mason P. *Dietary Supplements*. 4th ed. London, UK: Pharmaceutical Press; 2011.
- Pathak Y, ed. *Handbook of Nutraceuticals*. Boca Raton, FL: CRC Press; 2010.
- Stargrove MB, Treasure J, McKee DL. *Herb, Nutrient, and Drug Interactions: Clinical Implications and Therapeutic Strategies*. St. Louis, MO: Mosby Elsevier; 2008.
- Tracy TS, Kingston RL, eds. *Herbal Products: Toxicology and Clinical Pharmacology*. 2nd ed. Totowa, NJ: Humana Press; 2010.
- Ulbricht CE. *Natural Standard Herb and Supplement Guide*. St. Louis, MO: Mosby; 2010.

Online resources:

- American Botanical Council:
  - www.herbalgram.org
  - www.herbmed.org
- ConsumerLab: www.ConsumerLab.com
- Federal Trade Commission: www.ftc.gov
- Food and Drug Administration Dietary Supplements section: www.fda.gov/Food/DietarySupplements/default.htm
- National Institutes of Health Office of Dietary Supplements: http://ods.od.nih.gov
- National Sanitation Foundation (NSF):
  - Home page: www.nsf.org
  - Search for NSF Certified Dietary Supplements: www.nsf.org/certified/dietary
- Natural Medicines: https://naturalmedicines.therapeuticresearch.com
- Natural Products Association: www.npainfo.org
- Pharmacist's Letter: http://pharmacistsletter.therapeuticresearch.com
- QuackWatch: www.quackwatch.org
- US Pharmacopeia: www.usp.org

---

ment use in the medical record was found to be insufficient in a prospective study of interviewed patients.[6] Product description, product name, and frequency of use were often missing from documentation. In another investigation, reported use of a supplement 2 to 3 days prior to surgery was also not recorded in the medical record.[7]

Dickinson and colleagues surveyed physicians and nurses about their own use of supplements. They found that dietary supplements are used regularly by 37% to 59% of physicians and 59% of nurses, with most of those surveyed also recommending dietary supplements to their patients.[8,9]

Definitions

For purposes of this chapter, the ingredients that can be found in dietary supplements are divided into 3 groups based in part on the raw material sources. The first group comprise ingredients accepted as nutrients that have been recognized with Dietary Reference Intake (DRI) values (Table 19-2). The second group is herbal ingredients that contain parts or extracts of medicinal plants (Table 19-3). Lastly, are the other dietary supplement ingredients that are not officially recognized as nutrients and are not of botanical origin (Table 19-4). The official regulatory framework surrounding dietary supplements, including definitions, is important for better appreciating their role in patient care.

The controlling legal definition of *dietary supplement* is that which the US Congress included in DSHEA,[10] which amended the FDA authority under the Federal Food, Drug, and Cosmetic Act (FDCA).[11] This legal definition is broad and includes products taken by mouth that contain one or more of the following "dietary ingredients": a vitamin; a mineral; an herb or other botanical; an amino acid; a dietary substance for use by humans to supplement the diet by increasing the total dietary intake; or a concentrate, metabolite, constituent, extract, or combination of any ingredients previously described. A dietary supplement must be labeled as such and may be in tablet, capsule, powder, softgel, gelcap, or liquid form. *Supplement* means that the product is not represented for use as a conventional food or as a sole item of a meal or the diet.[12]

In addition to defining the term, Congress included dietary supplements under the general category of *foods* for purposes of the FDCA.[12] Hence, dietary supplements do not undergo the stringent and expensive premarket approval process required for prescription or over-the-counter drugs. Congress also excluded dietary supplements from the definition of *food additives*,[13] which means that manufacturers are exempt from the food additive premarket approval provisions of the FDCA as well.

In addition to the legal definition of dietary supplement, nutrition support clinicians and other healthcare providers should be aware of several other terms that may arise in a discussion of dietary supplements. For example, the National Institutes of Health (NIH) defines *complementary and alternative medicine* (CAM) as a group of diverse medical and healthcare systems, practices, and products that are not generally considered part of conventional medicine (also called *allopathic medicine*).[14] *Complementary medicine* refers to practices and products used together with conventional medicine, whereas *alternative medicine* refers to systems, practices, and products that are used as a substitute for conventional medicine. *Integrative medicine* (also called *integrated medicine*) refers to a practice that combines both conventional and CAM approaches for which there is evidence of safety and effectiveness.[14] The National Institute for Complementary and Alternative Medicine (NCCAM) is a branch of NIH that provides grants for research investigating whether CAM modalities have proven benefits. NCAAM also serves as an educational resource for the public.

TABLE 19-2 Common Nutrient Supplement Ingredients

| Ingredient Name | Common Uses[a] | Daily Dose[b] | Major Adverse Effects | | Comments |
			Side Effects	Interactions	
Arginine	Athletic performance, wound healing	2–3 g	GI discomfort, headache	Antihypertensives, blood thinners	Avoid use status post myocardial infarction; caution in hepatic/renal impairment.
Ascorbic acid	Wound healing	100–1000 mg	Diarrhea, kidney stones	Aspirin, estradiol, iron, indinavir	Dose cautiously in glucose-6-phosphate dehydrogenase deficiency; use with caution in renal impairment.
Biotin	Alopecia, brittle nails	300 mcg	NK	Antiepileptics	High-dose pantothenic acid reduces biotin absorption.
Calcium	Osteoporosis	400–2000 mg	Hypercalcemia, constipation	Bisphosphonates, digoxin, fluoroquinolones, levothyroxine	Use with caution if at risk for calcium oxalate stones.
Cholecalciferol	Osteoporosis	10–25 mcg (400–1000 IU)	Hypercalcemia, kidney stones	Antiepileptics	
Choline	Athletic performance, dementia	250–500 mg	GI discomfort	NK	Lecithin (phosphatidylcholine) has a less fishy odor.
Chromium	Diabetes, depression	200–500 mcg	Hypoglycemia	Insulin	Trivalent form and chloride salt are preferred.
Copper	Hypercholesterolemia	1–2 mg	GI discomfort	Penicillamine, iron, zinc	Available as chloride, acetate, or sulfate salt.
Folic acid	NTD prevention	400–1000 mcg	NK	Phenytoin, methotrexate	Assess vitamin B_{12} status. Supplementation >DRI may lead to inappropriate methylation, imposing health risks.
Iron	Fatigue	60–180 mg	GI discomfort, esophageal ulcers	ACE inhibitors	Fumarate or sulfate if inorganic. RDA is 8 mg for men and postmenopausal women and 18 mg for nonpregnant women.
Pyridoxine	PMS, depression	50–150 mg	Neuropathy	Isoniazid, hydralazine	Allergic reaction and photosensitivity are rare.
Selenium	CVD, rheumatoid arthritis, cancer	50–100 mcg	Hair loss, nail dystrophy	Clozapine	Sodium selenite or selenomethionine are preferred forms.
Taurine	Athletic performance, CVD	0.5–2 g	NK	NK	Nonprotein amino acid
Zinc	Diarrhea, wound healing	25–100 mg	Immunosuppression, anemia, and neuropathy from copper deficiency	Fluoroquinolones	Sulfate or chloride are preferred forms. RDA is 11 mg for men, 8 mg for women.

ACE, angiotensin-converting-enzyme; CVD, cardiovascular disease; DRI, Dietary Reference Intake; GI, gastrointestinal; NK, none known or not known; NTD, neural tube defect; PMS, premenstrual syndrome; RDA, Recommended Dietary Allowance.
[a]In addition to prevention/treatment of nutrient deficits.
[b]Elemental doses are listed for minerals.

TABLE 19-3 Popular Herbal Supplement Ingredients

Ingredient Name	Common Uses	Daily Dose	Major Adverse Effects	
			Side Effects	Interactions
Black cohosh (*Cimicifuga racemose*)	Menopausal symptoms	40–80 mg	Headache, GI discomfort	Tamoxifen
Chamomile (*Matricaria recutita*)	Indigestion; insomnia	400–1600 mg	Allergic reactions, drowsiness	Benzodiazepines
Echinacea (*Echinacea purpurea, Echinacea pallida, Echinacea angustifolia*)	Upper respiratory infection	600–1600 mg	Allergic reactions, headache, GI discomfort	Acetaminophen, steroids, and other immunosuppressants
Feverfew (*Tanacetum parthenium*)	Migraine prevention	125 mg	Allergic reactions, joint pain, mucositis, photosensitivity	NK
Garlic (*Allium sativum*)	Hyperlipidemia	600–900 mg	Bleeding, body odor, GI discomfort	Anticoagulants, saquinavir
Ginger (*Zingiber officinale*)	Nausea, vomiting	1000 mg	Heartburn	Anticoagulants
Ginkgo (*Ginkgo biloba*)	Vascular insufficiency	80–240 mg	Allergic reactions, bleeding, GI discomfort	Anticoagulants
Ginseng (*Panax ginseng, Panax quinquefolius*)	Panacea	100–200 mg	Headache, insomnia, GI discomfort	Antihypertensives
Goldenseal (*Hydrastis canadensis*)	Dyspepsia, diarrhea	400–800 mg	GI discomfort, hypoglycemia, mucositis, photosensitivity	Anticoagulants
Green tea (*Camellia sinensis*)	Weight loss	100–750 mg	Stimulant	Warfarin
Hawthorn (*Crataegus monogyna*)	Heart failure	160–900 mg	GI discomfort, headache, insomnia	Antihypertensives, digoxin
Milk thistle (*Silybum marianum*)	Liver disease	200–400 mg	Anaphylaxis, GI discomfort	NK
Saw palmetto (*Serenoa repens*)	Benign prostatic hyperplasia	320 mg	Dry mouth, GI discomfort, headache	NK
St. John's wort (*Hypericum perforatum*)	Depression	240–1800 mg	Dry mouth, GI discomfort, confusion, hypomania, photosensitivity	Antiepileptics, cyclosporine, digoxin, indinavir, oral contraceptives, triptans, warfarin
Valerian (*Valeriana officinalis*)	Anxiety; insomnia	400–1200 mg	Drowsiness	Benzodiazepines

GI, gastrointestinal; NK, none known.

Both conventional and CAM practitioners may use dietary supplements as part of a patient's biologically based treatment. What defines a dietary supplement product is the legal definition (as previously described), not who recommends it.

Naturopathy is a medical system that aims to support the body's ability to heal itself through dietary and lifestyle changes with therapies including the use of herbal supplements, massage, and joint manipulation.[14] *Phytotherapy* is the science of using plant-based medicines to prevent or treat illness.[15]

The terms *nutraceutical* and *functional food* are often used in the context of dietary supplements. *Nutraceutical* can refer to nutrients or other active food ingredients delivered in a pharmaceutical dosage form. By contrast, an active ingredient delivered within a food matrix, whether added or natural, may be considered a *functional food;* these functional food ingredients may be nutrients, herbals, or other compounds.[16] For example, vitamin C tablets might be described as a nutraceutical, whereas orange juice may be considered a functional food because it is high

TABLE 19-4 Other Popular Supplement Ingredients

Ingredient Name	Common Uses	Daily Dose	Major Adverse Effects[a]		Comments
			Side Effects	Interactions	
Beta-carotene	Cardiovascular disease	5–15 mg	Diarrhea, joint pain	Colestipol, ethanol, orlistat	Avoid in smokers (increased risk of lung cancer and cardiovascular mortality).
Chitosan	Hypercholesterolemia	1.3 g	Bleeding, GI discomfort, hypoglycemia	Antiplatelets	Avoid in people with shellfish allergy; may interfere with vitamin absorption.
Chondroitin	Osteoarthritis	800–1200 mg	GI complaints	Warfarin	May be natural (cartilage, trachea) or synthetic.
Coenzyme Q	Hypertension, heart failure	100–600 mg	Headache, fatigue	Warfarin	Synthesized by body; decreases with age.
Creatine	Muscle mass/strength	2–5 g	GI complaints, muscle cramps, renal impairment reported	Caffeine	Synthesized by body; influences creatinine levels.
Curcumin	Wound healing, inflammation	NK	GI irritation (usually when combined with black pepper)	NK	A component of turmeric.
Fish oils	Cardiovascular disease	1–4 g	Anticoagulant	Antiplatelets	Contents may vary with fish sources used.
Glucosamine	Osteoarthritis	1500 mg	GI complaints, proteinuria	Antiplatelets, diuretics	Source may be natural (shellfish).
Lutein	Ocular disorders	2–20 mg	NK	NK	Carotenoid found in a variety of foods.
Lycopene	Cancer, cardiovascular disease	2–30 mg	GI discomfort	Antiplatelets	Carotenoid found in tomato products.
Melatonin	Sleep disturbances	0.5–5 mg	Dysphoria, headache, infertility	Antiepileptics, sedatives, warfarin	Pineal gland hormone.
MSM	Allergic rhinitis, osteoarthritis	0.5–2.5 g	GI discomfort	NK	An oxidation product of dimethyl sulfoxide.
Resveratrol	Cancer, cardiovascular disease	NK	NK	Antiplatelets	Oral bioavailability unclear.

GI, gastrointestinal; MSM, methylsulfonylmethane; NK, none known or not known.
[a]Data on adverse effects and interactions are limited for this category of dietary supplements.

in vitamin C. The Academy of Nutrition and Dietetics (AND) defines *functional foods* as foods that "move beyond necessity to provide additional health benefits that may reduce disease risk and/or promote optimal health." According to AND, this definition would include conventional foods, modified foods (fortified, enriched, or enhanced), medical foods, and foods for special dietary use, such as infant foods and weight loss foods.[17] Notably, the terms *nutraceutical* and *functional food* have no legal meaning under the FDCA, and the FDA has regulatory authority over nutraceutical and functional food products either as dietary supplements or as foods.[18]

Dietary supplements are also distinguished from medical foods, such as enteral nutrition formulas. The Orphan Drug Act legally defines *medical food* as a "food which is formulated to be consumed or administered enterally under the supervision of a physician and which is intended for the specific dietary management of a disease or condition for which distinctive nutritional requirements, based on recognized scientific principles, are established by medical evaluation."[19] The original reasoning behind orphan drugs and this subcategory of orphan foods was to ease premarket development costs for those products not anticipated to recoup costs due to minimal need.[20] Examples include liquid protein and other modular components used in enteral nutrition, some oral nutritional drinks, and a few vitamin products approved for use as medical foods. Medical foods are exempt from both food labeling[21] and dietary supplement labeling requirements. Therefore, even though a medical food product might look like a dietary supplement in terms of content, different regulations apply because it is labeled as a medical food.

Homeopathy is a system of medicine that originated in Europe in the late 18th century. It is based on the "principle of similars," or "like cures like," which is described by practitioners of homeopathy as the observation that while high doses of pharmacologically active substances cause symptoms when administered to healthy people, those same substances when prepared in very dilute form may relieve similar symptoms in conditions resulting from different etiologies.[22] Homeopathic remedies are not dietary supplements under the legal definition of the FDCA. Although 2 products may contain similar ingredients, they may also be subject to different regulations depending on whether the product is officially recognized as a homeopathic medicine or a dietary supplement. Articles listed in the official Homeopathic Pharmacopeia of the United States are categorized as drugs by the FDCA.[23] These products have official monographs that provide drug information in the Homeopathic Pharmacopeia of the United States.[22] However, whereas the premarket approval process for most new drugs is governed by the FDA, the homeopathic products' premarket approval process is controlled by the Homeopathic Pharmacopeia Convention of the United States, which is comprised of scientists and clinicians trained in homeopathy.[22]

Regulatory Issues

US Food and Drug Administration Oversight

Under the DSHEA, the manufacturer is responsible for ensuring that a dietary supplement is safe before it is marketed. The FDA is responsible for taking action against an unsafe product and its manufacturer after it reaches the market. Generally, manufacturers do not need to register dietary supplement products with the FDA nor obtain FDA approval before producing or selling dietary supplements unless the product contains a new dietary ingredient (NDI).[24] NDI refers to any ingredient not previously marketed in the United States before the enactment of the DSHEA (October 15, 1994).[25] A dietary supplement product on the market is considered *adulterated* if it contains an ingredient that was not present in the food supply prior to the DSHEA or a known ingredient that has been chemically altered and the manufacturer markets it without giving prior notification to the FDA.[26] If a product includes an ingredient formerly unknown to the food supply, the manufacturer must make an NDI submission to the FDA that includes premarket safety data. The agency has rejected some submissions for failure to adequately identify the ingredient or failure to provide sufficient safety information.[27] For more information on premarket notification requirements for NDIs, see the FDA's online guidance.[28] In addition, compilations of dietary supplement regulations are available for reference.[29,30]

History of Federal Dietary Supplement Regulation

The Pure Food and Drug Act of 1906 prohibited "adulterated or misbranded" products from reaching consumers. The FDCA (1938) required products to be safe, and subsequent amendments created the requirement of efficacy.[14] In the 1960s and early 1970s, the FDA attempted to increase regulation of vitamin and mineral formulations under its authority to regulate special dietary foods.[31] In 1966, the FDA issued regulations that created several new requirements for vitamins and mineral formulations, including the requirement that products carry a statement that "there is no scientific basis for recommending the routine use of dietary supplements."[29] In response to strenuous objections, these regulations were stayed, and the agency eventually revoked them. In response to the FDA's attempts to assert its control over the dietary supplement industry, critics supported legislation that would severely limit the FDA's role in regulating dietary supplements. In 1976, amendments to the FDCA substantially limited the agency's authority to regulate the composition of dietary supplements.[31]

The FDA again attempted to increase regulation of dietary supplements in the 1990s. The Nutritional Labeling and Education Act (NLEA) of 1990 addressed the regulation of labeling and claims of food and food products, including dietary supplements. At that time, a review of over-the-counter products revealed a lack of safety and efficacy documentation, which meant that many dietary supplement products would have to be pulled from store shelves.[14] The dietary supplement industry argued that herbs, botanicals, and their components would not have been adequately quantified on labels under the nutrition labeling rules of the NLEA.[32] Further debate resulted in the Dietary Supplement Act of 1992, which delayed the NLEA and exempted dietary supplements from the purview of the legislation.

This legislative history is the backdrop for the Congress passing the DSHEA in 1994 despite strong objection from the FDA. Passage of the DSHEA established an inclusive definition of dietary supplements, which covers a wide range of products. Dietary supplements were relegated to the category of "foods," not drugs or food additives, both of which require submission of premarket safety data to the FDA. Congress specifically allowed structure/function claims that previously would have made the product a drug for regulatory purposes. This allowance placed the burden on the FDA to show that a product is unsafe after it is already being sold instead of requiring the manufacturer to demonstrate safety prior to a product's sale.[31] While the legislative intent was to improve access to dietary supplements for consumers and prevent burdensome and time-consuming premarket requirements, a consequence has been that dietary supplements are less regulated than medications and food additives.

Despite the length of time that the DSHEA has been in place, several studies demonstrate that the public does not understand how dietary supplements are regulated; in particular, they believe that the FDA or another government agency approves dietary supplements before they can be sold.[33] Safety considerations have led to recommending a return to more stringent regulation.[34]

Labeling Requirements and Claims

Labeling Requirements

The DSHEA amended the FDCA to add specific requirements for dietary supplement labels and ingredient declarations.[35] The FDA has jurisdiction to promulgate rules to prevent the misbranding of dietary supplements. These rules, which have been in effect since 1999, require dietary supplements to carry a Supplement Facts label that meets specific requirements.[36] Among other requirements, Daily Values must be listed for dietary ingredients present in a significant amount and for which a daily consumption value has been established. This daily reference value (ie, the Daily Value) does not necessarily reflect the Recommended Dietary Allowance (RDA) or Adequate Intake (AI) level for those nutrients that have DRIs. If no Daily Value has been established for an ingredient, the ingredient must still be listed but identified as having no such recommendation.[35] The label must also contain contact information identifying a "responsible person" who can receive serious adverse event reports.[37] Manufacturers must ensure that product label information is truthful and not misleading.[22] For a complete description of labeling and claims requirements, see the FDA's *Dietary Supplement Labeling Guide* intended for industry.[17]

Under federal law, scientific literature from a peer-reviewed publication that is used in connection with the sale of a dietary supplement is exempt from labeling requirements if the report is reprinted in its entirety; is not false or misleading; does not promote a particular manufacturer or brand; is presented with other items on the same subject matter to give a balanced view of available scientific information; if displayed in an establishment, is physically separate from the dietary supplements; and does not have appended to it any other information.[38] This provision is referred to as the *third-party literature exemption*, but there is no requirement that the publication be prepared by an independent party with no financial interest in the successful marketing and sale of the product.[31]

In addition to federal regulations, states may have additional laws regarding the labeling and sale of dietary supplements. For example, the New York State Attorney General investigated several retailers for violating New York law by falsely labeling dietary supplements and selling adulterated herbals,[39] including supplements containing wheat, which could be harmful to those with wheat allergy, celiac disease, or gluten sensitivity.

Claims

Federal law allows dietary supplements to carry a variety of different types of claims. Some require approval by the FDA prior to use and some do not. All must comply with pertinent statutes and regulations. Three types of claims—nutrient content, structure/function, and health—are described subsequently, but many other types exist. A complete description of all types may be found on the FDA's website.[17]

Nutrient Content Claims

Manufacturers are required to accurately describe the nutrient content of a dietary supplement. If claims regarding the content do not meet statutory requirements, the product may be deemed *misbranded* within the meaning of the FDCA.[40] A product is misbranded if any of the following are true:

- The labeling fails to list (1) the name of each ingredient in the supplement and (2) the quantity of each ingredient or, if it contains a proprietary blend, the total quantity of all the ingredients in the blend.
- The product is a botanical product and the labeling fails to identify the part of the plant from which the ingredient is derived.
- The product is purported to conform to the specifications of an official compendium but fails to do so.
- The product fails to have the identity and strength that the supplement is represented to have or fails to meet the quality, purity, or compositional specifications based on the assay or method the supplement purports to meet.

Structure/Function Claims (Statements of Nutritional Support)

Under the FDCA, *drugs* are defined as articles intended for use in the diagnosis, cure, mitigation, treatment, or prevention of a disease and articles (other than food) intended to affect the structure or any function of the body.[23] However, the DSHEA specifically allows dietary supplements to make structure/function claims if they meet certain statutory criteria, including a disclaimer statement that the product is not intended to prevent or cure a disease. Before the DSHEA, herbal supplements (but not vitamin/mineral supplements) were classified as drugs if they made structure/function claims.[31]

These structure/function claims, or statements of nutritional support, tend to be nonspecific (eg, "helps support the immune system"). Premarket notification or approval by the FDA is not required to use these types of claims. The label can include one of these claims if either of the following is true:

- The benefit is related to a classic nutrient-deficiency disease, describes the role of the ingredient in affecting structure or function in humans, and characterizes the mechanism by which the ingredient acts to maintain such structure or function.
- The claim describes general well-being from consumption of a nutrient or dietary ingredient; the statement is truthful and not misleading and contains the following disclaimer in full: "This statement has not been evaluated by the FDA. This product is not intended to diagnose, treat, cure, or prevent any disease."[41]

Health Claims

A *health claim* is an explicit or implied characterization of a relationship between a substance and a disease or a health-related condition. This type of claim requires significant scientific agreement and must be authorized by the FDA. A health claim describes the effect a substance has on reducing the risk of or preventing a disease (eg, "calcium may reduce the risk of osteoporosis"). By contrast, a structure/function claim describes the role of a substance intended to maintain the structure or function of the body (eg, "calcium for bone and colon health") and does not require approval by the FDA before use.[42,43]

As noted earlier, although homeopathic remedies (eg, cold remedies) may contain the same ingredients as a dietary supplement, they are not recognized legally as dietary supplements. Therefore, homeopathic remedies can make more specific claims about treating or curing illness than dietary supplements without having to demonstrate scientific evidence to the FDA.[44]

Advertising and Promotion

The FTC is responsible for ensuring that dietary supplement advertising is truthful, not misleading, and based on sound scientific evidence. The FTC publishes an *Advertising Guide for Industry* to assist those who sell or market dietary supplements with compliance.[45] The FTC can send warning letters to companies making potentially misleading statements in their advertisements. If a clinician believes advertising is false, misleading, or without scientific proof, complaints can be filed online with the FTC (www.ftc.gov/complaint). In 2010, it was reported that over the past decade the FTC had brought more than 100 law enforcement actions challenging claims about the effectiveness of a wide variety of supplements, including cold and flu products, weight loss products, and supplements claiming to treat serious diseases, including cancer and AIDS.[46] For a discussion of current actions brought by the FTC against Internet supplement advertisers, see the FTC press releases found on the FTC website.

However, despite the FTC's role in preventing deceptive advertising, the public is inundated with marketing about dietary supplements that may not be accurate or based in science. The advertising and sale of dietary supplements on the Internet is common in today's economy and estimated to account for at least 4% of total dietary supplement sales.[47] When dietary supplement advertisements dominate search engine results, consumers and health professionals may be challenged to find resources that provide reliable information. Several sources are available (Table 19-1), and some perform better than others.[48]

Adolescents have been identified as a group at risk for susceptibility to questionable advertising in fashion, sports, and lifestyle magazines because they reportedly desire to improve their physical appearance or performance and because teenagers often identify with celebrities and sports figures.[49] One study of advertising in magazines with a high adolescent readership showed problems with the accuracy of information about dietary supplements in these publications.[46]

Product Quality

The quality of dietary supplement products has long been an area of concern given the minimal regulation of dietary supplements since the passage of the DSHEA in 1994. The DSHEA gave the FDA the authority to promulgate rules to prevent dietary supplement products of poor quality.[50] However, rules relating to CGMPs for dietary supplements took time to develop. The final rule governing CGMPs was published in June of 2007, but compliance dates exempted smaller manufacturers until June 2010.[51,52] For a complete history of dietary supplement CGMPs, see the FDA's website.[53] Prior to adoption of the final rule, general food Good Manufacturing Practices applied to dietary

supplements; however, unlike foods, most dietary supplements are taken in the form of tablets, gelcaps, and capsules, which means the physiological processes involved in taking supplements can be very different from food intake.

The CGMPs require that process controls are in place at each step of the manufacturing process, regardless of whether one company or multiple firms are involved, to ensure that the product contains what it purports to contain. These controls include establishing and meeting specifications to ensure that the finished supplement contains the correct ingredient, purity, strength, and composition intended consistently and reliably each time.[52] While establishing standardized CGMPs for dietary supplements is an important step in promoting product quality, the onus remains on the manufacturer to ensure that these processes are established and being followed. The FDA has limited resources to inspect manufacturing plants and products for compliance with CGMPs. However, if a violation is found, the agency can take steps to remove the offending product from the market. (See Practice Scenario 19-1 for discussion of an adulterated dietary supplement.)

Practice Scenario 19-1

Question: What steps would you take in the case of a woman who is admitted to the hospital with unexplained rapid heartbeat and high blood pressure and indicates that she used weight loss supplements in the recent past?

Scenario: A 45-year-old woman with a history of obesity and fluctuating weight is admitted for unexplained hypertension and tachycardia. She says she has used a weight loss product that is labeled "100% natural." The dietitian reviews the label and confirms the "100% natural" claim but notes that the label does not list any ingredients known to cause the patient's symptoms. A call to the hospital pharmacist identifies the product as a dietary supplement and not a drug. After searching online for further product information, the dietitian locates the US Food and Drug Administration (FDA) website and discovers that the FDA has warned consumers about tainted weight loss products containing sibutramine, a prescription medication that was taken off the market in 2010. The supplement used by this patient is one of the products identified as containing sibutramine.

Intervention: The dietitian informs the patient to stop taking the supplement and explains the rationale for stopping. The dietitian also discusses with the medical team the results of the search and the advice given to the patient and reports the adverse event using the FDA's MedWatch Safety Information and Adverse Event Reporting Program (www.fda.gov/medwatch/report.htm).

Answer: (1) Discuss the supplement with the pharmacist. (2) Investigate supplement on the FDA's website and other reliable sites (refer to Table 19-1). (3) Communicate all information to the patient and medical team. (4) Report the adverse event on MedWatch.

Rationale: The FDA has reported incidents of weight loss products marketed as "100% natural" being adulterated with prescription medications including sibutramine, which was removed from the market in 2010 for safety reasons. Sibutramine is known to substantially increase blood pressure and/or pulse rate in some patients and may present a significant risk for patients with a history of coronary artery disease, congestive heart failure, arrhythmias, and stroke. Sibutramine may also interact with medications in a life-threatening way.

Adverse Event Reporting

In 2006, Congress amended the FDCA to require dietary supplement manufacturers to report any serious adverse events that come to their attention to the FDA.[54,55] A *serious adverse event* is defined as an event that either results in death, a life-threatening experience, inpatient hospitalization, a persistent or significant disability or incapacity, or a congenital anomaly or birth defect, or any event that requires a medical or surgical intervention to prevent one of these outcomes.[55] If a consumer or clinician reports such an event to the manufacturer identified on the label of the suspect product, the manufacturer is bound by law to file a report of the event to the FDA through the agency's MedWatch reporting system.[55] At this point, the agency can take appropriate steps to investigate the product and consider requiring the manufacturer to remove it from store shelves, if appropriate. However, submission of a serious adverse event report by a manufacturer does not constitute an admission that the product caused the event.[55]

Only serious events, as defined by law, require this type of reporting to the FDA. While manufacturers must keep records of both serious and nonserious events for 6 years and make them available to the FDA if the plant is inspected, nonserious events are not reported publicly for healthcare professionals to review. For example, if a product causes mild rash in many people but no hospital admissions or other serious event criteria apply, the general public is not given access to this information. Because of this reporting system and the lack of premarket testing reports, the availability of minor adverse reaction data is limited with dietary supplements. Clinicians who believe a patient's illness or injury might be related to the use of a dietary supplement should report the event directly to the FDA. Previously reported adverse events are also published on the FDA's website for review by clinicians.[56]

In February 2010, Senators John McCain (R-AZ) and Byron Dorgan (D-ND) introduced a bill that proposed to amend the FDCA to tighten regulation of dietary supplements on the basis that these products may pose safety risks unknown to consumers.[57] While this bill did not become law, it reflected the efforts of those who believe increased regulation of dietary supplements would benefit the public. The bill would have required dietary supplement facilities to register with the FDA and obligated manufacturers to submit a compilation of all nonserious adverse events to the FDA.

Efficacy of Dietary Supplements

Given the diversity of dietary supplement ingredients, one cannot generalize about the clinical efficacy of all dietary supplements as a group. Thousands of marketed products contain countless ingredients, often in a variety of combinations. Data on efficacy vary with the individual ingredient(s) in a product. As with any therapeutic intervention, the value of a dietary supplement ingredient or a specific combination of ingredients in a dietary supplement product is based on an evaluation of known benefits and risk.

For the patients' benefit, clinicians should thoroughly and critically evaluate research data before making recommendations about incorporating a dietary supplement into clinical practice. The trials used to evaluate clinical efficacy should meet accepted criteria for a well-designed study. Well-designed clinical intervention studies provide the highest level of data to support the effectiveness of therapeutic interventions. Once published, such studies can provide information on indications, contraindications, dosing, and monitoring of a dietary supplement. Because national regulatory frameworks for dietary supplements vary, it is important to pay close attention to the description of the pharmaceutical quality of the product used in each study.

Epidemiologic data and case reports on the use of a dietary supplement ingredient are less valuable than research trial data in making clinical decisions about efficacy. Information on traditional use—including dietary patterns that include a given component—cannot necessarily be extrapolated to the use of dietary supplement ingredients in a pharmaceutical regimen. Common uses of popular dietary supplement ingredients (Tables 19-2, 19-3, and 19-4) are supported by widely varying levels of evidence. Although the body of peer-reviewed literature studying the use of individual dietary supplement ingredients or specific combinations of ingredients is growing, many marketed products are not yet supported by evidence. Differentiating the available evidence from the marketing hype is important for consumers and clinicians alike.[58] Ideally, adequate efficacy data would be available to evaluate whether a dietary supplement does what the claims say it does. However, once a product is in the marketplace, a patient could choose to use it even in the absence of any supporting data. In such a case, it would be valuable to know that the product is at least reasonably safe and of high quality. (See Practice Scenario 19-2 for an example of questionable use of a dietary supplement.)

Practice Scenario 19-2

Question: What advice would you give to the medical team treating a young woman admitted with a severe Crohn's disease flare who refuses conventional medications in favor of using aloe vera?

Scenario: A 25-year-old woman with an established history of Crohn's disease, a body mass index of 17.5, and a weight loss of 10 pounds over the last 3 months is admitted to the hospital with an acute Crohn's disease flare and iron deficiency anemia. In taking her history, she tells you she is refusing anti-inflammatory medications in favor of natural dietary supplements because of the potential side effects of the medications. She is taking aloe vera on the advice of a natural medicine practitioner. The medical team assumes taking aloe vera orally is not harmful and agrees to allow the patient a trial period of treatment with the aloe vera. The patient and team mutually agree that if her condition does not improve, the patient will try conventional medications used for treating Crohn's disease. The team asks you for information on the appropriate dosage of oral aloe vera.

Intervention: Tell the team that oral aloe vera is relatively contra-indicated given the patient's current presentation.

Answer: (1) Research information on oral aloe vera use. (2) Communicate results of search to patient and team. (3) Recommend against its use in this patient.

Rationale: Aloe vera is used topically to treat minor wounds, minor burns, and other dermatological conditions. Its traditional use in oral form is for managing constipation, for which there is supporting scientific evidence. There is no convincing evidence of any benefit of oral aloe vera for inflammatory bowel disease; its use has not been compared with conventional treatments for Crohn's disease. Risks of oral aloe vera supplementation include exacerbating abdominal pain, cramping, diarrhea, and significant electrolyte imbalances. The risk of harm outweighs any potential benefit, and the medical team should be advised that oral aloe vera is not safe for this patient.

Safety of Dietary Supplements

Given the presence of biologically active ingredients, the safety issues for dietary supplements share many similarities with the issues for more closely regulated pharmaceutical products, but dietary supplements also involve a few unique safety concerns. As with other pharmaceutical products, adverse effects resulting from the intrinsic (ie, labeled) ingredients may occur. These effects may be predictable and dose-related; unexpected allergic or idiosyncratic reactions; or interactions with prescribed medication. The risk to the patient may vary by age, sex, genetics, nutritional status, conditions or disorders, and treatments. Adverse effects may influence any organ system—for example, the influence of a supplement containing kava on the liver may range from mild transient transaminitis to fulminant hepatic failure, or influence of ginkgo on the skin may range from a self-limited rash to exfoliative dermatitis.

Safety evaluation based on epidemiologic data or traditional use data may fall short of identifying or predicting potential adverse effects. The doses, matrixes, and chronicity of exposure using pharmaceutical dosage forms may mean that outcomes from using these products are unlike outcomes associated with traditional use, findings from epidemiologic data, or even results from short-term, clinical intervention trials. Unfortunately, well-designed and adequately powered clinical trials to evaluate adverse effects of dietary supplements are uncommon.[59] As a result, adverse effects of dietary supplements are not as well characterized, recognized, or reported as they are with medications. When adverse effects are identified, reported, and documented, it is not always clear whether the findings can be attributed to the labeled ingredients or to poor product quality. In either case, knowledge about the potential harm a dietary supplement may cause a patient allows for informed decision-making about the product's use. Some ingredients are recognized to have risks that outweigh benefits (Table 19-5).

TABLE 19-5 Dietary Supplement Ingredients Where Risk Outweighs Benefit[a]

Ingredient Name	Potential Danger
Androstenedione	Carcinogenicity
Bitter orange *(Citrus aurantium)*	Cardiotoxicity, hypertension
Blue-green algae	Hepatotoxicity, neurotoxicity
Blue cohosh *(Caulophyllum thalictroides)*	Cardiotoxicity, hypertension
Calamus *(Acorus calamus)*	Carcinogenicity, nephrotoxicity
Chaparral *(Larrea tridentata)*	Hepatotoxicity
Coltsfoot *(Tussilago farfara)*	Carcinogenicity, hepatotoxicity
Comfrey *(Symphytum* spp.)	Carcinogenicity, hepatotoxicity
Dong quai *(Angelica sinensis)*	Anticoagulant, carcinogenicity
Ephedra [ma huang] *(Ephedra sinica)*[a]	Cardiotoxicity, hepatotoxicity
Germander *(Teucrium chamaedrys)*	Hepatotoxicity
Germanium	Nephrotoxicity
Kava *(Piper methysticum)*	Hepatotoxicity
Lobelia *(Lobelia inflata)*	Coma, hepatotoxicity, neurotoxicity
Pennyroyal *(Hedeoma pulegioides; Mentha pulegium)*	Multiorgan dysfunction, neurotoxicity, abortifacient
St. John's Wort *(Hypericum perforatum)*	Multiple drug interactions by interfering with liver's microsomal mixed oxidase enzyme system
Sassafras *(Sassafras albidum)*	Genotoxicity, hepatocarcinogenicity, abortifacient
Skullcap *(Scutellaria* spp.)	Hepatotoxicity
Snakeroot or boneset *(Eupatorium perfoliatum)*	Carcinogenicity, hepatotoxicity, nephrotoxicity
Valerian root *(Valeriana officinalis)*	Hepatotoxicity
Wormwood *(Artemisia absinthium)*	Neurotoxicity
Yohimbe *(Pausinystalia yohimbe)*	Cardiotoxicity

[a]Ephedra is banned for sale in the United States by the US Food and Drug Administration (FDA). All other ingredients listed in this table are commercially available in stores and pharmacies and online. Note the advisory warnings on FDA's Food and Dietary Supplement Division (http://www.fda.gov/Food/DietarySupplements).

The safety of multi-ingredient products is not always known because the study of such products has been limited.[60] To determine the maximum safe levels of dietary supplement ingredients, one must account for the interindividual variability of intake of foods fortified with nutrients or other ingredients.[61] This risk assessment approach can be most easily conducted for nutrient ingredients. Toxicological data on many of the plant sources of herbal ingredients are still lacking.[62]

In sum, the incidence of adverse effects with a dietary supplement product or ingredient is difficult to ascertain because the United States has a voluntary system of reporting that captures very few events and there is little valuable denominator data on overall use.[63] Some of the best data come from poison control centers, with estimates of about 30% to 40% of referred dietary supplement exposures being associated with adverse effects.[60] About one-half of calls to poison control centers concerning dietary supplement exposures described symptoms, with 62% of these considered "probably" associated with the supplement.[64] Dietary supplements ranked second behind antidepressants in adverse-reaction hospitalizations following exposures as evaluated by poison control centers.[65] Adverse effects related to dietary supplement interactions with medications are not always delineated, but they need to be taken into account. Dietary supplements and herbals are a leading cause of liver injury and account for 20% of the cases of hepatotoxicity in the United States.[66] Many herbals that are linked to liver injury; for example, the weight loss supplements containing green tea extracts may be associated with acute hepatitis. Multi-ingredient dietary supplements and body building supplements containing anabolic steroids that can cause hepatotoxicity are other common culprits.[67]

At least 43% of ambulatory adults regularly use dietary supplements concurrently with prescription medicine, but dietary supplement information is not always included in medication histories in institutional or community settings.[68] Among adults using prescription drugs, 32% to 39% are also taking a dietary supplement.[69,70] Among patients with 2 or more chronic medications, 44% reported use of herbal dietary supplements.[65] Among women age 75 years and older using prescription medication, 60% combined them with dietary supplements.[5] An estimated 12% to 45% of individuals using dietary supplement products with prescription drugs are at risk for a drug-supplement interaction, with 6% to 29% of these interactions considered potentially serious or clinically significant.[71-74]

Approximately 90% of dietary supplement users thought that pharmacists should routinely be checking for interactions.[67] The information on documented interactions or potential interactions is limited but continues to grow.[72,75] These may occur within the gastrointestinal lumen, but they are more likely occur at the level of transporters and metabolizing enzymes found in the intestinal epithelium and the liver. Many of the dietary polyphenols as well as botanicals found in dietary supplement products are substrates for—or influence expression and activity of—drug transporters and drug metabolizing enzymes.[76-82] For example, soy isoflavones (eg, daidzein, genistein) can significantly upregulate 2 drug transporters and 5 enzymes.[83,84] Also, catechins found in green tea can significantly influence drug transporters in entero-cytes and hepatocytes.[85] Nutrient transporters (eg, thiamin, folic acid) can also be reduced by polyphenols.[86] Even specific probiotic strains may play a role in altering transporter function responsible for drug and nutrient absorption.[87] Cautious interpretation and extrapolation from in vitro and in vivo data are necessary until more human data become available.

In contrast to prescription and nonprescription medication, dietary supplements may be associated with adverse effects that are extrinsic to the labeled ingredients. This problem relates to the quality of the product and may be caused by misidentification of the raw material or ingredients, or the presence of impurities, which may be introduced by adulteration (eg, prescription drugs), substitution (eg, different plant), or contamination (eg, heavy metals, pesticides). CGMPs are intended to reduce the likelihood of this group of adverse effects.

Plant-derived (ie, botanical) ingredients can vary widely in their chemical content, depending in part on soil and environmental conditions. Quality assurance of dietary supplement products containing botanical ingredients should take Good Agricultural Practices into account, with manufacturers requiring an independent certificate of analysis for all raw materials purchased (botanical or otherwise) that provide thorough documentation of composition including concentrations of any contaminants.[88] The ability to analyze dietary supplement ingredients containing or extracted from plant sources is improving. To monitor the quality of these herbal ingredients requires validated and adopted standard assays for chemical constituents (ie, marker compounds) as well as evaluation of contaminants.[89-91]

Ideally, quality control methods would occur with raw materials as well as finished products.[87] Any manufacturing practice that cannot confirm the identity, purity, strength, and quality of a dietary supplement product falls short of maximizing patient safety. Multiple independent testing programs that provide data on quality of dietary supplements are accessible to the public. Manufacturers may choose to submit their products for independent testing, and the results are published in reports available to consumers. However, only a small proportion of products on the market are independently tested. Independent testing programs include the US Pharmacopeia Dietary Supplement Verification Program, ConsumerLab.com, the National Sanitation Foundation, and the Natural Products Association (formerly the National Nutritional Foods Association), which offers a third-party CGMP certification program specific to dietary supplements that includes the FDA CGMP requirements. Aside from general tests and assays, many dietary supplement ingredients have officially recognized monographs in the US Pharmacopeia that can be used to better identify high-quality products.[92]

The Clinician's Role and Implications for Nutrition Support Practice

Open dialogue between clinicians and patients, including regular discussions with patients about their medications and dietary supplements, is vital in communicating health-related information. It is recommended that clinicians have a good working knowledge of common dietary supplements based on validated sources of information.[93] One goal is to support informed decision making by the patient. Another goal is to prevent adverse outcomes associated with dietary supplement use, keeping in mind that the risk for adverse reactions is increased for individuals receiving concurrent drug therapy or undergoing surgery. The involved clinician should be willing to evaluate the dietary supplement literature and report any observed adverse effects, including interactions with other therapies, when needed.[92] Of patients regularly using dietary supplements, 93% think it is important for their healthcare providers to be knowledgeable about them; however, only about half felt that their providers actually were familiar with such products.[67]

For a practitioner to be able to counsel patients on the use of dietary supplements, he or she first needs to be familiar with common ingredients, their safety and efficacy, and any potential interactions between the supplements and medications. Clinicians should frequently ask patients about supplement use; collect data on the patient's current or proposed use of vitamins, minerals, herbals, and other dietary supplements, including the specific regimen and the reason/indication for each product used; and carefully evaluate indications, dosing, and safety and efficacy data. The assessment of the patient's intended or current use of supplements provides the clinician an opportunity to counsel the patient on safety issues related to supplement use. Clinicians should approach the subject of supplement use with a "buyers beware" perspective. Documenting the patient's use of supplements in the health record allows practitioners to continually monitor the patient for potential adverse reactions. Patients who have taken their supplements consistently with other medications should be counseled to check with a provider before making any changes in dose or discontinuing use of the product. One study demonstrated that certain ethnic groups (eg, Asian Americans and Hispanics) may be less likely to disclose dietary supplement use to healthcare providers.[69] The authors suggest that this is associated with limited English-language ability and lower socioeconomic status, which may inhibit members of these groups from seeking medical attention. Other potential influences on patient disclosure include the responses from their healthcare provider—negative responses may discourage patients from speaking openly about supplement use.[69] Deficits in consumer knowledge about dietary supplement safety, efficacy, and regulation can be significantly improved through education by clinicians.[31]

Given the limited evidence on safety and efficacy, clinicians have had little guidance in directing patient use of dietary supplements. Weiger et al developed a systems approach to guiding clinicians to "recommend," "accept," or "discourage" dietary supplement use.[94] A recommendation for a specific dietary supplement should be based on evidence that supports its efficacy and safety. Supplement acceptance can be considered if evidence of the efficacy of the product is questionable but its safety has been established. Clinicians should discourage use of supplements when evidence demonstrate a lack of efficacy and potential harm, but they should give this advice in a professional manner to foster open communication and not cast dispersions or judgment.[95]

Among the oncology populations, patients may opt for alternative treatments instead of conventional therapy.

Michaud and colleagues have presented an algorithm for evaluating dietary supplement use in oncology patients, which may also be applied to other medical situations.[96] Oral supplement products increase the potential risk for interactions between drug and nondrug therapies for oncology patients. Under safety review, each supplement should be evaluated to identify any ingredients that may have antioxidant, anticoagulant, procoagulant, immune modulator, or hormonal properties, particularly if there are established safety concerns or known drug interactions. If the supplement potentially has any of these characteristics, the clinician should address the patient's risk level. Even if the safety concern is only hypothetical concern or based on questionable data, individuals at risk should be discouraged from using the product. If the supplement seems to pose no risk to the patient's safety, clinicians should proceed to evaluate the efficacy of the product. If there is decisive evidence for lack of efficacy, use of the product should be discouraged. If convincing evidence supports efficacy, use of the product may be recommended. When efficacy evidence is lacking or questionable, clinicians must use clinical judgment to assess whether use of the supplement is acceptable. Supplements falling into this category may warrant continued follow-up and especially close monitoring.[95]

AND recommends that dietetics professional consider several factors before they decide to sell supplements.[97] Providers should avoid selling products that are beyond their scope of practice or are not compliant with institutional policies regarding sales and distribution of dietary supplements. They should acknowledge the patient's choice and avoid any potential bias in persuading patients to choose specific dietary supplements. Accurate and relevant educational information should be included when providing/selling dietary supplements. If the providers gain financial revenue from the sale of the product(s), they need to disclose this fact to their patients via face-to-face interaction or in written documentation that is easily understood and readily available. Information about comparable products on the market should also be presented. Legal issues, including malpractice, are a concern for providers who choose to sell dietary supplements. It is further recommended that providers have a grasp of federal and state regulations pertaining to licensure and business practices.

Recommendations for individual patients do not preclude setting institutional protocols or policies that address dietary supplements. The Joint Commission has set forth recommendations for health-system formulary implementation on the use of dietary supplements, but it is otherwise silent on specifics.

The American Society of Health-System Pharmacists (ASHP) has issued clinical practice recommendations on the use of dietary supplements in response to the increased frequency of use.[98] Because of safety concerns, ASHP discourages use of supplements in situations where irrevocable consequences may occur, such as use in conjunction with immune suppression, chemotherapy, HIV infection, anticoagulation therapy, or use of hormonal contraceptives. Health-system formularies should have established criteria for inclusion of dietary supplements, and these products should undergo the same scrutiny as prescription and nonprescription medications to decrease institutional liability. ASHP suggests discontinuing use of patient self-administered dietary supplements on admission, especially as diagnostic workup continues. Allowing patient dietary supplement use during hospital admission should require documentation in the medical record, including a physician order and the supplement name. In addition, a pharmacist should review and verify the ordered supplement before dispensing it.[97] The safety of hospitalized patients may be compromised if written policies about dietary supplements are inadequate.[99] (See Practice Scenario 19-3 for an example of dealing with dietary supplements in an inpatient setting.)

Practice Scenario 19-3

Question: What dietary supplement would you recommend for a patient with heart failure and with history of gastric bypass surgery 5 years earlier?

Scenario: A 57-year-old man presented with new onset mild heart failure, leukopenia, and peripheral neuropathy. He reported that he had never been fully compliant with advice to take a multivitamin with minerals and a calcium supplement following his gastric bypass procedure. The team immediately ordered the oral multivitamin supplement on the hospital formulary and ordered a laboratory micronutrient panel for bariatric patients to check for deficiencies (ie, thiamin, vitamin B$_{12}$, vitamin C, vitamin D, iron, copper, selenium, and zinc). The results of the panel revealed deficiencies of thiamin, copper, zinc, and vitamin D. The neurology team is concerned with the patient's neuropathy and calls the nutrition support clinician to ask whether the formulary micronutrient product contains the necessary amount of copper for repletion. The clinician checks with the pharmacy for the supplement label information and learns that the current formulary product supplied by the wholesaler to the pharmacy and dispensed contains the following:

- Vitamin A (no beta-carotene): 5000 IU
- Thiamin mononitrate: 1.5 mg
- Riboflavin: 2 mg
- Niacinamide: 20 mg
- Pyridoxine: 0.1 mg
- Calcium pantothenate: 1 mg
- Vitamin C: 37.5 mg
- Vitamin D: 400 IU

The clinician quickly realizes that this supplement is not the appropriate multivitamin/mineral product for the patient. The content of vitamin A (salt not described) exceeds the Dietary Reference Intake (DRI) of 900 mcg (5000 IU = 1500 mcg); the content of pyridoxine, pantothenic acid, and vitamin C are below the DRIs; and the form of vitamin D is not described for the dose (400 IU = 10 mcg).

Intervention: Initially, the nutrition support clinician recommends a complete therapeutic multivitamin/mineral preparation. She also investigates the product on formulary to determine the product composition and identify whether it contains adequate amounts and forms of the nutrients to replete the identified deficiencies. Additionally, she considers the costs and benefits of repleting individual deficiencies using single ingredient products of appropriate dose and salt.

Answer: (1) Identify a therapeutic multivitamin/mineral product containing adequate amounts to meet the patient's specific needs. (2) Communicate the information to the patient and the team. (3) Consider approaching the institution to add this standardized product to the formulary, knowing that patients with certain nutrient deficiencies may require amounts greater than the DRI.

Rationale: The composition of the formulary oral micronutrient supplement did not meet the patient's needs. The patient was deficient in copper, which the supplement available on formulary did not contain. An individual oral copper supplement containing 2 to 8 mg of copper that is not the sulfide or oxide forms would be most appropriate. A set of criteria for selecting an appropriate multivitamin/mineral product should be determined and shared with the purchasing officer.

Summary

The popularity of dietary supplement products containing nutrient, herbal, and/or other ingredients remains unabated. The well-informed nutrition support clinician understands what constitutes a dietary supplement and how these products are regulated. Whenever required to do so, the responsible clinician will determine clinical effectiveness and safety of specific dietary supplement ingredients through a careful review of evidence-based compilations and the primary literature. Patients should be supported in making fully informed decisions about dietary supplements.

References

1. Kantor ED, Rehm CD, Du M, White E, Giovannucci EL. Trends in dietary supplement use among us adults from 1999-2012. *JAMA*. 2016;316(14):1464–1474. doi:10.1001/jama.2016.14403.
2. Mullin GE. Time for more regulation of dietary supplements? The Hill blog. http://thehill.com/blogs/congress-blog/healthcare/238010-time-for-more-regulation-of-dietary-supplements. Accessed January 20, 2016.
3. Council for Responsible Nutrition. Fact sheet: Dietary supplements—safe, beneficial and regulated. Revised June 2016. http://www.crnusa.org/resources/dietary-supplements-safe-beneficial-and-regulated. Accessed January 20, 2017.
4. Gahche J, Bailey R, Burt V, et al. *Dietary Supplement Use Among U.S. Adults has Increased Since NHANES III (1988-1994)*. NCHS data brief no 61. Hyattsville, MD: National Center for Health Statistics; 2011. https://www.cdc.gov/nchs/products/databriefs/db61.htm. Accessed January 20, 2017.
5. Qato DM, Alexander GC, Conti RM, et al. Use of prescription and over-the-counter medications and dietary supplements among older adults in the United States. *JAMA*. 2008;300:2867–2878.
6. Chhay C, Rynes R, Kajimura-Beck M, et al. Alternative medicine use in a community hospital. *Am J Health Syst Pharm*. 2002; 59:2452–2453.
7. Cockayne NL, Duguid M, Shenfield GM. Health professionals rarely record history of complementary and alternative medicines. *Br J Clin Pharmacol*. 2004;59:254–258.
8. Dickinson A, Boyon N, Shao A. Physicians and nurses use and recommend dietary supplements: report of a survey. *Nutr J*. 2009;8:29.
9. Dickinson A, Shao A, Boyon N, et al. Use of dietary supplements by cardiologists, dermatologists and orthopedists: report of a survey. *Nutr J*. 2011;10:20.

10. Pub Law No. 103-417, 108 Stat 4325 (1994).
11. USC 321 et seq.
12. USC 321(ff).
13. USC 321(s).
14. National Center for Complementary and Alternative Medicine. Complementary, alternative, or integrative health: what's in a name? Updated June 28, 2016. http://nccam.nih.gov/health/whatiscam/#definingcam. Accessed January 20, 2017.
15. Morrow K. Food and nutrient delivery: complementary and integrative medicine and dietary supplementation. In: Mahan LK, Raymond JL, eds. *Krause's Food, Nutrition, & Diet Therapy*. 14th ed. St. Louis, MO: Saunders Elsevier; 2016.
16. Boullata JI. Dietary supplements. In: Rolandelli RH, Bankhead R, Boullata J, et al, eds. *Clinical Nutrition: Enteral and Tube Feeding*. 4th ed. Philadelphia, PA: Elsevier Saunders; 2005:248–264.
17. Hasler CM, Brown AC; American Dietetic Association. Position of the American Dietetic Association: functional foods. *J Am Diet Assoc.* 2009;109:735–746.
18. US Food and Drug Administration. Dietary supplement labeling guide, April 2005. Updated July 2016. http://www.fda.gov/Food/GuidanceRegulation/GuidanceDocumentsRegulatoryInformation/DietarySupplements/ucm2006823.htm. Accessed January 20, 2017.
19. 21 USC 360ee.
20. Bankhead R, Boullata J, Brantley S, et al., A.S.P.E.N. Board of Directors. Enteral nutrition practice recommendations. *JPEN J Parenter Enteral Nutr.* 2009;33:122–167.
21. 21 CFR 101.9.
22. Borneman JP, Field RI. Regulation of homeopathic drug products. *Am J Health Syst Pharm.* 2006;63:86–91.
23. 221 USC 321(g).
24. US Food and Drug Administration. Dietary supplements. Updated April 4, 2016. http://www.fda.gov/Food/DietarySupplements. Accessed January 20, 2017.
25. 21 USC 350b.
26. 21 CFR 190.6.
27. McGuffin M, Young AL. Premarket notifications of new dietary ingredients: a ten-year review. *Food Drug Law J.* 2004;59:229.
28. US Food and Drug Administration. Chapter VII. Premarket notification of new dietary ingredients, April 2005. Updated May 27, 2015. http://www.fda.gov/Food/GuidanceRegulation/GuidanceDocumentsRegulatoryInformation/DietarySupplements/ucm070614.htm. Accessed January 20, 2017.
29. Allport-Settle MJ. Dietary Supplements: Current Good Manufacturing Practice, Labeling and Pre-market Notification. Willow Springs, NC: PharmaLogika; 2010.
30. US Pharmacopeia. *USP Dietary Supplements Compendium: The Authoritative Reference*. Rockville, MD: US Pharmacopeia Convention; 2012.
31. Hutt PB, Merrill RA, Grossman LA, eds. *Food and Drug Law: Cases and Materials*. 3rd ed. New York: Foundation Press; 2007:246–268.
32. Dickinson A. History and overview of DSHEA. *Fitoterapia*. 2011;82:5–10.
33. Dodge T, Litt D, Kaufman A. Influence of the Dietary Supplement Health and Education Act on consumer beliefs about the safety and effectiveness of dietary supplements. *J Health Commun.* 2011;16:230–244.
34. Rogovik AL, Vohra S, Goldman RD. Safety considerations and potential interactions of vitamins: should vitamins be considered drugs? *Ann Pharmacother.* 2010;44:311–324.
35. USC 343(q)(5)(F).
36. *Federal Register* 1997;62(184):49825-49858.
37. USC 343(y).
38. USC 343-2.
39. Kaplan S. GNC, Target, Wal-Mart, Walgreens accused of selling adulterated "herbals." *Washington Post*. Feb 3, 2016. https://www.washingtonpost.com/news/morning-mix/wp/2015/02/03/gnc-target-wal-mart-walgreens-accused-of-selling-fake-herbals. Accessed January 20, 2017.
40. USC 343(s).
41. USC 343(r).
42. USC 101.14.
43. 421 CFR 101.93.
44. Anonymous. In from the cold. *Nutr Action Health Letter*. 2011:10–11.
45. US Federal Trade Commission. Dietary supplements: an advertising guide for industry. April 2001. https://www.ftc.gov/tips-advice/business-center/guidance/dietary-supplements-advertising-guide-industry. Accessed January 20, 2017.
46. US Federal Trade Commission. FTC submits statement to Congress on deceptive marketing of dietary supplements, May 2010. https://www.ftc.gov/news-events/press-releases/2010/05/ftc-submits-statement-congress-deceptive-marketing-dietary. Accessed January 20, 2017.
47. Saldanha LG, Dwyer JT, Andrews KW, et al. Online dietary supplement resources. *J Am Diet Assoc.* 2010;110:1427–1431.
48. Clauson KA, Polen HH, Peak AS, et al. Clinical decision support tools: personal digital assistant versus online dietary supplement databases. *Ann Pharmacother.* 2008;42:1592–1599.
49. Shaw P, Zhang V, Metalinos-Katsaras E. A content analysis of the quantity and accuracy of dietary supplement information found in magazines with high adolescent readership. *J Altern Complement Med.* 2009;15:159–164.
50. USC 342(g).
51. CFR 111.1.
52. *Federal Register* 2007;72(121):34752-34800.
53. US Food and Drug Administration. Guidance for industry: Current Good Manufacturing Practice for dietary supplements. http://www.fda.gov/Food/GuidanceRegulation/CGMP/ucm079496.htm. Accessed November 14, 2016.
54. Stat 3469 2006.
55. USC 379aa-1.
56. US Food and Drug Administration. Dietary supplement alerts and safety information. September 2016. http://www.fda.gov/Food/RecallsOutbreaksEmergencies/SafetyAlertsAdvisories. Accessed January 20, 2017.
57. US Library of Congress. Bill summary and status, 111th Congress (2009–2010), S.3002, Feb 2010. http://thomas.loc.gov/cgi-bin/bdquery/z?d111:S.3002. Accessed September 1, 2011.
58. Temple NJ. The marketing of dietary supplements in North America: the emperor is (almost) naked. *J Altern Complement Med.* 2010;16:803–806.
59. Lobb A. Science of weight loss supplements: compromised by conflicts of interest? *World J Gastroenterol.* 2010;16(38):4880–4882.
60. Higgins JP, Tuttle TD, Higgins CL. Energy beverages: content and safety. *Mayo Clin Proc.* 2010;85(11):1033–1041.
61. Dufour A, Wetzler S, Touvier M, et al. Comparison of different maximum safe levels in fortified foods and supplements using a probabilistic risk assessment approach. *Br J Nutr.* 2010;104:1848–1857.
62. Fu PP, Chiang H-M, Xia Q, et al. Quality assurance and safety of herbal dietary supplements. *J Environ Sci Health Part C.* 2009;27:91–119.
63. Gardiner P, Sarma DN, Dog TL, et al. The state of dietary supplement adverse event reporting in the United States. *Pharmacoepidemiol Drug Saf.* 2008;17:962–970.
64. Palmer M, Haller C, McKinney P, et al. Adverse events associated with dietary supplements: an observational study. *Lancet.* 2003;361:101–106.

65. Vassilev ZP, Chu AF, Ruck B, et al. Evaluation of adverse drug reactions reported to a poison control center between 2000 and 2007. *Am J Health Syst Pharm.* 2009;66:481–487.

66. Navarro V, Khan I, Björnsson E, Seeff LB, Serrano J, Hoofnagle JH. Liver injury from herbal and dietary supplements. *Hepatology.* 2017;65(1):363–373. doi:10.1002/hep.28813.

67. Zheng EX, Navarro VJ. Liver injury from herbal, dietary, and weight loss supplements: a review. *J Clin Transl Hepatol.* 2015;3(2):93–98. doi:10.14218/JCTH.2015.00006.

68. Braun LA, Tiralongo E, Wilkinson JM, et al. Perceptions, use and attitudes of pharmacy customers on complementary medicines and pharmacy practice. *BMC Complement Altern Med.* 2010;10:38.1–38.7.

69. Slone Epidemiology Center at Boston University. Patterns of medication use in the United States, 2006. http://www.bu.edu /slone/files/2012/11/SloneSurveyReport2006.pdf. Accessed January 20, 2017.

70. Mehta DH, Gardiner PM, Phillips RS, et al. Herbal and dietary supplement disclosure to health care providers by individuals with chronic conditions. *J Altern Complement Med.* 2008;14:1263–1269.

71. Peng CC, Glassman PA, Trilli LE, et al. Incidence and severity of potential drug-dietary supplement interactions in primary care patients: an exploratory study of 2 outpatient practices. *Arch Intern Med.* 2004;164:630–636.

72. Lee AH, Ingraham SE, Kopp M, et al. The incidence of potential interactions between dietary supplements and prescription medications in cancer patients at a Veterans Administration hospital. *Am J Clin Oncol.* 2006;29:178–182.

73. Sood A, Sood R, Brinker FJ, et al. Potential for interactions between dietary supplements and prescription medications. *Am J Med.* 2008;121:207–211.

74. Loya AM, González-Stuart A, Rivera JO. Prevalence of polypharmacy, polyherbacy, nutritional supplement use and potential product interactions among older adults living on the United States-Mexico border: a descriptive, questionnaire-based study. *Drugs Aging.* 2009;26:423–436.

75. Chan L-N. Interaction of natural products with medication and nutrients. In: Boullata JI, Armenti VT, eds. *Handbook of Drug-Nutrient Interactions.* 2nd ed. New York: Humana Press; 2010:341–366.

76. Nabekura T, Kamiyama S, Kitagawa S. Effect of dietary chemopreventive phytochemicals on P-glycoprotein function. *Biochem Biophys Res Comm.* 2004;327:866–870.

77. Morris ME, Zhang S. Flavonoid-drug interactions: effects of flavonoids on ABC transporters. *Life Sci.* 2006;78:2116–2130.

78. Shim C-K, Cheon E-P, Kang KW, et al. Inhibition effect of flavonoids on monocarboxylate transporter 1 (MCT1) in Caco-2 cells. *J Pharm Pharmacol.* 2007;59:1515–1519.

79. Cermak R. Effect of dietary flavonoids on pathways involved in drug metabolism. *Expert Opin Drug Metab Toxicol.* 2008;4:17–35.

80. Volak LP, Ghirmai S, Cashman JR, et al. Curcuminoids inhibit multiple human cytochromes P450, UDP-glucuronosyltransferase, and sulfotransferase enzymes, whereas piperine is a relatively selective CYP3A4 inhibitor. *Drug Metab Disp.* 2008;36:1594–1605.

81. Sergent T, Dupont I, Van Der Heiden E, et al. CYP1A1 and CYP3A4 modulation by dietary flavonoids in human intestinal Caco-2 cells. *Toxicol Lett.* 2009;191:216–222.

82. Chen Y, Liu W-H, Chen B-L, et al. Plant polyphenol curcumin significantly affects CYP1A2 and CYP2A6 activity in healthy, male Chinese volunteers. *Ann Pharmacother.* 2010;44:1038–1045.

83. Peng WX, Li HD, Zhou HH. Effect of daidzein on CYP1A2 activity and pharmacokinetics of theophylline in healthy volunteers. *Eur J Clin Pharmacol.* 2003;58:237–241.

84. Li Y, Mezei O, Shay NF. Human and murine hepatic sterol-12-α-hydroxylase and other xenobiotic metabolism mRNA are upregulated by soy isoflavones. *J Nutr.* 2007;137:1705–1712.

85. Roth M, Timmermann BN, Hagenbuch B. Interactions of green tea catechins with organic anion-transporting polypeptides. *Drug Metab Disp.* 2011;39:920–926.

86. Martel F, Monteiro R, Calhau C. Effect of polyphenols on the intestinal and placental transport of some bioactive compounds. *Nutr Res Rev.* 2010;23:47–64.

87. Chen H-Q, Shen T-Y, Zhou Y-K, et al. *Lactobacillus plantarum* consumption increases PepT1-mediated amino acid absorption by enhancing protein kinase C activity in spontaneously colitic mice. *J Nutr.* 2010;140:2201–2206.

88. Singh SK, Jha SK, Chaudhary A, et al. Quality control of herbal medicines by using spectroscopic techniques and multivariate statistical analysis. *Pharm Biol.* 2010;48(2):134–141.

89. Waksmundzka-Hajnos M. Modern high performance liquid chromatography in the analysis of phytochemicals. *J AOAC Int.* 2011;94:1–3.

90. Chen P, Harnly JM. Flow injection mass spectroscopic fingerprinting and multivariate analysis for differentiation of three *Panax* species. *J AOAC Int.* 2011;94:90–99.

91. Zhou L, Duan C, Wang M, et al. Analysis of residues of 81 pesticides on Ginkgo leaves using QuEChERS sample preparation and gas chromatography/mass spectrometry. *J AOAC Int.* 2011;94:313–321.

92. US Pharmacopeia Convention. *United States Pharmacopeia/ National Formulary, Edition 34/29.* Rockville, MD: US Pharmacopeia Convention; 2011.

93. Glisson JK, Walker LA. How physicians should evaluate dietary supplements. *Am J Med.* 2010;123:577–582.

94. Weiger WA, Smith M, Boon H, et al. Advising patients who seek complementary and alternative medical therapies for cancer. *Ann Intern Med.* 2002;137:889–903.

95. Ben-Arye E, Attias S, Levy I, Goldstein L, Schiff E. Mind the gap: disclosure of dietary supplement use to hospital and family physicians. *Patient Educ Couns.* 2017;100(1):98–103. doi:10.1016/j. pec.2016.07.037.

96. Michaud LB, Phillps-Karpinski J, Jones KL, et al. Dietary supplements in patients with cancer: risks and key concepts, part 1. *Am J Health Syst Pharm.* 2007;64:369–381.

97. Thompson C, Diekman C, Saurubin-Fragakis A, et al. Guidelines regarding the recommendation and sale of dietary supplements. *J Am Diet Assoc.* 2002;102:1158–1164.

98. American Society of Health-System Pharmacists. ASHP statement on the use of dietary supplements. *Am J Health Syst Pharm.* 2004;61:1707–1711.

99. Gardiner P, Phillips RS, Kemper KJ, et al. Dietary supplements: inpatient policies in US children's hospitals. *Pediatrics.* 2008;121:e775–e781.

PART III

NUTRITION SUPPORT OF SPECIFIC STATES

20 Pregnancy and Lactation

Kris M. Mogensen, MS, RD-AP, LDN, CNSC, and Miriam Erick, MS, RD, LDN, CDE

CONTENTS

Acknowledgments: Catherine Cimbalik, RN, RD, CNSC, and James D. Paauw, MD, PhD, were the authors of this chapter for the second edition.

Objectives

1. Describe nutrition requirements for pregnancy and lactation.
2. Identify special considerations for assessing nutrition status in pregnancy.
3. Determine indications for enteral nutrition (EN) and parenteral nutrition (PN) in pregnancy and lactation, and understand the decision process for selecting enteral and venous access devices.
4. Identify nutrition monitoring parameters that are altered by pregnancy.

Test Your Knowledge Questions

1. Which of the following statements is true regarding the nutrition status of the pregnant woman and its impact on the fetus?
   A. Obese pregnant women should lose weight during pregnancy to improve fetal outcomes.
   B. The fetus is a "perfect parasite," and the nutrition status of the mother is of no consequence.
   C. Appropriate weight gain for women of all body mass index (BMI) ranges is essential to fetal health.
   D. Poor maternal health and nutrition status has only short-term impact on the fetus.
2. Which of the following statements about energy needs during pregnancy is true?
   A. Energy requirements are the same for pregnant and nonpregnant women.
   B. Energy needs are increased only during the second and third trimesters of pregnancy.
   C. Compared with nonobese women, energy requirements are lower for obese women to promote weight loss during pregnancy.
   D. Energy goals should only focus on nonprotein energy intake.
3. Which of the following parameters is appropriate for monitoring glycemic control of pregnant women receiving nutrition support?
   A. Urine glucose
   B. Urine lactic acid
   C. Serum glucose
   D. Serum insulin

Test Your Knowledge Answers

1. The correct answer is **C**. Appropriate weight gain for women of all BMI ranges is essential to fetal health. Inadequate or excessive maternal weight gain can lead to poor fetal outcomes. Weight gain below recommended targets set by the Institute of Medicine (IOM; now the Health and Medicine Division of the National Academies of Science, Engineering, and Medicine) in 2009 has been associated with low birth weight (LBW) infants.[1] Obese women who lost weight during pregnancy had twofold greater odds of LBW infants and 1.8 greater odds of small-for-gestational age (SGA) infants. Excessive weight gain increases the odds of gestational hypertension or preeclampsia, macrosomia, and a decrease in the infant's 5-minute appearance, pulse, grimace, activity, and respiration (APGAR) scores.[2]
2. The appropriate answer is **B**. Energy requirements in pregnancy increase in the second and third trimesters.[3] Most women do not need to increase energy intake in the first trimester, although underweight women may be encouraged to do so.
3. The correct answer is **C**. Serum glucose levels must be strictly monitored during pregnancy to avoid the possible detrimental effects of neonatal hyperglycemia and hyperinsulinemia. The presence of glucose in a pregnant woman's urine is not abnormal and therefore does not necessarily indicate the presence of maternal diabetes.[4] The presence of lactic acid in the urine is typically observed during strenuous exercise and has no value in terms of monitoring glycemic control.

Background

Good maternal nutrition is essential for positive fetal outcomes. Inadequate maternal weight gain affects fetal growth and increases the risk of delivering a LBW infant. In addition, maternal micronutrient deficiencies may also impact fetal outcomes. After delivery, good maternal nutrition must continue to ensure adequate infant growth and development during breastfeeding as well as maintenance of good nutrition status of the mother.

Achieving adequate nutrition intake can be challenging when a pregnant woman cannot take adequate oral nutrition, as in cases of severe hyperemesis gravidarum. Pregnant women with medical conditions that affect digestion and absorption, such as cystic fibrosis or inflammatory bowel disease (IBD), may require EN or PN to ensure adequate nutrition to support fetal growth. In addition, women with pre-existing metabolic diseases such as phenylketonuria or maple syrup urine disease require specialized nutrition planning before conception and close monitoring and adjustment of the nutrition plan throughout the pregnancy.[5] Discussion of pregnancy in women with genetic and metabolic conditions is beyond the scope of this chapter. Patients with these conditions may require the attention of the nutrition support clinician along with the genetic-metabolic team.

This chapter reviews physiological changes during a healthy pregnancy and proposes an approach to nutrition assessment that focuses on malnutrition in pregnancy and the determination of the woman's nutrition needs during pregnancy and lactation. It also addresses indications for EN and PN, special considerations for nutrition support during pregnancy, and some disease-specific considerations.

Maternal Weight Gain in Pregnancy

Appropriate maternal weight gain is an important component of a positive fetal outcome. Weight gain is spread among multiple compartments of the body, in varying amounts. Table 20-1 outlines components of weight gain for singleton and multiple pregnancies.[6] In its 2009 guidelines, IOM recommended weight gain goals by pregravid BMI.[7] Table 20-2 outlines these recommendations for singleton pregnancies.[7] Weight gain guidelines with anticipated fetal weight for women pregnant with multiples are outlined in Table 20-3.[8] Clinicians should be aware that recommendations for triplets and quadruplets are based on much smaller numbers of pregnancies than singleton and twin pregnancies and, thus, should be used more cautiously.[8] Siega-Riz and colleagues[1] conducted a systematic review evaluating outcomes of maternal weight gain according to the IOM recommendations and found strong evidence associating weight gain below the recommendations and LBW infants.

TABLE 20-1 Components of Pregnancy Weight Gain

Compartment	Weight Gain, lb (% Total Weight Gain)			
	Singleton	Twins	Triplets	Quadruplets
Gestational				
Fetus	8 (22%–32%)	10–16 (26%–27%)	12–18 (20%–24%)	12–20 (17%–25%)
Amniotic fluid	2–3 (8%–12%)	4–6 (10%–11%)	6–8 (8%–10%)	10–12 (14%–15%)
Placenta	2–3 (8%–12%)	4–6 (10%–11%)	6–8 (8%–10%)	10–12 (14%–15%)
Maternal				
Breast tissue	2–3 (8%–12%)	3–5 (8%–8.5%)	3–5 (5%–7%)	3–5 (4%–6%)
Uterus	2–5 (8%–14%)	3–8 (8%–13%)	3–8 (5%–10%)	3–8 (4%–10%)
Blood volume	4 (11%–16%)	8 (13%–21%)	8–10 (13%–14%)	8–10 (11%–12%)
Adipose	5–9 (20%–26%)	6–10 (16%–17%)	10–12 (16%–17%)	10–12 (14%–15%)
Muscle mass	Not described	Not described	Not described	Not described
Total, lb	**25–35**	**38–59**	**58–75**	**70–80**

Source: Adapted with permission from reference 6: Luke B. Nutrition for multiples. *Clin Obstet Gynecol.* 2015;58:585–610. doi:10.1097/GRF.0000000000000117.

TABLE 20-2 Recommended Weight Gain Based on Prepregnancy Body Mass Index

Prepregnancy BMI	Recommended Weight Gain Range, lb	Rate of Weight Gain for 2nd and 3rd Trimesters, mean (range), lb/wk
<18.5	28–40	1 (1–1.3)
18.5–24.9	25–35	1 (0.8–1)
25.0–29.9	15–25	0.6 (0.5–0.7)
>30	11–20	0.5 (0.4–0.6)

BMI, body mass index.
Source: Adapted with permission from reference 7: Institute of Medicine and National Research Council. *Weight Gain During Pregnancy: Reexamining the Guidelines.* Washington, DC: National Academies Press; 2009.

TABLE 20-3 Summary of Data on Multiple Gestations and Maternal Weight Gain

	Singleton[a]	Twins[b]	Triplets[c]	Quadruplets[d]
Gestation, weeks	38–41	36–38	34–35	31–33
Birth weight				
Average, g	3700–4000	2500–3800	1900–2200	1500–1800
LBW, %	6	50	90	98
VLBW, %	1	10	32	75
Maternal weight gain				
At 24 weeks, lb	12	24	36	50
Total, lb	25–35	40–45	50–60	60–80

LBW, low birth weight (<2500 g); VLBW, very low birth weight (<1500 g).
[a]Sample size = 3,851,109 infants.
[b]Sample size = 97,064 infants.
[c]Sample size = 4233 infants.
[d]Sample size = 360 infants.
Source: Data are from reference 8.

Obesity

For women with preexisting obesity, it may be tempting to limit weight gain to amounts below the IOM recommendations. However, this choice may have detrimental consequences for the fetus. Although maternal obesity alone is a risk factor for infant mortality, very low weight gain is also a risk factor for infant mortality.[9] Cox Bauer and associates[2] found that obese women who lost weight during pregnancy had twofold greater odds of having a LBW infant and 1.8 greater odds of having an SGA infant. Conversely, excessive weight gain beyond the IOM recommendations was also problematic, increasing the odds of gestational hypertension or pre-eclampsia, macrosomia, and a decrease in 5-minute APGAR scores.[2] Planning for appropriate weight gain and avoiding weight loss or excessive weight gain are important aspects of managing the obese pregnant patient.

Multiple Births

The most recent data from the *National Vital Statistics Reports* state that the twin birth rate in the United States reached a record high in 2014, resulting in 1 of every 30 babies born being a twin. For 2014, there were 135,336 twin births, 4233 triplet births, 246 quadruplet births, and 47 quintuplets and higher order births.[10] Women with multiple pregnancies are at high risk for premature delivery and SGA infants. The weight gain guidelines in Table 20-3 should be followed for women pregnant with multiple births to promote appropriate fetal growth; however, as stated previously, these recommendations are based on small numbers of triplet and quadruplet pregnancies and should be interpreted and implemented with caution.[8]

Nutrition Assessment

As with all other clinical conditions, a comprehensive nutrition assessment is the first step in nutrition care for a pregnant patient. The assessment should include evaluation of the patient's pregravid nutrition status as well as her current status. The outcome of conception is influenced by preconception and gestation nutrition, absence or presence of complications from the fetal compartment (eg, discordant growth in twin or triple gestations), and the absence or presence of acute maternal disease (eg, viral infections such as Ebola, mumps, measles, and Zika; bacterial infections). In addition, other nutrition challenges may occur during pregnancy, such as pre-existing maternal metabolic conditions (eg, diabetes, obesity), chronic illnesses that affect digestion and absorption (eg, IBD), and acute events (eg, motor vehicle crash or cerebral vascular accident). All of these factors may affect a patient's nutrition status and nutrition requirements. Many of these situations are not common, and, because there is a paucity of published case reports, clinicians in these situations have little published data for guidance.

Assessment of Pregravid Nutrition Status

When assessing a pregnant woman, clinicians should aim to identify any nutrition deficiencies that existed prior to pregnancy. This part of the nutrition assessment includes careful evaluation of the pregravid weight status, which can be challenging when an accurate pregravid weight is not be available and the clinician must rely upon a patient's recall of her most recent weight prior to pregnancy.

When pregnancies are unplanned, determining the timing of the last menstrual cycle and the true, non-fluid-overloaded, pregravid weight may be more challenging. Also, women whose pregnancies are unplanned may not have optimized their own nutrition status to adequately bear the additional metabolic burden of pregnancy. In the United States, approximately 45% of pregnancies were unintended in 2011, as compared with 51% in 2008.[11] The rates of unintended pregnancies declined by 18% between 2008 and 2011, from 54 to 45 per 1000 US women and girls ages 15 to 44 years. The rates of unintended pregnancies were 2 to 3 times the national average for women and girls whose incomes were below or within 199% of the federal poverty level. Rates of unintended pregnancy were also substantially above average for those who were unmarried, those who did not have a high school education, and Hispanics.[11]

Women with significant comorbidities may have more frequent pregravid medical monitoring and an accurate weight may be available from their medical records. Clinicians can also use pregravid percentage of ideal body weight, BMI, and weight change prior to pregnancy to help evaluate pregravid nutrition status, identify malnutrition, and set weight gain goals for the pregnancy. Review of pregravid laboratory values such as hemoglobin, hematocrit, and mean corpuscular volume helps evaluate patients for anemia.

Assessment of Current Nutrition Status

The nutrition support clinician may see a pregnant patient at any stage during her pregnancy, and the appropriate nutrition assessment process will depend on stage of pregnancy. Pregnant patients may have signs of malnutrition, but those signs may not be easily categorized by the malnutrition characteristics identified by the Academy of Nutrition and Dietetics (AND) and the American Society for Parenteral and Enteral Nutrition (ASPEN).[12] As described in detail in Chapter 9, ASPEN and AND categorize malnutrition by its etiological context: acute illness or injury, chronic illness, or social or environmental circumstances. Any of these contexts can be relevant in pregnancy (eg, trauma, IBD, or severe financial limitations leading to limited access to food). ASPEN and AND also identify several individual characteristics that may support a diagnosis of malnutrition: insufficient energy intake, weight loss, loss of muscle mass, loss of subcutaneous fat, localized or generalized fluid accumulation, and diminished functional status.[12] These characteristics can be evaluated in the pregnant patient, but interpretation may present challenges and there is no current, validated tool specifically for evaluating malnutrition in pregnant women. Therefore, this section reviews evaluation of each characteristic in the context of pregnancy.

Insufficient Energy Intake

A detailed diet history is an important part of evaluating the adequacy of energy and protein intake. In addition to the basic diet history, the clinician should also ask questions about vitamin supplements (especially prenatal vitamins), mineral supplementation (eg, iron supplementation), and use of other supplements (eg, herbal supplements). Information about the patient's support system for food shopping and meal preparation is helpful. For the acutely ill pregnant patient, the clinician should evaluate how long the patient was *nil per os* status or restricted to clear liquids.

Weight Loss

Evaluation of weight change in the pregnant woman can be very challenging. Some pregnant women (eg, those with severe hyperemesis gravidarum or patients with active IBD with extremely limited oral intake) lose weight below their pregravid weight. The nutrition support clinician should compare current weight to the pregravid weight and compare the current weight to the expected weight gain for the patient's stage of pregnancy. The Centers for Disease Control and Prevention offer weight tracking tools that can assist with this process.[13] This practice is not noted in the current published malnutrition characteristics, but it can give the clinician a sense of how "behind" a patient is in her expected weight gain. As stated previously, inadequate maternal weight gain is associated with LBW and SGA infants.

Evaluation of Muscle Mass, Subcutaneous Fat, and Edema

Muscle mass, subcutaneous fat, and edema can be evaluated during the nutrition-focused physical examination. Like other malnourished patients, malnourished pregnant patients may exhibit no wasting, profound wasting, or varying degrees of fat and muscle wasting.

Edema, particularly in the lower extremities, is a common problem starting in the second trimester of pregnancy.[14] The clinician must interpret this complication with great care to determine whether the edema is related to malnutrition, a "normal" part of pregnancy, or the beginning of fluid accumulation associated with the onset of early pre-eclampsia.

Functional Status

There are no validation studies of changes in functional status in pregnant women. Therefore, it may be difficult to evaluate this change using a validated tool. Measures of handgrip strength could be attempted for appropriate patients, but it is not known whether the interpretation of such measures should change during pregnancy.

Micronutrient Status

In addition to evaluating the 6 characteristics for determining presence or absence of malnutrition, clinicians should assess pregnant women for specific micronutrient concerns that can affect the woman's health and pregnancy outcomes. Iron deficiency is common in pregnancy and should be evaluated and corrected if present. In addition, deficiency of other micronutrients (particularly folate, vitamin B_{12}, calcium, and zinc) may have a negative impact on fetal growth. These deficiencies may also contribute to long-range health consequences for the child, including impaired neurologic development and diseases such as hypertension and diabetes in adulthood.[15] Micronutrient requirements and the consequences of deficiencies and excess are discussed in greater detail later in this chapter.

Specific disease states or clinical conditions increase the risk of preexisting micronutrient deficiencies. For example, women who have had bariatric surgery may see an increase in fertility after weight loss[16] and may become pregnant unexpectedly. Micronutrient deficiencies are more prevalent in Roux-en-Y gastric bypass (RYGB) patients compared with sleeve gastrectomy patients. Monitoring recommendations have been published and should be followed to ensure that all micronutrient deficiencies are corrected.[17] If an RYGB patient becomes pregnant unexpectedly, vitamin B_{12}, folate, vitamin D, and an iron panel should be checked as soon as feasible and deficiencies should be promptly corrected. Pregnant women with a history of malabsorptive disorders, such as cystic fibrosis, IBD, or short bowel syndrome, are also at risk for micronutrient deficiencies and require close examination and monitoring. Physical signs and symptoms of micronutrient deficiencies as well as deficiencies in the initial surveillance levels may prompt additional assessment of micronutrient status.

Determining Nutrition Requirements

General guidelines for determining energy, carbohydrate, fat, protein, fluid, and micronutrient requirements are covered in Chapters 2, 3, 5, 6, 7, and 8, respectively. This section discusses specific considerations for pregnancy.

Energy

Multiple methods are available to determine energy requirements in pregnancy (see Table 20-4).[3,18] All methods take into consideration that additional energy is required to support normal body composition changes in pregnancy (eg, increased development of fetal, uterine, and mammary tissue and increased maternal fat deposition) and the increased metabolism associated with these tissues. The equations vary in complexity. Some equations estimate energy needs based on height, weight, and activity level, and add additional calories for weight gain.[3] Others are simple calorie-per-kilogram methods.[18] Energy requirements are generally calculated using pregravid weight or ideal body weight. The overall energy "cost" of pregnancy has been reported to be approximately 78,000 kcal.[19] However, it is important to note that additional energy is generally not required in the first trimester, and increased energy goals for weight gain should be applied in the second and third trimesters. Unfortunately, no research is available to guide recommendations for severely underweight pregnant women, who may require additional energy for weight gain throughout the pregnancy, including the first trimester.

There are little data to guide calculations for energy delivery in pregnant women undergoing metabolic stress. In pregnant women with trauma, burn, severe sepsis, or other illness that may contribute to hypermetabolism, predictive equations may underestimate energy requirements. Serial indirect calorimetry measurements (see Chapter 2) are beneficial to guide the energy prescription during times of severe illness during pregnancy. In the absence of indirect calorimetry, the clinician could consider use of standard equations for the acute illness and then add additional energy for the appropriate trimester. Close monitoring of weight gain and the health of the fetus

TABLE 20-4 Equations to Determine Energy Requirements in Pregnancy

Age Group	Type of Pregnancy	Recommendation
IOM recommendations		
14–18 y	Singleton	EER + Pregnancy Energy Deposition Where: • EER = 135.3 − (30.8 × A) + PA × [(10.0 × Wt) + (934 × Ht)] + 25 • PA = 1.00 for sedentary PAL; 1.16 for low active PAL; 1.31 for active PAL; 1.56 for very active PAL • Pregnancy energy deposition = 0 kcal for 1st trimester; 340 kcal for 2nd trimester; 452 kcal for 3rd trimester
≥19 y	Singleton	EER + Pregnancy Energy Deposition Where: • EER = 354 − (6.91 × A) + PA × [(9.36 × Wt) + (726 × Ht)] • PA = 1.00 for sedentary PAL; 1.12 for low active PAL; 1.27 for active PAL; 1.45 for very active PAL • Pregnancy energy deposition = 0 kcal for 1st trimester; 340 kcal for 2nd trimester; 452 kcal for 3rd trimester
AND recommendations		
All ages	Singleton	Use IOM guidelines
All ages	Multiples	• BMI <18.5: 42–50 kcal per kg pregravid weight • BMI 18.5–24.9: 40–45 kcal per kg pregravid weight • BMI >25: 30–35 kcal per kg pregravid weight

A, age (years); AND, Academy of Nutrition and Dietetics; BMI, body mass index; EER, Estimated Energy Requirement (kcal/d); Ht, height (meters); IOM, Institute of Medicine; PA, physical activity coefficient; PAL, physical activity level (sedentary: ≥1.0 to <1.4; low active: ≥1.4 to <1.6; active: ≥1.6 to <1.9; very active: ≥1.9 to <2.5); Wt, weight (kg).
Source: Data are from references 3 and 18.

are essential during this time. Serial fetal ultrasound may be beneficial, but discovery of intrauterine growth restriction, depending on the severity, may demonstrate that fetal harm has already been done.[20]

Protein

Changes in protein metabolism can be seen within weeks of conception,[21] and whole body protein turnover increases in the second and third trimesters of pregnancy.[3] The IOM report on protein requirements states that in a singleton pregnancy with a 12.5-kg weight gain and a 3.3-kg fetus, there is accretion of 148 g nitrogen (approximately 925 g protein); this protein accretion is divided among the fetus (440 g), uterus (166 g), expanded maternal blood volume (81 g), placenta (100 g), extracellular fluid (135 g), and amniotic fluid (3 g).[3] One can assume that these accretions are greater with multiples. Ziegler et al[22] conducted a landmark study of fetal body composition and found that as gestation advanced, the percentage of fetal body water decreased while protein, fat, carbohydrate, and minerals were accrued. Table 20-5 summarizes recommendations for protein intake in healthy pregnant women.[3,18]

Recent work by Elango and Ball[21] suggest that protein requirements in pregnancy may be higher than the amounts recommended by the IOM. Using the minimally invasive indicator amino acid oxidation method, they found that protein requirements are 1.2 g/kg/d in early pregnancy and 1.52 g/kg/d in late pregnancy. Adequacy of protein delivery seems to have a "sweet spot," with excessively low or high protein intake posing potential for harm.[23] Inadequate protein intake may lead to poor growth and development, but excessive protein delivery may also be harmful. In early work by Rush and colleagues,[24] the addition of high-protein supplements to prenatal diets (470 kcal and 40 g protein vs 322 kcal and 6 g protein vs no supplementation) in addition to the usual oral diet was associated with higher rates of early premature births and neonatal deaths. However, in a study of individual nutrition rehabilitation in pregnancies of lower socioeconomic groups of women in Montreal, Canada, Higgins et al[25] demonstrated that 100 g protein per day provided the best outcome as measured by reduced numbers of LBW infants in singleton pregnancies. More recent studies of high-protein intake

during pregnancy have shown long-range negative impacts (eg, insulin resistance, hypertension, and higher adult BMI) in offspring.[23,26]

In some clinical cases, protein requirements are greater than normal. Pregnant women with complications arising from trauma, burn, or major surgery may benefit from increased protein delivery, and pregnant women receiving high-dose steroid therapy may require higher protein intake to offset catabolism associated with this therapy. There are little data to guide protein provision in the complicated pregnant patient. Therefore, as with energy, the clinician should plan to give patients additional protein during times of metabolic stress and monitor closely whether growth and development of the fetus are appropriate.

Carbohydrate

Carbohydrate is required in the oral diet or nutrition support regimen because some tissues (the brain and red blood cells) can only use glucose for energy. In pregnancy, patients also require carbohydrates as a source of energy to meet the demands to support weight gain. The IOM set the Recommended Dietary Allowance (RDA) for carbohydrate in pregnancy at 175 g/d. The fetus can use both glucose and ketoacids generated by the mother for energy, but fetal use of free fatty acids is limited.[3]

Carbohydrate has a greater effect on blood glucose levels compared with other macronutrients (see Chapter 3). In a normal pregnancy, consumption of a high-carbohydrate meal results in postprandial hyperglycemia and hyperinsulinemia, which provides a constant supply of glucose to the fetus.[27] Pregnant women tend to have decreased premeal and fasting blood glucose levels, which likely reflects the constant glucose uptake by the placenta as well as altered hepatic gluconeogenesis.

Prolonged hyperglycemia may be seen in gestational diabetes as well as other conditions, such as metabolic stress; this problem may also affect women receiving steroid therapy. In pregnancy, prolonged hyperglycemia can lead to excess transfer of glucose across the placenta. During the second trimester, progesterone, estrogen, human placental lactogen, growth hormone, and cortisol levels all rise, which may lead

TABLE 20-5 Protein Requirements in Pregnancy for Healthy Women

Institution/Society	Recommendation
Institute of Medicine	• Singleton: – RDA (1.1 g/kg/d) *or* – Maintenance protein requirements + 25 g/d • Multiples: Maintenance protein requirements + 50 g/d (starting in the 2nd trimester)
Academy of Nutrition and Dietetics	• Singleton: No specific protein recommendation • Multiples: – 20% of total kcal *or* – Maintenance protein requirements + 50 g/d

RDA, Recommended Dietary Allowance.
Source: Data are from references 3 and 18.

to increased insulin resistance and decreased insulin sensitivity. These factors contribute to the development of gestational diabetes.[28] Hyperglycemia in the pregnant woman will lead to fetal hyperglycemia and hyperinsulinemia, which are detrimental to the fetus. In the early stages of pregnancy, chronically elevated fetal blood glucose levels are associated with fetal anomalies and increased risk of miscarriage. In later stages of pregnancy, poor maternal glucose control is associated with increased risk of fetal macrosomia, which may result in birth trauma and an increased rate of cesarean deliveries.[29-32] Poor maternal glucose control is also associated with increased risk of stillbirth,[33] and hyperglycemia impairs oxygen delivery to the fetus.[34] Given these complications, relatively tight glucose control is advocated. For women with diabetes (type 1 or gestational diabetes), the target fasting blood glucose is 95 mg/dL or lower, the 1-hour postprandial blood glucose target is 140 mg/dL or less, and the 2-hour postprandial blood glucose goal is 120 mg/dL or less.[35] These targets are also important to follow for pregnant women requiring nutrition support.

Inadequate carbohydrate intake during pregnancy can also be harmful and may lead to ketonemia or ketonuria. Ketone bodies have a negative effect on embryogenesis[36] and the behavior and intellectual development of offspring in childhood.[37] When planning a nutrition support regimen, clinicians must aim to provide adequate carbohydrate to prevent ketonemia. In general, this goal may be achieved by providing the RDA for carbohydrate (175 g/d), but that amount of carbohydrate may not be sufficient for the metabolically stressed pregnant patient or in situations of multiple gestations.

Fat

Adequate fat intake in pregnancy supports fetal growth and development. The fetus has a significant increase in fat deposition in the second half of gestation, and fat accounts for 16% of the fetus' body weight at term.[38] Appropriate essential fatty acid intake is important for fetal growth and lung maturation as well as production of fetal phosphatidylglycerol, pulmonary surfactant, and myelin. There is no formal recommendation for total fat intake in pregnancy, but a reasonable starting point would be approximately 20% to 35% of energy, as suggested by the IOM Dietary Reference Intakes (DRIs).[3] In addition, the IOM set the Adequate Intake (AI) for linoleic acid at 13 g/d and the AI for α-linolenic acid at 1.4 g/d.[3] The relevance of ω-3 fatty acids, particularly docosahexaenoic acid (DHA), during pregnancy has received significant attention because DHA plays an important role in fetal brain and central nervous system development, which occurs at a rapid pace during the third trimester of pregnancy.[39] Proposed benefits of DHA supplementation include improved infant visual acuity, postnatal growth, cognitive development, and prevention of allergies and asthma; in the mother, DHA may potentially lower incidence of gestational hypertension and peripartum depression. A recent systematic review found that fish oil supplementation had no significant effect on markers for any of these potential benefits.[40] However, consensus guidelines recommend at least 200 mg DHA in the diet for both pregnant and lactating women.[41]

Lipid metabolism changes during pregnancy, and transient hyperlipidemia is common. Free fatty acids, triglycerides, and cholesterol are all elevated during pregnancy, particularly during late stages of pregnancy.[29,42] Of note, triglyceride levels may rise 150% and cholesterol may rise from 125% to 150% of prepregnancy levels without any adverse sequelae.[43] Maternal hypertriglyceridemia results from several factors, including enhanced adipose tissue lipolysis, which increases the amount of substrate available to the liver for triglyceride synthesis; reduced lipoprotein lipase activity in extrahepatic tissues; and increased chylomicron formation from dietary fat intake.[44]

Fluid

Intravascular, interstitial, and intracellular fluid compartments increase during pregnancy. Adequate fluid should be provided to meet requirements needed to support these normal physiological changes. The AI for fluid for pregnant women is 3 L/d, with approximately 2.3 liters from beverages and the rest coming from water contained in food.[45] An individual's fluid requirements may be greater or less than the AI, depending on the patient's volume status, need for fluid restriction (eg, the pregnant woman with heart failure), or need for replacement of losses (eg, a patient with severe diarrhea with IBD). Care must be taken to avoid dehydration, which may be associated with a reduction in amniotic fluid volume. This reduction is reversible if treated appropriately, but oligohydramnios (amniotic fluid less than expected for gestational age) may lead to fetal deformation, umbilical cord compression, and death.[46]

Micronutrients

Clinicians may be most familiar with the need for increased folic acid during pregnancy, but requirements for practically all vitamins and minerals increase during pregnancy relative to the nonpregnant state. Tables 20-6 and 20-7 list vitamin and mineral requirements in normal pregnancy, respectively;[47-51] requirements for healthy adults are more generally discussed in Chapter 8.

Micronutrient Deficiencies

Inadequate micronutrient intake may have a profound impact on fetal growth and development, and may affect length of gestation. Vitamin A deficiency during pregnancy is strongly associated with growth restriction, eye abnormalities, and impaired vision in children.[52] Women at particular risk for vitamin A deficiency include those with a history of fat malabsorption and those with a prior history of bariatric surgery.

Vitamin D deficiency is highly prevalent in pregnant women and can contribute to neonatal hypocalcemia and early onset of rickets (along with inadequate calcium intake).[53] A recent study evaluating vitamin D supplementation in pregnancy found that women with vitamin D levels equal to or greater than 40 ng/mL had lower risk of preterm birth compared with those with levels of 20 ng/mL or less.[54]

Vitamin K deficiency is a cause of chondrodysplasia punctate (CDP). In a recent case series of 8 women (7 with hyperemesis gravidarum and 1 with Crohn's disease) with vitamin K deficiency, all 8 offspring had characteristics of CDP, which include stippled epiphyses, hypoplasia of the nasal cartilages,

TABLE 20-6 Dietary Reference Intakes for Vitamins in Pregnancy and Lactation

Vitamin (Type of DRI)	Pregnancy			Lactation		
	Age ≤18 y	Age 19–30 y	Age 31–50 y	Age ≤18 y	Age 19–30 y	Age 31–50 y
A, mcg (RDA)	750	770	770	1200	1300	1300
D, IU (RDA)	600	600	600	600	600	600
E, mg (RDA)	15	15	15	19	19	19
K, mcg (AI)	75	90	90	75	90	90
Vitamin C, mg (RDA)	80	85	85	115	120	120
Thiamin (B_1), mg (RDA)	1.4	1.4	1.4	1.4	1.4	1.4
Riboflavin (B_2), mg (RDA)	1.4	1.4	1.4	1.6	1.6	1.6
Pyridoxine (B_6), mg (RDA)	1.9	1.9	1.9	2.0	2.0	2.0
Niacin, mg (RDA)	18	18	18	17	17	17
Pantothenic acid, mg (AI)	6	6	6	7	7	7
Biotin, mcg (AI)	30	30	30	35	35	35
Folate, mcg (RDA)	600	600	600	500	500	500
Vitamin B_{12}, mcg (RDA)	2.6	2.6	2.6	2.8	2.8	2.8

AI, Adequate Intake; DRI, Dietary Reference Intake; RDA, Recommended Dietary Allowance.
Source: Data are from references 47–51.

and abnormal distal digits.[55] Risk factors for vitamin K deficiency during pregnancy include hyperemesis gravidarum, IBD, celiac disease, prior bariatric surgery, pancreatitis, liver disease, renal disease, use of medications that may interfere with vitamin K (coumarin derivatives, antibiotics, antiepileptics), autoimmune disorders, and alcohol use during pregnancy.[55]

Inadequate folic acid intake is a known risk factor for neural tube defects (NTDs). Since food manufacturers started fortifying flour with folic acid in the late 1990s, the incidence of NTDs has decreased by up to 50%.[56] Supplementation with folic acid outside of the normal diet remains important in prenatal care, particularly for women who have had a prior pregnancy with an NTD, women taking medications with antifolate activity, obese women (especially with history of bariatric surgery), women who are actively smoking or have significant exposure to passive smoking, and those with diabetes.[17,56]

Iron deficiency anemia is one of the most common deficiencies during pregnancy, with a reported prevalence of 38% of pregnant women.[57] Women with IBD, celiac disease or have a history of bariatric surgery carry additional risk for iron deficiency. Iron deficiency during pregnancy has been associated with increased incidence of fetal growth restriction, premature birth, and fetal death.[58] In addition, new research is emerging correlating maternal iron deficiency with impaired cognitive development in offspring.[59] As previously stated, pregnant women should be screened for iron deficiency and receive adequate repletion (which may be oral or intravenous [IV] iron, depending on gastrointestinal [GI] function) if necessary.

Zinc deficiency may lead to preterm birth and may prolong labor.[60] It may contribute to restricted fetal growth and development, central nervous system abnormalities, and congenital malformations.[15,60–63]

Iodine is crucial for brain development. Severe iodine deficiency is classically associated with cretinism, and mild iodine deficiency has been associated with developmental impairments.[64] A recent study of 141 women living in Washington, DC, revealed marginal iodine status and evidence of mild hypothyroidism.[65] Clinicians should be aware of this problem and ensure that patients achieve adequate iodine intake through use of fortified foods (eg, iodized salt) or appropriate supplements.

Micronutrient Toxicities

Micronutrient toxicities may also have an adverse effect on the fetus, with vitamin A being the main micronutrient of concern. Vitamin A intake in excess of 10,000 IU/d or 0.5 to 1.5 mg 13-cis retinoic acid (isotretinoin) per kg has been associated with a high incidence of spontaneous abortions and birth defects.[66,67] Similar abnormalities can be caused by large daily doses of retinyl esters or retinol in amounts greater than 6,000 RE or 20,000 IU.[52,68,69]

Additional Micronutrient Supplementation Considerations in Pregnancy

DRIs are intended for healthy individuals with normal digestive and absorptive capacity (see Chapter 8). Individuals with underlying diseases or altered GI anatomy that may affect digestion and absorption may have different micronutrient requirements above and beyond the DRI. For pregnant women requiring nutrition support, EN formulations may not contain the same sources or combinations of vitamins and minerals found in foods, which may change exactly how

TABLE 20-7 Dietary Reference Intakes for Minerals in Pregnancy and Lactation

Mineral (Type of DRI)	Pregnancy			Lactation		
	Age ≤18 y	Age 19–30 y	Age 31–50 y	Age ≤18 y	Age 19–30 y	Age 31–50 y
Calcium, mg (RDA)	1300	1000	1000	1300	1000	1000
Magnesium, mg (RDA)	400	350	360	360	310	320
Phosphorus, mg (RDA)	1250	700	700	1250	700	700
Iron, mg (RDA)	27	27	27	10	9	9
Chromium, mg (AI)	29	30	30	44	45	45
Copper, mcg (RDA)	1000	1000	1000	1300	1300	1300
Iodine, mcg (RDA)	220	220	220	290	290	290
Manganese, mg (AI)	2	2	2	2.6	2.6	2.6
Selenium, mcg (RDA)	60	60	60	70	70	70
Zinc, mg (RDA)	12	11	11	13	12	12

AI, Adequate Intake; DRI, Dietary Reference Intake; RDA, Recommended Dietary Allowance.
Source: Data are from references 47–51.

much is absorbed. The DRIs for pregnancy are designed for women taking an oral diet who have normal intestinal absorption processes. Therefore, the appropriate dosing of micronutrients in PN may be different from the DRI levels; research in this area is lacking. Because of these concerns, pregnant women receiving nutrition support must be monitored very closely for any signs and symptoms of micronutrient deficiencies or excess.

Nutrition Support Therapy for the Pregnant Patient

Enteral Nutrition

EN has been used successfully in pregnant women. Indications for EN in this population are the standard ones: any situation in which the patient has a functional GI tract but cannot take adequate oral nutrition. Examples of situations when EN might be used in pregnancy include hyperemesis gravidarum, multiple gestation, trauma, or critical illness (see Complications and Specific Clinical Challenges in Pregnancy, later in this chapter).

Enteral Access

The selection of enteral access requires careful consideration of the duration of therapy as well as the type of feeding tube device (see Chapter 12). A nasoenteric tube, which can generally remain in place for 6 to 8 weeks, is an appropriate feeding tube for short-term EN. It carries the risk of reflux and aspiration in pregnant women for 2 reasons. First, gastric emptying is delayed and lower esophageal sphincter (LES) tone is decreased in pregnancy.[70] Second, a nasoenteric tube will prevent the LES from closing completely, allowing for reflux of gastric contents into the esophagus. Maximum efforts should be taken to decrease the risk of aspiration, which could lead to serious complications such as pneumonia and even death (see Chapter 13).

Gastrostomy tubes or jejunostomy tubes may be considered for long-term EN.[71-77] These tubes may reduce the risk of reflux and aspiration but are more invasive than nasoenteric tubes and pose other risks. Extrapolation from reports of other fluoroscopic procedures during pregnancy suggest that fluoroscopic tube placement practice is safe with appropriate radiation shielding.[78-81] In a case series of 5 pregnant women with severe hyperemesis gravidarum who underwent surgical jejunostomy insertion between 12 and 26 weeks' gestation (mean 14 weeks), 1 patient required jejunostomy insertion for 2 consecutive pregnancies, for a total of 6 insertions. Five of six women gained weight, and all pregnancies ended with term deliveries (2 LBW infants). The only tube complications were late dislodgment in 2 patients (tubes were replaced via the established tract).[81] In a case report, a woman with intractable hyperemesis had an open gastrostomy tube (for drainage and decompression) and feeding jejunostomy tube inserted at 26 weeks after 3 nasogastric feeding tubes failed in a 2-day period. Premature contractions began 30 minutes after the tubes were placed, and contractions were tocolyzed.[77]

Formula Selection

The process for selecting an enteral formula for the pregnant patient requiring EN is similar to the process for nonpregnant patients (see Chapter 11). A polymeric formula is appropriate for patients with adequate digestive and absorptive capacity. If the patient has heart failure, renal failure, or another complication leading to volume overload or need for a fluid restriction, a concentrated enteral formula may be selected. Because constipation is often a problem in pregnancy (25% to 45% of pregnant women experience this complication[70]), a fiber-containing formula should be considered. Clinicians should carefully review micronutrient delivery at the goal volume and compare the amounts provided to the DRIs for pregnancy to ensure that micronutrient needs are met. Additional micronutrient supplementation may be required if the micronutrient delivery from formula will not meet the patient's needs or if the patient requires repletion of a deficiency.

Enteral Nutrition Infusion

Determining the appropriate infusion method will depend on the tube location and the patient's clinical status (see Chapter 10).

Enteral Nutrition Monitoring and Complications

Monitoring of EN and management of enteral feeding complications are covered in Chapters 10, 12, and 13. Recommendations in this chapter are appropriate for the pregnant woman receiving EN. The nutrition support clinician must consider interventions for complications carefully, as some interventions are not appropriate in pregnancy. For example, diarrhea is a common complication associated with EN. In the nonpregnant patient, antidiarrheals may be prescribed if the diarrhea is not caused by infection. Prior to prescribing antidiarrheal medications to a pregnant patient, the clinician should consult with a pharmacist and carefully evaluate the risks to the fetus. Use of loperamide in early pregnancy has been associated with increased risk of congenital malformations, hypospadias, placenta previa, large-for-gestational age fetus, and need for cesarean section.[82] Bismuth subsalicylates and diphenoxylate with atropine are both contraindicated during pregnancy because they are known teratogens.[70]

As mentioned previously, constipation is a common problem in pregnancy. In addition to the use of a fiber-containing enteral formula and assuring adequate fluid intake, stool softeners may be required to treat this complication.

Parenteral Nutrition

Indications

As with any other patient requiring nutrition support, EN is the preferred mode of therapy. However, in some cases, EN is not feasible and PN must be used (see Chapter 14). For example, when EN is contraindicated in pregnant women, PN may be used in cases of severe hyperemesis gravidarum, IBD complications, intestinal stricture, or other clinical complications. ASPEN has recently published guidelines for PN use, which are applicable to pregnant women.[83] PN has many risks, and the risks and benefits must be weighed carefully in the pregnant patient. However, fear of complications should not delay initiation of PN in a patient who truly requires it.

Safety of Parenteral Nutrition in Pregnancy

PN can be safe during pregnancy and can support healthy outcomes in women with underlying disorders that limit their ability to tolerate oral or enteral nutrition or digest and absorb nutrients.[84-88] Two recently published reports recount the experiences of pregnant women with long-term PN requirements and their pregnancy outcomes. Theilla and colleagues[87] focused on the safety of home PN during pregnancy in 9

pregnancies in 7 home PN-dependent patients (4 with short bowel syndrome and prior home PN dependence for a mean of 6.4 years; 1 with antiphospholipid antibody syndrome with severe hyperemesis who started PN 2 months into the pregnancy; 1 with ulcerative colitis who started PN 3 months into the pregnancy; and 1 with anorexia nervosa who started PN 3 months into the pregnancy). Complications related to the home PN included 3 catheter-related infections in 2 women. Complications associated with pregnancy included dyspnea and palpitations in 1 patient during the first trimester; edema and cervical insufficiency in 2 patients, urinary tract infection in 1 patient, sciatica in 2 patients, and heartburn in 2 patients during the second trimester; and edema in 2 patients in the third trimester. There were no reports of hyperglycemia, and 1 patient had hypoglycemia after completing the PN cycle for the day, requiring extension of the cycle from 12 to 18 h/d. Overall, the women had appropriate weight gain and, in general, delivered normal weight infants without significant complications related to nutrition.

Billiauws and colleagues[88] reported a case series of 21 pregnancies in 15 women with intestinal failure and PN dependence. They found that 67% of the patients had a complication related to the pregnancy, including preeclampsia, postpartum hemorrhage, and thrombosis. Half of the patients had a complication related to their underlying disease during the pregnancy, and 33% of the patients had a complication related to the PN. Negative infant outcomes included 45% of infants were LBW, 29% were hypotrophic, and 19% had other complications (3 cases of respiratory distress syndrome and 1 cardiopulmonary arrest). There was 1 intrauterine death of unclear etiology. Infants were followed for a median of 4 years, and no severe complications were reported in early childhood. Chronic intestinal pseudo-obstruction was suspected in 2 infants who were born to mothers with that condition. Continued monitoring of the offspring will be important to evaluate the impact of PN during pregnancy on long-term outcomes during growth and development.

Peripheral vs Central Parenteral Nutrition

Once the decision has been made to initiate PN, the route of delivery must be considered (see Chapter 14). For the pregnant patient, both peripheral PN and central PN have risks and benefits that must be considered. To reduce the risk of thrombophlebitis during infusion via peripheral vein, the maximum osmolarity of peripheral PN is usually 900 mOsm/L.[89] Because of this restriction, the amino acid and dextrose concentrations are fairly low, and the patient must be able to tolerate a large volume of this solution to receive maintenance energy requirements. Therefore, peripheral PN may not provide adequate energy to support growth and development of the fetus. It could be used as a bridge therapy while central venous access is obtained to allow for central PN.

Central PN allows for provision of full energy and protein requirements in a reduced volume. The concentrated solution generally has an osmolarity greater than 900 mOsm/L and therefore requires central venous access for administration. A common central venous catheter used to administer PN for short-to-intermediate courses (eg, 2 to 12 weeks) is the peripherally inserted central catheter (PICC). It generally requires ultrasound for insertion and is simple to insert at the bedside (in contrast to tunneled catheters or implantable ports, which require insertion in interventional radiology or the surgical suite). PICCs seem less risky compared with other types of central venous access. However, in a retrospective review of 66 pregnant women with a total of 84 PICCs inserted, Cape and colleagues identified a high complication rate, particularly for bacteremia (6.7 cases per 1000 PICC days) and thrombosis (2.7 cases per 1000 PICC days).[90] This study does not imply that PICCs should never be used in pregnant women. Instead, clinicians should carefully select the most appropriate therapy and type of central venous access in this population, and take extra precautions if a PICC is required for any therapy.

Parenteral Nutrition Composition

As with any patient requiring PN, the final composition of a PN solution for a pregnant patient will be calculated based on her energy, protein, and fluid requirements. Chapter 15 reviews general principles for the composition of PN formulations. Additionally, there are some special considerations when calculating PN goals for pregnant women.

Hyperglycemia is a significant risk in pregnancy,[28-34] and it is important to provide adequate carbohydrate to prevent ketonemia while avoiding hyperglycemia.[3] Clinicians should monitor the patient's blood glucose closely. Regular insulin may be added to the PN to achieve the target blood glucose of equal to or less than 140 mg/dL to avoid complications.[35] Adequate protein should be provided to support fetal growth and meet protein demands associated with the underlying disease or therapy. Lipid injectable emulsion (ILE) delivery should be calculated to ensure adequate provision of essential fats. In the United States, an ILE preparation that contains fish oil is now available (see Chapters 5 and 15). If the patient does not have a history of fish allergy, clinicians may want to consider using this product to ensure adequate provision of DHA.[91] One recent case report used this ILE in a pregnant woman dependent on long-term PN because of short bowel syndrome.[92]

Standard multivitamin and trace element preparations should be provided, and electrolytes adjusted to meet metabolic needs. The clinician must recognize that IV preparations of these additives may not be adequate to meet 100% of pregnancy requirements; therefore, additional supplementation may be required. Nutrients of concern include vitamin D, vitamin K, folic acid, calcium, magnesium, iron, iodine, and selenium.

Parenteral Nutrition Complications

Chapter 17 extensively reviews PN complications. A pregnant woman can have the same complications as any other patient receiving PN.

As discussed previously, glucose control is especially important in pregnancy. To avoid fetal complications, clinicians should closely monitor blood glucose levels in pregnant women receiving PN and provide regular insulin if necessary to keep blood glucose levels in the desirable range. Regular

insulin can be added to the PN admixture if the patient has significant insulin requirements.

Nutrition Monitoring

The monitoring of a patient's response to EN is reviewed in Chapter 10, and Chapter 14 addresses monitoring of patients receiving PN. A large part of nutrition support monitoring involves evaluating biochemical changes in response to the nutrition intervention. This assessment is challenging in pregnancy because alterations in blood volume and other pregnancy-related factors contribute to changes in electrolytes, circulating proteins, vitamins, and minerals. These changes vary by trimester. Table 20-8 compares normal ranges for selected laboratory test results in the 3 trimesters of pregnancy with nonpregnant values. Abbassi-Ghanavati and associates[93] provide a resource for many additional laboratory studies that may be evaluated during pregnancy.

Circulating proteins, primarily albumin and prealbumin, are poor indicators of nutrition status. Both are sensitive to inflammation, and low levels likely reflect severity of illness rather than malnutrition or poor response to nutrition therapy.[94] In pregnancy, albumin levels decrease as a result of changes in volume status as well as a shift in production of gamma-globulin to alpha- and beta-globulins.[95] Creatinine levels are lower in pregnancy than the nonpregnant population because of increased renal clearance. Pregnant women with a creatinine level equal to or greater than 0.9 mg/dL should be evaluated for possible developing renal insufficiency.[96] It is unclear whether protein delivery should be modified when renal function is reduced. For women receiving PN with ILE, a baseline triglyceride level should be checked and compared with normal values for her trimester of pregnancy.

Total iron-binding capacity (TIBC), serum iron, hemoglobin, and hematocrit levels may be used to assess iron status. A transferrin saturation of 16% or a serum iron level of less than 60 to 70 mcg/dL may indicate iron deficiency during pregnancy.[97] The National Research Council recommends that transferrin saturation in pregnancy be maintained above 20%.[98] Iron may be affected by factors other than nutrition during critical illness (for example, anemia of chronic disease where iron is sequestered in the liver). Compared with TIBC, serum ferritin concentration more accurately reflects the body's iron stores, and it may help to differentiate iron deficiency from dilutional changes in pregnancy. A serum ferritin concentration of 12 mcg/L is classified as iron deficiency; however, concentrations less than 35 mcg/L may indicate deficiency during a singleton pregnancy; values for multiples are not known. If a patient has a depressed serum hemoglobin concentration, low mean corpuscular volume, and low mean corpuscular hemoglobin concentration, a serum ferritin level should be checked to confirm iron deficiency. Generally, iron deficiency anemia may be indicated by serum hemoglobin and hematocrit levels less than 11.0 mg/dL and 33.0%, respectively, in the first trimester; 10.5 mg/dL and 32.0% in the second trimester; or 11.0 mg/dL and 33.0% in the third trimester.[99] IV iron may be required to correct deficiency in patients who cannot take oral iron; Auerbach and Deloughery provide guidelines for dosing in various clinical conditions, including pregnancy.[100]

TABLE 20-8 Selected Laboratory Values in Pregnancy by Trimester

	Normal Values			
	Nonpregnant	1st Trimester	2nd Trimester	3rd Trimester
Electrolytes and acid-base values				
Sodium, mEq/L	136–146	133–148	129–148	130–148
Potassium, mEq/L	3.5–5.0	3.6–5.0	3.3–5.0	3.3–5.1
Chloride, mEq/L	102–109	101–105	97–109	97–109
Bicarbonate, mmol/L	22–30	20–24	20–24	20–24
pCO_2, mm Hg	38–42	NR	NR	25–33
pO_2, mm Hg	90–100	93–100	90–98	92–107
Anion gap, mmol/L	7–16	13–17	12–16	12–16
pH	7.38–7.42 (arterial)	7.36–7.52 (venous)	7.40–7.52 (venous)	7.39–7.45 (arterial)
BUN, mg/dL	7–20	7–12	3–13	3–11
Creatinine, mg/dL	0.5–0.9	0.4–0.7	0.4–0.8	0.4–0.9
Calcium, mg/dL	8.7–10.2	8.8–10.6	8.2–9.0	8.2–9.7
Magnesium, mg/dL	1.5–2.3	1.6–2.2	1.5–2.2	1.1–2.2
Phosphate, mg/dL	2.5–4.3	3.1–4.6	2.5–4.6	2.8–4.6
Osmolality, mOsm/kg H_2O	275–295	275–280	276–289	278–280
Liver function tests and lipids				
Total bilirubin, mg/dL	0.3–1.3	0.1–0.4	0.1–0.8	0.1–1.1
Direct bilirubin, mg/dL	0.1–0.4	0–0.1	0–0.1	0–0.1
ALP, U/L	33–96	17–88	25–126	38–229
ALT, U/L	7–41	3–30	2–33	2–25
AST, U/L	12–38	3–23	3–33	4–32
Total protein, g/dL	6.7–8.6	6.2–7.6	5.7–6.9	5.6–6.7
Albumin, g/dL	4.1–5.3	3.1–5.1	2.6–4.5	2.3–4.2
Total cholesterol, mg/dL	<200	141–210	176–299	219–349
Triglycerides, mg/dL	< 150	40–159	75–382	131–453
Hematologic laboratory values				
Hemoglobin, g/dL	12–15.8	11.6–13.9	9.7–14.8	9.5–15
Hematocrit, %	35.4–44.4	31–41	30–39	28–40
MCV, mcm^3	79–93	81–96	82–97	81–99
WBC count, $\times10^3/mm^3$	3.5–9.1	5.7–13.6	5.6–14.8	5.9–16.9
Lymphocytes, $\times10^3/mm^3$	0.7–4.6	1.1–3.6	0.9–3.9	1.0–3.6
Platelets, $\times10^9/L$	165–415	174–391	155–409	143–429
Serum iron, mcg/dL	41–141	72–143	44–178	30–193
TIBC, mcg/dL	251–406	278–403	NR	359–609
TS, %	22–46	NR	18–92	9–98
Ferritin, ng/mL	10–150	6–130	2–230	0–116

ALP, alkaline phosphatase; ALT, alanine aminotransferase; AST, aspartate aminotransferase; BUN, blood urea nitrogen; MCV, mean corpuscular volume; NR, not reported; pCO_2, partial pressure of carbon dioxide; pO_2, partial pressure of oxygen; TIBC, total iron-binding capacity; TS, transferrin saturation; WBC, white blood cell. Source: Adapted with permission from reference 93: Abbassi-Ghanavati M, Greer LG, Cunningham FG. Pregnancy and laboratory studies. A reference table for clinicians. *Obstet Gynecol*. 2009;114:1326–1331. doi:10.1097/AOG.0b013e3181c2bde8.

Clinicians may use urine studies as part of the nutrition monitoring process. Glomerular filtration increases significantly in pregnancy beginning in the first trimester. The increases may result in glucosuria, which may be present in more than 50% of pregnant women.[4] Glucosuria is not necessarily related to maternal hyperglycemia, and urine glucose levels should not be used to diagnose diabetes or for monitoring glycemic status in pregnant women. The presence of ketones in the urine can be caused by inadequate hydration, hyperglycemia, or inadequate energy intake. Catabolic illness during pregnancy may also increase the risk of ketonuria. Monitoring urine ketones during the provision of nutrition support therapy is advisable so that energy and fluid intake from EN and/or PN may be adjusted appropriately. The presence of ketones should initially be checked daily and then as needed if weight loss, hyperglycemia, or another change in maternal status (eg, fever) might affect fluid requirements.

Nitrogen balance studies may help the clinician assess individual total nitrogen requirements (see Chapter 6), but published studies have demonstrated that nitrogen intake is often overestimated and nitrogen output can be underestimated.[21] It can be difficult to obtain a complete urine collection unless the patient has a urinary catheter in place, and the correction for insensible losses may be over- or underestimated depending on the patient's other losses (eg, large-volume diarrhea, enterocutaneous fistula losses, or skin sloughing in conditions such as Steven Johnson syndrome). If the clinician elects to conduct a nitrogen balance study, a positive balance of 4 to 6 g nitrogen per day is ideal to support fetal growth and development. However, positive nitrogen balance may not be obtainable during the immediate period following acute illness, such as trauma or sepsis (see Chapters 23 and 24). Serial nitrogen balance studies (eg, weekly) could be monitored to evaluate trends in nitrogen balance.

Clinicians monitoring tolerance to EN and PN support should be familiar with normal changes in acid-base status (see Chapter 7) associated with pregnancy. During pregnancy, a chronic state of compensated respiratory alkalosis exists, and buffering capacity is decreased. The alteration is mostly caused by an increase in maternal respiratory rate and increased excretion of bicarbonate by the maternal kidneys; the result is that the maternal pH is maintained within normal limits. These changes facilitate the transfer of carbon dioxide from the fetus to the mother.

Transitional Feeding

In pregnancy, as in other conditions, the transition to EN or oral intake should be initiated and tolerated before the PN or EN is discontinued (see Chapters 10 and 14).

Lactation

Energy and Protein Requirements

Lactation is the process of producing nutritionally appropriate sustenance with immunologic benefit for the infant. It is a physiologically and metabolically demanding activity that occurs after the delivery of an infant. Energy is expended

TABLE 20-9 Energy and Protein Requirements for Lactation

	Requirement
Energy	• First 6 months postpartum: Prepregnancy EER + 330 kcal[a] • Second 6 months postpartum: Prepregnancy EER + 400 kcal[b]
Protein	• 1.3 g/kg/d *or* • Add 25 g/d to maintenance protein requirements

EER, Estimated Energy Requirement (see Table 20-4 for EER equations).
[a]330 kcal = 500 kcal for milk energy output – 170 kcal for weight loss.
[b]400 kcal is for milk energy output; no adjustment is made to support weight loss.
Source: Data are from reference 3.

for production of breast milk, and increased protein intake is required to ensure adequate protein content. The average "cost" of lactation (often referred to as the *milk energy output*) is approximately 500 kcal/d in the first 6 months postpartum and 400 kcal/d in the second 6 months postpartum (Table 20-9).[3] The milk energy output is calculated from production and energy density of human milk. The IOM suggests a mild degree of energy reduction to promote postpartum weight loss during the first 6 months of lactation. Milk production is in response to demand, and production is generally reduced in the second 6 months postpartum. Protein needs during lactation are also increased (Table 20-9). As previously stated, consensus guidelines recommend at least 200 mg DHA in the diet for lactating women.[41]

Composition of Breastmilk and Micronutrient Considerations

The nutrient content of breastmilk is not uniform. Lawrence and Lawrence have provided nutrient analysis of human breastmilk from well-nourished women, which changes in the initial month postpartum.[101] Nutrition content of breastmilk will vary based on maternal intake. If a mother was nutritionally compromised during her pregnancy, that may lead to suboptimal breastmilk quality.

Micronutrient requirements during lactation are summarized in Tables 20-6 and 20-7, earlier in the chapter. Lactating women may need to increase their intake of vitamin B_{12} and vitamin D to ensure adequate levels in breast milk. Women at risk for low vitamin B_{12} levels in breastmilk include impoverished women whose diet is low in animal protein, those with unsupplemented vegan diets, and those with a history of bariatric surgery (particularly those with poor adherence to vitamin supplementation).[102–104] The vitamin D concentration in breast milk of women taking 400 IU vitamin D per day in pregnancy is relatively low, leading to vitamin D deficiency in breastfed infants. The vitamin D activity in normal lactating women is known to be in the range of 5 to 80 IU, depending on the method of assay. The American Academy of Pediatricians and the IOM have endorsed supplementation with vitamin D to the nursing infant.[105] Compliance to this practice is poor, ranging from 2% to 19%.[105] In a US study supplementing nursing mothers with 400, 2400, or 6400 IU vitamin D₃ daily for 6 months showed supplementation with 6400 IU/d safely supplied breast milk with adequate vitamin D to meet the infant requirements and offered an alternative strategy to direct infant supplementation.[105] Breastmilk is low in vitamin K and iron.[106,107] Infants who are exclusively breastfed and who do not receive intramuscular vitamin K at birth are at risk for hemorrhagic disease of the newborn.[106,108] The exclusively breastfed preterm infant requires iron supplementation; term breastfed infants should not require iron supplementation until 4 to 6 months of age.[109,110]

Nutrition Support During Lactation

There is little information in the literature to guide nutrition support therapy for women who require nutrition support during lactation. In 2 recent reports of PN-dependent women with short bowel syndrome who had been maintained on PN through pregnancy and lactation, the women were able to support adequate growth and development of their infants with lactation.[86,92]

Complications and Specific Clinical Challenges in Pregnancy

Hyperemesis Gravidarum

Hyperemesis gravidarum is a complication distinct from the typical "morning sickness" associated with pregnancy. Occasional nausea and vomiting may occur in 85% of all pregnancies. In contrast, hyperemesis gravidarum is severe, intractable nausea and vomiting complicated by dehydration, electrolyte imbalance, ketosis, nutrition deficiencies and at least 5% weight loss; it affects 0.3% to 3% of total pregnancies.[111,112] The etiology of hyperemesis gravidarum is not fully understood, and research continues to identify causes and appropriate treatments. A recent case-control study found that women with hyperemesis gravidarum were more likely to report a history of allergies, anxiety disorder, dental cavities, depression, gynecologic disorder, immune disorder, migraine headaches, motion sickness, premenstrual syndrome, and temporomandibular joint disorder compared to those without hyperemesis gravidarum.[113] This knowledge may assist with risk screening. Symptoms start at 6 to 8 weeks of gestation and often resolve by 20 weeks, but nausea and vomiting can persist into the third trimester in about one-quarter of cases.[111,114]

Women with hyperemesis gravidarum are at risk for Wernicke's encephalopathy, acute kidney injury, liver dysfunction, and esophageal rupture. In addition, limitations in oral intake because of severe vomiting can contribute to the development of malnutrition. Maternal deaths related to hyperemesis gravidarum have been reported.[115] Risks to the fetus include higher risk of LBW, intrauterine growth restriction, preterm delivery, fetal and neonatal death, and neurodevelopmental delay.[115]

A recent systematic review provides guidance for managing hyperemesis gravidarum.[111] Initial management generally starts with basic interventions of small, frequent meals comprised of low-fat, high-carbohydrate foods and the avoidance

of trigger foods and foods with strong odors. If these interventions are unsuccessful, treatment may include supplemental vitamin B₆, ginger, and acupressure. The next line of therapy would be combined vitamin B₆/doxylamine, antihistamines, dopamine antagonists, serotonin antagonists, and IV fluids with or without diazepam. Finally, the last line of therapy would be corticosteroids, EN (or PN in severe cases), gabapentin, or transdermal clonidine (see Practice Scenario 20-1).[93,116]

Practice Scenario 20-1

Question: How do you decide when to initiate nutrition support for a patient with severe hyperemesis gravidarum?

Scenario: A 30-year-old woman who has experienced persistent severe nausea and emesis throughout the entire course of her pregnancy presents in her 17th week of gestation with weight loss, ongoing nausea and vomiting, and severe fatigue. The patient's height is 160 cm, and her pregravid weight was 56.8 kg, meaning her prepregnancy body mass index (BMI) was 22.2 and her prepregnancy ideal body weight was 52.3 kg (per the Hamwi formula). Her current weight is 48.1 kg. She had previously been admitted at week 14 with dehydration and weight loss (then weighing 50.8 kg) and was discharged after receiving 3 days of intravenous hydration and being able to tolerate a single meal of 2 slices of dry white toast and a cup of decaffeinated tea. Since being discharged, she was seen in the outpatient infusion clinic for hydration 2 days per week.

Physical examination shows that the patient has pale conjunctiva, and her oral cavity is dry. She has moderate temporal muscle and clavicular wasting; severe fat wasting at the triceps and prominent ribs. No edema is noted.

Her diet recall documents minimal oral intake since discharge 3 weeks ago. At best, she was only able to sip water throughout the day and eat plain white bread or a few saltine crackers daily. She is unable to tolerate her prenatal vitamin. Pertinent laboratory test results include the following:[93]

- Hemoglobin, 9.7 g/dL (nonpregnancy normal: 12–15.8 g/dL; second trimester normal: 9.7–14.8 g/dL)
- Hematocrit, 29% (nonpregnancy normal: 35.4%–44.4%; second trimester normal: 30%–39%)
- Mean corpuscular volume, 79 mcm³ (nonpregnancy normal: 79–93 mcm³; second trimester normal: 82–97 mcm³)
- Serum iron: 38 mcg/dL (nonpregnancy normal: 41–141 mcg/dL; second trimester normal: 44–178 mcg/dL)
- Total iron-binding capacity, 293 mcg/dL (nonpregnancy normal: 251–406; second trimester normal: not reported; first trimester normal: 278–403)

Intervention: Dextrose-containing intravenous fluid is initiated to hydrate patient until a nasogastric tube can be inserted. Once the nasogastric tube is placed, continuous enteral nutrition (EN) is initiated with an isotonic enteral formula. The patient is at risk for refeeding syndrome; therefore, EN is advanced slowly while serum levels of potassium, magnesium, and phosphorus are closely monitored, with aggressive repletion if levels are low. Supplemental thiamin and folic acid are provided for the first 3 to 5 days of feeding. The patient is monitored closely for signs and symptoms of heart failure.[116] Aggressive antiemetic therapy is provided during the initiation and advancement of enteral nutrition. Oral iron will be started once nausea and vomiting are controlled.

Answer: Because the patient is severely malnourished, nutrition support (EN in this case) should be started as soon as appropriate access can be obtained.

Rationale: This patient started out with a healthy BMI and her target weight gain was 25 to 35 pounds (11.4 to 15.9 kg). She has lost approximately 15% of her pregravid weight and now has a BMI of 18.8, with overt signs of fat and muscle wasting. At this point in her pregnancy, she should have gained approximately 2.3 kg from her pregravid weight, with a target weight of 59.1 kg at week 17 of her pregnancy. Using this weight, she is 19% below where she should be at this stage of her pregnancy; therefore, she is at high risk for refeeding syndrome. Her appearance and assessment of her laboratory values are consistent with iron deficiency. She can be categorized with severe malnutrition in the context of chronic disease because she has had hyperemesis gravidarum for more than 3 months, has had prolonged inadequate energy intake meeting less than 75% of her estimated needs for more than 1 month, has lost 15% of her pregravid weight in approximately 4 months, and has severe fat wasting and moderate muscle wasting. In addition, she is iron deficient. The patient requires initiation of EN to stabilize her weight, with the eventual goal to support appropriate weight gain and correction of nutrition deficiencies. If the patient demonstrates intolerance of EN for a prolonged period of time (eg, more than 7 days) and is still unable to tolerate and oral diet, parenteral nutrition should be considered.

For some women, the severity of hyperemesis gravidarum has prompted termination of the pregnancy; in a survey of 808 women with hyperemesis gravidarum, 15.2% had at least 1 termination because of hyperemesis gravidarum, and 6.1% had multiple terminations.[117] Another survey of 610 women, 377 with hyperemesis gravidarum and 233 without, 18% of women with hyperemesis gravidarum reported posttraumatic stress symptoms associated with their pregnancies, and compared with those without hyperemesis gravidarum, reported significantly more negative outcomes, including inability to breastfeed, missed time from work or school, lost job (or had to leave employment), and experienced marital and financial difficulties.[118]

In addition to the negative impact on the mother, hyperemesis gravidarum poses risks for the fetus. Women with hyperemesis gravidarum tend to have smaller infants overall, have more SGA infants, and shorter gestations.[115,119–121] In a literature review of Wernicke's encephalopathy as a result of hyperemesis gravidarum, 16 of 49 cases experienced spontaneous abortion and 2 of 49 cases had fetal death, for a 37% fetal loss rate. The authors suggested that thiamin deficiency may have played a role in this high fetal loss rate.[122] Nutrition support clinicians can play a major role in the management of hyperemesis gravidarum. Severe vomiting has been associated with thiamin depletion; therefore, it is essential that patients are given IV thiamin along with IV

fluid (particularly if dextrose-containing IV fluids are used) to prevent Wernicke's encephalopathy or Wernicke-Korsakoff syndrome (Practice Scenario 20-2). Thiamin repletion (generally 100 mg/d) should be provided with IV fluids.[112,122] An IV multivitamin could also be included, as the patient has likely had inadequate micronutrient intake for a prolonged period of time. Van Stuijvenberg and colleagues[123] documented that the intake of most nutrients by women with hyperemesis gravidarum fell below the 50% of the DRI, and 60% of patients had suboptimal levels of thiamin, riboflavin, vitamin B6, and vitamin A.

Practice Scenario 20-2

Question: How do you prevent an adverse neurologic outcome when initiating nutrition support in a patient with severe intractable hyperemesis gravidarum?

Scenario: The insertion of a nasogastric tube in the patient from Practice Scenario 20-1 is delayed because of lack of availability in interventional radiology. She continues to have severe nausea and vomiting, and she continues to receive hydration with intravenous (IV) fluid containing 5% dextrose, infusing at 125 mL/h. She is prescribed an oral prenatal vitamin but promptly vomits after taking it. On hospital Day 2, she becomes confused and starts to exhibit short-term memory loss. Physical examination reveals nystagmus and gait ataxia that was not present on her admission examination.

Intervention: The patient is given 100 mg thiamin intravenously and prescribed 100 mg IV thiamin daily for the next 2 days.

Answer: Dextrose or other carbohydrate repletion should not proceed until supplemental thiamin is provided first. The classic triad of Wernicke's encephalopathy caused by thiamin deficiency is confusion, ophthalmoplegia, and ataxia. If a patient with hyperemesis gravidarum develops these symptoms, prompt thiamin replacement should be provided.

Rationale: Patients with prolonged severe vomiting are at risk for Wernicke's encephalopathy. This condition is usually precipitated by provision of glucose without prior or concurrent thiamin supplementation.

If the patient's response to the therapies outlined in the recent systematic review by McParlin et al[111] mentioned previously are minimal, nutrition support initiation should be considered. The comprehensive nutrition assessment will help guide decision-making regarding when to consider EN vs PN. Ideally, EN would be the starting point for nutrition support. However, if a patient is severely malnourished and well below her pregravid weight with little nutrition reserve, it may be prudent to initiate PN early as a bridge to obtaining enteral access and transitioning to EN.

The literature to support the use of EN as a way to improve nausea and vomiting with hyperemesis gravidarum is limited to individual case reports and small case series.[78,124–126] The

MOTHER trial (Maternal and Offspring outcomes after Treatment of HyperEmesis by Refeeding) is in progress to evaluate early nasogastric tube feeding to optimize treatment of hyperemesis gravidarum.[127] Once the patient has stopped vomiting and electrolytes are stable, a small-bore feeding tube may be inserted and gastric feedings with an isotonic enteral formula can be initiated at a low rate with slow advancement to the calculated goal as long as nausea is not worsened and there is no vomiting or diarrhea.[126] Gastric residual volumes (GRVs) should not be checked in patients with a small-bore feeding tube because of the risk of tube clogging (see Chapter 13). As long as the patient can report nausea, fullness, or other GI discomfort, there should be no need to check GRVs. Antiemetics can be used concurrently with EN to minimize retching and decrease the risk of tube dislodgment and aspiration. Vaisman and colleagues[78] noted that it took 48 hours of nasojejunal feeding to reduce vomiting, and complete cessation occurred after an average of 5 days of enteral feeding. Lord and Pelletier[128] reported success with nasogastric feeding in a series of 26 patients with hyperemesis gravidarum. The patients received intermittent EN over 4 to 6 gravity-drip feedings via a small-bore nasoenteric feeding tube. The mean time to resolution of emesis was 4.5 days and the mean time to stabilize and promote weight gain was 3.6 days. The mean duration of EN was 7 weeks. Of interest, the patients required frequent replacement of the nasogastric feeding tubes, with a report of 2.7 feeding tubes per patient.[128] In general, nasojejunal feeding should be considered in patients with poor tolerance to gastric feeding.[126] For patients requiring long-term enteral access, a percutaneous endoscopic gastrostomy with or without jejunal extension tube or direct feeding jejunostomy may need to be considered.[71-76] If the patient is unable to tolerate EN or has a contraindication to enteral access, PN should then be considered. For patients with severe malnutrition, clinicians may want to consider PN earlier in the clinical course, particularly if there are delays in obtaining enteral access (see Figure 20-1).

Management of the Pregnant Trauma Patient

Medical and nutrition support of pregnant trauma patients are especially challenging because catecholamines released in response to stress cause increased nutrient catabolism and vasoconstriction of the placental vasculature, thereby reducing the nutrient and oxygen supplies to the fetus. The nutrition needs to support maternal illness together with demands of the growing fetus are difficult to estimate. Requirements for nutrients are likely to be altered by trauma, but the degree of alteration depends on the nature and extent of the injury. In the few published case reports of pregnant trauma patients receiving nutrition support, various methods for estimating energy requirements in the absence of indirect calorimetry were used.[75,129-132] In these cases, energy delivery ranged from 2000 to 3000 kcal/d. Indirect calorimetry is a valuable tool for

determining the resting energy expenditure of the maternal-fetal unit so that under- or overfeeding can be prevented. If indirect calorimetry is not available, traditional equations that estimate the needs of critically ill patients can be used with 200 to 300 kcal/d added for pregnancy; this pregnancy energy deposition is slightly below the recommendations to support weight gain in a healthy pregnancy because the energy expenditure from activity while recovering from trauma would most likely be low and it is important to avoid overfeeding the critically ill patient.[133] Weight gain goals would remain the same as in a healthy pregnancy. However, accurate weights can be difficult to obtain in the intensive care unit, where weight gain may reflect volume resuscitation, rather than true weight gain. The initial estimation for protein requirements can be calculated

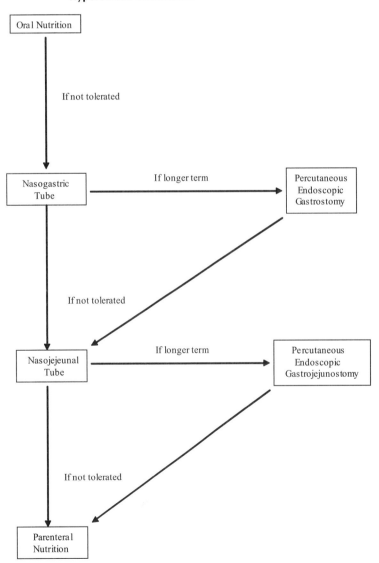

FIGURE 20-1 Algorithm for Preference of Route of Nutrition Support in Hyperemesis Gravidarum

If severe malnutrition is present, parenteral nutrition should be considered earlier in the patient's course to allow for correction of deficiencies while enteral access options are pursued.

by using the same methods for nonpregnant patients, beginning with 1.5 to 2.0 g/kg pregravid weight.[133]

As with any other critically ill patient, EN is preferred over PN. Methods to insert enteral feeding tubes have been discussed previously in this chapter; pregnant patients requiring mechanical ventilation may have an orogastric tube inserted for EN. The guidelines for enteral formula choice in critical illness from ASPEN and the Society of Critical Care Medicine should be followed; a specialty enteral formula is likely not necessary unless the patient has significant organ dysfunction, such as acute kidney injury, and requires an electrolyte modified enteral formula.[133] A multivitamin with minerals should be provided daily as well as additional folic acid; additional iron may also be required. Glucose control should be managed as discussed previously. Because of the risk for bowel obstruction with the use of insoluble fiber use in critically ill patients, a soluble fiber supplement and appropriate stool softeners and laxatives should be used to ensure regular stool output.

Other Considerations in Pregnancy

With improvements in therapies for IBD, short bowel syndrome, other GI motility disorders, chronic pancreatitis, cystic fibrosis, and genetic metabolic disorders, patients are living longer and clinicians may encounter long-term EN or PN patients who become pregnant. With little in the literature to guide management of these patients, nutrition support clinicians should work closely with the obstetrician to determine the optimal route of feeding, implementation of the nutrition plan, and close monitoring of the patient's nutrition status and fetal growth.

Conclusion

Nutrition support during pregnancy poses many challenges to the nutrition support clinician, particularly given the limitations in data available to guide the assessment and management process for these high-risk patients. Careful assessment of nutrition status, close monitoring of response to nutrition therapy, and frequent communication with the patient's obstetrician is important to promote positive outcomes for the patient and the fetus.

References

1. Siega-Riz AM, Viswanathan M, Moos M, et al. A systematic review of outcomes of maternal weight gain according to the Institute of Medicine recommendations: birthweight, fetal growth, and postpartum weight retention. Am J Obstet Gynecol. 2009;201:339, e1–e14.
2. Cox Bauer CM, Bernhard KA, Greer DM, Merrill DC. Maternal and neonatal outcomes in obese women who lose weight during pregnancy. J Perinatol. 2016;36:278–283.
3. Institute of Medicine, Food and Nutrition Board. Dietary Reference Intakes for Energy, Carbohydrate, Fiber, Fat, Fatty Acids, Cholesterol, Protein and Amino Acids. Washington, DC: National Academies Press; 2002.
4. Davison JM, Hytten FE. The effect of pregnancy on the renal handling of glucose. Br J Obstet Gynaecol. 1975;82:374–381.
5. Wessel AE, Mogensen KM, Rohr F, et al. Management of a woman with maple syrup urine disease during pregnancy, delivery, and lactation. JPEN J Parenter Enteral Nutr. 2015;39:875–879.
6. Luke B. Nutrition for multiples. Clin Obstet Gynecol. 2015;58:585–610. doi:10.1097/GRF.0000000000000117.
7. Institute of Medicine and National Research Council. Weight Gain During Pregnancy: Reexamining the Guidelines. Washington, DC: National Academies Press; 2009.
8. Luke B. What is the influence of maternal weight gain on the fetal growth of twins? Clin Obstet Gynecol. 1998;41:57–64.
9. Bodner LM, Siminerio LL, Himes KP, et al. Maternal obesity and gestational weight gain are risk factors for infant death. Obesity. 2016;24:290–498.
10. Hamilton BE, Martin JA, Osterman MJK, Curtin SC, Mathews TJ. Births: final data for 2014. Natl Vital Stat Rep. 2015;64:1–4.
11. Finer BL, Bolna MR. Declines in unintended pregnancy in the United States, 2008–2011. N Engl J Med. 2016;374:843–852.
12. White JV, Guenter P, Jensen G, et al. Consensus statement: Academy of Nutrition and Dietetics and American Society for Parenteral and Enteral Nutrition: characteristics recommended for the identification and documentation of adult malnutrition (undernutrition). JPEN J Parenter Enteral Nutr. 2012;36:275–283.
13. Centers for Disease Control and Prevention. Weight gain during pregnancy. Updated October 14, 2016. https://www.cdc.gov/reproductivehealth/maternalinfanthealth/pregnancy-weight-gain.htm. Accessed March 7, 2017.
14. Cho S, Atwood JE. Peripheral edema. Am J Med. 2002;113:580–586.
15. Christian P, Stewart CP. Maternal micronutrient deficiency, fetal development, and the risk of chronic disease. J Nutr. 2010;140:437–445.
16. Milone M, De Placidio G, Sosa Fernandez LM, et al. Incidence of successful pregnancy after weight loss interventions in infertile women: a systematic review and meta-analysis of the literature. Obes Surg. 2016;26:443–451.
17. Isom KA, Andromalos L, Ariagno M, et al. Nutrition and metabolic support recommendations for the bariatric patient. Nutr Clin Pract. 2014;29:718–739.
18. Kaiser LL, Campbell CG; Academy Positions Committee Workgroup. Practice paper of the Academy of Nutrition and Dietetics. Nutrition and lifestyle for a healthy pregnancy outcome. J Acad Nutr Diet. 2014;114(7):1099–1103.
19. Thomson AM, Hytten FE. Calorie requirements in human pregnancy. Proc Nutr Soc. 1961;20–76–83.
20. Dall'Asta A, Brunelli V, Prefumo F, Frusca T, Lees CC. Early onset fetal growth restriction. Matern Health Neonatol Perinatol. 2017;3:2. doi:10.1186/s40748-016-0041-x.
21. Elango R, Ball RO. Protein and amino acid requirements during pregnancy. Adv Nutr. 2016;7(Suppl):839S–844S.
22. Ziegler EE, O'Donnell AM, Nelson ST, Fomon SJ. Body composition of the reference fetus. Growth. 1976.40:329–341.
23. Blumfield ML, Collins CE. High-protein diets during pregnancy: healthful or harmful for offspring? Am J Clin Nutr. 2014;100:993–995.
24. Rush D, Stein Z, Susser M. A randomized controlled trial of prenatal nutritional supplementation in New York City. Pediatrics. 1980;65:683–697.
25. Higgins AC, Moxley JE, Pencharz PB, Mikolainis D, Dubois S. Impact of the Higgins Nutrition Intervention Program on birth weight: a within-mother analysis. J Am Diet Assoc. 1989;89:1097–103.
26. Maslova E, Rytter D, Bech BH, et al. Maternal protein intake during pregnancy and offspring overweight 20 y later. Am J Clin Nutr. 2014;100:1139–1148.
27. MacBurney M, Matarese LE. Pregnancy. In: Matarese L, Gottschlich MM, eds. Contemporary Nutrition Support Practice. 2nd ed. Philadelphia, PA: Saunders; 2003:337–343.

28. Catalano PM, Kirwan JP, de Mouzon SH, King J. Gestational diabetes and insulin resistance: role in short- and long-term implications for mother and fetus. *J Nutr.* 2003;133(Suppl):1674S–1683S.

29. Butte NF. Carbohydrate and lipid metabolism in pregnancy: normal compared with gestational diabetes mellitus. *Am J Clin Nutr.* 2000;71(Suppl):1256S–1261S.

30. Turok DK, Ratcliffe SD, Baxley EG. Management of gestational diabetes mellitus. *Am Fam Physician.* 2003;68:1767–1772.

31. Christoffersson M, Rydhstroem H. Shoulder dystocia and brachial plexus injury: a population-based study. *Gynecol Obstet Invest.* 2002;53:42–47.

32. Hod M, Bar K, Peled Y, et al. Antepartum management protocol. Timing and mode of delivery in gestational diabetes. *Diabetes Care.* 1998;21(Suppl 2):B113–B117.

33. Rosenstein MG, Cheng YW, Snowden JM, et al. The risk of stillbirth and infant death stratified by gestational age in women with gestational diabetes. *Am J Obstet Gynecol.* 2012;206:309, e1–e309.

34. Mimouni FB, Sheffer GM, Mandel D. The infant of the diabetic mother: short-term implications. In: Langer O, ed. *The Diabetes in Pregnancy Dilemma: Leading Change with Proven Solutions.* 2nd ed. Shelton, CT: People's Medical Publishing House–USA; 2015: 99–108.

35. American Diabetes Association. Management of diabetes in pregnancy. *Diabetes Care.* 2017;40(Suppl 1):S114–S119.

36. Weigensberg M, Sobel R, Garcia-Palmer F, Freinkel N. Temporal differences in vulnerability to fuel mediated teratogenesis. *Diabetes.* 1988;37(Suppl 1):85A.

37. Rizzo T, Metzger BE, Burns WJ, Burns K. Correlations between antepartum maternal metabolism and child intelligence. *N Engl J Med.* 1991;325:911–916.

38. Kimura RE. Lipid metabolism in the fetal-placental unit. In: Cowett RM, ed. *Principles of Perinatal-Neonatal Metabolism.* 2nd ed. New York: Springer-Verlag; 1998:389.

39. Lauritzen L, Brambilla P, Mazzocchi A, et al. DHA effects in brain development and function. *Nutrients.* 2016;8:6.

40. Newberry SJ, Chung M, Booth M, et al. *Omega-3 Fatty Acids and Maternal and Child Health: An Updated Systematic Review.* Rockville, MD: Agency for Healthcare Research and Quality; 2016. https://www.effectivehealthcare.ahrq.gov/ehc/products/610/2321/omega-3-maternity-report-161027.pdf. Accessed July 12, 2017.

41. Koletzko B, Lien E, Agostoni C, et al. The roles of long-chain polyunsaturated fatty acids in pregnancy, lactation, and infancy: review of current knowledge and consensus recommendations. *J Perinat Med.* 2008;36:5–14.

42. Hachey DL. Benefits and risks of modifying maternal fat intake in pregnancy and lactation. *Am J Clin Nutr.* 1994;59(2 Suppl): 454S–464S.

43. Everson GT. Liver problems in pregnancy: distinguishing normal from abnormal hepatic changes. *Medscape Women's Health.* 1998;3:3.

44. Herrera E, Gomez-Coronado D, Lasuncion MA. Lipid metabolism in pregnancy. *Biol Neonate.* 1987;51:70–77.

45. Institute of Medicine. *Dietary Reference Intakes for Water, Potassium, Sodium, Chloride, and Sulfate.* Washington, DC: National Academies Press; 2005.

46. Lindower JB. Water balance in the fetus and neonate. *Semin Fetal Neonatal Med.* 2017;22:71–75.

47. Institute of Medicine. *Dietary Reference Intakes for Vitamin A, Vitamin K, Arsenic, Boron, Chromium, Copper, Iodine, Iron, Manganese, Molybdenum, Nickel, Silicon, Vanadium, and Zinc.* Washington, DC: National Academies Press; 2001.

48. Institute of Medicine. *Dietary Reference Intakes for Calcium and Vitamin D.* Washington, DC: National Academies Press; 2010.

49. Institute of Medicine. *Dietary Reference Intakes for Vitamin C, Vitamin E, Selenium, and Carotenoids.* Washington, DC: National Academies Press; 2000.

50. Institute of Medicine. *Dietary Reference Intakes for Thiamin, Riboflavin, Niacin, Vitamin B6, Folate, Vitamin B12, Pantothenic Acid, Biotin, and Choline.* Washington, DC: National Academies Press; 2000.

51. Institute of Medicine. *Dietary Reference Intakes for Calcium, Phosphorus, Magnesium, Vitamin D, and Fluoride.* Washington, DC: National Academies Press; 1997.

52. Worthington-Roberts B, Williams SR. Appendix A: vitamins and minerals and pregnancy outcome. In: Worthington-Roberts BS, Williams SR, eds. *Nutrition in Pregnancy and Lactation.* 6th ed. St. Louis, MO: Times Mirror/Mosby; 1997:480–486.

53. Schoenmakers I, Pettifor JM, Pena-Rosas J-P, et al. Prevention and consequences of vitamin D deficiency in pregnant and lactating women and children: a symposium to prioritise vitamin D on the global agenda. *J Steroid Biochem Mol Biol.* 2016;164:156–160.

54. Wagner CL, Baggerly C, McDonnell S, et al. Post-hoc analysis of vitamin D status and reduced risk of preterm birth in two vitamin D pregnancy cohorts compared with South Carolina March of Dimes 2009–2011 rates. *J Steroid Biochem Mol Biol.* 2016;155: 245–251.

55. Toriello HV, Erick M, Alessandri JL, et al. Maternal vitamin K deficient embryopathy: association with hyperemesis gravidarum and Crohn disease. *Am J Med Genet.* 2013;161(A):417–429.

56. Chitayat D, Matsui D, Amitai Y, et al. Folic acid supplementation for pregnant women and those planning pregnancy: 2015 update. *J Clin Pharmacol.* 2016;56:170–175.

57. Camaschella C. New insights into iron deficiency and iron deficiency anemia. *Blood Rev.* 2017. Epub ahead of print Feb 13, 2017. doi:10.1016/j.blre.2017.02.004.

58. Yip R. Significance of an abnormally low or high hemoglobin concentration during pregnancy: special consideration of iron nutrition. *Am J Clin Nutr.* 2000;72(Suppl):272S–279S.

59. Cao C, O'Brien KO. Pregnancy and iron homeostasis: an update. *Nutr Rev.* 2013;71:35–51.

60. Ota E, Mori R, Tobe-Gai R, et al. Zinc supplementation for improving pregnancy and infant outcome. *Cochrane Database Syst Rev.* 2015;(2):CD000230.

61. Pathak P, Kapil U. Role of trace elements zinc, copper and magnesium during pregnancy and its outcome. *Indian J Pediatr.* 2004; 71:1003–1005.

62. Vohr BR, Poggi Davis E, Wanke CA, Krebs NF. Neurodevelopment: the impact of nutrition and inflammation during preconception and pregnancy in low-resource settings. *Pediatrics.* 2017; 139(Suppl):S38–S49.

63. Moghimi M, Ashrafzadeh S, Rassi S, Naseh A. Maternal zinc deficiency and congenital abnormalities in newborns. *Pediatrics Internat.* 2017;59:443–446.

64. Ahmed RG. Maternal iodine deficiency and brain disorders. *Endocrin Metab Syndr.* 2016;5:1.

65. Stagnaro-Green A, Dodo-Isonaige E, Pearce EN, Spencer C, Gaba ND. Marginal iodine status and high rate of subclinical hypothyroidism in Washington DC women planning conception. *Thyroid.* 2015;25:1151–1154.

66. Rothman KJ, Moore LL, Singer MR, et al. Teratogenicity of high vitamin A intake. *N Engl J Med.* 1995;333:1369–1373.

67. Lammer EJ, Chen DT, Hoar RM, et al. Retinoic acid embryopathy. *N Engl J Med.* 1985;313:837–841.

68. Costas K, Davis R, Kim N, et al. Use of supplements containing high-dose vitamin A—New York state, 1983–1984. *JAMA.* 1987; 257:1292–1297.

69. Bernhart IB, Dorsey DJ. Hypervitaminosis A and congenital renal anomalies in a human infant. *Obstet Gynecol.* 1974;43:750–755.

70. Body C, Christie JA. Gastrointestinal diseases in pregnancy. Nausea, vomiting, hyperemesis gravidarum, gastroesophageal reflux disease, constipation, and diarrhea. *Gastroenterol Clin North Am.* 2016;45:267–283.

71. Irving PM, Howell RJ, Shidrawi RG. Percutaneous endoscopic gastrostomy with a jejunal port for severe hyperemesis gravidarum. *Eur J Gastroenterol Hepatol.* 2004;16:937–939.

72. Pendlebury J, Phillips F, Ferguson A, Ghosh S. Successful pregnancy in a patient with chronic intestinal pseudo-obstruction while on ambulatory percutaneous endoscopic gastrostomy feeding. *Eur J Gastroenterol Hepatol.* 1997;9:711–713.

73. Shaheen NJ, Crosby MA, Grimm IS, Isaacs K. The use of percutaneous endoscopic gastrostomy in pregnancy. *Gastrointest Endosc.* 1997;46:564–565.

74. Serrano P, Velloso A, Garcia-Luna PP, et al. Enteral nutrition by percutaneous endoscopic gastrojejunostomy in severe hyperemesis gravidarum: a report of two cases. *Clin Nutr.* 1998;17:135–139.

75. Koh ML, Lipkin EW. Nutrition support of a pregnant comatose patient via percutaneous endoscopic gastrostomy. *JPEN J Parenter Enteral Nutr.* 1993;17:384–387.

76. Wejda BU, Soennichsen B, Huchzermeyer H, et al. Successful jejunal nutrition therapy in a pregnant patient with apallic syndrome. *Clin Nutr.* 2003;22:209–211.

77. Erick M. Nutrition via jejunostomy in refractory hyperemesis gravidarum. A case report. *J Am Diet Assoc.* 1997;97:1154–1156.

78. Vaisman N, Kaidar R, Levin I, Lessing JB. Nasojejunal feeding in hyperemesis gravidarum—a preliminary study. *Clin Nutr.* 2004;23:53–57.

79. Kahaleh M, Hartwell GD, Arseneau KO, et al. Safety and efficacy of ERCP in pregnancy. *Gastrointest Endosc.* 2004;60:287–292.

80. Damilakis J, Theocharopoulos N, Perisinakis K, et al. Conceptus radiation dose and risk from cardiac catheter ablation procedures. *Circulation.* 2001;104:893–897.

81. Saha S, Loranger D, Pricolo V, Degli-Esposti S. Feeding jejunostomy for the treatment of severe hyperemesis gravidarum: a case series. *JPEN J Parenter Enteral Nutr.* 2009;33:529–534.

82. Källén B, Nilsson E, Otterblad Olausson P. Maternal use of loperamide in early pregnancy and delivery outcome. *Acta Paediatr.* 2008;97:541–545.

83. Worthington P, Balint J, Bechtold M, et al. When is parenteral nutrition appropriate? *JPEN J Parenter Enteral Nutr.* 2017;41:324–377.

84. Russo-Stieglitz KE, Levine AB, Wagner BA, Armenti TV. Pregnancy outcomes in patients requiring parenteral nutrition. *J Maternal-Fetal Med.* 1999;8:164–167.

85. Campo M, Albinana S, Garcia-Burguillo A, et al. Pregnancy in a patient with chronic intestinal pseudoobstruction on long term parenteral nutrition. *Clin Nutr.* 2000;19:455–457.

86. Borbolla Foster A, Dixon S, Tyrrell-Price J, Trinder J. Pregnancy and lactation during long-term total parenteral nutrition: a case report and literature review. *Obstet Med.* 2016;9:181–184.

87. Theilla M, Lawinski M, Cohen J, et al. Safety of home parenteral nutrition during pregnancy. *Clin Nutr.* 2017;36:288–292.

88. Billiauws L, Armengol Debeir L, Poullenot F, et al. Pregnancy is possible on long-term home parenteral nutrition in patients with chronic intestinal failure: results of a long term retrospective observational study. *Clin Nutr.* 2017;36:1165–1169.

89. Boullata JI, Gilbert K, Sacks G, et al. A.S.P.E.N. clinical guidelines: parenteral nutrition ordering, order review, compounding, labeling, and dispensing. *JPEN J Parenter Enteral Nutr.* 2014;38:334–377.

90. Cape AV, Mogensen KM, Robinson MK, Carusi DA. Peripherally inserted central catheter (PICC) complications during pregnancy. *JPEN J Parenter Enteral Nutr.* 2014;38:594–600.

91. Smoflipid (lipid injectable emulsion), for intravenous use. Prescribing information. Lake Zurich, IL: Fresenius Kabi; May 2016.

92. Buchholz BM, Ruland A, Kiefer N, et al. Conception, pregnancy, and lactation despite chronic intestinal failure requiring home parenteral nutrition. *Nutr Clin Pract.* 2015;30:807–814.

93. Abbassi-Ghanavati M, Greer LG, Cunningham FG. Pregnancy and laboratory studies. A reference table for clinicians. *Obstet Gynecol.* 2009;114:1326–1331. doi:10.1097/AOG.0b013e3181c2bde8.

94. Jensen GL. Malnutrition and inflammation—"burning down the house": inflammation as an adaptive physiologic response versus self-destruction. *JPEN J Parenter Enteral Nutr.* 2015;39:56–62.

95. Mendenhall HW. Serum protein concentrations in pregnancy. *Am J Obstet Gynecol.* 1970;106:388–399.

96. Cunningham GF, Gant NF, Leveno KJ, et al. Assessment of renal disease during pregnancy. In: *Williams Obstetrics.* 21st ed. New York: McGraw-Hill; 2001:1252–1253.

97. Institute of Medicine. *Dietary Reference Intakes. Vitamin A, Vitamin K, Arsenic, Boron, Chromium, Copper, Iodine, Iron, Manganese, Molybdenum, Nickel, Silicon, Vanadium, and Zinc.* Washington, DC: National Academies Press; 2001.

98. National Research Council. *Laboratory Indices of Nutritional Status in Pregnancy.* Washington, DC: National Academy of Science; 1978.

99. Centers for Disease Control and Prevention. Recommendations to prevent and control iron deficiency in the United States. *MMWR Morb Mortal Wkly Rep.* 1998;47:1–36.

100. Auerbach M, Deloughery T. Single-dose iron for iron deficiency: a new paradigm. *Hematology Am Soc Hematol Educ Program.* 2016;1:57–66.

101. Lawrence RA, Lawrence RM. Appendix A: composition of human milk. In: Lawrence RA, Lawrence RM, eds. *Breastfeeding: A Guide for the Medical Profession.* 8th ed. Philadelphia, PA: Elsevier; 2016:765.

102. Akcaboy M, Malbora B, Zorlu P, et al. Vitamin B12 deficiency in infants. *Indian J Pediatr.* 2015;82:619–624.

103. Honzik T, Adamovicova M, Smolka V, et al. Clinical presentation and metabolic consequences in 40 breastfed infants with nutritional vitamin B12 deficiency: what have we learned? *Eur J Paediatr Neurol.* 2010;14:488–495.

104. Sunil S, Santiago VA, Gougeon L, et al. Predictors of vitamin adherence after bariatric surgery. *Obes Surg.* 2017;27:416–423.

105. Hollis BW, Wanger CL, Howard CR, et al. Maternal versus infant vitamin D supplementation during lactation: a randomized controlled trial. *Pediatrics.* 2015;136:625–634.

106. Greer FR. Are breast-fed infants vitamin K deficient? *Adv Exp Med Biol.* 2001;501:391–395.

107. Friel JK. There is no iron in human milk. *J Pediatr Gastroenterol Nutr.* 2017;64:460–464.

108. Enz R, Anderson RS. A blown pupil and intracranial hemorrhage in a 4 week old: a case of delayed onset vitamin K bleeding, a rare "can't miss" diagnosis. *J Emerg Med.* 2016;51:164–167.

109. Greer FR. How much iron is needed for breastfeeding infants? *Curr Pediatr Rev.* 2015;11:298–304.

110. Baker RD, Greer FR, Committee on Nutrition. Clinical report: diagnosis and prevention of iron deficiency and iron-deficiency anemia in infants and young children (0–3 years of age). *Pediatrics.* 2010;126:1040–1050.

111. McParlin C, O'Donnell A, Robson SC, et al. Treatments for hyperemesis gravidarum and nausea and vomiting in pregnancy: a systematic review. *JAMA.* 2016;316:1392–1401.

112. Goodwin TM. Hyperemesis gravidarum. *Obstet Gynecol Clin North Am.* 2008;35:401–417.

113. Tian R, MacGibbon K, Martin B, Mullin P, Fejzo M. Analysis of pre- and post-pregnancy issues in women with hyperemesis gravidarum. *Auton Neurosci.* 2017;202:73–78.

114. Einarson RT, Piwko C, Koren G. Quantifying the global rates of nausea and vomiting of pregnancy: a meta-analysis. *J Popul Ther Clin Pharmacol.* 2013;20:e171–e183.

115. Fejzo MS, MacGibbon K, Mullin PM. Why are women still dying from nausea and vomiting of pregnancy? *Gynecol Obstet Case Rep.* 2016;2:25.

116. Solomon SM, Kirby DF. The refeeding syndrome: a review. *JPEN J Parenter Enteral Nutr.* 1990;14:90–97.

117. Poursharif B, Korst LM, MacGibbon KW, et al. Elective pregnancy termination in a large cohort of women with hyperemesis gravidarum. *Contraception.* 2007;76:451–455.

118. Christodoulou-Smith J, Gold JI, Romero R, et al. Posttraumatic stress symptoms following pregnancy complicated by hyperemesis gravidarum. *J Matern Fetal Neonatal Med.* 2012;25:632–636.

119. Koudijs HM, Savitri AI, Browne JL, et al. Hyperemesis gravidarum and placental dysfunction disorders. *BMC Pregnancy Childbirth.* 2016;16:374.

120. Bailit JL. Hyperemesis gravidarum: epidemiological findings from a large cohort. *Am J Obstet Gynecol.* 2005;193:811–814.

121. Paauw JD, Bierling S, Cook C, Davis AT. Hyperemesis gravidarum and fetal outcome. *JPEN J Parenter Enteral Nutr.* 2005;29:93–96.

122. Chiossi G, Neri I, Cavazzuti M, Basso G, Facchinetti F. Hyperemesis gravidarum complicated by Wernicke encephalopathy: background, case report, and review of the literature. *Obstet Gynecol Surv.* 2006;61:255–268.

123. Van Stuijvenberg ME, Schabort I, Labadarios D, Nel JT. The nutritional status and treatment of patients with hyperemesis gravidarum. *Am J Obstet Gynecol.* 1995;172:1585–1591.

124. Boyce RA. Enteral nutrition in hyperemesis gravidarum: a new development. *J Am Diet Assoc.* 1992;92:733–736.

125. Hsu JJ, Clark-Glena R, Nelson DK, Kim CH. Nasogastric enteral feeding in the management of hyperemesis gravidarum. *Obstet Gynecol.* 1996;88:343–346.

126. van de Ven CJM. Nasogastric enteral feeding in the management of hyperemesis gravidarum. *Lancet.* 1997;349:445–446.

127. Grooten IJ, Mol BW, van der Post JAM, et al. Early nasogastric tube feeding in optimizing treatment for hyperemesis gravidarum: the MOTHER randomised controlled trial (Maternal and Offspring outcomes after Treatment of HyperEmesis by Refeeding). *BMC Pregnancy Childbirth.* 2016;16:22.

128. Lord LM, Pelletier K. Management of hyperemesis gravidarum with enteral nutrition. *Pract Gastroenterol.* 2008;63:15–31.

129. Landye ST. Successful enteral nutrition support of a pregnant, comatose patient: a case study. *J Am Diet Assoc.* 1988;88:718–720.

130. Smith BK, Rayburn WF, Feller I. Burns and pregnancy. *Clin Perinatol.* 1983;10:383–398.

131. Wong M, Apodaca CC, Markenson MG, Yancey M. Nutrition management in a pregnant comatose patient. *Nutr Clin Pract.* 1997;12:63–67.

132. Aderet NB, Cohen I, Abramowicz JB, et al. Traumatic coma during pregnancy with persistent vegetative state. Case report. *Br J Obstet Gynaecol.* 1984;91:939–941.

133. McClave SA, Taylor BE, Martindale RG, et al. Guidelines for the provision and assessment of nutrition support therapy in the adult critically ill patient: Society of Critical Care Medicine (SCCM) and American Society for Parenteral and Enteral Nutrition (A.S.P.E.N.). *JPEN J Parenter Enteral Nutr.* 2016;40:159–211.

21 | Wound Healing

Mary Ellen Posthauer, RDN, CD, LD, FAND, and Mary Marian, DCN, RDN, CSO, FAND

CONTENTS

Acknowledgment: Joyce K. Stechmiller, PhD, ACNP-BC, FAAN, was the author of this chapter for the second edition.

Objectives

1. Describe the process of wound healing with specific focus on the requirements for macro- and micronutrients.
2. Describe the incidence and etiology of chronic wounds.
3. Discuss the nutrition care process as it relates to individuals at risk for and experiencing poor wound healing.
4. Specify nutrition support interventions to augment healing of chronic wounds.

Test Your Knowledge Questions

1. What are the goals for protein support for adults with delayed healing of pressure injuries/ulcers?
   A. Provide adequate protein: 0.8 g/kg/d
   B. Provide adequate protein: 1.0 to 1.2 g/kg/d
   C. Provide adequate protein: 1.25 to 1.5 g/kg/d
   D. Provide adequate protein: 0.6 g/kg/d
2. Which of the following should be offered to provide elemental zinc for pressure injuries/ulcers healing?
   A. Zinc sulfate: 220 mg/d
   B. Zinc gluconate: 84 mg/d
   C. Daily multivitamin with minerals supplement
   D. Zinc chloride: 170 mg/d
3. All wounds begin as acute wounds. Which of the following distinguishes an acute wound from a chronic wound?
   A. An acute wound will generally heal within 2 to 3 days, whereas a chronic wound will likely take 7 to 10 days to heal.
   B. Acute wounds are related to an initial injury, whereas chronic wounds develop due to an underlying pathological process.
   C. The microenvironments of the 2 types of wounds are different, with acute wounds having fewer inflammatory mediators present.
   D. Both B and C.

Test Your Knowledge Answers

1. The correct answer is **C**. The goal for protein support for patients with pressure injuries/ulcers is 1.25 to 1.5 g protein per kg body weight per day.[1,2]
2. The correct answer is **C**. Zinc supplementation is recommended only for patients with confirmed zinc deficiencies, and adequate levels can be achieved with a daily multivitamin with minerals supplement. For patients with normal levels of zinc, supplementation offers no benefit and may result in zinc toxicity.[2]
3. The correct answer is **D**. Wound healing progresses in a predictable series of events. However, when disruptions in the healing process occur, they lead to poor wound healing and the presence of a chronic wound. An acute wound tends to heal within 4 weeks, although there is no strict timetable for when a wound will heal. Acute wounds occur due to an initial insult but can become chronic, typically because of abnormalities in underlying pathophysiology. The microenvironment is very different between acute and chronic wounds. Chronic wounds are characterized by a disruption in the sequence of expected healing events or prolonged inflammatory metabolism.[1] There are also distinct differences at the molecular level of chronic wounds; increased levels of inflammatory cytokines, such as tumor necrosis factor-α, interleukin-1, and interleukin-6, and proteases, such as matrix metalloproteinases (particularly matrix metalloproteinase-2 and matrix metalloproteinase-9), are evident in chronic wound fluid. This results in an inhibition of fibroblast and endothelial cell proliferation and function, as well as decreased levels of tissue inhibitors of metalloproteinases. Increased bacterial burden (tissue bacterial levels exceed 100,000 CFU per gram of tissue) and altered keratinocyte function as well as extracellular matrix degradation have also been implicated in chronic wounds.[3,4]

Introduction

Wound healing is a complex process that involves a cascade of events to repair and heal damaged tissue. Interruptions in the healing process can lead to wounds becoming chronic and difficult to heal, which can be debilitating and costly. Although estimates vary depending on the types of wounds counted, chronic wounds are reportedly experienced by up to 4.5 million Americans; pressure injuries/ulcers, diabetic ulcers, and vascular ulcers are the most common types.[3,4] The incidence of chronic wounds is also expected to increase as the aging and diabetes populations grow.[3] Healthcare costs associated with treatment of chronic wounds are approximately 2% to 3% of the healthcare budget in developed nations.[3] Effective management involves (1) identifying the factors that are adversely affecting healing and (2) instituting best practices to eliminate or overcome identified barriers to effective care. Given the complexities associated with wound care today, an interdisciplinary team approach is often required to obtain the best clinical outcomes, and many facilities now have wound care teams.

Skin as an Organ

The skin is the largest organ of the human body. It functions as a protective barrier from external environmental factors and helps maintain homeostasis internally.[4] The layers of the skin include the epidermis, or outermost layer; the dermis, which is the thickest tissue layer of the skin; the basement membrane, which separates the epidermis from the dermis; and the hypodermis, or the superficial fascia, which rests beneath the dermis and covers the muscle, ligaments, tendon, and bone that reside beneath these layers of skin.[4]

The epidermis is comprised mostly of keratinocytes in several strata of various stages of maturation. This layer of skin does not contain nerve endings or blood vessels, but it is responsible for epithelialization (skin closure) of wounds.

The dermis provides the supportive matrix upon which the epidermis sits and is composed of various connective tissue elements, such as collagen fibers, elastic fibers, ground substance, mast cells, macrophages, lymphocytes, fat cells, fibroblasts, hair follicles, nerve endings, sweat glands, and blood vessels.[4,5] Ground substance—a gelatinous material composed largely of water, glycoproteins, glycosaminoglycans, and proteoglycans—plays a role in connective tissue similar to that of plasma in blood.[4,5] The fibroblast, the most common cell found in connective tissue, is responsible for secreting the essential elements of the extracellular matrix, such as collagen. The various types of collagen and other components of the extracellular matrix secreted by the fibroblasts are necessary for wound bed epithelialization or granulation of full thickness or partial thickness wounds that extend past the epidermal layer. Thus, the dermis provides critical components of the immune response for the complex processes of wound healing.[4,5]

An alteration in the skin's integrity is considered a wound and may be caused by injury (including pressure), disease, surgery, or environmental factors.[4] Chronic, recalcitrant or nonhealing wounds represent a significant health, economic, and quality-of-life burden to individuals as well as to society in general. To review how wounds typically heal, one must examine basic wound and tissue physiology. Partial thickness wounds are shallow wounds involving full or partial epidermal loss and partial loss of the dermal layer. Full-thickness wounds involve total loss of both epidermal and dermal layers, extending to at least the subcutaneous tissue layer and possibly as deep as the fascia, muscle layer, and the bone.[4,5]

including platelet-derived growth factor and transforming growth factor-β, they slowly replace the neutrophils.[7,8] Cytokines and other enzymes needed for the wound healing process are released by macrophages that have been transformed from monocytes.[8] During the inflammatory phase, which typically lasts between 4 and 6 days following tissue injury, the foundation is set with granulation tissue, and the removal of cellular debris and other foreign materials prepares the site for healing and the second phase of healing, the proliferative phase.[9]

The need for energy, protein, and micronutrients (including vitamins C, E, and K, iron, selenium and copper) increases during the inflammatory phase.[7,8] Energy expenditure is greater

Acute vs Chronic Wounds

Acute wounds, such as cuts, surgical incisions, and skin tears, are generally repaired and healed in a stepwise and predictable process that occurs over a few days or a few weeks. *Chronic wounds* are defined as wounds that have not healed within 12 weeks of the initial injury.[5] Chronic wounds often begin as minor acute wounds, but they become chronic because various factors that adversely affect the healing process—including infection, malnutrition, medications, the presence of comorbidities, and so on—delay healing.[5,6]

Phases of Wound Healing and Role of Nutrition

The healing process involves 3 phases: the inflammatory, proliferative, and maturation phases (see Figure 21-1).[1-6]

Inflammatory Phase

The inflammatory phase begins immediately following an acute injury to the tissue and is accompanied by the classic signs of tissue damage, including rubor (redness), heat, swelling, and pain.[7,8] Platelets and other coagulation substrates together create a fibrin clot that facilitates hemostasis and provides a protective barrier. Damage to the tissue and vasculature orchestrates a cascade of events that initiates the wound repair and healing process, beginning with the release of inflammatory mediators that attract neutrophils and monocytes to the wound.[7,8] Neutrophils arrive within 6 to 12 hours after the initial injury. Over the next 24 hours and for the next several days (ie, 3 to 7 days), leukocytes and monocytes arrive; attracted to the injured tissue through chemotaxis substrates,

FIGURE 21-1 Phases of Wound Healing

Hemostasis/Inflammation
Occurs immediately after injury.

Coagulation pathways → Blood coagulation, clot formulation and breakdown, PDGF released

Proinflammatory pathways → Cytokine signaling, vasodilation, edema, increased metabolism → Signaling/synthesis of macrophages, TNF-α, TIMP, IL-1 and IL-2, MMPs, etc

Proliferative Phase
Also known as "Constructive Phase"; occurs around Day 4–Day 14.

Fibroblast proliferation, collagen synthesis, matrix formation, epithelialization

Angiogenesis stimulated by cytokines results in formation of new capillaries in the wound bed

Maturation Phase
Also known as "Remodeling Phase"; occurs from Day 8 until 12 months.

Collagen cross-linking, wound contraction, increased scar tissue tensile strength, and wound closure

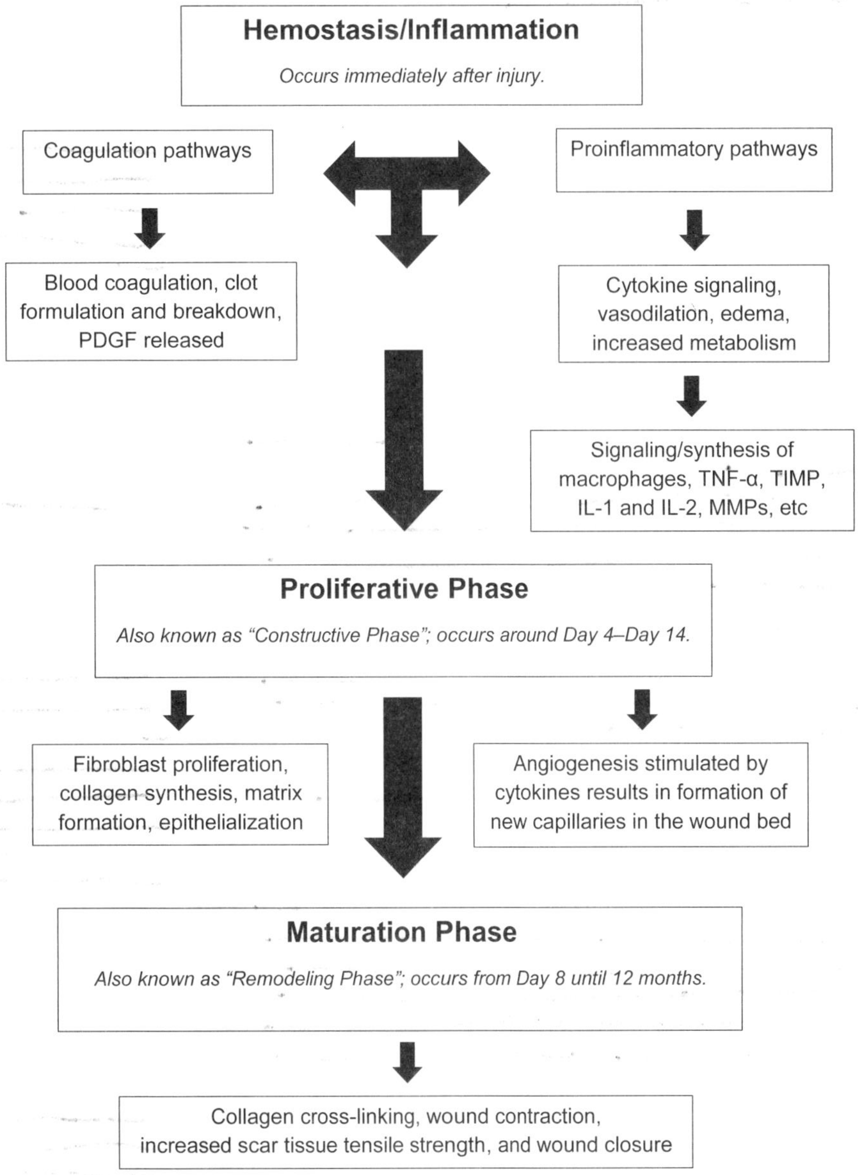

IL, interleukin; MMP, matrix metalloproteinase; PDGF, platelet-derived growth factor; TIMP, tissue inhibitors of metalloproteinases; TNF-α, tumor necrosis factor-α.
Source: Data are from references 1–6.

because of increased cell proliferation, protein synthesis, and production of biochemical mediators involved in the wound healing phases.[6,7] Inadequate energy intake and malnutrition are associated with poor wound healing.

Amino acids and proteins are considered the building blocks for tissue growth and repair after injury and therefore affect all phases on healing. The inflammatory process, cell proliferation, production of granulation tissue, production of growth factors, keratinization, and so on, all depend on an adequate supply of protein.[6,7] Delayed immunity, increased risk for infectious complications, sarcopenia, and malnutrition are all possible adverse outcomes related to inadequate protein intake.[6-9]

Vitamin C plays an important role in wound healing. Maintaining a balance between reactive oxygen species (ROS) and anti-inflammatory substrates depends on optimal levels of vitamin C.[8-10] ROS play a critical role in the disposal of bacteria and wound debris; however, healthy tissues may also be damaged when ROS are overproduced.[8-10] Antioxidants such as vitamin C can promote homeostasis by detoxifying ROS and protecting neutrophils by quenching intracellular ROS.[8-10] The formation of granulation tissues results from the differentiation of fibroblasts and collagen. The presence of vitamin C in the extracellular environment protects the neutrophils, fibroblasts, and collagen, thereby allowing the wound healing process to transition from the inflammatory to the proliferative phase.[8-10] Vitamin C also helps maintain homeostasis at the wound site by promoting the inflammatory phase while participating in the regulation of ROS production and oxidative damage.[8-10]

Formation of fibrin and blood clots involves vitamin K and calcium.[8,9] Fibrin clot formation depends on clotting factors, and vitamin K serves as a cofactor in the enzymatic activation of the clotting factors prothrombin VII, IX, and X.[8] Calcium plays an essential role in binding the clotting factors to tissues at the injury site.[8]

Wound "clean-up" also depends on both cellular and humoral immune responses during the inflammatory phase as debris and foreign agents are removed.[8,11] Poor zinc status can adversely affect B and T lymphocyte production, leading to delayed wound healing.[11] The production of granulation tissue also reportedly increases zinc requirements.[8,11] However, delays in wound healing can result with excess zinc intake, causing zinc toxicity and impairments in neutrophil and lymphocyte function.[12] Lymphocyte synthesis can also be reduced with copper deficiency in the face of excess zinc intake.[12]

During the inflammatory phase, adequate intake of vitamins A and D is important. Vitamin A is necessary for the synthesis of immune cells such as monocytes and macrophages.[8,9] A deficiency of vitamin D may impair immune function because vitamin D enhances phagocytosis and the bactericidal action of macrophages.[13,14] T cell production and proliferation can also be suppressed due to vitamin D deficiency.[13,14]

Proliferative Phase

Following the inflammatory phase, the proliferative (constructive) phase begins within 3 to 4 days after the initial injury. This phase may then continue for up to 2 weeks.[5-8] In this phase, 3 key changes occur: epithelization, granulation and angiogenesis.[1,7]

Epithelization begins at the wound margin or at the basement membrane level.[1,8,9] Activated platelets and macrophages stimulate epithelization through the release of epidermal growth factor and transforming growth factor-α. Keratinocyte growth factors are produced by the fibroblasts and, together with interleukin-6, promote keratinocyte migration over the wound bed, forming a protective barrier.[1,7-9] Moreover, fibroblasts proliferate and begin synthesizing collagen, reticulin, and elastin—critical components for healing the wound and establishing the extracellular matrix.[1,7-9] Fibroblast growth factor and tumor growth factor-β released from the macrophages and platelets stimulate fibroblastic development.[1,7-9]

Epithelialization is influenced by many factors, including medications (eg, anti-inflammatories), hypoxemia, and nutritional deficiencies.[1,8,9] Phagocyte production of biochemical substrates necessary for epithelialization is inhibited by anti-inflammatory agents; cellular energy production required for wound healing is reduced with hypoxemia; and cellular migration into the wound can be negatively affected with inadequate zinc intake due to reduced matrix metalloproteinase activity.[1,11]

Granulation tissue is comprised of new capillaries and veins, fibroblasts, macrophages, and new deposits of collagen particles.[1,8,9] Granulation tissues form as the fibroblasts migrate from the outer edges of the wound, proliferate, and synthesize collagen. Through angiogenesis and neovascularization, new capillaries infiltrate the granulation tissue, thereby allowing the fibroblasts to proliferate. Angiogenesis and neovascularization allow for the delivery of nutrients and cytokines to the wound site while the metabolic wastes are removed.[1,8,9]

As the proliferative phase evolves, fibroblasts are also transformed into myofibroblasts, which have contractile actin fibers necessary for wound contraction—the final process in the constructive phase—which is needed for wound closure as the wound edges move inward.[1,8,9] Although initiated during the proliferative phase, wound contraction is not completed until the maturation phase.[1,8,9]

Vitamins A and C and the minerals zinc and iron are necessary for fibroblastic, collagen, and protein matrix synthesis.[1,8,15] In this phase, vitamin A promotes collagen synthesis and facilitates epithelization.[8] Vitamin A may also reverse the negative impact of corticosteroids on wound healing.[8] Vitamin C is essential for collagen formation.[1,8,10] Inadequate intake leads to poor vitamin C stores, which quickly become depleted, thereby negatively affecting collagen production.[10] Interestingly, some studies have found that patients with signs of mild scurvy experience normal wound healing, comparable to patients without scurvy.[10] Furthermore, high-dose supplementation of vitamin C has not been found to enhance healing rates in some patients exhibiting vitamin C deficiency. This finding may be related to the fact that only 10 to 20 mg of vitamin C per day is needed to prevent scurvy.[8,10]

Protein requirements associated with wound healing have been extensively investigated, and, in general, diets higher in protein result in improved healing.[1,2] Diets with adequate amounts of protein ensure the availability of the various amino acids needed for repair and healing in the proliferative phase. The amino acid methionine, which is converted to cysteine, serves as a cofactor in the enzymatic reactions needed for collagen synthesis; methionine also contains sulfur, which is necessary to form the cross-linked collagen fibrils. The amino acids arginine and glutamine are thought to be "conditionally essential" during this phase of healing.[1,8,9] Collagen and tissue synthesis require arginine for wound strength.[1,8,9] Antioxidant benefits are also derived from arginine through the formation of nitric oxide.[7] T cell stimulation and response also rely on arginine.[1,8,9] Glutamine is an important source of fuel for rapid turnover of cells, such as neutrophils, macrophages, and lymphocytes, which occurs in both the inflammatory and proliferative phases of wound healing.[1] Glutamine also serves as key antioxidant (as glutathione) that participates in promoting a balance of ROS.[1,7,8]

Vitamin D provides a number of pleiotropic benefits, including cellular differentiation and proliferation.[13,14] Lower vitamin D levels have been reported in patients with chronic wounds such as venous ulcers and diabetic foot ulcer.[13,14] While it is unclear whether vitamin D insufficiency results in delayed wound healing, a recent prospective, placebo-controlled, double-blinded study conducted by Burkiewicz and colleagues found that patients supplemented with 50,000 IU vitamin D weekly for 2 months demonstrated a trend toward statistical significance in reduced ulcer size compared with the placebo group.[14]

Iron serves a vital role in the enzymatic hydrolysis of lysyl, and prolyl in the formation of collagen requires the participation of iron as a cofactor.[1,8] Moreover, iron is important for hemoglobin synthesis. The delivery of adequate oxygen via hemoglobin is essential in wound healing and collagen synthesis, fibroblastic proliferation, and angiogenesis, as well as epithelization.[1,8] Iron deficiency anemia can thus impair wound healing by effecting the integrity of the collagen produced.[5] Iron needs may also increase during the proliferative phase because DNA synthesis is greater during this time.[7-9]

Maturation Phase

During the maturation (remodeling) phase, collagen synthesis, tissue regeneration, and wound contraction continue and can persist for many years.[7-9] During remodeling, collagen is resynthesized, reabsorbed, and reorganized into a more organized format to increase the tensile strength and scar formation.[7-9] Matrix metalloproteinase collagenolysis also achieves a steady state with collagen production.[7-9] Additionally, scar tissue is remodeled, the capillaries dissolve, and the scar tissue gains strength—although, at best, wounds regain only about 80% of their original tensile strength.[7-9]

"Dysfunctional" wound healing occurs when the previous described steps in the wound healing process are adversely affected or inhibited. A prolonged inflammatory state, reduced availability of growth factors, and increased bioburden contribute to wound chronicity.[6] Further contributors include underlying disease (eg, diabetes mellitus), prolonged bleeding during the inflammatory phase, inadequate availability of nutrients and blood supply, prescribed drugs, hypoxemia, and inadequate nutrient intake.[1-3] As described previously, adequate energy, protein and micronutrient intake is critical for normal wound repair and healing.[5-8]

Medical Management

Chronic poor-healing wounds often require a variety of treatment modalities, such as compression therapy, wound debridement, advanced wound dressings, topical wound care creams and ointments, medications, mechanical treatment using topical negative pressure wound therapy (eg, vacuum-assisted closure [VAC]), hyperbaric oxygen therapy, bioengineered skin, and skin grafts; surgery may also be required in some cases to encourage tissue repair and healing.[16] To promote optimal healing, wounds must remain clean and free of debris and bioburden.[7,16] Ideally, the wound dressing facilitates healing by promoting a moist wound environment and absorbing any excess exudate while also allowing gaseous exchange and protecting the wound site from microorganism contamination.[5,16] Multiple types of dressings with various functions are available for use during the different phases of healing. For example, some open dressings, including wet-to-dry dressings, are used to debride the wound whereas semi-open dressings have a fine mesh gauze that is impregnated with ointments that allow fluid to be pass through to a secondary dressing. These types of dressings do not adhere to the wound bed, thus reducing discomfort and pain during dressing changes.[8,16] VAC, also known as a *wound VAC*, is used to remove inflammatory substrates, excess interstitial fluid, and edema to promote improvements in tissue oxygenation.[8,16] Wound VACs are also associated with reduced infection and promotion of wound granulation.[8] These modalities are largely reserved for large, poor-healing wounds that are difficult to close surgically.

Chronic Wounds

Incidence/Prevalence

Roughly 2% of the US adult population has at least 1 chronic wound.[16] Pressure injuries/ulcers and lower extremity ulcers, including diabetic foot ulcers, venous ulcers, and arterial ulcers, are the most common chronic wounds diagnosed; other types of chronic wounds may involve burns, skin cancer, fistulas, nonhealing surgical wounds, radiation wounds, and dermatitis or vasculitis wounds (Figure 21-2).[17]

The percentage of individuals with pressure ulcers/injuries in a healthcare setting varies widely depending on how the data are measured. Prevalence is a measure of the number of cases of pressure ulcers/injuries at a specific time. Incidence measures the number of new pressure ulcers/injuries in individuals without an ulcer/injury at baseline and is a better indication of quality of care.[2]

Malnutrition is a contributing factor for the development of pressure injuries/ulcers and poor wound healing, which is of concern because an estimated 12% to 50% of hospitalized patients are malnourished.[18] Fry noted that preexisting malnutrition was a positive predictive variable for pressure ulcer after a major surgery, which is designated as a type of "never event," a term used by the Centers for Medicare and Medicaid Services (CMS) to deny payment for costs associated with select complications of patient care that could be prevented.[19]

FIGURE 21-2 Wound Categories

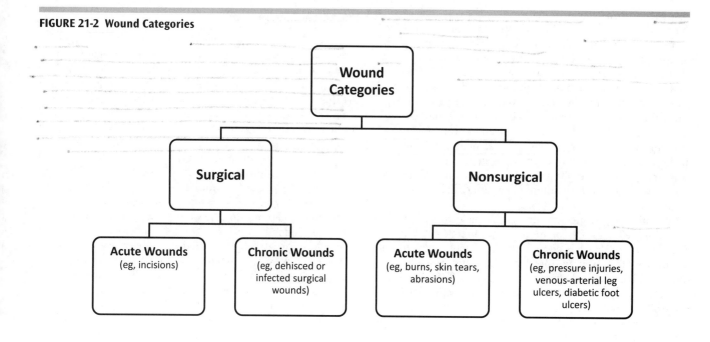

Risk Factors

A number of factors increase the risk for pressure injuries/ulcers, including malnutrition, weight-bearing pressure, shear, friction, old age, immobility, incontinence, hyperglycemia, poor perfusion, and comorbidities, including catabolic injury and illness.[1,3] Anorexia, early satiety, and inadequate nutrient intake can also increase the risk.[6,8] Body mass index (BMI) outside of the normal range is also associated with an increased risk—individuals with a BMI less than 18.5 or greater than 30 are more likely to develop pressure injuries/ulcers than normal-weight individuals.[20] Because there is no single index that identifies patients with malnutrition, completion of a comprehensive nutrition assessment is essential (see Chapter 9).

Economic Consequences

The economic costs of providing care for nonhealing chronic wounds is staggering—approximately $50 billion annually—with costs increasing when the number of comorbid conditions present increases.[16] Pressure injuries/ulcers reportedly are the second most common adverse event in medical facilities.[21] Starting in 2008, CMS stopped reimbursing inpatient medical facilities for care for stage 3 and stage 4 pressure injuries/ulcers that develop during the inpatient stay, as well as other preventable hospital-acquired conditions (ie, "never events").[21] Cost estimates for treating pressure injuries/ulcers range from $9.1 billion to 11.5 billion annually.[21]

Terminology

The National Pressure Ulcer Advisory Panel (NPUAP) announced a terminology change following the February 2016 consensus conference. The term *pressure injury* replaces *pressure* *ulcers* in the NPUAP injury staging system (see Table 21-1).[22] The change in terminology more accurately describes pressure injuries in both intact skin and ulcerated skin. In the previous staging system, *stage I* and *deep tissue injury* described injured intact skin, whereas the other stages described open ulcers. This older vocabulary led to confusion because the definitions for each of the stages referred to all types of pressure injuries as *pressure ulcers*.[22]

Venous Ulcers, Diabetic Foot Ulcers, and Other Chronic Wounds

Wounds of the lower extremities are common and can have debilitating consequences, including increased morbidity, prolonged disability, pain, discomfort, and significant economic burdens to both the patient and the healthcare system.[3,21–24] Moreover, many of these wounds tend to be chronic and slow to heal, which significantly increases the risk for amputation of the affected area.[3] Venous leg ulcers (also known as *stasis* or *varicose ulcers*) are the most common type of chronic wound that develops in the lower extremities, although diabetic foot ulcers and pressure injuries/ulcers are also problematic.[3,21–24] Among the patients at risk for venous ulcers are older adults with a history of deep vein thrombosis and previous surgery for varicose veins. The ulcerations drain moderate amounts of protein-rich exudate and are painful and debilitating. Improved patient outcomes have been achieved by the use of interdisciplinary teams, surgical interventions, compression systems, and adequate nutrition.[1,25]

Diabetes affects millions of people around the world. Healing of wounds is impaired in individuals with diabetes. Patients with diabetes are at risk for developing nonhealing diabetic foot ulcers, which are a significant complication of diabetes and can result in lower leg amputations. The treatment of diabetic foot

TABLE 21-1 National Pressure Ulcer Advisory Panel Terminology for Pressure Injuries

Term	Definition
Pressure injury	Localized damage to the skin and underlying soft tissue, usually over a bony prominence or related to a medical or other device. The injury can present as intact skin or an open ulcer and may be painful. The injury occurs as a result of intense and/or prolonged pressure or pressure in combination with shear. The tolerance of soft tissue for pressure and shear may also be affected by microclimate, nutrition, perfusion, comorbidities, and condition of the soft tissue.
Stage 1 pressure injury	Intact skin with a localized area of nonblanchable erythema, which may appear differently in darkly pigmented skin. Presence of blanchable erythema or changes in sensation, temperature, or firmness may precede visual changes. Color changes do not include purple or maroon discoloration; these may indicate deep tissue pressure injury.
Stage 2 pressure injury	Partial-thickness loss of skin with exposed dermis. The wound bed is viable, pink or red, and moist, and may also present as an intact or ruptured serum-filled blister. Adipose (fat) is not visible and deeper tissues are not visible. Granulation tissue, slough, and eschar are not present. These injuries commonly result from adverse microclimate and shear in the skin over the pelvis and shear in the heel. This stage should not be used to describe moisture-associated skin damage (MASD) including incontinence-associated dermatitis (IAD), intertriginous dermatitis (ITD), medical adhesive–related skin injury (MARSI), or traumatic wounds (skin tears, burns, abrasions).
Stage 3 pressure injury	Full-thickness loss of skin, in which adipose (fat) is visible in the ulcer and granulation tissue and epibole (rolled wound edges) are often present. Slough and/or eschar may be visible. The depth of tissue damage varies by anatomical location; areas of significant adiposity can develop deep wounds. Undermining and tunneling may occur. Fascia, muscle, tendon, ligament, cartilage, and/or bone are not exposed. If slough or eschar obscures the extent of tissue loss, this is an unstageable pressure injury.
Stage 4 pressure injury	Full-thickness skin and tissue loss with exposed or directly palpable fascia, muscle, tendon, ligament, cartilage, or bone in the ulcer. Slough and/or eschar may be visible. Epibole (rolled edges), undermining, and/or tunneling often occur. Depth varies by anatomical location. If slough or eschar obscures the extent of tissue loss, this is an unstageable pressure injury.
Unstageable pressure injury	Full-thickness skin and tissue loss in which the extent of tissue damage within the ulcer cannot be confirmed because it is obscured by slough or eschar. If slough or eschar is removed, a stage 3 or stage 4 pressure injury will be revealed. Stable eschar (ie, dry, adherent, intact without erythema or fluctuance) on the heel or ischemic limb should not be softened or removed.
Deep tissue pressure injury	Intact or nonintact skin with localized area of persistent nonblanchable deep-red, maroon, or purple discoloration or epidermal separation revealing a dark wound bed or blood-filled blister. Pain and temperature change often precede skin color changes. Discoloration may appear differently in darkly pigmented skin. This injury results from intense and/or prolonged pressure and shear forces at the bone-muscle interface. The wound may evolve rapidly to reveal the actual extent of tissue injury or may resolve without tissue loss. If necrotic tissue, subcutaneous tissue, granulation tissue, fascia, muscle, or other underlying structures are visible, this indicates a full thickness pressure injury (unstageable, stage 3 or stage 4). Do not use *deep tissue pressure injury* to describe vascular, traumatic, neuropathic, or dermatologic conditions.

Source: Adapted from reference 22: NPUAP Staging System: http://www.npuap.org/resources/educational-and-clinical-resources/npuap-pressure-injury-stages. Accessed May 8, 2017. Used with permission of the National Pressure Ulcer Advisory Panel, June 4, 2017.

ulcers requires adequate nutrition to stabilize blood glucose levels, proper wound care, prevention and treatment of inflammation and infection, and off-loading pressure.[26]

Etiology of Delayed Healing

Chronic wounds exhibit distinct differences from acute wounds and often require a variety of interventions to promote healing; continued monitoring of nutrition status and intake is also essential to facilitate wound recovery.[1,8,9,27,28]

Chronic inflammatory conditions, poor wound care, increased bioburden, and altered keratinocyte function, as well as extracellular matrix degradation, have also been implicated in chronic wounds.[25,26] *Bioburden* refers to the number of microorganisms present on a contaminated object or, in this context, in a wound. The production (or overproduction) of enzymes in the wound fluid of chronic wounds further complicates the healing process by breaking down the protein-rich collagen and matrix materials that are attempting to close the wound.[23,26]

Nutrition Screening and Assessment

Nutrition screening and assessment should be completed for individuals at risk for malnutrition or in the presence of a wound.[2,8] Initial screening identifies an individual at nutrition risk who may require a referral for a comprehensive nutrition assessment (see Chapter 9). Poor outcomes, including morbidity and mortality, are associated with malnutrition; therefore, the need to screen for and treat malnutrition is imperative. Individuals should be screened for malnutrition and pressure injury risk on admission to any healthcare setting and reassessed periodically as their conditions change.[2,29] The screening tool used should be validated, reliable, and applicable to the population group being screened. A cross-sectional study by Langkamp-Henken and colleagues of older men with pressure injuries who resided in residential care facilities found a positive correlation between use of the Mini Nutritional Assessment (MNA) and clinical indicators for the injuries.[30] A German study comparing the nutrition status of individuals with and without pressure injuries noted that the MNA was easy to use to assess individuals with pressure injuries and multiple comorbidities.[31] A pilot study in an outpatient wound care clinic included a convenience study of 105 individuals with at least 1 active wound. Data collected from the convenience sample of outpatients with wounds were used to determine which of the proposed items was most strongly associated with malnutrition as assessed by the Scored Patient-Generated Subjective Global Assessment. The MEAL scale was initiated; it included the 4 factors that proved to be statistically significant out of the 18 factors suspected to associate malnutrition with chronic wounds. Additional studies are needed to establish the validity and reliability of this nutrition screening tool.[32] The Braden pressure ulcer risk assessment scale is widely used to screen for pressure injury risk in adults in all settings and includes a subscale for nutrition risk that has been validated.[33]

Once identified, the individual at nutrition or malnutrition risk should be referred to a registered dietitian nutritionist to complete a comprehensive nutrition assessment, define a nutrition diagnosis, and determine individualized nutrition interventions based on the specific information identified in the nutrition assessment (see Chapter 9). The comprehensive nutrition assessment reviews all pertinent data: anthropometric measurements, biochemical data, nutrition-focused physical examination, diet history, and interviews with the individual and/or caregiver. Using this information, nutrition diagnoses or problems are identified, nutrient requirements are estimated, and nutrition intervention(s) are planned and implemented.

Nutrition Considerations

Several studies demonstrate that malnutrition adversely affects wound healing and adequate nutrition is required for healing to occur.[19,34-37] The following sections discuss the current nutrition recommendations for individuals with acute and chronic wounds, including the function of specific nutrients in the healing process. Table 21-2 summarizes the 2014 clinical practice nutrition guidelines for pressure injuries/ulcers copublished by NPUAP, European Pressure Ulcer Advisory Panel (EPUAP), and Pan Pacific Pressure Injury Alliance (PPPIA).[2]

TABLE 21-2 2014 National Pressure Ulcer Advisory Panel/European Pressure Ulcer Advisory Panel/Pan Pacific Pressure Injury Alliance Recommendations for Nutrition Assessment and Treatment

Recommendation	Strength of Evidence	Strength of Recommendation[a]
Nutrition screening		
1. Screen nutritional status for each individual at risk of or with a pressure ulcer:	C	Probably do it
• at admission to a healthcare setting;		
• with each significant change of clinical condition; and/or		
• when progress toward pressure ulcer closure is not observed.		
2. Use a valid and reliable nutrition-screening tool to determine nutritional risk.	C	Probably do it
3. Refer individuals screened to be at risk of malnutrition and individuals with an existing pressure ulcer to a registered dietitian or an interprofessional nutrition team for a comprehensive nutrition assessment.	C	Probably do it
Nutrition assessment		
1. Assess the weight status of each individual to determine weight history and identify significant weight loss (5% in 30 days or 10% in 180 days).	C	Probably do it
2. Assess the individual's ability to eat independently.	C	Probably do it
3. Assess the adequacy of total nutrient intake (ie, food, fluid, oral supplements, and enteral/parenteral feeds).	C	Definitely do it
Care planning		
1. Develop an individualized nutrition care plan for individuals with or at risk of a pressure ulcer.	C	Probably do it
2. Follow relevant and evidence-based guidelines on nutrition and hydration for individuals who exhibit nutritional risk and who are at risk of pressure ulcers or have an existing pressure ulcer.	C	Probably do it

TABLE 21-2 *(continued)*

Recommendation	Strength of Evidence	Strength of Recommendation[a]
Energy intake		
1. Provide individualized energy intake based on underlying medical condition and level of activity.	B	Probably do it
2. Provide 30–35 kcal/kg body weight for adults at risk of a pressure ulcer who are assessed as being at risk of malnutrition.	C	Probably do it
3. Provide 30–35 kcal/kg body weight for adults with a pressure ulcer, who are assessed as being at risk of malnutrition.	B	Probably do it
4. Adjust energy intake based on weight change or level of obesity. Adults who are underweight or who have had significant unintended weight loss may need additional energy intake.	C	Definitely do it
5. Revise and modify/liberalize dietary restrictions when limitations result in decreased food and fluid intake. These adjustments should be made in consultation with a medical professional and managed by a registered dietitian whenever possible.	C	Probably do it
6. Offer fortified foods and/or high-calorie, high-protein oral nutritional supplements between meals if nutritional requirements cannot be achieved by dietary intake.	B	Definitely do it
7. Consider enteral or parenteral nutritional support when oral intake is inadequate. This must be consistent with the individual's goals.	C	Probably do it
Protein intake		
1. Provide adequate protein for positive nitrogen balance for adults assessed to be at risk of a pressure ulcer.	C	Probably do it
2. Offer 1.25–1.5 g protein/kg body weight daily for adults at risk of a pressure ulcer who are assessed to be at risk of malnutrition, when compatible with goals of care, and reassess as condition changes.	C	Probably do it
3. Provide adequate protein for positive nitrogen balance for adults with a pressure ulcer.	B	Probably do it
4. Offer 1.25–1.5 g protein/kg body weight daily for adults with an existing pressure ulcer who are assessed to be at risk of malnutrition, when compatible with goals of care, and reassess as condition changes.	B	Probably do it
5. Offer high-calorie, high-protein nutritional supplements in addition to the usual diet to adults with nutritional risk and pressure ulcer risk, if nutritional requirements cannot be achieved by dietary intake.	A	Probably do it
6. Assess renal function to ensure that high levels of protein are appropriate for the individual.	C	Definitely do it
7. Supplement with high-protein, arginine, and micronutrients for adults with a pressure ulcer category/stage III or IV or multiple pressure ulcers when nutritional requirements cannot be met with traditional high-calorie and protein supplements.	B	Probably do it
Hydration		
1. Provide and encourage adequate daily fluid intake for hydration for an individual assessed to be at risk of or with a pressure ulcer. This must be consistent with the individual's comorbid conditions and goals.	C	Definitely do it
2. Monitor individuals for signs and symptoms of dehydration, including change in weight, skin turgor, urine output, elevated serum sodium, and/or calculated serum osmolality.	C	Probably do it
3. Provide additional fluid for individuals with dehydration, elevated temperature, vomiting, profuse sweating, diarrhea, or heavily exuding wounds.	C	Definitely do it
Vitamins and minerals		
1. Provide/encourage individuals assessed to be at risk of pressure ulcer to consume a balanced diet that includes good sources of vitamins and minerals.	C	Definitely do it
2. Provide/encourage an individual assessed to be at risk of a pressure ulcer to take vitamin and mineral supplements when dietary intake is poor or deficiencies are confirmed or suspected.	C	Probably do it
3. Provide/encourage an individual with a pressure ulcer to consume a balanced diet that includes good sources of vitamins and minerals.	B	Definitely do it
4. Provide/encourage an individual with a pressure ulcer to take vitamin and mineral supplements when dietary intake is poor or deficiencies are confirmed or suspected.	B	Probably do it

Note: The recommendations in this section of the guideline are predominantly for adult individuals and have been derived from evidence conducted in adult populations. "The recommendations in this guideline are a general guide to clinical practice, to be implemented by qualified health professionals subject to their clinical judgment of each individual case and in consideration of the patient consumer's personal preferences and available resources. The guidelines should be implemented in a culturally aware and respectful manner in accordance with the principles of protection, participation and partnership."

[a]"Strength of recommendation indicates the confidence the health professional can place in each recommendation, with consideration to the strength of supporting evidence; clinical risk versus benefits; cost effectiveness; and system implications." The overall aim of the strength of recommendations is to help health professionals prioritize interventions—strong positive recommendation = definitely do it; weak positive recommendation = probably do it.

Source: Reprinted from reference 2: National Pressure Ulcer Advisory Panel, European Pressure Ulcer Advisory Panel, and Pan Pacific Pressure Injury Alliance. Used with permission of the National Pressure Ulcer Advisory Panel, June 4, 2017.

Energy Requirements

Adequate energy is essential for optimal wound healing, specifically for cell metabolism, anabolism, collagen formation, nitrogen retention, and angiogenesis.[6-8,28] Estimated energy needs should be individualized based on age, comorbidities, body weight, activity level, severity and number of wounds, stage in the healing process, nutrition status, basal metabolic rate, and level of physiological stress (see Chapter 2). For example, as healthy adults age, they experience an age-related decline in energy intake and appetite.[38-41] However, the acute inflammatory response related to pressure injuries and wounds increases the energy requirement for all adults.

Obese individuals are at risk for immune incompetence, wound infections, and delayed wound healing. Adipose tissue exerts additional burden on dependent tissues and causes vascular obstruction, which can impair blood flow and delivery of essential nutrients to the wound.[41,42] In critically ill obese adults, providing adequate energy in catabolic states is often problematic and may require indirect calorimetry for more accurate determination of energy needs.[43] Blood glucose control should be maximized for individuals with diabetes mellitus or corticosteroid-induced hyperglycemia. Uncontrolled blood glucose is associated with impairment of the production of leukocytes. This problem has implications for the healing process, risk for infection, and impaired wound healing.[44] Strict therapeutic dietary restriction may not be appropriate for obese individuals, those with diabetes mellitus, or frail older adults when the limitations result in decreased food and fluid intake that may delay healing.[28,45] The risk vs the benefits of restrictions should be considered and discussed with the individual, and modifications considered until the wound heals. Chapters 34, 35, and 36 address nutrition care for obese, diabetic, and older patients, respectively.

A recommended energy guideline for adults with a pressure injury/ulcer who are assessed as being at risk for malnutrition is 30 to 35 kcal per kg body weight per day.[2] NPUAP/EPUAP/PPPIA 2014 guidelines recommend that energy intake be adjusted based on weight change or level of obesity and note that individuals who have had significant unintended weight loss may need additional energy intake.[2] A meta-analysis by Cereda found that individuals with pressure injuries had increased energy expenditure compared with controls and were usually characterized as having negative nitrogen balance. The prediction of resting energy expenditure using the Harris-Benedict equation underestimated energy expenditure by 10%. The authors recommended 30 kcal/kg/d for individuals with pressure injuries.[46]

The types and amount of food the patient consumes daily should be periodically reviewed to ensure that energy and protein intake meets the requirements determined in the nutrition assessment. Fortified foods or oral nutritional supplements should be offered between meals to combat unintended weight loss and achieve positive outcomes.[2,6]

Protein Requirements

As discussed in Chapter 6, protein is vital for growth and maintenance of cells, promotes positive nitrogen balance, and provides structure. It is essential for fluid balance, blood clotting, hormone and enzyme production, and immune function. Protein is responsible for the inflammatory response, fibroblast proliferation, collagen production, and angiogenesis, all of which are necessary for wound healing. All stages of healing require adequate protein for wound closure, and increased protein levels have been linked to improved healing rates.[47-50]

The Recommended Dietary Allowance (RDA) for protein in healthy adults is 0.8 g/kg/d.[51] In general, older adults require more protein than younger adults to offset the inflammatory and catabolic conditions associated with acute and chronic diseases that occur with aging.[52] The PROT-AGE study group recommends 1.2 to 1.5 g/kg/d for older adults with acute or chronic disease.[52] Loss of lean body mass (LBM) occurs with aging and is accelerated in hypermetabolic conditions such as wound healing. Since LBM is metabolically active and contains all of the body's protein, any loss of LBM is harmful. Demling noted, with a LBM loss of 20%, the competition for protein between LBM restoration and wound healing is equal and consequentially the wound healing rate slows.[53] Demling's recommendations include increasing energy intake by 50% above normal daily needs and increasing protein to 1.5 g/kg/d.[53] For adults with pressure injuries/ulcers, the NPUAP/EPUAP/PPPIA guidelines recommend 1.25 to1.5 g/kg/d.[2]

Arginine

Arginine has been studied for its potential to enhance wound healing.[54,55] In healthy volunteers and rodents, studies have shown that arginine supplementation will enhance wound strength and collagen deposition in artificial incisional wounds.[54,55]

Arginine promotes the transport of amino acids into the tissues, supports the synthesis of cellular of protein, stimulates insulin secretion, and serves as a precursor of nitric acid formation. Studies have found that supplementing with additional energy, protein, arginine, and micronutrients promotes healing both in nonmalnourished and malnourished individuals when done in addition to standard wound treatment. In a randomized controlled trial (RCT), nonmalnourished adults with stage 3 and stage 4 pressure injuries/ulcers received either a high-calorie, high-protein, arginine-containing, and micronutrient-rich (vitamins C and E, zinc, copper) formula or a nonfortified formula between meals for 8 weeks.[56] There was a significant reduction in wound size for those drinking the enriched supplement vs the control group.[56] In a multicenter RCT, Cereda and colleagues evaluated use of the same enriched formula with 200 malnourished adults with stage 2, 3, or 4 pressure injuries/ulcers. Individuals consuming the intervention formula had a 40% greater reduction in wound size compared with the control group.[57] Both studies suggest that the efficacy of these nutrients in wound healing is likely synergistic since there is no evidence supporting an independent effect when the supplemented nutrients are given alone.[57] In another RCT conducted by Cereda and colleagues, 56 individuals with pressure injuries received either a standard house diet plus a 500 kcal (400 mL/d), high-protein (40 g) supplement with 15% (6 g) of amino acids as arginine, 500 mg vitamin C, and 18 mg zinc, or, if on enteral nutrition (EN), a feeding enriched with arginine, zinc, and ascorbic acid.[58] The control group received either the standard house diet plus an energy-dense (500 kcal), protein-rich (40 g) oral formula or, if receiving EN, a standard tube feeding formulation. After 12 weeks, those receiving the intervention formula had a greater reduction in wound size.[58] These intervention studies have led multiple organizations, including NPUAP, EPUAP, and PPPIA, to recommend supplements enriched with protein, arginine, and micronutrients for adults with stage 3 or 4 or multiple pressure injuries/ulcers when traditional high-calorie, high-protein supplements do not meet nutrition requirements and facilitate wound healing.[2] No research examining the use of arginine alone as a supplement to promote wound healing has demonstrated efficacy.

Hydration

Adequate hydration contributes to good skin turgor, perfusion, and oxygenation of tissue and is an important factor in the prevention and treatment of skin breakdown.[6–8,26] Dehydration impairs oxygen delivery to wounded tissues.[6–8,26] Individuals with elevated temperatures, vomiting, profuse sweating, diarrhea, or heavily draining wounds or other extraneous fluid losses (such as ostomies or fistulas) require additional fluid to compensate for fluid that is lost. Clinicians should monitor each patient's hydration status by checking for signs and symptoms of dehydration, such as decreased skin turgor, dry mucous membranes, decreased urine output, darker-than-normal urine, elevated serum sodium, or increased calculated osmolality.[2,6–8]

There are a variety of approaches to calculate fluid requirements. Tannenbaum and colleagues reviewed the various approaches commonly used and recommend that energy-based methods are less likely to overestimate water needs.[59] Thus, they recommend starting with this approach, rather than using weight-based calculations (eg, 35 mL/kg), if the clinician is concerned about overhydration. Patients with severe cardiac or kidney distress are among those who should be monitored for fluid overload. Chapter 7 discusses fluid requirements in greater detail.

Micronutrients

As noted earlier in the chapter and summarized in Table 21-3 several micronutrients are essential to wound healing.[1,2,8] The NPUAP/EPUAP/PPPIA guidelines recommend a multivitamin with minerals be considered when an individual with a pressure injury is not consuming a balanced diet or a deficiency is suspected or confirmed.[2] Refer to Chapter 8 for additional information on micronutrient requirements and signs and symptoms of toxicity or deficiency.

Vitamin A

Vitamin A is a fat-soluble vitamin that plays a role in protein synthesis, collagen formation, immune function, and the maintenance for the epithelium.[7,8] Impaired collagen synthesis with delayed wound healing may occur with high doses of glucocorticoids, which may cause a vitamin A deficiency.[7,8]

However, there is no evidence of benefit from vitamin A supplementation for healing wounds or pressure injuries/ulcers. Sources of vitamin A are widespread in foods, and adequate amounts can be obtained when individuals consume a balanced diet.

Vitamin C

Vitamin C is essential for tissue repair and regeneration and is a cofactor in the hydroxylation of proline and lysine in collagen formation. It aids in the absorption of iron, the activation of copper, and protein metabolism, and it plays an important role in immune function. Since scar tissue cannot form without collagen, vitamin C deficiency can delay wound healing and may increase the risk of infection.[60] The RDA for vitamin C is 90 mg/d for men and 75 mg/d for women. Because of the high oxidative damage of nicotine, an additional 35 mg/d is recommended for those who use tobacco products.[61]

A double-blind RCT did not demonstrate any positive effect on wound healing in adults supplemented with 1 g vitamin C per day compared with adults given 10 mg/d.[62] While 70% to 90% of oral vitamin c is absorbed at a moderate rate of 30 to 189 mg/d, absorption for doses greater than 1 g/d declines to less than 50%. Because ascorbic acid is a water-soluble vitamin, the excess vitamin C is excreted in the urine.[60–63]

Excess vitamin C may cause oxalate deposits in bone or soft tissues. Therefore, the National Kidney Foundation recommends no more than 60 to 100 mg of vitamin C supplements per day for individuals with chronic kidney disease.[64]

Vitamin E

Vitamin E is an antioxidant that is responsible for normal fat metabolism and collagen synthesis. Several recent studies demonstrated a synergistic effect on pressure injury healing when vitamin E is combined with other antioxidants in an energy-dense, oral supplement enriched with arginine and zinc.[56,57]

Zinc

Zinc is an essential trace mineral necessary for cell replication and growth; it is a cofactor for collagen and protein synthesis and proliferation of inflammatory cells and epithelial cells.[6–8,65] There is no accurate, practical, and cost-effective method for assessing zinc status. Plasma and serum zinc levels are the most common methods of zinc assessment, but they do not necessarily reflect zinc status because zinc is widely distributed throughout the body as a component of proteins.[66] Health professionals must use clinical judgment and fully assess the individual's dietary intake, potential losses, and conditions that may negatively affect zinc status. Zinc deficiencies occur secondary to gastrointestinal (GI) surgery and diseases that impair intestinal absorption and/or increase zinc losses, such as celiac disease, cystic fibrosis, inflammatory bowel disease, and Crohn's disease.[67] Chronic diarrhea and exudate from large wounds also can lead to zinc losses.[66]

The RDA for zinc is 11 mg/d for men and 8 mg/d for women, which can easily be achieved by the consumption of foods with high-quality protein, such as meat, fish, or eggs.

TABLE 21-3 Role of Micronutrients in Wound Healing

	Function in Wound Healing	Effects of Deficiency or Toxicity
Vitamin A	• Maintains integrity of epithelial and mucosal surfaces • Stimulates fibroblasts, which increase collagen synthesis; cross-linking and remodeling of collagen • Antagonizes inhibitory effects of glucocorticoids	• Vitamin A deficiency is associated with widespread alterations in immune function (altered epithelial and mucosal surfaces, T and B cell function, and antibody response). • Deficiency increases risk of infection (diarrheal and respiratory). • In patients with vitamin A deficiency, impaired collagen synthesis with delayed wound healing may occur with high doses of glucocorticoids.
Vitamin E	• Antioxidant, which when combined in a high-calorie oral nutritional supplement enriched with arginine, zinc and other antioxidants, promotes healing • Inhibits collagen synthesis, decreases tensile strength of wounds	• No clinically significant effects of vitamin E deficiency on wound healing are known.
Vitamin C	• Required for fibroblast maturation as well as hydroxylation of proline and lysine in collagen synthesis • Required for angiogenesis • Affects immune function (leukocyte function and complement production)	• Vitamin C deficiency is associated with reduced wound tensile strength and increased wound dehiscence due to impaired fibroblast and collagen maturation. • Deficiency may contribute to increased capillary fragility and angiogenesis with increased wound hemorrhage. • Old wounds may break down in very severe vitamin C deficiency.
Vitamin K	• Cofactor for synthesis of prothrombin and clotting factors VII, IX, and X	• If vitamin K is deficient, excessive bleeding can occur in wounds and predispose patients to wound infection.
Iron	• Cofactor in hydroxylation of lysine and proline for collagen synthesis • Oxygen transport to wounded tissue • Component of many enzymes (eg, required in oxidative burst of phagocytosis)	• When low hemoglobin concentration is due to iron deficiency anemia, it may be a factor in tissue hypoxia and impair wound healing if compensatory mechanisms cannot maintain adequate tissue perfusion. • Impaired hydroxylation of collagen due to iron deficiency is rarely seen in clinical practice. • Iron deficiency may contribute to impaired immune response (T cell and phagocytic function).
Zinc	• Component of many enzyme systems (eg, various growth factors, synthesis of fibroblasts, DNA, and RNA) • Affects multiple aspects of immune function • Production of metalloproteinases is zinc-dependent	• Zinc deficiency is associated with impaired wound strength (decreased fibroblast proliferation, collagen synthesis, and rate of epithelialization). • Depressed immunity is seen even in mild deficiency; susceptibility to a variety of pathogens is increased. • Zinc deficiencies occur secondary to diseases that impair intestinal absorption and/or increase zinc losses. • Zinc toxicity can have adverse effects on wound healing and the immune system, including impaired neutrophil and lymphocyte function.
Copper	• Essential for collagen cross-linking • Competes for the same bonding site as zinc on the albumin molecule	• Copper deficiency is rare, but high doses of oral zinc can interfere with copper absorption and cause copper deficiency and anemia.

Source: Data are from references 1, 2, and 8.

Oral or enteral supplements recommended for wound healing usually contain additional zinc, vitamin C, and other micronutrients to meet estimated needs (see Chapter 11).[68]

High doses of zinc above the Tolerable Upper Intake Level (40 mg/d for adults) is not recommended because it can adversely affect copper status, resulting in anemia.[68] Zinc is associated with copper- and calcium-binding interactions that reduce availability of these nutrients for wound healing.[69] Zinc toxicity can have adverse effects on wound healing and the immune system. Impaired neutrophil and lymphocyte function has been observed in men receiving 150 mg of oral, elemental zinc twice a day for 6 weeks.[12]

Individuals with chronic leg ulcers may have abnormal zinc metabolism and low serum zinc levels, and zinc sulfate has been suggested as a treatment.[70] However, research has not proved that the general use of zinc sulfate is effective in individuals with chronic leg ulcers or arterial or venous ulcers.[71,72] For patients receiving parenteral nutrition (PN), the recommended dose for zinc is 2.5 to 4 mg/d for patients in noncatabolic states and 4.5 to 6 mg/d for severely injured patients. For individuals with small intestinal fluid loss, an additional 12.2 mg zinc per liter of fluid loss and 17.1 mg zinc per kg of stool output or ileostomy drainage is recommended.[73] In severe deficiency states, zinc supplements can be continuously infused over 24 hours at 50 to 100 mg/d if well tolerated; close monitoring of response is recommended.[73]

Nutrition Support

The goals for nutrition support for individuals with chronic wounds are to restore and/or maintain adequate nutrition status, enhance wound healing and immune function, and reduce susceptibility to wound infection.[6–8,26] Nutrition interventions are based on a comprehensive nutrition assessment in concert with a skin risk assessment that determines the severity of the wounds as well as the size and staging of any pressure injuries/ulcers that may be present.

Early recognition of a depleted nutritional state and an aggressive nutrition regimen may help prevent delays in the healing of pressure injuries/ulcers.[6–8,26] A variety of strategies are available for meeting the increased nutrition needs during wound healing, including use of nutrient-dense foods or commercially prepared, over-the-counter, oral nutritional supplements, EN, and PN. When the GI tract can be used, strategies to augment oral intake should be employed first. Patients may be given high-protein and energy-dense nutritional supplements to help meet daily goals of 30 to 35 kcal/kg/d for energy, 1.2 to 1.5 g/kg/d for protein, and the Dietary Reference Intakes for micronutrients.[2,6,7] Increasing protein intake either through protein supplements, sip feedings, or conventional food has a beneficial effect on the healing rate.[6–8] If oral intake is inadequate, EN or PN may be recommended if consistent with the individual's plan of care. The discussion with the individual and/or surrogate should include the risks and benefits of enteral or parenteral feeding.[2]

Commercial supplements fortified with protein, arginine, and various micronutrients, including vitamin C and zinc, have been found to provide some advantages that promote wound healing.[50,56–58,74–76] Langer and Fink published a 2014 systematic review of nutrition interventions for the prevention and treatment of pressure injuries/ulcers and concluded that research on whether nutritional supplements enriched with these various nutrients promote wound healing should be interpreted with caution because the studies were very small, included heterogeneous patient populations with high dropout rates, and examined several types of oral nutritional supplements.[77] The authors noted that this conclusion should not be interpreted to mean that nutrition interventions have no effect on pressure injury/ulcer healing. Instead, they emphasized that individuals at risk of malnutrition and those who are malnourished should receive assessment and intervention.

The use of fortified commercial supplements to produce positive clinical outcomes such as reducing infectious complications, wound dehiscence, and length of hospital stay has been investigated in the surgical population. Osland and coauthors compared the use of pharmaconutrition supplements with arginine-dominated components and standard formulas and concluded that the arginine-enriched supplements improved these clinical outcomes in patients undergoing elective GI surgeries when provided either peri- or postoperatively as oral supplements or as EN support.[78] The Society of Critical Care Medicine (SCCM) and the American Society for Parenteral and Enteral Nutrition (ASPEN) recommend the use of these immune-modulating formulations for surgical and trauma patients.[79] Moreover, in patients with an open abdomen without bowel injury, EN reduces the time to abdominal fascial closure, reduces fistula formation, and decreases intra-abdominal complications and mortality compared with standard therapy, particularly when patients are fed within 24 to 48 hours following admission to the intensive care unit (ICU).[80] For patients with burns, EN should be initiated whenever possible within 4 to 6 hours following ICU admission.[79] Refer to Chapters 24 and 37 for further information on nutrition support therapy for patients with trauma, burns, and surgical complications.

In patients who are unable to achieve 60% of their energy and protein requirements with EN alone after 7 to 10 days, the SCCM/ASPEN guidelines recommend using supplemental PN.[78] PN should also be considered when patients who are at high nutrition risk or malnourished and nutrition support is indicated but EN is not feasible.[79] Further research using RCTs is needed to determine the nutrition needs of patients with specific types of chronic wounds.

Monitoring of Wound Healing and Outcomes

Regular assessment of the wound (ie, monitoring) is necessary to determine the effectiveness of care and clinical outcomes, including the progression of tissue granulation formation, changes in wound size and depth, and eventual wound closure and healing. Outcomes of care are based on a complete patient history, initial assessment, and regular follow-up assessments.[6–8] The patient and wound should be monitored for signs of improvement, infection, or complications. A complete wound assessment should be performed to determine progress. Realistic and clearly defined goals of care help achieve the desired outcomes. Figure 21-3 outlines the process of patient and wound assessment, development of goals, plan of care, and monitoring with outcomes and evaluation.

The goals of therapy are different for different types of wounds. Therefore, the first step in the assessment process is to classify the wound (Figure 21-2). Wounds are commonly categorized by the cause (surgical vs nonsurgical) and whether the wound is chronic or acute. The depth of the wound is also considered. Superficial or partial-thickness wounds are expected to heal in less time than deeper, full-thickness wounds that are associated with complications. There are wound classification systems for chronic wounds of the lower limbs. For example, diabetic and venous ulcers are graded according to clinical signs, etiologic classification, anatomical distribution, and

FIGURE 21-3 Process of Care for Patient and Wound Healing Assessment

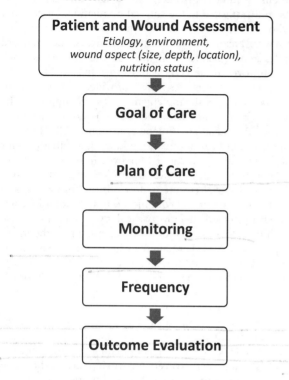

depth. A wound assessment and monitoring model considers close evaluation of the wound bed, size, wound edges, and surrounding skin.[6–8] A recommended approach for wound bed assessment uses the TIME acronym: *t*issue characteristics, *i*nfection, *m*oisture, and *e*dges of the wound described elsewhere.[6–8] This approach is widely used in the clinical setting as a helpful guide for including all aspects of the wound bed in the monitoring of wound healing.

Throughout the process and progress of wound healing, adequate nutrition, as previously described, is requisite for tissue granulation, reduction in wound size and depth, and wound closure. Practice Scenarios 21-1 and 21-2 discuss the approach to nutrition support in the healing of chronic wounds (pressure ulcers) and acute wounds (surgical wounds).[2,6–8,28,51]

Practice Scenario 21-1

Question: What are the protein and energy recommendations for stage 2 and stage 3 pressure injuries/ulcers in a malnourished individual receiving enteral nutrition (EN) support?

Scenario: A 72-year-old woman was admitted to the hospital with a history of hypertension, decompensated congestive heart failure, and dysphagia due to a stroke. On admission, her height was 63 inches, she weighed 104 pounds, and she had a Braden scale score of 14. A swallowing evaluation by the speech language pathologist was completed on Day 2, and tube feeding was initiated the same day. Based on the hospital EN protocol,

the tube feeding was progressed to goal rate. On Day 3, a stage 2 pressure injury/ulcer was observed on her coccyx. On Day 5, a stage 3 coccyx pressure injury/ulcer (4 cm × 5 cm × 6 cm) was observed with exudates consisting of moderate amounts of serous drainage from the wound. The wound bed was covered with yellow slough, and a tissue culture revealed a wound infection with gram-negative organisms.

Intervention: The nutrition support clinician determined that the tube feeding order met the estimated needs for the patient.

Answer: A chronic pressure injury with an active infection results in increased physiological stress that would increase dietary protein needs. Age, immobility, and chronic disease states are all risk factors for protein-energy malnutrition. The outcome for healing can be accomplished by the following:[2]
- Provide 30 to 35 kcal/kg/d.
- Provide 1.2 to 1.5 g protein per kg per day.
- Ensure that 100% of the Dietary Reference Intakes for vitamins and minerals is supplied in the enteral formula provided.
- Provide adequate hydration and monitor fluid status.
- Monitor nutrition status and individualize the nutrition care plan as appropriate.

The goals for EN support for individuals with pressure injuries/ulcers are to restore or maintain adequate nutrition status, enhance wound healing and immune function, and reduce susceptibility to wound infection.[6–8]

Practice Scenario 21-2

Question: What are the recommendations for energy, protein, and micronutrients in a patient with an acute surgical wound?

Scenario: A 78-year-old man with chronic obstructive pulmonary disease was admitted to the surgical intensive care unit following prostate surgery. Despite spontaneous breathing trials each morning, the patient was unable to be weaned from the ventilator. Because the patient could not resume oral feedings while on the ventilator, enteral nutrition (EN) was initiated on Day 3 to meet the need for adequate nutrients for surgical wound healing.

Intervention: The patient was started on EN support with goals based on the nutrition assessment, including a multivitamin once daily. The Recommended Dietary Allowance for protein in healthy adults is 0.8g/kg/d.[51] The nutrition support clinician determined the additional nutrition needs for wound healing, documented the information in the medical record, and obtained the order from the physician.

Answer: A surgical patient intubated postoperatively with acute wounds and comorbidities has increased requirements for protein and energy.

Rationale: A common energy prescription guideline for optimal wound healing is 30 to 35 kcal/kg/d.[2] Older adults (those 65 years of age or older) have an increased protein requirement of 1 g/kg/d to maintain a positive nitrogen balance.[6,8,28] The optimal micronutrient intake to promote wound healing is unknown. What is known is that all nutrients potentially are important to wound healing; energy, protein, arginine, water, vitamins A, C, and E, and minerals play a critical role in the process of wound healing.

References

1. Sherman AR, Barkley M. Nutrition and wound healing. *J Wound Care*. 2011;20(8):357–367.

2. National Pressure Ulcer Advisory Panel, Europe Pressure Ulcer Advisory Panel, Pan Pacific Pressure Injury Alliance. *Prevention and Treatment of Pressure Ulcers: Clinical Practice Guideline*. Perth, Australia: Cambridge Media; 2014.

3. Frykberg RG, Banks J. Challenges in the treatment of chronic wounds. *Adv Wound Care*. 2015;4(9):560–582.

4. Demidova-Rice TN, Hamblin MR, Herman IM. Acute and impaired wound healing: pathophysiology and current methods for drug delivery, part 1: normal and chronic wounds: biology, causes, and approaches to care. *Adv Skin Wound Care*. 2010;25(7):304–314.

5. Mustoe TA, O'Shaughnessy K, Kloeters O. Chronic wound pathogenesis and current treatment strategies: a unifying hypothesis. *J Plast Reconstr Surg*. 2006;117:35–41.

6. Quain AM, Khardori NM. Nutrition in wound care management: a comprehensive overview. *Wounds*. 2015;27(12):327–335.

7. Dryden SV, Shoemaker WG, Kim JH. Wound management and nutrition for optimal wound healing. *Atlas Oral Maxillofacial Surg Clin N Am*. 2013;21:37–47.

8. Wild T, Rahbarnia A, Killner M, Sobotka L, Eberlein T. Basics in nutrition ad wound healing. *Nutrition*. 2010;26(9):862–866.

9. Moores J. Vitamin C: a wound healing perspective. *Br J Community Nurs*. 2013;(Suppl): S6, S8–S11.

10. Lazareth I, Hubert S, Michon-Pasturel U, Priollet P. Vitamin C deficiency and leg ulcers: a case control study. *J Mal Vasc*. 2007; 32:96–99.

11. Walsh CT, Sandstead HH, Prasad AD, et al. Zinc: health effects and research priorities for the 1990s. *Environ Health Perspect*. 1994;102 (Suppl 2):S5–S46.

12. Chandra RK. Excessive intake of zinc impairs immune responses. *JAMA*. 1984;252:1443–1446.

13. Morán-Auth Y, Penna-Martinez M, Shoghi F, Ramos-Lopez E, Badenhoop K. Vitamin D status and gene transcription in immune cells. *J Steroid Biochem Mol Biol*. 2013;136:83–85.

14. Burkiewicz CC, Guadagnin FA, Skare TL, et al. Vitamin D and skin repair: a prospective, double-blind and placebo controlled study in the healing of leg ulcers. *Rev Col Bras Cir*. 2012;39(5):401–407.

15. Powers JG, Higham C, Broussard K, Phillips TJ. Wound healing and treating wounds: chronic wound care and management. *J Am Acad Dermatol*. 2016;74(4):607–625.

16. Fife CE, Carter MJ, Walker D, Thomson B. Wound care outcomes and associated cost among patients treated in US outpatient wound centers: data from the US Wound Registry. *Wounds*. 2012; 24(1):10–17.

17. Agale SV. Chronic leg ulcers: epidemiology, aetiopathogenesis, and management. *Ulcers*. 2013;(2013). doi:10.1155/2013/413604.

18. Williams JZ, Barbul A. Nutrition and wound healing. *Crit Care Nurs Clin North Am*. 2012;24:179–200.

19. Fry D, Pine M. Patient characteristics and the occurrence of never events. *Arch Surg*. 2010;145(2):148–151.

20. Hyun S, Li X, Vermillion B, et al. Body mass index and pressure ulcers: improved predictability of pressure ulcers in intensive care patients. *Am J Crit Care*. 2014;23(6):494–501.

21. Centers for Medicare and Medicaid Services. Proposed changes to the hospital inpatient prospective payment systems and fiscal year 2009. April 30, 2008. http://www.cms.hhs.gov/AcuteInpatientPPS /IPPS/itemdetail.asp?filterType=none&filterByDID=0&sortByDID =4&. Accessed August 8, 2016.

22. National Pressure Ulcer Advisory Panel. NPUAP Pressure Injury Stages. http://www.npuap.org/resources/educational-and-clinical -resources/npuap-pressure-injury-stages. Accessed May 8, 2017.

23. Spentzouris G, Labropoulos N. The evaluation of lower-extremity ulcers. *Semin Intervent Radiol*. 2009;26(4):286–295.

24. Jones V, Harding K, Stechmiller JK, et al. Acute and chronic wound healing. In: Baranoski S, Ayello E, eds. *Wound Care Essentials: Practice Principles*. 3rd ed. Baltimore, MD: Wolters Kluwer, Lippincott Williams & Wilkins; 2012:83–100.

25. Cowan L, Stechmiller JK, Phillips P, et al. Science of wound healing: translation of bench science into advances for chronic wound care. In Krasner D, Sibbald G, Rodeheaver G, eds. *Chronic Wound Care: A Clinical Source Book for Healthcare Professionals*. 5th ed. King of Prussia, PA: Health Management Publications; 2014.

26. Guo S, DiPietro LA. Factors affecting wound healing. *J Dental Res*. 2010;89:223–229.

27. Chen YT, Chang CC, Shen JH, Lin WN, Chen MY. Demonstrating a conceptual framework to provide efficient wound management service for a wound care center in a tertiary hospital. *Medicine (Baltimore)*. 2015;94(44):e1962.

28. Wounds International. International best practice guidelines: wound management in diabetic foot ulcers. 2013. http://www .woundsinternational.com/media/best-practices/_/673/files /dfubestpracticeforweb.pdf. Accessed July 20, 2016.

29. Horn SD, Bender SA, Ferguson ML, et al. The National Pressure Ulcer Long-Term Care Study: pressure ulcer development in long-term care residents. *J Am Geriatr Soc*. 2004;52:359–367.

30. Langkamp-Henken BJ, Hudgens JK, Stechmiller JK, Herrlinger-Garcia KA. Mini-Nutritional Assessment and screening scores are associated with nutritional indicators in elderly people with pressure ulcers. *J Am Diet Assoc*. 2005;105(10):1590–1596.

31. Hengstermann SA Fischer E, Steinhagen-Thiessen E, Schulz RJ. Nutrition status and pressure ulcer: what we need for nutrition screening. *JPEN J Parenter Enteral Nutr*. 2007;31(4):288–294.

32. Fulton J, Evans B, Miller S, Blasiole KN, et al. Development of a nutrition screening tool for an outpatient wound center. *Adv Skin Wound Care*. 2016;29(3):136–142.

33. Braden Risk Assessment Scale. http://www.education.woundcare strategies.com/coloplast/resources/BradenScale.pdf Accessed May 8,2017.

34. Banks MD, Bauer JD, Graves N, Ash S, Malnutrition and pressure ulcer risk in adults in Australian health care facilities, *Nutrition*. 2010;29:896–901.

35. Iizaka S, Okuwa M, Sugama J, Sanada H. The impact of malnutrition and nutrition-related factors on the development and severity of pressure ulcers in older patients receiving home care. *Clin Nutr*. 2010;29(1):47–53.

36. Verbrugghe M, Beeckman D, Van Hecke A, et al. Malnutrition and associated factors in nursing home residents: a cross-sectional, multi-centre study. *Clin Nutr*. 2013;32:438–443.

37. Litchford MD, Dorner B, Posthauer ME. Malnutrition as a precursor of pressure ulcers. *Adv Wound Care*.2014;3(1):54–63.

38. Langer G, Schloemer G, Knerr A, et al. Nutritional interventions for preventing and treating pressure ulcers. *Cochrane Database Syst Rev*. 2003;(4):CD003216.

39. Thomas DR. Anorexia: Etiology, epidemiology and management in older people. *Drugs Aging*. 2009;26(7):557–570.

40. Chernoff R. Normal aging, nutritional assessment, and clinical practice. *Nutr Clin Pract*. 2003;18:12–20.

41. Shipman A Millington G, Obesity and the skin. *Br J Dermatol*. 2001;165(4):743–750.

42. Baugh N, Zuelzer H, Meador J, Blankinship J. Wound wise: wounds in surgical patients who are obese. *Am J Nurs*. 2007; 107(6):40–50.

43. Frankenfield D, Roth-Yousey L, Compher C. Comparison of predictive equations for resting metabolic rate in healthy nonobese and obese adults: a systematic review. *J Am Diet Assoc*. 2005; 105(5):775–789.

44. Lioupis MD. Effects of diabetes mellitus on wound healing: an update. *J Wound Care*. 2005;14(2):84–86.

45. Dorner B, Friedrich EK, Posthauer ME. Position paper of the American Dietetic Association: individualized nutrition approaches for older adults in healthcare communities. *J Am Diet Assoc*. 2010;110(10):1549–1553.

46. Cereda E, Klersy C, Rondanelli M, Caccialanza R. Energy balance in patients with pressure ulcers: a systematic review and meta-analysis of observational studies. *J Am Diet Assoc*. 2011;111(12): 1868–1876.

47. Stratton RJ, Ek M, Engfer M, et at. Enteral nutritional support in prevention and treatment of pressure ulcers: a systematic review and meta-analysis. *Ageing Res Rev*. 2005;4(3):422–450.

48. Trans Tasman Dietetic Wound Care Group. Evidence based practice guidelines for the nutritional management of adults with pressure ulcers. 2011. www.ttdwcg.org. Accessed July 7, 2016.

49. Lee SK, Posthauer ME, Dorner B, et al. Pressure ulcer healing with a concentrated, fortified, collagen protein hydrolysate supplement: a randomized controlled trial. *Adv Skin Wound Care*. 2006;19(2):92–96.

50. Ohura TT, Nakajo S, Okada S, Omura K, Adachi K. Evaluation of effects of nutrition intervention on healing of pressure ulcers and nutritional states (randomized controlled trial). *Wound Repair Regen*. 2011;19(3):330–336.

51. Institute of Medicine. *Dietary Reference Intakes for Energy, Carbohydrates, Fiber, Fat, Protein, and Amino Acids (Macronutrients)*. Washington, DC: National Academies Press; 2005.

52. Bauer J, Biolo G, Cederholm T, et al. Evidence-based recommendations for optimal protein intake for older people: a position paper form the PROT-AGE Study Group. *J Am Med Dir Assoc*. 2013;14:542–559.

53. Demling RH. Nutrition, anabolism and the wound healing process: an overview. *ePlasty*. 2009;9:65–94.

54. Barbul A, Lazarou S, Efron DT, et al. Arginine enhances wound healing and lymphocyte immune responses in humans. *Surgery*. 1990;108:331–337.

55. Kavalukas S, Barbul A. Nutrition and wound healing: an update. *Plast Reconstr Surg*. 2010;127(Suppl):38S–43S.

56. van Anholt RD, Sobotka L, Meijer EP, et al. Specific nutritional support accelerates pressure ulcer healing and reduces wound care intensity in non-malnourished patients. *Nutrition*. 2010;26: 867–872.

57. Cereda E, Klersy C, Serioli M, et al; OligoElement Sore Trial Study Group. A nutritional formula enriched with arginine, zinc, and antioxidants for the healing of pressure ulcers: a randomized trial. *Ann Intern Med*. 2015;162(3):167–174.

58. Cereda E, Gini A, Pedrolli C, Vanotti A. Disease-specific, versus standard, nutritional support for the treatment of pressure ulcers in institutionalized older adults: a randomized controlled trial. *J Am Geriatr Soc*. 2009;57(8):1395–1402.

59. Tannenbaum SL, Castellanos VH, Arheart KL. Current formulas for water requirements produce different estimates. *JPEN J Parenter Enteral Nutr*. 2012;36:299–305.

60. Ronchetti IP, Quaglino D, Bergamini G. Ascorbic acid and connective tissue. In: *Subcellular Biochemistry. Volume 25: Ascorbic Acid: Biochemistry and Biomedical Cell Biology*. New York: Plenum Press; 1996.

61. Institute of Medicine. *Dietary Reference Intakes for Vitamin C, Vitamin E, Selenium, and Carotenoids*. Washington, DC: National Academies Press, 2000.

62. ter Riet G, Kessels AG, Knipschild PG. Randomized clinical trial of ascorbic acid in the treatment of pressure ulcers. *J Clin Epidemiol*. 1995;48(12):1453–1460.

63. Jacob RA, Sotoudeh G. Vitamin C function and status in chronic disease. *Nutr Clin Care*. 2002;5:66–74.

64. National Kidney Foundation. Nutrition in CKD: current guidelines. https://www.kidney.org/professionals/guidelines/guidelines_commentaries/nutrition-ckd. Accessed July 19, 2016.

65. Hambidge KM, Krebs NF. Zinc deficiency: a special challenge. *J Nutr*. 2007;137:1101–1105.

66. Prasad AS. Zinc deficiency: its characterization and treatment. *Met Ions Biol Syst*. 2004;41:103–137.

67. Naber TH, van den Hamer CJ, Baadenhuysen H, Jansen JB. The value of methods to determine zinc deficiency in patients with Crohn's disease. *Scand J Gastroenterol*. 1998;33:514–523.

68. Institute of Medicine. *Dietary Reference Intakes for Vitamin A, Vitamin K, Arsenic, Boron, Chromium, Copper, Iodine, Iron, Manganese, Molybdenum, Nickel, Silicon, Vanadium, and Zinc*. Washington, DC: National Academies Press; 2001.

69. Willis MS, Monaghan SA, Miller ML, et al. Zinc-induced copper deficiency: a report of three cases initially recognized on bone marrow examination. *Am J Clin Pathol*. 2005;123:125–131.

70. Lansdown AB, Mirastschijski U, Stubbs N, Scanlon E, Agren MS. Zinc in wound healing: theoretical, experimental, and clinical aspects. *Wound Repair Regen*. 2007;15:2–16.

71. Wilkinson EA, Hawke CI. Does oral zinc aid the healing of chronic leg ulcers? A systematic literature review. *Arch Dermatol*. 1998;134:1556–1560.

72. Wilkinson EA, Hawke CI. Oral zinc for arterial and venous leg ulcers. *Cochrane Database Syst Rev*. 2000;(2):CD001273.

73. Jeejeebhoy K. Zinc: an essential trace element for parenteral nutrition. *Gastroenterology*. 2009;137(5 Suppl):S7–S12.

74. Wolman SL, Anderson GH, Marliss EB, et al. Zinc in total parenteral nutrition: requirements and metabolic effects. *Gastroenterology*. 1979;76(3):458–467.

75. Desneves KJ, Todorovic BE, Cassar A, et al. Treatment with supplementary arginine, vitamin C and zinc in patients with pressure ulcers: a randomized controlled trial. *Nutr Clin Care*. 2005; 24:979–987.

76. Blass SC, Goost H, Tolba R, et al. Time to wound closure in trauma patients with disorders in wound healing is shortened by supplements containing antioxidant micronutrients and glutamine. *Clin Nutr*. 2012;21:469–475.

77. Langer G, Fink A. Nutritional interventions for preventing and treating pressure ulcers. *Cochrane Database Syst Rev*. 2014;(6): CD003216.

78. Osland E, Hossain MG, Khan S, Memon MA. Effect of timing of pharmaconutrition (immunonutrition) administration on outcomes of elective surgery for gastrointestinal malignancies: a systematic review and meta-analysis. *JPEN J Parenter Enteral Nutr*. 2014.38(1):53–69.

79. McClave SA, Taylor BE, Martindale RG, et al. Guidelines for the provision and assessment of nutrition support therapy in the adult critically ill patient: Society of Critical Care Medicine (SCCM) and American Society for Parenteral and Enteral Nutrition (A.S.P.E.N.). *JPEN J Parenter Enteral Nutr*. 2016;40(2):159–211.

80. Burlew CC, Moore EE, Cuschieri J, et al. Who should we feed? Western Trauma Association multi-institutional study of enteral nutrition in the open abdomen after injury. *J Trauma Acute Care Surg*. 2012;73(6):1380–1387.

22 Neurologic Impairment

Barbara Magnuson Woodward, PharmD, CNSC, Douglas R. Oyler, PharmD, BCCCP, Kathryn Ruf, PharmD, BCPS, Natalia Bailey, MS, RD, CD, and Jimmi Hatton Kolpek, PharmD, FCCP, FCCM, FNAP

CONTENTS

Acknowledgment: Aaron M. Cook, PharmD, BCPS, was a contributor to this chapter for the second edition.

Objectives

1. Discuss energy and protein assessment in patients with acute neurologic injury, such as traumatic brain injury (TBI), spinal cord injury (SCI), and stroke.
2. Explain current clinical approaches to glucose, sodium, and fluid resuscitation and the use of immunonutrition in acute neurologic injury.
3. Describe common nutrition-related challenges inherent in the acute rehabilitation of the neurologically injured patient.
4. Understand energy and protein assessment and other nutrition-related challenges in patients with chronic neurologic diseases.

Test Your Knowledge Questions

1. Which of the following is most strongly correlated with improved mortality in TBI?
   A. Strict avoidance of parenteral nutrition (PN)
   B. Early initiation of nutrition
   C. High protein content in nutrition formula
   D. Supplementation of vitamins C and E
2. Which of the following commonly used medications in TBI is not associated with a reduction in measured energy expenditure?
   A. Propranolol
   B. Mannitol
   C. Pentobarbital
   D. Rocuronium
3. Metabolic changes following SCIs depend on the level of cord injury and the extent of injuries. Which of the following statements is true?
   A. The energy expenditure following SCI is approximately 48% higher than that following TBI.
   B. To accurately assess the energy requirements for a patient with SCI, multiply the resting energy expenditure (calculated with the Harris-Benedict equation) by an injury factor of 1.6 and then again by an activity factor of 1.2.
   C. A modified body mass index (BMI) scale has been proposed for individuals with SCI, with healthy normal categorized as BMI 18 to 22.
   D. Patients with chronic SCI require approximately 30 to 33 kcal/kg/d depending on their physical activity.
4. Which of the following statements regarding a subarachnoid hemorrhage (SAH) is false?
   A. High doses of folic acid should be administered to reduce the likelihood of a second hemorrhagic stroke.
   B. Energy expenditure is higher for patients with SAH than for those with ischemic stroke.
   C. Concentrated enteral nutrition (EN) may be necessary if fluid intake is restricted to minimize cerebral edema.
   D. Bedside or formal swallow studies should be performed to confirm that the patient does not have dysphagia before an oral diet is initiated.

Test Your Knowledge Answers

1. The correct answer is **B**. Of the choices, only early initiation of nutrition has been associated with improved outcomes. EN is preferred in patients with TBI because of the general benefits associated with it, but available evidence does not suggest a strong correlation between PN provision and worsened outcome in TBI (answer A is incorrect). Protein needs are increased after trauma, but provision of high-protein nutrition is not directly correlated with outcomes in TBI (answer C is incorrect). While supplementation of antioxidants is likely beneficial for neurologic recovery after TBI, vitamin replacement has not changed mortality (answer D is incorrect).
2. The correct answer is **B**. Propranolol, pentobarbital, and all neuromuscular antagonists have been shown to reduce energy expenditure after administration (answers A, C, and D are incorrect). Mannitol does not affect energy expenditure.
3. The correct answer is **C**. Energy expenditure following SCI has been repeatedly reported to be almost 48% lower than following TBI. Most patients with SCI will expend 5% to 15% more energy than estimated with the Harris-Benedict equation, and, therefore, Harris-Benedict equation should not be multiplied by extreme injury or activity factors. In the chronic phase, patients with SCI are at risk for obesity and related disorders such as diabetes and cardiovascular disease. Generally, these patients require approximately 20 to 23 kcal/kg/d, depending on their physical activity. A modified proposed BMI scale suggests a normal healthy BMI be 18 to 22.
4. The correct answer is **A**. The VITATOPS study concluded that daily folic acid and vitamin B_6 and B_{12} supplements did not reduce the recurrence of an ischemic stroke.[1] Recent studies show the SAH is likely more hypermetabolic than the ischemic stroke. Concentrated enteral formulas may be indicated if the patient has a free water or total fluid restriction to minimize cerebral edema. The Joint Commission dropped mandatory dysphagia screening from their core measures as of January 2010, but such screening remains part of many stroke quality programs to ensure that no dysphagia is present prior to advancing an oral diet.[2]

Introduction

The central nervous system (CNS) acts as a regulator of nutrient intake. It does so via internal signaling mechanisms that maintain homeostasis of blood glucose and electrolytes and by triggering awareness of hunger and thirst. In CNS injury, these normal physiological functions become disrupted. The severity of this disruption depends on the acuity and magnitude of the brain insult. Acute TBI and stroke generate immediate consequences on nutrition intake and metabolic parameters. Chronic, degenerative diseases of the brain can also cause significant nutrition complications, which gradually become evident as the disease progresses. Residual neurologic function often changes over time, generating different nutrition concerns depending on the stage of CNS recovery.

Numerous factors are pertinent when evaluating nutrition support in a neurologically impaired patient. Nutrition assessment provides the basis for nutrition interventions, in both the acute care and rehabilitation settings. TBI and SCI often affect young, healthy men; in contrast, malnutrition and concomitant diseases are more common in patients with acute stroke or Parkinson's disease. Independent of the initial diagnosis, the extent of neurologic recovery following CNS injury is a common, primary factor to consider when determining nutrition recommendations. Nutrition support is no longer considered adjunctive in the critical care population; rather, it is understood to be therapy to attenuate the metabolic response to stress, prevent metabolic oxidative stress, and modulate the immune response.[3] Nutrition therapy continues to be a vital component in the acute and long-term rehabilitation populations for continued healing and further prevention of malnutrition.

This chapter reviews the nutrition support therapies for a variety of neurologic impairments, beginning with the acute critical phases of TBI, SCI, and stroke. Equally important to the initial therapies provided in the intensive care unit (ICU) are the therapies provided during the acute rehabilitation phase of injury recovery. This chapter also addresses distinctive nutrition challenges associated with several chronic neurologic disease states, including amyotrophic lateral sclerosis (ALS), epilepsy, and Parkinson's disease.

Nutrition in Acute Traumatic Brain Injury

Nutrition Requirements

TBI is a heterogeneous injury that drastically varies in etiology, clinical presentation, severity, and pathophysiology. In general, the acute phase of TBI can be categorized as a hypermetabolic, catabolic one that is proportional to the severity of injury.[4] The subsequent rapid depletion of muscle mass and immunosuppression have been associated with increased morbidity,[5,6] and early provision of nutrition has been proposed as a preventive measure.[7] At present, the Brain Trauma Foundation (BTF) guidelines provide no level 1 recommendations regarding nutrition in TBI.[8]

The primary benefits of adequate nutrition support in the trauma patient are threefold: prevention of protein malnutrition, modulation of the immune response, and preservation of gastrointestinal (GI) structure and function.[9] If exogenous energy is not supplied to the acutely injured patient with a severe stress response, the requirements are ultimately met through skeletal muscle proteolysis followed by breakdown of visceral and circulating proteins, which has a direct effect on immune function.[10] Specific types of amino acid supplementation (discussed under "Immunonutrition," later in this section) may have a direct role in ameliorating critical illness–mediated immunosuppression.[11] Administration of early EN has been shown to help prevent GI dysfunction that may occur as a result of neuroendocrine reflexes and ischemia/reperfusion injuries as well as multiple concomitant interventions in critical care (eg, abdominal surgery and medication therapy with some types of H_2-antagonists and opioids).[12]

Depending on the severity of TBI, concomitant injuries, and medical management, measured energy expenditure can vary from 87% to 200% of the energy expenditure estimated by using the Harris-Benedict equation (the predictive equation most studied in the TBI literature).[13] Use of neuromuscular blocking agents (NMBAs), nonselective beta-blockers, morphine, and barbiturates is associated with reductions in measured energy expenditure (discussed under "Pharmacological Therapies," later in this section).[14-18] Where available, use of indirect calorimetry (IC) to estimate energy needs is strongly encouraged.[3] If IC is unavailable or impractical to use, estimating energy requirements to be 140% of what the Harris-Benedict equation predicts is recommended by the BTF, American Association of Neurological Surgeons, and Congress of Neurological Surgeons.[19] Protein requirements are in the range of 1.3 to 2.5 g/kg/d.[20,21] See Chapter 2 for a broader discussion of IC and predictive energy equations. See Chapter 6 for additional information on protein.

Finally, multiple alterations occur in the productions of hormonal and inflammatory mediators, including growth hormone, adrenocorticotropin-releasing hormone, cortisol, prolactin, glucagon, vasopressin, and catecholamines.[22] Lower concentrations of zinc, magnesium, and insulin-like growth factor 1 (IGF-1) may also worsen outcomes after TBI. Supplementation with zinc and IGF-1 has been shown to improve some outcomes after TBI.[23,24] Table 22-1 highlights major metabolic alterations after TBI.[23,25-27]

Role of Nutrition Support

Outcomes for patients with TBI are likely better correlated to the timing of nutrition than the route of nutrition. A recent Cochrane review analyzed 11 prospective trials involving patients with TBI, including 7 studies that addressed the timing of nutrition support (total N = 284 patients). In those 7 trials, provision of early (within 24 to 72 hours of injury) nutrition support was associated with a trend toward reduced mortality when compared with late (within 3 to 5 days) nutrition support (risk ratio [RR] = 0.67; 95% confidence interval [CI], 0.41–1.07).[28]

The importance of early nutrition is further illustrated in a recent retrospective database review conducted by the BTF, wherein patients who received no nutrition within 5 and 7

TABLE 22-1 Metabolic Alterations After Traumatic Brain Injury

Diminished Concentrations in CNS Injury	Elevated Concentrations in CNS Injury
Albumin	Alpha-1 acid glycoprotein
Insulin-like growth factor-1	C-reactive protein
Iron	Ceruloplasmin
Prealbumin	Interleukin-1
Thyroxine	Interleukin-6
Thyroid-stimulating hormone	Vasopressin (in SIAD)
Transferrin	Cortisol (acute injury)
Vasopressin (in diabetes insipidus)	Growth hormone (acute injury)
Zinc	
Cortisol (chronic injury)	
Growth hormone (chronic injury)	

CNS, central nervous system; SIAD, syndrome of inappropriate antidiuresis.
Source: Data are from references 23 and 25–27.

days after isolated severe TBI with or without polytrauma had a 2- and 4-fold increased likelihood of death, respectively, when compared with patients who received nutrition within each time frame.[29] Furthermore, the risk of mortality increased by 30% to 40% with each 10 kcal/kg decrease in the amount of nutrition provided, even after the analysts controlled for other predictors of mortality.

A meta-analysis by Wang and colleagues evaluated EN vs PN in patients sustaining TBI and showed no significant difference in outcomes.[30] In fact, PN was associated with nonsignificant reductions in mortality (RR = 0.61; 95% CI, 0.34–1.09), poor outcome (RR = 0.73; 95% CI, 0.51–1.04), and infectious complications (RR = 0.89; 95% CI, 0.66–1.22). Of note, most mortality (28/41) and poor outcome events (49/63) occurred in studies that randomly assigned patients to early PN vs late EN, and infectious complications data were strongly driven by pneumonia rates.[30]

A recent retrospective study found an increased risk of pneumonia in 90 patients with severe TBI (Glasgow Coma Scale less than 8) who were fed enterally; notably, 70% of the patients in this study received EN via an orogastric or nasogastric tube.[31] However, in light of the well-known benefits of EN when compared with PN, clinicians are urged to start EN as soon as possible following TBI to maximize its benefits. Given the poor outcomes associated with delayed nutrition in the TBI population, a low threshold for using PN if a patient does not tolerate EN is advised.

Special Considerations

Sodium

Hyponatremia (serum sodium less than 135 mEq/L) is common in patients in neurosurgical ICUs and contributes to wors-

ening cerebral edema, intracranial pressure elevations, and death from herniation.[32] A serum sodium concentration of less than 130 mEq/L has been associated with a 60-fold increase in case fatality rate.[33] TBI is a common cause of the syndrome of inappropriate antidiuresis (SIAD), which results in euvolemic hyponatremia. Because of the euvolemia and normal urine volume, SIAD is often difficult to detect before clinical symptoms manifest unless the patient's serum sodium concentration is monitored. Because SIAD is typically transient, fluid restriction is the primary method of treatment; however, caution should be used in the acute phase of neurologic insult because volume restriction may be inappropriate.[34] Pharmacological treatment with demeclocycline, sodium supplementation, or vasopressin antagonists should only be used in refractory cases.

Cerebral salt wasting (CSW) is a rare hypovolemic hyponatremia characterized by increased natriuresis; like SIAD, CSW is usually transient after TBI.[35] CSW is a diagnosis of exclusion and should only be considered in hypovolemic patients when another cause of natriuresis is not identified. CSW should be managed with intravenous (IV) sodium supplementation. In both SIAD and CSW, hyponatremia should be corrected no faster than 10 to 12 mEq/L/d to avoid central pontine myelinolysis.[36]

Diabetes insipidus is a hypernatremic state characterized by a deficiency in vasopressin (neurogenic), lack of response to vasopressin (nephrogenic), or accelerated degradation of vasopressin (gestational).[37] Neurogenic diabetes insipidus is the most common type; damage to the hypothalamus or posterior pituitary, usually as a result of rotational forces sustained in motor vehicle collisions, reduces central vasopressin production leading to neurogenic diabetes insipidus after TBI.[38] Supplementation of salt-free water and replacement of vasopressin or analogues can reduce serum sodium to normal levels. As with hyponatremia, hypernatremia should be corrected no faster than 10 to 12 mEq/L/d to avoid worsening of cerebral edema.

Hyperglycemia

Hyperglycemia following TBI has been linked to poor neurologic outcomes,[39] but the role of glucose in secondary injury has not been elucidated. Hyperglycemia may induce lactic acidosis as well as endothelial dysfunction and cerebrovascular changes during ischemia and reperfusion. Additionally, hyperglycemia enhances neutrophil transmigration across the blood-brain barrier and, along with tumor necrosis factor, activates production of interleukin-8.[40] The impact of hyperglycemia on its own, weighed against the risk of inadequate provision of nutrition, has not been evaluated. At present, the maintenance of serum glucose in patients with TBI is expected to be similar to maintenance for other critically ill populations.[41] (Refer to Chapter 34 for more information on managing hyperglycemia in critical illness.)

Pharmacological Therapies

Pharmacological therapies used as part of the care of a patient with TBI can have important implications for nutrition support therapy. Table 22-2 provides a list of medications

<table>
<tr><td colspan="2">**TABLE 22-2 Medication Considerations in Traumatic Brain Injury**</td></tr>
<tr><td>Medication</td><td>Nutrition Implications</td></tr>
<tr><td>Barbiturates</td><td>May reduce energy requirements. Combine with bowel regimen.</td></tr>
<tr><td>Carbamazepine</td><td>Avoid combining suspension with water or other medication diluents (forms rubbery precipitate). Monitor for hyponatremia.</td></tr>
<tr><td>Corticosteroids</td><td>Monitor for hyperglycemia.</td></tr>
<tr><td>Demeclocycline</td><td>Avoid combination with divalent cations (eg, magnesium, calcium) or EN.</td></tr>
<tr><td>Mannitol</td><td>Monitor for hypokalemia, hypomagnesemia, hypovolemia.</td></tr>
<tr><td>NMBAs (eg, rocuronium, cisatracurium)</td><td>May reduce energy requirements.</td></tr>
<tr><td>Phenytoin</td><td>Caution combining suspension with EN (diminished/delayed absorption. Hold EN at least 1–2 hours before and after administration).</td></tr>
<tr><td>Propofol</td><td>10% lipid emulsion provides 1.1 kcal/mL.</td></tr>
<tr><td>Propranolol</td><td>May reduce energy requirements.</td></tr>
</table>

EN, enteral nutrition; NMBA, neuromuscular blocking agent.
Source: Data are from references 14, 18, 42, and 43.

that may affect nutrition support or subsequent monitoring.[14,18,42,43] Many medications may cause electrolyte abnormalities, and several others can reduce energy expenditure to varying degrees.

Based on numerous recent studies,[44–46] propranolol therapy in the acute phase of TBI may soon be used more frequently. Propranolol administration has been shown to reduce measured energy expenditure by 5% to 18%, likely related to a reduction in response to circulating catecholamines.[14,15] Morphine, which may be used for analgesia or to mediate symptoms of paroxysmal sympathetic hyperactivity (PSH), can reduce energy expenditure by up to 8%.[16] For management of PSH, morphine and propranolol may be used concomitantly,[47] and it is plausible that their effects on energy expenditure are additive.

Pentobarbital may be used to reduce intracranial pressure after TBI, primarily by reducing cerebral blood volume and cerebral metabolism.[42] Dempsey and colleagues found that induction of pharmacological coma using pentobarbital reduced energy expenditure by up to 32% compared with no barbiturate therapy (86% ± 28% vs 126% ± 36% of predicted energy expenditure using Harris-Benedict equation; P <0.01).[17]

NMBAs have also been used to reduce intracranial pressure after TBI and can affect energy requirements. In 18 patients with severe head injury receiving pancuronium, NMBA administration reduced energy expenditure to basal levels independent of morphine use, body temperature, and feeding.[18] A smaller study of patients receiving midazolam and vecuronium or pancuronium showed a reduction of energy expenditure to levels below what the Harris-Benedict equation predicted, similar to energy expenditure levels seen with barbiturate therapy.[48]

Immunonutrition

Immunonutrition is the supplementation of specific nutrients—mainly arginine, glutamine, ω-3 fatty acids, and antioxidants—with the intent of immunomodulation. Because immune function in critical illness is heterogeneous among patients and among patient groups,[49] broad conclusions about the safety or efficacy of various components of immunonutrition in critically ill patients should be avoided.

Arginine

L-arginine is required for regulation of cerebral blood flow, extracellular matrix remodeling, and energy production.[50] Low circulating levels of arginine have been postulated to be a critical component of the development of the persistent inflammation, immunosuppression, and catabolism syndrome after critical illness.[11] After severe TBI, plasma levels of arginine and metabolic byproducts (citrulline, ornithine, urea, proline, and 4-hydroxyproline) are significantly decreased; these alterations in plasma arginine and metabolites may contribute to secondary injury following TBI.[51] Importantly, the decrease in plasma arginine seems to occur through a different mechanism that in other models of critical illness (eg, sepsis), where the L-arginine nitric oxide pathway seems to be hyperactive.[52] (Refer to Chapter 23 for more information on sepsis.)

Despite an abundance of theoretical evidence, clinical research has not found that arginine supplementation in trauma and TBI improves outcomes. A recent systematic review of 8 studies enrolling 372 patients indicated that pharmaconutrition did not improve infection, hospital length of stay, or mortality outcomes.[53] Seven of these studies (n = 300 patients) included arginine as part of the nutrition formula.

Of theoretical concern is the ability of L-arginine to be converted to nitric oxide, which may react with reactive oxygen species to form peroxynitrite. However, this reaction is likely more related to levels of nitric oxide synthase as opposed to arginine supplementation.[54]

Glutamine

Glutamine plays a central role in nitrogen transport and is fuel for the rapidly dividing cells of the gut and immune system.[55] Low plasma glutamine concentration at ICU admission is an independent risk factor for post-ICU mortality in critically ill patients.[56] The mechanism underlying this association with mortality is currently unknown.

Despite the association of low plasma glutamine concentration with poor outcomes, early provision of glutamine did not improve these outcomes in a large-scale study of critically ill patients.[57] However, in this study, only 2.5% of patients were admitted with trauma; given the heterogeneity of critically ill patients, extrapolation of these results to the TBI population should be done with extreme caution.

Theoretically, glutamine supplementation may increase cerebral glutamate concentration, which may act to worsen secondary injury through N-methyl-D-aspartate (NMDA) receptor agonism.[22] The available evidence to date does not support this hypothesis. A recent study of 12 patients with severe TBI who were given IV glutamine supplementation showed an increase only in plasma and cerebrospinal fluid (CSF) concentrations of glutamine and alanine; CSF glutamate concentrations significantly *decreased* during and after glutamine infusions.[58] No signs of potential glutamate-mediated cerebral injury were noted.

ω-3 Fatty Acids

The human brain is 60% lipid by dry weight, and docosahexaenoic acid (DHA) comprises 50% of neuronal membrane phospholipids.[59] Because of its extreme flexibility, DHA is abundant in neuronal synapses. Additionally, both DHA and eicosapentaenoic acid (EPA) have the ability to transform into neuroprotective metabolites that protect against oxidative stress, tissue inflammation, and synaptic degradation.[60,61] Following TBI, existing DHA and EPA are converted to neuroprotectins and resolvins, which upregulate antiapoptotic cascades and expression of receptor families involved in tissue repair,[62,63] thereby improving neurologic outcomes in animal models or with preinjury supplementation.[64-66] No clinical trial data regarding post-TBI ω-3 supplementation in humans are presently available.

Antioxidants

Lipid peroxidation biomarkers—such as thiobarbituric acid–reactive substances, protein carbonyls, and 8-iso-prostagladin $F_{2\alpha}$—are increased following TBI and have been correlated with clinical outcomes.[67] Oxidative stress following TBI may lead to excitotoxicity, mitochondrial dysfunction, apoptosis, autophagy, cerebral edema, and inflammation.[68] To attenuate this response, a number of antioxidant substances have been evaluated, including ω-3 fatty acids, ascorbic acid, and α-tocopherol.[69,70]

Plasma ascorbic acid levels are suppressed following head trauma.[71] Supplementation of ascorbic acid may protect neurons from NMDA-induced excitotoxicity and lipid peroxidation.[72] Furthermore, ascorbic acid supplementation may be beneficial because ascorbic acid transport through the sodium-dependent vitamin C transporter may be altered in TBI, and the ability of cells to maintain high levels of intracellular ascorbic acid may be reduced.

α-Tocopherol is the major peroxyl radical scavenger in in lipid membranes.[73] Preinjury supplementation has been shown to be beneficial in rat models of TBI, and ascorbic acid supplementation may reduce α-tocopheroxyl to improve α-tocopherol levels.[69] In a study of 100 patients with severe TBI, supplementation of 400 IU of intramuscular vitamin E per day significantly improved mortality and Glasgow Outcomes Score at discharge compared with placebo.[70]

At present, available information is insufficient to recommend specific dosing strategies of any pharmaconutrient to patients with TBI. Additionally, evidence is lacking regarding the clinical benefits of supplementation. However, given the significant amount of theoretical evidence supporting the use of pharmaconutrition in the trauma population, its use is recommended in patients with TBI,[3] and exogenous supplementation of ω-3 fatty acids, ascorbic acid, and vitamin E should be considered as recommended in the 2016 American Society for Parenteral and Enteral Nutrition (ASPEN) and Society of Critical Care Medicine (SCCM) guidelines for the provision and assessment of nutrition support therapy in the adult critically ill patient.[3] Practice Scenario 22-1 explores the use of phramaconutrition and other aspects of an optimal nutrition support regimen for a patient with acute TBI.[3,19,20]

Practice Scenario 22-1

Question: What is the optimal nutrition support regimen for a patient in the acute phase of a traumatic brain injury (TBI)?

Scenario: A 35-year-old woman was admitted with a severe TBI after a motor vehicle collision. She has multiple other orthopedic injuries, including a left femur fracture, right 3–7 rib fractures, and a right humerus fracture. Her presenting Glasgow Coma Score was 7T, and she has remained intubated because of her neurologic status. The nutrition support clinician is asked to evaluate the patient's current enteral nutrition (EN) regimen and recommend changes if necessary. The patient is receiving a 1.2 kcal/mL formula at a rate of 60 mL/h through a postpyloric small-bore feeding tube and is tolerating it well. The nutrition assessment notes:
- Height: 162.5 cm
- Weight: 62 kg
- Enteral formula: 1.2 kcal/mL, 54 g protein per liter, and 809 mL free water per liter administered at rate of 60 mL/h.
- Medications: Enteral administration of 100 mg phenytoin suspension every 8 hours, with enteral feeds held for 1 hour before and 1 hour after each dose; enteral administration of 100 mg docusate twice daily; 30 mg enoxaparin administered subcutaneously twice daily; enteral administration of 20 mg famotidine twice daily; and 10 mg propofol per mL lipid emulsion as a continuous infusion running at 25 mcg/kg/min.

Intervention: Tube feedings are changed to an immune-modulating formulation (1.5 kcal/mL, 94 g protein per liter, 770 mL free water per liter, an ω-6 to ω-3 fatty acid ratio of 1.4:1, 18.7 arginine per liter, and 8.1 g glutamine per liter) at a rate of 55 mL/h. The patient's phenytoin administration is changed to 150 mg twice daily so the EN will need to be held for only 4 hours per day. At a rate of 55 mL/h for 20 hours per day, her nutrition support will provide 1650 kcal and 103.4 g protein per day. Additionally, she will receive 245 kcal/d from propofol.

Answer: Because of the variability in energy expenditure associated with TBI and the patient's medication regimen, indirect calorimetry (IC) should be performed to determine energy requirements. If IC is not done, the patient's energy requirements may be roughly estimated to be 1921 kcal/d, 40% more than the Harris-Benedict equation would predict.[19] Approximately 1.3 to 2.5 g protein per kg body weight should be given per day (80 to 155 g/d for this patient). Immunonutrition and medication therapy (eg, propofol, phenytoin) should be considered.

Rationale: This patient's predicted energy expenditure, as estimated by the Harris-Benedict equation, is 1372 kcal/d. Accounting for an approximate 40% increase in energy expenditure associated with TBI,[19] she may require 1921 kcal/d (31 kcal/kg/d). However, given the wide variability in measured energy expenditure associated with TBI and the unknown effect of propofol administration on energy expenditure, IC is recommended to accurately determine the patient's energy requirements.

The energy from 25 mg propofol per day is calculated as follows:

$$\frac{25 \text{ mcg propofol}}{\text{kg} \times \text{min}} \times 62 \text{ kg} \times \frac{60\text{min}}{\text{h}} \times \frac{24\text{ h}}{\text{d}} \times \frac{1 \text{ mg propofol}}{1000 \text{ mcg propofol}}$$
$$\times \frac{1 \text{ mL propofol}}{10 \text{ mg propofol}} \times \frac{1.1\text{kcal}}{\text{mL propofol}} = 245 \text{ kcal}$$

Because phenytoin suspension requires separation from EN by 1 hour, each administered phenytoin dose results in 2 hours of nutrition missed. By changing phenytoin administration to twice daily, EN can be administered for 20 hours as opposed to 18. (Phenytoin suspension should not be given once daily because of the short half-life of the drug.)

Using a more energy-dense formula will reduce this patient's administered free water, which may prevent development of hyponatremia. Very energy-dense formulations (eg, 2 kcal/mL) may not provide adequate protein and typically require exogenous protein supplementation. Medication administration, specifically of powder packets, typically requires additional free water to administer, which may negate the benefit of an energy-dense formulation. For that reason, a 1.5 kcal/mL solution is chosen. At a rate of 55 mL/h for 20 hours, this formula provides 1650 kcal/d (26.6 kcal/kg) vs the 1296 kcal/d (20.9 kcal/kg) the patient previously received from EN.

Estimations of protein requirements vary from 1.3 g/kg[21] to more than 2 g/kg[20] and are likely affected by concomitant disease states. Given this patient's polytrauma, it may be reasonable to administer a dose of protein even higher than the proposed dose of 1.67 g/kg. With the current formula providing 94 g/L, the patient will receive 103.4 g protein per day over 20 hours (vs the 58.3 g/d she was receiving previously). As discussed in the chapter, immune-modulating formulations should be considered for traumatically injured patients;[3] the benefits of ω-3 supplementation in the setting of propofol administration are unknown.

Nutrition in Acute Spinal Cord Injury

Isolated SCI patients have nutrition needs distinct from those of patients with TBI. The physiological rationale for such a difference has been attributed to the difference in neuronal connectivity and stimuli, which results in energy expenditure being lower in patients with SCI than in those with TBI.[74,75]

Nutrition Requirements

IC measurements for patients after SCI, rather than use of predictive equations, is supported as a level II recommendation in the American Association of Neurological Surgeons and Congress of Neurological Surgeons SCI guidelines.[74] No validated predictive equation best determines the SCI energy expenditure.[75] Use of the Harris-Benedict equation with an injury factor of 1.6 and activity factor of 1.2 was initially supported in a 1979 landmark paper by Long and colleagues to estimate post-SCI energy needs.[76] However, using such approach has been found to overestimate energy requirements.[77] See Chapter 2 for a general discussion of IC and equations used to predict energy needs.

In a study of 7 patients with TBI and 7 with SCI, the SCI population had 48% lower energy needs than the patients with TBI. Patients with SCI were also found to have a measured energy expenditure that was 56% of what was predicted by the equation proposed by Long and colleagues.[77]

Extent of injury seems to affect energy needs in patients with SCI. Measured resting energy expenditure is lower in patients with higher and more complete SCIs.[74,78]

Interestingly, patients with SCI seem to have lower-than-predicted metabolic needs long after the acute stages of injury. Bauman and colleagues studied energy expenditure in 13 sets of adult twins with 1 twin having an SCI and the other as a control.[79] All SCIs occurred 3 to 26 years before the study. The investigators reported that energy expenditure remained low for years following SCI. The measured energy expenditure for the participants with SCI was, on average, 15% less than the energy requirement predicted by the Harris-Benedict equation, and the mean energy requirement for this group was approximately 20.4 kcal/kg. Monroe and colleagues evaluated 10 male subjects with SCI that had occurred at least 2 years before the study. They concluded that the individuals with SCI expended significantly lower daily energy than the control subjects. The lower energy expenditure in those with SCI was explained by lower levels of physical activity, lower resting metabolic rate, and the thermogenic effect of food.[80]

Persistent nitrogen losses have been noted after SCI. This loss seems to be independent of nutrition support high in protein (2 g/kg/d) and energy.[81] The nitrogen loss peaks have been described at about 3 weeks, and ongoing loss may last for 7 weeks.[82,83] Guideline recommendations focus on meeting energy and nitrogen needs, rather than attempting to achieve a nitrogen balance.[74] Protein requirements immediately following SCI are estimated to be 1.5 to 2 g/kg/d.[74]

Role of Nutrition

Currently, no data are available to validate that early EN (within 72 hours of injury) improves neurologic outcome after SCI. However, such an approach is regarded as safe and is a level III recommendation in the SCI guidelines based on 2 studies.[74] Dvorak and colleagues compared patients receiving early EN (initiated less than 72 hours after SCI) vs late EN (initiated more than 120 hours after SCI) and found no differences in nutrition status, feeding complications, days on mechanical ventilation, infection, or length of stay.[84] A retrospective review also noted a lack of complications with early EN.[85]

No specific recommendations have been made for the ideal nutrition formulation for patients with SCI.[74]

Special Considerations

Nutrition support after SCI may be complicated by many factors. For example, SCI-related autonomic dysfunction may lead to paralytic ileus or neurogenic bowel and may further affect the patient's ability to feed.[82]

Glycemic Control

Initial increases in hepatic gluconeogenesis and initial changes in insulin response may result increased lactic acid production and neurotoxicity from increased glucose substrate availability.[82] This problem could be further complicated by post-SCI methylprednisolone protocols, which are used less frequently than in the past and are no longer recommended in current guidelines.[86-89]

As in TBI, hyperglycemia in SCI may be deleterious and must be aggressively managed in the acute phase of the injury.[82] IV or subcutaneous insulin therapy may be used both acutely and chronically to control blood glucose. However, optimal glycemic targets and the effects of intensive insulin therapy for the SCI population remain largely unknown, and specific guidelines for glycemic control are lacking.[90]

Vitamin D Deficiency

Vitamin D deficiency has also been noted in SCI. It can result in hyperparathyroidism and increased bone resorption.[82,91]

Obesity and Cardiovascular Disease

Long-term management of SCI patients requires special attention to this population's elevated risk of obesity and cardiovascular disease.[92,93] A modified BMI scale has been proposed for individuals with SCI, with normal weight defined as a BMI of 18 to 22, overweight as a BMI of 22 to 25, and obesity as a BMI of more than 25.[93] In a study of 73 individuals with SCI that occurred at least 1 year earlier, Groah reported that nearly 70% of the participants were overweight when assessed using the modified scale; this study also noted deficient intake of some vitamins, minerals, and macronutrients.[94] Another study evaluated 7959 veterans with SCI and reported that almost 53% were obese or overweight as defined by the standard BMI categories (overweight: BMI, 25.0 to 29.9; obesity: BMI, 30 or greater).[95] When the BMI scale was adjusted for people with SCI to define overweight as a BMI between 23 and 27 and obesity as a BMI of greater than or equal to 28, 68% of subjects were classified as overweight or obese.[95]

General energy recommendations for weight maintenance in quadriplegic patients are 20 to 22 kcal/kg/d or 55% to 90% of the energy goal estimated by the Harris-Benedict equation.[96] For paraplegics, energy recommendations are increased slightly to 22 to 24 kcal/kg/d (80% to 90% of the estimate calculated from the Harris-Benedict equation).[96]

Pressure Ulcers

Individuals with SCI in long-term care have protein requirements comparable to those for healthy individuals (0.8 to 1 g protein per kg ideal body weight per day). The estimated protein requirement should be increased if the patient has decubitus ulcers.[3] Estimates for the incidence of pressure ulcers in patients with SCI are quite high (25% to 66%). Notably, patients with higher level lesions are more likely to develop pressure ulcers.[97-99]

In 2009, the National Pressure Ulcer Advisory Panel and European Pressure Ulcer Advisory Panel published guidelines for patients with pressure ulcers, recommending adequate intake of protein (1.25 to 1.5 g/kg/d) and energy (30 to 35 kcal/kg/d), sufficient daily fluid, and vitamin and mineral supplementation if intake is poor or deficiencies are suspected.[100] The guidelines also recommend a consultation with a dietitian to ensure the patient's nutrition needs are being met.[97,100]

Nutrition in Acute Stroke

Each year, more than 795,000 people in the United States have a stroke.[101] Stroke is the fifth leading cause of death in United States. Although more than 80% of patients with stroke survive, many have serious long-term disabilities.[101] Nearly 87% of stroke cases are ischemic, and less than 13% are hemorrhagic, intracerebral, or subarachnoid.[101]

Dysphagia

Besides gross neuromotor and cognitive dysfunction, 78% of stroke patients may experience various aspects of dysphagia. Most patients regain full swallow recovery within a few weeks, but others may take much longer or do not completely recover swallow function.[102]

Dysphagia should be assessed and addressed immediately because swallowing difficulty can contribute to complications of care, including aspiration pneumonia, malnutrition, prolonged rehabilitation, and increased mortality.[103,104] The Joint Commission dropped the dysphagia screening from the core patient care measures in 2010, but many stroke centers continue to require dysphagia screening before any oral intake, including food, fluid, or medications, can be initiated.[2] Patients experiencing dysphagia after a stroke have an increased risk of developing dehydration, pneumonia, and possibly chronic malnutrition.[105]

Al-Khaled and colleagues screened more than 9000 acute ischemic stroke patients within 24 hours of admission and reported that 25.1% of patents had dysphagia, which independently correlated with increases in mortality (odds ratio [OR] = 3.2; 95% CI, 2.4–4.2; $P <0.001$) and disability (OR = 2.3; 95% CI, 1.8–3.0; $P <0.001$) at 3 months after the stroke.[106] Patients with dysphagia had a higher rate of pneumonia than those without (29.7% vs 3.7%; $P <0.001$). Screening for dysphagia within 24 hours of admission was associated with decreased risk of stroke-related pneumonia (OR = 0.68; 95% CI, 0.52–0.89; $P = 0.006$) and disability at discharge (OR = 0.60; 95% CI, 0.46–0.77; $P <0.001$).[106]

Several mechanisms are available for informal bedside screening for dysphagia.[107] Cummings published a successful, easy-to-use dysphagia screening tool that nurses can use to quickly identify dysphagia.[108] Campbell and associates have presented a facility-developed Nursing Bedside Dysphagia Screen as a valid and reliable tool to help identify patients with stroke who are at risk for aspiration pneumonia.[109]

Trained personnel should frequently assess stroke patients for dysphagia and evaluate the aspiration risk with the goal to return to "normal" oral consumption. A modified barium swallow evaluation remains the gold standard to diagnose oropharyngeal dysphagia and should be performed when dysphagia is suspected.[110]

Role of Nutrition Support

When the patient has dysphagia or is unable to maintain volitional intake, nutrition via an enteral access device should be considered because oral nutritional supplements alone may not provide adequate nutrition. The 2005 Feed or Ordinary Diet (FOOD) trial was a series of 3 multicenter, randomized controlled trials that evaluated the use of oral nutritional supplements following a stroke in 4023 patients in 125 hospitals in 15 countries.[111] The FOOD trial findings showed no beneficial outcomes to support the routine use of oral nutritional supplements to well-nourished hospitalized patients following a stroke.[111] However, because the FOOD trial studied a well-nourished population, its finding may not apply to patients with a predisposition to or existing protein-energy malnutrition; these patients may see positive results from the routine use of oral nutritional supplements.

Qualified clinicians should use a validated tool, such as Nutrition Risk in Critically Ill (NUTRIC) or Nutrition Risk Screening (NRS-2002), to assess all stroke patients admitted to the ICU for nutrition risk.[112,113] The 2016 ASPEN and SCCM guidelines recommend that EN be initiated within 24 to 48 hours of admission for all critically ill patients at high nutrition risk and for others with anticipated prolonged *nil per os* (nothing by mouth) status.[3] Most stroke patients should tolerate EN and not require PN unless they have preexisting physical or physiological impediments to EN.

EN should be advanced to the optimal rate or volume with added modulars as needed within 24 to 72 hours of initiation. In a study of patients with acute stroke and dysphagia, Zheng et al compared those who received early EN with those fed by orally by their family and found that the group receiving early EN had better nutrition status and reduced nosocomial infection and mortality rates after 21 days.[114] In a study of 273 comatose acute stoke patients, Yamada found that the use of early PN along with a 20% glucose solution via a feeding tube was beneficial but also recommended that early PN not be administered for longer than 10 days because switching to EN after initial PN contributed to better nutrition recovery than the extended use of PN.[115]

Most stroke patients tolerate EN with a gastric feeding access, commonly with a bedside-placed nasogastric feeding tube. A bridle may be used to secure the nasally inserted tube to deter unintentional dislodgement.[116–119] The feeding tube should be diverted to the small bowel if the patient is at risk for aspiration of gastric contents.[3]

Prospective randomized studies have not been done on the optimal timing of placement of percutaneous endoscopic gastrostomy (PEG) tubes or gastrostomy tubes (G-tubes). Therefore, timing is based on clinical judgment, experience, and patient condition. The American Stroke Association recommends that a secure G-tube be considered when EN is expected to be necessary for more than 4 weeks.[120] Many acute rehabilitation hospitals and long-term care facilities require a more secure type of enteral access before the patient is transferred. However, a G-tube or PEG tube does not prevent complications from aspirations of oral pharyngeal secretions, and placement carries some risk; therefore, selection of appropriate candidates for G-tube placement is important.

The FOOD trial reported that early EN was associated with an absolute reduction in risk of death of 5.8% and a reduction in death and poor outcome of 1.2%; however, in stroke patients with dysphagia, early PEG placement/feeding was associated with increased risk of death or poor outcome compared with nasogastric feedings.[121]

Conversely, Geeganage and colleagues reviewed 33 studies with 6779 participants from the Cochrane Library stroke group and reported that data were insufficient to make specific recommendations on the effects of swallow therapy, feeding, and nutrition support on functional outcome and death in patients with dysphagia following stroke. The review reported that, compared with G-tube feeding, nasogastric feeding reduced treatment failures and GI bleeding, and nasogastric feeding had higher nutrition delivery for long-term therapy. Nutritional supplementation was associated with fewer pressure sores and increased energy and protein intake.[122]

Limited physical activity, dysphagia, aspiration, constipation, adverse effects of anticholinergic drugs, depression, and skin breakdown all contribute to nutrition complications in the stroke population. Jiang et al investigated risk factors that predicted short-term mortality in poststroke patients with persistent dysphagia following a PEG placement.[123] The 3 risk factors associated with increased risk for mortality for PEG insertion were age, American Society of Anesthesia score, and pre–PEG insertion serum albumin levels.[123] Jiang and colleagues suggest that assessment of patients for these 3 risk factors could help identify patients likely to survive more than 3 months following a PEG insertion.[123]

Healthcare providers should inform patients and family members that the G-tube or PEG tube is not necessarily a permanent form of feeding access and can be easily removed when dysphagia resolves.[124,125] See Chapter 12 for additional information on enteral access devices.

Nutrition Requirements

Energy requirements of stroke patients may vary depending on whether the acute stroke is ischemic or hemorrhagic. IC is the gold standard for determining the energy requirements.[3] No equation has been validated to precisely determine the energy expenditure for the stoke population, and estimating the degree of hypermetabolism following stroke remains controversial.

Finestone and colleagues prospectively evaluated 91 first-event ischemic and hemorrhagic stroke patients, comparing measured and estimated energy requirements of this population.[126] On average, the measured energy expenditure was 107% to 114% above the energy requirement estimated by the Harris-Benedict equation and did not significantly change over a 90-day period. Based on their findings, the authors concluded that the stroke patient population shows a lack of a hypermetabolic response following injury. Their measurements did not significantly vary between ischemic and hemorrhagic stroke patients, but it should be noted that 84% of patients studied had ischemic stroke and SAH patients were excluded.[126]

Bardutzky also reported a lack of hypermetabolism following a stroke and found that measured energy expenditure closely correlated to estimates using the Harris-Benedict equation.[127] Nagano et al compared several predictive equations in patients with ischemic stroke and reported the Harris-Benedict equation provided the prediction closest to energy expenditure measured by IC.[128]

Two studies suggest that hemorrhagic stroke patients elicit a more hypermetabolic response than those with ischemic stroke.[129,130] Esper et al measured energy expenditure in 14 nontraumatic intracerebral, intraventricular, and SAH patients who exhibited a hypermetabolic response. The median measured energy expenditure was 126% (range: 101% to 170%) above the estimate from the Harris-Benedict equation.[129] Frankenfield and associates compared energy expenditures of 30 ischemic stroke, 36 hemorrhagic stroke, and 32 TBI patients.[130] The ischemic stroke population was the least hypermetabolic, likely because these patients had a lower incidence of fever and lower average body temperature. The hemorrhagic stroke population exhibited a hypermetabolic state with measurements similar to those of the TBI population. Both stroke types were accurately predicted by the Penn State equation 72% of the time.[130,131] See Chapter 2 for additional information on the Penn State equation.

Kasuya et al reported severe hypermetabolism in 36 patients following SAH, with measured energy expenditures ranging from 139% ± 32% to 198% ± 78% of the resting energy expenditure predicted by the Harris-Benedict equation.[132] The highest energy needs of these SAH patients occurred at Day 10 following injury (coinciding with the typical apex of vasospasm risk).[132] Badjatia and coauthors prospectively observed 229 patients following SAH.[133] They defined the inflammatory-mediated hypercatabolic response following SAH as a ratio of C-reactive protein to transthyretin (prealbumin).[133] This ratio correlated with a negative nitrogen balance and overall poor outcome at 3 months. In this cohort, 53 patients (23%) developed hospital-acquired infections following SAH.[133] Lower energy intake (less than 11.3 kcal/kg/d; P = 0.02) and greater negative nitrogen balance (more than –8.8 g/d; P = 0.001) were both associated with the development of hospital-acquired infections in these patients.

Based on available data, the energy requirements following an ischemic stroke are likely close to estimated basal metabolic needs as determined by the Harris-Benedict equation or Penn State equation. Data suggest that patients with hemorrhagic stroke, especially SAH, have elevated energy needs as compared with estimates of basal metabolic requirements.

Energy needs will change as the patient recovers and will reflect whether the patient participates in rehabilitation physical therapy or remains with limited physical activity. Nutrition support should be reassessed and adjusted to minimize excessive or unnecessary weight gain or weight loss, prevent micronutrient and macronutrient deficiencies, and address any skin breakdown that occurred following the stroke. Use of a nutrition-focused physical examination can help identify any new onset of malnutrition.

Protein requirements should be determined by assessing the patient's prestroke nutrition status and renal and liver function immediately following the stroke. The recommended protein goals range from 1 to 1.5 g/kg/d.[134] Prealbumin and albumin often decline secondary to brain injury as an acute-phase response; therefore, neither prealbumin nor albumin accurately assesses nutrition status in the immediate poststroke and critically ill patient.[3] Evidence of protein-energy malnutrition, recent weight loss, or wounds or skin breakdown indicate a higher protein requirement. Patients requiring hemodialysis or continuous renal replacement therapy also have increased protein requirements.[3,135] Clinicians should monitor ongoing changes in protein requirements and adjust the protein in feedings accordingly, until the patient consumes nutritionally adequate oral intake.

Refeeding syndrome, a rapid depletion of serum potassium, magnesium, and phosphorus, can occur in the stroke population when nutrition support, specifically carbohydrates, is initiated.[136] This phenomenon most frequently occurs after aggressive EN or PN is initiated following a hypermetabolic injury, after prolonged underfeeding, and in chronically malnourished or alcoholic patients. The depleted serum electrolytes, especially phosphorus, make it difficult to wean the patient from the ventilator. Severe hypokalemia and hypomagnesemia can result in deleterious cardiac, GI, and mental status changes. Frequent initial electrolyte monitoring and aggressive thiamin and electrolyte replacement protocols help avoid refeeding syndrome in the critically ill stroke population.[136]

Most stroke patients tolerate a standard polymeric enteral formula with 1 to 1.5 kcal/mL unless malabsorption or a GI disease was present prior to the stroke.[134] de Aguilar-Nascimento and associates reported that, compared with standard casein protein formulas, a whey protein formula may contribute to decreased inflammation following an ischemic stroke.[137]

If hypernatremia protocols aim for serum sodium ranges of 140 to 150 mEq/L to minimize cerebral edema, a concentrated enteral formula with 1.5 to 2 kcal/mL may be appropriate to provide less free water. Once the free-water restriction is liberated, modifying the enteral formula to a more-dilute feeding of 1.2 to 1.5 kcal/mL provides more free water continuously without the need for large bolus free-water administration, which can contribute to GI intolerance. To avoid dehydration, more-dilute formulas with 0.8 to 1.2 kcal/mL can meet all necessary daily free-water needs for patients who require long-term EN.

Clinicians should assess whether patients receive the Recommended Daily Intake (RDI) of vitamins/minerals from EN. A multivitamin with minerals can be given daily if the total volume of enteral formula does not provide 100% of the RDI. Crushable multivitamin-multimineral tablets often provide more vitamins and minerals than prepackaged liquid preparations. Supplements of individual micronutrients may be appropriate if they are not included in the EN regimen or if patients experience excessive losses.

The VITATOPS study evaluated 8164 patients and concluded that daily folic acid and vitamin B_6 and B_{12} supplements did not reduce the recurrence of an ischemic stroke.[1] In a meta-analysis of 18 trials with 57,143 individuals, Zhang and colleagues also found that high-dose B vitamin supplementation was not associated with a lower risk of stroke.[138,139] Further studies are needed to provide evidence about high-dose vitamin/mineral therapies and their effect on secondary stroke prevention.

Practice Scenario 22-2 describes a nutrition support regimen that meets the needs of a patient with dysphagia after an ischemic stroke.[126,127,134]

Practice Scenario 22-2

Question: What is the appropriate nutrition support regimen for a patient with dysphagia following an ischemic stroke?

Scenario: A 64-year-old woman (weight, 63 kg; height, 165 cm) presented to the emergency department with a potential stroke 8 hours after her first symptoms of a sudden fall, right-side weakness, facial droop, and slurred speech. Computed tomography of the head revealed left middle cerebral artery thrombus and was negative for hemorrhage. The patient did not receive tissue plasminogen activator (tPA) in the emergency department because the timing was beyond the window when tPA provides benefit. Her past medical history included chronic obstructive pulmonary disease (COPD), hypertension, hyperlipidemia, and cataracts. Because of her history of COPD, the patient could not be extubated from mechanical ventilation for 8 days after a thrombectomy. She had residual weakness and slurred speech, and she failed a bedside swallow evaluation after extubation. Laboratory data included blood glucose, 122 mg/dL, and albumin, 3.3g/dL.

Intervention: A nutrition support consult was ordered. A nasal feeding tube was placed on Day 2 in the intensive care unit. Indirect calorimetry (IC) indicated energy expenditure of 1390 kcal/d. A standard polymeric enteral formula (1.2 kcal/mL and 60 g protein per liter) was ordered to be adminstered at 50 mL/h to provide 1440 kcal/d and 72 g protein per day. Medications were administered enterally. Once maintenance intravenous fluids were stopped, free water was supplemented at 200 mL 4 times daily.

Answer: Enteral nutrition via a nasoenteric feeding tube with energy requirement directed by IC is appropriate in this scenario. The patient's protein needs were 63 to 95 g/d (1 to 1.5 g/kg/d).[126,127,134]

Rationale: When a patient has had a stroke and experiences dysphagia that prevents oral intake, the nutrition support regimen must meet the patient's needs for energy, protein, micronutrients, and fluids.

Dysphagia and Oral Intake

Not all stroke patients demonstrate dysphagia severe enough to necessitate EN. Dysphagia can present as oropharyngeal or esophageal dysfunction, and, therefore, proper diagnosis and management are critical to avoid aspiration, malnutrition, and acute and chronic dehydration. A speech and language pathologist can determine the dysphagia etiology and recommend appropriate strategies to avoid or minimize aspiration. These therapists and other qualified clinicians should teach patients and caregivers about interventions and swallowing techniques and can recommend a variety of dysphagia diets to be used as the patient recovers or transitions off EN.

The National Dysphagia Diet, published in 2002 by the American Dietetic Association, defined a standardized terminology for specific dietary texture modifications and liquid viscosities.[140] The National Dysphagia Diet has 3 levels of modified diets and 4 levels of liquid viscosity. The level 1 diet is pureed (homogenous, very cohesive, and pudding-like in texture, requiring very little chewing ability). The level 2 diet is mechanically altered (cohesive, moist, semisolid foods, requiring some chewing) and is followed by the advanced level 3 diet (soft foods that require more chewing).[140] Liquid consistencies are spoon-thick viscous, honey-thick viscous, nectar-like viscous, and thin liquids.[141] Once cleared to consume oral nutrition, the patient with the most severe dysphagia initiates the level 1 diet, progresses toward levels 2 and 3, and eventually resumes a regular diet if the dysphagia has resolved.

Nutrition in Acute Neurologic Injury Rehabilitation

Preadmission Considerations

Early initiation of rehabilitation after acute neurologic injury is cost effective and has significant effects on outcome measures and lifetime care costs for patients with stroke or TBI.[142,143] Patients with SCI, TBI, or stroke who qualify for acute rehabilitation are transferred within the first few weeks following the initial injury. Acute rehabilitation facilities accept patients who have the potential to respond to intensive therapy targeting progress toward activities of daily living. Patients participate in multiple sessions of physical therapy, occupational therapy, and, if applicable, speech and language therapy for 3 to 6 hours per day for a 2- to 6-week period. Interdisciplinary teams of therapists, nurses, physicians, and pharmacists work closely with families and patients to set functional recovery goals.

Baseline cognitive and physical function affects decisions on medications and nutrition care regimens employed in the acute rehabilitation period. Well-designed studies of nutrition requirements during this transition period are needed. As patients make progress, their energy requirements, supplement needs, routes of nutrition intake, and medications continually evolve. Risks of malnutrition are affected by preinjury nutrition status, the effectiveness of nutrition during acute care, and any cognitive and physical limitations associated with the neurologic injury.

Baseline Nutrition Status on Admission

On admission to the acute rehabilitation facility, the patient's baseline weight, BMI, and standard nutrition-related laboratory data must be assessed and documented.[144] Liver function tests are important because medications used in rehabilita-

tion may exacerbate preexisting inflammation from hepatitis or other injury mechanisms. Medications and the nutrition history should be examined for potential confounding of nutrition recommendations during the rehabilitation program (Table 22-3).[14,18,42,43,120,145] Effective nutrition strategies require collaborative discussions between dietitians and other

TABLE 22-3 Medication Considerations in Long-Term and Acute Care Rehabilitation

Medication Type or Name	Indication	Nutrition Considerations
Atypical antipsychotics (quetiapine)	Agitation/aggression	Weight gain; increased appetite; metabolic changes in glucose, triglycerides, and cholesterol; dysphagia; drug interaction with erythromycin; potential for prolonged QT interval
Amantadine	Cognitive stimulation	Altered GI motility, appetite reduction; avoid oral potassium supplements; may decrease GI stimulation response to erythromycin
Bromocriptine	Cognitive stimulation	Altered GI motility; appetite reduction; elevated AST, ALT, and alkaline phosphatase levels
Levodopa/carbidopa	Cognitive stimulation	Drug interactions: vitamin B_6 stimulation of carbidopa metabolism; metoclopramide; iron
Methylphenidate	Cognitive stimulation/attention	Decreased appetite; weight loss; herbal supplement interactions
Donepezil	Attention/memory	Altered GI motility; decreased appetite; weight loss
Atomoxetine	Attention	Altered GI motility; weight loss; decreased appetite
Lisdexamfetamine	Attention	Altered GI motility; weight loss; decreased appetite; drug interactions with potassium citrate, magnesium supplements; sodium bicarbonate; caffeine; and herbal supplements
Selective serotonin reuptake inhibitors (sertraline, citalopram)	Depression	Hyponatremia; SIAD; altered GI motility; may cause hepatoxicity; interactions with multiple herbal supplements, metoclopramide, erythromycin
Melatonin	Sleep	May alter glucose tolerance
Trazodone	Sleep	Hyponatremia; SIAD; hepatoxicity; altered GI motility; interactions with erythromycin, chondroitin, ω-3 supplements, and multiple herbal supplements
Topiramate	Headache	Metabolic acidosis; hypokalemia; hyperammonemic encephalopathy; decreased appetite; weight loss; altered GI motility; taste changes; interactions with metoclopramide, herbal supplements
Baclofen (oral/intrathecal routes available)	Spasticity	Altered GI motility; weight gain; interactions with magnesium citrate, metoclopramide, and herbal supplements
Tizanidine	Spasticity	Constipation; elevated AST/ALT levels; vomiting; interactions with caffeine, herbal supplements, and metoclopramide
Dantrolene	Spasticity	Hepatoxicity; nausea; diarrhea; interactions with herbal supplements, metoclopramide
Benzodiazepines (diazepam, clonazepam)	Spasticity	Altered GI motility; elevated AST/ALT levels; appetite changes; interactions with metoclopramide, herbal supplements
Gabapentin	Neuropathic pain; spasticity	Altered GI motility; weight gain; interactions with iron supplements, magnesium, herbal supplements, and metoclopramide
Botulinum toxin	Spasticity	Dysphagia; nausea; interaction with magnesium
Warfarin	Stroke guidelines,[120] deep vein thrombosis	Interactions with erythromycin, orlistat, coenzyme Q, fish oils, herbal supplements, and vitamin K from nutritional formula, oral supplements, and oral diet components

ALT, alanine transaminase; AST, aspartate transaminase; GI, gastrointestinal; SIAD, syndrome of inappropriate antidiuresis.
Source: Data are from references 14, 18, 42, 43, 120, and 145.

members of the interdisciplinary team. Therapists are key partners in mobilizing patients to avoid decubiti development, introduce physical activities to stimulate hunger, and educate patients on methods to restore oral intake when possible. Maintaining communication among team members facilitates optimal nutrition intake as the patient progresses throughout the rehabilitation program.

Nutrition Goals During Acute Rehabilitation

Nutrition adequacy as a predictive component affecting rehabilitation outcomes is not routinely captured in database models used in research.[146,147] Traditional endpoints such as weight gain, improved anthropometrics, or metabolic improvements are not readily accessible in these data sets. Functional independence measures of motor and comprehension progress during rehabilitation include feeding scores. Recently, data from the Traumatic Brain Injury Model Systems National Database were retrospectively examined to create a prognostic model for rehabilitation admission factors affecting discharge destination.[147] Feeding and bowel and bladder management scores were significantly lower in participants discharged to another institution compared with those returning to a private residence. Although feeding did not become a final predictive factor in the proposed model, these results highlight the importance of addressing nutrition goals throughout the acute rehabilitation stay.[148]

Energy goals should be adjusted during rehabilitation to create a balanced postinjury diet that maintains muscle mass and allows the patient to participate in activities of daily living once transferred to home. Measurement of energy expenditure by IC is not routinely done in acute rehabilitation. Predictive equations have not been validated in TBI, stroke, and SCI patients participating in acute rehabilitation.

In ventilator-dependent SCI patients, multiplying the estimated energy requirement calculated from the Harris-Benedict equation by an activity factor of 1.1 and a stress factor of 1.2 provided a strong correlation between measured and predicted energy expenditures.[149] Acute SCI and TBI patients followed over a 3-week inpatient period (nonrehabilitation) showed marked differences in energy and nitrogen balance.[77] Intake of less than 20 nonprotein kcal/kg/d and mean protein intakes less than 1 g/kg/d resulted in positive energy balance for patients with SCIs, but nitrogen balance remained negative. In contrast, TBI patients fed more than 25 nonprotein kcal/kg/d and mean protein intakes greater than 1 g/kg/d were in negative energy and nitrogen balance.[77] These data demonstrate the persistent risk of muscle loss in both SCI and TBI patients as well as a stark difference in the energy demands between these populations.

Total daily energy expenditure after SCI is reduced by 12% to 54%, depending on injury level, activity, and lean body mass.[93] Mean energy expenditures of 22.7 kcal/kg/d and 27.9 kcal/kg/d were measured in tetraplegic and paraplegic rehabilitation patients, respectively.[78] Patients gained 1.7 kg/wk when the diet was not controlled and more than 1700 kcal/d were consumed.

Recently, older SCI subjects in acute rehabilitation reported energy intakes higher than 1900 kcal/d and protein intake greater than 70g/d.[150] Nutrition intake was identified as a modifiable risk factor for obesity-related complications affecting this population.[150] This study also reported energy and protein intake in patients with TBI, new onset stroke, and Parkinson's disease during acute rehabilitation. Energy intake was greater than 1500 kcal/d for individuals with TBI and 1400 kcal/d for those who had a stroke and for patients with Parkinson's disease. Protein intake was greater than 61 g/d for patients with TBI and greater than 55 g/d for the stroke and Parkinson's disease patients. Subjects in the SCI group were younger than those in the TBI, stroke, or Parkinson's disease groups and were identified as the group at highest risk for overeating.[150]

Although overeating creates risks for SCI patients, poor intake may increase the risk of pressure ulcers. When pressure ulcer incidence was examined in SCI patients, a higher percentage of underweight patients developed pressure ulcers compared to healthy weight, overweight or obese patients with SCI.[151] Monitoring weekly weight changes throughout the rehabilitation program is useful in guiding adjustments in energy requirements.

When selecting enteral formula for patients in acute rehabilitation, nutrition support clinicians should consider the patient's higher demand for protein replacement; products designed to delivery higher protein content may be preferable. The evidence on specialized enteral formulas, branched-chain amino acids, glutamine, arginine, and fish oil supplements is insufficient to support routine use of these products during acute rehabilitation of patients with neurologic injuries.

Limited studies in neurologic patients during acute rehabilitation suggest that total energy intake should be controlled.[150] Using admission body weights for SCI, TBI, stroke, and Parkinson's disease patients, average energy intake ranged between 19.2 and 24.4 kcal/kg.[150] Macronutrient formulation tolerance may be monitored by routine testing of blood chemistries, prealbumin, hepatic function, and triglycerides.

Special Considerations

Hormonal Issues

Pituitary dysfunction has the potential to significantly affect the metabolic tolerance and traditional monitoring parameters of the nutrition regimen.[152] The growth hormone–IGF-1 system is altered following brain injury.[23,24] Dysfunction of sodium homeostasis is common. Hypothyroidism is a common finding in patients with TBI.[35-37] Thyroid replacement, growth hormone, and sodium modulators may affect patients' responses to a nutrition regimen and the monitoring of that regimen.

Protein Loss

Continued protein losses up to 2 months' postinjury with negative nitrogen balances have been reported in SCI patients.[153] Collecting urine to measure nitrogen loss in patients with SCI can be a challenge unless catheters are in place. Incontinence episodes may also complicate assessment of urinary nitrogen loss in patients with other types of neurologic injuries. Serial anthropometrics or body mass analysis may be informative options for assessing protein dosing adequacy and muscle maintenance for some patients.

Formula Efficacy and Gastrointestinal Tolerance

The assessment of formula effectiveness must include careful examination of GI intolerance, which can significantly limit participation in physical therapy and predispose patients to other complications.

Micronutrient Deficiencies

Micronutrient deficiencies reported in patients with neurologic injuries include folic acid, zinc, selenium and, most recently, vitamin D.[24,154,155] Reduced concentrations in vitamin D have been reported in SCI and TBI patients in acute and outpatient rehabilitation settings.[156,157] In 101 acute rehabilitation patients, 77% were deficient in vitamin D at admission.[156] In addition to osteopenia, muscle weakness, and impaired physical function, vitamin D deficiencies were associated with higher in-hospital mortality in neurocritical care patients.[158]

Vitamin D may act as a "neurosteroid," and replacement should be considered for acute rehabilitation patients with neurologic injuries.[155] Patients with serum 25-hydroxyvitamin D concentrations below 20 ng/mL should be treated with 6000 IU cholecalciferol daily or 50,000 IU once a week for 8 weeks to achieve a serum 25-hydroxy vitamin D level greater than 30 ng/mL.[159] Once stabilized, patients should receive maintenance cholecalciferol doses of 1500 to 2000 IU/d.[159]

Weight Management

The long-term nutrition goal for patients with neurologic injury is to provide a diet optimized for weight management given the projected activity level of the patient.[160] Patients with SCI and stroke have reported changes in muscle mass when diets are not modified. In a multicenter longitudinal study, 5 years after discharge from acute inpatient rehabilitation, 56% to 75% of SCI patients were classified as overweight or obese.[161,162] Obesity increases the risks of medical complications, rehospitalization, and poor functional outcomes.[150] Educating patients and caregivers about dietary modification strategies to include more protein, less fat, and controlled carbohydrates may help reduce long-term metabolic complications.

Fluid Therapy

Fluid therapy can be a unique challenge in the acute rehabilitation population. Independent intake goals for oral ingestion of electrolyte water products, protein shakes, and normal food allow the patient to manage daily fluid totals. After patients have a stroke or TBI, challenges with movement and memory may significantly affect independent intake. Patients are at risk for dehydration, and administration of fluid bolus by nursing is often required. Dehydration is exacerbated by activities or infections as well as limited oral intake. If dehydration is not addressed, patients are at increased risk of renal insults when

antibiotics (eg, vancomycin, penicillin), nonsteroidal pain medications, or diuretics are administered. Dosing adjustments for maintenance medications may also be required to prevent dehydration.

Accurate fluid monitoring may be difficult because the collection and measurement of urine output are often imprecise in the acute rehabilitation setting. Medical complications of neurologic injury include urinary retention, constipation, and diarrhea.[74,82,163] When setting fluid therapy goals, clinicians should consider the patient's functional status for bladder and bowel. As patient independence increases, normalizing routines for bladder and bowel emptying is encouraged, but that can make the collection of urine for measurement impractical. Nonambulatory patients may have poor bladder control and require incontinence pads. Urinalysis results for specific gravity and sodium are useful for guiding fluid intake adjustments. This assessment becomes particularly important when patients receive desmopressin for sodium management following TBI.[22,36] Hypotension or dizziness from poor fluid management may increase fall risks in this predisposed patient population.

Dysphagia

Nutrition-related strategies are affected by the patient's swallowing status and goals for achieving improvement in activities of daily living. Patients with higher levels of SCI are at greater risk of dysphagia complications and may experience altered taste, smell, or appetite.[164] Gastrostomy devices may be required to achieve nutrition goals until patients stabilize effective oral intake. Enteral formulations may be delivered via existing PEG tubes in many cases, and clinicians deciding whether to remove these devices will consider return of swallowing skills during or following acute rehabilitation.[165] Bolus dosing is often used during rehabilitation and avoids the use of cumbersome poles that affect ambulation. In a prospective multicenter observational study of patients with severe TBI, those with weight loss at 3 months after injury and continued PEG requirements for feeding were at increased risk of complications and poor outcome independent of injury severity.[166]

Optimally, patients progress to oral diets. However, they may still require energy and protein supplements for some time. Dysphagia assessments and training by speech and language therapists facilitate patients' advancement to oral diets. Despite a report that dysphagia diets did not improve intake compared with regular diets following acute stroke, neurologic rehabilitation patients must be cautiously assessed before regular diets are introduced.[167] Once swallowing tests confirm that an oral diet can be safely introduced, clinicians can design formal progress plans to guide individualized recovery of eating skills.

Medications and Dietary Supplements

Use of probiotics, stool softeners, pain medications, cognitive stimulants, anticoagulants, mood modulators, and chronic maintenance medications creates complex medication regimens for neurologically impaired patients.[163,168] Preinjury and rehabilitation admission medications should be routinely reviewed for potential interactions with nutrition treatment goals and monitoring endpoints.

Clinicians should ask patients and families to identify any nonprescription medications or herbal supplements used by the patient, because these products may potentially interact with prescription medications used following neurologic injury. Information on drug-herbal interactions is available from the National Center for Complementary and Integrative Health,[169] MedlinePlus from the National Library of Medicine,[170] and pharmacy medication resources. See Chapter 19 for more information and resources on dietary supplements.

Appetite stimulants (eg, megestrol, dronabinol, mirtazapine, cyproheptadine) should only be recommended after review for potential drug interactions.

Use of methylene blue for assessment of aspiration risks with EN is no longer recommended. If it is used, clinicians must be aware that some routine medications have serious interactions with this agent.

Chronic Neurologic Diseases

Inpatient nutrition therapy for patients with chronic neurologic diseases presents considerable challenges. Patients may be more prone to having dysphagia, nutrition deficiencies, and drug-nutrient interactions. Special care is needed when assessing patients with these disease states.

Amyotrophic Lateral Sclerosis

ALS (also known as *Lou Gehrig's disease*) is a rapidly progressing, degenerative motor neuron disease that results in significant muscle weakness and atrophy.

Weight Loss and Malnutrition

Approximately 75% of patients with ALS will experience bulbar involvement, which includes the muscles that control speech, swallowing, and chewing and can lead to substantial weight loss. Causes of weight loss in patients with ALS include dysphagia, upper limb motor difficulties, weakness of tongue and other oropharyngeal muscles, loss of appetite, dyspnea, depression, and hypermetabolism.[171-174] Malnutrition is an independent prognostic factor of ALS survival, with an 8-fold increase in risk of death when the patient is of poor nutrition status.[175-177] Malnutrition is defined as greater than 10% loss of body weight during the course of illness, in conjunction with BMI less than 18 for adults between the ages of 18 and 65 years or BMI less than 20 for patients older than 65 years.[178] Approximately 16% to 53% of patients with ALS are malnourished.[179,180] With every weight loss of 5% from the time of diagnoses, there is a twofold increase in mortality.[172] Early nutrition intervention in patients with ALS has been shown to maintain good nutrition status for a longer period of time.[181]

Dysphagia

An estimated 81% of patients with ALS experience dysphagia and may require modified diet textures and thickened liquids.[177,178] Patients may be unable to meet their nutrient needs via diet alone, and many require EN. EN administered by PEG tubes often replaces or augments an oral diet, and PEG tube placement earlier in the disease process is more effective in preserving nutrition status for a longer period of time.[171,178,182] The American Academy of Neurology ALS practice parameters recommend PEG tube placement while forced vital capacity is more than 50% of predicted value or when the patient has dysphagia or a BMI less than 20 or loses 5% to 10% of usual body weight.[183]

Energy and Protein Requirements

When determining nutrition needs, the clinician should assess the stage of progression of ALS, because patients initially are in energy balance.[173] As ALS progresses, the resting metabolic rate increases, and patients typically experience an energy deficit.[173] The Mifflin–St. Jeor and Harris-Benedict equations have been shown to be the most accurate methods to estimate energy needs, with the Harris-Benedict equation being the most practical.[173] Some research supports increasing the calculated resting energy expenditure by 10% when determining energy needs for patients with ALS.[173,178] Genton and colleagues recommend estimating energy needs to be 120% greater than basal energy expenditure measured by IC, and 130% greater than energy requirements predicted by the Harris-Benedict equation.[180] As patients with ALS lose muscle mass, the ratio of organ mass to muscle mass increases, which increases the amount of energy per kg fat-free mass.[178] Because of these changes, patients with ALS may require 34 to 35 kcal/kg/d.[178] Protein requirements for this patient population range from 0.8 to 1.2 g/kg/d.[172,183]

Approximately 50% of patients with ALS are hypermetabolic; the reason for the hypermetabolism is unknown.[174,178] Theoretically, with the loss and atrophy of muscle mass, reduced physical activity, and denervation, the ALS patient should have a reduced metabolic demand, but this has not been demonstrated.[178] Several theories have been proposed to explain why this patient population is hypermetabolic, including variations of increased work of both skeletal and respiratory muscles because of muscle loss or increased spasticity, and mitochondrial dysfunctions.[174,178]

Micronutrient Requirements

The role of antioxidants and other micronutrients in ALS is not fully understood, although several studies have been done. Creatine monohydrate, coenzyme Q_{10}, selenium, and vitamins C, E, and D have been studied in relation to slowing the progression of ALS, but no large-scale studies have reported definitive benefits. At this time, recommendations cannot be made regarding micronutrient supplementation in patients with ALS.[178,183]

Epilepsy/Seizures

The ketogenic diet—which has been well documented as a therapy for controlling seizures in the pediatric population—is being used with increasing frequency and success in the adult population.[184-188] The exact antiepileptic mechanism of action of the ketogenic diet is unknown. Several theories suggest it is related to changes in the nerve cell lipid membranes or neurotransmitter production.[189]

Specific energy needs are not addressed in the literature on epilepsy. However, to decrease frequency of seizures, a 4:1 ratio of fat to carbohydrate and protein is recommended; this ratio can be titrated down as the disease state stabilizes.[184,190]

Many medications contain carbohydrates, which must be considered as dietary goals for carbohydrate intake are set. See Table 22-4 for a list of ingredients with carbohydrates.[191]

A modified Atkins diet (a 1:1 ratio fat to protein and carbohydrate) can be used once a patient's seizure frequency is more stable. The modified Atkins diet has shown to reduce seizures in adult and adolescent patients with drug-resistant epilepsy.[187]

Compliance with the ketogenic and modified Atkins diets by patients who can take an oral diet is low because the diets are unpalatable and rigid.[187,192] Extreme diet modifications should be used in conjunction with anticonvulsant therapy prescribed by the medical team.

Antiepileptic therapy can increase vitamin D elimination; however, a study compared patients with epilepsy and those without the disease, and both groups had equally low levels of vitamin D.[193] Recommendations for micronutrient supplementation in adults who are on the ketogenic diet would be premature because of the lack of studies that address this subject. Only a limited number of case reports have been published

TABLE 22-4 Carbohydrate and Noncarbohydrate Ingredients

Carbohydrate ingredients:
- Glycerin
- Maltodextrin
- Magnasweet
- Organic acids: ascorbic acid, citric acid, lactic acid
- Propylene glycol
- Sugars: dextrose, fructose, glucose, lactose, sucrose, sugar, palm sugar, agave nectar, cane syrup, cane juice, corn syrup, honey
- Sugar alcohols: erythritol, isomalt, glycerol, mannitol, maltitol, sorbitol, xylitol
- Starches: cornstarch, hydrogenated starch hydrolysates (HSH), pregelatinized starch, sodium starch glycolate

Noncarbohydrate ingredients:
- Asulfamine potassium (AceK)
- Aspartame
- Carboxymethylcellulose
- Cellulose
- Hydroxymethylcellulose
- Magnesium stearate
- Microcrystalline cellulose
- Polyethylene glycol
- Saccharine
- Superose
- Stevia (rebiana)

Source: Adapted with permission from reference 191: The Charlie Foundation for Ketogenic Therapies. Carb/non-carb ingredients. http://www.charliefoundation .org/resources-tools/resources-3/low-carb/item/1137-carbohydrate-non -carbohydrate-ingredients. Copyright ©2016 The Charlie Foundation.

about this patient population. More research is needed before definitive nutrition recommendations can be made.

See Practice Scenario 22-3 for discussion of the use of EN for an adult patient with intractable seizures.[172–176,187,188,190,192,194–198]

Practice Scenario 22-3

Question: How can the ketogenic diet (via enteral formula) be used as a therapy for intractable seizures?

Scenario: A 27-year-old male patient is admitted from an outside hospital with refractory generalized convulsive status epilepticus. He is on mechanical ventilation and has been in a pentobarbital coma for nearly 2 weeks, in addition to receiving multiple antiepileptic drugs. The cause of seizures is still being investigated; however, in the meantime, the clinical team would like to try using the ketogenic diet to decrease the frequency of seizures.

Intervention: The physician adjusts intake of pentobarbital and dextrose-containing medications (including propofol, which contains glycerol), and the patient is to be put on a 48-hour fast. The following initial laboratory tests are done:
- Baseline beta-hydroxybutyrate level
- Fasting lipid panel
- Aspartate transaminase (AST)/alanine transaminase (ALT)
- Prealbumin
- C-reactive protein
- Vitamin C
- Zinc
- 25-hydroxyvitamin D
- Carnitine (total, acyl)
- Lactic acid
- Pyruvic acid

Triglyceride and cholesterol levels are normal, indicating that the high-fat ketogenic diet will not pose undue risk of cardiovascular complications or pancreatitis. The clinicians evaluate the patient's energy needs, because the provision of protein will be deficient on this diet. They initiate a ketogenic enteral formula with a 4:1 ratio of fat to protein and carbohydrate and monitor the following laboratory test results: beta-hydroxybutyrate daily, antiepileptic drug levels every other day, and glucose every 4 hours. Lipid levels and a liver panel are checked weekly.

Answer: A ketogenic enteral formula can be considered in refractory seizure disorder and should be monitored for safety and efficacy after initiation.

Rationale: Although the mechanism by which seizures are controlled with the ketogenic diet is largely unknown, there are several theories. One common theory suggests that the increase in ketones and decrease in glucose levels in the brain increases γ-aminobutyric acid uptake, which then increases adenosine-mediated neuronal inhibition as well as activity of adenosine triphosphate (ATP)–sensitive potassium channels, thereby decreasing the firing of neurons as well as the excitability during seizures.[188]

Commonly used in children with well-documented success, the ketogenic diet has been emerging as an effective therapy for intractable seizures in adults; however, data are scarce on its use in the adult population.[172-176] The ketogenic diet is not commonly used in adults because of the difficulty of maintaining the 4:1 ratio of fat to protein and carbohydrate.[190,192,194] In addition, the diet is deficient in protein, and weight loss is common.[187,195]

The 4:1 ratio of fat to protein and carbohydrate is difficult to maintain, in part because many medications contain carbohydrates as fillers or suspensions (see Table 22-4). Prior to starting the patient on the diet, the medical team needs to strictly control dextrose-containing medications (including topical medications) and items (such as mouthwash) that provide carbohydrates. Administering additional carbohydrates may prevent ketosis.

Monitoring of laboratory test values is important to ensure that ketosis is achieved; the most accurate data are beta-hydroxybutyrate levels (as opposed to urine levels of ketones).[196] Monitoring laboratory values on a regular basis also ensures that the patient does not have emerging problems such as hepatic steatosis, pancreatitis, or critically low blood glucose levels.[196-198] Lower glucose levels should be tolerated while the patient is in ketosis. However, if glucose levels are less than 50 mg/dL, the patient should be given either 15 mL apple juice via the feeding tube or 50 mL of intravenous 5% dextrose in water at 100 mL/h. Lipid levels and a liver panel should be checked weekly. If triglyceride and cholesterol levels are above normal, the dietitian and medical team should reevaluate the safety of a high-fat diet to consider the patient's cardiac status and pancreatitis risk.

Parkinson's Disease

Information regarding macro- and micronutrient requirements in Parkinson's disease is limited. Several factors affect the nutrition status of patients with Parkinson's disease, and weight fluctuations are common in the population.[199] In the beginning stages of the disease, body weight increases, likely due to a decrease in motor function. As the disease progresses, weight loss occurs. It is theorized that the metabolic rate increases because of worsening rigidity and dyskinesia.[199] In addition to increased energy needs, individuals with Parkinson's disease may experience dysphagia, which can further impair nutrition status.[200] EN via a nasogastric tube is recommended for short-term nutrition support if the patient cannot meet nutrition needs by oral diet alone; PEG tubes are recommended when long-term EN is required.[200]

Common micronutrient deficiencies in Parkinson's disease have not been identified. Therefore, recommendations regarding supplementation cannot be made. One study suggested that vitamin D may be neuroprotective in Parkinson's disease, but the investigators did not make recommendations regarding vitamin D supplementation.[199]

The interaction between carbidopa/levodopa drug therapy and protein intake is well documented. The medication and protein compete for transport into the small intestine and blood-brain barrier.[199] Fluctuations in absorption of levodopa can affect motor function, and this drug therapy has been associated with decreased intake of protein.[199]

Constipation is common in patients with Parkinson's disease, and fiber and fluid intake are encouraged.[199] Higher levodopa requirements have been associated with increased constipation, and diet management is recommended.[199]

Other Neurologic Conditions

Other neurologic diseases, such as multiple sclerosis, muscular dystrophy, Alzheimer's disease, and dementia, can affect nutrition status. The literature on nutrient needs, micronutrient deficiencies, and unique metabolic issues in these conditions is limited. More research is clearly needed to determine how to optimize nutrition status and establish guidelines for medical nutrition therapy specific to these disease states.

Patients with chronic neurologic conditions may be more prone to malnutrition because of declining cognition, dysphagia, motor difficulties, and other comorbidities common to advancing neurologic diseases. Nutrition therapy is paramount to improving outcomes and, in some cases, decreasing mortality. See Chapter 36 for more information on dementia.

References

1. VITATOPS Trial Study Group. B vitamins in patients with recent transient ischaemic attack or stroke in the VITAmins TO Prevent Stroke (VITATOPS) trial: a randomised, double-blind, parallel, placebo-controlled trial. *Lancet Neurol.* 2010;9(9):855–865.
2. Poisson SN, Josephson SA. Quality measures in stroke. *Neurohospitalist.* 2011;1(2):71–77.
3. Taylor BE, McClave SA, Martindale RG, et al. Guidelines for the provision and assessment of nutrition support therapy in the adult critically ill patient: Society of Critical Care Medicine (SCCM) and American Society for Parenteral and Enteral Nutrition (A.S.P.E.N.). *Crit Care Med.* 2016;44(2):390–438.
4. Clifton GL, Robertson CS, Choi SC. Assessment of nutritional requirements of head-injured patients. *J Neurosurg.* 1986;64(6):895–901.
5. Quattrocchi KB, Issel BW, Miller CH, Frank EH, Wagner FC Jr. Impairment of helper T-cell function following severe head injury. *J Neurotrauma.* 1992;9(1):1–9.
6. Wolach B, Sazbon L, Gavrieli R, Broda A, Schlesinger M. Early immunological defects in comatose patients after acute brain injury. *J Neurosurg.* 2001;94(5):706–711.
7. Young B, Ott L, Twyman D, et al. The effect of nutritional support on outcome from severe head injury. *J Neurosurg.* 1987;67(5):668–676.
8. Carney N, Totten AM, O'Reilly C, et al. Guidelines for the management of severe traumatic brain injury. 4th ed. Brain Trauma Foundation. 2016. https://braintrauma.org/uploads/03/12/Guidelines_for_Management_of_Severe_TBI_4th_Edition.pdf.
9. Todd SR, Kozar RA, Moore FA. Nutrition support in adult trauma patients. *Nutr Clin Pract.* 2006;21(5):421–429.
10. Cerra FB. Hypermetabolism, organ failure, and metabolic support. *Surgery.* 1987;101(1):1–14.
11. Gentile LF, Cuenca AG, Efron PA, et al. Persistent inflammation and immunosuppression: a common syndrome and new horizon for surgical intensive care. *J Trauma Acute Care Surg.* 2012;72(6):1491–1501.
12. McClave SA, Heyland DK. The physiologic response and associated clinical benefits from provision of early enteral nutrition. *Nutr Clin Pract.* 2009;24(3):305–315.
13. Foley N, Marshall S, Pikul J, Salter K, Teasell R. Hypermetabolism following moderate to severe traumatic acute brain injury: a systematic review. *J Neurotrauma.* 2008;25(12):1415–1431.

14. Chiolero RL, Breitenstein E, Thorin D, et al. Effects of propranolol on resting metabolic rate after severe head injury. *Crit Care Med.* 1989;17(4):328–334.

15. Robertson CS, Clifton GL, Grossman RG. Oxygen utilization and cardiovascular function in head-injured patients. *Neurosurgery.* 1984;15(3):307–314.

16. Raurich JM, Ibanez J. Metabolic rate in severe head trauma. *JPEN J Parenter Enteral Med.* 1994;18(6):521–524.

17. Dempsey DT, Guenter P, Mullen JL, et al. Energy expenditure in acute trauma to the head with and without barbiturate therapy. *Surg Gynecol Obstet.* 1985;160(2):128–134.

18. McCall M, Jeejeebhoy K, Pencharz P, Moulton R. Effect of neuromuscular blockade on energy expenditure in patients with severe head injury. *JPEN J Parenter Enteral Med.* 2003;27(1):27–35.

19. Brain Trauma Foundation; American Association of Neurological Surgeons; Congress of Neurological Surgeons; Joint Section on Neurotrauma and Critical Care; Bratton SL, et al. Guidelines for the management of severe traumatic brain injury. XII. Nutrition. *J Neurotrauma.* 2007;24(Suppl 1):S77–S82.

20. Dickerson RN, Pitts SL, Maish GO, et al. A reappraisal of nitrogen requirements for patients with critical illness and trauma. *J Trauma Acute Care Surg.* 2012;73(3):549–557.

21. Chapple LA, Chapman MJ, Lange K, Deane AM, Heyland DK. Nutrition support practices in critically ill head-injured patients: a global perspective. *Crit Care (London).* 2016;20:6.

22. Cook AM, Peppard A, Magnuson B. Nutrition considerations in traumatic brain injury. *Nutr Clin Pract.* 2008;23(6):608–620.

23. Hatton J, Rapp RP, Kudsk KA, et al. Intravenous insulin-like growth factor-I (IGF-I) in moderate-to-severe head injury: a phase II safety and efficacy trial. *J Neurosurg.* 1997;86(5):779–786.

24. Young B, Ott L, Kasarskis E, et al. Zinc supplementation is associated with improved neurologic recovery rate and visceral protein levels of patients with severe closed head injury. *J Neurotrauma.* 1996;13(1):25–34.

25. Young AB, Ott LG, Beard D, Dempsey RJ, Tibbs PA, McClain CJ. The acute-phase response of the brain-injured patient. *J Neurosurg.* 1988;69(3):375–380.

26. Loan T. Metabolic/nutritional alterations of traumatic brain injury. *Nutrition (Burbank).* 1999;15(10):809–812.

27. Schneider M, Schneider HJ, Stalla GK. Anterior pituitary hormone abnormalities following traumatic brain injury. *J Neurotrauma.* 2005;22(9):937–946.

28. Perel P, Yanagawa T, Bunn F, Roberts I, Wentz R, Pierro A. Nutritional support for head-injured patients. *Cochrane Database Syst Rev.* 2006(4):CD001530.

29. Hartl R, Gerber LM, Ni Q, Ghajar J. Effect of early nutrition on deaths due to severe traumatic brain injury. *J Neurosurg.* 2008;109(1):50–56.

30. Wang X, Dong Y, Han X, Qi XQ, Huang CG, Hou LJ. Nutritional support for patients sustaining traumatic brain injury: a systematic review and meta-analysis of prospective studies. *PloS One.* 2013;8(3):e58838.

31. Azim A, Haider AA, Rhee P, et al. Early feeds not force feeds: enteral nutrition in traumatic brain injury. *J Trauma Acute Care Surg.* 2016.

32. Fraser JF, Stieg PE. Hyponatremia in the neurosurgical patient: epidemiology, pathophysiology, diagnosis, and management. *Neurosurgery.* 2006;59(2):222–229.

33. Anderson RJ, Chung HM, Kluge R, Schrier RW. Hyponatremia: a prospective analysis of its epidemiology and the pathogenetic role of vasopressin. *Ann Intern Med.* 1985;102(2):164–168.

34. Ellison DH, Berl T. Clinical practice. The syndrome of inappropriate antidiuresis. *N Engl J Med.* 2007;356(20):2064–2072.

35. Singh S, Bohn D, Carlotti AP, et al. Cerebral salt wasting: truths, fallacies, theories, and challenges. *Crit Care Med.* 2002;30(11):2575–2579.

36. Sterns RH. Disorders of plasma sodium—causes, consequences, and correction. *N Engl J Med.* 2015;372(1):55–65.

37. Qureshi S, Galiveeti S, Bichet DG, Roth J. Diabetes insipidus: celebrating a century of vasopressin therapy. *Endocrinology.* 2014;155(12):4605–4621.

38. Capatina C, Paluzzi A, Mitchell R, Karavitaki N. diabetes insipidus after traumatic brain injury. *J Clin Med.* 2015;4(7):1448–1462.

39. Rovlias A, Kotsou S. The influence of hyperglycemia on neurological outcome in patients with severe head injury. *Neurosurgery.* 2000;46(2):335–342.

40. Kinoshita K, Tanjoh K, Noda A, et al. Interleukin-8 production from human umbilical vein endothelial cells during brief hyperglycemia: the effect of tumor necrotic factor-alpha. *J Surg Res.* 2008;144(1):127–131.

41. Finfer S, Chittock DR, Su SY, et al. Intensive versus conventional glucose control in critically ill patients. *N Engl J Med.* 2009;360(13):1283–1297.

42. Magnuson B, Hatton J, Zweng TN, Young B. Pentobarbital coma in neurosurgical patients: nutrition considerations. *Nutr Clin Pract.* 1994;9(4):146–150.

43. 198. Doak KK, Haas CE, Dunnigan KJ, et al. Bioavailability of phenytoin acid and phenytoin sodium with enteral feedings. *Pharmacotherapy.* 1998;18(3):637–645.

44. Murry JS, Hoang DM, Barmparas G, et al. Prospective evaluation of early propranolol after traumatic brain injury. *J Surg Res.* 2016;200(1):221–226.

45. Mohseni S, Talving P, Thelin EP, et al. the effect of beta-blockade on survival after isolated severe traumatic brain injury. *World J Surg.* 2015;39(8):2076–2083.

46. Schroeppel TJ, Sharpe JP, Magnotti LJ, et al. Traumatic brain injury and beta-blockers: not all drugs are created equal. *J Trauma Acute Care Surg.* 2014;76(2):504–509.

47. Rabinstein AA, Benarroch EE. Treatment of paroxysmal sympathetic hyperactivity. *Curr Treat Opt Neurol.* 2008;10(2):151–157.

48. Osuka A, Uno T, Nakanishi J, et al. Energy expenditure in patients with severe head injury: controlled normothermia with sedation and neuromuscular blockade. *J Crit Care.* 2013;28(2):218. e219–213.

49. Mizock BA. Immunonutrition and critical illness: an update. *Nutrition (Burbank).* 2010;26(7–8):701–707.

50. Cherian L, Hlatky R, Robertson CS. Nitric oxide in traumatic brain injury. *Brain Pathol (Zurich).* 2004;14(2):195–201.

51. Jeter CB, Hergenroeder GW, Ward NH, Moore AN, Dash PK. Human traumatic brain injury alters circulating L-arginine and its metabolite levels: possible link to cerebral blood flow, extracellular matrix remodeling, and energy status. *J Neurotrauma.* 2012;29(1):119–127.

52. Duke T, South M, Stewart A. Activation of the L-arginine nitric oxide pathway in severe sepsis. *Arch Dis Child.* 1997;76(3):203–209.

53. Marik PE, Zaloga GP. Immunonutrition in critically ill patients: a systematic review and analysis of the literature. *Intens Care Med.* 2008;34(11):1980–1990.

54. Hall ED, Wang JA, Miller DM. Relationship of nitric oxide synthase induction to peroxynitrite–mediated oxidative damage during the first week after experimental traumatic brain injury. *Exp Neurol.* 2012;238(2):176–182.

55. Novak F, Heyland DK, Avenell A, Drover JW, Su X. Glutamine supplementation in serious illness: a systematic review of the evidence. *Crit Care Med.* 2002;30(9):2022–2029.

56. Rodas PC, Rooyackers O, Hebert C, Norberg A, Wernerman J. Glutamine and glutathione at ICU admission in relation to outcome. *Clin Sci (London).* 2012;122(12):591–597.

57. Heyland D, Muscedere J, Wischmeyer PE, et al. A randomized trial of glutamine and antioxidants in critically ill patients. *N Engl J Med.* 2013;368(16):1489–1497.

58. Nageli M, Fasshauer M, Sommerfeld J, et al. Prolonged continuous intravenous infusion of the dipeptide L-alanine- L-glutamine significantly increases plasma glutamine and alanine without elevating brain glutamate in patients with severe traumatic brain injury. *Crit Care (Lond)*. 2014;18(4):R139.

59. Crawford MA. The role of essential fatty acids in neural development: implications for perinatal nutrition. *Am J Clin Nutr*. 1993;57(5 Suppl):703S–709S.

60. Bazan NG. Neuroprotectin D1 (NPD1): a DHA-derived mediator that protects brain and retina against cell injury-induced oxidative stress. *Brain Pathol (Zurich)*. 2005;15(2):159–166.

61. Niemoller TD, Stark DT, Bazan NG. Omega-3 fatty acid docosahexaenoic acid is the precursor of neuroprotectin D1 in the nervous system. *World Rev Nutr Diet*. 2009;99:46–54.

62. Kim HY, Akbar M, Lau A, Edsall L. Inhibition of neuronal apoptosis by docosahexaenoic acid (22:6n-3). Role of phosphatidylserine in antiapoptotic effect. *J Biol Chem*. 2000;275(45):35215–35223.

63. Bazan NG. Cell survival matters: docosahexaenoic acid signaling, neuroprotection and photoreceptors. *Trends Neurosci*. 2006; 29(5):263–271.

64. Wu A, Ying Z, Gomez-Pinilla F. Dietary omega-3 fatty acids normalize BDNF levels, reduce oxidative damage, and counteract learning disability after traumatic brain injury in rats. *J Neurotrauma*. 2004;21(10):1457–1467.

65. Mills JD, Hadley K, Bailes JE. Dietary supplementation with the omega-3 fatty acid docosahexaenoic acid in traumatic brain injury. *Neurosurgery*. 2011;68(2):474–481.

66. Shin SS, Dixon CE. Oral fish oil restores striatal dopamine release after traumatic brain injury. *Neurosci Lett*. 2011;496(3):168–171.

67. Yu GF, Jie YQ, Wu A, Huang Q, Dai WM, Fan XF. Increased plasma 8-iso-prostaglandin F2alpha concentration in severe human traumatic brain injury. *Clin Chimica Acta*. 2013;421:7–11.

68. Hohl A, Gullo Jda S, Silva CC, et al. Plasma levels of oxidative stress biomarkers and hospital mortality in severe head injury: a multivariate analysis. *J Crit Care*. 2012;27(5):523.e511–529.

69. Yang J, Han Y, Ye W, et al. Alpha tocopherol treatment reduces the expression of Nogo-A and NgR in rat brain after traumatic brain injury. *J Surg Res*. 2013;182(2):e69–77.

70. Razmkon A, Sadidi A, Sherafat-Kazemzadeh E, et al. Administration of vitamin C and vitamin E in severe head injury: a randomized double-blind controlled trial. *Clin Neurosurg*. 2011;58:133–137.

71. Polidori MC, Mecocci P, Frei B. Plasma vitamin C levels are decreased and correlated with brain damage in patients with intracranial hemorrhage or head trauma. *Stroke*. 2001;32(4):898–902.

72. Rice ME. Ascorbate regulation and its neuroprotective role in the brain. *Trends Neurosci*. 2000;23(5):209–216.

73. Terentis AC, Thomas SR, Burr JA, Liebler DC, Stocker R. Vitamin E oxidation in human atherosclerotic lesions. *Circ Res*. 2002;90(3): 333–339.

74. Dhall SS, Hadley MN, Aarabi B, et al. Nutritional support after spinal cord injury. *Neurosurgery*. 2013;72(Suppl 2):S255–S259.

75. Nevin AN, Steenson J, Vivanti A, Hickman IJ. Investigation of measured and predicted resting energy needs in adults after spinal cord injury: a systematic review. *Spinal Cord*. 2016;54(4):248–253.

76. Long CL, Schaffel N, Geiger JW, Schiller WR, Blakemore WS. Metabolic response to injury and illness: estimation of energy and protein needs from indirect calorimetry and nitrogen balance. *JPEN J Parenter Enteral Med*. 1979;3(6):452–456.

77. Kolpek JH, Ott LG, Record KE, et al. Comparison of urinary urea nitrogen excretion and measured energy expenditure in spinal cord injury and nonsteroid-treated severe head trauma patients. *JPEN J Parenter Enteral Med*. 1989;13(3):277–280.

78. Cox SA, Weiss SM, Posuniak EA, et al. Energy expenditure after spinal cord injury: an evaluation of stable rehabilitating patients. *J Trauma*. 1985;25(5):419–423.

79. Bauman WA, Spungen AM, Wang J, Pierson RN. The relationship between energy expenditure and lean tissue in monozygotic twins discordant for spinal cord injury. *J Rehabil Res Dev*. 2004;41(1):1–8.

80. Monroe MB, Tataranni PA, Pratley R, et al. Lower daily energy expenditure as measured by a respiratory chamber in subjects with spinal cord injury compared with control subjects. *Am J Clin Nutr*. 1998;68(6):1223–1227.

81. Rodriguez DJ, Clevenger FW, Osler TM, Demarest GB, Fry DE. Obligatory negative nitrogen balance following spinal cord injury. *JPEN J Parenter Enteral Med*. 1991;15(3):319–322.

82. Dionyssiotis Y. Malnutrition in spinal cord injury: more than nutritional deficiency. *J Clin Med Res*. 2012;4(4):227–236.

83. Cooper IS, Hoen TI. Metabolic disorders in paraplegics. *Neurology*. 1952;2(4):332–340.

84. Dvorak MF, Noonan VK, Belanger L, et al. Early versus late enteral feeding in patients with acute cervical spinal cord injury: a pilot study. *Spine (Philadelphia)*. 2004;29(9):E175–E180.

85. Rowan CJ, Gillanders LK, Paice RL, Judson JA. Is early enteral feeding safe in patients who have suffered spinal cord injury? *Injury*. 2004;35(3):238–242.

86. Hurlbert RJ, Hadley MN, Walters BC, et al. Pharmacological therapy for acute spinal cord injury. *Neurosurgery*. 2013;72(Suppl 2): S93–S105.

87. Bracken MB, Collins WF, Freeman DF, et al. Efficacy of methylprednisolone in acute spinal cord injury. *JAMA*. 1984;251(1):45–52.

88. Bracken MB, Shepard MJ, Collins WF, et al. A randomized, controlled trial of methylprednisolone or naloxone in the treatment of acute spinal-cord injury. Results of the Second National Acute Spinal Cord Injury Study. *N Engl J Med*. 1990;322(20):1405–1411.

89. Bracken MB, Shepard MJ, Holford TR, et al. Administration of methylprednisolone for 24 or 48 hours or tirilazad mesylate for 48 hours in the treatment of acute spinal cord injury. Results of the Third National Acute Spinal Cord Injury Randomized Controlled Trial. National Acute Spinal Cord Injury Study. *JAMA*. 1997;277(20):1597–1604.

90. Godoy DA, Di Napoli M, Rabinstein AA. Treating hyperglycemia in neurocritical patients: benefits and perils. *Neurocrit Care*. 2010; 13(3):425–438.

91. Bauman WA, Zhong YG, Schwartz E. Vitamin D deficiency in veterans with chronic spinal cord injury. *Metabolism*. 1995;44(12): 1612–1616.

92. Cragg JJ, Noonan VK, Krassioukov A, Borisoff J. Cardiovascular disease and spinal cord injury: results from a national population health survey. *Neurology*. 2013;81(8):723–728.

93. Gater DR. Obesity after spinal cord injury. *Phys Med Rehabil Clin N Am*. 2007;18(2):333–351.

94. Groah SL, Nash MS, Ljungberg IH, et al. Nutrient intake and body habitus after spinal cord injury: an analysis by sex and level of injury. *J Spinal Cord Med*. 2009;32(1):25–33.

95. Weaver FM, Collins EG, Kurichi J, et al. Prevalence of obesity and high blood pressure in veterans with spinal cord injuries and disorders: a retrospective review. *Am J Phys Med Rehabil*. 2007;86(1):22–29.

96. Jacobs DG, Jacobs DO, Kudsk KA, et al. Practice management guidelines for nutritional support of the trauma patient. *J Trauma*. 2004;57(3):660–678.

97. Kruger EA, Pires M, Ngann Y, Sterling M, Rubayi S. Comprehensive management of pressure ulcers in spinal cord injury: current concepts and future trends. *J Spinal Cord Med*. 2013;36(6):572–585.

98. Regan MA, Teasell RW, Wolfe DL, et al. A systematic review of therapeutic interventions for pressure ulcers after spinal cord injury. *Arch Phys Med Rehabil*. 2009;90(2):213–231.

99. Fuhrer MJ, Garber SL, Rintala DH, Clearman R, Hart KA. Pressure ulcers in community-resident persons with spinal cord

injury: prevalence and risk factors. *Arch Phys Med Rehabil.* 1993; 74(11):1172–1177.

100. Dorner B, Posthauer ME, Thomas D; National Pressure Ulcer Advisory Panel. The role of nutrition in pressure ulcer prevention and treatment: National Pressure Ulcer Advisory Panel white paper. *Adv Skin Wound Care.* 2009;22(5):212–221.

101. Mozaffarian D, Benjamin EJ, Go AS, et al. Heart disease and stroke statistics—2015 update: a report from the American Heart Association. *Circulation.* 2015;131(4):e29–e322.

102. Martino R, Foley N, Bhogal S, et al. Dysphagia after stroke: incidence, diagnosis, and pulmonary complications. *Stroke.* 2005; 36(12):2756–2763.

103. FOOD Trial Collaboration. Poor nutritional status on admission predicts poor outcomes after stroke: observational data from the FOOD trial. *Stroke.* 2003;34(6):1450–1456.

104. George BP, Kelly AG, Schneider EB, Holloway RG. Current practices in feeding tube placement for US acute ischemic stroke inpatients. *Neurology.* 2014;83(10):874–882.

105. Crary MA, Carnaby GD, Shabbir Y, Miller L, Silliman S. Clinical variables associated with hydration status in acute ischemic stroke patients with dysphagia. *Dysphagia.* 2016;31(1):60–65.

106. Al-Khaled M, Matthis C, Binder A, et al. Dysphagia in patients with acute ischemic stroke: early dysphagia screening may reduce stroke-related pneumonia and improve stroke outcomes. *Cerebrovasc Dis (Basel).* 2016;42(1–2):81–89.

107. Jeyaseelan RD, Vargo MM, Chae J. National Institutes of Health Stroke Scale (NIHSS) as an early predictor of poststroke dysphagia. *PM R.* 2015;7(6):593–598.

108. Cummings J, Soomans D, O'Laughlin J, et al. Sensitivity and specificity of a nurse dysphagia screen in stroke patients. *Medsurg Nurs.* 2015;24(4):219–222, 263.

109. Campbell GB, Carter T, Kring D, Martinez C. Nursing bedside dysphagia screen: is it valid? *J Neurosci Nurs.* 2016;48(2):75–79.

110. Brady S, Donzelli J. The modified barium swallow and the functional endoscopic evaluation of swallowing. *Otolaryngol Clin North Am.* 2013;46(6):1009–1022.

111. Dennis MS, Lewis SC, Warlow C. Routine oral nutritional supplementation for stroke patients in hospital (FOOD): a multicentre randomised controlled trial. *Lancet.* 2005;365(9461):755–763.

112. Coltman A, Peterson S, Roehl K, Roosevelt H, Sowa D. Use of 3 tools to assess nutrition risk in the intensive care unit. *JPEN J Parenter Enteral Med.* 2015;39(1):28–33.

113. Rahman A, Hasan RM, Agarwala R, et al. Identifying critically-ill patients who will benefit most from nutritional therapy: further validation of the "modified NUTRIC" nutritional risk assessment tool. *Clin Nutr.* 2016;35(1):158–162.

114. Zheng T, Zhu X, Liang H, et al. Impact of early enteral nutrition on short term prognosis after acute stroke. *J Clin Neurosci.* 2015;22(9):1473–1476.

115. Yamada SM. Too early initiation of enteral nutrition is not nutritionally advantageous for comatose acute stroke patients. *J Nippon Med Sch.* 2015;82(4):186–192.

116. McGinnis C. The feeding tube bridle: one inexpensive, safe, and effective method to prevent inadvertent feeding tube dislodgement. *Nutr Clin Pract.* 2011;26(1):70–77.

117. Mahoney C, Rowat A, Macmillan M, Dennis M. Nasogastric feeding for stroke patients: practice and education. *Br J Nurs.* 2015;24(6):319–320.

118. Bechtold ML, Nguyen DL, Palmer LB, et al. Nasal bridles for securing nasoenteric tubes: a meta-analysis. *Nutr Clin Pract.* 2014;29(5):667–671.

119. Puricelli MD, Newberry CI, Gov-Ari E. Avulsed nasoenteric bridle system magnet as an intranasal foreign body. *Nutr Clin Pract.* 2016;31(1):121–124.

120. Jauch EC, Saver JL, Adams HP, et al. Guidelines for the early management of patients with acute ischemic stroke: a guideline for healthcare professionals from the American Heart Association/ American Stroke Association. *Stroke.* 2013;44(3):870–947.

121. Dennis MS, Lewis SC, Warlow C. Effect of timing and method of enteral tube feeding for dysphagic stroke patients (FOOD): a multicentre randomised controlled trial. *Lancet.* 2005;365(9461): 764–772.

122. Geeganage C, Beavan J, Ellender S, Bath PM. Interventions for dysphagia and nutritional support in acute and subacute stroke. *Cochrane Database Syst Rev.* 2012;10:CD000323.

123. Jiang YL, Ruberu N, Liu XS, et al. Mortality trend and predictors of mortality in dysphagic stroke patients postpercutaneous endoscopic gastrostomy. *Chinese Med J.* 2015;128(10):1331–1335.

124. Kejariwal D, Bromley D, Miao Y. The "cut and push" method of percutaneous endoscopic gastrostomy tube removal in adult patients: the Ipswich experience. *Nutr Clin Pract.* 2009;24(2):281–283.

125. Karakus SC, Celtik C, Koku N, Ertaskin I. A simple method for percutaneous endoscopic gastrostomy tube removal: "tie and retrograde pull." *J Pediatr Surg.* 2013;48(8):1810–1812.

126. Finestone HM, Greene-Finestone LS, Foley NC, Woodbury MG. Measuring longitudinally the metabolic demands of stroke patients: resting energy expenditure is not elevated. *Stroke.* 2003; 34(2):502–507.

127. Bardutzky J, Georgiadis D, Kollmar R, Schwarz S, Schwab S. Energy demand in patients with stroke who are sedated and receiving mechanical ventilation. *J Neurosurg.* 2004;100(2):266–271.

128. Nagano A, Yamada Y, Miyake H, Domen K, Koyama T. Comparisons of predictive equations for resting energy expenditure in patients with cerebral infarct during acute care. *J Stroke Cardiovasc Dis.* 2015;24(8):1879–1885.

129. Esper DH, Coplin WM, Carhuapoma JR. Energy expenditure in patients with nontraumatic intracranial hemorrhage. *JPEN J Parenter Enteral Med.* 2006;30(2):71–75.

130. Frankenfield DC, Ashcraft CM. Description and prediction of resting metabolic rate after stroke and traumatic brain injury. *Nutrition (Burbank).* 2012;28(9):906–911.

131. Frankenfield DC, Coleman A, Alam S, Cooney RN. Analysis of estimation methods for resting metabolic rate in critically ill adults. *JPEN J Parenter Enteral Med.* 2009;33(1):27–36.

132. Kasuya H, Kawashima A, Namiki K, Shimizu T, Takakura K. Metabolic profiles of patients with subarachnoid hemorrhage treated by early surgery. *Neurosurgery.* 1998;42(6):1268–1274.

133. Badjatia N, Fernandez L, Schlossberg MJ, et al. Relationship between energy balance and complications after subarachnoid hemorrhage. *JPEN J Parenter Enteral Med.* 2010;34(1):64–69.

134. Corrigan ML, Escuro AA, Celestin J, Kirby DF. Nutrition in the stroke patient. *Nutr Clin Pract.* 2011;26(3):242–252.

135. McCarthy MS, Phipps SC. Special nutrition challenges: current approach to acute kidney injury. *Nutr Clin Pract.* 2014;29(1):56–62.

136. Parli SE, Ruf KM, Magnuson B. Pathophysiology, treatment, and prevention of fluid and electrolyte abnormalities during refeeding syndrome. *J Infus Nurs.* 2014;37(3):197–202.

137. de Aguilar-Nascimento JE, Prado Silveira BR, Dock-Nascimento DB. Early enteral nutrition with whey protein or casein in elderly patients with acute ischemic stroke: a double-blind randomized trial. *Nutrition (Burbank).* 2011;27(4):440–444.

138. Zhang C, Chi FL, Xie TH, Zhou YH. Effect of B-vitamin supplementation on stroke: a meta-analysis of randomized controlled trials. *PloS One.* 2013;8(11):e81577.

139. Zhang C, Wang ZY, Qin YY, Yu FF, Zhou YH. Association between B vitamins supplementation and risk of cardiovascular outcomes: a cumulative meta-analysis of randomized controlled trials. *PloS One.* 2014;9(9):e107060.

140. Diniz PB, Vanin G, Xavier R, Parente MA. Reduced incidence of aspiration with spoon-thick consistency in stroke patients. *Nutr Clin Pract*. 2009;24(3):414–418.

141. Leder SB, Judson BL, Sliwinski E, Madson L. Promoting safe swallowing when puree is swallowed without aspiration but thin liquid is aspirated: nectar is enough. *Dysphagia*. 2013;28(1):58–62.

142. Andelic N, Ye J, Tornas S, et al. Cost-effectiveness analysis of an early-initiated, continuous chain of rehabilitation after severe traumatic brain injury. *J Neurotrauma*. 2014;31(14):1313–1320.

143. Griesbach GS, Kreber LA, Harrington D, Ashley MJ. Post-acute traumatic brain injury rehabilitation: effects on outcome measures and life care costs. *J Neurotrauma*. 2015;32(10):704–711.

144. Laven GT, Huang CT, DeVivo MJ, et al. Nutritional status during the acute stage of spinal cord injury. *Arch Phys Med Rehabil*. 1989;70(4):277–282.

145. Lexicomp Online. 2016. https://online.lexi.com. Accessed September 1, 2016.

146. Malec JF, Kean J. Post-inpatient brain injury rehabilitation outcomes: report from the National OutcomeInfo Database. *J Neurotrauma*. 2016;33(14):1371–1379.

147. Greenwald BD, Hammond FM, Harrison-Felix C, et al. Mortality following traumatic brain injury among individuals unable to follow commands at the time of rehabilitation admission: a National Institute on Disability and Rehabilitation Research traumatic brain injury model systems study. *J Neurotrauma*. 2015;32(23):1883–1892.

148. Eum RS, Seel RT, Goldstein R, et al. Predicting institutionalization after traumatic brain injury inpatient rehabilitation. *J Neurotrauma*. 2015;32(4):280–286.

149. Barco KT, Smith RA, Peerless JR, Plaisier BR, Chima CS. Energy expenditure assessment and validation after acute spinal cord injury. *Nutr Clin Pract*. 2002;17(5):309–313.

150. Pellicane AJ, Millis SR, Zimmerman SE, Roth EJ. Calorie and protein intake in acute rehabilitation inpatients with traumatic spinal cord injury versus other diagnoses. *Topics Spinal Cord Inj Rehabil*. 2013;19(3):229–235.

151. Tian W, Hsieh CH, DeJong G, Backus D, Groah S, Ballard PH. Role of body weight in therapy participation and rehabilitation outcomes among individuals with traumatic spinal cord injury. *Arch Phys Med Rehabil*. 2013;94(4 Suppl):S125–S136.

152. Bondanelli M, Ambrosio MR, Cavazzini L, et al. Anterior pituitary function may predict functional and cognitive outcome in patients with traumatic brain injury undergoing rehabilitation. *J Neurotrauma*. 2007;24(11):1687–1697.

153. Rodriguez DJ, Benzel EC, Clevenger FW. The metabolic response to spinal cord injury. *Spinal Cord*. 1997;35(9):599–604.

154. Pontes-Arruda A, Martins LF, de Lima SM, et al. Enteral nutrition with eicosapentaenoic acid, gamma-linolenic acid and antioxidants in the early treatment of sepsis: results from a multicenter, prospective, randomized, double-blinded, controlled study: the INTERSEPT study. *Crit Care (London)*. 2011;15(3):R144.

155. Groves NJ, McGrath JJ, Burne TH. Vitamin D as a neurosteroid affecting the developing and adult brain. *Annu Rev Nutr*. 2014;34:117–141.

156. Pellicane AJ, Wysocki NM, Mallinson TR, Schnitzer TJ. Prevalence of 25-hydroxyvitamin D deficiency in the acute inpatient rehabilitation population and its effect on function. *Arch Phys Med Rehabil*. 2011;92(5):705–711.

157. Pellicane AJ, Wysocki NM, Schnitzer TJ. Prevalence of 25-hydroxyvitamin D deficiency in the outpatient rehabilitation population. *Am J Phys Med Rehabil*. 2010;89(11):899–904.

158. Guan J, Karsy M, Brock AA, et al. A prospective analysis of hypovitaminosis D and mortality in 400 patients in the neurocritical care setting. *J Neurosurg*. 2016:1–7.

159. Holick MF, Binkley NC, Bischoff-Ferrari HA, et al. Evaluation, treatment, and prevention of vitamin D deficiency: an Endocrine Society clinical practice guideline. *J Clin Endocrinol Metab*. 2011;96(7):1911–1930.

160. Powell D, Affuso O, Chen Y. Weight change after spinal cord injury. *J Spinal Cord Med*. 2016:1–8.

161. de Groot S, Post MW, Hoekstra T, et al. Trajectories in the course of body mass index after spinal cord injury. *Arch Phys Med Rehabil*. 2014;95(6):1083–1092.

162. de Groot S, Post MW, Postma K, Sluis TA, van der Woude LH. Prospective analysis of body mass index during and up to 5 years after discharge from inpatient spinal cord injury rehabilitation. *J Rehabil Med*. 2010;42(10):922–928.

163. Kitzman P, Cecil D, Kolpek JH. The risks of polypharmacy following spinal cord injury. *J Spinal Cord Med*. 2016:1–7.

164. Bryce T. Spinal cord injury. In *Braddom's Physical Medicine and Rehabilitation*. 5th ed. Philadelphia, PA: Elsevier; 2015:1095–1136.

165. Rahnemai-Azar AA, Rahnemaiazar AA, Naghshizadian R, Kurtz A, Farkas DT. Percutaneous endoscopic gastrostomy: indications, technique, complications and management. *World J Gastroenterol*. 2014;20(24):7739–7751.

166. Godbolt AK, Stenberg M, Jakobsson J, et al. Subacute complications during recovery from severe traumatic brain injury: frequency and associations with outcome. *BMJ Open*. 2015;5(4):e007208.

167. Foley N, Finestone H, Woodbury MG, Teasell R, Greene-Finestone L. Energy and protein intakes of acute stroke patients. *J Nutr Health Aging*. 2006;10(3):171–175.

168. Bhatnagar S, Iaccarino MA, Zafonte R. Pharmacotherapy in rehabilitation of post-acute traumatic brain injury. *Brain Res*. 2016;1640(A):164–179.

169. National Center for Complementary and Integrative Health. Herbs at a glance. November 21, 2016. https://nccih.nih.gov/health/herbsataglance.htm. Accessed February 2, 2017.

170. US National Library of Medicine. Medline Plus. https://medlineplus.gov. Accessed February 2, 2017.

171. Benstead T, Jackson-Tarlton C, Leddin D. Nutrition with gastrostomy feeding tubes for amyotrophic lateral sclerosis in Canada. *Can J Neurol Sci*. 2016:1–5.

172. Salvioni CC, Stanich P, Almeida CS, Oliveira AS. Nutritional care in motor neurone disease/amyotrophic lateral sclerosis. *Arq Neuropsiquiatr*. 2014;72(2):157–163.

173. Kasarskis EJ, Mendiondo MS, Matthews DE, et al. Estimating daily energy expenditure in individuals with amyotrophic lateral sclerosis. *Am J Clin Nutr*. 2014;99(4):792–803.

174. Bouteloup C, Desport JC, Clavelou P, et al. Hypermetabolism in ALS patients: an early and persistent phenomenon. *J Neurol*. 2009;256(8):1236–1242.

175. Desport JC, Preux PM, Truong TC, et al. Nutritional status is a prognostic factor for survival in ALS patients. *Neurology*. 1999;53(5):1059–1063.

176. Marin B, Desport JC, Kajeu P, et al. Alteration of nutritional status at diagnosis is a prognostic factor for survival of amyotrophic lateral sclerosis patients. *J Neurol Neurosurg Psychiatr*. 2011;82(6):628–634.

177. Park Y, Park J, Kim Y, Baek H, Kim SH. Association between nutritional status and disease severity using the amyotrophic lateral sclerosis (ALS) functional rating scale in ALS patients. *Nutrition (Burbank)*. 2015;31(11–12):1362–1367.

178. Braun MM, Osecheck M, Joyce NC. Nutrition assessment and management in amyotrophic lateral sclerosis. *Phys Med Rehabil Clin N Am*. 2012;23(4):751–771.

179. Piquet MA. [Nutritional approach for patients with amyotrophic lateral sclerosis]. *Rev Neurol (Paris)*. 2006;162(Suppl 2): 4S177–4S187.

180. Genton L, Viatte V, Janssens JP, Heritier AC, Pichard C. Nutritional state, energy intakes and energy expenditure of amyotrophic lateral sclerosis (ALS) patients. *Clin Nutr.* 2011;30(5):553–559.

181. Morassutti I, Giometto M, Baruffi C, et al. Nutritional intervention for amyotrophic lateral sclerosis. *Minerva Gastroenterol Dietol.* 2012;58(3):253–260.

182. Mitsumoto H, Davidson M, Moore D, et al. Percutaneous endoscopic gastrostomy (PEG) in patients with ALS and bulbar dysfunction. *Amyotroph Lateral Scler Other Motor Neuron Disord.* 2003;4(3):177–185.

183. Greenwood DI. Nutrition management of amyotrophic lateral sclerosis. *Nutr Clin Pract.* 2013;28(3):392–399.

184. Selter JH, Turner Z, Doerrer SC, Kossoff EH. Dietary and medication adjustments to improve seizure control in patients treated with the ketogenic diet. *J Child Neurol.* 2015;30(1):53–57.

185. Thakur KT, Probasco JC, Hocker SE, et al. Ketogenic diet for adults in super-refractory status epilepticus. *Neurology.* 2014;82(8):665–670.

186. Thammongkol S, Vears DF, Bicknell-Royle J, et al. Efficacy of the ketogenic diet: which epilepsies respond? *Epilepsia.* 2012;53(3): e55–59.

187. Payne NE, Cross JH, Sander JW, Sisodiya SM. The ketogenic and related diets in adolescents and adults—a review. *Epilepsia.* 2011;52(11):1941–1948.

188. Klein P, Janousek J, Barber A, Weissberger R. Ketogenic diet treatment in adults with refractory epilepsy. *Epilepsy Behav.* 2010; 19(4):575–579.

189. Martin K, Jackson CF, Levy RG, Cooper PN. Ketogenic diet and other dietary treatments for epilepsy. *Cochrane Database Syst Rev.* 2016;2:CD001903.

190. Shorvon S, Ferlisi M. The treatment of super-refractory status epilepticus: a critical review of available therapies and a clinical treatment protocol. *Brain.* 2011;134(10):2802–2818.

191. Charlie Foundation for Ketogenic Therapies. Carb/non-carb ingredients. http://www.charliefoundation.org/resources-tools/resources-3/low-carb/item/1137-carbohydrate-non-carbohydrate-ingredients. Accessed January 22, 2017.

192. Mosek A, Natour H, Neufeld MY, Shiff Y, Vaisman N. Ketogenic diet treatment in adults with refractory epilepsy: a prospective pilot study. *Seizure.* 2009;18(1):30–33.

193. Nagarjunakonda S, Amalakanti S, Uppala V, Rajanala L, Athina S. Vitamin D in epilepsy: vitamin D levels in epilepsy patients, patients on antiepileptic drug polytherapy and drug-resistant epilepsy sufferers. *Eur J Clin Nutr.* 2016;70(1):140–142.

194. Ye F, Li XJ, Jiang WL, Sun HB, Liu J. Efficacy of and patient compliance with a ketogenic diet in adults with intractable epilepsy: a meta-analysis. *J Clin Neurol (Seoul).* 2015;11(1):26–31.

195. Wusthoff CJ, Kranick SM, Morley JF, Christina Bergqvist AG. The ketogenic diet in treatment of two adults with prolonged nonconvulsive status epilepticus. *Epilepsia.* 2010;51(6):1083–1085.

196. Zupec-Kania B. *Professional's Guide to the Ketogenic Diet.* Santa Monica, CA: Ketogenic Seminars, The Charlie Foundation; 2014.

197. Gimenez-Cassina A, Martinez-Francois JR, Fisher JK, et al. BAD-dependent regulation of fuel metabolism and K(ATP) channel activity confers resistance to epileptic seizures. *Neuron.* 2012; 74(4):719–730.

198. Klein P, Tyrlikova I, Mathews GC. Dietary treatment in adults with refractory epilepsy: a review. *Neurology.* 2014;83(21):1978–1985.

199. Barichella M, Cereda E, Cassani E, et al. Dietary habits and neurological features of Parkinson's disease patients: implications for practice. *Clin Nutr.* Epub ahead of print July 5, 2016. doi:10.1016/j.clnu.2016.06.020.

200. Stavroulakis T, McDermott CJ. Enteral feeding in neurological disorders. *Pract Neurol.* 2016.

23 Sepsis and Critical Illness

Robert G. Martindale, MD, PhD, Jayshil J. Patel, MD, Thomas J. Herron, MD, and Panna A. Codner, MD, FACS

CONTENTS

Acknowledgments: Keith Miller, MD, and Laszlo Kiraly, MD, were contributors to this chapter for the second edition.

Objectives

1. Understand working definitions of *infection*, *sepsis*, and *septic shock*.
2. Describe the physiology and pathophysiology of inflammation and its effect on metabolism.
3. Review the enteral and parenteral routes of feeding and the pros and cons of each.
4. Describe the quantity and quality of appropriate macronutrients in the septic patient.
5. Delineate options for feeding the septic patient.
6. Describe nutrition adjuncts that may improve outcomes in septic patients.
7. Recognize the impact of nutrition support in host immunity.

Test Your Knowledge Questions

1. Which of the following characterizes the current understanding of systemic inflammatory response?
   A. Overstimulated immune system
   B. Mixture of immune stimulation and suppression
   C. Initial immune suppression followed by stimulation
   D. Immune suppression
2. Why is hemodynamic stability an important consideration before initiating enteral nutrition (EN)?
   A. To avoid overfeeding.
   B. Hemodynamic instability is an indication for parenteral nutrition (PN).
   C. Gastrointestinal (GI) perfusion may be compromised.
   D. Patients cannot absorb any nutrients when they are underresuscitated.
3. What is the best reason to conservatively prescribe energy in nutrition support regimens?
   A. Glycemic control
   B. To facilitate permissive underfeeding
   C. Cost containment
   D. To achieve goal infusions more efficiently

Test Your Knowledge Answers

1. The correct answer is **B**. Current understanding of systemic inflammatory response has evolved from interpreting the condition as one of an overstimulated immune system and altered metabolic reaction to infection and trauma to a combination, depending on clinical and individual attributes, of both overstimulation of metabolic and immune responses as well as a compensatory reaction causing immune metabolic suppression. In fact, decreased immunity may predominate, depending on the source of inflammation, the timing, and the clinical status of the patient.
2. The correct answer is **C**. GI perfusion is compromised during septic states, particularly in conditions of hemodynamic instability. Feeding into the GI tract may initiate an ischemic event. Once adequately resuscitated, enteral feeding may help preserve GI perfusion. In any case, EN should be started as early as possible under conditions of hemodynamic stability.
3. The correct answer is **A**. In critical care populations, hyperglycemia is associated with adverse outcomes, including increased incidence of infections. Conservative energy prescription, including a gradual increase of infusion rates to goal energy requirements, assists in controlling serum glucose levels.

Background

Sepsis continues to be a major healthcare problem in the United States. From 2000 to 2012, the rate of hospitalization doubled.[1] Sepsis is the 11th leading cause of death in the United States, and this figure does not include the common diagnoses of pneumonia and influenza.[2] Sepsis accounts for 10% of all admissions to the intensive care unit (ICU) in US hospitals and remains the leading cause of hospital deaths.[3] In a study of 8 academic tertiary care centers,

the hospital-wide incidence of sepsis syndrome was 2.0 ± 0.2 cases per 100 admissions, or 2.8 ± 0.2 per 1000 patient-days, and patients in the ICU accounted for 59% of sepsis cases.[4] A retrospective analysis in the surgical ICU indicated that in 78% of the patients who died of sepsis and multiple system organ failure, the main source of infection was either the respiratory or GI tract.[5] According to the Centers for Disease Control and Prevention, the most common sources of sepsis in adults patients being admitted with a sepsis diagnosis are infections of the lung (35%), urinary tract (25%), GI system (11%), and skin (11%).[6] Anti-infective agents have had little impact on mortality in sepsis in the last century.[7] Most of the decrease in mortality from sepsis resulted from public health measures such as immunization, establishment of public health departments, and the pasteurization of milk.[7] The major influence of antibiotics has, in fact, been to change the sources of bacteria causing sepsis from exogenous environmental sources to endogenous sources. Specialized nutrition therapy including appropriate nutrient substrate prescription delivered at the most suitable time and via the optimal route significantly influences the endogenous microbial population (microbiome), and sepsis and its treatment dramatically affect the quantity and variety of bacteria as well as their virulence. Many investigators now suspect that the microbiome can become a "pathobiome" in many ICU conditions, including sepsis.[8] See Chapter 4 for further discussion of gut microbiota.

This chapter discusses our current understanding of nutrition therapy in sepsis and infection, and the multiple benefits appropriate nutrition intervention can offer in sepsis management.

Definitions

The term *sepsis* has traditionally been used to encompass a spectrum of diseases ranging from systemic inflammatory response syndrome (SIRS) to severe sepsis and multiple organ failure. Sepsis is no longer considered a disease with a specific definition but a group of diseases based on the predisposition of the patient, the severity of insult, the physiological or pathophysiological response of the host, the number of organs involved, and the extent of their involvement. The terms *sepsis*, *infection*, and *inflammation* are commonly misused in the critically ill population. Standardized definitions of these and related terms were first published in 1992 by the American College of Chest Physicians[9] and have since been updated.[10] *Sepsis* is properly defined as life-threatening organ dysfunction caused by a dysregulated host response to infection. *Septic shock* refers to a subset of sepsis in which profound circulatory, cellular, and metabolic abnormalities are associated with a greater risk of mortality than with sepsis alone. These definitions help to clarify the differences between *sepsis* and *infection* and can be readily applied to patients in different stages of infection or inflammation.

Sepsis is the systemic response to infection. Historically, the term *sepsis* described a life-threatening condition characterized by fever, tachycardia, tachypnea, and organ dysfunction, and it was frequently associated with shock and death. It was also often associated with a bacterial, fungal, or viral infection, which could be either localized or systemic in nature. However, other conditions, such as severe trauma, pancreatitis, hemorrhage, ischemia, and burn injury, can produce the same clinical findings in the absence of an identified infectious source. This constellation of fever, tachycardia, tachypnea, and organ dysfunction has come to be known as *SIRS*, a clinical syndrome that can be caused by a variety of insults, including sepsis.

The exact definition of *sepsis* varies, but the term generally refers to the presence or presumed presence of an infectious source accompanied by SIRS, as described previously. *Septic shock* is associated with hemodynamic instability, which is primarily refractory hypotension with systolic peak pressures less than 90 mm Hg, mean arterial pressures less than 65 mm Hg, or a drop of greater than 40 mm Hg from baseline. These blood pressures are unresponsive to crystalloid volume resuscitation of at least 20 to 40 mL/kg.[4,11,12]

Pathophysiology

The metabolic response to sepsis is in many ways similar to the response that follows major surgery or trauma (see Chapter 24). Both responses are characterized by increases in energy expenditure, protein catabolism, and oxidation of stored lipids along with significant alterations in the body's ability to metabolize carbohydrate.[13]

A series of events involving multiple organ systems are required for the progression from localized infection to sepsis and septic shock. The initial reaction of the host is localized to the site of infection or injury. The process begins with cellular activation at the endothelial level of macrophages, monocytes, and neutrophils. Various microbial components, such as cell wall structures, proteins, or deoxyribonucleic acid, bind to specific receptors on the surface of white cells called *pattern recognition receptors*, including toll-like receptors and others.[14] These cells then start a cascade of events, including activation of the complement system leading to vasodilatation and increased capillary permeability, which leads to increased interstitial fluid, and chemoattractants in the local area. Additional macrophages are attracted to the area; these, in turn, orchestrate the intensity of the inflammatory response. In the presence of infection, the macrophages undergo accelerated phagocytic activity with elaboration of tumor necrosis factor (TNF), interleukin (IL)-1, IL-2, IL-6, and multiple other proinflammatory cytokines, which can, if in high enough concentration, "spill over" into the systemic circulation to influence the entire systemic response. Once systemic activation has begun, microvascular coagulation is noted; platelets, mast cells, and local vasodilators result in generalized edema, accelerated oxygen free radical production, and eventual organ injury. This initial septic response is proinflammatory. This proinflammatory phase is immediately followed by a compensatory anti-inflammatory response.[2,7,15] Virtually all major organs are involved, but disruption in cardiac, pulmonary, renal, and hepatic function is most commonly observed clinically. Although it would appear at first glance that the systemic response is destructive to the host, these systemic manifestations of the "septic response" are in effect related to attempts to contain or eliminate the infection.[2,7] It is only when the cascade of events becomes overwhelming to the host that it is destructive and not protective. It is important to remember that immune suppression is a major part of the later phases of sepsis, making this period a perfect target for nutrition intervention.[7]

The hallmark of the management of sepsis includes the timely use of appropriate antimicrobial agents and early drainage or removal of purulent foci (source control) to achieve rapid bacterial or fungal eradication. Support of the septic patient also includes administration of early, goal-directed therapy with crystalloid and colloid solutions, blood products (including red blood cells and fresh frozen plasma), inotropic and vasoactive agents, and mechanical ventilation to ensure hemodynamic stability and oxygenation of vital tissues.[7,16,17] Data also support intense management of hyperglycemia, with targets of no greater than 180mg/dL, and corticosteroids for the appropriate patient.[7]

The understanding of sepsis has become somewhat more complicated than described previously as an initial proinflammatory phase followed by compensatory anti-inflammatory stage. In fact, anti-inflammatory cytokines (IL-4 and IL-10) may predominate rather than proinflammatory cytokines (TNF-α, IL-2, interferon-γ), depending on the initial stimulus of inflammation, polymorphisms in genes for cytokines, and clinical status, including age. Thus, susceptible patients may be immune suppressed, causing host inability to eradicate the pathogen adequately.[7] Outcome in sepsis is extremely difficult to predict or affect because the timing of intervention is so variable in relation to the host inflammatory response.[13] To date, attempts to blockade of targeted mediators of the inflammatory response have been uniformly unsuccessful.[2,18] Over 30 years of dedicated efforts to reverse sepsis with various broad-spectrum antibiotics (alone or in combination) and monoclonal antibodies have, at best, shown only modest benefit and, in fact, have been harmful in some cases.[2] Appropriate nutrition therapy during sepsis and severe infections is essential because it plays a key role in modulating the inflammatory response, maintaining immune function, abrogating skeletal muscle catabolism, improving wound healing, and maintaining GI and pulmonary mucosal barrier function.

Metabolic Responses During Sepsis

Carbohydrate Metabolism

Under normal conditions, glucose homeostasis is regulated by several control mechanisms to match the uptake and production of glucose (see Chapter 3). These mechanisms maintain "normal" blood glucose concentrations under a wide range of conditions. However, hyperglycemia and significant insulin resistance are clinical characteristics uniformly found in sepsis. Proinflammatory cytokines potentiate the release of catabolic hormones (glucagon, catecholamines, and cortisol). These catabolic hormones stimulate glycogenolysis and gluconeogenesis to mobilize glucose. Glucagon-stimulated glycogenolysis, for example, is one of the most sensitive and reproducible metabolic effects of hormones on any tissue.[19,20] Following the onset of sepsis, glycogen stores are depleted within hours, and endogenous lipid and protein become the major source of oxidative energy substrate.[21] However, mobilization and oxidation of lipid from endogenous adipose stores is impaired during sepsis, as discussed below.

Sepsis results in hyperglycemia secondary to alterations in endogenous glucose production, decreased glucose uptake, and insulin resistance.[21,22] Moderate or severe infection is associated with a 150% to 200% increase in the glucose production rate, and circulating glucose levels tend to be correspondingly high. Dahn and colleagues reported hepatic glucose production in trauma and sepsis is six-fold greater than in trauma alone.[23] Gluconeogenesis increases with progressive organ failure, as does the level and production of gluconeogenic precursors (lactate, pyruvate, alanine, and glycerol). As sepsis progresses, reduced splanchnic blood flow and severe end-stage hepatic dysfunction eventually lead to decreased glucose production and hypoglycemia at the final stages of life.

Protein Metabolism

Although protein breakdown and synthesis both continue to occur at accelerated rates during sepsis, patients remain in generalized net-negative nitrogen balance for variable periods even after the inciting insult has been resolved.[21] The accelerated peripheral muscle protein breakdown noted in sepsis is accompanied with diminished amino acid uptake by muscle, leading to the net flux of amino acids away from the periphery to the liver.[24] The ureagenesis rate and the synthesis rates of creatinine, uric acid, and ammonia are all increased. All are excreted in increased amounts in the urine during sepsis. The nitrogen loss of severe sepsis complicating recovery from trauma may exceed 30 g/d.[24,25] The primary sites of this amino acid efflux are from the "labile" amino acid pools in skeletal muscle, connective tissue, and unstimulated gut. It is important to keep in mind that mammalian species have no "storage" of protein and that any protein utilized during catabolic stress of any kind comes at the expense of other tissues that are more labile. During sepsis, hepatic uptake of amino acids and hepatic protein synthesis are increased, which allows a substrate for gluconeogenesis and production of acute-phase proteins. However, the increase in hepatic protein synthesis is not uniform. Although serum concentrations of positive acute-phase proteins, such as haptoglobin and C-reactive protein, increase in response to stress, synthesis of negative acute-phase proteins, such as albumin and prealbumin, falls.[26] This concept is often referred to as *hepatic reprioritization.*

Under these catabolic circumstances, patients who receive adequate exogenous amino acids to maintain production of acute-phase proteins are more likely to survive.[27] Nonetheless, adequate nutrition support can only attenuate the response and will not completely ablate the catabolic effects and response.[27] In an elaborate series of metabolic studies by Plank and colleagues, 13.5% of total body protein in septic patients was lost in the first 21 days following a single septic or traumatic insult even though the patients received adequate nutrition support. The metabolic rate was still elevated above baseline at 21 days.[26] These studies have since been confirmed using more sophisticated tracer technology now available.[28]

As the systemic response to sepsis progresses, protein catabolism increases, and the failure of synthetic processes to keep up with the breakdown rate results in severe losses of skeletal

protein. In an unfed, stressed patient, up to 250 g of lean body mass will be broken down each day.[20] Some of the amino acids thus mobilized provide oxidative substrate for gluconeogenesis; however, even in the face of seemingly adequate exogenous glucose supplies, there is obligate mobilization of amino acids.[20] In addition to supplying amino acid for acute-phase protein synthesis, a driving force for the mobilization of amino acids during sepsis is thought to be the host attempting to provide glutamine to enterocytes, leukocytes, and rapidly dividing cells.[29] Unfortunately, prolonged catabolism of skeletal muscle protein compromises respiratory function, impairs wound healing, exacerbates immunosuppression, accelerates the loss of strength and endurance necessary for recovery, and increases ventilator-dependency time and ICU stay, the risk of thromboembolic disease, recovery time, and mortality incidence.[30] Refer to Chapter 6 for further discussion of protein catabolism in critical illness.

Lipid Metabolism

The catabolic hormones epinephrine, norepinephrine, and glucagon are the predominant stimulators of the hydrolysis of stored triglycerides (lipolysis) via direct stimulation of hormone-sensitive lipase. In early sepsis, catabolic hormones outweigh the effects of anabolic hormones such as insulin and growth hormone and result in the breakdown of stored triglycerides to glycerol and free fatty acids (FFAs).[31] In addition to the increased rate of lipolysis of peripheral adipose stores observed in sepsis, intracellular transport metabolism is also affected.[31] The ability of the cell to transport long-chain FFAs from the cytosol into mitochondria via the acylcarnitine carrier is impaired. Consequently, long-chain FFA esters accumulate within the cell and can directly inhibit the function of pyruvate dehydrogenase complex, which will result in intracellular acidosis and the accumulation of lactate and pyruvate.[32,33] This process is a major reason for the decrease in aerobic respiration and the cells' ability to use the Krebs cycle for efficient energy production. Furthermore, in addition to impaired FFA utilization, sepsis impairs ketogenesis. Keto acids are an important source of oxidative fuel for several organs during starvation. Finally, the activity of lipoprotein lipase, which is responsible for the conversion of triglycerides to FFAs in peripheral cells, is suppressed in sepsis. Consequently, hyperlipidemia, hyperglycemia, hyperlactatemia, and high levels of circulating β-hydroxybutyrate often are observed in severe sepsis.[31,32]

Nutrition Assessment in Sepsis and Critical Care

Traditional methods of nutrition assessment are less useful in the septic or critically ill patient than in the general hospitalized patient. Critically ill patients experience significant fluid shifts and metabolic abnormalities related to the inflammatory response that deem anthropometric and biochemical measures unreliable. Hepatically synthesized proteins such as albumin and prealbumin are commonly misused in severely ill patients as markers of nutrition status when, in fact, they are at best surrogate markers. The changes in serum levels noted are indicative of reprioritization of hepatic protein synthesis and increased vascular permeability during the inflammatory response.[26] In addition, an inability to obtain nutrition history from the patient directly makes it difficult to collect and interpret nutrition assessment data. A thorough weight and diet history must often be pieced together from the available medical record history and reports from family members. In absence of validated tools for assessment in sepsis and septic shock, the Society of Critical Care Medicine (SCCM) and American Society for Parenteral and Enteral Nutrition (ASPEN) recommend that clinicians evaluate weight loss and nutrition history prior to admission, level of disease severity, and GI function.[34] Thereafter, an ongoing meticulous review of the patient's current physical and metabolic status—including weight changes; findings from abdominal examinations; GI function; evidence of wounds; line, drain, and tube placements; ventilation parameters; vital signs; hemodynamics; and laboratory values—provides the information necessary to apply the appropriate nutrition intervention.

Energy Expenditure

Literature evaluating energy expenditure in sepsis has been limited by heterogeneity of the populations studied and the rather loose definitions of sepsis used in most studies. Elaborate metabolic studies following the onset of sepsis in patients with peritonitis indicated that resting energy expenditure progressively increases over the first 7 days and remains elevated for up to 21 days even when the sepsis has been adequately addressed and treated.[26] These data are partially clouded by the thermogenic influence of the nutrition delivery itself, which is noted when nutrition support is started. The very early stages of sepsis are also characterized by decreased mitochondrial energy utilization.[35] The clinical importance of this early phase, however, is largely unknown.

In summary, metabolism during sepsis is associated with a significant increase in energy expenditure estimated to be 20% to 60% above basal energy expenditure.[26] The increase in energy expenditure is associated with amplified protein muscle catabolism, as well as an increased reliance on lipid stores for oxidative fuel. Initially, these metabolic alterations may be beneficial to mobilize adequate endogenous substrate to support the immune and wound healing processes; however, when they are prolonged, they become detrimental to host survival. This supply may be even more important after the early phase of sepsis as the cellular "machinery" recovers. Although PN support cannot attenuate the rate of catabolism, EN and use of anti-inflammatory lipids (eicosapentaenoic acid [EPA] and docosahexaenoic acid [DHA]) can attenuate the catabolic response to stress.[36] Supplying substrates for enhanced acute-phase protein synthesis has the potential to improve conditions for enhanced survival. Emerging evidence suggests that delivery of exogenous protein or amino acid supplementation improves recovery in critical illness.[37,38] Many of the patients included in these studies were septic, but studies of septic patients exclusively have not been done.

Route of Feeding

Early administration of EN has been shown to offer outcome benefits in critical care populations when compared with PN.[34,39–41] Numerous mechanisms have been proposed to explain the benefits observed with EN, including maintenance of mucosal integrity, attenuation of the hyperdynamic metabolic response, improved visceral blood flow, support for the gut-associated lymphoid tissue (GALT), and others.

The GI tract and liver are susceptible to ischemia during sepsis secondary to the shunting of blood flow away from the splanchnic bed. Gut ischemia, in turn, leads to mitochondrial dysfunction, mucosal acidosis, progressive cell injury, and death.[42–44] Practitioners are often concerned that EN may increase the ischemic injury during states of decreased perfusion of the splanchnic organs in septic patients, especially if the patient is receiving vasoactive medications.[42] Laboratory evidence provides support for the opposing view: namely, that EN provides protection and even enhances perfusion during septic states.[45] For example, Gosche and colleagues used in vivo microvascular techniques to examine the effect of mucosally applied glucose on intestinal microvascular blood flow during *Escherichia coli* sepsis in the rat.[46] Blood flow was rapidly restored to above-baseline values after glucose was added, showing that the hyperemia induced by direct application of glucose to the mucosal surface of the small intestine is able to overcome the flow-restrictive effect of gram-negative bacteremia. The authors suggest that this direct hyperemic effect of transmucosal absorption of nutrients on the intestinal microvasculature is a factor that accounts for the improved maintenance of mucosal integrity associated with EN.[46] In 2010, Khalid and associates reported the results of early enteral feeding in more than 1000 patients who required ventilation for over 48 hours and vasopressors to maintain blood pressure. The investigators showed a decrease in mortality in those patients fed early despite the use of pressors.[47]

Generally, vasopressors shunt flow away from the splanchnic bed, although not all types of vasopressors have the same influence on the visceral blood flow, and each agent must be considered in relation to the clinical situation in which it is being used.[42] Revelly and colleagues evaluated EN in a group of hemodynamically unstable, critically ill patients requiring vasoactive medications and concluded that vasopressors increased visceral blood flow and that nutrient absorption was not adversely influenced.[48] Nonetheless, because splanchnic circulation is one of the major vascular beds affected by vasoactive agents, even at low doses, care must be taken when providing EN to patients in septic shock.[44] The vasoconstrictive effects of vasopressors may prevent a normal increase in splanchnic blood flow during enteral feeding, even though the GI tract may seem to be functional and without evidence of paralytic ileus. Restriction of splanchnic blood flow can lead to an ischemic state and result in jejunal feeding associated small bowel necrosis.[49–52]

Several approaches can be taken to maximize gut function in sepsis and inflammatory states such as critical illness.[34] They include maintaining visceral perfusion, which can usually be done by providing adequate resuscitation; glycemic control; correction of acidosis and electrolyte abnormalities; minimizing the use of anticholinergic medications, narcotics, and other medications that decrease intestinal motility; and instituting EN, even at low rates, within the first 24 to 48 hours of the onset of SIRS or sepsis. Additionally, the microbiome has recently come to the attention of the critical care community as an important factor in prevention and therapy in sepsis.[53] Currently available data support enteral feeding in the septic patient, but only after the patient has been adequately volume resuscitated and is at goal perfusion pressures.[17,52] Most clinicians rightfully approach the feeding of the resuscitated septic patient still requiring vasoactive agents with trepidation. These patients need close monitoring and frequent examinations to ensure that they do not develop the devastating complications of bowel ischemia. The ASPEN/SCCM guidelines recommend trophic feeding (10 to 20 kcal/h or 500 kcal/d) for the initial phase of sepsis, advancing as tolerated after 24 to 48 hours to greater than 80% of target energy goal over the first week.[34]

One of the foremost benefits of EN may be the prevention of serious infections.[34,54] However, once sepsis has been well established, EN is not proven to prevent further infection. For example, if EN is delayed until 4 to 6 days after the onset of injury, sepsis, or ICU admission, as in the study of ICU patients by Eyer and colleagues, it does not prevent progression to multiple organ system dysfunction or alter the risk of mortality.[55] Prior to the Elke study, evaluations of EN in patients with sepsis were rare.[41] Most papers addressing the benefits of enteral feeding are in mixed critical care populations, with only a portion of the studied patients having sepsis.

As discussed previously in this chapter, the enteral route is the preferred route of administration of nutrition therapy in critically ill patients whenever feasible.[34,54,56] However, during sepsis, EN may be complicated by lack of access or by GI dysfunction. Lack of access (see Chapter 12) should not be used as an excuse for not utilizing the GI tract. Numerous protocols have achieved 75% to 80% success rates in obtaining enteral access in severely ill patients.[57,58] Furthermore, centers with protocols including tube placement and promotility agents have demonstrated significantly higher nutrition adequacy and lower utilization of PN in critically ill patients.[60] When true GI intolerance or dysfunction prevents adequate nutrient delivery via the enteral route, PN should be considered. The institution of PN when EN is not tolerated is controversial, but starting PN earlier than 5 to 7 days has not proven to be of benefit.[34,56] If low infusion rates of EN can be safely administered, EN can be combined with PN to try to maintain gut mucosal integrity and GALT.[59-61] Despite the theoretical benefits of PN, a large randomized trial comparing ICU patients treated with early (48 hours) vs late (8 days) PN noted higher mortality, organ failure, and infections in the early group.[62] When a patient is in the acute phase of severe sepsis, the ASPEN/SCCM guidelines suggest not using exclusive PN or supplemental PN in conjunction with EN regardless of patient's degree of nutrition risk.[34] Practice Scenarios 23-1[63] and 23-2 address EN and PN use in patients with sepsis.

Practice Scenario 23-1

Question: What is the best approach to enteral nutrition (EN) initiation and feeding in an acutely septic trauma patient?

Scenario: A 58-year-old man was involved in a motorcycle collision and brought to the emergency department for evaluation.

Workup revealed a brain injury and bilateral rib fractures, pulmonary contusions, and a moderate spleen injury. The spleen injury was managed nonoperatively. No nutrition therapy was started. He required intubation for worsening mental status and hypoxia. After 48 hours of ventilator support, the patient developed a fever of 38.7°C and hypotension. His minute ventilation was 15 liters. A chest x-ray revealed a left lower lobe infiltrate. He was started on vasopressors and antibiotics. That morning, he had a blood pressure of 80/60 mm Hg despite moderate doses of norepinephrine and vasopressin. A nutrition consult was obtained because of the lack of nutrition delivery in the past 48 hours. His height was 175 cm, and his weight was 80 kg.

Intervention: Feeding was not initiated immediately because the patient was unstable. The patient was further resuscitated, and his vasopressor requirement decreased. Tube feeding was started at a low rate (20 mL/h). Frequent examinations were performed to ensure that the patient was tolerating the regimen. By the next day, the patient's hemodynamics were much improved. The tube feeds were advanced at a rate of 20 mL every 4 hours to the goal rate of 100 mL/h.

Answer: The patient's energy requirement was estimated by the Penn State equation to be approximately 2300 kcal/d (see Chapter 2).[63] His estimated protein requirement was approximately 140 g/d (1.8 g/kg/d). An immune-enhancing (isotonic, lactose-free, low-residue) tube feeding formulation was selected because of his history of trauma and sepsis. The specialized formula provided about 60 g protein per liter; therefore, a final goal rate of 100 mL/h would meet the patient's estimated nutrition needs. EN should not be started in the setting of acutely worsening hemodynamics. Once the patient's status improved, feeding was started carefully and advanced.

Rationale: Enteral tube feeds could have been started shortly after admission. The patient likely had an orogastric tube placed shortly after endotracheal intubation. Given the evidence for early tube feeding (within less than 48 hours), admission would have been an ideal time to start EN. Starting tube feeds earlier also gives clinicians the opportunity to "troubleshoot" patients who may not tolerate initial regimens (prokinetic agents, postpyloric tubes, etc). The patient required further stabilization with resuscitation. Good communication with the intensive care unit team allowed nutrition therapy to be started quickly.

Practice Scenario 23-2

Question: What is the best approach to parenteral nutrition (PN) initiation and feeding in an acutely septic patient?

Scenario: A 74-year-old woman was admitted with a 3-day history of diarrhea, abdominal pain, and lethargy. She had an extremely tender abdomen and a history of type 2 diabetes mellitus and atrial fibrillation. Laboratory examination indicated her blood glucose level was 542 mg/dL and white blood cell count was 22,100 cells/mm³. Given her status and examination results, she was taken to the operating room, where the surgery team found 100 cm of nonviable infarcted jejunum and performed a small bowel anastomosis. After surgery, the patient initially improved but then had high fevers and a high white blood cell count. A computed tomography scan was performed 7 days postoperatively, revealing a fluid collection around the anastomosis. The patient was taken to the operating room, her anastomosis was repaired, and drains were placed. Her blood cultures grew *Escherichia coli* and *Pseudomonas aeruginosa*. She was begun on broad-spectrum antibiotics. She improved at first but soon developed evidence of a proximal small bowel fistula from her surgically placed drains.

Intervention: PN was selected over enteral nutrition (EN) because the patient had a proximal intestinal fistula, diarrhea, and sepsis. A predictive equation was used to calculate her energy requirement. After several days, indirect calorimetry was used to reevaluate her energy needs.

Answer: This patient had not received nutrition for more than 7 days and was malnourished. EN would not be absorbed reliably, and PN would offer the best chance of her fistula closing spontaneously. Her estimated energy expenditure using the Mifflin-St. Jeor predictive equation was 1650 kcal/d (see Chapter 2). Her protein requirements were approximately 1.5 g/kg/d. A mixed-fuel system was preferable because the patient was hyperglycemic and dextrose alone was inadequate to provide enough energy. In addition to hyperglycemia, she was likely insulin resistant, as is the case in most septic patients. Furthermore, infusion of more than 5 mg/kg/min would likely exceed maximal glucose oxidation and lead to no additional protein synthesis. Exogenous lipids can be effectively used as a fuel source during sepsis. The patient received 1700 kcal with 1.5 g/kg of amino acid from PN and tolerated it well. During the next 3 days post surgery, her body temperature and white blood cell count gradually decreased. Her blood glucose level was maintained below 180 mg/dL. Indirect calorimetry was performed 5 days after surgery and observed to be 1150 kcal. To improve hyperglycemia and avoid other deleterious effects of overfeeding, the decision was made to lower the energy level of PN. The patient's nutrition status was monitored using daily weights, in-and-out fluid records, and serum glucose and electrolyte levels. Indirect calorimetry was repeated once or twice weekly as part of monitoring.

Rationale: The patient was at significant risk for complications secondary to her comorbidities and malnutrition. Her gut could not be reliably used, and PN was selected. She was given an increased protein allowance because of her wound and sepsis. Her energy requirements were estimated, reassessed, and then adjusted throughout her course of care.

Timing of Nutrition Support

The optimal time to start nutrition support is influenced by a host of factors, including age, premorbid conditions, route of nutrient delivery, metabolic state, and organ function.[64,65] As previously noted, literature evaluating nutrition support for critically ill patients has analyzed heterogeneous populations in which some but not all patients have sepsis. Nevertheless,

these studies yield important concepts for feeding the patient with sepsis.[20] The reported benefits of early EN are, among others, prevention of adverse structural and functional alterations in the mucosal barrier, augmentation of visceral blood flow, and enhancement of local and systemic immune response.[34,39,40] Three meta-analyses of the clinical benefits of early EN have reported reduced infections and shorter length of hospital stay with minimal risk and virtually no increase in major morbidity.[39,40,66] Despite these acknowledged benefits, nutrition support remains suboptimal in a significant percentage of critically ill patients.

Given that the early initiation of nutrition support is the superior and accepted practice, a multidisciplinary approach to determining appropriate timing in the individual patient cannot be overemphasized. This strategy entails the combined efforts of all involved healthcare providers while recognizing the unique skills and expertise that each team member brings to the care of the patient.

Enteral feeding should not proceed until appropriate resuscitation has been undertaken. Resuscitation remains a cornerstone of the 3-armed approach to the management of sepsis: source control, early antibiotic administration, and resuscitation. Early and aggressive resuscitation, or "early goal-directed therapy," involves the placement of invasive lines, including central venous catheters with continuous venous oxygen saturation monitoring, arterial lines, and so on, to evaluate the overall volume status of the patient. Fluid resuscitation is continued with set central venous pressure goals, at which point vasopressor medications are added in the hypotensive (mean arterial pressures less than 65 mm Hg), vasodilated patient.[17] A single laboratory or hemodynamic parameter signaling the successful resuscitation of the critically ill patient in shock remains elusive. Generally, clinicians use trends in hemodynamic parameters, including mean arterial pressures, central venous pressures, and vasopressor requirements, in conjunction with urine output, arterial base deficit, serum lactate, and venous oxygen saturations, to determine the relative success of resuscitation. Splanchnic circulation increases by as much as 40% to 60% in the setting of enteral feeding and increases the metabolic demand required of the GI tract.[54] If supply falls short of demand, rare but devastating complications can ensue. Fortunately, nonocclusive mesenteric ischemia (NMI) remains an uncommon complication following the early initiation of enteral feeding in the underresuscitated patient. NMI is a low flow state that most commonly affects the distribution of the superior mesenteric artery, which can result in irreversible ischemia and necrosis of the associated small and large bowel. Hypovolemia and underresuscitation can exaggerate the already hypoperfused and dysregulated splanchnic circulation in the setting of sepsis. Enteral feeding in the hemodynamically unstable patient should be undertaken with extreme caution. Treatment of NMI is usually supportive. Hemodynamic status is optimized, and intra-arterial vasodilators can be used as an adjunct. Patients that go on to require laparotomy and resection of nonviable bowel have very poor outcomes, with mortality rates as high as 80%.[67] Following resuscitation and assuming no other absolute contraindication to enteral feeding (ie, bowel obstruction), EN should be initiated as soon as possible.

Reports suggest that bowel sounds and evidence of bowel function (ie, passing flatus or stool) are not required for EN.[34,68] Waiting for these signs before initiating nutrition support can contribute to further delays in feeding. In a randomized trial, Suehiro and associates initiated oral feeding within 48 hours of gastrectomy, thereby demonstrating a proof of concept with regards to early feeding without awaiting traditional predictors of tolerance.[69] They reported no increase in morbidity and successfully reduced hospital stays. A meta-analysis examining 15 studies and 1240 patients with GI anastomoses demonstrated reduced postoperative complications when patients were fed within 24 hours of operation.[66] Other meta-analyses specifically in ICU and trauma patients report significant decreases in mortality and infectious complications.[70,71]

The SCCM/ASPEN guidelines recommend that critically ill patients receive EN therapy within 24 to 48 hours of making the diagnosis of severe sepsis/septic shock, as soon as resuscitation is complete and the patient is hemodynamically stable.[34] Although the benefits of early EN have been reported in many populations, feeding immediately after the initial diagnosis of sepsis yields a distinct set of problems. The proportion of ICU patients with GI dysfunction ranges from 30% to 70%, depending on the diagnosis, premorbid conditions, ventilation mode, medications, and metabolic state.[65,72] Proposed mechanisms of ICU and postoperative GI dysfunction can be separated into 3 general categories: mucosal barrier disruption, altered motility, and atrophy of the mucosa and GALT. Barrier disruption seems to be most commonly associated with splanchnic hypoperfusion, which is precipitated by numerous factors in the critical care setting and immediate postoperative period, including hypovolemia, increased catecholamines, increased proinflammatory cytokines, and decreased cardiac output. The net results are reduced mucosal blood flow and barrier disruption, altered GI motility, and changes in the bacterial flora and virulence of the organisms.[73–76] In sepsis, specific protein interactions continue to be more fully elucidated. Membrane toll-like receptors have been implicated in altered motility, with resultant changes in intestinal bacterial flora and the potential for translocation. Lipopolysaccharide, or endotoxin, has been demonstrated to stimulate toll-like receptor-4, resulting in impaired smooth muscle function in the GI tract, which may contribute to dysmotility.[77]

Kalff and colleagues described the mechanism that induces postoperative ileus.[73] Although it is not a septic model, similar mechanisms are extrapolated. In an elaborate series of human and animal studies, these investigators described the sequence of events following bowel manipulation. Following visceral manipulation, activation of transcription factors is noted, with upregulation of intracellular adhesion molecule-1 on the endothelium of the muscularis vessels. Leukocyte extravasation into the muscularis occurs, with resultant upregulation of inducible nitric oxide synthase, cyclooxygenase-2, IL-6, and signal transducer and activator of transcription-3 protein phosphorylation. This inflammatory focus then decreases contractile response and alters electrical activity, resulting in ileus.

As previously stated, recent approaches to maximize gut function in the postoperative and critical care settings include maintenance of visceral perfusion; glycemic control; electrolyte correction; early EN; and minimization of medications that alter GI function, such as anticholinergic agents, narcotics, and high-dose vasopressors.[68] GI intolerance should be continually reassessed and can manifest clinically in a variety of forms, including abdominal distension, increased gastric residual volumes or nasogastric output, abdominal pain, or diarrhea. The segmental contractility of the GI tract should be assessed because dysmotility can be focal (affecting predominately either the proximal or distal bowel) or diffuse. Impaired gastric and proximal GI motility can be addressed efficiently through the placement of postpyloric feeding tubes, which can be done successfully at the bedside in more than 80% of patients.[78]

Prokinetic agents can be utilized early and are helpful in some patients. Erythromycin acts on motilin receptors, resulting in increased motility, although its use may be limited by tachyphylaxis. Metoclopramide, a 5-HT(4) receptor agonist, works via cholinergic stimulation and is most efficacious in the proximal gut. Several peripherally acting mu opioid antagonists are available and have demonstrated some success in the setting of dysmotility associated with narcotic administration in the postoperative setting.[79] No single prokinetic agent will have uniform success in the ICU, and the factors contributing to GI dysmotility in each patient must be considered. Clinicians should exercise caution when using prokinetic agents in patients at high risk for bowel necrosis or obstruction.

In the ICU and postoperative settings, early EN using standardized protocols is associated with little morbidity and a GI tolerance rate in the 70% to 85% range.[59] When Barr and colleagues implemented a standardized, evidence-based enteral feeding protocol, they reported shortened duration of mechanical ventilation and reduced mortality.[57]

Complications of Enteral Nutrition in the Intensive Care Unit

In addition to the previously discussed problems of NMI and GI intolerance, other complications of nutrition support include aspiration and feeding tube malplacement. These complications are not specific to patients with sepsis but are commonly encountered in the ICU and warrant mention.

Aspiration can cause significant respiratory compromise and is likely related to an increased incidence of pneumonia. In addition to serial reassessment of the need for analgesics and sedatives, simple maneuvers such as electrolyte correction, elevation of the head of the bed, and routine oropharyngeal care can dramatically reduce the incidence of aspiration and pneumonia (see Chapter 13). Once again, the level of infusion in patients receiving enteral support can also be important. In a retrospective review, Metheny and associates demonstrated that the incidence of aspiration events was 12%, 13%, and 18% lower as the position of the feeding tube was advanced to the first, second, third, and fourth portions of the duodenum, respectively, when compared with feeding in the stomach.[80] This information suggests that postpyloric feeding should be the goal in patients who are at high risk for aspiration.[34] However, most literature does not suggest a clear benefit to routine postpyloric feeding for pneumonia prevention in all patients in the ICU.[34,81]

Complications associated with nasoenteric feeding tube placement include malpositioning of the tube into the respiratory tract, epistaxis, tube clogging, sinusitis, and displacement of an appropriately placed tube. Clinicians should confirm positioning of the tube by radiographic assessment prior to the initiation of feeding (see Chapter 12). Patients requiring prolonged enteral access (more than 4 weeks) should be evaluated for potential percutaneous gastric or jejunal access; complications of these procedures are discussed elsewhere.[82]

Complications of Parenteral Nutrition in the Intensive Care Unit

In patients with clear contraindications to EN or who present with preexisting malnutrition, PN may be appropriate. Several studies have demonstrated an increased risk of infectious complications in patients receiving PN, but the exact etiology is unknown. Newer trials have shown diminishing differences between the risk for complications with EN vs PN. The most common nosocomial infection associated with PN remains catheter-related bloodstream infection (CRBSI) because central venous access is required for administration. In a prospective trial, patients receiving PN had superior glycemic control but were 4 times as likely to develop CRBSI as their counterparts receiving EN.[83] Preventive measures taken to avoid this complication (eg, appropriate education with regards to sterile technique, hand hygiene, prudent choices of insertion sites, and meticulous line care) reduce the incidence of CRBSI in the ICU.[84]

Nutrition Requirements

Energy

Estimating energy requirements in patients with sepsis is difficult. As previously noted, energy expenditure studies report increases of 20% to 60% over basal expenditure.[26] The patient's ability to utilize the energy delivered in the early phases of sepsis is a second issue.[25] The methods for estimating energy requirements for septic and critically ill patients are evolving, as illustrated by the concept of hypocaloric or "permissive underfeeding" in the first few days of care in critically ill populations.[85-87] Several studies in critically ill obese patients have used a hypocaloric, high-protein regimen with beneficial outcomes.[87,88] The morbidly obese population is often treated separately in terms of energy prescriptions in the ICU (see Chapter 35). Generally, extreme energy restriction (less than 20% of estimated energy goals) has been cited as detrimental to the critically ill patient.[89] A teleological argument for permissive underfeeding during times of severe illness and stress states that a relative "anorexia of illness" develops with significant infection and that supply of nutrients during this period induces a more proinflammatory state, which then exacerbates the condition. This concept has led several investigators to hypothesize that hypocaloric feeding in the early phases of critical illness and sepsis may be beneficial to patients. Retrospective and prospective studies have evaluated energy delivery and outcome, suggesting a possible benefit for relative hypocaloric feeding regimens.[90,91] The earlier trials may have had numerous confounding factors. Specifically, the

retrospective studies tended to include healthier patients without prescribed nutrition therapy in the hypocaloric groups, thus improving their mortality. Currently, energy delivery in the range of 20 to 30 kcal/kg/d is considered safe for critically ill patients (excluding the morbidly obese). However, more recent trials have examined the association of outcomes and energy deficit in critically ill patients. Villet and associates observed that patients with a negative total energy balance had worse outcomes at 1 week.[92] In a larger multi-institutional ICU study, Heyland and associates grouped patients by proportion of prescribed nutrition support received.[93] This study demonstrated decreased mortality in patients receiving a larger proportion of their prescribed nutrition support. These newer data suggest a benefit to full delivery of nutrition support throughout the hospital course. Interestingly, even with aggressive delivery protocols, the energy delivered in the ICU is often about 80% of the prescribed amount.[94] In actual practice, this rate of delivery results in hypocaloric nutrition despite best efforts to meet the patient's energy goal.

Carbohydrate

Glucose oxidation is increased in sepsis and, to a certain extent, can provide the appropriate route of disposal for exogenously administered glucose.[95] The infusion of glucose is not associated with significant activation of the sympathetic nervous system and therefore carries a negligible thermogenic response.[96] In an elaborate series of studies, Wolfe and colleagues concluded that nonprotein energy provision in patients with sepsis should be largely in the form of carbohydrate, with exogenous insulin added to stimulate cellular protein anabolism.[97] However, glucose administration rates greater than 4 to 6 mg/kg/min result in excess lipogenesis and lead to hyperglycemia. Carbohydrate administration should supply 50% to 60% of the total energy prescription to avoid exceeding the maximum contribution of glucose oxidation and contributing to excess lipogenesis.[95]

Excess carbohydrate administration is also more likely to result in poor control of blood glucose levels. Studies have investigated strict control of blood glucose levels between 80 and 110 mg/dL in the ICU population. The first large prospective randomized trials demonstrated that critically ill patients whose blood glucose was strictly controlled had shorter ICU stays, decreased in-hospital mortality rates, and 46% fewer episodes of septicemia compared with ICU patients whose blood glucose levels were in the 180 to 200 mg/dL range.[22] In a subsequent study by the same investigators, significant hepatic mitochondrial abnormalities were noted in the control group that did not receive meticulous glucose control. The mitochondrial abnormalities noted in these critically ill populations no doubt have significance in the patients' ability to oxidize nutrient substrates.[98] However, a larger ICU trial with longer follow-up demonstrated a higher mortality in the group receiving very strict blood glucose control.[99] In the wake of these findings, there has been a shift to moderation in glucose control in the ICU. Carbohydrate administration and glucose control continue to be moving targets in the care of the critically ill (see Chapter 34 for further discussion of glycemic control in critical illness).

Lipid

Exogenous lipids can be effectively used as a fuel source during sepsis, although the optimal composition of the various lipid sources is controversial.[32,100] Two characteristics of lipids make them a valuable energy source for patients with sepsis. First, lipids are energy-dense, containing 9 kcal/g. Therefore, lipids deliver more energy in less volume than carbohydrate or protein, which is advantageous for patients in whom volume restriction is important (eg, in the setting of renal failure or pulmonary edema). Second, the respiratory quotient is lower for lipids than carbohydrates (0.7 vs 1.0). This finding implies that lipid oxidation produces less carbon dioxide than the metabolism of carbohydrates does and may therefore reduce blood concentrations of carbon dioxide. Theoretically, this outcome seems appealing, but no prospective, randomized studies have shown significant benefit of high-fat diets in the patient with sepsis.

In critical care and sepsis patients, the amount of lipid injectable emulsions (ILEs) should not exceed 1.0 g/kg/d if soybean oil (18-carbon, ω-6 fatty acid) is the source of lipid. In 2016, Smoflipid became available in the United States and seems likely to replace the soy-based lipids. Smoflipid emulsion contains 30% soybean oil, 30% medium-chain triglycerides, 25% olive oil and 15% fish oil.[32,101] See Chapters 5 and 15 for further information on ILE products.

Guidelines for enteral lipid delivery are similar to those for parenteral lipid provision. The usual lipid goal (1.0 g/kg/d) can be liberalized when enteral lipids include lipid substrates containing ω-3 fatty acids, medium-chain fatty acids, and short-chain fatty acids. As discussed previously, the route and makeup of the lipid substrate is critical, and a mixture of lipid fuels should be delivered whenever possible. Sepsis results in a decrease in cellular ability to transport long-chain fatty acids across the mitochondrial membrane secondary to a sepsis-induced alteration in the acylcarnitine carrier.[32] Medium-chain fatty acids do not require carnitine for transport into the mitochondria.[102] Data supporting benefits of short-chain fatty acids (butyrate and propionate) produced from the bacterial fermentation of soluble fibers in the GI lumen have been extensively reported.[103,104] Benefits range from maintaining optimal GI mucosal membrane integrity to systemically enhancing immune function via receptors on multiple cell types including white blood cell lines.[105]

When ω-3 fatty acids are delivered as fish oils (DHA and EPA), they have beneficial effects in patients with sepsis, including modulation of leukocyte function and regulation of cytokine release through nuclear signaling and gene expression.[106,107] Leukotrienes, thromboxane, and prostaglandins derived from ω-6 fatty acids are proinflammatory compared with metabolites associated with the ω-3 fatty acids.[108] EPA and DHA lipids have been reported to enhance the production of a group of prostaglandin derivatives called *specialized proresolving molecules*,[101,109] which play a role in accelerating the resolution of the proinflammatory state. Abundant data report the influence of EPA and DHA on nuclear signaling and gene expression.[110] For example, polyunsaturated fatty acids interact with various nuclear receptor proteins such as peroxisome proliferator-activated receptor, which then alters nuclear

factor-kappa B (NF-κB) and gene expression. By decreasing NF-κB migration into the nucleus, ω-3 fatty acids downregulate the proinflammatory response to stressful stimuli.[108] The route of delivery of ω-3 fatty acids may also be of importance. Utilizing the enteral route, approximately 2 to 3 days are required to achieve adequate ω-3 fat levels in the cellular membrane to elicit the beneficial effects on the prostaglandin cascade. However, when given parenterally, a clinically relevant response can be achieved in 1 to 3 hours, depending on the dose and tissue being evaluated.[111,112] In a randomized trial in 661 patients receiving intravenous ω-3 PN admixtures, Heller and colleagues found a decrease in antibiotic use, shorter length of hospital stay, and a trend toward lowering mortality.[113] Respiratory failure is common in patients with sepsis. EPA has been recently reported to have beneficial influence on preventing the loss of diaphragm function in sepsis.[114] In addition, one report suggests that EPA can enhance resistance to gram-negative pathogens such as Pseudomonas.[115] Multiple prospective trials have demonstrated improved mortality and lung-related outcomes in the setting of acute lung injury/acute respiratory distress syndrome with the use of formulas containing EPA, DHA, and antioxidants.[116–119] However, a larger prospective trial found no benefit when patients with lung injury were treated with supplemental fatty acids and antioxidants.[120] This discrepancy highlights the need for further research in regards to method of delivery of these adjuncts. These reports are consistent with the concept that EPA and DHA can be thought of as not just passively modulating the inflammatory process but as actively involved in the resolution of inflammation. While the use of enteral formulations containing anti-inflammatory lipids (primarily EPA and DHA) can be used as pharmacologic agents to modulate the hyperdynamic/hypermetabolic response and outcomes in septic and critically ill patients, conflicting data in the literature prevented the ASPEN/SCCM Guidelines from making a recommendation for use of anti-inflammatory lipid formulas at this time.[34]

Other general functions of lipids important to nutrition support include carrying fat-soluble vitamins, forming structural units in cell membranes, providing precursors to eicosanoids, cytokine production, and interaction with gene expression (see Chapter 5).[32,111,113] The optimal lipid for the septic patient remains to be determined, but a blend of ω-3 and ω-6 lipid sources would certainly seem to be more appropriate for critically ill and septic patients than the predominant ω-6 source provided by the soy-based ILEs widely used in the United States.[113,121]

Protein

Optimal protein delivery during sepsis is estimated to be between 1.5 and 2 g/kg/d and possibly even up to 2.5 g/kg/d in selected cases.[20,24] However, protein requirements may be higher in patients with excessive nitrogen losses, such as those with burns and large open wounds.[122] Recent data also support increasing protein requirements in patients with sepsis during tight glucose control. Conversely, the amount and quality of protein required may be altered for patients with hepatic and acute renal failure (see Chapters 27 and 29). Data support the use of whey and casein protein sources in critically ill populations.[123-125] The biological value, protein efficiency ratio, and net protein utilization all are superior for whey and casein compared with soy.

Arginine and Glutamine

The use of amino acids supplements to improve outcome or limit morbidity and mortality in the critically ill and septic populations is controversial.[126] Arginine and glutamine have been the most extensively studied.

Regarding arginine, one school of thought indicates that arginine is potentially toxic,[127] whereas others posit that arginine is deficient in patients with sepsis and should be supplemented.[128] Arginine is critical in the nitric oxide production pathway. Arginine levels are also dramatically reduced in the septic state.[129] Nitric oxide has been reported to have numerous beneficial effects, including decrease in hepatic and splanchnic injury following ischemic insult, increasing myocardial perfusion, and preventing endothelial damage via platelet and leukocyte adherence changes noted in sepsis.[127-132] On the other hand, investigators have feared that increasing arginine levels with supplementation could lead to worsening hypotension and outcomes secondary to uncontrolled nitric oxide production. However, in a small study of patients with severe sepsis, large-dose L-arginine infusion did not have hemodynamic consequences.[133] In the clinical setting, one published study demonstrated dramatically increased mortality with arginine-containing enteral feeding vs PN in a subgroup analysis of a small number of patients with sepsis.[134] However, several trials studying arginine formulas demonstrated improved outcomes for general ICU patients, including those with sepsis.[135,136] The largest trial published on septic patients specifically demonstrated a mortality benefit with the use of arginine formula.[137] As noted previously, enterally feeding the patient with severe sepsis or septic shock must be done cautiously. However, recent prospective trials delivering arginine to septic patients has shown no harm. Additional arginine seems to at least partially overcome the elevated asymmetric dimethyl arginine, which causes vasoconstriction, consequently improving perfusion to underperfused tissues.[138-141] Several investigators in the area theorize that arginine may be deficient in sepsis. Although the overwhelming bulk of the current literature suggests that arginine-containing formulas are safe and might reduce complications in sepsis, the ASPEN/SCCM guidelines recommend use of an arginine/fish oil formula only in surgical ICU patients and do not recommend their routine use in patients with sepsis alone.[34]

Glutamine, like arginine, is considered conditionally essential in the stressed individual. Sepsis results in a rapid and precipitous drop in both plasma and muscle glutamine concentrations.[142] Over the past 20 years, glutamine has been reported to offer a number of biochemical and clinical benefits, including maintenance of acid-base balance, provision of primary fuel for rapidly proliferating cells (ie, enterocytes and lymphocytes), integrity of GI mucosa, decreased clinical infections and gram-negative bacteremia, synthesis of glutathione and arginine, lowering of insulin resistance and inflammatory response, and function as a key substrate for

gluconeogenesis.[132,143,144] Furthermore, glutamine can induce heat shock protein,[145] a class of cellular chaperone proteins that support appropriate protein folding as they come off the ribosome. These proteins prevent poorly folded intracellular proteins from irreversible degradation by endogenous cellular proteolytic enzyme systems.[146] Thus, by increasing production of heat shock protein, supplemental glutamine enhances the ability of cells to protect themselves from subsequent stress. Singleton and associates reported in a septic animal model that glutamine could decrease lung injury and mortality.[147] In a randomized controlled trial in ICU patients, of which 71% were septic, glutamine supplementation resulted in a 24% decrease in mortality.[148] These results are supported by a meta-analysis of glutamine use in the ICU, which found reduced length of hospital stay, lower infectious complications in surgical patients, and improved mortality in critically ill patients.[149] However, glutamine utilization in the ICU setting has come under new scrutiny with the publication of the REDOX trial.[150] In this large, multicenter clinical trial investigators observed that patients supplemented with glutamine and antioxidants had a higher mortality. The patients with the increased mortality were primarily those with renal or multiorgan failure. Because this trial showed potential harm and others showed no benefit with glutamine supplementation, the ASPEN/SCCM guidelines recommend that clinicians not supplement severely ill ICU patients with enteral or parenteral glutamine.[34]

Antioxidants

Evidence indicates that sepsis significantly increases production of reactive oxygen species (ROS) by multiple cell lines.[151] Oxidant injury occurs with loss of balance between endogenous antioxidant defenses and cellular production of ROS. ROS generated by activated phagocytic cells results in a host of signal transduction and gene activation events, resulting in a proinflammatory state. Free radicals may injure cell membranes directly by forming lipid peroxides or may damage intracellular proteins, nucleic acids, and organelles, leading to cell death.[151]

During normal physiological conditions and inspiration of 21% oxygen, humans have adequate defenses against ROS produced in routine metabolic processes. Cellular injury occurs when overproduction of ROS overwhelms the host's ability to detoxify the generated ROS. Once the endogenous antioxidant defenses, such as glutathione, superoxide dismutase, and antioxidant vitamins, are overwhelmed, injury occurs.[152]

The appropriate composition of an antioxidant cocktail for the septic population has yet to be determined. To date, at least 22 randomized, prospective trials of various antioxidants in severely stressed and septic patients have been reported with variable results, most showing benefit.[142] For example, Nathens and colleagues reported in a large prospective, randomized trial of 595 ICU patients (91% trauma) that the addition of 3 g intravenous vitamin C per day and 3000 IU enterally delivered vitamin E could decrease ICU stay and ventilator time.[153] In a study of high-risk trauma patients before and after initiation of an antioxidant protocol, Collier and associates found a modest mortality benefit after implementation of the protocol.[154] Several trials have investigated selenium supplementation specifically in patients with sepsis.[155-159] Most of these studies demonstrated some benefit. A notable exception is the study by Forceville and colleagues,[159] which used doses of up to 4000 mcg. Based on the current literature, moderate selenium doses around 500 mcg/d may have a mortality benefit for the septic population. Larger prospective trials are needed to confirm the benefit and address dosing specifics.

The optimal duration of antioxidant therapy in critical illness or sepsis is unknown. Published protocols have had a range from 7 to 28 days. Although there are no clear data comparing different intervals, a logical approach would be to continue therapy as long as the patient is at high risk for infectious complications (ie, for the duration of the ICU admission).

The literature suggests that clinicians provide at least the Recommended Dietary Allowances of antioxidant vitamins and trace elements to critically ill patients throughout hospitalization. However, the ASPEN/SCCM guidelines did not make a definitive recommendation for selenium, zinc, or antioxidant supplementation specifically in sepsis.[34]

Host Immunity

The progression from sepsis to septic shock and, ultimately, death results from the imbalance of a vast array of interrelated hormones, cytokines, altered substrate utilization, and the subsequent host response to the infection. Renowned physician Lewis Thomas described inflammation as follows: "Our arsenals for fighting off bacteria are so powerful . . . that we are more in danger from them than the invaders."[160]

The development of malnutrition is rapid in the critically ill and septic patient because of the complex metabolic changes induced by cytokine mediators and a wide array of hormones. Malnutrition is clearly linked to derangements in both humoral and cellular immunity, resulting in increased susceptibility to infection.[76,161] Many studies indicate that adequate nutrition is necessary to support a functional immune system and reduce septic morbidity and mortality.[7,161,162]

If appropriate nutrition support is not maintained during the management of sepsis, the gut can fail, contributing to multiple organ failure.[163,164] Gut failure is manifested as feeding intolerance as well as loss of the gut barrier to intestinal flora. The results of a prospective study investigating associations between bacterial translocation, gastric microflora, and septic morbidity in critically ill patients indicate that proximal gut colonization is associated with both increased bacterial translocation and septic morbidity.[165,166]

Bacterial translocation from the intestinal lumen to gut lymphatics or the portal venous system most likely occurs in all individuals, but it is not clinically significant in the immune-competent host.[167] Destruction of translocated bacteria in mesenteric lymph nodes depends on the immunological function of the host and individual bacterial virulence factors. Studies have suggested that early EN may protect the mucosal barrier from dysfunction.[168,169] In addition to the nutrients previously discussed as having potentially beneficial effects in septic patients, the administration of probiotics to maintain a "healthy" microbiome has recently shown promise in sepsis in immunocompromised hosts.[170,171]

At the present time, no specific biological immune modulators (eg, antibodies to E5 and HA-1A moieties of gram-negative cell walls, to IL-2 receptors, or to soluble TNF-α receptor) or pharmacological therapies (eg, naloxone, pentoxifylline, bradykinin antagonists, and N-acetylcysteine), with the exception of drotrecogin alfa (activated), have improved survival of septic patients.[1,13] Maintenance of host immunity is still the most valuable defense to reduce septic complications and mortality. Nutrition support, possibly including the use of immune-modulating nutrients via EN and PN, is one of the most effective ways to reach this goal.

References

1. Hall MJ, Williams SN, DeFrances CJ, Golosinskiy A. Inpatient care for septicemia or sepsis: a challenge for patients and hospitals. *NCHS Data Brief.* 2011(62):1–8.
2. Kochanek KD, Xu J, Murphy SL, Minino AM, Kung HC. Deaths: preliminary data for 2009. *Natl Vital Stat Rep.* 2011;59(4):1–51.
3. Yende S, Austin S, Rhodes A, et al. Long-term quality of life among survivors of severe sepsis: analyses of two international trials. *Crit Care Med.* 2016;44(8):1461–1467.
4. Sands KE, Bates DW, Lanken PN, et al. Epidemiology of sepsis syndrome in 8 academic medical centers. *JAMA.* 1997;278(3):234–240.
5. Manship L, McMillin RD, Brown JJ. The influence of sepsis and multisystem and organ failure on mortality in the surgical intensive care unit. *Am Surg.* 1984;50(2):94–101.
6. Centers for Disease Control and Prevention. Making health care safer: think sepsis. Time matters. *CDC Vital Signs.* August 23, 2016. http://www.cdc.gov/vitalsigns/sepsis/infographic.html#graphic. Accessed July 10, 2017.
7. Hotchkiss RS, Karl IE. The pathophysiology and treatment of sepsis. *N Engl J Med.* 2003;348(2):138–150.
8. Krezalek MA, Skowron KB, Guyton KL, et al. The intestinal microbiome and surgical disease. *Curr Probl Surg.* 2016;53(6):257–293.
9. Bone RC, Balk RA, Cerra FB, et al. Definitions for sepsis and organ failure and guidelines for the use of innovative therapies in sepsis. The ACCP/SCCM Consensus Conference Committee. American College of Chest Physicians/Society of Critical Care Medicine. *Chest.* 1992;101(6):1644–1655.
10. Singer M, Deutschman CS, Seymour CW, et al. the third international consensus definitions for sepsis and septic shock (Sepsis-3). *JAMA.* 23 2016;315(8):801–810.
11. Calandra T, Cohen J, International Sepsis Forum definition of infection in the ICUCC. The International Sepsis Forum consensus conference on definitions of infection in the intensive care unit. *Crit Care Med.* 2005;33(7):1538–1548.
12. Levy MM, Fink MP, Marshall JC, et al. 2001 SCCM/ESICM/ACCP/ATS/SIS International Sepsis Definitions Conference. *Crit Care Med.* 2003;31(4):1250–1256.
13. Rice TW, Bernard GR. Therapeutic intervention and targets for sepsis. *Annu Rev Med.* 2005;56:225–248.
14. Cinel I, Opal SM. Molecular biology of inflammation and sepsis: a primer. *Crit Care Med.* 2009;37(1):291–304.
15. Rosenthal MD, Vanzant EL, Martindale RG, Moore FA. Evolving paradigms in the nutritional support of critically ill surgical patients. *Curr Probl Surg.* 2015;52(4):147–182.
16. Dellinger RP, Carlet JM, Masur H, et al. Surviving Sepsis Campaign guidelines for management of severe sepsis and septic shock. *Crit Care Med.* 2004;32(3):858–873.
17. Rivers E, Nguyen B, Havstad S, et al. Early goal-directed therapy in the treatment of severe sepsis and septic shock. *N Engl J Med.* 2001;345(19):1368–1377.

18. Meisner M. Biomarkers of sepsis: clinically useful? *Curr Opin Crit Care.* 2005;11(5):473–480.

19. Rusavy Z, Sramek V, Lacigova S, et al. Influence of insulin on glucose metabolism and energy expenditure in septic patients. *Crit Care.* 2004;8(4):R213–R220.

20. Martindale RG, Nishikawa R, Siepler JK. The metabolic response to stress and alterations in nutrient metabolism. In: Shikora SA MR, ed. *Nutritional Considerations in the Intensive Care Unit: Science, Rationale and Practice*: Dubuque, IA: Kendall Hunt; 2002:11–20.

21. Plank LD, Hill GL. Sequential metabolic changes following induction of systemic inflammatory response in patients with severe sepsis or major blunt trauma. *World J Surg.* 2000;24(6):630–638.

22. van den Berghe G, Wouters P, Weekers F, et al. Intensive insulin therapy in critically ill patients. *N Engl J Med.* 2001;345(19):1359–1367.

23. Dahn MS, Mitchell RA, Lange MP, Smith S, Jacobs LA. Hepatic metabolic response to injury and sepsis. *Surgery.* 1995;117(5):520–530.

24. Shaw JH, Wildbore M, Wolfe RR. Whole body protein kinetics in severely septic patients. The response to glucose infusion and total parenteral nutrition. *Ann Surg.* 1987;205(3):288–294.

25. Streat SJ, Beddoe AH, Hill GL. Aggressive nutritional support does not prevent protein loss despite fat gain in septic intensive care patients. *J Trauma.* 1987;27(3):262–266.

26. Plank LD, Connolly AB, Hill GL. Sequential changes in the metabolic response in severely septic patients during the first 23 days after the onset of peritonitis. *Ann Surg.* 1998;228(2):146–158.

27. Cerra FB. Hypermetabolism, organ failure, and metabolic support. *Surgery.* 1987;101(1):1–14.

28. Liebau F, Norberg A, Rooyackers O. Does feeding induce maximal stimulation of protein balance? *Curr Opin Clin Nutr Metab Care.* 2016;19(2):120–124.

29. Ziegler TR, Bazargan N, Leader LM, Martindale RG. Glutamine and the gastrointestinal tract. *Curr Opin Clin Nutr Metab Care.* 2000;3(5):355–362.

30. Rosenthal MD. Moore FA. Persistent inflammatory, immunosuppressed, catabolic syndrome (PICS): a new phenotype of multiple organ failure. *J Adv Nutr Hum Metab.* 2015;1(1):e784. doi:10.14800/janhm.784.

31. Martinez A, Chiolero R, Bollman M, et al. Assessment of adipose tissue metabolism by means of subcutaneous microdialysis in patients with sepsis or circulatory failure. *Clin Physiol Funct Imaging.* 2003;23(5):286–292.

32. Hasselmann M, Reimund JM. Lipids in the nutritional support of the critically ill patients. *Curr Opin Crit Care.* 2004;10(6):449–455.

33. Bansal V, Syres KM, Makarenkova V, et al. Interactions between fatty acids and arginine metabolism: implications for the design of immune-enhancing diets. *JPEN J Parenter Enteral Nutr.* 2005;29(1 Suppl):S75–S80.

34. McClave SA, Taylor BE, Martindale RG, et al. Guidelines for the provision and assessment of nutrition support therapy in the adult critically ill patient: Society of Critical Care Medicine (SCCM) and American Society for Parenteral and Enteral Nutrition (A.S.P.E.N.). *JPEN J Parenter Enteral Nutr.* 2016;40(2):159–211.

35. Ruggieri AJ, Levy RJ, Deutschman CS. Mitochondrial dysfunction and resuscitation in sepsis. *Crit Care Clin.* 2010;26(3):567–575.

36. Martindale RG, McClave SA, Vanek VW, et al. Guidelines for the provision and assessment of nutrition support therapy in the adult critically ill patient: Society of Critical Care Medicine and American Society for Parenteral and Enteral Nutrition: Executive Summary. *Crit Care Med.* 2009;37(5):1757–1761.

37. Hoffer LJ, Bistrian BR. Appropriate protein provision in critical illness: a systematic and narrative review. *Am J Clin Nutr.* 2012;96(3):591–600.

38. Nicolo M, Heyland DK, Chittams J, Sammarco T, Compher C. Clinical outcomes related to protein delivery in a critically ill population: a multicenter, multinational observation study. *JPEN J Parenter Enteral Nutr.* 2016;40(1):45–51.

39. Marik PE, Zaloga GP. Early enteral nutrition in acutely ill patients: a systematic review. *Crit Care Med.* 2001;29(12):2264–2270.

40. Heyland DK, Dhaliwal R. Early enteral nutrition vs. early parenteral nutrition: an irrelevant question for the critically ill? *Crit Care Med.* 2005;33(1):260–261.

41. Elke G, Kuhnt E, Ragaller M, et al. Enteral nutrition is associated with improved outcome in patients with severe sepsis. A secondary analysis of the VItrial. *Med Klin Intensivmed Notfmed.* 2013;108(3):223–233.

42. Zaloga GP, Roberts PR, Marik P. Feeding the hemodynamically unstable patient: a critical evaluation of the evidence. *Nutr Clin Pract.* 2003;18(4):285–293.

43. Clemmesen O, Ott P, Larsen FS. Splanchnic metabolism in acute liver failure and sepsis. *Curr Opin Crit Care.* 2004;10(2):152–155.

44. McClave SA, Chang WK. Feeding the hypotensive patient: does enteral feeding precipitate or protect against ischemic bowel? *Nutr Clin Pract.* 2003;18(4):279–284.

45. Moore-Olufemi SD, Kozar RA, Moore FA, et al. Ischemic preconditioning protects against gut dysfunction and mucosal injury after ischemia/reperfusion injury. *Shock.* 2005;23(3):258–263.

46. Gosche JR, Garrison RN, Harris PD, Cryer HG. Absorptive hyperemia restores intestinal blood flow during *Escherichia coli* sepsis in the rat. *Arch Surg.* 1990;125(12):1573–1576.

47. Khalid I, Doshi P, DiGiovine B. Early enteral nutrition and outcomes of critically ill patients treated with vasopressors and mechanical ventilation. *Am J Crit Care.* 2010;19(3):261–268.

48. Revelly JP, Tappy L, Berger MM, et al. Early metabolic and splanchnic responses to enteral nutrition in postoperative cardiac surgery patients with circulatory compromise. *Intensive Care Med.* 2001;27(3):540–547.

49. Myers JG, Page CP, Stewart RM, et al. Complications of needle catheter jejunostomy in 2,022 consecutive applications. *Am J Surg.* 1995;170(6):547–551.

50. Schunn CD, Daly JM. Small bowel necrosis associated with postoperative jejunal tube feeding. *J Am Coll Surg.* 1995;180(4):410–416.

51. Smith-Choban P, Max MH. Feeding jejunostomy: a small bowel stress test? *Am J Surg.* 1988;155(1):112–117.

52. Marvin RG, McKinley BA, McQuiggan M, Cocanour CS, Moore FA. Nonocclusive bowel necrosis occurring in critically ill trauma patients receiving enteral nutrition manifests no reliable clinical signs for early detection. *Am J Surg.* 2000;179(1):7–12.

53. Krezalek MA, DeFazio J, Zaborina O, Zaborin A, Alverdy JC. The shift of an intestinal "microbiome" to a "pathobiome" governs the course and outcome of sepsis following surgical injury. *Shock.* 2016;45(5):475–482.

54. Zaloga GP. Parenteral nutrition in adult inpatients with functioning gastrointestinal tracts: assessment of outcomes. *Lancet.* 2006;367(9516):1101–1111.

55. Eyer SD, Micon LT, Konstantinides FN, et al. Early enteral feeding does not attenuate metabolic response after blunt trauma. *J Trauma.* 1993;34(5):639–644.

56. Jacobs DG, Jacobs DO, Kudsk KA, et al. Practice management guidelines for nutritional support of the trauma patient. *J Trauma.* 2004;57(3):660–679.

57. Barr J, Hecht M, Flavin KE, Khorana A, Gould MK. Outcomes in critically ill patients before and after the implementation of an evidence-based nutritional management protocol. *Chest.* 2004;125(4):1446–1457.

58. Kozar RA, McQuiggan MM, Moore EE, et al. Postinjury enteral tolerance is reliably achieved by a standardized protocol. *J Surg Res.* 2002;104(1):70–75.

59. Heyland DK, Cahill NE, Dhaliwal R, et al. Impact of enteral feeding protocols on enteral nutrition delivery: results of a multicenter observational study. *JPEN J Parenter Enteral Nutr.* 2010;34(6):675–684.

60. Alpers DH. Why, how, and to which part of the gastrointestinal tract should forced enteral feedings be delivered in patients? *Curr Opin Gastroenterol.* 2004;20(2):104–109.

61. Hammarqvist F. Can it all be done by enteral nutrition? *Curr Opin Clin Nutr Metab Care.* 2004;7(2):183–187.

62. Casaer MP, Mesotten D, Hermans G, et al. Early versus late parenteral nutrition in critically ill adults. *N Engl J Med.* 2011;365(6):506–517.

63. Frankenfield DC, Coleman A, Alam S, Cooney RN. Analysis of estimation methods for resting metabolic rate in critically ill adults. *JPEN J Parenter Enteral Nutr.* 2009;33(1):27–36.

64. Lewis SJ, Egger M, Sylvester PA, Thomas S. Early enteral feeding versus "nil by mouth" after gastrointestinal surgery: systematic review and meta-analysis of controlled trials. *BMJ.* 2001;323(7316):773–776.

65. Mutlu GM, Mutlu EA, Factor P. Prevention and treatment of gastrointestinal complications in patients on mechanical ventilation. *Am J Respir Med.* 2003;2(5):395–411.

66. Osland E, Yunus RM, Khan S, Memon MA. Early versus traditional postoperative feeding in patients undergoing resectional gastrointestinal surgery: a meta-analysis. *JPEN J Parenter Enteral Nutr.* 2011;35(4):473–487.

67. Park WM, Gloviczki P, Cherry KJ, et al. Contemporary management of acute mesenteric ischemia: factors associated with survival. *J Vasc Surg.* 2002;35(3):445–452.

68. Caddell KA, Martindale R, McClave SA, Miller K. Can the intestinal dysmotility of critical illness be differentiated from postoperative ileus? *Curr Gastroenterol Rep.* 2011;13(4):358–367.

69. Suehiro T, Matsumata T, Shikada Y, Sugimachi K. Accelerated rehabilitation with early postoperative oral feeding following gastrectomy. *Hepatogastroenterology.* 2004;51(60):1852–1855.

70. Doig GS, Heighes PT, Simpson F, Sweetman EA, Davies AR. Early enteral nutrition, provided within 24 h of injury or intensive care unit admission, significantly reduces mortality in critically ill patients: a meta-analysis of randomised controlled trials. *Intensive Care Med.* 2009;35(12):2018–2027.

71. Doig GS, Heighes PT, Simpson F, Sweetman EA. Early enteral nutrition reduces mortality in trauma patients requiring intensive care: a meta-analysis of randomised controlled trials. *Injury.* 2011;42(1):50–56.

72. Schmidt H, Martindale R. The gastrointestinal tract in critical illness: nutritional implications. *Curr Opin Clin Nutr Metab Care.* 2003;6(5):587–591.

73. Kalff JC, Turler A, Schwarz NT, et al. Intra-abdominal activation of a local inflammatory response within the human muscularis externa during laparotomy. *Ann Surg.* 2003;237(3):301–315.

74. Ritz MA, Fraser R, Tam W, Dent J. Impacts and patterns of disturbed gastrointestinal function in critically ill patients. *Am J Gastroenterol.* 2000;95(11):3044–3052.

75. Alverdy J, Zaborina O, Wu L. The impact of stress and nutrition on bacterial-host interactions at the intestinal epithelial surface. *Curr Opin Clin Nutr Metab Care.* 2005;8(2):205–209.

76. Ayala A, Chung CS, Grutkoski PS, Song GY. Mechanisms of immune resolution. *Crit Care Med.* 2003;31(8 Suppl):S558–S571.

77. Scirocco A, Matarrese P, Petitta C, et al. Exposure of toll-like receptors 4 to bacterial lipopolysaccharide (LPS) impairs human colonic smooth muscle cell function. *J Cell Physiol.* 2010;223(2):442–450.

78. Gatt M, MacFie J. Bedside postpyloric feeding tube placement: a pilot series to validate this novel technique. *Crit Care Med.* 2009;37(2):523–527.

79. Wolff BG, Michelassi F, Gerkin TM, et al. Alvimopan, a novel, peripherally acting mu opioid antagonist: results of a multi-

center, randomized, double-blind, placebo-controlled, phase III trial of major abdominal surgery and postoperative ileus. *Ann Surg.* 2004;240(4):728–735.

80. Metheny NA, Stewart BJ, McClave SA. Relationship between feeding tube site and respiratory outcomes. *JPEN J Parenter Enteral Nutr.* 2011;35(3):346–355.

81. Marik PE, Zaloga GP. Gastric versus post-pyloric feeding: a systematic review. *Crit Care.* 2003;7(3):R46–R51.

82. Itkin M, DeLegge MH, Fang JC, et al. Multidisciplinary practical guidelines for gastrointestinal access for enteral nutrition and decompression from the Society of Interventional Radiology and American Gastroenterological Association (AGA) Institute, with endorsement by Canadian Interventional Radiological Association (CIRA) and Cardiovascular and Interventional Radiological Society of Europe (CIRSE). *Gastroenterology.* 2011;141(2):742–765.

83. Matsushima K, Cook A, Tyner T, et al. Parenteral nutrition: a clear and present danger unabated by tight glucose control. *Am J Surg.* 2010;200(3):386–390.

84. Kim JS, Holtom P, Vigen C. Reduction of catheter-related bloodstream infections through the use of a central venous line bundle: epidemiologic and economic consequences. *Am J Infect Control.* 2011;39(8):640–646.

85. Heyland DK, Dhaliwal R, Drover JW, Gramlich L, Dodek P, Canadian Critical Care Clinical Practice Guidelines Committee. Canadian clinical practice guidelines for nutrition support in mechanically ventilated, critically ill adult patients. *JPEN J Parenter Enteral Nutr.* 2003;27(5):355–373.

86. Zaloga GP, Roberts P. Permissive underfeeding. *New Horiz.* 1994;2(2):257–263.

87. Grimble RF. Dietary manipulation of the inflammatory response. *Proc Nutr Soc.* 1992;51(2):285–294.

88. McGinnis C, Fischer J, Larson G. Nutrition support in the morbidly obese, critically ill patient. *Nutr Clin Pract.* 2004;19(3):290–296.

89. Rubinson L, Diette GB, Song X, Brower RG, Krishnan JA. Low caloric intake is associated with nosocomial bloodstream infections in patients in the medical intensive care unit. *Crit Care Med.* 2004;32(2):350–357.

90. Krishnan JA, Parce PB, Martinez A, Diette GB, Brower RG. Caloric intake in medical ICU patients: consistency of care with guidelines and relationship to clinical outcomes. *Chest.* 2003;124(1):297–305.

91. McCowen KC, Friel C, Sternberg J, et al. Hypocaloric total parenteral nutrition: effectiveness in prevention of hyperglycemia and infectious complications—a randomized clinical trial. *Crit Care Med.* 2000;28(11):3606–3611.

92. Villet S, Chiolero RL, Bollmann MD, et al. Negative impact of hypocaloric feeding and energy balance on clinical outcome in ICU patients. *Clin Nutr.* 2005;24(4):502–509.

93. Heyland DK, Cahill N, Day AG. Optimal amount of calories for critically ill patients: depends on how you slice the cake! *Crit Care Med.* 2011;39(12):2619–2626.

94. Heyland DK, Cahill NE, Dhaliwal R, et al. Enhanced protein-energy provision via the enteral route in critically ill patients: a single center feasibility trial of the PEPuP protocol. *Crit Care.* 2010;14(2):R78.

95. Long CL. Fuel preferences in the septic patient: glucose or lipid? *JPEN J Parenter Enteral Nutr.* 1987;11(4):333–335.

96. Carlson GL, Gray P, Arnold J, Little RA, Irving MH. Thermogenic, hormonal and metabolic effects of intravenous glucose infusion in human sepsis. *Br J Surg.* 1997;84(10):1454–1459.

97. Wolfe RR. Substrate utilization/insulin resistance in sepsis/trauma. *Baillieres Clin Endocrinol Metab.* 1997;11(4):645–657.

98. Vanhorebeek I, De Vos R, Mesotten D, Wouters PJ, De Wolf-Peeters C, Van den Berghe G. Protection of hepatocyte mitochon-

drial ultrastructure and function by strict blood glucose control with insulin in critically ill patients. *Lancet.* 2005;365(9453): 53–59.

99. NICE-SUGAR Study Investigators; Finfer S, Chittock DR, et al. Intensive versus conventional glucose control in critically ill patients. *N Engl J Med.* 2009;360(13):1283–1297.

100. Garnacho-Montero J, Ortiz-Leyba C, Jimenez-Jimenez FJ, et al. Clinical and metabolic effects of two lipid emulsions on the parenteral nutrition of septic patients. *Nutrition.* 2002;18(2):134–138.

101. Serhan CN. Pro-resolving lipid mediators are leads for resolution physiology. *Nature.* 2014;510(7503):92–101.

102. Calabrese C, Myer S, Munson S, Turet P, Birdsall TC. A cross-over study of the effect of a single oral feeding of medium chain triglyceride oil vs. canola oil on post-ingestion plasma triglyceride levels in healthy men. *Altern Med Rev.* 1999;4(1):23–28.

103. Kamarul Zaman M, Chin KF, Rai V, Majid HA. Fiber and prebiotic supplementation in enteral nutrition: a systematic review and meta-analysis. *World J Gastroenterol.* 2015;21(17):5372–5381.

104. Bengmark S, Martindale R. Prebiotics and synbiotics in clinical medicine. *Nutr Clin Pract.* 2005;20(2):244–261.

105. Bengmark S. Synbiotics and the mucosal barrier in critically ill patients. *Curr Opin Gastroenterol.* 2005;21(6):712–716.

106. Calder PC, Grimble RF. Polyunsaturated fatty acids, inflammation and immunity. *Eur J Clin Nutr.* 2002;56(Suppl 3):S14–S19.

107. Sweeney B, Puri P, Reen DJ. Modulation of immune cell function by polyunsaturated fatty acids. *Pediatr Surg Int.* 2005;21(5): 335–340.

108. Mayer K, Grimm H, Grimminger F, Seeger W. Parenteral nutrition with n-3 lipids in sepsis. *Br J Nutr.* 2002;87(Suppl 1):S69–S75.

109. Martindale RG, Warren MM, McClave SA. Does the use of specialized proresolving molecules in critical care offer a more focused approach to controlling inflammation than that of fish oils? *Curr Opin Clin Nutr Metab Care.* 2016;19(2):151–154.

110. Calder PC. n-3 polyunsaturated fatty acids and inflammation: from molecular biology to the clinic. *Lipids.* 2003;38(4):343–352.

111. Roy CC, Bouthillier L, Seidman E, Levy E. New lipids in enteral feeding. *Curr Opin Clin Nutr Metab Care.* 2004;7(2):117–122.

112. Mayer K, Gokorsch S, Fegbeutel C, et al. Parenteral nutrition with fish oil modulates cytokine response in patients with sepsis. *Am J Respir Crit Care Med.* 2003;167(10):1321–1328.

113. Heller AR, Rossler S, Litz RJ, et al. Omega-3 fatty acids improve the diagnosis-related clinical outcome. *Crit Care Med.* 2006; 34(4):972–979.

114. Supinski GS, Vanags J, Callahan LA. Eicosapentaenoic acid preserves diaphragm force generation following endotoxin administration. *Crit Care.* 2010;14(2):R35.

115. Tiesset H, Pierre M, Desseyn JL, et al. Dietary (n-3) polyunsaturated fatty acids affect the kinetics of pro- and anti-inflammatory responses in mice with *Pseudomonas aeruginosa* lung infection. *J Nutr.* 2009;139(1):82–89.

116. Pontes-Arruda A, Aragao AM, Albuquerque JD. Effects of enteral feeding with eicosapentaenoic acid, gamma-linolenic acid, and antioxidants in mechanically ventilated patients with severe sepsis and septic shock. *Crit Care Med.* 2006;34(9):2325–2333.

117. Gadek JE, DeMichele SJ, Karlstad MD, et al. Effect of enteral feeding with eicosapentaenoic acid, gamma-linolenic acid, and antioxidants in patients with acute respiratory distress syndrome. Enteral Nutrition in ARDS Study Group. *Crit Care Med.* 1999; 27(8):1409–1420.

118. Singer P, Theilla M, Fisher H, et al. Benefit of an enteral diet enriched with eicosapentaenoic acid and gamma-linolenic acid in ventilated patients with acute lung injury. *Crit Care Med.* 2006; 34(4):1033–1038.

119. Grau-Carmona T, Moran-Garcia V, Garcia-de-Lorenzo A, et al. Effect of an enteral diet enriched with eicosapentaenoic acid,

gamma-linolenic acid and anti-oxidants on the outcome of mechanically ventilated, critically ill, septic patients. *Clin Nutr.* 2011;30(5):578–584.

120. Rice TW, Wheeler AP, Thompson BT, et al. Enteral omega-3 fatty acid, gamma-linolenic acid, and antioxidant supplementation in acute lung injury. *JAMA.* 2011;306(14):1574–1581.

121. Serhan CN. Novel eicosanoid and docosanoid mediators: resolvins, docosatrienes, and neuroprotectins. *Curr Opin Clin Nutr Metab Care.* 2005;8(2):115–121.

122. Verbruggen SC, Coss-Bu J, Wu M, et al. Current recommended parenteral protein intakes do not support protein synthesis in critically ill septic, insulin-resistant adolescents with tight glucose control. *Crit Care Med.* 2011;39(11):2518–2525.

123. Lefton J, Lopez PP. Macronutrient requirements: carbohydrate, protein, and lipid. In: Cresci GA, ed. *Nutritional Support for the Critically Ill Patient: A Guide to Practice.* Boca Raton, FL: Taylor and Francis; 2005:99–108.

124. Katsanos CS, Kobayashi H, Sheffield-Moore M, Aarsland A, Wolfe RR. A high proportion of leucine is required for optimal stimulation of the rate of muscle protein synthesis by essential amino acids in the elderly. *Am J Physiol Endocrinol Metab.* 2006;291(2):E381–E387.

125. Tipton KD, Elliott TA, Cree MG, et al. Ingestion of casein and whey proteins result in muscle anabolism after resistance exercise. *Med Sci Sports Exerc.* 2004;36(12):2073–2081.

126. Furst P, Stehle P. What are the essential elements needed for the determination of amino acid requirements in humans? *J Nutr.* 2004;134(6 Suppl):1558S–1565S.

127. Heyland DK, Samis A. Does immunonutrition in patients with sepsis do more harm than good? *Intensive Care Med.* 2003;29(5): 669–671.

128. Luiking YC, Poeze M, Dejong CH, Ramsay G, Deutz NE. Sepsis: an arginine deficiency state? *Crit Care Med.* 2004;32(10):2135–2145.

129. Davis JS, Anstey NM. Is plasma arginine concentration decreased in patients with sepsis? A systematic review and meta-analysis. *Crit Care Med.* 2011;39(2):380–385.

130. Suchner U, Heyland DK, Peter K. Immune-modulatory actions of arginine in the critically ill. *Br J Nutr.* 2002;87(Suppl 1): S121–S132.

131. Chiarla C, Giovannini I, Siegel JH. Plasma arginine correlations in trauma and sepsis. *Amino Acids.* 2006;30(1):81–86.

132. Grimble RF. Immunonutrition. *Curr Opin Gastroenterol.* 2005; 21(2):216–222.

133. Luiking YC, Poeze M, Deutz NE. Arginine infusion in patients with septic shock increases nitric oxide production without haemodynamic instability. *Clin Sci (Lond).* 2015;128(1):57–67.

134. Bertolini G, Iapichino G, Radrizzani D, et al. Early enteral immunonutrition in patients with severe sepsis: results of an interim analysis of a randomized multicentre clinical trial. *Intensive Care Med.* 2003;29(5):834–840.

135. Caparros T, Lopez J, Grau T. Early enteral nutrition in critically ill patients with a high-protein diet enriched with arginine, fiber, and antioxidants compared with a standard high-protein diet: the effect on nosocomial infections and outcome. *JPEN J Parenter Enteral Nutr.* 2001;25(6):299–309.

136. Atkinson S, Sieffert E, Bihari D. A prospective, randomized, double-blind, controlled clinical trial of enteral immunonutrition in the critically ill. Guy's Hospital Intensive Care Group. *Crit Care Med.* 1998;26(7):1164–1172.

137. Galban C, Montejo JC, Mesejo A, et al. An immune-enhancing enteral diet reduces mortality rate and episodes of bacteremia in septic intensive care unit patients. *Crit Care Med.* 2000;28(3): 643–648.

138. Luiking YC, Poeze M, Ramsay G, Deutz NE. Reduced citrulline production in sepsis is related to diminished de novo argi-

nine and nitric oxide production. *Am J Clin Nutr.* 2009;89(1): 142–152.

139. Kao CC, Bandi V, Guntupalli KK, et al. Arginine, citrulline and nitric oxide metabolism in sepsis. *Clin Sci (Lond).* 2009;117(1): 23–30.

140. Boger RH. The pharmacodynamics of L-arginine. *J Nutr.* 2007; 137(6 Suppl 2):1650S–1655S.

141. Zhou M, Martindale RG. Immune-modulating enteral formulations: optimum components, appropriate patients, and controversial use of arginine in sepsis. *Curr Gastroenterol Rep.* 2007;9(4): 329–337.

142. Coeffier M, Dechelotte P. The role of glutamine in intensive care unit patients: mechanisms of action and clinical outcome. *Nutr Rev.* 2005;63(2):65–69.

143. Wischmeyer PE, Lynch J, Liedel J, et al. Glutamine administration reduces gram-negative bacteremia in severely burned patients: a prospective, randomized, double-blind trial versus isonitrogenous control. *Crit Care Med.* 2001;29(11): 2075–2080.

144. Newsholme P, Procopio J, Lima MM, Pithon-Curi TC, Curi R. Glutamine and glutamate: their central role in cell metabolism and function. *Cell Biochem Funct.* 2003;21(1):1–9.

145. Ziegler TR, Ogden LG, Singleton KD, et al. Parenteral glutamine increases serum heat shock protein 70 in critically ill patients. *Intensive Care Med.* 2005;31(8):1079–1086.

146. Macario AJ, Conway de Macario E. Sick chaperones, cellular stress, and disease. *N Engl J Med.* 2005;353(14):1489–1501.

147. Singleton KD, Serkova N, Beckey VE, Wischmeyer PE. Glutamine attenuates lung injury and improves survival after sepsis: role of enhanced heat shock protein expression. *Crit Care Med.* 2005; 33(6):1206–1213.

148. Griffiths RD, Jones C, Palmer TE. Six-month outcome of critically ill patients given glutamine-supplemented parenteral nutrition. *Nutrition.* 1997;13(4):295–302.

149. Novak F, Heyland DK, Avenell A, Drover JW, Su X. Glutamine supplementation in serious illness: a systematic review of the evidence. *Crit Care Med.* 2002;30(9):2022–2029.

150. Heyland D, Muscedere J, Wischmeyer PE, et al. A randomized trial of glutamine and antioxidants in critically ill patients. *N Engl J Med.* 2013;368(16):1489–1497.

151. Macdonald J, Galley HF, Webster NR. Oxidative stress and gene expression in sepsis. *Br J Anaesth.* 2003;90(2):221–232.

152. Heyland DK, Dhaliwal R, Suchner U, Berger MM. Antioxidant nutrients: a systematic review of trace elements and vitamins in the critically ill patient. *Intensive Care Med.* 2005;31(3):327–337.

153. Nathens AB, Neff MJ, Jurkovich GJ, et al. Randomized, prospective trial of antioxidant supplementation in critically ill surgical patients. *Ann Surg.* 2002;236(6):814–822.

154. Collier BR, Giladi A, Dossett LA, et al. Impact of high-dose antioxidants on outcomes in acutely injured patients. *JPEN J Parenter Enteral Nutr.* 2008;32(4):384–388.

155. Zimmermann T, Albrecht S, Kuhne H, et al. [Selenium administration in patients with sepsis syndrome. A prospective randomized study]. *Med Klin (Munich).* 1997;92(Suppl 3):S3–S4.

156. Angstwurm MW, Schottdorf J, Schopohl J, Gaertner R. Selenium replacement in patients with severe systemic inflammatory response syndrome improves clinical outcome. *Crit Care Med.* 1999;27(9):1807–1813.

157. Angstwurm MW, Engelmann L, Zimmermann T, et al. Selenium in Intensive Care (SIC): results of a prospective randomized, placebo-controlled, multiple-center study in patients with severe systemic inflammatory response syndrome, sepsis, and septic shock. *Crit Care Med.* 2007;35(1):118–126.

158. Mishra V, Baines M, Perry SE, et al. Effect of selenium supplementation on biochemical markers and outcome in critically ill patients. *Clin Nutr.* 2007;26(1):41–50.

159. Forceville X, Laviolle B, Annane D, et al. Effects of high doses of selenium, as sodium selenite, in septic shock: a placebo-controlled, randomized, double-blind, phase II study. *Crit Care.* 2007;11(4):R73.

160. Thomas L. *The Lives of a Cell: Notes of a Biology Watcher.* New York: Viking Press; 1974.

161. Riedemann NC, Guo RF, Ward PA. The enigma of sepsis. *J Clin Invest.* 2003;112(4):460–467.

162. Martindale RG, Cresci G. Preventing infectious complications with nutrition intervention. *JPEN J Parenter Enteral Nutr.* 2005;29(1 Suppl):S53–S56.

163. Moore EE, Moore FA, Harken AH, et al. The two-event construct of postinjury multiple organ failure. *Shock.* 2005;24(Suppl 1):71–74.

164. Wheeler AP, Bernard GR. Treating patients with severe sepsis. *N Engl J Med.* 1999;340(3):207–214.

165. Shimizu K, Ogura H, Goto M, et al. Altered gut flora and environment in patients with severe SIRS. *J Trauma.* 2006;60(1):126–133.

166. MacFie J, O'Boyle C, Mitchell CJ, et al. Gut origin of sepsis: a prospective study investigating associations between bacterial translocation, gastric microflora, and septic morbidity. *Gut.* 1999; 45(2):223–228.

167. De-Souza DA, Greene LJ. Intestinal permeability and systemic infections in critically ill patients: effect of glutamine. *Crit Care Med.* 2005;33(5):1125–1135.

168. Magnotti LJ, Deitch EA. Burns, bacterial translocation, gut barrier function, and failure. *J Burn Care Rehabil.* 2005;26(5):383–391.

169. MacFie J. Enteral versus parenteral nutrition: the significance of bacterial translocation and gut-barrier function. *Nutrition.* 2000; 16(7–8):606–611.

170. Besselink MG, Timmerman HM, van Minnen LP, Akkermans LM, Gooszen HG. Prevention of infectious complications in surgical patients: potential role of probiotics. *Dig Surg.* 2005;22(4):234–244.

171. Madden JA, Plummer SF, Tang J, et al. Effect of probiotics on preventing disruption of the intestinal microflora following antibiotic therapy: a double-blind, placebo-controlled pilot study. *Int Immunopharmacol.* 2005;5(6):1091–1097.

24 Trauma, Surgery, and Burns

David C. Evans, MD, FACS, PNS, and Bryan R. Collier, DO, FACS, CNSC

CONTENTS

Acknowledgments: Material from the first and second editions was contributed by Robert G. Martindale, PhD, MD, Gail Cresci, MS, RD, LD, CNSD, Michele Gottschlich, PhD, RD, LD, CNSD, Theresa Mayes, RD, LD, Jill R. Cherry-Bukowiec, MD, MS, FACS, Mary E. (Beth) Mills, MS, RD, CNSC, LDN, and Charles Mueller, PhD, RD, CD, CNSD.

Objectives

1. Recognize how injury and inflammation alter metabolism.
2. Differentiate injury-related malnutrition from starvation-related malnutrition.
3. Assess nutrition risk and determine nutrient requirements for trauma, surgery, and burn patients.
4. Discuss the role of parenteral, enteral, and oral nutrition therapy in trauma, burn, and surgical patients.

5. Select the best adjunct nutrition therapies for the trauma, surgical, and burned patient.
6. Describe perioperative strategies to optimize outcomes for the elective surgical patient.

Test Your Knowledge Questions

1. Which of the following is the most important benefit to starting early enteral nutrition (EN) after trauma?
   A. Addressing protein-energy malnutrition before it is severe
   B. Preventing negative nitrogen balance
   C. Modulating the immune process and supporting the gastrointestinal (GI) tract
   D. Preventing severe hyperglycemia
2. For routine colon surgery, which of the following components of Enhanced Recovery After Surgery (ERAS) protocols contributes to the improved outcomes?
   A. Keeping the patient *nil per os* (NPO) after midnight to avoid aspiration on induction of general anesthesia
   B. Providing glucose-rich supplementation 6 and 2 hours prior to surgery
   C. Using high-dose oral protein supplements
   D. Using probiotics to restore normal intestinal flora after surgery
3. Which of the following are *not* thought to benefit burn wound healing?
   A. Vitamin C supplementation
   B. Calcium
   C. Protein delivery of 1.5 to 2 g/kg/d
   D. Zinc supplementation

Test Your Knowledge Answers

1. The correct answer is **C**. Negative nitrogen balance frequently occurs despite adequate energy provision because of the counterregulatory hormone and cytokine changes that occur from traumatic insult. Epinephrine, glucagon, and growth hormones are elevated, resulting in increased lipolysis and increased glycerol and free fatty release. Circulating levels of insulin are elevated in most metabolically stressed patients, but the responsiveness of tissues, especially skeletal muscle, to insulin is severely blunted. Insulin resistance is believed to be caused by the effects of the counterregulatory hormones and causes hyperglycemia regardless of nutrition provision. The hormonal milieu normalizes only after the injury or metabolic stress has resolved. By providing early EN, the cytokine storm and counterregulatory hormone secretion are attenuated. As a result, critically ill patients experience fewer infections despite not obtaining protein and energy goals within the first few days of nutrition provision.
2. The correct answer is **B**. The principles of a perioperative plan to improve outcomes in elective colon surgery have included avoiding starvation, limiting intravenous (IV) fluids, and increasing mobility. Providing a carbohydrate-enhanced drink preoperatively as part of a complex perioperative plan has improved outcomes. Patients consuming 800 mL of a carbohydrate-rich liquid (100 g carbohydrate) at midnight and 400 mL 2 hours before the surgical

intervention demonstrate a faster recovery, fewer infectious complications, and no increased aspirations. By providing this fluid and nutritional supplementation without a preoperative bowel prep, patients received less IV fluid, which improved recovery. In addition, a decrease in insulin resistance has been observed and associated with decreased complications and mortality. While oral nutritional supplements and probiotic use both have potential benefits, neither is currently standard in ERAS protocols.
3. The correct answer is **B**. Numerous studies have evaluated nutrients in the critically ill; however, few have focused on burn patients. Vitamin C and zinc have been demonstrated to promote healing in burn patients. Protein delivery to maintain positive nitrogen balance is crucial to burn wound healing.

Background

Incidence

In the United States, injury represents the most common cause of death between the ages of 1 and 44 years, accounting for almost 200,000 deaths per year. In addition, over 2.5 million hospitalizations occur annually in the United States.[1]

Overall, mortality has improved after trauma and major surgery; however, patients who survive critical illness often experience the morbidity related to protein-energy malnutrition. Two major nutrition tenets that must be addressed when treating patients who are admitted to various surgical wards and critical care units and undergo one or more surgical interventions. The first tenet is that these patients will be in negative nitrogen balance and suffer weight loss, weakness, and a long duration of rehabilitation prior to return to baseline.[2] The second tenet is that early administration of nutrition and nutritional supplements is needed as the patient is being admitted and going to the operating room within minutes of evaluation in the emergency department. These early decisions could affect the risk of surgical infections and hospital length of stays, as well as the time the patient spends returning to baseline.[3-5]

Severity of Injury

Trauma can be differentiated as blunt vs penetrating injury, with burns considered separately. The severity of trauma and burns has been described with multiple scoring systems (eg, Injury Severity Score, Glasgow Coma Scale, and total body surface area [TBSA] burn affected) that attempt to not only predict mortality but also predict who will benefit from aggressive nutrition therapy.

In general, all trauma and burn patients undergo a systemic inflammatory response syndrome (SIRS), which entails the presence of 2 out of 4 abnormal systems (heart rate, respiratory rate, temperature, and white blood cell count). When at least 2 SIRS criteria are met, the local injury of trauma or burn is producing a systemic reaction.[6] During this "flow" phase, originally described by Cuthbertson, amino acid mobilization occurs for gluconeogenesis, immunologic properties, and the initiation of healing. The magnitude of the flow phase or

SIRS suggests the degree of inflammation.[7] SIRS is associated with higher risk of death (infectious and noninfectious), and patients who survive tend to have a greater negative nitrogen balance, longer hospital stays, more weight loss, and a more difficult time returning to their previous level of function.[8]

Physiological Response to Stress

Neuroendocrine Response and Systemic Inflammation

The immediate goal following major trauma is to maintain oxygen delivery and diminish the *systemic* inflammation that is a result of the insult. Although nutrition support is often considered on posttrauma Days 1 to 3, clinicians must begin considering access and initiation of various modes of nutrition support (enteral tube feeds, immunomodulating formulas, antioxidants, etc) as soon as resuscitation is complete. Otherwise, the goal of early (within 24 hours of insult) EN and antioxidant provision will not be achieved, thereby potentiating worse outcomes.[9,10] However, aggressive nutrition provision has potential, albeit low, risks (ie, small bowel necrosis) that must be considered after complete resuscitation.

After injury, the neuroendocrine and cytokine response activates a cascade of events resulting in what has been termed the *systemic inflammatory response*, which was described previously

(see also Chapter 23). The response includes an increase in heart rate and minute ventilation to meet tissue demands for increased oxygen requirements. In addition, a rapid shift occurs from a state of storing protein, lipid, and glycogen to a catabolic state with mobilization of these nutrients for energy utilization. There is a direct correlation between the severity of the injury and the degree of substrate mobilization. Tissue catabolism is mediated through the release of cytokines such as tumor necrosis factor; interleukins-1, -2, and -6; and counterregulatory hormones such as epinephrine, norepinephrine, glucagon, and cortisol.[11] These hormones are labeled *counterregulatory* because they oppose the effects of insulin and other anabolic hormones. Circulating levels of insulin are elevated in most metabolically stressed patients, but the responsiveness of tissues, especially skeletal muscle, to insulin is severely blunted. This relative insulin resistance is believed to be caused by the effects of counterregulatory hormones (Figure 24-1).[12] The hormonal milieu normalizes only after the injury or metabolic stress has resolved (see Chapter 23).

With appropriate resuscitation maneuvers, the SIRS abates. These maneuvers include source control (hemorrhage control, controlling bowel content spillage, debriding necrotic tissues) and oxygen delivery (ventilator management, fluid and vasopressor resuscitation). In the last decade, nutrition support literature has focused the benefit(s) of nutrition support toward

FIGURE 24-1 Mechanisms of Hyperglycemia During States of Stress and Inflammation

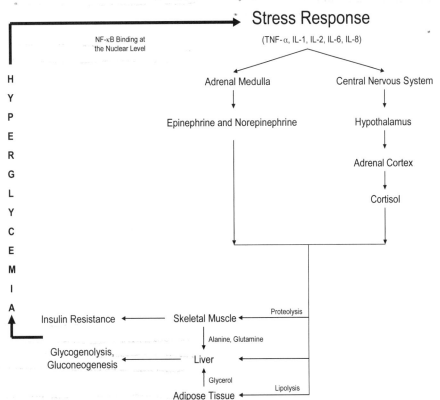

IL, interleukin; NF-κB, nuclear factor kappa B; TNF-α, tumor necrosis factor alpha.
Data are from reference 12.

FIGURE 24-2 Key Components in the Treatment of Systemic Inflammatory Response Syndrome

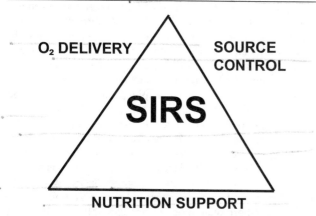

Effective treatment of systemic inflammatory response syndrome (SIRS) requires a focus on 3 strategies: the delivery of oxygen (O₂) to vital tissues, source control (control of bleeding, necrotic, and infected tissues), and provision of nutrition support. Control of the patient's global inflammatory response is crucial for achieving euglycemia.

reducing systemic inflammation (Figure 24-2). Primarily, this support comes in the form of early (less than 36 hours after insult) initiation of EN.[3,10,13] Current evidence suggests that energy and protein goals need not be met initially. These early nutrition therapies are less likely to address protein-energy malnutrition and more likely to address the modulation of the immune function.[14] Even in extreme cases such as the open abdomen or exposed bowel, EN has been shown to lead to improved outcomes.[15]

Reperfusion Injury/Low-Flow States

Significant insults, such as sepsis and hemorrhage, decrease splanchnic blood flow and increase oxygen consumption. In human studies, removing as little as 3% to 5% of the blood volume can result in a 50% to 70% shunt of visceral blood flow.[16] Other events, such as routine general anesthesia and midline abdominal incisions can lower visceral blood flow by approximately 40% to 50%.[17] Gut ischemia can lead to mitochondrial disruption, mucosal acidosis, progressive cell injury, and cell destruction (see Chapter 23). Mucosal acidosis, a measure of reduced intraoperative splanchnic perfusion, is associated with exaggerated local and systemic immune responses, increased intestinal permeability, an increase in septic complications, and a trend toward increased multiorgan dysfunction syndrome.[18] The presence of luminal nutrients increases GI blood flow, a phenomenon termed *postprandial hyperemia*.[19]

Inadequate splanchnic blood flow is thought to play a pivotal role in the development of multiorgan dysfunction syndrome. When splanchnic perfusion is compromised, feeding that increases intestinal metabolic demand poses a theoretical risk of intestinal ischemia.[20] In these conditions, some suggest that EN may cause nonocclusive bowel necrosis.[21] Nonocclusive bowel necrosis has an estimated incidence of approximately 0.3% in the intensive care unit (ICU) and remains a concern.[22]

Increased blood flow associated with EN protects the gut mucosa in most patients despite the risk of bowel necrosis. Several investigators using large and small animal models of shock states have reported that nutrient delivery enhances visceral blood perfusion in these low-flow states.[23-28] In addition, clinical and laboratory evidence suggests that EN is not necessarily contraindicated with the use of vasoactive agents.[22] However, care must be taken in providing EN to patients in shock (see Chapter 23). In a review of the literature of jejunal feeding associated with small bowel necrosis, virtually all patients experienced distention, and half had pneumatosis, abdominal pain, hypotension, and increased nasogastric output.[29] Use of EN in hemodynamically unstable or low-flow state, critically ill patients requires consideration of the feeding location, delivery rate, and bowel motility. Use of EN in such patients should be conservative (low infusion rate) until they are adequately resuscitated, with the EN advanced only when the patient demonstrates tolerance. Following adequate resuscitation, EN may protect the GI tract, especially the mucosa, from relatively low levels of ischemia.

Malnutrition in the Intensive Care Unit

Traditionally, malnutrition has been defined on the basis of inadequate intake or starvation. Malnutrition related to stress or trauma differs from starvation-related malnutrition in that the former stems from increased resting energy expenditure and tremendous mobilization of protein deposits. Such a process is driven by systemic inflammation.

Inflammation has gained recognition as the prime factor in the pathophysiology of chronic disease states. Whether the inflammation is acute or chronic, it promotes cytokine-driven protein catabolism of the skeletal muscle.[30] This systemic inflammation can drive catabolism to the severity of affecting cardiac mass and function.[31] Once muscle is catabolized to the degree that it alters functional level, malnutrition is typically considered present. However, when this level of skeletal muscle depletion is observed in the outpatient setting or in patients with chronic inflammatory states, severe protein-energy malnutrition is noted and aggressive measures to address the disease state and the malnutrition are warranted. Unfortunately, inflammation and its metabolic consequences start immediately, rapidly depleting even the well-nourished critically injured or ill patient. This inflammatory response and subsequent protein catabolism provide the environment for adverse outcomes.

Changes to the nomenclature of malnutrition highlight our understanding of the links between inflammatory metabolism and catabolic depletion of body habitus. Terminology specifies the nomenclature of *acute disease–* or *injury-related malnutrition* to acknowledge the phenomenon of elevated resting energy expenditure, increased nitrogen excretion, and subsequent increased energy and protein requirements.[32] This phenomenon occurs over the first hours to days after the patient is admitted. However, this inflammation and subsequent nitrogen excretion continue for weeks to months after the patient is discharged from the ICU (Figure 24-3).[33] In addition, this inflammation, which continues to drive the protein catabolism, exacerbates the anorexia that prevents appropriate intake.

FIGURE 24-3 Metabolic Response to Injury and Illness: Estimation of Energy and Protein Needs from Indirect Calorimetry and Nitrogen Balance

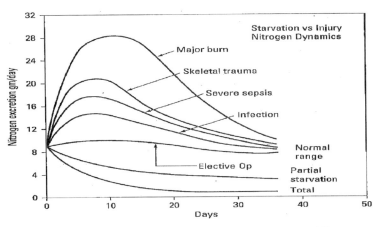

Reprinted with permission from reference 33: Long CL, Schaffel N, Geiger JW, Schiller WR, Blakemore WS. Metabolic response to injury and illness: estimation of energy and protein needs from indirect calorimetry and nitrogen balance. *JPEN J Parenter Enteral Nutr.* 1979;3(6):452–456.

Nutrition Assessment

Screening and Anthropometrics

Up to 40% of hospitalized patients are malnourished, and malnutrition has been linked to immunosuppression, impaired wound healing, increased hospital costs, longer hospital stays, and even increased mortality.[34]

Multiple national advisory organizations mandate screening for malnutrition risk within 24 to 48 hours of hospital admission followed by nutrition assessment (when required) and timely nutrition intervention. Such practice has been identified as a national standard by the Joint Commission and by the Academy of Nutrition and Dietetics/American Society for Parenteral and Enteral Nutrition (ASPEN) consensus statement (see Chapter 9).[32] Multiple nutrition screening tools have been developed for hospitalized populations; however, most patients requiring admission to a hospital for trauma, surgery, or burns have increased energy and protein requirements, putting them at increased risk for malnutrition, as previously described. The risk is especially significant for critically ill patients in a surgical ICU.

The 2016 Society of Critical Care Medicine (SCCM)/ ASPEN guidelines recommend assessment using the Nutrition Risk Screening (NRS-2002) or Nutrition Risk in Critically ill (NUTRIC) scoring systems to identify patients who would benefit from nutrition therapy.[35] While many patients who undergo emergency surgery have pre-existing malnutrition, most trauma and burn patients do not. NRS-2002 attempts to account for both preexisting malnutrition (eg, weight loss, decreased food intake) and severity of illness (ie, type of injury, APACHE II score), whereas NUTRIC focuses on severity of illness. Additional validation of these scores in various populations is still needed.

Surgical ICU patients typically fall into 3 main categories: postoperative major elective surgery, major injury (eg, burns and trauma), and serious sepsis. The patients who undergo major elective surgery are often moderately depleted of body protein preoperatively because of their disease process. In addition, these patients can lose approximately 5% of body protein (43 g/d) during the first 2 weeks postoperatively.[36,37] Up to 20% of total body protein is metabolized in critically ill patients in the first 3 weeks following trauma or illness.[38] The severity of illness can be compounded by preexisting medical conditions, such as liver disease and associated alcohol abuse, renal dysfunction, cardiac failure, obesity, pulmonary dysfunction and failure requiring mechanical ventilation, and diabetes. All of these factors contribute to nutrition risk. Additionally, extensive wounds, infections, and burns significantly increase the body's energy requirements.

These conditions not only place patients at increased risk of malnutrition but also make assessment of body composition and energy and protein requirements challenging. In such patients, nutrition assessment data (eg, medical/surgical history, medication, nutrition intake) is often obtained from family members or caregivers. Generally, anthropometric data such as height and weight are not valuable as an index of functional capacity or metabolic health in critically/ acutely ill patients.[39] Resuscitative fluids and capillary permeability cause generalized body edema, anasarca, and elevated body weights. Hill demonstrated that over a 4-week period, critically ill patients had a net accumulation of 4.7 to 12.5 liters of fluid.[37] Therefore, body weight measured in the ICU is not a valid indicator of body cell mass. Often, weight must be estimated using historical information provided by family members, with consideration of clinical events affecting body compartment fluid shifts. Ideally, weight changes should be monitored weekly. Acute weight changes are most likely due to fluid shifts, as 1 liter of fluid is equal to 1 kg body weight.[40] Loss of limb(s), bulky dressings, and other attached supportive materials required for critical care must be factored into interpretation of body weight. See Chapter 9 for additional information on nutrition assessment.

Biochemical Measures

Protein biochemical markers traditionally used in nutrition assessment, such as albumin, prealbumin, transferrin, and retinol-binding protein, do not accurately reflect the nutrition status of critically ill patients but are negative acute-phase response proteins.[35] During liver dysfunction, inflammation, and physical stress, the liver decreases the synthesis of transport proteins and increases the synthesis of positive acute-phase response proteins such as C-reactive protein.[41] Additionally, fluid shifts and increased vascular permeability change the proportion of fluid to protein, effectively altering the measured concentration of serum proteins. Therefore, in patients with acute illness, inflammation, or injury (such as in the early postoperative period and in trauma and burn patients), transport proteins cannot reliably be regarded as a marker of nutrition status, but can only be interpreted as a marker of severity of illness and inflammation.[35] This concept is illustrated in Practice Scenario 24-1.[22]

Practice Scenario 24-1

Question: How does the clinician prescribe nutrition therapy for a complex burn patient?

Scenario: A 39-year-old man involved in a house fire was transferred from the emergency department to the burn unit within 4 hours after injury. Physical assessment revealed an injury involving 75% total body surface area burn, 60% full thickness. Although the patient's lungs were clear, bronchoscopy via the endotracheal tube showed significant erythema in the airways. In addition, the ratio of partial pressure of oxygen in arterial blood to fraction of inspired oxygen (PaO_2:FiO_2) of 280 was diagnostic for inhalation injury. The patient was measured to be 178 cm in height and weighed 78 kg (dry weight) per bed scale. A nasogastric tube was connected to intermittent low wall suction. Bowel sounds were absent in all 4 quadrants. Intravenous resuscitative fluids were provided to maintain urine output at 30 to 50 mL/h.

Intervention: Within 6 hours of admission, an enteric feeding tube was placed into the proximal duodenum and its location confirmed with x-ray. Once adequate urine output was accomplished and cardiopulmonary resuscitation was complete, a high-protein enteral formula was started and increased to goal over the next 72 hours. Because the patient required multiple surgeries, enteral nutrition (EN) was provided through the immediate perioperative period. Once the patient tolerated oral intake, EN was cycled to a 12-hour nighttime regimen. EN was discontinued when the patient consistently received greater than 60% of nutrition requirements via oral intake.

Answer: The patient's energy requirement (measured energy expenditure) was determined by indirect calorimetry (IC) to be 2886 kcal/d. Protein needs were estimated at 20% to 25% of this energy goal, which correlates to 144 to 180 g of protein per day. As energy needs change over the course of treatment, protein needs are adjusted accordingly. The patient required a product that provides high-biological-value intact protein. The total nonprotein energy-to-nitrogen ratio of the selected product should be low (100:1 or less). The formula should also be moderately low in fat. The presence of arginine, glutamine, and ω-3 fatty acids in the formulation should be considered (see Chapter 11). Because burn patients need a large volume of fluid, a 1.6 to 2.0 kcal/mL formula was not considered. Osmolality was not a significant factor in the decision about formula type.

For the first week off the ventilator, the patient consumed mostly liquids with a few bites of solids. Over the next week, he gradually improved, consuming approximately 25% of energy needs orally. At this point, tube feedings were withheld 1 hour before and 1 hour during mealtimes. When his oral energy intake improved to 75% of goal, EN was discontinued. The patient's intake continued to improve; however, approximately 25% of his intake was met by high-energy oral supplements.

Rationale: Energy need is influenced by numerous variables (see Chapter 2). IC incorporates the stage of recovery as well as changes in clinical status and, therefore, is the best tool for determining energy requirements. However, many facilities lack access to IC measurement. Alternatively, predictive equations are used in critical care populations. Refer to Chapter 2 for a discussion of these equations.

In general, protein amounting to 20% to 25% of energy is recommended. This percentage translates to about 2.5 g/kg of protein per day in the early postburn course, and up to 4 g/kg/d during the extended flow period.

A growing number of institutions are safely providing continuous enteral feedings to burn patients in the perioperative period.[22] The EN regimen is minimally interrupted and nutrient provision is maximized.

Nutrition Requirements

Determination of Requirements

Assessment of nutrition requirements can be quite difficult in critically ill patients.[42] The 2016 SCCM/ASPEN guidelines provide updated and specific recommendations for commonly encountered disease states.[35] Critical illness and its treatment can profoundly alter metabolism and significantly increase or decrease energy expenditure. Determination of energy expenditure is necessary to ensure that energy needs are provided without over- or underfeeding (see Chapter 2). Overfeeding is associated with many complications including hepatic steatosis, hyperglycemia, and pulmonary compromise. Prolonged periods of undernutrition can lead to poor wound healing, impaired organ function, altered immunologic status, and increased risk of mortality. To adequately assess a patient's nutrition requirements, one must first determine the amount of energy needed to meet the patient's daily energy expenditure.

Energy

The clinical gold standard for determining energy (caloric) requirements is by measurement with an indirect calorimeter (sometimes referred to as a "metabolic cart"). Indirect calorimetry (IC) measures energy expenditure through analysis of respiratory gases (oxygen consumption, carbon dioxide production) and uses a modified Weir equation to determine energy expenditure.[43] Although IC is considered the gold standard, with the best accuracy for measuring energy requirements in the clinical setting, it is expensive to perform routinely, and many facilities do not have the technology or trained personnel to conduct the studies. Also, IC may be less accurate under a variety of circumstances that commonly affect critically ill patients, such as those receiving 60% fraction of inspired oxygen in a gas mixture or those with leaking chest tubes or endotracheal tubes in which the ventilated gas is not completely captured. See Chapter 2 for additional information on IC.

Most institutions do not have access to a metabolic cart and rely instead on predictive equations to determine energy requirements. Early in the 20th century, Harris and Benedict developed one of the first widely accepted predictive equations derived from metabolic research performed on healthy men and women with no extremes of weight or age. More than 200 predictive equations have been reported in the literature since then, and many of these equations are currently in use. As medicine has evolved over the last century, ICUs have come to manage patients who are older, more critically ill, and recovering from more invasive surgery. Patients are surviving tremendous trauma and burn injuries. Through research, we now have a better understanding of how these processes alter metabolic demands. We have responded to these changes by adding modifiers to the Harris-Benedict equation and by creating new equations in attempt to better estimate energy requirements of specific populations. Despite these efforts, no single equation can be routinely recommended as the best predictor of energy needs. A detailed description of these equations is provided in Chapter 2.

Despite slightly more accurate equations, estimating energy requirements in surgical, critically ill, injured, and burn patients is challenging. The estimates are often inaccurate, particularly in very obese patients, very underweight patients, and patients with acute or chronic liver disease. These findings are reflected in the 2016 SCCM/ASPEN guidelines,[35] which recommend using IC to measure resting energy expenditure in these patient populations when it is available (see Chapter 2). Even when energy requirements are accurately determined, most ICU patients do not receive their estimated energy needs.[44]

One of the most important aspects of monitoring a patient receiving EN or parenteral nutrition (PN) is to assess delivery of estimated nutrition needs. An astute clinician should evaluate whether the patient has attained prescribed enteral feeding goals. If not, the nutrition support team should determine impediments, troubleshoot, and develop new recommendations for attainment of goals. Clinicians have used many methods to improve the daily amounts of energy and protein provided to patients. Examples include compensatory goal feeding rate increases, avoidance of unnecessary cessation of tube feedings for repositioning patients, reduction in the time patients with protected airways are made NPO prior to procedures or surgeries, and the bridling of feeding tubes.[45-47] Heyland and colleagues developed and validated a new feeding protocol (known as "the PEPuP protocol") that increased protein delivery by 14% and energy by 12% in a multicenter trial.[48] This protocol, which is driven by the bedside nurse, uses daily volume-based goals, liberalizes the gastric residual volume threshold, and initiates protein supplementation with motility agents on Day 1 of a patient's ICU stay. Another method to promote adequate enteral provision is early initiation of EN infusion after percutaneous endoscopic gastrostomy (PEG) tube placement. In adults, current practice recommendations indicate that after a PEG tube is placed, it may be used for feeding within 2 hours instead of the routine 24-hour delay.[49]

Protein

Despite optimal nutrition support, patients sustaining major injury lose a large amount of protein via wound exudate and urine during the first 10 days following injury (approximately 110 g/d).[36] Surgical ICU patients often have preexisting nutrition depletion as a result of other medical conditions (eg,

diabetes, renal failure, cancer, or hepatic failure), multiple operations, or prolonged admissions. Large losses of lean body mass (approximately 150 g/d) typically occur in septic patients despite aggressive nutrition support sufficient to result in a gain in total body fat.[36] Because of the increased protein loss that is associated with critical illness and injury, protein needs are elevated. Although catabolism is not reversed by provision of energy and protein, the protein synthetic rate is partially responsive to amino acid infusion.[50,51] The current recommendation for stressed patients, including those with burns, is that 20% to 25% of total nutrient intake be provided as protein. This proportion equates to roughly 1.5 to 2.0 g/kg/d, with the higher range to promote nitrogen equilibrium, or at least minimize nitrogen deficit. Administration of 2 g protein per kg of ideal body weight per day has been suggested for obese patients (body mass index equal to or greater than 30). In patients with large surface area burns, higher protein loads (3 to 4 g/kg/d) may be required.[52,53] Protein administration exceeding these amounts has not been shown to be beneficial and, in fact, may cause azotemia.[54] It has also been suggested that ICU patients receiving continuous renal replacement therapy should receive 2.0 to 2.5 g protein per kg per day to overcome protein losses in the dialysate.[55] See Chapter 6 for further discussion of protein requirements.

Nitrogen balance has historically been used as an indicator of the adequacy of whole body protein delivery, calculated by measuring the amount of nitrogen provided as nutrition support (protein intake) and subtracting the total body nitrogen loss (see Chapter 9). A positive nitrogen balance would indicate that the patient is receiving enough nitrogen to meet or exceed the body's demand. However, in acute illness, injury, and burn, it can be difficult to quantify all sources of protein loss (stool, wounds, abdominal drains, urine, dialysate, etc).[56] Additionally, in the early stages of a severe burn, injury, postoperative setting, or sepsis, patients are severely catabolic. Until their catabolic drive has passed, a positive nitrogen balance may not be achievable due to intrinsic protein synthesis and breakdown cycles. Therefore, measuring nitrogen balance to determine adequacy of nutrient delivery is infrequently performed in the clinical setting.

Carbohydrate

Glucose is the primary fuel for the central nervous system and blood cells, with a minimum of about 120 g/d necessary to maintain central nervous system function. In the metabolically stressed adult, the maximum rate of glucose oxidation is 4 to 7 mg/kg/min, roughly equivalent to 400 to 700 g/d in a 70-kg person.[57] In the hypermetabolic patient, a large portion of oxidized glucose is derived from amino acid substrates via gluconeogenesis yielding up to 2 to 3 mg/kg/min of glucose. This endogenous production is poorly suppressed by exogenous glucose administration. Therefore, providing large amounts of exogenous carbohydrate can cause hyperglycemia and hyperinsulinemia. Complications of excess glucose administration include hyperosmolar states, excess carbon dioxide production, hepatic steatosis, and hyperglycemia.[54]

Studies have found admission hyperglycemia to be a prognostic indicator in trauma patients, with elevations correlating with increased morbidity and mortality.[58–60] Insulin therapy, where patients are kept normoglycemic with continuous insulin infusion, has been shown to prevent excessive inflammation in critically ill patients.[61] In a single-institution, prospective randomized controlled trial (RCT) performed on parenterally fed surgical patients in Leuven, Belgium, Van den Berghe and colleagues initially found significant benefit from maintaining tight glucose control (blood glucose concentration of 80 to 110 mg/dL [4.4 to 6.1 mmol/L]) in cardiac surgery patients.[62] However, subsequent studies failed to show benefit in general surgery or vascular surgery patients. Results from these later studies, such as the international, multicenter Normoglycemia in Intensive Care Evaluation-Survival Using Glucose Algorithm Regulation (NICE-SUGAR) trial, differed from the Van den Berghe trial, demonstrating increased morbidity and mortality when glucose levels were tightly controlled in mixed ICU patients (who were mostly fed enterally).[63,64] In addition, the Efficacy of Volume Substitution and Insulin Therapy in Severe Sepsis multicenter trial was stopped early because of concerns of an unacceptably high incidence of hypoglycemia.[65] Because of these findings and similar findings in smaller trials, a more moderate blood glucose control regimen, such as less than 180 mg/dL (10 mmol/L) is recommended.[35,66]

Fat

Lipid metabolism is altered in critically ill patients because of alterations in hormonal and cytokine mediators.[67–69] Enhanced mobilization of adipose tissue triglyceride stores, despite increased plasma levels of glucose and insulin, is characteristic of the metabolic response to severe stress.[70] Linoleic acid and α-linolenic acid are essential fatty acids required for proper body metabolism and are routinely provided to all critically ill patients. However, research to determine how much and which lipid preparation should be provided to critically ill patients is ongoing.

Polyunsaturated fatty acids are major structural components of cell membranes. The main types of polyunsaturated fatty acids are ω-6 (linoleic acid [18:2 n-6]), and ω-3 (α-linolenic acid [18:3 n-3]). Both ω-6 and ω-3 fatty acids are converted to biologically active long-chain triglycerides (eicosanoids). The ω-6 eicosanoids (such as arachidonic acid [20:4 n-6] and docosapentaenoic acid [22:5 n-6]) tend to have proinflammatory and prothrombotic effects. ω-3 polyunsaturated fatty acids (such as eicosapentaenoic acid [20:5 n-3] and docosahexaenoic acid [22:6 n-3]) tend to produce anti-inflammatory and antithrombotic effects. Multiple studies have concluded that critically ill patients receiving EN formulas with high concentrations of ω-3 polyunsaturated fatty acids from fish oil had decreased infection rates, hospital length of stay, and mortality.[35] Medium-chain triglycerides are attractive because they are small and water-soluble and can be absorbed without requiring bile salts. Most available commercial EN formulations contain mixtures of both long-chain triglycerides and medium-chain triglycerides. Most patients in the United States receive soy-based lipid injectable emulsions that have a high percentage of ω-6 long-chain triglycerides. New lipid emulsions such as mixtures of soybean, olive, and fish oils are widely used around the world but were only introduced into the US market in 2016 (see Chapter 5).

Fluid and Electrolytes

Surgery, trauma, and burns disrupt normal fluid and electrolyte homeostasis as a result of resuscitative fluid delivery and fluid compartmental shifts. Isosmotic fluids such as normal saline or balanced electrolyte solutions (eg, lactated Ringer's) are typically used for fluid and electrolyte replacement. When these solutions are used as maintenance, 5% dextrose is typically added as an energy source for several purposes, including protein sparing, prevention of ketosis, and maintenance of stable glucose levels.

Calculations of resuscitation and maintenance fluid requirements for early burn patients have been well described. The most commonly used method to determine adult fluid resuscitation requirements is the Parkland formula, traditionally used for patients with greater than 15% TBSA second- and third-degree burns. The formula calls for 4 mL of lactated Ringer's for each kilogram of body weight multiplied by the TBSA. One half of this total amount is administered in the first 8 hours after the burn. The remaining amount is administered over the subsequent 16 hours, followed by maintenance fluids. Inhalational injury results in additional fluid needs and is often estimated as another 10% of TBSA. Monitoring urine output is an essential part of providing fluid to thermal injury patients, as adequate hydration should result in a minimum of 0.3 to 0.5 mL/kg/h.[71] Rates of fluid administration should be adjusted to ensure adequate fluid volume resuscitation. Clinicians should also be aware that overresuscitation of fluids can increase morbidity and mortality in these patients by increasing the chances of respiratory failure, total body edema, and abdominal and/or extremity compartment syndromes. Respiratory failure is of greatest concern in inhalation injuries and in the patient who suffers both burn and traumatic injuries (such as pulmonary contusions). Many institutions have begun to incorporate colloid administration into their burn resuscitation protocols in efforts to reduce "fluid creep" (a phenomenon where burn patients receive progressively increasing crystalloid fluid resuscitation) and avoid adverse outcomes associated with excessive fluid administration.

Pediatric burn centers also often use the Parkland formula; however, they use a goal urine output of 1 to 2 mL/kg/h in patients weighing less than 30 to 50 kg.[71] Colloid administration has also been described in the pediatric population.

The large-volume fluid resuscitations required in burn victims can lead to electrolyte imbalances. Electrolyte levels should be monitored closely and replaced when necessary. Electrolytes can be safely provided for critically ill adult patients in doses specified in Table 24-1. See Chapter 7 for further discussion of fluid and electrolytes.

Vitamins, Trace Elements, and Minerals

Currently, there are no specific guidelines regarding vitamin and mineral requirements in the critically ill patient. Presumably, micronutrient needs are increased after injury because of increased metabolic demands. However, objective data to support specific recommendations for supplementation are lacking.

The antioxidant vitamins and minerals have received the most recent attention. Oxidative metabolites or reactive oxygen species are theoretically overproduced during critical illness (eg, trauma, surgery, reperfusion injury, acute respiratory distress syndrome, infection, and burns). Release of cytokines and initiation of an acute-phase response most likely mediate this response.[72] Reactive oxygen species induce tissue injury through peroxidation of plasma membranes, oxidation of critical enzymatic or structural proteins, induction of apoptosis, and activation of nuclear factor kappa B, leading to the induction of genes critical to the initiation and perpetuation of the systemic inflammatory response. Along with increased levels of reactive oxygen species, decreased levels of circulating vitamins C and E have been found after surgery, trauma, burns, sepsis, and long-term PN.[73-77] Several retrospective and prospective studies, specifically in trauma patients, have demonstrated that antioxidant supplementation with vitamin C, vitamin E, and selenium improves outcomes,[9,78] and the 2016 SCCM/ASPEN guidelines supports use of antioxidants because of a mortality benefit.[35] However, the REducing Deaths due to OXidative Stress (REDOXS) study suggests that extremely high doses of glutamine and antioxidants may be harmful,[79] and these results have dampened enthusiasm for use of selenium and glutamine as antioxidants in most critically ill patients. Notably, the REDOXS study contained relatively low numbers of trauma and surgical patients.[79]

Current recommendations for critically ill patients are to provide, at minimum, the Dietary Reference Intakes (DRIs) for vitamins and minerals.[80] EN formulations meet DRIs when provided at specified volumes. If those volumes are not tolerated, patients may require additional supplementation enterally or intravenously—keeping in mind that supratherapeutic doses present the risk of adverse effects and toxicity.

A daily multivitamin is recommended for burn patients whose burns are less than 20% TBSA and burn patients undergoing delayed reconstructive procedures.[81] For those whose burns are greater than 20% TBSA, daily supplements including a multivitamin, 20,000 IU vitamin A, and 220 mg zinc plus twice daily doses of 500 mg ascorbic acid (vitamin C) are recommended, and supplemental selenium and copper may be considered if levels are low. Large doses of oral vitamin C and zinc may cause nausea or vomiting; therefore, delivery in suspension for tube feeding is advisable.[81]

Hypovitaminosis D is common in critically ill patients and has been associated with increased mortality. Therefore, clinical monitoring with appropriate vitamin D supplementation may be warranted.[82] Further studies are needed before the true efficacy of vitamin D replacement in the critically ill can be determined.[83-86] See Chapter 8 for further discussion of micronutrients.

Route of Nutrition Support

When patients are unable to consume adequate nutrients (at least 60% of nutrition needs) orally, EN or PN should be considered. EN is the preferred route of feeding for critically ill patients and should be initiated in the hemodynamically stable patient within 24 to 48 hours of admission.[35] In the past several years, the emphasis in critical care nutrition has moved away from PN toward EN. PN has been lifesaving in short bowel syndrome and intestinal failure, and has been successful in reversing malnutrition in many disease states (see Chapter 14). However, the narrow risk/benefit ratio for PN limits its use in critically ill patients in an ICU setting. PN has also been associated with an increased incidence of hyperglycemia, adding to patient immunocompromise with decreased neutrophil chemotaxis, phagocytosis, oxidative burst, and superoxide production. Comparisons of PN to EN have revealed that PN is associated with increasing the metabolic stress response, alterations in gut flora, gut atrophy, and contributing to systemic immunocompromise (see Chapter 16).[35]

Assessment of the patient's disease state, the extent of functional GI anatomy, the expected duration of EN support, and the ability to safely access the GI tract (via radiologic, surgical, or endoscopic techniques) should be considered when selecting an enteral access device.[87] (See Chapter 12 for additional information on enteral access devices.) The 2016

TABLE 24-1 Electrolyte Recommendations for Critically Ill Patients

Electrolyte	Daily Needs	Reasons for Increased Needs	Reasons for Decreased Needs
Sodium	70–100 mEq	Loop diuretics, cerebral salt wasting, wound losses	Hypertension, fluid overload
Potassium	70–100 mEq	Refeeding syndrome, diuretic therapy, amphotericin wasting, wound losses	Renal failure
Chloride	80–120 mEq	Wound or prolonged gastric losses	Acid-base balance
Phosphorus	10–30 mmol	Refeeding syndrome	Renal failure
Magnesium	8–24 mEq	Refeeding syndrome, diuretic therapy, gastrointestinal or wound losses	—
Calcium	5–20 mEq	Wound losses, receiving blood products	—

Source: Adapted from Cresci GA, Martindale RG. Nutrition support in trauma. In: Gottschlich MM, ed. *The Science and Practice of Nutrition Support: A Case-Based Core Curriculum.* Dubuque, IA: Kendall/Hunt Publishing; 2001:445–464. Reproduced with permission of Kendall/Hunt Publishing Company.

SCCM/ASPEN practice guidelines for the ICU patient population indicate that either gastric or small bowel feeding is acceptable. Neither the presence nor absence of bowel sounds nor evidence of passage of flatus or stool is required prior to the initiation of EN feeding.[35]

In meta-analyses comparing PN with EN after trauma, PN has been associated with a higher relative risk of infection, even accounting for catheter sepsis, complication rates, and mortality.[88,89] Two prospective RCTs[5,10] compared early EN to early PN in trauma patients and found that patients randomly assigned to receive EN had reduced major septic complications (abdominal abscesses and pneumonia) compared with those assigned to no supplemental feeding or PN. A study by the same investigators of trauma patients showed a blunting of the hepatic stress response, with higher constitutive proteins and lower acute-phase proteins in the EN group than in the PN group.[13] These findings were later confirmed in patients who were randomly assigned to either early EN (initiated in less than 24 hours) or early PN.[3] Those receiving early EN experienced significantly fewer major septic complications (eg, pneumonias, intra-abdominal abscesses, and line sepsis) than those receiving PN (14% vs 38%). Severely injured patients and those with penetrating injuries were most likely to benefit from EN. A subsequent meta-analysis of 8 prospective RCTs comparing EN and PN in a total of 230 high-risk surgical patients found that the enterally fed trauma patients had significantly fewer septic complications.[10] Given the overwhelming data, EN should be given primary consideration for all trauma, surgery, and burn patients with an intact GI system.[35]

In the previously well-nourished patient, PN support should be reserved and initiated only after efforts to provide nutrition via the enteral route have failed to advance EN to meet 60% of target goal energy for 7 to 10 days.[35] Exceptions to the delay of PN initiation are made for patients who (1) have preexisting severe malnutrition, (2) cannot receive EN, and (3) are expected to undergo elective major upper GI surgery. For these patients, the 2016 ASPEN/SCCM guidelines recommend that 5 to 7 days of preoperative PN be provided with continued PN postoperatively. However, if EN was contraindicated and the malnourished GI surgery patient did not receive preoperative PN, ASPEN and SCCM recommend, based on limited data, that initiation of PN be delayed postoperatively for 5 to 7 days if EN continues to be contraindicated. PN provided for fewer than 5 days has not shown benefit.[35]

Enteral Nutrition Access

The early initiation of EN can be challenging because not all GI access methods are suitable for the critically ill patient (see Chapter 12). The optimal access site for EN in critically ill patients is not yet clear. As described previously, clinicians must make decisions based on the clinical condition and individual needs of each patient. When patients are unstable, transporting them to radiology or endoscopy suites may be too risky, and they may not tolerate procedures at the bedside.[90] Many studies report successful early EN in trauma patients with the use of a feeding jejunostomy tube placed at the time of laparotomy.[13] However, only some critically ill or trauma patients require laparotomy, and this method is rarely used.

Gastric Access

While it is easy to obtain gastric access, critically ill patients fed gastrically may be predisposed to aspiration, regurgitation, and reflux. Many critically ill, injured, and postoperative patients have delayed gastric emptying, potentially limiting their ability to tolerate gastric feedings.[91,92] In the medical/surgical ICU, approximately 40% to 79% of gastrically fed patients exhibit some degree of upper digestive intolerance caused by impaired gastric emptying.[93,94] Many diagnoses commonly seen in the ICU (eg, pneumonia, pancreatitis, sepsis, peritonitis, elevated intracranial pressures, and altered hemodynamics) are associated with gut dysmotility.[95] Careful monitoring and use of promotility agents may improve tolerance.

However, delayed gastric emptying and gastric feeding in critically ill patients do not automatically lead to pulmonary aspiration. Studies have shown that while the risk of aspiration decreases as the level of formula infusion descends the GI tract, similar rates of pneumonia are seen whether patients are fed in the stomach or small bowel.[96] These results are limited by small sample sizes and lack of determination as to whether patients aspirated tube feeding formula or their own oral secretions. Regurgitation and pulmonary aspiration may occur despite extremely low gastric residuals (30 to 35 mL).[97] Some authors advocate small bowel feeding in critically ill patients because it is associated with decreased gastroesophageal reflux, reduced aspiration, an increase in nutrient delivery, and a shorter time to achieve desired nutrient delivery.[98]

Small Bowel Access

A clinically rational approach to EN in the critically ill patient population is to feed into the small bowel in patients at high risk for aspiration and gut dysmotility. High-risk patients include those who have undergone major intra-abdominal surgery, those who have had a previous episode of aspiration or emesis, those with persistent high gastric residuals (greater than 500 mL), those who are unable to protect the airway, and those who require prolonged supine or prone positioning. Blind bedside placement of a small-bore feeding tube has a 1% to 2% airway placement risk with a significant mortality risk.[99] Electromagnetic-guided and video-guided techniques have emerged that allow bedside placement with positional confirmation without use of radiology or need for patient transport. The electromagnetic-guided technique of small bowel feeding tube placement in a nurse- or dietitian-driven protocol has been reported to decrease complications.[100] These developments can decrease costs and improve accessibility of small bowel feeding with success rates ranging from 80% to 95% when trained personnel follow a protocol for bedside placement.[101,102]

Transitioning to Oral Nutrition

Clinicians should strive to transition patients to partial or full oral nutrition whenever the patient's clinical course will permit. Nighttime cycling of EN may be considered when patients are meeting more than 60% of the energy goal by the oral route prior to discontinuing EN. To maximize intake, oral dietary restrictions are discouraged.[103]

Perioperative Nutrition

Perioperative nutrition support can be divided into 4 principal categories: preoperative PN, preoperative EN, postoperative PN, and postoperative EN. Postoperative PN and EN are the more important groups because surgery often cannot (and should not) be delayed.[35] However, surgeons have recognized the association between nutrition status and morbidity and mortality for many years. In 1936, Studley reported that chronic peptic ulcer patients undergoing gastrectomy had a 3.5% mortality rate if they had 20% preoperative weight loss and a 33% mortality rate with greater than 20% preoperative weight loss.[104] In fact, recognition of this problem drove Rhoads's efforts that led to the development of PN.[105]

Parenteral vs Enteral Nutrition

In 1991, a prospective trial randomly assigned 395 preoperative malnourished patients to receive PN or not.[106] Results of the study demonstrated that severely malnourished patients benefited from preoperative PN, with significant reductions in noninfectious complications. Patients who were only borderline or mildly malnourished had higher infection rates when PN was used. Jie and associates published their experience using NRS-2002 scores to identify malnourished patients who benefited from preoperative PN.[107] Preoperative nutrition support (mostly PN) in severely malnourished patients (NRS-2002 score of 5 or higher) reduced complication occurrences from 51% to 26% of surgical patients.

Trials have also compared early postoperative PN and EN in surgical populations, most notably trauma and acute pancreatitis populations. In general, the trauma studies have reported fewer postoperative infections, improved protein or nitrogen balance studies, and shorter hospital stays in subjects who received EN. Patients with pancreatitis who received EN had fewer infections, experienced decreased hospitalization, and had faster disease resolution.[108-111] Early postoperative feeding (within 24 hours) whether by oral or enteral route is increasingly practiced and is associated with reduced complications, no increase in anastomotic leak rates, and only small increases in nausea and vomiting.[103]

Compared with research on preoperative PN, research on preoperative EN is relatively scarce. In 1984, an Indian group reported reduced postoperative mortality and wound infections in malnourished subjects receiving EN for 10 days before surgery vs controls (who received a routine hospital diet).[112] Gastric and colorectal cancer patients randomly assigned to PN or EN for 10 days before surgery had a significant decrease in postoperative intra-abdominal abscesses, with the groups receiving either form of preoperative nutrition compared with controls who went directly to surgery.[113]

Two meta-analyses of 9 studies concluded that preoperative PN had no effect on mortality, but it was associated with increased morbidity (mostly septic complications).[88,114] The latest SCCM/ASPEN guidelines recommend that PN should be reserved and initiated only after the first 7 days of hospitalization in patients without preadmission malnutrition.[35]

Enhanced Recovery After Surgery Protocols

The Enhanced Recovery After Surgery (ERAS) group has introduced an elaborate pre- and postoperative care program. The objectives of the program are to avoid starvation, decrease the physiological stress of surgery (which induces insulin resistance), and limit postoperative IV fluids, while optimizing pain control, GI function, and mobilization.[115] Collectively, the objectives aim to decrease insulin resistance, which has been shown in multiple studies to be associated with increased complications (such as infections, increased hospitalization, and mortality).[116]

The nutrition components to the ERAS program are progressive. The first component is to avoid preoperative fasting. Solid meals are provided up until 6 hours before surgery. In addition, 800 mL (approximately 100 g and 400 kcal) of a carbohydrate-rich, clear liquid is given at midnight and 400 mL of the same formula is given again 2 hours before the surgical intervention. The ERAS pathway meta-analysis (452 patients) demonstrated a decrease in complications (infectious and noninfectious) by approximately 50%, and a 2.5-day reduction in length of hospitalization, with no change in readmissions (in view of earlier discharges) or mortality (from aspiration) when the program is used.[117,118]

By providing the preoperative carbohydrate nutrition/fluid administration in combination and withholding a routine bowel prep, patients receive a smaller volume of IV fluids and experience fewer postoperative complications (such as wound dehiscence).[119-121] As adherence to the program increased to over 70%, symptoms, morbidity, hospital length of stay, and readmissions all improved.[121] ERAS was originally designed for elective colon resection patients. Emerging evidence suggests that these protocols are also applicable to other types of operations and even emergency surgery.[122]

Enteral Formula Selection

The appropriate selection of an EN formula following injury requires individualized consideration of the patient's age, GI function, clinical condition, nutrient requirements, and tolerance, as well as the product's efficacy and cost. Relevant to patients with trauma, surgery, and burns is the emergence of EN products formulated to modulate the immune system, wound healing, inflammation, and/or organ function.[103,123-126] Despite considerable research, such formulas continue to be the subject of controversy (see Chapter 11). Practice Scenario 24-2 describes clinical exercises involved in the selection of appropriate enteral products for trauma patients.[35,127-129]

Practice Scenario 24-2

Question: How does the practitioner prescribe nutrition therapy for a complex trauma patient?

Scenario: A 42-year-old man sustained a sternal fracture, right rib fractures, pulmonary contusion, lumbar spine fracture (L1–L3), open pelvic fracture, left femur fracture, right open tibia/fibula fractures, right open ankle fracture, right sinus fracture, and closed head injury from a motor vehicle collision. After stabilization in the emergency department, he arrived in the shock/trauma intensive care unit chemically sedated and intubated. The patient was wearing a cervical collar and because of his spinal injury was in a supine position and was under log roll–only orders. Chest radiograph showed fluffy infiltrates in the right lung. A neurologic examination revealed a Glasgow Coma Scale score of 10. The patient had an orogastric tube for low intermittent wall suction and was receiving intravenous fluids of normal saline at 120 mL/h.

Intervention: A member of the nutrition support team placed a feeding tube at bedside, passing the tube through the mouth instead of the naris because of the patient's sinus fracture. Abdominal radiograph confirmed that the tube position was in the fourth portion of the duodenum. An immune-enhancing formula was initiated at 30 mL/h within 24 hours of admission, after resuscitation was complete. The goal regimen was achieved on posttrauma Day 4, approximately 72 hours after enteral nutrition (EN) was initiated.

Answer: After resuscitation, it is imperative to provide an initial tube feed prescription (approximately 50% of energy goal) within 24 to 48 hours. To avoid an ongoing protein-energy deficit, goals for nutrition should subsequently be met within the first week of admission.

Rationale: While most patients are suited for a standard, isotonic enteral feeding formula, a disease-specific formula may be indicated for some. Commercially available immune-modulating formulas contain combinations of added arginine, ω-3 fatty acids, and nucleotides. Numerous prospective, randomized controlled trials have studied the efficacy and safety of immune-modulating formulations in a variety of clinical settings, including trauma.[127–129] These studies have documented that trauma patients receiving immunonutrition formula had fewer nosocomial infections, reduced intra-abdominal abscesses and multiple organ failure, decreased days receiving antibiotics, and decreased hospital length of stay when compared to standard formulas.

The patient is at risk for gastric feeding intolerance, reflux, and pulmonary aspiration because of supine positioning, high fraction of inspired oxygen in a gas mixture, and absence of bowel sounds. Additionally, the patient will require multiple surgical interventions in the forthcoming days. Studies indicate that patients fed postpylorically do not necessarily have a decrease in gastroesophageal regurgitation, time to achieve nutrition goals, or increased nutrient delivery. However, patients who may require multiple interruptions to feeding for procedures, such as surgical interventions, may benefit from postpyloric feeds to reduce the preoperative *nil per os* time required by anesthesia. For most critically ill patients, EN via the stomach is safe.[35]

Indirect calorimetry provides the most accurate determination of energy requirements. If logistics and resources do not allow for the use of indirect calorimetry, the clinicians caring for this patient may consider recommendations for moderately to severely injured patients, which are to provide 25 to 30 kcal/kg/d or 120% to 140% of the energy expenditure derived from predictive equations, and to meet high protein requirements (1.5 to 2 g/kg/d).[35]

Immunonutrition as Enteral or Oral Supplementation

The 2016 SCCM/ASPEN guidelines recommend the use of continuously administered enteral immunonutrition formulations with supplemental ω-3 fatty acids and arginine in postoperative and trauma ICU patients.[35] Plasma arginine levels are reported to drop by 50% or more within hours of trauma or surgery and remain depressed for days to weeks.[130] Arginine is crucial to T lymphocyte function, nitric oxide production, and formation of collagen—all of which contribute to recovery after surgery. Lipid mediators derived from eicosapentaenoic acid and docosahexaenoic acid (resolvins, protectins, and maresins) have potent proresolving, anti-inflammatory, and neuroprotective properties, and have been found to play a role in the repair and resolution of inflammation.

Immunonutrition oral supplements have also been studied in surgical patients. Numerous studies have found beneficial effects, but inconsistencies in study design make the interpretation of results challenging. Most studies and a 2015 meta-analysis by Song and colleagues have suggested that perioperative immunonutrition (meaning both pre- and postoperative immunonutrition) is the superior strategy.[131]

Studies of preoperative immunonutrition supplements have often been difficult to interpret because of inconsistencies in study design, but a pragmatic quality improvement project demonstrated a reduction in length of stay and trend toward reduction in adverse events in more than 3000 patients in Washington state.[132] A meta-analysis has suggested that standard high-protein oral supplements can achieve results similar to immunonutrition, reducing complications when used in advance of surgery.[133] Many studies of preoperative immunonutrition supplements have been done in cancer patients, who often experience some level of moderate malnutrition, but the studies have not typically examined whether the supplements have a specific impact in malnourished patients. Patients with severe malnutrition will likely require enteral or parenteral supplementation for preoperative optimization.

Burns

European Society for Clinical Nutrition and Metabolism guidelines report insufficient data to recommend routine supplementation of ω-3 fatty acids, arginine, glutamine, or nucleotides in burn patients.[134] However, these guidelines recommend that the trace elements copper, selenium, and zinc be supplemented at higher than standard doses in this patient population.[135] Daily doses of 40.4 mcmol copper, 2.9 mcmol selenium, and 406 mcmol zinc for 30 days after burn injury have been associated with a reduction in the length of hospital stay and the number of bronchopneumonic infections.[134]

Vitamin C functions as a cofactor in many enzymes, including those involved with wound healing and recovery such as the hydroxylation of collagen and cortisol.[136] In burn patients, treatment with high-dose vitamin C (up to 66 mg/kg/h for 48 hours) has been advocated to diminish fluid resuscitation.[137,138] Further investigation is required to define clinical benefit and optimal doses for supplementation.[138]

Data are insufficient in burn patients to support routine use of immunonutrients (such as arginine and fish oil) in combination therapies or for individual supplementation. However, many institutions use immunonutrition in burns despite the paucity of evidence.[82] One high-quality study does suggest that glutamine has a mortality benefit in burn populations, and this topic is being investigated in a large, ongoing RCT.[139] The 2016 SCCM/ASPEN guidelines recommended not adding glutamine to EN for any critically ill until additional evidence is available.[35] Questions remain regarding the ideal dosage, timing, and duration of therapy. Large RCTs have suggested no benefit to enteral or parenteral glutamine in a mostly medical ICU population—particularly in high doses—and burns are one of the few areas where glutamine supplementation is still considered as a possible intervention.[79]

References

1. US Centers for Disease Control and Prevention. Injury in the US: 2013 Chartbook. http://www.cdc.gov/injury. Accessed November 7, 2016.

2. Wilmore DW. Alterations in protein, carbohydrate, and fat metabolism in injured and septic patients. *J Am Coll Nutr.* 1983;2(1):3–13.

3. Kudsk KA, Croce MA, Fabian TC, et al. Enteral versus parenteral feeding. Effects on septic morbidity after blunt and penetrating abdominal trauma. *Ann Surg.* 1992;215(5):503–511.

4. Kudsk KA, Minard G, Croce MA, et al. A randomized trial of isonitrogenous enteral diets after severe trauma. An immune-enhancing diet reduces septic complications. *Ann Surg.* 1996; 224(4):531–540.

5. Moore FA, Moore EE, Jones TN, McCroskey BL, Peterson VM. TEN versus TPN following major abdominal trauma—reduced septic morbidity. *J Trauma.* 1989;29(7):916–922.

6. American College of Chest Physicians/Society of Critical Care Medicine. Consensus conference: definitions for sepsis and organ failure and guidelines for the use of innovative therapies in sepsis. *Crit Care Med.* 1992;20(6):864–874.

7. Cuthbertson DP. Second annual Jonathan E. Rhoads Lecture. The metabolic response to injury and its nutritional implications: retrospect and prospect. *JPEN J Parenter Enteral Nutr.* 1979; 3(3):108–129.

8. Malone DL, Kuhls D, Napolitano LM, McCarter R, Scalea T. Back to basics: validation of the admission systemic inflammatory response syndrome score in predicting outcome in trauma. *J Trauma.* 2001;51(3):458–463.

9. Collier BR, Giladi A, Dossett LA, Dyer L, Fleming SB, Cotton BA. Impact of high-dose antioxidants on outcomes in acutely injured patients. *JPEN J Parenter Enteral Nutr.* 2008;32(4):384–388.

10. Moore FA, Feliciano DV, Andrassy RJ, et al. Early enteral feeding, compared with parenteral, reduces postoperative septic complications. The results of a meta-analysis. *Ann Surg.* 1992;216(2):172–183.

11. Gabay C, Kushner I. Acute-phase proteins and other systemic responses to inflammation. *N Engl J Med.* 1999;340(6):448–454.

12. Collier B, Dossett LA, May AK, Diaz JJ. Glucose control and the inflammatory response. *Nutr Clin Pract.* 2008;23(1):3–15.

13. Moore EE, Moore FA. Immediate enteral nutrition following multisystem trauma: a decade perspective. *J Am Coll Nutr.* 1991; 10(6):633–648.

14. Todd SR, Kozar RA, Moore FA. Nutrition support in adult trauma patients. *Nutr Clin Pract.* 2006;21(5):421–429.

15. Burlew CC, Moore EE, Cuschieri J, et al. Who should we feed? A Western Trauma Association multi-institutional study of enteral nutrition in the open abdomen after injury. *J Trauma.* 2012;73(6): 1380–1388.

16. Ohri SK, Somasundaram S, Koak Y, et al. The effect of intestinal hypoperfusion on intestinal absorption and permeability during cardiopulmonary bypass. *Gastroenterology.* 1994;106(2): 318–323.

17. Fink MP. Adequacy of gut oxygenation in endotoxemia and sepsis. *Crit Care Med.* 1993;21(2 Suppl):S4–S8.

18. Holland J, Carey M, Hughes N, et al. Intraoperative splanchnic hypoperfusion, increased intestinal permeability, downregulation of monocyte class II major histocompatibility complex expression, exaggerated acute phase response, and sepsis. *Am J Surg.* 2005;190(3):393–400.

19. Matheson PJ, Wilson MA, Garrison RN. Regulation of intestinal blood flow. *J Surg Res.* 2000;93(1):182–196.

20. Ceppa EP, Fuh KC, Bulkley GB. Mesenteric hemodynamic response to circulatory shock. *Curr Opin Crit Care.* 2003;9(2):127–132.

21. Marvin RG, McKinley BA, McQuiggan M, Cocanour CS, Moore FA. Nonocclusive bowel necrosis occurring in critically ill trauma patients receiving enteral nutrition manifests no reliable clinical signs for early detection. *Am J Surg.* 2000;179(1):7–12.

22. Gottschlich MM, Jenkins ME, Mayes T, et al. The 2002 Clinical Research Award. An evaluation of the safety of early vs delayed enteral support and effects on clinical, nutritional, and endocrine outcomes after severe burns. *J Burn Care Rehabil.* 2002;23(6): 401–415.

23. Bortenschlager L, Roberts PR, Black KW, Zaloga GP. Enteral feeding minimizes liver injury during hemorrhagic shock. *Shock.* 1994;2(5):351–354.

24. Gielkens HA, van Oostayen JA, Onkenhout W, Lamers CB, Masclee AA. Effect of amino acids on mesenteric blood flow in humans. *Scand J Gastroenterol.* 1997;32(12):1230–1234.

25. Gosche JR, Garrison RN, Harris PD, Cryer HG. Absorptive hyperemia restores intestinal blood flow during *Escherichia coli* sepsis in the rat. *Arch Surg.* 1990;125(12):1573–1576.

26. Inoue S, Lukes S, Alexander JW, Trocki O, Silberstein EB. Increased gut blood flow with early enteral feeding in burned guinea pigs. *J Burn Care Rehabil.* 1989;10(4):300–308.

27. Kazamias P, Kotzampassi K, Koufogiannis D, Eleftheriadis E. Influence of enteral nutrition–induced splanchnic hyperemia on the septic origin of splanchnic ischemia. *World J Surg.* 1998; 22(1):6–11.

28. Purcell PN, Davis K Jr, Branson RD, Johnson DJ. Continuous duodenal feeding restores gut blood flow and increases gut oxygen utilization during PEEP ventilation for lung injury. *Am J Surg.* 1993;165(1):188–193.

29. Schunn CD, Daly JM. Small bowel necrosis associated with postoperative jejunal tube feeding. *J Am Coll Surg.* 1995;180(4): 410–416.

30. Jensen GL, Bistrian B, Roubenoff R, Heimburger DC. Malnutrition syndromes: a conundrum vs continuum. *JPEN J Parenter Enteral Nutr.* 2009;33(6):710–716.

31. Hill AA, Plank LD, Finn PJ, et al. Massive nitrogen loss in critical surgical illness: effect on cardiac mass and function. *Ann Surg.* 1997;226(2):191–197.

32. Jensen GL, Mirtallo J, Compher C, et al. Adult starvation and disease-related malnutrition: a proposal for etiology-based diagnosis in the clinical practice setting from the International Consensus Guideline Committee. *JPEN J Parenter Enteral Nutr.* 2010; 34(2):156–159.

33. Long CL, Schaffel N, Geiger JW, Schiller WR, Blakemore WS. Metabolic response to injury and illness: estimation of energy and protein needs from indirect calorimetry and nitrogen balance. *JPEN J Parenter Enteral Nutr.* 1979;3(6):452–456.

34. Barker LA, Gout BS, Crowe TC. Hospital malnutrition: prevalence, identification and impact on patients and the healthcare system. *Int J Environ Res Public Health.* 2011;8(2):514–527.

35. McClave SA, Taylor BE, Martindale RG, et al. Guidelines for the provision and assessment of nutrition support therapy in the adult critically ill patient: Society of Critical Care Medicine (SCCM) and American Society for Parenteral and Enteral Nutrition (A.S.P.E.N.). JPEN J Parenter Enteral Nutr. 2016;40(2):159–211.

36. Hill GL. Jonathan E. Rhoads Lecture. Body composition research: implications for the practice of clinical nutrition. JPEN J Parenter Enteral Nutr. 1992;16(3):197–218.

37. Hill GL. Implications of critical illness, injury, and sepsis on lean body mass and nutritional needs. Nutrition. 1998;14(6): 557–558.

38. Plank LD, Hill GL. Sequential metabolic changes following induction of systemic inflammatory response in patients with severe sepsis or major blunt trauma. World J Surg. 2000;24(6):630–638.

39. Winkler M. Nutrition assessment and monitoring. In: Cresci G, ed. Nutrition Support for the Critically Ill Patient: A Guide to Practice. Boca Raton, FL: CRC Press; 2005:71–81.

40. Cresci G. Nutrition assessment and monitoring. In: Shikora S, Martindale R, Schwaitzberg S, eds. Nutritional Considerations in the Intensive Care Unit. Dubuque, IA: Kendall/Hunt Publishing; 2002:21–30.

41. Ritchie RF, Palomaki GE, Neveux LM, Navolotskaia O, Ledue TB, Craig WY. Reference distributions for the negative acute-phase serum proteins, albumin, transferrin and transthyretin: a practical, simple and clinically relevant approach in a large cohort. J Clin Lab Anal. 1999;13(6):273–279.

42. Flancbaum L, Choban PS, Sambucco S, Verducci J, Burge JC. Comparison of indirect calorimetry, the Fick method, and prediction equations in estimating the energy requirements of critically ill patients. Am J Clin Nutr. 1999;69(3):461–466.

43. Weir JB. New methods for calculating metabolic rate with special reference to protein metabolism. J Physiol. 1949;109(1-2):1–9.

44. McClave SA, Lowen CC, Kleber MJ, et al. Are patients fed appropriately according to their caloric requirements? JPEN J Parenter Enteral Nutr. 1998;22(6):375–381.

45. Lichtenberg K, Guay-Berry P, Pipitone A, Bondy A, Rotello L. Compensatory increased enteral feeding goal rates: a way to achieve optimal nutrition. Nutr Clin Pract. 2010;25(6):653–657.

46. Pousman RM, Pepper C, Pandharipande P, et al. Feasibility of implementing a reduced fasting protocol for critically ill trauma patients undergoing operative and nonoperative procedures. JPEN J Parenter Enteral Nutr. 2009;33(2):176–180.

47. Seder CW, Stockdale W, Hale L, Janczyk RJ. Nasal bridling decreases feeding tube dislodgment and may increase caloric intake in the surgical intensive care unit: a randomized, controlled trial. Crit Care Med. 2010;38(3):797–801.

48. Heyland DK, Murch L, Cahill N, et al. Enhanced protein-energy provision via the enteral route feeding protocol in critically ill patients: results of a cluster randomized trial. Crit Care Med. 2013;41(12):2743–2753.

49. Bankhead R, Boullata J, Brantley S, et al. Enteral nutrition practice recommendations. JPEN J Parenter Enteral Nutr. 2009;33(2): 122–167.

50. Cerra FB, Siegel JH, Coleman B, Border JR, McMenamy RR. Septic autocannibalism. A failure of exogenous nutritional support. Ann Surg. 1980;192(4):570–580.

51. Shaw JH, Wildbore M, Wolfe RR. Whole body protein kinetics in severely septic patients. The response to glucose infusion and total parenteral nutrition. Ann Surg. 1987;205(3):288–294.

52. Alexander JW, MacMillan BG, Stinnett JD, et al. Beneficial effects of aggressive protein feeding in severely burned children. Ann Surg. 1980;192(4):505–517.

53. Jacobs DG, Jacobs DO, Kudsk KA, et al. Practice management guidelines for nutritional support of the trauma patient. J Trauma. 2004;57(3):660–678.

54. Cerra FB. Hypermetabolism, organ failure, and metabolic support. Surgery. 1987;101(1):1–14.

55. Scheinkestel CD, Kar L, Marshall K, et al. Prospective randomized trial to assess caloric and protein needs of critically ill, anuric, ventilated patients requiring continuous renal replacement therapy. Nutrition. 2003;19(11-12):909–916.

56. Cheatham ML, Safcsak K, Brzezinski SJ, Lube MW. Nitrogen balance, protein loss, and the open abdomen. Crit Care Med. 2007; 35(1):127–131.

57. Wolfe RR, Allsop JR, Burke JF. Glucose metabolism in man: responses to intravenous glucose infusion. Metabolism. 1979;28(3): 210–220.

58. Collier B, Diaz J Jr, Forbes R, et al. The impact of a normoglycemic management protocol on clinical outcomes in the trauma intensive care unit. JPEN J Parenter Enteral Nutr. 2005;29(5):353–358.

59. Laird AM, Miller PR, Kilgo PD, Meredith JW, Chang MC. Relationship of early hyperglycemia to mortality in trauma patients. J Trauma. 2004;56(5):1058–1062.

60. Yendamuri S, Fulda GJ, Tinkoff GH. Admission hyperglycemia as a prognostic indicator in trauma. J Trauma. 2003;55(1):33–38.

61. Hansen TK, Thiel S, Wouters PJ, Christiansen JS, Van den Berghe G. Intensive insulin therapy exerts antiinflammatory effects in critically ill patients and counteracts the adverse effect of low mannose-binding lectin levels. J Clin Endocrinol Metab. 2003;88(3):1082–1088.

62. Van den Berghe G, Wouters P, Weekers F, et al. Intensive insulin therapy in the critically ill patient. N Engl J Med. 2001;345(19): 1359–1367.

63. Finfer S, Chittock DR, Su SY, et al. Intensive versus conventional glucose control in critically ill patients. N Engl J Med. 2009; 360(13):1283–1297.

64. Griesdale DE, de Souza RJ, van Dam RM, et al. Intensive insulin therapy and mortality among critically ill patients: a meta-analysis including NICE-SUGAR study data. CMAJ. 2009;180(8): 821–827.

65. Brunkhorst FM, Engel C, Bloos F, et al. Intensive insulin therapy and pentastarch resuscitation in severe sepsis. N Engl J Med. 2008;358(2):125–139.

66. Egi M, Finfer S, Bellomo R. Glycemic control in the ICU. Chest. 2011;140(1):212–220.

67. Carpentier YA, Scruel O. Changes in the concentration and composition of plasma lipoproteins during the acute phase response. Curr Opin Clin Nutr Metab Care. 2002;5(2):153–158.

68. Gottschlich MM, Alexander JW. Fat kinetics and recommended dietary intake in burns. JPEN J Parenter Enteral Nutr. 1987; 11(1):80–85.

69. Nordenstrom J, Carpentier YA, Askanazi J, et al. Free fatty acid mobilization and oxidation during total parenteral nutrition in trauma and infection. Ann Surg. 1983;198(6):725–735.

70. Shaw JH, Wolfe RR. An integrated analysis of glucose, fat, and protein metabolism in severely traumatized patients. Studies in the basal state and the response to total parenteral nutrition. Ann Surg. 1989;209(1):63–72.

71. Warden GD. Burn shock resuscitation. World J Surg. 1992; 16(1):16–23.

72. Goode HF, Webster NR. Free radicals and antioxidants in sepsis. Crit Care Med. 1993;21(11):1770–1776.

73. Crimi E, Liguori A, Condorelli M, et al. The beneficial effects of antioxidant supplementation in enteral feeding in critically ill patients: a prospective, randomized, double-blind, placebo-controlled trial. Anesth Analg. 2004;99(3):857–863.

74. Goode HF, Cowley HC, Walker BE, Howdle PD, Webster NR. Decreased antioxidant status and increased lipid peroxidation in patients with septic shock and secondary organ dysfunction. Crit Care Med. 1995;23(4):646–651.

75. Lemoyne M, Van GA, Kurian R, Jeejeebhoy KN. Plasma vitamin E and selenium and breath pentane in home parenteral nutrition patients. *Am J Clin Nutr.* 1988;48(5):1310–1315.

76. Louw JA, Werbeck A, Louw ME, et al. Blood vitamin concentrations during the acute-phase response. *Crit Care Med.* 1992; 20(7):934–941.

77. Schorah CJ, Downing C, Piripitsi A, et al. Total vitamin C, ascorbic acid, and dehydroascorbic acid concentrations in plasma of critically ill patients. *Am J Clin Nutr.* 1996;63(5):760–765.

78. Nathens AB, Neff MJ, Jurkovich GJ, et al. Randomized, prospective trial of antioxidant supplementation in critically ill surgical patients. *Ann Surg.* 2002;236(6):814–822.

79. Heyland D, Muscadere J, Wischmeyer PE, et al. A randomized trial of glutamine and antioxidants in critically ill patients. *N Engl J Med.* 2016;368(16):1489–1497.

80. Prelack K, Sheridan RL. Micronutrient supplementation in the critically ill patient: strategies for clinical practice. *J Trauma.* 2001; 51(3):601–620.

81. Gottschlich MM, Warden GD. Vitamin supplementation in the patient with burns. *J Burn Care Rehabil.* 1990;11(3):275–279.

82. Coffey R, Thomas S, Murphy CV, et al. clinical guide to nutrition therapy: one center's guide. *Austin J Emergency Crit Care Med.* 2015:2(6):id1036.

83. Klein GL, Langman CB, Herndon DN. Vitamin D depletion following burn injury in children: a possible factor in post-burn osteopenia. *J Trauma.* 2002;52(2):346–350.

84. Lee P, Nair P, Eisman JA, Center JR. Vitamin D deficiency in the intensive care unit: an invisible accomplice to morbidity and mortality? *Intensive Care Med.* 2009;35(12):2028–2032.

85. Lucidarme O, Messai E, Mazzoni T, Arcade M, du CD. Incidence and risk factors of vitamin D deficiency in critically ill patients: results from a prospective observational study. *Intensive Care Med.* 2010;36(9):1609–1611.

86. Melamed ML, Michos ED, Post W, Astor B. 25-hydroxyvitamin D levels and the risk of mortality in the general population. *Arch Intern Med.* 2008;168(15):1629–1637.

87. Ukleja A, Freeman KL, Gilbert K, et al. Standards for nutrition support: adult hospitalized patients. *Nutr Clin Pract.* 2010;25(4): 403–414.

88. Heyland DK, MacDonald S, Keefe L, Drover JW. Total parenteral nutrition in the critically ill patient: a meta-analysis. *JAMA.* 1998;280(23):2013–2019.

89. Koretz RL, Lipman TO, Klein S. AGA technical review on parenteral nutrition. *Gastroenterology.* 2001;121(4):970–1001.

90. Shirley PJ, Bion JF. Intra-hospital transport of critically ill patients: minimising risk. *Intensive Care Med.* 2004;30(8):1508–1510.

91. Heyland DK, Tougas G, Cook DJ, Guyatt GH. Cisapride improves gastric emptying in mechanically ventilated, critically ill patients. A randomized, double-blind trial. *Am J Respir Crit Care Med.* 1996;154(6 Pt 1):1678–1683.

92. Jooste CA, Mustoe J, Collee G. Metoclopramide improves gastric motility in critically ill patients. *Intensive Care Med.* 1999;25(5): 464–468.

93. Mentec H, Dupont H, Bocchetti M, et al. Upper digestive intolerance during enteral nutrition in critically ill patients: frequency, risk factors, and complications. *Crit Care Med.* 2001;29(10): 1955–1961.

94. Montejo JC. Enteral nutrition-related gastrointestinal complications in critically ill patients: a multicenter study. The Nutritional and Metabolic Working Group of the Spanish Society of Intensive Care Medicine and Coronary Units. *Crit Care Med.* 1999;27(8):1447–1453.

95. Mutlu GM, Mutlu EA, Factor P. GI complications in patients receiving mechanical ventilation. *Chest.* 2001;119(4): 1222–1241.

96. Neumann DA, DeLegge MH. Gastric versus small-bowel tube feeding in the intensive care unit: a prospective comparison of efficacy. *Crit Care Med.* 2002;30(7):1436–1438.

97. McClave SA, Lukan JK, Stefater JA, et al. Poor validity of residual volumes as a marker for risk of aspiration in critically ill patients. *Crit Care Med.* 2005;33(2):324–330.

98. Heyland DK, Drover JW, Dhaliwal R, Greenwood J. Optimizing the benefits and minimizing the risks of enteral nutrition in the critically ill: role of small bowel feeding. *JPEN J Parenter Enteral Nutr.* 2002;26(6 Suppl):S51–S55.

99. Prabhakaran S, Doraiswamy VA, Nagaraja V, et al. Nasoenteric tube complications. *Scand J Surg.* 2012;101(3):147–155.

100. Koopmann MC, Kudsk KA, Szotkowski MJ, Rees SM. A team-based protocol and electromagnetic technology eliminate feeding tube placement complications. *Ann Surg.* 2011;253(2): 287–302.

101. Cresci G, Martindale R. Bedside placement of small bowel feeding tubes in hospitalized patients: a new role for the dietitian. *Nutrition.* 2003;19(10):843–846.

102. Zaloga GP. Bedside method for placing small bowel feeding tubes in critically ill patients. A prospective study. *Chest.* 1991; 100(6):1643–1646.

103. Osland E, Yunus RM, Khan S, Memon MA. Early versus traditional postoperative feeding in patients undergoing resectional gastrointestinal surgery: a meta-analysis. *JPEN J Parenter Enteral Nutr.* 2011;35(4):473–487.

104. Studley HO. Percentage of weight loss: a basic indicator of surgical risk in patients with chronic peptic ulcer. *Nutr Hosp.* 2001;16(4):141–143.

105. Barker CF. Jonathan Rhoads, MD 1907–2002. *Ann Surg.* 2002; 235(5):740–744.

106. Perioperative total parenteral nutrition in surgical patients. The Veterans Affairs Total Parenteral Nutrition Cooperative Study Group. *N Engl J Med.* 1991;325(8):525–532.

107. Jie B, Jiang ZM, Nolan MT, et al. Impact of preoperative nutritional support on clinical outcome in abdominal surgical patients at nutritional risk. *Nutrition* 2012;28(10):1022–1027.

108. Abou-Assi S, Craig K, O'Keefe SJ. Hypocaloric jejunal feeding is better than total parenteral nutrition in acute pancreatitis: results of a randomized comparative study. *Am J Gastroenterol.* 2002;97(9):2255–2262.

109. McClave SA. Nutrition support in acute pancreatitis. *Gastroenterol Clin North Am.* 2007;36(1):65–74.

110. O'Keefe SJ, Broderick T, Turner M, Stevens S, O'Keefe JS. Nutrition in the management of necrotizing pancreatitis. *Clin Gastroenterol Hepatol.* 2003;1(4):315–321.

111. Olah A, Pardavi G, Belagyi T, Nagy A, Issekutz A, Mohamed GE. Early nasojejunal feeding in acute pancreatitis is associated with a lower complication rate. *Nutrition.* 2002;18(3):259–262.

112. Shukla HS, Rao RR, Banu N, Gupta RM, Yadav RC. Enteral hyperalimentation in malnourished surgical patients. *Indian J Med Res.* 1984;80:339–346.

113. von Meyenfeldt MF, Meijerink WJ, Rouflart MM, Builmaassen MT, Soeters PB. Perioperative nutritional support: a randomised clinical trial. *Clin Nutr.* 1992;11(4):180–186.

114. Heyland DK, Montalvo M, MacDonald S, et al. Total parenteral nutrition in the surgical patient: a meta-analysis. *Can J Surg.* 2001;44(2):102–111.

115. Fearon KC, Ljungqvist O, Von MM, et al. Enhanced recovery after surgery: a consensus review of clinical care for patients undergoing colonic resection. *Clin Nutr.* 2005;24(3):466–477.

116. Sato H, Carvalho G, Sato T, et al. The association of preoperative glycemic control, intraoperative insulin sensitivity, and outcomes after cardiac surgery. *J Clin Endocrinol Metab.* 2010; 95(9):4338–4344.

117. Varadhan KK, Lobo DN, Ljungqvist O. Enhanced recovery after surgery: the future of improving surgical care. *Crit Care Clin.* 2010;26(3):527–547.

118. Varadhan KK, Neal KR, Dejong CH, Fearon KC, Ljungqvist O, Lobo DN. The enhanced recovery after surgery (ERAS) pathway for patients undergoing major elective open colorectal surgery: a meta-analysis of randomized controlled trials. *Clin Nutr.* 2010;29(4):434–440.

119. Brandstrup B, Tonnesen H, Beier-Holgersen R, et al. Effects of intravenous fluid restriction on postoperative complications: comparison of two perioperative fluid regimens: a randomized assessor-blinded multicenter trial. *Ann Surg.* 2003;238(5):641–648.

120. Gustafsson UO, Hausel J, Thorell A, et al. Adherence to the enhanced recovery after surgery protocol and outcomes after colorectal cancer surgery. *Arch Surg.* 2011;146(5):571–577.

121. Lobo DN, Bostock KA, Neal KR, et al. Effect of salt and water balance on recovery of gastrointestinal function after elective colonic resection: a randomised controlled trial. *Lancet.* 2002; 359(9320):1812–1818.

122. Gan TJ, Thacker JK, Miller TE, Scott MJ, Holubar SD, eds. *Enhanced Recovery for Major Abdominopelvic Surgery.* West Islip, NY: Professional Communications; 2016.

123. Gadek JE, DeMichele SJ, Karlstad MD, et al. Effect of enteral feeding with eicosapentaenoic acid, gamma-linolenic acid, and antioxidants in patients with acute respiratory distress syndrome. Enteral Nutrition in ARDS Study Group. *Crit Care Med.* 1999;27(8):1409–1420.

124. Gottschlich MM, Jenkins M, Warden GD, et al. Differential effects of three enteral dietary regimens on selected outcome variables in burn patients. *JPEN J Parenter Enteral Nutr.* 1990; 14(3):225–236.

125. Nelson JL, DeMichele SJ, Pacht ER, Wennberg AK. Effect of enteral feeding with eicosapentaenoic acid, gamma-linolenic acid, and antioxidants on antioxidant status in patients with acute respiratory distress syndrome. *JPEN J Parenter Enteral Nutr.* 2003;27(2):98–104.

126. Pacht ER, DeMichele SJ, Nelson JL, Hart J, Wennberg AK, Gadek JE. Enteral nutrition with eicosapentaenoic acid, gammalinolenic acid, and antioxidants reduces alveolar inflammatory mediators and protein influx in patients with acute respiratory distress syndrome. *Crit Care Med.* 2003;31(2):491–500.

127. Brown RO, Hunt H, Mowatt-Larssen CA, Wojtysiak SL, Henningfield MF, Kudsk KA. Comparison of specialized and standard enteral formulas in trauma patients. *Pharmacotherapy.* 1994; 14(3):314–320.

128. Kudsk KA, Minard G, Croce MA, et al. A randomized trial of isonitrogenous enteral diets after severe trauma. An immune-enhancing diet reduces septic complications. *Ann Surg.* 1996; 224(4):531–540.

129. Weimann A, Bastian L, Bischoff WE, et al. Influence of arginine, omega-3 fatty acids and nucleotide-supplemented enteral support on systemic inflammatory response syndrome and multiple organ failure in patients after severe trauma. *Nutrition.* 1998; 14(2):165–172.

130. Zhu X, Herrera G, Ochoa JB. Immunosupression and infection after major surgery: a nutritional deficiency. *Crit Care Clin.* 2010;26(3):491–500.

131. Song GM, Tian X, Zhang L, et. al. Immunonutrition support for patients undergoing surgery for gastrointestinal malignancy: preoperative, postoperative, or perioperative? A Bayesian Network meta-analysis of randomized controlled trials. *Medicine* (Baltimore). 2015;94(29):e1225.

132. Thornblade LW, Varghese TK, Shi X, et al. Preoperative immunonutrition and elective colorectal resection outcomes. *Dis Colon Rectum.* 2017;60(1):68–75.

133. Hegazi RA, Hustead DS, Evans DC. Preoperative standard oral nutrition supplements vs immunonutrition: results of a systematic review and meta-analysis. *J Am Coll Surg.* 2014; 219(5):1078–1087.

134. Kreymann KG, Berger MM, Deutz NE, et al. ESPEN guidelines on enteral nutrition: intensive care. *Clin Nutr.* 2006;25(2):210–223.

135. Kurmis R, Parker A, Greenwood J. The use of immunonutrition in burn injury care: where are we? *J Burn Care Res.* 2010; 31(5):677–691.

136. Fukushima R, Yamazaki E. Vitamin C requirement in surgical patients. *Curr Opin Clin Nutr Metab Care.* 2010;13(6):669–676.

137. Kahn SA, Beers RJ, Lentz CW. Resuscitation after severe burn injury using high-dose ascorbic acid: a retrospective review. *J Burn Care Res.* 2011;32(1):110–117.

138. Kremer T, Harenberg P, Hernekamp F, et al. High-dose vitamin C treatment reduces capillary leakage after burn plasma transfer in rats. *J Burn Care Res.* 2010;31(3):470–479.

139. Garrel D, Patenaude J, Nedelec B, et al. Decreased mortality and infectious morbidity in adult burn patients given enteral glutamine supplements: a prospective, controlled, randomized clinical trial. *Crit Care Med.* 2003;31(10):2444–2449.

25 Pulmonary Disease

Karen S. Allen, MD, Leah A. Hoffman, PhD, RD, LD, CNSC, Kellie Jones, MD, Michelle Kozeniecki, MS, RD, CNSC, Jayshil J. Patel, MD, and Joseph West, MD

CONTENTS

Acknowledgment: Krista L. Turner, MD, FACS, was the author of this chapter for the second edition.

Objectives

1. Understand nutrition strategies for acute and chronic pulmonary failure as they relate to energy needs, mode and timing of nutrition support, and selection of optimal enteral nutrition (EN) or parenteral nutrition (PN).
2. Learn about nutrition requirements and nutrition's impact on disease outcome of chronic pulmonary diseases.
3. Understand nutrition strategies for patients with acute respiratory distress syndrome (ARDS).
4. Explore options for providing optimal micro- and macronutrients and best practices for nutrition support for patients with acute pulmonary failure.
5. Understand prevention strategies for aspiration and ventilator-associated pneumonia (VAP).

Test Your Knowledge Questions

1. The strategy of restricted fluid intake may decrease the number of days that patients require mechanical ventilation for which disease process?
   A. Traumatic brain injury (TBI)
   B. ARDS
   C. Pulmonary embolism (PE)
   D. Septic shock secondary to bacterial pneumonia
2. Which of the following does not help reduce VAP?
   A. Elevating the head of the bed to at least 45°
   B. Gastric ulcer prophylaxis and early PN
   C. Early mobility and decreased days on a mechanical ventilator
   D. Minimizing sedation and a daily sedation vacation
3. Which of the following should not be supplemented via EN to patients in pulmonary failure?
   A. Phosphorus
   B. Calcium
   C. Glutamine
   D. Magnesium

Test Your Knowledge Answers

1. The correct answer is **B**. Restricted fluid intake has decreased the number of days that patients with ARDS require mechanical ventilation and decreased the overall number of days in intensive care unit (ICU) for patients with ARDS. However, fluid restriction did not improve mortality for patients with ARDS. Evidence-based treatment for ARDS includes permissive hypercapnia as necessary to reduce the lung barotrauma, fluid restriction, early paralytics, and prone positioning. Fluid restriction has not been shown to make a clinically significant difference in patients with TBI or PE. Fluids should not be restricted in patients with septic shock; instead, these patients should be given aggressive fluid resuscitation.
2. The correct answer is **B**. VAP is a preventable disease in the ICU. Strategies to prevent or reduce the incidence of VAP include limiting mechanical ventilator time, sedation, and minimizing aspiration risk. Components of VAP "bundles" are typically implemented in the ICU setting and include elevating the head of the bed, early mobilization, minimal sedation, limiting mechanical ventilator time, and minimizing pooling of oral secretions. Early PN and gastric ulcer prophylaxis do not seem to decrease incidence of VAP.
3. The correct answer is C. Initial studies showed promising results regarding enteral glutamine supplementation and reduced mortality, but REDOX, a large randomized controlled trial (RCT), indicated that glutamine may potentially harm patients with pulmonary failure. The most recent guidelines (2016) from the Society of Critical Care Medicine (SCCM) and American Society for Parenteral and Enteral Nutrition (ASPEN) do not recommend the use of glutamine supplementation in general critical care patients.[1] Electrolytes should be monitored and replaced as necessary to maintain normal serum levels.

Introduction

Nutrition support is critical for patients with acute or chronic pulmonary disease. The use of nutrition support as a therapeutic modality for critically ill patients who experience pulmonary failure has been well studied in recent years. Pulmonary failure is associated with increased catabolism and, at times, decreased gut absorption. Nutrition support clinicians should individually design nutrition support for each patient to ensure it is nutritionally adequate without overfeeding and delivered safely. Malnutrition is a risk factor for pulmonary failure in the acute setting and can lead to worsening prognosis of chronic respiratory diseases. Patients with pulmonary diseases require nutrition risk assessment and screening. This chapter will focus mainly on nutrition support in the setting of acute pulmonary failure, as this is the most common situation for patients to encounter clinical nutrition support specialists. Additionally, the chapter will briefly highlight other types of pulmonary disease that can be affected by a patient's nutrition status.

Pulmonary Function

Pulmonary anatomy is primarily a series of airways, alveoli and capillaries, with the primary function of performing *gas exchange*, the exchange of inhaled oxygen for carbon dioxide (CO_2) that is produced during cellular respiration. Patency of the airways and preservation of the alveoli and capillary units throughout the lung is critical for proper function and adequate gas exchange.

Inhalation is an active process driven by a set of muscles that work in concert to bring air into the lung whereas expiration is a result of the elasticity of the lungs and ribcage. The primary respiratory muscles and driving force of inhalation are the diaphragm, a dome-like muscle situated between the abdomen and the thoracic cavity, and the intercostal muscles. Contraction of the diaphragm in conjunction with the intercostal muscles causes an expansion of the thoracic space creating a negative pressure and resultant inward airflow. The scalene and sternocleidomastoid muscles are accessory respiratory muscles and function when there is an increased work of breathing.

The lungs and rib cage have a natural elastic property. As a result, expiration, under normal conditions, is a passive process in which the diaphragm and intercostal muscles relax allowing the thoracic cavity to return to its normal resting state. In times of distress, primary and accessory muscles can aid in forced exhalation.

Gas exchange, the primary purpose of the lungs, takes place at the level of the alveoli and capillary units. Fick's law governs this diffusion process in that gas moves across the alveoli or capillary unit in proportion to the area of the unit and inversely proportional to the thickness of the unit. Therefore, the alveoli are in almost direct contact with the capillaries that surround them, allowing for a very thin membrane through which gases move. The progressive narrowing of airways into eventual alveoli allows for an increased surface area between capillaries and alveoli, increasing gas exchange

FIGURE 25-1 Lung Alveoli and Gas Exchange

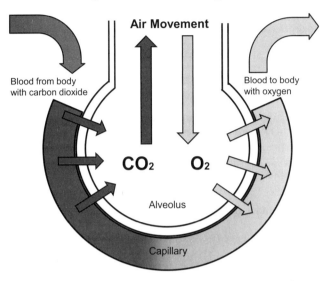

Lungs are comprised of numerous air sacs called *alveoli*. These sacs are surrounded by pulmonary capillaries. Blood flows into the pulmonary circulation that is high in carbon dioxide (CO_2) and low in oxygen (O_2). Inspired O_2 diffuses across the alveolar and capillary membranes to bind with red blood cells in the capillary (ie, oxygenation). CO_2 diffuses from the capillary into the alveolus where it is expired via the airway (ie, ventilation).

Oxygen and CO_2 diffusion is regulated by the partial pressure differences of each gas between the lung and venous blood. The large partial pressure difference between inhaled oxygen and oxygen in venous blood leads to a perfusion limited exchange of oxygen from the lung to the capillary. CO_2 diffusion works in the reverse and is limited secondary to higher partial pressures in venous blood compared to inhaled air in the lung (Figure 25-1). Critical illness, perfusion abnormalities, infection, poor nutrition, and other factors can all affect the pulmonary system and cause shifts in normal physiology leading to gas exchange abnormalities.

Modes of Respiratory Support

The failure of any of the components of the respiratory system may result in the patient requiring additional support in the form of supplemental oxygen or ventilator support (either noninvasive or invasive). If the patient develops mild hypoxemia, is conscious, and is not in moderate to severe respiratory distress (frequently judged by accessory muscle use), oxygen delivered by nasal cannula or mask may be sufficient until the patient recovers. Common causes of hypoxemia are pulmonary edema, pneumonia, inflammation, and chronic pulmonary diseases.

Hypoventilation leads to CO_2 retention (hypercapnia). In this situation, the patient may require noninvasive ventilator support, which involves positive airway pressure ventilation via an airtight mask as well as supplemental oxygen therapy. Common causes of hypercapnia include obstructive pulmonary disease, sleep apnea, obesity leading to a collapse of the upper airways (also referred to as *obesity hypoventilation syndrome*), or respiratory muscle weakness.

Invasive modes of ventilator support are required for patients who develop more severe hypoxemia or hypercapnia, fail to respond to the previously described treatment methods, or experience prolonged respiratory distress. Invasive ventilation requires an endotracheal tube placed into the patient's trachea and provides complete pulmonary support via a mechanical ventilator. The principles of managing mechanical ventilation varies based on the set respiratory rate (RR), tidal volumes (TV), inspiratory pressure, positive end expiratory pressure, inspiratory and expiratory times, and the fraction of inspired oxygen (FIO_2). Each of these factors may be manipulated based on the patient's underlying pathophysiology (hypoxic vs hypercapnic respiratory failure), lung compliance, patient ventilator synchrony, and operator experience. Table 25-1 outlines the most commonly used pulmonary mechanics terms and modes of mechanical ventilation. However, a full discussion of mechanical ventilation is outside the scope of this chapter.

Pulmonary Disease

Types of Respiratory Failure

There are 4 types of respiratory failure. Type I is hypoxemic respiratory failure and occurs when the partial pressure of oxygen (PaO_2) in arterial blood is less than 60 mm Hg. Simply stated, this type of respiratory failure is secondary to a failure of oxygen exchange and typically occurs at the level of the alveoli (Figure 25-1). Mechanisms for type I respiratory failure include diffusion defect (ie, underlying lung disease), a ventilation-perfusion mismatch (eg, pneumonia), hypoventilation when it leads to low oxygen levels (eg, opiate intoxication), and shunt physiology (eg, severe ARDS). Regardless of the etiology, insufficient alveoli oxygen leads to reduced arterial hemoglobin oxygen saturation (SaO_2) and therefore reduced tissue oxygenation (hypoxia).

Type II is hypercapnic respiratory failure (high body CO_2 levels), which occurs when the partial pressure of arterial carbon dioxide ($PaCO_2$) is elevated and causes blood pH to be less than 7.37. Hypercapnia occurs from either too much CO_2 production through increased cellular respiration secondary to increased overall metabolic function (sepsis, fever, overfeeding) or decreased alveolar ventilation causing decreased CO_2 gas exchange. Common causes for type II respiratory failure include exacerbations of chronic obstructive pulmonary disease (COPD), opiate overdose, chest wall defects, or decreased respiratory muscle function, which may be related to conditions such as amyotrophic lateral sclerosis or muscular dystrophy.

Type III is mixed hypoxemic-hypercapnic respiratory failure, which is commonly encountered in the perioperative setting because of anesthesia. This form of respiratory failure is always acute and frequently secondary to atelectasis (a complete or partial collapse of lung segments). Atelectasis is exacerbated in patients who have obstructive sleep apnea or morbid obesity.

TABLE 25-1 Pulmonary Disease Terminology

Respiratory mechanics terms:

- Respiratory rate (RR): Frequency of respiration; the number of breaths delivered per minute.
- Tidal volume (TV): The volume of gas delivered during a breath.
- Minute ventilation: The TV multiplied by the RR.
- Vital capacity: The volume of change of the lung between full inspiration and maximal expiration.
- Forced expiratory volume in 1 second (FEV_1): The volume of gas an individual can forcibly exhale in the first second of a maximal breath.
- Forced vital capacity (FVC): The total volume of gas an individual can forcibly exhale from a maximal breath.
- FEV_1/FVC ratio: The forced expiratory volume of 1 second divided by the FVC. A ratio <0.7 indicates that a patient has an obstructive lung disease.
- Lung compliance: The relationship of volume of gas and pressure of the lung (V/P); the lung's ability to stretch and expand. Diseased lungs frequently have poor compliance, which may increase the work of breathing.

Mechanical ventilator terminology and modes:

- Mechanical ventilator: A machine designed to provide all or part of the work to move gas into and out of the lungs to meet the body's respiratory requirements.
- Positive end expiratory pressure (PEEP): A positive pressure applied at the end of expiration during mechanical ventilation to prevent alveolar collapse and subsequent barotrauma.
- Volume control: The delivery of a predetermined inspiratory volume despite changing lung compliance or respiratory muscle activity. The pressure in the lungs will vary with this type of breath.
- Pressure control: The delivery of a predetermined inspiratory pressure throughout inspiration despite changing respiratory muscle activity. The volume of gas delivered (TV) with this type of breath varies depending on the lung compliance.
- Breath type: Two types of breath are possible with mechanical ventilation: (1) *mandatory* breath is an assisted breath delivered by the mechanical ventilator based on the set RR; (2) *spontaneous breath* may be assisted or unassisted and is a breath initially generated (triggered) by the patient.
- Plateau pressure: The pressure applied to small airways and alveoli during positive-pressure mechanical ventilation. It is measured during an inspiratory pause.
- Fraction of inspired oxygen (FIO_2): The fraction of oxygen in the space being measured or the concentration of oxygen in inspired air.
- Inspiratory time: The time from the start of inspiratory flow to the beginning of expiratory flow.
- Expiratory time: The time from the start of expiratory flow to the beginning of inspiratory flow. Typically, expiratory time is longer than inspiratory time.
- Patient ventilator asynchrony: A problem that occurs when the timing of the ventilator cycle is not simultaneous with the timing of the patient's respiratory cycle. It frequently increases the work of breathing for patients.

Type IV is shock-related respiratory failure. It can be caused by sepsis, hypovolemia (low blood volume), or cardiogenic shock. The presence of shock puts increased strain on the respiratory system and often subsequently leads to respiratory failure.

General Nutrition Considerations

Regardless of type, patients with respiratory failure may be at nutrition risk.[2] First, respiratory failure often necessitates placement of an artificial airway (eg, endotracheal tube) for mechanical ventilation. The presence of an artificial airway prevents volitional nutrition intake, leading to an energy deficit, thereby increasing morbidity.[3] Second, the underlying process leading to respiratory failure may induce protein catabolism, causing loss of diaphragmatic and intercostal muscle mass, impairing immunity, impairing wound healing, and increasing the risk for new infections. In addition, conditions leading to acute respiratory failure increase the risk for prolonged mechanical ventilation (PMV). Therefore, nutrition support is vital to reduce the energy deficit, modulate inflammation, augment immunity, and potentially mitigate downstream

consequences such as nosocomial infections. Nutrition support also protects patients by minimizing malnutrition and loss of lean body mass.

In addition, patients with pulmonary failure may simultaneously experience other medical insults, including surgery, trauma, sepsis, or acute cerebral vascular disease. Patients with multiple disease processes are often receiving ongoing resuscitation and need close monitoring for signs of intolerance to nutrition support, including hyper or hypoglycemia, gastrointestinal (GI) intolerance, and changing energy needs. Specialty formulas may benefit certain patients and should be considered in the appropriate setting. For example, trauma patients may benefit from immunonutrition; renal failure patients need close monitoring of electrolytes; and ARDS patients need reduced total fluid volume. Recommendations for these patients can be found in condition-specific chapters of this text.

Acute Respiratory Distress Syndrome

ARDS is a potentially severe form of type I respiratory failure. It is defined as follows by the Berlin criteria: (1) respiratory symptoms within 7 days of a known clinical insult (eg, pneumonia or sepsis) lead to (2) bilateral lung opacities on chest radiograph or computed tomography (CT) scan; (3) the respiratory failure and lung opacities are not explained by heart failure or fluid overload; and (4) an oxygenation impairment is present, as defined by the ratio of PaO_2 to FiO_2 (PaO_2:FiO_2), also known as the *P:F ratio*. Mild ARDS is a P:F ratio between greater than 200 mm Hg and less than or equal to 300 mm Hg; moderate ARDS is defined as a P:F ratio between greater than 100 mm Hg and less than or equal to 200 mm Hg; and severe ARDS is defined as a P:F ratio of less than or equal to 100 mm Hg.[4]

ARDS can be caused by direct and indirect lung injury. Common direct causes include gastric aspiration leading to pneumonia, and indirect causes include sepsis, trauma, and acute pancreatitis.[5] There are 3 phases of ARDS: exudative (0 to 7 days), proliferative (7 to 10 days), and fibrotic (more than 10 days).[6] The exudative phase is associated with widespread lung inflammation and injury, which causes proteinaceous fluid to leak into alveolar spaces, contributing to hypoxemia. Inflammatory mediators also induce a catabolic response culminating in protein breakdown. The consequential diaphragmatic weakness places the patient at risk for PMV.[7]

During the exudative phase of ARDS, extensive alveolar damage occurs via neutrophil accumulation, cytokine-mediated inflammation, and oxidant-mediated injury to the alveoli. Both ω-3 fatty acids (which are anti-inflammatory) and ω-6 fatty acids (which are proinflammatory) are released from the cell membranes. ω-3 fatty acids are polyunsaturated fatty acids found in cold-water fish, flaxseed, and canola oil; the 3 most important ω-3 fatty acids are α-linolenic acid (ALA), docosahexaenoic acid (DHA), and eicosapentaenoic acid (EPA). Modulation of the ω-3 and ω-6 fatty acid pathways by providing enteral immunonutrition with predominantly ω-3 fatty acids has been a focus of research to improve ARDS outcomes.[8]

Human studies using ω-3 fatty acids in ARDS have demonstrated variable outcomes. In a multicenter RCT, Gadek et al compared patients receiving EN enriched in EPA, DHA, γ-linolenic acid (GLA), and antioxidants vs an isonitrogenous isocaloric control formula. Patients receiving the enriched EN had improvements in oxygenation (from baseline), fewer days on ventilator support, and decreased length of ICU stay.[9] Notably, the control group received EN with a high amount of ω-6 fatty acids, which potentially widened the benefit for the experimental group receiving ω-3 fatty acids. In a small randomized trial by Parish et al, patients who received EN enriched only with ω-3 fatty acids demonstrated benefits in oxygenation and ventilator-free days.[10] Stapleton et al published work showing no benefit with EN enriched only with ω-3 fatty acids with regard to biomarkers of pulmonary or systemic inflammation, duration of mechanical ventilation, or mortality.[11,12]

The largest trial to date (N = 272 patients) evaluating ω-3 supplementation in EN for patients with ARDS was stopped early because of lack of efficacy and potential harm.[13] This study had potential confounders. First, there was a trend toward increased fluid balance in the study population, although this trend was not statistically significant. The study group's cumulative fluid balance was 2082 mL in the first 7 days of the study compared with 94 mL in the control group. In addition, the control group received a higher daily oral protein intake because the control supplement provided 20 g protein per day compared with the study supplement, which provided 3.8 g/d.[13]

A meta-analysis of 7 RCTs also failed to demonstrate benefit of ω-3 fatty acid supplementation in ARDS for mortality, ventilator-free days, and ICU-free days.[14] The RCTs of ω-3 fatty acids in ARDS have serious limitations. The trials lack homogeneity in ω-3 formulations and infusion methods, and the placebo formulas that are used may obscure results; the inclusion of other anti-inflammatory compounds in the study formula, duration of therapy, and primary outcomes also vary among studies.[9,15–18] Therefore, based on low-quality evidence, the SCCM/ASPEN 2016 nutrition therapy guidelines did not make a recommendation regarding the routine use of an enteral formulation characterized by an anti-inflammatory lipid profile in patients with ARDS (recommendation E3).[1]

Obstructive Lung Diseases

Obstructive lung diseases are characterized by airflow limitation (ie, patients have a difficult time exhaling) and can cause type I or type II respiratory failure. Common obstructive lung diseases include asthma, cystic fibrosis (CF), and COPD. Asthma is a chronic inflammatory disorder of the airways, which leads to recurrent but reversible episodes of airway obstruction and is manifested clinically by chest tightness, coughing, wheezing, and shortness of breath.[19] COPD is defined by the Global Initiative for Chronic Obstructive Lung Disease as a common, preventable, and treatable disease, characterized by persistent airflow limitation that is usually progressive and associated with an enhanced chronic inflammatory response in the airways and the lung to noxious particles or gases. Exacerbations and comorbidities contribute to the overall severity of COPD in individual patients.[20] COPD is the third leading cause of death in the United States.[21] It is staged according to degree of airflow limitation, as defined by forced expiratory volume in 1 second (FEV_1). The BODE index—characterized by (*B*) body mass index (BMI); (*O*) obstruction as assessed by FEV_1; (*D*) dyspnea as assessed by modified Medical Research Council score; (*E*) exercise capacity as measured by 6-minute walk distance—has been used to determine risk for death from COPD and may be a better indicator of prognosis than FEV_1 alone. In addition, the BODE index has been used to evaluate responses to medications and rehabilitation.[22,23]

Malnutrition associated with advanced lung disease (such as COPD) has been termed *pulmonary cachexia syndrome*, defined as a lean BMI of less than 17 in men and less than 14 in women.[24] Malnutrition in COPD may be as high as 60% among inpatients and 45% among outpatients.[25] Numerous factors account for malnutrition, including aging, hypoxemia, increased resting energy expenditure (REE), low-grade inflammation, and systemic treatment with glucocorticoids.[16] Malnutrition and cachexia in COPD reduce respiratory muscle function and increase 1-year mortality, hospital readmission rate, and length of hospital stay.[25,26] Once continuous involuntary body weight loss begins, the average survival time is 2.9 years.[26] Among COPD patients with acute exacerbations, malnutrition increases the risk for PMV.[27] (See Practice Scenario 25-1.[23,28])

Practice Scenario 25-1

Question: When are patients with chronic obstructive pulmonary disease (COPD) nutritionally at risk, and what interventions maybe considered?

Scenario: A 62-year-old woman with a history of COPD presents today with concerns of decreased exercise tolerance. She has had no recent COPD exacerbations, no change in her forced expiratory volume in 1 second (FEV$_1$), or other measures of respiratory function. She is compliant with her inhalers and has not required oral steroids or antibiotics in the past year. Data from her physical examination show no notable recent changes except that she has lost weight and her current body mass index (BMI) is 20. Upon questioning, she states that she is unable to eat large meals, because that makes her breathing worse.

Intervention: The patient is started on nutritional supplements as tolerated to increase daily energy intake to 1.3 times her resting energy expenditure (REE).[28] The supplements are divided into frequent small meals through the day. Appetite-enhancing drugs, such as megestrol, may also be considered.

Answer: This patient's weight changes are cause for concern. Low BMI (≤21) is associated with higher mortality in patients with COPD.[23] Although the overall evidence for nutritional supplementation is limited, efforts should be made to increase the patient's weight and BMI.

Rationale: Studies have shown increased mortality in patients with low BMI compared with subjects of normal weight, and, in severe COPD, BMI is a significant independent predictor of all-cause mortality. The exact cause of low BMI and fat-free mass in patients with COPD is not completely understood. Patients with COPD have increased REE, but the increased work of breathing cannot completely explain low body weight in these patients. Other factors contributing to poor nutrition status may include increased oxygen debt during respiratory effort, ongoing inflammation, and the inability to eat large amounts secondary to shortness of breath. Nutritional supplements have been shown to improve patients' general sense of well-being and breathlessness, but good data on mortality or long-term improvement in functional status are lacking.[28]

Restrictive Lung Diseases

Interstitial lung diseases (ILDs) are a heterogeneous group of disorders that are classified together because of similar radiographic, clinical, and pathological manifestations.[29] ILDs cause lung restriction (ie, limit expansion). There are numerous causes of ILD, including occupational and environmental agents, drug-induced etiologies, radiation-induced etiologies, connective tissue disorders, and idiopathic causes. ILDs commonly cause chronic hypoxemic respiratory failure. The prevalence of malnutrition is not well defined, likely because of the heterogeneity of ILD. Among lung transplant candidates, lean body mass depletion in idiopathic pulmonary fibrosis was associated with increasing hypoxemia.[30] The mechanisms for

pulmonary cachexia syndrome may be similar to those seen in COPD patients, and caused by hypoxemia, low-grade inflammation, and corticosteroid use.

Cystic Fibrosis

CF has a significant and ongoing disease burden for the US healthcare system. The median survival age has increased steadily over the last 2 decades and many patients are now surviving past the age of 40 years. Several factors can lead to malnutrition in patients with CF. Malnutrition from either pancreatic insufficiency or steatorrhea can be caused by malabsorption leading to nutrition deficiencies. These deficiencies may be additionally complicated by meconium ileus, which further reduces absorptive abilities.[31] Patients with CF also suffer from vitamin deficiencies secondary to malabsorption, which further complicate their disease and functional status. In addition to decreased nutrition intake, patients with CF have greater overall energy requirements than individuals without CF who are of similar height and weight. Given the decreased ability of patients with CF to maintain adequate nutrition, it is difficult for these patients to consistently meet their daily energy requirements.

Nutrition assessment in patients with CF is complicated because many do not reach their full growth potential, which means that BMI may not be as accurate of a measure of nutritional status in patients with CF as it is for the general population.[32] Many patients with CF have a low BMI when they reach adulthood—approximately 6% of pediatric patients with CF (younger than 18 years) have a BMI less than the 10 percentile for their age and sex, and most adult patients do not reach the peak median BMI of 23 until age 35 years.[33] These numbers highlight both the importance of maintaining adequate nutrition and the impact of ongoing malnutrition on patients with CF.

Patients with CF should be screened for malnutrition and vitamin deficiency at regular intervals (typically, at their quarterly physician visit). Malnutrition should be treated aggressively with oral supplements and placement of a long-term enteral access device (ie, percutaneous endoscopic gastrostomy tube) if necessary to meet energy requirements. The most common vitamin deficiencies are fat-soluble vitamins (vitamins A, E, D, and K) because patients with CF are prone to malabsorption secondary to pancreatic insufficiency. In addition to clinical screening for signs and symptoms of vitamin deficiency, patients should have their serum fat-soluble vitamin levels checked yearly. Patients with CF who have fat-soluble vitamin deficiencies should receive specifically formulated CF replacement supplements of these vitamins to help ensure adequate dosages.[34] CF is further discussed in Chapter 26.

Prolonged Mechanical Ventilation and Chronic Critical Illness

The Centers for Medicare and Medicaid Services define PMV as ventilator dependence for more than 21 days for at least 6 hours per day.[35] Preexisting lung diseases such as severe COPD, ILDs, and chronic hypercapnia may increase the risk for PMV. Acquired diseases (eg, ARDS) leading to ICU admission may also increase the risk for PMV. In one study, more than 40% of patients admitted to ICU for pneumonia, ARDS, neuromuscular disease, head trauma, or intracerebral hemorrhage had PMV.[36]

Chronic critical illness is defined as an ICU stay longer than 14 days with continued low-grade organ dysfunction.[37] Ventilator dependence and malnutrition are central components to chronic critical illness. A new phenotype of critical illness, called *persistent inflammatory and immunocompromised catabolic syndrome* (PICS) is emerging. PICS occurs in patients who survive acute critical illness and multiple organ failure, only to enter a state of chronic critical illness (after 14 days) characterized by low-grade organ dysfunction plus immune suppression with malnutrition, muscle weakness, recurrent infections, and poor wound healing.[9] Among patients with chronic critical illness, 30% to 50% deteriorate into PICS.[37] The role, timing, and impact of nutrition in this patient population are ongoing areas of research.[38,39]

Medication Considerations

Critically ill patients who experience respiratory failure are frequently placed on multiple medications, which may alter their nutrition care plan. Patients may receive multiple sedatives and/or be paralyzed to assist with patient ventilator synchrony and preserve respiratory function. Gut peristalsis is not inhibited by paralytic medications or sedatives; however, physical examinations may be difficult to do and signs of GI intolerance may be challenging to identify. Clinicians should consider these issues when starting EN and carefully evaluate patients for other clinical signs of GI intolerance, including abdominal distention or changes in stool frequency or caliber. An abdominal x-ray may be needed to fully evaluate potential constipation or ileus. The sedative propofol is delivered in a lipid emulsion, and many intravenous medications may be delivered in dextrose solutions; therefore, these medications should be considered when determining energy intake to avoid overfeeding.

Patients with respiratory failure frequently experience co-existing shock. These patients frequently receive catecholamine vasopressors administration. The use of EN when patients are receiving high doses of vasopressors is a subject of considerable debate because vasopressors could potentially cause bowel ischemia via splenic vasoconstriction. Direct evidence of this potential problem is lacking, and EN has been safely given in some studies when patients receive vasopressor administration.[40] Furthermore, there is no evidence showing what dose of vasopressor prohibits use of EN. Individual clinicians must rely on their experience and judgment until further evidence is available.

Nutrition Assessment

Physical Examination and Patient History

Nutrition assessment of patients with pulmonary failure is critical for improving outcomes. Malnourished patients exhibit expiratory muscle weakness and decreased chest wall expansion, and are at higher risk for pulmonary complications

following surgery.[41] Low BMI is a known risk factor for respiratory impairment and mortality in patients with COPD and chronic respiratory insufficiency.[23,42,43] In addition to BMI, assessment of body composition may help predict lung function impairments in the pulmonary failure population.[44]

The ASPEN and Academy of Nutrition and Dietetics consensus statement on identifying and documenting adult malnutrition includes discussion of the role of body composition assessment in diagnosing malnutrition. The consensus statement recommends that at least 2 of the following 6 characteristics be present for diagnosis of malnutrition: "insufficient energy intake, weight loss, loss of muscle mass, loss of subcutaneous fat, localized or generalized fluid accumulation that may sometimes mask weight loss, and diminished functional status as measured by handgrip strength."[45,46] The consensus statement recommends physical examination as a method to identify loss of muscle mass and loss of subcutaneous fat. The nutrition-focused physical examination should include assessment of fluid status; both fluid retention and dehydration are common in patients with pulmonary failure. In addition to physical examination, other methods of assessing body composition (especially to identify sarcopenia) shown to be appropriate for the respiratory failure population include use of preexisting CT scans, bioelectrical impedance analysis, and dual-energy x-ray absorptiometry.[47-49]

A thorough diet history for a patient with pulmonary failure may assist in identifying whether more in-depth measurements of body composition are appropriate. However, this history is often impossible to complete in the early assessment of a patient who requires mechanical ventilation. When possible, nutrition assessment should include the patient's history of recent weight loss, anorexia, shortness of breath while eating, and early satiety. Medications to note in this patient population include glucocorticoids, with special attention to potential adverse effects of hyperglycemia, poor wound healing, weight gain, and fluid retention.

Energy Requirements

Indirect calorimetry (IC) is the preferred method of determining an individual's REE and energy needs for a 24-hour period. IC must be correctly preformed for the resulting measurements to be accurate. Protocols should be developed for non-critically ill patients that account for the many factors affecting the assessment of resting metabolic rate. These factors include patient-controlled variables of time since last exercise, smoking, caffeine consumption, or eating. The procedure setting is also important because room temperature; body position; type of gas-collection device; and length of measurement can influence the results.[50] Similarly, clinicians must carefully evaluate the factors that can affect IC results in patients who are critically ill or receiving mechanical ventilation. Technical flaws in measurement technique as well as patient-specific factors such as the time since the last painful procedure, anesthesia, last feeding, body position, renal replacement therapy, involuntary movements, pain and analgesics, and concurrent nursing procedures can cause inaccurate IC results in the ICU.[51]

Mechanical ventilator settings may significantly influence IC results. The level of FIO_2 is important—an FIO_2 greater than

0.60 causes inaccuracy in the calculations required to determine the REE. In addition, air leaks (created either though a circuit failure or by a spontaneously breathing patient) in the mechanical ventilator circuit can cause measurement inaccuracy.[51] Finally, a patient's resting metabolic rate may change significantly over time; a one-time measurement is an insight into only that time point, not the entire course of the disease or even the entire course of a single hospitalization. The SCCM/ASPEN 2016 guidelines recommend evaluating energy expenditure more than weekly, although no specific time intervals are outlined (recommendations A3a and A3b).[1]

IC is not always available for energy needs assessment; a lack of equipment or trained personnel and patient-specific factors may preclude its use. In lieu of IC, clinicians may use equations to estimate energy needs but clinicians should understand the inherent limitations of such estimates. No equation includes consideration of all factors that may affect energy expenditure, and all equations may lead to over- or underfeeding an individual patient. For example, weight, a consideration in practically all equations to estimate energy requirements, may be falsely elevated by fluid retention, which would cause energy needs to be overestimated. Because no equation has been shown to be a universally effective guide to calculate energy requirements in critically ill adults, the SCCM/ASPEN 2016 guidelines do not recommend a single equation but instead encourage close monitoring of the individual's response to feeding and frequent (more than once per week) reassessment of the patient's energy and protein needs (recommendation A3b).[1] Each patient should be monitored for signs of under- and overfeeding. See Chapter 2 for a complete discussion of the energy prescription.

Underfeeding and Overfeeding

Prolonged underfeeding of patients with chronic respiratory disease may lead to deficits in lean body mass that may increase mortality, as previously noted.[26] Patients with COPD frequently have an increased REE secondary to their disease, although the exact etiology of this hypermetabolism is not fully understood. Clinicians should closely monitor the weight and BMI of patients with COPD and other types of chronic respiratory disease because these patients are at risk for developing pulmonary cachexia syndrome. Patients with weight loss should be encouraged to increase their daily energy intake.[28] These patients may benefit from additional supplementation of energy and protein. Use of smaller, more frequent doses to reduce early satiety and shortness of breath associated with eating may aid in compliance.

In critically ill patients, recent research has indicated that early, short-term trophic enteral feeding (low-dose feeding for 7 days before proceeding to full delivery of energy and protein) may result in less GI intolerance than full feeding in patients with acute lung injury or ARDS who are not at high nutrition risk.[52,53] However, accumulation of an energy deficit throughout a hospitalization has been associated with a greater risk of increased length of stay, complications, infections, days on antibiotics, and time on mechanical ventilation.[54] If trophic feeding is used as a strategy to minimize GI intolerance, the patient should be closely monitored and evaluated frequently to ensure that goals for energy and protein provision are safely met as soon as possible.[55]

Overfeeding in this population can also have negative effects. Overfeeding can cause hyperglycemia, lipogenesis, liver dysfunction, azotemia, fluid overload, and respiratory compromise including increased RR and decreased TV.[56,57] Patients demonstrating these symptoms should be evaluated for overfeeding, and their overall energy load should be appropriately reduced. All patients receiving propofol as a sedative (1.1 kcal/mL) and intravenous dextrose solutions should be carefully monitored for overall energy intake from these medications and nutrition support. Excessive energy intake can also lead to increased CO_2 production, which is particularly detrimental to patients with pulmonary failure because the work of breathing increases secondary to increased ventilation to remove excess CO_2.[58] This issue is discussed in more detail in the following section.

Nutrition Support

The SCCM/ASPEN 2016 guidelines address nutrition support therapy for patients with pulmonary failure (see Table 25-2).[1] The guidelines are intended to provide support for clinicians caring for the average patient with pulmonary failure and do not include all circumstances.

Macronutrients

Patients with pulmonary failure require similar carbohydrate, protein, and lipid nutrition as other critically ill patients. There is no reliable evidence to support augmentation of any of these components in EN for these patients. Most CO_2 production in critical illness is from metabolism by-products, not carbohydrate intake. However, excessive CO_2 production can occur when patients in the ICU are overfed. This problem is most likely to occur in patients receiving PN because there is no protective mechanism to prevent overfeeding when nutrition is provided via a venous catheter. Patients receiving EN will typically not tolerate excessive energy intake secondary to gastric distention, vomiting, and elevated gastric residuals.[59] Excessive CO_2 production can be detrimental to patients with pulmonary failure and may lead to PMV and hepatic steatosis. However, adjusting carbohydrate intake below the patient's energy requirements does little to decrease this risk and may lead to more harm secondary to underfeeding patients.

Micronutrients

Clinicians should closely monitor micronutrient status in patients with pulmonary failure and critical illness. Deficiencies in electrolytes, including phosphorus, calcium, and magnesium, can lead to diaphragm weakness and potentially prolong mechanical ventilator dependence. Electrolytes should therefore be monitored and replaced aggressively as needed. However, recent studies have shown that other micronutrients may actually be harmful for patients with pulmonary failure. The REDOX trial (2013) was the largest RCT to evaluate glutamine and antioxidant supplementation in patients with pulmonary failure and critical illness.[60] The study showed that

TABLE 25-2 Summary of SCCM/ASPEN 2016 Guidelines for Nutrition Support for Patients with Pulmonary Failure

Guideline	Recommendation Notation
Enteral nutrition:	
1. Standard polymeric formulas are preferred when initiating EN in the ICU setting.	E1
2. Disease-specific and specialty formulas should be avoided in patients with pulmonary failure in the medical ICU.	E3
3. High-fat/low-carbohydrate formulations designed to reduce CO_2 production should not be used in ICU patients with acute respiratory failure.	I1
4. Serum phosphate should be monitored closely and replaced as necessary.	I3
5. Fluid restriction and therefore energy-dense EN formulations may be considered for patients with acute respiratory failure.	I2
6. Immune-modulating enteral formulations with arginine, EPA, DHA, glutamine, and nucleic acid should not be used routinely for patients admitted to the medical ICU.	E2
7. Data regarding the use of anti-inflammatory lipid profile formulas in patients with ARDS and acute lung injury are conflicting. Therefore, there is no recommendation regarding these formulas.	E3
8. Trophic or full nutrition by EN is appropriate for patients with ARDS expected to have a duration of mechanical ventilation more than 72 hours as both strategies have similar outcomes during the first week of hospitalization.	C2
Parenteral nutrition:	
1. In patients with low nutrition risk (eg, NRS 2002 ≤3 or NUTRIC score ≤5), exclusive PN should be withheld during the first 7 days following ICU admission if the patient cannot maintain volitional intake and if early EN is not feasible.	G1
2. When EN is not feasible in patients determined to be at high nutrition risk (eg, NRS 2002 ≥5 or NUTRIC score ≥5) or severely malnourished, consider initiating exclusive PN as soon as possible following ICU admission.	G2
3. In patients at either low or high nutrition risk, consider use of supplemental PN after 7–10 days if the patient is unable to meet >60% of energy and protein requirements by the enteral route alone.	G3
4. Protocols and nutrition support teams should be utilized to help incorporate strategies to maximize efficacy and reduce associated risks of PN.	H1
5. In appropriate patients (those who are at high nutrition risk or severely malnourished) requiring PN, consider hypocaloric PN dosing (≤20 kcal/kg/d or 80% of estimated energy needs) with adequate protein (≥1.2 g/kg/d) initially over the first week of hospitalization in the ICU.	H2

ARDS, acute respiratory distress syndrome; ASPEN, American Society for Parenteral and Enteral Nutrition; CO_2, carbon dioxide; DHA, docosahexaenoic acid; EN, enteral nutrition; EPA, eicosapentaenoic acid; ICU, intensive care unit; NRS, Nutritional Risk Screening [assessment tool]; NUTRIC, Nutrition Risk in Critically ill [assessment tool]; PN, parenteral nutrition; SCCM, Society of Critical Care Medicine.
Adapted with permission from reference 1: McClave SA, Taylor BE, Martindale RG, et al. Guidelines for the provision and assessment of nutrition support therapy in the adult critically ill patient: Society of Critical Care Medicine (SCCM) and American Society for Parenteral and Enteral Nutrition (A.S.P.E.N.). *JPEN J Parenter Enteral Nutr.* 2016;40(2):159–211.

glutamine supplementation may be associated with harm, and there was no therapeutic benefit associated with antioxidant supplementation.

One condition that deserves some additional comment is refeeding syndrome because it leads to electrolyte depletion of which the hallmark is hypophosphatemia. Patients with significant vomiting or diarrhea, those undergoing major surgery, those with alcoholism, those receiving chemotherapy for malignancy, and those with poor oral intake prior to hospitalization are at risk for refeeding syndrome, particularly when admitted to the ICU. The etiology of the electrolyte depletion is secondary to the transcellular shifts following carbohydrate administration as well as overall body depletion during illness or poor oral intake. Phosphorus is an important component of cellular membranes, enzyme systems, and

adenosine triphosphate (ATP), which is vital to cellular energy production. Phosphate is also an essential component of 2,3-diphosphoglycerate (DPG), which is an enzyme involved in oxygen release from hemoglobin. A decrease in DPG results in decreased oxygen unloading from hemoglobin and subsequent decreased oxygen available for body tissues (ie, skeletal muscle and cardiac muscle).[61]

Refeeding syndrome is frequently seen within the first 2 to 3 days when patients are receiving saline dextrose infusion and PN, but it can also occur with EN, and patients at risk should be followed closely. Symptoms may be nonspecific but frequently include fatigue, dyspnea, hypoxia, anemia, palpitations, and cardiac dysfunction that may result in death if untreated. Serum levels of electrolytes should be closely monitored in patients at risk and should be replaced to normal levels. Slowly advancing PN or EN (typically beginning with approximately half of a patient's goal energy intake) over 2 to 3 days helps avoid refeeding syndrome. Finally, patients should also receive supplemental water-soluble B vitamins (in particular, thiamin) because these vitamins are likely also depleted in patients at risk for refeeding syndrome.[61] Monitoring and treatment of refeeding syndrome is illustrated in Practice Scenario 25-2.

Practice Scenario 25-2

Question: How should clinicians evaluate patients for refeeding syndrome and avoid its consequences?

Scenario: A 78-year-old man with a history of dementia is brought to the hospital and intubated secondary to altered mental status and pneumonia. According to his family, the patient has had a poor appetite at home for the past month, and he has lost some weight. He has a history of gastroesophageal reflux disease and congestive heart failure. He was previously admitted 6 months ago for pneumonia that was thought to be due to aspiration because he is unable to swallow effectively secondary to his dementia. His physical examination confirms cachexia but is otherwise as expected.

Intervention: The nursing staff place a small bowel feeding tube and begin enteral nutrition at 50% of the patient's goal energy intake.

Answer: This patient has a history of poor oral intake, weight loss, and swallowing difficulty, and his physical examination provides evidence of poor nutrition status. His feeding should be started at approximately one-half his goal energy intake (given the risk of refeeding syndrome) and advanced over the next 3 days. His electrolytes (particularly potassium, phosphate, and magnesium) should be closely monitored during this time. He should also have continuous cardiac monitoring because one of the most severe complications of refeeding syndrome is cardiac failure. Finally, he should also be given supplemental thiamin and multivitamin replacement.

Rationale: The patient is high risk for refeeding syndrome given his poor oral intake and weight loss. Other risk factors include vomiting, diarrhea, homelessness, alcoholism, and history of malignancy receiving chemotherapy. Patients with refeeding syndrome often experience vague symptoms related to muscle weakness, including syncope, dyspnea, hypoxia, and muscle aches or pain. Hypophosphatemia can cause neurologic symptoms in some cases. Symptoms include paresthesia, confusion, seizure, and muscle weakness (including diaphragm weakness leading to respiratory failure). Other symptoms may relate to fluid retention, which may cause systemic or pulmonary edema and, most concerning, cardiac dysfunction from volume overload. Finally, patients may experience acute cardiac rhythm changes that can result in ventricular arrhythmias and death. In patients at risk for refeeding syndrome, nutrition (enteral or parenteral) should be initiated slowly and titrated up to goal energy intake over approximately 72 hours. In additional, careful monitoring of the patient's volume status, cardiac rhythm, and serum electrolytes is important

to avoid complications and possible death. Electrolytes should be monitored frequently and replaced aggressively to normal levels. Patients should also receive thiamin replacement to avoid Wernicke's syndrome, which is characterized by the triad ophthalmoplegia, ataxia, and confusion.

Obesity

Data regarding increased complication rates for obese patients admitted to the ICU are variable. Several studies show increased complications, whereas others show no difference in complication rates. A meta-analysis indicates that a higher BMI is a risk factor for increased length of stay and longer duration of ventilator dependence but not mortality.[62] Studies of ICU practice patterns show that obese patients have delayed onset of nutrition support compared with other patients with similar diagnosis and level of critical illness.[63] Traditional nutrition assessment of albumin, BMI, and evaluation of subcutaneous fat does not accurately predict malnutrition or nutrition risk in obese patients.[63] Previous studies have shown that many hospitalized patients with a BMI greater than 25 show evidence of malnutrition compared with patients with normal BMI, and a higher BMI is considered a risk factor for malnutrition.[64,65] An elevated BMI should not be mistakenly used to determine that a patient has nutrition reserves during critical illness.

Although well-designed, large RCTs are lacking, there are guidelines and recommendations for nutrition support in obese critically ill patients. If possible, clinicians should use IC to determine energy requirements for obese patients receiving nutrition support. If IC is not available, the Penn State University 2010 predictive equation should be used to estimate energy requirements. Obese patients may also be considered for a hypocaloric, high-protein regimen. Typically, this regimen provides less than 14 kcal per kg actual body weight with 1.2 to 1.5 g protein per kg actual body weight. This guideline is based on comparative studies and case series; larger trials have not been done. However, the initial studies show overall favorable outcomes with decreased length of stay in the ICU and a trend toward decreased mechanical ventilator days.[66] See Chapter 2 for further discussion of the Penn State equation and Chapter 35 for more information on nutrition support for patients with obesity.

Enteral Nutrition

EN has multiple benefits for patients with pulmonary failure. EN has been shown to preserve gut mucosa and immune function as well as modulate stress in critically ill patients. EN specifically maintains the functional integrity of the gut by preserving tight junctions and maintaining villous height within the gut. It further acts to enhance immune function via support secretory immunoglobulin A–producing immunocytes (B cells and plasma cells) that compose the gut-associated lymphoid tissue.[67] EN may also provide gut prophylaxis against GI bleeding, which is a frequent complication of pulmonary failure and mechanical ventilator use.[68]

The evidence for best practice regarding the amount of EN given to patients with pulmonary failure is variable and remains debatable. Trophic feeds (the amount of substrate necessary to provide gut stimulation) have not been clearly defined, but they are typically thought to be 10 to 20 mL EN per hour. A large study published in 2012 (EDEN) compared full enteral feeding (defined in this study as 1300 kcal/d) and trophic feeding (400 kcal/d) during the first week of critical illness and found no differences in ventilator days, 60-day mortality, or infectious complications.[53] A follow-up study also showed no difference in patients' functional status 1 year following their critical illness.[69] However, the EDEN study exclusively enrolled patients with ARDS; therefore, the findings should not be applied broadly to all critically ill patients. Furthermore, the average BMI in the study was 29.9 in the trophic group and 30.4 in the full-feeding group; both BMI values are classified as overweight. Patients who are overweight are thought to potentially benefit from hypocaloric feeding (although they should also receive high amounts of protein) compared with normal-weight patients. Use of trophic feeding is further discussed in Practice Scenario 25-3.

Practice Scenario 25-3

Question: What patients are most appropriate for trophic feeds, and how should these feeds be implemented?

Scenario: A 52-year-old woman is admitted to the medical intensive care service for hypoxic respiratory failure. She has a history of type 2 diabetes and had a cholecystectomy approximately 10 years ago. Her body mass index is 28, and she was otherwise in good health prior to her admission. She is intubated and placed on mechanical ventilation in a prone position. Physical examination, chest x-ray, laboratory values, and echocardiogram confirm a diagnosis of acute respiratory distress syndrome (ARDS). A small bowel feeding tube is placed and confirmed in good position.

Intervention: The patient is started on enteral nutrition (EN) within 24 to 48 hours of her admission. Because she is a normal weight and otherwise healthy without evidence of significant nutrition risk or malnutrition, the patient may be considered for trophic feeding (400–800 kcal/d) given her diagnosis of ARDS. As with other enteral feeding, trophic feeding should not be delayed and clinicians should minimize interruptions.

Answer: Patients with ARDS may be fed trophically and may be safely fed in the prone position. Although there is no evidence comparing gastric vs small bowel access for EN, a small bowel feeding tube is typically preferred.

Rationale: Studies have shown that rates of ventilator-associated pneumonia for patients in the prone position are comparable to rates for patients in the supine. Recent evidence further suggests that EN via a gastric tube in prone position patients is safe and without additional complications. Although there are no studies of prone patients receiving prescribed trophic feeding through a small bowel tubes specifically, this nutrition support method is generally considered safe. Patients with ARDS have also been shown to have improved outcomes from fluid restriction and therefore may be better candidates for trophic feeding than other critically

ill patients. Trophic feeding should be advanced to full energy requirements by Day 7 because trophic feeding past this timeframe in ARDS patients has not been studied. Finally, trophic feeding should not be considered in patients who are either under- or overweight, because it has not been studied in these populations.

In the EDEN trial,[53] enteral feeding was well tolerated overall and not associated with significant adverse events. Patients with a functional gut should be started on EN once resuscitation is complete. Patients without ARDS should be advanced toward the goal feeding as tolerated. Clinicians may consider initial trophic feeding in patients with ARDS.

Parenteral Nutrition

The benefits of EN are well documented in multiple studies. Therefore, EN should always be the preferred route of nutrition support in critically ill patients with a functional gut. However, PN may be considered for patients who cannot tolerate EN. Evidence and guidelines about the optimal time to begin administration of PN vary. The European Society for Clinical Nutrition and Metabolism (ESPEN) suggests starting PN within 24 to 48 hours of admission if patients are not expected to fully tolerate EN by Day 3 of admission.[70] In contrast, the ASPEN/SCCM guidelines recommend holding PN for the initial 7 days of critical illness if the patient is not considered to be at nutrition risk.[1] The ESPEN guidelines are controversial, and a recent (2011) study from Europe suggests that early PN may be associated with increased infections and days of mechanical ventilator dependence.[71] See Chapter 17 for additional information on PN complications.

PN may be useful to reduce the energy debt in patients who cannot tolerate EN. Patients with a nonfunctioning gut may require PN to maintain energy requirements completely or as a supplement if EN fails to meet daily energy goals for a prolonged period. The exact timing, composition, and amount of PN that should be prescribed to critically ill patients with pulmonary failure requires further study. See Chapter 14 for an overview of PN and Chapter 15 for information on PN formulations.

Aspiration and Ventilator-Associated Pneumonia

Although EN has many protective benefits, aspiration pneumonia is a risk for patients with pulmonary failure. Rates of VAP have decreased in recent years, and the current US rate is estimated to be between 5% and 15%. However, mortality related to VAP is still high (around 10% depending on the patient population) and VAP increases the costs of care and lengths of hospital stays.[72] The pathogenesis of VAP can be difficult to determine, but it is thought to involve colonization of the oral pharynx, larynx, and upper esophagus with bacteria as well as microaspiration of secretions with bacteria. The placement of an endotracheal tube causes the trachea to be stented open and provides passage for secretions and bacteria into the lower respiratory tract.

Patients with pulmonary failure are at increased risk of VAP because of several factors: the placement of the endotracheal tube; the sedation and analgesia that are often used to facilitate treatment; patient positioning in a supine position; and gastric dysmotility. In addition, if patients are experiencing shock or have aggressive antibiotic regimens, they may have altered oral or GI flora that increases their risk of VAP.[72] Patients may also experience aspiration pneumonitis, a condition where gastric contents are aspirated into the respiratory tract but cause a chemical inflammation as opposed to a true infection. Finally, once patients recover from pulmonary failure and the endotracheal tube is removed, they remain at risk for aspiration and may have persistent dysphagia.

Hospitals should have an active program to prevent VAP in all ICU patients. Effective strategies focus on aspects of care that may prevent colonization and aspiration and minimize time on mechanical ventilation.[73] Table 25-3 lists VAP prevention guidelines.

Decreased aspiration and decreased gastroesophageal reflux may be achieved through a distally placed small bowel feeding tube with a nasogastric or orogastric tube used to decompress the stomach. This method is used frequently in practice, and some studies have shown decreased rates of VAP with jejunum-delivered EN compared with gastric or duodenal feeding.[74] However, in clinical practice, postpyloric feeding can be difficult to achieve, and the literature on nutrition support in patients with pulmonary failure typically indicates that gastric feeding is well tolerated. Patients in the EDEN trial (85%) were initially fed via a gastric tube, which was well tolerated and avoided delay in onset of EN.[53] Additional studies published in 2013 have shown that lack of monitoring gastric residual volumes did not change VAP rates in an open-label study.[75] More recently, an open-label trial showed no difference in VAP rates between gastric and duodenal delivery of EN.[76]

TABLE 25-3 Strategies for Prevention of Ventilator-Associated Pneumonia

---

- If possible, avoid intubation by using noninvasive means of respiratory support.

- Minimize sedation and analgesia as tolerated and needed for effective patient care, and, if possible, provide a daily sedation vacation.

- Maintain the patient's physical conditioning through early mobilization and in-bed exercise.

- Use continuous subglottic suctioning to decrease pooling of oral secretions.

- Elevate the head of the patient's bed by more than 45° when possible.

- Maintain the ventilator circuit by minimizing changes to the circuit unless it is soiled or malfunctioning.

- Decrease the patient's time on mechanical ventilator if possible.

- Provide oral care with chlorhexidine.

- Consider probiotic use in select patient populations.[a]

- Limit broad spectrum antibiotics.

---

[a]See Chapter 4 for a discussion of probiotics.

Patient positioning has previously been one of the main strategies for VAP prevention. The Centers for Disease Control and Prevention recommend that patients be placed in a semirecumbent position with the head of bed at 45°. Evidence regarding the overall impact of this intervention is limited, but it is simple to implement and conveys minimal patient risk. Patients with ARDS are, however, frequently placed in a prone position because recent evidence suggests this position improves outcomes for these patients.[77,78] Gastric feeding is thought to be poorly tolerated by patients in the prone position, but pneumonia rates are, overall, the same for patients in the prone vs supine position.[79,80] (One study did report higher rates of VAP in prone patients than in patients in a semirecumbent position.[81]) Small bowel enteral feeing may be better tolerated in patients who are prone to pneumonia, but no studies have explored this hypothesis. A recent small study shows that EN in critically ill prone patients on mechanical ventilation is feasible, safe, and not associated with an increased risk of GI complications.[78] Enteral feeding is generally considered safe in the prone position, but patients should be monitored closely for intolerance and aspiration.

References

1. McClave SA, Taylor BE, Martindale RG, et al. Guidelines for the provision and assessment of nutrition support therapy in the adult critically ill patient: Society of Critical Care Medicine (SCCM) and American Society for Parenteral and Enteral Nutrition (A.S.P.E.N.). *JPEN J Parenter Enteral Nutr.* 2016;40(2):159–211.

2. Heyland DK, Dhaliwal R, Jiang X, Day AG. Identifying critically ill patients who benefit the most from nutrition therapy: the development and initial validation of a novel risk assessment tool. *Crit Care.* 2011;15(6):R268.

3. Dvir D, Cohen J, Singer P. Computerized energy balance and complications in critically ill patients: an observational study. *Clin Nutr.* 2006;25(1):37–44.

4. ARDS Definition Task Force, Ranieri VM, Rubenfeld GD, et al. Acute respiratory distress syndrome: the Berlin definition. *JAMA.* 2012;307(23):2526–2533.

5. Tomashefski JF. Pulmonary pathology of the adult respiratory distress syndrome. *Clin Chest Med.* 1990;11(4):593–619.

6. Ware LB. Pathophysiology of acute lung injury and the acute respiratory distress syndrome. *Semin Respir Crit Care Med.* 2006; 27(4):337–349.

7. Levine S, Nguyen T, Taylor N, et al. Rapid disuse atrophy of diaphragm fibers in mechanically ventilated humans. *N Engl J Med.* 2008;358(13):1327–1335.

8. Garcia de Acilu M, Leal S, Caralt B, et al. The role of omega-3 polyunsaturated fatty acids in the treatment of patients with acute respiratory distress syndrome: a clinical review. *Biomed Res Int.* 2015;2015:653750.

9. Gadek JE, DeMichele SJ, Karlstad MD, et al. Effect of enteral feeding with eicosapentaenoic acid, gamma-linolenic acid, and antioxidants in patients with acute respiratory distress syndrome. Enteral Nutrition in ARDS Study Group. *Crit Care Med.* 1999; 27(8):1409–1420.

10. Parish M, Valiyi F, Hamishehkar H, et al. The effect of omega-3 fatty acids on ARDS: a randomized double-blind study. *Adv Pharm Bull.* 2014;4(Suppl 2):S555–S561.

11. Stapleton RD, Martin TR, Weiss NS, et al. A phase II randomized placebo-controlled trial of omega-3 fatty acids for the treatment of acute lung injury. *Crit Care Med.* 2011;39(7):1655–1662.

12. Patel J, Kha V, Butler D, Kozeniecki M, Martindale R, Allen K. Organ-specific nutrition: one for the history books or still an active player? *Curr Surg Rep.* 2016;4(8). doi:10.1007/s40137 -016-0149.

13. Rice TW, Wheeler AP, Thompson BT, et al. Enteral omega-3 fatty acid, gamma-linolenic acid, and antioxidant supplementation in acute lung injury. *JAMA.* 2011;306(14):1574–1581.

14. Zhu D, Zhang Y, Li S, Gan L, Feng H, Nie W. Enteral omega-3 fatty acid supplementation in adult patients with acute respiratory distress syndrome: a systematic review of randomized controlled trials with meta-analysis and trial sequential analysis. *Intensive Care Med.* 2014;40(4):504–512.

15. Pontes-Arruda A, Aragao AM, Albuquerque JD. Effects of enteral feeding with eicosapentaenoic acid, gamma-linolenic acid, and antioxidants in mechanically ventilated patients with severe sepsis and septic shock. *Crit Care Med.* 2006;34(9):2325–2333.

16. Singer P, Theilla M, Fisher H, et al. Benefit of an enteral diet enriched with eicosapentaenoic acid and gamma-linolenic acid in ventilated patients with acute lung injury. *Crit Care Med.* 2006;34(4):1033–1038.

17. Grau-Carmona T, Moran-Garcia V, Garcia-de-Lorenzo A, et al. Effect of an enteral diet enriched with eicosapentaenoic acid, gamma-linolenic acid and anti-oxidants on the outcome of mechanically ventilated, critically ill, septic patients. *Clin Nutr.* 2011;30(5):578–584.

18. Elamin EM, Miller AC, Ziad S. Immune enteral nutrition can improve outcomes in medical-surgical patients with ARDS: a prospective randomized controlled trial. *J Nutr Disord Ther.* 2012;2:109.

19. Global Initiative for Asthma (GINA). Global strategy for asthma management and prevention. 2016. http://ginasthma.org/2016 -gina-report-global-strategy-for-asthma-management-and -prevention. Accessed February 6, 2017.

20. Rennard S, Thomashow B, Crapo J, et al. Introducing the COPD Foundation guide for diagnosis and management of COPD, recommendations of the COPD Foundation. *COPD.* 2013;10(3):378–389.

21. Minino AM, Murphy SL, Xu J, Kochanek KD. Deaths: final data for 2008. *Natl Vital Stat Rep.* 2011;59(10):1–126.

22. Celli B, Goldstein R, Jardim J, Knobil K. Future perspectives in COPD. *Respir Med.* 2005;99(Suppl B):S41–S8.

23. Celli BR, Cote CG, Marin JM, et al. The body-mass index, airflow obstruction, dyspnea, and exercise capacity index in chronic obstructive pulmonary disease. *N Engl J Med.* 2004;350(10):1005–1012.

24. Wagner PD. Possible mechanisms underlying the development of cachexia in COPD. *Eur Respir J.* 2008;31(3):492–501.

25. Hoong JM, Ferguson M, Hukins C, Collins PF. Economic and operational burden associated with malnutrition in chronic obstructive pulmonary disease. *Clin Nutr.* Epub ahead of print 2016(July 18). doi:10.1016/j.clnu.2016.07.008.

26. Akner G, Larsson K. Undernutrition state in patients with chronic obstructive pulmonary disease. A critical appraisal on diagnostics and treatment. *Respir Med.* 2016;117:81–91.

27. Vitacca M, Clini E, Porta R, Foglio K, Ambrosino N. Acute exacerbations in patients with COPD: Predictors of need for mechanical ventilation. *Eur Respir J.* 1996;9(7):1487–1493.

28. Planas M, Alvarez J, Garcia-Peris PA. Nutritional support and quality of life in stable chronic obstructive pulmonary disease (COPD) patients. *Clin Nutr.* 2005;24(3):433–441.

29. Raghu G, Collard HR, Egan JJ, et al. An official ATS/ERS/JRS/ ALAT statement: Idiopathic pulmonary fibrosis: Evidence-based guidelines for diagnosis and management. *Am J Respir Crit Care Med.* 2011;183(6):788–824.

30. Schwebel C, Pin I, Barnoud D, et al. Prevalence and consequences of nutritional depletion in lung transplant candidates. *Eur Respir J.* 2000;16(6):1050–1055.

31. Lai H, Kosorok M, Laxova A, et al. Nutritional status of patients with cystic fibrosis with meconium ileus: a comparison with patients with and without meconium ileus and diagnosis early through neonatal screening. 2000;105(1):53–61.

32. Sheikh S, Zemel BS. Body composition and pulmonary function in cystic fibrosis. *Front Pediatr.* 2014;2:33. doi:10.3389/ fped2014.0033.

33. Cystic Fibrosis Foundation. 2013 Patient Registry Annual Data Report. https://www.cff.org/2013_CFF_Patient_Registry_Annual _Data_Report.pdf. Accessed February 6, 2017.

34. Boyle MP. Adult cystic fibrosis. *JAMA.* 2007;298(15):1787–1793.

35. Murray MJ, Kumar M, Gregory TJ, et al. Select dietary fatty acids attenuate cardiopulmonary dysfunction during acute lung injury in pigs. *Am J Physiol.* 1995;269(6 Pt 2):H2090–H2099.

36. Mancuso P, Whelan J, DeMichele SJ, et al. Dietary fish oil and fish and borage oil suppress intrapulmonary proinflammatory eicosanoid biosynthesis and attenuate pulmonary neutrophil accumulation in endotoxic rats. *Crit Care Med.* 1997;25(7):1198–1206.

37. Mancuso P, Whelan J, DeMichele SJ, et al. Effects of eicosapentaenoic and gamma-linolenic acid on lung permeability and alveolar macrophage eicosanoid synthesis in endotoxic rats. *Crit Care Med.* 1997;25(3):523–532.

38. MacIntyre NR, Epstein SK, Carson S, et al. Management of patients requiring prolonged mechanical ventilation: report of a NAM-DRC consensus conference. *Chest.* 2005;128(6):3937–3954.

39. Seneff MG, Zimmerman JE, Knaus WA, Wagner DP, Draper EA. Predicting the duration of mechanical ventilation: the importance of disease and patient characteristics. *Chest.* 1996;110(2):469–479.

40. Khalid I, Doshi P, DiGiovine B. Early enteral nutrition and outcomes of critically ill patients treated with vasopressors and mechanical ventilation. *Am J Crit Care.* 2010;19(3):261–268.

41. Lunardi AC, Miranda CS, Silva KM, Cecconello I, Carvalho CR. Weakness of expiratory muscles and pulmonary complications in malnourished patients undergoing upper abdominal surgery. *Respirology.* 2012;17(1):108–113.

42. Budweiser S, Heinemann F, Meyer K, Wild PJ, Pfeifer M. Weight gain in cachectic COPD patients receiving noninvasive positive-pressure ventilation. *Respir Care.* 2006;51(2):126–132.

43. Toth S, Tkacova R, Matula P, Stubna J. Nutritional depletion in relation to mortality in patients with chronic respiratory insufficiency treated with long-term oxygen therapy. *Wien Klin Wochenschr.* 2004;116(17–18):617–621.

44. Budweiser S, Meyer K, Jorres RA, Heinemann F, Wild PJ, Pfeifer M. Nutritional depletion and its relationship to respiratory impairment in patients with chronic respiratory failure due to COPD or restrictive thoracic diseases. *Eur J Clin Nutr.* 2008;62(3):436–443.

45. White JV, Guenter P, Jensen G, et al. Consensus statement: Academy of Nutrition and Dietetics and American Society for Parenteral and Enteral Nutrition: characteristics recommended for the identification and documentation of adult malnutrition (undernutrition). *JPEN J Parenter Enteral Nutr.* 2012;36(3):275–283.

46. White JV, Guenter P, Jensen G, et al. Consensus statement of the Academy of Nutrition and Dietetics/American Society for Parenteral and Enteral Nutrition: characteristics recommended for the identification and documentation of adult malnutrition (undernutrition). [erratum *J Acad Nutr Diet.* 2012;112(11):1899]. *J Acad Nutr Diet.* 2012;112(5):730–738.

47. Braunschweig CA, Sheean PM, Peterson SJ, et al. Exploitation of diagnostic computed tomography scans to assess the impact

of nutrition support on body composition changes in respiratory failure patients. *JPEN J Parenter Enteral Nutr.* 2014;38(7): 880–885.

48. Sheean PM, Peterson SJ, Gomez Perez S, et al. The prevalence of sarcopenia in patients with respiratory failure classified as normally nourished using computed tomography and subjective global assessment. *JPEN J Parenter Enteral Nutr.* 2014;38(7):873–879.

49. Engelen MP, Schols AM, Heidendal GA, Wouters EF. Dual-energy x-ray absorptiometry in the clinical evaluation of body composition and bone mineral density in patients with chronic obstructive pulmonary disease. *Am J Clin Nutr.* 1998;68(6):1298–1303.

50. Fullmer S, Benson-Davies S, Earthman CP, et al. Evidence Analysis Library review of best practices for performing indirect calorimetry in healthy and non-critically ill individuals. *J Acad Nutr Diet.* 2015;115(9):1417–1446.e2.

51. Schlein KM, Coulter SP. Best practices for determining resting energy expenditure in critically ill adults. *Nutr Clin Pract.* 2014;29(1):44–55.

52. Rice TW, Mogan S, Hays MA, et al. Randomized trial of initial trophic versus full-energy enteral nutrition in mechanically ventilated patients with acute respiratory failure. *Crit Care Med.* 2011;39(5):967–974.

53. National Heart, Lung, and Blood Institute Acute Respiratory Distress Syndrome Clinical Trials Network. Initial trophic vs full enteral feeding in patients with acute lung injury: the EDEN randomized trial. *JAMA.* 2012;307(8):795–803.

54. Villet S, Chiolero RL, Bollmann MD, et al. Negative impact of hypocaloric feeding and energy balance on clinical outcome in ICU patients. *Clin Nutr.* 2005;24(4):502–509.

55. McClave SA, Codner P, Patel J, et al. Should we aim for full enteral feeding in the first week of critical illness? *Nutr Clin Pract.* 2016;31(4):425–431. doi:10.1177/0884533616653809.

56. McClave SA, Lowen CC, Kleber MJ, et al. Are patients fed appropriately according to their caloric requirements? *JPEN J Parenter Enteral Nutr.* 1998;22(6):375–381.

57. McClave S, Lowen C, Kleber M, et al. Clinical use of the respiratory quotient obtained from indirect calorimetry. *JPEN J Parenter Enteral Nutr.* 2003;27(1):21–26.

58. Allen KS, Mehta I, Cavallazzi R. When does nutrition impact respiratory function? *Curr Gastroenterol Rep.* 2013;15(6):327. doi:10.1007/s11894-013-0327-3.

59. Plank L, Hill G. Energy balance in critical illness. *Proc Nutr Soc.* 2003;62: 545–552.

60. Heyland D, Muscedere MD, Wishmeyer P, et al. A randomized trial of glutamine and antioxidants in critically ill patients (REDOX). *N Engl J Med.* 2013;368(16):1489–1497.

61. Marinella M. Refeeding syndrome and hypophosphatemia. *J Intensive Care Med.* 2005;20(3):155–159.

62. Akinnusi ME, Pineda LA, El Solh AA. Effect of obesity on intensive care morbidity and mortality: a meta-analysis. *Crit Care Med.* 2008;36(1):151–158.

63. Borel AL, Schwebel C, Planquette B, et al. Initiation of nutritional support is delayed in critically ill obese patients: a multicenter cohort study. *Am J Clin Nutr.* 2014;100(3):859–866. doi:10.3945/ajcn.114.088187.

64. Agarwal E, Ferguson M, Banks M, et al. Nutritional status and dietary intake of acute care patients: results from the Nutrition Care Day Survey 2010. *Clin Nutr.* 2012;31:41–47.

65. Mudge AM, Ross LJ, Young AM, Isenring EA, Banks MD. Helping understand nutritional gaps in the elderly (HUNGER): a prospective study of patient factors associated with inadequate nutritional intake in older medical inpatients. *Clin Nutr.* 2011;30:320–325.

66. Choban P, Dickerson R, Malone A, Worthington P, Compher C; American Society for Parenteral and Enteral Nutrition. A.S.P.E.N. clinical guidelines: nutrition support of hospitalized adult patients with obesity. *JPEN J Parenter Enteral Nutr.* 2013;37(6):714–744. doi:10.1177/0148607113499374.

67. King BK, Kudsk KA, Li J, et al. Route and type of nutrition influence mucosal immunity to bacterial pneumonia. *Ann Surg.* 1999;229(2):272–278.

68. McClave SA, Chang WK. When to feed the patient with gastrointestinal bleeding. *Nutr Clin Pract.* 2005;20(5):544–550.

69. Needham DM, Dinglas VD, Bienvenu OJ, et al. One year outcomes in patients with acute lung injury randomised to initial trophic or full enteral feeding: prospective follow-up of EDEN randomised trial. *BMJ.* 2013;346:f1532. doi:10.1136/bmj.f1532.

70. Singer P, Berger MM, Van den Berghe G, et al. ESPEN guidelines on parenteral nutrition: intensive care. *Clin Nutr.* 2009;28:387–400.

71. Casaer M, Dieter M, et al. Early versus late parenteral nutrition in critically ill adults. *N Engl J Med.* 2011;365(6):506–551.

72. Klompas M, Branson R, Eichenwald C, et al. Strategies to prevent ventilator-associated pneumonia in acute care hospitals: 2014 update. *Infect Control Hosp Epidemiol.* 2014;35(suppl):S2.

73. McClave SA, DeMeo MT, DeLegge MH, et al. North American Summit on Aspiration in the Critically Ill Patient: consensus statement. *JPEN J Parenter Enteral Nutr.* 2002;26(6 Suppl):S80–S85.

74. Heyland DK, Drover JW, Dhaliwal R, et al. Optimizing the benefits and minimizing the risk of enteral nutrition in the critically ill: role of small bowel feeding. *JPEN J Parenter Enteral Nutr.* 2002;26(6 Suppl): S51–S55.

75. Reignier J, Mercier E, Le Gouge A, et al. Effect of not monitoring residual gastric volume on risk of ventilator-associated pneumonia in adults receiving mechanical ventilation and early enteral feeding. *JAMA.* 2013;309(3):249–256.

76. Davies AR, Morrison SS, Bailey MJ, et al. A multicenter, randomized controlled trial comparing early nasojejunal with nasogastric nutrition in critical illness. *Crit Care Med.* 2012;40(8):2342–2348.

77. Guérin C, Reignier J, Richard JC, Beuret P; PROSEVA Study Group, et al. Prone positioning in severe acute respiratory distress syndrome. *N Engl J Med.* 2013;368(23):2159–2168. doi:10.1056/NEJMoa1214103.

78. Saez de la Fuente I, Saez de la Fuente J, Quintana Estelles MD, et al. Enteral nutrition in patients receiving mechanical ventilation in a prone position. *JPEN J Parenter Enteral Nutr.* 2016;40(2): 250–255. doi:10.1177/0148607114553232.

79. Reignier J, Thenoz-Jost N, Fiancette M, et al. Early enteral nutrition in mechanically ventilated patients in the prone position. *Crit Care Med.* 2004;32(1):94–99.

80. Mancebo J, Fernandez R, Blanch L, et al. A multicenter trial of prolonged prone ventilation in severe acute respiratory distress syndrome *Am J Respir Crit Care Med.* 2006;173(11):1233–1239.

81. Alexiou VG, Ierodiakonou V, Dimopoulos G, et al. Impact of patient position on the incidence of ventilator pneumonia: a meta-analysis of randomized controlled trials. *J Crit Care.* 2009;24(4):515–522.

26 Gastrointestinal Disease

Lena B. Palmer, MD, MSCR, Rachael Janas, RD, CNSC, and Michael Sprang, MD

CONTENTS

Acknowledgments: David Frantz, MD, MS, Craig Munroe, MD, Carol Rees Parrish, MS, RD, Joseph Krenitsky, MS, RD, Kate Willcutts, MS, RD, CNSC, and Amy Fortune, RD, PA-C, were the authors of this chapter for the second edition.

Objectives

1. Outline common diseases of the stomach, small intestine, and colon and their associated nutrition-related complications.
2. Discuss nutrition assessment and dietary management of these disorders.
3. Discuss laboratory monitoring and medical management strategies to prevent and reduce complications from common gastrointestinal (GI) disorders.
4. Outline appropriate indications of enteral nutrition (EN) and parenteral nutrition (PN) support in many of these conditions.

Test Your Knowledge Questions

1. A 56-year-old man with long-standing history of type 2 diabetes mellitus presents with postprandial abdominal pain, nausea, and vomiting. His diabetes is uncontrolled despite the use of insulin, and his glycosylated hemoglobin A1C is 10%. He also has painful peripheral neuropathy in his legs as well as diabetic retinopathy. His GI symptoms have progressed over the past 6 months, and he now reports eating very little because he fears the abdominal pain and vomiting will worsen. The emesis occurs 30 minutes to 2 hours after eating, and it has the appearance of undigested food. A diagnostic upper endoscopy (EGD) is normal. Which diagnostic test is the ideal next step in determining the cause of his symptoms?
   A. Mesenteric Doppler ultrasound
   B. Gastric emptying scan
   C. Small bowel series/follow-through
   D. Abdominal computed tomography
2. A 35-year-old white woman presents to the clinic with diarrhea, weight loss, and abnormal liver function tests. Her primary care physician also noted that the patient was vitamin D and iron deficient with anemia. On physical examination, the patient has a very pruritic maculopapular rash with vesicular eruptions on her lower legs. An EGD is performed, and a mosaic pattern with nodularity is noted in the second portion of the duodenum. Which of the following is most likely cause of the patient's symptoms?
   A. Crohn's disease
   B. Celiac disease
   C. Whipple disease
   D. Peptic ulcer disease
3. A 19-year-old woman with a history of Crohn's ileitis since the age of 13 years presents for ongoing care. She has been on several medications for Crohn's disease over the course of her diagnosis. Her disease is isolated to the terminal 30 cm of her ileum and ileocecal valve. Despite adequate medication compliance and dosing, her disease remains active. She complains of 4 to 5 loose, watery stools a day, bloating, and mild abdominal pain. She has a microcytic anemia, signs of fat and lean muscle wasting, and osteopenia. She is determined to have failed medical management and undergoes an ileocecectomy. Which of the following vitamins is she most likely to eventually need to take as a supplement?
   A. Folate
   B. Vitamin B_{12}
   C. Vitamin A
   D. Vitamin E

Test Your Knowledge Answers

1. The correct answer is **B**. This patient already has signs of end-organ damage from the uncontrolled diabetes (peripheral neuropathy, retinopathy), which means he likely has diabetic gastroparesis. Postprandial abdominal pain, nausea, and vomiting of food that was just consumed are common symptoms of diabetic gastroparesis. All the

diagnostic tests listed as options could be reasonable steps in the diagnosis, but a gastric emptying scan is the most valuable initial test as it is used to confirm the presence of delayed gastric emptying.

2. The correct answer is **B**. The patient has classic celiac disease. In addition to the mosaic pattern seen on endoscopy, the patient has both vitamin D and iron deficiency, findings consistent with celiac disease. The rash on the legs likely represents dermatitis herpetiformis, a finding that is pathognomonic but not always present. Abnormal liver function tests and abdominal pain are also commonly seen in celiac disease.

3. The correct answer is **B**. The terminal ileum is one of the most commonly affected sites in Crohn's disease. As the terminal ileum is the primary site of vitamin B_{12} absorption, many Crohn's patients with resection of the terminal ileum will eventually require supplemental vitamin B_{12}.

Background

N utrition status and the digestive tract are inescapably linked. Research into digestive diseases has also produced some of the earliest evidence-based nutrition recommendations. To optimize patient care, nutrition support clinicians need to thoroughly understand the digestive process and the interactions between GI pathology and nutrition (see Chapter 1). The most common GI disorders and their nutrition-related ramifications are presented here.

Motility Disorders

Gastroparesis

Gastroparesis, or delayed gastric emptying, is also known as *gastric stasis* or *diabetic gastropathy* or *enteropathy* (in patients with diabetes mellitus). Gastroparesis has many etiologies (Table 26-1).[1,2] The most common of these are diabetes mellitus, postvagotomy syndrome, postviral gastroparesis, and narcotics or other agents that slow motility. Clinically, gastroparesis will wax and wane, depending on the underlying etiology.

Symptoms of gastroparesis range from mild to severely debilitating and can be life-threatening. In severe cases, patients can develop severe dehydration and electrolyte imbalances such as hypokalemia and hypochloremia associated with emesis. Patients with protracted symptoms can require an alternate means of nutrition and hydration to combat weight loss and dehydration. During this period, early nutrition support can reverse significant malnutrition. Many patients with refractory gastroparesis related to a postviral or a posttraumatic condition may eventually be able to resume adequate oral intake.[3]

Diagnostic testing to confirm gastroparesis in patients with consistent symptoms involves a motility test, such as a gastric emptying study. A gastric emptying study measures retained contents of solid food in the stomach over 4 hours. International control values using a low-fat meal have been established.[1] Defined cutoff values at scheduled intervals at 0, 1, 2 and 4 hours during the test can suggest elevated retention of food and can be diagnostic for gastroparesis. Retention of more than 10% of food at 4 hours is considered diagnostic for

TABLE 26-1 Clinical Conditions Associated with Gastroparesis

Mechanical obstruction:
- Duodenal ulcer
- Pancreatic carcinoma or pseudocyst
- Gastric carcinoma
- Superior mesenteric artery syndrome

Metabolic/endocrine disorders:
- Diabetes mellitus
- Hypothyroidism
- Hyperthyroidism
- Hyperparathyroidism
- Adrenal insufficiency (Addison disease)

Acid-peptic disease:
- Gastric ulcer
- Gastroesophageal reflux disease

Gastritis:
- Atrophic gastritis
- Viral gastroenteritis

Surgery:
- Vagotomy
- Lung transplant
- Antrectomy
- Subtotal gastrectomy
- Roux-en-Y gastrojejunostomy
- Fundoplication

Disorders of gastric smooth muscle:
- Scleroderma
- Polymyositis
- Muscular dystrophy
- Amyloidosis
- Chronic idiopathic pseudo-obstruction
- Dermatomyositis
- Systemic lupus erythematosus

Psychogenic disorders:
- Anorexia
- Bulimia
- Depression

Neuropathic disorders:
- Parkinson's disease
- Paraneoplastic syndrome
- Central nervous system disorders
- High cervical cord lesions (C4 and above)

Source: Data are from references 1 and 2.

delayed gastric emptying. Liquid testing is not recommended because the results do not accurately represent functional gastric motility. For the test to be valid, the patient must not be taking motility-slowing agents and must undergo a sufficient washout period.

Small Bowel Motility Disorders

Motility disorders are not limited to the stomach; they can also involve the small bowel.[4] The etiologies of small bowel dysmotility affecting the central, autonomic, and enteric nervous system or the smooth muscle, lamina propria and/or submucosa of the intestine can be neuropathic, myopathic, immune, or infiltrative. Examples of systemic disorders that can affect small bowel motility include amyloidosis, systemic sclerosis and scleroderma, mitochondrial myopathies, paraneoplastic syndromes, and other rare infiltrative disorders such as Chagas disease (an intestinal infection with *Trypanosoma cruzi*). *Chronic intestinal pseudo-obstruction* (CIPO) refers to intestinal motility disorders that demonstrate signs of a mechanical obstruction (intestinal dilation, air-fluid levels) on radiographic imaging in the absence of an overt mechanical obstruction as the cause. The symptoms and treatment of gastroparesis and small bowel dysmotility overlap significantly, with the latter being more difficult to manage through dietary modification alone. Clarification of the underlying etiology of the dysmotility and targeted medical therapy or cessation of the offending agent will guide the initial treatment approach.

Nutrition Assessment

Nutrition screening and evaluation of patients with motility disorders help to distinguish the adequately nourished patient who can tolerate further GI evaluation from a malnourished patient who requires immediate nutrition support. Unintentional weight loss over time is probably the most important noninvasive parameter by which to determine overall nutrition status. A thorough diet history can help identify those patients for whom diet manipulation may be advantageous. For example, a patient who develops nausea while eating 3 large meals per day may benefit by simply instituting smaller, more frequent meals. In contrast, the patient with severe gastroparesis who has significant vomiting after ingestion of water may require gastric decompression and enteral jejunal feeding to provide symptom relief, nutrients, fluids, and medications. When obtaining a diet history, to the clinician should evaluate the following:

- Changes in appetite and nausea, vomiting, or diarrhea
- Problems chewing or swallowing, which can affect one's ability to ingest certain foods
- The patient's typical daily dietary intake
- The use of supplemental nutrition (oral, enteral, or parenteral)
- Food intolerances or allergies
- Use of supplements, such as vitamins, minerals, herbs, or protein powders
- Use of stool-bulking agents or laxatives
- History of severe constipation
- Medications known to slow gastric emptying (Table 26-2)[2,5]

Medical Management

Prokinetics

Antiemetics and prokinetic agents may reduce symptoms in patients with significant nausea and vomiting; empiric trials can be used to evaluate the effects of these medications in specific individuals.[6,7] Scheduled dosing (vs as-needed dosages) and liquid preparations or suppositories provide the most

TABLE 26-2 Medications Known to Delay Gastric Emptying

- Aluminum-containing antacids
- Anticholinergics
- Atropine
- Beta-agonists
- Calcitonin
- Calcium channel blockers
- Dexfenfluramine
- Diphenhydramine
- Ethanol
- Glucagon
- Interleukin-1
- L-Dopa
- Lithium
- Octreotide
- Ondansetron
- Narcotics
- Nicotine
- Potassium salts
- Progesterone
- Selective serotonin reuptake inhibitors
- Sucralfate
- Tricyclic antidepressants

Source: Data are from references 2 and 5.

consistent symptom control in the setting of active symptoms of nausea and vomiting. Metoclopramide is one of the most commonly used prokinetics because of its rapid onset of action and efficacy. Longer term use of metoclopramide is limited by a low but real risk of irreversible tardive dyskinesia. For this reason, the medication carries a black box warning, and the risks and benefits need to be weighed regarding its use for more than 12 weeks. Other prokinetic medications include intravenous erythromycin; however, this medication is limited by tachyphylaxis when taken orally, and it can lose efficacy rapidly. Domperidone has been used with some success, but this medication is not currently commercially available in the United States except in restricted programs. In the past, cisapride was an additional option; however, this drug has been withdrawn from the US market in all but very limited programs because it is associated with cardiac arrhythmias. Although all of these options and others, such as octreotide, have been attempted in patients with small bowel motility disorders and CIPO, results are inconsistent and disappointing.[4]

Surgical Procedures

Investigators have explored multiple surgical interventions for gastroparesis, including gastric electrical stimulator placement, botulinum toxin injection, pyloroplasty, gastrectomy, and decompressive gastrostomy placement. The Enterra gastric electrical stimulator is proposed to improve symptoms of nausea, vomiting, and quality of life, without objective improvement in gastric emptying studies through enhanced relaxation of the stomach and decreased sensitivity to distension. Conclusions from studies on the efficacy of this device are conflicting; it seems to be most effective in diabetic gastroparesis.[8] Botulinum injection into the pylorus to cause relaxation and improve emptying has been tried as an alternative. Although studies have shown some improvement in gastric emptying study results, botulinum was not associated with significant improvement in symptoms when compared to placebo.[9] More invasive surgical interventions, including gastrojejunostomy and pyloroplasty, have been used but have only shown success in a very select subset of patients. Alternatively, gastrostomy placement for decompression and jejunal feeding tube placement has been used to alleviate symptoms and provide nutrition support, but data regarding efficacy and outcomes are limited.

Nutrition Management

The primary treatment for gastroparesis beyond treating the underlying cause is dietary modification. Dietary modification focuses on eating multiple small meals throughout the day; these meals should be limited in fat and fiber content,

both of which can slow gastric emptying. In more severe cases, patients tolerate liquids better than solids, and these patients may require a liquid diet, at least initially.

Oral Nutrition

Patients and clinicians alike prefer nutrition via the oral route. If the patient is not malnourished, a trial of dietary manipulation is worthwhile (Table 26-3).[10] Patients should keep a food diary to help determine actual oral intake. During the trial, it is prudent to define a target weight goal and the time frame over which this goal must be achieved. If patients maintain their weight while on an oral diet, no further intervention is required. However, those who lose weight may require enteral support.

Enteral Nutrition

When significant malnutrition prevails despite maximal diet manipulation, a trial of EN should be pursued. Most clinicians

---

TABLE 26-3 Summary of Oral Nutrition Intervention in the Patient with Gastroparesis

1. Advise patients to eat smaller, more frequent meals.
2. Use more liquid calories.
   - If solid foods cause increased symptoms, begin with a liquid/pureed diet to promote gastric emptying.
   - If symptoms increase over the course of the day, try solid food meals in the morning, switching to more liquid meals later in the day.
   - Chew foods well.
   - Suggest that the patient sit up during meals and for 1 to 2 hours afterward.
3. Glucose control:
   - If gastroparesis is a result of diabetes mellitus, maximize glucose control.
   - Monitor the need to change the timing or the overall requirements for insulin in order to have consistent delivery of nutrients with optimal total calories ingested.
   - Expect an increase in insulin requirements because improved symptom control will likely result in an increase in total calories ingested.
   - In general, dietary restrictions (eg, diabetic or heart healthy diets) should be lifted during the trial.
4. Medications:
   - Prokinetics and antiemetics should be given in regular scheduled doses (rather than "as needed") and may be best tolerated in liquid form.
   - Avoid use of medications that alter gastric motility.[a]
   - Review and delete any "unnecessary" medications.
5. Fat:
   - Fat in liquids should be tolerated; before restricting them, implement steps 1 to 4.
6. Fiber:
   - Fiber, fermented by small intestine bacteria if present in significant amounts, may cause gas, cramping, and bloating, aggravating symptoms of gastroparesis.
   - If bezoar formation is a concern, avoid the following high-fiber foods and medications: Oranges, persimmons, coconuts, berries, green beans, figs, apples, sauerkraut, brussels sprouts, potato peels, and legumes; fiber supplements such as Metamucil, Perdiem, Benefiber, Fibercon, Citrucel, etc.
7. Treat small intestinal bacterial overgrowth (SIBO) if suspected/symptomatic.
8. Monitor and replace as needed: iron, vitamin B_{12}, vitamin D, and calcium.
   - If the patient is significantly malnourished, a daily standard vitamin/mineral elixir can be used for 1 month or longer or until stores are replete.
   - If patient has gastric intolerance to iron, try smaller doses; some is better than none. Liquid iron may be a better choice in some patients. Consider giving iron with vitamin C.

[a]Refer to Table 26-2.
Adapted from reference 10 with permission from University of Virginia Health System, Nutrition Support Traineeship Syllabus; Charlottesville, VA; updated July 2016. www.ginutrition.virginia.edu.

prefer a trial of nasojejunal feeding to assess tolerance before enteral access is endoscopically or surgically placed. Unfortunately, patients may dislodge the nasojejunal tube with a bout of emesis. Nasogastric-jejunal tubes, which allow gastric venting concomitantly with jejunal feedings, are also used; however, patient acceptance of these tubes is poor because the tube's large diameter causes discomfort. Patients should remain *nil per os* (NPO) during initiation of EN until tolerance is established. NPO status will ensure that intolerance to oral intake is not mistaken to be EN intolerance. Finally, in patients with significant weight loss, clinicians should anticipate refeeding syndrome and initiate EN judiciously.[11]

Long-Term Enteral Access

Long-term jejunal access can be achieved by various methods, including percutaneous endoscopic gastrostomy (PEG)/jejunostomy, separate venting PEG with a percutaneous endoscopic jejunostomy, or a surgical jejunostomy.[12] Motility specialists do not agree on the best approach to feed patients with motility disorders who require EN. Further clinical trials may help determine whether one technique is better than others with regard to patient preference, symptom improvement, and complications.

Formula Selection/Delivery

Available evidence suggests that most patients with motility disorders—including those with diabetes mellitus—tolerate standard, polymeric formulas.[13] Because the stomach is bypassed, a formula that contains fiber may be tolerated; however, indigestible fiber may aggravate symptoms if small intestinal bacterial overgrowth (SIBO) is a chronic problem. (SIBO is discussed later in this chapter.)

The small bowel is volume sensitive and generally does not tolerate bolus feeding. Jejunal feeding may be administered via a cycled pump or gravity infusion, typically for 8 to 14 hours. Enteral feedings do not need to be diluted. The flow rate can be increased from 125 to 160 mL/h as tolerated; some patients may tolerate rates even greater than 160 mL/h. Intolerance of jejunal EN is variable in patients with gastroparesis. Often, the adverse effects associated with EN can be explained physiologically and are relatively simple to resolve.[14]

Parenteral Nutrition

PN is rarely necessary for the patient with gastroparesis and should be considered a last resort for patients with a functional GI tract distal to the stomach. Exceptions include patients with CIPO, end-stage scleroderma, or other dysmotility disorders that involve both the small bowel and the stomach.

Complications

Micronutrient Deficiencies

Intolerance to various foods, as well as malabsorption, can lead to nutrient deficiencies. Although intolerances can often be managed with dietary manipulation, nutrient deficiencies—particularly those resulting in anemia and metabolic bone disease—require ongoing monitoring and supplementation.

Iron

Iron deficiency anemia is common in this patient population, and the etiology is likely multifactorial. First, many patients with gastroparesis limit iron-rich foods (eg, red meat) because they do not tolerate these foods. Second, acid reflux, which is often associated with gastroparesis, is commonly treated with acid-suppressive medications such as proton pump inhibitors (PPIs). The reduced gastric acidity impairs the conversion of dietary ferric iron to the more absorbable ferrous form.[15] Third, elevated gastric pH and poor motility can increase the risk of developing SIBO, which can significantly decrease duodenal iron absorption.

Iron deficiency must be carefully monitored in patients receiving jejunal EN because the duodenum (the primary site for iron absorption) is bypassed.[15] Serum ferritin is an accurate indicator of iron stores over time, but it is an acute-phase reactant and should therefore be checked in the nonacute setting.[16] Oral iron supplementation is the preferred method of replacement and is available as ferrous sulfate, gluconate, or fumarate.[17] Iron is constipating, and attention to symptoms and prompt treatment are important to prevent worsening symptoms. Taking iron with a beverage containing vitamin C, which is acidic, will enhance iron absorption.[5] See Chapter 8 for additional information on iron deficiency and supplementation.

Vitamin B$_{12}$

Some patients with gastroparesis have a history of gastric resection and therefore are at risk for vitamin B$_{12}$ deficiency. Vitamin B$_{12}$ deficiency can take several years to develop, and the clinical features of B$_{12}$ deficiency are nonspecific and often absent in deficient patients. Baseline and periodic monitoring, in addition to supplementation when necessary, are therefore important. See Chapter 8 for additional information on B$_{12}$ deficiency and supplementation.

Vitamin D

Osteoporosis affects patients with gastroparesis and a history of subtotal gastrectomy. Evaluation of 25-hydroxyvitamin D (25-OHD) levels (not 1,25-dihydroxyvitamin D [1,25-OH$_2$D]) and bone mineral density (BMD) is important. After the intestine absorbs vitamin D, it is rapidly converted to 25-OHD in the liver. In vitamin D–deficient states, calcium levels drop, resulting in hyperparathyroidism and the release of parathyroid hormone, which increases the rate at which the limited 25-OHD is converted to 1,25-OH$_2$D. As a result, calcium bone loss increases despite the finding of a normal level of 1,25-OH$_2$D. Patients with metabolic bone disease are recommended to take 1500 mg of elemental calcium and 800 IU of vitamin D daily. To maximize absorption, calcium should be administered in single doses no greater than 500 mg.

Hyperglycemia

Hyperglycemia—especially if serum glucose levels are widely fluctuating—can cause transient gastroparesis in some patients; however, this delayed emptying responds to normalization of serum glucose levels.[2,18] In addition, hyperglycemia has been shown to attenuate the prokinetic effect of erythromycin.[19] Glycemic control must be evaluated at the initial nutrition assessment and monitored continually. Periodic monitoring of glycosylated hemoglobin A1C ensures that optimal glucose control is maintained over time.

Small Intestinal Bacterial Overgrowth

Patients with GI motility disorders are at a higher risk of developing SIBO,[20] which is discussed below.

Bezoar Formation

Bezoars, which are retained concretions of indigestible foreign material, accumulate in the stomach and may be caused by indigestible food material (phytobezoars) or medications (pharmacobezoars). Patients with altered GI motility are at an increased risk for bezoar formation. The symptoms associated with bezoars often mimic those of gastroparesis: patients may experience early satiety, nausea, and vomiting. Fiber intake and some medications have been implicated in the formation of bezoars.[20] Treatment of gastric phytobezoars includes enzymatic therapies such as cellulase and lavage with or without endoscopic intervention.[21] Infusions of Coca-Cola or acetylcysteine have also seemed to be effective in case studies.[22–25] Use of meat tenderizer that contains papain—a protease with broad activity—has been reported in the literature, but meat tenderizer should be avoided because papain breaks down normal tissue and its use is associated with peptic ulcer disease, esophagitis, and gastritis. Long-term prokinetic therapy to treat and prevent bezoar formation may also be beneficial. In refractory cases, surgery to remove the bezoar provides definitive treatment.

Small Intestinal Bacterial Overgrowth

A wide variety of bacteria colonize the small intestine. Ordinarily, the concentration of bacteria in the small bowel is several orders of magnitude lower than the concentration found in the colon. Multiple factors prevent the overgrowth of bacteria within the small intestine, including gastric acid, intestinal peristalsis, the ileocecal valve, bile acids, the enteric immune system, and pancreatic enzyme secretion.[26] Clinical conditions that impair any of these defenses may allow bacteria to proliferate within the small bowel (Table 26-4). Patients with GI motility disorders are at a higher risk of developing SIBO.[26] It was traditionally thought to occur primarily in the setting of surgical blind loops, small bowel diverticula, or in small bowel motility disorders. However, research has demonstrated that SIBO is also common in the setting of diarrhea-predominant irritable bowel syndrome, end-stage liver disease, exocrine pancreatic insufficiency (EPI), and even in end-stage kidney failure.[27–31] Bacterial colonization of the small bowel results in deconjugation of bile salts and impaired micelle formation, which

TABLE 26-4 Risk Factors for Small Intestinal Bacterial Overgrowth

Impaired motility:
- Vagotomy
- Diabetic neuropathy
- Gastroparesis

Small bowel dysmotility:
- Hypothyroidism
- Chronic intestinal pseudo-obstruction
- Scleroderma
- Radiation enteritis/fibrosis
- Amyloidosis

Impaired immune function:
- Chronic immunosuppression
- Immune deficiency syndrome
- Diabetes mellitus
- Cirrhosis

Anatomical defects:
- Duodenal or jejunal diverticula
- Strictures/obstructions/adhesions
- Gastrocolic/jejunal-colic fistulas
- Resection of the ileocecal valve
- Blind loops (Billroth II, Roux-en-Y, Whipple, etc)
- Crohn's disease

Other:
- Hypochlorhydria/achlorhydria
- Atrophic gastritis
- Pancreatic insufficiency
- Postcholecystectomy

causes fat malabsorption. Intestinal bacteria can also degrade brush border glycoproteins, including disaccharidases, which can impair carbohydrate metabolism or induce lactose intolerance.[32] Intestinal bacteria can also compete with the host for available nutrients. SIBO can produce an inflammatory process that impairs nutrient absorption, or it can cause a protein-losing enteropathy.[33] Bacterial metabolism produces short-chain fatty acids (SCFAs). SCFAs may decrease luminal pH, denature intestinal enzymes, and increase the overall osmotic load. The result is rapid gut transit, maldigestion, and malabsorption.

The symptoms of SIBO include gas, bloating, abdominal distension and discomfort, nausea, diarrhea, weight loss, and an overall decline in nutrition status. The possibility of SIBO is often underappreciated in patients with another GI pathology. Testing for and treatment of SIBO should be considered in those patients who have persistent GI symptomatology despite adequate therapy of their primary GI disorder.

Diagnosis

A noninvasive hydrogen breath test is the most common way to assay for SIBO. The patient is administered an oral sugar load (either lactulose or glucose), and hydrogen gas (a byproduct of bacterial sugar metabolism) is measured in the expelled breath at scheduled intervals. An early increase in hydrogen production suggests an increased quantity of bacteria prior to the expected colonic arrival and is diagnostic of SIBO. This test has limitations, including the fact that a subset of patients produces methane gas as an alternative to the hydrogen. Accurate assessment of this population requires additional equipment to detect the methane, and that equipment is not as commonly available. An additional, less commonly available test includes radiolabeled carbon incorporated into xylose, which can then be measured in the expelled carbon dioxide. The traditional gold standard test for SIBO is a small bowel aspirate and culture. This test is invasive (requiring EGD) and fraught with technical challenges in both obtaining the fluid and processing it correctly. In practice, clinicians may empirically treat for SIBO based on symptoms and an underlying diagnosis that would predispose the patient to SIBO.

Treatment

Enteral antibiotics are the treatment of choice for SIBO.[26,34] The most frequently used antibiotics have been metronidazole, ciprofloxacin, amoxicillin/clavulanate, or doxycycline. As an alternative, rifaximin is being used with increasing frequency.[35] Patients may sometimes require retreatment or cyclic antibiotics for persistent SIBO symptoms or recurrence.

Celiac Disease

Celica disease, also known as *celiac sprue, nontropical sprue,* and *gluten-sensitive enteropathy,* is a T lymphocyte immune disorder causing small intestinal inflammation and villous flattening.[36,37] The intestinal injury seen in celiac disease causes malabsorption, and it is triggered by the ingestion of gluten and other protein antigens in wheat, barley, and rye. Celiac disease is not the same as wheat allergy, which is an immunoglobulin E (IgE)–mediated, true food allergy (see section on food allergies, later in this chapter). The exact triggers leading to the manifestation of celiac disease in susceptible individuals are unknown; however, there is a strong genetic predisposition in patients who carry the HLA-DQ2 and DQ8 loci that encode part of the major histocompatibility complex, the system involved in differentiating "self" and "nonself."[38,39] Indeed, HLA-DQ2/DQ8 inheritance is seen in more than 98% of all patients with celiac disease. The lack of this genetic predisposition is helpful in ruling out celiac disease, but HLA-DQ2/DQ8 is a common genetic variant, found in approximately 30% to 50% of the general population, the vast majority of whom do not have celiac disease.[39,40]

Celiac disease is a worldwide disorder with considerable regional variation in prevalence. The highest incidence of celiac disease is in the North African Berber population (5.6%), and the lowest incidences are seen in certain South American, sub-Saharan African, and South Asian countries.[41] Celiac disease is significantly underdiagnosed and underrecognized in the United States; a population-based study estimated a prevalence of 0.71% and suggested that approximately 70% of affected individuals were unaware of their diagnosis.[42] Celiac disease is more prevalent than Crohn's disease, ulcerative colitis (UC), and cystic fibrosis (CF) combined, affecting approximately 1.8 million United States adults. However, the often mild and subtle symptoms are easily overlooked by patients

and providers, and, currently, the estimated time to diagnosis in the United States is 11 years.[37]

Diagnosis

History and Physical Examination

The wide array of symptoms and varying severity of celiac disease make its timely diagnosis problematic. See Table 26-5 for the clinical features of celiac disease. The classic symptoms of diarrhea, steatorrhea, and weight loss are often not present.[43] In many cases, abdominal bloating and indigestion may be the main manifestation of the disease, and some patients report constipation.

Dermatitis herpetiformis is a bullous skin rash pathognomonic for celiac disease, affecting 10% to 20% of patients. About 20% of patients with dermatitis herpetiformis exhibit recognizable clinical symptoms of celiac disease,[37] whereas nearly 100% will have varying degrees of enteropathy found in biopsies of the small intestine.[36] Medical therapy for dermatitis herpetiformis exists; however, only a gluten-free diet will clear both the intestinal and skin lesions.[37]

Some patients with celiac disease exhibit no overt intestinal symptoms, and extraintestinal manifestations, such as unexplained iron deficiency or abnormal serum transaminases (aspartate aminotransferase/alanine aminotransferase), may be the only clue to the diagnosis.[41,44,45] Also, celiac disease is seen at a higher frequency in conjunction with several other disorders (see Table 26-6). Many of these disorders are other autoimmune conditions associated with the same genetic predisposition, such as type 1 diabetes mellitus.

Serological Testing

Serology testing is the first-line diagnostic test used to screen patients for celiac disease. While several different serologic markers have been identified, antitissue transglutaminase–immunoglobulin A (TTG-IgA) is currently the most widely recommended initial screening test because of its high sensitivity, specificity, and reliability.[44,46] In patients with selective immunoglobulin A (IgA) deficiency, the most common immunodeficiency in humans, TTG-IgA may result in a false negative because of low overall levels of IgA. Many celiac panels also measure total IgA levels. If an IgA deficiency is identified in

---

TABLE 26-5 Clinical Features Encountered in Celiac Disease

- Diarrhea, weight loss, and failure to thrive
- Recurrent abdominal pain and bloating
- Iron deficiency anemia
- Macrocytic anemia (folate or B$_{12}$)
- Short stature
- Osteopenia, bone pain, and pathological fractures
- Infertility and adverse reproductive outcomes
- Recurrent aphthous stomatitis
- Elevated serum transaminases
- Fatigue
- Depression

TABLE 26-6 Disorders Associated with Celiac Disease

- Type 1 diabetes mellitus
- Autoimmune thyroid disease
- Hyper- and hypothyroidism
- Dermatitis herpetiformis
- Addison disease
- Autoimmune hepatitis
- Systemic lupus erythematosus
- Connective tissue disease
- Sjögren syndrome
- Atrophic gastritis
- Autoimmune thyroid disease
- Alopecia
- Rheumatoid arthritis
- Primary biliary cirrhosis
- Down syndrome
- Turner syndrome
- William syndrome
- Congenital heart defects
- Immunoglobulin A deficiency
- Psoriasis

a patient, endomysial antibodies, antitissue transglutaminase–immunoglobulin G (IgG) and IgG–deamidated gliadin peptide testing should be ordered. A patient's serum serology levels fall quickly after he or she starts a gluten-free diet; therefore, it is essential that patients with suspected celiac disease have serology tests before they eliminate gluten. Additionally, TTG-IgA testing may not be reliable in children younger than 2 years because the IgA system has not fully developed. For this reason, alternative serologic testing may be needed in this age group.[47]

Small Bowel Biopsy

Serologic testing is an important initial screening tool, but it is not adequate to confirm the diagnosis of celiac disease. An EGD to obtain biopsies of the proximal small intestine is required to confirm the celiac disease diagnosis in all adult patients with positive serology screening tests.

Small bowel biopsy is not without limitations: multiple biopsies (6 to 8) from the proximal duodenum including the bulb are required, as is correct orientation of the sample on the slide, which must be read by a pathologist trained in identifying celiac disease.[46] Patients must consume a sufficient amount of gluten before the procedure to ensure that inflammation will be present in the biopsy specimens. If the patient has already been on a gluten-limited or gluten-free diet, the endoscopy should be delayed, and the patient should consume at least 3 g or a generous serving of gluten daily (eg, a couple of slices of bread, a serving of pasta, a muffin, or another baked good) for 6 to 8 weeks or until symptoms develop.

Nutrition Management

The only treatment for celiac disease is lifelong elimination of gluten. Even small amounts of gluten can lead to mucosal changes on intestinal biopsy.[48] Gluten is found in food products containing wheat, rye, and barley, and ingredients derived from those grains can be found in a wide array of unsuspected items such as frozen vegetables, soy sauce, ketchup, ice cream, and processed deli meats. Additional sources of hidden gluten come in the form of medications (both prescription and over-the-counter), cosmetics, toothpaste, and products that are processed in facilities that also process gluten-containing products, where cross-contamination may occur.[49,50] While the Codex Alimentarius, the international code that defines food standards, adopted a definition of gluten-free products as those products containing less than 20 parts per million of gluten (less than 20 mg of gluten per kg of food), studies have shown that many products labeled gluten-free may contain excess levels of gluten.[51]

Oats contain an antigenic protein (avenin), but patients with celiac disease often do not react to oats in the way they react to the proteins in wheat, barley, and rye.[52] However, given the extensive amount of cross-contamination between oat and gluten-containing grains, the inclusion of oats in the gluten-free diet remains controversial.[52] In patients with stable celiac disease, the decision to include oats should be determined on an individual basis by the clinician and patient.[44]

Patients may initially experience lactose intolerance. However, many people with celiac disease can resume intake of lactose-containing foods after approximately 1 month on a strict gluten-free diet, after the mucosa has begun to heal.

Patients should be referred early to a dietitian with expertise in celiac disease; the longer the interval between diagnosis and nutrition counseling, the greater the chance the patient will receive misinformation from family, friends, and the online sources.[53] Many surveys have described the dissatisfaction of patients with celiac disease when they encounter physicians or dietitians not well trained in the nutrition management of celiac disease, only to find that support groups provide the most accurate and helpful information.[54,55] The clinician should be sensitive to the emotional, lifestyle, and relationship infringements that a gluten-free diet imposes—such as challenging food situations at work, school, or social events; grocery shopping; or when traveling or going out to eat—and the unwanted attention this diet sometimes brings.[56]

In patients with newly diagnosed celiac disease, baseline levels of folate, ferritin, 25-OHD, vitamin A, and vitamin B$_{12}$ should be checked, especially in those who have diarrhea or significant weight loss. Initial use of a therapeutic vitamin/mineral supplement may be important while initiating a gluten-free diet. The micronutrient levels should be rechecked in 2 to 3 months to ensure efficacy of supplementation.

Symptomatic improvement is expected within 2 weeks in 70% to 95% of patients after the initiation of a gluten-free diet.[45,57] However, histology may not recover completely for months to years, despite clinical normalization. Serology antibody titers should be negative after 4 to 6 months on a strict gluten-free diet, although elevated TTG-IgA levels may persist because of various causes. See Table 26-7 for a summary of important aspects of celiac disease management.[58]

Patients with celiac disease rarely need nutrition support. For patients who fail to respond to a gluten-free diet and are at

TABLE 26-7 Key Elements for Managing Patients with Celiac Disease

- **C**onsultation with a dietitian skilled in celiac disease
- **E**ducation about the disease
- **L**ifelong adherence to a gluten-free diet
- **I**dentification and treatment of nutrition deficiencies
- **A**ccess to an advocacy group
- **C**ontinuous long-term follow-up by a multidisciplinary team

Source: Data are from reference 58.

significant nutrition risk, a trial of a gluten-free oral or enteral feeding as the sole source of intake may be beneficial (and diagnostic). This intervention will help to determine a true refractory patient vs the patient who is inadvertently including gluten in his or her diet. In severe cases, an elemental diet may even be worthwhile, at least initially.[59]

Complications

Patients with newly diagnosed celiac disease should be evaluated for nutrition deficiencies.[60] The classic presentation of celiac disease has been described as a patient with significant weight loss, diarrhea (steatorrhea), and iron deficiency. In addition, celiac disease is associated with an increased risk of deficiencies of fat-soluble vitamins, zinc, magnesium, and folate.[37,61] Vitamin B12 deficiency, which was once thought to be uncommon in celiac disease, was found in up to 41% of patients in a prospective study.[62]

Iron deficiency may be the sole manifestation of celiac disease in the absence of diarrhea; in fact, iron deficiency anemia is the most common clinical presentation of celiac disease, and it resolves after initiation of a gluten-free diet.[45,63,64] Up to 8% of cases of iron deficiency anemia resistant to oral iron supplementation can be attributed to celiac disease.[65]

Metabolic Bone Disease

Osteoporosis is another consequence of untreated celiac disease, affecting up to 75% of patients.[66] The causes are multifactorial and include decreased calcium absorption precipitating secondary hyperparathyroidism, increased bone resorption turnover and loss, malabsorption of vitamin D and calcium, and inadequate intake from avoidance of milk products because of lactose intolerance. Furthermore, the patient may never have achieved peak bone mass at baseline.

Vitamin D and BMD should be measured in all adults after initial diagnosis of celiac disease.[67] In patients with demonstrable bone loss, aggressive intervention is warranted. Improved BMD was seen in patients with celiac disease after 1 year on a gluten-free diet with standard amounts of oral calcium and cholecalciferol.[66]

Adverse Reproductive Outcomes

Infertility and other adverse reproductive outcomes have long been associated with celiac disease, although not all studies demonstrate the association. Early observational studies examined the prevalence of celiac disease in women presenting for infertility evaluation in tertiary care centers. A meta-analysis of observational studies published between 1966 and 2013 showed an association between fertility and undiagnosed celiac disease but failed to identify an increased risk of infertility among women with known celiac disease.[68] Dhalwani and colleagues examined a large, prospective, population-based database of health records for over 2 million British women of childbearing years and found that rates of newly diagnosed fertility problems were no different in women with or without celiac disease except in the age group 25 to 29 years.[69] Although the association of infertility with celiac disease remains controversial, other adverse reproductive outcomes such as miscarriage, preterm delivery, low birth weight, and intrauterine growth restriction have also been associated with celiac disease. When young women of childbearing age are compliant with a gluten-free diet, these risks decrease.[70]

Microscopic Colitis

Microscopic colitis and celiac disease share many common features, and up to 30% of patients with celiac disease have microscopic colitis.[71] These patients often present with watery diarrhea despite negative celiac disease serology tests and good compliance with the gluten-free diet. Diagnosis requires a full colonoscopy with an adequate number of mucosal biopsies taken throughout the colon. Histologically, a T lymphocyte–predominant inflammatory infiltrate is found in the lamina propria of the colonic mucosa. Some patients have a prominent subepithelial collagen band and are diagnosed with collagenous colitis. Management of microscopic colitis is not standardized and can be done with a variety of medical therapies, including mesalamine, budesonide, and bismuth subsalicylate. Unfortunately, a gluten-free diet does not control microscopic colitis.

Asplenia, Small Intestinal Bacterial Overgrowth, and Lactose Intolerance

Celiac disease confers functional asplenia, and pneumococcal vaccination is recommended to decrease the risk of infection.[46] SIBO is also common, and it presents an important consideration in the differential of patients with seemingly refractory celiac disease. In those patients who present with diarrhea/steatorrhea, lactose restriction might be beneficial for a short period. The villous blunting seen in celiac disease can cause a temporary deficiency in brush border lactase, thus leading to lactose intolerance. Some patients with symptoms attributed to lactose intolerance may ultimately be diagnosed with untreated celiac disease.[48]

Refractory Celiac Disease and Malignancies

True refractory celiac disease is a rare complication of celiac disease.[72] The most common cause of seemingly refractory celiac disease is noncompliance or inadvertent gluten ingestion. In fact, the single most important threat to disease remission is dietary noncompliance, with rates reported at 50% to 80%.[49,73] Therefore, in nonresponders, intentional or inadvertent gluten

TABLE 26-8 Conditions with Similar Symptoms to Celiac Disease

- Agammaglobulinemia
- Acquired immunodeficiency syndrome enteropathy
- Amyloidosis
- Autoimmune enteropathy
- Bacterial overgrowth
- Eosinophilic gastroenteritis
- Giardiasis
- Inflammatory bowel disease
- Intestinal allergy to nongluten proteins such as milk, egg, or soy
- Intestinal lymphangiectasia
- Intestinal lymphoma
- Irritable bowel syndrome
- Lactose intolerance
- Microscopic colitis
- Pancreatic insufficiency
- Tropical sprue
- Whipple disease

ingestion must be excluded. If symptoms persist with adherence to a gluten-free diet, consider reevaluating the celiac disease diagnosis after 6 to 9 months. Collagenous sprue, ulcerative jejunitis, and small bowel T cell lymphoma may have symptoms similar to those of celiac disease. Table 26-8 lists conditions and symptoms that can mimic celiac disease. Clinicians must rule out celiac disease "mimics" when evaluating a patient with seemingly refractory sprue.

There are 2 types of refractory celiac disease: type 1, where the hallmark is a polyclonal expansion of T lymphocytes in the lamina propria of the small intestine, and type 2, which is a monoclonal expansion of T lymphocytes. While both are considered lymphoproliferative disorders, type 1 carries a better prognosis, with 80% to 96% of treated patients surviving therapy after 5 years.[74] Patients with type 2 refractory celiac disease fare much worse, with a 5-year survival rate of 44% to 56%.[74] Type 2 refractory celiac disease is rare, and therapy is similar to chemotherapy for lymphoproliferative disorders.

Inflammatory Bowel Disease

Crohn's Disease

Crohn's disease is characterized by transmural inflammation of the digestive tract anywhere from the mouth to the anus. The precise etiology of Crohn's disease remains unknown. Evidence indicates that inflammation results from excessive T helper cell type 1 response to bacteria within normal GI flora. No single test is absolute for the diagnosis of inflammatory bowel disease. Diagnosis of inflammatory bowel disease is based on a combination of symptoms, endoscopic findings, and biopsy results. Newer markers for inflammation such as fecal calprotectin are used with increased frequency in the assessment of inflammatory bowel disease.[75] Serological markers for inflammatory bowel disease such as anti–*Saccharomyces*

cerevisiae antibodies and anti–neutrophil cytoplasmic antibodies are insensitive and remain controversial because they are not confirmatory for the diagnosis.[76]

Nutrition Assessment

Malnutrition occurs frequently in patients with inflammatory bowel disease. An estimated 65% to 75% of inpatients and more than 50% of outpatients with Crohn's disease experience significant weight loss.[77] Weight loss is caused by decreased oral intake in response to abdominal pain, diarrhea, nausea, or small bowel strictures. Patients can develop sitophobia (fear of eating) because of their previous experiences with diarrhea, abdominal pain, or oral pain with food intake.[77] Finally, malabsorption may contribute to malnutrition in patients with extensive intestinal resection(s).

Energy and Protein Requirements

Energy expenditure is not significantly elevated in patients with inactive Crohn's disease.[78] Resting energy expenditure is increased during active inflammation, but total energy expenditure is not significantly elevated—perhaps because physical activity decreases during periods of disease exacerbation.[79] Standard predictive equations may be used to estimate energy requirements with appropriate adjustments for activity level and comorbidities (see Chapter 2). Initial feedings should be provided to malnourished patients at a decreased energy level to reduce the incidence of refeeding syndrome.[10]

Protein requirements may be elevated in Crohn's disease because of increased losses related to intestinal inflammation or fistulas. Patients in the postoperative setting or those with short bowel syndrome (SBS) may benefit from an increase in protein intake. Protein recommendations for those with Crohn's disease are 1 to 1.5 g/kg,[80] although no randomized trials have investigated optimal protein intake in this population. See Chapter 30 for additional information on SBS.

Nutrition Intervention

Fiber

No specific dietary fiber regimen has been proven effective in Crohn's disease. Patients with stricturing Crohn's disease often follow a low-fiber diet. Clinicians should not routinely advise patients to restrict fiber intake in the absence of stricturing disease, as a low-fiber diet can be associated with decreased intake of fruits and vegetables, which, in turn, decreases vitamin and mineral intake. Additionally, evidence on the role of fiber in improving inflammatory bowel disease outcomes is increasing.[81]

Lactose

Evidence is insufficient to support withholding lactose-containing foods in patients with Crohn's disease who are not symptomatic after ingestion of normal amounts of lactose. A study by Park and coworkers has suggested that the incidence of lactose intolerance in patients with Crohn's disease is not increased compared with the general public, based on jejunal lactase levels.[82] In contrast, 2 studies of breath hydrogen in response to lactose ingestion documents a significantly increased incidence of lactose intolerance in patients with Crohn's disease vs healthy controls.[83,84] The clinical significance of this increased breath hydrogen response is unclear—many patients with lactose intolerance and Crohn's disease tolerate normal amounts of dairy products.[85]

Fish Oil

Fish oils are rich in ω-3 fatty acids, which have antiinflammatory effects through their ability to modify production of prostaglandins, leukotrienes, and thromboxanes. The results of studies with fish oil supplements in Crohn's disease remain conflicting. A prior systematic review and meta-analysis concluded that data are insufficient to recommend the use of ω-3 fatty acids for maintenance of remission in inflammatory bowel disease.[86]

Enteral Nutrition

In patients with Crohn's disease and adequate bowel length, EN effectively reverses malnutrition and supports growth (in pediatric patients). EN is significantly more efficacious than placebo in children and should be considered as first-line therapy.[87] However, EN is not as effective as corticosteroid therapy in inducing remission in adults. Elemental, semielemental, and polymeric formulas are not significantly different in terms of effectiveness.[88,89] Reduced-fat formulas may be more effective than formulas with increased amounts of long-chain triglycerides, but formulas with increased amounts of medium-chain triglycerides provided remission rates that were the same as the rates for low-fat formulas.[90,91] Controlled trials have demonstrated no clinical benefit of supplemental glutamine or glutamine-rich enteral formulas for patients with inflammatory bowel disease.[92-94] See Practice Scenario 26-1 for an example of EN used to treat Crohn's disease.

Practice Scenario 26-1

Question: Is it appropriate to place a percutaneous endoscopic gastrostomy (PEG) tube in a patient with Crohn's disease and short bowel syndrome (SBS)?

Scenario: A 31-year-old man with a history of inflammatory bowel disease comes to the outpatient clinic for a nutrition consultation. Ten years ago, he underwent a total abdominal colectomy with end-ileostomy after presenting with "abdominal sepsis." At first, he was thought to have ulcerative colitis based on pancolonic involvement of the inflammatory process. However, 3 years later he presented to the emergency department with abdominal pain. Conservative measures with pain medications and fluids were unsuccessful. Evidence of small bowel disease was seen on computed tomography scan. The diagnosis for the patient was changed to Crohn's enteritis. He was started on corticosteroids and an aminosalicylic acid compound with partial resolution of symptoms.

Over the next 12 months, the patient seemed to improve after switching to stronger immunosuppressive therapy with infliximab and azathioprine therapy. The patient presented again 2 years ago with severe pain, fever, decreased ostomy output, nausea, vomiting, and confusion. An abdominal film revealed Crohn's disease with a spontaneous bowel perforation. The patient became critically ill, requiring aggressive management with antibiotics and fluid volume resuscitation, and required an exploratory laparotomy. The patient required 10 units of blood intraoperatively, and an extensive small bowel resection was performed. Postoperatively, the patient was estimated to have approximately 200 cm of remaining small intestine, resulting in an end-jejunostomy. A central venous catheter was placed, and he was started on parenteral nutrition (PN). Although his weight fluctuated on PN, his main problem has been recurrent central line infections and the need to frequently replace his central line catheter. He presents now to the clinic for a nutrition consultation and further management.

Intervention: A PEG tube was placed and the patient was started on EN with a small-peptide/medium-chain triglyceride formula. Use of a small portable pump carried in a fanny pack allowed the patient to feed 24 hours a day. Gradually, over 4 months, the patient was weaned off PN. Oral intake was allowed ad lib, as tolerated by volume of ostomy output. The patient was encouraged to use oral rehydration solutions and small frequent meals with no fat restriction, separating fluid intake from the solid meals. Six months later, his weight is stable at 10 pounds over his ideal body weight.

Answer: In the past, Crohn's disease was thought to be a relative contraindication to placement of a PEG tube because physicians were concerned about creating an intentional gastrocutaneous fistula in a disease process characterized by fistula formation and intraperitoneal adhesions. Physicians were also wary of perforating an intervening loop of small bowel caught in an adhesion. In challenging cases, however, placement of a PEG tube may be the key strategy that allows the patient to finally achieve gut autonomy and wean off PN.

Rationale: Patients with severe Crohn's disease who require continued immunosuppressive therapy to keep the disease process in remission are at high risk for recurrent central line infections. The central line usually must be changed when an infection occurs. The patient may lose weight in the interim, and the risk of running out of intravenous access sites in the future increases. In the absence of disease activity in the remaining small bowel, gut autonomy may be achieved with as little as 70 to 90 cm of remaining small bowel in patients who still have their colon intact. In the absence of a colon, a greater length of small bowel is required (at least 120 to 150 cm) to achieve autonomy. In this patient, who should have enough bowel length to achieve autonomy, the remaining 200 cm of small bowel may be compromised by continued Crohn's disease activity and suboptimal absorption. While the patient is instructed to follow diet recommendations for severe SBS, these measures may not be sufficient to achieve gut autonomy. Provision of a semi-elemental formula at a slow rate throughout the day optimizes efficiency of absorption.

Parenteral Nutrition

PN does not have a role as primary therapy in patients with Crohn's disease.[95,96] The indications for PN in Crohn's disease include SBS with malabsorption that cannot be medically and nutritionally managed, persistent small bowel obstruction, high-output fistulas or enteric fistula originating in a location that does not allow EN distal to the fistula site. It is also reasonable to provide perioperative PN support to severely malnourished patients for 1 to 2 weeks prior to surgery.[97]

Complications

Vitamin and Mineral Deficiencies

Patients with Crohn's disease are at risk for several micronutrient deficiencies. Iron deficiency anemia is frequently related to blood loss. However, iron supplements should not be provided unless a patient has a documented iron deficiency. Enteral iron supplements may exacerbate GI symptoms,[98] and parenteral iron carries an infrequent but real risk of anaphylactic reactions. Several studies indicate that parenteral iron is a more effective and better tolerated way to replete iron stores than enteral iron in patients with inflammatory bowel disease despite an increased risk of adverse events.[99]

Patients with Crohn's disease have a high incidence of hyperhomocysteinemia (associated with increased risk of cardiovascular disease) that is related to decreased serum levels of vitamin B_{12} and folate.[96,108] Ileal resections increase the risk of vitamin B_{12} deficiency, whereas use of methotrexate or sulfasalazine or decreased intake of leafy green vegetables increase the risk of folate deficiency. Additionally, patients with fat malabsorption associated with Crohn's are at increased risk of fat-soluble vitamin deficiency.

Patients with high-output enterocutaneous fistulas and those with frequent diarrhea are at increased risk of zinc deficiency.[101] Although inflammatory conditions can result in temporary decreases in serum zinc that may not represent a true deficiency, patients with excessive GI fluid losses or those with documented zinc deficiency should receive supplemental zinc. The chronic use of zinc supplementation has been associated with subsequent copper deficiency; therefore, copper stores should be monitored in patients who take long-term zinc supplements. See Chapter 8 for additional information on micronutrient assessment and supplementation.

Metabolic Bone Disease

Patients with Crohn's disease are at increased risk of osteopenia and osteoporosis. The estimated incidence of osteopenia in populations with Crohn's disease is between 35% and 40%.[102,103] Periodic exposure to corticosteroids is believed to be a primary etiology, although inflammatory cytokines and malabsorption also contribute. Supplemental calcium to reach a total daily intake of 1500 mg elemental calcium and 800 to 1000 IU of vitamin D per day is recommended to those with frequent use of corticosteroids. Supplemental calcium of 500 mg/d and

vitamin D of 400 IU/d for 2 years in patients with Crohn's disease resulted in a significant increase in BMD.[104]

A nutrient that is frequently underappreciated in terms of osteoporosis risk is vitamin K, which is essential to form osteocalcin. Populations with Crohn's disease have a decreased dietary intake of vitamin K,[105] and fat malabsorption may also contribute to vitamin K losses.

Kidney Stones

Patients with Crohn's disease are at increased risk of forming calcium oxalate kidney stones. The primary mechanism responsible for stone formation is competitive binding of calcium by malabsorbed fat and subsequent increased oxalate uptake in the colon. In the absence of a colon, there is no increased risk of calcium oxalate stones. Evidence to conclusively associate increased oxalate intake and kidney stone formation is weak,[106] and strict restriction of oxalate should not be routinely recommended unless the patient has SBS and an intact colon. Primary treatment for prevention involves copious hydration to support adequate urine output along with calcium supplementation to help bind oxalate.

Ulcerative Colitis

UC is a chronic inflammatory disease of the colon. The incidence of protein-energy malnutrition is lower in UC than in Crohn's disease because the primary nutrient absorptive area (small bowel) is not affected in UC.

There is no evidence to support the use of EN (elemental, semi-elemental, or polymeric) as primary therapy in the treatment of UC.[107] Two studies have demonstrated that EN is tolerated during acute flares of UC.[86,108] Gonzalez-Huix reported that polymeric EN maintained nutrition status with fewer infectious complications compared with PN during severe acute flares.[108] In this study, the rates of remission and need for surgery for patients receiving EN were similar to the rates for those who received PN. Patients who required surgery had significantly fewer postoperative infections after EN than those who received PN.

Nutrition Issues Specific to Ulcerative Colitis

The incidence of iron deficiency anemia related to GI blood loss is higher in UC than in Crohn's disease. Up to 80% of patients with UC may develop iron deficiency anemia.[109]

Patients with long-standing UC are known to be at increased risk of colon cancer. Therefore, folic acid adequacy has special relevance for these patients because of its link to cancer prevention. Two case control studies and a retrospective review have suggested that folate supplementation may have a protective role in cancer prevention in this patient population.[110]

The incidence of osteopenia reported in UC is 25% to 32%, which is somewhat less than that seen in Crohn's disease.[104] Recommendations for increased daily calcium and vitamin D intake are the same as those for Crohn's disease: 1500 mg of elemental calcium and 800 to 1000 IU of vitamin D.

SCFAs (butyrate, acetate, propionate) are fermented in the colon from dietary fiber by colonic microorganisms.

SCFAs serve as fuel for the colonocytes and promote water and sodium absorption in the colon (see Chapters 1 and 4).[98,111] Butyrate enemas reduced inflammation in UC, and, when combined with 5-aminosalicylic acid, resulted in more patients with remission than with 5-aminosalicylic acid alone.[111] However, this intervention is not widely used because of its limited availability. Increased dietary fiber increases colonic butyrate production, and several studies have found that using increased fiber diets or fiber supplements improves symptoms in UC.[112-114]

Cystic Fibrosis

CF, which is also discussed in Chapter 25, is an autosomal recessive genetic disease that currently affects around 30,000 people in the United States and more than 70,000 people worldwide.[115] The disease causes an accumulation of mucus in several organs, including the lungs, GI tract, pancreas, and reproductive system, because of a mutation in the CF transmembrane conductance regulator (CFTR).[115] Between 85% and 90% of patients with CF have EPI because of the buildup of mucus in pancreatic ducts, which prevents pancreatic enzymes from being adequately released during food digestion. This EPI leads to malabsorption with steatorrhea and a need for the addition of exogenous pancreatic enzyme replacement therapy (PERT). Thus, patients with CF are at a heightened risk for malnutrition because of EPI with malabsorption, increased energy requirements related to excessive work of breathing, and challenges with decreased appetite related to chronic infections and medication.[116,117]

Nutrition Assessment and Management

Ongoing nutrition assessment and intervention are crucial to ensure adequate growth in patients with CF, and appropriate nutrition care can also help to preserve lung function and body weight.[118] Comparison and cohort studies as well as CF registry data have shown a direct correlation between body mass index (BMI) and forced expiratory volume in 1 second (FEV$_1$): FEV$_1$ is positively affected by an increase in BMI up to 25.[118] Additionally, survival has been positively linked to a high-fat diet with adequate pancreatic enzyme supplementation compared with a low-fat diet and less pancreatic enzyme supplementation.[119] The Cystic Fibrosis Foundation recommends that pediatric patients achieve a weight-for-length status greater than the 50th percentile for their age and sex by age 2 years and maintain a BMI at or above the 50th percentile from age 2 to age 20 years. These goals are associated with improved pulmonary function later in life.[120] Adult patients 20 years and older should aim to maintain a BMI of 22 (women) or BMI of 23 (men) with limited unintentional weight loss.[121] Pulmonary function, anthropometrics, growth chart trends, nutrition status, and pancreatic activity are addressed at each clinic visit, often quarterly.

Fat-soluble vitamin status, an oral glucose tolerance test, dual-energy X-ray absorptiometry, and liver function tests are reviewed at least annually. A fecal elastase level is obtained after birth to assess pancreatic function and to determine whether the patient needs PERT. Patients who are deemed pancreatic sufficient at birth should be reassessed if they exhibit signs of malabsorption. Clinic visits often involve encounters with the physician, nurse, dietitian, social worker, and respiratory therapist. Endocrinology is another discipline that is often used in well-rounded care of patients with CF.[122,123]

Energy and Protein Requirements

Undernourishment is of concern in CF for several reasons:
- Resting energy expenditure is elevated because of the increased work of breathing with chronic inflammation and infection.[117]
- Fat malabsorption from EPI and dextrosuria from CF-related diabetes (CFRD) increase nutrient losses.[124]
- Patients often have poor appetites and therefore do not intake enough energy. Poor appetite may be related to gastroesophageal reflux, gastroparesis, altered smell and taste from sinusitis/nasal polyps, abdominal pain, SIBO, or constipation.[125]

The prevalence of undernutrition in patients with CF has led to the recommendation for 110% to 200% of estimated energy requirements with adjustment based on individual needs. Patients are strongly encouraged to increase the proportion of fat in their diets to 35% to 40% of daily energy intake (compared with the recommendation of less 30% of energy from fat for the general population), and unnecessary restrictions on diet are discouraged.[123] Patients with advanced lung disease who are candidates for lung transplant need even higher energy requirements, and predictive energy equations are shown to underestimate their energy needs. In advanced CF lung disease, indirect calorimetry is the gold standard for determining energy provision.[126]

Enteral Nutrition

For patients with CF who are unable to grow or maintain weight with food and oral supplement intake alone, it is common and advisable to place a gastrostomy tube for supplemental nutrition, and a jejunostomy tube if gastric feedings are not tolerated. EN is typically provided via nocturnal feeding with the aim to provide 50% to 75% of prescribed nutrition targets. Patients are then advised to meet the remainder of their energy targets via oral intake during the day.[127] The most optimal time for feeding tube placement is debatable; however, placement before the patient develops end-stage lung disease is ideal. When respiratory function declines, especially with advanced CF lung disease, patients are at increased risk for complications with feeding tube placement and have little to no success with weight gain at this time; the less severe the lung disease, the larger the benefit from supplemental EN is.[128,129]

Typically, a concentrated formula is ideal because it provides more nutrition in less volume, and a 1.5 kcal/mL or 2 kcal/mL enteral formula is often used. Depending on growth trends, the severity of malabsorption, and GI issues, patients may benefit from peptide-based EN formulation (elemental or semi-elemental), which has enzymatically hydrolyzed protein as well as greater than 50% of fat from medium-chain triglycerides.[120] See Practice Scenario 26-2.

Practice Scenario 26-2

Question: How can the nutrition and pulmonary status of a patient with cystic fibrosis (CF) be optimized when he or she is already consuming a hyperphagic diet?

Scenario: A 22-year-old man with a history of CF requiring supplemental oxygen presents to the clinic with an inability to gain weight and abdominal distension. Despite eating at least 1900 kcal/d (approximately 35 kcal/kg/d), the patient, who is 67 inches is tall, weighs only 118 pounds. With a body mass index (BMI) of 18.5, he remains underweight. The patient also complains of foul-smelling stools that "stick to the toilet bowl" and are yellow and oily in color and consistency. Alanine transaminase and aspartate transaminase levels are slightly above the upper limit of normal. A 72-hour fecal fat analysis reveals a fat content of 20 g per 24 hours (normal is less 7 g per 24 hours). The patient is vitamin D–deficient and is incidentally found to have an International Normalized Ratio of 1.4.

Intervention: The patient is started on pancreatic enzyme replacement therapy (PERT) with every meal and snacks with fat content. In addition to starting cholecalciferol to correct the vitamin D deficiency, serum levels of fat-soluble vitamins A, E, and K are checked, and vitamin K is found to be low. He is therefore started on oral phytonadione (vitamin K) replacement in addition to a multivitamin with increased levels of vitamins A, D, E, and K. After 2 months of PERT therapy, he feels better, but remains underweight. The patient and his clinicians decide to insert a percutaneous endoscopic gastrostomy tube and begin nightly supplemental enteral nutrition (EN). In 6 months, he gains 12 pounds, his BMI increases to 20, and his forced expiratory volume in 1 minute improves.

Answer: This patient has exocrine pancreatic insufficiency (EPI), a common problem in patients with CF, particularly those with compromised lung function (as indicated by his requirement for supplemental oxygen). Numerous factors contribute to malabsorption and increased metabolic demands, and nutrition requirements are usually greater than predicted based on weight and height.

Rationale: EPI is almost universally present to some degree in patients with CF and usually requires PERT as well as fat-soluble vitamin replacement. CF can also affect the liver, and mild abnormalities in liver enzymes can be seen. Nocturnal EN is a common intervention used to improve nutrition status, weight, and potentially lung function.

Complications

Exocrine Pancreatic Insufficiency

Because of mutations in the CFTR gene, mucus builds up in the pancreas, causing destruction of the acinar cells and inefficient or no release of pancreatic enzymes in about 85% to 90% of patients with CF.[122,130] Patients must therefore consume exogenous enzymes at the start of all fat-containing nutrition.

TABLE 26-9 Commercially Available Pancreatic Enzyme Replacement Therapy

- Porcine-derived oral capsules for oral intake or administration prior to tube feeding (Creon, Zenpep, Pancreaze, and Pertzye, which contains additional bicarbonate)
- Crushable powder tablets for use in tube feeding (Viokace)
- An external enzyme filtration device, which hydrolyzes fat outside the body before infusion via feeding tube (Relizorb)

The goal is for pancreatic enzymes to mix directly with the nutrition consumed to hydrolyze fat and thereby facilitate digestion and absorption. Prior to 2010, pancreatic enzymes were unregulated. However, since 2010, the US Food and Drug Administration must approve all prescribed enzymes for CF.[122,130] Currently, 3 forms of pancreatic enzymes are available (Table 26-9). In recent years, it has become increasingly common for patients to be given multiple types of enzyme for use with both oral intake and tube feeding.[122,130]

Fat-Soluble Vitamin Deficiencies

Fat malabsorption affects fat-soluble vitamin absorption as well. Patients with CF should be screened annually for deficiencies of vitamins A, D, E, and K. To obtain the most accurate levels, the following surveillance tests are recommended:[131,132]

- Vitamin A: Serum vitamin A level
- Vitamin D: 25-OHD level
- Vitamin E: α-tocopherol/cholesterol ratio or α-tocopherol/total serum lipid ratio
- Vitamin K: International Normalized Ratio or protein induced by vitamin K antagonist-II level

Patients are prescribed a specialty fat-soluble multivitamin in a water-miscible form that is taken daily with enzymes to help improve absorption. Additional supplementation of single vitamins may be necessary to achieve optimal levels.[131,133]

Distal Intestinal Obstructive Syndrome

Distal intestinal obstructive syndrome (DIOS) is characterized by a partial or full small bowel obstruction in the terminal ileum of patients with CF. The obstruction is caused by intestinal mucus accumulation mixing with stool. DIOS most commonly occurs in patients with pancreatic insufficiency and in those with a history of meconium ileus or previous DIOS episodes. This history as well as excessive fat malabsorption, post–organ transplant status, dehydration, and CFRD can be precursors to an episode of DIOS. An osmotic laxative bowel regimen can be used for prevention as well as maintenance of intestinal hydration. Additionally, osmotic laxatives in larger doses are the first-line treatment for an acute DIOS episode.[134]

Cystic Fibrosis–Related Diabetes

CFRD is a specific type of diabetes distinct from type 1 or type 2 diabetes mellitus, which occurs in 40% to 50% of adults with CF and around 20% of children with CF. CFRD does not usually occur before age 10 years. Therefore, an annual oral glucose tolerance test is recommended for CF patients who do not have CFRD. Management of CFRD involves insulin coverage with minimal diet restriction to promote growth or weight maintenance.[124]

Gastroparesis

Gastroparesis, described earlier in the chapter, can affect patients with CF. This condition can be secondary to diabetes (specifically CFRD in this population) and may also be related to phrenic nerve injury secondary to thoracic surgery (eg, lung transplant). Gastroparesis is one reason why a jejunostomy feeding tube may be used for supplemental nutrition as opposed to a gastrostomy tube.[135]

Protein-Losing Gastroenteropathy

Protein-losing gastroenteropathy (PLG) is not a specific disorder but a clinical syndrome seen as the result of several disorders with common pathophysiology. The hallmark of PLG is significant hypoalbuminemia and peripheral edema, which is often the initial indicator of the underlying problem. Pleural effusions, ascites, and pericardial effusions can also be present. PLG is associated with various disease states that result in a loss of serum proteins into the GI tract (Table 26-10).[136,137] PLG is thought to occur by 1 of 2 mechanisms: (1) disorders of the GI mucosa and (2) disorders of lymphatic flow.

Radiolabeled human serum albumin was once the gold standard for diagnosing PLG; however, given its technical difficulty and the requirement for radiation exposure, this method has been largely replaced with fecal measurement of alpha-1 antitrypsin clearance, with technetium 99m–labeled human serum albumin used as a confirmatory test if needed.[136,137] Alpha-1 antitrypsin is an endogenous protein synthesized by the liver. It has a molecular weight similar to albumin, but, unlike albumin, it is not degraded in the intestinal lumen, and it is not actively secreted, absorbed, or digested in a healthy GI tract, which makes it a good target to measure intestinal protein loss. However, it is degraded at a pH less than 3; therefore, patients undergoing alpha-1 antitrypsin clearance evaluation should take a PPI concomitantly to avoid false-negative results in those who are losing protein from the stomach mucosa.[138] In PLG, the GI loss of albumin and other plasma proteins occurs faster than the body can synthesize new proteins.[139] Consequently, the hypoalbuminemia cannot be reversed simply by providing additional protein to the patient.

The mainstay of PLG treatment is to treat the underlying disease, which is necessary in most cases of PLG. To address the protein loss specifically, dietary therapy is often the initial management strategy, specifically the restriction of long-chain fatty acids from the diet. The absorption of long-chain fatty acids increases intestinal lymph flow, thus increasing pressure in the intestinal lymphatics and resulting in further protein leakage into the intestinal lumen. A very low-fat diet (less than 20 g/d) may relieve pressure in the lymphatic system and decrease protein losses.[140] Alternatively, enteral formulations high in medium-chain fatty acids may be used. These fats are not absorbed through the lymphatics and are transported

TABLE 26-10 Disorders Associated with Protein-Losing Gastroenteropathies

Disorders of the mucosa:
- Without erosions or ulceration:
  — Acquired immunodeficiency syndrome–associated gastroenteropathy
  — Acute viral gastroenteritis
  — Allergic enteritis
  — Celiac disease
  — Collagenous colitis
  — Eosinophilic gastroenteritis
  — Hypertrophic hypersecretory gastropathy
  — Small intestinal bacterial overgrowth
  — Parasitic diseases: malaria, giardiasis, schistosomiasis, nematodiasis
  — Lymphocytic colitis
  — Tropical sprue
  — Vascular ectasia (gastric, colonic)
  — Whipple disease
- With erosions or ulceration:
  — Alpha-chain disease
  — Amyloidosis, Behçet disease
  — Carcinoid syndrome
  — Crohn's disease
  — Duodenitis
  — Erosive gastritis
  — Gastrointestinal carcinomas
  — Graft-vs-host disease
  — *Helicobacter pylori* gastritis
  — Idiopathic ulcerative jejunoileitis
  — Infectious diarrhea: *Clostridium difficile* infection, shigellosis
  — Kaposi sarcoma
  — Lymphoma
  — Neurofibromatosis
  — Ulcerative colitis
  — Waldenström macroglobulinemia

Disorders of lymphatic flow:
- Congestive heart failure
- Constrictive pericarditis
- Increased central venous pressure
- Intestinal endometriosis
- Intestinal lymphangiectasia (congenital, acquired)
- Lymphenteric fistula
- Lymphoma
- Mesenteric tuberculosis and sarcoidosis
- Mesenteric venous thrombosis
- Portal hypertensive gastroenteropathy
- Posttransplant lymphoproliferative disease
- Retroperitoneal fibrosis
- Sclerosing mesenteritis
- Systemic lupus erythematosus
- Whipple disease

Source: Data are from references 136 and 137.

across the mucosa directly into the portal system. Medium-chain fatty acids provide a source of energy, but they do not contain the essential fatty acids linoleic and α-linolenic acid; therefore, patients are at increased risk of essential fatty acid deficiency (EFAD) and fat-soluble vitamin deficiencies. The plasma triene-to-tetraene ratio is used to assess for EFAD, and the fat-soluble vitamins A, D, E, and K should be monitored.

PN may be indicated in those patients with failure to thrive or with no symptom improvement when receiving very low-fat EN. Because of the varied nature and infrequent occurrence of PLG, no randomized trials have been done to determine the optimum nutrition regimen. The goal is to help restore protein balance when possible. The available data are in the form of retrospective reviews, which suggest that both EN and PN therapy are effective ways to provide nutrition for some patients with PLG who cannot maintain adequate nutrition on an oral low-fat diet alone.[141]

Carbohydrate Maldigestion and Intolerance

Carbohydrate maldigestion is one of the most common disorders of the GI system. The prevalence of lactose intolerance varies greatly by race and ethnicity because of the variable expression of the lactase dehydrogenase enzyme in the brush border of the small intestine and numerous other factors, including the dose of ingested lactose, intestinal transit time, gut microbiota, and the presence of SIBO. Although almost all humans are born with the ability to split the lactase molecule into its 2 separate simple sugars, glucose and galactose, mucosal expression of the enzyme decreases as humans age, and up to 95% of adults of African and 99% of adults of South Asian descent cannot digest lactase.[142] In contrast, loss of lactase expression affects approximately 10% of people of Northern European descent, perhaps because people in this region adopted dairy cultivation thousands of years ago. Fructose intolerance is less common than lactose intolerance and not as well studied.[143]

Unabsorbed small molecule carbohydrates such as lactose and fructose in the intestinal lumen cause an osmotic gradient, thus bringing water into the intestine and contributing to diarrhea. Also, the commensal gut microbes ferment the simple sugars, creating hydrogen and methane gases, which are thought to be responsible for the uncomfortable bloating experienced by those with a carbohydrate intolerance. Recently, investigators have theorized that a class of simple sugars known as FODMAPs (fermentable oligo-, di-, and monosaccharides and polyols) cause symptoms of malabsorption and maldigestion, and FODMAPs have been demonstrated to exacerbate symptoms of irritable bowel syndrome. A low-FODMAPs diet has been proposed to help manage the uncomfortable symptoms.[144]

The diagnostic tests most often used to evaluate patients with suspected carbohydrate maldigestion are breath tests where subjects ingest a small amount of the substance in question then breathe into a collection system every 15 to 20 minutes thereafter for a period of 2 to 3 hours. Hydrogen and methane levels are measured, and the presence or absence of maldigestion is confirmed based on the rise in gas levels as well as patient-reported symptoms. These tests are noninvasive and inexpensive, but confounders make the interpretation of the tests difficult. Many practitioners eschew formal testing and instead recommend dietary elimination trials to determine the clinical effect of food elimination.

Food Allergies and Eosinophilic Esophagitis

Most true food allergies are IgE-mediated disorders of the adaptive immune system, and they result in classic symptoms of urticaria (hives), eczema, angioedema (mucosal swelling of the tongue, lips, face, and other mucous membranes), and sometimes vomiting and diarrhea. Respiratory distress is caused by swelling of the oropharynx and epiglottis that compromises oxygen intake into the lungs, swelling of the bronchial mucosa that limits oxygen diffusion into the bloodstream, and bronchospasm. *Anaphylaxis* is the term for the respiratory compromise and cardiovascular collapse caused by food allergies, and it is a medical emergency that requires immediate treatment. Most patients at risk for an anaphylactic reaction are advised to carry autoinjecting epinephrine "pens" to begin treatment immediately if they are unexpectedly exposed to an allergen. In the United States, food allergies are estimated to affect anywhere from 3 million to 38 million people, depending on whether prevalence is measured by allergy testing or self-report and whether children or adults are studied.[145] The allergens in 8 foods—wheat, eggs, soy, dairy (cow's milk), peanuts, tree nuts, fish, and shellfish— are responsible for 90% of all food allergies in the United States.[145]

While most true food allergies are IgE-mediated and result in the classic symptoms described above, there are other mixed-IgE-mediated, non-IgE-mediated, or cell-mediated immune reactions to food allergens. Celiac disease (described earlier) is a type of non-IgE-mediated immune reaction to food. Food protein enterocolitis syndrome (FPIES, also known as cow's milk protein enterocolitis), oral allergy syndrome, eosinophilic esophagitis (EoE), and eosinophilic gastroenteritis (EoG) are additional examples.[145] FPIES is mostly seen in children who are weaning from breast milk or formula. Affected infants experience vomiting and bloody diarrhea. Treatment for FPIES is avoidance of the allergen, and most infants will eventually grow out of it. Oral allergy syndrome occurs when a person who is allergic to certain environmental pollens has a reaction to food with a similar chemical structure. This syndrome can usually be managed by cooking the culprit food items, thus denaturing the protein antigen and rendering it nontoxic. A syndrome that often affects health care workers is latex-fruit syndrome. Like oral allergy syndrome, it is seen in those who have a latex allergy and then develop symptoms of anaphylaxis when they consume fruit with very similar protein antigens. Cross-reactive fruits include kiwi, tomato, peach, potato, chestnut, banana, avocado, fig, bell pepper, mango, and possibly cucumbers, papaya, jackfruit, cassava, turnips, and zucchini.[146-149]

EoE and EoG are rare but increasing in prevalence. In EoE and EoG, affected patients can have a wide spectrum of symptoms ranging from dysphagia and food impaction (the most common presenting features of EoE) to bloating, diarrhea, and malabsorption. Mucosal biopsies show a dense eosinophilic infiltrate; indeed, the diagnostic criteria for EoE and EoG requires greater than 15 eosinophils per high-powered field.[150] The cellular mechanisms underlying EoE and EoG are not fully delineated; however, they show features of both IgE-mediated and non-IgE-mediated processes.[145] Medical treatment usually employs courses of topical steroid therapy (swallowed fluticasone or budesonide capsules). Systemic steroid therapy seems to be less effective. Unfortunately, the rate of relapse is high, and steroid-sparing medical therapies are not available.

Given the refractory nature of EoE and EoG and their occurrence in children where long-term steroid therapy has significant downsides, dietary therapy has been studied and is successful in most affected individuals. Exclusive EN with an elemental formula is effective at inducing remission in affected patients; however, the disease relapses with reintroduction of solid foods.[151] Additionally, exclusive elemental EN is not a practical therapy for extended use, and the formula is exceedingly expensive and unpalatable. Research on targeted elimination-diet therapy based on allergy testing was initially disappointing, with less than 50% of subjects responding. Greatly improved success has been seen with diets that empirically eliminate the 6 most common food triggers: wheat, dairy, soy, eggs, fish/shellfish, and nuts. The so-called 6-food elimination diet has been shown to be effective in up to 70% of patients with EoE.[152] Modifications of this diet that eliminate 4 or sometimes 2 foods (wheat and dairy, the 2 most common inciting agents) are also successful and may increase patient compliance.[153] Medical nutrition therapy has given patients with these rare disorders options for management that allow them to experience a better quality of life without the concern of the significant adverse effects of long-term steroid therapy.

References

1. Tougas G, Eaker EY, Abell TL, et al. Assessment of gastric emptying using a low-fat meal: establishment of international control values. Am J Gastroenterol. 2000;95(6):1456–1462.
2. Horowitz M, Harding PE, Maddox AF, et al. Gastric and oesophageal emptying in patients with type 2 (non-insulin-dependent) diabetes mellitus. Diabetologia. 1989;32(3):151–159.
3. Naftali T, Yishai R, Zangen T, Levine A. Post-infectious gastroparesis: clinical and electerogastrographic aspects. J Gastroenterol Hepatol. 2007;22(9):1423–1428.
4. Stanghellini V, Cogliandro RF, de Giorgio R, et al. Chronic intestinal pseudo-obstruction: manifestations, natural history and management. Neurogastroenterol Motil. 2007;19(6):440–452.
5. Hallberg L, Brune M, Rossander-Hulthen L. Is there a physiological role of vitamin C in iron absorption? Ann N Y Acad Sci. 1987;498:324–332.
6. American Gastroenterological Association medical position statement: nausea and vomiting. Gastroenterology. 2001;120(1):261–263.
7. Abell TL, Bernstein RK, Cutts T, et al. Treatment of gastroparesis: a multidisciplinary clinical review. Neurogastroenterol Motil. 2006;18(4):263–283.
8. Camilleri M, Parkman HP, Shafi MA, Abell TL, Gerson L. Clinical guideline: management of gastroparesis. Am J Gastroenterol. 2013;108(1):18-37.
9. Friedenberg FK, Palit A, Parkman HP, Hanlon A, Nelson DB. Botulinum toxin A for the treatment of delayed gastric emptying. Am J Gastroenterol. 2008;103(2):416–423.
10. University of Virginia Health System, Nutrition Support Traineeship Syllabus. Charlottesville, VA; updated July 2016. www.ginutrition.virginia.edu.
11. McCray S, Parrish CR. Refeeding the malnourished patient: lessons learned. Pract Gastroenterol. 2016;40(9):27–37.
12. Palmer LB, McClave SA, Bechtold ML, et al. Tips and tricks for deep jejunal enteral access: modifying techniques to maximize success. Curr Gastroenterol Rep. 2014;16(10):409.
13. Parrish CR. Nutritional considerations in the patient with gastroparesis. Gastroenterol Clin N Am. 2015;44(1):83–95.
14. Parrish CR. Enteral feeding: the art and the science. Nutr Clin Pract. 2003;18(1):76–85.
15. Radigan A. Post-gastrectomy: managing the nutrition fall-out. Pract Gastroenterol. 2004;28(6):63–75.
16. Pawson R, Mehta A. Review article: the diagnosis and treatment of haematinic deficiency in gastrointestinal disease. Aliment Pharmacol Ther. 1998;12(8):687–698.
17. Harju E. Metabolic problems after gastric surgery. Int Surg. 1990;75(1):27–35.
18. MacGregor IL, Gueller R, Watts HD, Meyer JH. The effect of acute hyperglycemia on gastric emptying in man. Gastroenterology. 1976; 70(2):190–196.
19. Rayner CK, Su YC, Doran SM, et al. The stimulation of antral motility by erythromycin is attenuated by hyperglycemia. Am J Gastroenterol. 2000;95(9):2233–2241.
20. Bilimoria KY, Bentrem DJ, Ko CY, et al. Validation of the 6th edition AJCC Pancreatic Cancer Staging System: report from the National Cancer Database. Cancer. 2007;110(4):738–744.
21. Sanders MK. Bezoars: from mystical charms to medical and nutritional management. Pract Gastroenterol. 2004;28(1):37–50.
22. Hayashi K, Ohara H, Naitoh I, et al. Persimmon bezoar successfully treated by oral intake of Coca-Cola: a case report. Cases J. 2008;1(1):385.
23. Lin CS, Tung CF, Peng YC, et al. Successful treatment with a combination of endoscopic injection and irrigation with Coca-Cola for gastric bezoar-induced gastric outlet obstruction. J Chinese Med Assoc. 2008;71(1):49–52.
24. Silva FG, Goncalves C, Vasconcelos H, Cotrim I. Endoscopic and enzymatic treatment of gastric bezoar with acetylcysteine. Endoscopy. 2002;34(10):845.
25. Schlang HA. Acetylcysteine in removal of bezoar. JAMA. 1970; 214(7):1329.
26. DiBaise JK. Small intestinal bacterial overgrowth: nutritional consequences and patients at risk. Pract Gastroenterol. 2008;32(12).
27. Lin HC. Small intestinal bacterial overgrowth: a framework for understanding irritable bowel syndrome. JAMA. 2004;292(7): 852–858.
28. Teo M, Chung S, Chitti L, et al. Small bowel bacterial overgrowth is a common cause of chronic diarrhea. J Gastroenterol Hepatol. 2004;19(8):904–909.
29. Strid H, Simren M, Stotzer PO, et al. Patients with chronic renal failure have abnormal small intestinal motility and a high prevalence of small intestinal bacterial overgrowth. Digestion. 2003; 67(3):129–137.
30. Gunnarsdottir SA, Sadik R, Shev S, et al. Small intestinal motility disturbances and bacterial overgrowth in patients with liver cirrhosis and portal hypertension. Am J Gastroenterol. 2003; 98(6):1362–1370.
31. Trespi E, Ferrieri A. Intestinal bacterial overgrowth during chronic pancreatitis. Curr Med Res Opin. 1999;15(1):47–52.
32. Toskes PP, Giannella RA, Jervis HR, Rout WR, Takeuchi A. Small intestinal mucosal injury in the experimental blind loop syndrome. Light- and electron-microscopic and histochemical studies. Gastroenterology. 1975;68(5 Pt 1):1193–1203.

33. Su J, Smith MB, Rerknimitr R, Morrow D. Small intestine bacterial overgrowth presenting as protein-losing enteropathy. *Dig Dis Sci.* 1998;43(3):679–681.

34. Di Stefano M, Miceli E, Missanelli A, Corazza GR. Treatment of small intestine bacterial overgrowth. *Eur Rev Med Pharmacol Sci.* 2005;9(4):217–222.

35. Di Stefano M, Malservisi S, Veneto G, Ferrieri A, Corazza GR. Rifaximin versus chlortetracycline in the short-term treatment of small intestinal bacterial overgrowth. *Aliment Pharmacol Ther.* 2000;14(5):551–556.

36. Fasano A, Catassi C. Current approaches to diagnosis and treatment of celiac disease: an evolving spectrum. *Gastroenterology.* 2001;120(3):636–651.

37. Murray JA. The widening spectrum of celiac disease. *Am J Clin Nutr.* 1999;69(3):354–365.

38. US National Library of Medicine Genetics Home Reference. Human leukocyte antigens. 2016. https://ghr.nlm.nih.gov/primer/genefamily/hla. Accessed September 2, 2016.

39. Cassinotti A, Birindelli S, Clerici M, et al. HLA and autoimmune digestive disease: a clinically oriented review for gastroenterologists. *Am J Gastroenterol.* 2009;104(1):195–217.

40. Sollid LM, Lie BA. Celiac disease genetics: current concepts and practical applications. *Clin Gastroenterol Hepatol.* 2005; 3(9):843–851.

41. Gujral N, Freeman HJ, Thomson AB. Celiac disease: prevalence, diagnosis, pathogenesis and treatment. *World J Gastroenterol.* 2012;18(42):6036–6059.

42. Rubio-Tapia A, Ludvigsson JF, Brantner TL, Murray JA, Everhart JE. The prevalence of celiac disease in the United States. *Am J Gastroenterol.* 2012;107(10):1538–1544.

43. Crowe SE. In the clinic. Celiac disease. *Ann Intern Med.* 2011; 154(9):ITC5-1–ITC5-15.

44. Alaedini A, Green PH. Narrative review: celiac disease: understanding a complex autoimmune disorder. *Ann Intern Med.* 2005;142(4):289–298.

45. Hill ID, Dirks MH, Liptak GS, et al. Guideline for the diagnosis and treatment of celiac disease in children: recommendations of the North American Society for Pediatric Gastroenterology, Hepatology and Nutrition. *J Pediatr Gastroenterol Nutr.* 2005;40(1):1–19.

46. Rubio-Tapia A, Hill ID, Kelly CP, Calderwood AH, Murray JA. ACG clinical guidelines: diagnosis and management of celiac disease. *Am J Gastroenterol.* 2013;108(5):656–676.

47. Husby S, Koletzko S, Korponay-Szabo IR, et al. European Society for Pediatric Gastroenterology, Hepatology, and Nutrition guidelines for the diagnosis of coeliac disease. *J Pediatr Gastroenterol Nutr.* 2012;54(1):136–160.

48. Duggan JM, Duggan AE. Systematic review: the liver in coeliac disease. *Aliment Pharmacol Ther.* 2005;21(5):515–518.

49. Ciacci C, Cirillo M, Cavallaro R, Mazzacca G. Long-term follow-up of celiac adults on gluten-free diet: prevalence and correlates of intestinal damage. *Digestion.* 2002;66(3):178–185.

50. Case S. *Gluten-Free Diet: A Comprehensive Resource Guide.* Regina, Canada: Case Nutrition Consulting; 2006.

51. Lee HJ, Anderson Z, Ryu D. Gluten contamination in foods labeled as "gluten free" in the United States. *J Food Protect.* 2014; 77(10):1830–1833.

52. Comino I, Moreno Mde L, Sousa C. Role of oats in celiac disease. *World J Gastroenterol.* 2015;21(41):11825–11831.

53. Case S. The gluten-free diet: how to provide effective education and resources. *Gastroenterology.* 2005;128(4 Suppl 1):S128–S134.

54. Zarkadas M, Cranney A, Case S, et al. The impact of a gluten-free diet on adults with coeliac disease: results of a national survey. *J Hum Nutr Diet.* 2006;19(1):41–49.

55. Green PHR, Stavropoulos SN, Panagi SG, et al. Characteristics of adult celiac disease in the USA: results of a national survey. *Am J Gastroenterol.* 2001;96(1):126–131.

56. Sverker A, Hensing G, Hallert C. "Controlled by food"—lived experiences of coeliac disease. *J Hum Nutr Diet.* 2005;18(3): 171–180.

57. Murray JA, Watson T, Clearman B, Mitros F. Effect of a gluten-free diet on gastrointestinal symptoms in celiac disease. *Am J Clin Nutr.* 2004;79(4):669–673.

58. Farrell RJ, Kelly CP. Celiac sprue. *N Engl J Med.* 2002; 346(3):180–188.

59. Mandal A, Mayberry J. Elemental diet in the treatment of refractory coeliac disease. *Eur J Gastroenterol Hepatol.* 2001;13(1):79–80.

60. Vici G, Belli L, Biondi M, Polzonetti V. Gluten free diet and nutrient deficiencies: a review. *Clin Nutr (Edinburgh).* 2016;35(6): 1236–1241.

61. Caruso R, Pallone F, Stasi E, Romeo S, Monteleone G. Appropriate nutrient supplementation in celiac disease. *Ann Med.* 2013; 45(8):522–531.

62. Dahele A, Ghosh S. Vitamin B12 deficiency in untreated celiac disease. *Am J Gastroenterol.* 2001;96(3):745–750.

63. Fasano A, Berti I, Gerarduzzi T, et al. Prevalence of celiac disease in at-risk and not-at-risk groups in the United States: a large multicenter study. *Arch Intern Med.* 2003;163(3):286–292.

64. Murray JA. Celiac disease in patients with an affected member, type 1 diabetes, iron-deficiency, or osteoporosis? *Gastroenterology.* 2005;128(4 Suppl 1):S52–S56.

65. Hoffman RJ, Dhaliwal G, Gilden DJ, Saint S. Clinical problem-solving. Special cure. *N Engl J Med.* 2004;351(19):1997–2002.

66. Corazza GR, Di Stefano M, Maurino E, Bai JC. Bones in coeliac disease: diagnosis and treatment. *Best Pract Res Clin Gastroenterol.* 2005;19(3):453–465.

67. National Institutes of Health Consensus Development Conference statement on celiac disease, June 28-30, 2004. *Gastroenterology.* 2005;128(4 Suppl 1):S1–S9.

68. Lasa JS, Zubiaurre I, Soifer LO. Risk of infertility in patients with celiac disease: a meta-analysis of observational studies. *Arq Gastroenterol.* 2014;51(2):144–150.

69. Dhalwani NN, West J, Sultan AA, Ban L, Tata LJ. Women with celiac disease present with fertility problems no more often than women in the general population. *Gastroenterology.* 2014;147(6): 1267–1274.

70. Tersigni C, Castellani R, de Waure C, et al. Celiac disease and reproductive disorders: meta-analysis of epidemiologic associations and potential pathogenic mechanisms. *Hum Reprod Update.* 2014;20(4):582–593.

71. Park T, Cave D, Marshall C. Microscopic colitis: A review of etiology, treatment and refractory disease. *World J Gastroenterol.* 2015;21(29):8804–8810.

72. Abdulkarim AS, Murray JA. Celiac disease. *Curr Treat Gastroenterol.* 2002;5(1):27–38.

73. Ciclitira PJ, Ellis HJ, Lundin KE. Gluten-free diet—what is toxic? *Best Pract Res Clin Gastroenterol.* 2005;19(3):359–371.

74. Nijeboer P, van Wanrooij RL, Tack GJ, Mulder CJ, Bouma G. Update on the diagnosis and management of refractory coeliac disease. *Gastroenterol Res Pract.* 2013;2013:518483.

75. Henderson P, Casey A, Lawrence SJ, et al. The diagnostic accuracy of fecal calprotectin during the investigation of suspected pediatric inflammatory bowel disease. *Am J Gastroenterol.* 2012; 107(6):941–949.

76. Sandborn WJ, Loftus EV, Jr., Colombel JF, et al. Evaluation of serologic disease markers in a population-based cohort of patients with ulcerative colitis and Crohn's disease. *Inflamm Bowel Dis.* 2001;7(3):192–201.

77. Krok KL, Lichtenstein GR. Nutrition in Crohn disease. *Curr Opin Gastroenterol.* 2003;19(2):148–153.

78. Chan AT, Fleming CR, O'Fallon WM, Huizenga KA. Estimated versus measured basal energy requirements in patients with Crohn's disease. *Gastroenterology.* 1986;91(1):75–78.

79. Stokes MA, Hill GL. Total energy expenditure in patients with Crohn's disease: measurement by the combined body scan technique. *JPEN J Parenter Enteral Nutr.* 1993;17(1):3–7.

80. Eiden K. Nutritional considerations in inflammatory bowel disease. *Pract Gastroenterol.* 2003;27(5).

81. Shah ND, Limketkai BN. Low residue vs. low fiber diets in inflammatory bowel disease: evidence to support vs. habit? *Pract Gastroenterol.* 2015;49(7).

82. Park RH, Duncan A, Russell RI. Hypolactasia and Crohn's disease: a myth. *Am J Gastroenterol.* 1990;85(6):708–710.

83. von Tirpitz C, Kohn C, Steinkamp M, et al. Lactose intolerance in active Crohn's disease: clinical value of duodenal lactase analysis. *J Clin Gastroenterol.* 2002;34(1):49–53.

84. Mishkin B, Yalovsky M, Mishkin S. Increased prevalence of lactose malabsorption in Crohn's disease patients at low risk for lactose malabsorption based on ethnic origin. *Am J Gastroenterol.* 1997;92(7):1148–1153.

85. Pironi L, Callegari C, Cornia GL, et al. Lactose malabsorption in adult patients with Crohn's disease. *Am J Gastroenterol.* 1988; 83(11):1267–1271.

86. Klaassen J, Zapata R, Mella JG, et al. [Enteral nutrition in severe ulcerative colitis. Digestive tolerance and nutritional efficiency]. *Rev Med Chil.* 1998;126(8):899–904.

87. Ruemmele FM, Veres G, Kolho KL, et al. Consensus guidelines of ECCO/ESPGHAN on the medical management of pediatric Crohn's disease. *J Crohns Colitis.* 2014;8(10):1179–1207.

88. Griffiths AM, Ohlsson A, Sherman PM, Sutherland LR. Meta-analysis of enteral nutrition as a primary treatment of active Crohn's disease. *Gastroenterology.* 1995;108(4):1056–1067.

89. Makola D. Elemental and semi-elemental formulas: are they superior to polymeric formulas? *Pract Gastroenterol.* 2005;29(12): 59–72.

90. Gassull MA, Fernandez-Banares F, Cabre E, et al. Fat composition may be a clue to explain the primary therapeutic effect of enteral nutrition in Crohn's disease: results of a double-blind randomised multicentre European trial. *Gut.* 2002;51(2):164–168.

91. Sakurai T, Matsui T, Yao T, et al. Short-term efficacy of enteral nutrition in the treatment of active Crohn's disease: a randomized, controlled trial comparing nutrient formulas. *JPEN J Parenter Enteral Nutr.* 2002;26(2):98–103.

92. Akobeng AK, Miller V, Stanton J, Elbadri AM, Thomas AG. Double-blind randomized controlled trial of glutamine-enriched polymeric diet in the treatment of active Crohn's disease. *J Pediatr Gastroenterol Nutr.* 2000;30(1):78–84.

93. Den Hond E, Hiele M, Peeters M, Ghoos Y, Rutgeerts P. Effect of long-term oral glutamine supplements on small intestinal permeability in patients with Crohn's disease. *JPEN J Parenter Enteral Nutr.* 1999;23(1):7–11.

94. Ockenga J, Borchert K, Stuber E, et al. Glutamine-enriched total parenteral nutrition in patients with inflammatory bowel disease. *Eur J Clin Nutr.* 2005;59(11):1302–1309.

95. Goh J, O'Morain CA. Review article: nutrition and adult inflammatory bowel disease. *Aliment Pharmacol Ther.* 2003;17(3):307–320.

96. Guidelines for the use of parenteral and enteral nutrition in adult and pediatric patients. *JPEN J Parenter Enteral Nutr.* 2002; 26(1 Suppl):1SA–138SA.

97. Detsky AS, Baker JP, O'Rourke K, et al. Predicting nutrition-associated complications for patients undergoing gastrointestinal surgery. *JPEN J Parenter Enteral Nutr.* 1987;11(5):440–446.

98. Erichsen K, Ulvik RJ, Nysaeter G, et al. Oral ferrous fumarate or intravenous iron sucrose for patients with inflammatory bowel disease. *Scan J Gastroenterol.* 2005;40(9):1058–1065.

99. Bonovas S, Fiorino G, Allocca M, et al. Intravenous versus oral iron for the treatment of anemia in inflammatory bowel disease: a systematic review and meta-analysis of randomized controlled trials. *Medicine.* 2016;95(2):e2308.

100. Chowers Y, Sela BA, Holland R, et al. Increased levels of homocysteine in patients with Crohn's disease are related to folate levels. *Am J Gastroenterol.* 2000;95(12):3498–3502.

101. Wolman SL, Anderson GH, Marliss EB, Jeejeebhoy KN. Zinc in total parenteral nutrition: requirements and metabolic effects. *Gastroenterology.* 1979;76(3):458–467.

102. Vestergaard P. Prevalence and pathogenesis of osteoporosis in patients with inflammatory bowel disease. *Minerva Med.* 2004; 95(6):469–480.

103. Schulte CM. Review article: bone disease in inflammatory bowel disease. *Aliment Pharmacol Ther.* 2004;20(Suppl 4):S43–S49.

104. Siffledeen JS, Fedorak RN, Siminoski K, et al. Randomized trial of etidronate plus calcium and vitamin D for treatment of low bone mineral density in Crohn's disease. *Clin Gastroenterol Hepatol.* 2005;3(2):122–132.

105. Duggan P, O'Brien M, Kiely M, McCarthy J, Shanahan F, Cashman KD. Vitamin K status in patients with Crohn's disease and relationship to bone turnover. *Am J Gastroenterol.* 2004; 99(11):2178–2185.

106. Taylor EN, Curhan GC. Oxalate intake and the risk for nephrolithiasis. *J Am Soc Nephrol.* 2007;18(7):2198–2204.

107. Gassull MA. Nutrition and inflammatory bowel disease: its relation to pathophysiology, outcome and therapy. *Dig Dis (Basel).* 2003;21(3):220–227.

108. Gonzalez-Huix F, Fernandez-Banares F, Esteve-Comas M, et al. Enteral versus parenteral nutrition as adjunct therapy in acute ulcerative colitis. *Am J Gastroenterol.* 1993;88(2):227–232.

109. Wilson A, Reyes E, Ofman J. Prevalence and outcomes of anemia in inflammatory bowel disease: a systematic review of the literature. *Am J Med.* 2004;116(Suppl 7A):44S–49S.

110. Diculescu M, Ciocirlan M, Ciocirlan M, et al. Folic acid and sulfasalazine for colorectal carcinoma chemoprevention in patients with ulcerative colitis: the old and new evidence. *Romanian J Gastroenterol.* 2003;12(4):283–286.

111. Vernia P, Annese V, Bresci G, et al. Topical butyrate improves efficacy of 5-ASA in refractory distal ulcerative colitis: results of a multicentre trial. *Eur J Clin Invest.* 2003;33(3):244–248.

112. Seidner DL, Lashner BA, Brzezinski A, et al. An oral supplement enriched with fish oil, soluble fiber, and antioxidants for corticosteroid sparing in ulcerative colitis: a randomized, controlled trial. *Clin Gastroenterol Hepatol.* 2005;3(4):358–369.

113. Hallert C, Bjorck I, Nyman M, et al. Increasing fecal butyrate in ulcerative colitis patients by diet: controlled pilot study. *Inflamm Bowel Dis.* 2003;9(2):116–121.

114. Fernandez-Banares F, Hinojosa J, Sanchez-Lombrana JL, et al. Randomized clinical trial of Plantago ovata seeds (dietary fiber) as compared with mesalamine in maintaining remission in ulcerative colitis. Spanish Group for the Study of Crohn's Disease and Ulcerative Colitis (GETECCU). *Am J Gastroenterol.* 1999;94(2):427–433.

115. Cystic Fibrosis Foundation. About cystic fibrosis. https://www.cff.org/What-is-CF/About-Cystic-Fibrosis. Accessed August 9, 2016.

116. Solomon M, Bozic M, Mascarenhas MR. Nutritional issues in cystic fibrosis. *Clin Chest Med.* 2016;37(1):97–107.

117. Culhane S, George C, Pearo B, Spoede E. Malnutrition in cystic fibrosis: a review. *Nutr Clin Pract.* 2013;28(6):676–683.

118. Stephenson AL, Mannik LA, Walsh S, et al. Longitudinal trends in nutritional status and the relation between lung function and

BMI in cystic fibrosis: a population-based cohort study. *Am J Clin Nutr.* 2013;97(4):872–877.

119. Corey M, McLaughlin FJ, Williams M, Levison H. A comparison of survival, growth, and pulmonary function in patients with cystic fibrosis in Boston and Toronto. *J Clin Epidemiol.* 1988;41(6):583–591.

120. Yen EH, Quinton H, Borowitz D. Better nutritional status in early childhood is associated with improved clinical outcomes and survival in patients with cystic fibrosis. *J Pediatr.* 2013;162(3):530–535.e531.

121. Cystic Fibrosis Foundation. *Cystic Fibrosis Foundation Patient Data Registry.* Bethesda, MD: Cystic Fibrosis Foundation; 2009.

122. Stallings VA, Stark LJ, Robinson KA, Feranchak AP, Quinton H. Evidence-based practice recommendations for nutrition-related management of children and adults with cystic fibrosis and pancreatic insufficiency: results of a systematic review. *J Am Diet Assoc.* 2008;108(5):832–839.

123. Borowitz D, Baker RD, Stallings V. Consensus report on nutrition for pediatric patients with cystic fibrosis. *J Pediatr Gastroenterol Nutr.* 2002;35(3):246–259.

124. Moran A, Brunzell C, Cohen RC, et al. Clinical care guidelines for cystic fibrosis-related diabetes: a position statement of the American Diabetes Association and a clinical practice guideline of the Cystic Fibrosis Foundation, endorsed by the Pediatric Endocrine Society. *Diabetes Care.* 2010;33(12):2697–2708.

125. Nasr SZ, Drury D. Appetite stimulants use in cystic fibrosis. *Pediatr Pulmonol.* 2008;43(3):209–219.

126. Hollander FM, Kok A, de Roos NM, Belle-van Meerkerk G, van de Graaf EA. Prediction equations underestimate resting energy expenditure in patients with end-stage cystic fibrosis. *Nutr Clin Pract.* 2017;32(1):116–121.

127. Matel JL. Nutritional management of cystic fibrosis. *JPEN J Parenter Enteral Nutr.* 2012;36(1 Suppl):60S–67S.

128. Oliver MR, Heine RG, Ng CH, Volders E, Olinsky A. Factors affecting clinical outcome in gastrostomy-fed children with cystic fibrosis. *Pediatr Pulmonol.* 2004;37(4):324–329.

129. Bradley GM, Carson KA, Leonard AR, Mogayzel PJ, Oliva-Hemker M. Nutritional outcomes following gastrostomy in children with cystic fibrosis. *Pediatr Pulmonol.* 2012;47(8):743–748.

130. Berry AJ. Pancreatic enzyme replacement therapy during pancreatic insufficiency. *Nutr Clin Pract.* 2014;29(3):312–321.

131. Maqbool A, Stallings VA. Update on fat-soluble vitamins in cystic fibrosis. *Curr Opin Pulm Med.* 2008;14(6):574–581.

132. Sathe MN, Patel AS. Update in pediatrics: focus on fat-soluble vitamins. *Nutr Clin Pract.* 2010;25(4):340–346.

133. Tangpricha V, Kelly A, Stephenson A, et al. An update on the screening, diagnosis, management, and treatment of vitamin D deficiency in individuals with cystic fibrosis: evidence-based recommendations from the Cystic Fibrosis Foundation. *J Clin Endocrinol Metab.* 2012;97(4):1082–1093.

134. Colombo C, Ellemunter H, Houwen R, et al. Guidelines for the diagnosis and management of distal intestinal obstruction syndrome in cystic fibrosis patients. *J Cyst Fibros.* 2011;10(Suppl 2):S24–S28.

135. Pauwels A, Blondeau K, Mertens V, et al. Gastric emptying and different types of reflux in adult patients with cystic fibrosis. *Aliment Pharmacol Ther.* 2011;34(7):799–807.

136. Karbach U, Singe CC, Ewe K. Simplified determination of intestinal protein excretion based on alpha 1-antitrypsin clearance. *Zeitschrift Gastroenterol.* 1988;26(3):169–173.

137. Chiu NT, Lee BF, Hwang SJ, et al. Protein-losing enteropathy: diagnosis with (99m)Tc-labeled human serum albumin scintigraphy. *Radiology.* 2001;219(1):86–90.

138. Greenwald DA. Protein-losing gastroenteropathy. In: Feldman MD, Friedman LS, Brandt LJ, eds. *Sleisenger and Fordtran's Gastrointestinal and Liver Disease.* 10th ed. Philadelphia, PA: Saunders; 2016:464–470.

139. Takeda H, Ishihama K, Fukui T, et al. Significance of rapid turnover proteins in protein-losing gastroenteropathy. *Hepatogastroenterology.* 2003;50(54):1963–1965.

140. McCray S, Parrish CR. When chyle leaks: nutrition intervention. *Pract Gastroenterol.* 2004;28(5).

141. Aoyagi K, Iida M, Matsumoto T, Sakisaka S. Enteral nutrition as a primary therapy for intestinal lymphangiectasia: value of elemental diet and polymeric diet compared with total parenteral nutrition. *Dig Dis Sci.* 2005;50(8):1467–1470.

142. Deng Y, Misselwitz B, Dai N, Fox M. Lactose intolerance in adults: biological mechanism and dietary management. *Nutrients.* 2015;7(9):8020–8035.

143. Fedewa A, Rao SS. Dietary fructose intolerance, fructan intolerance and FODMAPs. *Curr Gastroenterol Rep.* 2014;16(1):370.

144. Nanayakkara WS, Skidmore PM, O'Brien L, Wilkinson TJ, Gearry RB. Efficacy of the low FODMAP diet for treating irritable bowel syndrome: the evidence to date. *Clin Exp Gastroenterol.* 2016;9:131–142.

145. Boyce JA, Assa'ad A, Burks AW, et al. Guidelines for the diagnosis and management of food allergy in the United States: report of the NIAID-sponsored expert panel. *J Allerg Clin Immunol.* 2010;126(6 Suppl):S1–S58.

146. Wongrakpanich S, Klaewsongkram J, Chantaphakul H, Ruxrungtham K. Jackfruit anaphylaxis in a latex allergic patient. *Asian Pac J Allerg Immunol.* 2015;33(1):65–68.

147. Vlaicu PC, Rusu LC, Ledesma A, et al. Cucumber anaphylaxis in a latex-sensitized patient. *J Investig Allergol Clin Immunol.* 2011;21(3):236–239.

148. Pereira C, Tavares B, Loureiro G, Lundberg M, Chieira C. Turnip and zucchini: new foods in the latex-fruit syndrome. *Allergy.* 2007;62(4):452–453.

149. Ibero M, Castillo MJ, Pineda F. Allergy to cassava: a new allergenic food with cross-reactivity to latex. *J Investig Allergol Clin Immunol.* 2007;17(6):409–412.

150. Furuta GT, Katzka DA. Eosinophilic esophagitis. *N Engl J Med.* 2015;373(17):1640–1648.

151. Wechsler JB, Schwartz S, Amsden K, Kagalwalla AF. Elimination diets in the management of eosinophilic esophagitis. *J Asthma Allerg.* 2014;7:85–94.

152. Lucendo AJ. Meta-analysis-based guidance for dietary management in eosinophilic esophagitis. *Curr Gastroenterol Rep.* 2015;17(10):464.

153. Gonzalez-Cervera J, Lucendo AJ. Eosinophilic esophagitis: an evidence-based approach to therapy. *J Investig Allergol Clin Immunol.* 2016;26(1):8–18.

27 Liver Disease

Valentina Medici, MD, Mardeli Saire Mendoza, MD, and Matthew R. Kappus, MD

CONTENTS

Acknowledgments: Thomas H. Frazier, MD, Benjamin E. Wheeler, MD, Craig J. McClain, MD, and Matthew Cave, MD, were the authors of this chapter in the second edition.

Objectives

1. Understand the pathogenesis of various liver diseases, with an emphasis on how pathogenesis relates to nutrition and malnutrition.
2. Review the challenges of assessing nutrition status in patients with liver disease and identify possible solutions to these problems.
3. Identify important micronutrient deficiencies and toxicities in patients with liver disease.
4. Determine the energy and protein requirements for patients with both acute and chronic liver diseases.
5. Identify and learn how to address barriers to the delivery of nutrition in patients with liver disease.

Test Your Knowledge Questions

1. Which of the following is an accurate marker of nutrition status in all patients with chronic liver disease with portal hypertension?
   A. Serum prealbumin
   B. Retinol-binding protein
   C. Anthropometry
   D. None of the above
2. Which of the following statements is false regarding alcoholic hepatitis?
   A. Virtually all patients with alcoholic hepatitis have some degree of malnutrition.
   B. The severity of liver disease generally correlates with the degree of malnutrition.
   C. Energy intake correlates with mortality.
   D. Protein delivery should be reduced to prevent portal systemic encephalopathy (PSE).
3. Which of the following statements is true regarding parenteral nutrition (PN) in the care of the inpatient with liver disease?
   A. There is no role for PN in nutrition in liver disease.
   B. PN should be initiated in all hospitalized patients with liver disease.
   C. If a patient cannot tolerate enteral feeding, PN can provide necessary nutrition, but it should be discontinued in favor of enteral nutrition (EN) as soon as possible.
   D. When a patient cannot tolerate EN, he or she should receive PN for the duration of the hospitalization.

Test Your Knowledge Answers

1. The correct answer is **D**. There are no consistently accurate measures of malnutrition in patients with significant liver disease. Visceral proteins such as albumin, prealbumin, and retinol-binding protein are made in the liver and better correlate with the severity of liver disease rather than the degree of malnutrition. Anthropometry can be inaccurate in the setting of edema and/or ascites.
2. The correct answer is **D**. The Veterans Health Administration (VA) Cooperative Studies Program demonstrated that virtually all patients with alcoholic hepatitis have some degree of malnutrition. In addition, the severity of liver disease generally correlated with the degree of malnutrition. Study subjects consuming more than 3000 kcal/d had almost no mortality, whereas those consuming less than 1000 kcal/d had greater than 80% mortality. Thus, food intake correlated with 6-month mortality. Protein requirements in patients with alcoholic hepatitis are increased, and the delivery of protein is not a significant precipitant of PSE. Protein restriction is rarely required in alcoholic hepatitis (or any other liver disease, for that matter) and should only be considered in the setting of PSE refractory to medical treatment.
3. The correct answer is **C**. The goal should always be to provide EN to patients with liver disease. In certain patients, such as those without a functional gut, it is necessary to provide PN. PN should be continued for the briefest period possible. EN is *always* preferred to PN when enteral feeding is possible.

Background

Nutrition support for patients with liver disease is a complex topic. The liver is pivotal in many metabolic processes. It normally has considerable metabolic reserve, but patients with decompensated liver disease can develop significant nutritional deficiencies. A complicating factor for providing nutrition support is the tremendous variability in the causes and severity of liver disease among patients. In addition, traditional methods of assessing nutrition status are often unreliable. These issues make it difficult to provide a "blanket" recommendation for nutrition therapy in liver disease patients.

Perfused by both the portal vein and hepatic artery, the liver has a unique dual blood supply and consists of multiple cell types having differing functions. Hepatocytes make up over 80% of the total liver mass and play a critical role in (1) the metabolism of amino acids and ammonia; (2) the detoxification of a variety of drugs, vitamins, and hormones; and (3) biochemical oxidation reactions. Hepatic Kupffer cells, the largest reservoir of fixed macrophages in the body, play a protective role against gut-derived toxins that have escaped into the portal circulation. These cells are major producers of cytokines, which can markedly influence nutrition status. The liver also contains hepatic stellate cells, which play an important role in collagen formation following liver injury and are the major storehouse for vitamin A in the body. There are a host of additional cell types located in the liver, each with distinctive functions (eg, bile duct epithelium in bile flow; sinusoidal endothelial cells in adhesion molecule expression and endocytosis).

The liver plays an essential role in the metabolism of proteins, carbohydrates, and fats. Plasma proteins, nonessential amino acids, urea (for ammonia excretion), glycogen, and critical hormones such insulin-like growth factor 1 are synthesized in the liver. The liver is also a chief site for the metabolism of fatty acids. In addition, bile from the liver is needed for fat absorption from the intestine. Thus, a properly functioning liver is imperative for achieving and maintaining appropriate nutrition status.

Acute hepatitis is usually a self-limited liver disease characterized by the elevation of serum transaminases (alanine aminotransferase [ALT] and aspartate aminotransferase [AST]). Acute hepatitis is most frequently caused by a viral infection, medication/toxicant, Wilson disease, or shock. Malnutrition and the presence of chronic liver diseases, such as nonalcoholic fatty liver disease (NAFLD), may predispose patients to acute liver injury. The functional reserve of the liver is so great that 80% to 90% of liver cells must be injured before physiologic functions are impaired. Destruction of a large proportion of the hepatocytes results in acute liver failure, which is characterized by rapid deterioration in hepatic synthetic function (eg, jaundice, coagulopathy, hypoalbuminemia) and manifestations of portal hypertension, primarily hepatic encephalopathy (HE). Signs and symptoms of HE can range from subtle behavioral changes to disorientation and deep coma (Table 27-1).[1] Chronic liver disease is characterized by prolonged liver inflammation, with infiltration of lymphocytes, plasma cells, and hepatocytes apoptosis. In the long term, there may be deposition of fibrosis and ultimately development of cirrhosis.

TABLE 27-1 Clinical Stages of Hepatic Encephalopathy

Stage	Signs and Symptoms
Minimal	No clinical manifestations but abnormal results on psychometric testing
Grade I	Altered sleep pattern, mild confusion, short attention span
Grade II	Lethargy, moderate confusion, agitation
Grade III	Marked confusion, incoherent speech, arousable by pain
Grade IV	Coma, unarousable, unresponsive to pain

Source: Data are from reference 1.

Pathogenesis and Nutrition-Related Aspects of Liver Disease

Two epidemics are fueling the most recent increase in the prevalence of chronic liver disease, namely, hepatitis C virus and NAFLD/nonalcoholic steatohepatitis (NASH). Approximately 2% of Americans are infected with hepatitis C virus.[2] NAFLD, the hepatic manifestation of metabolic syndrome/insulin resistance, has become the most common liver disease in the United States.[3] Both of these diseases can progress to cirrhosis in a significant percentage of patients. In addition, excess alcohol ingestion remains among the most common etiologies of liver disease and is frequently associated with malnutrition. Cirrhosis, characterized by dense collagen accumulation, or fibrosis, may lead to end-stage (or decompensated) liver disease, which may also be accompanied by synthetic dysfunction and portal hypertension as well as hepatocellular carcinoma (HCC). However, in its early stages, chronic liver disease may be asymptomatic. Serologic tests may reveal abnormal liver enzymes in either a hepatocellular (AST/ALT) or a cholestatic pattern (alkaline phosphatase). Progressive fibrosis develops in some, but not all, patients with chronic liver disease resulting in cirrhosis.

Liver disease has multiple etiologies (Table 27-2). Although often difficult to diagnose, patients with advanced liver disease are often at risk for malnutrition.[4] Local and systemic neurohormonal mechanisms are likely involved in causing delayed gastric emptying, small bowel dysmotility and bacterial overgrowth, and constipation.[5-9] Further complicating this picture are increased renal losses of micronutrients, such as zinc, in conditions such as alcoholic liver disease (ALD).[10]

Maldigestion and malabsorption may occur in liver disease and may play an important role in causing malnutrition. Typical gastrointestinal (GI) disturbances in liver disease include dysgeusia, anorexia, nausea, and early satiety. Concomitant complications typical of liver disease such as upper GI bleeding, PSE, and sepsis also cause prolonged periods of poor oral intake. Dietary management of fluid retention with salt and water restriction and carbohydrate and lipid restrictions used in patients with diabetes mellitus, chronic pancreatic insufficiency, and cholestatic liver disease can all affect diet palatability and severely restrict patients' food choices.

TABLE 27-2 Causes of Liver Disease

- Toxins:
  - Ethanol
  - Medications
  - Industrial chemicals (vinyl chloride)
  - Aflatoxins
  - Other (eg, Amanita sp. mushroom)
- Metabolic causes:
  - Obesity (NAFLD)
  - Wilson disease
  - Hemochromatosis
  - Alpha-1 antitrypsin deficiency
- Infections:
  - Viral infections (eg, hepatitis A, B, C, E)
  - Bacterial and mycobacterial infections (eg, brucellosis, tuberculosis)
- Immune-mediated causes:
  - Autoimmune hepatitis
  - PBC
  - PSC
  - Sarcoidosis
- Other:
  - Budd-Chiari syndrome
  - Amyloidosis
  - HCC

HCC, hepatocellular carcinoma; NAFLD, nonalcoholic fatty liver disease; PBC, primary biliary cholangitis; PSC, primary sclerosing cholangitis.

Impaired lipid metabolism is multifactorial in liver disease. Decreased intraluminal bile salts, small bowel bacterial overgrowth, coexistent pancreatic insufficiency or intestinal disease (inflammatory bowel disease, celiac disease), and mucosal vascular hypertension and edema can worsen maldigestion and malabsorption. Cholestatic liver disorders are associated with decreased intraluminal concentration of bile salts, resulting in malabsorption of lipids and lipid-soluble vitamins.[11]

The loss of glycogen stores that occurs in patients with advanced liver disease predisposes them to enter a starvation state within a few hours of fasting.[12,13] That can lead to peripheral muscle proteolysis to provide amino acids for gluconeogenesis, thus contributing to protein malnutrition. Liver disease patients with portal hypertension and ascites and those with acute alcoholic hepatitis are at increased risk of developing a hypermetabolic state (resting energy expenditure [REE] greater than 110% of its expected value), which also contributes to overall malnutrition.[14-16]

Dysregulated cytokine metabolism (eg, elevated tumor necrosis factor [TNF]) is well documented in many forms of liver disease.[17] Low-grade endotoxemia, facilitated by portal hypertension and gut bacterial translocation, leads to increases in proinflammatory cytokines and further affects nutrient management and overall metabolism.[18] Increased levels of cytokines have been postulated to cause many of the metabolic and nutrition-related abnormalities observed in liver disease, especially in acute alcoholic hepatitis and in chronic decompensated liver disease.[17] Thus, abnormalities such as fever, anorexia, muscle breakdown, and wasting and altered mineral metabolism are likely to be at least partially cytokine mediated.

Despite the increased frequency of malnutrition in patients with chronic liver disease, one cannot assume that all of these patients are at nutrition risk. Moreover, obesity and metabolic syndrome are increasingly recognized as major causes of abnormal liver enzymes and can also coexist with and worsen liver diseases of other etiologies. Consequently, both undernutrition and obesity play important roles in liver disease. For this reason, an accurate assessment of nutrition status in patients with liver disease is essential. Patients with ALD are also at risk for complications of alcohol use such as pancreatitis and myopathy. It is not clear, however, what contribution a diminished nutrition status plays in the incidence of these complications. Although the role of nutrition in the pathogenesis, progression, and treatment of specific forms of liver disease (Table 27-2) is beyond the scope of this chapter, some etiologies deserve special focus because they are prevalent or closely linked to nutrition. These include ALD, NFALD, viral hepatitis, hemochromatosis, Wilson disease, and cholestatic diseases, including primary sclerosing cholangitis (PSC) and primary biliary cholangitis (PBC; previously known as *primary biliary cirrhosis*).

Alcoholic Liver Disease

The liver is the main organ responsible for ethanol metabolism; other organs, such as the stomach, contribute to a much lesser degree. The pathogenesis is complex and involves numerous mechanisms that are variably well understood. Acetaldehyde (one of the main products of oxidative metabolism of ethanol) is postulated to play an etiologic role in ALD. Another major mechanism implicated in the pathogenesis of ALD is the increased intestinal permeability, related to protein-energy malnutrition (PEM). Altered intestinal permeability causes translocation from the intestine to the hepatocytes of the endotoxin lipopolysaccharide (LPS), a component of gram-negative intestinal bacteria outer wall. LPS activates the Toll-like receptor and TNF-α pathways with increased inflammation. Other mechanisms—including oxidative stress (through both direct injury and cell signaling); mitochondrial dysfunction; hypoxia; impaired proteasome function; abnormal metabolism of methionine, S-adenosylmethionine (SAM or SAMe), and folate; Kupffer cell activation; dysregulated cytokine production; immune responses to altered hepatocellular proteins; and genetic/epigenetic mechanisms—are all thought to be involved in the development and progression of ALD.[19] Importantly, many of the mechanisms are directly modifiable through nutrition interventions (eg, oxidative stress).

The most extensive studies involving interactions between nutrition status and liver disease have been in patients with ALD. The most detailed of these studies derive from the VA Cooperative Studies Program in patients with alcoholic hepatitis.[20-24] In these and other studies, malnutrition is a major complication of ALD. Importantly, malnutrition worsens clinical outcomes in ALD, and nutrition support improves nutrition status and may improve clinical outcomes (Practice Scenario 27-1).[20-25]

Practice Scenario 27-1

Question: How important is enteral nutrition (EN) in the management of acute alcoholic hepatitis?

Scenario: A 55-year-old man with a past medical history of alcoholism presents with a 2-week history of nausea, vomiting, increasing abdominal girth, and jaundice. Until 2 weeks ago, the patient was drinking a fifth of vodka per day, but he has been unable to tolerate anything by mouth during the past 2 weeks. A physical examination reveals scleral icterus, jaundice, and a tense abdomen with a positive fluid wave consistent with ascites. The patient's memory is normal, and there is no asterixis. His weight is 70 kg and his height is 173 cm. Diagnostic studies, including laboratory and radiologic investigations, reveal severe alcoholic hepatitis, normal renal function, and new-onset ascites. The original diet order is a 2-g sodium diet. Over the next 48 hours, despite aggressive supportive care and corticosteroids, the patient develops worsening renal function consistent with hepatorenal syndrome, and an assessment of oral diet intake reveals the patient is consuming 10% of goal energy and protein.

Intervention: Given the inadequacy of the patient's energy and protein intake, nasogastric access (tube feeding for enteral feeding) is obtained and the patient is started on a standard polymeric enteral formula. EN is increased slowly with close attention to his risk for refeeding syndrome. By Day 5 of the hospitalization, the patient is receiving 1.2 times his resting energy expenditure per day and tolerating 1.5 g of protein per kilogram of dry weight per day. Over the next several days, the patient begins tolerating oral feeding and tube feeding is stopped. One week later, he is discharged in stable condition on an oral diet.

Answer: Early and aggressive EN improves outcomes in patients with alcoholic hepatitis. Nasoenteral access is generally required given the many obstacles to enteral feeding in patients with severe liver disease (eg, anorexia, nausea, vomiting). These patients are at risk for refeeding syndrome.

Rationale: The Veterans Health Administration Cooperative Studies Program demonstrated that virtually all patients with alcoholic hepatitis have some degree of malnutrition.[20-24] In addition, the severity of liver disease generally correlated with the degree of malnutrition. Study subjects consuming orally more than 3000 kcal/d had near zero mortality, whereas those consuming less than 1000 kcal/d had greater than 80% mortality. Thus, food intake correlated with 6-month mortality. A major multicenter study demonstrated that nutrition via enteral feeding tube, when compared with corticosteroids, has similar short-term mortality rates, improved 1-year mortality rates, and reduced infectious complications.[25] Restricting protein is not recommended in alcoholic hepatitis (or any other liver disease, for that matter) and should only be implemented in the setting of PSE refractory to medical treatment.

The first of the VA Cooperative Studies (Study #119) established that nearly every patient with alcoholic hepatitis had some degree of malnutrition.[22] This study categorized 284 patients with complete nutrition assessments into groups with mild, moderate, or severe alcoholic hepatitis (based on clinical and biochemical parameters). Mean alcohol consumption among all patients was 228 g per day (about 16 alcoholic drinks per day, assuming that 1 drink contains 14 grams of alcohol), with almost 50% of energy intake coming from alcohol. As a result, although energy intake for many patients was adequate, intake of protein was often deficient. The severity of liver disease generally correlated with the severity of malnutrition. Similar data were generated in a follow-up VA study on alcoholic hepatitis (Study #275).[24]

In both of these studies, patients were carefully monitored by a dietitian and encouraged to eat a balanced, 2500-kcal hospital diet. In the second study, patients in the therapy arm of the protocol also received oxandrolone 80 mg/d and an oral nutrition support product high in branched-chain amino acids (BCAAs). Energy intake correlated in a stepwise fashion with 6-month mortality data. Those patients who consumed less than 1000 kcal/d had greater than 80% 6-month mortality, whereas those who voluntarily consumed more than 3000 kcal/d had virtually no mortality.[20] Furthermore, the degree of malnutrition correlated with the development of serious complications such as encephalopathy, ascites, and hepatorenal syndrome.[20] Although it is possible that nutrition prevented mortality, it is also possible that the inability to eat was simply a marker of disease severity. Nonetheless, many centers provide EN support to patients with severe acute alcoholic hepatitis who are unable to voluntarily consume sufficient energy. A study showed that EN supplementation via tube feeding providing 2000 kcal/d for 28 days in patients with severe alcoholic hepatitis was associated with improved outcome when compared with steroids. In particular, patients on supplemental nutrition and patients who received steroids had similar mortality rates during treatment, but patients who received steroids had higher long-term mortality at 1-year follow-up due to increased risk of infections.[25] Other studies present more controversial findings. Adding intensive EN (via feeding tube for 14 days) to methylprednisolone for the treatment of severe alcoholic hepatitis did not improve survival when compared with conventional nutrition and methylprednisolone.[26] A meta-analysis on 262 patients with ALD revealed no difference in mortality when special nutrition therapy was compared with a normal, balanced diet.[27] In patients with alcoholic cirrhosis, EN via nasogastric tube was not associated with improved survival or nutrition status compared with conventional treatment.[28] The discrepancies among these data may be related to the different patient populations studied and the varying degrees of severity of liver disease. They also highlight the importance of evaluating critically the role of nutrition support in alcoholic hepatitis.

In the VA Cooperative Studies, the chronic, alcohol-consuming control population without liver disease also frequently had some degree of PEM. This contradicts other data indicating that only those with alcoholism and underlying liver disease demonstrated significant PEM. The VA studies evaluated patients with acute alcoholic hepatitis; however, patients with stable alcoholic cirrhosis without alcoholic hepatitis have been studied as well. One such investigation of patients with compensated alcoholic cirrhosis (not actively drinking) revealed indicators of malnutrition almost as severe

as those in patients with alcoholic hepatitis, including body mass index (BMI), which may not be a very reliable parameter in this population); pyridoxal phosphate; and red blood cell folate levels.[29] ALD is characterized by several specific nutritional deficiencies, including folate, vitamin B_{12} (cobalamin), B_1 (thiamin), and B_6 (pyridoxine), which should be regularly checked and eventually supplemented. Supplemental micronutrients such as SAM and zinc have a potential therapeutic role in ALD (see the discussion of complementary and alternative medicine [CAM] agents later in this chapter).

Nonalcoholic Fatty Liver Disease and Nonalcoholic Steatohepatitis

An estimated 65% of Americans are either overweight or obese. Some estimates predict that close to 100% of Americans will be overweight by the year 2030, placing them at increased risk for development of metabolic syndrome. See Chapter 35 for additional discussion of the prevalence of obesity.

NAFLD, the hepatic manifestation of metabolic syndrome, occurs when inappropriate hepatic management of lipids results in the abnormal accumulation of fat in the hepatocytes. This phenomenon, although not completely understood, seems to be a consequence of increased free fatty acid (FFA) delivery to the liver from visceral sources coupled with hyperinsulinemia-related inadequate formation, and the export of very low-density lipoproteins out of the hepatocyte.

Although steatosis alone does not usually result in progressive fibrosis, approximately 10% to 20% of patients with NAFLD experience a "second hit," of unknown nature, that induces an inflammatory response to the fat-laden hepatocytes. This inflammation, in turn, can lead to liver cell injury, death, and replacement by scarring (fibrosis). As this necroinflammatory response progresses, it can, and frequently does, lead to cirrhosis. NASH-related cirrhosis can lead to liver failure and has been associated with the development of HCC. Of note, liver cancer is often detected in NASH at a later stage and can develop also in the absence of cirrhosis.[30] NASH-related cirrhosis is among the most frequent indications for liver transplant.

Most, but not all, NAFLD/NASH patients are obese. As with other obese patients, nutrition assessment is often challenging and complicated, and standard estimates of nutrition needs based on weight and anthropometric measurements are often misleading (see Chapters 2, 9, and 35). Additionally, patients with NAFLD/NASH often have type 2 diabetes and varying degrees of diabetic nephropathy and associated proteinuria, which can lead to low serum albumin levels.

When a patient's fatty liver disease advances to cirrhosis with serologic hepatic dysfunction, hepatic production of proteins is often impaired. Furthermore, because cirrhosis often results in a catabolic state, a patient's nutrition needs, especially with respect to protein requirements, can be underestimated. Patients with cirrhotic NASH can be malnourished and protein deprived despite being obese. In addition, sarcopenia, or low skeletal muscle, is a frequent finding in patients with NAFLD. Given that the skeletal muscle is the primary tissue for glucose metabolism, sarcopenia could explain the insulin resistance in NAFLD. Recent studies showed an association between sarcopenia and the stage of liver fibrosis.[31]

Evidence indicating that specific dietary components play a role in the development/progression of NAFLD is continually emerging. Mechanisms such as lipotoxicity, oxidative stress, endotoxemia, dysregulated cytokines/adipokines, and alterations in gut microflora seem to be involved in triggering both steatosis and steatohepatitis. These mechanisms are also linked with specific dietary habits (eg, obesity, high-fat diets, high-fructose corn syrup, diets low in ω-3 fatty acids). High-fat diets have often been implicated in NAFLD. In fact, many animal models use a high-fat diet (71% of energy from fat) to induce NAFLD.[32] Importantly, high-fat diets result in multiple metabolic derangements that likely play an etiologic role in NAFLD, including oxidative stress, alterations in postprandial triglyceride metabolism, increased TNF-α, circulating FFAs, and insulin resistance.

Although the amount of dietary fat certainly seems to be important in the development of NAFLD, evidence is emerging that the type and ratios of dietary fats can also contribute. An increased fat intake with an excessive amount of ω-6 fatty acids has been implicated in promoting necroinflammation.[33] On the other hand, a diet containing medium-chain triglycerides (MCTs) in the absence of long-chain triglycerides has been reported to be hepatoprotective.[34] There are also studies demonstrating the role of fructose in the pathogenesis of NAFLD.[35,36] Specific sources of fructose, such as soft drinks, have also been implicated. Animal studies have confirmed that high-fructose diets induce metabolic syndrome with intrahepatic accumulation of triglycerides. In these models, fructose-induced NAFLD was associated with intestinal bacterial overgrowth (IBO) and increased intestinal permeability, subsequently leading to an endotoxin-dependent activation of hepatic Kupffer cells and increased levels of monocyte chemotactic protein 1 and TNF-α.[37,38] Fructose consumption, estimated through a questionnaire administered to 427 patients with fatty liver, was associated with more severe hepatic fibrosis and inflammation.[39]

Diet and physical activity for weight reduction and weight loss surgery for extreme obesity are the current standard recommendations for the treatment of NAFLD. Recent evidence indicates that intensive lifestyle intervention in patients with type 2 diabetes can reduce steatosis and the incidence of NAFLD.[40] Energy restriction can result in significant changes in both liver fat and volume within a few days. Another area of increasing interest is the use of low-carbohydrate diets in NAFLD. A low-carbohydrate, ketogenic diet in patients with NASH led to significant weight loss and histologic improvement of fatty liver disease at 6 months.[41] Dietary avoidance of lipogenic, simple sugars (ie, fructose) seems to be universally recommended. A reduction in the consumption of sweetened beverages can also lead to significant weight loss because total energy intake decreases.[42] The Mediterranean diet, which is rich in monounsaturated fatty acids, is probably effective for NASH, although large studies testing this hypothesis are lacking.[43] Regarding physical activity, vigorous and moderate exercise are similarly beneficial in improving hepatic triglyceride content, as demonstrated by proton magnetic resonance spectroscopy, and the change seems to be partly related to the effect of exercise on weight loss.[44] Similarly, it has been shown that aerobic exercise can improve hepatic steatosis and stiffness in NAFLD.[45] Weight loss by bariatric surgery attenuates both steatosis and

steatohepatitis, but data supporting improvements in fibrosis are limited.[46] Despite intensive research, the US Food and Drug Administration (FDA) has not approved any therapy for NAFLD. However, the Pioglitazone vs Vitamin E vs Placebo for the Treatment of Nondiabetic Patients with Nonalcoholic Steatohepatitis (PIVENS) trial demonstrated a benefit with vitamin E therapy (800 IU/d),[47] which has become standard practice in many areas of the United States. The PIVENS study is further discussed in the Complementary and Alternative Medicine section of this chapter. Some initial promising results indicate that probiotics and their potential to modify the intestinal microbiota are associated with improvement in liver enzymes, hepatic steatosis, and fibrosis in patients with NASH.[48,49] See Chapter 4 for additional information on probiotics and the gut microbiota.

Patients with NASH-related decompensated cirrhosis pose other challenges. Because of the catabolic nature of cirrhosis, these patients are often significantly malnourished with protein deficits, even if they are obese.[50,51] Although weight reduction is still beneficial, all efforts should be made to ensure adequate protein is supplied. As is the case with patients with cirrhosis in general, limiting protein intake to subnormal levels is rarely, if ever, indicated in patients with NAFLD. In fact, data are emerging that high protein intake may lead to better outcomes in patients with cirrhosis with liver failure.[16,52]

Viral Hepatitis

Viral hepatitis consists of 5 distinct entities (A to E). Hepatitis A is an RNA virus that is transmitted via the fecal-oral route. It is an uncommon infection in the United States, but it is more prevalent in other parts of the world in areas of low socioeconomic status, such as Africa, Asia (excluding Japan), the Mediterranean basin, Eastern Europe, the Middle East, Mexico, Central and South America, and parts of the Caribbean. In the United States, hepatitis A infection is most often encountered in individuals who have emigrated from or traveled to these locations without receiving appropriate vaccinations. This virus does not cause chronic infection. Management of acute hepatitis A infection consists of supportive care; there are no specific recommendations for dietary restrictions or nutrition interventions, aside from abstinence from alcohol intake.

Hepatitis B is a DNA virus that is transmitted most commonly via perinatal, percutaneous, and sexual routes. The disease is endemic in sub-Saharan Africa and Asia, where up to 25% of the population have an active hepatitis B infection. Rates of infection in the United States are substantially lower, where 0.1% to 0.2% of the population has chronic hepatitis B infection, and 200,000 to 300,000 new cases of hepatitis B infection occur annually.[53] In the United States, most cases of hepatitis B infection can be attributed to intravenous (IV) drug use and high-risk sexual practices. Low rates in developed countries are largely due to preventive measures, specifically, vaccination against the virus. In young, otherwise healthy individuals, the virus will be cleared with complete recovery 95% to 99% of the time. The infection is more likely to become chronic in newborns who contract the virus during birth and in young children who contract the virus. The disease will become chronic in 1% to 5% of adults that contract the virus.[53] Chronic infection can cause inflammation and

© 2017 ASPEN, www.nutritioncare.org

hepatic cellular carcinoma

fibrosis leading to cirrhosis. Among the types of viral hepatitis, chronic hepatitis B virus infection is associated with the highest risk for the subsequent development of HCC. Concomitant exposure to dietary aflatoxins, particularly in Asia, has been associated with a greater risk for the development of cirrhosis and HCC in patients with hepatitis B.[54] Preliminary liver cancer chemoprevention trials have been performed in these patients using broccoli extracts, which are shown to activate the antioxidant response element.[55]

Hepatitis C is the most common blood-borne infection in the United States, where an estimated 3.2 million people have chronic hepatitis C infection.[56] The peak incidence of the disease occurs in individuals between the ages of 40 and 49 years. Approximately 30,000 new cases are diagnosed each year, with most infections having been contracted decades prior to presentation.[56] Infection with hepatitis C is most commonly acquired via IV drug use, but it also occurs in transfusion recipients (most often those who received transfusions prior to 1992), hemodialysis patients, Vietnam veterans, and healthcare workers who are stuck with infected needles. Sexual and perinatal transmission of the disease is far less common.[56] Hepatitis C usually results in chronic infection, and an estimated 20% of chronically infected patients will develop cirrhosis within 20 to 25 years. Acute hepatitis C is typically asymptomatic, although signs such as fever, nausea, and jaundice can occur 1 to 3 months after exposure.[57] Hepatitis C infection is often associated with hepatic steatosis, type 2 diabetes, and features of metabolic syndrome, and these entities seem to be interconnected in a vicious cycle: hepatitis C virus is directly involved in the development of diabetes, and diabetes and insulin resistance are independent factors for the development of NASH and progression of fibrosis.[58]

Supplement use is common with chronic hepatitis C infection. In the most rigorously designed study to date, highly purified silymarin (milk thistle) was found to have no effect on liver enzymes in patients with chronic hepatitis C infection, but the use of this over-the-counter supplement remains widespread.[59] Since 2014, the treatment of hepatitis C infection has been revolutionized by the FDA approval of oral antiviral agents that can achieve sustained virologic response with high rates.[60] Interestingly, evidence from multiple clinical trials indicates that hepatitis C eradication with new oral antiviral treatments (eg, simeprevir and sofosbuvir) is associated with improved glycemic control and normalization of glycosylated hemoglobin.[61] In contrast, multiple studies demonstrate vitamin D deficiency in patients with chronic hepatitis C infection of all stages of liver disease severity.[62] Similarly, vitamin D supplementation increases sustained virologic response (cure) rates in patients on hepatitis C virus therapy with pegylated interferon and ribavirin.[63] Likewise, preliminary studies indicate that SAM may lead to increased sustained viral response rates.[64] However, the appropriateness of clinical use of vitamin D or SAM is currently uncertain given the recent introduction of anti–hepatitis C virus direct agents.

Hereditary Hemochromatosis

Hereditary hemochromatosis is a genetic disorder of iron overload that classically occurs as an autosomal recessive disorder in individuals heterozygous for the C282Y mutation in the human hemochromatosis (HFE) gene. The disease is common, with an incidence of 1 in 250 people. Penetrance is incomplete, with clinical disease presenting more commonly in males of Northern European descent.[65] The resulting iron accumulation affects the liver, as well as the heart, endocrine system, and musculoskeletal systems. The disease results in cirrhosis in its late stages. However, if the disease is caught before the onset of cirrhosis, it can essentially be cured. The most effective treatment for hemochromatosis is therapeutic phlebotomy, initially scheduled weekly, with maintenance phlebotomy performed as need based on serum ferritin levels.[66] Patients with hereditary hemochromatosis must limit dietary iron intake and alcohol consumption. Ethanol intake greater than 60 g/d (about 5 drinks/d) is associated with increased rates of cirrhosis.[66] In a study of HFE (-/-) mice accumulating hepatic iron similarly to patients with hereditary hemochromatosis and receiving oral ethanol, a corn oil–based diet improved markers of oxidative stress, inflammation, and hepatic fibrosis.[67] Individuals with hereditary hemochromatosis should also avoid excess vitamin C–specific supplementation because vitamin C may increase dietary iron absorption. All patients with hemochromatosis must avoid supplements containing iron, especially when not receiving phlebotomies. The American Association for the Study of Liver Diseases guidelines specify that dietary restrictions are not necessary during treatment because the amount of iron removed by phlebotomies largely balances out any amount of oral intake of dietary iron.[68]

Wilson Disease

Wilson disease is an autosomal recessive disease caused by mutations affecting the biliary copper transporter ATP7B. More than 500 known possible mutations affect the ATP7B gene, with resulting impairment of copper trafficking within the hepatocytes and its reduced biliary excretion. Wilson disease can have various phenotypes. In more than 50% of cases, it presents with hepatic involvement, which includes hepatic steatosis, chronic hepatitis, cirrhosis, and acute liver failure with hemolysis. The remaining presentations have neurologic and psychiatric signs and symptoms, characterized by resting tremors similar to Parkinson's disease, rigidity, ataxia, and dystonia. Psychiatric manifestations include depression, worsening school and sport performance, and sexual disinhibition.

Wilson disease occurs in 1 out of 30,000 people and usually becomes clinically apparent before the age of 40 years.[69] A variety of tests (serum ceruloplasmin, 24-hour urine copper, slit-lamp eye examination, and liver biopsy with hepatic copper quantification) are used to diagnose suspected Wilson disease.[70] Treatment involves the use of chelating agents to remove tissue copper and allow copper excretion in the urine. The chelating agents used most often are trientine and penicillamine. Trientine is becoming the preferred choice because of the growing evidence of multiple adverse effects associated with the use of penicillamine.[71] Patients receiving penicillamine therapy require the replacement of vitamin B6.

The FDA has also approved zinc acetate administered at the dosage of 50 mg of elemental zinc daily for the treatment of Wilson disease. Providers should also consider concomitant intake of oral supplements with additional zinc content. Zinc induces intestinal metallothionein, which leads to reduced dietary copper absorption. Zinc should be provided on empty stomach, at least 1 hour before or 2 hours after a meal to ensure adequate absorption. A study of German and Polish patients demonstrated that there may be more "nonresponders" to zinc than chelation therapy.[72] However, a previous analysis on a Polish cohort did not show any difference in survival between those receiving zinc sulfate and those prescribed penicillamine.[73]

Patients with Wilson disease should also be instructed to avoid foods high in copper, including liver, chocolate, mushrooms, shellfish, and nuts.[70] These dietary restrictions should be followed strictly, especially during the first year after the diagnosis.

Cholestatic Liver Diseases

In contrast to the aforementioned hepatocellular liver diseases, PBC and PSC are the most prevalent etiologies of chronic cholestatic liver disease. Cholestatic liver diseases pose unique challenges in nutrition. In PBC, the initial damage occurs in the biliary tree because of T cell–mediated destruction of the intrahepatic bile ducts. Over time, the damage becomes severe enough to cause cholestasis, which results in a universal endpoint of cirrhosis and end-stage liver disease.[74] The disease most commonly presents with pruritus and alkaline phosphatase elevation in middle-aged women. Striking hypercholesterolemia may accompany PBC, but hypercholesterolemia in PBC has not been definitively linked to increased atherosclerosis. The only approved treatment in the United States for PBC is ursodeoxycholic acid (UDCA), which alters bile cholesterol composition.[75]

PSC is characterized by inflammation and sclerosis of the intrahepatic and/or extrahepatic bile ducts. PSC has a more rapid and severe course than PBC, with the median time from diagnosis to time of death ranging between 9 and 12 years. As PSC progresses, complete obstruction of the biliary tree occurs, leading to cirrhosis and the development of end-stage liver disease.[71] PSC has been associated with both inflammatory bowel disease and autoimmune hepatitis (especially in children). PSC carries an increased risk of cholangiocarcinoma; estimates of risk are between 8% and 15% over a patient's lifetime.[76] UDCA does not seem to be an effective treatment for PSC.[77,78] Endoscopic treatment (endoscopic retrograde cholangiography) of dominant biliary strictures may be performed to exclude cholangiocarcinoma and to relieve obstruction. Interestingly, the gut microbiota, as assessed by analysis of stool samples, is different and characterized by reduced bacterial diversity in patients with PSC compared with healthy subjects.[79] Even though these findings are preliminary, they may indicate a future strategy in the care of PSC based on the manipulation of the intestinal flora.

Regardless of its etiology, chronic cholestasis may cause calcium and lipid-soluble vitamin malabsorption. Fat malabsorption is usually associated with a decrease in dietary calcium absorption and an increase in oxalate absorption because FFAs bind to calcium in the digestive tract, making it unavailable for absorption. Calcium malabsorption may be worsened by vitamin D deficiency. The liver usually activates vitamin D into its active compound, 1,25-dihydroxyvitamin D. Most patients with chronic cholestasis have osteoporosis, but osteomalacia is rare. These bone problems are known as *metabolic bone disease* and are responsible for significant morbidity. Calcium usually binds oxalates in the intestine; therefore, fatty acid malabsorption results in an increase in free oxalates that are easily absorbed and predispose the patient to kidney stones. In PBC, 23% of patients have a decrease in their vitamin K plasma levels, which does not correlate with the prothrombin time.[80] Deficiencies of vitamins A, D, and E are usually present along with vitamin K deficiency. The prevalence of fat-soluble vitamin deficiencies correlates with bilirubin levels.

In chronic cholestatic diseases, such as PBC and PSC, oral supplementation of fat-soluble vitamins (A, D, E, and K) may be necessary, especially if steatorrhea is present. Oral supplements and tube feeding products should be high in energy and protein but low in fat. Consideration should be given to water-miscible formulations of fat-soluble vitamins. Oral calcium supplements are also recommended. The progression of PBC-related osteodystrophy can be slowed by supplementing with calcium, 1,25-dihydroxyvitamin D, and calcitonin.[81] In patients with weight loss, supplements containing MCT oil can be given to provide extra energy because MCTs do not need bile acids to be absorbed.

Malnutrition in Chronic Liver Disease

There is a high prevalence of PEM in cirrhosis, which appears to correlate more closely with the severity rather than the etiology of the chronic liver disease.[82-84] The literature reports malnutrition in 34% to 82% patients with alcoholic cirrhosis.[23] In patients with nonalcoholic cirrhosis, the prevalence of PEM ranges from 27% to 87%.[23] Because of the difficulties with nutrition assessment in cirrhosis, these prevalence figures are based on anthropometric data only.

In general, malnutrition in cirrhosis has many causes, which can be classified into 3 groups: (1) causes that limit oral intake; (2) causes that decrease the digestion and absorption of nutrients; and (3) causes that interfere with the metabolism of nutrients (Table 27-3). Most patients with cirrhosis have GI symptoms, such as anorexia, early satiety secondary to ascites, taste dysfunction, nausea, and vomiting, that limit their nutrient intake. In 1991, McCullough and Tavill reported the he prevalence of weight loss, nausea, and anorexia among patients with cirrhosis to be 60%, 55%, and 87%, respectively.[85] Taste abnormalities have been associated with zinc and magnesium deficiencies.[86] Steatorrhea (fat malabsorption) has been reported in 40% of patients with cirrhosis, and 10% have severe steatorrhea (more than 6 g of fat in the stool per day), usually caused by concomitant pancreatic insufficiency. Adverse effects of medications and diets with excessive protein and salt restriction seem to be common causes of malnutrition in cirrhosis, but studies evaluating the magnitude of these problems are not available.

Regardless of the etiology of cirrhosis, poor nutrition status is associated with a poor prognosis for survival in decompensated patients as well as those awaiting liver transplantation

TABLE 27-3 Causes of Malnutrition in Cirrhosis

- Decreased oral intake related to the following:
  - Anorexia
  - Nausea
  - Vomiting
  - Early satiety
  - Taste abnormalities
  - Alcohol abuse
  - Iatrogenic problems associated with restrictive diets or NPO status
  - Medications
- Maldigestion and malabsorption:
  - Fat malabsorption due to cholestasis or chronic pancreatitis
  - Water-soluble vitamin malabsorption related to alcohol abuse
  - Calcium and fat-soluble vitamin malabsorption due to cholestasis
- Metabolic abnormalities:
  - Glucose intolerance
  - Increased protein and lipid catabolism similar to sepsis
  - Trauma or other catabolic states
- Associated renal diseases:
  - Urinary micronutrient losses
  - Hepatorenal syndrome
  - Viral hepatitis–associated glomerulonephritis (MPGN in hepatitis C virus, MGN in hepatitis B virus)

MGN, membranous glomerulonephritis; MPGN, membranoproliferative glomerulonephritis; NPO, *nil per os* (nothing by mouth).

and those undergoing abdominal surgery.[87,88] Whether PEM is an independent predictor of survival or just a reflection of the severity of liver insufficiency is still a subject of controversy.

Energy Expenditure in Chronic Liver Disease

Patients with chronic liver disease can develop serious metabolic abnormalities that mimic a state of catabolism similar to sepsis or trauma.[85] Measurements of the basal energy expenditure in patients with cirrhosis are not significantly different from those of healthy controls when energy expenditure is expressed in kilocalories per kilogram of body weight.[89–91] The Harris-Benedict equation does not accurately predict REE in most patients with cirrhosis,[90] and, in general, predictive equations perform poorly in patients with liver diseases.[92–94] The presence of ascites has been noted to increase REE by 10%.[95] Given that body cell mass is decreased even in early stages of cirrhosis, the energy expenditure per unit of metabolically active tissue is thought to be increased. In a recent study of male patients with cirrhosis, most patients were hypermetabolic according to measured REE, and those who were hypermetabolic weighed less and had a greater proportion of fat-free mass than those who were not hypermetabolic.[96]

Regardless of the absolute rates of energy expenditure, the type of fuel preferred by patients with cirrhosis is altered.

After an overnight fast, these patients have significantly lower respiratory quotients than controls. This finding indicates that patients with cirrhosis use more fat as a fuel, which is similar to what occurs in healthy subjects after 72 hours of starvation.[91] In other words, the metabolism of patients with cirrhosis after an overnight fast mimics that of starving controls. However, as opposed to a starving patient in whom the energy expenditure decreases over time, cirrhotic patients continue to have normal or increased energy expenditures, leading to progressive loss of muscle and fat mass and resulting in chronic, disease-related malnutrition.

Metabolism in Chronic Liver Disease

Studies of carbohydrate metabolism in cirrhosis have shown that the prevalence of glucose intolerance in cirrhosis is high.[97] In addition, in end-stage liver disease, hypoglycemia is also frequently observed. The pathogenesis of this abnormality is not well defined, but it seems to be caused by a postreceptor intracellular abnormality in both the liver and muscle. Associated with this insulin resistance are (1) the decreased storage of glycogen in the liver and muscle and (2) the early use of lipids and protein as fuel sources, manifested as a low respiratory quotient. Abnormalities in lipid metabolism have also been described in cirrhosis. The levels of fatty acids and ketone bodies are increased, and there is an increase in ketone body production.[85] There is evidence of impairment of fatty acid storage in the form of triglycerides, which is likely caused by lipoprotein lipase inhibition and a decrease in the availability of glycerol phosphate in the adipocyte. This imbalance between fat synthesis and catabolism results in depletion of the reserves in adipose tissue. In addition, leptin levels in patients with cirrhosis are inappropriately elevated for their fat mass.[98] This excessive leptin production by the adipose tissue is postulated to decrease appetite and increase energy expenditure in these patients. Both insulin resistance and hepatic steatosis have been associated with hepatitis C infection and with viral replication and resistance to antiviral therapy.

Perhaps the most remarkable metabolic abnormality of patients with end-stage liver disease is in amino acid metabolism. Urine nitrogen losses are increased in cirrhotic patients with a normal renal function, suggesting a catabolic state. The catabolism of protein is increased and fails to decrease normally in response to feeding.[99] In cirrhosis, the plasma levels of BCAAs (leucine, valine, and isoleucine) are low, and the levels of aromatic amino acids (phenylalanine, tyrosine, and tryptophan) are high. This serum amino acid imbalance is also seen in sepsis and trauma, and it is probably mediated by an alteration in the balance between insulin and other regulatory hormones.

The role of skeletal muscle in amino acid metabolism has gained prominence. Skeletal muscle constitutes the largest metabolic organ of the body and actively takes up BCAAs that are used to synthesize glutamine and alanine. These amino acids are, in turn, released into the bloodstream and taken up by the liver to become the substrates for hepatic gluconeogenesis. Glutamine is a carrier for ammonia that is converted to urea by the liver and excreted by the kidneys. In cirrhosis, excessive glutamine is synthesized in the skeletal muscle while hepatic urea synthesis is impaired. That leads to an increase in renal glutamine uptake and constitutes a back-up mechanism for ammonia elimination through the kidneys. Studies have shown that cirrhotic patients with decreased skeletal muscle mass are more prone to develop HE.[100] This finding underscores the importance of preserving the skeletal muscle mass in patients with cirrhosis as a means of preventing chronic HE.

In summary, patients with cirrhosis have decreased carbohydrate use and storage capacity plus an increase in fat and protein catabolism, which lead to a chronic catabolic state and the depletion of protein and lipid reserves. These abnormalities, combined with a decrease in food intake and nutrient absorption, constitute the basis of the pathogenesis of PEM in end-stage liver disease. Without question, dysregulated cytokine levels are intimately involved in many of the metabolic and nutrition abnormalities observed in liver disease, especially in acute alcoholic hepatitis and in more decompensated liver disease.[17] More specifically, patients with cirrhosis have increased levels of TNF and interleukin (IL)-1 and IL-6, which have catabolic effects in muscle, adipose tissue, and the liver.[101] Endotoxin produced by intestinal gram-negative bacteria are often present in the blood of patients with cirrhosis.[102] Patients with cirrhosis have an increase in intestinal permeability that allows the leakage of endotoxin from the intestine to the lymphatics and the bloodstream. Endotoxin triggers the release of cytokines and nitric oxide, which may be mediators of the catabolic state as well as the hyperdynamic circulation associated with cirrhosis.[103]

Nutrition Assessment

As the previous data suggest, a proper assessment of nutrition status in patients with liver disease is important but challenging. Several issues make a nutrition assessment in these patients difficult (Table 27-4).

Height and weight are normally a good starting point for a nutrition assessment, but patients with liver disease may have a normal or greater than normal BMI and still have decreased protein and muscle mass because excess fluid, such as ascites, can increase weight without increasing protein stores. Because the excess fluid weight provides no structural protein for strength and activities of daily living, it makes a physical examination in a patient with liver disease essential. In this examination, the clinician must determine whether the patient has muscle wasting in the extremities, the upper body, and the temporal areas despite a weight greater than the ideal weight. Note that dry weight should be used in the nutrition assessment, and it can be estimated based on the severity of ascites. Estimate that 3 to 5 kg of ascitic weight is added to the euvolemic weight for mild ascites, 7 to 9 kg for moderate ascites, and 14 to 15 kg for severe ascites.[104] Alternatively, the lowest recent body weight or ideal body weight can be used. Triceps skinfold and midarm muscle area are not reliable markers of nutrition status in liver disease; however, functional measures like handgrip strength are predictive of nutrition status in liver disease.[105,106]

Laboratory values can also be misleading in patients with liver disease. When liver disease is ongoing, albumin and prealbumin levels may be moderately or very low, even in the presence of good nutrition status;[107] therefore, these measures are not relevant to nutrition status. One method of determining muscle mass is to collect a 24-hour urine sample for creatinine. A normal value of 18 mg per kilogram of ideal weight in women and 23 mg per kilogram of ideal weight in men would suggest normal muscle mass, and below-normal values would suggest decreased muscle mass. This technique is limited to patients with normal renal function and requires an accurate 24-hour urine collection, which can be challenging in an ambulatory setting.

TABLE 27-4 Nutrition Assessment in Advanced Liver Disease

Method	Reliable	Unreliable
BMI		X
Plasma proteins: albumin, prealbumin		X
Delayed skin reactions and total lymphocyte count		X
24-h creatinine:height ratio	X (only with normal renal function)	
BIA		X
Anthropometry: triceps skinfold and midarm muscle area	X	
SGA		X
RFH-NPT	X[a]	
CT/MRI scans	X	
DXA	X	
Handgrip strength	X	

BIA, bioelectric impedance analysis; BMI, body mass index; CT, computed tomography; DXA, dual x-ray absorptiometry; MRI, magnetic resonance imaging; RFH-NPT, Royal Free Hospital–Nutritional Prioritizing Tool; SGA, Subjective Global Assessment.
[a]Needs further validation.

The Subjective Global Assessment (SGA) has been extensively evaluated in patients with cirrhosis,[108] and a revised version has been proposed for liver transplant candidates.[109] This method evaluates patient performance during daily activities and includes a physical examination. However, although relatively easy to apply, the SGA tends to underestimate the severity of malnutrition in patients with cirrhosis and it does not predict the outcome reliably.[106,110,111]

A physical and functional examination is essential in assessing the nutrition status of patients with liver disease. A promising tool is the Royal Free-Hospital–Nutritional Prioritizing Tool (RFH-NPT) (Figure 27-1),[112] which is based on

FIGURE 27-1 Royal Free Hospital–Nutritional Prioritizing Tool (RFH-NPT)

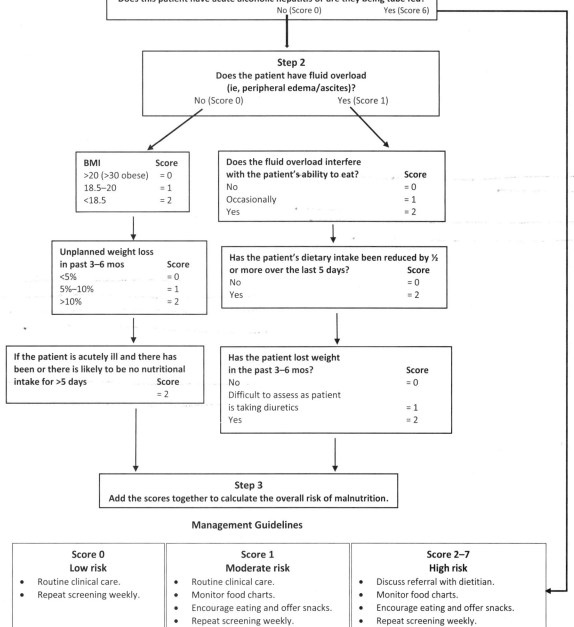

BMI, body mass index.

Source: Adapted from reference 112: Amodio P, Bemeur C, Butterworth R, et al. The nutritional management of hepatic encephalopathy in patients with cirrhosis: International society for hepatic encephalopathy and nitrogen metabolism consensus. *Hepatology*. 2013;58(1):325–336. doi:10.1002/hep.26370. Reproduced with permission from John Wiley and Sons.

BMI, presence of edema, dietary intake, and recent weight loss. The scoring system is fast and easy to apply, but the method needs validation.[113] In general, traditional methods of nutrition status assessment should be used with caution in patients with cirrhosis.[114]

Dual X-ray absorptiometry measures fat, lean, and bone mass, and some initial data indicate its potential utility in patients with liver diseases.[115] Computed tomography or magnetic resonance imaging scans can assess the presence of sarcopenia with high accuracy, but no specific cutoff points have been established in patients with cirrhosis and these procedures expose patients to the risks of radiations and contrast.[116]

Provision of Nutrients to Patients with Liver Disease

Patients with Compensated Liver Disease

Interest in nutrition therapy in cirrhosis began when Patek and colleagues[117] showed that patients who ate a nutritious diet had improved 5-year outcomes compared with control subjects consuming an inadequate diet. Although these patients had ALD, several recent studies further support the concept of improved outcomes with nutrition support in patients with cirrhosis due to any cause. Hirsch and associates[118] demonstrated that outpatients supplementing their diet with an EN support product (1000 kcal, 34 g protein) had significantly improved protein intake and significantly fewer hospitalizations. These investigators then provided an oral supplement to outpatients with alcoholic cirrhosis and observed an improvement in nutrition status and immune function.[118] In the VA Cooperative Study on nutrition support in ALD, mortality was improved with the combination of the anabolic steroid oxandrolone plus EN supplementation in patients who had moderate PEM.[20] Those with severe malnutrition did not significantly benefit from this therapy, possibly because their disease was so severe that no intervention could improve their outcomes. Studies by Kearns and colleagues[119] showed that patients with ALD who were hospitalized for treatment and given an EN supplement via a feeding tube had significantly improved serum bilirubin levels and liver function as assessed by antipyrine clearance. A multicenter, randomized study of EN vs steroids in patients with alcoholic hepatitis showed similar overall short-term results.[25] Moreover, those receiving EN (rich in BCAAs) had better long-term outcomes with fewer infection-related deaths. Thus, nutrition supplementation clearly improved nutrition status and, in some instances, hepatic function and other indicators of outcome in cirrhosis.

There is a long tradition of protein restriction for patients with advanced liver disease who also have HE. However, this tradition has no solid scientific basis, and recent studies do not support this approach. In a prospective, randomized study, Cordoba et al[120] treated 30 patients with cirrhosis who had episodic overt HE with either a low-protein EN formula (with increased protein every 3 days [0 g, then 12 g, 24 g, and 48 g]) or a normal protein EN formula (1.2 g/kg/d) from the first day. Both formulas provided 30 kcal/kg/d. The outcome of HE was similar with both formulas. In a second study, Gheorghe and associates[121] treated 153 consecutive cirrhotic patients with overt HE with a diet providing 30 kcal/kg/d and 1.2 g of protein per kilogram per day, divided in 5 meals from 8:00 AM to 10:00 PM. In most patients, the HE improved, with the best results seen in the patients with more severe HE.[121] HE should be treated with FDA-approved medications, such as lactulose or rifaximin, if needed. If the HE persists despite maximal medical therapy and an evaluation for other causes of changes in mentation, then a BCAA-enriched supplemental formula (via tube feeding, if not contraindicated, or oral supplementation) can be administered to help meet the patient's nitrogen needs. These studies highlight the need to maintain energy intake in patients with liver disease at 25 to 30 kcal/kg/d via enteral feeds and, more specifically, the importance of maintaining protein intake at 1.0 to 1.5 g/kg/d (Table 27-5).[122]

Patients with Decompensated Liver Disease

Patients with decompensated liver disease can be very challenging to manage because of the presence of ascites,

---

TABLE 27-5 Nutrition Therapy in Cirrhosis

- Early assessment of nutrition status along with regular follow-up.
- Total energy can be estimated by the following formula: $1.2-1.4 \times$ REE (kcal/d).
- Protein requirement: 1.0–1.5 g/kg/d.[a]
- Fat requirement: 30%–40% of nonprotein energy.
- Replace vitamins and minerals as needed.
- Alcoholic liver disease: Supplement mainly vitamins B_1, B_6, and B_{12}, folate, and zinc.
- Cholestatic liver diseases (PBC, PSC): Supplement mainly fat-soluble vitamins (A, D, E, and K).
- Nonalcoholic steatohepatitis: Ensure adequate diabetes and hyperlipidemia management; supplement vitamin D as needed.
- Other chronic liver diseases (hepatitis C, hepatitis B, autoimmune hepatitis): supplement vitamins and minerals as needed.
- Use enteral supplementation (ie, tube feeds) to complement other EN (may use PN for shortest time possible if necessary and only if EN through GI tract is contraindicated).

EN, enteral nutrition; GI, gastrointestinal; PBC, primary biliary cholangitis; PN, parenteral nutrition; PSC, primary sclerosing cholangitis; REE, resting energy expenditure.

[a]A patient's actual body weight may be affected by edema and ascites. Dry weight should be used to determine body weight–based nutrient needs, and it can be estimated based on the severity of ascites. For mild ascites, estimate that 3 to 5 kg of ascitic weight is added to the euvolemic weight. For moderate ascites, estimate 7 to 9 kg, and, for severe ascites, estimate 14 to 15 kg. The patient's lowest recent body weight or ideal body weight can also be used as an estimate of dry weight.

encephalopathy, and the increased frequency of diminished renal function. *Decompensated cirrhosis* is defined as cirrhosis with ascites and/or encephalopathy. Liver chemistries usually show albumin levels less than 3 g/dL and total bilirubin greater than 2.5 mg/dL. Patients with PSE may experience behavioral changes, reversal of sleep pattern, slurred speech, disorientation, or coma (Table 27-1). The nutrition requirements mentioned earlier in this chapter apply to the decompensated patient, but it is more difficult to provide proper nutrition to patients with decompensated liver disease (see Practice Scenario 27-2).[12,123,124]

Practice Scenario 27-2

Question: What are the nutrition recommendations for a patient with decompensated cirrhosis, and what is the appropriate meal schedule to provide optimal nutrition to the outpatient with chronic liver disease?

Scenario: A 57-year-old woman with a history of cirrhosis secondary to primary biliary cholangitis (PBC) presents to the clinic for a consultation regarding her nutrition and ongoing issues with advanced liver disease. The patient states that she has had trouble maintaining her muscle strength despite her best efforts to eat an appropriate amount. The patient states that she feels progressively weaker and believes that she has been losing muscle mass. In addition, the patient reports that her husband notices that she tends to function more slowly in the mornings. She is also experiencing worsening ascites and edema. The patient has never received any education regarding proper nutrition in the setting of her liver disease. She requests that some intervention be made to help her maintain or increase her weight, control her fluid retention, and to improve her mentation.

Intervention: The patient is started on a diet consisting of 3 meals per day, including an early-morning meal. She is encouraged to consume breakfast as soon after rising as possible. In addition, the patient begins to eat 3 snacks per day, as well as a late-night, high-protein snack before going to bed. For her ascites and peripheral edema, she dietary sodium restriction (2000 mg/d) is recommended. Over the course of the next 6 months, the patient gains 5 pounds and notes improvement in her strength and mentation.

Answer: Nutrition is essential to improve both lean muscle mass and overall function in patients with liver disease. This patient needed to be educated regarding the importance of consuming an appropriate number of calories and the benefits of consuming 3 meals per day, beginning with an early-morning breakfast, plus 3 small snacks in between meals and a late-night snack before bed. This eating plan can improve her overall functioning and, more importantly, increase lean muscle mass. In addition, because the patient has PBC, it is important to check her levels of fat-soluble vitamins (A, D, E, and K). Their absorption depends on intraluminal solubilization by bile acids and adequate bile flow.

Rationale: An important component of the dietary management of the patient with advanced liver disease is to minimize periods

without food intake because patients rapidly enter starvation mode, with decreased glucose oxidation and increased protein and fat catabolism.[123] To prevent this problem, the diet should include at least 4 feedings (meals and snacks) per day. The first feeding should be early in the morning, and the last can be a bedtime supplement. The early breakfast improves cognitive function in patients with subclinical (minimal) hepatic encephalopathy, and the bedtime supplement improves body protein stores.[124] Importantly, an improvement in muscle mass with nighttime supplements was demonstrated by Plank et al,[12] who randomly assigned 103 patients with cirrhosis to receive 2 cans of Ensure Plus (710 kcal with 26 g of protein) or 2 cans of Diabetic Resource (500 kcal with 30 g of protein) either during the day or at bedtime for a total of 12 months. Patients who received supplements at bedtime gained lean muscle mass (2 kg) over 12 months,[12] demonstrating the importance of late-night snacking in maintaining muscle mass in patients with cirrhosis.

If patients fail to achieve on their own the recommended energy intake of 1.2 to 1.4 times REE and 1.0 to 1.5 g protein per kg, supplemental EN in the form of nasogastric or orogastric tube feeds should be considered.[114,122] Some initial data seem to indicate that dairy and vegetables are preferable sources of proteins compared with animal proteins because the former are better tolerated and may more effectively help eliminate ammonia in the case of PSE.[125,126]

EN is preferred over PN because EN costs less, avoids the risk of sepsis associated with the PN line, preserves the integrity of the gut mucosa, and can prevent bacterial translocation and multiple organ failure. Moreover, PN can, in some instances, cause liver disease as one of its complications.

If EN is not possible, PN can be used. However, it is important to return to the enteral route as soon as the small bowel shows evidence of recovered function. PN can be started with a standard amino acid formula in amounts that are increased until nitrogen needs are met. If the patient develops PSE, standard therapy with FDA-approved medications should be given. If the patient still cannot tolerate the amount of amino acids needed to satisfy nitrogen requirements, the standard amino acid formulation can be replaced by a BCAA-enriched solution specifically designed for liver disease.[127,128] Patients do not usually require either PN or BCAA-enriched formulas, and the primary goal is always aggressive EN (Practice Scenario 27-3).[106] Of note, the American Society for Parenteral and Enteral Nutrition guidelines for critically ill patients state that there is no evidence to support the use of BCAAs in the comatose intensive care unit patient who is already receiving standard treatment for HE.[129]

Practice Scenario 27-3

Question: What are the appropriate nutrition interventions to institute in a malnourished inpatient with liver disease?

Scenario: A 60-year-old man with hepatitis C cirrhosis is admitted with portal systemic encephalopathy. In addition to his encephalopathy, a physical examination reveals ascites, bitemporal wasting, and muscle atrophy. The patient is admitted, and a nasoenteric tube is placed for enteral access and the administration of lactulose and rifaximin. An interview with the patient's wife reveals that the patient has had a poor appetite for several years, and particularly in the last 3 to 4 weeks. He is currently on lactulose and rifaximin at home, but he does not take any additional nutritional supplements, including no vitamin or mineral supplements.

Intervention: This patient shows characteristic signs of malnutrition (bitemporal wasting and muscle atrophy). In addition, his ascites and encephalopathy reveal that he has decompensated disease. As such, the patient is started on enteral tube feeding with additional protein modules to provide 1.2 g protein per kilogram per day. The patient is also given nutritional supplements, including oral zinc.

Answer: Patients with malnutrition caused by their liver disease require the early institution of nutritional supplementation, including adequate provision of specific micronutrients (vitamins and trace elements) and optimization of protein intake via oral supplements (drinks), if tolerated. Patients with liver disease are likely to have protein-energy malnutrition. Adequate energy and protein must be given as soon as possible. In addition, patients with liver disease are typically deficient in a variety of vitamins and minerals. Supplementation of these vitamins and minerals should also be a priority.

Rationale: If patients are unable to achieve on their own the recommended energy intake of 1.2 to 1.4 times their resting energy expenditure and the protein goal of 1.0 to 1.5 g/kg/d, supplemental enteral nutrition via a nasogastric tube should be considered.[106] Zinc is an essential trace element that participates in cellular function through hundreds of zinc proteins, including zinc metalloenzymes and critical zinc transcription factors. Zinc may be a helpful adjunctive therapy in hepatic encephalopathy.

Complementary and Alternative Medicine Agents

A recent major change in therapy for liver disease has been the use of CAM, including supplementation with individual nutrients. According to the Centers for Disease Control and Prevention, more than 40% of the US population uses CAM.[130] Furthermore, patients with chronic disease processes, such as cirrhosis, are frequent users of CAM.[131] However, as discussed in Chapter 19, patients frequently do not report CAM use to physicians. A variety of forms of CAM have been used effectively to treat or prevent liver injury in animal models, and preliminary data with some agents suggest efficacy in human liver disease. Clinicians must be aware of the potential benefits and toxicities of these agents and should demand well-designed, randomized controlled trials (RCTs) of such products. In this chapter, the specific CAM agents that will be reviewed in relation to liver disease include vitamin E, glutathione (GSH) prodrugs and antioxidant cocktails, SAM and betaine, silymarin (milk thistle), and other herbals. Selected vitamin and mineral deficiencies frequently complicating chronic liver disease are also discussed.

Vitamin E

Vitamin E is a potent antioxidant that is widely used as a nutritional supplement. Depressed serum and hepatic levels of vitamin E have been documented in patients with ALD and in experimental models of liver disease. Vitamin E has been used extensively to protect against experimental models of liver injury, such as that induced by carbon tetrachloride via the inhibition of nuclear factor kappa B (NF-κB) activation.[132] Hill and associates[133] treated human peripheral blood monocytes and rat Kupffer cells in vitro with vitamin E, inhibiting both NF-κB activation and TNF production. Vitamin E also inhibits the activation of hepatic stellate cells and collagen production in vitro.

Vitamin E was initially reported to have beneficial effects in some, but not all studies of patients with fatty liver (NASH).[47,134,135] A pilot study in children showed improvement in liver enzymes, and a study from Japan showed that vitamin E not only improved liver enzymes but also decreased serum levels of the profibrotic cytokine transforming growth factor beta.[134,135] Notably, a study in patients with alcoholic hepatitis showed improvement in hyaluronic acid, a marker of fibrosis. However, that study did not demonstrate improvement in mortality.[136] The most important and compelling vitamin E data are from the PIVENS trial, a large multicenter National Institutes of Health–funded study, which assigned 247 adults with NASH (without diabetes) to receive pioglitazone at a dose of 30 mg/d (80 subjects), vitamin E at a dose of 800 IU/d (84 subjects), or placebo (83 subjects) for 96 weeks.[47] Vitamin E therapy, as compared with placebo, was associated with a significantly higher rate of improvement in NASH (43% vs 19%; $P = 0.001$). Compared with placebo, serum alanine and aspartate aminotransferase levels were reduced with vitamin E and with pioglitazone ($P < 0.001$ for both comparisons). No treatment demonstrated an improvement in fibrosis. Subjects who received pioglitazone gained more weight than those who received vitamin E or placebo. In conclusion, vitamin E improved liver histology and liver enzymes and was not associated with the weight gain seen with pioglitazone; at this time, 800 IU of vitamin E is the preferred "drug" therapy for nondiabetic NASH patients at some centers.

Glutathione Prodrugs and Combined Antioxidants

GSH is a tripeptide synthesized from glutamate, cysteine, and glycine. GSH, in its reduced form, is the main nonprotein thiol in cells and has an important role in the detoxification of electrophiles and in protection against reactive oxygen toxicity, including protection against intracellular free radicals, reactive oxygen intermediates, and several endogenous and exogenous toxins.[137] GSH also protects against toxicity from certain drugs (eg, acetaminophen). GSH cannot be taken up by hepatocytes, but a number of pharmacologic agents have been devised to enhance intracellular pools (eg, N-acetylcysteine [NAC], 2-oxothiazolidine-4-carboxylic acid). There are 2 distinct intercellular GSH pools: cytosolic (approximately 80%) and mitochondrial (approximately 20%). Mitochondrial GSH detoxifies hydrogen peroxide and other organic peroxides produced in mitochondria. Chronic alcohol consumption has been reported to deplete GSH levels.[118] Moreover, alcohol causes a marked depletion of GSH in the mitochondrial pool, with at least part of that depletion attributed to its impaired transport from the cytosolic pool. This depletion renders hepatocytes more vulnerable to oxidative stress. The molecular basis for the impaired GSH transport into mitochondria is unclear, but it has been reported that exogenous SAM—but not NAC or other pro-GSH molecules—restores mitochondrial function, enhances mitochondrial transport, and corrects mitochondrial GSH deficiency.

GSH precursors also can regulate the production of proinflammatory cytokines, such as TNF and IL-8, by Kupffer cells and monocytes, with increased GSH levels decreasing cytokine production.[138] This regulation of cytokine production occurs, at least in part, through the inhibition of the oxidative-stress–sensitive transcription factor NF-κB, which plays a central role in LPS-stimulated TNF production.

The GSH precursor NAC has been used clinically for decades to treat acute acetaminophen overdose, with good results when it is administered early (optimally within 12 hours of acetaminophen ingestion). A recent study evaluated the effects of IV NAC on transplant-free survival in patients with non-acetaminophen-related acute liver failure.[139] The 173 patients received either NAC or a placebo. In patients with early stage non-acetaminophen-related acute liver failure, NAC improved transplant-free survival. This important study supports the use of IV NAC in patients with acute liver failure.

Combined trials of antioxidants that not only increase GSH but also provide other antioxidant effects have not shown efficacy in patients with chronic ALD. In contrast to administering exogenous antioxidants, an alternative approach uses CAM agents (broccoli extracts) to stimulate the endogenous production of antioxidants. This approach has been evaluated in preliminary HCC chemoprevention studies in Asian patients exposed to aflatoxins.[55] Thus, there is a scientific rationale for an antioxidant approach, but defining appropriate clinical populations and establishing doses seem to be major challenges.

S-Adenosylmethionine and Betaine

Elevated methionine and decreased methionine clearance represent possible therapeutic targets for liver disease, especially ALD. In animal models of liver injury, decreased levels of SAM and elevated levels of S-adenosylhomocysteine are regularly observed. In human studies of alcoholic hepatitis and cirrhosis, abnormal hepatic gene expression occurs and contributes to decreased hepatic SAM, cysteine, and GSH levels. Rodent and primate studies demonstrate that SAM depletion occurred in early stages of fatty liver infiltration in ALD, and decreased SAM concentration, liver injury, and mitochondrial damage could be reversed with SAM supplementation.[140] SAM attenuated oxidative stress and hepatic stellate cell activation in an ethanol-LPS–induced fibrotic rat model.[141] Most importantly, a double-blind RCT was performed in 123 patients with alcoholic cirrhosis treated with SAM (1200 mg/d, orally) or

placebo for 2 years.[142] When patients with Child class C cirrhosis were excluded from the analysis, the overall mortality/liver transplantation rate was significantly greater in the placebo group than in the SAM group (20% vs 12%), and differences between the 2-year survival curves (defined as the time to death or liver transplantation) of the 2 groups were also statistically significant. A subsequent Cochrane review of SAM and ALD could not find evidence supporting or refuting the use of SAM for patients with ALD.[143] A more recent study did not show any improvement of liver enzymes and liver histology after 6 months of SAM supplementation in patients with various severity of ALD. The study was probably underpowered to detect a difference, but it is the only study that compared liver pathology before and after treatment.[144] Further studies and long-term, high-quality RCTs are clearly needed.

Betaine (trimethylglycine) is a key nutrient in humans and is obtained from a variety of foods and nutritional supplements. In the liver, betaine can transfer 1 methyl group to homocysteine to form methionine. This process removes toxic metabolites (homocysteine and S-adenosylhomocysteine), restores SAM levels, reverses steatosis, prevents apoptosis, and reduces both damaged protein accumulation and oxidative stress. Betaine also appears to attenuate alcoholic steatosis by restoring phosphatidylcholine generation via the phosphatidylethanolamine methyltransferase pathway.[145] However, the most definitive human trial thus far (in NASH patients) showed no benefit.[146]

Zinc

Zinc is an essential trace element that participates in cellular function through hundreds of zinc proteins, including zinc metalloenzymes and critical zinc transcription factors. Zinc deficiency can present as angular (perioral) cheilosis, muscle cramps, and neurosensory defects, and it has been well examined in liver disease.[147,148] An altered zinc metabolism with zinc deficiency and decreased serum zinc is noted in most forms of clinical liver disease, especially ALD. Stress/inflammation caused by a variety of factors, including LPS/TNF, also leads to an internal redistribution of zinc, with loss of zinc from some tissues (deficiency) and redirection to other tissues or organs, including the liver. Importantly, zinc deficiency was shown to be induced by oxidative stress, in which thiol oxidation of zinc-finger transcription factors resulted in zinc loss, leading to a loss of DNA-binding activity.[149–151]

A study from Kang and Zhou and colleagues[151] provides major insights into the molecular mechanisms of altered zinc metabolism in the development and progression of experimental ALD, with important potential therapeutic implications for ALD and other forms of chronic liver disease. In both acute and chronic alcohol-induced hepatotoxicity, alcohol intake and oxidative stress disrupt tight junctions in the intestine, leading to the translocation of bacterial products such as endotoxin.[147,149] Endotoxin activates Toll-like receptor 4 and TNF production, with subsequent oxidative stress and liver injury. Endotoxin and TNF also play critical roles in liver fibrosis. The disruption of tight-junction proteins occurs not only in the intestine but also in the lung and likely at the blood-brain barrier, thus potentially predisposing the patient to lung injury and HE.[147] Zinc treatment in experimental animals with ALD attenuated the increased gut permeability, endotoxemia, TNF production, oxidative stress, and liver injury, while improving the activity of key zinc transcription factors.[147,150,151] Thus, zinc supplementation targets most postulated mechanisms for the development of ALD and certain other forms of chronic liver disease, such as NAFLD.

A human pilot trial also suggests that zinc may stabilize or cause the regression of hepatic fibrosis.[152] In this trial, polaprezinc, a synthetic, zinc-containing compound with 34 mg of elemental zinc, was administered daily for 24 weeks to patients with chronic hepatitis or cirrhosis, and the zinc-supplemented patients significantly improved their serum zinc levels and markers of fibrosis.[152] Zinc may also be effective in the treatment of HE.[153] The preliminary results of a small RCT in patients with cirrhosis, elevated ammonia levels, and low zinc serum levels showed that, compared with no supplementation, zinc supplementation of total 150 mg/d for 3 months was effective in reducing blood ammonia levels.[154] Both supplemented and nonsupplemented patients continued with their standard treatment based on BCAA and lactulose.

There are no strict parameters for zinc replacement. Zinc can be replaced in patients with liver disease as 50 mg elemental zinc by mouth. If higher doses are used, copper deficiency with cytopenia may ensue.

Silymarin

Silymarin, the active ingredient extracted from *Silybum marianum* (also known as *milk thistle*), was shown in experimental animals to protect against multiple types of liver injury, including those induced by carbon tetrachloride, acetaminophen, and iron overload, and, very importantly, mushroom poisoning.[155] It is probably the most widely used form of CAM in the treatment of liver disease, perhaps because it has a good safety profile, has been extensively investigated in multiple forms of experimental liver injury in animals, and is associated with some positive results in humans. Clinically, it has been suggested to have hepatoprotective effects in various forms of toxic hepatitis, fatty liver, cirrhosis, ischemic injury, and viral-induced liver disease.[155] It has antioxidant activities, protects against lipid peroxidation, and has anti-inflammatory and antifibrotic effects. However, large, controlled trials of silymarin performed in Europe have had variable results,[156,157] and the results of a Cochrane analysis questioned the beneficial effects of milk thistle for patients with alcoholic and/or hepatitis B or C virus liver diseases and highlighted the lack of high-quality evidence to support this intervention.[158]

Branched-Chain Amino Acids

The use of oral BCAAs can be a consideration in the management of individuals with cirrhosis. Investigators have studies the effects of BCAA supplementation on HE, survival, and HCC. In a study by Hayaishi and colleagues,[159] high doses of oral BCAAs (12 g/d) were given to individuals with cirrhosis and no history of HCC. After 6 months of therapy, the patients receiving BCAAs had a lower incidence of HCC, as well as

fewer medical complications related to their cirrhosis.[159] An RCT showed that BCAA supplementation reduces the incidence of HCC, but this effect was limited to obese patients with cirrhosis and hepatitis C infection.[160] Additional support for BCAA supplementation was demonstrated in a multicenter RCT involving the administration of a 12 g/d dose of BCAAs vs diet therapy for 2 years. Patients given high-dose BCAAs were found to have an improved quality of life, increased event-free survivals, and improved serum albumin concentrations.[161] In a study by Fan et al,[162] benefits were also seen in patients undergoing a partial hepatectomy for HCC. The patients were given 14 days of IV nutrition therapy that consisted of 35% BCAAs. When compared with a control group undergoing the same procedure, the group receiving BCAAs had decreased postoperative morbidity, including less weight loss, less ascites, and fewer infectious complications.[162] In a multicenter, randomized study, 1-year oral supplementation with BCAAs was compared with lactalbumin or maltodextrin in 174 patients with advanced cirrhosis. The results indicated that BCAA supplementation reduced the primary outcome (a combination of deaths, number of hospital admissions, and hospital lengths of stay). However, the BCAA group was also characterized by a high dropout rate (about 15%) because of poor compliance.[163] It is important to note the great heterogeneity in the modalities (oral powders or IV) and doses of BCAA supplementation in the reported studies. This variability limits our ability to draw definitive conclusions about the routine clinical use of BCAAs.

Probiotics

Emerging evidence suggests the gut microbiome plays an important role in the pathogenesis of liver disease and its complications. There is growing interest in the therapeutic effects of probiotics related to their capacity to produce antimicrobial substances and enhance protective mechanisms in the gut epithelium, avoiding adherence of pathogenic bacteria and thereby protecting against IBO and translocation. Probiotics can also modulate local and systemic oxidative and inflammatory responses (see Chapter 4).[164]

Increased IBO and intestinal permeability in patients with NAFLD[165] promote the delivery of gut-derived microbial products to the liver. In an experimental model of NASH, this phenomenon evokes a local inflammatory response and leads to steatosis, inflammation, and fibrosis.[49,166] Most clinical trials of probiotics in patients with NAFLD strongly suggest improvements in liver enzymes, oxidative stress, and inflammatory markers.[49,166-168] Interestingly, one of these studies showed reductions in the amount of hepatic steatosis, insulin resistance, and NASH activity index.[167] A recent meta-analysis of 4 RCTs supported these findings.[168]

ALD is associated with IBO and enteric dysbiosis. As the liver disease decompensates further, dysbiosis worsens, the intestinal mucosal barrier becomes defective, and the local host immune system becomes compromised, resulting in many of the complications seen in advanced liver disease such as systemic endotoxemia,[169] spontaneous bacterial peritonitis (SBP), and HE. Evidence shows that probiotics improve liver function and inflammatory and oxidative markers in alcohol-induced liver injury.[170,171]

We know that patients with HE also have significant dysbiosis.[172] Recent RCTs revealed that probiotics were effective in primary prevention[173] and secondary prevention of overt HE.[174] Finally, a meta-analysis of 496 patients showed that probiotics are effective in preventing overt HE development in patients with liver cirrhosis.[175]

However, even though probiotics can reduce endotoxemia, their use as an adjuvant to antibiotics for SBP prophylaxis has not been proven successful.[176] Evidence regarding portal hypertension is conflicting, and few RCTs have investigated the relationship between probiotics and hemodynamics in cirrhosis. In half of the studies that have been done, the probiotic medical food VSL#3 did not reduce portal pressure in patients with compensated or decompensated cirrhosis, but reduction in plasma aldosterone suggested a possible beneficial effect.[177,178] However, another study showed improvement in the hepatic, systemic hemodynamics and serum sodium levels in patients with cirrhosis who took VSL#3.[179] Recently, an RCT showed that adjunctive probiotics to propranolol treatment decreased hepatic venous pressure gradient in cirrhotic patients with large esophageal varices.[180]

However, it is important to note that the types, dosages, and duration of probiotic treatment vary widely among studies. Therefore, it is not possible to draw final conclusions about their use in the routine clinical practice. Table 27-6 summarizes the major studies on probiotics in fatty liver, hepatitis C, and ALD.[49,165,167,181–183]

Management of Various Micronutrient Problems Complicating Cirrhosis

Issues related to vitamin E and zinc are discussed in the previous section on CAM. Other micronutrients of concern in patients with cirrhosis include vitamin D, vitamin A, thiamin, iron, and manganese.

A substantial number of patients with liver disease, regardless of etiology, are known to be deficient in vitamin D.[184] This fact should prompt an assessment of vitamin D status in the form of a serum 25-hydroxyvitamin D level. Although guidelines for the replacement of vitamin D in liver disease have not been completely delineated, replacement to achieve a 25-hydroxyvitamin D level greater than 32 ng/mL has been suggested[185] and 2000 IU daily of vitamin D_3 with 1200 to 1500 mg of calcium per day are generally effective in achieving this goal.[114] Patients with cholestatic liver diseases may be at particularly high risk for vitamin D deficiency.

Vitamin A deficiency presents primarily in cholestatic liver diseases and decompensated cirrhosis and is associated with increased risk of HCC.[186] Vitamin A deficiency in patients with cholestatic liver diseases can be addressed with dietary supplements of vitamin A of 15,000 IU daily.[187] Children with cholestatic liver diseases may require up to 25,000 IU of vitamin A for 4 to 12 weeks.[188] Of note, there is an increased risk of hepatic toxicity and long bone fractures with high-dose vitamin A supplementation. Therefore, vitamin A levels should be checked before starting supplementation.

Thiamin deficiency may be a complication of chronic alcoholism or bariatric surgery.[189] This deficiency increases the risk of serious neurologic consequences, specifically Wernicke encephalopathy, and should be treated aggressively. A recommended protocol includes 500 mg of thiamin intravenously, infused over 30 minutes, 3 times daily for 2 consecutive days followed by 250 mg intravenously or intramuscularly once daily for 5 days, in combination with other B vitamins.[190] At the end of parenteral supplementation protocol, oral thiamin supplementation should be continued at the dose of 100 mg/d.

Iron deficiency anemia may occur in some patients with chronic GI blood loss due to portal hypertensive gastropathy or gastric antral vascular ectasia. Iron should be replaced in these patients.[161]

TABLE 27-6 Clinical Studies on the Use of Probiotics in Common Liver Diseases

Reference	Sample Size	Treatment	Duration
Aller et al[165]	28 patients with NAFLD	500 million CFU of *Lactobacillus bulgaricus* and *Streptococcus thermophilus* daily	12 weeks
Eslamparast et al[49]	52 patients with NAFLD	200 million CFU of *L. casei, L. rhamnosus, S. thermophilus, Bifidobacterium breve, L. acidophilus, B. longum,* and *L. bulgaricus,* plus FOS and probiotic cultures and a vegetable capsule twice a day	28 weeks
Loguercio et al[181]	36 patients with chronic hepatitis C, 20 patients with alcoholic cirrhosis, 22 patients with NAFLD	450 billion bacteria *(S. thermophilus, B. breve, B. longum, B. infantis, L. acidophilus, L. plantarum, L. casei, L. bulgaricus),* 2 capsules twice a day	12 weeks
Malaguarnera et al[167]	66 patients with NASH	*B. longum* plus FOS	24 weeks
Vajro et al[182]	20 children with NAFLD	12 billion CFU *L. rhamnosus* strain GG daily	8 weeks
Wong et al[183]	20 patients with NASH	200 million CFU *L. plantarum, L. deslbrueckii, L. acidophilus, L. rhamnosus,* and *B. bifidum* twice a day, plus FOS, cellulose, magnesium stearate, silica, and milk	24 weeks

CFU, colony-forming units; FOS, fructooligosaccharides; NAFLD, nonalcoholic fatty liver disease; NASH, nonalcoholic steatohepatitis.

When recommending supplements to patients, it may be helpful to recommend supplements with low or no manganese content. Patients with cirrhosis may present manganese accumulation in the basal ganglia, and it may contribute to their encephalopathy.[191,192]

Monitoring and Treating Complications

Many of the complications of liver disease can be effectively managed as long as signs and symptoms are appropriately monitored. Monitoring can begin with basic physical examination findings. Patients with decompensated liver disease often have ascites that are easily assessed by increased abdominal girth. Assessment of weight loss and BMI is affected by the presence of ascites. Therefore, it is important to estimate the BMI using dry weight. Clinicians can use serial measurements of midarm muscle circumference to evaluate changes in muscle mass, whereas functional changes can be assessed by measuring changes in handgrip strength.[193]

Simple nutrition interventions can decrease the occurrence of ascites. Institution of a sodium-limited diet (2 g/d) is an important step in preventing the recurrence of ascites.[194] Hypervolemic hyponatremia is common in patients with cirrhosis, but fluid restriction is not necessary in treating most patients because severe hyponatremia (serum sodium less than 125 mmol/L) is relatively rare.[194] Practice guidelines indicate that fluid restriction for serum sodium less than 125 mmol/L is reasonable.[194] In patients with cirrhosis and hyponatremia who are receiving EN, 2 kcal/mL formulas may be used.

Furthermore, patients with decompensated cirrhosis present several unique challenges to the delivery of EN. Patients in a hepatic coma will likely require nasoenteric tube placement for the delivery of medications as well as nutrition. Thrombocytopenia and coagulopathy typically accompany decompensated liver disease, and, in this setting, epistaxis may complicate nasoenteric tube placement. If a patient with compromised airway protection due to HE experiences epistaxis, it can result in aspiration. Furthermore, tubes can be inadvertently displaced in patients with HE. The authors' practice is to carefully place soft-tipped, fine-bore nasogastric tubes, often accompanied by commercially available, magnetic string-type bridles, in these patients. Unless patients have a history of epistaxis and/or significant thrombocytopenia (platelets less than 20,000/mcL) or coagulopathy (international normalized ratio greater than 1.5), we do not routinely transfuse platelets or fresh frozen plasma prior to a nasoenteric tube placement. Anecdotally, we have administered topical vasoconstrictor sprays (such as oxymetazoline) intranasally prior to tube placement to reduce the likelihood of epistaxis. Although we could find no published data to support this practice, Katz and colleagues reported that oxymetazoline prevented epistaxis prior to nasotracheal intubation.[195]

A second potential problem confounding nasoenteric tube placement is esophageal varices. The risk that the placement of a soft-tipped, fine-bore nasally or orally placed feeding tube will precipitate variceal hemorrhage (in nonbleeding varices) is low and should typically not contraindicate tube placement.[196] An important exception occurs during (or immediately following the treatment of) bleeding gastroesophageal varices. Bleeding esophageal varices are typically managed by an endoscopic band ligation. A tube could, theoretically, prematurely dislodge the band from the varices and precipitate rebleeding. There is also a theoretical risk that EN could increase intestinal blood flow and portal pressures. Although a small study found an increased risk of rebleeding when EN was initiated within 72 hours of variceal hemorrhage,[197] other authors advise holding EN for the first 48 hours.[166]

Mortality with percutaneous endoscopic gastrostomy (PEG) tube placement is high in patients with cirrhosis, and especially in those with ascites.[198] Therefore, PEG tubes are contraindicated in patients with ascites. Patients with liver disease may also be intolerant of intragastric feeding due to nausea, vomiting, or increased gastric residuals. Although these problems may necessitate alteration in the delivery of nutritional supplementation, they should not lead to cessation of nutrition support. These issues with intragastric feeding can be addressed with use of postpyloric tube feeds.

Summary

Liver disease encompasses a heterogeneous group of disorders with diverse clinical outcomes ranging from acute hepatitis, acute liver failure, asymptomatic chronic elevation of liver enzymes, compensated cirrhosis, and end-stage liver disease. In many cases, poor nutrition has been linked to the pathogenesis and progression of liver disease. Likewise, data indicate that nutrition therapy may favorably affect the course of liver disease in many cases. Therefore, nutrition support clinicians have a unique opportunity to improve the lives of these patients.

References

1. Vilstrup H, Amodio P, Bajaj J, et al. Hepatic encephalopathy in chronic liver disease: 2014 practice guideline by the American Association for the Study of Liver Diseases and the European Association for the Study of the Liver. *Hepatology.* 2014;60(2): 715–735.
2. Mohd Hanafiah K, Groeger J, Flaxman AD, Wiersma ST. Global epidemiology of hepatitis C virus infection: new estimates of age-specific antibody to HCV seroprevalence. *Hepatology.* 2013;57(4): 1333–1342.
3. Younossi ZM, Stepanova M, Afendy M, et al. Changes in the prevalence of the most common causes of chronic liver diseases in the United States from 1988 to 2008. *Clin Gastroenterol Hepatol.* 2011;9(6):524–530.
4. Santolaria F, Perez-Manzano JL, Milena A, et al. Nutritional assessment in alcoholic patients: its relationship with alcoholic intake, feeding habits, organic complications and social problems. *Drug Alcohol Depend.* 2000;59(3):295–304.
5. Galati JS, Holdeman KP, Bottjen PL, Quigley EM. Gastric emptying and orocecal transit in portal hypertension and end-stage chronic liver disease. *Liver Transpl Surg.* 1997;3(1):34–38.
6. Galati JS, Holdeman KP, Dalrymple GV, Harrison KA, Quigley EM. Delayed gastric emptying of both the liquid and solid components of a meal in chronic liver disease. *Am J Gastroenterol.* 1994;89(5):708–711.
7. Kalaitzakis E. Gastrointestinal dysfunction in liver cirrhosis. *World J Gastroenterol.* 2014;20(40):14686–14695.
8. Thuluvath PJ, Triger DR. Autonomic neuropathy and chronic liver disease. *Q J Med.* 1989;72(268):737–747.

9. Quigley EM. Gastrointestinal dysfunction in liver disease and portal hypertension: gut-liver interactions revisited. *Dig Dis Sci.* 1996;41(3):557–561.

10. Yoshida Y, Higashi T, Nouso K, et al. Effects of zinc deficiency/zinc supplementation on ammonia metabolism in patients with decompensated liver cirrhosis. *Acta Med Okayama.* 2001;55(6):349–355.

11. Camilleri M, Gores GJ. Therapeutic targeting of bile acids. *Am J Physiol Gastrointest Liver Physiol.* 2015;309(4):G209–G215.

12. Plank LD, Gane EJ, Peng S, et al. Nocturnal nutritional supplementation improves total body protein status of patients with liver cirrhosis: a randomized 12-month trial. *Hepatology.* 2008;48(2):557–566.

13. Swart GR, Zillikens MC, van Vuure JK, van den Berg JW. Effect of a late evening meal on nitrogen balance in patients with cirrhosis of the liver. *BMJ.* 1989;299(6709):1202–1203.

14. Dolz C, Raurich JM, Ibanez J, et al. Ascites increases the resting energy expenditure in liver cirrhosis. *Gastroenterology.* 1991;100(3):738–744.

15. Muller MJ, Lautz HU, Plogmann B, et al. Energy expenditure and substrate oxidation in patients with cirrhosis: the impact of cause, clinical staging and nutritional state. *Hepatology.* 1992;15(5):782–794.

16. Guglielmi FW, Panella C, Buda A, et al. Nutritional state and energy balance in cirrhotic patients with or without hypermetabolism: multicentre prospective study by the "Nutritional Problems in Gastroenterology" Section of the Italian Society of Gastroenterology (SIGE). *Dig Liver Dis.* 2005;37(9):681–688.

17. McClain CJ, Song Z, Barve SS, Hill DB, Deaciuc I. Recent advances in alcoholic liver disease. IV. Dysregulated cytokine metabolism in alcoholic liver disease. *Am J Physiol Gastrointest Liver Physiol.* 2004;287(3):G497–G502.

18. McClain CJ, Barve S, Deaciuc I, Kugelmas M, Hill D. Cytokines in alcoholic liver disease. *Semin Liver Dis.* 1999;19(2):205–219.

19. Sleisenger MH, Feldman M, Friedman LS, Brandt LJ. *Sleisenger and Fordtran's Gastrointestinal and Liver Disease: Pathophysiology, Diagnosis, Management.* 9th ed. Philadelphia, PA: Saunders/Elsevier; 2010.

20. Mendenhall C, Roselle GA, Gartside P, Moritz T. Relationship of protein calorie malnutrition to alcoholic liver disease: a reexamination of data from two Veterans Administration Cooperative Studies. *Alcohol Clin Exp Res.* 1995;19(3):635–641.

21. Mendenhall CL, Tosch T, Weesner RE, et al. VA Cooperative Study on Alcoholic Hepatitis. II: prognostic significance of protein-calorie malnutrition. *Am J Clin Nutr.* 1986;43(2):213–218.

22. Mendenhall CL, Anderson S, Weesner RE, Goldberg SJ, Crolic KA. Protein-calorie malnutrition associated with alcoholic hepatitis. Veterans Administration Cooperative Study Group on Alcoholic Hepatitis. *Am J Med.* 1984;76(2):211–222.

23. Mendenhall CL, Moritz TE, Roselle GA, et al. Protein energy malnutrition in severe alcoholic hepatitis: diagnosis and response to treatment. The VA Cooperative Study Group #275. *JPEN J Parenter Enteral Nutr.* 1995;19(4):258–265.

24. Mendenhall CL, Moritz TE, Roselle GA, et al. A study of oral nutritional support with oxandrolone in malnourished patients with alcoholic hepatitis: results of a Department of Veterans Affairs Cooperative Study. *Hepatology.* 1993;17(4):564–576.

25. Cabre E, Rodriguez-Iglesias P, Caballeria J, et al. Short-and long-term outcome of severe alcohol-induced hepatitis treated with steroids or enteral nutrition: a multicenter randomized trial. *Hepatology.* 2000;32(1):36–42.

26. Moreno C, Deltenre P, Senterre C, et al. Intensive enteral nutrition is ineffective for patients with severe alcoholic hepatitis treated with corticosteroids. *Gastroenterology.* 2016;150(4):903–910.

27. Antar R, Wong P, Ghali P. A meta-analysis of nutritional supplementation for management of hospitalized alcoholic hepatitis. *Can J Gastroenterol.* 2012;26(7):463–467.

28. Dupont B, Dao T, Joubert C, et al. Randomised clinical trial: enteral nutrition does not improve the long-term outcome of alcoholic cirrhotic patients with jaundice. *Aliment Pharmacol Ther.* 2012;35(10):1166–1174.

29. Gloria L, Cravo M, Camilo ME, et al. Nutritional deficiencies in chronic alcoholics: relation to dietary intake and alcohol consumption. *Am J Gastroenterol.* 1997;92(3):485–489.

30. Piscaglia F, Svegliati-Baroni G, Barchetti A, et al. Clinical patterns of hepatocellular carcinoma in nonalcoholic fatty liver disease: a multicenter prospective study. *Hepatology.* 2016;63(3):827–838.

31. Koo BK, Kim D, Joo SK. Sarcopenia is an independent risk factor for non-alcoholic steatohepatitis and significant fibrosis. *J Hepatol.* 2017;66(1):123–131.

32. Lieber CS, Leo MA, Mak KM, et al. Model of nonalcoholic steatohepatitis. *Am J Clin Nutr.* 2004;79(3):502–509.

33. Cortez-Pinto H, Jesus L, Barros H, et al. How different is the dietary pattern in non-alcoholic steatohepatitis patients? *Clin Nutr.* 2006;25(5):816–823.

34. Lieber CS, DeCarli LM, Leo MA, et al. Beneficial effects versus toxicity of medium-chain triacylglycerols in rats with NASH. *J Hepatol.* 2008;48(2):318–326.

35. Lim JS, Mietus-Snyder M, Valente A, Schwarz JM, Lustig RH. The role of fructose in the pathogenesis of NAFLD and the metabolic syndrome. *Nat Rev Gastroenterol Hepatol.* 2010;7(5):251–264.

36. Ouyang X, Cirillo P, Sautin Y, et al. Fructose consumption as a risk factor for non-alcoholic fatty liver disease. *J Hepatol.* 2008;48(6):993–999.

37. Spruss A, Kanuri G, Wagnerberger S, et al. Toll-like receptor 4 is involved in the development of fructose-induced hepatic steatosis in mice. *Hepatology.* 2009;50(4):1094–1104.

38. Sanchez-Lozada LG, Mu W, Roncal C, et al. Comparison of free fructose and glucose to sucrose in the ability to cause fatty liver. *Eur J Nutr.* 2010;49(1):1–9.

39. Abdelmalek MF, Suzuki A, Guy C, et al. Increased fructose consumption is associated with fibrosis severity in patients with nonalcoholic fatty liver disease. *Hepatology.* 2010;51(6):1961–1971.

40. Lazo M, Solga SF, Horska A, et al. Effect of a 12-month intensive lifestyle intervention on hepatic steatosis in adults with type 2 diabetes. *Diabetes Care.* 2010;33(10):2156–2163.

41. Tendler D, Lin S, Yancy WS, et al. The effect of a low-carbohydrate, ketogenic diet on nonalcoholic fatty liver disease: a pilot study. *Dig Dis Sci.* 2007;52(2):589–593.

42. Zivkovic AM, German JB, Sanyal AJ. Comparative review of diets for the metabolic syndrome: implications for nonalcoholic fatty liver disease. *Am J Clin Nutr.* 2007;86(2):285–300.

43. Kontogianni MD, Tileli N, Margariti A, et al. Adherence to the Mediterranean diet is associated with the severity of non-alcoholic fatty liver disease. *Clin Nutr.* 2014;33:678–683.

44. Zhang HJ, He J, Pan LL, et al. Effects of moderate and vigorous exercise on nonalcoholic fatty liver disease: a randomized clinical trial. *JAMA Intern Med.* 2016;176(8):1074–1082.

45. Oh S, So R, Shida T, et al. High-intensity aerobic exercise improves both hepatic fat content and stiffness in sedentary obese men with nonalcoholic fatty liver disease. *Sci Rep.* 2017;7:43029.

46. Rafiq N, Younossi ZM. Effects of weight loss on nonalcoholic fatty liver disease. *Semin Liver Dis.* 2008;28(4):427–433.

47. Sanyal AJ, Chalasani N, Kowdley KV, et al. Pioglitazone, vitamin E, or placebo for nonalcoholic steatohepatitis. *New Engl J Med.* 2010;362(18):1675–1685.

48. Alisi A, Bedogni G, Baviera G, et al. Randomised clinical trial: the beneficial effects of VSL#3 in obese children with non-alcoholic steatohepatitis. *Aliment Pharmacol Ther.* 2014;39(11):1276–1285.

49. Eslamparast T, Poustchi H, Zamani F, et al. Synbiotic supplementation in nonalcoholic fatty liver disease: a randomized, double-

blind, placebo-controlled pilot study. *Am J Clin Nutr*. 2014; 99(3):535–542.

50. Dickerson RN. Hypocaloric, high-protein nutrition therapy for critically ill patients with obesity. *Nutr Clin Pract*. 2014;29(6): 786–791.

51. Choban PS, Flancbaum L. Nourishing the obese patient. *Clin Nutr*. 2000;19(5):305–311.

52. Ney M, Abraldes JG, Ma M, et al. Insufficient protein intake is associated with increased mortality in 630 patients with cirrhosis awaiting liver transplantation. *Nutr Clin Pract*. 2015;30(4): 530–536.

53. Lok AS, McMahon BJ. Chronic hepatitis B. *Hepatology*. 2007; 45(2):507–539.

54. Wild CP, Montesano R. A model of interaction: aflatoxins and hepatitis viruses in liver cancer aetiology and prevention. *Cancer Lett*. 2009;286(1):22–28.

55. Yates MS, Kensler TW. Keap1 eye on the target: chemoprevention of liver cancer. *Acta Pharmacol Sin*. 2007;28(9):1331–1342.

56. Armstrong GL, Wasley A, Simard EP, et al. The prevalence of hepatitis C virus infection in the United States, 1999 through 2002. *Ann Intern Med*. 2006;144(10):705–714.

57. Conry-Cantilena C, VanRaden M, Gibble J, et al. Routes of infection, viremia, and liver disease in blood donors found to have hepatitis C virus infection. *N Engl J Med*. 1996;334(26):1691–1696.

58. Ballestri S, Nascimbeni F, Romagnoli D, et al. Type 2 diabetes in non-alcoholic fatty liver disease and hepatitis C virus infection—liver: the "musketeer" in the spotlight. *Int J Mol Sci*. 2016; 17(3):355.

59. Fried M, Navarro V, Afdhal N, et al. A randomized, placebo-controlled trial of oral silymarin (milk thistle) for chronic hepatitis C: final results of the SYNCH multicenter study. *Hepatology*. 2011;54(Suppl 1):119A.

60. Hull MW, Yoshida EM, Montaner JS. Update on current evidence for hepatitis C therapeutic options in HCV mono-infected patients. *Curr Infect Dis Rep*. 2016;18(7):22.

61. Vanni E, Bugianesi E, Saracco G. Treatment of type 2 diabetes mellitus by viral eradication in chronic hepatitis C: myth or reality? *Dig Liver Dis*. 2016;48(2):105–111.

62. Mateos-Muñoz B, Devesa-Medina MJ, Matía-Martín MP, et al. The relation of fibrosis stage with nutritional deficiencies and bioelectrical impedance analysis of body composition in patients with chronic hepatitis C. *Ann Hepatol*. 2016;15(4):492–500.

63. Gutierrez JA, Parikh N, Branch AD. Classical and emerging roles of vitamin D in hepatitis C virus infection. *Semin Liver Dis*. 2011; 31(4):387–398.

64. Feld JJ, Modi AA, El-Diwany R, et al. S-adenosyl methionine improves early viral responses and interferon-stimulated gene induction in hepatitis C nonresponders. *Gastroenterology*. 2011; 140(3):830–839.

65. Pietrangelo A. Hereditary hemochromatosis—a new look at an old disease. *N Engl J Med*. 2004;350(23):2383–2397.

66. Adams PC. Review article: the modern diagnosis and management of haemochromatosis. *Aliment Pharmacol Ther*. 2006; 23(12):1681–1691.

67. Tan TC, Crawford DH, Jaskowski LA, et al. A corn oil-based diet protects against combined ethanol and iron-induced liver injury in a mouse model of hemochromatosis. *Alcohol Clin Exp Res*. 2013;37(10):1619–1631.

68. Bacon BR, Adams PC, Kowdley KV, et al; American Association for the Study of Liver Diseases. Diagnosis and management of hemochromatosis: 2011 practice guideline by the American Association for the Study of Liver Diseases. *Hepatology*. 2011;54(1):328–343.

69. Ala A, Walker AP, Ashkan K, et al. Wilson's disease. *Lancet*. 2007; 369(9559):397–408.

70. Roberts EA, Schilsky ML. A practice guideline on Wilson disease. *Hepatology*. 2003;37(6):1475–1492.

71. Medici V, Trevisan CP, D'Incà R, et al. Diagnosis and management of Wilson's disease: results of a single center experience. *J Clin Gastroenterol*. 2006;40(10):936–941.

72. Weiss KH, Gotthardt DN, Klemm D, et al. Zinc monotherapy is not as effective as chelating agents in treatment of Wilson disease. *Gastroenterology*. 2011;140(4):1189–1198, e1181.

73. Członkowska A, Tarnacka B, Litwin T, et al. Wilson's disease—cause of mortality in 164 patients during 1992–2003 observation period. *J Neurol*. 2005;252(6):698–703.

74. Kaplan MM, Gershwin ME. Primary biliary cirrhosis. *N Engl J Med*. 2005;353(12):1261–1273.

75. Corpechot C, Carrat F, Bahr A, et al. The effect of ursodeoxycholic acid therapy on the natural course of primary biliary cirrhosis. *Gastroenterology*. 2005;128(2):297–303.

76. Maggs JR, Chapman RW. Sclerosing cholangitis. *Curr Opin Gastroenterol*. 2007;23(3):310–316.

77. Kim WR, Therneau TM, Wiesner RH, et al. A revised natural history model for primary sclerosing cholangitis. *Mayo Clin Proc*. 2000;75(7):688–694.

78. Lindor KD, Kowdley KV, Luketic VA, et al. High-dose ursodeoxycholic acid for the treatment of primary sclerosing cholangitis. *Hepatology (Baltimore, MD)*. 2009;50(3):808–814.

79. Kummen M, Holm K, Anmarkrud JA, et al. The gut microbial profile in patients with primary sclerosing cholangitis is distinct from patients with ulcerative colitis without biliary disease and healthy controls. *Gut*. 2016;66(4):611–619.

80. Kowdley KV, Emond MJ, Sadowski JA, Kaplan MM. Plasma vitamin K1 level is decreased in primary biliary cirrhosis. *Am J Gastroenterol*. 1997;92(11):2059–2061.

81. Floreani A, Zappala F, Fries W, et al. A 3-year pilot study with 1,25-dihydroxyvitamin D, calcium, and calcitonin for severe osteodystrophy in primary biliary cirrhosis. *J Clin Gastroenterol*. 1997;24(4):239–244.

82. Sarin SK, Dhingra N, Bansal A, Malhotra S, Guptan RC. Dietary and nutritional abnormalities in alcoholic liver disease: a comparison with chronic alcoholics without liver disease. *Am J Gastroenterol*. 1997;92(5):777–783.

83. Caregaro L, Alberino F, Amodio P, et al. Malnutrition in alcoholic and virus-related cirrhosis. *Am J Clin Nutr*. 1996;63(4):602–609.

84. DiCecco SR, Wieners EJ, Wiesner RH, et al. Assessment of nutritional status of patients with end-stage liver disease undergoing liver transplantation. *Mayo Clin Proc*. 1989;64(1):95–102.

85. McCullough AJ, Tavill AS. Disordered energy and protein metabolism in liver disease. *Semin Liver Dis*. 1991;11(4):265–277.

86. Madden AM, Bradbury W, Morgan MY. Taste perception in cirrhosis: its relationship to circulating micronutrients and food preferences. *Hepatology*. 1997;26(1):40–48.

87. Kalman DR, Saltzman JR. Nutrition status predicts survival in cirrhosis. *Nutr Rev*. 1996;54(7):217–219.

88. Selberg O, Bottcher J, Tusch G, et al. Identification of high-and low-risk patients before liver transplantation: a prospective cohort study of nutritional and metabolic parameters in 150 patients. *Hepatology*. 1997;25(3):652–657.

89. Heymsfield SB, Waki M, Reinus J. Are patients with chronic liver disease hypermetabolic? *Hepatology*. 1990;11(3):502–505.

90. Shanbhogue RL, Bistrian BR, Jenkins RL, et al. Resting energy expenditure in patients with end-stage liver disease and in normal population. *JPEN J Parenter Enteral Nutr*. 1987;11(3):305–308.

91. Merli M, Riggio O, Romiti A, et al. Basal energy production rate and substrate use in stable cirrhotic patients. *Hepatology*. 1990; 12(1):106–112.

92. Martincevic I, Mouzaki M. Resting energy expenditure of children and adolescents with nonalcoholic fatty liver disease.

JPEN J Parenter Enteral Nutr. Epub 2016(July 12). doi:10.1177/0148607116658761.

93. Carpenter A, Ng VL, Chapman K, et al. Predictive equations are inaccurate in the estimation of the resting energy expenditure of children with end-stage liver disease. *JPEN J Parenter Enteral Nutr.* 2017;41(3):507–511.

94. Teramoto A, Yamanaka-Okumura H, Urano E, et al. Comparison of measured and predicted energy expenditure in patients with liver cirrhosis. *Asia Pac J Clin Nutr.* 2014;23(2):197–204.

95. Campillo B, Bories PN, Pornin B, Devanlay M. Influence of liver failure, ascites, and energy expenditure on the response to oral nutrition in alcoholic liver cirrhosis. *Nutrition.* 1997;13(7–8):613–621.

96. Prieto-Frías C, Conchillo M, Payeras M, et al. Factors related to increased resting energy expenditure in men with liver cirrhosis. *Eur J Gastroenterol Hepatol.* 2016;28(2):139–145.

97. Petrides AS, Vogt C, Schulze-Berge D, Matthews D, Strohmeyer G. Pathogenesis of glucose intolerance and diabetes mellitus in cirrhosis. *Hepatol.* 1994;19(3):616–627.

98. McCullough AJ, Bugianesi E, Marchesini G, Kalhan SC. Gender-dependent alterations in serum leptin in alcoholic cirrhosis. *Gastroenterology.* 1998;115(4):947–953.

99. Mullen KD, Denne SC, McCullough AJ, et al. Leucine metabolism in stable cirrhosis. *Hepatol.* 1986;6(4):622–630.

100. Mullen KD, Weber FL. Role of nutrition in hepatic encephalopathy. *Semin Liver Dis.* 1991;11(4):292–304.

101. Khoruts A, Stahnke L, McClain CJ, Logan G, Allen JI. Circulating tumor necrosis factor, interleukin-1 and interleukin-6 concentrations in chronic alcoholic patients. *Hepatology (Baltimore, MD).* 1991;13(2):267–276.

102. Bigatello LM, Broitman SA, Fattori L, et al. Endotoxemia, encephalopathy, and mortality in cirrhotic patients. *Am J Gastroenterol.* 1987;82(1):11–15.

103. Guarner C, Soriano G, Tomas A, et al. Increased serum nitrite and nitrate levels in patients with cirrhosis: relationship to endotoxemia. *Hepatol.* 1993;18(5):1139–1143.

104. Krenitsky J. Nutrition update in hepatic failure. *Pract Gastroenterol.* 2014;128:47–55.

105. Gaikwad NR, Gupta SJ, et al TH. Handgrip dynamometry: a surrogate marker of malnutrition to predict the prognosis in alcoholic liver disease. *Ann Gastroenterol.* 2016;29(4):509–514.

106. Alvares-da-Silva MR, Reverbel da Silveira T. Comparison between handgrip strength, Subjective Global Assessment, and prognostic nutritional index in assessing malnutrition and predicting clinical outcome in cirrhotic outpatients. *Nutrition.* 2005;21(2):113–117.

107. Lieber CS. Relationships between nutrition, alcohol use, and liver disease. *Alcohol Res Health.* 2003;27(3):220–231.

108. Detsky AS, McLaughlin JR, Baker JP, et al. What is Subjective Global Assessment of nutritional status? *JPEN J Parenter Enteral Nutr.* 1987;11(1):8–13.

109. Hasse J, Strong S, Gorman MA, et al. Subjective Global Assessment: alternative nutrition-assessment technique for liver-transplant candidates. *Nutrition.* 1993;9(4):339–343.

110. Figueiredo FA, Perez RM, Freitas MM, et al. Comparison of three methods of nutritional assessment in liver cirrhosis: Subjective Global Assessment, traditional nutritional parameters, and body composition analysis. *J Gastroenterol.* 2006;41(5):476–482.

111. Tandon P, Low G, Mourtzakis M, et al. A model to identify sarcopenia in patients with cirrhosis. *Clin Gastroenterol Hepatol.* 2016;14(10):1473–1480.

112. Amodio P, Bemeur C, Butterworth R, et al. The nutritional management of hepatic encephalopathy in patients with cirrhosis: International society for hepatic encephalopathy and nitrogen metabolism consensus. *Hepatol.* 2013l;58(1):325–336. doi:10.1002/hep.26370.

113. Arora S, Mattina C, McAnenny C, et al. The development and validation of a nutritional prioritizing tool for use in patients with chronic liver disease. *J Hepatol.* 2012;56(Suppl 2):S241.

114. Johnson TM, Overgard EB, Cohen AE, et al. Nutrition assessment and management in advanced liver disease. *Nutr Clin Pract.* 2013;28(1):15–29.

115. Barbu EC, Chiţu-Tişu CE, Lazăr M, et al. Body composition changes in patients with chronic hepatitis C. *J Gastrointest Liver Dis.* 2016;25(3):323–329.

116. Tandon P, Mourtzakis M, Low G, et al. Comparing the variability between measurements for sarcopenia using magnetic resonance imaging and computed tomography imaging. *Am J Transplant.* 2016;16(9):2766–2767.

117. Patek AJ, Post J, Ratnoff OD, et al. Dietary treatment of cirrhosis of the liver; results in 124 patients observed during a ten year period. *JAMA.* 1948;138(8):543–549.

118. Hirsch S, de la Maza MP, Gattas V, et al. Nutritional support in alcoholic cirrhotic patients improves host defenses. *J Am Coll Nutr.* 1999;18(5):434–441.

119. Kearns PJ, Young H, Garcia G, et al. Accelerated improvement of alcoholic liver disease with enteral nutrition. *Gastroenterology.* 1992;102(1):200–205.

120. Cordoba J, Lopez-Hellin J, Planas M, et al. Normal protein diet for episodic hepatic encephalopathy: results of a randomized study. *J Hepatol.* 2004;41(1):38–43.

121. Gheorghe L, Iacob R, Vadan R, et al. Improvement of hepatic encephalopathy using a modified high-calorie, high-protein diet. *Rom J Gastroenterol.* 2005;14(3):231–238.

122. Brown Bowman BA, Russell R. *Present Knowledge in Nutrition.* 9th ed. Washington, DC: International Life Sciences Institute; 2006.

123. Owen OE, Trapp VE, Reichard GA, et al. Nature and quantity of fuels consumed in patients with alcoholic cirrhosis. *J Clin Invest.* 1983;72(5):1821–1832.

124. Vaisman N, Katzman H, Carmiel-Haggai M, et al. Breakfast improves cognitive function in cirrhotic patients with cognitive impairment. *Am J Clin Nutr.* 2010;92(1):137–140.

125. Bessman AN, Mirick GS. Blood ammonia levels following the ingestion of casein and whole blood. *J Clin Invest.* 1958;37(7):990–998.

126. Greenberger NJ, Carley J, Schenker S, et al. Effect of vegetable and animal protein diets in chronic hepatic encephalopathy. *Am J Dig Dis.* 1977;22(10):845–855.

127. Marchesini G, Bianchi G, Merli M, et al. Nutritional supplementation with branched-chain amino acids in advanced cirrhosis: a double-blind, randomized trial. *Gastroenterology.* 2003;124(7):1792–1801.

128. Charlton M. Branched-chain amino acid-enriched supplements as therapy for liver disease: Rasputin lives. *Gastroenterology.* 2003;124(7):1980–1982.

129. McClave SA, Taylor BE, Martindale RG, et al. Guidelines for the provision and assessment of nutrition support therapy in the adult critically ill patient: Society of Critical Care Medicine (SCCM) and American Society for Parenteral and Enteral Nutrition (A.S.P.E.N.). *JPEN J Parenter Enteral Nutr.* 2016;40(2):159–211.

130. Barnes PM, Bloom B, Nahin R. Complementary and alternative medicine use among adults and children: United States, 2007. *Natl Health Stat Rep.* 2008;(12):1–23.

131. Corey RL, Rakela J. Complementary and alternative medicine: risks and special considerations in pretransplant and posttransplant patients. *Nutr Clin Pract.* 2014;29(3):322–331.

132. Liu SL, Degli Esposti S, Yao T, et al. Vitamin E therapy of acute CCl4-induced hepatic injury in mice is associated with inhibition of nuclear factor kappa B binding. *Hepatol.* 1995;22(5):1474–1481.

133. Hill DB, Devalaraja R, Joshi-Barve S, et al. Antioxidants attenuate nuclear factor-kappa B activation and tumor necrosis factor-alpha production in alcoholic hepatitis patient monocytes and rat Kupffer cells, in vitro. *Clin Biochem.* 1999;32(7):563–570.

134. Lavine JE. Vitamin E treatment of nonalcoholic steatohepatitis in children: a pilot study. *J Pediatr.* 2000;136(6):734–738.

135. Hasegawa T, Yoneda M, Nakamura K, et al. Plasma transforming growth factor-beta1 level and efficacy of alpha-tocopherol in patients with non-alcoholic steatohepatitis: a pilot study. *Aliment Pharmacol Ther.* 2001;15(10):1667–1672.

136. Mezey E, Potter JJ, Rennie-Tankersley L, et al. A randomized placebo controlled trial of vitamin E for alcoholic hepatitis. *J Hepatol.* 2004;40(1):40–46.

137. Lauterburg BH, Velez ME. Glutathione deficiency in alcoholics: risk factor for paracetamol hepatotoxicity. *Gut.* 1988;29(9):1153–1157.

138. Pena LR, Hill DB, McClain CJ. Treatment with glutathione precursor decreases cytokine activity. *JPEN J Parenter Enteral Nutr.* 1999;23(1):1–6.

139. Lee WM, Hynan LS, Rossaro L, et al. Intravenous N-acetylcysteine improves transplant-free survival in early stage non-acetaminophen acute liver failure. *Gastroenterology.* 2009;137(3):856–864, e851.

140. Lieber CS. S-Adenosyl-L-methionine and alcoholic liver disease in animal models: implications for early intervention in human beings. *Alcohol.* 2002;27(3):173–177.

141. Karaa A, Thompson KJ, McKillop IH, et al. S-adenosyl-L-methionine attenuates oxidative stress and hepatic stellate cell activation in an ethanol-LPS-induced fibrotic rat model. *Shock.* 2008;30(2):197–205.

142. Mato JM, Camara J, Fernandez de Paz J, et al. S-adenosylmethionine in alcoholic liver cirrhosis: a randomized, placebo-controlled, double-blind, multicenter clinical trial. *J Hepatol.* 1999;30(6):1081–1089.

143. Rambaldi A, Gluud C. S-adenosyl-L-methionine for alcoholic liver diseases. *Cochrane Database Syst Rev.* 2006;(2):CD002235.

144. Medici V, Virata MC, Peerson JM, et al. S-adenosyl-L-methionine treatment for alcoholic liver disease: a double-blinded, randomized, placebo-controlled trial. *Alcohol Clin Exp Res.* 2011;35(11):1960–1965.

145. Kharbanda KK, Mailliard ME, Baldwin CR, et al. Betaine attenuates alcoholic steatosis by restoring phosphatidylcholine generation via the phosphatidylethanolamine methyltransferase pathway. *J Hepatol.* 2007;46(2):314–321.

146. Abdelmalek MF, Sanderson SO, Angulo P, et al. Betaine for nonalcoholic fatty liver disease: results of a randomized placebo-controlled trial. *Hepatology.* 2009;50(6):1818–1826.

147. Joshi PC, Mehta A, Jabber WS, et al. Zinc deficiency mediates alcohol-induced alveolar epithelial and macrophage dysfunction in rats. *Am J Respir Cell Mol Biol.* 2009;41(2):207–216.

148. McClain CJ, Antonow DR, Cohen DA, et al. Zinc metabolism in alcoholic liver disease. *Alcohol Clin Exp Res.* 1986;10(6):582–589.

149. Zhong W, McClain CJ, Cave M, Kang YJ, Zhou Z. The role of zinc deficiency in alcohol-induced intestinal barrier dysfunction. *Am J Physiol Gastrointest Liver Physiol.* 2010;298(5):G625–G633.

150. Kang X, Zhong W, Liu J, et al. Zinc supplementation reverses alcohol-induced steatosis in mice through reactivating hepatocyte nuclear factor-4alpha and peroxisome proliferator-activated receptor-alpha. *Hepatology.* 2009;50(4):1241–1250.

151. Zhou Z, Kang X, Jiang Y, et al. Preservation of hepatocyte nuclear factor-4alpha is associated with zinc protection against TNF-alpha hepatotoxicity in mice. *Exp Biol Med* (Maywood). 2007;232(5):622–628.

152. Takahashi M, Saito H, Higashimoto M, et al. Possible inhibitory effect of oral zinc supplementation on hepatic fibrosis through downregulation of TIMP-1: a pilot study. *Hepatol Res.* 2007;37(6):405–409.

153. Takuma Y, Nouso K, Makino Y, et al. Clinical trial: oral zinc in hepatic encephalopathy. *Aliment Pharmacol Ther.* 2010;32(9):1080–1090.

154. Katayama K, Saito M, Kawaguchi T, et al. Effect of zinc on liver cirrhosis with hyperammonemia: a preliminary randomized, placebo-controlled double-blind trial. *Nutrition.* 2014;30(11–12):1409–1414.

155. Luper S. A review of plants used in the treatment of liver disease: part 1. *Altern Med Rev.* 1998;3(6):410–421.

156. Ferenci P, Dragosics B, Dittrich H, et al. Randomized controlled trial of silymarin treatment in patients with cirrhosis of the liver. *J Hepatol.* 1989;9(1):105–113.

157. Pares A, Planas R, Torres M, et al. Effects of silymarin in alcoholic patients with cirrhosis of the liver: results of a controlled, double-blind, randomized and multicenter trial. *J Hepatol.* 1998;28(4):615–621.

158. Rambaldi A, Jacobs BP, Iaquinto G, et al. Milk thistle for alcoholic and/or hepatitis B or C virus liver diseases. *Cochrane Database Syst Rev.* 2005;(2):CD003620.

159. Hayaishi S, Chung H, Kudo M, et al. Oral branched-chain amino acid granules reduce the incidence of hepatocellular carcinoma and improve event-free survival in patients with liver cirrhosis. *Dig Dis.* 2011;29(3):326–332.

160. Muto Y, Sato S, Watanabe A, et al; Long-Term Survival Study (LOTUS) Group. Overweight and obesity increase the risk for liver cancer in patients with liver cirrhosis and long-term oral supplementation with branched-chain amino acid granules inhibits liver carcinogenesis in heavier patients with liver cirrhosis. *Hepatol Res.* 2006;35(3):204–214.

161. Muto Y, Sato S, Watanabe A, et al. Effects of oral branched-chain amino acid granules on event-free survival in patients with liver cirrhosis. *Clin Gastroenterol Hepatol.* 2005;3(7):705–713.

162. Fan ST, Lo CM, Lai EC, et al. Perioperative nutritional support in patients undergoing hepatectomy for hepatocellular carcinoma. *N Engl J Med.* 1994;331(23):1547–1552.

163. Marchesini G, Bianchi G, Merli M, et al. Nutritional supplementation with branched-chain amino acids in advanced cirrhosis: a double-blind, randomized trial. *Gastroenterology.* 2003;124(7):1792–1801.

164. Esposito E, Iacono A, Bianco G, et al Probiotics reduce the inflammatory response induced by a high-fat diet in the liver of young rats. *J Nutr.* 2009;139(5):905–911.

165. Miele L, Valenza V, La Torre G, et al Increased intestinal permeability and tight junction alterations in nonalcoholic fatty liver disease. *Hepatology.* 2009;49(6):1877–1887.

166. Aller R, De Luis DA, Izaola O, et al. Effect of a probiotic on liver aminotransferases in nonalcoholic fatty liver disease patients: a double blind randomized clinical trial. *Eur Rev Med Pharmacol Sci.* 2011;15(9):1090–1095.

167. Malaguarnera M, Vacante M, Antic T, et al. Bifidobacterium longum with fructo-oligosaccharides in patients with non alcoholic steatohepatitis. *Dig Dis Sci.* 2012;57(2):545–553.

168. Ma YY, Li L, Yu CH, et al. Effects of probiotics on nonalcoholic fatty liver disease: a meta-analysis. *World J Gastroenterol.* 2013;19:6911–6918.

169. Bauer TM, Schwacha H, Steinbrückner B, et al. Small intestinal bacterial overgrowth in human cirrhosis is associated with systemic endotoxemia. *Am J Gastroenterol.* 2002;97(9):2364–2370.

170. Kirpich IA, Solovieva NV, Leikhter SN, et al. Probiotics restore bowel flora and improve liver enzymes in human alcohol-induced liver injury: a pilot study. *Alcohol.* 2008;42(8):675–682.

171. Stadlbauer V, Mookerjee RP, Hodges S, et al. Effect of probiotic treatment on deranged neutrophil function and cytokine

responses in patients with compensated alcoholic cirrhosis. *J Hepatol.* 2008;48(6):945–951.

172. Liu Q, Duan ZP, Ha DK, et al. Synbiotic modulation of gut flora: effect on minimal hepatic encephalopathy in patients with cirrhosis. *Hepatology.* 2004;39(5):1441–1449.

173. Lunia MK, Sharma BC, Sharma P, et al. Probiotics prevent hepatic encephalopathy in patients with cirrhosis: a randomized controlled trial. *Clin Gastroenterol Hepatol.* 2014;12(6):1003–1008.

174. Agrawal A, Sharma BC, Sharma P, et al. Secondary prophylaxis of hepatic encephalopathy in cirrhosis: an open-label, randomized controlled trial of lactulose, probiotics, and no therapy. *Am J Gastroenterol.* 2012;107(7):1043–1050.

175. Xu J, Ma R, Chen LF, et al. Effects of probiotic therapy on hepatic encephalopathy in patients with liver cirrhosis: an updated meta-analysis of six randomized controlled trials. *Hepatobiliary Pancreat Dis Int.* 2014;13(4):354–360.

176. Pande C, Kumar A, Sarin SK. Addition of probiotics to norflox-acin does not improve efficacy in the prevention of spontaneous bacterial peritonitis: a double-blind placebo-controlled randomized-controlled trial. *Eur J Gastroenterol Hepatol.* 2012;24(7):831–839.

177. Jayakumar S, Carbonneau M, Hotte N, et al. VSL#3® probiotic therapy does not reduce portal pressures in patients with decompensated cirrhosis. *Liver Int.* 2013;33(10):1470–1477.

178. Tandon P, Moncrief K, Madsen K, et al. Effects of probiotic therapy on portal pressure in patients with cirrhosis: a pilot study. *Liver Int.* 2009;29(7):1110–1115.

179. Rincón D, Vaquero J, Hernando A, et al. Oral probiotic VSL#3 attenuates the circulatory disturbances of patients with cirrhosis and ascites. *Liver Int.* 2014;34(10):1504–1512.

180. Gupta N, Kumar A, Sharma P, et al. Effects of the adjunctive probiotic VSL#3 on portal haemodynamics in patients with cirrhosis and large varices: a randomized trial. *Liver Int.* 2013;33(8):1148–1157.

181. Loguercio C, Federico A, Tuccillo C, et al. Beneficial effects of a probiotic VSL#3 on parameters of liver dysfunction in chronic liver diseases. *J Clin Gastroenterol.* 2005;39(6):540–543.

182. Vajro P, Mandato C, Licenziati MR, et al. Effects of Lactobacillus rhamnosus strain GG in pediatric obesity-related liver disease. *J Pediatr Gastroenterol Nutr.* 2011;52(6):740–743.

183. Wong VW, Won GL, Chim AM, et al. Treatment of nonalcoholic steatohepatitis with probiotics: a proof-of-concept study. *Ann Hepatol.* 2013;12(2):256–262.

184. Barchetta I, Angelico F, Del Ben M, et al. Strong association between non-alcoholic fatty liver disease (NAFLD) and low 25(OH) vitamin D levels in an adult population with normal serum liver enzymes. *BMC Med.* 2011;9(1):85.

185. Pappa HM, Bern E, Kamin D, et al. Vitamin D status in gastrointestinal and liver disease. *Curr Opin Gastroenterol.* 2008;24(2):176–183.

186. Chang WT, Ker CG, Hung HC, et al. Albumin and prealbumin may predict retinol status in patients with liver cirrhosis. *Hepatogastroenterology.* 2008;55(86-87):1681–1685.

187. Institute of Medicine. Vitamin K. In: *Dietary Reference Intakes for Vitamin A, Vitamin K, Arsenic, Boron, Chromium, Copper, Iodine, Iron, Manganese, Molybdenum, Nickel, Silicon, Vanadium, and Zinc.* Washington, DC: National Academies Press; 2000:162–196.

188. Feranchak AP, Sokol RJ. Medical and nutritional management of cholestasis in infants and children. In: Suchy FJ, Sokol RJ, Balistreri WF, eds. *Liver Disease in Children.* 3rd ed. New York: Cambridge University Press; 2007:190–231.

189. Zahr NM, Kaufman KL, Harper CG. Clinical and pathological features of alcohol-related brain damage. *Nat Rev Neurol.* 2011;7(5):284–294.

190. Cook CC, Hallwood PM, Thomson AD. B Vitamin deficiency and neuropsychiatric syndromes in alcohol misuse. *Alcohol.* 1998;33(4):317–336.

191. Inoue E, Hori S, Narumi Y, Fujita M, et al. Portal-systemic encephalopathy: presence of basal ganglia lesions with high signal intensity on MR images. *Radiology.* 1991;179(2):551–555.

192. Layrargues GP, Shapcott D, Spahr L, et al. Accumulation of manganese and copper in pallidum of cirrhotic patients: role in the pathogenesis of hepatic encephalopathy? *Metab Brain Dis.* 1995;10(4):353–356.

193. Tandon P, Raman M, Mourtzakis M, et al. A practical approach to nutritional screening and assessment in cirrhosis. *Hepatology.* 2017;65(3):1044–1057.

194. Runyon BA. Management of adult patients with ascites due to cirrhosis: an update. *Hepatology.* 2009;49(6):2087–2107.

195. Katz RI, Hovagim AR, Finkelstein HS, et al. A comparison of cocaine, lidocaine with epinephrine, and oxymetazoline for prevention of epistaxis on nasotracheal intubation. *J Clin Anesth.* 1990;2(1):16–20.

196. Hebuterne X, Vanbiervliet G. Feeding the patients with upper gastrointestinal bleeding. *Curr Opin Clin Nutr Metab Care.* 2011;14(2):197–201.

197. de Ledinghen V, Beau P, Mannant PR, et al. Early feeding or enteral nutrition in patients with cirrhosis after bleeding from esophageal varices? A randomized controlled study. *Dig Dis Sci.* 1997;42(3):536–541.

198. Baltz JG, Argo CK, Al-Osaimi AM, et al. Mortality after percutaneous endoscopic gastrostomy in patients with cirrhosis: a case series. *Gastrointest Endosc.* 2010;72(5):1072–1075.

28 Pancreatitis

Kristine Krueger, MD, Stephen A. McClave, MD, FASPEN, FASGE, FACN, AGAF, and Robert G. Martindale, MD, PhD

CONTENTS

Acknowledgments: Carol Rees Parrish, MS, RD, and Joseph Krenitsky, MS, RD, were contributors to this chapter for the second edition.

Objectives

1. Understand that acute and chronic pancreatitis represent a continuum of injury from inflammation to the pancreas.
2. Recognize how pancreatitis etiology is shaped by genetic predisposition, environmental factors, lifestyle choices, and response to medical/surgical treatment.
3. Learn the role of enteral nutrition (EN) in maintaining gut integrity, modulating immune responses, and attenuating the disease process of acute pancreatitis.
4. Describe the use of parenteral nutrition (PN) in severe acute pancreatitis in patients who cannot tolerate EN.
5. Review management strategies to minimize or reverse deterioration of nutrition status in chronic pancreatitis.

Test Your Knowledge Questions

1. A nutrition support clinician was consulted on the second day of hospitalization about a patient who presented with severe acute pancreatitis and required mechanical ventilation. A recent, dynamic contrast-enhanced computed tomography (CT) scan revealed necrosis involving 30% of the pancreatic gland and a small (4-cm) pseudocyst in the tail of the gland. Which of the following should the clinician recommend?
   A. Continue *nil per os* (NPO) status with no enteral tube feeding, noting that the necrosis may require surgical intervention.
   B. Start the patient on PN because the patient is mechanically ventilated and has a pseudocyst.
   C. Place a nasojejunal tube and begin enteral tube feeding, providing no more that 10 to 20 mL/h.
   D. Place a nasojejunal tube, begin tube feeding, and advance to the nutrition goal over the first 24 to 48 hours.
2. Which of the following nutrition regimens is appropriate for a patient with less than 2 Ranson criteria and an Acute Physiologic Assessment and Chronic Health Evaluation II (APACHE II) score of less than 9 (nonsevere) who has no pancreatic necrosis on a CT scan?
   A. Begin volume resuscitation, provide narcotic analgesia, and advance to an oral diet as soon as it is tolerated.
   B. Begin PN in the first 24 hours of admission because the patient has acute pain.
   C. Keep the patient NPO for at least 7 days.
   D. Use PN in the first 24 hours, and then switch to an oral diet.
3. Which of the following is true?
   A. The immune response of the gut remains intact when a patient is maintained on PN.
   B. The immune response of the gut remains intact when a patient is maintained on EN.
   C. Loss of gut integrity may allow bacteria of gut origin to infect distant organ sites, but this issue is improved with bowel rest.
   D. Enteral feedings should be stopped if the ileus is noted radiographically.

Test Your Knowledge Answers

1. The correct answer is **D**. Complications such as pancreatic ascites, fistulas, and pseudocysts are part of the natural disease course of acute pancreatitis. Information mostly from retrospective case series indicates that the use of the enteral route is safe and allows for the resolution of these complications in most circumstances. The patient has severe pancreatitis and should therefore benefit from EN.
2. The correct answer is **A**. Patients with mild to moderate pancreatitis may be supported with intravenous (IV) fluid resuscitation and analgesia without added specialized nutrition support.
3. The correct answer is **B**. Loss of gut integrity has been demonstrated in patients hospitalized for pancreatitis who are maintained on PN and gut disuse while awaiting surgery.

Over time, the villi in these patients become shortened, then lost. In contrast to pancreatitis patients who receive enteral tube feeding, pancreatitis patients placed on PN with gut disuse have greater exposure to endotoxins and greater oxidant stress. Clinicians should assess clinical signs of feeding intolerance because radiographic information on ileus may be misleading.

Acute Pancreatitis

Pathophysiology

Regardless of the etiology of pancreatitis, trypsin released into the acinar cytoplasm by premature activation from its zymogen trypsinogen activates tumor necrosis factor alpha, interleukins 1 and 6, and a host of other proinflammatory cytokines. Activation of these agents results in recruitment of inflammatory cells to the pancreas as well as systemic release of bradykinins and cytokines that can cause end-organ damage to the lung and kidney. This cascade of inflammation peaks 24 to 36 hours after the inciting event and can lead to organ failure within several days.[1-3] By about 72 hours, the acute inflammatory cascade has usually abated. It is impossible to predict which patients will progress to multiorgan failure, as neither the etiology nor the serum enzyme elevations are correlative.

Nutrition status of the patient is important to outcomes. Poorer outcomes are associated with alcoholism, states of starvation, undernutrition (reduced protective proteolytic enzymes), and chronic underlying inflammatory states, including obesity. Furthermore, the risk of severe acute pancreatitis is 2 to 3 times higher in obese than nonobese subjects.[4-7]

Alcohol abuse is commonly associated with both acute and chronic pancreatitis. The pathophysiology is complex, with ethanol sensitizing the pancreas to injury and additional factors triggering overt pancreatitis. Pancreatic mitochondria play a crucial role in many of the pathologic pathways leading to apoptosis and cell necrosis. In the ducts, degraded proteins may calcify to form pancreatic stones. Ductal stones further the damage by inhibiting the flow of secretions into the duodenum. As discussed later in this chapter, forms of pancreatitis with an alcohol-related and/or genetic etiology are commonly associated with ductal stones, strictures, and outflow obstruction.

Incidence

In the United States, the incidence of acute pancreatitis is estimated to be 40 cases per 100,000 adult-years, with conservative estimated cost in excess of $2.5 billion.[8] With advancing age in Western countries, as well as increasing rates of obesity, the incidence of gallstone-associated, biliary pancreatitis is steadily increasing.[9]

Etiology

Alcohol abuse, gallstones, and idiopathic causes account for 90% of cases of acute pancreatitis; other causes include drugs, autoimmune and tropical diseases, infection, hypertriglyceridemia, hereditary factors, and malignancy.[10] Age, country of origin, and gender influence causality, with alcohol-related pancreatitis more common in men and gallstone-associated pancreatitis more common in women.[9–11] Gallstone-induced pancreatitis remains the most common worldwide etiology, although gallstone pathophysiology varies considerably.[12]

Alcohol-induced pancreatitis represents a significant proportion of all cases of acute pancreatitis in industrialized societies, and particularly in men. Notably, the amount of alcohol intake associated with alcoholic pancreatitis is greater than the amount associated with alcoholic liver disease; consuming between 50 and 150 g ethanol per day for 6 to 12 years can lead to chronic pancreatitis.[13,14] Patients with acute pancreatitis attacks due to alcohol typically present with chronic pancreatic scarring, which can be demonstrated by imaging. This observation has led to the sentinel acute pancreatitis event (SAPE) hypothesis, which suggests that virtually any etiology of acute pancreatitis, if severe enough, may lead to underlying scarring and end-organ damage. Furthermore, recurrent bouts of acute pancreatitis lead to cumulative damage and result in chronic pancreatitis.[15]

Up until the last decade, many acute pancreatitis cases were attributed to idiopathic causes. This etiology makes it more difficult to select an effective treatment (eg, cholecystectomies with or without selective sphincterotomies, abstinence from alcohol, lipid-lowering medications) to prevent recurrent acute pancreatitis and progression to chronic pancreatitis. Today, enhanced molecular and genetic studies have improved the identification of autoimmune and genetic etiologies, and fewer cases are considered idiopathic in origin.

Autoimmune-induced pancreatitis is usually associated with less-severe acute attacks, small duct disease, or silent disease that can eventually lead to chronic pancreatitis with malabsorption.[16] The risk of autoimmune pancreatitis is greater in women than men; other risk factors include autoimmune diseases such as thyroid disease, type 1 diabetes mellitus, celiac disease, lupus, rheumatoid arthritis, and inflammatory bowel disease.

Hereditary causes of pancreatitis include mutations of the cystic fibrosis transmembrane conductance regulator (CFTR), cationic trypsinogen (PRSS1), pancreatic secretory trypsin inhibitor (SPINK 1), and trypsinogen-degrading enzyme chymotrypsin (CTRC) genes.[17] A detailed family history, paying particular attention to the patient's age at presentation, may help identify individuals at risk for hereditary causes. Patients with a family history that suggests a genetic cause can be referred to specialized centers for management and treatment. People with hereditary pancreatitis, particularly with PRSS1 mutations, have a marked increased risk of pancreatic cancer (upward of 30% lifetime risk)[18] and require intense screening with referral for pancreatectomy and islet cell transplantation.[19,20]

Clinical Signs and Symptoms

Acute pancreatitis is defined by the onset of severe epigastric pain, which often radiates into the left abdomen and midback. Nausea, vomiting, and anorexia are associated symptoms. Amylase levels become elevated within the initial hours of the pancreatitis bout. Elevations in serum lipase levels usually follow;

they can often reach or exceed 2 to 3 times the upper limits of normal. However, the absolute elevation of the enzymes does not correlate with the severity of an individual episode of acute pancreatitis. In fact, enzyme elevations may not be dramatic for recurrent attacks, especially in patients with chronic pancreatitis. Also, amylase and lipase elevations may not definitively indicate pancreatitis, unless tests to evaluate pancreatic-specific isoenzymes are ordered. Both amylase and lipase are cleared from serum by the kidneys and may therefore be elevated if secretion is impaired, and many organs other than the pancreas (including the oral mucosa, tongue, small intestine, ovaries, and muscle) produce amylase and lipase.

Concomitant elevation of liver enzymes, including aspartate aminotransferase, alanine aminotransferase, and alkaline phosphatase, or liver enzyme levels that wax and wane with bouts of abdominal pain are highly suggestive of a biliary etiology.[10,21] In patients whose pancreatitis has a biliary cause, the onset of acute pain is associated with intake of a fatty meal, and symptoms may include colicky right upper quadrant to right subscapular pain that is about as severe as kidney colic or labor pains. Episodes of colic last from 20 minutes to several hours as the stones/biliary debris migrate from the cystic duct to the common duct with obstruction of the sphincter of Oddi and pain from the stretch of the biliary tree. Standing or walking can alleviate the pressure associated with stone passage. Increased hydrostatic pressure from obstruction as well as enzyme activation from the mixing of bile acids and enzymes in the ducts causes local inflammation. CT scans of the abdomen may show predominant edema at the pancreatic head, although diffuse inflammation may also occur if the inflammatory cascade is severe. Small stones often pass, and the colicky pain is relieved but replaced by continuous, duller pain from pancreatic inflammation. CT scans may also show dilated bile ducts with retained common duct stones that were too large to pass through the sphincter.

Nonbiliary causes of acute pancreatitis are associated with pain that steadily increases for hours and then remains constant. Ileus caused by contiguous inflammation results in further midabdominal pain with distention and vomiting. Bowel sounds may be absent or diminished on physical examination, and patients usually want to sit very still because movement exacerbates pain.

Assessment of Disease Severity and Medical Management

To optimally manage patients and prevent complications, clinicians need to determine the severity of the acute event as soon as possible (Table 28-1). Useful tools for determining disease severity include CT scans to assess necrosis (discussed in the next section on imaging and endoscopic interventions); Ranson, Imrie, and APACHE II scores; multiorgan failure or systemic inflammatory response syndrome (SIRS) criteria; and blood tests to check for elevations of C-reactive protein. Among the scoring methods, APACHE II is most predictive of both severity and clinical outcomes.[22,23]

To date, there is no specific treatment for acute pancreatitis. Therefore, management is largely expectant and supportive when cases are mild to moderate. Patients who present with

TABLE 28-1 Differentiating Degrees of Pancreatitis

	Mild/Moderate Pancreatitis	Severe Pancreatitis
APACHE II score	≤9	≥10
Ranson criteria	≤2	≥3
CT scan	No necrosis	Necrosis
Mortality	0%	19%
PO diet in 7 days	81%	0%
Management	Supportive	EN/PN and ICU

APACHE II, Acute Physiologic Assessment and Chronic Health Evaluation II; CT, computed tomography; EN, enteral nutrition; ICU, intensive care unit; PN, parenteral nutrition; PO, *per os* (oral).

8 or more APACHE II criteria, more than 3 Ranson criteria, or indication of an acute, single-organ failure (eg, a creatinine level of 2 mg/dL when baseline was 1 mg/dL) have more severe disease and are best managed in the intensive care unit (ICU). Early recognition of SIRS can prompt adequate management with intravascular volume replacement, which may serve to prevent or reduce ischemic end-organ damage related to hypoperfusion and changes in microvascular blood flow induced by the inflammatory cascade. Although debates and studies comparing the benefits of colloid vs crystalloid solutions are ongoing, prompt volume resuscitation serves as the most important initial therapy.[24] The most beneficial management strategies for severe acute pancreatitis involve ICU admission, delaying CT scans, implementing early and adequate EN, avoiding prophylactic antibiotics, and treating local complications (see Figure 28-1).[25-27]

FIGURE 28-1 Algorithm for Nutrition Management of Acute Pancreatitis

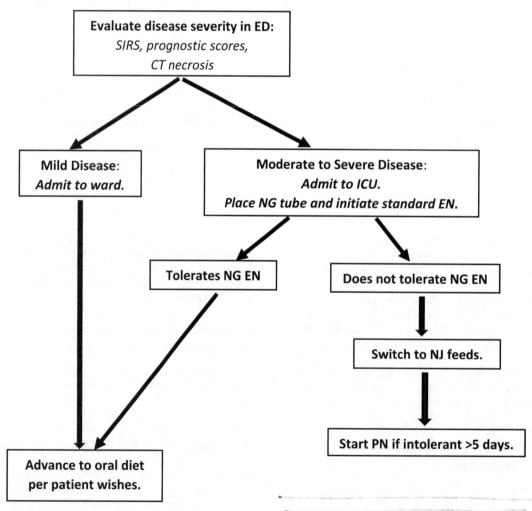

CT, computed tomography; ED, emergency department; EN, enteral nutrition; ICU, intensive care unit; NG, nasogastric; NJ, nasojejunal; PN, parenteral nutrition; SIRS, systemic inflammatory response syndrome.

Imaging and Endoscopic Interventions

Imaging methods for the pancreas include standard, external-beam abdominal ultrasound; regular plain films; CT scans; magnetic resonance imaging (MRI); magnetic resonance cholangiopancreatography (MRCP); endoscopic ultrasound (EUS); and endoscopic retrograde cholangiopancreatography (ERCP). Each technique provides different information about acute and chronic pancreatitis. EUS and ERCP are used therapeutically as well as for diagnosis.

Standard, external-beam abdominal ultrasound is readily available and routinely performed; however, findings do not correlate with severity of disease. Although gallstones in the gallbladder can be seen easily in an ultrasound, stones retained in the common bile duct and pancreatic cysts are often missed because of artifacts from an overlying gas- and fluid-filled bowel. Regular, plain films might show ileus, but the presence of calcifications varies even in chronic disease.

Pancreas-protocol, contrast-enhanced CT scanning is most helpful for determining the presence of pancreatic necrosis, ductal obstruction, presence or absence of acute fluid collections, pseudocysts, or pancreatic abscess. CT scans can be used to grade as acute pancreatitis as follows:[26]

- Grade A: Normal-appearing pancreas
- Grade B: Focal or diffuse enlargement of the pancreas
- Grade C: Pancreatic gland abnormalities accompanied by mild parapancreatic inflammatory changes
- Grade D: Fluid collection in a single location, usually within the anterior pararenal space
- Grade E: 2 or more fluid collections near the pancreas, or gas either within the pancreas or within parapancreatic inflammation

A score between 0 and 4 may then be assigned to the CT grade (A = 0 points through E = 4 points) and combined with a score for the degree of necrosis (less than 33% necrosis = 2 points; 33% to 50% necrosis = 4 points; and greater than 50% necrosis = 6 points). A total score equal to or greater than 7 has been associated with increased mortality.[27]

The timing of CT scanning is important. CT scanning before adequate volume resuscitation may worsen contrast-associated renal injury and may underdiagnose the severity of pancreatitis, as necrosis may not be radiographically present until after 72 hours. Moreover, pancreatic abscess is usually a late complication, occurring in the second week or later post severe acute pancreatitis.

MRI scanning does not expose the patient to ionizing radiation and can offer exquisite soft tissue characterization, and MRCP is a useful and noninvasive way to verify or exclude the possible presence of retained common duct stones and identify aberrant or variant ductal anatomy.[28,29] Information from these imaging techniques can help the clinicians tailor planned interventions, such as ERCP to remove stones, or perform sphincterotomy.[30]

EUS, an endoscopic procedure providing ultrasound examination of the pancreas through the gastric wall, has advanced the diagnosis and management of pancreatic disease more than any other single modality in the last 2 decades. Diagnostic EUS can reveal both biliary and pancreatic ductal stones, evaluate pancreatic solid and cystic masses, stage lymph nodes, and use imaging criteria to diagnose chronic pancreatitis.[31] Therapeutic EUS techniques are used to drain pseudocysts, assess cyst contents (for tumor markers, mucin, amylase), and perform fine-needle aspiration for cytology in suspicious lesions.[32] EUS is typically performed after resolution of the acute attack. Percutaneous or endoscopic drainage of acute fluid collections or sampling of early encapsulated fluid collections may also be necessary to diagnose or treat infected necrosis or pancreatic abscess. These techniques help tailor medical management with antibiotics and can prompt surgical management for debridement in select cases.[33]

ERCP provides direct cannulation of the pancreas and biliary ducts. It is generally avoided during acute inflammation of the pancreas, but it is clearly beneficial to treat patients with ascending cholangitis or retained common duct stones. Performance of sphincterotomy and/or placement of a temporary biliary stent for ductal decompression and use of systemic antibiotics will result in prompt clinical improvement of sepsis in most patients who would otherwise have high mortality. Definitive bile duct stone removal and elective cholecystectomy can be delayed until pancreatitis and sepsis fully resolve.[34] ERCP with stenting of pancreatic duct disruptions is highly beneficial in the management of pancreatic ascites and pleural effusions.[35,36] ERCP with measurement of the pressure at the sphincter of Oddi (manometry) performed by expert endoscopists is useful to determine causality in idiopathic pancreatitis. In a series of 1241 patients who were initially classified as having idiopathic pancreatitis, sphincter of Oddi dysfunction was found in 40% and pancreas divisum in 18.8%.[37] Over the last several decades, improvement in ERCP techniques have proved its value for the definitive diagnosis and management for a multitude of acute and pancreatic diseases, including sphincter of Oddi dysfunction, gallstones, smoldering or recurrent acute pancreatitis, and pancreas divisum, and for selected cases of chronic pancreatitis complicated by symptomatic pseudocysts, pancreatic duct leaks, dominant ductal strictures, or intraductal stones.[34,38-42] A major indication for endoscopic therapy is the need for long-term relief of bile duct strictures that occur as a complication of fibrosis in the pancreatic head from chronic pancreatitis.[43]

Value of Antibiotic Use

A recent systematic review and meta-analysis has determined that prophylactic antibiotics are of no benefit in most cases of acute severe pancreatitis.[44] Current recommendations are to reserve use of antibiotics to patients with ascending cholangitis or documented infections. Antibiotics may be used selectively during ERCP if ductal obstruction cannot be relieved; otherwise, prophylactic antibiotics are not beneficial.[45]

Clinical Outcomes

Patients presenting with acute pancreatitis usually improve over several days without significant morbidity or mortality. With initial recovery and then definitive management of the underlying cause, progression to chronic disease may be avoided. When severe acute pancreatitis occurs, patients are at greater risk for organ failure, infection, or even death. These risks are influenced by the adequacy of fluid resuscitation, the presence and extent of necrosis within the gland, the degree of organ failure, pancreatic necrosis, and underlying patient comorbidities including obesity, diabetes, and septic complications.

The clinical course and resolution of severe acute pancreatitis can be complicated by damage to pancreatic and surrounding tissue and the secondary response to this injury. Ultimately, even without complications of pseudocysts, a single severe attack may result in chronic scarring, with acute or chronic pancreatic exocrine insufficiency and transient or chronic damage to the islets of Langerhans with resultant diabetes. However, chronic disease with end-organ damage most often is the result of recurrent, acute or relapsing acute pancreatitis.

Nutrition Concerns

Patients with mild acute pancreatitis and no infectious complications have increased metabolic stress and greater demand for nutrition support. Although they are often kept NPO to rest the pancreas, they typically have sufficient energy stores to recover in a short period of time. Weight loss from muscle catabolism is generally minimal in these patients.

In contrast, patients with severe acute pancreatitis are hypermetabolic, with a hyperdynamic disease process that is similar to sepsis,[46,47] including oxidative stress, exaggerated catabolism, and SIRS, which leads to rapid deterioration of nutrition status (see Table 28-2). Energy expenditure may be 139% of that predicted by the Harris-Benedict equation, and protein catabolism may be marked.[48] Sepsis complicating pancreatitis can further increase energy expenditure. With muscle catabolism, ureagenesis is accelerated, and glutamine levels are decreased in muscle and serum.[49]

Nutrition decline in acute pancreatitis can also result from reduced oral intake due to abdominal pain, nausea, vomiting, ileus, or being kept from eating to rest the pancreas (pancreatic rest is discussed later in this chapter). Even if the patient is eating, reduced enzyme output may cause maldigestion and malabsorption of luminal nutrients, and excessive protein loss may be caused by steatorrhea, pancreatic fistulas, or inflammation of peritoneal and retroperitoneal surfaces (see Table 28-2).

Stress hyperglycemia from transient insulin resistance occurs in 40% to 90% of patients with severe acute pancreatitis.[50,51] Hyperglycemia risk is related to the degree of pancreatic inflammation, especially necrosis, and is exaggerated in individuals with obesity or prediabetes. Damage to inflamed islet cells leads to decreased insulin production and impaired fat metabolism, with hypertriglyceridemia resulting from inadequate glucose control and downregulation of lipoprotein lipase in hyperglycemia.[52,53] When hypertriglyceridemia is secondary to poor glucose control, achieving adequate glycemic control is essential to decrease serum triglyceride levels.[54]

Electrolyte and micronutrient alterations are common in patients with acute pancreatitis, and hypocalcemia may occur in up to 25% of cases.[52] The reduction in the serum calcium level is related to decreased parathyroid hormone release, increased calcitonin levels, and decreased magnesium levels, with hypoalbuminemia and saponification of calcium with unabsorbed free fatty acids being a devastating occurrence in a minority of patients.[52]

Role of the Gut and Benefits of Enteral Nutrition

EN can offer many benefits to the patient with acute pancreatitis. The provision of as little as 20% total daily energy as EN in a patient with severe pancreatitis helps maintain gut integrity by preventing increases in gut permeability and keeping the functional tight junctions between the intestinal epithelial cells closed (see Table 28-3).[55-57] EN stimulates blood flow to the gut, which ameliorates or prevents ischemic/reperfusion injury. EN also stimulates the release of secretory immunoglobulin A and bile salts, which coat bacteria and prevent their adherence to the intestinal epithelium.[55-57] EN maintains the

TABLE 28-2 Factors Causing Deterioration of Nutrition Status in Acute and Chronic Pancreatitis

	Acute Pancreatitis	Chronic Pancreatitis
Hypermetabolism	++	+
Skeletal muscle catabolism	++	+
Increased oxidative stress	++	+
Reduced oral intake	++	+
Nausea, vomiting	++	+
Impaired carbohydrate and fat metabolism	++	+
Abdominal pain	++	++
Food aversion	++	++
Protein loss (via diarrhea, fistulas, inflammation)	++	++
Delayed gastric emptying	+	++
Continued alcohol abuse	+	++
Maldigestion, malabsorption	+	++
Gastric outlet obstruction	+	++

+ moderate frequency/degree of severity; ++ significant frequency/degree of severity.

TABLE 28-3 Benefits of Early Enteral Feeding in Acute Severe Pancreatitis

- Maintains gut integrity (reduces bacterial challenge)
- Sets the tone for systemic immunity (downregulates immune response)
- Attenuates oxidative stress
- Lessens disease severity
- Promotes a faster resolution of the disease process
- Reduces complications: fewer infections and less need for surgical interventions, shorter hospital length of stays, and possibly fewer multiple organ failures

mass of gut-associated lymphoid tissue, which in turn supports the mass of mucosal-associated lymphoid tissue at distant organ sites.[58,59]

EN also supports the role of commensal bacteria, which prevent colonization of the gut by pathogenic organisms.[55,60] Colonization of the gut with commensal organisms may reduce the likelihood for contact-dependent activation of intestinal epithelial cells by pathogenic organisms. Such a process can lead to increases in gut permeability from cell apoptosis and opening of the tight junctions, activation of neutrophils, and the release of inflammatory cytokines.[55,60] A small study suggested that a probiotic preparation may potentiate the action of commensal bacteria.[61] However, a subsequent, large, multicenter randomized study demonstrated no decrease in infectious complications and a significantly increased mortality from ischemic bowel from a high-dose multispecies probiotic preparation given in severe pancreatitis.[62] Refer to Chapter 4 for further discussion of probiotics.

Complications of pancreatitis (such as the presence of pseudocyst, abscess, or ascites) are not a contraindication to EN. EN may be provided as long as the patient demonstrates feeding tolerance. Compared with PN, the provision of EN attenuates the stress response in patients.[63] In cases of severe acute pancreatitis, patients who receive EN demonstrate increases in antioxidant capacity, faster decreases in C-reactive protein levels, and faster resolution of SIRS when compared with patients who receive PN.[63] In a comparative randomized trial, Abou-Assi and colleagues found that time to resolution of the disease process—as evidenced by reduction of abdominal pain, normalization of amylase, and successful advancement to an oral, clear liquid diet—was reduced by half with the use of EN compared with PN.[64] According to 2 meta-analyses involving 7 prospective randomized trials of patients admitted for acute pancreatitis, the use of early EN reduced the number of infections by as much as 52%, shortened hospital stay by as much as 4 days, cut in half the need for surgical interventions, and reduced the incidence of organ failure when compared with the use of PN.[65,66] The safety of jejunal EN has been well documented in 10 prospective, randomized trials, with the superiority of EN over PN being demonstrated for every study endpoint related to clinical outcome, including days to normalization of amylase, days to oral diet, length of hospitalization, length of stay in the ICU, percentage of nosocomial infection, and mortality.[63,64,67–74]

Pancreatic Rest

Opinions about the need for pancreatic rest and its overall clinical significance have changed dramatically in recent decades. Formerly, clinicians believed that early use of the gut would increase the risk for complications, including pancreatic abscess. However, prospective, randomized controlled trials have failed to confirm this hypothesis.[65,66] Instead, the clinical consequences of early use of enteral route lead to 1 of 3 possible scenarios: (1) a clinically silent increase in pancreatic enzyme output; (2) an uncomplicated exacerbation of symptoms in about 20% of cases; or (3) a significant exacerbation of symptoms, with an increase in SIRS seen in 4% of cases.[67,75] According to reports from the literature, efforts

to promote pancreatic rest via nasogastric suction, somatostatin therapy, and acid reduction are ineffective and have no impact on clinical outcomes.[49] This information suggests that pancreatic rest to basal unstimulated levels is not necessary, and reduced output to subclinical levels may be sufficient. The concept of putting the pancreas to rest and using the gut are not incompatible; both may be accomplished simultaneously in the same patient and are likely dependent on the types of nutrients delivered as well as the entry point of nutrients into the gut.

Nutrition Support Options

Options for nutrition support include standard therapy, where the patient remains NPO until able to tolerate an oral diet; placement of nasogastric or nasojejunal tube for delivery of EN; and placement of a central or peripherally placed central venous catheter to infuse PN for those patients intolerant of EN. The choice among these options is determined by disease severity and whether the degree of SIRS warrants admission to the ICU. Intestinal permeability is greater in patients with severe pancreatitis than in patients with mild pancreatitis and controls with no pancreatic disease.[76]

Although cumulative studies have clearly shown that EN is superior to PN in severe acute pancreatitis, few studies have specifically compared EN or PN to standard therapy. In a small study in patients admitted with acute pancreatitis, Powell and colleagues randomly assigned patients to EN vs standard therapy. The overall stress response (as suggested by decreases in tumor necrosis factor, interleukin-6, and C-reactive protein levels) was lower in the patients receiving EN than in those assigned to the standard therapy; however, the duration of therapy was only 4 days and the differences did not reach statistical significance.[77] Pupelis and associates published 2 studies of patients requiring surgery for complications of acute pancreatitis who were randomly assigned to EN or standard therapy postoperatively. Aggregating from these 2 studies of 71 patients, a trend toward reduced mortality was seen in those receiving EN compared with those assigned to standard therapy.[78,79] In a trial by the Dutch Pancreatitis Study Group, patients with acute pancreatitis were randomly assigned to early EN or an "on-demand" oral diet.[80] The participants purportedly had severe pancreatitis, but 80% of them were managed on a medical ward, and not in an ICU, which indicates they actually had moderately severe pancreatitis. Approximately 70% of the patients assigned to the on-demand group tolerated an oral diet by the fourth day, and outcomes in the 2 groups were the same. The findings from this trial imply that early EN should be initiated if the patient's SIRS response is severe enough to require ICU admission (especially if the patient is placed on mechanical ventilation). On the other hand, when patients are admitted to the medical ward, attempts to advance to oral diet should be made and EN initiated only after 4 days if the oral diet is unsuccessful.[80]

The patients with the greatest need for nutrition support are those with severe disease, which increases catabolism, inflammation, infectious risk, and malabsorption. APACHE scores greater than 10 and Ranson scores greater than 3 predict which patients are most likely to have severe necrotizing

---

TABLE 28-4 Initiating Enteral Nutrition in Severe Acute Pancreatitis

- Ensure hemodynamic stability (off pressors, adequate mean arterial pressure) before starting enteral nutrition.
- Initiate nutrition support by continuous or bolus infusion to meet daily energy and protein requirements:
  - Estimate energy requirements with indirect calorimetry, if available, or use 25 kcal/kg/d as energy goal.
  - Estimated protein requirements are 1.5 g/kg/d.
- Provide mixed-fuel regimen (protein, fat, and carbohydrate).
- Monitor tolerance closely; do not stop feeds due to diarrhea.
- Keep head of bed elevated to 30° to prevent aspiration.

TABLE 28-5 Enteral Formula Selection in Severe Acute Pancreatitis

- Standard polymeric formula may be used in most patients.
- If patient has signs of intolerance (increased pain, fever, or white blood cell count in association with increases in serum amylase and serum lipase), switch to elemental, very low–fat formula or switch to a semi-elemental formula with small peptides and medium-chain triglycerides.
- If patient has signs of malassimilation (diarrhea and/or steatorrhea), switch to semi-elemental formula with small peptides and medium-chain triglycerides and check stool for *Clostridium difficile* toxin.

---

pancreatitis.[81,82] In these patients, the provision of EN is more likely to positively affect outcomes. In contrast, patients with mild to moderate pancreatitis are less likely to have improved outcomes with EN and may be supported with IV fluids and narcotic analgesia and then advanced to oral diet as tolerated. It is recommended that patients who require EN undergo placement of an enteral feeding tube and have EN initiated within 48 to 72 hours of admission, after establishment of hemodynamic stability (see Table 28-4).[65] When EN is indicated, gastric access is usually much easier to achieve than jejunal access. Clinical trials comparing gastric vs jejunal EN feeding show no difference in tolerance or delivery of EN.[83–86]

Not all patients will tolerate EN, particularly if they have significant ileus or gastroparesis, and some patients may therefore require PN to prevent severe malnutrition and deleterious effects of acute starvation. When PN is indicated, initiation may need to be delayed until after the 5th day of hospitalization. In a study from China, patients were randomly assigned to PN or standard therapy after they underwent a complete fluid resuscitation, and nutrition was then started within 48 hours. Compared with standard therapy, the provision of PN at this point (presumably several days after the peak of inflammation) had a favorable impact on outcomes by reducing mortality, overall complications, pancreatic infection, and hospital length of stay. Outcomes were even better for a third group of patients in the study who received PN supplemented with parenteral glutamine.[87]

Enteral Nutrition Formula Selection

Standard polymeric enteral feeding formulas may be used in patients with acute pancreatitis. Several of the studies that demonstrated the superiority of EN over PN used polymeric formulas.[63,79,88] Also, in a small study (36 healthy volunteers), Kaushik and colleagues found that polymeric formulas infused 40 to 60 cm distal to the ligament of Treitz inhibited pancreatic secretions better than PN.[89]

Patients with extensive pancreatic necrosis or those demonstrating signs of maldigestion/malabsorption may benefit from a semi-elemental or elemental feeding. Before these types of formulas are selected, the most common causes of

diarrhea (sorbitol-containing medications and *Clostridium difficile* infection) should be excluded (see Chapter 13). A review of 127 patients with complicated pancreatitis receiving jejunal feeding revealed that 30% had a positive fecal fat test results indicating steatorrhea.[90] Fat delivered in the proximal small intestine (jejunum) may inhibit intestinal transit; therefore, peptide-based, semi-elemental feeds are often the preferred choice, although standard feeds may be trialed if tolerated. Some patients may tolerate and absorb nutrients from a formula with a high proportion of medium-chain triglycerides (MCTs). However, few trials have adequately compared tolerance to or benefits from specific types of enteral formulas (see Table 28-5).[91] Additional information on the nutrient composition of enteral formulas is found in Chapter 11.

Troubleshooting Enteral Nutrition

Patients intolerant of enteral feedings may have increased abdominal pain or exacerbation of SIRS. In these circumstances, clinicians should first recheck the position of the feeding tube or advance it further beyond the ligament of Treitz. In a study by McClave and colleagues,[67] a patient tolerant of jejunal infusion of formula flared with an exacerbation of SIRS when the same formula was infused into the stomach after the tube was displaced proximally. In a study by Louie and associates, the presence of prolonged ileus (more than 6 days) predicted the need for PN.[69] In other studies, over 50% of patients tolerated EN when the duration of ileus was limited to 5 days or less, and EN was tolerated in 92% of patients with ileus for less than 2 days.[92,93]

Macronutrient Balance in Parenteral Nutrition

When PN is indicated, a mixed-fuel solution of carbohydrate (dextrose), protein, and lipids is recommended.[94,95] Lipid injectable emulsions (ILEs) do not exacerbate the symptoms of pancreatitis unless the condition is caused by hypertriglyceridemia. Hypertriglyceridemia-induced pancreatitis generally occurs only in susceptible individuals with serum triglycerides greater than 1000 mg/dL, and an ILE can be safely started when triglyceride levels decrease below 400 mg/dL. If the quantity of lipids in PN is limited to less than 1 g/kg and glucose control is maintained, the risk for hypertriglyceridemia during PN is diminished.[96]

When hypertriglyceridemia occurs in the setting of pancreatitis, it is frequently related to familial dyslipidemia and or hyperglycemia.[97] Nonetheless, clinicians ordering and instituting PN need to monitor all patients for the possible occurrence of hypertriglyceridemia.

Resumption of Oral Intake

To assess a patient's readiness to resume oral intake, clinicians consider the absence or reduction in pain, reduction in need for parenteral narcotics to control pain, absence of vomiting, findings on CT scan (if obtained), and biochemical markers. Starting the transition to oral intake with a liquid diet does not seem advantageous. In patients with moderate to severe disease or complications such has sterile necrosis or pseudocyst, clinicians are more conservative with dietary advancement. Extending the period of jejunal tube feedings and NPO status offers no benefit over the standard care of "resume oral intake as tolerated."[90,98] Although low-fat diets are often recommended for patients recovering from pancreatitis, allowing patients the freedom to choose when to resume eating and self-select foods may decrease the length of hospitalization without increasing the rate of relapse or abdominal pain (see Practice Scenario 28-1).[99–101]

Practice Scenario 28-1

Question: How should the patient with severe acute pancreatitis receive nutrition support?

Scenario: A 57-year-old woman was admitted with a sudden acute onset of bilateral, upper quadrant abdominal pain, nausea, and vomiting accompanied by fever. Initial laboratory results revealed amylase 450 U/L (normal: 40–140 U/L) and lipase 2200 U/L (normal: 24–400U/L), findings consistent with acute pancreatitis, and her Acute Physiologic Assessment and Chronic Health Evaluation II (APACHE II) score was 16. Over the first 12 hours of hospitalization, the patient developed respiratory distress and hypoxemia, requiring placement on mechanical ventilation. The patient was 62 inches tall and weighed 165 pounds (body mass index: 30.2). Her temperature was 103° F, her blood pressure was 100/70 mm Hg, and her heart rate of 135 bpm. The patient's abdomen was distended, and bowel sounds were hypoactive. She had voluntary guarding, and examination of her extremities revealed mild edema. Current medications included acetaminophen, a proton pump inhibitor, meperidine, and promethazine hydrochloride. Initial laboratory tests revealed the following: white blood cell (WBC) count, 21,000/mL; hemoglobin, 10.5 g/dL; hematocrit of 32.8%; blood urea nitrogen, 55 mg/dL; creatinine, 2.5 mg/dL; serum potassium, 3.4 mmol/L; sodium, 155 mmol/L; glucose, 186 mg/dL; albumin, 3.0 g/dL; and calcium, 7.8 mg d/L. The patient underwent a computed tomography (CT) scan, which revealed an enlarged, edematous pancreas; necrosis involving 35% of the gland; surrounding inflammatory changes; and free fluid in the lesser sac. An abdominal

ultrasound revealed a prominent common bile duct with possible choledocholithiasis. The patient's urinalysis was remarkable for increased specific gravity but provided no evidence of infection. Blood cultures and a urine culture were negative; however, the patient was placed on antibiotics to cover biliary sepsis. The patient was admitted to the intensive care unit, and a central line was placed. She was started on intravenous volume resuscitation with normal saline.

Intervention: On Day 2 of admission, the patient underwent endoscopic retrograde cholangiopancreatography with sphincterotomy and stent placement, which produced copious pus. At the end of the procedure, she had a small-bore orojejunal tube placed while under fluoroscopy, with the feeding ports distal to the ligament of Treitz. Antibiotics were started for the bacterial cholangitis and planned for a short course (1 to 3 days) until drainage was effectively achieved with stenting.

Answer: With a feeding tube placed well below the ligament of Treitz, a standard polymeric formula may be initiated. Hypocaloric feedings would be appropriate in a patient with a body mass index of 30, and the use of a high-nitrogen, 1.0-kcal/mL formula would help meet her energy and protein goals. A reduced-electrolyte, "renal" formula should not be necessary unless clinically relevant hyperkalemia occurs on a standard formula. The patient's acute kidney injury was related to inflammatory mediators and sepsis from cholangitis and should resolve with aggressive hydration. Given the severity of the pancreatitis and extensive necrosis, the patient might require a semi-elemental diet or very low–fat elemental formula to prevent steatorrhea. If the patient experienced distention or nausea, the decompression of endogenous gastric and or biliary secretions with a nasogastric or orogastric tube might be necessary. Finally, the patient was at increased risk for transient or long-term hyperglycemia; therefore, her glucose levels and serum triglycerides required close monitoring. Insulin should be used for glycemic control if needed.

Rationale: The patient presented with classic acute biliary pancreatitis, complicated by necrosis and bacterial cholangitis. She had an early systemic inflammatory response and 3 Ranson criteria (WBC count greater than 16,000/mL; lactate dehydrogenase greater than 350 IU/L; serum calcium less than 8 mg/dL) and her admission APACHE II score indicated severe pancreatitis. The CT scan showed more than 30% necrosis of the pancreas, and there was evidence of multiorgan failure (lung, kidney). Given the severe pancreatitis, the patient had an increased chance for complications and a low likelihood of advancing to oral diet within 7 days. For these reasons, a jejunal tube was placed and EN was initiated as soon as possible after adequate hydration and hemodynamic stability were achieved.

Chronic Pancreatitis

In chronic pancreatitis, the gland has ultrastructural changes including irreversible loss of exocrine and endocrine mass with replacement of the stroma by fibrous tissue, with or without a lymphocytic inflammatory cell infiltrate. It is an insidious, debilitating, and costly disorder that diminishes quality of life for patients and their families.

Epidemiology

The reported yearly incidence of chronic pancreatitis in the United States varies from 3 to 8 cases per 100,000 people,[102] and men represent 73% to 91% of cases.[13] The gender difference is most likely related to alcoholism, as the vast majority of individuals with alcoholic-induced chronic pancreatitis are men. Worldwide, the incidence of chronic pancreatitis is rising. The increase is likely explained by the growing prevalence of alcohol use as well as improved diagnostic techniques.

The US healthcare cost burden of chronic pancreatitis is difficult to measure because of the associated comorbidities, such as diabetes, smoking-related disease, and alcoholic liver disease, but it has been estimated to be close to $3 billion.[103] Among all digestive disorders, pancreatitis ranked eighth in the United States in overall healthcare costs to society and seventh in hospital admissions and charges.[103]

The US mortality rate for chronic pancreatitis is approximately 50% within 20 to 25 years of onset.[13] Also, the incidence of pancreatic cancer in patients with chronic pancreatitis is 3 to 5 times greater than in the general US population.[104]

Etiology

The belief that the acute and chronic forms of pancreatitis are separate diseases should be abandoned now that we know that a single SAPE can result in chronic end-organ damage.[15] However, it still holds true that repeated insults (ie, bouts of acute pancreatitis) result in cumulative damage. Thus, the causes of chronic pancreatitis include recurrent overt or subclinical acute pancreatitis, while genetic and environmental factors also play a significant etiological role in the ongoing inflammation.

Tobacco smoking quadruples a patient's risk of acute pancreatitis progressing to chronic pancreatitis. The mechanisms for smoking injury are likely multifactorial, from the vasoconstrictive effects of nicotine and resulting oxidative stress, to direct toxic effects of volatile hydrocarbons and the myriad of chemicals created with combustion.[105] Cigarette smoke contains greater than 4000 compounds, with nitrosamines and nicotine primarily implicated in pancreatic secretion and premature zymogen activation. Smoking is also independently associated with an increased risk for pancreatic cancer, with or without underlying chronic pancreatitis.[105]

Genetic factors can influence outcomes of acute pancreatitis, increase the rate of progression to chronic pancreatitis, and significantly elevate one's risk for pancreatic cancers. Mutations of CFTR, PRSS1, SPINK1, CTRC, calcium-sensing receptor, and gamma-glutamyltransferase 1 genes have been linked to acute and chronic pancreatitis.[17] Recently, polymorphisms in genes other than those involved with intrapancreatic trypsin regulation, including the Claudin-2 and carboxypeptidase A1 genes, have also been associated with pancreatitis.[106]

In chronic pancreatitis, persistent inflammation increases the risk of pancreatic cancer, and, depending on the genetic mutation as well as the underlying immune response of the

patient,[107] cancer risk can be 100 times greater than in the general population. Early identification of relatives for genetic counseling and strict avoidance of cancer risk cofactors, including smoking and alcohol use, are strongly advised. Biomarkers have not yet been identified for screening and identification of early pancreatic cancers.

Although alcohol use is the leading cause of chronic pancreatitis worldwide, less than 10% of individuals categorized as heavy alcohol drinkers develop the disease, which suggests that underlying genetic or epigenetic factors are involved in the disease etiology.[13] As previously noted, hypertriglyceridemia (triglyceride level greater than 1000 mg/dL) is associated with acute pancreatitis, and recurrent bouts can lead to chronic pancreatitis if serum triglycerides are not adequately controlled by medication. Patients at increased risk for hypertriglyceridemia-induced pancreatitis include those with type I, IV, or V hyperlipoproteinemia, diabetes mellitus, alcohol abuse, obesity, or pregnancy.[107-109]

Chronic pancreatitis can occur as a sequelae of biliary tract disorders. However, this etiology is involved in a minority of cases, as patients with such disorders typically undergo definitive management (cholecystectomy, stone removal, sphincterotomy, and so on) to avoid recurrent acute pancreatitis and progression to chronic pancreatitis. Autoimmune pancreatitis is another rare cause of chronic pancreatitis.

Clinical Presentation and Pathophysiology

Chronic pancreatitis is a progressive inflammatory process initiated by a sentinel event and often involving repeated bouts of acute injury. As structural changes occur over time, functional alterations follow, including exocrine and endocrine deficiencies. After an initial episode of acute pancreatitis, 10% of patients develop chronic pancreatitis; 36% of patients with recurrent acute pancreatitis develop the chronic form.[110,111]

A hallmark feature of chronic pancreatitis is abdominal pain.[112] Many patients report acute exacerbations of pain superimposed on chronic dull pain, while others report chronic, unrelenting pain or intermittent pain. A minority have no pain at all. Most patients who develop pancreatic exocrine and endocrine deficiency leading to malabsorption and maldigestion will lose weight, and weight loss may also be secondary to sitophobia (fear of pain with eating). The amount of weight loss varies; patients with small duct disease, diabetes, or autoimmune causes may not lose any weight. The degree of glandular damage and replacement by fibrosis predicates the development of pancreatitis-related malabsorption or diabetes, which may take many decades to develop or may never occur.[113] Additional complications may include bile duct stricture, portal hypertension due to prolonged "trapped" bile duct, duodenal stricture, pseudocysts, and pancreatic fistulas and ascites.[13]

Nutrition Concerns

Like acute pancreatitis, recurrent flares of chronic pancreatitis can deteriorate nutrition status by increasing energy and protein requirements, discouraging oral intake, and causing greater nutrient losses.[114] The possible complications from chronic pancreatitis can set the stage for progressive malnutrition. Patients with recurrent or continuous abdominal pain may have anorexia,[115] or they may decrease intake to avoid exacerbating symptoms of pain or nausea; some follow fat-restricted diets (either prescribed or self-imposed).[116,117] Furthermore, pseudocysts can cause duodenal obstruction or gastric outlet obstruction. Also, patients may experience gastric dysmotility from pain medication use or diabetes or develop exocrine or endocrine deficiency over time. The prevalence of gastroparesis among patients with chronic pancreatitis is 44%, and exocrine insufficiency occurs in about 50% of patients.[118] The latter complication typically develops 10 to 12 years after onset of chronic pancreatitis, when substantial proportion of acini are destroyed.

Exocrine insufficiency manifests as diarrhea, steatorrhea, and malassimilation, with multiple physiologic derangements secondary to pancreatic acinar damage.[119] Steatorrhea is defined as the quantitative appearance of more than 7 g fat per day after consuming 100 g dietary fat. Historically, gold-standard testing for steatorrhea required feeding individuals diet with 100 g fat per day and collecting stool for 1 or 3 days. Today, most clinical practices use the fecal elastase-1 (FE1) test, which is reliable, patient-friendly, and relatively inexpensive. It requires a single, excreted stool sample for enzyme-linked immunosorbent assay detection of FE1, a human pancreas–specific proteolytic enzyme that is not degraded during its passage through the gut. An FE1 value less than 200 mcg per gram of stool indicates pancreatic exocrine insufficiency.

Maldigestion increases the risk for vitamin and trace mineral deficiencies. Although vitamin B_{12} deficiency is uncommon in chronic pancreatitis, it can occur from loss of the pancreatic enzymes required to cleave the R-protein from intrinsic factor so B_{12} can later be absorbed in the terminal ileum.[120] Patients with chronic pancreatitis are also at risk for malabsorption of the fat-soluble vitamins (A, D, E, and K). Reports of actual overt, clinical deficiencies are uncommon for vitamin K, whereas osteomalacia related to vitamin D deficiency, severe eye defects from vitamin A deficiency and neurologic problems related to vitamin E deficiency have been reported in extreme cases. The consequences of subclinical biochemical deficiencies are not clear.[121]

The bone mineral density of patients with chronic pancreatitis has been shown to be markedly decreased compared with controls,[122] and, in a recent systematic review of osteoporosis in chronic pancreatitis, two-thirds of patients had osteopenia or osteoporosis.[123] Vitamin D deficiency may play a role in osteoporosis in chronic pancreatitis, but other factors to consider include poor diet, systemic inflammation, smoking, and malabsorption of other nutrients (eg, magnesium, calcium). Dual-emission x-ray absorptiometry can be used to identify patients with chronic pancreatitis who might require nutrition interventions to proactively maximize bone health.

In alcoholic chronic pancreatitis, long-term ethanol use can contribute to zinc, magnesium, thiamin, and folate deficiencies. These problems are caused by reduced intake of food in favor of alcohol as well as changes in absorption related to alterations in gut microbacteria and damage to the gut endothelium. Continued alcohol consumption is itself an independent risk factor for malnutrition. Magnesium is an important

mineral in bone density and homeostasis.[124] Alcohol intake has been shown to reduce absorption of magnesium and increase renal excretion of magnesium.[125] Serum magnesium concentrations are a poor indicator of magnesium deficiency because 60% of the mineral is bound to bone. In a small clinical trial using an IV loading test, 10 of 13 patients with chronic pancreatitis had magnesium deficiency.[126] Ongoing clinical trials of zinc supplementation in subjects with alcoholic liver disease show improved nutrition status, with decreased infections and liver injury attributed to improved gut immunologic and barrier function (see Chapter 27).[127] Zinc and magnesium supplementation in pancreatitis for prevention of infection or improved bone mineral density has not been formerly studied.

Diabetes mellitus is the major late sequelae of chronic pancreatitis and is an independent risk factor for mortality in patients with chronic pancreatitis.[128] In a prospective study of 500 patients with chronic pancreatitis, the cumulative rates of diabetes mellitus since the onset of chronic pancreatitis were 50% and 83% at 10 and 25 years, respectively.[128] Patients with chronic pancreatitis and diabetes may have wildly fluctuating glucose levels and a propensity for hypoglycemia.[119,129] Diabetes alone may contribute further to developing gastroparesis.

Medical and Surgical Treatment

Identifying the underlying etiology of chronic pancreatitis helps clinicians provide a targeted therapeutic approach to avoid recurrent attacks and disease exacerbation. Patients should strictly avoid any identified environmental/external causes, such as alcohol or cigarette use. When patients abstain, symptoms tend to progress more slowly; with cessation of alcohol, 75% of patients can achieve symptomatic relief or modest improvement.[130]

As noted earlier, pain is the hallmark clinical symptom of chronic disease and debilitates many patients with chronic pancreatitis.[112] Recognizing whether the pain is nocioceptive (mediated by activation of normal pain pathways), neuropathic (abnormal response to pain stimuli), or psychogenic is essential for appropriate management.[131] Treatments include adjuvant analgesics such as gabapentin, nonsteroidal anti-inflammatory agents, and narcotics. Narcotic analgesic use is often required, but patients may need increasingly larger doses to achieve comfort. Tachyphylaxis can also lead to hyperalgesia with increased opiate dosing, and side effects from opiates, including nausea, vomiting and constipation, escalate. Neurolysis by anesthesiologists or gastroenterologists using EUS to ablate sympathetic nerve fibers has not been shown to have long-term benefits and may result in complicating diarrhea as a side effect of interruption of the parasympathetic/vagal nerve functioning.

Surgical treatments for chronic pancreatitis are selectively available, with retrospective reports showing amelioration of pain post ductal decompression and establishment of effective ductal drainage. ERCP with stenting beyond dominant strictures that provides relief of pain may help identify patients who would benefit from definitive surgery.[40,41] Surgeries with reasonable outcomes include the lateral pancreatojejunostomy (Puestow procedure) and selective procedures to remove segmentally diseased pancreatic portions. Total pancreatectomy followed by islet cell transfusion may be offered to a select minority of patients with chronic pancreatitis.[19,20]

The use of micronutrient antioxidants has emerged as a potentially beneficial treatment to reduce ongoing inflammation and glandular damage. Pain from chronic pancreatitis could theoretically be relieved or reduced by decreasing oxidative stress and pancreatic inflammation. A recent study from India evaluating daily doses of an antioxidant cocktail containing 600 mcg organic selenium, 0.54 g ascorbic acid, 9000 IU beta-carotene, 270 IU alpha-tocopherol (vitamin E), and 2 g methionine concluded that the supplement was effective in relieving abdominal pain in patients with chronic pancreatitis.[132] In a double-blind, randomized placebo-controlled trial of 70 patients with painful chronic pancreatitis largely due to alcohol intake, administration of antioxidants did not reduce pain or improve quality of life.[133] A recent Cochrane review of 12 randomized controlled studies, including 6 that were double-blind, placebo-controlled trials, included 585 participants with chronic pancreatitis.[134] Pain was described in 11 of 12 trials as slightly improved in participants who took antioxidants compared with the control group. Adverse events deemed to be related to ingestion of the antioxidants occurred in 16% of patients. The authors concluded that better designed studies are required before definitive recommendations for use of antioxidants in chronic pancreatitis can be made.[134]

Nutrition Management

Fat-Controlled Diets

In some patients, modifications of oral intake may reduce abdominal pain and reverse early changes of malnutrition. Although high-fat diets are more likely than high-carbohydrate diets to induce pancreatic enzyme secretions, no randomized trials have investigated a low-fat vs high-fat diet in this patient population. Low-fat diets could accelerate the energy deficit; therefore, a comparative trial is warranted.

When compared with a standard enteral formula, an enteral formulation containing MCTs and hydrolyzed peptides decreased cholecystokinin levels and pancreatic stimulation in normal volunteers, and the specialized formula improved persistent pain in a small group of patients with chronic pancreatitis.[135] However, participants with chronic pancreatitis were not tried on a standard enteral formula for comparison. In a small study of patients with severe pancreatic insufficiency, Caliari and colleagues[136] found that MCTs were absorbed better than long-chain triglycerides but required pancreatic enzymes for optimal absorption. The authors concluded that no advantage is to be expected from replacing usual dietary fats with MCTs if pancreatic supplements are used. In a study by Singh and associates of 60 malnourished patients with chronic pancreatitis,[117] dietary counseling was as effective as the use of an oral liquid supplement enriched with MCTs in improving pain and measures of nutrition status.

Enteral Nutrition

Patients with a refractory disease course who are unable to eat or regain weight may require EN. Gastric feeding may be tried first, and jejunal feeding may be an option for those who do not tolerate gastric enteral feeding. Feeds via a nasogastric or nasojejunal tube may be sufficient until oral intake is resumed. In retrospective studies, the use of prolonged nasojejunal feedings was compared with placement on an oral diet and resulted in fewer complications, less need for surgical intervention, and fewer readmissions to the hospital.[137,138] If patients require long-term enteral feeding, delivery may be via percutaneous endoscopic gastrostomy (PEG), PEG with jejunal tube extension (PEGJ), direct percutaneous endoscopic jejunostomy (DPEJ), or laparoscopically placed jejunostomy.[139] In one case series, long-term enteral feeding through a PEGJ or DPEJ tube over 6 months resulted in a significant reduction in the incidence of abdominal pain (96% before EN vs 24% after 6 months receiving EN), and in the number of patients requiring narcotic analgesia (91% before EN vs 28% after 6 months receiving EN).[98]

In patients with pancreatic insufficiency, pancreatic enzymes may be used with standard enteral products. However, the microspheres are difficult to administer via the feeding tube, and it may therefore be more cost-effective to use semi-elemental or elemental products instead of standard formulas (see Practice Scenario 28-2).[140,141] Pancreatic enzyme supplementation is discussed further in the next section.

Practice Scenario 28-2

Question: What are appropriate criteria for the use of nutrition support in a patient with chronic pancreatitis?

Scenario: A 42-year-old man was admitted for the sixth time this year with an exacerbation of chronic abdominal pain. His prior imaging, including endoscopic retrograde cholangiopancreatography and endoscopic ultrasound, demonstrated a diffusely diseased pancreas. The patient had a history of chronic ethanol abuse and admitted to an episode of binge drinking 1 week before admission. On review of systems, the patient complained of soft, runny, "greasy" stools with increased bloating. He reported a penetrating, deep epigastric pain, radiating to the back, which was made worse by eating; extreme thirst, frequent urination, nausea, and anorexia since his abdominal pain had worsened. Physical examination revealed a thin, white man who looked older than his stated age. His height was 68 inches, and he weighed 128 pounds (body mass index: 19.8), down from his original weight of 153 pounds 1 year prior. Current laboratory tests for the patient revealed a normal leukocyte count, with a mild elevation in alkaline phosphatase and a mildly elevated bilirubin level. The patient had normal amylase and lipase values, most likely because of his calcified pancreas and insufficient functional pancreatic tissue for synthesizing and secreting these enzymes. Repeated glucose levels were greater than 250 mg/dL with a glycated hemoglobin (HbA1c) of 10. Diabetes mellitus had not been clinically apparent in this patient until this admission.

Intervention: Jejunal feedings were initiated at a refeeding level early in the hospital admission.

Answer: Appropriate nutrition support for this patient includes a trial of nasojejunal feeding at home, which will provide the opportunity to determine a response to this management strategy. More permanent enteral access would be achieved by percutaneous endoscopic gastrostomy with jejunal tube extension (PEGJ) or direct percutaneous endoscopic jejunostomy (DPEJ) placement. This procedure may be performed in the outpatient setting and should not be difficult in a thin patient with no previous abdominal scars, surgeries, or ascites. The successful placement of a DPEJ or PEGJ and the initiation of jejunal feeds would be expected to improve nutrition status, increase the likelihood for symptomatic relief, and reduce the frequency for subsequent hospitalizations in the future. This patient is at a significant risk for refeeding syndrome, particularly while his hyperglycemia is brought under control.[140] He will need to be started at a refeeding level of between 15 and 20 kcal/kg while his glucose is carefully controlled. Electrolytes will need to be carefully monitored and replaced. Ultimately, this patient may need more than 35 kcal/kg/d to achieve weight gain with good glycemic control and adequate hydration. Current pancreatic enzyme preparations cannot be used with jejunal feeding tubes without significant clogging potential. Therefore, the patient will need to concomitantly take enzymes by mouth during feeds throughout the day, or he will need a semi-elemental formula. If the patient has persistent steatorrhea and failed clinical response, he may need an elemental product.

Rationale: Although pancreatic enzymes are recommended to help with absorption and reduce steatorrhea, they are unlikely to control this patient's pain or anorexia. His persistent weight loss in the setting of continued oral (gastric) intake indicates that he is an appropriate candidate for jejunal enteral nutrition.[141]

Pancreatic Enzyme Supplementation

Pancreatic enzyme supplementation is used to maximize absorption in patients with significant malabsorption from chronic pancreatitis, but it does not completely prevent steatorrhea.[142] Additionally, a meta-analysis of studies evaluating whether supplementation with high doses of pancreatic enzymes provides pain relief concluded that supplementation has not been shown to reduce pain.[143]

Enzymes used for malabsorption typically contain various concentrations of lipase, protease, and amylase. The dose of enzymes to treat steatorrhea should approximate 10% of what a normal pancreas would produce and achieve maximum efficacy at a pH between 7 and 8. Taking 30,000 lipase units orally per meal will usually provide the required adult dose.[116]

Enteric-coated preparations resist degradation by gastric acid and are absorbed after passage into the small bowel. These products require a luminal pH greater than 5. If uncoated enzymes are used, gastric acid suppression (eg, use of proton pump inhibitors, H2 blockers, or bicarbonate tablets) can prevent inactivation of the supplemented enzymes. Enteric-coated enzymes are designed to avoid this problem, but bicarbonate secretion may be insufficient to neutralize gastric acid entering the proximal small bowel unless concomitant acid suppression is used.[144] Bile acids will also be denatured at an acidic pH, adding to the problem of malabsorption.

Enzymes should be taken with, or just before, meals and snacks so they are timed to be present when the food passes into the small bowel.[145] Enteric-coated supplements should not be crushed or chewed.

Poor tolerance of enzyme supplements may occur in some patients with symptoms of nausea, bloating, cramping, or altered bowel habits. Clinicians should monitor patients for tolerance to and compliance with the supplementation regimen and may prescribe a different enzyme or dose as needed. Use of a prokinetic agent may be appropriate for some patients if slow gastric emptying is an issue. Fat restriction or a trial of MCT oil may be necessary if malabsorptionpersists.[146]

References

1. Saluja AK, Steer MLP. Pathophysiology of pancreatitis: role of cytokines and other mediators of inflammation. *Digestion.* 1999; 60 (Suppl 1):S27–S33.

2. Norman JG. New approaches to acute pancreatitis: role of inflammatory mediators. *Digestion.* 1999;60(Suppl 1):S57–S60.

3. Lankisch PG, Apte M, Banks PA. Acute pancreatitis. *Lancet.* 2015; 386(9988):85–96; erratum in *Lancet.* 2015;386(10008):2058.

4. O'Leary DP, O'Neill D, McLaughlin P, O'Neill S, Myers E, Maher MM, Redmond HP. Effects of abdominal fat distribution parameters on severity of acute pancreatitis. *World J Surg.* 2012;36(7): 1679–1685.

5. Sempere L, Martinez J, de Madaria E, et al. Obesity and fat distribution imply a greater systemic inflammatory response and a worse prognosis in acute pancreatitis. *Pancreatology.* 2008;8(3): 257–264.

6. Evans AC, Papachristou GI, Whitcomb DC. Obesity and the risk of severe acute pancreatitis. *Minerva Gastroenterol Dietol.* 2010; 56(2):169–179.

7. Chen SM, Xiong GS, Wu SM. Is obesity an indicator of complications and mortality in acute pancreatitis? An updated meta-analysis. *J Dig Dis.* 2012;13(5):244–251.

8. Khan AS, Latif SU, Eloubeidi MA. Controversies in the etiologies of acute pancreatitis. *JOP.* 2010;11(6):545–552.

9. Tonsi AF, Bacchion M, Crippa S, Malleo G, Bassi C. Acute pancreatitis at the beginning of the 21st century: the state of the art. *World J Gastroenterol.* 2009;15(24):2945–2959.

10. Whitcomb DC. Clinical practice. Acute pancreatitis. *N Engl J Med.* 2006;354(20):2142–2150.

11. Satoh K, Shimosegawa T, Masamune A, et al. Nationwide epidemiological survey of acute pancreatitis in Japan. *Pancreas.* 2011; 40(4):503–507.

12. Cucher D, Kulvatunyou N, Green DJ, Jie T, Ong ES. Gallstone pancreatitis: a review. *Surg Clin North Am.* 2014;94(2):257–280.

13. Jupp J, Fine D, Johnson CD. The epidemiology and socioeconomic impact of chronic pancreatitis. *Best Pract Res Clin Gastroenterol.* 2010;24(3):219–231.

14. Braganza JM, Lee SH, McCloy RF, et al. Chronic pancreatitis. *Lancet.* 2011;377(9772):1184–1197.

15. Whitcomb DC, Yadav D, Adam S, et al. Multicenter approach to recurrent acute and chronic pancreatitis in the United States: the North American Pancreatitis Study 2 (NAPS2). *Pancreatology.* 2008;8(4–5):520–531.

16. Gardner TB, Chari ST. Autoimmune pancreatitis. *Gastroenterol Clin North Am.* 2008;37(2):439–460.

17. Mounzer R, Whitcomb DC. Genetics of acute and chronic pancreatitis. *Curr Opin Gastroenterol.* 2013;29(5):544–551.

18. Weiss FU. Pancreatic cancer risk in hereditary pancreatitis. *Front Physiol.* 2014;5:70.

19. Witkowski P, Savari O, Matthews JB. Islet autotransplantation and total pancreatectomy. *Adv Surg.* 2014;48:223–233.

20. Bellin MD, Schwarzenberg SJ, Cook M, Sutherland DE, Chinnakotla S. Pediatric autologous islet transplantation. *Curr Diab Rep.* 2015;15(10):67.

21. Swaroop VS, Chari ST, Clain JE. Severe acute pancreatitis. *JAMA.* 2004;291(23):2865–2868.

22. Papachristou GI, Muddana V, Yadav D, et al. Comparison of BISAP, Ranson's, APACHE-II, and CTSI scores in predicting organ failure, complications, and mortality in acute pancreatitis. *Am J Gastroenterol.* 2010;105(2):435–441.

23. Kuo DC, Rider AC, Estrada P, Kim D, Pillow MT. Acute pancreatitis: what's the score? *J Emerg Med.* 2015;48(6):762–770.

24. Pavlidis P, Crichton S, Lemmich Smith J, et al. Improved outcome of severe acute pancreatitis in the intensive care unit. *Crit Care Res Pract.* 2013;2013:897107.

25. Russell PS, Mittal A, Brown L, et al. Admission, management and outcomes of acute pancreatitis in intensive care. *ANZ J Surg.* 2016(Mar 28). doi:10.1111/ans.13498.

26. Balthazar EJ, Freeny PC, van Sonneberg E. Imaging and interventions in acute pancreatitis. *Radiology.* 1994;193:297–306.

27. Banks PA. Practice guidelines in acute pancreatitis. *Am J Gastroenterol.* 1997;92:377–386.

28. Busireddy KK, Al Obaidy M, Ramalho M, et al. Pancreatitis-imaging approach. *World J Gastrointest Pathophysiol.* 2014;5(3):252–270.

29. O'Neill E, Hammond N, Miller FH. MR imaging of the pancreas. *Radiol Clin North Am.* 2014;52(4):757–777.

30. Darge K, Anupindi S. Pancreatitis and the role of US, MRCP and ERCP. *Pediatr Radiol.* 2009;39(Suppl 2):S153–S157.

31. Albashir S, Stevens T. Endoscopic ultrasonography to evaluate pancreatitis. *Cleve Clin J Med.* 2012;79(3):202–206.

32. Tashima CW, Sandha GS. Endoscopic ultrasound in the diagnosis and treatment of pancreatic disease. *World J Gastroenterol.* 2014;20(29):9976–9989.

33. Tyberg A, Karia K, Gabr M, et al. Management of pancreatic fluid collections: a comprehensive review of the literature. *World J Gastroenterol.* 2016;22(7):2256–2270.

34. Riff BP, Chandrasekhara V. The role of endoscopic retrograde cholangiopancreatography in management of pancreatic diseases. *Gastroenterol Clin North Am.* 2016;45(1):45–65.

35. Pai CG, Suvarna D, Bhat G. Endoscopic treatment as first-line therapy for pancreatic ascites and pleural effusion. *J Gastroenterol Hepatol.* 2009;24(7):1198–1202.

36. Larsen M, Kozarek R. Management of pancreatic ductal leaks and fistulae. *J Gastroenterol Hepatol.* 2014;29(7):1360–1370.

37. Fischer M, Hassan A, Sipe BW, et al. Endoscopic retrograde cholangiopancreatography and manometry findings in 1,241 idiopathic pancreatitis patients. *Pancreatology.* 2010;10(4):444–452.

38. Somani P, Navaneethan U. Role of ERCP in patients with idiopathic recurrent acute pancreatitis. *Curr Treat Options Gastroenterol.* 2016;14(3):327–339.

39. Das R, Yadav D, Papachristou GI. Endoscopic treatment of recurrent acute pancreatitis and smoldering acute pancreatitis. *Gastrointest Endosc Clin N Am.* 2015;25(4):737–748.

40. Attasaranya S, Abdel Aziz AM, Lehman GA. Endoscopic management of acute and chronic pancreatitis. *Surg Clin North Am.* 2007;87(6):1379–1402.

41. Elmunzer BJ. Endoscopic approaches to pancreatic disease. *Curr Opin Gastroenterol.* 2016;32:422–428.

42. Gurusamy KS, Pallari E, Hawkins N, Pereira SP, Davidson BR. Management strategies for pancreatic pseudocysts. *Cochrane Database Syst Rev.* 2016;(4):CD011392.

43. Sakai Y, Tsuyuguchi T, Ishihara T, et al. Long-term prognosis of patients with endoscopically treated postoperative bile duct stricture and bile duct stricture due to chronic pancreatitis. *J Gastroenterol Hepatol.* 2009;24(7):1191–1197.

44. Wittau M, Mayer B, Scheele J, et al. Systematic review and meta-analysis of antibiotic prophylaxis in severe acute pancreatitis. *Scand J Gastroenterol.* 2011;46(3):261–270.

45. Brand M, Bizos D, O'Farrell P. Antibiotic prophylaxis for patients undergoing elective endoscopic retrograde cholangiopancreatography. *Cochrane Database Syst Rev.* 2010;(10):CD007345.

46. Di Carlo V, Nespoli A, Chiesa R, et al. Hemodynamic and metabolic impairment in acute pancreatitis. *World J Surg.* 1981;5:329–339.

47. Shaw JH, Wolfe RR. Glucose, fatty acid, and urea kinetics in patients with severe pancreatitis. *Ann Surg.* 1986;204:665–672.

48. Dickerson RN, Vehe KL, Mullen JL, Feurer ID. Resting energy expenditure in patients with pancreatitis. *Crit Care Med.* 1991;19:484–490.

49. Helton WS. Intravenous nutrition in patients with acute pancreatitis. In: Rombeau JL, ed. *Clinical Nutrition: Parenteral Nutrition.* Philadelphia, PA: Saunders; 1990:442–461.

50. Marulendra S, Kirby D. Nutrition support in pancreatitis. *Nutr Clin Pract.* 1995;10:45–53.

51. Havala T, Shronts E, Cerra F. Nutritional support in acute pancreatitis. *Gastroenterol Clin North Am.* 1989;18:525–542.

52. Kohn CL, Brozenec S, Foster PF. Nutritional support for the patient with pancreatobiliary disease. *Crit Care Nurs Clin North Am.* 1993;5:37–45.

53. Kovár J, Fejfarová V, Pelikánová T, Poledne R. Hyperglycemia downregulates total lipoprotein lipase activity in humans. *Physiol Res.* 2004;53:61–68.

54. Mesotten D, Swinnen JV, Vanderhoydonc F, Wouters PJ, Van den Berghe G. Contribution of circulating lipids to the improved outcome of critical illness by glycemic control with intensive insulin therapy. *J Clin Endocrinol Metab.* 2004;89:219–226.

55. DeWitt RC, Kudsk KA. The gut's role in metabolism, mucosal barrier function, and gut immunology. *Infect Dis Clin North Am.* 1999;13:465–481.

56. Kagnoff MF. Immunology of the intestinal tract. *Gastroenterology.* 1993;105:1275–1280.

57. Jabbar A, Chang WK, Dryden GW, McClave SA. Gut immunology and the differential response to feeding and starvation. *Nutr Clin Pract.* 2003;18:461–482.

58. Targan SR, Kagnoff MF, Brogan MD, Shanahan F. Immunologic mechanisms in intestinal diseases. *Ann Intern Med.* 1987;106:853–870.

59. Dobbins WO. Gut immunophysiology: a gastroenterologist's view with emphasis on pathophysiology. *Am J Physiol.* 1982;242:G1–G8.

60. Alverdy JC, Laughlin RS, Wu L. Influence of the critically ill state on host-pathogen interactions within the intestine: gut-derived sepsis redefined. *Crit Care Med.* 2003;31:598–607.

61. Oláh A, Belágyi T, Issekutz A, Gamal ME, Bengmark S. Randomized clinical trial of specific lactobacillus and fibre supplement to early enteral nutrition in patients with acute pancreatitis. *Br J Surg.* 2002;89(9):1103–1107.

62. Besselink MG, van Santvoort HC, Buskens E, et al. Probiotic prophylaxis in predicted severe acute pancreatitis: a randomised, double-blind, placebo-controlled trial. *Lancet.* 2008;371(9613):651–659.

63. Windsor AC, Kanwar S, Li AG, et al. Compared with parenteral nutrition, enteral feeding attenuates the acute phase response and improves disease severity in acute pancreatitis. *Gut.* 1998;42:431–435.

64. Abou-Assi S, Craig K, O'Keefe SJ. Hypocaloric jejunal feeding is better than total parenteral nutrition in acute pancreatitis: results of a randomized comparative study. *Am J Gastroenterol.* 2002;97:2255–2262.

65. McClave SA, Chang WK, Dhaliwal R, Heyland DK. Nutrition support in acute pancreatitis: a systematic review of the literature. *JPEN J Parenter Enteral Nutr.* 2006;30:143–156.

66. Marik PE, Zaloga GPL. Meta-analysis of parenteral nutrition versus enteral nutrition in patients with acute pancreatitis. *BMJ*. 2004;328:1407–1412.
67. McClave SA, Greene LM, Snider HL, et al. Comparison of the safety of early enteral vs parenteral nutrition in mild acute pancreatitis. *JPEN J Parenter Enteral Nutr*. 1997;21:14–20.
68. Kalfarentzos F, Kehagias J, Mead N, et al. Enteral nutrition is superior to parenteral nutrition in severe acute pancreatitis: results of a randomized prospective trial. *Br J Surg*. 1997;84:1665–1669.
69. Louie B, Noseworthy T, Hailey D, et al. Enteral or parenteral nutrition for severe pancreatitis: a health technology assessment. *JPEN J Parenter Enteral Nutr*. 2002;26(suppl):S32.
70. Gupta R, Patel K, Calder PC, et al. A randomised clinical trial to assess the effect of total enteral and total parenteral nutritional support on metabolic, inflammatory and oxidative markers in patients with predicted severe acute pancreatitis (APACHE II > or = 6). *Pancreatology*. 2003;3:406–413.
71. Petrov MS, Kukosh MV, Emelyanov NV. A randomized controlled trial of enteral versus parenteral feeding in patients with predicted severe acute pancreatitis shows a significant reduction in mortality and in infected pancreatic complications with total enteral nutrition. *Dig Surg*. 2006;23(5–6):336–345.
72. Doley RP, Yadav TD, Wig JD, et al. Enteral nutrition in severe acute pancreatitis. *JOP*. 2009;10(2):157–162.
73. Wu XM, Ji KQ, Wang HY, et al. Total enteral nutrition in prevention of pancreatic necrotic infection in severe acute pancreatitis. *Pancreas*. 2010;39(2):248–251.
74. Casas M, Mora J, Fort E, et al. Total enteral nutrition vs. total parenteral nutrition in patients with severe acute pancreatitis. *Rev Esp Enferm Dig*. 2007;99(5):264–269.
75. O'Keefe SJ, Broderick T, Turner M, et al. Nutrition in the management of necrotizing pancreatitis. *Clin Gastroenterol Hepatol*. 2003;1:315–321.
76. Ammori BJ, Leeder PC, King RF, et al. Early increase in intestinal permeability in patients with severe acute pancreatitis: correlation with endotoxemia, organ failure, and mortality. *J Gastrointest Surg*. 1999;3:252–262.
77. Powell JJ, Murchison JT, Fearon KC, et al. Randomized controlled trial of the effect of early enteral nutrition on markers of the inflammatory response in predicted severe acute pancreatitis. *Br J Surg*. 2000;87:1375–1381.
78. Pupelis G, Austrums E, Jansone A, et al. Randomised trial of safety and efficacy of postoperative enteral feeding in patients with severe pancreatitis: preliminary report. *Eur J Surg*. 2000;166:383–387.
79. Pupelis G, Selga G, Austrums E, Kaminski A. Jejunal feeding, even when instituted late, improves outcomes in patients with severe pancreatitis and peritonitis. *Nutrition*. 2001;17:91–94.
80. Bakker OJ, van Brunschot S, van Santvoort HC, et al. Early versus on-demand nasoenteric tube feeding in acute pancreatitis. *N Engl J Med*. 2014;371:1983–1993.
81. Corfield AP, Cooper MJ, Williamson RC, et al. Prediction of severity in acute pancreatitis: prospective comparison of three prognostic indices. *Lancet*. 1985;2:403–407.
82. Wilson C, Heath DI, Imrie CW. Prediction of outcome in acute pancreatitis: a comparative study of APACHE II, clinical assessment and multiple factor scoring systems. *Br J Surg*. 1990;77:1260–1264.
83. Eatock FC, Chong P, Menezes N, et al. A randomized study of early nasogastric versus nasojejunal feeding in severe acute pancreatitis. *Am J Gastroenterol*. 2005;100:432–439.
84. Kumar A, Singh N, Prakash S, Saraya A, Joshi YK. Early enteral nutrition in severe acute pancreatitis: a prospective randomized controlled trial comparing nasojejunal and nasogastric routes. *J Clin Gastroenterol*. 2006;40(5):431–434.
85. O'Keefe SJ. Jejunal feeding is the best approach to early enteral feeding in patients with acute pancreatitis. *AGA Perspectives*. 2006;2:5–19.
86. Eckerwall GE, Axelsson JB, Andersson RG. Early nasogastric feeding in predicted severe acute pancreatitis: a clinical, randomized study. *Ann Surg*. 2006;244(6):959–965.
87. Xian-LI H, Qing-Jiu M, Jian-Guo L, et al. Effect of total parenteral nutrition (TPN) with and without glutamine dipeptide supplementation on outcome in severe acute pancreatitis (SAP). *Clin Nutr*. 2004;1(Suppl):43–47.
88. Modena JT, Cevasco LB, Basto CA, Vicuna AO, Ramirez MP. Total enteral nutrition as prophylactic therapy for pancreatic necrosis infection in severe acute pancreatitis. *Pancreatology*. 2006;6:58–64.
89. Kaushik N, Pietraszewski M, Holst JJ, O'Keefe SJ. Enteral feeding without pancreatic stimulation. *Pancreas*. 2005;31:353–359.
90. Makola D, Krenitsky J, Parrish C, et al. Efficacy of enteral nutrition for the treatment of pancreatitis using standard enteral formula. *Am J Gastroenterol*. 2006;101(10):2347–2355.
91. Lin HC, Zhao XT, Wang L. Jejunal brake: inhibition of intestinal transit by fat in the proximal small intestine. *Dig Dis Sci*. 1996;41(2):326–329.
92. Cravo M, Camilo ME, Marques A, Pinto Coneia J. Early tube feeding in acute pancreatitis: a prospective study. *Clin Nutr*. 1989;8(suppl):S14.
93. Schneider H, Boyle N, McCluckie A, Beal R, Atkinson S. Acute severe pancreatitis and multiple organ failure: total parenteral nutrition is still required in a proportion of patients. *Br J Surg*. 2000;87:362–373.
94. Stabile BE, Borzatta M, Stubbs RS, et al. Intravenous mixed amino acids and fats do not stimulate exocrine pancreatic secretion. *Am J Physiol*. 1984;246:G274–G280.
95. Burns GP, Stein TA. Pancreatic enzyme secretion during intravenous fat infusion. *JPEN J Parenter Enteral Nutr*. 1987;11:60–62.
96. Willcutts K, Krenitsky J, Banh L, et al. Is monitoring of serum triglycerides indicated in all parenterally fed patients? [abstract] *Nutr Clin Pract*. 2005;20:142.
97. Ewald N, Hardt PD, Kloer HU. Severe hypertriglyceridemia and pancreatitis: presentation and management. *Curr Opin Lipidol*. 2009;20(6):497–504.
98. Giger U, Stanga Z, DeLegge MH. Management of chronic pancreatitis. *Nutr Clin Pract*. 2004;191:37–49.
99. Moraes JM, Felga GE, Chebli LA, et al. A full solid diet as the initial meal in mild acute pancreatitis is safe and results in a shorter length of hospitalization: results from a prospective, randomized, controlled, double-blind clinical trial. *J Clin Gastroenterol*. 2010;44(7):517–522.
100. Teich N, Aghdassi A, Fischer J, et al. Optimal timing of oral refeeding in mild acute pancreatitis: results of an open randomized multicenter trial. *Pancreas*. 2010;39(7):1088–1092.
101. Eckerwall GE, Tingstedt BB, Bergenzaun PE, Andersson RG. Immediate oral feeding in patients with mild acute pancreatitis is safe and may accelerate recovery: a randomized clinical study. *Clin Nutr*. 2007;26(6):758–763.
102. Braganza JM, Dormandy TL. Micronutrient therapy for chronic pancreatitis: rationale and impact. *JOP*. 2010;11(2):99–112.
103. Everhart JE, Ruhl CE. Burden of digestive diseases in the United States Part III: liver, biliary tract, and pancreas. *Gastroenterology*. 2009;136:1134–1144.
104. Andersson R, Tingstedt B, Xia J. Pathogenesis of chronic pancreatitis: a comprehensive update and a look into the future. *Scand J Gastroenterol*. 2009;44(6):661–663.
105. Greer JB, Thrower E, Yadav D. Epidemiologic and mechanistic associations between smoking and pancreatitis. *Curr Treat Options Gastroenterol*. 2015;13(3):332–346.

106. Ravi KV, Nageshwar RD. Genetics of acute and chronic pancreatitis: an update. *World J Gastrointest Pathophysiol.* 2014;5(4): 427–437.

107. Inman KS, Francis AA, Murray NR. Complex role for the immune system in initiation and progression of pancreatic cancer. *World J Gastroenterol.* 2014;20(32):11160–11181.

108. Lloret Linares C, Pelletier AL, Czernichow S, et al. Acute pancreatitis in a cohort of 129 patients referred for severe hypertriglyceridemia. *Pancreas.* 2008;37(1):13–20.

109. Tsuang W, Navaneethan U, Ruiz L, et al. Hypertriglyceridemic pancreatitis: presentation and management. *Am J Gastroenterol.* 2009;104(4):984–991.

110. Sankaran SJ, Xiao AY, Wu LM, et al. Frequency of progression from acute to chronic pancreatitis and risk factors: a meta-analysis. *Gastroenterology.* 2015;149(6):1490–1500.

111. Yadav D, O'Connell M, Papachristou GI. Natural history following the first attack of acute pancreatitis. *Am J Gastroenterol.* 2012; 107(7):1096–1103.

112. Lieb JG, Forsmark CE. Review article: pain and chronic pancreatitis. *Aliment Pharmacol Ther.* 2009;29(7):706–719.

113. Barrett KE, Boitano S, Barman SM, Brooks HL. Overview of gastrointestinal function and regulation and digestion and absorption. In: Barrett KE, Barman SM, Boitano S, Brooks H, eds. *Review of Medical Physiology.* 23rd ed. New York: Lange Medical Books/ McGraw-Hill; 2010:467–478.

114. Duggan S, O'Sullivan MO, Feehan S, et al. Nutrition treatment of deficiency and malnutrition in chronic pancreatitis: a review. *Nutr Clin Pract.* 2010;25:362–370.

115. Ammann RW, Muellhaupt B. The natural history of pain in alcoholic chronic pancreatitis. *Gastroenterology.* 1999;116:1132–1140.

116. Domínguez-Muñoz JE. Pancreatic enzyme replacement therapy for pancreatic exocrine insufficiency: when is it indicated, what is the goal and how to do it? *Adv Med Sci.* 2011;56(1):1–5.

117. Singh S, Midha S, Singh N, Joshi YK, Garg PK. Dietary counseling versus dietary supplements for malnutrition in chronic pancreatitis: a randomized controlled trial. *Clin Gastroenterol Hepatol.* 2008;6(3):353–359.

118. Chowdhury RS, Forsmark CE, Davis RH, et al. Prevalence of gastroparesis in patients with small duct chronic pancreatitis. *Pancreas.* 2003;26:235–238.

119. Krishnamurty DM, Rabiee A, Jagannath SB, Andersen DK. Delayed release pancrelipase for treatment of pancreatic exocrine insufficiency associated with chronic pancreatitis. *Ther Clin Risk Manag.* 2009;5(3):507–520.

120. Taubin HL, Spiro HM. Nutritional aspects of chronic pancreatitis. *Am J Clin Nutr.* 1973;26:367–373.

121. Duggan SN, Smyth ND, O'Sullivan M, et al. The prevalence of malnutrition and fat-soluble vitamin deficiencies in chronic pancreatitis. *Nutr Clin Pract.* 2014;29(3):348–354. doi:10.1177 /0884533614528361.

122. Dujsikova H, Dite P, Tomandl J, Sevcikova A, Precechtelova M. Occurrence of metabolic osteopathy in patients with chronic pancreatitis. *Pancreatology.* 2008;8:583–586.

123. Duggan SN, Smyth ND, Murphy A, et al. High prevalence of osteoporosis in patients with chronic pancreatitis: a systematic review and meta-analysis. *Clin Gastroenterol Hepaotol.* 2014;12(2): 219–228.

124. Ryder KM, Shorr RI, Bush AJ, et al. Magnesium intake from food and supplements is associated with bone mineral density in healthy older white subjects. *J Am Geriatr Soc.* 2005;53(11): 1875–1880.

125. Abbott L, Nadler J, Rude RK. Magnesium deficiency in alcoholism: possible contribution to osteoporosis and cardiovascular disease in alcoholics. *Alcohol Clin Exp Res.* 1994;18(5):1076–1082.

126. Papazachariou IM, Martinez-Isla A, Efthimiou E, Williamson RN, Girgis SI. Magnesium deficiency in patients with chronic pancreatitis identified by an intravenous loading test. *Clin Chim Acta.* 2000;302(1–2):145–154.

127. Mohammad MK, Zhou Z, Cave M, Barve A, McClain CJ. Zinc and liver disease. *Nutr Clin Pract.* 2012;27(1):8–20.

128. Malka D, Hammel P, Sauvanet A, et al. Risk factors for diabetes mellitus in chronic pancreatitis. *Gastroenterology.* 2000;119: 1324–1332.

129. Latifi R, McIntosh JK, Dudrick SJ. Nutritional management of acute and chronic pancreatitis. *Surg Clin North Am.* 1991;71: 579–595.

130. Trapnell JE. Chronic relapsing pancreatitis: a review of 64 cases. *Br J Surg.* 1979;66:471–475.

131. Cruciani RA, Jain S. Pancreatic pain: a mini review. *Pancreatology.* 2008;8(3):230–235.

132. Bhardwaj P, Garg PK, Maulik SK, et al. A randomized controlled trial of antioxidant supplementation for pain relief in patients with chronic pancreatitis. *Gastroenterology.* 2009;136(1):149–159.

133. Siriwardena JK, Mason JM, Sheen AJ, Makin AJ, Shah NS. Antioxidant therapy does not reduce pain in patients with chronic pancreatitis: the ANTIPIPATE study. *Gastroenterology.* 2012;143(3): 655–663.

134. Ahmed Ali U, Jens S, Busch OR, et al. Antioxidants for pain in chronic pancreatitis. *Cochrane Database Syst Rev.* 2014;(8): CD008945.

135. Shea JC, Bishop MD, Parker EM, et al. An enteral therapy containing medium-chain triglycerides and hydrolyzed peptides reduces postprandial pain associated with chronic pancreatitis. *Pancreatology.* 2003;3:36–40.

136. Caliari S, Benini L, Sembenini C, et al. Medium-chain triglyceride absorption in patients with pancreatic insufficiency. *Scand J Gastroenterol.* 1996;31(1): 90–94.

137. Hamvas J, Schwab R, Pap A. Jejunal feeding in chronic pancreatitis with severe necrosis. *JOP.* 2001;2:112–116.

138. Gonzalez C, Silverman W. The impact of prolonged nasojejunal tube feeding in patients with refractory pancreatitis and abdominal pain: a five year retrospective review. *Gastroenterology.* 2003;124:A401.

139. O'Keefe SJ. A guide to enteral access procedures and enteral nutrition. *Nat Rev Gastroenterol Hepatol.* 2009;6(4):207–215.

140. McCray S, Walker S, Parrish CR. Much ado about refeeding. *Pract Gastroenterol.* 2004;28(12):26.

141. Al-Omran M, Albalawi ZH, Tashkandi MF, Al-Ansary LA. Enteral versus parenteral nutrition for acute pancreatitis. *Cochrane Database Syst Rev.* 2010;(1):CD002837.

142. Waljee AK, Dimagno MJ, Wu BU, et al. Systematic review: pancreatic enzyme treatment of malabsorption associated with chronic pancreatitis. *Aliment Pharmacol Ther.* 2009;29(3):235–246.

143. Brown A, Hughes M, Tenner S, et al. Does pancreatic enzyme supplementation reduce pain in patients with chronic pancreatitis: a meta-analysis. *Am J Gastroenterol.* 1997;92:2032–2035.

144. Graham DY. Pancreatic enzyme replacement: the effect of antacids or cimetidine. *Dig Dis Sci.* 1982;27(6):485–490.

145. Quatrara B. FDA-approved pancreatic enzyme replacement therapy. *Practical Gastroenterol.* 2011;35(5):19.

146. Berry AJ. Pancreatic enzyme replacement therapy during pancreatic insufficiency. *Nutr Clin Pract.* 2014;29(3):312–321.

29 Renal Disease

Menaka Sarav, MD, and Csaba P. Kovesdy, MD

CONTENTS

Acknowledgments: Robert Wolk, PharmD, and Charles J. Foulks, MD, FACP, FACN, were the authors of this chapter for the second edition.

Objectives

1. Describe the anatomical features and physiological function of the kidney.
2. Define and understand diagnosis of acute kidney injury (AKI) and chronic kidney disease (CKD).
3. Review the nutrition requirements of patients with AKI and CKD, and discuss how requirements change once dialysis is initiated.
4. Construct a parenteral nutrition (PN) formula that considers the metabolic changes that occur in AKI.

Test Your Knowledge Questions

1. Which of the following metabolic alterations is most commonly observed in AKI?
   A. Decreased energy expenditure
   B. Metabolic acidosis
   C. Decreased serum magnesium concentration
   D. Metabolic alkalosis
2. Which of the following parenteral amino acid preparations is most appropriate for a dialysis-dependent patient with renal failure?
   A. Essential amino acids only
   B. Nonessential amino acids only
   C. Mixtures of essential and nonessential amino acids
   D. High branched-chain amino acids (BCAAs)
3. Which of the following is a measurement of body iron stores?
   A. Total iron-binding capacity (TIBC)
   B. Ferritin
   C. Transferrin
   D. Ceruloplasmin
4. What percentage of instilled dextrose is typically absorbed from peritoneal dialysate with a 6-hour dwell time?
   A. 25%
   B. 50%
   C. 75%
   D. 100%

Test Your Knowledge Answers

1. The correct answer is **B**. In AKI, a metabolic acidosis develops from organic and inorganic acid accumulation. Serum potassium concentrations increase as obligate renal clearance is reduced.
2. The correct answer is **C**. Essential and nonessential amino acids are lost via dialysis solutions used for hemodialysis (HD) and peritoneal dialysis (PD). The ability to synthesize nonessential amino acids is reduced in patients with acute renal insufficiency. Therefore, a solution containing both essential and nonessential amino acids is preferred in this clinical setting. Enriched BCAA solutions have been studied in AKI and have not been shown to improve clinical outcomes.
3. The correct answer is **B**. Ferritin is a serum protein that binds iron and serves as a reliable indicator of total iron stores. Low levels of this protein are typically seen with iron deficiency anemia, whereas high values occur with iron overload from an excessive intake of iron or the presence of hemochromatosis. Ferritin is an acute-phase protein and is also increased with acute inflammatory diseases of the liver. In CKD, ferritin should be greater than 100 ng/dL and the transferrin saturation (TSAT) should be greater than 20%. TIBC is a measure of serum iron and various proteins that transport iron within the circulation. A saturation index for these proteins is a measure of the available iron within the bloodstream. Transferrin is a circulating transport protein that carries iron that can be used in hematopoiesis. Ceruloplasmin is a copper transport protein, which possess ferroxidase activity that is important for binding of recycled and stored iron to transferrin.
4. The correct answer is **C**. In 6 hours, approximately 75% to 80% of the instilled dextrose of the dialysate solution is absorbed. This dextrose can be a significant source of energy.

Background

The kidney is responsible for clearing nitrogenous waste, regulating volume status, and maintaining electrolyte levels and acid-base balance. It also eliminates certain drugs and synthesizes and metabolizes certain hormones. Impairment or loss of these functions can have a profound effect on the metabolic and nutrition status of patients. In AKI, increases in protein and energy requirements parallel those seen in patients who experience trauma, serious infection, and other acute inflammatory illnesses. On the other hand, CKD patients may experience a series of metabolic changes that lead to protein-energy wasting (PEW), which is "a state of decreased body stores of protein and energy fuels."[1]

The advent of renal replacement therapy (RRT) has vastly improved the management of AKI and CKD. RRT takes over a portion of the function of the failing kidneys to remove the fluid and waste products and makes it possible to provide adequate protein and energy to patients with AKI or CKD. When provided in sufficient amounts, nutrition support could reverse PEW (in the absence of injury, inflammation, or the presence of cancer), reduce nutrition-related complications, and perhaps improve overall survival in patients with kidney disease.[2] This chapter reviews the physiological changes that occur in patients with a decreased glomerular filtration rate (GFR), examines the impact of RRT on these changes, discusses the nutrition requirements of patients with impaired renal function, and addresses how to apply these principles to the provision of nutrition support.

Normal Renal Function

The kidneys are 2 fist-sized organs located in the retroperitoneal space and are attached to the lower portion of the aorta and vena cava by the renal arteries and veins, respectively.[3] Each kidney is composed of approximately 1 million nephrons, which are the functional units of the kidney. Each nephron includes (1) the glomerulus, through which blood is filtered; (2) the proximal tubule, through which various substances are actively or passively reabsorbed, secreted, or metabolized; (3) the loop of Henle and the distal tubules, which are involved in fluid and electrolyte regulation; and (4) the collecting duct, where the urine is concentrated.[4] Most fluid and solute reabsorption occurs by active transport in the proximal and distal tubule, or by passive transport, which relies on the development of an osmotic gradient that varies along the length of the loop of Henle and collecting duct. The entire process results in the formation of urine, an ultrafiltrate of the plasma. The nephron also functions in conjunction with the liver to clear the plasma of metabolic end products, including urea, creatinine, uric acid, and organic and inorganic acids. Electrolytes (sodium, potassium, chloride), minerals (calcium, phosphorus, magnesium), and micronutrients (zinc, selenium) are filtered through the glomeruli and may be reabsorbed or excreted, depending on the metabolic needs of the body.[3,5] Small nutrients that are filtered through the glomerulus, such as glucose, small proteins, amino acids, and vitamins, are reabsorbed by active transport in the proximal tubule.[3] Other functions include gluconeogenesis, regulation of calcium–phosphorus balance, vitamin activation and metabolism, hormone synthesis and elimination, and drug metabolism and clearance.

GFR is usually accepted as the best overall index of kidney function in health and disease. The level of GFR and its magnitude of change over time are vital to the detection of kidney disease, understanding its severity, and making decisions about diagnosis, prognosis, and treatment. GFR is measured using plasma or urinary clearance of exogenous filtration markers such as inulin. This method is very cumbersome and is only used in research studies when very accurate estimation of renal function is necessary.[6] In clinical practice, GFR is usually estimated from endogenous filtration markers.

Serum creatinine is the most commonly measured endogenous filtration marker. It is an amino acid derivative that is generated from the breakdown of creatine in muscle, distributed throughout total body water, and excreted by the kidneys, primarily by glomerular filtration. Although the serum creatinine level is primarily affected by the GFR, it is to a smaller degree affected by other physiological processes, such as tubular secretion, generation, and extrarenal excretion of creatinine. Because of the multiple factors that affect the serum creatinine levels, particularly the variation in creatinine generation with regards to change in muscle mass, the cutoff for normal serum creatinine concentration differs among groups. Because of the wide normal range for serum creatinine in most clinical laboratories, GFR must decline to approximately half the normal level before the serum creatinine concentration rises above the upper limit of normal. Therefore, the estimated GFR, which combines the serum level with other demographic factors, provides more information than the serum creatinine value alone.

Three commonly used equations for estimating GFR or creatinine clearance are the Chronic Kidney Disease Epidemiology Collaboration (CKD-EPI) creatinine equation,[7] Modification of Diet in Renal Disease (MDRD) Study equation,[8] and Cockcroft and Gault equation.[9] All 3 equations use serum creatinine in combination with age, sex, weight, and/or race to estimate GFR and, therefore, improve on several of the limitations of using serum creatinine alone.[10,11] All creatinine-based estimating equations are limited by (1) use of serum creatinine as a filtration marker, as there are non-GFR factors that influence serum creatinine; (2) decreased accuracy at higher levels of estimated GFR; and (3) non-steady-state conditions for the filtration marker when GFR is changing.

The CKD-EPI equation[7] was developed in 2009 using a diverse population. It estimates GFR from serum creatinine, age, sex, and race, normalized to body surface area. The CKD-EPI equation is as accurate as the MDRD Study equation (currently reported by most laboratories) in the subgroup with estimated GFR less than 60 mL/min/1.73 m[2] and substantially more accurate in the subgroup with estimated GFR greater than 60 mL/min/1.73 m[2]. It is the equation recommended in the Kidney Disease: Improving Global Outcomes (KDIGO), Chronic Kidney Disease Guidelines.[12]

The 4-variable MDRD Study equation[8] was developed in 1999 using data from 1628 patients with CKD that measured GFR from approximately 5 to 90 mL/min/1.73 m[2]. It estimates GFR adjusted for body surface area and is more accurate than GFR estimated by the Cockcroft and Gault formula. The MDRD Study equation was re-expressed in 2005 for use with a standardized serum creatinine assay, which yields 5% lower values for serum creatinine concentration.

The Cockcroft and Gault formula[9] was developed in 1973 using data from 249 men with creatinine clearance from approximately 30 to 130 mL/min. It is not adjusted for body surface area, but it incorporates body weight. The Cockcroft and Gault formula is no longer recommended for use because it has not been expressed using standardized creatinine values.

Acute Kidney Injury

Definition, Incidence, and Impact of Acute Kidney Injury

AKI is defined as an abrupt decline in kidney function over hours to days that leads to a reduction of both glomerular filtration and tubular function.[13,14] Clinically, the diagnosis and the severity of the AKI are determined by observing a rise in the serum creatinine often in association with a decrease in urine output (Table 29-1).[15,16] Based on the severity of the AKI, a number of complications may occur, including hyperkalemia, hyperphosphatemia, glucose intolerance, fluid overload, acidosis, and azotemia.[13,17] The causes of AKI may be divided into 3 broad categories depending on the injury: prerenal, postrenal, and intrinsic. Prerenal AKI results when there is reduced renal blood flow, which can be caused by any renal hypoperfusion, such as volume depletion, congestive heart failure, shock, acute myocardial injury, nephrotic syndrome, or cirrhosis. Postrenal AKI is caused by a blockage of the urinary drainage, such as ureteral obstruction or prostatic hypertrophy.[18,19] Intrinsic AKI occurs with a direct injury to the kidney, such as with glomerulonephritis, acute tubular necrosis, allergic interstitial nephritis, vasculitis, or thrombotic microangiopathy.

AKI occurs in approximately 0.37% to 5% of all hospitalized patients and is most often caused by a combination of events, including sepsis, hypotension, and exposure to nephrotoxic drugs and therapeutic agents.[13,20,21] AKI is associated with a 30% to 80% mortality rate. Death is usually the result of multisystem organ failure or uncontrolled sepsis and is

TABLE 29-1 KDIGO Clinical Practice Guideline Definition of Acute Kidney Injury

AKI is defined as any of the following *(not graded)*:
- Increase in SCr by ≥0.3 mg/dL (≥26.5 mcmol/L within 48 hours);
- Increase in SCr by ≥1.5 times baseline, which is known or presumed to have occurred within the prior 7 days; or
- Urine volume <0.5 mL/kg/h for 6 hours.

Stages of AKI

Stage	Serum Creatinine	Urine Output
1	1.5–1.9 times baseline *Or* ≥0.3 mg/dL (≥26.5 mcmol/L) increase	<0.5 mL/kg/h for 6–12 hours
2	2.0–2.9 times baseline	<0.5 mL/kg/h for ≥12 hours
3	3.0 times baseline *Or* Increase in serum creatinine to ≥4.0 mg/dL (≥353.6 mcmol/L) *Or* Initiation of renal replacement therapy *Or* In patients <18 years, decrease in eGFR to <35 mL/min/1.73m^2	<0.3 mL/kg/h for ≥24 hours *Or* Anuria for ≥12 hours

AKI, acute kidney injury; eGFR, estimated glomerular filtration rate; KDIGO, Kidney Disease: Improving Global Outcomes; SCr, serum creatinine.
Source: Adapted from Table 2 in reference 15: KDIGO clinical practice guideline for acute kidney injury. *Kidney Int Suppl.* 2012;2:1–138. http://www.kdigo.org/clinical_practice_guidelines/pdf/KDIGO%20AKI%20Guideline.pdf. Accessed May 4, 2017. Reproduced with permission from Elsevier.

generally not directly related to the renal failure, per se.[3,5,13] AKI that occurs in patients in the intensive care unit (ICU) carries a higher mortality than AKI that occurs in patients who are not receiving care in an ICU.[22]

Metabolic Abnormalities Associated with Acute Kidney Injury

Patients with AKI occasionally are both hypermetabolic and hypercatabolic as a result of the neurohumoral responses associated with acute injury.[20] Table 29-2 lists the metabolic complications that occur in AKI, which include the loss of glucose homeostasis, muscle wasting, protein catabolism, electrolyte imbalance, and the development of metabolic acidosis.[21,23]

Protein catabolism can result in an accumulation of several byproducts of protein metabolism. The accumulation of blood urea nitrogen is referred to as *azotemia*. Besides urea, creatinine, aromatic and aliphatic amines, guanidines, and indoles are elevated in the blood of patients with AKI compared with those with normal kidney function.[24] Tissue catabolism also releases intracellular electrolytes, such as potassium, phosphorus, magnesium, and protein-bound acids, such as sulfuric acid (from sulfur-containing methionine and cysteine) and hydrochloric acid (from the chloride salt amino acids).[24] This accumulation can lead to metabolic acidosis and electrolyte imbalance. Metabolic acidosis increases skeletal muscle release of BCAAs that are preferentially used for gluconeogenesis and worsening protein catabolism.[25]

TABLE 29-2 Metabolic Complications of Acute Kidney Injury and Chronic Kidney Disease

System	Metabolic Complications
Endocrine	Glucose intolerance (insulin resistance, hyperglycemia), renal osteodystrophy, secondary hyperparathyroidism, amenorrhea, infertility
Cardiovascular	Lipid abnormalities (hypercholesterolemia, hypertriglyceridemia), hypertension, atherosclerosis
Gastrointestinal	Anorexia, nausea, and vomiting; altered taste acuity; gastroenteritis; peptic ulceration; ascites; decreased protein and amino acid synthesis
Renal	Azotemia, volume expansion and contraction, electrolyte imbalances (dysnatremia, hyperkalemia, hyperphosphatemia, hypocalcemia, metabolic acidosis)
Other	Anemia, vitamin deficiencies

Nutrition support plays an important role in the setting of AKI and may influence the patient's clinical course and, ultimately, clinical outcome.[13,26-28] Some authors have suggested that nutrition support may promote renal functional recovery.[25,26,29] Sufficient nutrition may decrease the degree of protein catabolism and decrease the severity of negative nitrogen balance.[21,26,27] Although it might seem necessary to achieve a positive nitrogen balance to enhance survival in patients with AKI, achieving adequate energy balance and neutral nitrogen balance seems to be more important. As with all forms of nutrition support, the success of this therapy depends on the ability to reverse or control the patient's underlying illness, and positive protein balance is hard to attain in AKI patients until all acute inflammatory processes are controlled.

Chronic Kidney Disease

Definition, Incidence, and Impact of Chronic Kidney Disease

CKD is defined as abnormalities of kidney structure or function, present for more than 3 months, with implication for health. Based on the KDIGO 2012 guidelines, CKD is classified based on estimated GFR (GFR stages 1 to 5) and albuminuria (stages 1 to 3), as follows:[30]

- GFR stage 1 (normal or high): GFR equal to or greater than 90 mL/min/1.73 m^2
- GFR stage 2 (mildly decreased): 60–89 mL/min/1.73 m^2
- GFR stage 3a (mildly to moderately decreased): 44–59 mL/min/1.73 m^2
- GFR stage 3b (moderately decreased): 30–44 mL/min/1.73 m^2
- GFR stage 4 (severely decreased): 15–29 mL/min/1.73 m^2
- GFR stage 5 (kidney failure): less than 15 mL/min/1.73 m^2
- Albuminuria stage 1 (normal to mildly increased): less than 30mg/g (3 mg/mmol)
- Albuminuria stage 2 (moderately increased): 30–300 mg/g (3–30 mg/mmol)
- Albuminuria stage 3 (severely increased): greater than 300 mg/g (30 mg/mmol)

A "heat map" has been generated that combines the GFR and albuminuria stages, thus providing a simplified tool for risk assessment and, in turn, prognosis.[30] For example, GFR stage 3 + Albuminuria stage 3 has a higher risk for poor prognosis when compared with GFR stage 3 + Albuminuria stage 1. Clinicians can use these risk categories to describe and prioritize efforts for treatments and follow-up.

According to data from the US Renal Data System (USRDS) public health surveillance, CKD affects 14.8% US population.[31] People with diabetes mellitus and hypertension account for 65% to 80% of all new cases of CKD.[5,21,32] The remaining cases occur in patients with primary renal diseases such as a glomerulonephritis, adult polycystic kidney disease, or progressive CKD from a preceding episode of AKI, as well as genitourinary obstruction.

If a patient has CKD, the remaining nephrons increase their workload in an attempt to maintain the highest level of renal function possible. This increase in single-nephron GFR results in intraglomerular hypertension, stretching of the mesangial supporting cells, and an increase in oxygen-free radicals and other inflammatory metabolic products, which then cause progressive scarring of the remaining glomeruli.[33]

Metabolic Abnormalities Associated with Chronic Kidney Disease

Many of the metabolic complications of CKD are similar to those seen with AKI (Table 29-2). These complications include impaired electrolyte clearance, abnormal acid-base status, and altered fluid status.[3] The metabolic changes that occur in CKD have a profound influence on mineral and bone metabolism. CKD results in altered levels of serum phosphate, vitamin D, calcium, parathyroid hormone (PTH) and fibroblast growth factor 23 (FGF23); the increased levels of serum phosphate, PTH, and FGF23 contribute to the increased cardiovascular mortality in CKD patients. Anemia is common and is in part caused by decreased erythropoietin (EPO) synthesis, a decrease in the erythrocyte life span, and nutrient deficiencies (in particular, iron deficiency).

In addition to the metabolic abnormalities noted above, PEW is the result of multiple mechanisms inherent to CKD, including poor nutrition, systemic inflammation, hormonal derangements, comorbidities, the dialysis procedure, and other consequences of uremic toxicity.[1,34,35] Anorexia, dietary restrictions, depression, and inability to obtain or prepare food lead to decreased protein and energy intake. Resistance to growth hormone and insulin-like growth factor-1, testosterone deficiency, and low thyroid hormone lead to decreased anabolism. Diabetes, congestive heart failure, depression, coronary heart disease, and peripheral vascular disease are common comorbidities that can complicate nutrition status in CKD. RRT may reverse uremia, residual metabolic derangements, inflammation, and comorbid conditions; however, the dialysis procedure itself may allow PEW to develop or worsen because of nutrient loss into dialysate, dialysis-related inflammation and hypermetabolism, and loss of residual renal function. PEW may cause infection, cardiovascular disease, frailty, and depression, but these complications may also increase the extent of PEW.[35] These factors should be considered when developing a nutrition program for individuals with CKD.

Renal Replacement Therapy

Although the rate of all-cause mortality remains higher for patients on dialysis than for the general population, the life expectancy of patients with end-stage renal disease (ESRD) has gradually improved since the introduction of RRT via dialysis in the 1960s. RRT replaces the nonendocrine function of the kidney in ESRD patients. Dialysis modalities include HD, either in a dialysis center or at home, as well as PD, such as continuous ambulatory PD or automated PD.[3,5] The decision to perform dialysis and the modality of dialysis depends on a number of factors, including the availability and convenience of the modality, the patient's comorbid conditions, socioeconomic and dialysis-center factors, the patient's home situation, and the patient's ability to tolerate volume shifts. In 2009, the USRDS[36] showed that 94% of prevalent ESRD patients were treated with in-center HD and 6% with

PD. This modality distribution is distinctive to the United States; in other countries, PD is more popular. Compared with in-center HD, PD may provide relatively short-term survival benefits but comparable or decreased survival after the first few years. Comorbidities such as heart failure or diabetes may attenuate the early relative benefit associated with PD. For patients in the ICU with tenuous hemodynamics and inability to tolerate large volume shifts, continuous renal replacement therapy (CRRT) can be used. The major advantage of CRRT is the slower, gentler rate of solute or fluid removal. The type of RRT affects the nutrient requirements and metabolic complications of the patient.

Hemodialysis

HD is highly effective in treating uremia and other metabolic complications associated with AKI and ESRD.[3,5] While this therapy can be provided in-center or at home, in-center HD accounts for the majority of all RRT used to manage patients with ESRD. Dialysis is used in ESRD to maintain fluid and electrolyte balances, and to prevent the accumulation of nitrogen waste products. This form of dialysis can also remove a variety of medications that would otherwise be excreted by the kidney and thus prevents the accumulation and potentially toxic effects of these drugs. In HD, blood is removed from a venous catheter or arteriovenous fistula and is pumped through a filter that contains a semipermeable membrane.[37] A dialysate solution is pumped through the filter on the other side of the membrane in the opposite direction. The dialysate is an isotonic sodium chloride solution with calcium, magnesium, potassium, bicarbonate, and dextrose. Modern dialysis machines allow hypertonic concentrations of sodium to be attained that can stabilize the blood pressure in some patients receiving HD who are prone to the development of hypotension across the HD procedure. The countercurrent flow of dialysate to blood increases dialysis efficiency. Solutes such as urea, creatinine, and potassium are cleared by diffusion or convective transport, and, in general, molecular substances with a size less than 5000 Da can be efficiently removed with HD. Excess volume is removed by the application of a pressure gradient across the dialysis membrane. HD removes amino acids and small peptides from the blood, with losses as high as 10 to 13 g per HD session.[38] HD also removes some water-soluble vitamins (such as vitamin C and pyridoxine), minerals (magnesium and phosphorus), and electrolytes. Calcium, potassium, sodium, and bicarbonate concentrations in the dialysate can be adjusted as needed based on the patient's condition. In-center HD is typically administered 3 to 4 hours per day, 3 days per week to provide effective RRT.

Peritoneal Dialysis

PD is useful for the management of CKD.[39,40] Although this form of RRT is quite effective, only 6% of dialysis patients in the United States use PD because of access problems, difficulty complying with the prescription and thus achieving adequate clearance of solute, the potential for peritonitis, and hyperglycemia.[3] PD has the advantage of being relatively "low-tech," portable, and useful for home therapy.[3] The peritoneum acts as a semipermeable membrane where solute and water cross between the blood and peritoneal fluid. Elevated concentrations of urea and other solutes pass from the blood into the dialysate, which is initially free of urea. Potassium, urea, glucose, and other electrolytes pass between the peritoneal capillaries and the dialysate by diffusion based on the concentration gradient.[5] Hypokalemia can occur on occasion because most commercially available solutions do not contain potassium. To prevent or treat hypokalemia, oral supplementation of potassium may be needed, or potassium can be added to the dialysate, usually in amounts ranging from 3 to 5 mEq/L of solution.

Water crosses from the blood to the dialysate as the result of a glucose-mediated osmotic pressure gradient that is provided by using a dextrose-based dialysis solution. Commercially prepared dialysis solutions contain dextrose in concentrations of 1500 to 4250 mg/dL, which is considerably higher than the normal serum glucose of 60 to 110 mg/dL. As water moves from the blood into the peritoneal dialysate, solutes transfer to the peritoneal fluid based on their size and electrical charge. This transfer is termed *convection* or *solvent drag* and is responsible for a large part of the clearance of small molecules from the uremic patient receiving PD.

Although PD is not as efficient as HD per unit of time in removing solutes and water from the body, its application on a continuous basis allows it to be as effective as HD as a chronic therapy. Continuous ambulatory PD is the most commonly used form of PD.[39] Adult patients will typically instill (and drain) 2 to 3 liters of dialysate 4 to 5 times each day, with dwell times of 4 to 6 hours. Another form of PD is continuous cycling PD (CCPD), which uses a cycling machine that automatically fills and drains the patient's abdomen of dialysate, usually during the nighttime while the patient sleeps. The machine is set up with the appropriate amount of peritoneal dialysate, and the patient connects to the dialysate circuit. The cycler warms the peritoneal fluid, measures and delivers the prescribed amount of dialysis fluid, controls the time that the dialysate dwells in the abdomen, and drains the abdomen of dialysate over a preselected time period. CCPD was originally prescribed as a procedure that drained the patient's abdomen at the end of the sleep cycle, leaving no fluid during the daytime; however, many, if not most CCPD patients will leave the last dwell in place during the day; some patients also require a manual exchange of dialysate, as if the patient were on continuous ambulatory PD.

PD can provide a significant glucose load to the patient via the dialysate. The amount absorbed depends on the volume infused, the dwell time, the dialysate dextrose concentration, and the condition of the patient's peritoneal membrane.[40] The energy derived from the dialysate dextrose must be considered when formulating a nutrition care plan. Protein and amino acid losses via PD can be significant and typically range from 5 to 24 g/d.[41] Protein losses can be higher if therapy is complicated by peritonitis. PD is effective in removing electrolytes, trace elements, and vitamins, and it is inefficient at removing medications.

Patients receiving PD can remain ambulatory, provide their own care, and have reduced dietary restrictions because their waste products are constantly filtered. Patients with heart disease experience fewer complications with PD than with HD because fluid shifts with PD are not as rapid as those that occur with HD. Common complaints related to PD include bloating, abdominal fullness, and loss of appetite from the indwelling dialysate.

Continuous Renal Replacement Therapies

CRRT is ideal for patients who are unable to tolerate standard HD.[42,43] Although HD remains the most common form of dialysis used during AKI, CRRT has become the preferred method of dialysis for ICU patients with AKI in many centers. The major advantage of CRRT is the slower rate of solute or fluid removal per unit of time. Thus, CRRT is generally better tolerated than HD therapy because many of the complications of HD are related to the rapid rate of solute and fluid loss. However, CRRT is not a widely available treatment option because it is more labor intensive for the hospital staff, requires regular monitoring of hemodynamic status and fluid balance, involves continuous anticoagulation, and is a more expensive mode of therapy. CRRT involves either diffusion or filtration based treatments that operate in a continuous mode.

Continuous veno-venous hemofiltration (CVVH), continuous veno-venous hemodialysis and continuous veno-venous hemodiafiltration are forms of CRRT currently used for the therapy of unstable ICU patients in the United States. Of these, CVVH is the most commonly used procedure. All of these therapies require a specialized filtration or diafiltration membrane that is highly permeable to fluid, electrolytes, minerals, and certain drugs. Because of this permeability, solutes can be removed by convection. This process can require large volumes of replacement fluid to maintain adequate circulating blood volume. The filters are expensive, and patients require continuous anticoagulation because clotting of the extracorporeal circuit is a frequent occurrence. However, trained ICU staff can maintain the procedure, and the provision of enteral and parenteral feeding solutions is made easier because volume overload and electrolyte imbalances can be easily corrected during the CRRT, thus avoiding common changes that need to be made during intermittent HD, such as fluid and electrolyte restrictions. The decision to use a particular form of CRRT vs HD relies on the experience and comfort of the attending physician and nursing staff with a particular form of RRT. Although CRRT usually runs continually for 24 hours, there are variations of the CRRT that can run for 12 to 14 hours, which might be advantageous for facilities that want to use CRRT during the daytime, when more staff are available.

Sustained low-efficiency dialysis (SLED) is a modified HD treatment that uses low blood flow rates, low dialysate flow rates, and an extended dialysis time (usually 8 to 24 hours). SLED is an emerging technique with multiple advantages: it can achieve adequate solute and volume removal while causing less hemodynamic instability than conventional HD, and it does not require special equipment other than standard HD equipment.[3]

The effectiveness of SLED and CRRT makes it possible to provide nutrition support without the need to restrict protein or fluid to a great degree.[44] Patients with AKI can have increased protein needs because of the associated inflammatory response to the renal failure or other comorbid conditions.[1,45] CRRT allows increased protein to be given to patients.[46] The amount of dialysis delivered to a patient should be designed to remove the metabolic wastes created from catabolism and nutrition support. The nutrition regimen should never be designed to decrease the need for dialysis.

Nutrition Assessment

Depending in part on the method used or the population studied, malnutrition is prevalent in 40% to 70% of patients with ESRD.[47–49] Malnutrition in these patients has been associated with increased mortality and morbidity. In the MDRD Study, the small but significant decreases in some nutrition indices, together with the decrease in protein and energy intake in all patient groups, strongly suggest the need for frequent nutrition monitoring in all renal patients;[50] ideally, nutrition deficiencies should be identified before they become clinically relevant. Periodic nutrition assessment is necessary to determine the appropriateness of the nutrition support regimen and the patient's response to therapy.[27] The standard methods for assessment of nutrition status may be limited in renal failure patients because these parameters may be altered by kidney disease. In addition to the causes of AKI or CKD, any associated complications need to be noted as they may be relevant to the assessment of malnutrition in renal failure patients. Table 29-3 shows the multiple nutrition assessment parameters that have been recommended by the various guideline committees.[27,35,51,52]

Assessment of dietary intake and dietary compliance by a skilled registered dietitian may help determine a patient's total protein and energy intake and provide insight into the distribution of the macronutrient and micronutrient intake.[1,45] However, it important to note that typical dietary assessment methods provide poor estimates of absolute energy intake, and energy estimation equations in the CKD population are of limited validity; therefore, such assessment techniques are unlikely to yield valid information regarding energy balances unless the patient's intake is very poor or excessive.

The validity and reliability of assessing more objective parameters, such as visceral store using serum albumin, are now being challenged. Several studies have demonstrated that a low serum albumin concentration in CKD and dialysis patients is strongly associated with cardiovascular disease and mortality.[53–56] However, when adjusted for inflammatory markers such as C-reactive protein, serum albumin loses it predictive value, showing that inflammation itself is the stronger predictor for poor outcome.[57–59] Besides protein intake, several other factors affect serum albumin levels (inflammation, catabolic and anabolic processes, age, underlying comorbid conditions such as diabetes mellitus, external protein losses, and fluid overload), making serum albumin a nonspecific marker for malnutrition and a poor prognostic indicator.

Nitrogen balance is discussed in detail in Chapter 6. Its application in CKD, especially in patients with ESRD, is limited.

Anthropometry measurements may be influenced multiple factors unrelated to nutrition. Body weight and body mass

TABLE 29-3 Recommended Nutrition Assessment Parameters for Patients with Renal Disease

Guideline Committee (Reference)	Nutrition Assessment Parameters
NKF KDOQI 2000 (45)	Recommended: Dietary interview and/or diary, serum albumin, dry weight, SGA, nPNA. Optional: Prealbumin, midarm muscle circumference, DXA, serum creatinine, creatinine index.
ESPEN 2009 (51)	Consider SGA.
ASPEN 2010 (27)	Consider SGA with serum albumin.
ISRNM 2013 (35)	In CKD: • Screening: Serum albumin, weight, BMI, MIS, DPI, DEI. • Assessment: Serum prealbumin, SGA, anthropometrics.
SCCM/ASPEN 2016 (52)	Assessment in ICU: NUTRIC score or NRS 2002.

ASPEN, American Society for Parenteral and Enteral Nutrition; BMI, body mass index; CKD, chronic kidney disease; DEI, dietary energy intake; DPI, dietary protein intake; DXA, dual-energy x-ray absorptiometry; ESPEN, European Society for Clinical Nutrition and Metabolism; ICU, Intensive care unit; ISRNM, International Society of Renal Nutrition and Metabolism; MIS, malnutrition inflammation score; NKF KDOQI, National Kidney Foundation Kidney Disease Outcomes Quality Initiative; nPNA, normalized protein nitrogen appearance; NRS 2002, Nutrition Risk Screening 2002; NUTRIC, Nutrition Risk in Critically Ill; SCCM, Society of Critical Care Medicine; SGA, Subjective Global Assessment.

index could be affected by increased fluid retention in patients with renal failure; however, changes over time in these 2 parameters may provide valuable information. Midarm muscle circumference, which is used as a surrogate for total body protein and lean body mass, is limited by age, gender, and edema.

Body composition measurements may represent a "gold standard" for evaluating nutrition status, but they are tedious to use on a daily basis and are usually reserved for research purposes. Available technologies are becoming more complex, which allows for greater accuracy in measuring body composition. Body impedance analysis is widely used to assess total body water, intracellular water, and lean body mass, but the results should be interpreted with caution in patients with body water changes. Better results have been obtained with dual-energy x-ray absorptiometry (DXA), especially if serial measurements are required; however, DXA is expensive and is not available for routine clinical practice.

Several nutrition screening and assessment tools are available for use in patients with renal disease. The Subjective Global Assessment (SGA), which scores 7 items in the patient's medical history and 4 items from the clinical findings, is a well-validated tool for screening for malnutrition.[60–62] Although the SGA scores are determined in a subjective manner, it is the only screening tool recommended by all the guideline committees for non-ICU CKD patients (see Table 29-3). Another method, the malnutrition-inflammation score (MIS), was proposed by Kalantar-Zadeh and associates as a nutrition screening tool for HD patients.[63] Using components of the conventional SGA, the MIS is a comprehensive scoring system that has been shown to have significant associations with prospective hospitalization and mortality, as well as measures of nutrition, inflammation, and anemia in HD patients. The MIS may be superior to the conventional SGA, as well as to individual laboratory values, as a predictor of dialysis outcome and an indicator of malnutrition and inflammation in the maintenance HD population.[64] In the critical care setting, the American Society for Parenteral and Enteral Nutrition (ASPEN) and Society of Critical Care Medicine[52] recommend using the Nutrition Risk in Critically Ill (NUTRIC) and Nutrition Risk Screening 2002 (NRS 2002) screening tools.

Nutrition Requirements

Providing adequate energy, protein, and electrolytes to meet the needs of patients with CKD can both minimize the metabolic complications associated with the loss of renal function and retard the progression of renal disease.[21,32,65] Table 29-4 lists the nutrition requirements for adults with CKD or AKI.[16,27,35,66]

Energy

Energy needs for patients with AKI and CKD are similar to those of patients without renal impairment. Typically, energy needs do not increase appreciably with decreased renal function alone.[26] Rather, the physiological stress of associated medical conditions and surgical interventions increases the energy needs of patients with AKI or CKD. For patients with AKI, 20 to 30 kcal/kg/d is recommended, based on KDIGO 2012 guidelines,[66] and the recommendation for dialysis or nondialysis dependent CKD patients is 30 to 35 kcal/kg/d.[35] Conditions such as severe sepsis, respiratory failure, and other hypercatabolic conditions may increase energy requirements to 30 to 45 total kcal/kg/d.[67] It is important to understand that the energy requirements per kilogram of body weight are greatly influenced by body composition because lean body mass uses more energy than fat mass. In summary, energy needs for patients with AKI and CKD are similar to those of patients without renal dysfunction and must be adjusted based on the severity of their illness, comorbid conditions, and type of dialysis.[24,67]

Indirect calorimetry (IC) is recommended for determining energy needs in patients with impaired renal function.[27] As explained in Chapter 2, IC is a noninvasive means for measuring the oxygen consumed compared with the carbon dioxide

TABLE 29-4 Nutrition Recommendations for Adults with Kidney Disease[a]

	Nondialysis CKD	PD	HD	CRRT	AKI
Energy[b,c]	30–35 kcal/kg/d	30–35 kcal/kg/d, including energy from dialysate	30–35 kcal/kg/d	30–35 kcal/kg/d; may need to consider energy from dialysate carbon but that may be offset by CRRT-induced hypothermia	20–30 kcal/kg/d
Protein[b]	0.6–0.8 g/kg/d; 1 g/kg/d in illness[d]	1.2 g/kg/d[d]	>1.2 g/kg/d[d]	≥2.5 g/kg/d in CRRT	0.8–0.1 g/kg/d in noncatabolic AKI without dialysis; 1.0–1.5 g/kg/d in AKI on RRT
Fluid[e]	Oliguric: Usually not restricted unless CHF or hyponatremia; as tolerated	Oliguric: Usually not restricted unless CHF or hyponatremia; as tolerated	Oliguric: Usually not restricted unless CHF or hyponatremia; as tolerated	May have very high needs; monitor closely for fluid balance	Anuric: 1–1.2 L/d Oliguric: Usually not restricted unless CHF or hyponatremia; as tolerated
Sodium	2–2.3 g/d, as tolerated	2–2.3 g/d, as tolerated	2–2.3 g/d, as tolerated	As tolerated	As tolerated
Calcium	1.5 g/d	<2 g/d	<2 g/d	Monitor closely and replete as needed	—
Potassium	<40 mg/kg/d if serum level is elevated	No restriction as hyperkalemia is not usually an issue	<40 mg/kg/d if serum level is elevated	Monitor closely and replete as needed	As tolerated
Phosphate	800–1000 mg/d; use binders if elevated	800–1000 mg/d; use binders if elevated	800–1000 mg/d; use binders if elevated	No restriction needed for CRRT; monitor for hypophosphatemia as CRRT is phosphate depleting	—
Magnesium	DRI[f]	DRI[f]	DRI[f]	Monitor levels closely and replete as needed	DRI[f]
Vitamins	DRI[f]	DRI[f]	DRI[f]	Standard additive	—
Vitamins C	—	75–100 mg/d	75–100 mg/d	—	—
Pyridoxine	—	5 mg/d	—	—	—
Folic acid	—	1 mg/d	1 mg/d	—	—
Vitamin D	Aim for levels similar to general population	Aim for levels similar to general population	Aim for levels similar to general population	Aim for levels similar to general population	Aim for levels similar to general population
Trace elements	DRI	DRI	DRI	Standard additive	—
Iron	Supplement as needed[g]	Supplement as needed[g]	Supplement as needed[g]	Supplement as needed[g]	Supplement as needed[g]

AKI, acute kidney injury; CHF, congestive heart failure; CKD, chronic kidney disease; CRRT, continuous renal replacement therapy; DRI, Dietary Reference Intake; HD, hemodialysis; PD, peritoneal dialysis; RRT, renal replacement therapy.
[a]All recommendations are based on ideal body weight.
[b]Initial needs. Needs are increased with dialysis/stress/hypercatabolic states.
[c]Based on physical activity level. In sedentary adults, recommended energy intake is 30 kcal/kg/d.
[d]>50% of high biological value protein.
[e]Standard needs; may need to be adjusted based on individual needs.
[f]Initially; adjust based on serum levels.
[g]For anemia, follow iron/ferritin status.
Source: Data are from references 16, 27, 35, and 66.

expired and then calculating the patient's resting metabolic rate.[68] Because IC has limited availability and may be expensive, predictive equations are commonly used to calculate energy needs.[68] For either AKI or CKD, energy requirements can also be calculated using the Harris-Benedict equation for resting energy expenditure and an appropriate stress factor.[69] However, more recent studies have shown that a population-specific predictive energy equation may be more useful in CKD and dialysis-dependent patients.[70-72] These findings need to be interpreted with caution and must be validated with further research in a larger CKD patient population. An adjusted body weight should be used for patients who weigh more than 120% of their ideal body weight. Patients with CKD receiving HD or PD may have PEW and may require energy sufficient for weight gain if they are underweight. For optimal management of CKD, dietary modification should be an integral part of patient care. Energy recommendations for obese patients with CKD are complicated and involve creation of an individualized dietary plan with adjustment of overall energy intake to promote weight loss, yet maintain good nutrition status.[73]

Macronutrient distribution and fluid needs must be considered when determining an appropriate PN regimen or choosing an enteral tube feeding formula. Energy requirements are usually met by providing a balanced formula that provides protein (10% to 15% of total energy), carbohydrate (55% to 70% of total energy), and fat (20% to 30% of total energy). Excessive energy from lipids should be avoided to minimize risk of hypertriglyceridemia caused by diminished clearance rates in CKD. Fluid restriction is often necessary when renal failure is associated with oliguria or anuria. When nutrition support is provided via tube feeding, concentrated enteral formulas, which provide 1.5 to 2.0 kcal/mL, are generally preferred.

Energy delivery from RRT must be considered when deciding amounts to provide via enteral and parenteral solutions. PD can provide a significant amount of energy (up to 500 to 1000 kcal/d).[74] Methods that can be used for estimating energy uptake from PD are discussed elsewhere.[75,76] CRRT can also be an indirect source of energy for patients with renal failure. CRRT solutions contain a small amount of glucose, and a substantial glucose load can be delivered with replacement fluids (up to 20 L/d).[44] The energy from the dextrose load should be calculated and included as part of the patient's total energy goal from carbohydrate; in other words, to maintain a stable dextrose intake, the dextrose provided in the PN solution or the enteral nutrition (EN) formula should be decreased to account for the energy from dextrose in the replacement fluid. The amount of glucose transferred across the dialysis membrane can range from 35% to 45% or higher, depending on the dextrose concentration, dialysate flow rate, and the blood glucose concentration.[44] As an example, a 1 L/h dialysate flow at a concentration of 1.5% and a 40% uptake provides about 500 kcal/d, as illustrated in the following equation:[44]

Energy from Dialysate = Flow Rate (L/h) × 24 hours
    × Dextrose Concentration (g/L) × % Uptake
    × 3.4 kcal/g (Energy from Dextrose)
    = 1 L/h × 24 hours × 15 g Dextrose/L × 40%
    × 3.4 kcal/g = 490 kcal/d

Use of dextrose-containing dialysate with a physiological concentration of dextrose (0.1% to 0.15%) or no dextrose may provide a better strategy to reduce energy intake and minimize problems with glucose control.[44]

Patients may experience hyperglycemia or inappropriate weight gain if the energy from glucose received during PD or CRRT is not considered. The energy provided from both the dialysate and replacement fluid should be subtracted from the targets for energy from carbohydrate provided in PN or from EN feedings. Adjusting the EN feeding rate to provide less energy may also decrease the amount of protein supplied; therefore, supplemental protein powder may be needed.

Glucose losses may occur in the ultrafiltrate fluids removed by CRRT.[77] Glucose losses into the dialysate are equivalent to the serum blood glucose concentration against which they are dialyzed.[78] These losses should be calculated because the PN solution dextrose concentrations or EN formula rates may need to be increased to compensate for the loss of the dextrose in the dialysate.

Protein

Low-protein diets (0.6 to 0.8 g/kg) have historically been recommended for patients with impaired renal function to reduce uremic symptoms, slow the progression of renal dysfunction, and obviate or delay the need for dialysis.[21,24,27,33] Although protein restriction can slow the progression of renal dysfunction in some patients with CKD, there is no evidence that these diets provide any benefit in AKI. In fact, patients with AKI should be fed the amount of protein and energy needed by their overall condition. A recent study showed that very-low-protein diets (0.3 mg/kg/d) supplemented with ketoanalogue of amino acid delays the progression of kidney disease when compared with a low-protein diet (0.6 mg/kg/d).[79] This study is interesting, but, at this point, evidence is insufficient to recommend a very-low-protein diet.[80] Patients with kidney disease receiving dialysis need additional protein because of losses that occur through the dialysate.[21,33] Recommended protein requirements for patients receiving HD and PD are greater than 1.2 g/kg/d (Table 29-4).[35] The amounts of amino acids and small peptides lost during CRRT depend on the method used. However, the differences in amounts lost between methods are not significant.[81] Protein requirements for adults receiving CRRT are at least 1 g/kg/d and may be as high as 2.5 g/kg/d because small peptide and amino acid losses can be high.[27,44,69] However, the losses with SLED are minimally increased over those losses from standard HD. In one study, 11 critically patients with AKI treated with CRRT and receiving PN had serum levels of amino acids that were below normal range until protein intake reached 2.5 g/kg/d.[78]

The use of amino acids in AKI is controversial. In 1973, Abel and colleagues conducted the first randomized controlled trial (RCT) of intravenous (IV) essential amino acids (EAA) vs hypertonic glucose in patients with AKI and showed that patients treated with EAA were more likely to recover from AKI. No lethal complications of the EAA solution were reported. The study was limited because it excluded critically ill patients and included only surgical patients with AKI.[29] Subsequent RCTs studying EAA supplementation did not show benefit in terms of nitrogen balance, rate or frequency of AKI recovery, or survival.[82-87] A meta-analysis of 8 studies did not demonstrate a mortality benefit with EAA, as compared with a standard amino acid infusion, in patients with AKI.[88] Therefore, the 2010 ASPEN clinical guidelines for nutrition support in adult acute renal failure recommend using a standard amino acid solution for patients with AKI.[37]

Fluid and Sodium Requirements

Fluid status must be closely monitored in all patients with renal failure. Urine, gastrointestinal (GI), and insensible losses should be considered when determining fluid requirements. Typical adults with normal kidney function require 1200 to 2500 mL/d to maintain fluid balance. The need for fluid restriction often depends on the presence of oliguria or anuria. Patients who are anuric, defined as urine output of less than 50 mL/d, are typically fluid restricted to 1000 to 1200 mL/d, which reflects usual daily insensible water losses.[5] Somewhat larger volumes of fluid may be tolerated in patients with oliguria, which is defined as urine output greater than 50 mL/d but less than 500 mL/d.[5] Concentrated EN or PN solutions are often required to facilitate these restrictions. Concentrated formulas may not be necessary in nonoliguric patients or those receiving RRT.[23,25] Oliguria often leads to a decrease in urine sodium and potassium losses. In general, sodium or water should not be restricted in patients with nonoliguric AKI unless there is evidence of volume overload or hyponatremia. Patients with oliguric AKI will require sodium restriction once normovolemia has been attained. Water should be restricted only for patients with hyponatremia. Occasionally, patients undergoing CRRT or during the diuretic phase of AKI must be given fluid in excess of maintenance needs. Fluid losses can be as high as 20 L/d in CRRT; therefore, fluid replacement is important for fluid balance.[44,77] Fluid therapy adjustments should be determined by daily measurements of intake and output, weight, and serum sodium.

Electrolytes and Minerals

Patients with impaired renal function lose the ability to maintain normal serum concentrations of sodium, potassium, phosphate, and magnesium because of impaired excretion. Before nutrition support is instituted, tissue catabolism typically leads to elevated serum potassium, magnesium, and phosphate concentrations because the intracellular concentrations of these electrolytes are high. Serum levels of potassium, magnesium and phosphate must be closely monitored during nutrition support, and their amounts in enteral and parenteral solutions may need to be limited. If nutrition support occurs in the setting of protein anabolism, concentrations of these electrolytes may decline within the first few days of feeding. The degree of anabolism and catabolism must be considered when determining electrolyte requirements and setting electrolyte doses. In patients who are not severely malnourished or whose feeding has been stabilized, electrolyte requirements are generally low and depend on renal and GI losses. Electrolytes should be adjusted based on the regular measurement of serum levels.[27]

RRT can be effective in clearing potassium, sodium, and magnesium. Potassium content of the HD or PD solutions can be adjusted to maintain normal serum levels. With CRRT, electrolyte clearance may be high, and electrolyte supplementation may be necessary.[67,77] Serum electrolytes should be measured frequently throughout the therapy period and repleted as needed. Hypophosphatemia is a common complication of CRRT because the dialysate does not contain phosphorus. When formulating nutrient solutions (ie, the solution volume, dextrose, and amino acid concentrations, and additive amounts needed), it useful to know the type of RRT used and the amount of fluid removed. Premixed dialysate and replacement fluids are available to meet electrolyte and fluid needs but not mineral needs. Standard vitamin and mineral (trace element) packages should be provided to patients receiving CRRT to meet the Recommended Daily Intake and replace losses in the dialysate.[28,77] Table 29-4 lists the suggested ranges for electrolyte and mineral requirements.

Mineral Bone Disease

In healthy individuals, serum concentrations of phosphorus and calcium are maintained through the interaction of 3 hormones: PTH, 1,25-dihyrdroxyvitamin D (calcitriol; the active metabolite of vitamin D), and FGF23. These hormones act on 3 primary target organs: bone, kidney, and intestine. The kidneys play a critical role in maintaining normal serum calcium and phosphorus concentrations; thus, derangements in mineral metabolism are common in patients with CKD. Abnormalities are initially observed in patients with estimated GFR of less than 60 mL/min/1.73 m^2 and are nearly uniform as the estimated GFR becomes less than 30 mL/min/1.73 m^2. With the progressive development of CKD, the body attempts to maintain normal serum concentrations of calcium and phosphorus with altered production of calcitriol, PTH, and FGF23. Disturbances of mineral metabolism include hyperparathyroidism, phosphate retention, hypocalcemia, and vitamin D deficiency. Life expectancy in patients with CKD is limited by the development of mineral abnormalities and is associated with bone loss, fractures, cardiovascular disease, immune suppression, and increased mortality.

Increased PTH concentrations are generally the first clinically measured abnormality observed in patients with evolving CKD.[89] Increases in PTH concentrations in the early stages of the CKD are an adaptive mechanism to help maintain the serum calcium and phosphorus concentrations in the normal range. In addition to the increase in PTH, there is also an early increase in FGF23 concentrations,[90] as well as a decrease in calcitriol.[89] It is not until the development of CKD stages 4 and 5 that measurable abnormalities of calcium and phosphorus become apparent.[89]

Calcium

There are no data to support an increased risk of mortality or fracture with increasing serum calcium concentrations in patients with CKD stages 3 and 4. However, studies have been done in dialysis patients, with variability in the range at which hypercalcemia becomes significantly associated with increased all-cause mortality.[63,91-94] With regard to hypocalcemia, it is unclear at which level of calcium deficiency the relative risk for mortality increases.[91,92]

In CKD, the total amount of elemental calcium intake should not exceed 2000 mg/d, which includes both nutrition intake and medications (calcium-based binders). Hypercalcemia, as evidenced by a corrected calcium level greater than 10.2 mg/dL for patients with stage 5 CKD, may be treated by several measures, including decrease in total calcium intake (nutrition provision and medication adjustments), decrease or discontinuation of vitamin D preparations, and/or a decrease in calcium dialysate. Serum calcium levels are considered a poor indicator of calcium balance, and patients with advanced CKD can develop a positive calcium balance with consequent vascular and soft tissue calcifications without significant elevations in serum calcium levels. Low calcium levels (less than 8.4 mg/dL) should be corrected in patients exhibiting clinical symptoms of deficiency.[95,96]

Phosphorus

Epidemiologic data suggest that serum phosphorus levels above normal are associated with increased morbidity and mortality in patients with CKD. In patients with CKD stages 2 through 5 who are not undergoing dialysis, higher concentrations of serum phosphorus, even within the normal range, have been associated with increased risk of all-cause or cardiovascular mortality.[97] Multiple studies in patients on dialysis have had similar results, although with slight differences in the degree of hyperphosphatemia at which phosphorus becomes significantly associated with increased mortality.[63,91,92,94] Thus, there are clear epidemiologic data to support that patients with lower serum concentrations of phosphorus do better. Unfortunately, no study has demonstrated that lowering the serum phosphorus concentration to a specific value leads to improved outcomes. A meta-analysis found that the greatest effect of the parameters of mineral metabolism on mortality was phosphorus, followed by PTH.[98] The restriction of phosphorus to 800 to 1200 mg/d is based on either elevated serum phosphorus or plasma intact PTH levels. Further management of elevated serum phosphorus often includes calcium-, noncalcium-, or nonaluminum-based phosphate binders.[95,96] Calcium-based binders include calcium carbonate, calcium acetate, and calcium citrate. These agents are effective at reducing hyperphosphatemia while also being a source of calcium in CKD patients.[99] Calcium citrate should only be used in patients who are not taking or who are not exposed to aluminum salts, including the use of aluminum cookware. Noncalcium, nonaluminum binders, such as sevelamer carbonate, lanthanum carbonate, and newer iron-based binders (eg, succroferric oxyhydroxide, and ferric citrate), are also effective and are used in adults when there is a concern for soft tissue calcification.[99]

An important consideration regarding strategies to improve dietary protein intake in ESRD patients is the potential increase of phosphorus intake. Although strictly limiting dietary phosphorus intake may indirectly lead to increased risk for PEW, unrestricted protein intake will undoubtedly increase phosphorus load. Epidemiologic data indicate that a combination of decreased serum phosphorus and increased protein intake had the best outcomes in HD patients, whereas a combination of low serum phosphorus and protein intake had the worst outcomes. Therefore, dietary recommendations to improve protein intake should take into account the phosphorus content of the specific protein sources and other phosphorus-containing nutrients. Another important source of dietary phosphorus is the phosphorus contained in additives and preservatives from processed food.[1,45] Also, the use of phosphate binders with meals reduces the severity of hyperphosphatemia, which facilitates the use of more dietary protein.[100] In that context, a small RCT indicated that the source of protein (ie, vegetarian diet leading lower serum phosphorus levels) has a significant effect on phosphorus homeostasis in patients with CKD.[37] This finding is likely related to the fact that the phosphorus from animal protein is better absorbed than the phosphorus from plant proteins.

Vitamin D

Vitamin D deficiency in patients with CKD has generally been defined as having calcidiol (25-hydroxyvitamin D) levels of less than 30 ng/mL.[101] Several other investigators have found widespread vitamin D insufficiency in CKD, although not all investigators have identified a relationship with CKD stage.[89,102-104] Vitamin D deficiency in patients with CKD stages 3 and 4 is associated with increased PTH.[103-105] Vitamin D deficiency has also been associated with mortality in incident dialysis patients,[106] and increased cardiovascular events in patients receiving PD.[107] These data have led KDIGO[12] to recommend that calcidiol levels be measured but conclude that there are insufficient data to suggest an optimal level in CKD patients; however, KDIGO notes that there is also no reason to assume that CKD patients would require different levels for nonendocrine effects of calcidiol. Furthermore, there is a lack of definitive studies demonstrating that treatment with vitamin D leads to improvement in secondary hyperparathyroidism or other diseases common in patients with CKD.

Regulation of mineral metabolism is predominately related to circulating calcitriol (activated vitamin D) levels, which mediate cellular function via both nongenomic and genomic mechanisms. Calcitriol facilitates the uptake of calcium in intestinal and renal epithelium, directly suppresses PTH synthesis,[108,109] and is important for normal bone turnover.[110,111] The predominant source of the circulating calcitriol concentrations is from activation of calcidiol in the kidney by PTH, whereas FGF23 inhibits the activation. Other factors that are involved in the regulation of calcitriol include low calcium and low phosphorus.[112] Elevated serum levels of PTH raise serum calcitriol levels, which results in a rise in serum calcium; then, calcitriol feeds back on the parathyroid gland, decreasing PTH secretion, thus completing the typical endocrine feedback loop. As CKD progresses, calcitriol production progressively decreases.[89]

Parathyroid Hormone

PTH has long been considered a surrogate marker for bone disease, and the ability to predict low and high turnover bone disease was the rationale for the target range of 150 to 300 pg/mL in the Kidney Disease Outcomes Quality Initiative guidelines for CKD stage 5D.[101] However, the assay used for those analyses is no longer available, and subsequent studies have demonstrated that PTH levels within a range of 150 to 300 pg/mL are not predictive of underlying bone histology.[113] Similar to other biochemical measures of mineral bone disease in CKD, observational studies have found an association of all-cause mortality with various levels of PTH, with concentrations greater than 600 pg/mL being associated with increased mortality.[93,94,114] One study showed an increased risk of all-cause mortality with PTH concentrations approaching 400 pg/mL.[63] Based on these observational data, and limitations associated with various PTH assays, the KDIGO guidelines suggest that target PTH concentrations be assay-specific and should range between 2 and 9 times the upper limit of normal for the PTH assay being utilized. The recommendations also advise clinicians to interpret values within that range by evaluating trends and intervene if the trends are going up or down.[12] However, no RCTs have tested the hypothesis that treatment to achieve specific PTH targets results in improved outcomes.

Changes in ionized calcium are the immediate signal for the parathyroid gland to secrete PTH. The PTH-calcium relationship is very tightly regulated, such that a very small decrease in the serum ionized calcium concentration will cause a maximal PTH secretion and vice versa.[115] The parathyroid gland is able to sense changes in the ionized serum calcium concentration via the activity of the calcium-sensing receptor,[116] which directly inhibits PTH secretion. PTH maintains normal serum calcium concentrations through both direct and indirect actions. PTH directly increases serum calcium via increasing bone resorption and increasing renal tubular calcium absorption. PTH indirectly increases serum calcium by increasing renal synthesis of calcitriol, which is responsible for absorption of calcium from the GI tract.

Fibroblast Growth Factor 23

FGF23 is a phosphate-regulating hormone that is secreted by bone cells. Both PTH and FGF23 inhibit renal tubular phosphate reabsorption. In the setting of residual kidney function, the actions of both PTH and FGF23 maintain phosphorus balance by increasing excretion of phosphorus. With progressive loss of kidney function, these hormones no longer significantly affect renal phosphorus excretion. In this situation, increased levels of PTH may now have a negative effect on phosphorus balance because elevated concentrations of PTH lead to increased bone resorption, and thus increase serum phosphorus levels by moving it out of the bone mineral. As renal dysfunction worsens, FGF23 levels continue to rise progressively.

The 2009 KDIGO guideline[12] and the 2010 KDIGO commentary[117] agree that the control of calcium, phosphorus, low vitamin D, and PTH is central to the management of secondary hyperparathyroidism. A retrospective study showed that being out of target for any of these parameters is associated with an increased risk of mortality. Furthermore, when more parameters are out of control, the associated risk for mortality is higher.[118]

Acid-Base Balance

Acidosis occurs in AKI and CKD because of loss of normal acid excretion or loss of bicarbonate.[23] Under normal circumstances, the body generates 1 mEq of acid per kg of body weight each day as a result of the metabolism of a normal diet. Inflammation with its associated catabolism coupled with an excessive dietary protein intake may lead to the development of metabolic acidosis in patients with advanced CKD. This metabolic acidosis can lead to further protein breakdown, bone reabsorption, and a decrease in the responsiveness of adrenergic beta-receptors. Bicarbonate therapy is recommended for patients with CKD with a serum bicarbonate less than 22 mEq/L or in acutely ill patients with a bicarbonate less than 10 to 15 mEq/L.[119]

Sodium bicarbonate can be given intravenously when the enteral route is not available. When using a bicarbonate infusion for severe metabolic acidosis, close attention should be paid to serum potassium and calcium levels. Potassium levels can drop because or cell shifts, and ionized calcium levels decrease because of excess binding of calcium to albumin. Bicarbonate forms an insoluble precipitate with calcium in PN solutions. Acetate is an acceptable salt to be used with PN solutions. A dialysate with a 40 mEq/L bicarbonate concentration is frequently used for HD. Oral citrate should be used with caution in patients with CKD and ESRD because it can markedly increase GI aluminum absorption and cause aluminum toxicity.[5]

Vitamins

Vitamin requirements are not well established for patients with AKI or CKD.[25] Generally, vitamins are supplemented in amounts that provide the Dietary Reference Intake (DRI). Supplementation of water-soluble vitamins is recommended for all dialysis patients.[67,69] Supplementation of other vitamins may also be occasionally required, depending on the patient's clinical condition and RRT use (see Table 29-4).

Water-Soluble Vitamins

The exact requirements for water-soluble vitamins in renal failure are unknown. The DRI amounts for healthy people are recommended for CKD and ESRD. The clearance of the water-soluble vitamins is increased with RRT. Requirements for these vitamins are met when adequate amounts of enteral tube feeding are given and with standard parenteral multiple vitamin preparations. A water-soluble vitamin supplement should be given to patients on renal-restricted diets. Patients receiving dialysis may also need supplements of other vitamins because of nutrient loss in the dialysate in combination with poor intake and altered metabolism. Vitamin requirements for patients receiving CRRT tend to mirror those of HD patients.

Vitamin C losses may be significant in both HD and PD.[120,121] Vitamin C at doses of 100 mg/d have been recommended for adults receiving RRT.[122,123] However, doses greater than 200 mg/d have led to elevated blood oxalate levels, which can result in deposition of oxalate in the heart, kidney, and blood vessels, and precipitate acute pseudogout.[67,123]

Some authors recommend folate supplementation because serum folate levels have been found to be low in patients with CKD receiving HD or PD, and the concentration of folate in HD and PD dialysis effluent has been found to be high. However, actual tissue levels may not be low because normal concentrations have been found in white and red blood cells.[124] Therefore, the need to supplement folic acid has remained controversial in renal disease. The elderly patient with AKI is at higher risk for folate deficiency.[24] If a patient's folate is assessed, it should be measured as red blood cell folate, which is more representative of body stores.

Pyridoxine (B$_6$) has been studied extensively in HD. Normal levels have been reported in granulocytes and serum, but reduced enzyme activity suggests a functional deficiency.[125] Patients receiving PD have also been shown to have reduced enzyme activity. In addition, reduced pyridoxine activity can lead to increased oxalate formation.[126] Pyridoxine supplementation of 5 mg/d or 50 mg 3 times a week has been advised in patients receiving PD, but this recommendation remains controversial. Elderly patients with AKI are at higher risk for a pyridoxine deficiency.[24]

Patients receiving HD may be deficient in thiamin; however, supplementation does not seem to improve enzyme activity in these patients. Thiamin losses have been reported in patients receiving PD.[127] Supplementation of riboflavin (B$_2$), biotin, niacin (B$_3$), and pantothenic acid does not seem necessary for patients receiving HD, because these vitamins are not cleared by HD.[127] Similar data on these vitamins are not available for PD.

Fat-Soluble Vitamins

Fat-soluble vitamin excesses or deficiencies should not pose a problem during AKI because of the short-term nature of this illness. Therefore, DRI guidelines should be followed for AKI. Standard enteral formulas and parenteral multiple vitamin preparations are adequate for most patients with AKI and CKD.[28] Patients receiving PN should be given vitamin K in sufficient amounts each week, as would be done for any other patient receiving PN.[19] Vitamin A levels are not typically monitored in patients with CKD.[69] Supplements should not be provided if RRT is not used because excessive amounts of vitamin A can lead to toxicity.[69] If signs of hypervitaminosis A, such as visual disturbances, abnormal liver function tests, irritability, and fatigue occur, vitamin A supplements may need to be withheld.[24]

Trace Elements

Trace mineral requirements in patients with renal impairment are not well established.[25] Some trace elements (zinc, selenium, chromium, and iodine) are normally excreted by the kidneys.[128] Excess accumulation of trace elements is unlikely because losses also occur through the GI tract.[129] Commercially prepared enteral formulas and parenteral trace element solutions are generally well tolerated because they provide normal amounts of these substances. Because trace elements are protein-bound, one would imagine that supplementation would not be required in RRT; however, this supposition does

not seem to be valid.[130] Of interest is the application of inductively coupled plasma-mass spectrometry techniques in evaluations of copper, selenium, zinc, manganese, and nickel in a large group of patients receiving HD and age-matched controls.[131] Patients receiving HD were found to have significantly lower concentrations of selenium, zinc, and manganese and significantly higher concentrations of nickel when compared with controls. Further research employing these techniques may give insight on trace element imbalances and clinical monitoring needs.

Zinc

Low serum zinc levels have been demonstrated in patients receiving PD.[129] Low zinc levels are most likely the result of compartmental shifts from plasma to the intracellular space. Although patients with symptomatic zinc deficiency have reported improved taste acuity and improved appetite following supplementation, more information is required before routine zinc supplementation can be recommended prophylactically for all patients receiving PD.[24]

Aluminum

Aluminum toxicity can occur in patients with CKD stage 4 or stage 5, with or without RRT.[24,95] Aluminum excess can lead to osteodystrophy, anemia, and encephalopathy. The best method for management of aluminum excess is to restrict its intake. Toxicity has become a less common problem since dialysate solutions are now commercially prepared with water devoid of aluminum, and PN solutions do not contain protein hydrolysates. Furthermore, aluminum-based phosphate binders have been replaced with calcium- and noncalcium-based binders. One potential venue for aluminum accumulation is the use of parenteral vitamin preparations. Prudence in product selection and proper plasma monitoring of aluminum levels may be warranted.

The diagnosis of aluminum toxicity is based on the baseline serum aluminum levels followed by deferoxamine-stimulated serum aluminum level. The test is considered positive if the serum aluminum levels increase by more than 50 mcg/L. If the initial serum aluminum level is greater than 200 mcg/L, a deferoxamine stimulation test should not be performed because the stimulation can cause fatal neurotoxicity.[95] Treatment of aluminum toxicity involves stopping all the aluminum-containing drugs and HD 6 times per week for 4 to 6 weeks until the aluminum level drops below 200 mcg/L; if levels do not improve, IV desferoxamine may be needed.

Iron

Many patients with CKD and ESRD have iron deficiency anemia because of decreased red blood cell survival, GI blood loss from angiodysplasia, bone marrow toxicity caused by elevated serum PTH levels, diminished oral intake, and losses through repeated laboratory testing of blood (such losses may range from 30 to 90 mL per month). Inflammation is also an important factor associated with anemia in CKD, as inflammatory markers affect iron metabolism and, indirectly, hemoglobin levels.[132] Iron status should be assessed by measuring serum iron, TIBC, iron saturation, and ferritin.[133,134] Ferritin levels must be interpreted with caution because many patients have chronic low-grade inflammation, which can cause elevated ferritin values independent of iron status.[134,135] Serum transferrin is less reliable in patients with CKD because of metabolic abnormalities, such as malnutrition and altered protein metabolism, seen with renal failure.[136] In patients with ESRD, iron dosing should be sufficient to maintain adequate ferritin and iron saturation.[135,136] Iron is necessary to ensure the effectiveness of EPO, a hormone given to patients with CKD to improve red cell production and reduce anemia.[134,135] Iron supplementation is recommended if serum ferritin levels are less than 100 ng/dL. The goal of therapy is a serum ferritin level greater than 100 ng/dL and a TSAT greater than 20%.[137] EPO will be ineffective with a serum ferritin level less than 100 ng/dL and a TSAT less than 20%. For CKD patients with anemia who are not on iron or erythropoietin-stimulating agent (ESA) therapy, a trial of IV iron for 1 to 3 months should be tried if TSAT is less than 30% and ferritin is less than 500 ng/mL, to assess for an increase in hemoglobin prior to starting ESA.[66] Iron should be held if serum ferritin levels exceed 500 ng/mL. Excess iron could worsen sepsis by potentiating the growth of certain bacteria and inhibiting neutrophil phagocytic activity. The goal of iron therapy in adults is to maintain the serum hemoglobin at 10 to 11 g/dL.[136,137]

HD may significantly affect iron status because of the blood loss in the dialyzer circuit and catheter, anticoagulant-related blood loss, and increased fragility of the red blood cells.[136,138] Patients with ESRD receiving PD may also require supplemental iron, although iron does not seem to be lost in the PD dialysate.[134,136] Oral iron is generally preferred, if tolerated, because of the potential complications associated with IV iron. Iron sulfate and other iron salts are available as tablets or as a liquid for oral/enteral therapy. However, ESRD patients frequently receive calcium salts, phosphate binders, proton pump inhibitors, and other medications that might impair iron absorption. If EPO is being used, oral iron usually cannot replete and maintain the body's iron stores in patients with CKD who are receiving HD.[137,138] Iron can be given parenterally, and that is the most commonly applied form in chronic HD patients. IV iron dextran has the potential for inciting an anaphylaxis. Therefore, a test dose must always be given before regular dosing begins.[136] Newer forms of IV iron, such as iron sucrose and sodium ferric gluconate complex, are associated with less risk of life-threatening adverse reactions such as hypotension and anaphylaxis. Injectable iron can be given during HD 3 times a week, typically intravenously, at varying intervals.[134] Iron may need to be withheld when sepsis is suspected or documented because of its potential detrimental effect on the control of infection.[129,136]

Carnitine

Serum carnitine levels may be reduced in dialysis because carnitine seems to be lost in HD and PD.[67,139] Carnitine deficiency can lead to intradialytic hypotension, cardiomyopathy, skeletal muscle weakness, and anemia.[140] The mechanism by which carnitine deficiency contributes to anemia or hyporesponsiveness to EPO is unknown. Patients with CKD who are receiving dialysis have shown improved exercise tolerance and well-being with carnitine supplementation.[141] Oral carnitine is not recommended for EPO-treated patients with CKD who are receiving dialysis because of its limited bioavailability and lack of demonstrated efficacy.[138,142] Although carnitine supplementation seems to be safe, there is no strong evidence that supplementation of carnitine in dialysis patient improves muscle wasting, cardiomyopathy, exercise capacity, or intradialytic symptoms. Currently, there is insufficient evidence for the use of carnitine in dialysis patients.

Nutrition Therapy

Oral Diets

A typical diet for a patient with CKD not receiving RRT restricts protein and phosphorus and may restrict sodium and potassium.[32] Restricted intake of meat, dairy, and egg products reduces protein, acid, and phosphorus intake. Phosphorus in oral diets for adults with CKD not receiving dialysis should be restricted to 800 to 1200 mg/d. Potassium restriction includes limiting high-potassium fruits, fruit juices, and vegetables. Processed foods tend to be high in sodium, potassium, and phosphorus; therefore, restricting processed food is a potential target for avoiding these nutrients. Fluid restriction should be based on weight changes, fluid status, and urine output. In patients with CKD, protein intake is initially limited to 0.6 to 0.8 g/kg/d.[32] Intense nutrition intervention early in CKD reduces the risk of diabetes, hypertension, anemia, and dyslipidemias, and may delay the progression of renal dysfunction in some patients.[32]

Enteral Nutrition

Standard enteral formulas tend to deliver a substantial amount of fluid, electrolytes, and phosphorus. Disease-specific renal enteral formulas for CKD patients are concentrated to reduce volume and have lower potassium, phosphorus, and sodium concentrations (see Chapter 11). Maintenance HD patients with albumin levels equal to or less than 3.5 g/dL who received monitored intradialytic oral nutritional supplements showed survival and lower hospitalizations compared with similar, matched patient controls.[143,144] It should be noted that these studies did not compare supplements to real food. See Chapter 10 for a detailed discussion of indications for EN.

Formulas designed for patients with CKD not on dialysis are usually not necessary for patients with CRRT because the large volume of fluid and electrolytes removed by CRRT reduces the need for fluid restriction and increases the need for increased electrolyte supplementation. Because of the hypercatabolism seen with AKI, standard formulas may be a better option unless the patient is fluid restricted. Practice Scenario 29-1 discusses EN use in a malnourished patient receiving chronic HD.

Practice Scenario 29-1

Question: What is the best approach to nutrition support in a hospitalized malnourished patient receiving hemodialysis (HD)?

Scenario: MR is a 66-year-old woman who has been admitted with a diagnosis of a left lower lobe pneumonia and acute respiratory failure with hypoxemia. She has been receiving HD for 6 years. In the last 9 months, she has had multiple episodes of vascular access stenosis and clotting, which has resulted in the placement of central HD catheters while her vascular access has been revised. She has had 4 bacteremic episodes requiring intravenous antibiotics and has had recurring *Clostridium difficile* enterocolitis during this time. She has lost 10.2 kg of body weight and now weighs 60 kg. Her last 3 monthly urea reduction ratios have been 55%, 50%, and 57% (adequate dialysis urea reduction ratio is greater than 65%). The renal dietitian has documented inadequate energy and protein intake for the last 2 months. MR's serum albumin has fallen from 3.5 g/dL 3 months ago to 2.2 g/dL today, indicating an underlying inflammatory state. Her daily oral intake over the last month has been 1 can of Glucerna, part of a tuna sandwich, and some cookies. Physical examination shows loss of temporal, masseter, and interosseous muscles. She has little subcutaneous fat. She has an infected arteriovenous graft in the right upper arm and a left subclavian HD catheter. Her abdomen is soft with good bowel sounds. Her laboratory test results include blood urea nitrogen, 118 mg/dL; creatinine, 3.4 mg/dL; calcium, 7.8 mg/dL; potassium, 3.2 mEq/L; and phosphorus, 3.2 mg/dL. Her white blood cell count is elevated with a left shift, and blood cultures are positive at 12 hours for gram-positive cocci in pairs. She is placed on broad spectrum antibiotics. She is also committed to daily HD that represents a 25% increase over her outpatient procedures.

Intervention: The patient is started on a standard enteral formula via nasoenteric feeding tube with precautions taken to prevent refeeding syndrome.

Answer and Rationale: The patient has been malnourished for the past 3 months. The malnutrition is a complication of chronic underdialysis and recurrent inflammatory illness from vascular access thrombosis, infection, and repeated surgeries. It is unlikely that diet stimulants will work or that she will take adequate oral supplements. Intradialytic parenteral nutrition and parenteral nutrition are not indicated because MR has a functional gastrointestinal tract. An enteral tube should be placed as soon as her respiratory status is stabilized. Because she will receive daily dialysis, a concentrated feeding solution is not needed. The patient is at high risk of the refeeding syndrome and the use of a "renal" formula is not indicated. Her protein requirements are 1.2 g/kg/d or greater, with more than 50% of this protein being of high biological value; her total energy requirement is in the range of 30 to 35 kcal/kg/d.

Because refeeding syndrome is likely, the enteral feeding should be started at a slow rate and increased every 12 hours until the goal rate is reached. Laboratory test data on electrolyte levels, including phosphorus and calcium, should be obtained after the enteral feeding is initiated, and electrolyte levels should

be measured frequently thereafter. Before the enteral feeding is begun, the patient should receive enteral thiamin because her intake predisposes her to thiamin deficiency. She should also receive oral renal multivitamins. After stabilization of her medical, dialysis, and nutrition status, the enteral feeding should be changed to a nocturnal or postprandial regimen, and oral intake should be encouraged. Her diet should be liberalized to a totally select diet. She will require nutrition support for several weeks.

Parenteral Nutrition

If nutrition requirements cannot fully be met with EN or if the GI tract is nonfunctional, then PN should be used.[67] Fluid restriction requires concentration of the admixture and restriction of sodium chloride. IV lipid emulsion is commonly used daily to meet the patient's energy needs while controlling the amount of fluid administered. Patients receiving HD are fluid restricted, but CRRT may allow liberalization of the fluid restriction and can simplify the PN formula. Overall intake and output, weight changes, and renal function should be assessed daily and fluids adjusted accordingly. Electrolytes should be adjusted based on the severity of renal failure, status of RRT, and other medical conditions.[24,67] Water-soluble vitamins should be given, but fat-soluble vitamins other than vitamin K should be restricted in short-term PN (less than 8 weeks). Trace element supplementation is not needed in patients with AKI who receive blood products or in those in whom oral intake is restricted less than 2 weeks. If needed, a trace element solution should be given once every 1 to 2 weeks. There are no data to guide this recommendation, and each center may have its own supplementation guidelines. Specifically, selenium deficiency is to be avoided. Chromium, manganese, and copper deficiency are quite unlikely to occur in short-term PN (less than 6 to 8 weeks) unless the patient remains hypercatabolic for an extended period of time (eg, burn patient with multiple debridements and grafts). See Practice Scenario 29-2 for an example of PN administration for a patient with AKI.[35,40]

Practice Scenario 29-2

Question: How do you formulate a parenteral nutrition (PN) solution for a hospitalized patient with nonoliguric acute kidney injury (AKI) who is not going to be starting renal replacement therapy (RRT)?

Scenario: A 67-year-old man recently underwent repair of an abdominal aortic aneurysm. He was admitted to the hospital 2 days before surgery with intense abdominal pain that was unrelated to meals or physical activity. On postoperative Day 4, he developed respiratory failure and required intubation for mechanical ventilation and intravenous vasopressor support. On postoperative Day 5, his urine output rapidly declined, and he became oliguric (making less than 500 mL of urine in 24 hours) with a continued increase in the serum creatinine. The nutrition support team was consulted. He was eating normally until 2 days before his admission, and he had little intake postoperatively. His height was 175.3 cm and he weighed 79.3 kg (usual weight, 75 kg; ideal weight, 72 kg). On postoperative Day 6, his abdomen was distended and tympanic to percussion, and bowel sounds were not audible on auscultation. An abdominal x-ray showed dilated loops of small and large bowel with air-fluid levels in the small bowel. Laboratory values were as follows: potassium, 5.2 mEq/L; blood urea nitrogen (BUN), 38 mg/dL; creatinine, 4.6 mg/dL (baseline, 1.0 mg/dL); and albumin, 2.3 g/dL. Other laboratory values were normal. The patient remained on nil per os (nothing by mouth) orders.

Intervention: This patient was started on PN. The PN was fluid restricted and supplemented as appropriate for a patient who would not be immediately started on dialysis.

Answer: PN was indicated because of presumed small bowel obstruction. Volume should be restricted in a PN solution for a patient in AKI who is not receiving dialysis. Generally, a concentrated admixture should be used. The volume to be given must account for ongoing fluid loss (urine output, nasogastric output, and insensible fluid losses) and subtract for intravenous medications, drips, and antibiotics. The total energy provided should be in the range of 20 to 30 kcal/kg/d (approximately 2000 kcal/d) with total protein of 0.8 to 1 g/kg/d (approximately 72 g/d). Standard amino acids should be provided.

When PN is started, it should provide half of the estimated energy needs on the first day to assess the patient's tolerance to the dextrose load and reduce shifts in electrolytes and minerals related to refeeding syndrome. The initial prescription for this patient was 40 g of amino acids, 1000 kcal with 70% of the nonprotein energy as dextrose and 30% as lipid. Electrolytes should be provided based on the serum concentrations. If the serum sodium concentration is normal and patient is euvolemic, it is appropriate to add sodium chloride sufficient to mimic 0.45% saline solution (roughly 70 to 77 mEq/L). Reduced amounts of phosphorus and magnesium should be provided because of the elevated creatinine unless the patient is hypophosphatemic or hypomagnesemic. As this patient had no intake for more than 8 days, he was at risk for refeeding syndrome with hypophosphatemia and hypokalemia. In general, provision of phosphorus at 10 mM per 1000 kcal delivered is sufficient to begin PN. Again, phosphorus concentrations should be monitored daily, especially if refeeding syndrome is a concern.

Potassium should be routinely checked after the start of PN. Although the patient has mild hyperkalemia, potassium should not be held. Potassium should be administered at 10 to 20 mEq per 1000 kcal supplied. In this case, it would be prudent to start with 5 mEq per 1000 kcal and to measure the potassium concentration 6 to 8 hours after starting the PN and increase as needed, especially if refeeding syndrome is a concern. The PN regimen should include 10 mL/d standard multivitamin injection/week. Trace elements should be provided if the patient has been on PN for more than 2 weeks. Serum glucose, electrolytes, calcium, phosphorus, and magnesium should be monitored closely. If the patient is hyperglycemic, regular insulin should be added to the PN and increased daily as needed. In general, 6 to 10 units of insulin per 1000 kcal delivered represents a safe starting point for the addition of insulin. (See Chapter 34 for additional discussion of insulin use in nutrition support.)

Rationale: This patient would benefit from nutrition support because he did not have any nutrition for more than 8 days. Patients with severe injury without adequate oral intake for 5 to 7 days should receive either enteral nutrition or PN. In this particular case, PN would be the best method of nutrition support because the patient has a nonfunctional gastrointestinal tract. The physicians decided that RRT was not required at that time because the patient's BUN was well below 100 mg/dL, fluid accumulation was mild with an increase in weight of only 4.3 kg since admission, and electrolyte abnormalities were only slight. Therefore, PN was planned without dialysis. The need to restrict fluid is based on assessment of a patient's fluid status. In this case, the patient's weight was increased from his preoperative weight because of accumulation of fluids administered during surgery and fluid retention from AKI. His preoperative dry weight should be used to calculate estimated protein and energy requirements. His estimated energy requirements would be based on the standard of the Harris-Benedict equation, which predicts the basal energy requirement of 1200 kcal.[40] The activity factor would be 1.1, which is used for a hospitalized patient unless the patient is very active. When determining the stress factor to use with the equation, the underlying medical condition—not the AKI—is the primary consideration. Using a stress factor of 1 to 1.3, the estimated total energy expenditure is 1300 to 1700 kcal/d. This estimate is consistent with the International Society of Renal Nutrition and Metabolism recommendation of 20 to 30 kcal/kg/d.[35] For patients with AKI who do not need dialysis, 0.8 to 1 g of protein initially is recommended. This patient would need his full requirement (1.5 to 1.8 g/kg) but might need to be tapered up to that amount, based on tolerance. As the patient stabilizes, the protein provided should be increased as tolerated and, hopefully, as renal function returns. Starting PN at half of the estimated energy requirement facilitates evaluation of tolerance to the dextrose load. The initial prescription for this patient was 40 g amino acids and 1000 kcal, with 70% of the nonprotein energy as dextrose and 30% as lipid. Electrolytes should be provided based on the electrolyte serum levels and current renal function. Additives should include sodium and calcium as needed. Typically, in renal dysfunction, reduced amounts of potassium, phosphorus, and magnesium would be provided. The amounts of electrolytes administered should be adjusted in response to changes in serum creatinine, renal function, and the amount of losses. In this patient, potassium supplementation was held because of the increased serum level. As the potassium level drops in response to utilization, anabolism, and improving renal function, additional potassium will be needed. A standard AKI PN regimen could include a standard multivitamin injection of 10 mL/d and standard trace element package daily to meet basic needs. The patient's needs allowed only specific water-soluble vitamins to be given, and trace elements were held. If the patient were being dialyzed, then additional protein and supplements might be required.

Intradialytic Parenteral Nutrition

Intradialytic PN (IDPN) has been used for malnourished patients with inadequate oral intake when oral/enteral supplementation was ineffective and standard PN was not indicated.[145] The goal of IDPN is to provide additional energy and protein to the malnourished patient receiving HD during dialysis; the volume of IDPN administered can be removed immediately by increasing the ultrafiltration rate during the dialysis procedure.[146] The volume of IDPN solutions typically ranges from approximately 350 to 1000 mL per dialysis treatment.[146-148]

IDPN solutions are comprised of dextrose, amino acids, and lipid emulsion.[146-148] Optimal composition of IDPN solutions has not been defined. An IDPN solution generally provides approximately 300 to 1200 kcal and 1.2 to 1.4 g of protein per kg per HD treatment.[146-148] The delivery of increased protein will necessitate changes to ensure dialysis adequacy. Acidosis because of increased protein 88 provision may occur and should be corrected if observed. Glucose monitoring before, during, and after IDPN is necessary, and the addition of short-acting insulin during therapy may be necessary. The energy from protein and lipid generally prevents post-IDPN hypoglycemia as long as large amounts of exogenous insulin are avoided. Lipids are used to provide an increase in energy intake with minimal effect on volume delivery and hyperglycemia. Although there is concern lipid delivery in dialysis patients may have adverse effects related to preexisting hyperlipidemia, possible carnitine deficiency, and possible free fatty acid toxicity, these problems have not been reported and do not seem to occur. Clinical and physical monitoring is necessary for identification and correction of electrolyte and fluid imbalance.[149]

Most information on the efficacy of IDPN is from small studies or anecdotal reports.[148,150] Some studies have demonstrated improved protein synthesis, reduced proteolysis, and improved energy metabolism, as well as increased serum albumin and weight gain.[146-148] Nutrition improvements in one study did not extend to patients with behavioral health issues that involved poor nutrition intake.[139] IDPN is not recommended for routine use at this time. It is an expensive therapy with multiple risks, and it has not clearly been shown to be associated with improved quality of life or survival.

References

1. Fouque D, Kalantar-Zadeh K, Kopple J, et al. A proposed nomenclature and diagnostic criteria for protein-energy wasting in acute and chronic kidney disease. *Kidney Int.* 2008;73:391–398.
2. Cheu C, Pearson J, Dahlerus C, et al. Association between oral nutritional supplementation and clinical outcomes among patients with ESRD. *Clin J Am Soc Nephrol.* 2013;8(1):100–107. doi:10.2215/CJN.13091211.
3. Brady HR, Clarkson MR, Lieberthal W. Acute kidney injury. In: Brenner BM, ed. *The Kidney.* 8th ed. New York; 2007:1215–1292.
4. Formation of urine by the kidney. In: Guyton A, ed. *Basic Human Physiology.* Philadelphia, PA: Saunders; 1971:271–287.
5. Elderstein LER, Schrier RW. Acute kidney injury. In: Schrier RW, ed. *Renal and Electrolyte Disorders.* 6th ed. Philadelphia, PA: 2004:401–455.
6. Traynor J, Mactier R, Geddes CC, Fox JG. How to measure renal function in clinical practice. *BMJ.* 2006;333(7571):733–737.
7. Levey AS, Stevens LA, Schmid CH, et al. A new equation to estimate glomerular filtration rate. *Ann Intern Med.* 2009;150(9):604–612.
8. Levey AS, Coresh J, Greene T, et al. Expressing the Modification of Diet in Renal Disease Study equation for estimating glomerular filtration rate with standardized serum creatinine values. *Clin Chem.* 2007;53(4):766–772.
9. Cockcroft DW, Gault MH. Prediction of creatinine clearance from serum creatinine. *Nephron.* 1976;16:31–41.
10. Earley A, Miskulin D, Lamb EJ, Levey AS, Uhlig K. Estimating equations for glomerular filtration rate in the era of creatinine standardization: systematic review. *Ann Intern Med.* 2012; 156(11):785–795.
11. Chronic Kidney Disease Epidemiology Collaboration. Creatinine based equations. http://ckdepi.org/equations/creatinine-based-equations. Accessed April 14, 2017.
12. Kidney Disease: Improving Global Outcomes (KDIGO) CKD-MBD Work Group. KDIGO clinical practice guideline for the diagnosis, evaluation, prevention, and treatment of chronic kidney disease–mineral and bone disorder (CKD-MBD). *Kidney Int Suppl.* 2009;(113):S1–S130. doi:10.1038/ki.2009.188.
13. Strejc JM. Considerations in the nutritional management of patients with acute kidney injury. *Hemodial Int.* 2005;9:135–142.
14. Bellomo R, Ronco C, Kellum JA, et al. Acute kidney injury: definition, outcome, measures, animal models, fluid therapy and information technology needs: the Second International Consensus Conference of the Acute Dialysis Quality Initiative (ADQI) Group. *Crit Care.* 2004;8:R204.
15. Kidney Disease: Improving Global Outcomes (KDIGO). KDIGO clinical practice guideline for acute kidney injury. *Kidney Int Suppl.* 2012;2:1–138. http://www.kdigo.org/clinical_practice_guidelines/pdf/KDIGO%20AKI%20Guideline.pdf. Accessed May 4, 2017.
16. Palevsky PM, Liu KD, Brophy PD, et al. KDOQI US Commentary on the 2012 KDIGO clinical practice guideline for acute kidney injury. *Am J Kidney Dis.* 2013;61(5):649–672. doi:10.1053/j.ajkd.2013.02.349.
17. Thurau K. Pathophysiology of the acutely failing kidney. *Clin Exp Dial Apheresis.* 1983;7:9–24.
18. Star R. Treatment of acute kidney injury. *Kidney Int.* 1998;54: 1817–1831.
19. Wolk R, Stokowski R, Yorgin P. Nutrition support in the pediatric renal failure patient. In: Merritt RJ, ed. *A.S.P.E.N. Nutrition Support Practice Manual.* Silver Spring, MD: American Society for Parenteral and Enteral Nutrition; 1998;18.1–18.13.
20. Kopple JD. Dietary protein and energy requirements in ESRD patients. *Am J Kidney Dis.* 1998;32(Suppl):97S–104S.
21. Seidner D, Dweik R, Gupta B. Nutrition support in liver, pulmonary and renal disease. In: Shikora S, Blackburn G, eds. *Nutrition Support: Theory and Therapeutics.* New York: Chapman & Hall; 1997:336–357.
22. Friedericksen DV, Van der Merwe L, Hattingh TL, Nel DG, Moosa MR. Acute kidney injury in the medical ICU still predictive of high mortality. *South Afr Med J.* 2009;99(12):873–875.
23. Caravaca F, Arrobas M, Pizarro J, Esparrago JF. Metabolic acidosis in advanced renal failure: differences between diabetic and non-diabetic patients. *Am J Kidney Dis.* 1999;33:892–898.
24. Kopple JD. Nutritional therapy in kidney failure. *Nutr Rev.* 1981; 39:193–206.
25. O'Connell TM. The complex role of branched chain amino acids in diabetes and cancer. *Metabolites.* 2013;3(4):931–945.
26. Abel R. Nutritional support in patients with acute kidney injury. *J Am Coll Nutr.* 1983;2:33–44.
27. Brown RO, Compher C. ASPEN clinical guidelines: nutrition support in adult acute and chronic renal failure. *JPEN J Parenter Enteral Nutr.* 2010;34(4):366–377.
28. Cano N, Fiaccadori E, Tesinsky P, et al. ESPEN guidelines on enteral nutrition in acute kidney injury. *Clin Nutr.* 2006;25:295–310.
29. Abel RM, Beck CH, Abbott WM, et al. Improved survival from acute renal injury after treatment with intravenous essential

L-amino acids and glucose: results of a prospective, double-blind study. *N Engl J Med.* 1973;288:695–699.

30. Kidney Disease: Improving Global Outcomes (KDIGO). KDIGO 2012 clinical practice guideline for the evaluation and management of chronic kidney disease. *Kidney Int Suppl.* 2013;3:1–163. http://www.kdigo.org/clinical_practice_guidelines/pdf/CKD/KDIGO_2012_CKD_GL.pdf. Accessed January 16, 2013.

31. US Renal Data System. Chapter 1: CKD in the general population. In: USRDS Annual Data Report 2016. https://www.usrds.org/2016/view/v1_01.aspx. Accessed May 4, 2017.

32. Kent PS. Integrating clinical nutrition practice guidelines in chronic kidney disease. *Nutr Clin Pract.* 2005;20:213–217.

33. Walser M, Mitch WW, Maroni BJ, Kopple JD. Should protein intake be restricted in predialysis patients? *Kidney Int.* 1999;55:771–777.

34. Dukkipati R, Kopple JD. Causes and prevention of protein-energy wasting in chronic kidney failure. *Semin Nephrol.* 2009;29(1):39–49. doi:10.1016/j.semnephrol.2008.10.006.

35. Ikizler TA, Cano NJ, Franch H, et al. Prevention and treatment of protein energy wasting in chronic kidney disease patients: a consensus statement by the International Society of Renal Nutrition and Metabolism. *Kidney Int.* 2013;84(6):1096–1107. doi:10.1038/ki.2013.147.

36. US Renal Data System. Annual data report 2009. https://www.usrds.org/atlas09.aspx. Accessed April 14, 2017.

37. Carvana R, Keep D, Kozeny G, et al. Isolated ultrafiltration. In: Nissenson A, Fine R, eds. *Dialysis Therapy.* 2nd ed. Philadelphia, PA: Hanley & Belfus; 1993:104–107.

38. Wolfson M, Jones MR, Kopple JD. Amino acid losses during hemodialysis with infusion of amino acids and glucose. *Kidney Int.* 1982;21:500–506.

39. Schoenfeld P. Care of the patient on peritoneal dialysis. In: Cogan M, Schoenfeld P, eds. *Introduction to Dialysis.* 2nd ed. New York: Churchill Livingstone; 1991:181–240.

40. Khanna R, Nolph K, Oreopoulos D. In: *The Essentials of Peritoneal Dialysis.* Boston, MA: Kluwer Academic Publishing; 1993:81,93–94.

41. Blumenkrantz MJ, Gahl GM, Kopple JD, et al. Protein loss during peritoneal dialysis. *Kidney Int.* 1981;19:593–602.

42. Uchino S, Kellum JA, Bellomo B, et al. Acute kidney injury in critically ill patients: a multinational, multicenter study. *JAMA.* 2005;294(7):813–818.

43. Bock KR. Renal replacement therapy in pediatric critical care medicine. *Curr Opin Pediatr.* 2005;17(3):368–371.

44. Wooley JA, Btaiche IF, Good KL. Metabolic and nutritional aspects of acute kidney injury in critically ill patients requiring continuous renal replacement therapy. *Nutr Clin Pract.* 2005;20:176–191.

45. Clinical practice guidelines for nutrition in chronic renal failure. K/DOQI, National Kidney Foundation. *Am J Kidney Dis.* 2000;35(6;Suppl 2):S1–S140.

46. Orlando Regional Healthcare. *Principles of Continuous Renal Replacement Therapy: Self-Training Manual.* Orlando, FL: Orlando Regional Healthcare, 2005.

47. Blumenkrantz MJ, Kopple JD, Gutman RA, et al. Methods for assessing nutritional status of patients with renal failure. *Am J Clin Nutr.* 1980;33:1567–1585.

48. Ikizler TA, Hakim RM. Nutrition in end-stage renal disease. *Kidney Int.* 1996;50:343–357.

49. Kopple JD. Pathophysiology of protein-energy wasting in chronic renal failure. *J Nutr.* 1999;129(1S Suppl):247S–251S.

50. Levey AS, Green T, Beck GJ, et al. Dietary protein restriction and the progression of chronic renal disease: what have all of the results of the MDRD study shown? Modification of Diet in Renal Disease Study group. *J Am Soc Nephrol.* 1999;10(11):2426–2439.

51. Cano NJ, Aparicio M, Brunori G, et al. ESPEN guidelines on parenteral nutrition: adult renal failure. *Clin Nutr.* 2009;28(4):401–414. doi:10.1016/j.clnu.2009.05.016.

52. McClave SA, Taylor BE, Martindale RG, et al. Guidelines for the provision and assessment of nutrition support therapy in the adult critically ill patient: Society of Critical Care Medicine (SCCM) and American Society for Parenteral and Enteral Nutrition (A.S.P.E.N.). *JPEN J Parenter Enteral Nutr.* 2016;40(2):159–211.

53. Lowrie EG, Lew NL. Death risk in hemodialysis patients: the predictive value of commonly measured variables and an evaluation of death rate differences between facilities. *Am J Kidney Dis.* 1990;15:458–482.

54. Pifer TB, McCullough KP, Port FK, et al. Mortality risk in hemodialysis patients and changes in nutritional indicators: DOPPS. *Kidney Int.* 2002;62:2238–2245.

55. Foley RN, Parfrey PS, Harnett JD, et al. Hypoalbuminemia, cardiac morbidity, and mortality in end-stage renal disease. *J Am Soc Nephrol.* 1996;7:728–736.

56. Owen WF, Lew NL, Liu Y, Lowrie EG, Lazarus JM. The urea reduction ratio and serum albumin concentration as predictors of mortality in patients undergoing hemodialysis. *N Engl J Med.* 1993;329:1001–1006.

57. Yeun JY, Levine RA, Mantadilok V, Kaysen GA. C-Reactive protein predicts all-cause and cardiovascular mortality in hemodialysis patients. *Am J Kidney Dis.* 2000;35:469–476.

58. Noh H, Lee SW, Kang SW, et al. Serum C-reactive protein: a predictor of mortality in continuous ambulatory peritoneal dialysis patients. *Perit Dial Int.* 1998;18:387–394.

59. Iseki K, Tozawa M, Yoshi S, Fukiyama K: Serum C-reactive protein (CRP) and risk of death in chronic dialysis patients. *Nephrol Dial Transplant.* 1999;14:1956–1960.

60. Detsky AS, Baker JP, Mendelson RA, et al. Evaluating the accuracy of nutritional assessment techniques applied to hospitalized patients: methodology and comparisons. *JPEN J Parenter Enteral Nutr.* 1984;8:1539.

61. Persson C, Sjoden PO, Glimelius B. The Swedish version of the Patient-Generated Subjective Global Assessment of nutritional status: gastrointestinal vs urological cancers. *Clin Nutr.* 1999;18:71–77.

62. Julien JP, Combe C, Lasseur C. Subjective Global Assessment of nutrition a useful diagnostic tool for nurses. *EDTNA/ERCA J.* 2001;27:193–196.

63. Kalantar-Zadeh K, Kuwae N, Regidor DL, et al. Survival predictability of time-varying indicators of bone disease in maintenance hemodialysis patients. *Kidney Int.* 2006;70(4):771–780.

64. Kalantar-Zadeh K, Kopple JD, Block G, Humphreys MH. A malnutrition-inflammation score is correlated with morbidity and mortality in maintenance hemodialysis patients. *Am J Kidney Dis.* 2001;38(6):1251–1263.

65. Stratton RJ, Bircher G, Fouque D, et al. Multinutrient oral supplements and tube feeding in maintenance dialysis: a systematic review and meta-analysis. *Am J Kidney Dis.* 2005;46(3):387–405.

66. Kidney Disease: Improving Global Outcomes. KDIGO 2012 clinical practice guideline for the evaluation and management of chronic kidney disease. *Kidney Int Suppl.* 2013;3:1–163. http://www.kdigo.org/clinical_practice_guidelines/pdf/CKD/KDIGO_2012_CKD_GL.pdf. Accessed January 16, 2013.

67. Druml W, Kerdorf HP. Parenteral nutrition in patients with renal failure—guidelines on parenteral nutrition. *German Med Sci.* 2009;7:1–11.

68. Hipskind P, Glass C, Charlton D, Nowak D, Daasarathy S. Do handheld calorimeters have a role in assessment of nutrition

needs in hospitalized patients? A systematic review of the literature. *Nutr Clin Pract.* 2011;26(4);426–433.

69. A.S.P.E.N. Board of Directors. Guidelines for the use of parenteral and enteral nutrition in adult and pediatric patients. *JPEN J Parenter Enteral Nutr.* 2002;26(1 Suppl):78SA–80SA.

70. Byham-Gray LD. Weighing the evidence: energy determinations across the spectrum of kidney disease. *J Ren Nutr.* 2006;16(1):17–26.

71. Byham-Gray L, Parrott JS, Ho WY, et al. Development of a predictive energy equation for maintenance hemodialysis patients: a pilot study. *J Ren Nutr.* 2014;24(1):32–41. doi:10.1053/j.jrn.2013.10.005.

72. Vilar E, Machado A, Garrett A, et al. Disease-specific predictive formulas for energy expenditure in the dialysis population. *J Ren Nutr.* 2014;24(4):243–251. doi:10.1053/j.jrn.2014.03.001.

73. Anderson CA, Miller ER. Dietary recommendations for obese patients with chronic kidney disease. *Adv Chronic Kidney Dis.* 2006;13(4):394–402.

74. Manji S, Shikora S, McMahon M, et al. Peritoneal dialysis for acute kidney injury: overfeeding resulting from dextrose absorbed during dialysis. *Crit Care Med.* 1990;18:29–31.

75. Wideroe TE, Sneby LC, Berg KJ, et al. Intraperitoneal insulin absorption during intermittent and continuous peritoneal dialysis. *Kidney Int.* 1983;23:22–28.

76. Mactier RA, Khanna R, Twardowski Z, Moore H, Nolph KD. Contribution of lymphatic absorption to loss of ultrafiltration and solute clearances in continuous ambulatory peritoneal dialysis. *J Clin Invest.* 1987;80(5):1311–1316. doi:10.1172/JCI113207.

77. Weisen P, Van Overmeire L, Delanaye P, et al. Nutrition disorders during acute kidney injury and renal replacement therapy. *JPEN J Parenter Enteral Nutr.* 2011;35(2):217–222.

78. Scheinkestel CD, Adams F, Mahony L, et al. Impact of increasing parenteral protein loads on amino acid levels and balance in critically ill anuric patients on continuous renal replacement therapy. *Nutrition.* 2003;19:733–740.

79. Garneata L, Stancu A, Dragomir D, Stefan G, Mircescu G. Ketoanalogue-supplemented vegetarian very low-protein diet and CKD progression. *J Am Soc Nephrol.* 2016;27(7):2164–2176. doi:10.1681/ASN.2015040369.

80. Fouque D, Chen J, Chen W, et al. Adherence to ketoacids/essential amino acids-supplemented low protein diets and new indications for patients with chronic kidney disease. *BMC Nephrol.* 2016;17(1):63. doi:10.1186/s12882-016-0278-7.

81. Maxvold NJ, Smoyer WE, Custer JR, Bunchman TE. Amino acid loss and nitrogen balance in critically ill children with acute kidney injury: a prospective comparison between classic hemofiltration and hemofiltration with dialysis. *Crit Care Med.* 2000;28(4):1161–1165.

82. Lopez Martinez J, Caparros T, Perez Picouto F, Lopez Diez F, Cereijo E. [Parenteral nutrition in septic patients with acute renal failure in polyuric phase.] [Article in Spanish.] *Rev Clin Esp.* 1980;157(3):171–177.

83. Singer P. High-dose amino acid infusion preserves diuresis and improves nitrogen balance in non-oliguric acute renal failure. *Wien Klin Wochenschr.* 2007;119(7-8):218–222.

84. Abel RM, Abbott WM, Fischer JE. Acute kidney injury: treatment without dialysis by total parenteral nutrition. *Arch Surg.* 1971;103:513–514.

85. Feinstein E, Blumenkrantz M, Healy M, et al. Clinical and metabolic responses to parenteral nutrition in acute kidney injury: a controlled double-blind study. *Medicine.* 1981;60:124–137.

86. Feinstein EI, Kopple JD, Silberman H, Massry SG. Total parenteral nutrition with high or low nitrogen intakes in patients with acute kidney injury. *Kidney Int.* 1983;16(Suppl):S319–S323.

87. Mirtallo JM, Schneider PJ, Mavko K, et al. A comparison of essential and general amino acid infusions in the nutritional support of patients with compromised renal function. *JPEN J Parenter Enteral Nutr.* 1982;6:109–113.

88. Li Y, Tang X, Zhang J, Wu T. Nutritional support for acute kidney injury. *Cochrane Database Syst Rev.* 2012;(8):CD005426.

89. Levin A, Bakris GL, Molitch M, et al. Prevalence of abnormal serum vitamin D, PTH, calcium, and phosphorus in patients with chronic kidney disease: results of the study to evaluate early kidney disease. *Kidney Int.* 2007;71(1):31–38.

90. Westerberg PA, Linde T, Wikström B, et al. Regulation of fibroblast growth factor-23 in chronic kidney disease. *Nephrol Dial Transplant.* 2007;22(11):3202–3207.

91. Block GA, Klassen PS, Lazarus JM, et al. Mineral metabolism, mortality, and morbidity in maintenance hemodialysis. *J Am Soc Nephrol.* 2004;15(8):2208–2218.

92. Tentori F, Blayney MJ, Albert JM, et al. Mortality risk for dialysis patients with different levels of serum calcium, phosphorus, and PTH: the Dialysis Outcomes and Practice Patterns Study (DOPPS). *Am J Kidney Dis.* 2008;52(3):519–530. doi:10.1053/j.ajkd.2008.03.020.

93. Kimata N, Akiba T, Pisoni RL, et al. Mineral metabolism and haemoglobin concentration among haemodialysis patients in the Dialysis Outcomes and Practice Patterns Study (DOPPS). *Nephrol Dial Transplant.* 2005;20(5):927–935.

94. Young EW, Albert JM, Satayathum S, et al. Predictors and consequences of altered mineral metabolism: the Dialysis Outcomes and Practice Patterns Study. *Kidney Int.* 2005;67(3):1179–1187.

95. National Kidney Foundation. K/DOQI clinical practice guidelines for bone metabolism and disease in chronic kidney disease. *Am J Kidney Dis.* 2003;42(Suppl 3):S1–S201.

96. McCann L. Nutrient calculations. In: *Pocket Guide to Nutrition Assessment of the Renal Patient.* 3rd ed. New York: National Kidney Foundation; 1998:4–5.

97. Kestenbaum B, Sampson JN, Rudser KD, et al. Serum phosphate levels and mortality risk among people with chronic kidney disease. *J Am Soc Nephrol.* 2005;16(2):520–528.

98. Covic A, Kothawala P, Bernal M, et al. Systematic review of the evidence underlying the association between mineral metabolism disturbances and risk of all-cause mortality, cardiovascular mortality and cardiovascular events in chronic kidney disease. *Nephrol Dial Transplant.* 2009;24(5):1506–1523. doi:10.1093/ndt/gfn613.

99. National Kidney Foundation. Guideline 6: use of phosphate binders in CKD. KDOQI clinical practice guidelines for bone metabolism and disease in children with chronic kidney disease. 2011. http://www2.kidney.org/professionals/KDOQI/guidelines_pedbone. Accessed April 14, 2017.

100. Shinaberger CS, Greenland S, Kopple JD, et al. Is controlling phosphorus by decreasing dietary protein intake beneficial or harmful in persons with chronic kidney disease? *Am J Clin Nutr.* 2008;88(6):1511–1518. doi:10.3945/ajcn.2008.26665.

101. Kidney Disease Outcomes Quality Initiative (K/DOQI) Group. K/DOQI clinical practice guidelines for management of dyslipidemias in patients with kidney disease. *Am J Kidney Dis.* 2003;41(4 Suppl 3):S1–S91.

102. González EA, Sachdeva A, Oliver DA, Martin KJ. Vitamin D insufficiency and deficiency in chronic kidney disease. A single center observational study. *Am J Nephrol.* 2004;24(5):503–510.

103. LaClair RE, Hellman RN, Karp SL, et al. Prevalence of calcidiol deficiency in CKD: a cross-sectional study across latitudes in the United States. *Am J Kidney Dis.* 2005;45(6):1026–1033.

104. Elder G, Mackun K. 25-Hydroxyvitamin D deficiency and diabetes predict reduced BMD in patients with chronic kidney disease. *J Bone Miner Res.* 2006;21(11):1778–1784.

105. Tomida K, Hamano T, Mikami S, et al. Serum 25-hydroxyvitamin D as an independent determinant of 1-84 PTH and bone mineral density in non-diabetic predialysis CKD patients. *Bone.* 2009;44(4):678–683. doi:10.1016/j.bone.2008.11.016.

106. Wolf M, Shah A, Gutierrez O, et al. Vitamin D levels and early mortality among incident hemodialysis patients. *Kidney Int.* 2007;72(8):1004–1013.

107. Wang AY, Lam CW, Sanderson JE, et al. Serum 25-hydroxyvitamin D status and cardiovascular outcomes in chronic peritoneal dialysis patients: a 3-y prospective cohort study. *Am J Clin Nutr.* 2008;87(6):1631–1638.

108. Silver J, Naveh-Many T, Mayer H, Schmelzer HJ, Popovtzer MM. Regulation by vitamin D metabolites of parathyroid hormone gene transcription in vivo in the rat. *J Clin Invest.* 1986;78(5):1296–1301.

109. Brown AJ, Ritter CS, Knutson JC, Strugnell SA. The vitamin D prodrugs 1alpha(OH)D2, 1alpha(OH)D3 and BCI-210 suppress PTH secretion by bovine parathyroid cells. *Nephrol Dial Transplant.* 2006;21(3):644–650.

110. Goltzman D, Miao D, Panda DK, Hendy GN. Effects of calcium and of the vitamin D system on skeletal and calcium homeostasis: lessons from genetic models. *J Steroid Biochem Mol Biol.* 2004;89-90(1-5):485–489.

111. Anderson PH, Atkins GJ. The skeleton as an intracrine organ for vitamin D metabolism. *Mol Aspects Med.* 2008;29(6):397–406. doi:10.1016/j.mam.2008.05.003.

112. Shimada T, Yamazaki Y, Takahashi M, et al. Vitamin D receptor-independent FGF23 actions in regulating phosphate and vitamin D metabolism. *Am J Physiol Renal Physiol.* 2005;289(5):F1088–F1095.

113. Barreto FC, Barreto DV, Moysés RM, et al. K/DOQI-recommended intact PTH levels do not prevent low-turnover bone disease in hemodialysis patients. *Kidney Int.* 2008;73(6):771–777. doi:10.1038/sj.ki.5002769.

114. Block GA, Hulbert-Shearon TE, Levin NW, Port FK. Association of serum phosphorus and calcium x phosphate product with mortality risk in chronic hemodialysis patients: a national study. *Am J Kidney Dis.* 1998;31(4):607–617.

115. Goodman WG, Belin T, Gales B, et al. Calcium-regulated parathyroid hormone release in patients with mild or advanced secondary hyperparathyroidism. *Kidney Int.* 1995;48(5):1553–1558.

116. Brown EM, Gamba G, Riccardi D, et al. Cloning and characterization of an extracellular Ca(2+)-sensing receptor from bovine parathyroid. *Nature.* 1993;366(6455):575–580.

117. Uhlig K, Berns JS, Kestenbaum B, et al. KDOQI US commentary on the 2009 KDIGO clinical practice guideline for the diagnosis, evaluation, and treatment of CKD-mineral and bone disorder (CKD-MBD). *Am J Kidney Dis.* 2010;55(5):773–799. doi:10.1053/j.ajkd.2010.02.340.

118. Danese MD, Belozeroff V, Smirnakis K, Rothman KJ. Consistent control of mineral and bone disorder in incident hemodialysis patients. *Clin J Am Soc Nephrol.* 2008;3(5):1423–1429. doi:10.2215/CJN.01060308.

119. Brito-Ashurst I, Varagunam M, Raftery MJ, Yaqoob MM. Bicarbonate supplementation slows progression of CKD and improves nutritional status. *J Am Soc Nephrol.* 2009;20(9):2075–2084. doi:10.1681/ASN.2008111205.

120. Ono K. The effect of vitamin C supplementation and withdrawal on the mortality and morbidity of regular hemodialysis patients. *Clin Nephrol.* 1989;31:31–34.

121. Pru C, Eaton J, Kjellstrand C. Vitamin C intoxication and hyperoxalemia in chronic hemodialysis patients. *Nephron.* 1985;39:112–116.

122. Makoff R, Gonick H. Renal failure and the concomitant derangement of micronutrient metabolism. *Nutr Clin Pract.* 1999;14:238–246.

123. Tarng DC, Wei YH, Huan TP, et al. Intravenous ascorbic acid as an adjuvant therapy for recombinant erythropoietin in hemodialysis patients with hyperferritinemia. *Kidney Int.* 1999;55:2477–2486.

124. Bamonti-Catena F, Buccianti G, Porcella A, et al. Folate measurements in patients on regular hemodialysis treatment. *Am J Kidney Dis.* 1999;33:492–497.

125. Blumberg A, Hanck A, Sander G. Vitamin nutrition in patients on continuous ambulatory peritoneal dialysis (CAPD). *Clin Nephrol.* 1983;20;244–250.

126. Marangella M, Vitale C, Petrarulo M, et al. Pathogenesis of severe hyperoxalaemia in Crohn's disease-related renal failure on maintenance haemodialysis: successful management with pyridoxine. *Nephrol Dial Transplant.* 1992;7:960–964.

127. Jagadha V, Deck J, Halliday W, Smyth H. Wernicke's encephalopathy in patients on peritoneal dialysis or hemodialysis. *Ann Neurol.* 1987;21:78–89.

128. Baumgartner TG. Trace elements in clinical nutrition. *Nutr Clin Pract.* 1993;8:251–263.

129. Fournier A, Corvazier M, Man W. Skin test sensitivity in zinc deficient patients in hemo- and peritoneal dialysis [abstract]. *Artif Organ.* 1989;13;296.

130. Hsieh YY, Shen WS, Lee LY, et al. Long-term changes in trace elements in patients undergoing chronic hemodialysis. *Biol Trace Elem Res.* 2006;109(2):115–121.

131. Lyon TD, Fell GS, Hutton RC, Eaton AN. Evaluation on inductively coupled argon plasma mass spectrometry (ICP-Ms) for simultaneous multielement trace analysis in clinical chemistry. *J Anal Atom Spectrom.* 1998;3:265–271.

132. De Francisco AL, Stenvinkel P, et al. Inflammation and its impact on anaemia in chronic kidney disease: from haemoglobin variability to hyporesponsiveness. *NDT Plus.* 2009;2(Suppl 1):i18–i26.

133. Nissenson A, Strobos J. Iron deficiency in patients with renal failure. *Kidney Int.* 1999;69(Suppl):S18–S21.

134. Macdougall I. Strategies for iron supplementation: oral versus intravenous. *Kidney Int.* 1999;69(Suppl):S61–S66.

135. Kaltwasser J, Gottschalk R. Erythropoietin and iron. *Kidney Int.* 1999;69(Suppl):S49–S56.

136. Fishbane S. Iron treatment: impact of safety issues. *Am J Kidney Dis.* 1998;32(6 Suppl):S152–S156.

137. National Kidney Foundation: KDOQI clinical practice guidelines for anemia of chronic kidney disease: update 2000. *Am J Kidney Dis.* 2001;37(Suppl 1):S182–S238.

138. Chertow GM, Mason PD, Vaage-Nilsen O, Ahlmen J. On the relative safety of parenteral iron formulations. *Nephrol Dial Transplant.* 2004;19:1571–1575.

139. Feinstein E. Nutritional therapy in maintenance hemodialysis. In: Nissenson A, Fine R, eds. *Dialysis Therapy.* Philadelphia, PA: Hanley and Belfus; 1993:181–201.

140. Berns JS, Mosenkis A. Pharmacologic adjuvants to epoetin in the treatment of anemia in patients on hemodialysis. *Hemodial Int.* 2005;9:7–22.

141. Bartel L, Hussey J, Elson C, et al. Depletion of heart and skeletal muscle carnitine in the normal rat by peritoneal dialysis. *Nutr Res.* 1981;1:261–266.

142. Schreiber B. Levocarnitine and dialysis: a review. *Nutr Clin Pract.* 2005;20:218–243.

143. Lacson E Jr, Wang W, Zebrowski B, Wingard R, Hakim RM. Outcomes associated with intradialytic oral nutritional supplements in patients undergoing maintenance hemodialysis: a quality improvement report. *Am J Kidney Dis.* 2012;60:591–600.

144. Cheu C, Pearson J, Dahlerus C, et al. Association between oral nutritional supplementation and clinical outcomes among patients with ESRD. *Clin J Am Soc Nephrol.* 2013;8:100–107.

145. Ikizler TA. Protein and energy: recommended intake and nutrient supplementation in chronic dialysis patients. *Semin Dialy.* 2004;17(6):471–478.

146. Cano N. Intradialytic parenteral nutrition: where do we go from here? *J Ren Nutr.* 2004;14:3–5.

147. Pupim LB, Flakoll PJ, Brouillette JR, et al. Intradialytic parenteral nutrition improves protein and energy homeostasis in chronic hemodialysis patients. *J Clin Invest.* 2002;110(4):483–492.

148. Charry N, Shalansky K. Efficacy of intradialytic parenteral nutrition in malnourished hemodialysis patients. *Am Soc Health Syst Pharm.* 2002;59:1736–1741.

149. Moore E, Celano J. Challenges of providing nutrition support in the outpatient dialysis setting. *Nutr Clin Pract.* 2005;20:202–212.

150. Orellana P, Juarez-Congelosi M, Goldstein SL. Intradialytic parenteral nutrition treatment and biochemical marker assessment for malnutrition in adolescent maintenance hemodialysis patients. *J Ren Nutr.* 2005;15(3):312–317.

30 Short Bowel Syndrome

Berkeley N. Limketkai, MD, PhD, Ryan T. Hurt, MD, PhD, and Lena B. Palmer, MD, MSCR

CONTENTS

Acknowledgments: Sherry Tarleton, RD, CNSC, and John K. DiBaise, MD, FACG, were the authors of this chapter for the second edition.

Objectives

1. Describe potential causes, symptoms, and complications associated with short bowel syndrome (SBS).
2. Learn diverse nutrition-related strategies to optimize fluid, electrolyte, and nutrient balance in SBS.
3. Become familiar with the medical and surgical management of SBS.

Test Your Knowledge Questions

1. Which of the following answers best reflects dietary modifications that may prevent the development of nephrolithiasis-related renal failure?
   A. A calcium-restricted diet with increased free-water intake
   B. A low-fat diet with adequate phosphorus repletion and increased free-water intake
   C. A low-fat and oxalate- and calcium-restricted diet
   D. A low-fat, oxalate-restricted diet and adequate hydration

2. Because of the malabsorptive process present in SBS, patients have a high risk for micronutrient deficiencies. Which of the following answers is correct regarding the monitoring and repletion of micronutrients in SBS?
   A. If patients are receiving parenteral nutrition (PN), there is no reason to monitor micronutrients because the PN should satisfy all micronutrient needs.
   B. Micronutrients should be checked periodically. Micronutrients can usually be repleted via the oral route.
   C. Micronutrients should be checked monthly. Repletion should be administered in high doses both intravenously and orally.
   D. Micronutrients should be checked annually, and all micronutrients should be repleted intravenously because patients with SBS cannot absorb micronutrients administered orally.

3. Which of the following answers best describes how a clinician determines the most appropriate feeding route (ie, oral, enteral, parenteral, or a combination) for a patient with SBS?
   A. All patients with SBS need lifelong PN; if their energy and protein needs are met with PN, they can eat whatever they want for comfort.
   B. To avoid the risk of PN-associated complications, PN should always be discontinued as soon as oral intake or enteral nutrition (EN) is initiated.
   C. The nutrition regimen should be individualized to meet the needs of the particular person.
   D. Insurance reimbursement plays the major role in deciding the feeding route.

4. Which of the following characteristics of an initial enteral feeding regimen would be most appropriate for a patient with SBS?
   A. A fiber-free, energy-dense formula administered via bolus infusion
   B. A hydrolyzed, elemental formula that is high in medium-chain triglyceride (MCT) oil
   C. An isotonic, polymeric, fiber-containing formula administered via continuous gastric infusion
   D. A semi-elemental, peptide-based formula administered nocturnally

Test Your Knowledge Answers

1. The correct answer is **D**. Patients with SBS who have fat malabsorption and an intact colon are at risk for oxalate kidney stones. Calcium normally binds to oxalate—a substance found naturally in many foods—in the colon, thus preventing oxalate's absorption. In the setting of fat malabsorption, calcium will bind to excess fat entering the colon, leaving the oxalates free to be absorbed into the bloodstream and excreted via the kidney, thus forming oxalate kidney stones. A low-fat, oxalate-restricted diet plays a key role in the prevention of oxalate kidney stones. The use of a calcium supplement or consumption of food that is high in calcium may also help to bind the oxalate and facilitate its excretion in the feces.

2. The correct answer is **B**. Patients with SBS are at risk for deficiencies of micronutrients (vitamins, minerals, trace elements) and essential fatty acids. There are no formal guidelines regarding the monitoring and repletion of micronutrients in this patient population. Nevertheless, micronutrients and an essential fatty acid profile should be checked at least annually, and interventions to replete deficient micronutrients should be done. Abnormal micronutrient levels should be monitored on a quarterly basis. Although some micronutrients can be increased in the PN solution, not all micronutrients will be able to be added to the PN solution because of formula stability issues or because the nutrient does not come in single-unit doses. Fortunately, adequate micronutrient supplementation can be provided orally, although the regimen will need to be tailored to meet the patient's increased needs. Some micronutrients are available for either intramuscular or intravenous (IV) administration.

3. The correct answer is **C**. Many nutrition support options are available. The best option will depend on the patient's bowel anatomy, length of time since surgery, current weight, laboratory test data, and hydration status. The most appropriate nutrition regimen should be individualized to meet the needs of the particular person. As the adaptation process progresses and the patient becomes more stable, nutrition support may be decreased as tolerated.

4. The correct answer is **C**. When initiating enteral feedings in a patient with SBS, it is important that the formula be isotonic. Polymeric formulas are generally well tolerated. Gastric feeding may result in less diarrhea than small bowel feeding. The inclusion of soluble fiber may also be beneficial because it can slow gastric emptying, enhance adaptation, and provide an energy source in those patients who have a colon. Slow initiation of feedings administered via continuous gastric infusion as opposed to bolus administration may be better tolerated.

Background

The small bowel plays a central role in nutrient, fluid, and electrolyte absorption. SBS is a chronic condition characterized by a compromise in these intestinal functions because of extensive small bowel resection. Clinical manifestations often include chronic diarrhea, dehydration, electrolyte abnormalities, macro- and micronutrient deficiencies, and weight loss. While the length of residual small bowel contributes to the severity of SBS, other related factors (eg, bowel segment, time since last bowel resection, health of the residual intestinal mucosa, presence or absence of a colon, and diet) can strongly influence net intestinal absorption. SBS therefore represents a spectrum of disease, ranging from intestinal sufficiency to insufficiency and failure. Intestinal insufficiency indicates a reduction in absorptive ability that requires an increase in oral fluid or nutrient intake to maintain nutrient, fluid, and electrolyte balance. Intestinal failure involves a more severe compromise of intestinal function that requires additional support with EN, parenteral hydration, and/or PN.

The symptoms associated with SBS may be nonspecific, although the underlying mechanisms that drive these symptoms will differ based on anatomical and physiological factors. As such, management of SBS requires a personalized plan of nutrition-related, medical, and/or surgical interventions to optimize nutrient, fluid, and electrolyte balance, while also improving the patient's quality of life. In this chapter, we discuss the etiology of SBS, anatomical and physiological considerations, related complications, nutrition interventions, and rehabilitation strategies.

Causes of Short Bowel Syndrome

SBS is a relatively rare condition, although the true incidence and prevalence are unknown. Some epidemiologic estimates can be inferred from patients receiving home PN or from those who undergo intestinal transplantation. In the United States, an early estimate of the prevalence of home PN use was 120 per million residents, of whom approximately 10% to 20% had SBS.[1] This estimate does not include SBS patients who never or no longer required PN, so the true prevalence would be even higher. Between 2000 and 2013, 78% of the 937 intestinal transplants done in the United States were for SBS.[2]

The etiologies of SBS in children and adults generally differ. Children with SBS tend to develop it early in life because of congenital malformations or severe infections at birth. Common indications of small bowel resection in children include gastroschisis, intussusception, and necrotizing enterocolitis. Adults, on the other hand, tend to develop SBS after serial or massive small bowel resections related to conditions that develop later in life, such as Crohn's disease, mesenteric vascular insufficiency, postsurgical complications, malignancy, and trauma.[3]

Crohn's disease is a chronic inflammatory disorder of the gastrointestinal (GI) tract with a high risk of requiring small bowel resection. Individuals who undergo small bowel resection are subsequently at a high risk of requiring repeat resections, eventually leading to the development of anatomical SBS. Moreover, in the presence of active intestinal inflammation, the residual length of *functional* (healthy) intestine may be even shorter. Crohn's disease used to be the most common cause of SBS, but this etiology has recently become less common with the advent of powerful immunosuppressive therapies.[4,5]

More recently, surgical complications have become one of the more common causes of SBS. Surgical complications may include inadvertent trauma to the small bowel, vascular injury, postoperative fistulas, infections, and bowel obstruction from adhesions that prompt repeat surgery with possible resection.

Other causes of SBS stem from massive resection related to mesenteric vascular events, trauma, malignancy, radiation enteritis, or severe intestinal dysmotility. Prolonged occlusion of the mesenteric vasculature can lead to ischemia and subsequent intestinal necrosis. Major abdominal trauma, such as motor vehicle collisions or gunshot wounds, may lead to extensive small bowel damage. Large or metastatic abdominal tumors may require heavy debulking and resection. Radiation enteritis can involve long segments of small bowel, while severe and debilitating intestinal dysmotility (eg, chronic intestinal pseudo-obstruction) may prompt surgical resection to reduce small bowel transit time.

Knowing the etiology of the patient's SBS helps the clinician understand nonanatomical limitations of the residual small bowel, while targeting therapies with these considerations in mind. For instance, the patient with SBS from Crohn's disease may require aggressive control of inflammation to not only improve absorptive function of the residual small bowel but also reduce the risk of additional resection. Patients with SBS from mesenteric ischemia may be at risk for recurrent vascular events and need thoughtful medical prophylaxis. Knowledge of the patient's history of cancer would be vital data when considering whether growth factors are appropriate as part of intestinal rehabilitation therapy.

Anatomical and Physiological Considerations

The normal small bowel length in an adult ranges from 400 to 800 cm (average 630 cm for men and 590 cm for women).[6] The duodenum comprises between 25 to 40 cm of the proximal small bowel, while the jejunum and ileum respectively comprise approximately 60% and 40% of the remaining small bowel. By definition, SBS involves an anatomical reduction in the length of the small bowel, which results in a decrease in the surface area for intestinal absorption. The estimated surface area of the healthy small bowel is equivalent to half a badminton court, which permits the small bowel to absorb a daily average of 6 to 8 liters of fluid.[7] Because of the small bowel's impressive functional reserve, clinically significant symptoms do not typically appear until three-fourths of the original small bowel has been resected.

Nonetheless, the mechanism for intestinal malabsorption in SBS is more complex than the mere reduction in bowel length or surface area; the types of bowel segments involved in SBS also influence the patient's prognosis for achieving nutrition-related autonomy. There are 3 common anatomical variants of SBS, based on remaining bowel segments: (1) jejunoileocolonic anastomosis; (2) jejunocolonic anastomosis; and (3) end jejunostomy. On average, SBS patients with all segments of small bowel and a colon in continuity (jejunoileocolonic anastomosis) have the best prognosis and need at least 30 cm of residual small bowel to realistically wean off PN.[8] SBS patients with a jejunocolonic anastomosis need at least 60 cm of residual small bowel, whereas those with an end jejunostomy need at least 100 cm of small bowel. The end jejunostomy variant is the most difficult to manage and the most likely to require permanent PN.

The proximal 100 cm of the jejunum is the primary site of carbohydrate, protein, and water-soluble vitamin absorption.[9] Fat absorption occurs over a longer length of small bowel. The intercellular junctions along the jejunal epithelia are relatively porous, thus permitting rapid flow of fluids and nutrients across the epithelium and the generation of an isoosmolar jejunal content. As a result, the concentration of sodium in jejunostomy fluid is about 100 mEq/L (range: 90 to 140 mEq/L). Sodium absorption in the jejunum can only occur against a concentration gradient and is coupled to the absorption of glucose.[10] In contrast to the jejunum, the ileum has tighter intercellular junctions.[10] The active transport of sodium chloride allows for significant fluid reabsorption and the ability to concentrate the contents of the ileum.

The terminal ileum is the primary site of carrier-mediated absorption of vitamin B_{12} and enterohepatic recirculation of bile.[11] When less than approximately 100 cm of terminal ileum is resected, upregulated hepatic synthesis of bile can compensate for the losses from unrecycled bile. The bile that enters the colon interferes with colonic fluid absorption, which leads to watery diarrhea. On the other hand, when more than 100 cm of terminal ileum is resected, the amount of unrecycled bile loss exceeds the maximum rate of hepatic synthesis of bile, leading to bile insufficiency, fat malabsorption, and steatorrhea. The terminal ileum is also important for the enteric hormone feedback mechanism. Massive resection leads to gastric hypersecretion, accelerated gastric emptying, and more rapid gut transit.[12] Gastric hypersecretion and "dumping" contribute to an increased volume and rate of fluid flow into the duodenum, and the lower effluent pH may interfere with pancreatic enzyme activity.[13]

Although it is commonly believed that the ileocecal valve is beneficial in slowing transit, this benefit has not been observed in studies of small bowel transit after right hemicolectomy.[14] Nonetheless, resection of the ileocecal valve may promote retrograde transit of colonic bacteria into the small bowel, leading to bacterial overgrowth. This pathology can cause microscopic mucosal injury, alteration in bile salt absorption, and overall intestinal malabsorption.

The presence or absence of the colon plays a significant role in the patient's symptoms and prognosis. The colon primarily serves to absorb water from stool and helps reduce the risk of dehydration. Similar to the ileum, the proximal colon produces enteroglucagon, neurotensin, and peptide YY, which are responsible for modulating intestinal transit time.[15,16] (See Chapter 1.) The colon is also the site for bacterial fermentation of fiber and malabsorbed carbohydrates into short-chain fatty acids (SCFAs), which can provide up to an additional 1000 kcal/d.[17]

Intestinal Adaptation

Following surgical resection, the residual small bowel undergoes a process of adaptation to compensate for anatomical and functional losses. Intestinal adaptation is characterized by changes in structure (eg, increase in villous height, crypt cell depth, enterocyte number) and function (eg, modifications of the brush border fluidity, permeability, up- or downregulation of carrier-mediated transport, and deceleration in transit rate). These processes are mediated by a host of luminal factors, including nutrients, enteric hormones, growth factors, and GI peptides. Intestinal adaptation occurs over 1 to 2 years and is associated with progressive improvement in nutrient and fluid absorption. The ileum possesses the most potential for intestinal adaptation, followed by the colon. The duodenum and

jejunum otherwise have less potential for adaptation. These phenomena are among the reasons why the types of residual bowel variably influence the eventual patient's ability to achieve nutrition autonomy.

Complications

SBS patients are at high risk for developing complications related to the altered bowel anatomy and function (Table 30-1), medical comorbidities, long-term use of PN, and adverse effects from medical or surgical interventions.

Fluid, Electrolyte, and Nutritional Deficiencies

Because of a compromise in intestinal absorption, untreated patients with SBS often experience dehydration, electrolyte abnormalities, micronutrient deficiencies, and protein-energy malnutrition. Large-volume diarrhea leads to significant water loss and electrolyte wasting. Hydration strategies can be tailored for a goal urine output of more than 1 L/d and a urinary sodium concentration greater than 20 mEq/L.

Common electrolyte abnormalities include hypokalemia, hypomagnesemia, and hypocalcemia. Hypomagnesemia can occur because of (1) loss of magnesium-absorbing gut, (2) the binding of magnesium by unabsorbed fatty acids, and (3) sodium/water depletion that leads to secondary hyperaldosteronism with subsequent urinary magnesium losses.[18] Hypomagnesemia, in turn, can lead to hypocalcemia related to impaired parathyroid hormone (PTH) release.[19] The correction of sodium depletion is critical in treating hypomagnesemia. If severe hypomagnesemia persists, parenteral magnesium may be necessary.

Vitamin B_{12} is primarily absorbed in the terminal ileum and typically requires supplementation when at least 50 cm of terminal ileum has been resected.[20] Loss of the ileum, gastric hypersecretion, its effects on the R protein, and/or bacterial overgrowth can all contribute to vitamin B_{12} deficiency.

Fat-soluble vitamin and essential fatty acid deficiencies are also commonly encountered. Supplemental zinc and, occasionally, selenium may be required in the presence of excessive stool losses.

TABLE 30-1 Bowel-Related Complications in Short Bowel Syndrome

- Malabsorptive diarrhea
- Malnutrition
- Fluid and electrolyte disturbances
- Micronutrient deficiency
- Essential fatty acid deficiency
- Small bowel bacterial overgrowth
- D-lactic acidosis
- Oxalate nephropathy
- Renal dysfunction
- Metabolic bone disease
- Acid peptic disease
- Anastomotic ulceration/stricture
- Bowel obstruction

For patients who primarily rely on long-term PN as their source of hydration and nutrition, improperly formulated PN can lead to electrolyte, micronutrient, and essential fatty acid deficiencies. Although PN can provide the requisite electrolytes for physiological function, parenteral vitamin and mineral supplementation typically only contains a subset of what is needed to meet daily requirements. Some components, such as iron, cannot be added to the PN admixture because of incompatibility. These components can nonetheless be provided as an infusion separate from the PN formulation. The frequency of electrolyte and micronutrient monitoring will depend on the stability of the patient's levels.

Hepatobiliary Complications

Patients with SBS who depend on long-term PN are at risk for intestinal failure–associated liver disease, also known as PN–associated liver disease (PNALD). This syndrome encompasses 1 or more disorders, including cholestasis, hepatic steatosis, and cirrhosis. Putative mechanisms include excess energy intake that results in hepatic steatosis, phytosterol exposure from soybean-based lipid emulsions, and micronutrient toxicities that can cause hepatic injury.[21] Moreover, the reduction in oral intake and cholecystokinin secretion can lead to cholestasis. Diminished gallbladder contractility, altered bilirubin metabolism, and cholesterol supersaturation increase the risk of cholelithiasis and biliary obstruction. Nutrition deficiencies, in the context of SBS, and bacterial overgrowth are additional factors associated with PNALD. Strategies to reduce the risk of PNALD include trophic enteral feedings, cyclical PN, moderation of the lipid dose in soybean-based lipid emulsions, and close monitoring for mineral toxicities.

Nephrolithiasis

Normally, dietary oxalate binds to calcium and is excreted in the stool. However, in the presence of fat malabsorption, fatty acid anions compete with oxalate anions to bind to available calcium. The excess and unbound oxalate are absorbed in the colon and filtered in the kidneys. The high concentration of serum oxalate couples with relative dehydration, metabolic acidosis, and hypomagnesemia in patients with SBS to facilitate oxalate stone formation in the kidneys.[22] For this reason, patients who retain a colon are advised to consume a low-fat, low-oxalate diet; increase calcium intake; and remain well hydrated to minimize the risk of oxalate nephrolithiasis.

Metabolic Bone Disease

Patients with SBS are at high risk for developing osteopenia or osteoporosis because of compromised calcium and vitamin D absorption and secondary hyperparathyroidism. They are also at risk for developing osteomalacia from defective mineralization of newly formed bone (organic bone matrix deposition, but poor calcification). Mechanisms are multifactorial, including increased activation of osteoclasts by inflammatory cytokines, use of medications such as corticosteroids, inadequate minerals in PN formulation, and defective absorption and

processing of calcium, phosphorous, vitamin D, magnesium, and zinc.[22]

Other Complications

Long-term use of central venous catheters, as needed for PN, can lead to vascular injury and thromboses. Long-term use of these catheters also poses a nontrivial risk of central line–associated bloodstream infections (CLABSI). Other complications to consider include significant cost of care, increased health care utilization, concurrent infections (eg, risk of *Clostridium difficile* infections from recurrent hospitalizations), complications from surgical interventions, and marked reduction in the quality of life. All-cause mortality rates for patients with SBS are also high, as extrapolated from studies that evaluated long-term PN use: 6% at 1 year and 20% at 4 years.[23] Mortality rates among SBS patients with nutrition autonomy are less clear.

Nutrition Assessment

Preliminary Assessment

A thorough assessment of patients with SBS is essential for maintaining their nutrition, hydration, and overall health. Important nutrition information to collect include dietary preferences and practices, appetite, GI symptoms, weight changes, and potential manifestations of micronutrient deficiencies. (See Chapter 8 for additional information on assessment of micronutrient deficiencies.) Other important historical elements include the use of supplemental nutrition (eg, EN, PN), central and enteral access devices (eg, date placed, type and number of infections, and material of catheter [silicone vs polyurethane]), and nutrition support complications (eg, PNALD, CLABSI). The physical assessment should focus on signs of dehydration and malnutrition. Although the type of insurance coverage (eg, Medicare, Medicaid, private) should not dictate care recommendations for patients, it should be investigated because requirements for EN or PN coverage may vary depending on the patient's insurance plan.

An audit of the patient's total energy intake, micro- and macronutrient intake, and fluid balance can be estimated from a combination of diet recall, food log, reported EN use, and PN formulation order.[24] A baseline assessment of fluid intake, urine output, and stool output should be performed for at least 24 hours, but preferably over 3 to 5 days, to estimate the enteral and fluid balance. Documentation of intestinal fluid and urine loss relative to oral intake may be required by some insurers to support PN use. Finally, given the high level of motivation and education required of the patient to adhere to the complex dietary, fluid, and medical treatments prescribed, clinicians should inquire about the patient's education, motivation, support system, and potential economic or other barriers. See Chapter 9 for general information about the nutrition assessment process.

Given the impact of the residual bowel anatomy on outcomes, the clinician performing the nutrition assessment should elicit information on the site of resection, residual bowel length, condition of the residual bowel, presence of the colon, presence of the ileocecal valve, presence and location of any ostomies, and anatomical bowel complications (eg, anastomotic strictures, chronic obstruction, fistulas). Operative reports commonly indicate the length of *resected* small bowel, but the documentation often lacks data on the length of the *remaining* small bowel. The latter information is more important when assessing prognosis, providing counseling, and obtaining insurance coverage for PN. Measurements begin at the duodenojejunal flexure (ligament of Treitz) and end at the ileocecal valve.[25] When an operative report is unavailable or does not document the remaining bowel length, a barium contrast small bowel series can roughly estimate the residual bowel length and delineate other structural features, such as bowel dilatation, intestinal transit time, and strictures or fistulas.

Long-Term Monitoring

Although the evidence for serial laboratory monitoring is poor, recently published international guidelines for the management of chronic intestinal failure recommend routine assessment of electrolytes (including calcium, magnesium, and phosphorus), vitamins, minerals, and trace elements.[22] The frequency of monitoring differs among professional societies and varies even more widely in clinical practice.

A metabolic profile and complete blood counts should be monitored frequently to ensure adequate hydration and assess for any trends toward anemia or renal insufficiency. Vitamins and trace minerals should be monitored at least annually, and monitoring of these micronutrients should be done more frequently for patients receiving PN. If deficiencies are found, more frequent monitoring and vigilant replacement are indicated. In particular, levels of fat-soluble vitamins (A, D, E, and sometimes K), vitamin B_{12}, folate, iron, zinc, and copper should be assessed.[26] (See Chapter 8 for information on assessment of micronutrient status.) Several studies have also indicated that patients with SBS who receive PN are at risk for vitamin C deficiency.[22] Insurance companies may require a 72-hour fecal fat assessment of patients on a daily diet of at least 50 g fat, but ideally 100 g, to document fat malabsorption.

Clinicians should periodically assess the patient's urine and stool output to ensure net positive hydration and balanced nutrition. If a patient has less than 1 liter of urine output per day and serial weight loss, the clinician should intervene.[27] A sudden increase in stool or ostomy output requires further investigation.[28] Excessive loss of sodium through GI secretions leads to hypotension and prerenal azotemia. Hyperaldosteronism is common in this patient population and may decrease sodium losses in the urine. Sodium concentrations are lower in a jejunostomy effluent than an ileostomy effluent (90 vs 120 mEq/L, respectively), although net jejunostomy sodium losses are often greater because of the higher volume of stool output.[29] Random urine sodium levels can be used to monitor hydration status and detect sodium depletion. Urine sodium less than 5 to 10 mmol/L indicates maximal sodium conservation, and hence, sodium depletion. The urine sodium should be maintained at a concentration greater than 20 mmol/L. The ratio of blood urea nitrogen (BUN) to creatinine may also provide a measure of hydration status.[30]

Clinicians should routinely assess the patient's liver function profile. Positive trends in the alkaline phosphatase, transaminases, and bilirubin may suggest PN-related cholestasis and hepatic injury. An elevated alkaline phosphatase in the absence of abnormal transaminases and/or bilirubin is not uncommon. If it occurs, consider fractionating the alkaline phosphatase to determine the relative contribution of the liver and bone in the elevated levels. This step helps assess for metabolic bone disease as a cause of the abnormal laboratory test result.

Patients on long-term PN should have periodic assessments of their calcium, phosphorus, vitamin D, magnesium, and PTH levels. An elevated serum PTH level, a marker of insufficient vitamin D levels and increased bone turnover, is useful to identify patients who need more intensive management. Assessment of bone density using a dual energy x-ray absorptiometry scan should be performed in all patients with SBS regardless of PN need and repeated every 2 to 3 years, or annually if the patient is osteoporotic.

Nutrition Intervention

The goal of nutrition intervention is to maintain adequate nutrition and hydration to support bodily functioning and overall health. Given the wide range of factors influencing absorption and metabolism in patients with SBS, nutrition goals should be tailored to the individual. There is little consensus on how to determine "adequate" nutrition goals, and several methods exist to estimate energy needs, including indirect calorimetry, bioelectrical impedance, and predictive equations.[31,32] (See Chapter 2 for more information on methods to estimate energy requirements.) Although clinicians generally agree that nutrition interventions are vital in the management of SBS, there is a surprising paucity of data confirming their utility and efficacy. However, several practice principles can guide clinicians in treating patients with SBS.

Oral Nutrition

Most stable adult patients with SBS absorb about one-half to two-thirds of the energy that healthy individuals absorb. Patients who achieve nutrition autonomy from PN or EN may need to increase their dietary intake by at least 50% (and up to 400%) above their estimated needs.[33] The increased quantity of food tends to be best tolerated when consumed throughout the day in 5 or 6 meals. The types of food consumed are also important, as described in the following sections. Table 30-2 summarizes general dietary management principles.

Dietary Macronutrients

Stimulation of the residual bowel with macronutrient exposure is an important part of the adaptive process. Historically, some practitioners believed that use of continuous enteral elemental or semi-elemental nutrition maximized absorption of fluid and nutrients in patients with newly acquired SBS, but it is now accepted that patients with SBS should consume whole food diets and/or use a polymeric formula for maximum intestinal stimulation and adaptation.[29]

TABLE 30-2 Diet Recommendations in Short Bowel Syndrome

	Colon in Continuity	End Jejunostomy	Additional Considerations
Energy	35–45 kcal/kg/d; may need up to 60 kcal/kg/d	35–45 kcal/kg/d; may need up to 60 kcal/kg/d	• Due to hyperphagia, patients may need to eat more than normal (pre-SBS) to compensate for potential nutrient malabsorption. • Eat 5–6 small meals evenly spaced throughout the day.
Carbohydrate	50%–60% of daily energy goal	20%–40% of daily energy goal	• Limit simple sugars. • Include complex carbohydrates (starches).
Protein	1.5–2.0 g/kg/d or 20%–30% of daily energy goal	1.5–2.0 g/kg/d or 20%–30% of daily energy goal	• Choose high-quality, lean protein.
Fat	20%–30% of daily energy goal	40%–60% of daily energy goal	• Patient may need 72-hour fecal fat test if going home on PN. • Choose essential fatty acids as main component of oral fat intake. • May consider MCT oil if patient has fat malabsorption.
Fiber	10–15 g/d (adjust per patient tolerance)	10–15 g/d (adjust per patient tolerance)	• Individuals with stool output >3L/d should have 5–10 g soluble fiber daily.
Fluid	Isotonic/hypotonic	Isotonic/slightly hypotonic, high-sodium ORS	• Separate liquids from solids. • Avoid simple sugars. • Sip throughout the day. • Use commercial or homemade ORS.
Oxalate	Low-oxalate diet	No restriction necessary	• Include high-calcium food or calcium citrate supplement with meals to bind oxalate and alkalinize the urine.
Lactose	Do not restrict if tolerated	Do not restrict if tolerated	• Dairy foods provide protein, calcium, and vitamin D.
Sodium	Encourage liberal use of salt	Encourage liberal use of salt	• Patients experience increased sodium losses.

MCT, medium-chain triglyceride; ORS, oral rehydration solution; PN, parenteral nutrition; SBS, short bowel syndrome.

Carbohydrates

Basic dietary management strategies differ based on the presence or absence of a colon. In a field where few high-quality trials exist, a management strategy for SBS patients with a colon that possesses good supportive evidence is a diet high in complex carbohydrates and starches. In patients with a colon, a diet of complex carbohydrates and starches (50% to 60% of ingested macronutrients) in combination with low-fat foods (20% to 30% of ingested macronutrients) increases the amount of energy absorbed, decreases wet weight lost, may decrease diarrhea, contributes to greater SCFA production in the colon, and shows a higher percentage of absorption by macronutrient status (up to 96% absorption of ingested carbohydrates vs approximately 50% of fats or proteins).[34] This diet also results in a reduction in steatorrhea, oxalate absorption, and magnesium and calcium loss.

In contrast, a high-carbohydrate, low-fat diet in SBS patients without a colon does not seem to improve absorption.[35] As a constant proportion of dietary fat is absorbed in patients with an end jejunostomy, more is absorbed when more is consumed. However, higher fractions of long-chain fats can worsen divalent cation loss (magnesium and calcium) in the stool of patients with end jejunostomies.[22]

In both patients with and without a colon, complex carbohydrates are preferred to simple sugars. Complex carbohydrates, including starches, reduce osmotic load, can be converted to useful energy sources in the colon, and may exert a positive effect on the adaptation process.[36,37] In the intestine, starches are broken down more slowly than simple sugars, thus improving tolerance. A diet high in simple carbohydrates exerts a high osmotic load, pulling water into the lumen, and precipitating increased fluid and nutrient losses.[38] Concentrated sugars, fruit juices, sodas, and some nutrient supplements should be avoided in this patient population. Lactose is generally well tolerated and should not be restricted unless the patient is clearly intolerant, as milk-based products provide an important source of energy and calcium.[22,39]

Colonic Salvage and Soluble Fiber

Soluble fiber (eg, pectin, psyllium) and some starches can be converted to SCFA by colonic bacterial fermentation and used as energy, a process called "colonic salvage."[17] The importance of the colon in contributing to energy needs of patients with SBS has been demonstrated in numerous studies.[34] One study showed a benefit of untreated oat flakes (a source of soluble fiber) in reducing fecal output in some patients with SBS;[40] the effect was not as common among patients with an end ileostomy.[41] The addition of pectin, a source of soluble fiber, can also augment SCFA production in the colon and contribute to colonic salvage of energy.[36]

Protein

Because nitrogen absorption is least affected by the decreased absorptive surface in SBS, dietary protein goals do not generally need to be adjusted. Protein composition should range from 1.5 to 2.0 g/kg or 20% to 30% of the energy goal. The use of peptide-based EN is unnecessary.

Dietary Fats

Because MCTs are absorbed from both the small and large intestine and do not require digestion by pancreatic enzymes for absorption, they may be useful as an alternative energy source in the presence of bile acid or pancreatic insufficiency.[42] However, MCTs are generally not well tolerated in the long term, have a slightly lower energy density than long-chain triglycerides (LCTs) (8.3 vs 9 kcal/g), do not contain essential fatty acids, exert a greater osmotic load in the small bowel, and have less stimulatory effect on adaptation compared with LCTs. The provision of essential fatty acids (linoleic acid [ω-6 fatty acid] and linolenic acid [ω-3 fatty acid]), found in such substances as safflower and soybean oils, is important because deficiencies are common, particularly in the setting of low-fat diets and fat malabsorption.[43] Polyunsaturated fats are a major source of essential fatty acids and should be encouraged.

Oxalate

Nephrolithiasis from calcium oxalate stones can occur in patients with SBS who have an intact colon.[44] To reduce the risk of this complication, patients should consume a diet low in oxalate while maintaining a urine output of more than 1.2 L/d.[26,28,29] Moreover, oral calcium supplements of 800 to 1200 mg/d, in divided doses not exceeding more than 500 mg, can compete with fatty acids to bind oxalate. Patients may find adherence to low-oxalate diets to be difficult, highlighting the importance of longitudinal guidance by multidisciplinary teams.

Oral Hydration

The optimal fluid components of the diet depend on the remaining bowel anatomy (Table 30-3). The osmolality, sodium content, and glucose content of the fluid are important considerations, because inappropriate fluids will exacerbate fluid losses in SBS. *Osmolality* refers to the concentration of particles, molecules, and ions in the fluid. If a fluid is isotonic, it has the same concentration as blood and extracellular fluid (290 to 300 mOsm/L). Hyperosmolar fluids (greater than 350 mOsm/L) are concentrated and pull fluid from enterocytes in an attempt to dilute the luminal contents, thus contributing to a net secretion of fluid and electrolytes and leading to dehydration and diarrhea. For this reason, fruit juices and beverages with concentrated sugars should be restricted. In contrast, hypoosmolar fluids (eg, water, alcohol, tea, coffee) do not contain the sodium or glucose concentrations necessary to optimally facilitate fluid absorption in the small bowel and may also lead to dehydration if consumed in large amounts by a patient with an end jejunostomy.

Fluid is normally secreted into the intestinal lumen during digestion. This fluid is typically isoosmotic with blood because of its increased concentration of sodium. A healthy individual will secrete 20 to 30 g of sodium per day via intestinal secretions. Homeostasis occurs by reabsorption of the sodium by the intestine, and intestinal luminal sodium and

TABLE 30-3 Fluid Recommendations in Short Bowel Syndrome

Type of Fluid	Colon in Continuity	End Jejunostomy	Examples of Fluid Type
Isoosmolar (isotonic)	Patients with <50% of a colon may benefit from ORS.	ORS should be main source of hydration.	• Homemade ORS recipes • Milk • Diluted juice (at least 50% water) • Some enteral formulas • Commercial ORS
Hyperosmolar	Should be avoided.	Should be avoided.	• Fruit juice • Sugar-containing soft drinks and powdered drink mixes • Nutritional supplement beverages (eg, Ensure, Boost, Carnation Instant Breakfast)
Hypo-osmolar	May be tolerated.	Restrict to 4–6 oz/d.	• Water • Sugar-free soft drinks and powdered drink mixes • Decaffeinated tea and coffee

ORS, oral rehydration solution.

glucose play important roles in promoting fluid absorption.[45] Glucose absorption occurs by multiple mechanisms. The first step involves active transport of both glucose and sodium together by the sodium glucose cotransporter (SGLT1). Once inside the enterocyte, glucose is further transported across the basolateral membrane by facilitated glucose transporter type 2 (GLUT2). The sodium gradient is maintained by the sodium-potassium pump in the basolateral membrane of the enterocyte. Therefore, co-ingestion of glucose and sodium in a strict ratio is important for maximizing fluid absorption in the small intestine. This ratio is the basis for oral rehydration solutions (ORS). Because of segmental differences in water and sodium absorption, SBS patients without a colon often require the use of a slightly hypoosmotic (200 to 300 mOsm/L) or isotonic glucose-electrolyte ORS to enhance fluid absorption and reduce secretion. In contrast, most patients with a colon can maintain adequate hydration without excessive fluid loss by ingesting hypotonic fluids.[46] If excessive fluid loss is a problem, the patient may need a glucose-based, slightly low–osmolarity ORS. Use of an ORS will promote fluid absorption, help reduce diarrhea, and optimize hydration status. Importantly, ORS should be used to *maintain* adequate hydration but not used to salvage large fluid losses; therefore, patients are usually advised to consume ORS slowly throughout the day. Patients may need 2 to 3 liters of ORS daily to maintain hydration status. The optimal sodium concentration of ORS to promote jejunal absorption is 90 to 120 mEq Na⁺ per liter.[47] Because this concentration is higher than most traditional beverages, ORS may be unpalatable to patients. Palatability can be improved by starting with a lower volume, usually 1 L/d, and advising patients to sip slowly over the course of the day (Table 30-4). Commercial ORS products are available and may be more palatable than homemade solutions, but they may be too expensive for daily use. It is very important to counsel patients that commercial sport drinks are *not* acceptable substitutes for ORS, as these products usually contain less sodium and more sugar than patients need for enhanced absorption. An additional common misuse of ORS is in patients with high ostomy output. For these patients, the ostomy output must be controlled before ORS is used, as it will simply add to the fluid losses. Whereas a basic ORS contains sodium, chloride, and glucose, the solution can also be enhanced with potassium and magnesium in patients who need supplementation with these electrolytes. An alternative option would be to deliver ORS as a nocturnal infusion, first via a nasogastric tube and then, if the infusion is successful, through a gastrostomy tube.

TABLE 30-4 Tips for Improving Successful Use of Oral Rehydration Solutions

- Start slow. Start with 1 L/d and increase as tolerated.
- Keep ORS chilled.
- Flavor with sugar-free sweeteners or low-sodium broth.
- Sip ORS throughout the day. Drink ORS separately from food.
- ORS may be used as flushes or continuously via an indwelling feeding tube.

ORS, oral rehydration solution.

This option may allow some patients to avoid IV fluids.[27] Additionally, patients should be encouraged to use salt liberally and to ingest solids and liquids separately to avoid increasing the osmolarity of the ingested fluids.[48] See Practice Scenario 30-1 and Chapter 26 for additional information on assessing and maximizing hydration.

Practice Scenario 30-1

Question: How can the hydration status of a patient with short bowel syndrome (SBS) be optimized when he or she already seems to be consuming an abundance of oral fluids?

Scenario: A 53-year-old woman is admitted to the hospital for dehydration. She has a complex past surgical history including pancolonic ulcerative colitis status after a total proctocolectomy with an ileal pouch anal anastomosis. Her health over the years has been complicated by the development of enterocutaneous fistulas and recurrent small bowel obstructions resulting in multiple additional operations, ultimately leaving her with less than 200 cm of small bowel and an end jejunostomy. She has had about 20% unintentional weight loss since her last surgery (current body mass index is 21) and reports high-volume ostomy output and low urine output. She has been advised to increase her fluid intake and use oral nutritional supplements. Prior to admission, she collected 2 days of information regarding her fluid intake, urine output, and ostomy output: fluid intake was greater than 3 L/d; ostomy output was about 4 L/d; and urine output was 200 mL/d.

Intervention: On admission, intravenous (IV) hydration is initiated, oral hypotonic fluids are restricted to 4 to 6 oz/d, and the patient is educated about an appropriate short bowel diet and the use of an oral rehydration solution (ORS). After 72 hours, the IV hydration is discontinued and the patient sips 2.5 liters of ORS (235 mOsm/L; 70 mEq sodium per liter) throughout the day. These maneuvers result in a decrease in ostomy output to less than 2 L/d and an increase in urine output to about 1 L/d.

Answer: Education regarding appropriate food and beverage choices is imperative in all patients with SBS. Limiting hypoosmotic beverages and hyperosmotic food and beverages is important to optimize fluid and nutrient absorption and minimize stool losses in this population. Despite the large volume of fluid and energy ingested by this patient, dehydration and weight loss occurred because of poor food and beverage choices.

Rationale: This patient had been consuming fluids high in sugar. Simple sugars should be limited in the diet of persons with SBS because of their osmotic effect. The osmotic effect refers to the process whereby a substrate load attracts water because of the body's compensatory mechanism to decrease the concentration, thereby resulting in diarrhea in certain clinical circumstances such as SBS. The intake of simple sugars should be restricted in this setting. The risk that hypoosmotic "free" fluid intake will increase fluid loss is high for patients with SBS who do not have a colon. In these patients, the ingestion of free fluids results in net secretion of sodium into the intestinal lumen in an attempt to reach sodium balance. The secretion of fluid follows the sodium, resulting in increased luminal volume and increased stool output. An ORS, which is a high-sodium/low-sugar beverage, may help promote the net absorption of sodium and fluid across the bowel wall, thus limiting stool volume and improving hydration status and urine output. Commercial ORS products are available, as are inexpensive homemade recipes. These ORS solutions are slightly hypoosmotic (200 to 300 mOsm/L), which avoids the detrimental osmotic effects of hyperosmotic fluids and the fluid losses of hypoosmotic "free" fluid intake.

Enteral Nutrition

EN can be a valuable addition to the management strategies of SBS patients, particularly in the adaptation period. A small, randomized crossover trial (N = 15) of EN, oral feeding, or a combination of both in patients with SBS demonstrated increased intestinal absorption when both EN and oral feeding were used compared with oral feeding alone.[49] EN may be initiated during the acute phase following extensive resection or later when attempts to wean the patient off PN have stalled. In the acute setting, the EN rate should be advanced slowly to avoid increased stool output and further aggravation of fluid and electrolyte disturbances. Slow continuous infusion into the stomach, rather than a bolus administration or infusion directly into the small bowel, is advised to maximize intestinal transit time, improve nutrient contact time and absorption, and reduce diarrhea. Overnight tube feeding allows for the maximal use of the gut while enabling normal activities and an oral diet during the day. Use of an isotonic polymeric formula is recommended;[22] however, some patients may need a semi-elemental formula. Elemental formulas should be avoided because of their hypertonicity, expense, and lack of evidence supporting any benefits over standard formulas.[35,50,51] For reasons previously described, fiber-containing formulas may be advantageous in patient with SBS who have an intact colon. Keep in mind that concurrent PN and EN use poses potential challenges, such as increased workload for the patient, fatigue, and insurance coverage issues.

Parenteral Nutrition

Many patients with SBS need PN, but the duration of their need varies based on several factors (Table 30-5 and Practice Scenario 30-2). Intestinal adaptation improves intestinal absorption over time, thus permitting some patients to eventually wean off PN. The anatomy, length, and integrity of residual small bowel are strong predictors of long-term PN need. As mentioned earlier, patients with SBS who have all segments of small bowel and colon in continuity (jejunoileocolonic anastomosis) have the best prognosis and likely need at least 30 cm of residual small bowel to wean off PN.[8] Those with a jejunocolonic anastomosis need at least 60 cm of residual small bowel, and those with an end jejunostomy need at least 100 cm of small bowel. A prognostic biomarker of intestinal function is citrulline, a nonessential amino acid found to correlate with eventual independence from PN when serum levels are greater than 15 to 20 mcmol/L.[52]

TABLE 30-5 Clinical Factors That Predict Likelihood of Eventual Weaning from Parenteral Nutrition

- Retained segments of small bowel
- Length of residual small bowel
- Integrity of residual small bowel
- Presence of a colon
- Presence of an ileum/ileocecal valve
- Absence of residual mucosal disease in the bowel
- Degree to which intestinal adaptation has occurred
- Duration of time on parenteral nutrition
- Nutrition status prior to attempted weaning from parenteral nutrition
- Fasting plasma citrulline level

Practice Scenario 30-2

Question: What is the most appropriate feeding route for a patient with short bowel syndrome (SBS) who has severe malnutrition and failure to thrive and cannot or will not eat?

Scenario: A 20-year-old developmentally delayed woman is evaluated in the gastroenterology clinic for a failure to thrive. Her anthropometric measurements are height 160 cm, weight 31 kg, and body mass index 12. She has a history of SBS following surgical resection of most of her small intestine due to complications that occurred after an appendectomy 1 year ago; she now has approximately 80 cm of small intestine from the ligament of Treitz anastomosed to her ascending colon. She has been advised to eat a high-calorie diet and include extra desserts and snacks to optimize weight gain; however, because of severe diarrhea, she has been avoiding all oral intake. Examination reveals a cachectic woman who appears to be much older than her stated age.

Intervention: The patient is admitted to the hospital where she is evaluated by the nutrition support service. Parenteral nutrition (PN) is initiated along with the appropriate monitoring of electrolytes and hydration status. The patient and her family are educated on an appropriate diet for SBS and fluid goals. She is also started on antidiarrheal and antisecretory agents, which decrease her stool output substantially. However, she continues to refuse to eat for fear of worsening the diarrhea. Therefore, the team decides to also slowly initiate enteral nutrition (EN) via gastrostomy tube.

Answer: PN is the most appropriate initial feeding method in this patient given the severity of her malnutrition and the severe diarrhea that has caused her to avoid oral intake. The addition of EN support may also be useful to facilitate bowel adaptation while the patient is avoiding oral intake and may eventually allow for an easier transition off the PN once the patient's overall condition has improved.

Rationale: PN may meet all energy, hydration, macronutrient, and micronutrient needs while the patient's bowel is undergoing adaptation and the oral diet and medical management program is being optimized. As the patient's symptoms and nutrition status improve, transitioning to an enteral and/or oral diet may allow for the eventual discontinuation of the PN support. In the scenario described, EN may be useful to facilitate bowel adaptation because the patient refuses to eat. Bowel adaptation may occur over 2 or more years and the luminal nutrients provided by the EN are important for improving the mucosal structure and function of the gut. Concomitant EN support is unnecessary or can be discontinued if the patient can consume an adequate oral diet. If the patient were to go home on both EN and PN, the patient's ability to safely receive both forms of nutrition support must be evaluated and approval must be obtained to ensure insurance coverage.

Most commercial insurers cover PN, but Medicare has strict criteria regarding medical necessity for home PN use. To qualify for a diagnosis of SBS, the patient must have a residual small bowel of 5 feet (154.2 cm) or less. Providers must be familiar with reimbursement guidelines to avoid discharge delays and excessive financial burdens for patients who do not meet the strict criteria and thus have their claims retroactively denied. The Medicare Coverage Database (www.cms.gov /medicare-coverage-database) provides detailed information.

Although PN can be initiated in the home setting, most patients with SBS are not medically appropriate for a home start because their fluid and electrolyte needs are tenuous and they are at high risk for refeeding syndrome. Patients usually require 3 to 5 days of inpatient monitoring as they start PN. Most home patients infuse PN for 10 to 12 hours overnight to allow time off during the day to participate in desired activities; therefore, it is common to convert the initial continuous PN infusion to a "cycled" rate prior to discharge. Frequent nocturnal urination can be an uncomfortable adverse effect of nighttime infusions; if this problem occurs, review the PN prescription for potential excess fluid volume and consider lengthening the infusion time. Backpacks to transport the PN solution and the IV pump are also available to allow daytime infusion with increased mobility. See Chapter 38 for additional information about home nutrition support.

After PN is initiated, it should be periodically adjusted to meet the patient's fluid, electrolyte, energy, protein, and micronutrient needs. In the presence of a high ostomy output, fluid, potassium, magnesium, and zinc losses can increase and would need vigilant monitoring and repletion. The amount of PN can be decreased when the patient tolerates oral nutrition without excessive stool or ostomy output and manifests appropriate weight maintenance or gain. When calculating PN volume and content, clinicians should monitor changes in the patient's weight, energy levels, laboratory test data, stool or ostomy output, urine output, and complaints of thirst. As previously noted, the SBS patient on PN remains at risk for micronutrient deficiencies; therefore, micronutrient levels require periodic monitoring and supplementation should be used in addition to PN.[30]

Parenteral Hydration

Occasionally, patients may attain gut autonomy for macronutrients but still require parenteral fluid supplementation despite optimization of diet and ORS supplementation. This scenario is not uncommon in patients with an end jejunostomy, given the jejunum's limited ability to reabsorb fluid and electrolytes. In these patients, parenteral fluids are necessary if the stool output consistently exceeds fluid intake. During the hot summer months, patients receiving PN overnight may also require additional parenteral hydration during the day. The IV fluid is commonly provided as a liter of normal saline infused over a couple of hours once daily as needed. The contents of the fluid may include only sodium chloride, or dextrose, other electrolytes (eg, potassium and magnesium), vitamins, and bicarbonate may occasionally be added.

Psychosocial Support

Patient support groups, such as the Oley Foundation (www .oley.org), are important sources of information on practical topics (eg, body image, travel). Education and support may reduce the risk of complications and enhance survival and the quality of life for the patient receiving either EN or PN support.

Intestinal Rehabilitation

Intestinal rehabilitation emphasizes a combination of nutrition-related and medical strategies to reduce or eliminate the need for PN and intestinal transplantation.[53] Given the need for major dietary, lifestyle, and medication changes to successfully reduce PN dependence, intestinal rehabilitation requires strong motivation and perseverance from patients. Patient education and ongoing support are critical to enhance compliance with the care plan.

Table 30-5 lists several clinical factors useful in predicting whether patients with SBS can eventually wean off PN. From the outset, clinicians should help patients set realistic expectations and goals about the feasibility of partially or completely weaning off PN. Diverse dietary, fluid, and medication strategies should be employed to optimize intestinal absorption before PN weaning begins. Some strategies may include a reduction of meal sizes with an increase in number of meals (while achieving equal or greater total energy intake per day), restriction of fluid intake during meals, reduced consumption of hypertonic fluids, use of ORS for hydration, titration of antidiarrheal medications, and consideration of intestinotrophic agents. Before PN is reduced, patients should also meet certain criteria, including adequate hydration (urine output greater than 1 L/d), ability to consistently consume at least 80% of daily energy goals, weight stability or weight gain, stability of serum electrolyte levels, and positive enteral balance (oral fluid intake minus stool and urine output greater than 500 mL/d) (Table 30-6).[30] PN reductions are typically empirically determined, requiring an iterative series of energy/ volume reductions and follow-up nutrition assessments. PN reductions can occur by modestly decreasing the amount of energy per day, modestly decreasing the overall volume per day (eg, 10%), or reducing the number of days of PN. An optimal interval for evaluating the impact of PN reduction has not been defined. Once every 1 to 2 weeks seems generally appropriate, but the evaluation period needs to be individualized for each patient. If the patient tolerates the PN reduction

TABLE 30-6 Factors to Consider Before Weaning Patients from Parenteral Nutrition

Factor	Criteria to Consider
Hydration	Consider PN reductions only if (1) the patient consistently achieves the daily fluid intake goal; and (2) urine output exceeds 1 L/d and is at least 0.5 mL/kg/h on nights without PN. If urine output cannot be easily measured, serum creatinine, BUN, urine sodium, and osmolarity can be used as surrogate measures of hydration.
Energy goal	The patient should meet at least 80% of the energy goal without symptoms that limit oral intake.
Body weight	The patient should be able to maintain a stable body weight (eg, no more than 1.5 kg loss of body weight between PN reductions).
Laboratory values	Serum electrolytes with or without supplementation should remain stable.
Enteral balance (oral fluid intake minus stool and urine output)	The balance should be positive (>500 mL/d).

BUN, blood urea nitrogen; PN, parenteral nutrition.

and continues to meet the aforementioned criteria, further PN reduction can again be attempted. This process continues until the patient has either discontinued PN or reached a point of nutrition and hydration instability despite optimized intestinal rehabilitation strategies. Although the occasional patient may successfully discontinue PN without the gradual weaning strategy, this approach is not recommended for the patient with SBS who has been receiving PN for an extended period.

Medications

Most medications are absorbed within the first 50 cm of the jejunum and can be used in patients with SBS; however, delayed-release medications should be avoided. The most important medications in the patient with SBS are acid-suppression, antimotility, and antisecretory agents. Patients need histamine type 2 receptor antagonists and proton pump inhibitors soon after extensive intestinal resection to reduce the risk of ulcer development. These medications additionally help reduce the volume of gastric secretions and the detrimental effects of low pH fluid on the function of digestive enzymes.

Antidiarrheal agents work mainly to reduce intestinal motility, but they can also slightly reduce intestinal secretions. Commonly used agents include loperamide, diphenoxylate/atropine, codeine, and tincture of opium. The use of codeine and tincture of opium tends to be limited by their sedating effect, potential for addiction when used long term, and cost. Because of these adverse effects, we typically recommend loperamide and diphenoxylate/atropine as first-line pharmacological agents in SBS. We generally start with loperamide, because diphenoxylate/atropine crosses the blood-brain barrier and possesses anticholinergic effects. Because loperamide enters the enterohepatic circulation, which is disrupted in patients with SBS who do not have an ileum, these patients frequently need high doses of this medication. Patients can be instructed to open loperamide capsules or crush tablets, mix them in sugar-free applesauce, and take them 30 minutes prior to meals and at bedtime. This strategy enhances the absorption of the medication; patients who take whole tablets or capsules often report seeing them in their stool or ostomy bags. In the setting of SBS, these agents seem to be most effective when administered before meals and at bedtime. Loperamide may have synergistic effects with codeine or diphenoxylate/atropine.[54,55]

Clonidine, which can be administered transdermally, may help reduce high-output stool losses via its effects on intestinal motility and secretion.[56] However, its use is limited in clinical practice because of the risk of hypotension and rebound hypertension.

Ox bile supplements and the synthetic conjugated bile acid cholylsarcosine have been investigated as potential agents to improve the depleted bile salt pool without aggravating stool losses, and they have been shown to beneficially affect fat absorption.[57,58] However, these agents are not readily available for use.

The use of bile acid sequestrants, such as cholestyramine, may worsen steatorrhea and fat-soluble vitamin losses in patients with SBS. These medications should generally be avoided.[11]

Pancreatic function is reduced in patients with SBS receiving PN only when there is no concomitant enteral/oral diet and, potentially, during the hypersecretory period if no antisecretory medications are used. There is a theoretical concern that anatomical alterations in SBS would lead to poor mixing of ingested nutrients and endogenous pancreatic enzymes. However, no evidence currently supports the usefulness of pancreatic enzyme supplementation in SBS.

Octreotide reduces the production of a variety of GI secretions and slows jejunal transit.[59] Open-label studies suggest a clinical benefit of both short-acting and long-acting forms of octreotide;[60,61] however, this beneficial effect is often short lasting, and octreotide has not been shown to improve absorption or lead to the elimination of the need for PN. Octreotide increases risk for cholelithiasis, is expensive, and has the potential to inhibit bowel adaptation; therefore, the use of this agent should be reserved for patients with large-volume stool losses in whom fluid and electrolyte management is problematic and refractory to first-line therapies. Octreotide should be avoided in the early adaptation stage.[62]

Patients with SBS, particularly those lacking an ileocecal valve, are at increased risk for developing small intestinal bacterial overgrowth (SIBO), which, in turn, leads to bloating and diarrhea. A brief course of antibiotics (eg, rifaximin) may help improve symptoms. Patients with recurrent SIBO may occasionally need prolonged, rotating courses of antibiotics. Use of probiotics has theoretical benefits, although the supporting evidence is currently sparse.

Trophic Factors

Trophic factors are pharmacological agents developed to maximize intestinal absorption and adaptation, while reducing or eliminating the need for PN. Investigations in humans have focused on the use of trophic substances, such as nutrient (eg, glutamine) and growth factors (eg, growth hormone [GH] and glucagon-like peptide 2 [GLP-2]). Glutamine is an amino acid that is a primary energy source for the enterocyte and has been shown to prevent mucosal atrophy and deterioration of gut permeability in patients receiving PN.[63] In a small, randomized controlled crossover study of patients with SBS, no difference in small bowel morphology, transit time, D-xylose absorption, or stool output was seen.[64] Nevertheless, a synergistic role of glutamine with GH has been suggested. In a prospective randomized controlled study of recombinant human GH and an optimized diet with or without glutamine in 41 PN-dependent patients with SBS (most with colon in continuity), PN requirements were significantly reduced in all groups studied at the end of the 4-week treatment period.[65] However, the extent of reduction was greatest in the group in which GH was administered in addition to the diet, and, 12 weeks later, glutamine and the PN reduction remained significantly diminished in only the GH with the glutamine group. GH is not currently commercially available in the United States.

A GLP-2 analog (teduglutide) is the only drug approved by the US Food and Drug Administration for SBS patients requiring home PN support. In addition to direct structural improvements of the bowel during intestinal adaptation, GLP-2 or teduglutide has improved gastric emptying and intestinal transit, and reduced gastric and bowel secretions in SBS.[55] A randomized controlled study involving 86 patients with SBS receiving home PN compared the efficacy of teduglutide and placebo at reducing more than 20% of PN volume.[66] More participants in the teduglutide arm (63%) than the placebo arm (30%) experienced a reduction in PN use; the mean reductions for the 2 groups were 4.4 and 2.3 liters, respectively. In an extension trial of 52 weeks, only 4 participants (7.7%) achieved independence from home PN. In this study, all but 2 of the participants reported adverse effects, with the most common being headache, nausea, vomiting, and abdominal pain.[67] Patients started on teduglutide need to have stoma sites monitored (because they can increase in size) and colonoscopies performed at baseline and at regular intervals (because of the potential for polyp growth).[55] Teduglutide is contraindicated for patients with a previous history of malignancy because it can potentially stimulate growth of neoplasms.[55]

Glucagon-like peptide 1 (GLP-1) is secreted by the L cells of the ileum and has been potentially linked to intestinal transit through the ileal brake mechanism.[68] In addition, GLP-1 exerts a glucose-dependent insulinotropic effect and lowers blood glucose levels.[68] GLP-1 analogs have been used for the treatment of diabetes. In a small case series, 5 patients with SBS and less than 90 cm of bowel remaining (4 of the patients had colon in continuity) were placed on the GLP-1 agonist exenatide for 1 month. At the end of the 1-month treatment phase, 3 could wean off home PN.[69] In a subsequent small study of 9 patients with SBS, combined GLP-1 and GLP-2 administration had greater additive effects on intestinal absorption than either agent had individually.[70] Establishing the role of GLP-1 in the treatment of patients with SBS will require larger clinical trials.

Surgery

Because additional surgery is likely in many patients with SBS, the goals of subsequent operations should be to preserve as much bowel as possible and maximize the function of the remaining bowel whenever possible. Examples of such operations include surgeries that restore intestinal continuity, relieve obstruction, repair fistulas, and eliminate diseased bowel. Autologous bowel reconstruction refers to nontransplant surgical procedures that attempt to maximize the function of the SBS patient's existing intestines.[71] The choice of surgery is influenced by the existing bowel length, function, and caliber, and can be divided into procedures that optimize function (eg, lengthen, taper) or slow transit (eg, reversed segment). These procedures should only be considered after the initial adaptive period (2 years), when the patient is stable, and nutrition and medical management has been maximized.

Intestinal transplantation may be considered in patients with SBS who have a lifelong need for PN or when complications of PN arise, such as liver disease, loss of vascular access sites, or recurrent episodes of life-threatening catheter sepsis.[72] Intestinal transplantation can be performed in isolation, in combination with liver transplantation, or in combination with transplantation of multiple organs. Outcomes following intestinal transplantation have improved considerably with the development of more potent immunosuppressant medications and improvements in surgical techniques and postoperative care.[2,73] Nevertheless, graft survival rates remain significantly lower than patient survival rates, and a considerable percentage of patients with a functioning graft may still require PN.

References

1. Howard L, Ament M, Fleming CR, Shike M, Steiger E. Current use and clinical outcome of home parenteral and enteral nutrition therapies in the United States. *Gastroenterology*. 1995; 109(2):355–365.
2. Limketkai BN, Orandi BJ, Luo X, Segev DL, Colombel JF. Mortality and rates of graft rejection or failure following intestinal transplantation in patients with vs without Crohn's disease. *Clin Gastroenterol Hepatol*. 2016;14(11):1574–1581.
3. Dabney A, Thompson J, DiBaise J, Sudan D, McBride C. Short bowel syndrome after trauma. *Am J Surg*. 2004;188(6):792–795.
4. Scott NA, Leinhardt DJ, O'Hanrahan T, Finnegan S, Shaffer JL, Irving MH. Spectrum of intestinal failure in a specialised unit. *Lancet*. 1991;337(8739):471–473.
5. Lal S, Teubner A, Shaffer JL. Review article: intestinal failure. *Aliment Pharmacol Ther*. 2006;24(1):19–31.

6. Underhill BM. Intestinal length in man. *BMJ.* 1955;2(4950): 1243–1246.

7. Helander HF, Fandriks L. Surface area of the digestive tract— revisited. *Scand J Gastroenterol.* 2014;49(6):681–689.

8. Messing B, Crenn P, Beau P, et al. Long-term survival and parenteral nutrition dependence in adult patients with the short bowel syndrome. *Gastroenterology.* 1999;117(5):1043–1050.

9. Borgstrom B, Dahlqvist A, Lundh G, Sjovall J. Studies of intestinal digestion and absorption in the human. *J Clin Invest.* 1957; 36(10):1521–1536.

10. Fordtran JS, Rector FC, Jr., Carter NW. The mechanisms of sodium absorption in the human small intestine. *J Clin Invest.* 1968;47(4):884–900.

11. Hofmann AF, Poley JR. Role of bile acid malabsorption in pathogenesis of diarrhea and steatorrhea in patients with ileal resection. I. Response to cholestyramine or replacement of dietary long chain triglyceride by medium chain triglyceride. *Gastroenterology.* 1972;62(5):918–934.

12. Williams NS, Evans P, King RF. Gastric acid secretion and gastrin production in the short bowel syndrome. *Gut.* 1985;26(9): 914–919.

13. Cortot A, Fleming CR, Malagelada JR. Improved nutrient absorption after cimetidine in short-bowel syndrome with gastric hypersecretion. *N Engl J Med.* 1979;300(2):79–80.

14. Fich A, Steadman CJ, Phillips SF, et al. Ileocolonic transit does not change after right hemicolectomy. *Gastroenterology.* 1992; 103(3):794–799.

15. Nightingale JM, Kamm MA, van der Sijp JR, et al. Gastrointestinal hormones in short bowel syndrome. Peptide YY may be the "colonic brake" to gastric emptying. *Gut.* 1996;39(2):267–272.

16. Pironi L, Stanghellini V, Miglioli M, et al. Fat-induced ileal brake in humans: a dose-dependent phenomenon correlated to the plasma levels of peptide YY. *Gastroenterology.* 1993;105(3):733–739.

17. Nordgaard I, Hansen BS, Mortensen PB. Importance of colonic support for energy absorption as small-bowel failure proceeds. *Am J Clin Nutr.* 1996;64(2):222–231.

18. Horton R, Biglieri EG. Effect of aldosterone on the metabolism of magnesium. *J Clin Endocrinol Metab.* 1962;22:1187–1192.

19. Anast CS, Winnacker JL, Forte LR, Burns TW. Impaired release of parathyroid hormone in magnesium deficiency. *J Clin Endocrinol Metab.* 1976;42(4):707–717.

20. Booth CC. The metabolic effects of intestinal resection in man. *Postgrad Med J.* 1961;37:725–739.

21. Buchman AL, Iyer K, Fryer J. Parenteral nutrition-associated liver disease and the role for isolated intestine and intestine/liver transplantation. *Hepatology.* 2006;43(1):9–19.

22. Pironi L, Arends J, Bozzetti F, et al. ESPEN guidelines on chronic intestinal failure in adults. *Clin Nutr.* 2016;35(2):247–307.

23. Howard L, Malone M. Current status of home parenteral nutrition in the United States. *Transplant Proc.* 1996;28(5):2691–2695.

24. Matarese LE, Steiger E. Dietary and medical management of short bowel syndrome in adult patients. *J Clin Gastroenterol.* 2006;40(Suppl 2):S85–S93.

25. Nightingale JM, Bartram CI, Lennard-Jones JE. Length of residual small bowel after partial resection: correlation between radiographic and surgical measurements. *Gastrointest Radiol.* 1991; 16(4):305–306.

26. Sundaram A, Koutkia P, Apovian CM. Nutritional management of short bowel syndrome in adults. *J Clin Gastroenterol.* 2002;34(3):207–220.

27. Nauth J, Chang CW, Mobarhan S, et al. A therapeutic approach to wean total parenteral nutrition in the management of short bowel syndrome: three cases using nocturnal enteral rehydration. *Nutr Rev.* 2004;62(5):221–231.

28. Bambach CP, Robertson WG, Peacock M, Hill GL. Effect of intestinal surgery on the risk of urinary stone formation. *Gut.* 1981;22(4):257–263.

29. Wilmore DW. Indications for specific therapy in the rehabilitation of patients with the short-bowel syndrome. *Best Pract Res Clin Gastroenterol.* 2003;17(6):895–906.

30. DiBaise JK, Matarese LE, Messing B, Steiger E. Strategies for parenteral nutrition weaning in adult patients with short bowel syndrome. *J Clin Gastroenterol.* 2006;40(Suppl 2):S94–S98.

31. Skallerup A, Nygaard L, Olesen SS, et al. Can we rely on predicted basal metabolic rate in patients with intestinal failure on home parenteral nutrition? *JPEN J Parenter Enteral Nutr.* 29 2016.

32. Lawinski M, Singer P, Gradowski L, et al. Predicted versus measured resting energy expenditure in patients requiring home parenteral nutrition. *Nutrition.* 2015;31(11–12):1328–1332.

33. Jeppesen PB, Mortensen PB. Intestinal failure defined by measurements of intestinal energy and wet weight absorption. *Gut.* 2000;46(5):701–706.

34. Nordgaard I, Hansen BS, Mortensen PB. Colon as a digestive organ in patients with short bowel. *Lancet.* 1994;343(8894):373–376.

35. McIntyre PB, Fitchew M, Lennard-Jones JE. Patients with a high jejunostomy do not need a special diet. *Gastroenterology.* 1986; 91(1):25–33.

36. Atia A, Girard-Pipau F, Hebuterne X, et al. Macronutrient absorption characteristics in humans with short bowel syndrome and jejunocolonic anastomosis: starch is the most important carbohydrate substrate, although pectin supplementation may modestly enhance short chain fatty acid production and fluid absorption. *JPEN J Parenter Enteral Nutr.* 2011;35(2):229–240.

37. Tappenden KA. Mechanisms of enteral nutrient-enhanced intestinal adaptation. *Gastroenterology.* 2006;130(2 Suppl 1):S93–99.

38. Barrett JS, Gearry RB, Muir JG, et al. Dietary poorly absorbed, short-chain carbohydrates increase delivery of water and fermentable substrates to the proximal colon. *Aliment Pharmacol Ther.* 2010;31(8):874–882.

39. Arrigoni E, Marteau P, Briet F, et al. Tolerance and absorption of lactose from milk and yogurt during short-bowel syndrome in humans. *Am J Clin Nutr.* 1994;60(6):926–929.

40. Pagoldh M, Eriksson A, Heimtun E, et al. Effects of a supplementary diet with specially processed cereals in patients with short bowel syndrome. *Eur J Gastroenterol Hepatol.* 2008;20(11): 1085–1093.

41. Jeppesen PB, Mortensen PB. Significance of a preserved colon for parenteral energy requirements in patients receiving home parenteral nutrition. *Scand J Gastroenterol.* 1998;33(11):1175–1179.

42. Jeppesen PB, Mortensen PB. The influence of a preserved colon on the absorption of medium chain fat in patients with small bowel resection. *Gut.* 1998;43(4):478–483.

43. Jeppesen PB, Hoy CE, Mortensen PB. Deficiencies of essential fatty acids, vitamin A and E and changes in plasma lipoproteins in patients with reduced fat absorption or intestinal failure. *Eur J Clin Nutr.* 2000;54(8):632–642.

44. Nightingale JM, Lennard-Jones JE, Gertner DJ, Wood SR, Bartram CI. Colonic preservation reduces need for parenteral therapy, increases incidence of renal stones, but does not change high prevalence of gall stones in patients with a short bowel. *Gut.* 1992;33(11):1493–1497.

45. Lin R, Murtazina R, Cha B, et al. D-glucose acts via sodium/ glucose cotransporter 1 to increase NHE3 in mouse jejunal brush border by a Na$^+$/H$^+$ exchange regulatory factor 2-dependent process. *Gastroenterology.* 2011;140(2):560–571.

46. Matarese LE, O'Keefe SJ, Kandil HM, et al. Short bowel syndrome: clinical guidelines for nutrition management. *Nutr Clin Pract.* 2005;20(5):493–502.

47. Sladen GE, Dawson AM. Interrelationships between the absorptions of glucose, sodium and water by the normal human jejunum. *Clin Sci.* 1969;36(1):119–132.

48. Nightingale JM, Lennard-Jones JE, Walker ER, Farthing MJ. Oral salt supplements to compensate for jejunostomy losses: comparison of sodium chloride capsules, glucose electrolyte solution, and glucose polymer electrolyte solution. *Gut.* 1992;33(6):759–761.

49. Joly F, Dray X, Corcos O, Barbot L, Kapel N, Messing B. Tube feeding improves intestinal absorption in short bowel syndrome patients. *Gastroenterology.* 2009;136(3):824–831.

50. Levy E, Frileux P, Sandrucci S, et al. Continuous enteral nutrition during the early adaptive stage of the short bowel syndrome. *Br J Surg.* 1988;75(6):549–553.

51. Bosaeus I, Carlsson NG, Andersson H. Low-fat versus medium-fat enteral diets. Effects on bile salt excretion in jejunostomy patients. *Scand J Gastroenterol.* 1986;21(7):891–896.

52. Fitzgibbons S, Ching YA, Valim C, et al. Relationship between serum citrulline levels and progression to parenteral nutrition independence in children with short bowel syndrome. *J Pediatr Surg.* 2009;44(5):928–932.

53. DiBaise JK, Young RJ, Vanderhoof JA. Intestinal rehabilitation and the short bowel syndrome: part 2. *Am J Gastroenterol.* 2004;99(9):1823–1832.

54. King RF, Norton T, Hill GL. A double-blind crossover study of the effect of loperamide hydrochloride and codeine phosphate on ileostomy output. *Aust N Z J Surg.* 1982;52(2):121–124.

55. Bechtold ML, McClave SA, Palmer LB, et al. The pharmacologic treatment of short bowel syndrome: new tricks and novel agents. *Curr Gastroenterol Rep.* 2014;16(7):392.

56. Buchman AL, Fryer J, Wallin A, et al. Clonidine reduces diarrhea and sodium loss in patients with proximal jejunostomy: a controlled study. *JPEN J Parenter Enteral Nutr.* 2006;30(6):487–491.

57. Little KH, Schiller LR, Bilhartz LE, Fordtran JS. Treatment of severe steatorrhea with ox bile in an ileectomy patient with residual colon. *Dig Dis Sci.* 1992;37(6):929–933.

58. Heydorn S, Jeppesen PB, Mortensen PB. Bile acid replacement therapy with cholylsarcosine for short-bowel syndrome. *Scand J Gastroenterol.* 1999;34(8):818–823.

59. Ladefoged K, Christensen KC, Hegnhoj J, Jarnum S. Effect of a long acting somatostatin analogue SMS 201-995 on jejunostomy effluents in patients with severe short bowel syndrome. *Gut.* 1989;30(7):943–949.

60. Nehra V, Camilleri M, Burton D, Oenning L, Kelly DG. An open trial of octreotide long-acting release in the management of short bowel syndrome. *Am J Gastroenterol.* 2001;96(5):1494–1498.

61. O'Keefe SJ, Haymond MW, Bennet WM, et al. Long-acting somatostatin analogue therapy and protein metabolism in patients with jejunostomies. *Gastroenterology.* 1994;107(2):379–388.

62. Sukhotnik I, Khateeb K, Krausz MM, et al. Sandostatin impairs postresection intestinal adaptation in a rat model of short bowel syndrome. *Dig Dis Sci.* 2002;47(9):2095–2102.

63. van der Hulst RR, van Kreel BK, von Meyenfeldt MF, et al. Glutamine and the preservation of gut integrity. *Lancet.* 1993;341(8857):1363–1365.

64. Scolapio JS, McGreevy K, Tennyson GS, Burnett OL. Effect of glutamine in short-bowel syndrome. *Clin Nutr.* 2001;20(4):319–323.

65. Byrne TA, Wilmore DW, Iyer K, et al. Growth hormone, glutamine, and an optimal diet reduces parenteral nutrition in patients with short bowel syndrome: a prospective, randomized, placebo-controlled, double-blind clinical trial. *Ann Surg.* 2005;242(5):655–661.

66. Jeppesen PB, Pertkiewicz M, Messing B, et al. Teduglutide reduces need for parenteral support among patients with short bowel syndrome with intestinal failure. *Gastroenterology.* 2012;143(6):1473–1481, e1473.

67. O'Keefe SJ, Jeppesen PB, Gilroy R, et al. Safety and efficacy of teduglutide after 52 weeks of treatment in patients with short bowel intestinal failure. *Clin Gastroenterol Hepatol.* 2013;11(7):815–823, e811–813.

68. Schirra J, Goke B. The physiological role of GLP-1 in human: incretin, ileal brake or more? *Regul Pept.* 2005;128(2):109–115.

69. Kunkel D, Basseri B, Low K, et al. Efficacy of the glucagon-like peptide-1 agonist exenatide in the treatment of short bowel syndrome. *Neurogastroenterol Motil.* 2011;23(8):739–e328.

70. Madsen KB, Askov-Hansen C, Naimi RM, et al. Acute effects of continuous infusions of glucagon-like peptide (GLP)-1, GLP-2 and the combination (GLP-1+GLP-2) on intestinal absorption in short bowel syndrome (SBS) patients. A placebo-controlled study. *Regul Pept.* 2013;184:30–39.

71. Hommel MJ, van Baren R, Haveman JW. Surgical management and autologous intestinal reconstruction in short bowel syndrome. *Best Pract Res Clin Gastroenterol.* 2016;30(2):263–280.

72. Buchman AL, Scolapio J, Fryer J. AGA technical review on short bowel syndrome and intestinal transplantation. *Gastroenterology.* 2003;124(4):1111–1134.

73. Smith JM, Skeans MA, Horslen SP, et al. OPTN/SRTR 2013 annual data report: intestine. *Am J Transplant.* 2015;15(Suppl 2):S1–S16.

31 Solid Organ Transplantation

Jeanette M. Hasse, PhD, RD, LD, FADA, CNSC,
and Laura E. Matarese, PhD, RDN, LDN, FADA, CNSC, FASPEN, FAND

CONTENTS

Objectives

1. Differentiate nutrition goals of the pre- and posttransplant phases.
2. Evaluate nutrition alterations associated with patients who have undergone solid organ transplantation.
3. Assess nutrition implications of immunosuppression.
4. Illustrate how posttransplant complications influence nutrient needs and options for the delivery of nutrition support.

Test Your Knowledge Questions

1. Which of the following is a contraindication for organ transplantation?
   A. Diabetes mellitus
   B. End-stage organ failure
   C. Active infection
   D. History of substance abuse

2. Which of the following immunosuppressive agents is nephrotoxic and can cause hyperkalemia, hypomagnesemia, and hyperglycemia?
   A. Sirolimus
   B. Prednisone
   C. Tacrolimus
   D. Mycophenolate mofetil
3. Which of the following best describes nutrient requirements during the acute posttransplant phase?
   A. Moderate energy, high protein
   B. High energy, low protein
   C. Moderate energy, low protein
   D. High energy, high protein
4. Which of the following should be part of a nutrition care plan for a patient during an acute rejection episode that is being treated with high-dose corticosteroids?
   A. Provide increased amounts of dietary carbohydrate and monitor for signs of fluid overload.
   B. Provide increased amounts of dietary fat and monitor for signs of hyperlipidemia.
   C. Provide increased amounts of dietary carbohydrate and monitor for signs of azotemia.
   D. Provide increased amounts of dietary protein and monitor for signs of hyperglycemia.

Test Your Knowledge Answers

1. The correct answer is **C**. A significant, active infection such as pneumonia is likely to worsen after transplantation once immunosuppression is initiated. Diabetes mellitus is not by itself contraindication for transplantation. In fact, diabetes mellitus is the indication for pancreas transplantation. However, if a potential transplant candidate has diabetes that is not well controlled, transplantation could be denied based on the transplant selection committee's criteria until glucose control is improved. End-stage organ failure that is not amenable to further medical or surgical treatment is an indication for transplantation. Finally, although active substance abuse is a contraindication for transplantation, transplantation may be considered if a candidate has demonstrated recovery.
2. The correct answer is **C**. In addition to these side effects, tacrolimus may also cause neurologic symptoms. The main metabolic effect of sirolimus is hyperlipidemia. Corticosteroids, such as prednisone, contribute to hyperglycemia but are not nephrotoxic and do not affect serum magnesium levels. The major nutrition-related side effects of mycophenolate mofetil are gastrointestinal (GI) side effects, including nausea, vomiting, and diarrhea.
3. The correct answer is **A**. Energy needs are only moderately elevated after transplantation unless complications such as sepsis occur. Protein requirements are significantly elevated due to an increased catabolic rate caused by surgery, stress, and corticosteroids.
4. The correct answer is **D**. Because corticosteroids accelerate the rate of protein catabolism, it is essential to provide adequate protein to reduce nitrogen loss. Hyperglycemia is also a common side effect of high-dose corticosteroids.

Hyperlipidemia is a long-term side effect of corticosteroids but is not usually a short-term complication.

Overview

Prevalence of Organ Transplantation

The field of organ transplantation continues to expand as the number of transplants performed increases each year, new medical advances are achieved, and the survival rate of recipients improves. Transplantation of organs such as the kidney, liver, pancreas, heart, lung, and intestine give recipients a second chance at life. According to the United Network of Organ Sharing (UNOS), the number of organ transplants in the United States increased from 15,001 in 1990 to 33,610 in 2016.[1] As of July 2017, there were 342 transplant centers in the United States and 117,175 individuals waiting for transplants.[1] Because of a limited supply of deceased donor organs, living donors comprised 18% of donors in 2016. Unfortunately, the number of individuals waiting for organ transplantation continues to exceed the number of those who undergo transplantation.

Indications for Organ Transplantation

Organ transplantation is indicated for individuals with decompensated end-stage organ failure. For recipients of liver, heart, and lung transplants, transplantation is lifesaving. Dialysis, insulin therapy, and parenteral nutrition (PN) are alternative treatments for patients with renal, pancreatic, and intestinal failure, respectively. Some patients with these ailments may develop life-threatening complications such as loss of dialysis or PN intravenous (IV) access. For these patients, the benefits of transplantation must outweigh the risks of continuing medical therapy, the surgical procedure, and long-term immunosuppression. In addition, transplantation should be expected to result in a longer lifetime for a transplant recipient than for patients without a transplant.

Contraindications for Organ Transplantation

Not all individuals with organ failure are transplant candidates. Contraindications for transplantation include active or latent infection, sepsis, malignancy (individuals with some primary liver malignancies that are confined to the liver are acceptable for liver transplantation), multisystem organ failure, active substance abuse, advanced age, frailty, severe obesity, active psychiatric or psychological pathology, lack of any social support posttransplant, or other systemic illnesses with a poor prognosis. Absolute contraindications are those factors that cannot be reversed and would never allow a patient to be a transplant candidate. For example, a patient with irreversible systemic illness would not be a transplant candidate. Other contraindications are considered relative if that factor by itself does not exclude a patient for transplantation or if that complication can be corrected or reversed. For example, each center determines body mass index (BMI) limitations for transplantation, but transplant selection committees typically take into consideration additional risk factors such as age, diabetes history, activity level, and other disease states when determining whether BMI will exclude a patient from transplantation. If other contraindications (eg, infection, frailty, lack of social support) could be reversed with treatment or interventions, the patient would be eligible for transplantation once those factors were corrected or eliminated.

Immunosuppression and Nutrition Side Effects

The introduction of effective immunosuppressive drugs revolutionized the field of transplantation and allowed for prolonged patient and graft survival. There are multiple immunosuppressive medications that can be used in combination to prevent and treat rejection. Some side effects of these drugs may affect nutrient intake or use (Table 31-1).[2,3] It is important to note interactions between immunosuppressive drugs and specific foods. Grapefruit, pomegranate, seville oranges, and star fruit are inhibitors of the cytochrome P450 3A4 pathway and can result in elevated concentrations of cyclosporine, tacrolimus, and sirolimus. For this reason, transplant recipients taking these medications should avoid those foods.

Phases of Transplantation and Associated Nutrition Implications

There are 3 main phases of transplantation: pretransplant, acute posttransplant, and chronic posttransplant. Each phase is characterized by its own medical and nutrition goals.

TABLE 31-1 Immunosuppressive Medications and Side Effects

Drug	Action	Side Effects
Calcineurin inhibitors		
Cyclosporine	• Inhibits cell-mediated immunity; inhibits T cell proliferation • Suppresses IL-2 production • Prevents γ-IFN release	• Gingival hyperplasia • Hirsutism • Hyperglycemia • Hyperkalemia • Hyperlipidemia • Hypertension • Hypomagnesemia • Nephrotoxicity • Neurotoxicity
Tacrolimus	• Suppresses T cell–mediated immunity and IL-2 production	• Alopecia • Hyperglycemia • Hyperkalemia • Hypertension • Hypomagnesemia • Nephrotoxicity • Neurotoxicity
Antimetabolites		
Azathioprine	• Interrupts DNA synthesis phase of lymphocyte proliferation	• Alopecia • Liver toxicity • Macrocytic anemia • Nausea, vomiting • Pancreatitis • Pancytopenia
Mycophenolate mofetil, mycophenolic acid	• Inhibits DNA synthesis and lymphocyte production • Inhibits antibody formation	• Cytopenia • Diarrhea, nausea, vomiting
mTOR Inhibitors		
Sirolimus	• Blocks the response of T cell and B cell activation by cytokines, which prevent cell-cycle progression and proliferation	• Aphthous ulcers • Delayed wound healing • Gastrointestinal disorders • Hyperlipidemia • Leukopenia • Pneumonitis

(continued)

TABLE 31-1 Immunosuppressive Medications and Side Effects *(continued)*

Drug	Action	Side Effects
Everolimus	• Blocks response to cytokine stimulation and thus reduces lymphocyte activation and proliferation	• Angioedema • Cytopenia • Delayed wound healing • GI distress • Hepatotoxicity • Hyperlipidemia • Hypertension • Infection • Mucositis/stomatitis • Nephrotoxicity • Peripheral edema • Pneumonitis
Corticosteroids		
Methylprednisolone, prednisone	• Have anti-inflammatory properties • Inhibit cell-mediated and, to a lesser degree, humoral immunity • Inhibit lymphocyte proliferation • Inhibit lymphokine production	• Adrenal insufficiency • Avascular necrosis of bone • Cataracts, glaucoma • Cushingoid features • Hyperglycemia • Hyperphagia • Hypertension • Impaired wound healing and increased infection risk • Mood disturbances • Osteoporosis • Peptic ulcer, GI bleed • Proximal myopathy • Psychosis • Sodium retention
Costimulation blockades		
Belatacept	• Binds to B7-1/B7-2 cells, blocking their ability to interact with CD28 and creating a negative inhibition on immune response	• Minimal side effects
Antibodies		
ATG	• Binds with lymphocytes, resulting in phagocytosis • Inhibits and destroys lymphocytes	• Fever and chills • Increased risk of infection, profound leukopenia, thrombocytopenia
Basiliximab	• Acts against the IL-2R-α chain (CD25) on activated T lymphocytes, and inhibits IL-2–mediated activation of lymphocytes	• Bronchospasm • Hypersensitivity reaction • Hypotension • Pulmonary edema • Tachycardia
Rituximab	• Targets and lyses B cells by binding to CD20	• Neutropenia • Thrombocytopenia
Alemtuzumab	• Targets CD52, a receptor on many immune cells	• Fever, chills • Flu-like symptoms • Pancytopenia

ATG, antithymocyte globulin; GI, gastrointestinal; IFN, interferon; IL, interleukin; mTOR, mammalian target of rapamycin.
Source: Data are from references 2 and 3.

Pretransplant Phase

The main goal of the pretransplant phase is to optimize the patient's condition to allow transplantation to be performed. One aspect of managing symptoms of end-stage organ failure is to provide appropriate medications to manage symptoms. Surgery or interventional procedures may be required; examples include placement of access for hemodialysis, vascular shunts to treat complications of portal hypertension, or ventricular assistance devices as a bridge to heart transplant. In the case of intestinal and multivisceral transplantation, the surgeon may resect diseased bowel to relieve pain until the donor organs become available and reduce the potential for further complications such as obstructions or infection.

The patient's nutrition status should be optimized during this period. There are 3 major nutrition goals during the pretransplant phase. First, the patient's nutrition status must be maintained or improved. Many patients awaiting transplantation are malnourished. Malnourished patients tend to have increased rates of posttransplant morbidity and mortality as well as longer hospital stays compared with well-nourished recipients.[4-13] Practice Scenario 31-1 highlights the etiology and treatment of pretransplant malnutrition.

Practice Scenario 31-1

Question: What conditions contribute to malnutrition in a transplant candidate?

Scenario: A 55-year-old man with ischemic cardiomyopathy is awaiting heart transplantation. His condition deteriorates, requiring admission to a cardiac intensive care unit. He receives continuous intravenous infusions of milrinone and dobutamine. He is upgraded to Status IA (highest priority) for a heart transplant. The patient has experienced a loss of 15% of his usual body weight over a 4- to 6-month period due to anorexia, early satiety, and persistent nausea. However, he has recently gained 10 pounds because of fluid retention. His serum sodium level is 132 mEq/L (normal range: 135 to 145 mEq/L), and his potassium level is 3.4 mEq/L (normal range: 3.5 to 5 mEq/L).

Intervention: A 2-g sodium diet is prescribed as well as potassium supplementation and anti-emetic medications. Despite addition of high-calorie, high-protein oral supplements, a calorie count indicates that the patient is only eating approximately 900 kcal and 40 g protein per day and he complains of ongoing nausea and intermittent vomiting. Because his estimated needs are 2000 kcal and 85 g protein per day, a nasointestinal tube is placed and a 2 kcal/mL formula is initiated at 20 mL per hour continuously. Daily tests of serum levels of potassium, magnesium, and phosphorus are ordered, and these electrolytes are supplemented as needed. In addition, multivitamin supplementation is initiated.

Answer: The cause of malnutrition in a transplant candidate is multifactorial. It can be caused by reduced intake (due to anorexia, early satiety, nausea and vomiting, taste changes, poor dentition, limited food availability, severe diet restrictions), increased needs

(due to acute or chronic illness), altered metabolism, or increased losses (e.g., frequent paracentesis, steatorrhea). In this case, the patient was unable to eat adequately despite being provided with additional food choices and supplements. A postpyloric feeding tube was chosen because of his history of persistent nausea and vomiting. Initiation of inotropes may improve gut perfusion and reduce gastrointestinal symptoms allowing gastric tube feedings. Sodium restriction and concentrated tube-feeding formula were chosen interventions because of the fluid retention and mild hyponatremia. Because the patient was malnourished, refeeding syndrome was suspected, so the tube feeding was advanced slowly and electrolytes were supplemented when serum levels were low. In addition to increased thiamin needs in the face of refeeding, patients receiving diuretic therapy (as with heart failure) are also at increased risk for thiamin deficiency requiring supplementation, in this case with a multivitamin.

Rationale: Patients with end-stage organ failure have many risk factors that can cause malnutrition. Early identification and treatment of these factors can help prevent deterioration of nutrition status. Aggressive nutrition interventions are warranted because of the adverse effect that malnutrition can have on posttransplant outcomes. Treatment of nutrition-related conditions (such as fluid retention, hyponatremia, and refeeding syndrome in this scenario) helps keep patients in an optimal condition for transplant.

The prevalence of obesity among transplant candidates is on the rise. While pretransplant obesity can adversely affect posttransplant outcomes,[14] there is some controversy as to whether obesity should preclude a patient from transplantation. Some transplant programs set upper weight limits whereby candidates may need to lose weight to be accepted for transplantation.

The effect of obesity on transplantation risks is specific to the type of transplanted organ. With regards to kidney transplantation, obese kidney transplant recipients tend to have more wound complications compared with nonobese transplant recipients.[15-18] Obesity has been linked to hyperlipidemia and coronary events post–kidney transplantation.[19] Some studies suggest that obesity is associated with delayed kidney graft function[20-22] or decreased graft survival.[21,22] However, other reports have not shown that obesity affects kidney graft survival.[17,18,23-25]

Obese patients undergoing pancreas transplant have also been shown to have complications. Some studies have demonstrated that obese pancreas recipients have a greater incidence of thrombosis of the pancreas allograft in addition to overall surgical and infectious complications vs nonobese patients.[26-28] In a large retrospective study, Bédat and colleagues investigated more than 21,000 pancreas transplant patients and concluded that obesity increased 90-day graft loss and short-term mortality. Obesity also increased long-term graft failure; however, underweight, not obesity, increased long-term mortality.[29]

In lung transplant recipients, obesity has been associated with an increased rate of posttransplant mortality.[4,30] A study of 5978 lung transplant recipients concluded that being either underweight or overweight adversely affects patient outcomes.[30] Likewise, obese cardiac transplant recipients are often reported to have reduced long-term survival and higher rates of rejection, coronary artery disease, postoperative infections, renal complications, and diabetes mellitus vs nonobese recipients.[31,32] However, not all studies have linked obesity with reduced survival, infection, or rejection in heart transplant recipients.[33]

In single-center studies of liver transplant recipients, results have been mixed with regard to the effect of pretransplant obesity on posttransplant outcomes. Several studies have analyzed transplant-specific databases to evaluate the effect of obesity in large cohorts. In one study that evaluated graft and patient survival in 23,675 liver transplants performed during a 9-year period from the UNOS database, obesity was associated with reduced long-term survival, mainly as a result of cardiovascular events.[34] Another study evaluating UNOS data in over 73,000 liver transplant patients concluded that body weight extremes (BMI less than 18.5 or equal to or greater than 40) adversely affect survival.[35] Bambha and associates determined in more than 45,000 patients that being overweight or obese did not affect patient or graft survival, but a BMI less than 18.5 in the presence of a low Model for End-Stage Liver Disease (MELD) score increased graft loss and patient mortality.[36] Similarly, Wong and colleagues analyzed results of more than 57,000 patients and determined that obesity did not affect survival; instead, diabetes mellitus with or without obesity adversely affected survival.[37] Finally, in a meta-analysis involving 72,212 nonobese and 2275 obese liver transplant recipients Saab and coauthors found no difference in obese vs nonobese survival rates.[38] However, when Saab et al categorized the cohorts of obese and nonobese patients and analyzed them according to diagnosis, obesity did reduce survival rates.[38]

Obesity is just one factor in determining transplant candidacy. Obese patients accepted for transplantation are generally free from multiple other comorbidities. Considering the careful selection of these obese patients, transplantation still seems to confer a survival benefit at least in kidney and liver transplantation when compared with waiting list mortality.[39–41] Recommendations are generally to (1) encourage weight loss in obese patients waiting for a transplant, (2) closely evaluate cardiovascular status in obese patients before transplantation, and (3) consider corticosteroid-withdrawal strategies after transplantation to reduce weight gain. Some centers may consider bariatric surgery as a weight loss option for morbidly obese transplant candidates or recipients, but there is no consensus on the role of bariatric surgery in this population. Enforcing quick weight loss in patients needing to lose weight to qualify for transplantation can exacerbate sarcopenia and actually increase transplant risk. Clinicians on the transplant team should consider collaborating with other services such as physical therapy to create a plan to help patients maintain optimal muscle stores during weight loss.

A second pretransplant goal is to provide appropriate nutrition therapy to help alleviate complications due to organ failure. For example, sodium restriction will help reduce fluid retention, potassium restriction treats hyperkalemia, and calcium and vitamin D supplementation may be necessary to prevent bone loss. Refer to Chapters 25, 27, 29, 30, and 34 for specific guidelines on medical nutrition therapy

for pulmonary failure, liver disease, renal disease, short bowel syndrome, and diabetes, respectively. See Practice Scenario 31-2 for an example of nutrition support required before combined liver and intestinal transplantation.

Practice Scenario 31-2

Question: What is the nutrition goal during the preoperative phase of a patient undergoing a combined liver and intestinal transplantation?

Scenario: The patient is a 45-year-old man with a past surgical history of Roux-en-Y bariatric surgery for morbid obesity 12 years ago. The patient had been noncompliant with his prescribed medications and vitamin supplementation. He presented to the emergency department with severe abdominal pain and was taken to the operating room where he had a resection of most of his remnant bowel due to small bowel volvulus with resulting ischemia. He currently has 40 cm of remaining small bowel ending in a jejunostomy. He was placed on parenteral nutrition (PN) for 16 months with aggressive micronutrient repletion and subsequently had several line-related infections with multiple new lines replaced. He also developed PN-associated liver disease, cirrhosis, and severe jaundice. The pretransplant liver biopsy demonstrated steatohepatitis and portal pericellular bridging fibrosis.

On examination, the patient is severely jaundiced and exhibits moderate-to-severe muscle wasting and deficits of adipose tissue. There is no lymphadenopathy. The chest is clear to auscultation bilaterally. The abdomen shows splenomegaly. The liver is felt off the costal margin and is irregular and slightly firm. There are hyperactive bowel sounds. Extremities are without edema. His height is 187.9 cm, and he weighs 72 kg. His serum laboratory values are as follows, with normal values shown parenthetically:

- Total bilirubin: 15.3 mg/dL (0.1–1.9 mg/dL)
- Alanine aminotransferase (ALT): 559 IU/L (8–37 IU/L)
- Aspartate aminotransferase (AST): 438 IU/L (10–34 IU/L)
- Alkaline phosphatase: 149 IU/L (44–147 IU/L)
- Gamma-glutamyl transpeptidase (GGT): 160 IU/L (0–51 IU/L)
- Sodium: 137 mEq/L (136–144 mEq/L)
- Potassium: 4.3 mEq/L (3.7–5.2 mEq/L)
- Chloride: 101 mEq/L (96–106 mmol/L)
- Carbon dioxide: 27 mmol/L (20–29 mmol/L)
- Glucose: 88 mg/dL (65–110 mg/dL)
- Blood urea nitrogen (BUN): 27 mg/dL (7–20 mg/dL)

Intervention: The patient's ostomy output is averaging 4 L/d. Three liters of PN infuse over 12 hours at night, and an additional 3 liters of normal saline are infused during the day to prevent dehydration and damage to the kidneys. Dextrose and amino acids are supplied as 275 g and 120 g, respectively. The lipid component is a mixture of soybean, medium-chain triglyceride, olive, and fish oils and is dosed at 120 g per week to supply essential fatty acids and minimize the deleterious effects of the lipid emulsion on the liver. Amounts of vitamins and trace elements are customized based on measured serum values. The preoperative dual-energy x-ray absorptiometry test reveals osteoporosis, and intravenous bisphosphonates are started. Additional calcium and phosphorus are added to the PN solution.

Answer: The goal during the preoperative state is to optimize nutrition status, preserve or improve hepatic and renal function, and keep the patient free from infection until organs become available. Therefore, the patient's PN formula was designed to provide adequate hydration to preserve renal function, and the macronutrient portion of the PN was designed to minimize the deleterious effects on the liver. All micronutrients were corrected based on serum values.

Rationale: Following transplantation, recipients must take high doses of immunosuppressants and other nephrotoxic drugs. Therefore, it is important to prevent damage to the kidney in the preoperative phase. It is also important to minimize any damage to the liver so that the patient does not go into liver failure before the transplant organs become available. In some cases, the liver damage can be reversed, allowing the patient to be transplanted with an isolated small bowel.

The third pretransplant nutrition goal (which is usually out of the control of the transplant team unless the organ is from a living donor) is to provide appropriate nutrition to the donor. The effect of feeding on the donated organ is probably more prominent in liver transplantation than in other types of organ transplantation because of the liver's role in glycogen and adenosine triphosphate storage. Furthermore, nutrition may be important to the outcomes of living donor transplants. Living donors are screened to exclude those who should not donate for medical reasons. Hypertension, diabetes mellitus, and obesity are 3 nutrition-related comorbidities that are scrutinized and often exclude potential donors.[42] Some potential donors may be required to lose weight prior to donation. Weight loss may be required to reduce their postoperative risks such as infection, or, in the case of liver donors, it may be necessary if the donor has hepatic steatosis. Hwang et al[43] reported that short-term weight loss (mean of 5.9% ± 2% body weight) in 9 living liver donors reduced the degree of steatosis (from 48.9% ± 25.6% to 20.0% ± 16.2% fat), allowing for successful liver donation. In a large, retrospective study of the UNOS database evaluating outcomes from 23,303 patients, neither donor obesity nor moderate steatosis affected outcomes after liver transplantation.[44]

Acute Posttransplant Phase

Immunosuppression must achieve a delicate balance to prevent rejection and infection. Most acute rejections occur within the first 3 months after transplantation. Infection is most common during this phase. For this reason, laboratory markers and physical signs of rejection and infection are monitored closely.

The main nutrition goals of the acute posttransplant phase are to establish adequate nutrient intake to replete lost nutrient stores; provide substrate to support the body's ability to fight infection; heal anastomoses and surgical wounds; and supply energy to allow a patient to participate in physical rehabilitation and activities of daily living. The route of nutrition support in the posttransplant phase depends in part on the patient's nutrition status and the route and adequacy of pretransplant nutrition. Figure 31-1 outlines a decision tree for selection of posttransplant nutrition.[45] General nutrition

support guidelines are discussed later in this chapter. Nutrition goals of an intestinal transplant patient are unique to this population and are highlighted in Practice Scenario 31-3.[44,46-51]

Chronic Posttransplant Phase

During the chronic posttransplant phase, clinicians should continually monitor the patient for signs of rejection and infection as well as the recurrence of the primary disease that caused the organ failure. Monitoring overall rehabilitation status and quality of life is equally important. The observed improvements in the cognitive, emotional, and psychosocial states following organ transplantation are fairly abstract and difficult to define. Improved health is a subjective state, and perceptions of an acceptable health state will vary from individual to individual.

Many patients develop long-term problems with obesity, hypertension, hyperlipidemia, osteoporosis, and diabetes mellitus. The nutrition goals of this phase are, therefore, to prevent or treat these complications and ensure adequate nutrition intake. See Practice Scenario 31-4 to understand some effects of the original pretransplant disease on posttransplant nutrition care.

Metabolic Aberrations Associated with Organ Transplantation

Physiologic stress associated with transplantation and the side effects of immunosuppressive agents cause changes in the metabolism of carbohydrates, lipids, and proteins.

Glucose Alterations

Hyperglycemia is the most common abnormality in glucose metabolism that occurs during the early posttransplant period. Causative factors include physiologic stress, infection, and medications. Corticosteroids increase serum glucose levels by inducing insulin resistance and influencing gluconeogenesis in the liver. In addition, corticosteroids decrease insulin receptor affinity in adipose tissue and muscle and cause defects at the postreceptor level.[52] Cyclosporine and tacrolimus (calcineurin inhibitors) inhibit pancreatic islet cell function and insulin secretion and cause insulin resistance; sirolimus also has these effects, although to a lesser degree than calcineurin inhibitors.[53,54] Cyclosporine and tacrolimus have greatly improved the outcomes of solid organ transplantation, but they have been implicated in the development of new-onset diabetes after transplant (NODAT).[55] The prevalence of NODAT is greater in patients treated with tacrolimus than cyclosporine. The overall rate of NODAT varies depending on the definition of diabetes, the organ transplant specified, and the time period after transplantation.[56] The main risk factors for NODAT are increased BMI, family history of diabetes, recipient older than 55 to 60 years of age, hepatitis C or cytomegalovirus infection, and treatment with tacrolimus, corticosteroids, or sirolimus.[57-59] Hypertriglyceridemia in liver transplant recipients with diabetes is an independent risk factor for posttransplantation impairment of glucose metabolism. With the increased prevalence of metabolic syndrome, the likelihood of developing NODAT also increases.[60]

FIGURE 31-1 Nutrition Support Algorithm for Solid Organ Transplant Recipients

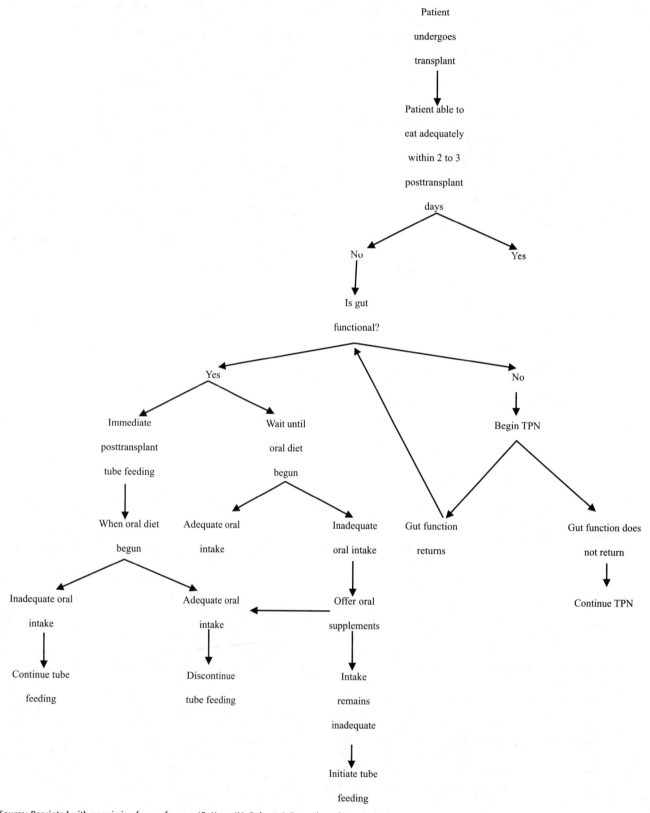

Source: Reprinted with permission from reference 45: Hasse JM, Roberts S. Transplantation. In: Rombeau JL, Rolandelli RH, eds. *Clinical Nutrition: Parenteral Nutrition.* 3rd ed. Philadelphia, PA: WB Saunders; 2001:529–561. Copyright Elsevier 2001.

Practice Scenario 31-3

Question: What is the nutrition goal during the postoperative phase of a patient who underwent intestinal transplantation?

Scenario: The patient is a 33-year-old woman who is status-post multivisceral (stomach, duodenum, small bowel) transplant for chronic intestinal pseudo-obstruction.

Intervention: Parenteral nutrition (PN) is initiated in the immediate postoperative phase. Within 3 days, there is the presence of ostomy effluent, flatulence, and bowel sounds. Enteral feeding with a low-potassium, polymeric formula is initiated at 5 mL/h while maintaining full PN. The PN is gradually decreased and eventually discontinued as the enteral formula rate is advanced and oral diet is started. The patient is started on a regular diet, and the enteral feedings are reduced as oral nutrition improves.

Answer and Rationale: Nutrition care for patients undergoing small bowel transplantation involves some unique considerations because the organ responsible for digestion and absorption is being transplanted. The nutrition goal is to transition the patient to an unrestricted diet. The transition phase is dynamic and often requires multiple concurrent feedings.[43] The protocols for nutrition management used to achieve this transition vary among transplant centers. The nutrition aspects of care have changed over the years as surgical techniques have evolved and experience has been gained in the care of these unique patients. Nutrient, fluid, and electrolyte requirements are met through a stepwise progression of transitions from PN to an oral diet. The transition to an unrestricted diet is fairly rapid after the surgery, but it is individualized for each patient. PN is reinstituted in the early postoperative phase to support the patient until the allograft is functional. However, the PN prescription changes dramatically from the prescription used during the preoperative phase. The patient no longer requires the large volumes of PN that were necessary to maintain hydration before transplantation. Depending on the center, enteral nutrition is initiated via a nasogastric tube, a nasoduodenal tube, a gastrostomy tube, or a jejunostomy tube before PN is discontinued. Enteral feedings are generally started at full strength and administered slowly at 5 to 10 mL/h. As the rate is advanced, the PN is gradually tapered.

The choice of enteral feeding formula remains somewhat controversial and will vary among centers.[46] Because the lymphatics are disrupted at the time of procurement of the organs, it has been hypothesized that a low-fat, predigested, or elemental formula would be necessary to prevent chylous accumulation. However, there are no data to suggest significant malabsorption of the intestinal allograft early after transplantation.[47] Although some centers use elemental, low-fat, or fat-free formulas in the first month following a transplant, other centers use polymeric formulas containing whole macronutrient components. Care should be given to the selection of a formula that is low in potassium because immunosuppressive medications may result in hyperkalemia.

An oral diet is usually started within the first 2 weeks after transplantation as the allograft begins to function. Gastric emptying and the subsequent potential risk of aspiration are carefully monitored by an abdominal examination and assessing for nausea or vomiting. As with the choice of enteral feeding, the use of a low-fat diet to reduce the risk of malabsorption and chylous ascites after an intestinal transplantation remains controversial. The low-fat approach is based solely on practice surveys during the early development of intestinal transplantation.[48,49] However, in each of these surveys, the reported risk of chylous ascites was low (less than 7%), and this early practice of limiting fat was based on minimizing the potential risk for this complication. Controlled trials to evaluate this theory are lacking. Spontaneous reconstitution of the lymphatic channels generally occurs within 1 month, thus indicating the self-limiting nature of fat malabsorption in the absence of chronic allograft damage.[50]

The time required to transition to an oral diet is variable and patient dependent. In one study, the mean time for enteral feeding initiation was 10.3 ± 6.9 days after transplantation (range: 3–35 days) and the mean time for discontinuation of PN was 30.8 ± 25 days posttransplantation (range: 9–132 days). Full clinical nutrition autonomy, whereby the patients were off all enteral and parenteral feedings and consuming an oral diet was achieved at a mean of 57 ± 36 days.[51]

Practice Scenario 31-4

Question: How does the pretransplant diagnosis affect posttransplant nutrition care?

Scenario: A 22-year-old man with a history of cystic fibrosis undergoes double lung transplant. He is 67 inches tall and weighs 135 pounds. The patient struggled before transplant to maintain his weight. The initial postoperative course is uneventful, so the patient is extubated and, in a couple of days, his diet is advanced to a high-energy, high-protein diet. A nutrition consult is requested for postoperative management of nutrition complications of cystic fibrosis.

Intervention: The dietitian obtains a detailed diet history from the patient. The recall reveals he was eating between 3000 and 3400 kcal/d prior to admission to maintain his weight. Double meat portions and high-energy, high-protein nutrition supplements between meals are ordered. Pancreatic enzymes are prescribed to be taken with meals. Vitamins A and D are supplemented along with a multivitamin.

Answer: Although a transplant may offer improved organ function, it does not necessarily "cure" other comorbidities or nutrition complications after transplantation. The cause of the patient's organ failure or other preexisting conditions will influence the nutrition care needed perioperatively because the conditions may not be corrected or cured by a transplant.

Rationale: In this scenario, lung transplantation improved the patient's lung function, but it did not correct or cure his cystic fibrosis and pancreatic insufficiency. The patient had malabsorption prior to the transplant, which would still be present after transplantation. In this scenario, using energy expenditure equations or even measuring resting energy expenditure is of limited value; predicting or measuring energy expenditure does not account for malabsorption, which is common among individuals with cystic fibrosis (see Chapters 25 and 26). It was important to resume the pancreatic enzymes to assist with absorption. Vitamin supplementation is recommended for transplant patients, and special formulations or high-dose supplementation are required for patients who are vitamin deficient. Vitamin levels should be rechecked in a couple of months to determine if the current supplement can restore vitamin levels to normal.

Just as this patient had contended with complications of his original disease after transplantation, so do other organ transplant recipients. Some conditions, such as malnutrition, ascites, edema, and so on, can resolve with time after transplantation, but patients will require appropriate therapy until these problems are resolved. Similarly, transplantation improves organ function but does not always rid the patient of the original disease that caused the failure, so that failure could happen again after transplant. Additional examples of conditions that may persist after transplantation include viral hepatitis, autoimmune liver disease, nonalcoholic steatohepatitis, primary sclerosing cholangitis in liver transplant recipients, and hypertension and diabetes mellitus in renal transplant recipients.

The main causative factors of NODAT can be classified as greater insulin resistance or impaired insulin secretion. Uremia, physical inactivity, obesity, and medications (corticosteroids, cyclosporine, tacrolimus, sirolimus) contribute to insulin resistance.[61] Reduced insulin secretion can be caused by perioperative stress, unhealthy diet habits, and medications (corticosteroids, cyclosporine, tacrolimus).[61]

Hyperglycemia in the postoperative period may be related to an increased risk of transplant rejection and infection. Some studies suggest that controlling intraoperative or postoperative glucose levels is associated with reduced transplant rejection[62-64] and infection rates[63,65] in kidney and liver transplant recipients. But other studies have not shown this association.[66,67] In fact, Hermayer and colleagues compared rates of rejection in patients who underwent intestinal transplantation and found that rates were higher with tight glycemic control (blood glucose 70 to 110 mg/dL) vs standard control (blood glucose 70 to 180 mg/dL).[66] These studies on glycemic control cannot be extrapolated to all transplant patients in all situations because the prevalence of pretransplant diabetes mellitus and presence of other comorbidities and complications in the study populations varied, and varying immunosuppression protocols were used. Furthermore, most of these studies were retrospective and used a variety of definitions for "tight" glucose control, with upper limits of 150 mg/dL to 200 mg/dL being considered "normal." In summary, the effect of postoperative hyperglycemia on outcomes in organ transplant recipients has not been conclusively determined. However, it seems reasonable to use a treatment approach that aims for optimal glucose control. The Society of Critical Care Medicine and American Society for Parenteral and Enteral Nutrition define optimal control in critically ill patients as blood glucose levels between 140 and 180 mg/dL.[68] IV insulin drips may be used in the acute posttransplant period when serum glucose levels are elevated. Treatment with long- and/or short-acting insulin may be required upon hospital discharge even in patients with no previous history of diabetes mellitus. However, as doses of immunosuppressant drugs are decreased and serum glucose levels improve, insulin doses may be decreased, converted to oral hypoglycemic agents, or discontinued.

Lipid Alterations

Hyperlipidemia is another common, long-term posttransplant problem affecting many patients who have undergone organ transplantation and is a risk factors for cardiovascular disease. Hyperlipidemia can be induced by immunosuppressive medications, particularly corticosteroids, cyclosporine, and sirolimus. Increased serum levels of total cholesterol, very low-density lipoprotein cholesterol, low-density lipoprotein (LDL) cholesterol, and triglycerides usually mark the pattern.[69] This effect is reduced when tacrolimus is used as the primary immunosuppressant. The Assessment of LEscol in Renal Transplantation study evaluated the effects of fluvastatin or placebo in lowering serum LDL cholesterol levels and reducing the risk for cardiac events in kidney transplant recipients.[70] Patients who received fluvastatin exhibited significantly lower serum total and LDL cholesterol levels than the control group, and achieved a reduction in cardiac death and nonfatal myocardial infarction. As a result, HMG-CoA reductase inhibitors (statins) have become standard management of posttransplantation hypercholesterolemia in patients who do not respond to lifestyle modifications.

Protein Alterations

Protein catabolic rate is accelerated after organ transplantation. The administration of corticosteroids is a main cause of increased protein oxidation. Protein losses from surgical drains, stomas, dialysis, and wounds also increase protein requirements. As corticosteroid doses are decreased or discontinued, the need for dietary protein may also decrease. Some transplant centers are using "steroid-free" immunosuppression regimens for certain transplant recipients. One could theorize that protein losses, and thus needs, would be lower with this type of regimen compared with catabolism associated with traditional steroid-containing treatment regimens. However, this hypothesis has yet to be studied.

Determining Nutrition Status

The best approach to assessing a transplant patient's nutrition status is to use a combination of objective and subjective parameters. Objective parameters may lack validity, specificity, or interrater reliability in this population. Table 31-2 summarizes the benefits and drawbacks of using different types of nutrition assessment parameters to assess transplant recipients. Refer to Chapter 9 for further discussion of nutrition assessment.

Nutrient Requirements

Energy

Organ transplant patients do not tend to be hypermetabolic unless secondary conditions such as sepsis are present. Factors

TABLE 31-2 Benefits and Drawbacks of Objective Nutrition Assessment Parameters When Assessing Organ Transplant Recipients

Parameter	Benefits	Drawbacks
Body weight	• Simple to perform • Reproducible • Low cost • Universal measurement	• Affected by body fluid changes • Does not account for alterations in body composition (lean body mass vs adipose tissue)
Anthropometric measurements	• Low cost • Portable	• Low interrater reliability • Influenced by a patient's fluid status • Low specificity
Functional tests (eg, handgrip strength, sit-to-stand test, 6-minute walk)	• Provides insight into level of frailty	• Can be affected by underlying disease or comorbidities (eg, shortness of breath, hepatic encephalopathy) • Not a direct measure of nutrition
Imaging tests such as DXA, CT scans, or MRI scans	• Total body DXA considered highly accurate to assess lean vs fat tissue • CT/MRI scans can assess fat vs muscle content at a single slice	• Increased cost • Not a bedside measurement • Entails radiation to the patient • Quantifying body mass on CT/MRI scans requires special software • CT/MRI scans look at single slice and require extrapolation to entire body
Other body composition measurements such as BIA, BIS, and air plethysmography	• BIA and BIS can be completed at bedside • Plethysmography highly accurate	• BIA affected by fluid status; BIA equation must be valid for population being evaluated • BIS considered more accurate than BIA but has not been validated in transplant patients or patients with fluid overload (eg, ascites) • Equipment for these tests are expensive and not available in most centers

BIA, bioelectrical impedance analysis; BIS, bioimpedance spectroscopy; CT, computed tomography; DXA, dual-energy x-ray absorptiometry; MRI, magnetic resonance imaging.

that influence resting energy expenditure include gender, age, pretransplant nutrition status, and medical condition. Three studies have evaluated energy needs following liver transplantation; the time period during which indirect calorimetry was performed varied from the 2nd to the 28th day posttransplant. Resting energy expenditure was 7% to 42% above predicted values using various predictive equations.[71–73] Absorption capability should also be considered in the final energy recommendation. This point is especially true for small bowel transplant recipients, because the transplanted intestine may have variable absorption capacity depending on the health and the state of infection and rejection of the graft, and for transplant recipients with cystic fibrosis and pancreatic insufficiency.

Generally, 70% of nonprotein energy in nutrition support regimens is provided by carbohydrates. Because posttransplant hyperglycemia is prevalent, blood glucose levels should be treated as discussed in Chapters 23 and 34.

Lipids fulfill the remainder of the nonprotein energy prescription. Most enteral and parenteral products contain ω-6 fatty acids. However, ω-3 fatty acids are theorized to benefit transplant recipients by decreasing inflammatory response, enhancing transplant tolerance, and improving graft function. One trial evaluated the use of an immune-enhancing enteral formula (containing fish oil, arginine, and nucleic acids) vs standard supplementation in liver transplant patients.[74] Fifty-two patients completed the immune-enhancing formula arm, and 49 patients completed the control arm. There were no differences between the groups with regard to rates of infection, rejection, and length of stay.[74] A meta-analysis attempted to look at effects of immunonutrition on liver transplant outcomes.[75] However, the analysis included 6 PN trials, and, because PN is not usually indicated for liver transplantation, it is difficult to apply any of the conclusions from such a meta-analysis. A Cochrane review on fish oil and kidney transplantation concluded that fish oil may mildly improve cardiovascular risk factors such as diastolic blood pressure and high-density lipoprotein cholesterol levels, but there are not adequate data to support that fish oil reduces cardiovascular disease risk or improves renal transplant function, rejection rates, or graft and patient survival rates.[76] Larger clinical trials are needed before the use of ω-3 fatty acids can be endorsed for regular use following transplantation.

Protein

Protein requirements are directly related to corticosteroid dose; nutrition status; stress state; losses from drains, stomas, and wounds; and requirements for wound healing (see Chapter 21 for more information on wound healing). Because corticosteroid doses are increased in the acute posttransplant phase and during rejection treatment, protein needs are higher in the acute phase (1.5 to 2 g per kg of estimated dry weight) vs the chronic posttransplant phase (1 g per kg). As mentioned earlier, some new antirejection regimens eliminate corticosteroids; theoretically, protein requirements would be lower in these circumstances than when regimens using corticosteroids are followed.

Fluid

Fluid requirements for transplant patients vary greatly depending upon volume status. Excess fluid administration and/or decreased urine output cause fluid overload. Renal insufficiency is common posttransplant, and the cause is multifactorial. Pretransplant renal insufficiency, surgical complications, and nephrotoxic medications all contribute to posttransplant renal insufficiency. Diarrhea, chest tubes, wounds, surgical drains, nasogastric drainage, ostomy output, and urine output are sources of fluid loss that commonly affect posttransplant fluid requirements.

Micronutrients

Posttransplant nutrient levels and requirements can be affected by many factors. Vitamins and mineral deficiencies may be caused by poor intake pretransplant, malabsorption related to disease state, extra losses, or altered metabolism (Table 31-3). Posttransplant medications can also influence micronutrient requirements as well as absorption and metabolism.

Selecting a Nutrition Support Route

Oral feeding is the preferred route of nutrition for organ transplant recipients. However, tube feeding and PN are needed occasionally as bridges to oral nutrition or during complications that prevent an oral diet. Major indications for tube feeding and PN are discussed in Chapters 10 and 14, respectively. An algorithm for nutrition support selection is featured in Figure 31-1. General nutrition support and monitoring guidelines for organ transplant recipients are highlighted in Table 31-4

TABLE 31-3 Factors That Contribute to Vitamin and Mineral Abnormalities in Organ Transplant Patients

Factor (Transplanted Organ)	Nutrient Alterations
Alcoholism	• Vitamins A, B_6, and B_{12}; niacin; thiamin; folate; magnesium; and zinc levels are decreased.
Antibiotics	• Vitamins E and K, and folate levels are decreased.
Bile drainage (liver)	• Copper loss is increased; fat-soluble vitamins may be malabsorbed.
Biliary obstruction, Wilson's disease (liver)	• Copper level may be increased.
Bleeding	• Iron loss is increased.
Calcineurin inhibitors	• Magnesium loss is increased.
Glucocorticoids	• Vitamin D and phosphorus levels are decreased. • Urinary loss of calcium is increased.
Hemochromatosis (liver)	• Iron stores are increased.
Liver failure (liver)	• Ability to activate vitamin D is decreased. • Vitamin K level is decreased.
Ostomy loss (small bowel), diarrhea	• Zinc loss is increased.
Refeeding syndrome	• Magnesium, phosphorus, thiamin, and potassium levels are decreased.
Renal failure	• Vitamin D, calcium, and phosphorus metabolism is abnormal. • Iron levels are decreased due to depressed erythropoietin. • Vitamin A level is increased. • Phosphorus and potassium levels may be increased in renal failure; levels can be altered depending on the type of dialysis and dialysate. • Excretion of magnesium and zinc is decreased. • Zinc level may be decreased in dialysis patients.
Steatorrhea	• Levels of vitamins A, D, E, and K are decreased. • Calcium level is decreased.
Wound	• Need for some vitamins (eg, A and C) and zinc may be increased to aid with healing.

Source: Reprinted with permission from reference 45: Hasse JM, Roberts S. Transplantation. In: Rombeau JL, Rolandelli RH, eds. *Clinical Nutrition: Parenteral Nutrition.* 3rd ed. Philadelphia, PA: WB Saunders; 2001:529–561. Copyright Elsevier 2001.

TABLE 31-4 General Posttransplant Nutrition Support Guidelines

Route of Nutrition	Usual Recommendations
Oral	• Liquid diet—once patient is extubated and assessed to be safe to swallow • General diet—once patient shows tolerance to liquid diet, diet is advanced to solid food • Carbohydrate-controlled diet—when serum glucose level is elevated • Sodium-restricted diet—when fluid retention is severe • Fluid restriction—when hyponatremia and fluid overload are present • Oral nutrition supplements—when intake of solid foods is inadequate • Vitamin/mineral supplement—to provide additional micronutrients

Enteral nutrition	• Formula:
	  – Usually a polymeric, high-nitrogen formula; can consider fiber-containing formulas
	  – Volume overload: concentrated formula
	  – Impaired digestion: semielemental or polypeptide formula
	• Feeding schedule—consider a cyclic tube-feeding schedule once an oral diet provides approximately 50% of the patient's needs

Parenteral nutrition	• Fluid—volume depends on intake and output • Amino acids—to meet increased protein requirements • Dextrose—may need to increase gradually if patient has diabetes mellitus or posttransplant hyperglycemia • Lipids—typically, aim for about 30% of nonprotein energy from lipids; may need to hold soy oil–based lipid emulsions if patient is septic • Electrolytes—adjust according to laboratory values; renal function is often impaired postoperatively and calcineurin inhibitors can cause hyperkalemia • Multiple vitamin infusion—daily • Trace elements—daily • Insulin—if serum glucose is elevated

TABLE 31-5 Approaches to Enteral Tube Feeding After Liver Transplantation

Approach	Drawbacks
Place feeding tube after transplantation only if it is determined that oral intake will be delayed or is inadequate.	Feeding is delayed while tube-feeding access is obtained. This delay is especially undesirable for patients who have severe complications or who are already malnourished.
Preselect patients who may benefit from tube feeding and place feeding tubes during surgery.	Predicting which patients will have posttransplant difficulties or delayed eating is difficult. If the decision to place feeding tubes is made based on nutrition status alone, patients who are well nourished but have significant posttransplant complications will lack access for tube feeding.
Place feeding tubes in all patients during surgery and begin tube feeding within 12 to 24 hours of surgery.	Some patients will require tube feeding for only a short period of time (2–3 days) before oral intake is adequate. Some tubes can become dislodged and may require replacement if oral intake does not meet needs.

Source: Data are from reference 82.

and are also discussed in the European Society for Parenteral and Enteral Nutrition guidelines.[77]

Several studies have shown that early postoperative tube feeding in liver transplant patients reduces infection rates when compared with no postoperative nutrition support or PN.[71,78–81] This benefit has been demonstrated in recipients of both deceased and living donor transplants. Tube-feeding options for liver transplant recipients are summarized in Table 31-5.[82]

Indications for PN in organ transplant patients include prolonged, active GI bleeding, ileus, and high-output intestinal fistula. In addition, PN is usually required initially after

small bowel transplantation and during periods of significant small bowel rejection or infection. When PN is required, several guidelines can be considered to determine the appropriate PN formula. First, the volume of the PN depends on overall fluid needs, as discussed previously. If a patient is volume overloaded or has limited urine output, concentrated forms of amino acids, dextrose, and fat emulsions should be used. On the other hand, additional volume may be required for the intestinal transplant patient with a high ostomy output. Electrolyte and micronutrient content of the PN solution should be individualized based on laboratory values. As mentioned earlier, glucose control is desired and patients may require an IV insulin drip or insulin in the PN formulation if serum glucose levels are elevated.

Transplant Complications and Nutrition Implications

Many potential posttransplant complications can directly or indirectly affect nutrition. Examples include rejection, preservation injury, delayed graft function, infection, surgical complications, hyperglycemia, hypertension, renal insufficiency, and electrolyte abnormalities. Interventions for many of these complications have a nutrition management component (Practice Scenario 31-5).[83]

Practice Scenario 31-5

Question: What are common early posttransplant complications and how do they influence decisions about nutrition or nutrition support?

Scenario: A 56-year-old woman undergoes kidney transplantation for end-stage renal disease due to hypertension. The patient has a history of metabolic syndrome marked by obesity, hyperlipidemia, hypertension, and diabetes mellitus. She had undergone gastric bypass several years earlier. Her current body mass index is 32. After undergoing kidney transplantation, her posttransplant course is unremarkable, and she is discharged 4 days after her transplant. Two weeks later, the patient is readmitted to the hospital with an elevated serum creatinine level, reduced urine output, and resultant weight gain. A kidney biopsy is performed, which confirms acute rejection. The patient is treated with corticosteroids. She also complains of redness at the incision site. The wound appears infected, and it is partially opened; a wound vacuum-assisted closure (VAC) is placed. Antibiotics are prescribed. The patient complains of nausea; she is eating only about half of her meals and is drinking ginger ale to reduce her nausea.

Intervention: When the corticosteroid treatment is initiated, an order is placed to measure blood glucose levels at the bedside before meals and at bedtime. Despite the patient receiving her usual dose of long-acting insulin, her blood glucose levels are elevated, ranging between 200 and 300 mg/dL. Short-acting insulin is given on a sliding scale, and her long-acting insulin dose is increased. She is encouraged to avoid highly concentrated sweets such as the ginger ale. An antinausea medicine is prescribed to be used on an as-needed basis. A high-protein oral supplement is ordered, and the patient is encouraged to eat the entrees at her meals.

Answer: Common posttransplant complications include rejection, infection, and technical/surgical complications. Each of these complications may require a change in the nutrition intervention, such as adjusting nutrient requirements, changing the mode of nutrient delivery, or prescribing insulin or another adjunct therapy.

Rationale: Antirejection medications are needed to prevent and treat transplant rejection, but antirejection medications have nutrition-related side effects (Table 31-1). Corticosteroids accelerate the protein catabolic rate and nitrogen loss. The mechanism of how tacrolimus and corticosteroids cause hyperglycemia was discussed earlier in this chapter. Often, serum glucose levels increase after a transplantation as a response to immunosuppressive medications and postoperative stress. New-onset diabetes after transplant can be transient. Glucose levels often return to normal several weeks posttransplant, and insulin therapy is not required long term. Infection is a potential posttransplant complication often potentiated by immunosuppressive medications. Malnourished patients may be more likely to develop infections than well-nourished patients. On the other hand, severely obese patients tend to have increased rates of wound infections. Antibiotics and antiviral and antifungal medications are usually given prophylactically during the early postoperative phase when immunosuppressive medications are at their highest doses. They are also administered when pathologic organisms are identified in wounds, urine, blood, or other body fluids. These medications may adversely affect appetite and taste and may cause nausea, vomiting, or diarrhea. These gastrointestinal symptoms may preclude a patient from eating adequate amounts. In addition, if a wound VAC is used for a wound (whether infected or not), it will remove protein-containing body fluids, thus requiring protein supplementation.[83]

Nutrition Monitoring

Monitoring a patient's nutrition progress includes an evaluation of body weight (including fluid fluctuations), intake and output, and laboratory parameters such as serum electrolytes, glucose, magnesium, phosphorus, and calcium. In addition to these objective parameters, an evaluation of the patient's ability to ambulate, eat adequately, perform activities of daily living, and heal wounds are all signs of recovery and progress. Anthropometric measurements and functional tests performed serially over time may provide information about body composition. Other methods of body composition such as computed tomography scans or dual-energy x-ray absorptiometry can be used to monitor long-term changes in muscle or fat mass but are usually only done for research purposes.

Summary

Organ transplantation is a medical therapy that can improve survival and quality of life in individuals with end-stage organ disease. The medical and surgical complexities of transplantation influence nutrition status and nutrient delivery. Nutrition therapy varies with transplant type, nutrition status, stage of transplant, function of organ, and presence of complications. Tailoring nutrition therapy based on these characteristics can help improve transplant outcomes.

References

1. United Network for Organ Sharing. Data. https://www.unos.org/data. Accessed July 14, 2017.
2. Allison TL. Immunosuppressive therapy in transplantation. *Nurs Clin N Am.* 2016;51:107–120.

3. Malat G, Culkin C. The ABCs of immunosuppression: a primer for primary care physicians. *Med Clin N Am.* 2016;100:505–518.

4. Allen JG, Arnaoutakis GJ, Weiss ES, et al. The impact of recipient body mass index on survival after lung transplantation. *J Heart Lung Transplant* 2010; 29:1026–1033.

5. Merli M, Giusto M, Gentili F, et al. Nutritional status: its influence on the outcome of patients undergoing liver transplantation. *Liver Int.* 2010;30(2):208–214.

6. Giusto M, Lattanzi B, Albanese C, et al. Sarcopenia in liver cirrhosis: the role of computed tomography scan for the assessment of muscle mass compared with dual-energy X-ray absorptiometry and anthropometry. *Eur J Gastroenterol Hepatol.* 2015;27(3):328–334.

7. Montano-Loza AJ, Meza-Junco J, Baracos VE, et al. Severe muscle depletion predicts postoperative length of stay but is not associated with survival after liver transplantation. *Liver Transpl.* 2014;20(6):640–648.

8. Masuda T, Shirabe K, Ikegami T, et al. Sarcopenia is a prognostic factor in living donor liver transplantation. *Liver Transpl.* 2014;20(4):401–407.

9. Krell RW, Kaul DR, Martin AR, et al. Association between sarcopenia and the risk of serious infection among adults undergoing liver transplantation. *Liver Transpl.* 2013;19(12):1396–1402.

10. Kaido T, Ogawa K, Fujimoto Y, et al. Impact of sarcopenia on survival in patients undergoing living donor liver transplantation. *Am J Transplant.* 2013;13(6):1549–1556.

11. Englesbe MJ, Patel SP, He K, et al. Sarcopenia and mortality after liver transplantation. *J Am Coll Surg.* 2010;211(2):271–278.

12. Molnar MZ, Czira ME, Rudas A, et al. Association of the malnutrition-inflammation score with clinical outcomes in kidney transplant recipients. *Am J Kidney Dis.* 2011;58(1):101–118.

13. Yost G, Gregory M, Bhat G. Short-form nutrition assessment in patients with advanced heart failure evaluated for ventricular assist device placement or cardiac transplantation. *Nutr Clin Pract.* 2014;29(5):686–691.

14. Heinbokel T, Floerchinger B, Schmiderer A, et al. Obesity and its impact on transplantation and alloimmunity. *Transplantation.* 2013;96(1):10–16.

15. Harris AD, Fleming B, Bromberg JS, et al. Surgical site infection after renal transplantation. *Infect Control Hosp Epidemiol.* 2015;36(4):417–423.

16. Fockens MM, Alberts VP, Bemelman FJ, van der Pant KA, Idu MM. Wound morbidity after kidney transplant. *Prog Transplant.* 2015;25(1):45–48.

17. Chung H, Lam VW, Yuen LP, et al. Renal transplantation: better fat than thin. *J Surg Res.* 2015;194(2):644–652.

18. Gusukuma LW, Harada KM, Baptista AP, et al. Outcomes in obese kidney transplant recipients. *Transplant Proc.* 2014;46(10):3416–3419.

19. De Lima JJ, Gowdak LH, de Paula FJ, et al. Coronary events in obese hemodialysis patients before and after renal transplantation. *Clin Transplant.* 2015;29(11):971–977.

20. Papalia T, Greco R, Lofaro D, et al. Impact of body mass index on graft loss in normal and overweight patients: retrospective analysis of 206 renal transplants. *Clin Transplant.* 2010;24(6):E241–E246.

21. Curran SP, Famure O, Li Y, Kim SJ. Increased recipient body mass index is associated with acute rejection and other adverse outcomes after kidney transplantation. *Transplantation.* 2014;97(1):64–70.

22. Cannon RM, Jones CM, Hughes MG, Eng M, Marvin MR. The impact of recipient obesity on outcomes after renal transplantation. *Ann Surg.* 2013;257(5):978–984.

23. Ditonno P, Lucarelli G, Impedovo SV, et al. Obesity in kidney transplantation affects renal function but not graft and patient survival. *Transplant Proc.* 2011;43(1):367–372.

24. Furriel F, Parada B, Campos L, et al. Pretransplantation overweight and obesity: does it really affect kidney transplant outcomes? *Transplant Proc.* 2011;43(1):95–99.

25. Pieloch D, Dombrovskiy V, Osband AJ, Lebowitz J, Laskow DA. Morbid obesity is not an independent predictor of graft failure or patient mortality after kidney transplantation. *J Ren Nutr.* 2014;24(1):50–57.

26. Sampaio MS, Reddy PN, Kuo HT, et al. Obesity was associated with inferior outcomes in simultaneous pancreas kidney transplant. *Transplantation.* 2010;89:1117–1125.

27. Hanish SI, Petersen RP, Collins BH, et al. Obesity predicts increased overall complications following pancreas transplantation. *Transplant Proc.* 2005;37:3564–3566.

28. Afaneh C, Rich B, Aull MJ, et al. Pancreas transplantation considering the spectrum of body mass indices. *Clin Transplant.* 2009;25:E520–E529.

29. Bédat B, Niclauss N, Jannot AS, et al. Impact of recipient body mass index on short-term and long-term survival of pancreatic grafts. *Transplantation.* 2015;99(1):94–99.

30. Lederer DJ, Wilt JS, D'Ovidio F, et al. Obesity and underweight are associated with an increased risk of death after lung transplantation. *Am J Respir Crit Care Med.* 2009;180:887–895.

31. Russo MJ, Hong KN, Davies RR, et al. The effect of body mass index on survival following heart transplantation: do outcomes support consensus guidelines? *Ann Surg.* 2010; 251:144–152.

32. Weiss ES, Allen JG, Russell SD, Shah AS, Conte JV. Impact of recipient body mass index on organ allocation and mortality in orthotopic heart transplantation. *J Heart Lung Transplant.* 2009; 28:1150–1157.

33. Macha M, Molina EJ, Franco M, et al. Pre-transplant obesity in heart transplantation: are there predictors of worse outcomes? *Scand Cardiovasc J.* 2009;43:304–310.

34. Nair S, Verma S, Thuluvath, PJ. Obesity and its effect on survival in patients undergoing orthotopic liver transplantation in the United States. *Hepatology.* 2002;35:105–109.

35. Dick AA, Spitzer AL, Seifert CF, et al. Liver transplantation at the extremes of the body mass index. *Liver Transpl.* 2009;15(8):968–977.

36. Bambha KM, Dodge JL, Gralla J, Sprague D, Biggins SW. Low, rather than high, body mass index confers increased risk for post-liver transplant death and graft loss: risk modulated by model for end-stage liver disease. *Liver Transpl.* 2015;21(10):1286–1294.

37. Wong RJ, Cheung R, Perumpail RB, Holt EW, Ahmed A. Diabetes mellitus, and not obesity, is associated with lower survival following liver transplantation. *Dig Dis Sci.* 2015;60(4):1036–1044.

38. Saab S, Lalezari D, Pruthi P, Alper T, Tong MJ. The impact of obesity on patient survival in liver transplant recipients: a meta-analysis. *Liver Int.* 2015;35(1):164–1170.

39. Glanton CW, Kao TC, Cruess, D, Agodoa LY, Abbott KC. Impact of renal transplantation on survival in end-stage renal disease patients with elevated body mass index. *Kidney Int.* 2003;63:647–653.

40. Pelletier SJ, Maraschio MA, Schaubel DE, et al. Survival benefit of kidney and liver transplantation for obese patients on the waiting list. *Clin Transpl.* 2003;77-88.

41. Gill JS, Lan J, Dong J, et al. The survival benefit of kidney transplantation in obese patients. *Am J Transplant.* 2013;13(8):2083–2090.

42. Bergen CR, Reese PP, Collins D. Nutrition assessment and counseling of the medically complex live kidney donor. *Nutr Clin Pract.* 2014;29(2):207–214.

43. Hwang S, Lee SG, Jang SJ, et al. The effect of donor weight reduction on hepatic steatosis for living donor liver transplantation. *Liver Transpl.* 2004;11:721–725.

44. Yoo HY, Molmenti E, Thuluvath PJ. The effect of donor body mass index on primary graft nonfunction, retransplantation rate,

and early graft and patient survival after liver transplantation. *Liver Transpl.* 2003;9:72–78.

45. Hasse JM, Roberts S. Transplantation. In: Rombeau JL, Rolandelli RH, eds. *Clinical Nutrition: Parenteral Nutrition.* 3rd ed. Philadelphia, PA: WB Saunders; 2001:529–561.

46. Mercer DF, Iverson AK, Culwell KA. Nutrition and small bowel transplantation. *Nutr Clin Pract.* 2014;29(5):615–620.

47. Kim J, Fryer J, Craig RM. Absorptive function following small intestinal transplantation. *Dig Dis Sci.* 1998;43:1925–1930.

48. Kaufman SS, Lyden ER, Brown CR, et al. Disaccharidase activities and fat assimilation in pediatric patients after intestinal transplantation. *Transplantation.* 2000;69:362–365.

49. Nour B, Reyes J, Tzakis A, et al. Intestinal transplantation with or without other abdominal organs: nutrition and dietary management of 50 patients. *Transplant Proc.* 1994;26:1432–1433.

50. Rovera G, Schoen R, Goldbach B, et al. Intestinal and multivisceral transplantation: dynamics of nutritional management and functional autonomy. *JPEN J Parenter Enteral Nutr.* 2003;27:252–259.

51. Matarese LE, Dvorchik I, Costa G, et al. Pyridoxal-5'-phosphate deficiency after intestinal and multivisceral transplantation. *Am J Clin Nutr.* 2009;89(1):204–209.

52. Marchetti P. New-onset diabetes after liver transplantation: from pathogenesis to management. *Liver Transpl.* 2005;11(6):612–620.

53. Araki M, Flechner SM, Ismail HR, et al. Posttransplant diabetes mellitus in kidney transplant recipients receiving calcineurin or mTOR inhibitor drugs. *Transplantation.* 2006;81(3):335–341.

54. Barlow AD, Nicholson ML, Herbert TP. Evidence for rapamycin toxicity in pancreatic β-cells and a review of the underlying molecular mechanisms. *Diabetes.* 2013;62(8):2674–2682.

55. Pham PT, Pham PC, Lipshutz GS, Wilkinson AH. New onset diabetes mellitus after solid organ transplantation. *Endocrinol Metab Clin North Am.* 2007;36:873–890.

56. Balla A, Chobanian M. New-onset diabetes after transplantation: a review of recent literature. *Curr Opin Organ Transplant.* 2009; 14:375–379.

57. Abe T, Onoe T, Tahara H, et al. Risk factors for development of new-onset diabetes mellitus and progressive impairment of glucose metabolism after living-donor liver transplantation. *Transplant Proc.* 2014;46(3):865–869.

58. Suarez O, Pardo M, Gonzalez S, et al. Diabetes mellitus and renal transplantation in adults: is there enough evidence for diagnosis, treatment, and prevention of new-onset diabetes after renal transplantation? *Transplant Proc.* 2014;46(9):3015–3020.

59. Einollahi B, Motalebi M, Salesi M, Ebrahimi M, Taghipour, M. The impact of cytomegalovirus infection on new-onset diabetes mellitus after kidney transplantation: a review on current findings. *J Nephropathol.* 2014;3:139–148.

60. Perito E, Lustig R, Rosenthal P. Metabolic syndrome components after pediatric liver transplantation: prevalence and the impact of obesity and immunosuppression. *Am J Transplant.* 2016;16(6): 1909–1916.

61. Hecking M, Werzowa J, Haidinger M, et al; European-New-Onset Diabetes After Transplantation Working Group. Novel views on new-onset diabetes after transplantation: development, prevention and treatment. *Nephrol Dial Transplant.* 2013;28(3):550–566.

62. Thomas MC, Moran J, Mathew TH, Russ GR, Rao MM. Early perioperative hyperglycemia and renal allograft rejection in patients without diabetes. *BMC Nephrology.* 2000;1:1.

63. Thomas MC, Mathew TH, Russ GR, Rao MM, Moran J. Early perioperative glycaemic control and allograft rejection in patients with diabetes mellitus: a pilot study. *Transplantation.* 2001;72(7): 1321–1324.

64. Wallia A, Parikh ND, Molitch ME, et al. Posttransplant hyperglycemia is associated with increased risk of liver allograft rejection. *Transplantation.* 2010;89(2):222–226.

65. Ammori JB, Sigakis M, Englesbe MJ, O'Reilly M, Pelletier SJ. Effect of intraoperative hyperglycemia during liver transplantation. *J Surg Res.* 2007;140(2):227–233.

66. Hermayer KL, Egidi MF, Finch NJ, et al. A randomized controlled trial to evaluate the effect of glycemic control on renal transplantation outcomes. *J Clin Endocrinol Metab.* 2012;97(12):4399–4406.

67. Ramirez SC, Maaske J, Kim Y, et al. The association between glycemic control and clinical outcomes after kidney transplantation. *Endocr Pract.* 2014;20(9):894–900.

68. McClave SA, Taylor BE, Martindale RG, et al. Guidelines for the provision and assessment of nutrition support therapy in the adult critically ill patient: Society of Critical Care Medicine (SCCM) and American Society for Parenteral and Enteral Nutrition (A.S.P.E.N.). *JPEN J Parenter Enteral Nutr.* 2016;40(2):159–211.

69. Bamgbola O. Metabolic consequences of modern immunosuppressive agents in solid organ transplantation. *Ther Adv Endocrinol Metab.* 2016;7(3):110–127.

70. Holdaas H, Fellström B, Jardine AG, et al; Assessment of LEscol in Renal Transplantation (ALERT) Study Investigators. Effect of fluvastatin on cardiac outcomes in renal transplant recipients: a multicentre, randomised, placebo-controlled trial. *Lancet.* 2003; 361(9374):2024–2031.

71. Hasse JM, Blue LS, Liepa GU, et al. Early enteral nutrition support in patients undergoing liver transplantation. *JPEN J Parenter Enteral Nutr.* 1995;19:437–443.

72. Plank LD, Metzger DJ, McCall JL, et al. Sequential changes in the metabolic response to orthotopic liver transplantation during the first year after surgery. *Ann Surg.* 2001;234:245–255.

73. Chen Y, Kintner J, Rifkin SK, Keim KS, Tangney CC. Changes in resting energy expenditure following orthotopic liver transplantation. *JPEN J Parenter Enteral Nutr.* 2016;40(6):877–882.

74. Plank LD, Mathur S, Gane EJ, et al. Perioperative immunonutrition in patients undergoing liver transplantation: a randomized double-blind trial. *Hepatology.* 2015;61(2):639–647.

75. Lei Q, Wang X, Zheng H, et al. Peri-operative immunonutrition in patients undergoing liver transplantation: a meta-analysis of randomized controlled trials. *Asia Pac J Clin Nutr.* 2015;24(4): 583–590.

76. Lim AK, Manley KJ, Roberts MA, Fraenkel MB. Fish oil for kidney transplant recipients. *Cochrane Database Syst Rev.* 2016;(8): CD005282. doi:10.1002/14651858.CD005282.pub3.

77. Weimann A, Braga M, Harsanyi L, et al. ESPEN guidelines on enteral nutrition: surgery including organ transplantation. *Clin Nutr.* 2006;25(2):224–244.

78. Rayes N, Seehofer D, Hansen S, et al. Early enteral supply of lactobacillus and fiber versus selective bowel decontamination: a controlled trial in liver transplant recipients. *Transplantation.* 2002;74(1):123–127.

79. Rayes N, Seehofer D, Theruvath T, et al. Supply of pre- and probiotics reduces bacterial infection rates after liver transplantation--a randomized, double-blind trial. *Am J Transplant.* 2005; 5(1):125–130.

80. Ikegami T, Shirabe K, Yoshiya S, et al. Bacterial sepsis after living donor liver transplantation: the impact of early enteral nutrition. *J Am Coll Surg.* 2012;214(3):288–295.

81. Kim JM, Joh JW, Kim HJ, et al. Early enteral feeding after living donor liver transplantation prevents infectious complications: a prospective pilot study. *Medicine (Baltimore).* 2015;94(44): e1771.

82. Hasse JM. Examining the role of tube feeding after liver transplantation. *Nutr Clin Pract.* 2006;21(3):299–311.

83. Hourigan LA, Linfoot JA, Chung KK, et al. Loss of protein, immunoglobulins, and electrolytes in exudates from negative pressure wound therapy. *Nutr Clin Pract.* 2010;25(5):510–516.

32 Human Immunodeficiency Virus Infection

Peter Wasserman, BSc, MA, David S. Rubin, MD, and Sorana Segal-Maurer, MD

CONTENTS

Objectives

1. Describe the epidemiology of the human immunodeficiency virus (HIV) pandemic globally and within the United States.
2. Discuss the transmission, diagnosis, and treatment of HIV infection and acquired immunodeficiency syndrome (AIDS)/HIV disease.
3. Identify the abnormalities of nutritional metabolism associated with HIV infection and combination antiretroviral therapy (cART).
4. Discuss diagnostic criteria and methodology, and treatment options for wasting syndrome, sarcopenia, osteopenia and osteoporosis, frailty phenotype, and dyslipidemia in patients with HIV infection.

Test Your Knowledge Questions

1. HIV infection is prevalent in which of the following populations?
   A. Men who have sex with men
   B. Urban heterosexuals in the lowest income strata
   C. Black and Hispanic/Latino Americans
   D. All of the above
2. Which of the following is the goal of antiretroviral therapy?
   A. To increase CD8+ T lymphocytes and decrease viral load (VL)
   B. To increase both CD4+ T lymphocytes and VL
   C. To increase CD4+ T lymphocytes and neutrophils
   D. To increase CD4+ T lymphocytes and decrease VL
3. Which of the following is predictive of the onset of wasting disease?
   A. Hypogonadism
   B. Hypermetabolism
   C. Decreased food intake
   D. All of the above

4. Which of the following is a central feature of HIV lipodystrophy?
   A. Abdominal obesity
   B. Increases in specific fat depots
   C. Subcutaneous adipose tissue loss
   D. All of the above
5. Hypertriglyceridemia is a frequent finding in which of the following patient populations?
   A. Febrile HIV+ patients with septicemia
   B. HIV+ patients with abdominal obesity receiving cART
   C. Patients with HIV infection and wasting disease
   D. All of the above

Test Your Knowledge Answers

1. The correct answer is **D**. The HIV epidemic in the United States is geographically concentrated with marked ethnic, social, and economic health disparities.
2. The correct answer is **D**. HIV infection leads to disease in the human host by depletion of CD4+ T-helper lymphocytes. Effective antiretroviral therapy suppresses viral replication. The level of viral replication is monitored clinically by quantitative polymerase chain reaction and reported as absolute and log copies per milliliter of serum sampled (VL). This number should decline with viral suppression. HIV does not infect CD8-cytolytic T lymphocytes and neutrophils.
3. The correct answer is **C**. Decreased food intake is predictive of the onset of wasting. Decreased activity or lethargy may initially compensate for hypermetabolism. Hypogonadism is not a uniform finding in all patients with involuntary weight loss or wasting.
4. The correct answer is **C**. Lipodystrophy is characterized by subcutaneous adipose tissue loss with visceral adipose

tissue sparing or accumulation. Subcutaneous adipose tissue loss is often most evident in the face, buttocks, and lower extremities. Lipodystrophic patients may also demonstrate insulin resistance in association with the loss of subcutaneous adipose tissue.

5. The correct answer is **D**. Hypertriglyceridemia may occur in association with wasting disease, as an adverse effect of antiretroviral medications, in association with abdominal adiposity, or during febrile response to bacterial infection as a host defense mechanism.

Background

Introduction

The first cases of AIDS in the United States were described over 35 years ago.[1] HIV-related mortality rates rose steadily through the 1980s and early 1990s, peaking in 1995. During that period, median survival following an AIDS diagnosis was 18 to 36 months. In the 7 years following the introduction of cART, HIV-related mortality declined by 65%.[2] Currently, the Centers for Disease Control and Prevention (CDC) estimate that more than 1.2 million people are living with HIV or AIDS in the United States.[3] Median survival for newly diagnosed patients initiating therapy is now estimated in decades.[4] Formidable challenges remain: insufficient HIV testing, persisting health inequities including access to care and life-years lost for patients in care, patient retention in care, and community burden of disease.[5-7] In addition, 1 in 5 people living with HIV is unaware of their infection and may unwittingly transmit the virus to others.[7] For many people unaware of their HIV infection, diagnosis and linkage to care continues to occur at presentation for the treatment of opportunistic infection(s) and/or wasting disease. Patients in care with long-term controlled HIV infection are at greater risk for age-related comorbidities (including acute myocardial infarction [AMI], hypertension, type 2 diabetes mellitus, and non-AIDS-defining cancers) than the general population.[8-10]

The Virus

HIV, the causative agent of AIDS in humans, is a zoonotic retrovirus of the lentivirus family. Of the 2 types of HIV, type 1 is distributed throughout the world (pandemic) and type 2 is found in sub-Saharan Africa, predominantly in west Africa (in addition to HIV-1).[11] HIV-1 is believed to have crossed over to the human population from chimpanzees, and the oldest documentation of human infection is a blood sample collected in 1959 in west-central Africa.[11] Of the 3 HIV-1 subgroups, group M accounts for most infections worldwide and has 10 identifiable clades or subtypes (A through H) based on genetic sequence diversity. Clade B virus predominates in western and central Europe, the Americas, Haiti, and Australia, whereas clade E predominates in Thailand. All clades are found in Africa. Molecular genetic tests currently used in North America may perform poorly on non–clade B virus. Therapeutic response to various antiretrovirals may be different among different clades and between HIV-1 and HIV-2.

Epidemiology of the HIV Pandemic

The Joint United Nations Programme and World Health Organization (WHO) estimate that 36.7 million people are infected with HIV worldwide.[12] Sub-Saharan Africa bears the greatest burden of disease, with an estimated prevalence of 25.6 million cases (Table 32-1).[12] Untreated or inadequately treated HIV infection has a case fatality rate that approaches 100%.

Prevention programs that target sexuality education, enable people to overcome stigma and discrimination, provide condoms, offer voluntary HIV counseling and testing, and make blood transfusions safer have been successful in lowering prevalence in several sub-Saharan countries.[13] Considerable progress in the provision of cART to persons with HIV infection has been made by national health services, the WHO, the President's Emergency Plan for AIDS Relief (PEPFAR), and the Global Fund to Fight to AIDS, Tuberculosis, and Malaria. The early initiation of cART has been shown to reduce the sexual transmission of HIV, providing public health as well as individual clinical benefits.[14] However, globally, less than

TABLE 32-1 Regional HIV/AIDS Statistics for 2015

Region	People Living with HIV Infection	New HIV Infections	People Living with HIV Receiving cART	AIDS-Related Mortality
Eastern and southern Africa	19.1 million	960,000	10.3 million	470,000
Western and central Africa	6.5 million	410,000	1.8 million	330,000
Asia and the Pacific	5.1 million	290,000	2.1 million	180,000
Latin America and the Caribbean	2.0 million	100,000	1.1 million	50,000
Eastern Europe and central Asia	1.5 million	190,000	321,800	47,000
Western and central Europe and North America	2.4 million	91,000	1.4 million	22,000
Global[a]	36.7 million	2.1 million	17 million	1.1 million

AIDS, acquired immunodeficiency syndrome; cART, combination antiretroviral therapy; HIV, human immunodeficiency virus.
[a]Differences in global and regional sums are because of rounding.
Source: Data are from reference 12.

half of people living with HIV infection at the end of 2015 were receiving cART (Table 32-1) and the integration of food support into HIV treatment programs remains inadequate.[13,15] Food insecurity (the limited or uncertain availability of nutritionally adequate, safe foods or the inability to acquire personally acceptable foods in socially acceptable ways) may lead to behaviors to obtain food that negatively impact community-dwelling HIV-infected patients' retention in care and cART adherence and increase HIV transmission.[13,15] For example, people experiencing food insecurity may migrate in search of work or engage in transactional sex.[13,15]

Worldwide, the majority of people with HIV infection are expected to progress to AIDS and succumb to opportunistic infections because they have limited access to care and live in nations with poor public health infrastructure. High mortality rates during what would normally be people's most productive years (prime age mortality) has a negative impact on population-level socioeconomic outcomes.

In 2014, over 1.2 million people were living with HIV infection in the United States.[2,3] Annually, 50,000 new infections occur and 14,000 people with diagnosed HIV infection die, leading to a net increase of 36,000 HIV-infected people.[2,3]

In the United States, the prevalence of HIV infection is greatest in the Northeast and South, with rates of 420.5 and 343.6 per 100,000 persons, respectively.[3] Southern states comprise 37% of the total US population but account for an estimated 44% of all people with HIV infection in the United States.[3,16] Rates of new HIV diagnoses per 100,000 people were 18.5 in the South compared to 14.2, 11.2, and 8.2 in the Northeast, West, and Midwest, respectively.[3,16] Of the 10 states with the highest rates of new HIV diagnoses, 8 are southern states, and all 10 of the metropolitan statistical areas with highest rates of new HIV diagnoses are in the South.[3,16]

In 2014, 81% of new adult and adolescent diagnoses of HIV infection were in males; 67% of the diagnoses were made in men who have sex with men (MSM), and most of the MSM diagnosed with HIV were young black men.[3] As such, health disparities in the United States are prominent in HIV acquisition. In 2014, 44% of HIV infections were diagnosed in black/African Americans, vs 27% in white/non-Hispanic Americans, and 17% in Hispanic/Latino Americans.[3] In contrast, black/African American, white/non-Hispanic, and Hispanic/Latino people comprise 13%, 65%, and 16% of the US population, respectively.[17] Young black MSM (ages 13 to 34 years) are the US subset most disproportionately affected by the epidemic, and are more likely to be unaware of their infection, and subsequently experience lower rates of linkage to and retention in care after diagnosis.[18] MSM, black, and Hispanic/Latino Americans are respectively 40, 8, and 3 times more likely to be HIV-infected than white/non-Hispanic heterosexual Americans.[6]

HIV prevalence in heterosexuals residing in urban areas is 6 times higher in the lowest income strata (vs the highest), regardless of ethnicity.[19] This finding, suggests that ethnicity may be a surrogate marker for socioeconomic status in surveillance data sets, and that poverty is a major determinant of risk for HIV infection in the United States. Poverty may place individuals at risk for HIV infection through high HIV density (prevalence greater than 2%), the presence of high-risk populations in their community, lack of education or resources,

or lack of access to healthcare.[20] In nonurban areas, stigma or sexual networks may mediate county-level disparities in HIV risk.[21] In clinical practice, health history should include key socioeconomic factors to avoid unfounded assumptions about biology or "culture" based on ethnicity.

Diagnosis

A definitive diagnosis of HIV infection is laboratory-based, uses serum or plasma specimens, and is made using HIV-1/2 antigen/antibody combination immunoassay, followed by HIV-1/HIV-2 antibody differentiation immunoassay.[22] The combination immunoassay detects the presence of HIV-1 and HIV-2 antibodies, and HIV-1 p24 antigen.[22] The inclusion of detection methodology for p24 antigen in fourth-generation immunoassays allows the diagnosis HIV-1 infection before the formation of detectable levels of antibodies (seroconversion).[22] If a specimen is reactive on the initial immunoassay but nonreactive or indeterminate on the antibody differentiation assay, HIV-1 nucleic acid testing is performed for resolution.[22] A diagnosis of AIDS may be made according to the CDC 1993 AIDS surveillance case definition (Table 32-2).[23]

TABLE 32-2 AIDS-Defining Events

- Cervical cancer (invasive)
- Coccidioidomycosis, disseminated
- Cryptococcosis, extrapulmonary
- Cryptosporidiosis, chronic intestinal (>1-month duration)
- Cytomegalovirus disease (other than liver, spleen, or lymph nodes)
- Cytomegalovirus retinitis (with loss of vision)
- Encephalopathy, HIV-related
- Herpes simplex: chronic ulcer(s) (>1-month duration) or bronchitis, pneumonitis, or esophagitis
- Histoplasmosis, disseminated
- Isosporiasis, chronic intestinal (>1-month duration)
- Kaposi sarcoma
- Lymphoma: Burkitt, or immunoblastic, or primary of brain (primary central nervous system lymphoma)
- *Mycobacterium avium* complex or disease caused by *M. kansasii*, disseminated
- Disease caused by *Mycobacterium tuberculosis*, any site (pulmonary or extrapulmonary)
- Disease caused by Mycobacterium, other species, or unidentified species, disseminated
- *Pneumocystis jiroveci (carinii)* pneumonia
- Pneumonia (recurrent)
- Progressive multifocal leukoencephalopathy
- Salmonella septicemia (recurrent)
- Toxoplasmosis of the brain (encephalitis)
- Wasting syndrome caused by HIV infection

AIDS, acquired immunodeficiency syndrome; HIV, human immunodeficiency virus.
Source: Adapted from reference 23: Centers for Disease Control and Prevention. 1993 revised classification system for HIV infection and expanded surveillance case definition for AIDS among adults and adolescents. *MMWR Morb Mortal Wkly Rep.* 1992;41:1–19.

Rapid, single-use point-of-care antigen/antibody combination tests have been approved for screening purposes by the US Food and Drug Administration (FDA). They require confirmation by laboratory-based testing, as described previously.[22]

Transmission

HIV is found in all body fluids except urine and sweat. Seminal fluids and blood are the most infectious. Transmission occurs when an uninfected host comes into contact with semen, blood, or blood-tinged body fluids (Table 32-3).[24] The patient's mode of HIV acquisition is denoted as the *risk factor* or *transmission category*. The most common form of HIV transmission worldwide is via heterosexual contact; however, in the United States, male-to-male sexual contact is the most common mode of transmission.[3] The risk of transmission is increased (1) when there is exposure to a large amount of virus (high VL) or a large amount of contaminated blood or body fluids; (2) if exposure is percutaneous or mucosal; or (3) if cutaneous exposure is of prolonged duration. The risk of sexual transmission is increased in the presence of sexually transmitted diseases (STDs), in uncircumcised men, and during receptive anal or receptive vaginal intercourse. The risk of maternal-fetal transmission is increased in the presence of high maternal VL, the prolonged rupture of membranes, the presence of STD ulcerations in the birth canal or genitals, and with breast feeding. Less than 1% of transmission occurs through occupational exposure.

The early treatment of HIV infection, with continuous suppression of VL in blood and genital fluids, can markedly decrease the risk of transmission. In the landmark multinational HIV Prevention Trials Network (HPTN) 052 trial, serodiscordant couples (where only 1 partner, the index partner, is HIV-infected) were randomly assigned to 2 study groups: a group in which the index participant received cART immediately at study enrollment (early cART) or a group in which administration of cART began when the index participant's health status reached a predetermined point (CD4 less than 250 cells per mm³ or AIDS-defining illness). In interim analyses after a median follow-up of 1.7 years, early cART was associated with a 96% lower risk of index-to-uninfected partner transmission.[25] At final analysis, median follow-up 5.5 years,

early cART was associated with a 93% lower risk of index-to-uninfected partner transmission.[25] Results from the trial informed the WHO guidelines, which now recommend the initiation of cART in individuals diagnosed with HIV infection irrespective of CD4 count.[26] The public health strategy of early cART for the reduction of HIV transmission is termed *treatment as prevention*, and delayed treatment is not recommended as a viable strategy.

Pre-exposure prophylaxis (PrEP)—daily regimen of oral fixed-dose tenofovir disoproxil fumarate and emtricitabine (Truvada)—is recommended for the prevention of HIV infection in people considered to be at risk, including sexually active MSM, uninfected partners in HIV-discordant heterosexual couples, intravenous (IV) drug users, and heterosexually active adults considered to be at substantial risk (ie, those with a recent bacterial STD).[27]

Immunopathogenesis

Mucosal exposure to HIV leads to the epithelial production of inflammatory cytokines and diminished barrier integrity, allowing viral entry into the body.[28] Acute HIV infection is marked by a rapid and severe loss of memory CD4+/CCR5+ T lymphocytes in gastrointestinal (GI) tissue.[29-31] Gut-associated lymphoid tissue (GALT) is a crucial component of the mucosal immune system and contains most of the body's memory CD4+ T lymphocytes.[32] The density of target cells within the lamina propria and GALT allows HIV to propagate rapidly, with severe and largely irreversible loss of gut CCR5 + CD4+ T cells occurring within days of HIV acquisition.[33-35] Early profound loss of CCR5+ CD4 + T cells is specific to the gut and precedes the loss of CD4 + T cells in systemic immune tissue (ie, blood, peripheral lymph nodes).[36] Persisting immune activation and the expression of proinflammatory chemokines and cytokines mark chronic HIV infection of GALT.[37-40] Fibrotic changes disrupting Peyer's patch architecture, as a result of inflammation, lead to impaired immunocyte regeneration and are associated with sustained depletion of CD4+ T cells and blunted reconstitution of CCR5+ CD4 + T cells.[41] Blunted regeneration of T lymphocytes may persist even when patients receive cART.[41]

Microbial translocation across the gut mucosa has been demonstrated by quantification of lipopolysaccharide and

TABLE 32-3 Modes of HIV Transmission

Route	Examples
Percutaneous	Contaminated transfusion, intravenous drug use sharing of needles, contaminated surgical or dental instruments, or during an occupational exposure
Mucous membrane	Sexual contact (vaginal, anal, or oral), occupational (eg, eye splash)
Cutaneous contact of nonintact skin with large volume of infected fluids and/or for a prolonged duration	Occupational contact with abraded skin
Maternal-fetal	Intrauterine, intrapartum (ie, during labor and delivery), postpartum (ie, breastfeeding)

Adapted from reference 24: Centers for Disease Control and Prevention. Transmission facts. http://www.cdc.gov/hiv/pubs/facts/transmission.htm. Accessed December 8, 2010.

16S rDNA (conserved DNA sequences common to gram-negative and gram-positive bacteria) in plasma from HIV-infected patients and is believed to participate in the activation of CD4+ T cells in spite of a lack of overt bacteremia.[42,43] Persistent immune activation ultimately leading to cell death is thought to contribute to the systemic depletion of CD4+ T cells in chronic HIV infection.[44,45]

Patients with secondary and/or opportunistic infections who initiate cART at low CD4 counts may experience a period of paradoxical clinical deterioration or immune reconstitution inflammatory syndrome (IRIS). IRIS is an inflammatory disorder caused by an enhanced antigen-specific immune response to a previously unseen (by the immune system) opportunistic or secondary infection. It is usually self-limited but can lead to permanent end-organ damage when a neurologic structure situated in a closed space is involved. Depending on the infective focus, the clinical presentation of IRIS may include lymphadenopathy, pulmonary infiltrates, headache, fever, and meningitis. In some instances, lymphadenopathy may lead to compartment syndromes requiring emergent treatment with anti-inflammatory agents (ie, corticosteroids). The patients at greatest risk for IRIS are those initiating cART who are also at risk for infection with granuloma-producing organisms (ie, mycobacteria or fungi) as well as infections within closed compartments (eg, cryptococcal meningitis).[46]

The Clinical Manifestation of Immunodeficiency

The natural history of HIV disease may begin with an initial retroviral syndrome, a flulike illness that may be accompanied by a variety of symptoms: rash, lymphadenitis, aseptic meningitis, and so on. The progressive loss of CD4 + T lymphocytes following establishment of infection leads to the deterioration of cell-mediated and humoral immunity and increased risk of opportunistic infection(s) or AIDS-defining malignances. For example, at a CD4 count of 200 to 500 cells/mm^3, patients may present with oral or vaginal candidiasis or reactivation of prior viral infections (ie, Herpes simplex or Herpes zoster) or bacterial infections (eg, Staphylococcus aureus or Pseudomonas aeruginosa). At CD4 counts less than 200 cells/mm^3, patients may present with opportunistic infections and AIDS-related malignancies. A diagnosis of AIDS is made whenever an HIV-infected person has a CD4 count less than 200 cells/mm^3 (or a CD4 cell percentage less than 14%) or is diagnosed with wasting syndrome or other AIDS-defining illness (Table 32-2). Wasting, hypogonadism or menstrual irregularities, nutrient malabsorption, and oropharyngeal candidiasis are prevalent in people with AIDS. A presumptive diagnosis of Candida esophagitis may be made in patients experiencing dysphagia or odynophagia.

Combination Antiretroviral Therapy

cART is recommended for all people with HIV infection, regardless CD4 count, to reduce HIV-associated morbidity and mortality as well as HIV transmission.[26,47,48] The goal of cART is to facilitate the reconstitution of CD4 + T lymphocytes by the long-term suppression of viral replication. The ability

of an antiretroviral regimen to suppress viral replication may be monitored by quantitative reverse transcription polymerase chain reaction (RT-PCR). VL is reported as copies per milliliter or log$_{10}$ copies per milliliter. Treatment-naïve patients initiating cART are expected to achieve VL reductions to below the limits of assay detection within 8 to 24 weeks and are expected to remain below the threshold of detection by quantitative RT-PCR during cART.[47] HIV clinicians usually monitor VL every 3 to 4 months in routine care.[47] Monitoring may be extended to intervals of 6 months in patients who have consistently demonstrated viral suppression and stable immunologic status for more than 2 years.[47]

Antiretroviral medications are prescribed in combination (2 or more classes) to prevent the emergence of resistant viruses. Several combinations have been coformulated as single-tablet regimens (STR), and the reduced pill burden has been associated with higher rates of patient adherence and viral suppression.[49] A therapeutic adherence rate of 95% or better is associated with three-fold lower all-cause mortality risk.[50] In practice, achievement of a 95% adherence rate means fewer than 2 missed doses per month. This level of therapeutic adherence is far greater than that required in the medical management of other chronic conditions.

There are 7 classes of FDA-approved antiretroviral medications for the treatment of HIV infection: nucleoside reverse transcriptase inhibitors (NRTIs), nucleotide reverse transcriptase inhibitors (NtRTIs), nonnucleoside reverse transcriptase inhibitors (NNRTIs), protease inhibitors (PIs), fusion inhibitors, coreceptor antagonists, and integrase strand transfer inhibitors (INSTIs). See Table 32-4 for currently approved drugs in these classes.[51,52] Each class inhibits a specific stage of HIV interaction with cell-surface receptors, viral membrane–to–cell membrane fusion, or intracellular viral replication (Figure 32-1).[53] Low-dose ritonavir and cobicistat are inhibitors of cytochrome 3A4 isoenzymes and are, therefore, used as pharmacokinetic enhancers for PIs or the integrase inhibitor elvitegravir.

The US Department of Health and Human Services and International Antiviral Society–USA Panel guidelines classify INSTI or ritonavir-boosted darunavir-based regimens as recommended for treatment-naïve, HIV-infected adults entering care.[47,54]

Nutritional Metabolism in the Modern cART Era

In the United States, approximately half of all people living with HIV infection are age 50 years or older, and about a quarter of incident HIV infections occur in people age 45 years or older.[3] Increasingly, newly diagnosed people with HIV/AIDS live in urban poverty areas and experience food and housing insecurity, as well as limited access to fresh, minimally processed foodstuffs.[19] These demographic data have profound implications for the nutritional care of people with HIV infection.

Prior to the advent of cART, wasting disease was the prominent nutrition-related issue in patients receiving care in high-income nations. Although wasting disease still occurs in association with deprivation, HIV infection has become a chronic condition for most patients in care in high-income nations.[3]

TABLE 32-4 Antiretroviral Medications

Generic Name (Brand Name; Abbreviation)	Form	Food Considerations	Forms for People with Swallowing Difficulties or Feeding Tubes[a]
Fixed-dose STRs			
efavirenz/emtricitabine/tenofovir DF (**Atripla**; EFV/FTC/TDF)	Tablet	Take 1 hour before food or on an empty stomach.	Do not crush.
rilpivirine/emtricitabine/tenofovir AF (**Odefsey**; RPV/FTC/TAF)	Tablet	Must be taken with a meal.	No data on crushing.
rilpivirine/emtricitabine/tenofovir DF (**Complera**; RPV/FTC/TDF)	Tablet	Must be taken with a meal.	No data on crushing.
elvitegravir/cobicistat/emtricitabine/ tenofovir disoproxil fumarate (**Stribild**; EVG/cobi/FTC/TDF)	Tablet	Take with food.	No data on crushing.
elvitegravir/cobicistat/emtricitabine/ tenofovir alafenamide (**Genvoya**; EVG/cobi/FTC/TAF)	Tablet	Take with food.	No data on crushing.
dolutegravir/abacavir/lamivudine (**Triumeq**; DTG/ABC/3TC)	Tablet	Preferable to take with food.	May be crushed and added to small amount of food or liquid; administer immediately.
INSTIs			
raltegravir (**Isentress**; RAL)	Tablet	Take with or without food.	100 mg/packet granular powder for oral suspension available.
dolutegravir (**Tivicay**; DTG)	Tablet	Preferable to take with food.	May be crushed and added to small amount of food or liquid, and administered immediately.
elvitegravir (**Vitekta**; EVG)	Tablet	Must be taken with food.	No data available.
Coreceptor antagonists			
maraviroc (**Selzentry**; MVC)	Tablet	Take with or without food.	No data available.
Coformulated NRTIs/NtRTIs[b]			
abacavir/lamivudine (**Epzicom**; EPZ)	Tablet	Take with or without food.	No data available.
zidovudine/lamivudine (**Combivir**; CBV)	Tablet	Take with or without food.	May be crushed and mixed with a small amount of semisolid food or liquid, which must be administered immediately.
abacavir/lamivudine/zidovudine (**Trizivir**; TRZ)	Tablet	Take with or without food.	Administer components: abacavir and lamivudine are available as oral solutions; zidovudine is available as a syrup.
emtricitabine/tenofovir DF (**Truvada**; TVD)	Tablet	Take with or after consuming food.	Tablets may be disintegrated in at least 100 mL water, orange juice, or grape juice and taken immediately.
emtricitabine/tenofovir AF (**Descovy**)	Tablet	Take with or without food.	No data available.
NRTIs/NtRTIs			
lamivudine (**Epivir**; 3TC)	Tablet	Take with or without food.	10 mg/mL oral solution available.
zidovudine (**Retrovir**; AZT or ZDV)	Tablet	Take with or without food.	50 mg/5mL syrup available.

(continued)

TABLE 32-4 Antiretroviral Medications *(continued)*

Generic Name (Brand Name; Abbreviation)	Form	Food Considerations	Forms for People with Swallowing Difficulties or Feeding Tubes[a]
abacavir (**Ziagen**; ABC)	Tablet	Take with or without food.	20 mg/mL oral solution available.
emtricitabine (**Emtriva**; FTC)	Capsule	Take with or without food.	10 mg/mL oral solution available.
tenofovir DF (**Viread**; TDF)	Tablet	Take with a meal.	40 mg/g powder for oral solution. Tablets may be disintegrated in at least 100 mL water, orange or grape juice, but have a bitter taste.
didanosine (**Videx EC**; DDI)	Capsule	Should be taken on empty stomach, 2 hours before or 2 hours after a meal.	4 g / 8-oz glass bottle pediatric powder for oral solution available.
stavudine (**Zerit**; D4T)	Capsule	Take without food or with a light meal.	1 mg/mL powder for oral solution available.
PIs			
darunavir (**Prezista**; DRV)	Tablet	Take with or after meal.	100 mg/mL oral suspension available.
fosamprenavir (**Lexiva**; FPV)	Tablet	Take with or without food.	50 mg/mL oral suspension available.
indinavir (**Crixivan**; IDV)	Capsule	Take without food; consume 1.5 L water per day to avoid nephrolithiasis.	None. Do not open capsules; stability is uncertain.
saquinavir (**Invirase**; SQV)	Tablet or capsule	Take within 2 hours of a full meal.	Capsules may be opened and powder suspended in either sugar syrup or sorbitol syrup (for patients with type 1 diabetes or glucose intolerance); must be coadministered with ritonavir.
atazanavir (**Reyataz**; ATZ)	Capsule	Take with or after food.	50 mg/packet oral powder available.
nelfinavir (**Viracept**; NFV)	Tablet	Take with a meal.	50 mg/g oral powder; or 625-mg or 250-mg tablets may be dissolved in water.
tipranavir (**Aptivus**; TPV)	Capsule	Take with or after food.	100 mg/mL oral solution available.
Coformulated PIs/PKEs			
darunavir/cobicistat (**Prezcobix**; DRV/cobi)	Tablet	Take with food or within 30 minutes of a meal.	None.
atazanavir/cobicistat (**Evotaz**; ATZ/cobi)	Tablet	Take with food.	None.
lopinavir/ritonavir (**Kaletra**; LPV/r)	Tablet	Take with or without food.	80mg/20mg per mL oral solution available.
NNRTIs			
etravirine (**Intelence**; ETR)	Tablet	Take following a meal.	None.
efavirenz (**Sustiva**; EFV)	Tablet or capsule	Take on an empty stomach.	None.

TABLE 32-4 Antiretroviral Medications *(continued)*

Generic Name (Brand Name; Abbreviation)	Form	Food Considerations	Forms for People with Swallowing Difficulties or Feeding Tubes[a]
nevirapine (**Viramune XR**; NVP)	Tablet	Take with or without food.	50 mg/5 mL Viramune oral suspension available.
rilpivirine (**Edurant**; RPV)	Tablet	Take with a meal.	None.
delavirdine (**Rescriptor**; DLV)	Tablet	Take with or without food.	100-mg tablets may be dissolved in water. 200-mg tablets may not be dissolved in water.
PKEs			
cobicistat (**Tybost**; cobi)	Tablet	Take with food.	None.
Ritonavir[c] (**Ritonavir**; RTV)	Tablet	Take with or after food.	80 mg/mL oral solution available.

INSTI, integrase strand transfer inhibitor; NNRTI, nonnucleoside reverse transcriptase inhibitor; NRTI, nucleoside reverse transcriptase inhibitor; NtRTI, nucleotide reverse transcriptase inhibitor; PI, protease inhibitor; PKE, pharmacokinetic enhancer; STR, single-tablet regimen.

[a]Data are from University of Liverpool. HIV drug interactions. http://www.hiv-druginteractions.org; and Immunodeficiency Clinic, Toronto General Hospital. http://hivclinic.ca.

[b]Class warning for lactic acidosis; consider in differential for nonspecific complaints of nausea, emesis, abdominal pain, fatigue, dyspnea, and weight loss.

[c]Originally developed as a PI.

FIGURE 32-1 The HIV Replication Cycle

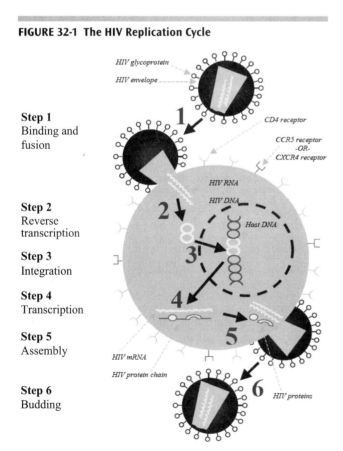

Step 1
Binding and fusion

Step 2
Reverse transcription

Step 3
Integration

Step 4
Transcription

Step 5
Assembly

Step 6
Budding

Source: Adapted from reference 53: US Department of Health and Human Services. AIDSinfo. The HIV cycle. May 2005. http://www.aidsinfo.nih.gov /contentfiles/HIVLifeCycle_FS_en.pdf.

Noninfectious comorbidities (eg, cardiovascular disease [CVD], osteopenia/osteoporosis, and sarcopenia/frailty) are now predominant in HIV medicine. They have a significant dietary component and are associated with aging.

Wasting Syndrome/Disease

History

Early in the HIV epidemic, wasting syndrome (disease) was often described in association with opportunistic infection and/or AIDS-related malignancies.[55] In 1987, the CDC defined *wasting syndrome* as an involuntary weight loss greater than 10% from baseline, chronic diarrhea or documented fever for more than 30 days, and associated weakness (asthenia). Before cART, the introduction of prophylaxis for *Pneumocystis carinii* (now known as *Pneumocystis jiroveci*) pneumonia (PCP) effectively diminished PCP as the predominant cause of AIDS-related morbidity and mortality, to be replaced by wasting syndrome. Despite the widespread availability of cART, wasting continues to occur and it remains an AIDS-defining event associated with morbidity and mortality.[56]

Epidemiology

In 2002, investigators documented wasting incidence rates as high as 10.6 per 100 patient-years in HIV-infected women attending an urban north American clinic, with estimated prevalence of 22.1%.[57] Other cohorts have documented wasting prevalence rates as high as 33%.[58] In the current decade, AIDS wasting remains prevalent in resource-constrained regions, particularly eastern and southern Africa.[59-61]

The development of well-tolerated and more potent anti-retroviral medications and STRs has led to better medical outcomes. This has likely led to a reduction in the prevalence of wasting syndrome in HIV-infected patients receiving care in high-income nations. However, no studies documenting this reduction have been published. Recent publications document prevalent food insecurity in community-dwelling HIV-infected people under care in North America.[54,62,63] In addition, people living with HIV infection in parts of the United States that have declined Medicaid expansion under the Affordable Care Act may not become aware of their infection until progression to AIDS, and substantive inequalities may, therefore, be embodied as wasting disease.

Wasting syndrome continues to be predictive of opportunistic infection, poor outcome, or mortality in patients initiating cART.[64,65] Loss of skeletal muscle and adipose tissue may lead to a patient's inability to execute the instrumental activities of daily living (IADLs), ensuing social isolation, and depression, all of which may be obstacles to therapeutic adherence.

Case Definition and Clinical Diagnosis

The definition of *wasting* has evolved in the years since the original 1987 CDC definition. Wasting is now defined by a combination of functional, body weight–based parameters, and mid–upper arm circumference, and other physical findings (Table 32-5). An evaluation of weight loss includes the degree of loss, whether the loss is acute or chronic, and the medical and psychological context (as weight loss may be statistically but not medically significant). For example, an overweight patient may achieve weight loss after entry into care with attention to food quality and regularly scheduled aerobic and resistance exercise. Such loss would not warrant intervention. On the other hand, when patients experience involuntary weight loss as well as diminished physical performance and well-being, these complaints require medical investigation and nutrition evaluation. In the classic investigation of semistarvation and refeeding, Keys and colleagues found that physical performance began to decline after a weight loss of greater than 10% in healthy, normal-weight volunteers.[66]

Analysis of body composition by the application of predictive equations to the measurement of body circumferences and skinfolds allows for the description of wasting disease and patients' recovery. Estimates of mid–upper arm or thigh skeletal muscle circumference from limb circumference and skinfold measurement–based equations correlate with skeletal muscle measurements by magnetic resonance imaging and long-term clinical outcomes.[67] These correlations have led to an appreciation of the importance of anthropometric evaluation in the routine care of HIV-infected patients.

Wasting Disease vs Uncomplicated Starvation

Severe undernutrition and famine have long been known to influence human susceptibility to infection and worsen the clinical course of infectious disease. Infectious disease may, in turn, blunt or prevent human physiological adaptation to diminished nutrient intake. The human species evolved in

TABLE 32-5 Clinical Findings Consistent with Wasting Disease[a]

Subjective:
- Lethargy
- Anorexia
- Loose-fitting clothes

Social history:
- Food insecurity

Physical function:
- Weakness
- Difficulty or inability to stand without assistance
- Chronic diarrhea

Vital signs:
- Unintentional weight loss[b]
  - >10%
  - >5% within 6 months
- BMI <18.5 or marked decline from usual BMI
- Mid–upper arm circumference <10th NHANES percentile

Physical findings:
- Head: Temporal wasting, periocular edema, or retro-orbital fat loss, prominent zygomatic arch
- Torso:
  - Subclavicular muscle loss, angular shoulders, visible articulations of ribs at junction with sternum
  - Sacral edema (in bed-rest/bed-bound patients)
- Extremities:
  - Diminished mass interosseous dorsalis when pressing thumb to forefinger
  - Diminished mass quadriceps femoris and vastus medialis when leg is bent at right angle
  - Delayed mid–upper arm skinfold return, loss of turgor
  - Lower extremity edema

BMI, body mass index; NHANES, National Health and Nutrition Examination Survey.
[a]Single findings may be consistent with wasting disease but not definitive per se.
[b]Note that individuals transitioning from highly structured environments providing regularly scheduled prepared meals and exercise programs to independent living (eg, the recently incarcerated) may experience weight loss unrelated to disease processes.

an environment of intermittent food availability ("feast or famine"). During starvation, the endocrine system and major metabolic pathways mount an evolutionarily appropriate adaptive response. Skeletal muscle, organ, and adipose tissue are subject to break down to yield substrate for energetic processes during starvation. Compensatory metabolic and constitutional changes occur in starvation to minimize the loss of skeletal muscle and organ parenchyma. Decreases in the insulin-to-glucagon ratio are believed to mediate these changes, and basal metabolic rate is reduced in an effort to bring total energy expenditure into balance with the energetic value of food intake. Individuals may experience lethargy (a reduction of voluntary energy expenditure) and present with flat affect. Fat is preferentially used directly for energy (including brain ketoacid use) and for the conversion of lactate and pyruvate to glucose (gluconeogenesis).[68,69] In muscle tissue, the use of fatty acids for energy reduces the breakdown of muscle fibers for the release of alanine, a primary gluconeogenic amino acid. This adaptation to preserve structural/functional proteins is known as *nitrogen sparing*. Death ensues from exhaustion of the 2 main energy depots (adipose tissue and skeletal muscle) and catabolism of organ parenchyma leading to organ system failure.

The inability to mount a compensatory metabolic response to undernutrition because of viral effect on metabolism is what distinguishes the HIV-infected patient experiencing undernutrition from the uninfected patient experiencing the same. Maladaptive metabolic abnormalities in the HIV-infected patient experiencing undernutrition include increased resting energy expenditure (REE), inappropriate substrate use, and the futile cycling of lipids.

Etiology and Pathogenesis of Wasting Disease

The etiology of wasting disease in a given patient is multifactorial. Wasting may be an effect of HIV infection, which in turn worsens a patient's clinical course by increasing vulnerability to other infectious disease and decreasing capacity for self-care. Conversely, the lesions of opportunistic infection may in turn lead to wasting disease. Mechanisms may include food insecurity, decreased food intake, and/or decreased nutrient assimilation related to the disease process, abnormal metabolism, and/or endocrine dysfunction. The identification of causation determines the appropriate therapeutic intervention(s) (Table 32-6).

Chronic undernutrition may be a consequence of food insecurity in association with large-scale social forces such as poverty or civil unrest, or it may be related to the constitutional manifestations of AIDS, profound fatigue, and impaired physical or cognitive function. The inability to consistently perform IADLs such as shopping for food and preparing meals may ensue from social, environmental, and/or biological causes. These factors singularly or in combination may all affect nutriture, disease course, and medical outcomes. HIV-infected

---

TABLE 32-6 Possible Nutrition-Related Interventions for Patients with Wasting Disease

- Consider use of an orexigenic agent.
- Address depression (social work, psychiatry, or chaplaincy consult).
- Help patients avoid food odors during periods of nausea (eg, serve meals in a well-ventilated room and/or serve cold foods).
- Consider ready-to-use peanut-based therapeutic food.
- Alter food texture, consistency, acidity, or temperature to facilitate intake.
- Manage electrolytes and fluids.
- Alter macronutrient content to facilitate drug absorption.
- Prescribe physiological testosterone replacement therapy (in hypogonadal male patients).
- Prescribe supraphysiological recombinant human growth hormone or anabolic-androgenic steroid therapy (usually outpatient only).
- Administer nutrition support by gastric or enteric tube.
- Administer intravenous alimentation.

---

patients often have a combination of these problems. Food insecurity may coexist with hunger or be experienced in the absence of hunger, and it may contribute to wasting or obesity.[70] The association of food insecurity with obesity, may seem counterintuitive, but food insecure patients may rely on inexpensive, energy-dense, ultraprocessed foods (manufactured combinations of multiple processed ingredients with cosmetic or sensory-intensifying additives, such as chicken "nuggets," fish "sticks," and sugar-sweetened beverages).

Prolonged decrease in energy intake is the proximate predictor and drive of wasting disease.[71] Decreased food intake may drive wasting despite compensatory lethargy, which attempts to bring total energy expenditure into balance with energy intake.[71] Negative energy balance with catabolism ensues when the patient can no longer achieve a sufficient compensatory decrease in total energy expenditure. Depression in a patient may manifest as anorexia and involuntary weight loss. Anorexia caused by systemic infection (eg, HIV viremia, bacteremia, disseminated opportunistic infection) is believed to ensue when proinflammatory cytokines such as interleukin (IL)-6 act on the central nervous system and viscera, mediating delayed gastric emptying and intestinal edema.

Compensatory lethargy may occur in wasting syndrome, but it is not accompanied by a decrease in basal metabolic rate or adaptive metabolic response to facilitate nitrogen sparing.[71,72] Therapeutically, the difference lies in the effect of refeeding, which alone reverses starvation but does not reverse AIDS wasting. In a seminal study, Grunfeld and colleagues assessed REE and 28-day weight trend in a cohort of HIV-infected patients.[71] REE increases of approximately 11% and 28% were documented in patients with HIV infection (HIV+) and AIDS or AIDS with active secondary infection (AIDS-SI), respectively.[71] The energy value of ad libitum food and beverage intake in AIDS-SI patients was 17% less than REE (energy intake–to-REE ratio less than 1.0), and the patients in this group lost weight during the study period. In this data set, decreased food intake and patients' inability to mount a compensatory decrease in basal metabolic rate (quantified as REE) were the primary predictors and drive of wasting disease, respectively.[71]

Dietary thermogenesis is the energy expended for nutrient absorption and assimilation. Patients with HIV infection experience both a temporal and quantitative change in diet-induced thermogenesis. In HIV infection, peak meal-induced thermogenesis occurs later, and the elevation is more prolonged. Patients with HIV infection and weight loss demonstrate greater increases than those with HIV infection alone.[73]

The futile cycling of fatty acids and increases in hepatic de novo lipogenesis may contribute to soft tissue wasting in people with HIV disease.[74] Approximately 30% of the energy value of glucose is lost if lipogenesis precedes its oxidation instead of its direct use for energy. In a patient experiencing wasting, such a conversion would be energetically inappropriate and contrasts sharply with the use of lipids for gluconeogenesis in uncomplicated starvation. Additionally, the expression of lipoprotein lipase may be diminished in peripheral tissue in association with elevated levels of interferon alpha, leading to a reduction in triglyceride clearance and hypertriglyceridemia.[75,76] However, isolated hypertriglyceridemia is not uniformly associated with (or predictive of) wasting syndrome.[76] Nevertheless, clinicians should check triglyceride levels in all HIV-infected patients when providing nutrition care and especially before the infusion of lipid-containing IV admixtures or emulsions.

Increase in whole body protein turnover (synthesis and degradation) has been documented in HIV-infected patients and is consistent with a hypermetabolic state. The fraction of total protein synthesis accorded to skeletal muscle is similar in asymptomatic HIV-infected and uninfected individuals.[77] Muscle protein synthesis represents a decreased fraction of whole body protein synthesis in individuals demonstrating AIDS wasting.[77] This finding suggests that patients with AIDS wasting have a diminished ability to use amino acids for synthetic pathways in skeletal muscle and/or there is increased competition from oxidative (energy-yielding) pathways or other tissue for amino acids (eg, hepatic or blood cell synthesis of immune effector proteins).

The investigative and therapeutic administration of cytokines, as well as the innate immune response to acute infection, has been associated with anorexia, fatigue, and malaise. For example, the administration of tumor necrosis factor (TNF)-α to study animals led to decreased gastric emptying, increased intestinal edema, and worsening anorexia.[78] Interestingly, the continued administration of TNF-α led to tolerance, as demonstrated by the animals' eventual resumption of oral intake.[78] In patients with AIDS wasting, plasma concentrations of TNF-α and IL-6 are elevated but do not reliably distinguish patients with wasting from HIV-infected patients without wasting.[79] The exact cause of anorexia is likely linked to cytokine milieu and not to a single factor.

Regardless of cause, when a patient can no longer achieve a compensatory decrease in total energy expenditure (leading to negative energy balance), the clinical impact is detrimental. The combination of an inability to maintain energy intake and increased REE (hypermetabolism) drives wasting. Patients are at highest risk for wasting during episodes of opportunistic or secondary infection(s) and/or malignancy. The mechanical (eg, oral and esophageal disease) and psychological (eg, depression) causes of diminished food intake require evaluation and treatment as needed.

The incidence of opportunistic infection and malignancies of the GI tract has declined with the widespread use of cART, but prevalence of these problems remains high in patients with immunodeficiency (CD4 count less than 200 cells/mm³). Intestinal infection may be marked by maldigestion, malabsorption, and diarrhea. Infections of the small and large bowel may disseminate to other organ systems and further compromise nutrition. Malabsorption is characterized by decreased nutrient absorption accompanied by fecal water and electrolyte loss. Malabsorption may occur in association with structural changes in small intestinal villi or obstruction of the lymphatics. For example, infection with the protozoal GI parasites *Cryptosporidium parvum* and *Enterocytozoon bieneusi* (microsporidia) results in partial atrophy of villi and diminished absorptive surface area (despite compensatory crypt hyperplasia). Moreover, immature enterocytes do not elaborate digestive and absorptive proteins, contributing to the loss of mucosal function. Infection with *Mycobacterium avium* complex results

in extensive macrophage infiltration of the lamina propria and lymphatics, leading to obstruction. The resulting diarrhea (eg, 4 or more bowel movements per day) may lead patients to eat less to reduce the frequency and urgency of bowel movements (thereby worsening wasting).

Both primary hypogonadism (testicular failure) and secondary hypogonadism (hypothalamic and/or pituitary failure) may occur in HIV-infected men.[80] In men with AIDS wasting syndrome, loss of lean body mass (LBM; ascertained by dual x-ray absorptiometry [DXA]), loss of skeletal muscle mass (calculated by measured urinary creatinine excretion on a meat-free diet), and decrease in exercise capacity were associated with low androgen levels.[81] Clinical investigators have documented biochemical hypogonadism prevalence rates of 19% in men demonstrating wasting and 24% in HIV-infected men older than 40 years in an observational cohort.[82,83]

Males with hypogonadism may present with complaints of depressed mood, decreased spontaneous erections, and reduced sexual desire or ideation (libido) in addition to weight or skeletal muscle loss. In serum, testosterone may be bioavailable (ie, free or loosely albumin-bound [readily dissociable]) or tightly bound by sex hormone–binding globulin (SHBG). SHBG may be increased in HIV infection, leading to a decrease in free testosterone levels while normal total testosterone levels are maintained. Therefore, hypogonadism in HIV-infected males is diagnosed by free, not total, testosterone levels. In addition to free testosterone, biochemical evaluation includes luteinizing hormone and follicle-stimulating hormone (to differentiate between primary and secondary hypogonadism), and prolactin (to identify hypothalamic and/or pituitary dysfunction). The patient's blood should be drawn for these assays in the early morning because of the circadian variation of serum testosterone levels. Medication review should include evaluation for patient's receipt of agents that suppress the hypothalamic pituitary gonadal axis, such as high-dose glucocorticoid therapy or long-acting opioid or methadone maintenance therapy. The diagnosis of hypogonadism should not be made during an acute illness. Transient downregulation of testosterone synthesis may occur during clinically active secondary or opportunistic infections.

Women with wasting disease may also experience reduced serum testosterone levels. Testosterone testing has not been standardized for women. However, several successful clinical trials of treatment with exogenous testosterone have been reported.[84,85] Levels of free testosterone in eumenorrheic women may be affected by the phases of the menstrual cycle, and the optimal long-term replacement dosage of testosterone for women has not been determined.[81] This usage remains investigational.[84–86]

Patients with wasting syndrome may demonstrate acquired growth hormone (GH) resistance. Studies of undernutrition and wasting disease in HIV-infected patients have identified a role for insulin-like growth factor-1 (IGF-1) in anabolism.[87,88] IGF-1 is produced by the liver in response to GH, and it works with GH in a synergistic manner on target tissues. IGF-1 upregulation of cellular metabolism and/or proliferation depends on the level of cellular differentiation. For example, GH and IGF-1 have a trophic effect on muscle cells, as demonstrated by increased myocyte synthesis of myofibrillar protein during exposure. IGF-1 production is downregulated in undernutrition and severe chronic illness, functioning as an adaptive mechanism to free amino acids and other substrates for critical processes. Investigators have documented elevated GH levels with inappropriately low IGF-1 levels in cohorts of hypogonadal and eugonadal HIV-infected men demonstrating wasting.[88] These findings are consistent with acquired GH resistance at the level of the liver in profound undernutrition and wasting disease, and they provide the rationale for treatment with supraphysiological doses of recombinant human growth hormone (rhGH).[89]

Clinical Encounter and Assessment

When investigating a complaint of wasting or involuntary weight loss, the clinician should evaluate the degree and rapidity of the weight change (ie, acute vs chronic), depression, and the patient's ability to perform IADLs. It is often helpful to ask patients for a pre-illness photograph, when they last remember being at their usual weight, and the last time they engaged in enjoyable activities or hobbies (Figure 32-2).

In patients with a CD4 count less than 100 cells/mm³, loss of appetite and weight may be the first signs of slowly progressive systemic opportunistic infections such as cytomegalovirus or *Mycobacterium avium* complex. In these patients, clinicians should pay attention to weight loss decrement, presence of fever, and presence and location of abdominal pain. Complaints of diarrhea may be evaluated by determining the change from usual bowel movement pattern (frequency), consistency, amount, or volume, and the presence of blood or mucus. For example, copious watery diarrhea may be associated with small bowel disease and mucus-containing, small-volume diarrhea with colonic disease.

Clinicians should be mindful of the social determinants of wasting disease. Food insecurity may be evaluated by using the US Department of Agriculture food security questionnaire

(6-item short form) or Radimer/Cornell questionnaire.[70,90] In many states, the Supplemental Nutrition Assistance Program (SNAP or "food stamps") application may be completed online or by mail. The ability to shop for and prepare meals as well as access to supermarkets and kitchen facilities should be evaluated. AIDS service organizations (ASOs) and dedicated government programs may provide home meal delivery, congregate meals, food pantries, or home attendants for shopping and cooking. Psychiatric counseling for depression and peer support groups may also be available through ASOs. However, patients frequently require an AIDS/HIV disease diagnosis and/or medical documentation of a medical condition that limits ambulation or cognition for home meal delivery or attendant care.

Nutrition-Focused Physical Examination

Patients with an HIV infection may present with wasting (involuntary loss of skeletal muscle and adipose tissue), sarcopenia (age-related loss of skeletal muscle mass and function), or lipodystrophy (focal or global loss of subcutaneous adipose tissue with the preservation of visceral adipose tissue and skeletal muscle). The nutrition-focused physical examination is essential in distinguishing between these clinical presentations.

Bilateral temporal wasting, retro-orbital fat mass wasting (lending a sunken appearance to the eyes), and the loss of Bichat's fat pads should be evaluated for during an examination of the head and neck. An oral examination should evaluate for missing dentition and oral mucosa ulcers (eg, aphthous or viral ulcers), malignancy (eg, Kaposi sarcoma), and fungal infections (eg, oral candidiasis), among other problems. Findings on inspection of the torso consistent with wasting include subclavicular muscle loss (with increased clavicle prominence), angular shoulders due to deltoid muscle loss (with increased acromion process prominence), and visible articulations of the ribs at the junction with the sternum. Waist circumference and the waist-to-hip ratio can help distinguish wasting from lipodystrophy syndrome, because the patient with wasting is unlikely to experience isolated fat loss in the face, extremities, and buttocks without significant abdominal fat loss. The loss of appendicular skeletal muscle and subcutaneous fat mass may be evaluated by measurement of mid–upper arm circumference and skinfold using the National Health and Nutrition Examination Survey percentiles for reference ranges.[91] Skeletal muscle may also be clinically evaluated by having the patient press the tips of his or her forefinger and thumb together and observing the mass of the interosseous dorsalis or by placing the patient's leg at a right angle and observing muscle mass at the insertion of the quadriceps femoris and the vastus medialis.

Bioelectrical impedance analysis (BIA) indirectly measures body composition using a 4-compartment model: LBM, which is

FIGURE 32-2 Wasting Treatment Strategies

Identify and treat underlying causes
- HIV infection
- Opportunistic infection(s)
- Depression
- Hypogonadism

Nutrition evaluation and interventions
- Diet quality, texture, and consistency
- Ready-to-use, peanut-based therapeutic foods
- Nonvolitional alimentation

Community-based interventions
- Home meal delivery program enrollment
- Food pantries and congregate meal sites
- Supplemental Nutrition Assistance Program enrollment

Pharmacological options
- Orexigenic agents
- Anabolic-androgenic steroids
- Growth hormone

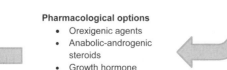

divided into body cell mass (BCM) and extracellular (interstitial) mass (ECM); fat mass; and osseous tissue.[92] BCM by weight is primarily skeletal muscle. Phase angle is a geometrical expression of the resistance and capacitance components of this assay. Ott and associates demonstrated that phase angles less than 5.6° and 4.8° were associated with diminished survival and nonsurvival, respectively, in the absence of cART.[93] In addition, the ratio of ECM to BCM of 1.3 or greater was associated with nonsurvival in the absence of cART.[93] Serial BIA will document weight loss or gain over time by soft tissue compartment, and will allow for the appreciation of each compartment's response to intervention(s) for wasting disease.

Medication Review

Polypharmacy is prevalent in HIV-infected people with access to care in North America and has been associated with impaired nutrition status, functional and cognitive deficits, and falls in the HIV-infected and general populations.[94-96] Medication review should include prescription and over-the-counter pharmaceuticals, as well as supplements and botanical (herbal) products. Certain botanical or supplemental products have negative drug interactions with cART (eg, garlic supplements, St. John's wort). Medications may require administration with a meal for absorption (eg, rilpivirine) or may interact with one another. Medications may also affect serum glucose, electrolyte, or lipid levels. Patients' routine meal composition and pattern should be identified and discussed. For example, a patient may think a cup of coffee and a doughnut or muffin are a meal, but this amount of food may not be adequate for drug absorption or the prevention of untoward GI side effects with certain medications (eg, atovaquone or ritonavir-boosted PIs). Patients should be counseled that certain foodstuffs negatively affect drug levels (eg, grapefruit contains furanocoumarins that irreversibly inhibit cytochrome P450 3A4). Patients with lactose intolerance may experience diarrhea from pharmaceutical formulations with lactose as an excipient. Clinicians should be familiar with the information contained in medication package inserts, such as food effect, drug interactions and metabolism, excipients, and data on the frequency of potential side effects.

The simplification of cART with STRs taken once daily, particularly elvitegravir/cobicistat/tenofovir disoproxil/ emtricitabine and rilpivirine/tenofovir disoproxil fumarate/ emtricitabine, is associated with higher rates of adherence and decreased risk of hospitalization.[97] cART adherence may be evaluated by asking patients if they have missed any doses within the past 7 days and if they have missed any doses in the past month. Most patients have good recall for the past 7 days, and an answer affirming recently missed doses may reveal problems that can be easily addressed (eg, by changing medication administration time from morning to evening, by having the patient position medication containers next to the coffee machine or toothbrush at home, or providing a 7-day pill box organizer with AM and PM compartments). An affirmative answer to the second part of the question about longer-term cART adherence (eg, "Yes, there was a week at the beginning of the month during which I didn't take my medications because . . .") may reveal problems related to refilling

prescriptions, such as insurance company prior authorizations, copays, or termination of coverage.

Social and Family History

Social history should include social determinants of health (eg, educational attainment, housing, access to kitchen facilities and supermarkets). Health-related behaviors should also be evaluated and documented in the nutrition consultation. The use of tobacco, alcohol, or other psychoactive substances and disordered sleeping habits may have quantitative and/or qualitative effects on food intake.[98] Prolonged bed rest and/ or a lack of weight-bearing exercise may negatively affect a patient's skeletal muscle, bone mineral density (BMD), and food intake.[99]

Evaluation of family history (3 generations for diabetes, premature CVD events in a first-degree relative, bone fragility fractures, end-stage renal disease, and cancer) may reveal potential intolerance of nutrition interventions or a need for additional testing. For example, a patient with a family history of diabetes may demonstrate glucose abnormalities while receiving megestrol acetate or rhGH. Patients with a family history of fragility fracture who have experienced wasting disease and low CD4 counts (additional risk factors) may be candidates for DXA to evaluate for BMD loss.

Clinical Management

Nutrition support of the wasted patient may include the following: the avoidance of food odors during periods of nausea, the alteration of foods (texture, consistency, acidity) to facilitate intake in the presence of oropharyngeal or esophageal lesions, ready-to-use therapeutic foods, orexigenic agents, electrolyte management, and feeding by intragastric or enteric tube or IV alimentation (Table 32-6). Nutrition interventions should focus on adequate nonprotein-energy and protein-energy intake, particularly during episodes of secondary or opportunistic infection; micronutrient adequacy; facilitating antimicrobial and/or antiretroviral absorption; and tolerance. Pharmaceutical agents are available to create the sensation of hunger, for physiological hormone replacement, and to promote preferential accrual of skeletal muscle (Table 32-7).

Orexigenic Agents

In recent years, with improved screening for HIV infection (opt-out and rapid antigen-antibody testing) and linkage to care, the use of orexigenic agents has markedly decreased because patients are frequently diagnosed at higher CD4 counts. Megestrol acetate (Megace or Megace ES oral suspension) is a synthetic progestin, related to progesterone, that has been shown to create the sensation of hunger and promote weight gain in patients with AIDS wasting syndrome.[100] Investigators have documented gains of fat and LBM in HIV-infected patients receiving megestrol acetate.[100] As a progestational steroid, megestrol acetate downregulates testosterone synthesis, and men may experience erectile dysfunction and/ or acceleration of wasting when use is prolonged. Other documented side effects include hyperglycemia, thromboembolic

TABLE 32-7 Medications for the Treatment of Wasting Disease

	Orexigenic Agents		Supraphysiological Hormone Administration	Physiological Testosterone Replacement			Anabolic-Androgenic Steroids	
	Megestrol Acetate	Dronabinol	Growth Hormone	Testosterone Gels	Testosterone Patch	Testosterone Enanthate	Nandrolone Decanoate	Oxandrolone
FDA indication specific for AIDS wasting	Yes	Yes	Yes	No	No	No	No	No
Route of administration	Oral	Oral	Subcutaneous injection	Topical	Topical	Intramuscular injection	Intramuscular injection	Oral
Dosage	800 mg daily (20-mL oral suspension)	2.5 mg twice daily (before lunch and dinner)	6 mg daily	Daily application[a]	5-mg patch daily[b]	200 mg every other week[c]	100–200 mg every other week[b]	20 mg daily[b]
Duration of clinical studies for AIDS wasting	12 weeks	6 weeks	12 weeks	Ongoing physiological replacement	Ongoing physiological replacement	At or above physiological level during dosing interval	12 weeks	8 weeks
Mechanism of effect	Increase intake	Increase intake	Promote protein synthesis, nitrogen retention	Restore physiological level, protein synthesis, nitrogen retention	Restore physiological level, protein synthesis, nitrogen retention	Promote protein synthesis, nitrogen retention	Promote protein synthesis, nitrogen retention	Promote protein synthesis, nitrogen retention
Clinical effect	Increased appetite	Increased appetite	Increased LBM and decreased fat (visceral subcutaneous)	Increased LBM	Increased LBM	Increased LBM	Increased LBM	Increased LBM[d]
Major side effects[e]	Hypogonadism, hyperglycemia, adrenal insufficiency	Dose-related euphoria, somnolence	Dose-related edema, insulin resistance, fat atrophy, arthralgias, myalgias	Application-site reaction, acne, peripheral edema	Application-site reaction, acne, peripheral edema	Gynecomastia acne, edema, excessive frequency and duration of penile erections	Testicular shrinkage, decreased HDL-C, acne, virilizing effects in women are possible, edema	Decreased HDL-C, hepatotoxicity, peliosis, hepatitis, reduced SHBG, virilizing effects in women are possible

AIDS, acquired immunodeficiency syndrome; FDA, US Food and Drug Administration; HDL-C, high-density lipoprotein cholesterol; LBM, lean body mass; SHBG, sex hormone–binding globulin.

[a]Indicated for replacement therapy in males; product testosterone concentrations differ—see package insert for dosages.
[b]Male dosage; female usage is investigational.
[c]Testosterone at replacement dosages in hypogonadal males.
[d]Requires resistance exercise for effect.
[e]Review package insert for complete information on side effects.

events, and adrenal insufficiency (due to some glucocorticoid activity).[101] Dosages are megestrol acetate oral suspension 20 mL to deliver 800 mg daily or bioequivalent Megace ES 5-mL oral suspension to deliver 625 mg daily.

Dronabinol (Δ-9-tetrahydrocannabinol or Marinol) is the active component of marijuana and is approved for the treatment of anorexia in patients with AIDS. Although not as potent as megestrol acetate, it does have mild antiemetic activity and a more benign side effect profile.[102] It has not been shown to consistently increase food intake or promote weight gain.[100,103] Potential side effects include psychotropic activity, drowsiness, and hypogonadism. Because of its long half-life, dronabinol may be dosed once daily at bedtime for those patients experiencing drowsiness as a side effect. The usual starting dosage is 2.5 mg orally twice daily or 5 mg orally once daily.

Anabolic-Androgenic Steroids

LBM accrual has been documented in HIV-infected men with AIDS wasting syndrome receiving long-term testosterone replacement therapy.[104,105] Several preparations are available for physiological testosterone replacement and include the transdermal patch, topical gel, or intramuscular (IM) injection. The testosterone patch (Androderm) is applied to the upper arm or buttocks to deliver 5 mg of testosterone daily. Transdermal delivery may also be achieved by topical gel (eg, Testim or AndroGel) with a dosage of 5 g of 1% testosterone gel 5 g to deliver 5 mg of testosterone when applied daily. Patients should be counseled that topical testosterone may be transferable by contact. This risk is an important issue for patients with female partners (especially pregnant ones) and/or those who are in close contact with children. Testosterone esters (eg, testosterone enanthate, an unmodified 17β-ester depot formulation) are available for IM injection with a dose of 200 mg every 2 weeks. Unlike daily dosing, this method results in perceptible peak and trough levels during the dosing interval instead of the steady-state physiological levels obtained with the use of gel or patch. Testosterone formulations for IM injection also carry a greater risk of polycythemia, especially in older men.

Pharmacological dosing of testosterone to achieve anabolic-androgenic effect on muscle tissue has been investigated in eugonadal men and women with involuntary weight loss and/or wasting disease. Nandrolone decanoate (19-normethyl-testosterone 17β-ester) is a depot formulation available for long-acting IM delivery of testosterone. It is FDA-approved for the treatment of anemia in chronic renal failure. Investigators have documented the association of its off-label use for AIDS wasting syndrome with increases in weight, LBM, and quality of life (QOL).[106,107] The usual IM dosage for the treatment of wasting syndrome is 100 to 200 mg every 2 weeks. The treatment of women with androgenic-anabolic steroids has been shown to result in LBM accrual without a loss of adipose tissue, but it remains investigational because of limited safety data.[108]

Oxandrolone (Oxandrin) is a 17α-methylated testosterone derivative for oral administration. Unlike nandrolone decanoate, it is FDA-approved for the treatment of weight loss caused by chronic infection. In a prospective randomized study, HIV-infected men who experienced a mean weight loss of 9% received oxandrolone 20 mg administered orally once daily.

Both arms of the study received testosterone enanthate (100 mg administered by IM injection once weekly) to suppress endogenous testosterone production and participated in a supervised progressive resistance exercise program. The patients in the oxandrolone arm demonstrated significantly greater increases in LBM and strength compared with patients in the control group.[109] Significant decreases in high-density lipoprotein cholesterol (HDL-C) cholesterol were also documented in the oxandrolone arm. Grunfeld and colleagues documented similar results in addition to the suppression of SHBG and total and free testosterone levels (subjects in this study were not receiving IM testosterone).[110] Low-density lipoprotein cholesterol (LDL-C) and transaminase levels were also significantly elevated in subjects receiving oxandrolone.[110] Orally ingested 17α-methylated testosterone analogs are subject to first-pass hepatic metabolism, and long-term use has been associated with hepatotoxicity, decreased serum SHBG and efficacy.[111] The identification of a single androgen receptor gene (and protein) suggests that, at bioequivalent dosages, all testosterone formulations have essentially the same physiological effects.[112] Therefore, nonorally administered testosterone therapy may be preferred to minimize the potential for hepatotoxicity.

Recombinant Human Growth Hormone

Once widely used, rhGH now has very limited application. Patients with wasting syndrome receiving rhGH (somatropin [Serostim]) at the supraphysiological dose of 6 mg (0.1 mg/kg/d) administered subcutaneously once daily for 12 weeks demonstrated increases in LBM and positive nitrogen balance during treatment.[113] Side effects may include edema, arthralgias, and myalgias that can be addressed by lowering dietary sodium intake, dose reduction, and/or the use of nonsteroidal anti-inflammatory agents. Other significant side effects include hyperglycemia and carpal tunnel syndrome. The evaluation of candidates for treatment with rhGH should include serum glucose for hyperglycemia and family history for diabetes mellitus. A 2-hour 75-g oral glucose tolerance test may be considered prior to initiation of rhGH therapy in candidates with a family history of diabetes mellitus or other risk factors. It is important to note that patients lose body fat while receiving rhGH (an undesired effect in patients with significant peripheral lipoatrophy).

Progressive Resistance and Aerobic Exercise

Eugonadal men diagnosed with AIDS wasting syndrome demonstrated increases in LBM and HDL-C at the completion of a 12-week supervised progressive resistance and aerobic exercise program.[114] An increase in cardioprotective HDL-C may be of benefit to HIV-infected patients with wasting and low CD4+ T cell count. CD4+ T cell count less than 500 cells/mm³ in HIV-infected outpatients is an independent risk factor for incident CVD events.[115]

Energy, Protein, and Electrolytes

Pharmacological intervention is of limited benefit in the absence of adequate alimentation. Alimentation may occur orally in response to hunger or appetite (volitional) or by feeding tube or IV infusion (nonvolitionally). The calculation of maintenance energy requirement includes basal metabolic rate and disease-related elevation, dietary thermogenesis, and voluntary activity. Additional energy for anabolism should be provided during nutritional rehabilitation at the convalescent stage. The Harris-Benedict predictive equation for basal metabolic rate is the most widely referenced in the literature and is useful when working without access to indirect calorimetry.[116] Refeeding should be initiated at less than the calculated energy requirement, slowly progressing toward goal intake over several days with patients' demonstration of tolerance.

Generally, HIV-infected patients have a higher protein requirement, which may be exacerbated during secondary or opportunistic infection due to increased synthesis of acute-phase immunologic (eg, complement and immunoglobulins), and hemostatic proteins. High-nitrogen feeding (1.5 to 1.8 g amino acids per kilogram of body weight) significantly improves nitrogen balance in patients with wasting syndrome receiving IV alimentation.[117] Investigators have also documented the maintenance of nutrient intake and decreased soft tissue catabolism in HIV-infected patients receiving nutrient-dense, ready-to-use therapeutic foods by mouth.[118,119] Nutrition outcomes are improved when food support is provided at earlier stages of wasting and with the initiation of cART.[120]

Patients with marked wasting disease may have profound electrolyte deficits and are at risk for refeeding syndrome. Sudden death due to arrhythmia and respiratory arrest during refeeding may occur when alimentation precipitates acute intravascular volume expansion, serum phosphate depletion, hypokalemia, and hypomagnesemia.[121] Electrolytes (eg, phosphorous, potassium, and magnesium) should be evaluated daily and replenished intravenously. Oral formulations of these electrolytes may be poorly tolerated due to dose-related cathartic effects (osmotic activity of these ions). Electrolyte normalization should commence before macronutrient-containing nutrition support begins. Patients with severe wasting or those with a history of chronic alcohol use may require a short course of IV thiamin before the initiation of refeeding. Orally administered cations (eg, calcium, magnesium, aluminum) may decrease the absorption of some antimicrobial agents (eg, azithromycin, levofloxacin), and coadministration should be avoided.

Sodium retention is a response to profound undernutrition and wasting disease. It may lead to a propensity to fluid overload during the early stages of refeeding. The syndrome of inappropriate antidiuresis may occur in patients with central nervous system or lung disease. As a result, fluid balance, urinary output, and urine electrolytes should be monitored during the nutrition support of these patients.

Glycated hemoglobin (A1C) may underestimate glycemia in HIV-infected people with lower CD4 counts or elevated mean corpuscular volumes as well as in those receiving abacavir.[122]

Vitamin D

Vitamin D deficiency and insufficiency are prevalent in HIV-infected as well as uninfected people in the United States.[123–125]

Risk factors for vitamin D deficiency include self-reported black or other non-white ethnicity, obesity, lower CD4 count, and treatment with antimycobacterials, anticonvulsants, or corticosteroids.[123–125] Severe vitamin D deficiency (less than 25 nmol/L) has been associated with receipt of the NNRTI efavirenz.[126] Vitamin D plays a crucial role in mediating the innate immune response to microbial pathogens, and deficiency has been associated with current and past tuberculosis infection, as well as latent tuberculosis infection.[127]

Hypovitaminosis D may manifest as lower extremity muscle weakness. Serum 25-hydroxyvitamin D (25[OH]D) should be routinely assayed in patients and supplemented as needed. In the absence of a serum 25(OH)D assay, lower extremity muscle weakness may be misattributed solely to skeletal muscle loss in wasted patients with hypovitaminosis D.

For people residing in North America, the Recommended Dietary Allowance and Tolerable Upper Intake Level for vitamin D are 600 and 4000 IU daily, respectively. Many experts recommend the maintenance of serum 25(OH)D concentration at approximately 75 nmol/L (30 ng/mL).[128] Patients with profound vitamin D deficiency may require a loading dose of 50,000 IU weekly for 8 weeks prior to maintenance supplementation.[128]

ω-3 Fatty Acid Enrichment

In patients with AIDS wasting without active secondary or opportunistic infection, investigators have documented the downregulation of hepatic triglyceride synthesis by dietary ω-3 fatty acid supplementation.[129] However, in a trial of an arginine and ω-3 fatty acid–enriched formula compared with a standard, protein- and energy-dense formula, HIV-infected patients receiving the enriched formula did not demonstrate superior anthropometric or immunologic parameters.[129]

Enteral Nutrition

HIV-infected patients who are candidates for tube feeding include those with neurologic disease (eg, progressive multifocal leukoencephalopathy), oropharyngeal or esophageal lesions, profound anorexia with or without nausea, or impaired gut function, and those who are unable to achieve significant volitional dietary intake. Intragastric feeding tubes are strongly preferred to minimize GI side effects and optimize medication absorption. Many antiretrovirals have food and pH requirements for absorption. The safety and benefit of nutrition by a gastrostomy tube in AIDS patients has been documented.[130] HIV-infected patients receiving nutrition by feeding tube demonstrated increases in both weight and BCM.[130,131] Medications administered by feeding tube should be evaluated for appropriate formulation or vehicle, the effect of coadministered drug excipients on their absorption (eg, buffers), and the effect of the excipients themselves (eg, lactose, oleic acid) on patient tolerance.

A potential complication of percutaneous endoscopic gastrostomy is buried bumper syndrome, in which the gastric bumper of the feeding tube migrates into or through the gastric wall, with accompanying severe complications. Loss of gastric wall mass in HIV-infected patients with wasting disease may contribute to risk for this complication, and severe abdominal pain in this setting requires endoscopic evaluation. Buried bumper syndrome may be prevented by checking the external bolster to ensure that it is not pressing against the skin too tightly (due to excessive tension between the internal and external bumpers), and rotating the tube 360° daily. Inability to rotate the gastric tube may be a sign of this syndrome.

Parenteral Nutrition

Patients with extensive small bowel disease, such as jejuno-ileitis, are candidates for IV alimentation (Practice Scenario 32-1[132-134]). These patients frequently demonstrate pan-malabsorption with the volume of diarrhea directly related to food intake by mouth. Opportunistic infections of the small bowel may lead to extensive small bowel erosion, ulceration, and edema or pseudo-obstruction, which precludes usage for enteral nutrition. Marked improvements in functional status (Karnofsky index), subjective feeling of health, and increases in total body weight and LBM have been documented in HIV-infected patients with wasting syndrome receiving IV alimentation.[135,136] Profoundly immunodeficient HIV-infected patients with wasting syndrome receiving a 2-month course of home infusion demonstrated a low rate of catheter-related septicemia (0.26 per 100 patient days).[135]

Practice Scenario 32-1

Question: When is intravenous (IV) alimentation warranted in a person with human immunodeficiency virus (HIV) disease?

Scenario: A 43-year-old man who has sex with men was recently diagnosed with HIV infection after admission to a local hospital with *Pneumocystis jiroveci* pneumonia. After being treated and discharged, he presented to the clinic for further management. On initial examination, he was noted to have orthostatic hypotension and was referred for admission to the hospital for IV hydration and management.

Upon further history, the patient revealed that he was having watery diarrhea, occasionally accompanied by blood, 6 or more times per day, as well as periumbilical and left lower-quadrant pain, and abdominal cramping, which was worse following meals. The patient also complained of odynophagia and anorexia, and had lost 20 pounds in the past 6 months. On questioning about his weight loss, he disclosed that he had been limiting his food intake for the last month to avoid urgent, "explosive" bowel movements and was occasionally soiling himself when away from home. He was 5 feet 7 inches tall, weighed 125 pounds, 76.2% of his usual weight and had a body mass index of 19.7. He has been spiking fevers to 103° Fahrenheit. Stool studies from his prior admission were unremarkable except for the presence of white blood cells. On physical examination, he demonstrated dry oral mucosa with no evidence of oral candidiasis or missing dentition, or lower extremity edema. His CD4 count was less than 50 cells/mm^3, and his serum potassium, magnesium and phosphorous levels were all low.

Visualization of the esophagus, small bowel, and colon revealed large, shallow ulcers in the distal esophagus, a small

ulcer in the antrum of the stomach, and several areas of erosion (loss of mucosal integrity), ulceration (deep lesions with necrotic tissue), and inflammation of the small bowel wall. Multiple areas of edema and erythema in addition to ulcers were also seen in the transverse and right colon. Histology (biopsy specimens) from all areas showed characteristic basophilic nuclear inclusion bodies with narrow clear halos consistent with diffuse cytomegalovirus enteritis/colitis with distal esophagitis and gastric involvement. The medical plan was for IV ganciclovir induction therapy for 21 to 28 days, with possible transition to oral valganciclovir, if gastrointestinal signs and symptoms resolved.

Intervention: The patient received IV hydration with dextrose 5%, 0.45% sodium chloride solution, and thiamin, potassium, magnesium, and phosphorous were repleted by IV administration. IV alimentation was subsequently initiated with 1.68 liters of an amino acid 5.0% (50 g/L), dextrose 10% (100 g/L) solution with electrolytes, infused at 70 mL/h continuous and a secondary IV infusion of 200 mL 20% lipid emulsion infused at 20 mL/h over 10 hours. The final concentration of dextrose in the solutions was advanced to 20% (200 g/L) over 1 week while serum phosphorus, potassium, and magnesium were monitored and repleted with bolus infusions as needed.

Answer: Parenteral nutrition was warranted in this patient with AIDS-related alimentary tract disease.

Rationale: The patient demonstrated signs, symptoms, and clinical findings consistent with extensive gastrointestinal disease and pan-malabsorption. Additionally, the resolution of pan-malabsorption was expected to require several weeks. Patients with severe wasting and dehydration are at significant risk for developing pneumothorax due to pleural puncture during central vein catheter insertion; therefore, adequate hydration should be achieved prior to this procedure.

To lessen the risk of refeeding (glucose)-induced acute thiamin deficiency, the patient received a loading dose of thiamin, in addition to the gradual correction of electrolyte deficits, prior to the initiation of IV alimentation. Acute thiamin deficiency in patients receiving PN may lead to lactic acidosis with urinary electrolyte losses, which may be clinically recognized by hypotension, change in patient's mental status, and Kussmaul's respiration.[132,133] In contrast to glucose-induced acute thiamin deficiency, the hypophosphatemia of refeeding syndrome is precipitated by an intracellular shift of electrolytes, in association with increased insulin secretion.[134]

Short-term infusion into a peripheral vein (peripheral parenteral nutrition [PPN]) is particularly effective in wasted patients receiving antimicrobials known to cause electrolyte losses or limited tolerance of food by mouth. PPN can deliver significant amounts of macronutrients per kilogram of body weight in these patients (with low body weight) while facilitating repletion and ongoing management of their electrolytes. PPN and provision of an oral diet are not mutually exclusive. We have observed a marked increase in appetite and oral intake after administration of PPN in wasted patients who initially present with profound electrolyte deficits and anorexia.

Sarcopenia

Background

Sarcopenia refers to age-associated loss of skeletal muscle mass and function (Table 32-8). Its onset is antecedent to frailty, and it may be associated with diminished health-related QOL.[137] It is characterized by the loss of skeletal muscle strength (force and torque), loss of protein (contractile unit) content, selective loss of type 2 (fast-twitch) motor units, intramyocellular lipid accumulation and toxicity, and intermuscular adipose tissue infiltration.[138,139] Over time, these age-related changes may lead to functional limitation and a predisposition to falls and long-bone fracture.

Etiology

Increased numbers of senescent cells (which secrete proinflammatory proteins), immunocyte activation, and chronic low-grade inflammation, characterize aging and chronic HIV infection.[44,140] The accumulation of senescent cells in tissue and inflammatory changes are thought to contribute to the loss of age-related organ system reserve capacity and functional decline.[140]

In addition to chronic low-grade inflammation, sarcopenia has been associated with several modifiable risk factors, including low serum levels of free testosterone in males, low 25(OH)D levels, lack of exercise (resistance and aerobic), prolonged bed rest, and tobacco or other substance use.[141,142]

Treatment

Preventive interventions and treatment for sarcopenia may target the modifiable risk factors associated with it. Assessment (Table 32-8) includes handgrip strength and the timed up-and-go test or timed walk (measurements of skeletal muscle voluntary strength and physical function). In midlife and older people, abnormalities in these measures are associated with diminished QOL and are predictive of falls, future disability, and the loss of independence.[137,143–146] These tests may be used to identify community-dwelling, HIV-infected people with strength or locomotor deficits, and for the evaluation of subsequent intervention(s) (ie, exercise). Regularly scheduled aerobic exercise with strength training has been shown to largely prevent age-associated intermuscular adipose tissue increase and attenuate muscle strength loss in older people.[147]

Free testosterone levels decline with age (by approximately 1.2% per year) in community-dwelling, midlife and older men (free testosterone decrement per decade does not seem to differ between HIV-infected and HIV-uninfected men).[148] However, HIV-infected men demonstrate significantly lower early-morning free testosterone levels when compared with HIV-uninfected males, consistent with loss of diurnal variation.[148]

Severe symptomatic testosterone deficiency has been associated with substantially higher risk of all-cause and cardiovascular-related mortality in community-dwelling, midlife and older men.[149] Severe deficiency was defined as total testosterone less than 231 ng/dL (8 nmol/L), free testosterone less than 63.5 pg/mL (220 pmol/L) and the presence of at least 3 sexual symptoms (infrequent sexual thoughts, poor morning erection, and erectile dysfunction).[149]

Older men typically maintain testosterone levels within the normal range. Chronic comorbidities, such as obesity or type 2 diabetes, are associated with symptomatic testosterone deficiency in men irrespective of age. There are intra- and interindividual differences in the free testosterone thresholds at which the signs and symptoms of deficiency may be experienced. This variability is due, in part, to differences in androgen receptor functionality and SHBG concentration. Patient assessment should be based on clinical presentation (eg, loss of skeletal muscle mass and sexual symptoms), aided by biochemical testing, and not the rigid application of a total testosterone threshold level for the "diagnosis" of testosterone deficiency.

Older men, with and without baseline mobility limitation, who received testosterone replacement therapy demonstrated gains in skeletal muscle mass and strength.[150,151] However, they did not demonstrate improvement in performance-based measures of physical function.[150,151] Other factors may be required for newly accrued or hypertrophied skeletal muscle tissue (from testosterone administration) to undergo the

TABLE 32-8 Sarcopenia vs Wasting Disease

	Sarcopenia	Wasting Disease
Physiology	Intrinsic 1% skeletal muscle loss/year after age 30 years	Complication of HIV or other infection or disease
Pathologic	Only at threshold level associated with loss of function	Always
Onset	Slow, over decades	Rapid, usually in association with other complications
Weight loss	Not always	Always
Tissue depots	Skeletal muscle loss (adipose tissue may be preserved or increased)	Lean body mass, including skeletal muscle, and adipose tissue lost
Histopathology	Selective loss of type 2 muscle fibers; increasing intermuscular adipose tissue	+/− type 2 muscle fiber loss in HIV infection in the absence of wasting
Metabolic	Decreased muscle protein synthesis prominent	Increased muscle protein catabolism prominent

neuromuscular adaptations that lead to improved physical function. Currently, testosterone administration for the treatment of sarcopenia remains an off-label use.

HIV-infected people with or without sarcopenia are often targeted by purveyors of herbal and dietary supplements. However, in 2013–2014, the use of these products accounted for 20% of the cases of liver injury documented by the National Institutes of Health–funded Drug-Induced Liver Injury Network.[152] A significant proportion of the cases were associated with the use of products marketed for "bodybuilding" or "performance (sexual) enhancement," which are often marketed online to midlife men.[152] These supplements frequently contain illicitly added synthetic testosterone derivatives, 5-phosphodiesterase inhibitors, corticosteroids, or other pharmaceutical agents.[152] Liver injury has also occurred in association with the use of herbal products (eg, green tea extract), vitamins or dietary supplements (eg, niacin or levocarnitine), and multi-ingredient nutritional supplements. Such products may be sold as "proprietary blends" or with little or no documentation of chemical composition and purity, making it difficult to identify the injurious substance with certainty.[152]

Patients receiving cART (largely metabolized by the liver) to suppress an otherwise lethal virus should be advised not to use herbal or dietary supplements. In addition to compromising the patient's ability to tolerate cART, the use of products such as creatine or other protein supplements or products for "muscle building" may perturb serum creatinine and calculated glomerular filtration rate values, leading to unnecessary workups to rule out kidney disease. Patients' use of illicitly obtained anabolic-androgenic steroids to increase skeletal muscle mass exposes them to additional risk for hepatitis C infection. Patients who are adamant about using supplements should be strongly encouraged to review their usage and drug interactions with knowledgeable clinicians. See Chapter 19 for additional information on the labeling, safety, and marketing of dietary supplements.

Osteopenia, Osteoporosis, and Fragility Fractures

Diagnosis

Fragility fracture (a fracture resulting from normal activity or a fall from less than standing height) is the clinical consequence of osteoporosis. Osteoporosis may be detected and diagnosed by DXA scan of bone. Osteoporosis and osteopenia are defined by T score: a comparison of the bone density of a patient age 50 years or older to that of a 25- to 35-year-old, gender- and ethnicity-matched reference population. A T score of −2.5 standard deviations (SD) in a subject age 50 years or older is considered osteoporotic. A T score of −1.0 SD is considered osteopenia. These scores correlate with increased risk of fracture in community-dwelling men and women.

Epidemiology

In large multicenter cohorts, the incidence of fragility fractures is higher in midlife and older HIV-infected male and female participants compared with those not infected.[153,154] In an evaluation of fracture prevalence that included young adults as well as midlife and older people, Triant and colleagues documented an increased prevalence of hip, vertebral, and wrist fractures in HIV-infected subjects compared with those without known HIV infection.[153] Women experienced higher rates of nontraumatic vertebral and wrist fractures, whereas men experienced higher rates of vertebral, hip, and wrist fractures.[155] The largest differences in fracture rates occurred in men younger than 40 or older than 60 years of age and women older than 50 years of age.[155]

Investigators in the Netherlands documented a high baseline prevalence of osteopenia (45%) and osteoporosis (6%) in treatment-naïve young men with primary HIV infection (positive RT-PCR/negative western blot).[156] Similarly, Duvivier and colleagues documented a 31% baseline prevalence of osteopenia in young, treatment-naïve, primarily male patients initiating cART.[157] The high prevalence of osteopenia and osteoporosis in young men with primary HIV infection who are treatment-naïve is highly suggestive of an overlap in risk factors for HIV acquisition with those for osteoporosis.

Etiology

Patients demonstrate a 2% to 6% loss of hip and spine BMD during the year following cART initiation (regardless of antiretroviral regimen) followed by stabilization.[158,159] The magnitude of bone loss in these patients is similar to that experienced by women during menopausal transition. However, subsequent stabilization is at an age-appropriate rate of BMD loss.[158,159] Investigators have found that approximately 12% to 16% of HIV-infected patients will progress from normal BMD to osteopenia or from osteopenia to osteoporosis.[160] Factors associated with clinical progression were male sex, current PI-containing regimen, and/or duration of PI exposure.[160] Low weight (or body mass index) are independently predictive of low BMD in individuals with HIV infection.[161,162] Other HIV-related factors associated with osteoporosis and fractures are hepatitis C or B co-infection, low CD4 count, prior AIDS, male hypogonadism and substance use.[143] The traditional risk factors prior fracture and falls—older age, white or non-black ethnicity, alcohol use, tobacco use, prolonged receipt of glucocorticoids, proton pump inhibitors, or anticonvulsants—may be overrepresented in HIV/AIDS clinical populations.[143]

At the tissue level, studies suggest that HIV and its treatment have direct independent effects on osteoclast activity, leading to a higher rate of bone remodeling (turnover).[163,164] At cART initiation, there is an initial increase in bone resorption markers with subsequent delay in compensatory increase in bone formation markers, consistent with a catabolic window. Immune activation and elevated levels of proinflammatory cytokines may also participate in the upregulation of osteoclast activity.[165] Bone marrow–derived mesenchymal stem cells may differentiate into either osteoblasts or adipocytes (within the bone marrow). Mesenchymal stem cells exposed ex vivo to sera from HIV-infected treatment-naïve patients were driven down an adipogenic differentiation pathway.[166] This finding suggests that exposure to HIV proteins may diminish the pool of osteoblast precursors and bone formation in people prior to treatment.[166]

Chronic immune activation by lipopolysaccharide due to HIV-mediated microbial translocation is believed to favor osteoclastogenesis and bone resorption.[167] B cell populations expressing receptor activator of nuclear factor kappa B ligand (RANKL; a cytokine favoring osteoclastogenesis) and activated T cell populations expressing proinflammatory cytokines in addition to RANKL are elevated in HIV-infected people, and correlate with BMD loss.[168,169]

Clinical and behavioral findings associated with BMD loss and osteoporosis (secondary causes) include vitamin D deficiency, low calcium intake, or high protein and/or sodium intake leading to urinary calcium losses, a lack of routine weight-bearing exercise, and low protein intake in older people. These modifiable risk factors are prevalent in people under care for HIV infection.[124,170]

Osteoporosis and osteopenia in HIV-infected patients likely result from an interplay of viral effect, a time-limited but irreversible drop in BMD with the initiation of cART, and traditional risk factors.

Clinical Management

Nutrition interventions for osteoporosis and osteopenia are first-line therapies for osteopenia/osteoporosis. These interventions include vitamin D supplementation in people with documented deficiency or insufficiency; calcium, preferably from food sources (1000 mg/d for men to age 70 years and women to age 50 years, 1200 mg/d for men 71 years and older and women 51 years and older), evaluation of dietary protein intake, and sodium reduction. Cessation of tobacco and recreational substance use, including marijuana (due to its association with falls), and alcohol misuse should also be the focus of clinical attention.[143,171] A propensity to fall because of diminished hip, knee, and ankle musculature often leads to fractures and loss of independence in older patients. Routine scheduled exercise may be preventive.[143] An affirmative answer to the question "Are you worried about falling?" is suggestive of need for therapeutic strength and balance training.

It has been suggested that calcium supplementation may increase CVD event risk. This hypothesis was based on data from a randomized trial (N = 1471), a meta-analysis and reanalysis of the Women's Health Initiative (WHI; which reported no association of calcium supplementation with CVD event risk) limited access data set, and another meta-analysis.[172-174] The WHI investigators did a subsequent analysis of their double-blind, randomized placebo-controlled trial (N = 36,282) with comparative analyses from the WHI prospective Observational Study (N = 68,719) and found calcium and vitamin D supplementation were not associated with CVD events.[175] In a subset of women who underwent cardiac computed tomography (CT), there was no association between supplementation and coronary artery calcium scores.[175] Similarly, calcium supplementation was not associated with CVD events in the Multi-ethnic Study of Atherosclerosis (N = 6236 men and women) or in the Nurses' Health Study Cohort (N = 74,245) after 24 years of follow-up.[176,177] However, calcium supplementation should be carefully evaluated in patients receiving thiazide diuretics because these agents reduce renal calcium excretion, leaving soft tissues and blood vessel walls among the alternative sites for its deposition.

Tenofovir has been redeveloped as an amidate prodrug, tenofovir alafenamide (FDA-approved in 2015) in place of the ester prodrug tenofovir disoproxil fumarate. People in phase 3 trials receiving cART containing the tenofovir amidate demonstrated smaller decrements in hip and spine BMD and renal function than those receiving the tenofovir ester.[178] Tenofovir alafenamide is more stable in blood, allowing for lower-dose administration and a reduction of systemic exposure to tenofovir.[179] Reduction of systemic exposure to tenofovir lowers the risk of the adverse events that have been associated with tenofovir disoproxil fumarate receipt, such as kidney injury, osteopenia, and osteoporosis.[180] Proximal tubular toxicity marked by proteinuria, normoglycemic glycosuria, hypophosphatemia, and/or hyperphosphaturia is the common pathogenic mechanism in the drug-associated bone and kidney injury. Urinary phosphate wasting (leading to its mobilization from bone) is indicated by a urine phosphate concentration greater than 5 to 10 mg/dL or greater than 100 mg/d, and a fractional excretion of phosphorous greater than 5% ([Urine Phosphate × Serum Creatinine] ÷ [Serum Phosphate × Urine Creatinine]).

Frailty Phenotype

Background

Successful aging is characterized by functional independence, social engagement, and the attenuation of age-related declines in strength and motor performance. HIV-infected patients have experienced a dramatic improvement in life expectancy. However, many people now aging with well-suppressed HIV infection have experienced AIDS wasting, opportunistic infection, intensive care unit admission, and antiretroviral-associated toxicity in the distant past. Consequently, some may have residual loss of physiological reserve capacity.[181,182]

Frailty was first described as a geriatric syndrome characterized by diminished physical function and loss of physiological reserve capacity that compromises an organism's ability to recover homeostatic equilibrium after acute stress and/or adapt to chronic internal or external stressors.[183] Its onset in community-dwelling older adults is predictive of disability, loss of independence, and mortality.[183] Similarly, in midlife and older adults living with HIV infection, functional impairment is associated with diminished skeletal muscle mass and BMD.[184]

Etiology

In HIV-infected people, frailty has been associated with elevations in markers of inflammation and immunosenescence: IL-6 and CD8+ T cells, respectively.[185] Whether HIV-associated inflammation amplifies the tissue-level effects of processes that have been linked to age-related changes, such as mitochondrial dysfunction, in midlife adults is an area of ongoing research.[186]

Case Definition and Epidemiology

The criteria for frailty that are operationalized for clinical research in HIV-infected populations add self-reported low

TABLE 32-9 Frailty Phenotype[a]

Criterion	Assay	Cutoff Points
Physical shrinkage	• "Since your last visit (3–6 months ago), have you had unintentional weight loss of at least 10 pounds?" *or* • Documented intercurrent weight loss >5%	"Yes"
Exhaustion	• "During the past 4 weeks, as a result of your physical health, have you had difficulty performing your work or other activities (eg, the activity took extra effort)?"	"Yes"
Low physical activity	• "Does your health now limit your ability to engage in vigorous activities, such as running, lifting heavy objects, or participating in strenuous sports?" *or* • Patient's LTPA energy expenditure	• "Yes, limited a lot." • Men: <383 kcal/wk[b] • Women <270 kcal/wk[b]
Slowness/gait speed	• 4.572-m timed walk at patient's usual pace (meters per second [m/s])	Women: • <0.65 m/s for height ≤1.59 m • <0.76 m/s for height >1.59 m Men: • <0.65 m/s for height ≤1.73 m • <0.76 m/s for height >1.73 m
Weakness	Grip strength (kg)	Women: • ≤17 kg for BMI ≤23 • ≤17.3 kg for BMI 23.1–26 • ≤18 kg for BMI 26.1–29 • ≤21 kg for BMI >29 Men: • ≤29 kg for BMI ≤24 • ≤30 kg for BMI 24.1–26 • ≤30 kg for BMI 26.1–28 • ≤32 kg for BMI >28

BMI, body mass index; LTPA, leisure time physical activity.
[a]Presentation with ≥3 criteria consistent with frailty phenotype; presentation with 1 or 2 criteria consistent with prefrailty.
[b]Energy expenditure from LTPA assessed using Minnesota Leisure Time Physical Activity Questionnaire. See reference 187: Pereira MA, FitzGerald SJ, Gregg EW, et al. A collection of physical activity questionnaires for health-related research. *Med Sci Sports Exerc.* 1997;29(6 Suppl):S1–S205.

physical activity, the constitutional symptoms of exhaustion and unintentional weight loss (physical shrinkage) to those of sarcopenia (Table 32-9).[143,182,184–186] The prevalence of frailty in HIV-infected MSM is approximately 12%, with statistically significant excess seen in those between the ages of 50 to 69 years.[182] Frailty incidence in HIV-infected cohorts was associated with depressive symptoms and a history of diabetes, as well as kidney disease, whereas higher education was protective.[182]

Clinical Management

No large randomized controlled trials have evaluated interventions for frailty in community-dwelling midlife and older adults with HIV infection. However, frailty has been associated with food insecurity and hypovitaminosis D in the aged general population, and with food insecurity in midlife HIV-infected individuals (Practice Scenario 32-2).[188–195]

Interventions for these problems are discussed earlier in this chapter. In the general population, the gait speed and chair rise time of older adults may be improved by strength training. Pilot studies of physical activity have demonstrated improvements in these measures in midlife and older HIV-infected adults.[184,185] Interestingly, HIV-infected people who exercised also demonstrated reductions in cellular markers of immune activation and serum markers of systemic inflammation.[196–198]

Practice Scenario 32-2

Question: A 67-year-old community-dwelling man who has sex with men and has well-suppressed HIV infection, longstanding CD4 reconstitution, and no active or clinically apparent comorbid disease is referred to you by his physician for evaluation of weight loss. What social determinants of health would you evaluate?

Scenario: On presentation, the patient is well groomed, although his clothes are loose-fitting and he ambulates with a cane. Past medical history indicates that he was diagnosed with HIV infection in 1995 during hospitalization for *Pneumocystis jiroveci* pneumonia. Medication history documents exposure to "Crixivan, d4T, and AZT in the late '90s." Social history documents that he lives alone in an apartment with full kitchen facilities and receives Social Security, and that his partner, who was his "only close friend," died 12 months ago. Upon further history, the patient discloses that he feels "down and fatigued" most of the time, finds no pleasure in the things he used to enjoy, such as baking pastries, and "even finds it difficult to concentrate when reading a novel." Subjective weight loss was 10 pounds over the last year. During the conversation about dietary intake, the patient states that he worries about his food running out before he gets enough money to buy more, often cannot afford to eat "proper meals," and sometimes eats less than he knows he should. He also states that he often finds it difficult to carry his food home from the store in one bag because "he needs the other hand for his cane."

Intervention: The patient qualifies for home meal delivery from an AIDS service organization (ASO) because of his mobility limitation and is enrolled in the program. Unfortunately, his income from Social Security exceeds the maximum income level for enrollment in the Supplemental Nutrition Assistance Program. The patient is also referred to an ASO program that provides social activities and congregate meals for older lesbian, gay, bisexual, and transsexual adults living with HIV infection. Because the patient reports ongoing symptoms consistent with depression, such as "feeling down," fatigue, and anhedonia, as well as weight loss, the metabolic support consult includes a recommendation for psychiatric evaluation.

Answer: Food insecurity, social isolation, anhedonia, mobility limitation, and likely depression related to the death of his partner are etiological factors in this patient's weight loss.

Rationale: Individuals aging with HIV infection have been found to have fragile social networks, with less than half of these adults having a partner, and the majority living alone.[191,192] Social isolation is more prevalent in HIV-infected older adults and has been associated with depressive symptoms, financial stress, food insecurity, and frailty.[193–195]

HIV-Associated Lipodystrophy Syndrome

Background

People aging with HIV infection today may demonstrate the stigmata of antiretroviral toxicity (ie, lipodystrophy) from regimens they received years ago. Additionally, in the United States, drug-class warnings persist in NRTI, NtRTI, and PI package inserts. Clinicians caring for people with HIV infection should be prepared to answer questions about lipodystrophy from patients initiating cART today and be able to identify its residual effects in older patients.

Lipodystrophy was a common complaint and physical finding in the first cART era. However, it has become an infrequent problem subsequent to the introduction of INSTIs, better-tolerated PIs, and NRTIs into clinical care, and the earlier diagnosis of HIV-infected patients at higher CD4 counts. The central feature of lipodystrophy in HIV-infected patients is selective and persisting subcutaneous adipose tissue loss.[199,200] Visceral adipose tissue is spared.[199,200] The accumulation of visceral adipose tissue may occur in HIV-infected patients with return to health following the initiation of modern cART or in otherwise healthy patients with well-suppressed virus. Lipodystrophy was strongly associated with first-generation NRTIs: the thymidine analogs zidovudine (AZT) and stavudine (d4T), and the adenosine analog didanosine (ddi). With decreased use of the thymidine analogs and ddi, the incidence of lipodystrophy in North America, the European Union, the United Kingdom, and Australia has markedly declined. However, use of these antiretrovirals may persist in resource-constrained regions.

Etiology and Pathogenesis

Biopsy of adipose tissue from lipodystrophic patients disclosed morphologic abnormalities and a reduction in mitochondrial DNA content in association with inflammatory change.[201–204] Inhibition of mitochondrial DNA polymerase γ by adenosine and thymidine analogs was believed to mediate their toxicity.[205] Mitochondria have multiple separate circularized genomes encoding respiratory chain proteins that are not encoded by nuclear chromosomal DNA. Dose reduction of respiratory chain proteins due to reduced mitochondrial DNA content likely led to mitochondrial dysfunction and adipocyte apoptosis (cell death) in patient's subcutaneous adipose tissue.

Mitochondrial toxicity has also been associated with hepatic steatosis, mild hyperlactatemia, and, rarely, with lactic acidosis.[206] While now a rare event, lactic acidosis is a potentially lethal complication most commonly encountered in obese female patients.[207] The prodrome of clinical lactic acidosis is nonspecific (eg, nausea, loss of appetite). Treatment includes the interruption of NRTIs and supplementation with thiamin and riboflavin to optimize mitochondrial function and biogenesis.

Evaluation and Diagnosis

Lipodystrophy is a clinical diagnosis based on physical findings. Subcutaneous adipose tissue volume is normally relatively constant in the absence of disease or prolonged undernutrition. Lipodystrophic loss of this tissue may be focal or generalized (eg, facial only, or facial and gluteal-femoral or head, trunk, and limbs). The most frequently affected areas are the face, buttocks, and thighs, and, lastly, the upper arms.

Facial adipose tissue loss is the most distressing stigmata of lipodystrophy for most patients. Facial lipoatrophy may be appreciated by noting a near total bilateral loss of Bichat's fat pads, manifesting as a visible subzygomatic notch, discernible zygomaticus major and minor muscles, prominent zygomatic arches and nasolabial skin fold. On examination, the abdomen may be firm because of subcutaneous adipose tissue loss, with relative sparing of omental and mesenteric adipocytes. Limb adipocyte content is primarily subcutaneous, and prominent vasculature ("cabling"), often accompanied by pseudomuscularity (visible muscle insertions and contours), is a frequent finding in afflicted patients. Atypical expansion of adipose tissue depots may be encountered; these changes include dorsocervical fat pad enlargement ("buffalo hump"), submandibular fat accumulation with loss of facial contour ("moon facies"), and marked female breast hypertrophy with thoracic-level back pain.[208-210]

Clinical Management

Antiretroviral regimen change to replace the thymidine analog or ddi with an alternative NRTI or NRTI-sparing regimen is an option for most patients. Improvements in lipoatrophy, although measurable, may take years to reach clinical significance.[211]

Cardiovascular Disease

Background

An increased rate of AMI has been observed in HIV-infected people compared with uninfected people of the same gender and similar age.[9] In high-income countries, CVD has become a major cause of morbidity and mortality in HIV-infected adults age 50 years or older.[212] A higher rate of AMI than that predicted by the Framingham equation has been documented by the Data Collection on Adverse Events of Anti-HIV Drugs (D:A:D) Study Group, an international pharmacosurveillance consortium.[213] More recently, the Veterans Aging Cohort demonstrated that HIV infection is associated with a 50% increased risk of AMI.[214] Adjudicated AMI events were higher in HIV-infected veterans ages 40 to 69 years vs demographically and behaviorally matched uninfected controls after adjustment for Framingham risk factors.[214] Excess risk of AMI is associated with direct HIV effect on atherosclerotic lesion burden, which is observable as internal carotid intima-media thickness by sonography, noncalcified plaque volume by CT angiography, and monocyte/macrophage activation and inflammatory activity by ^{18}F-fluourodeoxyglucose (FDG)–positron emission tomography (PET)/CT imaging, and dyslipidemia.[215]

Etiology

The natural history of an HIV infection is marked by proatherogenic lipid and lipoprotein changes. HDL-C is decreased early in HIV infection. Decline in HDL-C is followed by a later small decrease in LDL-C with an increase in the small-dense fraction (ie, very-low-density lipoprotein cholesterol [VLDL-C]). Small, dense LDL-C is believed to more easily penetrate blood vessel walls, where it undergoes oxidation and phagocytosis by macrophages, leading to atherosclerotic lesions. Progressive HIV disease (AIDS) may be accompanied by increases in serum triglyceride and VLDL-C. These proatherogenic changes in lipids and lipoproteins have been associated with increasing HIV-RNA levels (VL) and decreasing CD 4+ T cell count.[216] In 2 large studies of community-dwelling cohorts, current low CD4 count or detectable HIV viremia or low nadir CD4 count were independent risk factors for CVD events.[216,217]

Microbial translocation and macrophage activation have been linked to the progressive carotid intima-media thickening (expansion of the atheromatous lesions within the arterial wall) in patients receiving suppressive cART who demonstrate CD4 reconstitution.[218] In addition to their role as lipid scavengers, macrophages within the plaque lipid core may secrete matrix metalloproteases and procoagulant tissue factor. These secretions may lead to acute plaque rupture followed by clot formation, leading in turn to clinical events, including AMI. Glucose uptake by macrophages correlates with their inflammatory activity. [18]FDG, a glucose analog, may enter macrophages via glucose transporter proteins and undergo hexokinase-mediated phosphorylation (preventing egress), but it cannot proceed through glycolysis.[219]

Clinical investigators have demonstrated higher levels of arterial inflammation by [18]FDG-PET in midlife adults with well-suppressed HIV infection compared with Framingham risk score–matched controls who are not HIV-infected.[220] In people with no baseline CVD or cancer, receiving PET for oncologic evaluation, higher [18]FDG uptake in the ascending aorta was an independent predictor of CVD events.[221] These data strongly suggest that chronic immune activation, specifically macrophage activity within the lipid core of atherosclerotic plaques, contributes to the elevated risk of AMI and stroke documented in people living with HIV infection.

Data from the D:A:D prospective multicohort study suggests that specific older antiretrovirals (lopinavir-ritonavir, indinavir, didanosine, and abacavir) may also be associated with increased relative risk of CVD.[222,223] Although antiretroviral therapy use has been shown to be cardioprotective, clinical trial data sets and observational data from D:A:D suggest that some antiretrovirals may be slightly less cardioprotective than others.[222-224] Findings from observational studies suggest a possible association between abacavir exposure and increased relative risk of myocardial infarction; however, the data remain inconclusive.[225,226]

More importantly, analysis of D:A:D data sets demonstrated that traditional risk factors (tobacco use, male sex, higher BMI, older age, and dyslipidemia) are more strongly associated than either cART exposure or duration with CVD event risk.[227] Traditional risk factors, particularly tobacco use, may be overrepresented in people with HIV infection. The effect of traditional risk factors is often prominent in patients after the initiation of cART and may be referred to as a "return to health effect." Simply put, with the resolution of opportunistic infection(s) and constitutional symptoms with viral suppression, patients often demonstrate increases in weight, abdominal adiposity, total cholesterol, and LDL-C in association with return to usual dietary intake. Clinicians should counsel patients initiating cART to be mindful of the potential for untoward weight gain in association with sustained viral suppression and dietary indiscretions.

Clinical Evaluation

The absolute risk for a CVD events in an HIV-infected person may be estimated using the 2013 American College of Cardiology/American Heart Association (ACC/AHA) atherosclerotic CVD pooled cohort equations (http://tools.acc.org/ASCVD

-Risk-Estimator).[228,229] The ACC/AHA guidelines make no recommendations for or against the use of specific LDL-C targets for primary or secondary prevention.[228] However, other guidelines do recommend lowering LDL-C below certain levels (eg, <70 mg/dL in adults with CVD or those at very high risk).[230] These targets are supported by epidemiological and clinical trial data.[231–233] Assay of high-sensitivity C-reactive protein (hsCRP) and D-dimer may provide clinicians with additional information on a specific patient's CVD event risk.[234]

The Mediterranean Diet

The Mediterranean diet has demonstrated efficacy in primary and secondary prevention trials in individuals without known HIV infection.[235,236] A primary prevention trial of the Mediterranean diet documented reductions in hsCRP, improvement in markers of endothelial function, and improvement in insulin resistance.[237] Fiber intake has been inversely associated with insulin resistance, and higher polyunsaturated fat intake was positively associated with insulin resistance in HIV-infected patients.[238] In community-dwelling HIV-infected patients receiving cART, adherence to a Mediterranean diet was associated with better metabolic parameters and a lower risk for abdominal adiposity vs a typical Western diet.[239,240]

The Mediterranean diet is characterized by the following:

- Olive oil as the principal dietary fat
- Fish consumption 2 or more times a week
- Poultry consumed in moderate amounts
- A high intake of dark-green leafy and other vegetables
- Whole grain starches, beans, nuts, and seeds
- Dairy products (principally cheese and yogurt)
- Fresh fruit as the typical daily dessert
- Egg yolks limited to 4 per week
- Red meat consumed in low amounts
- Wine consumed in low-to-moderate amounts, normally with meals
- Low amounts of saturated fat (no more than 7% to 8% of energy), with total energy intake from dietary fat ranging from less than 25% to more than 35%

Clinicians should be mindful of guidelines for limiting adult sodium intake to less than 1500 mg/d and counsel patients accordingly. Patients should also be shown how to prepare familiar foods so they can fit into a Mediterranean diet. For example, collard greens (native to the Mediterranean region) are also a staple vegetable in the southern United States. Steamed and sautéed in extra-virgin olive oil with garlic, instead of being boiled with smoked ham or turkey wings for 2 hours, these greens are part of a cardioprotective diet. Clinicians should also be mindful of food costs, advising patients of farmer's markets that accept electronic benefits cards (SNAP) and suggesting that canned tuna or sardines packed in water (higher ω-3 fatty acid retention) are affordable fish options.

Multivitamins and discreet B vitamin and antioxidant supplementation are ineffective for primary or secondary CVD event and cancer prevention, and these supplements have no beneficial effect on cognitive performance, verbal memory, or all-cause mortality in community-dwelling adults.[241]

Indeed, vitamin E supplementation has been associated with increased all-cause mortality.[241] In a randomized, double-blind placebo-controlled trial in HIV-infected adults initiating cART in Uganda, multivitamin supplementation had no effect on CD4 reconstitution, weight gain, or QOL.[242]

HMG-CoA Reductase Inhibitors (Statins) and Fibrates

In the absence of contraindication, statins are first-line pharmacological treatment when elevated LDL-C and/or non-HDL-C are the predominant findings. HIV-infected people receiving statins have also demonstrated reductions in markers of immune activation, coronary plaque volume, and high-risk plaque morphology, as well as slower carotid intima-media thickness progression.[243–245] Generally, simvastatin and lovastatin are contraindicated in patients receiving PIs (in part because of the potential for cytochrome P450 3A4– and organic anion transporting polypeptide 1B1–mediated interactions), and pravastatin has the least lipid-lowering potency. In addition, pravastatin serum levels are increased by the PI darunavir, and pravastatin should be initiated at lowest possible dose when coadministration of these 2 drugs is required. The lowest possible dosages of atorvastatin or rosuvastatin (with careful monitoring) are more potent alternatives. Favorable modifications of atherogenic lipid profiles have been demonstrated by subjects receiving pitavastatin, and a potential advantage of this agent is its cytochrome P450–independent elimination. However, there are no data demonstrating a reduction in CVD events in people with or without HIV infection receiving pitavastatin.[246] Fibrates (gemfibrozil or fenofibrate) may be prescribed when hypertriglyceridemia is the predominant abnormality.

ω-3 Fatty Acids

Lovaza is a pharmaceutical grade ω-3 fatty acid supplement approved for the treatment of hypertriglyceridemia in HIV-uninfected people. A pilot study randomly assigned HIV-infected patients to receive ω-3 fatty acid supplementation (4 g/d orally) with diet and exercise counseling or diet and exercise counseling only. Participants in the supplementation group demonstrated statistically significant reductions in triglyceride levels at 1-month analysis.[247] Unfortunately, triglyceride reduction did not reach the National Cholesterol Education Program Expert Panel on Detection, Evaluation, and Treatment of High Blood Cholesterol in Adults goal level of below 150 mg/dL; LDL-C levels rose by 22% in the treatment group.[247] It should be noted that fibrates also increase LDL-C levels.[247] Of 26 subjects randomly assigned to receive ω-3 fatty acids, 2 withdrew from the study because of the unpleasant taste of the supplements and nausea (problems historically associated with fish oil supplementation).[247] No significant change in platelet function was observed.[247]

Conclusion

Increased testing and greater linkage to and retention in care, coupled with more tolerable and efficacious cART, have directly contributed to the increased longevity of people living with

HIV infection. Our current challenge is not only to optimize the safety of cART and deliver preventive care to newly diagnosed patients but also to treat and attempt to reverse potential adverse events associated with the use of older antiretroviral therapies (especially in patients who presented with profound immunodeficiency). Even patients with sustained viral suppression experience higher levels of chronic immune activation and inflammation than those who are uninfected with HIV. Dietary modifications, particularly the Mediterranean diet, and routine scheduled exercise have been shown to lessen markers of chronic inflammation, and these are interventions we can help our patients implement now. These interventions, along with smoking cessation counseling, avoidance of alcohol abuse and abuse of other substances (including recreational drugs), and weight management, universally benefit all patients. Helping this population to live and age well is the challenge before us.

References

1. Centers for Disease Control. Kaposi's sarcoma and Pneumocystis pneumonia among homosexual men—New York City and California. *MMWR Morb Mortal Wkly Rep.* 1981;30:305–308.
2. Centers for Disease Control and Prevention. Today's HIV/AIDS Epidemic. February 2016. https://www.cdc.gov/nchhstp/newsroom/docs/factsheets/todaysepidemic-508.pdf. Accessed June 8, 2016.
3. Centers for Disease Control and Prevention. HIV Surveillance Report, 2014, vol. 26. November 2015. http://www.cdc.gov/hiv/library/reports/surveillance. Accessed June 9, 2016.
4. Marcus JL, Chao CR, Leyden WA, et al. Narrowing the gap in life expectancy between HIV-infected and HIV-uninfected individuals with access to care. *J Acquir Immune Defic Syndr.* 2016;73(1):39–46.
5. Harrison KM, Song R, Zhang X. Life expectancy after HIV diagnosis based national HIV surveillance data from 25 states, United States. *J Acquir Immune Defic Syndr.* 2010;53(1):124–130.
6. Mermin J. The science and practice of HIV prevention in the United States. Centers for Disease Control and Prevention. Program and abstracts presented at 18th Conference on Retroviruses and Opportunistic Infections; February 27–March 2, 2011; Boston, MA: Plenary 1.
7. Skarbinski J, Rosenberg E, Paz-Bailey G, et al. Human immunodeficiency virus transmission at each step of the care continuum in the United States. *JAMA Intern Med.* 2015;175(4):588–596.
8. Freiberg MS, Chang CC, Kuller LH, et al. HIV infection and the risk of acute myocardial infarction. *JAMA Intern Med.* 2013;173:614–622.
9. Guaraldi G, Zona S, Brothers TD, et al. Aging with HIV vs. HIV seroconversion at older age: a diverse population with distinct comorbidity profiles. *PLoS One.* 2015;10(4):e0118531.
10. Robbins HA, Pfeiffer RM, Shiels MS, et al. Excess cancers among HIV-infected people in the United States. *J Natl Cancer Inst.* 2015;107(4):dju503.
11. Gao F, Bailes E, Robertson DL, et al. Origin of HIV-1 in the chimpanzee Pan troglodytes. *Nature.* 1999;397:436–441.
12. United Nations Programme on HIV/AIDS (UNAIDS). Global AIDS Update: UNAIDS 2016. http://www.who.int/hiv/pub/arv/global-AIDS-update-2016_en.pdf?ua=1. Accessed June 9, 2016.
13. United Nations Programme on HIV/AIDS (UNAIDS). On the fast track to end AIDS: UNAIDS: 2016 to 2021 strategy. http://www.unaids.org/sites/default/files/media_asset/20151027_UNAIDS_PCB37_15_18_EN_rev1.pdf 008;300:520–529. Accessed June 9, 2016.
14. Cohen MS, Chen YQ, McCauley M, et al. Prevention of HIV-1 infection with early antiretroviral therapy. *N Engl J Med.* 2011;365(6):493–505.
15. de Pee S, Grede N, Mehra D, Bloem MW. The enabling effect of food assistance in improving adherence and/or treatment completion for antiretroviral therapy and tuberculosis treatment: a literature review. *AIDS Behav.* 2014;18(Suppl 5):S531–S541.
16. Centers for Disease Control and Prevention. Issue brief: HIV in the southern United States. Updated May 2016. https://www.cdc.gov/hiv/pdf/policies/cdc-hiv-in-the-south-issue-brief.pdf. Accessed June 9, 2016.
17. US Census Bureau. Section 1: population. In *Statistical Abstract of the United States: 2012.* 131st ed. Washington DC: US Census Bureau; 2012:1–62.
18. Mathews DD, Herrick AL, Coulter RWS, et al. Running backwards: consequences of current HIV incidence rates for the next generation of black MSM in the United States. *AIDS Behav.* 2016;20:7–16.
19. Denning P, DiNenno E. Communities in crisis: is there a generalized HIV epidemic in impoverished urban areas of the United States? Poster presented at International Conference on AIDS; July 2010; Vienna, Austria.
20. Vaughan AS, Rosenberg E, Shouse L, Sullivan P. Connecting race and place: a county-level analysis of white, black, and Hispanic HIV prevalence, poverty, and level of urbanization. *Am J Public Health.* 2014;104(7):e77–e84.
21. Adimora AA, Schoenbach VJ, Martinson FE, et. Al. Social context of sexual relationships among rural African Americans. *Sex Transm Dis.* 2001;28(2):69–76.
22. Centers for Disease Control and Prevention and Association of Public Health Laboratories. Laboratory testing for the diagnosis of HIV infection: updated recommendations. June 27, 2014. http://dx.doi.org/10.15620/cdc.23447. Accessed June 14, 2016.
23. Centers for Disease Control and Prevention (CDC). 1993 revised classification system for HIV-infection and expanded surveillance case definition for AIDS among adults and adolescents. *MMWR Morb Mortal Wkly Rep.* 1992;41:1–19.
24. Centers for Disease Control and Prevention. Transmission facts. http://www.cdc.gov/hiv/pubs/facts/transmission.htm. Accessed December 8, 2010.
25. Cohen MS, Chen YQ, McCauley M, et al. Antiretroviral therapy for the prevention of HIV-1 Transmission. *N Engl J Med.* 2016;375(9):830–839.
26. World Health Organization. Guideline on when to start antiretroviral therapy and on pre-exposure prophylaxis for HIV. September 2015. http://apps.who.int/iris/bitstream/10665/186275/1/9789241509565_eng.pdf?ua=. Accessed September 7, 2016.
27. US Public Health Service. Preexposure prophylaxis for the prevention of HIV infection in the United States—2014: a clinical practice guideline. https://www.cdc.gov/hiv/pdf/guidelines/PrEPguidelines2014.pdf. Accessed September 7, 2016.
28. Nazli A, Chan O, Dobson-Belaire WN, et al. Exposure to HIV-1 directly impairs mucosal epithelial barrier integrity allowing microbial translocation. *PLoS Pathog.* 2010;6(4):1000852. doi:10.1371/journal.ppat.1000852.
29. Li Q, Duan L, Estes JD, et al. Peak SIV replication in resting memory CD4+ T cells depletes gut lamina propria CD4+ T cells. *Nature.* 2005;434:1148–1152.
30. Uchiyama J, Kishi S, Yagita H, et al. Fas ligand-mediated depletion of CD4 and CD8 lymphocytes by monomeric HIV-1-glycoprotein 120. *Arch Virol.* 1997;142:1771–1785.
31. Picker LJ, Hagen SI, Lum R, et al. Insufficient production and tissue delivery of CD4+ memory T cells in rapidly progressive simian immunodeficiency virus infection. *J Exp Med.* 2004;200:299–1314.

32. Dion ML, Poulin JF, Bordi R, et al. Human immunodeficiency virus infection rapidly induces and maintains a substantial suppression of thymocyte proliferation. *Immunity*. 2004;6:757–768.

33. Mattapallil JJ, Douek DC, Hill B, et al. Massive infection and loss of memory CD4+ T cells in multiple tissues during acute SIV infection. *Nature*. 2005;434:1093–1097.

34. Brenchley JM, Schacker TW, Ruff LE, et al. CD4+ T cell depletion during all stages of HIV disease occurs predominantly in the gastrointestinal tract. *J Exp Med*. 2004;200:749–759.

35. Mehandru S, Poles MA, Tenner-Racz K, et al. Primary HIV-1 infection is associated with preferential depletion of CD4+ T lymphocytes from effector sites in the gastrointestinal tract. *J Exp Med*. 2004;200:761–770.

36. Veazey RS, DeMaria M, Chalifoux LV, et al. Gastrointestinal tract as a major site of CD4+ T cell depletion and viral replication in SIV infection. *Science*. 1998;17;280(5362):427–431.

37. Eriksson K, Kilander A, Hagberg L, et al. Virus-specific antibody production and polyclonal B-cell activation in the intestinal mucosa of HIV-infected individuals. *AIDS*. 1995;9(7):695–700.

38. Levesque MC, Moody MA, Hwang KK, et al. Polyclonal B cell differentiation and loss of gastrointestinal tract germinal centers in the earliest stages of HIV-1 infection. *PLoS Med*. 2009;6(7):e1000107.

39. Olsson J, Poles M, Spetz AL, et al. Human immunodeficiency virus type 1 infection is associated with significant mucosal inflammation characterized by increased expression of CCR5, CXCR4, and beta chemokines. *J Infect Dis*. 2000;182(6):1625–1635.

40. McGowan I, Elliott J, Fuerst M, et al. Increased HIV-1 mucosal replication is associated with generalized mucosal cytokine activation. *J Acquir Immune Defic Syndr*. 2004;1;37(2):1228–1236.

41. Estes J, Baker JV, Brenchley JM, et al. Collagen deposition limits immune reconstitution in the gut. *J Infect Dis*. 2008;198(4):456–464.

42. Jiang W, Lederman MM, Hunt P, et al. Plasma levels of bacterial DNA correlate with immune activation and the magnitude of immune restoration in persons with antiretroviral-treated HIV infection. *J Infect Dis*. 2009;199(8):1177–1185.

43. Marchetti G, Bellistri GM, Borghi E, et al. Microbial translocation is associated with sustained failure in CD4+ T-cell reconstitution in HIV-infected patients on long-term highly active antiretroviral therapy. *AIDS*. 2008;22(15):2035–2038.

44. Brenchley JM, Price DA, Schacker TW, et al. Microbial translocation is a cause of systemic immune activation in chronic HIV infection. *Nat Med*. 2006;12(12):1365–1371.

45. Schacker TW, Nguyen PL, Beilman GJ, et al. Collagen deposition in HIV-1 infected lymphatic tissues and T cell homeostasis. *J Clin Invest*. 2002;110:1133–1139.

46. Akgün KM, Miller RF. Pathogenesis of the immune reconstitution inflammatory syndrome in HIV-infected patients. *Semin Respir Crit Care Med*. 2016;37(2):303–317.

47. Panel on Antiretroviral Guidelines for Adults and Adolescents. Guidelines for the use of antiretroviral agents in HIV-1-infected adults and adolescents. Department of Health and Human Services. http://www.aidsinfo.nih.gov/ContentFiles/AdultandAdolescentGL.pdf. Accessed September 8, 2016.

48. Lundgren JD, Babiker AG, Gordin F, et al. Initiation of antiretroviral therapy in early asymptomatic HIV infection *N Engl J Med*. 2015;373(9):795–807.

49. Sutton S, Magagnoli J, Hardin JW. Impact of pill burden on adherence, risk of hospitalization, and viral suppression in patients with HIV infection and AIDS receiving antiretroviral therapy. *Pharmacotherapy*. 2016;36(4):385–401.

50. Lima VD, Harrigan R, Bangsberg DR, et al. The combined effect of modern highly active antiretroviral therapy regimens and adherence on mortality over time. *J Acquir Immune Defic Syndr*. 2009;50(5):529–526.

51. University of Liverpool. HIV drug interactions. http://www.hiv-druginteractions.org. Accessed April 20, 2017.

52. Immunodeficiency Clinic, Toronto General Hospital. http://hivclinic.ca. Accessed April 20, 2017.

53. US Department of Health and Human Services. AIDSinfo. The HIV cycle. May 2005. http://www.aidsinfo.nih.gov/contentfiles/HIVLifeCycle_FS_en.pdf. Accessed April 20, 2017.

54. Günthard HF, Saag MS, Benson CA, et al. Antiretroviral drugs for treatment and prevention of HIV infection in adults: 2016 recommendations of the International Antiviral Society–USA Panel. *JAMA*. 2016;316(2):191–210.

55. Malebranche R, Arnoux E, Guerin JM, et al. Acquired immunodeficiency syndrome with severe gastrointestinal manifestations in Haiti. *Lancet*. 1983;2:873–878.

56. Siddiqui J, Phillips AL, Freedland ES, et al. Prevalence and cost of HIV-associated weight loss in a managed care population. *Curr Med Res Opin*. 2009;25(5):1307–1317.

57. Wasserman P, Segal-Maurer S, Rubin D. Significant prevalence of wasting among women on HAART 1997–2002 documented by bioelectrical impedance analysis. *Antiviral Ther*. 2002;7:L66.

58. Wanke CA, Silva M, Knox TA, et al. Weight loss and wasting remain common complications in individuals infected with human immunodeficiency virus in the era of highly active antiretroviral therapy. *Clin Infect Dis*. 2000;31:803–805.

59. Hadgu TH, Worku W, Tetemke D, Berhe H. Undernutrition among HIV positive women in Humera hospital, Tigray, Ethiopia 2013: antiretroviral therapy alone is not enough, cross sectional study. *BMC Public Health*. 2013;13:943.

60. Rawat R, Faust E, Maluccio JA, Kadiyala S. The impact of a food assistance program on nutritional status, disease progression, and food security among people living with HIV in Uganda. *J Acquir Immune Defic Syndr*. 20141;66(1):e15–e22.

61. Ford N, Shubber Z, Meintjes G, et al. Causes of hospital admission among people living with HIV worldwide: a systematic review and meta-analysis. *Lancet HIV*. 2015;2(10):e438–e444.

62. Anema A, Weiser SD, Fernandes KA. High prevalence of food insecurity among individuals receiving HAART in a resource-rich setting. *AIDS Care*. 2011;23(2):221–230.

63. Vogenthaler NS, Hadley C, Rodriguez AE, et al. Depressive symptoms and food insufficiency among HIV-infected crack users in Atlanta and Miami. *AIDS Behav*. 2011;15(7):1520–1526.

64. Marshall CS, Curtis AJ, Spelman T, et al. Impact of HIV-associated conditions on mortality in people commencing antiretroviral therapy in resource limited settings. *PLoS One*. 2013;8(7):e68445.

65. Zachariah R, Fitzgerald M, Massaquoi M, et al. Risk factors for high early mortality in patients on antiretroviral treatment in a rural district of Malawi. *AIDS*. 2006;20(18):2355–2360.

66. Keys A, Brozek J, Henschel A, et al. *The Biology of Human Starvation*. Minneapolis: University of Minnesota Press; 1950.

67. Scherzer R, Heymsfield SB, Lee D, et al. Decreased limb muscle and increased central adiposity are associated with 5-year all-cause mortality in HIV infection. *AIDS*. 2011;25(11):1405–1414.

68. Elia M. Hunger disease. *Clin Nutr*. 2000;19:379–386.

69. Cahill GF. Starvation in man. *N Engl J Med*. 1970;282:668–675.

70. Bickel G, Nord M, Price C, et al. *Guide to Measuring Household Food Security*. Revised ed. Alexandria, VA: US Department of Agriculture, Food and Nutrition; 2000.

71. Grunfeld C, Pang M, Shimizu L. Resting energy expenditure, caloric intake, and short term weight change in human immunodeficiency virus infection and the acquired immunodeficiency syndrome. *Am J Clin Nutr*. 1992;55:455–460.

72. Melchior JC, Salmon D, Rigaud D, et al. Resting energy expenditure is increased in stable, malnourished HIV-infected patients. *Am J Clin Nutr*. 1991;53:437–441.

73. Poizot-Martin I, Benourine K, Philibert P, et al. Diet-induced thermogenesis in HIV infection. *AIDS*. 1994;8:501–504.

74. Hellerstein MK, Grunfeld C, Wu K, et al. Increased de novo hepatic lipogenesis in human immunodeficiency virus infection. *J Clin Endocrinol Metab*. 1993;76:559–565.

75. Grunfeld C, Kotler DP, Shigenaga JK, et al. Circulating interferon-alpha levels and hypertriglyceridemia in the acquired immunodeficiency syndrome. *Am J Med*. 1991;90(2):154–162.

76. Grunfeld C, Kotler DP, Hamadeh R, et al. Hypertriglyceridemia in the acquired immunodeficiency syndrome. *Am J Med*. 1989; 86:27–31.

77. Yarasheski K, Zachweija J, Gischler J, et al. Increased plasma gln and Leu Ra and inappropriately low muscle protein synthesis rate in AIDS wasting. *Am J Physiol*. 1998;275(4 Pt 1):E577–E583.

78. Patton JS, Peters PM, McCabe J, et al. Development of partial tolerance to the gastrointestinal effects of high doses of recombinant tumor necrosis factor-alpha in rodents. *J Clin Invest*. 1987; 80:1587–1596.

79. Abad LW, Schmitz HR, Parker R, Roubenoff R. Cytokine responses differ by compartment and wasting status in patients with HIV infection and healthy controls. *Cytokine*. 2002;18(5):286–293.

80. Rochira V, Guarldi G. Hypogonadism in the HIV-infected man. *Endocrinol Metab Clin N Am*. 2014;43:709–730.

81. Grinspoon S, Corcoran C, Lee K, et al. Loss of lean body and muscle mass correlates with androgen levels in hypogonadal men with acquired immunodeficiency syndrome and wasting. *J Clin Endocrinol Metab*. 1996;81:4051–4058.

82. Rietschel P, Corcoran C, Stanley T, et al. Prevalence of hypogonadism among men with weight loss related to human immunodeficiency virus infection who were receiving highly active antiretroviral therapy. *Clin Infect Dis*. 2000;31:1240–1244.

83. Monroe AK, Dobs AS, Palella FJ, et al. Morning free and total testosterone in HIV-infected men: implications for the assessment of hypogonadism. *AIDS Res Ther*. 2014;11(1):6. doi:10.1186/1742-6405-11-6.

84. Dolan S, Wilkie S, Aliabadi N, et al. Effects of testosterone administration in human immunodeficiency virus–infected women with low weight: a randomized placebo-controlled study. *Arch Intern Med*. 2004;164:897–904.

85. Miller K, Corcoran C, Armstrong C, et al. Transdermal testosterone administration in women with acquired immunodeficiency syndrome wasting: a pilot study. *J Clin Endocrinol Metab*. 1998;83: 2717–2725.

86. Javanbakht M, Singh AB, Mazer NA, et al. Pharmacokinetics of a novel testosterone matrix transdermal system in healthy, pre-menopausal women and women infected with the human immunodeficiency virus. *J Clin Endocrinol Metab*. 2000;85: 2395–2401.

87. Smith WJ, Underwood LE, Clemmons DR. Effects of caloric restriction or protein restriction on insulin-like growth factor-1 (IGF-1) and IGF-binding proteins in children and adults. *J Clin Endocrinol Metab*. 1995;80:443–449.

88. Grinspoon S, Corcoran C, Stanley T, et al. Effects of androgen administration on the growth hormone-insulin-like growth factor 1 axis in men with acquired immunodeficiency syndrome wasting. *J Clin Endocrinol Metab*. 1998;83:4251–4256.

89. Scacchi M, Ida Pincelli A, Cavagnini F. Nutritional status in the neuroendocrine control of growth hormone secretion: the model of anorexia nervosa. *Front Neuroendocrinol*. 2003;24(3):200–224.

90. Weiser SD, Fernandes KA, Brandson EK, et al. The association between food insecurity and mortality among HIV-infected individuals on HAART. *J Acquir Immune Defic Syndr*. 2009;52(3): 342–349.

91. Centers for Disease Control and Prevention. National Center for Health Statistics. National Health and Nutrition Examination Survey (NHANES). https://www.cdc.gov/nchs/nhanes. Accessed April 9, 2017.

92. Lukaski HC, Bolonchuk WW, Hall CB, et al. Validation of tetrapolar bioelectrical impedance method to assess human body composition. *Appl Physiol*. 1986;60:1327–1332.

93. Ott M, Fischer H, Polat H, et al. Bioelectrical impedance analysis as a predictor of survival in patients with human immunodeficiency virus infection. *J Acquir Immune Defic Syndr Hum Retrovirol*. 1995;9:20–25.

94. Krentz HB, Gill MJ. The impact of non-antiretroviral polypharmacy on the continuity of antiretroviral therapy (ART) among HIV patients. *AIDS Patient Care STDS*. 2016;30(1):11–17.

95. Jyrkka J, Enlund H, Lavikainen P, et al. Association of polypharmacy with nutritional status, functional ability and cognitive capacity over a three-year period in an elderly population. *Pharmacoepidemiol Drug Saf*. 2010;20:514–522.

96. Erlandson KM, Plankey MW, Springer G, et al. Fall frequency and associated factors among men and women with or at risk for HIV infection. *HIV Med*. 2016;17(10):740–748.

97. Sutton SS, Hardin JW, Bramley TJ, D'Souza AO, Bennett CL. Single- versus multiple-tablet HIV regimens: adherence and hospitalization risks. *Am J Manag Care*. 2016;22(4):242–248.

98. Hendricks K, Gorbach S. Nutrition issues in chronic drug users living with HIV infection. *Addict Sci Clin Pract*. 2009;5(1):16–23.

99. Ferrando AA, Tipton KD, Bamman MM, Wolfe RR. Resistance exercise maintains skeletal muscle protein synthesis during bed rest. *J Appl Physiol*.1997;82(3):807–810.

100. Mwamburi DM, Gerrior J, Wilson IB, et al. Comparing megestrol acetate therapy with oxandrolone therapy for HIV-related weight loss: similar results in 2 months. *Clin Infect Dis*. 2004; 38:895–902.

101. Leinung M, Liporace R, Miller CH. Induction of adrenal suppression by megestrol acetate in patients with AIDS. *Ann Intern Med*. 1995;122:843–845.

102. Timpome JG, Wright DJ, Li N, et al. The safety and pharmacokinetics of single-agent and combination therapy with megestrol acetate and dronabinol for the treatment of HIV wasting syndrome. *AIDS Res Hum Retroviruses*. 1997;13:305–315.

103. Struwe M, Kaempfer SH, Geiger CJ, et al. Effect of dronabinol on nutritional status in HIV infection. *Ann Pharmacother*. 1993;27: 827–831.

104. Grinspoon S, Corcoran C, Anderson E, et al. Sustained anabolic effect of long-term androgen administration in men with AIDS wasting. *Clin Infect Dis*. 1999;28:634–636.

105. Bhashin S, Storer TW, Asbel-Sethi N, et al. Effects of testosterone replacement with a nongenital, transdermal system, Androderm, in human immunodeficiency virus-infected men with low testosterone levels. *J Clin Endocrinol Metab*. 1998;83:3155–3162.

106. Strawford A, Barbieri T, Neese R, et al. Effects of nandrolone decanoate therapy in borderline hypogonadal men with HIV-associated weight loss. *J Acquir Immune Defic Syndr Hum Retrovirol*. 1999;20:137–146.

107. Gold J, High HA, Li Y, et al. Safety and efficacy of treatment with nandrolone decanoate for treatment of wasting in patients with HIV infection. *AIDS*. 1996;10:745–752.

108. Mulligan K, Zackin R, Clark RA, et al. Effect of nandrolone decanoate therapy on weight and lean body mass in HIV-infected women with weight loss: a randomized double-blind placebo-controlled, multicenter trial. *Arch Intern Med*. 2005;165:578–585.

109. Strawford A, Barbieri T, van Loan M, et al. Resistance exercise and supraphysiologic androgen therapy in eugonadal men with HIV-related weight loss: a randomized controlled trial. *JAMA*. 1999;281:1282–1290.

110. Grunfeld C, Kotler DP, Dobs A, Bhasin S. Oxandrolone in the treatment of HIV-associated weight loss in men: a randomized,

double-blind, placebo-controlled study. *J Acquir Immune Defic Syndr.* 2006;41(3):304–314.

111. Wasserman P, Segal-Maurer S, Rubin D. Low sex-hormone binding globulin and testosterone levels in association with erectile dysfunction among human immunodeficiency virus-infected men receiving testosterone and oxandrolone. *J Sex Med.* 2008;5(1):241–247.

112. Lubahn D, Joseph DR, Sullivan PM, et al. Cloning of human androgen receptor complementary DNA and localization to the X chromosome. *Science.* 1988;240:327–330.

113. Schambelan M, Mulligan K, Grunfeld C, et al. Recombinant human growth hormone in patients with HIV-associated wasting: a randomized placebo-controlled trial. *Ann Intern Med.* 1996;125:873–882.

114. Grinspoon S, Corcoran C, Parlman K, et al. Effects of testosterone and progressive resistance training in eugonadal men with AIDS wasting. *Ann Intern Med.* 2000;133:348–355.

115. Lichtenstein KA, Armon C, Buchacz K, et al. Low CD4+ T cell count is a risk factor for cardiovascular disease events in the HIV outpatient study. *Clin Infect Dis.* 2010;51(4):435–437.

116. Harris JA, Benedict FG. *A Biometric Study of Basal Metabolism in Man.* Vol 2. Washington, DC: Carnegie Institution of Washington; 1919.

117. Selberg O, Suttmann U, Melzer A, et al. Effect of increased protein intake and nutritional status on whole-body protein metabolism in AIDS patients with weight loss. *Metabolism.* 1995;44:1159–1165.

118. Berneis K, Battegay M, Bassetti S, et al. Nutritional supplementation combined with dietary counseling diminish whole body protein catabolism in HIV infected patients. *Eur J Clin Invest.* 2000;1:87–94.

119. Fogaca H, Souza H, Carneiro AJ, et al. Effects of oral nutritional supplementation on the intestinal mucosa of patients with AIDS. *J Clin Gastroenterol.* 2000;30:77–80.

120. Ahoua L, Umutoni C, Huerga H, et al. Nutrition outcomes of HIV-infected malnourished adults treated with ready-to-use therapeutic food in sub-Saharan Africa: a longitudinal study. *J Int AIDS Soc.* 2011;14:2.

121. Nyirenda C, Zulu I, Kabagambe EK, et al. Acute hypophosphataemia in a patient starting antiretroviral therapy in Zambia—a new context for refeeding syndrome? *BMJ Case Rep.* 2009(Apr 3). doi:10.1136/bcr.07.2008.0469.

122. Monroe AK, Glesby MJ, Brown TT. Diagnosing and managing diabetes in HIV-infected patients: current concepts. *Clin Infect Dis.* 2015;60(3):453–462.

123. Zhang L, Tin A, Brown T, et al. Vitamin D deficiency and metabolism in HIV-infected and -uninfected men in the Multicenter AIDS Cohort Study (MACS). *AIDS Res Hum Retroviruses.* 2016(Nov). Epub ahead of print. doi:10.1089/aid.2016.0144.

124. Wasserman P, Rubin DS. Highly prevalent vitamin D deficiency and insufficiency in an urban cohort of HIV-infected men under care. *AIDS Patient Care STDs.* 2010;24(4):223–227.

125. Adeyemi OM, Agniel D, French AL, et al. Vitamin D deficiency in HIV-infected and HIV-uninfected women in the United States. *J Acquir Immune Defic Syndr.* 2011;57(3):197–204.

126. Weltz T, Childs K, Ibrahim F, et al. Efavirenz is associated with severe vitamin D deficiency and increased alkaline phosphates. *AIDS.* 2010;24(12):1923–1928.

127. Gibney KB, Mihrshahi S, Torresi J, et al. The profile of health problems in African immigrants attending an infectious disease unit in Melbourne, Australia. *Am J Trop Med Hyg.* 2009;80(5):805–811.

128. Ross CA, Manson JE, Abrams SA, et al. The 2011 report on Dietary Reference Intakes for calcium and vitamin D from the Institute of Medicine: what clinicians need to know. *J Clin Endocrinol Metab.* 2011;96(1):53–58.

129. Pichard C, Sudre P, Karsegard V, et al. A randomized double-blind controlled study of oral nutritional supplementation with arginine and omega-3 fatty acids in HIV-infected patients. Swiss HIV Cohort Study. *AIDS.* 1998;12:53–63.

130. Ockenga J, Suttmann U, Selberg O, et al. Percutaneous endoscopic gastrostomy in AIDS and control patients: risks and outcomes. *Am J Gastroenterol.* 1996;91:1817–1822.

131. Kotler DP, Tierney AR, Ferraro R, et al. Enteral alimentation and repletion of body cell mass in malnourished patients with acquired immunodeficiency syndrome. *Am J Clin Nutr.* 1991;53:149–154.

132. Hiffler L, Raqkotoambinina B, Lafferty N, Martinez Garcia D. Thiamine deficiency in tropical pediatrics: new insights into a neglected but vital metabolic challenge. *Front Nutr.* 3:16. doi:10.3389/fnut.2016.00016.

133. Nakasaki H, Ohta M, Soeda J, et al. Clinical and biochemical aspects of thiamine treatment for metabolic acidosis during total parenteral nutrition. *Nutrition.* 1997;13(2):110–117.

134. Maiorana A, Vergine G, Coletti V, et al. Acute thiamine deficiency and refeeding syndrome: similar findings but different pathogenesis. *Nutrition.* 2014;30:948–952.

135. Melchior JC, Chastang C, Gelas P, et al. Efficacy of 2-month total parenteral nutrition in AIDS patients: a controlled randomized prospective trial. *AIDS.* 1996;10:379–384.

136. Singer P, Rothkopf MM, Kvetan V, et al. Risks and benefits of home parenteral nutrition in acquired immunodeficiency syndrome. *JPEN J Parenter Enteral Nutr.* 1991;15:75–79.

137. Erlandson KM, Allhouse AA, Jankowski CM, et al. Relationship of physical function to quality of life among persons aging with HIV infection. *AIDS.* 2014;28(13):1939–1943.

138. Coen PM, Goodpaster BH, Role of intramyocellular lipids in human health. *Trends Endocrinol Metab.* 2012;23(8):391–398.

139. Delmonico MJ, Harris TB, Visser M, et al. Longitudinal study of muscle strength, quality, and adipose tissue infiltration. *Am J Clin Nutr.* 2009;90(6):1579–1585.

140. Baker DJ, Wijshake T, Tchkonia T, et al. Clearance of p16Ink4a-positive senescent cells delays ageing-associated disorders. *Nature.* 2011;479: 232–236.

141. Volpato S, Bianchi L, Chrubini A, et al. Prevalence and clinical correlates of sarcopenia in community-dwelling older people: application of the EWGSOP definition and diagnostic algorithm. *J Gerontol A Biol Sci Med Sci.* 2014;69(4):438–446.

142. Szulc P, Duboeuf F, Marchand F. Delmas PD. Hormonal and lifestyle determinants of appendicular skeletal muscle mass in men: the MINOS study. *Am J Clin Nutr.* 2004;80(2): 496-503.

143. Compston J. HIV infection and bone disease. *J Intern Med.* 2016;280(4):350–358.

144. Rantanen T, Guralnik JM, Foley D, et al. Midlife hand-grip strength as a predictor of old age disability. *JAMA.* 1999;281(6):558–560.

145. Richert L, Dehail P, Mercie P, et al. High frequency of poor locomotor performance in HIV-infected patients. *AIDS.* 2011; 25(6):797–805.

146. Guralnik JM, Ferrucci L, Pieper CF, et al. Lower extremity function and subsequent disability: consistency across studies, predictive models, and value of gait speed alone compared to the short physical performance battery. *J Gerontol.* 2000;55A(4):M221–M231.

147. Goodpaster BH, Chomentowski P, Ward BK, et al. Effects of physical activity on strength and skeletal muscle fat infiltration in older adults: a randomized controlled trial. *J Appl Physiol.* 2008;105(5):1498–1503.

148. Slama L, Jacobson LP, Xiuhong L, et al. Longitudinal changes over 10 years in free testosterone among HIV-infected and HIV-uninfected men. *J Acquir Immune Defic Syndr.* 2016;71(1):57–64.

149. Pye SR, Huhtaniemi IT, Finn JD, et al. Late-onset hypogonadism and mortality in aging men. *J Clin Endocrinol Metab.* 2014; 99(4):1357–1366.

150. Travison TG, Basaria S, Storer TW. et al. Clinical meaningfulness of changes in muscle performance and physical function associated with testosterone administration in older men with mobility limitation. *J Gerontol A Biol Sci Med.* 2011;66A(10):1090–1099.

151. Storer TW, Woodhouse L, Magliano L, et al. Changes in muscle mass, muscle strength and power, but not physical function are related to testosterone does in healthy older men. *J Am Geriatric Soc.* 2008;56(11):1991-1999.

152. Navarro V, Khan I, Björnsson E, et al. Liver injury from herbal and dietary supplements. *Hepatology.* 2017;65(1):363–373.

153. Sharma A, Shi Q, Hoover DR et al. Increased fracture incidence in middle-aged HIV-infected and HIV-uninfected women: updated results from the Women's Interagency HIV Study. *J Acquir Immune Defic Syndr.* 2015;70(1):54–61.

154. Womack JA, Goulet JL, Gibert C, et al. Increased risk of fragility fractures among HIV infected compared to uninfected male veterans. *PLoS One.* 2011;6(2):e17217.

155. Triant VA, Brown TT, Lee H, Grinspoon SK. Fracture prevalence among human immunodeficiency virus (HIV)-infected versus non-HIV-infected patients in a large U.S. healthcare system. *J Clin Endocrinol Metab.* 2008;93(9):3499–3504.

156. Grijsen ML, Vrouenraets SME, Steingrover R, et al. High prevalence of reduced bone mineral density in primary HIV-1 infected men. *AIDS.* 2010;24:2233–2238.

157. Duvivier C, Kolta S, Assoumou L, et al. Greater decrease in bone mineral density with protease inhibitor regimens compared with nonnucleoside reverse transcriptase inhibitor regimens in HIV-1 infected naïve patients. *AIDS.* 2009;23(7):817–824.

158. Brown TT, McComsey GA, King MS, et al. Loss of bone mineral density after antiretroviral therapy initiation, independent of antiretroviral regimen. *J Acquir Immune Defic Syndr.* 2009;51(5):554–561.

159. Gallant JE, Staszewski S, Pozniak AL, et al. Efficacy and safety of tenofovir DF vs satavudine in combination therapy in antiretroviral-naïve patients. *JAMA.* 2004;292(2):191–201.

160. Bonjoch A, Figueras M, Estany C, et al. High prevalence of and progression to low bone mineral density in HIV-infected patients: a longitudinal cohort study. *AIDS.* 2010;24;2827–2833.

161. Arnsten JH, Freeman R, Howard AA, et al. Decreased bone mineral density and increased fracture risk in aging men with or at risk for HIV infection. *AIDS.* 2007;21:617–623.

162. Guillemi S, Harris M, Bondy GP, et al. Prevalence of bone mineral density abnormalities and related risk factors in an ambulatory HIV clinic population. *J Clin Densitom.* 2010;13(4):456–461.

163. Yin MT, McMahon DJ, Ferris DC, et al. Low bone mass and high bone turnover in postmenopausal human immunodeficiency virus infected women. *J Clin Endocrinol Metab.* 2010;95:620–629.

164. Cotter AG, Sabin CA, Simelane S, et al. Relative contribution of HIV infection, demographics and body mass index to bone mineral density. *AIDS.* 2014;28(14):2051–2060.

165. McGinty T, Mirmonsef P, Mallon PWG, Landay AL. Does systemic inflammation and immune activation contribute to fracture risk in HIV? *Curr Opin HIV AIDS.* 2016;11:253–260.

166. Cotter EJ, Chew N, Powderly WG, Doran PP. HIV type 1 alters mesenchymal stem cell differentiation potential and cell phenotype ex vivo. *AIDS Res Hum Retroviruses.* 2011;27(2):187–199.

167. Abu-Amer Y, Ross FP, Edwards J, Teitelbaum SL. Lipopolysaccharide-stimulated osteoclastogenesis is mediated by tumor necrosis via its P55 receptor. *J Clin Invest.* 1997;100(6):1557–1567.

168. Tatanji K, Vunnava A, Sheth AN, et al. Dysregulated B cell expression of RANKL and OPG correlates with loss of bone mineral density in HIV infection. *PLoS Pathog.* 2014;10:e1004497.

169. Gazzola L, Bellistri GM, Tincati C, et al. Association between peripheral T-lymphocyte activation and impaired bone mineral density in HIV-infected patients. *J Transl Med.* 2013;11:51.

170. Guaraldi G, Orlando G, Squillace N, et al. Prevalence of secondary causes of osteoporosis in HIV-infected individuals. Program and abstracts presented at 8th International Workshop on Adverse Drug Reactions and Lipodystrophy in HIV; September 24–26, 2006; San Francisco, CA.

171. Sharma A, Hoover DR, Shi Q, et al. Longitudinal study of falls among HIV-infected women: results of the interagency HIV study. Program and abstracts presented at the 7th International Workshop on HIV and Aging; September 26–27, 2016; Washington., DC.

172. Bolland MJ, Barber PA, Doughty RN, et al. Vascular events in healthy older women receiving calcium supplementation: randomized controlled trial. *BMJ.* 2008;336(7638):262–266.

173. Bolland MJ, Avenell A, Baron JA, et al. Effect of calcium supplements on risk of myocardial infarction and cardiovascular events: meta-analysis. *BMJ.* 2010;341:c3691. doi:10.1136/bmj.c3691.

174. Bolland MJ, Grey A, Avenell A, Gamble GD, Reid IR. Calcium supplements with or without vitamin D and risk of cardiovascular events: reanalysis of the Women's Health Initiative limited access dataset and meta-analysis. *BMJ.* 2011;342:d2040. doi:10.1136/bmj.d2040.

175. Prentice RL, Pettinger MB, Jackson RD, et al. Health risks and benefits from calcium and vitamin D supplementation: Women's Health Initiative clinical trial and cohort study. *Osteoporos Int.* 2013;24(2):567–580.

176. Raffield LM, Agarwal S, Hsu FC, et al. The association of calcium supplementation and incident cardiovascular events in the Multi-ethnic Study of Atherosclerosis (MESA). *Nutr Metab Cardiovasc Dis.* 2016;26(10):899–907.

177. Paik JM, Curhan GC, Sun Q, et al. Calcium supplement intake and risk of cardiovascular disease in women. *Osteoporos Int.* 2014;25(8):2047–2056.

178. Wohl D, Oka S, Clumeck N, et al. A randomized, double-blind comparison of tenofovir alafenamide versus tenofovir disoproxil fumarate, each coformulated with elvitegravir, cobicistat, and emtricitabine for initial HIV-1 treatment: week 96 results. *J Acquir Immune Defic Syndr.* 2016;72(1):58–64.

179. Callebaut C, Stepan G, Tian Y, Miller MD. In vitro virology profile of tenofovir alafenamide, a novel oral prodrug of tenofovir with improved antiviral activity compared to that of tenofovir disoproxil fumarate. *Antimicrob Agents Chemother.* 2015;59(10):5909–5916.

180. Casado JL, Santiuste C, Vazquez M, et al. Bone mineral density decline according to renal tubular dysfunction and phosphaturia in tenofovir-exposed HIV-infected patients. *AIDS.* 2016;30(9):1423–1431.

181. Erlandson KM, Li X, Abraham AG, et al. Long-term impact of HIV wasting on physical function *AIDS.* 2016;30:445–454.

182. Althoff KN, Jacobson LP, Cranston RD, et al. Age, comorbidities, and AIDS predict a frailty phenotype in men who have sex with men. *J Gerontol A Biol Sci Med Sci.* 2014;69(2):189–198.

183. Xue QL. The frailty syndrome: definition and natural history. *Clin Geriatr Med.* 2011;27(1):1–15.

184. Erlandson KM, Allshouse AA, Jankowski CM, et al. Functional impairment is associated with low bone and muscle mass among persons aging with HIV infection. *J Acquir Immune Defic Syndr.* 2013;63(2):209–215.

185. Erlandson KM, Allshouse AA, Jankowski CM, et al. Association of functional impairment with inflammation and immune activation in HIV type 1-infected adults receiving effective antiretroviral therapy. *J Infect Dis.* 2013;208(2):249–259.

186. Kooij KW, Wit FW, Schouten J, et al. HIV infection is independently associated with frailty in middle-aged HIV type-1 infected individuals compared with similar but uninfected controls. *AIDS.* 2016;30:241–250.

187. Pereira MA, FitzGerald SJ, Gregg EW, et al. A collection of physical activity questionnaires for health-related research. *Med Sci Sports Exerc.* 1997;29(6 Suppl):S1–S205.

188. Smit E, Winters-Stone KM, Loprinzi PD, Tang AM, Crespo CJ. Lower nutritional status and higher food insufficiency in frail older US adults. *Br J Nutr.* 2013;110(1):172–178.

189. Wong YY, McCaul KA, Yeap BB. Hankey GJ. Flicker L. Low vitamin D status is an independent predictor of increased frailty and all-cause mortality in older men: the Health in Men Study. *J Clin Endocrinol Metab.* 2013;98(9):3821–3828.

190. Smit E, Wanke C, Dong K, et al. Frailty, food insecurity, and nutritional status in people living with HIV. *J Frailty Aging.* 2015; 4(4):191–197.

191. Shippy RA, Karpiak SE. The aging HIV/AIDS population: fragile social networks. *Aging Ment Health.* 2005;9(3):246–254.

192. Latkin CA, Van Tieu H, Fields S, et al. Social network factors as correlates and predictors of high depressive symptoms among black men who have sex with men in HPTN 061. *AIDS Behav.* 2016(Aug 1). Epub ahead of print.

193. Greysen SR, Horwitz LI, Covinsky KE, et al. Does social isolation predict hospitalization and mortality among HIV+ and uninfected older veterans? *J Am Geriatr Soc.* 2013;61(9):1456–1463.

194. Oppong Asante K. Social support and the psychological wellbeing of people living with HIV/AIDS in Ghana. *Afr J Psychiatry (Johannesbg).* 2012;15(5):340–345.

195. Hoogendijk EO, Suanet B, Dent E, Deeg DJ, Aartsen MJ. Adverse effects of frailty on social functioning in older adults: results from the Longitudinal Aging Study Amsterdam. *Mauritas.* 2016;83: 45–50.

196. Loiola de Souza PM, Jacob-Filho W, Santarem JM, Zomignan AA, Burattini NM. Effect of progressive resistance exercise on strength evolution of elderly patients living with HIV compared to healthy controls. *Clinics.* 2011;66(2):261–266.

197. Longo V, Bonato M, Bossolasco S, et al. Brisk walking improves inflammatory markers in cART-treated patients. Abstract 763 at 21st Conference on Retroviruses and Opportunistic Infections (CROI); March 3–6, 2014; Boston, MA.

198. Diraijal-Fargo S, Webel AR, Longenecker CT, et al. The effect of physical activity on cardiometabolic health and inflammation in treated HIV infection. *Antivir Ther.* 2016;21(3):237–245.

199. Bacchetti P, Gripshover B, Grunfeld C, et al. Fat distribution in men with HIV infection from the study of fat redistribution and metabolic change in HIV infection (FRAM). *J Acquir Immune Defic Syndr.* 2005;40:121–131.

200. Brown T, Wang Z, Chu H, et al. Longitudinal anthropometric changes in HIV-infected and HIV-uninfected men. *J Acquir Immune Defic Syndr.* 2006;43(3):356–362.

201. Hammond E, McKinnon E, Nolan D. Human immunodeficiency virus treatment-induced adipose tissue pathology and lipoatrophy: prevalence and metabolic consequences. *Clin Infect Dis.* 2010;51(5):591–599.

202. Bastard JP, Caron M, Vidal H, et al. Association between altered expression of adipogenic factor SREBP-1 in lipoatrophic adipose tissue from HIV-1 infected patients and abnormal adipocyte differentiation and insulin resistance. *Lancet.* 2002;359: 1026–1031.

203. Shikuma CM, Hu N, Milne C, et al. Mitochondrial DNA decrease in subcutaneous adipose tissue of HIV-infected individuals with peripheral lipoatrophy. *AIDS.* 2001;15:1801–1809.

204. Walker UA, Bickel M, Lutke Volksbeck SI, et al. Evidence of nucleoside analogue reverse transcriptase inhibitor-associated genetic and structural defects of mitochondria in adipose tissue of HIV infected patients. *J Acquir Immune Defic Syndr.* 2002;29:117–121.

205. Brinkman K, Smeitink JA, Romijn JA, Reiss P. Mitochondrial toxicity induced by nucleoside-analogue reverse-transcriptase

206. is a key factor in the pathogenesis of antiretroviral-related-lipodystrophy. *Lancet.* 1999;354:1112–1115.

206. Chariot P, Drogou I, de Lacroix-Szmania I, et al. Zidovudine-induced mitochondrial disorder with massive liver steatosis, myopathy, lactic acidosis, and mitochondrial DNA depletion. *J Hepatol.* 1999;30:156–160.

207. Gerard Y, Maulin L, Yazdanpanah Y, et al. Symptomatic hyperlactatemia: an emerging complication of antiretroviral therapy. *AIDS.* 2000;14:2723–2730.

208. Mallon PW, Wand H, Law M, et al. Buffalo hump seen in HIV-associated lipodystrophy is associated with hyperinsulinemia but not dyslipidemia. *J Acquir Immune Defic Syndr.* 2005;38: 156–162.

209. Gervasoni C, Ridolfo AL, Rovati L, et al. Maintenance of breast size reduction after mastoplasty and switch to a protease inhibitor-sparing regimen in an HIV-positive woman with highly active antiretroviral therapy-associated massive breast enlargement. *AIDS Patient Care STDS.* 2002;16:307–311.

210. Miller KK, Daly PA, Sentochk D, et al. Pseudo-Cushing's syndrome in human immunodeficiency virus-infected patients. *Clin Infect Dis.* 1998;27:68–72.

211. Martin A, Smith DE, Carr A, et al. Reversibility of lipoatrophy in HIV-infected patients 2 years after switching from a thymidine analogue to abacavir: the MITOX extension study. *AIDS.* 2004; 18:1029–1036.

212. Miller CJ, Baker JV, Bormann AM, et al. Adjudicated morbidity and mortality outcomes by age among individuals with HIV infection on suppressive antiretroviral therapy. *PLoS One.* 2014;9(4):e95061.

213. Friis-Moller N, Thiebaut R, Reiss P, et al. Predicting the risk of cardiovascular disease in HIV-infected patients: the data collection on adverse effects of anti-HIV drugs study. *Eur J Cardiovasc Prev.* 2010;17(5):491–501.

214. Burdo TH, Lo J, Abbara S, et al. Soluble CD163, a novel marker of activated macrophages, is elevated and associated with non-calcified coronary plaque in HIV-infected patients. *J Infect Dis.* 2011;204:1227–1236.

215. Nou E, Lo J, Grinspoon SK. Inflammation, immune activation, and cardiovascular disease in HIV. *AIDS.* 2016;30(10):1495–1509.

216. Lichtenstein KA, Armon C, Buchacz K, et al. Low CD4+ T cell count is a risk factor for cardiovascular disease events in the HIV outpatient study. *Clin Infect Dis.* 2010;51(4):435–447.

217. Lang S, Mary-Krause M, Simon A, et al. HIV replication and immune status are independent predictors of the risk of myocardial infarction in HIV-infected patients. *Clin Infect Dis.* 2012; 55(4):600–607.

218. Kelesidis T, Kendall M, Yang OO, Hodis HN, Currier JS. Biomarkers of microbial translocation and macrophage activation: association with progression of subclinical atherosclerosis in HIV-1 infection. *J Infect Dis.* 2012;206:1558–1567.

219. Joseph P, Tawakol A. Imaging atherosclerosis with positron emission tomography. *Eur Heart J.* 2016;37(39):2974–2980.

220. Subramanian S, Tawakol A, Burdo TH, et al. Arterial inflammation in patients with HIV. *JAMA.* 2012;308(4):379–386.

221. Figueroa AL, Abdelbaky A, Truong QA, et al. Measurement of arterial activity on routine FDG PET/CT images improves prediction of risk of future CV events. *JACC Cardiovasc Imaging.* 2013; 6(12):1250–1259.

222. Worm SW, Sabin C, Weber R, et al. Risk of myocardial infarction in patients with HIV infection exposed to specific individual antiretroviral drugs from the 3 major drug classes: the Data Collection on Adverse Events of Anti-HIV Drugs (D:A:D) Study. *J Infect Dis.* 2010;201:318–330.

223. Sabin CA, Reiss P, Ryom L, et al. Is there continued evidence for an association between abacavir usage and myocardial infarction

risk in individuals with HIV? A cohort collaboration. *BMC Med.* 2016;14:61. doi:10.1186/s12916-016-0588-4.

224. Stein JH, Ribaudo HJ, Hodis HN, et al. A prospective, randomized clinical trial of antiretroviral therapies on carotid wall thickness. *AIDS.* 2015;29(14):1775–1783.

225. Llibre JM, Hill A. Abacavir and cardiovascular disease: a critical look at the data. *Antiviral Res.* 2016;132:116–121.

226. Diallo YL, Ollivier V, Joly V, et al. Abacavir has no prothrombotic effect on platelets in vitro. *J Antimicrob Chemother.* 2016;71(12):3506–3509.

227. Friis-Mollner N, Reiss P, Sabin CA, et al. Class of antiretroviral drug and risk of myocardial infarction. *N Engl J Med.* 2007;356(17):1723–1735.

228. Goff DC, Lloyd-Jones DM, Bennett G, Coady S, et al. 2013 ACC/AHA guideline on the assessment of cardiovascular risk: a report of the American College of Cardiology/American Heart Association Task Force on Practice Guidelines. *J Am Coll Cardiol.* 2014;63(25 Pt B):2935–2959.

229. Crane HM, Nance R, Dellaney JA, et al. Comparing cardiovascular disease risk scores for use in HIV-Infected Individuals. Abstract 42: Conference on Retroviruses and Opportunistic Infections (CROI); February 22–25, 2016; Boston MA.

230. Jacobson TA, Ito MK, Maki KC, et al. National Lipid Association recommendations for patient-centered management of dyslipidemia: part 2-executive summary. *J Clin Lipidol.* 2014;8:473–488.

231. O'Keefe JA, Cordain L, Harris WH, Moe RM, Vogel R. Optimal low-density lipoprotein is 50 to 70 mg/dL: lower is better and physiologically normal. *J Am Coll Cardiol.* 2004;43(11):2142–2146.

232. Ridker PM, Danielson E, Fonseca FA, et al. Rosuvastatin to prevent vascular events in men and women with elevated C-reactive protein. *N Engl J Med.* 2008;359(21):2195–2207.

233. Packard C. Stezhka T. Did we IMPROVE-IT: thoughts on LDL targeting post-trial? *Expert Rev Cardiovasc Ther.* 2015;1395:465–466.

234. Woodward M, Rumley A, Welsh P, MacMahon S, Lowe G. A comparison of the associations between seven hemostatic or inflammatory variables and coronary heart disease. *J Thromb Haemost.* 2007;5:1795–1800.

235. deLongeril M, Salen P, Martin J, et al. Mediterranean diet, traditional risk factors, and the rate of cardiovascular complications after myocardial infarction: final report of the Lyon Diet Heart Study. *Circulation.* 1999;99:779–785.

236. Buckland G, Gonzalez CA, Aqudo A, et al. Adherence to the Mediterranean diet and risk of coronary heart disease in the Spanish EPIC Cohort Study. *Am J Epidemiol.* 2009;170(12):1518–1529.

237. Esposito K, Marfella R, Citotola M, et al. Effect of a Mediterranean-style diet on endothelial dysfunction and markers of vascular inflammation in the metabolic syndrome: a randomized trial. *JAMA.* 2004;292:1440–1446.

238. Hadigan C, Jeste S, Anderson EJ, et al. Modifiable dietary habits and their relation to metabolic abnormalities in men and women with human immunodeficiency virus infection and fat redistribution. *Clin Infect Dis.* 2001;33:710–717.

239. Tsiodras S, Poulia KA, Yannakoulia M. Adherence to Mediterranean diet is favorably associated with metabolic parameters in HIV-positive patients with the highly active antiretroviral therapy-induced metabolic syndrome and lipodystrophy. *Metabolism.* 2009;58(6):854–859.

240. Turcinov D, Stanley C, Rutherford GW, et al. Adherence to the Mediterranean diet is associated with a lower risk of body-shape changes in Croatian patients treated with combination antiretroviral therapy. *Eur J Epidemiol.* 2009;24(5):267–274.

241. Guallar E, Stranges S, Murlow C, Appel LJ. Enough is enough: stop wasting money on vitamin and mineral supplements. *Ann Intern Med.* 2013;159:850–851.

242. Guwatudde D, Wang M, Ezeamama AE, et al. The effect of standard dose multivitamin supplementation on disease progression in HIV-infected adults initiating HAART: a randomized double blind placebo-controlled trial in Uganda. *BMC Infect Dis* 2015;15:348. doi:10.1186/s12879-015-1082-x.

243. Funderberg NT, Jiang Y, Debanne SM, et al. Rosuvastatin reduces vascular inflammation and T-cell and monocyte activation in HIV-infected subjects on antiretroviral therapy. *J Acquir Immune Defic Syndr.* 2015;68(4):396–404.

244. Lo J, Lu MT, Ihenachor EJ, et al. Effects of statin therapy on coronary artery plaque volume and high-risk plaque morphology in HIV-infected patients with subclinical atherosclerosis: a randomized, double-blind, placebo-controlled trial. *Lancet HIV.* 2015;2(2):e52–e63.

245. Longenecker CT, Jiang Y, Debanne SM, et al. Rosuvastatin arrests progression of carotid intima-media thickness in treated HIV. Abstract 137: Conference on Opportunistic Infections and Retroviruses (CROI); February 23–26, 2015; Seattle, WA.

246. Wensel TM, Waldrop BA, Wensel B. Pitavastatin: a new HMG-CoA reductase inhibitor. *Ann Pharmacother.* 2010;44:507–514.

247. Wohl DA, Hsiao-chaun T, Busby M, et al. Randomized study of the safety and efficacy of fish oil (omega-3 fatty acid) supplementation with dietary and exercise counseling for the treatment of antiretroviral therapy-associated hypertriglyceridemia. *Clin Infect Dis.* 2005;41:1498–1504.

33 Cancer

Mary Marian, DCN, RDN, CSO, FAND, Todd Mattox, PharmD, BCNSP, and Valaree Williams, MS, RDN, CSO, FAND

CONTENTS

Acknowledgments: Robin Mendelsohn, MD, and Mark A. Schattner, MD, were the authors of this chapter for the second edition.

Objectives

1. Discuss the etiology and significance of malnutrition in cancer patients.
2. Identify nutrition abnormalities associated with cancer.
3. Review treatment options for medical nutrition therapy for cancer patients throughout the course of their disease.

Test Your Knowledge Questions

1. Which of the following is true about the mechanisms that promote weight loss and malnutrition in patients with cancer?
   A. Tumor-induced altered metabolism has been associated with increased energy expenditure.
   B. Inadequate nutrient intake and increased cytokine production can lead to weight loss.
   C. Some cancer patients demonstrate increased glucose turnover compared with non-tumor-bearing patients with simple starvation.
   D. All of the above.
2. Enteral nutrition (EN) is an appropriate therapy for which of the following patients?
   A. A well-nourished patient with colon cancer undergoing chemotherapy
   B. A severely malnourished gastric cancer patient with nausea and vomiting
   C. A moderately malnourished patient with head and neck cancer with dysphagia
   D. A well-nourished recipient of a hematopoietic stem cell transplant (HSCT)
3. Which of the following is true regarding a patient with newly diagnosed pancreatic cancer awaiting chemotherapy?
   A. A nutrition assessment should be performed.
   B. EN should be initiated because the patient will likely need nutrition support during chemotherapy.

C. Parenteral nutrition (PN) should be initiated because the patient will likely need nutrition support during chemotherapy.
D. PN should be initiated if surgical intervention is imminent.

Test Your Knowledge Answers

1. The correct answer is **D**. Early investigations suggested tumor-induced changes in metabolism caused increased energy expenditure and nitrogen loss. However, more recent investigations have demonstrated inconsistency with this response across a wide variety of cancer patient populations. Increased glucose turnover has been reported in cancer patients with weight loss, which is in stark contrast to non-tumor-bearing patients with simple starvation, who have decreased glucose turnover. Potential causes of metabolic abnormalities and weight loss in cancer patients include the presence of increased circulating cytokines, changes in hormones and neuropeptide levels, and tumor-derived products.

2. The correct answer is **C**. EN is indicated in patients undergoing anticancer therapies who are malnourished and who have a functional gastrointestinal (GI) tract. Nutrition support is not routinely indicated in patients undergoing treatment who are not malnourished. The patient with gastric cancer with nausea and vomiting has symptoms of gastric outlet obstruction and would require a further evaluation before EN could be initiated.

3. The correct answer is **A**. According to the American Society for Parenteral and Enteral Nutrition (ASPEN) guidelines, patients with cancer are nutritionally at risk and should undergo a nutrition screening to identify those who require formal nutrition assessment. Neither EN nor PN is routinely indicated in patients undergoing anticancer treatment who are not malnourished. The role of perioperative

PN is controversial, and it is not recommended for patients who are not malnourished.

Background

Trends and Impact of Cancer

Excluding individuals diagnosed with carcinoma in situ and skin cancers (basal or squamous cell), the annual incidence of new cancers in the United States is approximately 1.685 million cases, and cancer accounts for 1 in 4 of deaths in the United States annually.[1] Incidence rates have declined for a number of cancers, including lung and colorectal (in older adults), although rates have increased for other cancers, including leukemia and cancers of the liver, head/neck (in white males), pancreas, thyroid, cervix (in young women), endometrial tissue, and uterus.[1] When deaths are aggregated by age, cancer has surpassed heart disease as the leading cause of death for individuals under the age of 85 years.[1] Moreover, approximately 14.5 million adults in the United States have a personal history of cancer.[1]

The financial costs of cancer are enormous, both to patients and to society at large. The National Institutes of Health estimate that $263.8 billion was spent on cancer in 2013, with an estimated $124.6 billion spent on direct medical costs and $139.2 billion allocated to indirect mortality costs.[2] When compared to other causes of death, cancer represents the largest toll on the global economy because of years of life and productivity lost. And, as the US population continues to grow and age, this economic burden will undoubtedly continue to increase.[2]

Cancer and Nutrition Status

Unintended weight loss and progressive deterioration in nutrition status are common in the cancer population and often result in significant malnutrition.[3-5] While the exact prevalence of malnutrition in the oncology population is unknown, an estimated 20% to 80% of patients with cancer develop malnutrition at various times in the course of their illness.[4,5] Malnutrition (defined as "lack of proper nutrition") is associated with numerous adverse events, such as perioperative complications, poor tolerance of and delays in therapy, poorer quality of life (QOL), and increased morbidity and mortality.[4,5] Anorexia, early satiety, the presence of inflammatory and catabolic mediators, and a host of other factors, including oncologic treatments, contribute to the nutrition deterioration seen in cancer patients.[4,5] Screening for and diagnosing malnutrition in oncology patients is important because malnutrition can have an adverse impact on clinical outcomes.[3-6] In their landmark study, DeWys and colleagues reported that patients receiving chemotherapy who had lost weight prior to the initiation of treatment had decreased performance status and survival when compared with those without weight loss.[6] Furthermore, DeWys and associates emphasized the importance of an early assessment of nutrition status, because many patients have nutrition-related symptoms, such as weight loss, early satiety, poor appetite, and nausea, when diagnosed with cancer.[6]

Malnutrition in cancer patients is associated with longer length of hospital stay, increased cost, and increased morbidity and mortality, and it has been shown to make anticancer treatments less effective, leading to longer duration of treatment.[4,5]

Although any cancer survivor is at risk for developing malnutrition, patients with sarcomas, breast cancer, and hematologic cancers have the lowest risk whereas patients with colon, prostate, and lung cancers are at moderate risk. Malnutrition reportedly occurs at the highest frequency (over 80%) in patients with pancreatic, head/neck, and gastric cancers.[6-8] Studies reflect that malnutrition is not only affected by tumor type, location, grade, and stage but also by the anticancer therapy and patient characteristics, including age, gender, and other preexisting comorbidities such as diabetes and intestinal disorders.[9]

Not all cancer survivors develop malnutrition; however, when malnutrition is left untreated, many patients become cachectic.[6-8] Cachexia is a syndrome that is associated with several chronic conditions, manifested by not only severe weight loss but also significant loss of muscle and fat mass.[6-8] Multiple metabolic derangements play a key role in the development of cachexia.

Metabolic Alterations

Energy Expenditure

Early investigations suggested that tumor-induced metabolic abnormalities led to increased energy expenditure and nitrogen loss, resulting in weight loss and malnutrition. However, further studies revealed that this response is not consistent and have found resting energy expenditures (REEs) to vary widely.[10,11] In some studies, an association of energy expenditure with age, sex, height, weight, nutrition intake, nutrition status, or extent of tumor has not been observed, but other research has found that tumor stage and duration of disease, age, and gender affect energy expenditure.[10,11] Cao and colleagues found significant differences in the ratio of measured REE to fat-free mass in patients with esophageal, gastric, non-small-cell lung, and pancreatic cancer when compared with controls.[10]

Carbohydrate Metabolism

Many cancer patients exhibit glucose intolerance, which is thought to be caused by increased endogenous glucose production, increased resistance to both exogenous and endogenous insulin, and inadequate insulin release.[11,12] Other factors, including bed rest, weight loss, and sepsis, may also contribute to hyperglycemia in cancer as they do in other diseases.

This increase in glucose turnover and weight loss is not seen in non-tumor-bearing patients with simple starvation, who have decreased glucose turnover and weight loss.[13] Metabolically expensive futile cycles, such as the Cori cycle, likely also contribute to altered glucose metabolism in cancer patients.[13]

Tumor cells produce lactate, which is used as a substrate for gluconeogenesis in the Cori cycle and reconverted to glucose.[13] In initial studies, the increase in Cori cycle activity made a large contribution to increased energy expenditure in patients with metastatic disease and weight loss, but in subsequent studies an increase in the Cori cycle activity had only a minor role in the alterations of glucose metabolism.[13] Further research continues to identify other futile cycles.

Protein Metabolism

Cancer patients have increased protein turnover, which is thought to be caused by increased hepatic protein synthesis, increased muscle protein degradation, and impaired protein synthesis. During simple starvation in non-tumor-bearing patients, protein catabolism slowly decreases as the body attempts to preserve lean body mass (LBM). In contrast, protein turnover increases with the progression of disease and weight loss in some cancer patients.[13–16]

Increased protein breakdown in cancer patients involves at least 3 different proteolytic pathways: (1) lysosomal energy-dependent proteolysis (including cysteine proteases cathepsins B, H, and L, and aspartate proteases cathepsin D), which is mainly responsible for cell receptor and extracellular protein degradation; (2) calcium-dependent proteases (including calpains I and II), which are mainly involved in tissue injury, autolysis, and necrosis; and (3) the ubiquitin-proteasome–dependent pathway, which is adenosine triphosphate (ATP) dependent and works with the calpain system to break down myofilaments.[13] The ubiquitin-proteasome–dependent pathway is the most extensively studied and thought to be the predominant mechanism of protein breakdown, especially in patients with greater than 10% weight loss.[13–16]

Lipid Metabolism

The depletion of adipose tissue and lipid stores, which is caused by increased lipolysis and fatty acid oxidation, also contributes to weight loss in cancer patients.[13,16] Compared with cancer-free subjects and cancer patients without weight loss, cancer patients with weight loss have an increased turnover of both free fatty acids and glycerol.[13,16] Increased lipolysis has been attributed to multiple causes, including poor oral intake, stress response to illness leading to adrenal medullary stimulation and increased circulating catecholamine levels, insulin resistance, and the release of lipolytic factors produced by the tumor itself or by myeloid tissue cells.[13] Lipid-mobilizing factor (LMF) is a cachectic-inducing substrate produced by the tumor that seems to catalyze the mobilization of adipose tissue via cyclic adenylyl cyclase pathway–mediated process that facilitates the breakdown of glycerol and free fatty acids.[13–16] Cytokines such as tumor necrosis factor-α (TNF-α) have also been implicated as possible mediators of depleting lipid stores, although their precise role is unclear.[13–16] Continued loss of fat mass in conjunction with inadequate oral intake leads to malnutrition and the more serious state of cachexia.

Mediators of Altered Metabolism

Recent data demonstrate that various mediators including glycoproteins, proinflammatory cytokines, neurotransmitters, and neuropeptides induce a systemic inflammatory response leading to the characteristic metabolic derangements associated with cancer cachexia.

Glycoproteins

Two glycoproteins, proteolysis-inducing factor (PIF) and LMF, have been found to be important mediators of the cachexia seen in many patients with cancers.[11,13,15,16]

PIF, a 24-kDa molecular mass sulfated glycoprotein, is produced by human tumors and was found in the urine of patients with cancer (namely breast, colorectal, liver, lung, ovarian, and pancreatic) who were losing weight, but it was not in the urine of cancer patients who were maintaining their weight. Moreover, PIF levels did not seem to have an adverse impact on weight in patients with gastric or esophageal cancer.[15,16] In fact, PIF expression directly correlates with the severity of weight loss. PIF induces weight loss through multiple mechanisms. It has a direct effect on skeletal muscle by decreasing protein synthesis and increasing protein degradation by upregulating the ubiquitin-proteasome–dependent pathway. PIF also increases the expression of proinflammatory cytokines (ie, interleukin [IL]-6 and IL-8), which independently cause weight loss and induce the shedding of syndecans (transmembrane proteoglycans), which have been shown to be related to increased metastases and mortality.[9,12,13]

LMF, a glycoprotein produced by a variety of tumors, is identical to the plasma protein zinc-alpha2-glycoprotein (ZAG) and causes an increase in lipolysis.[13,15] LMF/ZAG has been shown to increase lipid mobilization and substrate use by increasing mitochondrial oxidative pathways in adipose tissue. In animal studies, LMF led to decreased body fat and weight independent of energy intake. Moreover, the degree of LMF activity correlates with the degree of weight loss and tumor burden.[9,12,13,15]

Proinflammatory Cytokines

Tumor Necrosis Factor-α

In animal studies, TNF-α promoted weight loss by inducing the enzyme lipoprotein lipase, which hydrolyzes fatty acids from plasma lipoproteins, stimulating lipolysis, and suppressing transcription.[17,18] Findings from human studies, however, are less consistent. Hypotheses to explain the disparity in results between animal and human models include differences in measuring techniques, fluctuations in TNF-α serum levels, or the short half-life of TNF-α. Also, some have proposed that perhaps TNF-α has a direct local effect before it circulates through the bloodstream.[13,15]

Interleukin 1, Interleukin 6, and Interferon Gamma

Animal models have shown IL-1, IL-6, and interferon gamma (IFN-γ) to be important mediators in cancer-related weight loss because they are associated with a variety of inflammatory metabolic abnormalities. Human studies, however, have been inconsistent.[13,15,17]

Neuropeptides

Neuropeptide Y (NPY) is a 36–amino acid neuropeptide found in the hypothalamus. NPY levels rise and stimulate feeding and decrease energy expenditure to restore energy balance during normal starvation. However, studies in tumor-bearing animals have shown that NPY levels are inappropriately low and do not have orexigenic (appetite-stimulating) effects. Data from human studies are very limited.[13,15]

Cancer cachexia may also be partly caused by orexigenic neuropeptides such as NPY and anorexigenic-stimulating neuropeptides such as proopiomelanocortin (POMC).[9,13] Alpha-melanocyte stimulating hormone (α-MSH), a product of POMC, induces anorexia by binding to 2 melanocortin receptors (Mc3r and Mc4r) in the hypothalamus. Studies in rats showed that Mc3r and Mc4r blockade to α-MSH binding reverses cancer anorexia in animals with cancer. The mechanism for tumor-induced upregulation in α-MSH is not clear, but it is likely mediated by cytokines (eg, IL-1, IL-6, TNF-α).[9,13,15]

Impact of Treatment Modalities

Treatment modalities for cancer include surgery, chemotherapy, radiation therapy, and biotherapies (eg, monoclonal antibodies, angiogenesis inhibitors). These treatment interventions can successfully eradicate the tumor, slow tumor growth, and reduce tumor size, but such modalities can also lead to profound, acute, and long-lasting adverse effects and nutrition-impact symptoms that impede oral intake and promote malnutrition. Additionally, digestion and absorption effects of cancer treatment may compound nutrition problems. Anorexia, dysphagia, early satiety, fatigue, mucositis, odynophagia, nausea, vomiting, diarrhea, constipation, and taste changes commonly occur during treatment and may persist after treatment has been completed.[3,11,13] As discussed later in this chapter, clinicians should perform a comprehensive nutrition assessment for all patients identified with malnutrition or a high risk for nutrition deterioration. This comprehensive assessment should uncover the presence of any nutrition-impact symptoms and provide strategies to improve and resolve any associated nutrition problems.

Impaired Energy Intake, Maldigestion, and Malabsorption

Changes in Taste and Appetite

Self-reported taste and smell alterations are prevalent in upward of 86% of cancer patients.[19] Many cancer patients complain of decreased ability to taste and diminished appetite, which are hypothesized to be related to proinflammatory cytokines and neuropeptide activity.[9] In addition, cancer treatments, including chemotherapy, radiation, and surgery, can lead to alterations in how foods taste, and these changes may persist for months after the completion of therapy. Taste and smell alterations can increase distress, reduce appetite, and contribute to poor nutrition status in cancer patients.

Learned Food Aversions

Cancer patients who receive chemotherapy or radiation therapy may develop food aversions. In a classic study, Bernstein

and associates tested children receiving chemotherapy associated with nausea and vomiting for a learned food aversion.[20] Their study had 3 groups: a group undergoing GI toxic chemotherapy who were given a novel ice cream flavor; a group undergoing GI toxic chemotherapy who were not given ice cream; and a control group who were not undergoing chemotherapy and were given ice cream. When tested later for aversions to this novel ice cream flavor, controls chose it 3 times more frequently than the experimental group, indicating a learned aversion in the children who had eaten the ice cream while undergoing chemotherapy. Similar findings have been reported in adults. The risk of developing a learned food aversion is directly related to the GI toxicity of the therapy.

Depression

Studies have reported that up to 58% of cancer patients have depressive symptoms and up to 38% experience major depression.[21] The mechanism is likely multifactorial and related to the stress of both the diagnosis and treatment as well as neurohumoral changes induced by the tumor. Factors that may be associated with increased risk for depression in patients with cancer include younger age (less than 50 years), a prior history of depression, and the presence of uncontrolled cancer symptoms.[21,22] Certain types of malignancies, including cancers of the head and neck, pancreas, breast, and lung, seem to be associated with increased incidence of depression.[21] As in patients without cancer, depression in patients with cancer is associated with impaired oral intake and malnutrition. A recent meta-analysis showed that depression predicted mortality in cancer patients.[23]

Disturbances of the Gastrointestinal Tract

Primary and secondary tumor involvement can lead to GI tract obstruction from intrinsic or extrinsic compression. Malignant bowel obstruction is often associated with GI and gynecological cancers. GI malignancies—namely, esophageal, gastric, intestinal, and pancreatic—frequently cause direct mechanical obstruction by the primary tumor. GI tract obstruction may also be caused by extrinsic compression on esophageal or other GI lumens by tumors, including lung cancer and malignant lymph nodes.[24] In addition, peritoneal disease can cause both mechanical obstruction and intestinal dysfunction without frank obstruction. Although acute obstruction presents with symptoms that require immediate medical attention, malignant obstruction develops slowly over time and causes a progressive decrease in food intake leading to weight loss and oral diet intolerance.[24] Recurrent episodes of intestinal obstruction are very common in cancer patients. Secondary malignant bowel obstruction is a disease with a poor prognosis. Multimodality treatments are available. However, there is no current consensus regarding the optimal treatment, and no strong evidence supports the efficacy of any specific treatment to improve QOL or prolong survival.[25]

In addition to GI obstructions, cancer patients can have altered intestinal motility. Altered GI motility is multifactorial, and contributors may depend on cancer origin. Factors include paraneoplastic phenomena, direct infiltration of tumor into the celiac plexus or vagus nerve, past GI surgery, and toxic effects of cancer treatments.[26] Tumors can also induce an immune-mediated destruction of components of the enteric nerve plexus, resulting in a paraneoplastic syndrome of gastroparesis and intestinal pseudo-obstruction. Lastly, the development of gastroparesis can also be influenced by comorbidities such as poorly controlled diabetes, hypothyroidism, and neuromuscular disorders as well as the use of medications that delay gastric emptying, including narcotics. Misdiagnosis of malignancy-associated gastroparesis as chemotherapy-induced emesis can lead to delays or dose reductions in potentially efficacious anticancer therapy administration.

Additional contributors to GI tract disturbances include prolonged postoperative ileus, radiation therapy, and medications. Prolonged postoperative ileus is common after surgical bowel resection. Patients treated with radiation therapy can experience both acute and chronic effects on GI motility. Medications, especially chemotherapeutic agents and narcotics, can alter GI motility. As with frank obstruction, disturbances in motility result in impaired oral intake and weight loss. The severity of dysmotility is directly correlated with the degree of malnutrition.[27,28]

Malabsorption

Normal nutrient absorption occurs in 3 phases: luminal processing, absorption into the intestinal mucosa, and transport into circulation.[29] (See Chapter 1.) Malabsorption can result from defects in any of the phases. In cancer patients, many factors may cause malabsorption, including adverse effects from chemotherapy, radiation therapy, surgery, or treatment-related medications; other medical conditions related to the malignancy or treatment; and infections. For example, surgical resection can result in altered intestinal transit time and reduction of intestinal absorptive surfaces, thereby contributing to malabsorption.

The presence of malignancy, chemotherapy after a cancer-related operation, and history of radiation therapy are associated with increased incidence of fistula formation.[30] Additionally, cancer, chemotherapy, and radiation therapy all hinder spontaneous healing of fistulas. The degree of malabsorption depends on the site and extent of the intestinal bypass. The most significant malabsorption is seen in gastrocolic (between the stomach and the large intestine), enterocolic (between the small intestine and the large intestine), enteroenteric (between the small intestine and the small intestine), and enterocutaneous (between the small bowel and the skin) fistulas.[31] Managing the nutrition of patients with such fistulas is difficult, and nutrition interventions must focus on replacing the ongoing loss of fluids, electrolytes, and minerals.

Extensive bowel resection frequently leads to small intestinal bacterial overgrowth (SIBO), which may contribute to malabsorption by damaging enterocytes. In patients with cancer, SIBO is usually caused by an anatomic abnormality such as a fistula, strictures, and surgical resections—most notably, surgically created blind loops, ileocecal resections (bacteria migrate from the colon to the small intestine), and gastric resections (in which the protective barrier from gastric acid is lost). Multiple studies have confirmed that most postgastrectomy patients have SIBO.[32] Lastly, malabsorption may be related to a protein-losing enteropathy, which has been associated with multiple malignancies, including gastric cancer, lymphoma, and melanoma, and is also a rare complication of chemotherapy and radiation therapy.

Nutrition Screening

In the acute care setting, nutrition screening of all patients within 24 hours of admission is mandatory. However, in the outpatient setting, screening for nutrition risk is not mandated. Nevertheless, a systematic nutrition screening program should be in place to triage and refer patients to the appropriate nutrition professionals.

The purpose of nutrition screening is to systematically identify oncology patients who are malnourished or are at risk for becoming malnourished. Although there is no widely accepted nutrition screening tool for use in cancer, an effective screening system is quick, easy, efficient, reliable, and inexpensive, and can be completed by any clinician. Nutrition screening identifies patients who may require a comprehensive nutrition assessment. Screening can also lead to a proactive, rather than reactive, approach to providing nutrition care. Because cancer patients may receive care over several weeks or months, and in many different treatment settings, nutrition screening should begin when the cancer is diagnosed and periodic rescreening should be done throughout the treatment period. Even patients who are initially identified to be at a low risk for becoming malnourished may develop nutrition-related issues during treatment that lead to a malnourished state.

Screening for the presence of nutrition-impact symptoms is essential for all cancer patients regardless of whether the patient is receiving curative or palliative treatment. Early detection of nutrition problems with the appropriate interventions employed can improve functional status and QOL.[33]

Multiple nutrition screening tools are available for use in the cancer patient population. Many nutrition screening programs use 2 simple parameters, unintended weight change and decreased intake/appetite, as screening parameters because these indices have been validated as indicators of nutrition status.[34-36] Regardless of the nutrition screening tools used, clinicians in the oncology setting must have a systematic approach in place for screening, triaging, and referring patients for appropriate nutrition assessment and nutrition care.

Nutrition Assessment

Patients with cancer who are identified as malnourished or at high nutrition risk should be referred to a nutrition professional (eg, registered dietitian nutritionist) with expertise in oncology. These patients should undergo a comprehensive nutrition assessment and receive an individualized nutrition prescription designed to maintain or improve the individual's nutrition status. They should then be reassessed at appropriate time points to avoid significant deteriorations in nutrition status.

The use of validated nutrition assessment tools has resulted in early identification and appropriate treatment of patients with moderate or severe malnutrition, which can reduce morbidity and mortality.[30,37,38] Unfortunately, malnutrition often goes unrecognized or undiagnosed because of confusion surrounding what are the best measures or indices to assess nutrition status.[39] Therefore, to standardize the approach to nutrition assessment, the Academy of Nutrition and Dietetics (AND) and ASPEN have published criteria that clinicians should use to diagnose and document malnutrition (see Chapter 9).[40] AND and ASPEN recommend using an etiology-based list of criteria for defining malnutrition that reflect not only the impact of inadequate nutrient intake but also the role of inflammation as an underlying factor.[40] In general, the definition of malnutrition as it relates to either the presence of acute or chronic disease applies when detecting malnutrition in the oncology population (see Chapter 9).[40]

The Patient-Generated Subjective Global Assessment (PG-SGA) is another common and accepted approach to diagnosing malnutrition in cancer patients. This methodology has been validated for use in the oncology population and endorsed by AND and ASPEN for assessing nutrition status.[36,41] Unlike the AND/ASPEN malnutrition framework, the PG-SGA asks the patient to report whether he or she is experiencing any nutrition-impact factors.[41] When using the AND/ASPEN malnutrition framework to assess a patient's nutrition status, the clinician should inquire during the diet history about the presence of any symptoms that may be impeding oral intake. Nutrition-impact symptoms—including anorexia, poor appetite, early satiety, constipation, diarrhea, malabsorption, dysphagia, mucositis, esophagitis, oral candidiasis, xerostomia, thick saliva, taste and smell changes, and fatigue—can vary depending on the disease site and treatment modalities.[3,8,11] Patients often have multiple symptoms, and effective management of these symptoms can positively affect comfort, weight maintenance, and tolerance of treatment. See Chapter 9 for a more in-depth discussion regarding nutrition screening and assessment.

Nutrition Therapies

There are 4 major modalities for nutrition therapy for patients with cancer: oral nutrition therapy, EN, PN, and pharmacological therapy.

Oral Nutrition Therapy

Oral nutrition interventions in cancer patients focus on diet modifications to (1) maintain nutrition intake despite nutrition-impact symptoms, (2) help patients regain weight, or (3) minimize weight loss. Interventions include adjusting meal delivery (eg, small, frequent meals), modifying energy and nutrient intake (eg, snacks, energy-dense foods, oral nutritional supplements), or changing the type or consistency of food (eg, liquids, mechanically altered diet). Most practitioners opt to first attempt to maximize oral nutrition therapy because this approach is simple and noninvasive.

Oral nutrition therapy is influenced by cancer disease site, treatment-related nutrition-impact symptoms, and GI impairment. The selection of dietary modifications is most appropriately based on the nature of the patient's GI impairment and the presence of nutrition-impact symptoms. For example, to

avoid symptoms of dumping syndrome after gastrectomy, a patient should consume small, frequent meals with energy-dense foods; separate intake of solids and fluids at meals; and reduce intake of simple carbohydrates and concentrated fats.[42] A patient with a partial small bowel obstruction should eat small, frequent meals with energy-dense foods and limited amounts of insoluble fiber.[43]

A 2012 systematic review and meta-analysis concluded that oral nutrition interventions increase nutrition intake and can improve some aspects of QOL in patients with cancer who are malnourished or are at nutrition risk, but these interventions do not seem to improve mortality.[44] If the issue is inadequate intake of energy and protein for any of the many reasons described previously, nutrition interventions will ideally focus on maximizing oral intake in an efficient and easy-to-tolerate manner. Many practitioners refer patients to a registered dietitian nutritionist for individualized medical nutrition therapy, including nutrition assessment, intervention, monitoring and evaluation.

Enteral Nutrition

EN is used when the oral feeding route is unavailable or not tolerated. In the oncology patient population, it is most commonly used for patients diagnosed with head and neck, gastric, esophageal, and pancreatic cancers.

Indications

EN is most appropriate for patients receiving active anticancer treatment who are malnourished and who are likely to be unable to ingest or absorb adequate nutrients for more than 7 to 14 days.[30] According to ASPEN clinical guidelines, patients undergoing major cancer-related surgeries do not benefit from routine use of EN.[30] Perioperative nutrition support may be beneficial in moderately or severely malnourished patients if administered for 7 to 14 days preoperatively, but the potential benefits must be weighed against potential risks, including the risks associated with delaying surgery. Nutrition support is not an appropriate routine addition to chemotherapy, radiation treatment, or cancer-related operations.[30]

When nutrition support is indicated, the enteral route is preferred over the parenteral route for patients with a functional GI tract and no other relative contraindications. EN uses the gut and normal physiological route of nutrition, which reduces the risk of bacterial translocation when compared with PN.[30] The prevalence of infectious complications and infectious morbidity is lower with EN than PN,[30] and, compared with PN, EN has been shown to reduce hospital length of stay[45] and lower incidence of hyperglycemia.[46] In addition to improved outcomes, EN is less expensive than PN.[46]

Enteral Access

Options for enteral access include nasogastric (NG) and other nasoenteric tubes for short-term use as well as tubes inserted directly into the stomach or small intestine, which may be used for longer periods. NG and other nasoenteric tubes can be placed at the bedside or intraoperatively; the placement methods for gastrostomy and jejunostomy tubes are more invasive. (See Chapter 12.)

Feedings into the stomach are typically well tolerated and physiologically similar to oral intake, and they provide flexibility in administration of feedings and formulas.[46] Postpyloric feedings are indicated in the presence of gastroparesis, gastric outlet or duodenal obstruction, or fistula proximal to the feeding tube location, and when aspiration of gastric contents is suspected.[46] Jejunal access is commonly used for patients requiring enteral access prior to anticipated esophagectomy, postoperatively after esophagectomy, and in the postoperative stage after gastric or pancreatic resection.[47] Clinicians should consider the short- and long-term treatment plan when determining the appropriate tube type and location for a patient.

Enteral Formula Selection

The selection of an appropriate feeding method depends on multiple factors, including location of the feeding tube, the patient's aspiration risk and GI function, and the ability of the patient or caregiver to use enteral feeding equipment. Insurance coverage, the cost of equipment, and the patient's lifestyle should also be considered. Bolus, intermittent or gravity, cyclic, and continuous methods of enteral administration are commonly used.

Types of enteral formula include standard, semi-elemental, elemental, and disease-specific formulas (see Chapter 11). When choosing a formula, clinicians should assess the patient's digestive and absorptive capacity, underlying medical conditions, metabolic requirements, lifestyle, and insurance coverage.

Researchers have investigated the potential positive effects of immune-modulating formulas on outcomes in cancer patients.[48-50] Four major nutrients—arginine, glutamine, ω-3 fatty acids, and polyribonucleotides—have been of particular interest and have been shown to alter immune response. Multiple meta-analyses have concluded that enteral immunonutrition reduces perioperative complications and shortens hospital length of stay when compared with standard EN but does not affect mortality.[48-50] Although these data initially seem to support use of immune-modulating formulations, clinicians should interpret the findings with caution for multiple reasons. First, the quality of the evidence to support these conclusions in the cancer patient population is low. With only a few exceptions, multiple randomized trials in patients with advanced metastatic cancer and cancer-associated anorexia/cachexia have not provided evidence that supplementation with eicosapentaenoic acid (EPA) improves clinical outcomes.[48-51] Similar large-scale studies with L-arginine and RNA nucleotides have not been published in patients with advanced cancer, and few studies have been done on formulas enhanced with single nutrients. Much of the research to date has lacked control groups, which limits evaluation of the relative costs and benefits of immunonutrition vs or standard EN. Also, the heterogeneity of individual studies limits their generalizability. Furthermore, when clinicians consider immunonutrition for their patients, they must evaluate cost issues as well as the lack of evidence that immune-modulating formulations improve mortality.

Immune-modulating formulations can be appropriate for some patients. In head and neck cancer patients undergoing surgery, use of arginine supplementation has been associated with fewer infections and shorter lengths of stay, suggesting a survival benefit.[51] The US Summit on Immune-Enhancing Enteral Therapy recommends that malnourished patients undergoing GI or major head and neck surgery receive 5 to 7 days of immune-enriched enteral feedings preoperatively.[52] ASPEN echoes these recommendations and suggests that immune-modulating enteral formulas containing mixtures of arginine, nucleic acids, and essential fatty acids may be beneficial in malnourished cancer patients undergoing major operations.[51]

Home Enteral Nutrition

Because many patients with cancer receive outpatient treatment and often require treatment for prolonged periods of time, home enteral nutrition (HEN) can be a valuable part of nutrition care. HEN may be provided if patients cannot meet nutrition needs via oral route, if EN is clinically indicated, and if the patient or caregiver is capable of safely delivering EN in the home setting. Clinical outcomes for these patients are largely dependent on the underlying cancer, but many patients can benefit from HEN. Complications are infrequent, with an overall complication rate of less than 0.4 per patient per year.[53] QOL has not been well studied in patients with cancer receiving HEN. Although the mere presence of a feeding tube is associated with a reduced QOL, diminished QOL is primarily attributed to the underlying disease and malnutrition that led to the tube placement. One study showed that a specialized nutrition support team reduces morbidity and the cost of HEN, which could help improve QOL.[54]

HEN may differ from feeding methods/schedules and formulas used during hospital admission. The nutrition support team should individualize the HEN care plan to suit the patient's cancer treatment schedule, nutrition needs, lifestyle, feeding environment, and preferences regarding nutrition. The location of the feeding tube, the patient's aspiration risk and GI function, the ability of the patient or caregiver to use enteral feeding equipment, insurance coverage, and out-of-pocket expenses also need to be considered.

Parenteral Nutrition

The role of PN as a supportive care modality in cancer patients has been historically controversial. Multiple reports have questioned whether the potential benefits of PN are greater than the potential risks, such as stimulation of tumor growth and other metabolic and infectious complications associated with PN use.[30,55-57] According to some reports, PN supports weight gain, increases body fat, and improves nitrogen balance, with minimal effect on LBM; however, compared with patients who do not have cancer, some cancer patients do not respond as well to PN, presumably because of tumor-induced altered metabolism.[30,56] Although PN has been associated with increased risk of infection and other complications, a recent meta-analysis comparing EN and PN in cancer patients reported no difference in nutrition support complications, major complications, or survival between the groups.[57] The EN group included both standard care and tube-fed patients. The infectious risk was significantly lower in the EN group; however, no difference was found between groups in a subgroup analysis of tube-feeding patients compared with PN patients nor standard care patients compared with PN patients.[57] EN remains the preferred route for nutrition support in cancer patients with a functional GI tract because of the other physiological and financial advantages.

Indications

PN is an option for cancer patients when aggressive nutrition support is a part of the individual's medical care plan and EN is contraindicated. Multiple investigations and subsequent systematic reviews and meta-analysis investigations have been conducted to better define appropriate candidates and appropriate timing for PN support.[30,55,56] Many of these investigations have been criticized for poor study design, small numbers of patients, inconsistent nutrition regimens, and the variations in tumor types, tumor stages, and nutrition status among the study subjects.[30,55,56] However, multiple reports have demonstrated that routine PN use in well-nourished cancer patients undergoing surgery, chemotherapy, or radiation therapy conveys no clear benefit.[30,56] Moderately to severely malnourished patients may benefit from perioperative PN if it is administered for 7 to 14 days before surgery. The potential benefits of nutrition support must outweigh the potential risks of delaying surgical treatment.[30,56] Stable, postoperative patients may be considered PN candidates after 7 to 10 days of inadequate nutrient intake related to enteral access complications or other GI complications resulting in gut failure.[56] Malnourished patients with GI toxicities resulting from other anticancer treatments may be considered potential candidates for PN therapy if the GI tract is expected to remain unusable for 7 to 14 days.[56]

Home Parenteral Nutrition

Cancer patients may receive home PN (HPN) for prolonged GI tract dysfunction caused by anticancer treatment or direct tumor effect.[58-61] Examples of conditions that may indicate HPN include short bowel syndrome, prolonged radiation enteritis, and high-output GI or pancreatic fistulas. Patients may also receive HPN for partial or complete bowel obstruction, which is frequently caused by carcinomatosis or recurrent abdominal tumors. Patients may or may not continue to receive anticancer treatment to resolve or palliate the underlying malignancy that is causing the GI disorder.

The goal of HPN for cancer patients is to improve QOL and, in some patients, provide nutrition support during outpatient anticancer treatment. However, the indications for PN support at home are not clear, and continue to evolve as newer cancer therapies become available; further trials are needed to examine the role of PN in patients with advanced cancers.[61] The most recent ASPEN guidelines suggest that palliative use of PN in terminally ill cancer patients is rarely indicated.[30] However, patients who are undergoing aggressive antineoplastic treatments, patients with a good performance status (Karnofsky Performance Scale Index score greater than 50), patients with

inoperable bowel obstruction; patients with minimal symptoms from disease involving major organs such as the brain, liver, and lungs; and patients with indolent disease progression are likely the best candidates for short-term PN. Usually, to qualify for reimbursement of HPN, patients must need PN for at least 3 months. Therefore, patients with a life expectancy of 40 to 60 days would not qualify.[30,59,61] (See Chapter 38 for additional information on reimbursement for home nutrition support.)

Pharmacotherapy

A variety of nutrients and medications, including hormones, appetite stimulants, and cytokine antagonists, have been used to counter metabolic abnormalities that cause inefficient nutrient use in patients with continued anorexia or unresponsive weight loss. However, success with use of available agents is extremely variable, and, in many patients with cancer, pharmacotherapy is minimally effective as an aggressive nutrition support intervention.[62] Although pharmacotherapy seems to positively affect appetite for many patients, other patients do not gain weight, and many patients receiving treatment for disease continue to lose weight. For many patients, weight gain may not be a reasonable goal. However, prevention of further weight loss and improved appetite or sense of well-being may be desirable and achievable goals for many patients. More recent data suggest that use of combination therapy may be more effective than a single-agent approach.[63]

Hormones

Ghrelin, a potent orexigenic peptide hormone produced by the stomach, has increased appetite and energy intake in normal individuals and in animal models of cancer cachexia.[64] A preliminary, very small investigation in 7 adults with cancer cachexia reported a marked increase in energy intake and reported no adverse effects.[65] An early concern regarding ghrelin use in cancer patients was promotion of cellular proliferation and invasion of certain types of cancer. However, a randomized, placebo-controlled, double-blind, double-crossover study demonstrated that ghrelin was safe and well tolerated, although it did not affect nutrition intake.[66]

The clinical utility of ghrelin is hindered by its short half-life and parenteral dosage form. Anamorelin is an investigational ghrelin-receptor agonist that can be administered orally that has demonstrated positive effects on appetite and LBM.[64,67] The efficacy and long-term safety of anamorelin as a treatment for cancer cachexia needs further study before routine use can be recommended.[68]

Melatonin, the major product of the pineal gland, has been found to have anticancer and anticachectic effects, which are possibly mediated by the inhibition of TNF production. Early investigations demonstrated that oral administration of 20 mg melatonin resulted in less weight loss and greater survival rates.[69] However, a recent investigation in adult patients with advanced lung or GI cancer reported contradictory results.[69] In this study, patients were randomly assigned to receive 20 mg melatonin or placebo. Appetite score, weight response, QOL, and other symptoms were evaluated. The investigation was closed after initial interim analysis because there were no differences in appetite, weight, other symptoms, or QOL between groups. Further studies are needed before melatonin can be recommended for routine use as a treatment for cancer cachexia.

Appetite Stimulants

Corticosteroids

Glucocorticoids are widely used for appetite stimulation. A single mechanism for appetite stimulation has not been identified, but several have been proposed, including hypothalamic-pituitary-adrenergic axis modulation, modulation of proinflammatory cytokines, reduction of peritumoral edema and tumor mass or function, and modulation of adrenergic activity in the dorsal horn.[70] Multiple investigations have reported improved appetite and QOL with corticosteroid therapy compared with placebo, but this effect is short lived (less than 4 weeks), and long-term corticosteroid use is associated with negative nitrogen balance, net calcium loss, glucose intolerance, and immunosuppression.[70]

Mercadante and colleagues reported that corticosteroid use successfully treated anorexia and other supportive care symptoms in patients whose life expectancy was very short.[71] These investigators studied 50 home hospice patients with advanced cancer after corticosteroid therapy was initiated for the treatment of symptoms such as weakness, anorexia, headache, drowsiness, nausea and vomiting, dyspnea, and confusion. Significant improvements occurred in all symptom categories except drowsiness. The most frequently used agent was dexamethasone, with a mean daily dose of 7 mg/d and a range of 4 to 16 mg/d. Similar results were reported in a prospective, randomized, double-blind, placebo-controlled investigation of dexamethasone in patients with advanced cancer.[72] Patients were randomly assigned to receive either dexamethasone 4 mg orally twice daily or placebo for 14 days. The treatment group had significant improvements in cancer-related fatigue, anorexia, and QOL.

In general, the risk of adverse effects, such as muscle wasting and immunosuppression, outweigh any nutrition-related advantage with the long-term use of corticosteroids.[70,73] However, terminal patients with poor performance status could be considered potential candidates for corticosteroid intervention because the positive pharmacological effects on other symptoms associated with end-stage cancer may outweigh the risks associated with the negative adverse effects.[73]

Anabolic Steroids

Anabolic agents are used to stimulate muscle anabolism. Multiple studies have investigated the use of anabolic agents in various clinical conditions and diseases, such as HIV infection and burns; however, very few published investigations characterize use of such agents in patients with cancer cachexia.[63] Loprinzi and associates studied the effect of the anabolic steroid fluoxymesterone on cancer cachexia in a double-blind, randomized comparison trial that included a progestational agent (megestrol acetate) and corticosteroid (dexamethasone).[74] The researchers assigned patients with advanced incurable cancer

and a history of weight loss or anorexia to receive megestrol acetate 800 mg/d, dexamethasone 0.75 mg orally 4 times daily, or fluoxymesterone 10 mg orally 2 times daily. Appetite, nausea, vomiting, drug toxicities, and QOL were evaluated. Fluoxymesterone had the least effect on appetite when compared with megestrol acetate, although megestrol acetate and dexamethasone had a similar effect. Differences in weight gain were not significant when megestrol acetate was compared with the other agents. However, the investigators identified a trend for improved weight gain when comparing megestrol acetate with fluoxymesterone and noted a similar trend for weight gain when dexamethasone was compared with megestrol acetate. There was no difference in QOL between the 3 agents. The dexamethasone group experienced a higher rate of drug discontinuation because of toxicities such as heartburn and insomnia compared to megestrol acetate, and the megestrol acetate group had a higher rate of venous thrombolic episodes compared with those who received dexamethasone.

Oxandrolone is an oral anabolic androgenic steroid approved by the US Food and Drug Administration (FDA) for counteracting the protein catabolism associated with long-term use of corticosteroids and for the relief of bone pain that frequently accompanies osteoporosis.[75] Oxandrolone also has an FDA orphan drug designation for use as an adjunctive therapy for AIDS patients with from HIV-wasting syndrome.[76] Very few studies have reported on the use of oxandrolone in cancer patients.[63] Lesser and colleagues investigated the effects of oxandrolone and megestrol acetate on LBM, weight, and QOL in patients with solid tumors and weight loss.[77] The researchers randomly assigned patients to receive either oxandrolone 10 mg twice daily or megestrol acetate 800 mg/d for 12 weeks and found a significant increase in weight in the megestrol acetate group compared with the oxandrolone group; however, there was a nonsignificant trend for increase in LBM in the oxandrolone group compared to the megestrol acetate group. No difference in QOL was found.

Oxandrolone is contraindicated for use in cancers that could be promoted by testosterone, such as prostate or male breast cancer.[75]

Progestins

Multiple investigations have reported appetite-stimulant activity associated with progestational agents such as megestrol acetate and medroxyprogesterone acetate (MPA).[63] Megestrol acetate has been investigated most frequently in randomized controlled trials of cancer patients. In numerous studies of patients with cancer and cachexia, progestational agents have improved appetite and ameliorated weight loss with maximal weight gain generally seen within 8 weeks. Several large, prospective studies of patients with cancer cachexia treated with megestrol acetate have demonstrated improved QOL, but a survival benefit has not been shown.[62] A recent Cochrane Database review reported that megestrol acetate had a beneficial effect on appetite improvement and a small effect on weight gain compared with placebo, but no difference in effect when compared with other drugs investigated in comparison trials.[78] The same review found that QOL with megestrol acetate was improved when compared with placebo, but no difference in QOL was identified when megestrol acetate was compared with other drugs investigated in comparison trials.[78] The mechanism for the effects of megestrol acetate on appetite is not completely understood, but it may be related to glucocorticoid activity. Progestins also induce the release of NPY from the hypothalamus and downregulate the synthesis and release of proinflammatory cytokines. Although the change in weight associated with megestrol acetate is thought to largely be related to increased adipose tissue and edema, emerging evidence indicates that megestrol acetate has antiproteolytic properties through inhibition of the ATP-ubiquitin–dependent proteolytic pathway.[79]

A more effective treatment for cancer cachexia may be MPA or megestrol acetate in combination with other agents. Mantovani and associates investigated MPA and megestrol acetate in a multiple-arm trial to determine the effects of therapy on LBM, REE, and fatigue.[80] Secondary end points included appetite, QOL, grip strength, Glasgow Prognostic Score for systemic inflammation, and proinflammatory cytokines. Patients were randomly assigned to 1 of 5 treatment groups. Group 1 received MPA or megestrol acetate, which were considered equivalent treatments. Group 2 received an oral supplement fortified with EPA. Group 3 received L-carnitine. Group 4 received thalidomide, and group 5 received the full study medication/supplement combination. In addition, all patients received a multicomponent antioxidant cocktail. Group 5 demonstrated a significant increase in LBM, a decrease in REE, improved fatigue, and a significant improvement in appetite. IL-6 levels significantly decreased in groups 4 and 5. Systemic inflammation and QOL improved in groups 3, 4, and 5. The authors concluded that the most effective treatment was a progestin in combination with the other medications and supplements as a multimodal intervention to counter tumor-induced altered metabolism associated with cancer cachexia.

Megestrol acetate is generally well tolerated and has fewer adverse effects than dexamethasone, but it can exacerbate underlying diabetes mellitus and rarely leads to adrenal suppression.[81,82] It may also be associated with a small increase in the risk for impotence in men, venous thrombolic episodes, and edema.

Cannabinoids

Cannabinoids have been investigated for antiemetic and appetite-stimulant properties in cancer patients.[83] Dronabinol is the synthetic oral form of tetrahydrocannabinol, which is the active agent in marijuana thought to be responsible for appetite-stimulating and antiemetic effects. The mechanism of action of dronabinol is not completely understood, but its activity is likely mediated by cannabinoid receptor–related processes.[84] A multicenter, phase III, randomized, double-blind, placebo-controlled clinical trial from the Cannabis-In-Cachexia-Study-Group found no difference in patients' appetite or QOL between dronabinol and placebo.[85] In addition, there were no differences in body weight between groups at baseline or week 6 or in weight loss. Another randomized trial of 469 patients with advanced cancer and cachexia compared dronabinol to megestrol acetate and demonstrated the latter agent to be superior for appetite improvement and weight

gain.[81] Furthermore, combination therapy with both agents was not superior to treatment with megestrol alone. Adverse effects reported in this investigation included dizziness, ataxia, and confusion. The potential adverse effects of dronabinol is further illustrated by a recent meta-analysis of investigations evaluating the effectiveness and tolerability of cannabis-based medications for chemotherapy-induced nausea and vomiting in adult cancer patients.[86] Patients who received cannabinoids had a higher chance of reporting dizziness, dysphoria, euphoria, "feeling high," and sedation. In addition, significantly more participants reported these adverse events with cannabinoids compared with prochlorperazine.

The role of medical marijuana for treatment of cancer cachexia is not clear.[83,87] Smoked or vaporized cannabis has not been well studied for effects on appetite or cachexia in cancer patients. However, clinical concerns with pulmonary administration of marijuana in cancer patients include potential for injury to large airways or increased symptoms of bronchitis, which may compromise oncologic treatments. In addition, immunocompromised patients who smoke marijuana may be at risk for invasive pulmonary aspergillosis because of natural aspergillus contamination. Given the risks and inconsistent clinical evidence, the routine use of dronabinol or medical marijuana as an appetite stimulant is not recommended.[63,87]

Cyproheptadine

Cyproheptadine is a potent histamine and serotonin antagonist that competes with histamine for H_1-receptor sites on effector cells in the GI tract, in blood vessels, and in the respiratory tract. Patients with advanced cancer received cyproheptadine 8 mg orally 3 times per day in a prospective, randomized, placebo-controlled trial and demonstrated a small subjective improvement in appetite but continued weight loss.[88] However, in patients with diarrhea and weight loss related to the carcinoid syndrome, cyproheptadine can result in significant weight gain.[89] The mechanism is likely direct blockade of the excess serotonin and histamine produced by the tumor. Cyproheptadine was investigated in children (ages 3.2 to 19.4 years) with cancer cachexia for effects on weight.[90] Cyproheptadine therapy was provided for at least 4 weeks; patients who continued to lose weight were eligible for a 4-week trial of megestrol acetate. Of the 66 patients evaluated, 50 responded to cyproheptadine (average weight gain of 2.6 kg) and 16 did not respond to cyproheptadine. In the latter group, 7 patients received megestrol treatment and 6 of them completed the additional 4-week trial. The 5 patients who responded to megestrol acetate therapy had an average weight gain of 2.5 kg. In this study, like in adult investigations, the most common adverse effects of cyproheptadine were insomnia, dry mouth, and drowsiness, which can problematic—especially in advanced cancer patients—by potentially worsening mental status. The routine use of cyproheptadine as an appetite stimulant is not recommended.

Olanzapine

Olanzapine is an atypical antipsychotic that blocks multiple neurotransmitters, including dopamine at D_1, D_2, D_3, and D_4

brain receptors; serotonin at $5\text{-}HT_{2a}$, $5\text{-}HT_{2c}$, $5\text{-}HT_3$, and $5\text{-}HT_6$ receptors; catecholamines at α_1 adrenergic receptors; acetylcholine at muscarinic receptors; and histamine at H_1 receptor dopaminergic and serotonin activities. Increased appetite and weight gain have been reported in non-tumor-bearing patients receiving olanzapine and are thought to be caused by a blockade of serotonin $5\text{-}HT_2$ and $5\text{-}HT_3$ receptors. Additional mechanisms have been proposed.[91] Improved weight gain, appetite, and QOL were reported in patients with advanced GI or lung cancer who received olanzapine and megestrol acetate compared with megestrol alone.[92] A more recent investigation in adult cancer patients assessed the effect of olanzapine on metabolic cytokine response and relationship to weight.[93] The authors reported no change in leptin, ghrelin, or growth hormone levels throughout the study period. They also found no relationship between cytokine response and weight. Further clinical data are needed before olanzapine can be recommended for routine use as a treatment for cancer cachexia.

Mirtazapine

Mirtazapine is a tetracyclic antidepressant that antagonizes presynaptic α_2–adrenergic receptors resulting in increased norepinephrine and serotonin release. Mirtazapine also antagonizes serotonin $5\text{-}HT_2$ and $5\text{-}HT_3$ receptors.[91] Mirtazapine has been investigated for its effects on pain, QOL, nausea, anxiety, insomnia, appetite, and weight gain in patients with advanced cancer. Improved appetite and QOL was reported in nondepressed patients with cancer-related cachexia or anorexia who received 15 to 30 mg mirtazapine in an open-label, single-institution phase II trial.[94] However, the effect on weight gain was variable. Further clinical data are needed before mirtazapine can be recommended for routine use as a treatment for cancer cachexia.

Cytokine Inhibitors

Cytokine inhibitors have the potential to be effective agents for treating cancer cachexia by modulating catabolic inflammatory conditions associated with anorexia and weight loss. Early experimental trials of monoclonal antibodies with anticytokine properties in patients with a variety of malignancies have demonstrated variable but promising results.[63] Thalidomide has been shown to counter TNF-α and IL-6 production, which are key inflammatory cytokines associated with metabolic abnormalities reported in patients with cancer cachexia.[63] Thalidomide was investigated as a potential treatment for weight loss in cancer patients in a randomized, placebo-controlled trial of 50 patients with pancreatic cancer. Patients were randomly assigned to receive thalidomide 200 mg/d or placebo for 24 weeks.[95] The authors reported thalidomide was well tolerated and effective at attenuating loss of weight and LBM. However, a recent meta-analysis of investigations of adult cancer patients who received thalidomide evaluated the effectiveness for treatment of cancer cachexia and identified adverse effects associated with treatment.[96] Adverse effects identified included peripheral neuropathy, paresthesia, rash/cutaneous reaction, somnolence, and venous thrombolic episodes. The authors reported inadequate evidence to

recommend routine clinical use of thalidomide for treatment of cancer cachexia.

Pentoxifylline, an orally available methylxanthine derivative used in the treatment of peripheral vascular disease, is a phosphodiesterase inhibitor that inhibits TNF-α synthesis by decreasing gene transcription. Animal models demonstrate that pentoxifylline inhibits the production of TNF-α. However, a trial that randomly assigned patients with a history of cancer-related anorexia or weight loss to receive pentoxifylline 400 mg 3 times daily or placebo demonstrated no difference in appetite or weight gain between the 2 groups.[97] Further investigations are necessary to better define the role of pentoxifylline as a routine treatment for cancer cachexia.

The ω-3 fatty acids EPA and docosahexaenoic acid (DHA) have been investigated in patients with cancer-related anorexia and weight loss.[63,98–100] Laboratory and clinical studies have shown that EPA has several potential anticachectic effects, including attenuation of protein degradation induced by PIF, inhibition of IL-6 production, and inhibition of tumor-derived LMF.[99] Initial uncontrolled trials of fish oil provided alone or as a part of a liquid nutritional supplement in patients with cancer cachexia reported positive effects on weight gain and performance status.[99] However, recent controlled trials have reported less favorable results. Patients with advanced GI and lung cancer with weight loss were randomly assigned to receive either 2 g EPA per day, 4 mg EPA per day, or placebo for 8 weeks.[98] No differences were found in survival or weight between groups. A recent meta-analysis based on 5 trials conducted prior to the previously described investigation concluded that data were insufficient to determine whether oral EPA is superior to placebo.[99] These results were confirmed in a subsequent systematic review of investigations of patients with cancer cachexia treated with EPA and DHA.[100] The authors compared 7 trials for outcome measures such as weight change, lean muscle mass change, survival, and QOL. They reported no statistically significant differences in any outcome measures for 6 trials, but 1 trial reported a positive effect on weight. Collectively, this body of research suggests a limited role for ω-3 fatty acids as a single-agent treatment for unintentional weight loss associated with cancer cachexia. However, the most recent ASPEN guidelines suggest ω-3 fatty acid supplementation may help stabilize weight in cancer patients on oral diets experiencing progressive, unintentional weight loss.[30]

Pharmacotherapy to Manage Nutrition-Impact Symptoms

Multiple nutrition-impact symptoms that impair oral intake, such as nausea and vomiting, mucositis, or delayed gastric emptying, may be managed with medication intervention (see Table 33-1).[8,101,102] Maximizing these therapies may improve oral intake and delay or prevent the need for EN or PN. However, use of some supportive care medications may negatively affect nutrition or metabolic management. For example, steroid therapy may adversely affect blood glucose control, and narcotic pain medications may contribute to the development or worsening of constipation or gastroparesis. Other supportive care drug therapies may cause drowsiness or GI distress,

TABLE 33-1 Selected Medications Used for Treatment of Nutrition-Impact Symptoms

Impact Symptom	Medications

Pain	• Opioid agonists:
	   – Morphine
	   – Hydromorphone
	   – Fentanyl
	   – Methadone
	   – Oxycodone
	   – Hydrocodone
	• Antidepressants:
	   – Tricyclic antidepressants (eg, amitriptyline, imipramine, nortriptyline)
	   – Duloxetine
	   – Venlafaxine
	• Anticonvulsants:
	   – Gabapentin
	   – Pregabalin
	• Corticosteroids (eg, dexamethasone)
	• Topical anesthetic agent (eg, lidocaine)
	• Nonopioid analgesics:
	   – Acetaminophen
	   – Nonsteroidal anti-inflammatory (eg, ibuprofen, celecoxib, topical diclofenac)

Nausea/ vomiting	• Antiemetics:
	   – Neurokinin-1 antagonists (eg, aprepitant, fosaprepitant)
	   – Serotonin antagonists (eg, ondansetron, granisetron, dolasetron)
	• Corticosteroids (eg, dexamethasone)
	• Atypical antipsychotic (eg, olanzapine)
	• Benzodiazepine (eg, lorazepam)
	• Phenothiazine (eg, promethazine)
	• Typical antipsychotic (eg, haloperidol)
	• Metoclopramide

Diarrhea	• Antidiarrheals:
	   – Loperamide
	   – Atropine-diphenoxylate
	   – Octreotide

Constipation	• Laxatives (lubricant, osmotic, saline, stimulant) • Opioid antagonists (eg, methylnaltrexone)
Fatigue	• Methylphenidate[a] • Modafinil[a]

[a]Investigational.
Source: Data are from references 8, 101, and 102.

which may adversely affect oral intake. Supportive care medications should be routinely reviewed for potential medication issues related to the nutrition care plan.

Effect of Nutrition on Tumor Growth

Animal studies have suggested that the glucose and essential nutrients in nutrition support may encourage tumor growth, and that the stimulation of hormones and growth factors in response to nutrition support may also promote tumors. The data in humans are conflicting. In their systematic review, Bossola and coauthors reviewed 14 studies that had investigated the impact of PN on tumor proliferation in cancer patients and concluded that data were inadequate to make any conclusions.[103] Overall, the average length of PN use in these studies was 6 to 7 days; 1 study used PN for 1 day. Additionally, lack of control groups, poor overall study methodology, and small sample sizes resulted in evidence that was insufficient to assess whether PN stimulates tumor growth.[103] Regarding the question of whether EN promotes tumor growth, only 3 studies with a total of 28 cancer patients met the inclusion criteria for the review by Bossola et al.[103] EN had no impact on tumor growth in 2 of these studies, whereas the third study, which was completed in 1986 with 6 patients, found that tumor growth increased in patients with head and neck cancers after 6 days of EN.[104-106] Further research is warranted to elucidate whether nutrition support therapies promote tumor proliferation.

Nutrition Management of Patients with Specific Cancers

Cancer of the Head and Neck

Head and neck cancer is the seventh most common cancer diagnosed in the United States and includes a variety of cancer sites, such as the lip, oral cavity (tongue, tonsil, soft/hard palate, etc), salivary glands, pharynx, larynx, nasal cavity, ear, and skull base. In the United States, more than 48,000 cases of head and neck cancer were expected to be diagnosed in 2016; many would be diagnosed at an advanced stage (stage III or IV).[1] Many of patients with head and neck cancer present with malnutrition at the time of diagnosis because of the location of the tumor and its adverse impact on chewing and swallowing; many of these patients also have a history of alcohol and tobacco use.[1] Up to 57% of patients with cancer of the head and neck have significant weight loss prior to beginning treatment, and 75% to 80% of patients will experience weight loss during the treatment period.[107] Moreover, the adverse effects of treatment can exacerbate malnutrition and promote life-threatening dehydration. The chemoradiation prescribed is a particularly toxic antineoplastic treatment regimen, which commonly results in xerostomia, alterations in taste, dysphagia, nausea, early satiety, fatigue, odynophagia, and severe mucositis. Deterioration in nutrition status can lead to increased treatment-related toxicities, diminished QOL, and interruptions and delays in treatment (which are associated with worse clinical outcomes).[107]

In head and neck cancer patients, clinicians may prophylactically place a percutaneous endoscopic gastrostomy (PEG) feeding tube, either before the initiation of radiation or at the time of surgical resection, for the treatment and prevention of malnutrition. A recent meta-analysis found a lower rate of nutrition-related emergency department visits and hospitalizations, less frequent interruptions in treatment, and less weight loss in patients receiving prophylactic PEG tube placement in comparison with reactive feeding tube placement, although the optimal timing of tube placement is still being debated.[108] Some clinicians are concerned that prophylactic placement of a PEG tube instead of reactively placing either a PEG or NG tube may promote long-term tube dependence and persistent dysphagia. However, there seems to be no long-term difference in return of swallow function between patients who receive a prophylactic PEG tube compared with those who receive an NG tube for EN.[108] Further prospective, randomized clinical trials with larger numbers of participants are needed to determine the clinical benefits of prophylactic feeding tube placement compared with reactive tube placement in patient with cancer.[108,109]

Very little evidence is available for recommending the best EN formula for use in patients with head and neck cancer. Standard polymeric formulas with 1.5 to 2 kcal/mL are typically used and are well tolerated. More concentrated formulations are used to provide adequate nutrition while limiting the number of feedings needed daily to achieve nutrient goals.

Multiple nutrition-impact symptoms, such as pain, dysphagia, early satiety, nausea, and constipation, can adversely affect the patient's ability to infuse adequate nutrition. Therefore, close monitoring and reassessment is required to effectively detect and treat these symptoms and ensure that the patient receives adequate nutrition. For example, the opioids that many patients require during radiation therapy can cause constipation and delayed gastric emptying.[109] These problems, in turn, can lead to a reduction in formula administration, weight loss, and dehydration.[109] Many studies have reported that patients being treated for head and neck cancer with a PEG or NG tube still lose weight, but none of these studies have discussed whether other nutrition-impact symptoms were identified and treated.[109]

For malnourished patients undergoing tumor resection, 7 to 10 days of preoperative EN support is associated with a reduction in morbidity and improved QOL.[110] Factors that have been shown to predict the need for perioperative EN include recent heavy alcohol use, tongue base involvement and surgery, pharyngectomy, composite resection, reconstruction with a myocutaneous flap, radiation therapy, tumor size, and moderately to poorly differentiated histology.[110] In patients with inoperable cancer, EN during palliative radiation therapy successfully maintained nutrition status and allowed more patients to return to their regular activities compared with those patients receiving only oral nutrition.[111] Most patients with head and neck cancer will regain their ability to eat and can have the PEG tube removed, although patients may depend on the feeding tube as a supplemental source of nutrition after commencement of treatment (the reported length of time that patients receive supplemental EN ranges from 53 days to over a year).[112,113] A significant minority of patients will have prolonged complete dependence on enteral feeding.[112,113] In these patients, complete EN can be safely provided via a PEG tube or a low-profile gastrostomy device indefinitely with few complications.

More than 90% of head and neck patients experience mucositis, a common nutrition-impact symptom associated with both chemotherapy and radiation.[114] Symptoms including severe oropharyngeal pain and mucosal ulceration that profoundly limit the individual's ability to consume food and liquids, adversely affect QOL, and may result in dose reduction and delays in treatment.[114] To limit the extent and severity of mucositis, good oral hygiene, opiate analgesics, nutrition support therapy providing adequate protein intake, and other strategies are employed.[108,114] Complementary strategies have been found to have significant benefits for reducing the severity of mucositis. In patients with head and neck cancer, the use of oral glutamine (30 g/d divided in 3 doses) has been reported to reduce the severity, time to onset, and duration of mucositis, and reduce weight loss.[115] Honey has also been shown to be beneficial in delaying the onset of mucositis, reducing the pain and severity of mucositis, and reducing weight loss as well as interruptions in treatment in patients with head and neck cancer.[116,117] To achieve the potential benefits, the patient should swish 20 mL of natural honey in his or her mouth to coat the oral mucosa and then swallow, 3 times daily.[117]

Cancer of the Esophagus

The American Cancer Society estimated that 16,910 new esophageal cancer cases would be diagnosed in the United States in 2016.[118] The disease is 3 to 4 times more common among men than women, with the lifetime risk in the United States being about 1 in 125 for men and 1 in 435 for women.[118] Esophageal cancer rates in the United States have been relatively stable for many years. The incidence of esophageal squamous cell carcinoma is decreasing in the United States whereas the incidence of adenocarcinoma arising from Barrett's esophagus is rising dramatically, although the rate of increase has slowed in the last few years.[119]

Overt symptoms of esophageal cancer rarely occur when disease is localized and in the early stages. As the cancer grows and advances, dysphagia and heartburn-like pain often occur and additional reported symptoms may include hoarseness, coughing, anorexia, and weight loss.[120] Dysphagia is the most common nutrition-impact symptom of esophageal cancer. Globally, over 70% of patients diagnosed with esophageal cancer present with weight loss and dysphagia.[121] Most patients with esophageal cancer (78.9%) are malnourished; postoperatively, up to 90% of patients lose at least 5% of body weight and 16% lose more than 15% of body weight because of the numerous negative effects esophageal cancer has on adequate nutrition intake.[122–123]

Treatment for esophageal cancer includes surgical resection, chemotherapy, radiation therapy, targeted therapy, and, frequently, a combination of these modalities. These therapies may impair oral intake and compound malnutrition. Radiation therapy results in nutrition-impact symptoms including anorexia, dysphagia, odynophagia, and heartburn. Late adverse effects of radiation to the esophagus may include strictures, stenosis, fibrosis, or necrosis. Nutrition-impact symptoms associated with chemotherapy regimens commonly used for esophageal cancer include nausea, vomiting, diarrhea, and mucositis.[124] Patients who receive concurrent chemotherapy and radiation therapy may experience the nutrition-impact symptoms associated with both treatments.

Esophagectomy and esophagogastrectomy surgeries alter digestion and absorption. Issues affecting nutrition status after esophagectomy surgery include gastroparesis and dysmotility, dumping syndrome, early satiety, and dysphagia. These issues can lead to decreased nutrition intake, weight loss, and malnutrition and nutrition deficiencies. After surgery, patients must make long-term adaptations to eating habits, such as consuming small, frequent meals on a schedule, eating slowly and chewing well, and avoiding foods that are poorly tolerated. Because eating patterns and habits are developed over decades, patients often struggle with postsurgical dietary limitations.

Options for the palliation of malignant dysphagia include dilation, placement of a self-expanding metal stent (SEMS), ablation therapy, chemotherapy or radiation therapy, and surgery. The choice of modality depends on the location of the disease, the stage of the tumor, the functional status of the patient, and physician expertise. Dilation is usually not considered a primary modality because its relief is temporary and most patients require repeat dilation within 1 to 2 weeks. SEMS has evolved as a common intervention for malignant dysphagia because it is a relatively easy procedure, is associated with minimal morbidity and mortality, and provides rapid palliation of dysphagia. Ablation therapies, including laser treatment, argon plasma coagulation, chemical injection of ethanol, and photodynamic therapy, are not widely available and are also associated with relatively high reintervention rates. Surgery for palliation of dysphagia is associated with very high morbidity and mortality rates and is therefore not usually recommended.[125] Additionally, anastomotic leaks and strictures can occur, preventing oral intake. Although tumor-related dysphagia hinders oral intake and can lead to malnutrition, the remaining GI tract is usually functional. EN via gastrostomy or jejunostomy is therefore an effective method of nutrition support in patients when EN is indicated (see Practice Scenario 33-1).

Practice Scenario 33-1

Question: What is the intervention of choice for the palliation of dysphagia associated with newly diagnosed esophageal cancer?

Scenario: A 55-year-old man with history of tobacco and alcohol use presented to his primary care physician with a 2-month history of dysphagia that initially began with dysphagia to solids and then progressed to liquids. He lost 10 pounds during this time. He did not report odynophagia, hoarseness, shortness of breath, abdominal pain, nausea, vomiting, or changes in his bowel habits. His physician referred him to a gastroenterologist, who performed an endoscopy and found a large, friable, partially obstructing mass in the distal esophagus; biopsies were positive for adenocarcinoma. The patient then underwent an endoscopic ultrasound for staging of the cancer and was found to have a stage III:T3N1M0 lesion (stage III, metastatic disease; T3, tumor invasion into the adventitia; N1, regional lymph node involvement; M0, no distant metastases).

Intervention: The patient underwent an endoscopic placement of a self-expanding metal stent (SEMS), resumed a mechanical soft diet, and was able to obtain adequate nutrition and gain weight.

Answer: SEMS is the treatment of choice for the palliation of malignant dysphagia, if feasible.

Rationale: Although dilation and ablative techniques are options, they only provide temporary relief and the patient would likely require frequent reinterventions. Given the high morbidity and mortality associated with surgery, a palliative esophagectomy is not recommended. SEMS is preferable over a percutaneous endoscopic gastrostomy tube because, although a percutaneous endoscopic gastrostomy tube will provide him with adequate nutrition, it would not relieve his dysphagia and could also delay treatment.

Feeding tubes may be placed for nutrition support in patients with esophageal cancer. EN may be utilized due to tumor-associated dysphagia in patients undergoing palliative cancer treatment, inadequate oral nutrition intake associated with current chemoradiation treatment or after esophagectomy surgery. EN also has been shown to promote weight maintenance during chemoradiation therapy, but it does not improve tolerance to treatment or survival.[126] The use of PN is not recommended for patients with esophageal cancer undergoing chemoradiation therapy.[127] PN is this population and treatment modality has not been shown to prevent weight loss or improve treatment effectiveness.[127]

Research findings are inadequate and data are mixed regarding the use EN via jejunostomy tube after esophagectomy. As they wait for additional evidence, many medical centers continue to use EN in patients with esophageal cancer undergoing esophageal surgical resection. EN is preferred over PN because EN is more physiological, is less costly, and has fewer complications.[128]

Cancer of the Stomach

The American Cancer Society estimated that 26,370 new gastric cancer cases would be diagnosed in the United States in 2016.[129] The disease is more common among older adults, with 6 out of 10 patients diagnosed with gastric cancer being age 65 years or older.[129] Gastric cancer is more commonly diagnosed in men than women.[129] The lifetime risk of gastric cancer in the United States is 1 in 111 people.[129] The incidence of gastric cancer has declined during the past 50 years in the United States; incidence rates are higher in other countries.[129]

Early satiety, heartburn or indigestion, abdominal pain and discomfort, nausea, vomiting, anorexia, and unintended weight loss are common symptoms of gastric cancer.[130] These symptoms often lead to reduced food intake, which may, in part, explain why malnutrition and weight loss occurs in more than 70% of people diagnosed with gastric cancer. Types of treatment include chemotherapy, biotherapy, radiation therapy, and surgery, or a combination of these modalities. The treatment plan considers the size, location, and stage of the disease as well as the patient's age and overall health. Each treatment modality can result in a unique set of adverse effects.

Surgical resection of gastric tumors results in several potential nutrition-related issues, including dietary intolerances, weight loss, and vitamin and mineral malabsorption. Gastric resection typically results in weight loss. Reported weight loss ranges from 10% to 30% of preoperative weight and has been attributed to inadequate oral intake, malabsorption, rapid intestinal transit time, and bacterial overgrowth.[131] Postsurgical issues can lead to long-term consequences including anemia and bone disease. Often, nutrient deficiencies develop months to years after gastric resection; therefore, ongoing monitoring and treatment of potential nutrition complications is necessary.

Digestion and absorption are affected by the altered anatomy of the GI tract after gastric resection. Symptoms of dumping syndrome are more prevalent after gastrectomy but often improve over time. The procedure can accelerate gastric emptying, which allows incompletely digested and hyperosmolar chyme to enter the small intestine.[121,132] Intestinal fluid rapidly increases in the small intestine to normalize osmolarity. High fluid volume along with hormonal and vasomotor changes can result in bloating, abdominal cramping, nausea, and dumping. Patients often experience increased symptoms of dumping syndrome after eating foods high in sugar; proper nutrition therapy can help relieve these symptoms.[42,133]

Dumping syndrome can be categorized as early or late. Early dumping syndrome (onset 10 to 30 minutes after eating) occurs in 75% of dumping syndrome cases. Symptoms of early dumping include epigastric fullness, nausea, vomiting, abdominal cramping, bloating, diarrhea, light-headedness, diaphoresis, a desire to lie down, pallor, and palpitations. Late dumping syndrome (onset 1 to 3 hours after meals) is thought to be the result of reactive hypoglycemia. Late dumping syndrome occurs in 25% of dumping syndrome cases. Symptoms include hunger, perspiration, tremors, and difficulty concentrating. Both the early and late forms of dumping syndrome can be improved with changes in eating habits and food choices.

The etiology of fat malabsorption after gastrectomy is multifactorial. Increased transit time prevents adequate mixing of food with digestive enzymes and bile salts, decreased enzyme production reduces the ratio of enzymes to food, and loss of the antrum and its sieving function allows for larger-than-normal food particles to empty into the jejunum and a resulting challenge for enzymes to attack.[134,135] Patients exhibiting signs and symptoms of fat maldigestion may be candidates for pancreatic enzyme replacement therapy.

Nutrition-related anemias resulting from vitamin B_{12}, folate, or iron deficiency are common in gastrectomy patients and often present as late complications of surgery. Baseline and periodic monitoring of markers of anemia is necessary to reduce the risk of potentially severe consequences.

After gastric resection, vitamin B_{12} malabsorption may occur because of decreased intrinsic factor and reduced gastric acidity, which impairs cleavage of protein-bound B_{12}.[135] Bacterial overgrowth and decreased oral intake of B_{12}-rich foods may also contribute to the deficiency.[136] Vitamin B_{12} deficiency can develop as early as 1 year after surgery and is more common in late postoperative states.[137] Vitamin B_{12} supplementation should be initiated if laboratory tests reveal a vitamin B_{12} deficiency. Supplementation may be delivered by mouth, intranasally, or intramuscularly.

Folate deficiency may develop after gastric surgery and will likely be related to malabsorption and impaired digestion.[136] Serum red blood cell folate is a better indicator of body folate

stores than serum folate and should be evaluated if a folate deficiency is suspected.[137]

Alterations in digestion and absorption are associated with iron deficiency in gastrectomy patients.[137] Reduced dietary iron intake may also play a role. Given the known postgastrectomy alterations in digestion and absorption of iron, clinicians should encourage patients to increase intake of iron-rich foods, with emphasis on sources of heme iron, which has greater bioavailability than nonheme iron. Ingestion of vitamin C may improve iron absorption. In some patients, strategies to maximize iron intake and absorption may not be adequate to prevent iron deficiency. Periodic and ongoing monitoring of serum iron stores is necessary to identify deficiency, and oral iron supplementation should be initiated as indicated.

The risk for osteoporosis is increased after gastrectomy because of changes in oral nutrition intake, malabsorption of calcium and vitamin D, absence of stomach acid, and lack of gastrocalcin production in stomach mucosa.[138] Several measures, including monitoring, diet adjustments, and lifestyle modifications, can be taken to lessen the risk for osteoporosis in this population. Dual-energy x-ray absorptiometry scanning is recommended every 2 years for individuals with low body mass index, significant weight loss, or other risk factors. Daily intake of 1500 mg calcium is encouraged and can be accomplished through intake of calcium-rich foods as tolerated and supplementation with calcium citrate in divided doses with equal to or less than 500 mg per dose.[138] Serum vitamin D levels should be routinely monitored with subsequent vitamin D supplementation as needed. Recommendations for lifestyle modifications to decrease osteoporosis risk include smoking cessation, limiting alcoholic beverage intake, and increasing weight-bearing exercises. A proactive approach to osteoporosis prevention is necessary for gastrectomy patients because of their increased risk.

Cancer of the Pancreas

The American Cancer Society estimated that 53,070 new pancreatic cancer cases would be diagnosed in the United States in 2016.[139] The lifetime risk of pancreatic cancer in the United States is 1 in 65 people.[139] Pancreatic cancer accounts for 3% of all new cancer diagnoses and 7% of all cancer deaths.[140] Based on data from 2006 to 2012, the 5-year survival rate for those diagnosed with pancreatic cancer is 7.7%.[140] Prognosis remains poor for all stages of this type of cancer.

Nutrition issues often present before the diagnosis of pancreatic cancer and include weight loss, poor appetite, mid-abdominal pain, malabsorption, delayed gastric emptying, jaundice, and diabetes. Symptoms of the disease and the effects of its common treatments increase the risk of malnutrition. Treatments for pancreatic cancer include surgery, chemotherapy, radiation therapy, and targeted therapies. Treatment for resectable pancreatic cancer may begin with surgery or involve neoadjuvant chemotherapy and/or chemoradiation prior to surgery. Chemotherapy is standard first-line therapy for unresectable, locally advanced, or metastatic pancreatic cancer. The stage of the cancer and the treatment modalities used influence nutrition status. In a prospective study of patients with adenocarcinoma of the pancreas, 70% of patients experienced weight loss at presentation, with 40% of patients reporting weight loss exceeding 10% of the stable weight.[141]

The only chance for cure is surgery. About 20% of patients are thought to have resectable disease. The types of surgeries commonly performed to resect pancreatic tumors are pancreaticoduodenectomy, total pancreatectomy and distal pancreatectomy. Pancreaticoduodenectomy and total pancreatectomy have greater implications for nutrition status than distal pancreatectomy. Most resectable tumors are in the head of the pancreas, and the surgery of choice for these tumors is a pancreaticoduodenectomy. In this procedure, the distal half of the stomach is removed, and the pancreas is transected (usually at the neck but by varying amounts; rarely, the entire gland may be removed); additionally, the entire duodenum and a few centimeters of the jejunum distal to the ligament of Treitz are resected. Evidence is conflicting about whether modification of the standard pancreaticoduodenectomy to spare the stomach and pylorus offers any long-term nutrition benefit.[142]

Regardless of the type of resection, individuals who are malnourished preoperatively are at a higher morbidity and mortality risk.[143] The role of perioperative nutrition is controversial. A systematic review of perioperative nutritional supplementation in patients undergoing pancreaticoduodenectomy concluded that most patients are nutritionally depleted at the time of surgery and that EN was superior to PN for nutrition support.[144] EN support may be used as indicated in the postoperative setting to aid with recovery and prevent nutrient deficiencies.

Most patients with pancreatic cancer have unresectable disease at the time of diagnosis or experience disease recurrence after surgery. These patients can experience partial or complete obstruction of the small bowel, gastric outlet, or duodenal outlet from tumor effect. Patients at risk for small bowel obstructions may benefit from instruction regarding diet (soft, low-fiber foods) and bowel management strategies.[145] SEMS is a safe and effective therapy for the palliation of gastric outlet obstruction in these patients and has multiple advantages over surgery, including increased clinical success, shorter time from procedure to initiation of oral intake, reduced morbidity, lower incidence of delayed gastric emptying, shorter hospital length of stay, and lower cost.[146] A recent study demonstrated that peritoneal disease is not a contraindication to enteral stenting in patients unless there are signs of multifocal obstruction.[147] If stenting or gastric bypass is not possible, insertion of a gastrostomy tube for drainage and jejunostomy tube for feeding may be appropriate.

Exocrine pancreatic insufficiency may be observed in patients with pancreatic and periampullary cancer at diagnosis, during chemotherapy and/or radiation treatments, and following surgery.[148] Studies indicate that 65% to 90% of patients with pancreatic cancer may have exocrine pancreatic insufficiency and malabsorption.[149,150] Malabsorption resulting in the need for pancreatic enzyme replacement therapy may also occur with resection of the GI tract, including gastric resection. Malabsorption can also be attributed to inadequate bile salts in the GI tract related to biliary obstruction. A low-fat diet and avoidance of gas-producing foods may reduce symptoms of biliary obstruction until the obstruction is resolved.[151]

Nutrition management is necessary to avoid weight loss and deficiencies of nutrients including vitamin B_{12}, iron, and fat-soluble vitamins.[152] Nutrient deficiencies may result from lack of nutrition intake or from malabsorption or maldigestion of nutrients. Malabsorption can lead to increased risk of fat-soluble vitamin and vitamin B_{12} deficiencies. With bypass of the duodenum and upper jejunum, the digestive processes through the stomach, duodenum, and pancreatobiliary system are disrupted. The duodenum and proximal jejunum are important sites for absorption of iron, folate, fatty acids, proteins, and trace elements; therefore, bypass of this part of the small bowel may result in impaired absorption of iron, calcium, zinc, copper, and selenium.[153] If supplementation of fat-soluble vitamins is necessary in the presence of malabsorption, water miscible forms of fat-soluble vitamins should be used.

Cancer of the Colon and Rectum

Despite the use of colonoscopies for early diagnosis, colon cancer is the third most common cause of cancer and the third most common cause of cancer-related mortality in the United States.[1] Surgical procedures to remove tumors are the primary mode of treatment for this type of cancer. More extensive resections (usually a total proctocolectomy) are performed in patients with underlying ulcerative colitis or hereditary colon cancer syndromes.

Resection of the right colon, including removal of the ileocecal valve and a portion of the terminal ileum, may be associated with watery diarrhea with multiple etiologies, including the loss of the breaking effect of the ileocecal valve, entry of increased amounts of bile salts into the colon with stimulation of water excretion into the colonic lumen (choleretic diarrhea), and impaired water and sodium absorption because of some loss of surface area in the colon.[154] Cholestyramine binds bile salts and often markedly attenuates the diarrhea. Resections of the left colon or rectum rarely have a significant impact on nutrition status.

The estimated prevalence of malnutrition in this patient population ranges from 8% to approximately 55%.[155] Despite this high prevalence, data regarding the role of nutrition support are lacking. Nutrition screening and assessment are recommended to identify patients who may benefit from the initiation of nutrition support to improve nutrition status.

Gynecologic Cancers

Gynecologic malignancies, most commonly ovarian cancer, and their multimodality therapies may be associated with severe malnutrition. Approximately 70% of ovarian cancer cases are diagnosed at an advanced stage. Symptoms of advanced gynecologic cancers include stomach and pelvic pain/pressure, early satiety, involuntary weight loss, and abdominal swelling. The choice of primary treatment depends on the cancer stage at diagnosis and usually includes a combination of surgery and chemotherapy; radiation therapy is sometimes used. Surgical resection of the primary tumor and other visible masses is recommended in most cases. Complete resection significantly improves survival, but it is difficult to achieve when the cancer is advanced.[156] Chemotherapy regimens may cause nutrition-impact symptoms, including nausea, vomiting, anorexia, mucositis, and diarrhea. Radiation therapy often results in diarrhea and fatigue.[157]

Patients with ovarian cancer may develop an intestinal obstruction during their illness. Intestinal surgery may be needed in 30% to 50% of advanced cases.[156] Malignant obstruction of the small or large bowel is common in advanced ovarian cancer and can be related to tumor location, radiation enteritis, carcinomatosis, or disease progression. Malignant obstructions may spontaneously resolve but often recur. Conservative management includes NG suction, bowel rest, symptom control via medications, and intravenous (IV) fluids.[158] Surgical treatment of malignant bowel obstruction in the setting of advanced disease may be an option, but it is associated with significant perioperative mortality and reobstruction rates. A meta-analysis found only low-quality evidence comparing surgery and medical management of bowel obstruction in ovarian cancer.[159] The evidence supporting prolonged survival after surgery is weak; therefore, the authors concluded the evidence was insufficient to yield any conclusions. An alternative treatment is to place a gastrostomy tube (ie, PEG) for drainage, decompression, and the palliation of symptoms.[160] This approach may successfully alleviate symptoms, but it does not resolve malnutrition.

The use of PN in advanced disease remains controversial and conflicting. Few studies have examined the benefits of PN for surgical patients with malignant bowel obstruction. One study reported a mean survival rate of 4 to 6 months and a 13% complication rate when PN was provided.[43] Therefore, the investigators concluded that PN should not be recommended in inoperable cases.[43]

A retrospective study at MD Anderson Cancer Center assessed the outcomes of concurrent chemotherapy and PN in the treatment of malignant small bowel obstruction and concluded that the efficacy of this treatment approach was low whereas the morbidity and mortality rate was high.[161] Although the use of HPN has not generally been shown to improve survival or QOL, it has been shown to improve nutrition status and QOL in a small subgroup of patients with a good performance status.[162] The decision to administer PN in these patients must be individualized to carefully select those who may benefit from PN.

Nutrition Support in Patients Undergoing Hematopoietic Stem Cell Transplantation

HSCT is a treatment for numerous disorders, including cancers of the blood, other malignancies, bone marrow–related diseases, and a variety of immunologic and genetic disorders.[163] The process involves the IV infusion of hematopoietic stem cells collected from bone marrow, peripheral blood, or placental cord blood into the patient after treatment with a cytoreductive conditioning regimen. An autologous transplant is the infusion of the patient's own stem cells, which were harvested before conditioning therapy. The infusion of stem cells from a histocompatible donor is an allogeneic transplant. The least common type of HSCT is a syngeneic transplant, where stem cells are harvested from an identical (monozygous) twin. Conventional HSCT recipients receive a pretransplant conditioning

regimen, which includes myeloablative doses or, in some cases, nonmyeloablative doses of chemotherapy and may or may not include total body irradiation, depending on the treatment plan.[163,164] Adverse effects and complications of HSCT depend on the conditioning regimen, age of the recipient at the time of the transplant, the presence of comorbid conditions, and the time between treatment and follow-up.[163,164] Allogeneic HSCT is associated with more frequent infectious and noninfectious complications. Infections may be caused by bacterial, fungal, or viral pathogens and can result in compromised organ function or organ failure. Other noninfectious complications, such as fluid and electrolyte abnormalities, sinusoidal obstruction syndrome, kidney injury, and compromised cardiopulmonary function, may be related to the conditioning regimen and other supportive care medications. Graft-vs-host disease is a particularly challenging complication that presents clinically as specific derangements in the skin, liver, and GI tract, which may result in altered nutrient requirements.[163,164] (See Practice Scenario 33-2.) Multiple nutrition-impact symptoms, such as nausea, vomiting, anorexia, dysgeusia, mucositis, and diarrhea, are associated with GI toxicities related to the conditioning regimen as well as infectious and noninfectious complications. Because of these potential and prevalent complications throughout the posttransplant period, all patients undergoing HSCT are at nutrition risk.

Practice Scenario 33-2

Question: When is nutrition support indicated in hematopoietic stem cell transplantation (HSCT) patients with graft-vs-host disease (GVHD)?

Scenario: A 50-year-old man presented with a 1-month history of fever, weight loss, bone pain, and easy bruising. His primary care physician evaluated routine chemistries and complete blood count, and the patient was found to have pancytopenia, with a low white blood cell count, low hemoglobin, and low platelets. A bone marrow biopsy was performed, which confirmed the diagnosis of acute myelogenous leukemia. He was treated with induction chemotherapy but did not respond. His brother was found to be a human leukocyte antigen match who could donate stem cells, and the patient underwent an allogeneic HSCT 2 months after diagnosis. His posttransplant course was complicated by prolonged inadequate oral intake related to severe mucositis, and PN was initiated. His mucositis slowly improved, and he tolerated an oral diet by posttransplant Day 14. PN support was subsequently discontinued. He engrafted on Day 21. On Day 45, he developed nausea, vomiting, and profuse diarrhea with an inability to tolerate oral intake. His weight had declined from 65 kg to 58 kg. An abdominal x-ray was negative for intestinal obstruction, and stool studies were negative for infection. He subsequently underwent a colonoscopy and upper endoscopy that confirmed severe GVHD of the gastrointestinal tract.

Intervention: Although GVHD treatment was initiated, intermittent nausea continued and diarrhea output ranged from 600 to 800 mL/d. PN support was reinitiated and provided 2000 kcal/d (35 kcal/kg) and 90 g protein per day (1.5 g/kg).

After 3 weeks, his diarrhea output steadily declined to less than 250 mL/d and he could tolerate adequate oral intake. The PN was discontinued.

Answer: Nutrition support is indicated in patients with moderate-to-severe GVHD with poor oral intake or malabsorption.

Rationale: Data supporting the use of nutrition support in patients with GVHD are sparse. No data indicate whether nutrition support leads to the resolution of GVHD. However, given that GVHD results in profound and prolonged nutrition compromise, it is appropriate to offer nutrition support in these patients.[30]

All HSCT patients should have a complete nutrition assessment (see Chapter 9) prior to transplant. Although the ideal nutrition assessment measurements for HSCT patients have not been defined, weight loss has been associated with a higher risk of nonrelapse mortality in adult HSCT patients.[30,163] When patients can continue adequate oral intake, HSCT centers often restrict them to low-microbial diets, which vary in their degree of sterility.[163] The objective of this type of diet is to avoid foods with high bacterial content to minimize the introduction of pathogenic organisms into the GI tract, but the degree of modification is highly variable. Many centers have adopted a more liberal low-microbial diet that allows patients to eat well-washed fruits and vegetables and only excludes extremely high-risk foods, such as unpasteurized dairy products, raw or undercooked meats, herbal products, aged cheeses, and unwashed, damaged, or moldy fruits and vegetables. Clinicians should educate patients and families about safe food-handling practices and high-risk foods to avoid.[30,164] Autologous graft patients usually follow these diets for 3 months after transplant; allogeneic patients may require a low-microbial eating plan for a year or more if they remain on immunosuppressive therapy. Supplementation with a general multivitamin and mineral supplement without iron is appropriate in view of these dietary restrictions.

Because evidence from investigations is inconsistent, the best route for nutrition support in patients who are unable to consume adequate nutrition orally is unclear.[30,164,165] Many patients are poor candidates for nasoenteric feedings early in the peritransplant period secondary to GI toxicities of the conditioning regimen. Some clinicians worry that use of nasoenteric feeding tubes in neutropenic and thrombocytopenic patients may increase their risk for infection, mucosal irritation, and bleeding; contribute to poor absorption of EN; or worsen GI symptoms associated with poor tolerance of an enteral formula. However, successful use of EN in allogeneic HSCT patients has been reported.[30,165,166] In some cases, patients required repeated tube placement to address malpositioning of the tube during emesis, and some patients required supplemental PN support because they did not tolerate goal volumes of EN.[166] Compared with EN, PN use in HSCT has been associated with higher rates of infectious complications in some studies, but the evidence is inconclusive.[30,167] The confounding data are reflected in the ASPEN recommendation that nutrition support is appropriate in patients undergoing HSCT who are malnourished and who are anticipated to be

unable to ingest or absorb adequate nutrients for a prolonged period of time (defined as 7 to 14 days).[30] PN therapy should be discontinued after engraftment or when the patient is able to consume adequate energy through EN or an oral diet. EN is recommended for patients with a functional GI tract.[30]

Energy requirements will vary with the patient's age, type of transplant, and clinical condition. In general, energy requirements are estimated to be 1.3 to 1.5 times the basal energy expenditure, or approximately 30 to 35 kcal/kg/d, for patients who are not critically ill. However, lower energy requirements of 25 to 30 kcal/kg/d have been suggested for those HSCT patients who are not severely malnourished.[168] The goal for protein intake should be 1.5 to 2 g/kg/d during the first 1 to 3 months after transplantation. Fluid goals must be tailored to the individual, and fluid intake from all sources (blood products, PN or EN, oral intake, IV medications, and fluids) must be carefully documented. Intake should be balanced against output.[164,168]

Glutamine supplementation has been investigated for its potential effect on multiple nutrition measurements and clinical outcomes in HSCT patients.[30,167,169,170] Evidence regarding whether glutamine has a positive effect on mucositis is conflicting. In addition, multiple studies have investigated the potential benefits of glutamine-enriched EN and PN in patients undergoing HSCT. Glutamine-enriched EN has not been shown to reduce morbidity and mortality in HSCT patients. PN-enriched glutamine has been shown to improve nitrogen balance, decrease the length of stay, and decrease morbidity. However, the results are not consistent across studies. The lack of consistent data on glutamine's effects on mucositis and outcomes for HSCT patients is reflected in multiple systematic reviews and guidelines statements. ASPEN recommendations conclude that parenteral glutamine may benefit patients undergoing HSCT, but there is no role for oral glutamine.[30] This recommendation is consistent with a 2009 Cochrane Collaboration review of nutrition support for bone marrow transplant patients.[167] While the 2014 Multinational Association of Supportive Care in Cancer/International Society of Oral Oncology (MASCC/ISOO) guidelines recommend no role for parenteral glutamine for management of mucositis, no guideline was given for oral glutamine because the evidence was deemed inadequate and/or conflicting.[169] Lastly, a 2011 Cochrane Collaboration review examined interventions for preventing oral mucositis in patients with cancer receiving treatment and reported there is no evidence of a benefit for oral glutamine for prevention of mucositis, but there is weak evidence, from small trials, that parenteral glutamine supplementation may help prevent severe mucositis.[170]

Further complicating the issue of glutamine supplementation is the lack of a commercially available parenteral glutamine formulation in the United States. Use of parenteral glutamine requires special manufacturing techniques not readily available in many institutional pharmacies. However, parenteral glutamine has been made available from several licensed pharmacies that extemporaneously compound glutamine crystalline powder under sterile conditions either as a separate parenteral solution or as a part of a crystalline amino acid solution. Recent FDA-mandated changes may create further obstacles to obtaining extemporaneously compounded glutamine-containing PN formulations. The FDA's Pharmacy Compounding Advisory Committee, which provides advice on scientific, technical, and medical issues concerning drug compounding, has recommended to not allow the use of alanyl-L-glutamine in compounding because of insufficient information to fully assess safety related to impurities of the product.[171]

Nutrition Support During Palliative Care

The use of EN and PN in patients with advanced incurable cancer is controversial and raises multiple ethical issues. Before the initiation of nutrition support in an advanced cancer patient, the clinician must consider the wishes of the patient and/or family, potential risks and benefits of the intervention, and the patient's prognosis of survival. See Chapter 39 for a detailed discussion of palliative care and nutrition support.

Most patients with advanced cancer do not benefit from nutrition intervention as defined by improved nutrition status, increased survival, or improved QOL. The adverse effects caused by nutrition support may actually worsen the patient's QOL and the overall palliative care of the patient. However, certain patient groups with advanced cancer and good performance status—such as those with inoperable, malignant bowel obstruction; those with minimal symptoms from disease involving major organs such as the brain, liver, or lungs; and those with relatively indolent disease progression—have demonstrated favorable response to EN or PN.[172]

Nutrition support is not usually indicated in patients with a prognosis of survival less than 3 months, although accurately predicting survival is frequently difficult. Good performance status, such as a Karnofsky score greater than 50, is also associated with better outcomes for palliative nutrition support.[58,173] If the patient is receiving palliative care at home, other issues that should be considered before determining suitability for home nutrition support, such as home environment, caregivers, and financial support, are similar to those for patients without cancer (see Chapter 38).

In general, cachexia, anorexia, and dehydration at the end of life are not uncomfortable. Patients near the end of life should be instructed to eat and drink as they desire, and restrictive diets should be discontinued. Sips of water, ice chips, and glycerin swabs can be used to palliate symptoms of thirst, dry mouth, and mucositis. All unnecessary medications should be discontinued, especially those that may exacerbate these symptoms (eg, anticholinergic medications).[174] The clinician should guide the patient and family in making decisions regarding goals of therapy, a timeline for reevaluating goals, and criteria for withdrawal of nutrition support.

References

1. National Cancer Institute. Cancer statistics. http://www.cancer.gov/about-cancer/understanding/statistics. Accessed June 1, 2016.
2. National Institutes of Health and National Cancer Institute. Research is saving lives. http://www.aaci-cancer.org/public-issues/pdf/NIH_Leave_Behind.pdf. Accessed June 2, 2016.
3. Nicolini A, Ferrari P, Masoni MC, et al. Malnutrition, anorexia and cachexia in cancer patients: a mini-review on pathogenesis and treatment. *Biomed Pharmacother*. 2013;67(8):807–817.
4. Rock CL, Doyle C, Demark-Wahnefried W, et al. Nutrition and physical activity guidelines for cancer survivors. *CA Cancer J Clin*. 2012;62(4):243–274.
5. Planas M, Alvarex-Hernandez J, Leon-Sanz M, et al. Prevalence of hospital malnutrition in cancer patients: a sub-analysis of the PREDyCES® study. *Support Care Cancer*. 2016;24(1):429–435.
6. DeWys WD, Begg C, Lavin PT, et al. Prognostic effect of weight loss prior to chemotherapy in cancer patients. *Am J Med*. 1980;69:491–497.
7. Hébuterne X, Lemarié E, Michallet M, et al. Prevalence of malnutrition and current use of nutrition support in patients with cancer. *JPEN J Parenter Enteral Nutr*. 2014;38(2):196–204.
8. Tong H, Isenring E, Yates P. The prevalence of nutrition impact symptoms and their relationship to quality of life and clinical outcomes in medical oncology patients. *Support Care Cancer*. 2009;17(1):83–90.
9. Tisdale MJ. Mechanisms of cancer cachexia. *Physiol Rev*. 2009;89(2):381–410.
10. Cao DX, Wu GH, Zhang B, et al. Resting energy expenditure and body composition in patients with newly detected cancer. *Clin Nutr*. 2010;29:72–77.
11. Mantovani G, Madeddu C. Cancer cachexia: medical management. *Support Care Cancer*. 2010;18:1–9.
12. Purcell SA, Elliott SA, Baracos VE, Chu Qs, Prado CM. Key determinants of energy expenditure in cancer and implications for practice. *Eur J Clin Nutr*. 2016(Jun 8). Epub ahead of print.
13. Fearon KC, Glass DJ, Guttridge DC. Cancer cachexia: mediators, signaling, and metabolic pathways. *Cell Metab*. 2012;16:153–166.
14. Aapro M, Arends J, Bozzetti F, et al. Early recognition of malnutrition and cachexia in the cancer patient: a position paper of a European School of Oncology Task Force. *Ann Oncol*. 2014;25(8):1492–1499.
15. Suzuki H, Asakawa A, Amitani H, Nakamura N, Inui A. Cancer cachexia-pathophysiology and management. *J Gastroenterol*. 2013;48:574–594.
16. Jatoi A, Foster N, Wieland B, et al. The proteolysis-inducing factor: in search of its clinical relevance in patients with metastatic gastric/esophageal cancer. *Dis Esophagus*. 2006;19:241–247.
17. Cariuk P, Lorite MJ, Todorov PT, et al. Induction of cachexia in mice by a product isolated from the urine of cachectic cancer patients. *Br J Cancer*. 1997;76:606–613.
18. Torelli G, Meguid M. Use of recombinant human soluble TNF receptor in anorectic tumor-bearing rats. *Am J Physiol Regul Integr Comp Physiol*. 1999;277:R850–R855.
19. Cohen J, Wakefield CE, Laing DG. Smell and taste disorders resulting from cancer and chemotherapy. *Curr Pharm Des*. 2016;22:2253–2263.
20. Bernstein IL, Borson S. Learned food aversion: a component of anorexia syndromes. *Psychol Rev*. 1986;93:462–472.
21. Massie MJ. Prevalence of depression in patients with cancer. *J Natl Cancer Inst Monogr*. 2004;32:57–71.
22. Walker J, Hansen CH, Martin P, et al. Prevalence, associations, and adequacy of treatment of major depression in patients with cancer: a cross-sectional analysis of routinely collected clinical data. *Lancet Psychiatry*. 2014;1:343–350.
23. Schneider S, Moyer A. Depression as a predictor of disease progression and mortality in cancer patients: a meta-analysis. *Cancer*. 2010;116:3304.
24. Ripamonti C, De Conno F, Ventafridda V, et al. Management of bowel obstruction in advanced and terminal cancer patients. *Ann Oncol*. 1993;4:15–21.
25. Chen JH, Huang TC, Chang PY, et al. Malignant bowel obstruction: a retrospective clinical analysis. *Mol Clinic Oncol*. 2014;2(1):13–18.

26. Donthireddy KR, Ailawadhi S, Nasser E, et al. Malignant gastroparesis: pathogenesis and management of an underrecognized disorder. *J Support Oncol.* 2007;5(8):355.

27. De Luis DA, Izaola O, Cuellar L, et al. Nutritional assessment: predictive variables at hospital admission related with length of stay. *Ann Nutr Metab.* 2006;50:394–398.

28. Schattner M, Shike M. Nutrition support of the patients with cancer. In: Shils ME, Shike M, eds. *Modern Nutrition in Health and Disease.* Philadelphia, PA: Lippincott Williams & Wilkins; 2006: 1290–1313.

29. Farrell JJ. Digestion and absorption of nutrients and vitamins. In: Feldman M, Friedman LS, Brandt LJ, eds. *Sleisenger and Fordtran's Gastrointestinal and Liver Disease.* 8th ed. Philadelphia, PA: Saunders Elsevier; 2006:2147.

30. August DA, Huhmann MB. A.S.P.E.N. clinical guidelines: nutrition support therapy during adult anticancer treatment and in hematopoietic cell transplantation. *JPEN J Parenter Enteral Nutr.* 2009;33:472–500.

31. Falconi M, Pederzoli P. The relevance of gastrointestinal fistulae in clinical practice: a review. *Gut.* 2001;49(Suppl 4):S2–S10.

32. Paik CN, Choi MG, Lim CH, et al. The role of small intestinal bacterial overgrowth in postgastrectomy patients. *Neurogastroenterol Motil.* 2011;23:e191–e196.

33. Tappenden KA, Quatrara B, Parkhurst ML, et al. Critical role of nutrition in improving quality of care: an interdisciplinary call to action to address adult hospital malnutrition. *JPEN J Parenter Enteral Nutr.* 2013;37:482–497.

34. Laky B, Janda M, Cleghorn G, Obermair A. Comparison of different nutritional assessments and body-composition measurements in detecting malnutrition among gynecologic cancer patients. *Am J Clin Nutr.* 2008;87:1678–1685.

35. Thoresen L, Fjeldstad I, Krogstad K, Kaasa S, Falkmer UG. Nutritional status of patients with advanced cancer: the value of using the subjective global assessment of nutritional status as a screening tool. *Palliat Med.* 2002;16:33–42.

36. Academy of Nutrition and Dietetics Evidence Analysis Library. Oncology nutrition. Malnutrition screening and nutrition assessment of adult oncology patients. http://www.andeal.org/topic .cfm?menu=5291&cat=4873. Accessed July 25, 2016.

37. Kruizenga HM, Tulder MW, Seidell JC, et al. Effectiveness and cost effectiveness of early screening and treatment of malnourished patients. *Am J Clin Nutr.* 2005;82:1082–1089.

38. Kyle UG, Kossovsky MP, Karsegard VL, Pichard C. Comparison of tools for nutritional assessment and screening at hospital admission: a population study. *Clin Nutr.* 2006;25:409–417.

39. Jensen GL, Bistrian B, Roubenoff R, Heimburger DC. Malnutrition syndromes: a conundrum vs. continuum. *JPEN J Parenter Enteral Nutr.* 2009;33(6):710–716.

40. White JV, Guenter P, Jensen G, Malone A, Schofield M. Consensus statement: Academy of Nutrition and Dietetics and American Society for Parenteral and Enteral Nutrition: characteristics recommended for the identification and documentation of adult malnutrition (undernutrition). *JPEN J Parenter Enteral Nutr.* 2012;36:275–283.

41. Isenring E, Cross G, Daniels L, Kellett E, Koczwara B. Validity of the malnutrition screening tool as an effective predictor of nutritional risk in oncology outpatients receiving chemotherapy. *Support Care Cancer.* 2006;14:1152-1156.

42. Van Beek AP, Emous M, Laville M, Tack J. Dumping syndrome after esophageal, gastric or bariatric surgery: pathophysiology, diagnosis and management. *Obesity Rev.* 2016;18(1):68–85. doi:10.1111/obr.12467.

43. Tuca A, Guell E, Martiniz-Losada E, Codorniu N. Malignant bowel obstruction in advanced cancer patient: epidemiology,

management, and factors influencing spontaneous resolution. *Cancer Manag Res.* 2012;4:159–169.

44. Baldwin C, Spiro A, Ahern R, Emery PW. Oral nutritional interventions in malnourished patients with cancer: A systematic review and meta-analysis. *J Natl Cancer Inst.* 2012;104:371–385.

45. Seres DS, Valcarcel M, Guillaume A. Advantages of enteral nutrition over parenteral nutrition. *Therap Adv Gastroenterol.* 2013; 6(2):157–167.

46. Maxim I, DeLegge MH, Fang JC, et al. Multidisciplinary practical guidelines for gastrointestinal access for enteral nutrition and decompression from the Society of Interventional Radiology and American Gastroenterological Association (AGA) Institute, with endorsement by Canadian Interventional Radiological Association (CIRA) and Cardiovascular and Interventional Radiological Society of Europe (CIRSE). *J Vasc Interv Radiol.* 2011; 22:1089–1110.

47. Gupta V. Benefits versus risks: a prospective audit. Feeding jejunostomy during esophagectomy. *World J Surg.* 2009;33:1432–1538.

48. Cerantola Y, Hubner M, Grass F, Demartines N, Schafer M. Immunonutrition in gastrointestinal surgery. *Br J Surg.* 2011;98(1):37–48.

49. Marik PE, Zaloga GP. Immunonutrition in high-risk surgical patients: a systematic review and analysis of the literature. *JPEN J Parenter Enteral Nutr.* 2010;34:378–386.

50. Marimuthu K, Varadhan KK, Ljungqvist O, Lobo DN. A meta-analysis of the effect of combinations of immune modulating nutrients on outcome in patients undergoing major open gastrointestinal surgery. *Ann Surg.* 2012;255:1060–1068.

51. McClave SA, Taylor BE, Martindale RG, et al. Guidelines for the provision and assessment of nutrition support therapy in the adult critically ill patient: Society of Critical Care Medicine (SCCM) and the American Society for Parenteral and Enteral Nutrition (A.S.P.E.N.). *JPEN J Parenter Enteral Nutr.* 2016;40(2):159–211.

52. Consensus recommendations from the US summit on immune enhancing enteral therapy. *JPEN J Parenter Enteral Nutr.* 2001; 25(suppl):S61–S62.

53. Schattner M, Barrera R, Nygard S, et al. Outcome of home enteral nutrition in patients with malignant dysphagia. *Nutr Clin Pract.* 2001;16:292–295.

54. Klek S, Szybinski P, Sierzega M, et al. Commercial enteral formulas and nutrition support teams improve the outcome of home enteral tube feeding. *JPEN J Parenter Enteral Nutr.* 2011;35: 380–385.

55. Mattox TW. Intravenous hyperalimentation and cancer: a historical perspective. *Nutr Clin Pract.* 2002;17:249–251.

56. Huhmann MB, August DA. Perioperative nutrition support in cancer patients. *Nutr Clin Pract.* 2012:27:586–592.

57. Chow R, Bruera E, Chiu L, et al. Enteral and parenteral nutrition in cancer patients: a systematic review and meta-analysis. *Ann Palliat Med.* 2016;5:30–41.

58. Vashi PG, Dahlk S, Popiel B, et al. A longitudinal study investigating quality of life and nutritional outcomes in advanced cancer patients receiving home parenteral nutrition. *BMC Cancer.* 2014;14:593.

59. Bozzetti F, Santarpia L, Pironi L, et al. The prognosis of incurable cachectic cancer patients on home parenteral nutrition: a multi-centre observational study with prospective follow-up of 414 patients. *Ann Oncol.* 2014;25:487–493.

60. Cotogni P, Pittiruti M, Barbero C, et al. Catheter-related complications in cancer patients on home parenteral nutrition: a prospective study of over 51,000 catheter days. *JPEN J Parenter Enteral Nutr.* 2013;37:375–383.

61. Mitchell J, Jatoi A. Parenteral nutrition in patients with advanced cancer: merging perspectives from the patient and healthcare provider. *Semin Oncol.* 2011;38:439–442.

62. Jatoi A. Weight loss in patients with advanced cancer: effects, causes, and potential management. *Curr Opin Support Palliat Care.* 2008;2:45–48.

63. Madeddu C, Mantovani G, Gramignano G, Macciò A. Advances in pharmacologic strategies for cancer cachexia. *Expert Opin Pharmacother.* 2015;16:2163–2177.

64. Esposito A, Criscitiello C, Gelao L, et al. Mechanisms of anorexia-cachexia syndrome and rational for treatment with selective ghrelin receptor agonist. *Cancer Treat Rev.* 2015;41:793–797.

65. Neary NM, Small CJ, Wren AM, et al. Ghrelin increases energy intake in cancer patients with impaired appetite: acute, randomized, placebo-controlled trial. *J Clin Endocrinol Metab.* 2004;89: 2832–2836.

66. Strasser F, Lutz TA, Maeder MT, et al. Safety, tolerability and pharmacokinetics of intravenous ghrelin for cancer-related anorexia/cachexia: a randomised, placebo-controlled, double-blind, double crossover study. *Br J Cancer.* 2008;98:300–308.

67. Zhang H, Garcia JM. Anamorelin hydrochloride for the treatment of cancer-anorexia/cachexia (CACS) in non-small cell lung cancer. *Expert Opin Pharmacother.* 2015;16:1245–1253.

68. Anker AD, Coats AJS, Morley JE. Evidence for partial pharmaceutical reversal of the cancer anorexia-cachexia syndrome: the case of anamorelin. *J Cachexia Sarcopenia Muscle.* 2015;6:275–277.

69. Del Fabbro E, Dev R, Hui D, Palmer L, Bruera E. Effects of melatonin on appetite and other symptoms in patients with advanced cancer and cachexia: a double-blind placebo-controlled trial. *J Clin Oncol.* 2013;31:1271–1276.

70. Yennurajalingam S, Bruera E. Role of corticosteroids for fatigue in advanced incurable cancer: is it a "wonder drug" or "deal with the devil"? *Curr Opin Support Palliat Care.* 2014;8:346–351.

71. Mercadante S, Fulfaro F, Casuccio A. The use of corticosteroids in home palliative care. *Support Care Cancer.* 2001;9:386–389.

72. Yennurajalingam S, Frisbee-Hume S, Palmer JL, et al. Reduction of cancer-related fatigue with dexamethasone: a double-blind, randomized, placebo-controlled trial in patients with advanced cancer. *J Clin Oncol.* 2013;31:3076–3082.

73. Radbruch L, Elsner F, Trottenberg P, Strasser F, Fearon K. *Clinical Practice Guidelines on Cancer Cachexia in Advanced Cancer Patients.* Aachen, Germany: Department of Palliative Medicine/European Palliative Care Research Collaborative; 2010.

74. Loprinzi CL, Kugler JW, Sloan JA, et al. Randomized comparison of megestrol acetate versus dexamethasone versus fluoxymesterone for the treatment of cancer anorexia/cachexia. *J Clin Oncol.* 1999;17:3299–3306.

75. Oxandrolone tablets USP [package insert]. http://www.accessdata.fda.gov/drugsatfda_docs/label/2006/076761lbl.pdf. Accessed July 31, 2016.

76. US Food and Drug Administration. Orphan drug designations and approvals. https://www.accessdata.fda.gov/scripts/opdlisting/oopd/listResult.cfm. Accessed July 31, 2016.

77. Lesser GJ, Case D, Ottery F. A phase III randomized study comparing the effects of oxandrolone (Ox) and megestrol acetate (Meg) on lean body mass (LBM), weight (wt) and quality of life (QOL) in patients with solid tumors and weight loss receiving chemotherapy. *J Clin Oncol.* 2008;26(Suppl).

78. Ruiz Garcia V, López-Briz E, Carbonell Sanchis R, Gonzalvez Perales JL, Bort-Marti S. Megestrol acetate for treatment of anorexia-cachexia syndrome. *Cochrane Database Syst Rev.* 2013;(3):CD004310.

79. Busquets S, Serpe R, Sirisi S, et al. Megestrol acetate: its impact on muscle protein metabolism supports its use in cancer cachexia. *Clin Nutr.* 2010;29(6):733–737.

80. Mantovani G, Macciò A, Madeddu C, et al. Randomized phase III clinical trial of five different arms of treatment in 332 patients with cancer cachexia. *Oncologist.* 2010;15:200–211.

81. Jatoi A, Windschitl HE, Loprinzi CL, et al. Dronabinol versus megestrol acetate versus combination therapy for cancer-associated anorexia: a North Central Cancer Treatment Group study. *J Clin Oncol.* 2002;20:567–573.

82. Nanjappa S, Thai C, Shah S, Snyder M. Megestrol acetate–induced adrenal insufficiency. *Cancer Control.* 2016;23:167–169.

83. Abrams DI, Guzman M. Cannabis in cancer care. *Clin Pharmacol Ther.* 2015;97:575–586.

84. Birdsall SM, Birdsall TC, Tims LA. The use of medical marijuana in cancer. *Curr Oncol Rep.* 2016;18:40.

85. Cannabis-In-Cachexia-Study-Group; Strasser F, Luftner D, et al. Comparison of orally administered cannabis extract and delta-9-tetrahydrocannabinol in treating patients with cancer-related anorexia-cachexia syndrome: a multicenter, phase III, randomized, double-blind, placebo-controlled clinical trial from the Cannabis-In-Cachexia-Study-Group. *J Clin Oncol.* 2006;24:3394–3400.

86. Smith LA, Azariah F, Lavender VTC, Stoner NS, Bettiol S. Cannabinoids for nausea and vomiting in adults with cancer receiving chemotherapy. *Cochrane Database Syst Rev.* 2015;(11):CD009464. doi:10.1002/14651858.CD009464.pub2.

87. Davis MP. Cannabinoids for symptom management and cancer therapy: the evidence. *J Natl Compr Canc Netw.* 2016;14:915–922.

88. Kardinal CG, Loprinzi CL, Schaid DJ, et al. A controlled trial of cyproheptadine in cancer patients with anorexia and/or cachexia. *Cancer.* 1990;65:2657–2662.

89. Moertel CG, Kvols LK, Rubin J. A study of cyproheptadine in the treatment of metastatic carcinoid tumor and the malignant carcinoid syndrome. *Cancer.* 1991;67:33–36.

90. Couluris M, Mayer JL, Freyer DR, et al. The effect of cyproheptadine hydrochloride (Periactin®) and megestrol acetate (Megace®) on weight in children with cancer/treatment-related cachexia. *J Pediatr Hematol Oncol.* 2008;30:791–797.

91. Davis MP, Khawam E, Pozuelo L, Lagman R. Management of symptoms associated with advanced cancer: olanzapine and mirtazapine. *Expert Rev Anticancer Ther.* 2002;2:365–376008;30:791–797.

92. Navari RM, Brenner MC. Treatment of cancer-related anorexia with olanzapine and megestrol acetate: a randomized trial. *Support Care Cancer.* 2010;18(8):951–956.

93. Naing A, Dalal S, Abdelrahim M, Wheler J, Hess K, et al. Olanzapine for cachexia in patients with advanced cancer: an exploratory study of effects on weight and metabolic cytokines. *Support Care Cancer.* 2015;23:2649–2654.

94. Riechelmann RP, Burman D, Tannock IF, et al. Phase II trial of mirtazapine for cancer-related cachexia and anorexia. *Am J Hosp Palliat Care.* 2010;27:106–110.

95. Gordon JN, Trebble TM, Ellis RD, et al. Thalidomide in the treatment of cancer cachexia: a randomised placebo controlled trial. *Gut.* 2005;54:447–448.

96. Reid J, Mills M, Cantwell M, et al. Thalidomide for managing cancer cachexia. *Cochrane Database Syst Rev.* 2012;(4):CD008664. doi:10.1002/14651858.CD008664.pub2.

97. Goldberg RM, Loprinzi CL, Mailliard JA, et al. Pentoxifylline for treatment of cancer anorexia and cachexia? A randomized, double-blind, placebo-controlled trial. *J Clin Oncol.* 1995;13: 2856–2859.

98. Fearon KC, Barber MD, Moses AG. Double-blind, placebo controlled, randomized study of eicosapentaenoic acid diets in patients with cancer cachexia. *J Clin Oncol.* 2006;24:3401–3407.

99. Dewey A, Baughan C, Dean TP, Higgins B, Johnson I. Eicosapentaenoic acid (EPA, an omega-3 fatty acid from fish oils) for the treatment of cancer cachexia. *Cochrane Database Syst Rev.* 2007;(1):CD004597. doi:10.1002/14651858.CD004597.pub2.

100. Mazzotta P, Jeney CM. Anorexia-cachexia syndrome: a systematic review of the role of dietary polyunsaturated Fatty acids in the

management of symptoms, survival, and quality of life. *J Pain Symptom Manage.* 2009;37:1069–1077.

101. Cherwin, CH. Gastrointestinal symptom representation in cancer symptom clusters: a synthesis of the literature. *Oncol Nurs Forum.* 2012;39:157–165.

102. National Comprehensive Cancer Network. NCCN guidelines for supportive care. https://www.nccn.org/professionals/physician _gls/f_guidelines.asp. Accessed September 12, 2016.

103. Bossola M, Pacelli F, Rosa, F, Tortorelli A, Battista G. Does nutrition support stimulate tumor growth in humans. *Nutr Clin Pract.* 2011:26:174–180.

104. Baron PL, Lawrence W, Chan WM, White FK, Banks WL. Effects of parenteral nutrition on cell cycle kinetics of head and neck cancer. *Arch Surg.* 1986;121(11):1282–1286.

105. Edstrom S, Westin T, Delle U, Lundholm K. Cell cycle distribution and ornithine decarboxylase activity in head and neck cancer in response to enteral nutrition. *Eur J Cancer Clin Oncol.* 1989;25(2):227–232.

106. Dionigi P, Jemos V, Cebrelli T, et al. Preoperative nutritional support and tumor cell kinetics in malnourished patients with gastric cancer. *Clin Nutr.* 1991;10(suppl):77–84.

107. Magnano M, Mola P, Machetta G, et al. The nutrition assessment of head and neck cancer patients. *Eur Arch Otorhinolaryngol.* 2015;272(12):3793–3799.

108. Zhang Z, Zhu Y, Ling Y, Zhang L, Wan H. Comparative effects of different enteral feeding methods in head and neck cancer patients receiving radiotherapy or chemoradiotherapy: a network meta-analysis. *Oncol Target Ther.* 2016;9:2897–2909.

109. Bossola M. Nutritional interventions in head and neck cancer patients undergoing chemoradiotherapy: a narrative review. *Nutrients.* 2015;7:265–276.

110. Schweinfurth JM, Boger GN, Feustel PJ. Preoperative risk assessment for gastrostomy tube placement in head and neck cancer patients. *Head Neck.* 2001;23(5):376–382.

111. Daly JM, Hearne B, Dunaj J, et al. Nutritional rehabilitation in patients with advanced head and neck cancer receiving radiation therapy. *Am J Surg.* 1984;148(4):514–520.

112. Koyfman SA, Adelstein DJ. Enteral feeding tubes in patients undergoing definitive chemoradiation therapy for head-and-neck cancer: a critical review. *Int J Radiation Oncol Biol Phys.* 2012;84 (3):581–589.

113. Prestwich RJ, Teo MT, Gilbert A, et al. Long-term swallow function after chemoradiotherapy for oropharyngeal cancer: the influence of a prophylactic gastrostomy or reactive nasogastric tube. *Clin Oncol* (R Coll Radiol). 2014;26:103–109.

114. Bonomi J, Batt K. Supportive management of mucositis and metabolic derangements in head and neck cancer patients. *Cancer.* 2015;7:1743–1757.

115. Sayles C, Hickerson SC, Bhat RR, et al. Oral glutamine in preventing treatment-related mucositis in adult patients with cancer: a systematic review. *Nutr Clin Pract.* 2016;31(2):171–179.

116. Cho HK, Jeong YM, Lee HS, Lee YJ, Hwang SH. Effects of honey on oral mucositis in patients with head and neck cancer: a meta-analysis. *Laryngoscope.* 2015;125(9):2085–2092.

117. Xu JL, Xia R, Sun ZH, et al. Effects of honey use on the management of radio/chemotherapy-induced mucositis: a meta-analysis of randomized controlled trials. *Int J Oral Maxillofac Surg.* 2016(Sep 3);pii:S0901-5027(16)30185-0. Epub ahead of print. doi:10.1016/j.ijom.2016.04.023.

118. American Cancer Society. Esophageal cancer facts and figures. http://www.cancer.org/cancer/esophaguscancer/detailedguide/ esophagus-cancer-key-statistics. Accessed July 29, 2016.

119. Pohl H, Sirovich B, Welch HG. Esophageal adenocarcinoma incidence: are we reaching the peak? *Cancer Epidemiol Biomarkers Prev.* 2010;19(6):1468.

120. National Cancer Institute. What you need to know about cancer of the esophagus. Revised March 2013. http://www.cancer .gov/publications/patient-education/wyntk-esophagus-cancer. Accessed July 29, 2016.

121. Lopes AB, Fagundes RB. Esophageal squamous cell carcinoma-precursor lesions and early diagnosis. *World J Gastrointest Endosc.* 2012;16;4(1):9–16.

122. Barker, LA, Gout BS, Crowe TC. Hospital malnutrition: prevalence, identification and impact on patients and the healthcare system. *Int J Environ Res Public Health.* 2011;8(2):514–527.

123. Bower MR, Martin RC. Nutritional management during neoadjuvant therapy for esophageal cancer. *J Surg Oncol.* 2009;100(1): 82–87.

124. Ilson DH. Esophageal cancer chemotherapy: recent advances. *Gastrointest Cancer Res.* 2008;2(2):85–92.

125. Javle M, Ailawadhi S, Yang GY, et al. Palliation of malignant dysphagia in esophageal cancer: a literature-based review. *J Support Oncol.* 2006;4(8):365–373.

126. Academy of Nutrition and Dietetics Evidence Analysis Library. Oncology: esophageal cancer: chemoradiation and use of enteral nutrition. http://www.andeal.org/topic.cfm?menu=5291&cat= 3239. Accessed July 5, 2016.

127. Academy of Nutrition and Dietetics Evidence Analysis Library. Oncology: esophageal cancer: parenteral nutrition in esophageal cancer. http://www.andeal.org/topic.cfm?menu=5291&cat= 3239. Accessed July 5, 2016.

128. Bozzetti F. Nutritional support in patients with oesophageal cancer. *Support Care Cancer.* 2010;18(Suppl 2):S41–S50.

129. American Cancer Society. Stomach cancer facts and figures. http://www.cancer.org/cancer/stomachcancer/detailedguide/ stomach-cancer-key-statistics. Accessed July 29, 2016.

130. Feig BW, Berger DH, Fuhrman GM, eds. *The MD Anderson Surgical Oncology Handbook.* 2nd ed. Philadelphia, PA: Lippincott Williams and Wilkins; 1999:478–483.

131. Radigan AE. Post-gastrectomy: managing the nutrition fall-out. *Pract Gastroenterol.* 2004;28:63–75.

132. Ligtheart-Melis GC, Weijs PJ, Te Boveldt ND, et al. Dietician-delivered intensive nutritional support is associated with a decrease in severe post-operative complications after surgery in patients with esophageal cancer. *Dis Esophagus.* 2013;26(6): 587–593.

133. Tack J, Arts J, Caenepeel P, De Wulf D, Bisschops R. Pathophysiology, diagnosis and management of postoperative dumping syndrome. *Nat Rev Gastroenterol Hepatol.* 2009;6(10):583–590.

134. Stael von Holstein C, Walther B, Ibrahimbegovic E, et al. Nutritional status after total and partial gastrectomy with Roux-en-Y reconstruction. *Br J Surg.* 1991;78:1084–1087.

135. Rosania R, Costanza C, Malfertheiner P, Venerito M. Nutrition in patients with gastric cancer: an update. *Gastrointest Tumors.* 2016;2(4):178–187.

136. Oh R., Brown DL. Vitamin B12 deficiency. *Am Fam Physician.* 2003;67(5):979–986.

137. Krenitsky JS, Decher N. Medical nutrition therapy for upper gastrointestinal disorders. In: Mahan LK, Escott-Stump S, Raymond JL, eds. *Krause's Food in the Nutrition Care Process.* 13th ed. St Louis, MO: Elsevier: 2011.

138. Carey S. Bone health after major upper gastrointestinal surgery. *Pract Gastroenterol.* 2013;115:46–55.

139. American Cancer Society. Pancreatic cancer facts and figures. http://www.cancer.org/cancer/pancreaticcancer/detailedguide/ pancreatic-cancer-key-statistics. Accessed July 29, 2016.

140. National Cancer Institute. SEER Stat Fact Sheets: Pancreatic Cancer. http://seer.cancer.gov/statfacts/html/pancreas.html. Accessed July 31, 2016.

141. Bachmann J, Ketterer K, Marsch C, et al. Pancreatic cancer related cachexia: influence on metabolism and correlation to weight loss and pulmonary function. *BMC Cancer.* 2009;9:255.

142. Diener MK, Fitzmaurice C, Schwarzer G, et al. Pylorus-preserving pancreaticoduodenectomy (PP Whipple) versus pancreaticoduodenectomy (classic Whipple) for surgical treatment of periampullary and pancreatic carcinoma. *Cochrane Database Syst Rev.* 2014;(11):CD006053.

143. Pappas S, Krzywda E, McDowell N. Nutrition and pancreaticoduodenectomy. *Nutr Clin Pract.* 2010;25(3):234–243.

144. Goonetilleke KS, Siriwardena AK. Systematic review of perioperative nutritional supplementation in patients undergoing pancreaticoduodenectomy. *JOP.* 2006;7(1):5–13.

145. McCallum P, Walsh D, Nelson KA. Can a soft diet prevent bowel obstruction in advanced pancreatic cancer? *Support Care Cancer.* 2002;10(2):174–175.

146. Shaw JM, Bornman PC, Krige JE, et al. Self-expanding metal stents as an alternative to surgical bypass for malignant gastric outlet obstruction. *Br J Surg.* 2010;97(6):872–876.

147. Mendelsohn RB, Gerdes H, Markowitz AJ, et al. Carcinomatosis is not a contraindication to enteral stenting in selected patients with malignant gastric outlet obstruction. *Gastrointest Endosc.* 2011;73(6):1135–1140.

148. Tempero MA, Arnoletti JP, Behrman S, et al. Pancreatic adenocarcinoma: clinical practice guidelines in oncology. *J Natl Compr Canc Netw.* 2010;8(9):972–1017.

149. Imrie CW, Connett G, Hall RI, Charnley RM. Review article: enzyme supplementation in cystic fibrosis, chronic pancreatitis, pancreatic and periampullary cancer. *Aliment Pharmacol Ther.* 2010;25(Suppl1):S1–S25.

150. Pezzilli R, Andriulli A, Bassi C, et al. Exocrine pancreatic insufficiency in adults: a shared position statement of the Italian association for the study of the pancreas. *World J Gastroenterol.* 2013;19(44):7930–7946.

151. Escott-Stump S. Hepatic, pancreatic and biliary disorders. In: *Nutrition and Diagnosis Related-Care.* 7th ed. Baltimore, MD: Lippincott Williams & Wilkins; 2012:471–518.

152. Ellison NM, Chevlen E, Still CD, Dubagunta S. Supportive care for patients with pancreatic adenocarcinoma: symptom control and nutrition. *Hematol Oncol Clin North Am.* 2002;16(1):105–121.

153. Decher N, Berry A. Post-Whipple: a practical approach to nutrition management. *Pract Gastroenterol.* 2012;108:30–42.

154. Denlinger CS, Barsevick AM. The challenges of colorectal cancer survivorship. *J Natl Compr Canc Netw.* 2009;7(8):883–894.

155. Barbosa LR, Lacerda-Filho A, Barbosa LC. Immediate preoperative nutritional status of patients with colorectal cancer: a warning. *Arq Gastroenterol.* 2014;51(4):331–336.

156. Burges A, Schmalfeldt B. Ovarian cancer: diagnosis and treatment. *Dtsch Arztebl Int.* 2011;108(38):635–641.

157. Bragalone DL. *Drug Information Handbook for Oncology.* Hudson, OH: Lexi-Comp; 2012.

158. Tsahalina E, Woolas RP, Carter PG, et al. Gastrostomy tubes in patients with recurrent gynaecological cancer and intestinal obstruction. *Br J Obstet Gynaecol.* 1999;106(9):964–968.

159. Kucukmetin A, Naik R, Galaal K, et al. Palliative surgery versus medical management for bowel obstruction in ovarian cancer. *Cochrane Database Syst Rev.* 2010;(7):CD007792.

160. Herman LL, Hoskins WJ, Shike M. Percutaneous endoscopic gastrostomy for decompression of the stomach and small bowel. *Gastrointest Endosc.* 1992;38(3):314–318.

161. Chouhan J, Gupta R, Ensor J, et al. Retrospective analysis of systemic chemotherapy and total parenteral nutrition for the treatment of malignant small bowel obstruction. *Cancer Med.* 2016; 5(2):239–247.

162. Cozzaglio L, Balsola F, Costentino F, et al. Outcome of cancer patients receiving home parenteral nutrition. Italian Society of Parenteral and Enteral Nutrition. *JPEN J Parenter Enteral Nutr.* 1997;21(6):339–342.

163. Akbulut G. Medical nutritional therapy in hematopoietic stem cell transplantation (HSCT). *Int J Hematol Oncol.* 2013;23:55–65.

164. Jaing TH. Complications of haematopoietic stem cell transplantation. *ISBT Sci Series.* 2011;6:332–336.

165. Lemal R, Cabrespine A, Pereira B, et al. Could enteral nutrition improve the outcome of patients with haematological malignancies undergoing allogeneic haematopoietic stem cell transplantation? A study protocol for a randomized controlled trial (the NEPHA study). *Trials.* 2015;16:136.

166. Seguy D, Duhamel A, Rejeb MB, et al. Better outcome of patients undergoing enteral tube feeding after myeloablative conditioning for allogeneic stem cell transplantation. *Transplantation.* 2012;94:287–294.

167. Murray SM, Pindoria S. Nutrition support for bone marrow transplant patients. *Cochrane Database Syst Rev.* 2009;(1):CD002920.

168. Fuji S, Einsele H, Savani BN, Kapp M. Systematic nutritional support in allogeneic hematopoietic stem cell transplant recipients. *Biol Blood Marrow Transplant.* 2015;1707–1713.

169. Lalla RV, Bowen J, Barasch A, et al. MASCC/ISOO clinical practice guidelines for the management of mucositis secondary to cancer therapy. *Cancer.* 2014;120:1453–1661.

170. Worthington HV, Clarkson JE, Bryan G, et al. Interventions for preventing oral mucositis for patients with cancer receiving treatment. *Cochrane Database Syst Rev.* 2011;(4): CD000978.

171. US Food and Drug Administration. Errata and Addendum to the FDA Briefing Document Pharmacy Compounding Advisory Committee 27-28 October 2015. www.fda.gov/downloads/AdvisoryCommittees/CommitteesMeetingMaterials/Drugs/PharmacyCompoundingAdvisoryCommittee/UCM466379.pdf. Accessed October 19, 2016.

172. Moynihan T, Kelly DG, Fisch MJ. To feed or not to feed: is that the right question? *J Clin Oncol.* 2005;23(25):6256–6259.

173. Mirhosseini N, Fainsinger RL, Baracos V. Parenteral nutrition in advanced cancer: Indications and clinical practice guidelines. *J Palliat Care.* 2005;8(5):914–918.

174. Akbulut G. New perspective for nutritional support of cancer patients: Enteral/parenteral nutrition. *Exp Ther Med.* 2011;2: 675–684.

34 Diabetes Mellitus

Renee Walker, MS, RD, LD, CNSC, Anne M. Tucker, PharmD, BCNSP, and Kim K. Birtcher, PharmD, MS, BCPS (AQ Cardiology), CDE, CLS

CONTENTS

Acknowledgments: Laura Newton, MA, RD, and W. Timothy Garvey, MD, were the authors of this chapter for the second edition.

Objectives

1. Describe the diagnosis, classification, and pathophysiology of diabetes mellitus.
2. Discuss the complications of uncontrolled hyperglycemia, particularly in hospitalized patients.
3. Describe the recommended glycemic targets for hospitalized patients.
4. Discuss the medications used for control of diabetes in hospitalized patients.
5. Review the nutrition assessment and management of patients with diabetes in the hospital and during transitions of care.

Test Your Knowledge Questions

1. What is the corrected sodium level when blood glucose is 340 mg/dL and current serum sodium is 129 mEq/L?
   A. 133 mEq/L
   B. 125 mEq/L
   C. 130 mEq/L
   D. 140 mEq/L
2. A patient is admitted to the medical intensive care unit (ICU) for sepsis and now requires the use of continuous intravenous (IV) insulin infusion for hyperglycemia management. What is the appropriate target glucose range for this patient?
   A. 80 to 110 mg/dL
   B. 100 to 150 mg/dL
   C. 140 to 180 mg/dL
   D. 150 to 200 mg/dL
3. A patient's glucose decreased from 180 mg/dL to 140 mg/dL when given 5 units of insulin lispro. Estimate the total daily insulin dose using the sensitivity factor and the rule of 1800.
   A. 8 units
   B. 40 units
   C. 187.5 units
   D. 225 units

Test Your Knowledge Answers

1. The correct answer is **A**. Hyperosmolarity from hyperglycemia shifts fluid from the intracellular to extracellular compartments, resulting in a dilutional decrease in sodium levels. Serum sodium concentrations decrease 1.6 mEq/L for every 100 mg/dL increase in serum glucose.[1] Corrected Serum Sodium = Measured Serum Sodium + [0.016 × (Serum Glucose – 100)].
2. The correct answer is **C**. The American Association of Clinical Endocrinologists (AACE) and American Diabetes Association (ADA) consensus statement on inpatient glycemic control[2] and ADA Standards for Medical Care 2016[3] recommend 140 to 180 mg/dL as the target glucose range for critically ill patients. In clinical studies, this range has been associated with positive outcomes and limited risk for hypoglycemic complications. This target range is also recommended for the general hospitalized patient population.[2,3]
3. The correct answer is **D**. To arrive at this answer, first calculate the sensitivity factor (the decline in blood glucose in mg/dL per unit of regular or rapid-acting insulin). If the glucose decreased 40 mg/dL (eg, from 180 to 140 mg/dL) following an injection of 5 units, the sensitivity factor is 8 (40/5 = 8). Since insulin lispro, a rapid-acting insulin, was used, the total daily dose may then be estimated using the rule of 1800: divide 1800 by the sensitivity factor. The patient will need a total daily insulin dose of 225 units (1800/8 = 225 units).

Introduction

Diabetes is prevalent and costly. In 2012, an estimated 29.1 million people (9.3% of the US population) had diabetes. Of these, 25.9% were 65 years of age or older, and approximately 28% were undiagnosed.[4] In the same year, an estimated 86 million Americans had prediabetes; however, 90% did not know they had this condition.[4] The economic impact of diabetes is also significant, with the direct and indirect treatment costs for diabetes estimated to be $245 billion in 2012.[4]

Because hyperglycemia has been associated with complications in the hospital and throughout a patient's lifetime, clinicians should focus on appropriate glycemic control.[3,4] Critical illness has been associated with insulin resistance and hyperglycemia in patients with diabetes, and stress hyperglycemia has been observed in patients with no medical history of diabetes. Hyperglycemia in the hospital has been linked to increased morbidity, mortality, and length of stay. Diabetes is the primary cause of new onset blindness, kidney failure, and nontraumatic lower-limb amputations in the United States. In addition, patients with diabetes are at an increased risk for cardiovascular disease.[4] Appropriate glycemic control can reduce complications both in the hospital[2] and over a patient's lifetime.[3]

This chapter will review the diagnosis, classification, and pathophysiology of diabetes, glycemic targets, approaches to glycemic management, and nutrition assessment and support, with an emphasis on the challenges associated with the care of hospitalized patients.

Diagnosis, Classification, and Pathophysiology

Diagnosis

Table 34-1 presents the ADA diagnostic criteria for diabetes and prediabetes.[3] The diagnosis of diabetes can be made by 4 different methods, with a few caveats. The glycated hemoglobin (A1C) test may be done in a fasting or nonfasting state, and it should be done by standardized assay performed in a certified laboratory (ie, not be done by finger-stick). The fasting glucose test should be done after the patient has gone at least 8 hours without energy intake. The oral glucose tolerance test (OGTT) should use a 75-g glucose load. In the absence of unequivocal hyperglycemia, an abnormal value from the A1C test, fasting blood glucose test, or OGTT must be confirmed on another day before diabetes is diagnosed. In contrast, a single random blood glucose in the diagnostic range for diabetes with the presence of symptoms (ie, polyuria, polydipsia, polyphagia, and unintended weight loss) may be used to diagnose diabetes. According to the ADA, the diagnosis of prediabetes can be made with 1 value in the diagnostic range for prediabetes using the A1C test, fasting glucose test, or OGTT.[3] According to the AACE and American College of Endocrinology (ACE), the diagnosis of prediabetes can be made using either the fasting glucose test or OGTT, but not the A1C test.[5] In addition, the AACE/ACE includes the presence of the metabolic syndrome as a diagnosis for prediabetes.[5]

Classification and Pathophysiology

Diabetes is a metabolic disorder characterized by hyperglycemia. It is associated with abnormalities in carbohydrate, fat, and protein metabolism. The classification scheme for diabetes is shown in Table 34-2.[3] Some individuals may not clearly fit in one clinical category of diabetes. For example, individuals with

TABLE 34-1 American Diabetes Association Diagnostic Criteria for Diabetes, Prediabetes, and Normoglycemia

	A1C	Fasting Glucose	2-hour Glucose During OGTT	Random Glucose
Diabetes	≥6.5%[a]	≥126 mg/dL[a] (7.0 mmol/L)	≥200 mg/dL[a] (11.1 mmol/L)	≥200 mg/dL (11.1 mmol/L) with symptoms
Prediabetes	5.7%–6.4%	Impaired fasting glucose: 100–125 mg/dL (5.6–6.9 mmol/L)	Impaired glucose tolerance: 140–199 mg/dL (7.8–11.0 mmol/L)	
Normoglycemia	<5.7%	<100 mg/dL (5.6 mmol/L)	<140 mg/dL (7.8 mmol/L)	

OGTT, oral glucose tolerance test.
[a]In the absence of unequivocal hyperglycemia, abnormal value must be confirmed on another day before giving diagnosis of diabetes.
Source: Data are from reference 3.

TABLE 34-2 American Diabetes Association Classification of Diabetes

Clinical Category	Characteristics
Type 1 diabetes	β cell destruction, absolute insulin deficiency
Type 2 diabetes	Progressive insulin secretory defect, insulin resistance
Gestational diabetes	Diagnosed during pregnancy, not clearly overt diabetes
Other types of diabetes	• Genetic defects in β cell function, insulin action • Diseases (eg, cystic fibrosis, Cushing's syndrome, hyperthyroidism, infections) • Drug- and chemical-induced (eg, atypical antipsychotics, protease inhibitors, transplant medications)

Source: Data are from reference 3.

no history of diabetes may develop acute hyperglycemia under conditions of severe stress (eg, critically ill individuals hospitalized due to infection, sepsis, trauma, or cardiovascular event).

Type 1 Diabetes

Type 1 diabetes was once known as insulin-dependent diabetes mellitus or juvenile-onset diabetes; however, the ADA has discouraged the use of this terminology. The initial diagnosis of type 1 diabetes is most common in children and adolescents, but type 1 diabetes may occur at any age. Individuals with type 1 diabetes are also vulnerable to other autoimmune disorders (eg, celiac sprue, autoimmune thyroid disease, and Addison's disease).[6]

Type 1 diabetes is caused by the autoimmune destruction of pancreatic β cells, leading to an absolute insulin deficiency. The rate of β cell destruction is variable: some individuals present with acute hyperglycemia and ketoacidosis, but others may preserve some insulin secretion for years before becoming dependent on exogenous insulin therapy.[6] Latent autoimmune diabetes of adults is an example of delayed onset diabetes. It generally presents in adults older than 40 years of age as a result of slow, progressive autoimmune β cell destruction and a slow decline in insulin secretion, with evidence of prediabetes for multiple years before the diagnosis of overt diabetes.[7]

Insulin and amylin are normally cosecreted.[8] With type 1 diabetes, hyperglycemia occurs in both the fasting and fed states through several mechanisms. With the absence of insulin, there is inadequate peripheral glucose uptake, continuing hepatic glucose production, and less storage of glucose in the liver as glycogen.[6] With the absence of amylin, gastric emptying times are accelerated and glucagon secretion is not suppressed.[8]

Individuals with type 1 diabetes require insulin to sustain life and prevent the development of diabetic ketoacidosis. During hospitalization, individuals with type 1 diabetes must receive insulin throughout each 24-hour period without cessation (eg, injections of basal long-acting or intermediate-acting insulin with or without bolus rapid-acting insulin; or continuous IV insulin therapy). Individuals with ketoacidosis require aggressive volume repletion (ie, initially normal saline, then normal or half-normal saline), continuous IV insulin, and potassium repletion. In addition, the clinician should seek and resolve or treat the precipitating events or disease processes.[9]

Type 2 Diabetes

Type 2 diabetes was once known as non–insulin-dependent diabetes or adult-onset diabetes; however, the ADA has discouraged the use of this terminology. Approximately 90% to 95% of all individuals with diabetes have type 2 diabetes. Some of the risk factors for developing type 2 diabetes include increasing age, overweight or obesity status, lack of physical activity, history of prediabetes, non-Caucasian race, and positive family history of type 2 diabetes.[6]

The pathophysiology of type 2 diabetes is complex, and several defects occur concurrently and contribute to hyperglycemia.[6] First, there is a combined progressive insulin secretory defect and insulin resistance. Type 2 diabetes results when insulin secretory capacity begins to fail, creating a state of relative insulin deficiency that can no longer compensate for insulin resistance. Insulin resistance may occur early in life and may be exacerbated by the development of obesity, particularly abdominal obesity. Insulin resistance places metabolic stress on β cells, which hypersecrete insulin to maintain glucose homeostasis. With time, the β cell mass and function progressively declines, resulting in less secretion of both insulin and amylin. Second, without adequate insulin, the insulin-mediated glucose uptake by skeletal muscles is not sufficient to reduce the glucose level. Third, insulin and glucagon secretion is not balanced as it would be for someone who does not have diabetes. Even though hyperglycemia and high circulating levels of insulin are present, hepatic glucose output rates are elevated because of high levels of glucagon and gluconeogenesis. Fourth, incretin activity declines. For the individual who does not have diabetes, incretin hormones, glucagon-like peptide 1 (GLP-1), and gastric inhibitory polypeptide (GIP) are secreted by the gut in response to food intake. With normal physiology, the secretion of incretin hormones promotes glucose-dependent insulin secretion, slows gastric emptying time, facilitates a feeling of satiety, and indirectly reduces glucagon secretion. The reduced incretin effect allows for accelerated gastric emptying, blunting of the feeling of satiety, and continued secretion of glucagon and release of glucose from the liver, thus exacerbating hyperglycemia. Medical therapy for diabetes addresses one or more of these metabolic defects to achieve glycemic control.[6]

Hyperglycemic hyperosmolar state can result when glucose levels rise above 600 mg/dL and are accompanied by severe dehydration and hyperosmolality without the development of pronounced ketoacidosis. Hyperglycemia develops because of increased gluconeogenesis, accelerated glycogenolysis, and impaired glucose utilization by the peripheral tissues. Infection is the most common precipitating intercurrent event; however, hyperglycemic hyperosmolar state may also be triggered by inadequate insulin therapy, certain medications, pancreatitis, myocardial infarction, or cerebrovascular accident. An older adult without access to free water or with an impaired thirst mechanism who has an intercurrent event would be most susceptible to the hyperglycemic hyperosmolar state. The hyperosmolar state may progress over several days to weeks and may produce varying degrees of obtundation or even coma. Treatment includes volume and potassium replacement, gradual reduction in hyperglycemia using continuous IV insulin infusion, and treatment of intercurrent illness or condition.[9]

Prediabetic Conditions

Prediabetes and metabolic syndrome are conditions that identify individuals at high future risk for the development of type 2 diabetes and cardiovascular disease events. These conditions also place individuals at higher risk for stress hyperglycemia and glucocorticoid-induced hyperglycemia during hospitalization. The first condition, prediabetes, includes individuals with increased glucose levels that are higher than the normal range but do not yet meet criteria for diabetes. Prediabetes can be diagnosed on the basis of an elevated A1C, impaired fasting glucose, or impaired glucose tolerance defined by the 2-hour post-OGTT glucose value (Table 34-1). The second condition, metabolic syndrome, is defined by a cluster of risk factors mechanistically related to insulin resistance, including abdominal obesity, dyslipidemia, elevated glucose level, elevated blood pressure, and systemic inflammation. Since metabolic syndrome confers risk for both diabetes and cardiovascular disease, it is sometimes referred to as *cardiometabolic disease*. The diagnostic criteria for metabolic syndrome from the National Cholesterol Education Program Adult Treatment Panel III,[10] the International Diabetes Federation,[11] and the World Health Organization[12] are shown in Table 34-3.

The treatment for prediabetes and metabolic syndrome is lifestyle modifications, including diet and exercise with a goal to achieve and sustain 5% to 10% weight loss to prevent or delay the diagnosis of diabetes and reduce cardiovascular risk. One of the symptoms used to diagnose metabolic syndrome is elevated glucose, so individuals may meet the criteria for both metabolic syndrome and prediabetes. The American Diabetes Association, American Association of Clinical Endocrinologists, and American College of Endocrinology suggest aggressive lifestyle interventions and potentially oral medications aimed to decrease blood glucose concentrations for individuals with metabolic syndrome and prediabetes.[3,13]

Gestational Diabetes

Gestational diabetes mellitus (GDM) refers to diabetes occurring during pregnancy in those without preexisting diabetes. GDM is becoming more prevalent in the United States and worldwide, and this trend is significant because uncontrolled diabetes during pregnancy confers increased risk and consequences to both the mother and the fetus, including increased rates of macrosomia, preeclampsia, cesarean section, and poor maternal-fetal outcomes. While most pregnancy-related diabetes cases are cases of GDM, the increase in obesity and overall diabetes rates has led to an increasing number of women of childbearing age diagnosed with type 2 diabetes before pregnancy and a corresponding rise in undiagnosed type 2 diabetes cases. For this reason, the ADA Standards of Medical Care recommend screening women with risk factors for diabetes at the first prenatal visit using standard diagnostic criteria.[3] Women found to have glucose intolerance at this screen should be assumed to have previously undiagnosed diabetes and managed similarly to pregnant women with known preexisting diabetes. For women not previously known to have diabetes or risk factors for diabetes, testing for GDM should occur during weeks 24 through 28 of the pregnancy, a period when sharp increases in insulin resistance occur. Insulin resistance observed during this time of pregnancy is driven by multiple factors and include increases in placental hormones, inflammation, and lipolysis, along with reduced adiponectin secretion.[14] When pregnant women with GDM are not able to overcome this insulin resistance through pancreatic insulin secretion, hyperglycemia results. Several methods exist to diagnosis GDM, including a 1-step 75-g OGTT[15] or 2-step approach consisting of a 50-g OGTT nonfasting screen followed by a 100-g fasting OGTT for those with a positive screen.[16] Both methods are supported by the ADA. Table 34-4 presents the diagnostic criteria for GDM.[3,15,17–19]

TABLE 34-3 Diagnostic Criteria for Metabolic Syndrome

Risk Factor/Trait	ATP III *Any 3 Out of 5 Risk Factors*	IDF *Abnormal Waist + 2 Risk Factors*	WHO *IFG or IGT + 2 Risk Factors*
Waist circumference	≥102 cm in men; ≥85 cm in women	Region specific: eg, ≥94 cm in males and ≥80 cm in Europid-origin women; ≥90 cm in males and ≥80 cm in South Asian, Chinese, and Japanese women	BMI >30 or waist-to-hip ratio >0.90 in men and >0.85 in women
Fasting triglycerides	≥150 mg/dL (1.7 mmol/L)	≥150 mg/dL (1.7 mmol/L) and/or use of medication for triglycerides	≥150 mg/dL (>1.7 mmol/L)
HDL cholesterol	<40 mg/dL (1.04 mmol/L) in men; <50 mg/dL (1.29 mmol/L) in women	<40 mg/dL (1.03 mmol/L) in men; <50 mg/dL (1.29 mmol/L) in women; and/or use of medication for HDL cholesterol	<35 mg/dL (0.9 mmol/L) in men; <39 mg/dL (1.0 mmol/L) in women
Blood pressure	Systolic ≥130 mmHg and/or diastolic ≥85 mmHg and/or use of medication for hypertension	Systolic ≥130 mmHg and/or diastolic ≥85 mmHg and/or use of medication for hypertension	Systolic ≥140 mmHg and/or diastolic ≥90 mmHg and/or use of medication for hypertension
Fasting glucose	≥100 mg/dL (5.6 mmol/L) and/or use of medication for hyperglycemia	≥100 mg/dL (5.6 mmol/L) and/or use of medication for hyperglycemia	IFG: fasting ≥100 mg/dL (5.6 mmol/L) and/or IGT: 2-hour 140–199 mg/dL (7.8–11.0 mmol/L)
Microalbuminuria			≥20 mcg/min ≥30 mg per g creatinine

ATP III, National Cholesterol Education Program Adult Treatment Panel III; BMI, body mass index; HDL, high-density lipoprotein; IDF, International Diabetes Foundation; IFG, impaired fasting glucose; IGT, impaired glucose tolerance; WHO, World Health Organization.
Source: Data are from references 10, 11, and 12.

TABLE 34-4 Diagnostic Criteria for Gestational Diabetes Mellitus[a]

IADPSG diagnostic criteria:
- 75-g, 1-h fasting OGTT: ≥1 abnormal values
- Fasting glucose ≥92 mg/dL (5.1 mmol/L)
- 1-h glucose ≥180 mg/dL (10.0 mmol/L)
- 2-h glucose ≥153 mg/dL (8.5 mmol/L)

ACOG screening criteria:
- 50-g, 1-h random OGTT
- 1-h glucose ≥140 mg/dL (≥7.8 mmol/L)
- Use of a lower threshold of 135 mg/dL (7.5 mmol/L) is recommended in high-risk ethnic populations

ACOG diagnostic criteria:
- 100-g, 3-h fasting OGTT: ≥2 abnormal values using the Carpenter/Coustan or NDDG scale.
- Carpenter/Coustan scale:
  - Fasting glucose ≥95 mg/dL (5.1 mmol/L)
  - 1-h glucose ≥180 mg/dL (10.0 mmol/L)
  - 2-h glucose ≥155 mg/dL (8.5 mmol/L)
  - 3-h glucose ≥140 mg/dL (7.8 mmol/L)
- NDDG scale:
  - Fasting glucose ≥105 mg/dL (5.8 mmol/L)
  - 1-h glucose ≥190 mg/dL (10.6 mmol/L)
  - 2-h glucose ≥165 mg/dL (9.2 mmol/L)
  - 3-h glucose ≥145 mg/dL (8.0 mmol/L)

ACOG, American Congress of Obstetricians and Gynecologists; IADPSG, International Association of Diabetes and Pregnancy Study Groups; NDDG; National Diabetes Data Group; OGTT, oral glucose tolerance test.
[a]Both IADPSG and ACOG recommend screening during weeks 24–28 of pregnancy.
Source: Data are from references 3, 15, and 17–19.

Glucose intolerance associated with GDM resolves in most women after delivery; however, women with a diagnosis of GDM are at increased risk for developing type 2 diabetes and obesity later in life. Therefore, the ADA recommends that another 75-g OGTT be done 6 to 12 weeks postpartum to identify persistent diabetes or prediabetes.[3] Lifetime monitoring for diabetes and prediabetes is recommended through use of A1C, 75-g OGTT, or fasting plasma glucose at least every 3 years.[3] More frequent of screening should be guided by the presence of associated risk factors for diabetes.

Stress-Related Hyperglycemia

Hyperglycemia that occurs during critical illness is referred to as *stress-related hyperglycemia, stress diabetes, diabetes of injury,* or *stress hyperglycemia.* Situations associated with stress-related hyperglycemia include sepsis, shock, acute myocardial infarction, cerebrovascular accidents, trauma, and burns. The AACE and ADA define hyperglycemia in hospitalized individuals as blood glucose concentrations greater than 140 mg/dL (7.8 mmol/L).[2,3] Stress-related hyperglycemia can occur in individuals without a previous diagnosis of diabetes and can also negatively influence glucose control in those with preexisting diabetes. For most individuals without a preadmission diabetes diagnosis, glucose homeostasis returns to normal after resolution of critical illness.

However, in a subset of individuals, a stress-related hyperglycemic event may reveal previously undiagnosed diabetes.

Multiple factors contribute to the development of stress-related hyperglycemia, but overall it seems to be due to complex interactions between counterregulatory hormones and cytokines during illness or injury. During severe physiological stress, increased production of the counterregulatory hormones glucagon, cortisol, growth hormone, and catecholamines promotes hyperglycemia through enhanced glycogenolysis and gluconeogenesis in the liver and inhibition of peripheral glucose uptake.[20] The systemic inflammatory response to stress leads to a release of proinflammatory cytokines (interleukin-1, interleukin-6, and tumor necrosis factor), augmenting hepatic gluconeogenesis and insulin resistance. Insulin resistance is a prominent contributor to stress hyperglycemia, and hyperinsulinemia in response to elevations in glucose production correlates with illness severity and mortality.[20,21] The increased rate of glucose production observed in stressed individuals is not responsive to exogenous glucose administration as seen with nonstressed individuals. Since endogenous insulin secretion is insufficient to maintain normoglycemia during stress-related hyperglycemia, IV insulin administration is commonly employed.

All critically ill individuals should be screened for other factors that can increase serum glucose concentrations. Occult or preexisting diabetes, cirrhosis, obesity, pancreatitis, and hypokalemia can all negatively affect glucose control and warrant optimal management. Use of parenteral nutrition (PN) with glucose infusion rates greater than 5 mg/kg/min promotes hyperglycemia in critically ill individuals.[22] Limiting energy intake while providing adequate protein is recommended to limit hyperglycemia and insulin resistance during the first week of ICU admission.[23] A thorough review of medications is needed to identify agents known to cause hyperglycemia. Such medications include corticosteroids, catecholamines, thiazide diuretics, immunosuppressant agents, atypical antipsychotics, and protease inhibitors.[24] Discontinuation of or reduction in patient exposure to offending medications and dilution of IV medications using saline-containing fluids instead of dextrose-containing fluids, whenever possible, aids in glucose management and reduction in insulin requirements.

Because of the increased hospital length of stay and high rates of morbidity and mortality associated with stress-related hyperglycemia, all hospitalized individuals should have routine glucose monitoring. For those with persistent serum glucose values greater than 180 mg/dL (10.0 mmol/L), insulin therapy should be initiated using validated, evidence-based insulin protocols in conjunction with appropriate treatment of the underlying stress-related event.[2,3]

Measures of Glycemic Control

The laboratory measures used to assess glycemic control and manage hyperglycemia in individuals with diabetes include fasting glucose, postprandial glucose, A1C, and glycemic variability.

Fasting Glucose

As noted earlier, the fasting glucose test should be done after at least 8 hours without intake of energy-containing foods and beverages.[3] A high fasting glucose level correlates with elevated rates of hepatic glucose production, and high fasting glucose levels contribute to A1C elevations of 8.5% or more.[25] Fasting glucose is an important parameter used to titrate doses of basal insulin.

Postprandial Glucose

Postprandial glucose should be assessed 1 to 2 hours after beginning a meal, snack, or OGTT.[3] Postprandial glucose elevations have a greater influence on A1C levels when diabetes is better controlled (when A1C values are less than 7.3%).[25] An elevated 2-hour post-OGTT glucose has been associated with increased risk of cardiovascular disease.[3] The postprandial glucose level, as well as the glucose level immediately preceding the next meal, is used to titrate doses of the bolus insulin doses (ie, rapid-acting or short-acting insulin), which are given prior to that meal. The postprandial glucose is a treatment target when the A1C is not at goal despite reaching fasting glucose goals.[3]

Glycated Hemoglobin

The A1C level is a measure of glucose levels during a 3-month period. It is highly correlated with the development of microvascular disease complications, and it is the most useful indicator of overall treatment efficacy.[3] For nonpregnant individuals, the ADA generally recommends a therapeutic target of A1C less than 7%.[3] A more stringent A1C target (eg, less than 6.5%) may be chosen for individuals with a recent diagnosis of diabetes, long life expectancy, and without cardiovascular disease or hypoglycemia;[3] a less stringent A1C target (eg, less than 8%) may be indicated for individuals with history of severe hypoglycemia, limited life expectancy, advanced micro- or macrovascular complications, extensive comorbid conditions, or long-standing diabetes.[3] In contrast, AACE/ACE established an A1C goal of 6.5% or less for those without concurrent illness and not at risk for hypoglycemia and an A1C goal of greater than 6.5% for those with concurrent illness and at risk for hypoglycemia.[5] An A1C level should be obtained when individuals with hyperglycemia are admitted to the hospital.[3] The clinician should suspect stress hyperglycemia for individuals admitted with hyperglycemia, a normal A1C, and no history of treatment for diabetes.[3] In addition, the A1C level is helpful in selecting optimal diabetes treatment regimens upon discharge from the hospital.

Glycemic Variability

Glucose variability is the magnitude in fluctuations in glucose levels over time. Glucose variability can be computed using frequent home glucose measurements or frequent glucose measurements in the hospital. There is some interest in managing glucose variability, particularly in critically ill individuals. Glycemic variability has been associated with increased risk of hypoglycemia, which is dangerous and should be avoided. Glycemic variability is also associated with oxidative stress and damage to vascular endothelium; however, glycemic variability needs to be studied further to discern the clinical implications of achieving low glucose variability as an independent contributor to positive patient outcomes.[26] The ADA has not yet provided recommendations on how to use glucose variability in practice.[3]

Diabetes Complications, Diabetes Outcomes, and Glycemic Control

Patients with diabetes may experience numerous serious complications. This section focuses on complications and patient outcomes related to hyperglycemia; targets for glycemic control to minimize complications in hospitalized patients; and the identification and treatment of hypoglycemia. Gastroparesis is discussed later in the chapter.

Vascular Complications

Hyperglycemia promotes microvascular and macrovascular complications of diabetes. The microvascular complications include retinopathy, nephropathy, and neuropathy, and the macrovascular complications include coronary artery, cerebrovascular, and peripheral vascular diseases.

As the A1C rises above 6.5% to 7%, the risk of microvascular complications increase progressively, and high fasting and postprandial glucose levels are risk factors for cardiovascular disease events. Clinical trials have consistently shown that intensive glycemic control effectively prevents microvascular disease complications.[27,28] Intensive therapy, initiated in early stages of diabetes with longer duration of follow-up, produced lower rates of cardiovascular disease events in individuals with type 1 diabetes[29,30] and type 2 diabetes.[31] In contrast, short-term studies in individuals with advanced disease did not demonstrate benefits of intensive therapy,[32,33] and 1 study demonstrated harm with intensive treatment.[34] As a result of these trials, the ADA modified the A1C targets based on individual characteristics.[3]

Other Complications Associated with Hyperglycemia

The presence of hyperglycemia in hospitalized individuals affects immune response and wound healing. Hyperglycemia (eg, glucose levels greater than 180 mg/dL) impairs the immunologic response by inducing abnormalities in granulocyte adhesion, chemotaxis, phagocytosis, and the intracellular killing of bacteria. When the glucose is controlled to levels less than 180 mg/dL, these functions and the clinical risk of infection are improved.[35,36] During hyperglycemia, the bactericidal activity in granulocytes and wound healing are impaired.

Hyperglycemia may also lead to glycosuria and an osmotic diuresis, resulting in the loss of water and electrolytes. With fluid and insulin therapy, electrolyte abnormalities can be accentuated, as fluid shifts between the intracellular and extracellular compartments accompanied by the net influx of potassium into cells.

Hyperglycemia and Inpatient Outcomes

Hyperglycemia, including that induced by nutrition support, is associated with increased morbidity and mortality in both critically and noncritically ill hospitalized patients leading to increased hospital length of stays and healthcare costs.[36–38] PN and enteral nutrition (EN) are independent risk factors for the development of hyperglycemia,[39–41] with PN providing the highest risk. The presence of hyperglycemia in patients receiving PN significantly increases mortality.[42–44]

Hyperglycemia during hospitalization increases the risk of infection, sepsis, poor wound healing, congestive heart failure, stroke, myocardial infarction, renal failure, transplant rejection, and prolonged mechanical ventilation and ICU length of stay in numerous patient populations.[2,20,42–47] Close monitoring and appropriate interventions to achieve optimal glycemic control should be undertaken to prevent or reverse such complications.

Glycemic Targets for Hospitalized Patients

Several notable studies regarding glycemic targets for hospitalized patients have focused on critically ill patients. The Leuven trials compared intensive glucose control with glucose targets of 80 to 110 mg/dL to standard care glucose targets of 180 to 200 mg/dL and found that patient outcomes were improved by using tight glucose control in both surgical and medical patients remaining in the ICU more than 3 days.[37,38] Subsequent randomized controlled trials during this time period and a related meta-analysis[43] similarly supported such therapy. However, as this practice was adopted and further research conducted, an increased risk of mortality due to induced hypoglycemia using intensive glucose control was uncovered.[47,48] Reasons for such discrepancies are unclear, but they are likely due to differences in the methods of glucose measurement, patient selection, glycemic variability, quality of hospital algorithms and policies, use of nutrition support, and the capability of the healthcare team to intensively use insulin without high risk for hypoglycemia.

In response to these findings, the AACE and ADA revised recommendations for glycemic targets (Table 34-5) in a consensus statement that recognizes the importance of glycemic control across the continuum of care and aims to identify reasonable, safe, and achievable glycemic targets and describe

potential procedures, protocols, and system approaches to facilitate implementation of the glycemic targets.[2] These glycemic targets continue to be supported by the ADA, the Endocrine Society, and the American Society for Parenteral and Enteral Nutrition (ASPEN).[3,49,50] For critically ill patients with hyperglycemia, continuous IV insulin infusion therapy should be initiated for glucose values greater than 180 mg/dL, with blood glucose values of 140 to 180 mg/dL being the goal. More stringent goals of 110 to 140 mg/dL may be appropriate for some ICU patients as long as these goals can be accomplished without significant hypoglycemia.[3] For noncritically ill patients, the premeal blood glucose target should be less than 140 mg/dL with random blood glucose targets (including postprandial) less than 180 mg/dL. Intensive glucose control in this subset of hospitalized individuals has not been studied and is therefore not recommended. Scheduled subcutaneous insulin is preferred for achieving and maintaining glucose control using a basal-bolus approach with correctional or supplemental insulin as needed. Point-of-care glucose monitoring should guide insulin therapy and be obtained at a frequency consistent with method of insulin administration chosen.[2,3]

Hypoglycemia

A serious complication related to hyperglycemia treatment is hypoglycemia, which can occur in patients with and without diabetes. Hypoglycemia is defined as any blood glucose value less than 70 mg/dL. Severe hypoglycemia is defined as a blood glucose value less than 40 mg/dL. Hypoglycemia is associated with increased mortality, hospital length of stay, and hospital costs.[48,51,52] Risk factors associated with hypoglycemia include type 1 diabetes, advanced age, malnutrition, increased severity of illness, renal impairment, liver failure, heart failure, previous history of severe hypoglycemic episodes, and autonomic neuropathy.[2,53–55] In-hospital practices associated with hypoglycemia include changes in nutrient delivery, including diet changes to *nil per os* (NPO [nothing by mouth]) or discontinuation of EN or PN; prolonged use of sliding-scale insulin regimens; failure to make adjustments in insulin based on glucose measurements or

TABLE 34-5 AACE/ADA Recommendations for Glycemic Targets and Treatment for Inpatient Glycemic Control

	Critically Ill Patients	Noncritically Ill Patients
Glycemic targets	• Maintain glucose 140–180 mg/dL. • Glucose <140 mg/dL may be appropriate in some patients. • Glucose <110 mg/dL is not recommended.	• Premeal glucose <140 mg/dL. • Random glucose <180 mg/dL. • Reassess therapy for premeal glucose <100 mg/dL. • Change therapy for premeal glucose <70 mg/dL.

Recommended treatment	• Initiate IV insulin infusion for any glucose ≥180 mg/dL.	• Scheduled subcutaneous insulin therapy with components:
		  – Basal
		  – Nutrition
		  – Correctional
		• Preference for rapid-acting insulins.
		• Prolonged use of sliding scale as sole therapy is discouraged.

AACE, American Association of Clinical Endocrinologists; ADA, American Diabetes Association; IV, intravenous.
Source: Data are from reference 2.

changes in medical therapy; poor timing of meals with insulin injections and glucose testing; transfer to different patient care teams; inpatient use of oral hypoglycemic agents; and errors in writing and/or dispensing of medication orders.[3,54,55]

To prevent hypoglycemia and limit potential complications, hospitals should develop protocols and adequately train personnel on the identification and treatment of hypoglycemia. Signs and symptoms of hypoglycemia include confusion, dizziness, shaking, sudden hunger, headaches, irritability, sweating, and elevated heart rate. Protocols should be designed for execution by nursing staff and include a prompt medication and treatment review for any patients with glucose values less than 70 mg/dL.[3] Glucose values less than 70 mg/dL should prompt intervention according to the hospital's approved hypoglycemia response algorithm, with immediate contact of the physician for a glucose value less than 40 mg/dL. Treatment should be based on the patient's condition and alertness. In conscious patients who are capable of oral intake, 15 to 20 g of rapid-acting carbohydrate (glucose gel or four 4-g glucose tablets) should be administered, with repeat carbohydrate administration in 15 minutes if glucose values continue to show hypoglycemia. In addition, a small meal or snack should be provided. If glucose gel or tablets are unavailable, other sources of approximately 15 g of carbohydrate can be used (eg, 8 oz nonfat milk; 4 to 6 oz orange or apple juice; 6 oz sugar-sweetened soda; or 1 tablespoon of sugar, honey, or syrup). If the patient is NPO status, IV access should be established with administration of 20 mL of 50% dextrose solution and initiation of 5% dextrose in water infusion at 100 mL/h. If the full 50 mL ampoule of the 50% dextrose is administered intravenously, the patient may experience "overshoot" hyperglycemia. For patients who are unresponsive or have an altered level of consciousness, 12.5 to 25 g dextrose (25 to 50 mL of a 50% dextrose solution) can be administered by IV push, with initiation of 5% dextrose in water infusion at 100 mL/h. If IV access is not promptly available, 1 mg glucagon may be administered intramuscularly for a total of 2 doses. Regardless of the hypoglycemia regimen used, blood glucose values should be rechecked at least every 15 minutes until the patient's glucose value is at least 80 mg/dL.

Medications to Control Diabetes

Oral Agents and Insulin

The treatment of diabetes in outpatient settings should be tailored to the needs of the specific patient. Patients with type 1 diabetes require insulin therapy. Some patients with type 1 diabetes may also receive mealtime pramlintide, which slows gastric emptying time. The treatment of type 2 diabetes is much more varied. Initially, a single oral agent may treat the patient; however, because of the progressive loss of β cell function and more complex pathophysiology of type 2 diabetes, the patient may need a combination of agents or insulin to adequately manage blood glucose. The ADA recommends metformin, in combination with lifestyle modifications (appropriate diet, physical activity, and weight control) as the initial therapy for patients with newly diagnosed type 2 diabetes.[3] Metformin decreases hepatic glucose production, increases insulin

sensitivity by increasing peripheral glucose uptake and utilization, and decreases intestinal absorption of glucose. The ADA recommends that metformin be combined with other therapy if the A1C target is not attained after 3 months of metformin monotherapy. Some patients may require triple-drug therapy or a combination of insulin and GLP-1 inhibitor to reach the A1C target.[3] Table 34-6 includes medications used to treat type 2 diabetes and their mechanism for glucose lowering.[3]

Insulin is usually the preferred treatment for hyperglycemia management during hospitalization,[3] particularly when patients are acutely ill or in the ICU setting. Insulin is the only therapy with the combined features of (1) rapid onset of action, (2) wide dosing range that may be adjusted to the changing needs for greater or lesser glucose-lowering effect, (3) flexible scheduling to adjust to nutrient intake, (4) multiple routes of administration (subcutaneous, IV), and (5) lack of drug-drug interactions. Oral agents, on the other hand, have slower onset of action, have fixed-doses that prevent rapidly adjusting to clinical needs, have adverse effects unrelated to the glycemic effects, and may interact with other medications; some oral agents (eg, metformin) may also interfere with administration of radiographic procedures employing iodinated dyes. For these reasons, oral agents should be discontinued and insulin therapy initiated when a patient who was taking oral agents to control glucose levels is admitted to the hospital.[3] Table 34-7 describes the categories of insulin preparations available for use in hospitalized patients. Figure 34-1 illustrates insulin time action curves; for simplification, an estimated curve is shown for the rapid-acting, intermediate-acting, and long-acting insulins collectively.

Intravenous Insulin Therapy

Continuous IV insulin infusion is the optimal method for achieving glycemic targets in critically ill patients. The ADA recommends that IV insulin infusions be administered based on validated written or computerized protocols, which allow for predefined adjustments that account for insulin dose and glycemic fluctuations.[3] IV insulin therapy should only be administered in ICUs or in special medical units staffed by experienced and trained personnel who can closely monitor the patient's response to IV insulin therapy. IV insulin therapy should not be administered on units where the patient would be at risk for undetected hypoglycemia. Human regular U-100 insulin is commonly used for IV insulin therapy. The US Food and Drug Administration has approved rapid-acting insulins (lispro U-100, aspart, and glulisine) for IV infusion, but there is no advantage to using any of these medications in place of regular insulin. Insulin lispro U-200, a rapid-acting insulin, should not be given by IV infusion.[56]

Because of the very short half-life of circulating insulin, continuous IV infusion of insulin allows for rapid dose adjustments based on patient status. In general, continuous IV insulin infusion may be initiated at 0.5 to 1 units/h, based on patient characteristics and hospital protocol. Patients experiencing insulin resistance may require a higher initial dose (2 or more units/h). The patient's glucose level should be monitored frequently (eg, at least once per hour initially) and the insulin infusion rate adjusted accordingly. Insulin is generally

TABLE 34-6 Medications Used to Treat Type 2 Diabetes

Class	Examples	Glucose-Lowering Mechanism
α-glucosidase inhibitors	acarbose, miglitol	• Reduce intestinal carbohydrate digestion and absorption
Biguanides	metformin	• Decrease hepatic glucose production • Increase insulin sensitivity by increasing peripheral glucose uptake and utilization • Decrease intestinal absorption of glucose
Bile acid sequestrant	colesevelam	• Unknown
Dipeptidyl peptidase-4 inhibitors	alogliptin, linagliptin, lixisenatide, saxagliptin, sitagliptin	• Inhibit degradation of endogenously produced GLP-1, GIP
Dopamine-2 agonists	bromocriptine	• Affect hypothalamic regulation of metabolism • Improve insulin sensitivity
GLP-1 analogs	albiglutide, dulaglutide, exenatide, liraglutide	• Increase glucose-dependent insulin secretion; decreases glucagon secretion • Slow gastric emptying time; increase satiety
Meglitinides	nateglinide, repaglinide	• Increase pancreatic insulin secretion without regard to blood glucose level
SGLT2 inhibitors	canagliflozin, dapagliflozin, empagliflozin	• Reduce reabsorption of glucose by the kidney • Increases glucose excretion in the urine
Sulfonylureas	glimepiride, glipizide, glyburide	• Increase pancreatic insulin secretion without regard to blood glucose level
Thiazolidinediones	pioglitazone, rosiglitazone	• Enhance insulin sensitivity

GIP, gastric inhibitory polypeptide; GLP-1, glucagon-like peptide 1; SGLT2, sodium-glucose cotransporter 2.
Source: Data are from reference 3.

placed in saline or half-normal saline (although other IV solutions can be used) at a concentration of 1 unit per 1 to 10 mL IV solution and infused using calibrated electronic volumetric pumps. Insulin infusion via a dedicated line and pump enables the healthcare team to vary the infusion rate independent of other IV solutions, including PN. Standard practice constitutes flushing 20 mL of the IV insulin solution through the tubing before connecting the tubing to the IV access catheter to the patient to occupy adherence sites for insulin on polyvinyl chloride tubing.[57]

The patient's glucose level should be checked every hour for up to 6 hours until stabilized at the target level, at which point the frequency of glucose testing may be reduced to once every 2 to 3 hours. The infusion rate may be increased or decreased depending on the glycemic response and hospital protocol. In patients who are NPO, the insulin infusion is primarily acting to restrain hepatic glucose production at a level that maintains the targeted glucose range and is analogous to basal insulin. When PN or continuous enteral feeding is initiated, the insulin infusion should be increased to manage both the hepatic glucose output and the glucose from nutrition. During PN or continuous enteral feeding, many patients will require approximately double the insulin infusion rate over the level needed while NPO. The insulin infusion rate should be decreased to the basal or NPO rate 30 to 60 minutes before the PN or enteral feeding is discontinued to accommodate the gradual decrease in insulin level. Insulin infusion rates

should be individualized to patient needs based on careful glucose monitoring.

Subcutaneous Insulin Injections

Subcutaneous Insulin Preparations

Subcutaneous basal insulin with bolus correction insulin is the preferred treatment regimen for noncritically ill patients who are NPO or have poor oral intake. An insulin regimen with subcutaneously administered basal (nutrition) insulin and a correction component is the preferred treatment for patients with good oral intake. (See "Basal-Bolus Insulin Therapy" section later in this chapter.)

The commercially available insulin products used in the hospital setting are also used in the outpatient setting. Some institutions may not have all insulin products on the formulary, which may require converting the patient from one insulin product to another during transitions in care between the outpatient and inpatient settings. It is important to monitor differences in response when interchanging insulin products during these transitions in care.

Insulin may be classified as basal or bolus insulin. Neutral protamine Hagedorn (NPH), glargine, detemir, degludec, and human regular U-500 are basal insulins. Usually basal insulin is injected once or twice a day, and is designed to achieve a steady state insulin level, with the main purpose

TABLE 34-7 Insulin Preparations

Class	Name	Brand (Manufacturer)	Onset	Peak	Duration	Comments
Intravenous preparations						
	Human regular U-100	Humulin R (Lilly)	Immediate	Immediate	<10 min	No clinical advantage for using rapid-acting insulin over regular insulin
	Aspart	Novolog (Novo Nordisk)	Immediate	Immediate	<10 min	
	Lispro U-100	Humalog (Lilly)	Immediate	Immediate	<10 min	
	Glulisine	Apidra (Sanofi)	Immediate	Immediate	<10 min	
Bolus (subcutaneous) preparations						
Rapid-acting	Lispro U-100, U-200	Humalog (Lilly)	5–15 min	30–90 min	<5 h	Used up to 15 min prior to meal or with meal
	Aspart	Novolog (Novo Nordisk)	5–15 min	30–90 min	<5 h	
	Glulisine	Apidra (Sanofi)	5–15 min	30–90 min	<5 h	
Short-acting	Human regular U-100	Humulin R (Lilly)	30–60 min	2–4 h	5–8 h	Used 30–60 min prior to meal
		Novolin R (Novo Nordisk)	30–60 min	2–4 h	5–8 h	
Basal (subcutaneous) preparations						
Intermediate-acting	Human NPH	Humulin N (Lilly) Novolin N (Novo Nordisk)	2–4 h	4–10 h	10–18 h	Used once or twice a day
	Human regular U-500	Humulin R U-500 (Lilly)	2-4 h	4-10 h	10–16 h	Used 2 or 3 times a day, before meals
Long-acting	Glargine U-100	Lantus (Sanofi)	2–4 h	None	20–24 h	Used once a day
	Glargine U-300	Toujeo (Sanofi)	6 h	None	24–36 h	Used once a day
	Detemir	Levemir (Novo Nordisk)	3–6 h	None	18–20 h	Used once or twice a day
	Degludec	Tresiba (Novo Nordisk)	1 h	None	>42 h	Used once a day
Mixed (subcutaneous) preparations						
Premixed	Human NPH/ regular	Humulin 70/30 (Lilly)	30–60 min	Dual	10–18 h	All mixed insulins have dual peaks reflecting the combination of rapid-/short-acting and intermediate-/long-acting insulins. Mixed insulins do not allow for independent manipulation of insulin components. Usually used twice a day.
		Novolin 70/30 (Novo Nordisk)	30–60 min	Dual	10–18 h	
		Humulin 50/50 (Lilly)	30–60 min	Dual	10–18 h	
		Humulin 70/30 (Lilly)	30–60 min	Dual	10–18 h	
	Lispro protamine/lispro	Humalog Mix 75/25 (Lilly)	5–15 min	Dual	10–18 h	
	Lispro protamine/lispro	Humalog Mix 50/50 (Lilly)	5–15 min	Dual	10-18 h	
	Aspart protamine/aspart	Novolog Mix 70/30 (Novo Nordisk)	5–15 min	Dual	10–18 h	

NPH, Neutral protamine Hagedorn.
Manufacturers may change products. Always check product labels or websites for current information.
Source: Data are from manufacturers, Eli Lilly and Company (https://www.lilly.com); Novo Nordisk (http://www.novonordisk-us.com), and Sanofi US (http://www.sanofi.us/l/us/en/index.jsp).

FIGURE 34-1 Insulin Time Action Curves

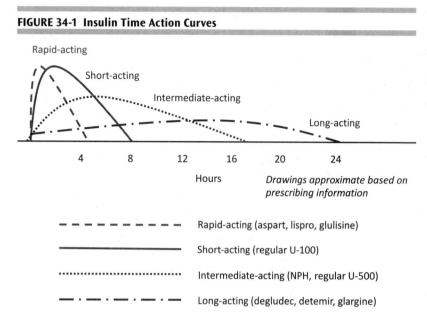

Hours

Drawings approximate based on prescribing information

‒ ‒ ‒ ‒ ‒ ‒ ‒   Rapid-acting (aspart, lispro, glulisine)

───────────   Short-acting (regular U-100)

·················   Intermediate-acting (NPH, regular U-500)

‒ · ‒ · ‒ · ‒ · ‒   Long-acting (degludec, detemir, glargine)

of controlling hepatic glucose output. Because the liver continuously produces glucose under fasting conditions, patients who are not eating or receiving nutrition support need to have basal insulin administered. Bolus insulin is given to achieve a peak insulin level after meals to coincide with rising postprandial glucose. Bolus insulin represents the nutrition or mealtime component of subcutaneous insulin therapy and is intended to lower plasma glucose by promoting tissue glucose uptake and nutrient metabolism following meals, as would occur physiologically with endogenous insulin secretory responses. Bolus insulins include rapid-acting insulins (lispro, aspart, and glulisine), with onset in 5 to 15 minutes, peak at 30 to 90 minutes, and duration of approximately 4 hours, and short-acting insulin (human regular), with onset in 30 to 60 minutes, peak at 2 to 4 hours, and duration of 5 to 8 hours. The combination of basal and bolus insulin can mimic physiological insulin production by providing insulin over 24 hours regardless of nutrient intake (basal) and insulin peaks for mealtime coverage (bolus). Rapid-acting and short-acting insulins can be used for the correctional component of therapy where an extra dose must be added to the prescheduled bolus when the premeal glucose is elevated.

There are also premixed insulin combinations of basal and bolus insulin in fixed-dose preparations, which could be used by patients who would have difficulty measuring or administering multiple insulin products. The fixed-dose ratios do not allow the clinician to independently adjust the basal and bolus insulin doses as needed for improving glycemic control. In hospitalized patients, it is generally advantageous to use basal and bolus insulins separately, as opposed to premixed formulations.

Sliding-Scale Insulin Therapy

Hyperglycemia in the inpatient hospital setting should not be managed solely with sliding-scale insulin.[3] In sliding-scale orders, a predetermined dose of regular or rapid-acting insulin is given subcutaneously in response to glucose values measured at predetermined time intervals. The sliding-scale approach is reactionary, because the insulin dose is always determined by the current glucose measurement. In addition, sliding-scale regimens do not mimic normal physiology. Often, the glucose measurements and insulin injections are done every 6 hours. The 6-hour interval is appropriate for regular insulin because it matches the duration of action of subcutaneously administered regular insulin. For rapid-acting insulin, it would be more appropriate to use an interval of every 4 hours, since the 4-hour time interval more closely matches the duration of action of rapid-acting insulin. If the rapid-acting insulin is scheduled every 6 hours, the patient will not have the effect of exogenous insulin for 1 or 2 hours leading up to the next glucose measurement. With sliding scales, insulin is usually not given when the glucose level declines below a predetermined level, leaving the patient without any exogenous insulin to restrain ongoing hepatic glucose production until the next glucose measurement. In summary, the use of sliding scales may put the patient at risk for wide fluctuations in glucose levels. AACE and the ADA recommend against prolonged use of sliding scales as the sole approach to insulin therapy.[2,3]

Basal-Bolus Insulin Therapy

For noncritically ill patients, the preferred approach for subcutaneous insulin administration is basal-bolus dosing. The basal-bolus approach mimics normal physiological insulin patterns of basal and meal-related insulin secretion in humans. For patients with adequate nutrition intake, the ADA recommends that patients receive the total daily dose of insulin as 3 components: basal insulin to control fasting glucose, bolus doses of regular or rapid-acting insulin before meals, and a correctional bolus dose added to the before-meal dose when premeal glucose levels exceed the targeted level.[3] For patients with poor oral intake or those who are NPO, the ADA recommends basal insulin and bolus doses of regular or rapid-acting insulin to "correct" blood glucose levels.[3]

Estimation of the Total Daily Insulin Dose

For hospitalized patients, the clinician should estimate the total daily insulin requirements using one of several methods. In the first method, the total daily insulin dose may be estimated from the number of units the patient required to control blood glucose in the outpatient setting. In the second method, for patients managed with IV insulin therapy, the total daily dose for subcutaneous insulin can be estimated as approximately 50% to 70% of the dose used intravenously to control blood glucose for 24 hours.[58,59] In the third method, the clinician may use formulas based on body weight to estimate the total daily insulin dose (type 1 diabetes: 0.3 to 0.5

units/kg/d; type 2 diabetes: 0.5 to 0.8 units/kg/d; very insulin-resistant type 2 diabetes and high-dose glucocorticoids: 0.9 to 1.5 units/kg/d). In the fourth method, the total daily insulin dose can be estimated using the assumptions from the 1500 rule or the 1800 rule (see more detailed explanation in the next section, "The 1500 Rule and 1800 Rule"). Each of these methods provides a reasonable starting estimation for total daily insulin dose that often must be altered based on careful monitoring of blood glucose.

After estimating the total daily insulin dose, begin by administering half of the estimated total daily dose as basal insulin. Basal insulin should not be held even if the patient is NPO because basal insulin controls hepatic glucose production throughout the 24-hour period. Administer the other half of the total daily dose as the sum of all bolus doses (nutrition) to be given at meal times. Assuming 3 isocaloric meals per day, one-sixth of the total daily dose (or one-third of the total bolus insulin) would be given at each meal. The basal dose can be titrated upward or downward based of the fasting morning glucose level, and each of the 3 premeal bolus doses are titrated to the glucose measured prior to the next meal. In addition to basal and bolus doses, a correctional dose of rapid-acting or short-acting insulin is added to each scheduled premeal dose.

The 1500 Rule and the 1800 Rule

The patient-specific correctional bolus dose, or sensitivity factor, may be calculated using the 1500 rule and the 1800 rule. The 1500 rule estimates the sensitivity factor or the point drop in glucose (mg/dL) for every 1 unit of regular insulin. The 1800 rule estimates the sensitivity factor or the point drop in glucose (mg/dL) for every 1 unit of rapid-acting insulin (lispro, aspart, or glulisine). These rules can be used to construct insulin-dosing algorithms for correctional doses of rapid- or short-acting insulin in the context of basal-bolus therapy.

To calculate the sensitivity factor for regular insulin, divide 1500 by the total daily insulin dose. For example, if the total daily insulin requirement is 60 units, the sensitivity factor is 25 (1500/60 = 25), predicting that the blood glucose level will decrease by 25 mg/dL for each unit of regular insulin given. If the premeal glucose is 195 mg/dL and the target is 120 mg/dL, the glucose needs to decrease by 75 mg/dL (195 – 120 = 75) to reach the target level. Therefore, 3 units of regular insulin (75/25 = 3) are needed to reduce the glucose level by the 75 mg/dL. The 3 units of regular insulin should be added to the scheduled insulin dose for that meal to bring the glucose into an acceptable range leading up to the next meal.

To calculate the sensitivity factor for rapid-acting insulin, the steps are similar but the sensitivity factor is calculated by dividing *1800* by the total daily insulin dose. For example, if the total daily insulin requirement is 60 units and rapid-acting insulin will be used as the bolus insulin, the sensitivity factor is 30 (1800/60 = 30), predicting that 1 unit of rapid-acting insulin will reduce blood glucose by 30 mg/dL. If the premeal glucose is 195 mg/dL and the target is 120 mg/dL, the glucose needs to decrease by 75 mg/dL (195 – 120 = 75) to reach the target level. In this case, 2.5 units of rapid-acting insulin (75/30 = 2.5) are needed to reduce the glucose level by the 75 mg/dL. The 2.5 units of rapid-acting insulin should be added to the scheduled insulin dose for that meal to bring the glucose into an acceptable range leading up to the next meal.

Nutrition Assessment

Patients with diabetes or hyperglycemia should receive a comprehensive nutrition assessment by a qualified clinician. This assessment should include a review of medical, nutrition, and medication histories as well as a nutrition-focused physical examination and evaluation of anthropometric and laboratory data.[60] The dietary history helps identify nutrient deficiencies or risk for deficiencies; unintended weight and appetite changes; nausea, vomiting, and diarrhea; use of supplements such as vitamins, minerals, or herbs; and chewing or swallowing issues. The clinician performing the assessment should pay close attention to the patient's diabetes-related medical history, including glucose control, self-monitoring practices, adherence to diet and lifestyle modifications, medications that could affect glucose levels or gastrointestinal (GI) function, and diabetes complications, as well as an assessment of the patient's educational needs as pertains to diabetes. The dose and administration schedule of oral hypoglycemic agents, insulin, or both should also be noted. During the physical examination, clinicians should carefully inspect skin integrity because patients with long-standing diabetes are particularly at risk for skin breakdown and poor wound healing.[61] (See Chapter 21 for more information on wound healing.)

Serum protein markers (ie, albumin, protein and transferrin) have poor utility as nutrition markers in acutely ill patients with diabetes. During acute illness, reprioritization of hepatic proteins occurs, resulting in decreased synthesis of negative acute-phase proteins (ie, albumin, prealbumin and transferrin) and increased synthesis of positive acute-phase proteins (ie, C-reactive protein).[23] These proteins are affected by injury, infection, and inflammation; thus, they are often better prognostic indexes than markers of nutrition status. Following trends in serum protein markers may be beneficial when evaluating the inflammatory response. Hyperglycemia and renal dysfunction due to diabetic nephropathy may also affect laboratory values. Prealbumin levels decrease with hyperglycemia and levels may be increased in patients with kidney disease because both prealbumin and retinol-binding protein are degraded in the kidney.[62] Following trends in these levels over time can provide valuable information regarding changes in a patient's clinical status.

Energy Requirements

Determining accurate energy requirements is necessary to avoid complications associated with intake. Indirect calorimetry remains the gold standard for measuring energy expenditure but is not always available or practical. In the absence of indirect calorimetry, predictive equations may be used to estimate energy requirements. More than 200 predictive equations exist. The appropriate equation to use depends on the availability of required patient data (eg, age, weight, height, minute ventilation, and maximum body temperature) and the population in which the equation was validated. Look to clinical guidelines published by professional organizations such as ASPEN, the Society of Critical Care Medicine (SCCM), and the Academy of Nutrition and Dietetics to help determine the best method to estimate energy requirements. No equation is 100% accurate, but they can provide a starting point from which clinical response may be monitored and nutrition therapy adjusted accordingly.[23] (See Chapter 2 for an expanded discussion of indirect calorimetry and predictive equations for determining energy requirements.)

Many patients with type 2 diabetes are obese, which further complicates estimation of energy requirements. Some predictive equations account and adjust for obesity while others do not.[63] Several organizations promote permissive hypocaloric feeding for patients with a body mass index (BMI) equal to or greater than 30. In this context, *hypocaloric* is defined as 65% to 70% of target energy requirements, 11 to 14 kcal per kg actual body weight if BMI is between 30 and 50, or 22 to 25 kcal per kg ideal body weight (IBW) if BMI is greater than 50.[23] While insulin sensitivity may be improved with some degree of weight loss, failure to receive more than 25% of estimated energy requirements is associated with a greater incidence of nosocomial infections.[64] A modest 5% weight loss achieved through daily energy reduction of 500 to 750 kcal/d has been associated with improved glycemic control, as well as a decrease in medication requirements.[3]

Overfeeding should be avoided in patients with diabetes or hyperglycemia because excessive energy intake can contribute to hyperglycemia and poor outcomes such as increased mortality, PN complications, risk for pneumonia and acute kidney injury, and impaired wound healing.[50,61] Other sources of energy intake—such as propofol (administered in a 10% lipid solution at 1.1 kcal/mL) or IV fluids/piggybacks containing dextrose—should be accounted for when determining the energy to be provided by nutrition support. Overall, the nutrition therapy goal is to provide adequate nutrition to meet the needs of patients while optimizing glucose control.

Protein Requirements

Protein requirements of patients with diabetes or hyperglycemia may vary depending on the severity of the disease or illness and the degree of malnutrition. The ideal amount of protein for optimal health and to improve outcomes is not known.[3] Generally, the normal protein recommendation used for healthy patients with diabetes is 0.8 to 1.0 g/kg/d or 15% to 20% of daily energy intake.[3,65,66] A patient's protein requirements may increase to 2 g/kg/d during stress or illness. For critically ill obese patients, protein needs should be based on IBW, particularly if the patient is receiving hypocaloric nutrition. If the patient's BMI is 30 to 40, the daily protein recommendation is 2 g per kg IBW; if the BMI is equal to or greater than 40, the daily protein recommendation is up to 2.5 g per kg IBW.[23] In patients with diabetic nephropathy (albuminuria and decreased glomerular filtration rate), protein intake of 0.8 g/kg/d is recommended. Providing protein below this level has not proven beneficial in altering glomerular filtration rate, cardiovascular risk, or glycemia.[3] In patients with type 2 diabetes, protein may increase insulin responses without affecting blood glucose; thus, carbohydrate-containing foods that are also high in protein should be avoided when correcting hypoglycemia.[67]

In critically ill patients with renal dysfunction, do not use protein restriction as a method of delaying the start of dialysis.[23]

Electrolytes

As insulin facilitates glucose entry into cells, hypophosphatemia and hypokalemia can develop from intercellular shifts of phosphorus and potassium. These electrolytes may need to be supplemented until levels are stabilized. Hyperglycemia contributes to a hyperosmolar state that results in the movement of fluid from the intracellular to the extracellular compartment and a dilutional decrease in the serum sodium level. For every 100 mg/dL increase in serum glucose concentration, the serum sodium concentration decreases 1.6 mEq/L.[1] The following equation is used to calculate corrected sodium for hyperglycemia:

$$\text{Corrected Serum Sodium} = \text{Measured Serum Sodium} + [0.016 \times (\text{Serum Glucose} - 100)]$$

Intervention to correct sodium levels related to hyperglycemia is unwarranted. Sodium levels will return to normal as hyperglycemia is corrected and insulin shifts glucose and water back into the intracellular compartment. Fluid and electrolyte status should be monitored closely, with supplementation given as needed to maintain adequate urine output and normal serum electrolyte levels.

Planning the Oral Diet

No single diet will suit everyone's eating patterns. Individuals with diabetes should be actively engaged in creating a treatment plan that will complement their lifestyle and accommodate their personal and ethnic food preferences while optimizing glycemic control.

Carbohydrate and Fiber Intake

Monitoring carbohydrate intake by carbohydrate counting, exchanges, or estimation, and adjusting medical therapy accordingly, is the key strategy in maintaining optimal glucose control. The minimum carbohydrate recommendation is 130 g/d.[66] As with protein, the optimal carbohydrate intake as a percentage of the total daily energy requirement is undefined. Using the glycemic index of food to plan food choices has been shown to be beneficial in reducing A1C levels for some people, but this benefit was not shown to apply to the those with type 2 diabetes.[3] People with diabetes (and others) should consume refined carbohydrates, added sugars, and sugar-sweetened beverages in moderation, while whole grains, legumes, fruits and vegetables are recommended. For individuals on scheduled insulin doses, their diets should focus on regularly scheduled meals with consistent carbohydrate content.[3] For some older adults and people with altered mentation or literacy issues, a simplistic approach to meal planning focused on healthy food choices and portion control is recommended.[3]

Fiber recommendations for people with diabetes are the same as for the general population: 14 g fiber per 1000 kcal consumed or 25 to 30 g/d.[68]

Dietary Fat and Cholesterol Intake

Limited research has been done on ideal fat intake in individuals with diabetes.[3] Emphasis on the type of fat rather than the amount of fat is recommended. Saturated fat intake should not exceed 10% of total energy intake and should be replaced with monounsaturated fats when the latter are available; *trans* fats should be avoided altogether.[3,68] Foods rich in ω-3 fatty acids (ie, fatty fish, nuts, and seeds) are encouraged to promote cardiovascular health.[3] Recommendations and dietary guidelines no longer include restrictions on dietary cholesterol.[68]

Sodium and Alcohol Guidelines

Reducing sodium consumption to less than 2300 mg/d may help lower blood pressure in some, but palatability, affordability and adherence must be factored in when determining whether this restriction is beneficial to particular individuals. Alcohol intake is permissible in moderation (1 drink per day for women and up to 2 drinks per day for men), but education about the increased risk for delayed hypoglycemia, especially for patients on diabetic medications, is warranted.[3]

Meal Planning and Weight Loss

For overweight and obese patients with type 2 diabetes, loss of 5% of body weight is recommended through interventions that focus on diet, activity, and behavioral changes that promote a daily energy deficit of 500 to 750 kcal. Diets containing the same amount of energy but different distributions of fat, carbohydrate, and protein content were shown to be equally effective in obtaining weight loss.[69-72] For weight loss of more than 5% in 3 months, medically supervised, high-intensity intervention coupled with a very low-calorie diet (less than 800 kcal/d) and meal replacement is recommended.[3] Benefits from weight loss may include reduction in A1C and triglyceride levels, decreased blood pressure, and reduction in medication needs. For patients with type 1 and type 2 diabetes, medical nutrition therapy involving multiple visits with a registered dietitian that involves the nutrition care process of nutrition assessment, nutrition diagnosis, nutrition intervention, and nutrition monitoring and evaluation will help achieve optimal glycemic control.[3,73]

Meal Planning in Hospitals and Long-Term Care Facilities

In hospitalized patients with diabetes, a consistent-carbohydrate meal-planning system, focusing on the total grams of daily carbohydrate, is often used as a key strategy for achieving optimal glucose control.[3] The diet order does not designate a specific energy intake level but rather specifies the amount of carbohydrate at each meal or snack, which may be stated as grams of carbohydrate or carbohydrate exchanges per meal. Typically, a consistent-carbohydrate meal plan provides between 1800 to 2000 kcal/d with 3 to 5 carbohydrate-servings per meal; each carbohydrate serving contains approximately 15 g carbohydrate. Use of this type of meal planning assists nursing in determining the amount of rapid-acting or short-acting insulin to administer at mealtime for the nutrition component of basal-bolus therapy.

If individuals are unable to meet their nutrition requirements through food, oral supplements may be used. Diabetes-specific nutritional supplements are available that limit carbohydrate content and result in lower glucose values following ingestion.

In long-term health care facilities, the ADA suggests tailoring diet to individual preferences, culture and personal goals. Older adults are more likely to have compromised nutrition status or dysphagia. In addition, risk for hypoglycemia is higher in this population due to altered renal function, variable intake, polypharmacy, and changes in intestinal absorption. A meal-planning system that emphasizes consistency in the timing and carbohydrate content of meals, rather than total energy, is recommended because undernutrition and inadequate intake are common in some institutionalized populations.[3] In these settings, medications can be adjusted to control glucose rather than restrict food intake or selection as nursing home residents have been found to eat better on less-restrictive diets.

Gastroparesis

Gastroparesis (delayed gastric emptying) can occur in individuals with diabetes when the vagus nerve, which controls GI motility, is damaged. Common signs and symptoms of gastroparesis include nausea, vomiting, early satiety, bloating, weight loss, and erratic glucose levels. Symptom severity and frequency may change over time. Gastroparesis is common in patients with type 1 diabetes whose glucose is poorly controlled, and it may also occur in patients with type 2 diabetes. Delayed gastric emptying may be aggravated by medications, specifically opioid therapy.

Treatment includes correcting hyperglycemia, which adversely affects the rate of gastric emptying. Low-fat, low-fiber diet interventions are implemented because fat delays gastric emptying and fiber is poorly digested. Meals should be small and frequent, patients should chew food well and remain upright 1 to 2 hours after meals. In some circumstances, patients may need soft, pureed, or liquid foods, which may be better tolerated because liquids empty from the stomach faster than solids. If a patient is vomiting, he or she may need supplemental fluid and electrolytes and close monitoring of hydration, electrolyte, and acid-base status is indicated. Certain medications such as metoclopramide and erythromycin may be used to stimulate gastric motility. An antiemetic may also be necessary to control nausea and vomiting. Other treatments that have been used in severe cases include implanted gastric neurostimulators (gastric pacemakers) and jejunostomy EN.[74-76]

Patients may require enteral feeding through a jejunostomy tube if their oral intake is insufficient or poorly tolerated. Jejunal feeding bypasses the stomach; therefore, the formula does not necessarily need to be low in fat. Formula selection should be based on the patient's individual needs, glucose control, and ability to tolerate the required volume of formula infused. One commonly used method is for the patient to receive continuous enteral feeding at night, which allows for oral intake during the day as tolerated. PN is rarely indicated for diabetic gastroparesis and should not be initiated unless other methods of nutrition support and pharmacotherapy have failed.[72] See Chapter 26 for additional information on gastroparesis.

Enteral Nutrition

EN is indicated in individuals who have a functioning GI tract but are unable or unwilling to meet energy and protein requirements via an oral diet. EN remains preferred to PN because EN provides physiological benefits such as attenuating the inflammatory response and is associated with fewer complications, particularly infectious risk and metabolic abnormalities. EN is also more cost effective than PN. (See Chapter 10 for more general information on EN.)

Formula Selection

When selecting an appropriate enteral formulation, multiple factors such as fluid, protein, and energy requirements, in addition to formula composition and cost should be considered.[77] (See Chapter 11.)

Products marketed as diabetes-specific enteral formulas are typically lower in carbohydrate and higher in fiber and fat than standard formulas; the protein contents of diabetes-specific and standard formulas are similar. Refer to Table 34-8 for more information on diabetes-specific enteral formula compositions.

Typical carbohydrate sources in standard enteral formulas are cornstarch, fiber, fructose, and oligosaccharides. Diabetes-specific formulas may contain slowly digestible carbohydrates such as isomaltulose and sucromalt. Unlike other carbohydrates where digestion starts in the mouth or stomach, digestion of these slowly digestible carbohydrates starts in the small intestine, with most digestion occurring in the duodenum.[78] Slowly digestible carbohydrates have a low glycemic index, and studies have found that their slower digestion and absorption rate reduce postprandial glycemic response.[79–85]

The quantity and fat sources in diabetes-specific formulas also differ from the standard enteral formulas. Fat sources in standard enteral formulas typically include canola, corn, medium chain triglyceride, safflower, sunflower, and soybean oils. Many of these fats are rich sources of ω-6 fatty acids (a family of polyunsaturated fatty acid), which may have a potential immunosuppressive effect if consumed in large amounts.[86,87] Diabetes-specific formulas contain monounsaturated fatty acids and ω-3 fatty acids as the primary fat sources to counter

TABLE 34-8 Select Diabetes-Specific Enteral Formulas

Product (Manufacturer)	Energy Density, kcal/mL	Carbohydrate, % kcal (Sources)	Protein, % kcal (Sources)	Fat, % kcal (Sources)	Fiber, g/L (Sources)
Diabetisource AC (Nestlé)	1.2	36 (corn syrup, pea puree, green bean puree, peach puree, fructose, tapioca dextrin, guar gum, maltodextrin)	20 (soy protein isolate, L-arginine, L-carnitine, taurine)	44 (canola oil, fish oil)	15.2 (FOS, Nutrisource, soy, vegetables, fruits)
Glucerna 1.0 (Abbott)	1	34.3 (maltodextrin, fructose)	16.7 (caseinate, L-carnitine, L-taurine)	49 (safflower oil, canola oil, soy lecithin)	14.4 (soy)
Glucerna 1.2 (Abbott)	1.2	35 (maltodextrin, isomaltulose, fructose, sucromalt)	20 (caseinate, soy protein isolate, milk protein concentrate, L-carnitine, taurine)	45 (safflower oil, canola oil, soy lecithin)	16.1 (scFOS, oat, soy)
Glucerna 1.5 (Abbott)	1.5	33 (maltodextrin, isomaltulose, fructose, sucromalt)	22 (caseinate, soy protein isolate, carnitine, taurine)	45 (safflower oil, canola oil, soy lecithin)	16.1 (scFOS, oat, soy)
Glytrol (Nestlé)	1	40 (maltodextrin, modified cornstarch, acesulfame potassium, sucralose)	18 (caseinate, taurine, L-carnitine)	42 (canola oil, safflower oil, MCT, soy lecithin)	15.2 (pea, gum acacia, FOS, inulin)

FOS, fructooligosaccharides; MCT, medium-chain triglyceride; scFOS, short-chain fructooligosaccharides.
Manufacturers may change product ingredients or nutritional content. Always check current product information.
Source: Data are from manufacturers' 2015–2016 product guides. Abbott Nutrition (https://abbottnutriton.com) and Nestlé Health Science (https://www.nestlehealthscience.us).

TABLE 34-9 Fat Sources in Enteral Nutrition

Type of Fat	Saturated Fat, %	Monounsaturated Fat, %	Polyunsaturated Fat, %
Canola oil	7	63	28
Corn oil	13	28	55
Safflower oil	8	75	13
Soybean oil	16	23	58
Sunflower oil, midoleic	9	57	29

Source: Data are from reference 88.

the immunosuppressive effect of ω-6 fatty acids. Enrichment of monounsaturated fatty acids in diabetes-specific formulas can exert favorable effects on insulin sensitivity and circulating lipid and lipoproteins.[80,81] Refer to Table 34-9 for more specifics on the sources of fat in enteral formulas.[88]

Use of a fiber-containing formula may assist with glucose control by improving the patient's insulin sensitivity as well as lowering the glycemic index of the formula. Soluble fiber can delay gastric emptying and decrease intestinal transit time, although this effect may not always be desirable, as in the case of a patient with gastroparesis. Formulas may also contain chromium supplementation; some studies have reported that formulas with added chromium improved glucose control and lipid levels in individuals with type 2 diabetes.[81,89,90]

Multiple studies comparing diabetes-specific enteral formulas with standard enteral formulas have found that the diabetes-specific products improved glycemic control by 12% to 21% and reduced insulin requirements by 26% to 71%.[79,80,82–84] A 2015 randomized controlled trial suggested that diabetes-specific formulas may also reduce the risk of acquired infections, ventilator-acquired pneumonia, and tracheobronchitis.[85] In addition, use of diabetes-specific EN was reported to reduce hospital length of stay by 0.88 days and decrease hospital costs by $2586 per patient when compared to standard EN.[91] Researchers found the positive results from diabetes-specific formulas are related to improved glycemic control from multiple factors: slowly digestible carbohydrate or reduced carbohydrate profile; higher protein content; differences in dietary fiber; and increased chromium supplementation.[79,81,82]

When compared to high-fat diabetes-specific enteral formulas, the diabetes-specific enteral formula with slowly digestible carbohydrate did not elevate postprandial triglyceride levels, and this benefit may therefore make it a preferred choice.[79] Findings suggest that the improved glycemic control seen with diabetes-specific formulas may also reduce cardiovascular complications when the formulas are used over the long term.[80] However, in critically ill patients, the higher fat content in diabetes-specific enteral formulas may further exacerbate delayed gastric emptying related to diabetic autonomic neuropathy, hemodynamic compromise, or medications affecting gastric motility. Providing postpyloric EN may improve EN tolerance in those with delayed gastric emptying.

Many of the studies on diabetes-specific enteral formulas were of short duration or conducted with nonacute or ambulatory patients.[79,81–84] Therefore, the results of these studies are not generalizable to acute-care or ICU patients. Studies investigating long-term use of diabetes-specific formulas are scarce. In addition, studies remain difficult to compare because of their small sample sizes and differences in populations studied, and most focused on type 2 diabetes.[23,50,92]

While diabetes-specific enteral formulas may be beneficial for some populations, no clear benefit has been demonstrated for *routine* use in ICU patients.[23,50,92] Therefore, use of diabetes-specific formulas should be determined on a case-by-case basis.

Delivery of Enteral Nutrition

In stable patients without gastric emptying abnormalities, enteral feeding may be initiated in the stomach using bolus or intermittent feeding. For most hospitalized patients, especially those who are critically ill, pump-assisted, continuous gastric enteral feeding results in improved tolerance. Small bowel feeding is recommended for patients at risk for aspiration or who have gastroparesis. Daily tolerance of EN should be evaluated using findings from physical examination, radiologic results, bowel movements, and patient complaints such as nausea or abdominal pain. Routine monitoring of gastric residual volumes (GRV) is no longer recommended in the ICU as data shows poor correlation with gastric emptying and incidence of pneumonia or aspiration.[23] For institutions that choose to continue to monitor GRV, the recommendation is to increase the GRV threshold at which EN is held to at least 500 mL.[23] Holding EN for GRV less than 500 mL without signs and symptoms of intolerance is not recommended.[23] Refer to Chapter 10 for more information on EN administration.

After EN is initiated, patients should be monitored closely for hypo- and hyperglycemia, GI intolerance, intake adequacy, hydration status, and alterations in laboratory data. For hospitalized patients receiving continuous EN, point-of-care glucose testing is recommended every 4 to 6 hours, and more frequent checks (every 1 to 2 hours) should be done when using an IV insulin infusion or with sudden cessation of EN regimen.[11] Clinicians should closely monitor the patient's electrolyte status because hypokalemia and hypophosphatemia can result from redistribution of electrolytes into the cells along with glucose, especially in those at risk for refeeding syndrome. Insulin doses are usually increased as EN is advanced to the goal feeding rate and glycemic control is achieved. Individuals who did not previously require insulin before enteral feeding may subsequently require insulin to achieve target glucose levels.

Insulin Therapy During Enteral Nutrition

As noted earlier, insulin therapy is often required to control hyperglycemia for patients with and without diabetes who are receiving EN. Clinicians should initiate insulin therapy when a patient's glucose levels are consistently equal to or greater than 180 mg/dL; the glycemic target is 140 to 180 mg/dL for hospitalized patients.[2,3] Many factors are considered when determining the appropriate insulin regimen, including the method of EN delivery (bolus/intermittent or continuous), the type and amount of enteral formula (diabetes-specific vs standard vs other specialized formulas), the level of patient care (ICU vs non-ICU), the patient's serum glucose values (and current A1C, if available), and specific patient factors such as diabetes type, weight, BMI, renal function, and nutrition status. The ADA and AACE advocate for the use of subcutaneous insulin regimens that provide basal, nutrition, and correction insulin coverage in hospitalized patients and continuous insulin infusions for select critically ill patients.[2,3]

Intermittent/Bolus Enteral Feeding

Basal-bolus insulin regimens typically work well for intermittent or bolus enteral feedings because this regimen mimics consistent meal patterns and provides standardized carbohydrate intake. Options for basal insulin include long-acting agents (glargine) administered once daily and intermediate-acting agents (NPH and detemir) administered twice daily. Starting doses of basal insulin are often based on the patient's prior basal insulin requirements at home or in the hospital prior to the start of EN. If the patient did not previously receive insulin therapy, the recommended approach is to start with 10 units of NPH or glargine insulin daily.[3] Subcutaneous rapid-acting insulin (aspart, lispro, or glulisine) or short-acting (human regular) insulin is administered before each enteral feeding to account for the carbohydrate content of the enteral formula. ADA and AACE guidelines recommend the use of rapid-acting insulins over human regular insulin because rapid-acting agents have a shorter onset of action, which allows for insulin administration immediately before or at the same time as enteral feedings, and shorter duration of action, which reduces the possibility of insulin stacking and hypoglycemia.[2,3] Dosing of rapid-acting insulin agents should be determined through prior home or hospital requirements or based on the amount of carbohydrate provided during EN feedings. Using the latter method, a starting point for dosing these agents is 1 unit of rapid-acting insulin for every 10 g carbohydrate, with adjustments made based on 2-hour postprandial glucose readings. Clinicians should use a standardized dosing protocol to provide supplemental doses of rapid-acting insulin agents to correct for hyperglycemia not covered by the basal-bolus insulin regimen. Use of commercially available preset mixtures of long- and short-acting insulins (75/25, 70/30, 50/50) mimicking a basal-bolus regimen through the use of fewer insulin injections has been studied during enteral feedings; however, these formulations are not generally used in the hospital because independent adjustment of basal (long- or intermediate-acting) and bolus/nutritional (short- or rapid-acting) components cannot be accomplished with these products.

Close monitoring of renal function status is necessary during insulin therapy, as the elimination of insulin will be reduced, resulting in prolonged insulin effects and increased risk for hypoglycemia. The Endocrine Society recommends a reduced initial total daily insulin dose for those with renal dysfunction.[49] Also, a study by Baldwin and colleagues illustrated that lower total daily doses of basal (insulin glargine) and bolus (insulin glulisine) insulins were equivalent in efficacy to standard total daily insulin dosing in noncritically ill individuals with renal dysfunction and resulted in 50% fewer episodes of hypoglycemia.[93] Hypoglycemia may also occur when enteral feedings are discontinued or held for procedures

or NPO status. In such cases, rapid- or short-acting insulin should not be administered. Use of long- or intermediate-acting insulin to provide the basal insulin component can be continued. Point-of-care glucose measurements every 4 to 6 hours or before each feeding and at bedtime are necessary because insulin doses may need to be titrated to accommodate multiple feeding times and changes in patient requirements or organ function to reach or maintain glycemic control.

Continuous Enteral Feeding

Patients receiving continuous EN require insulin therapy that accommodates the carbohydrate load being continuously absorbed. The insulin regimen should allow for incremental adjustments in the feeding rate while still maintaining good glycemic control. For critically ill patients in the ICU, continuous IV insulin infusions have been shown to be the ideal method to obtain glucose control. Continuous IV insulin infusions are titrated hourly based on point-of-care glucose readings to achieve target glucose levels. For facilities using continuous IV insulin infusions, the ADA and AACE recommend to use established, evidence-based written or computerized protocols and trained staff skilled in adjusting therapy in response to fluctuations in serum glucose and insulin doses.[2,3] Insulin protocols should provide clear, detailed instructions and algorithms for sudden interruptions or alterations in EN infusion (eg, diagnostic tests, procedures, intolerances, and nocturnal feedings) to prevent untoward events. When scheduled EN interruptions occur or when enteral feedings are discontinued without transition to oral intake or PN, insulin needs should be determined as if the patient is NPO. For example, the insulin infusion rate could be reduced to the basal rate 30 to 60 minutes before discontinuation of enteral feedings to allow for the biological effects of the higher insulin rate to deactivate. Another way to prevent hypoglycemia when EN is stopped is to maintain a 5% dextrose infusion at a keep-open rate (ie, 5 to 10 mL/h) while the EN is infusing and increase the dextrose infusion to 30 to 40 mL/h when the enteral feeding is held. A 10% dextrose solution may also be used. Glucose monitoring should be continued regardless of EN infusion.

In the non-ICU setting and in hospitals that do not use continuous IV insulin infusions, subcutaneous insulin injections using a basal-bolus approach (as described previously in the "Intermittent/Bolus Enteral Feeding" section) are recommended to manage hyperglycemia. In the non-ICU setting, subcutaneous injections of rapid-acting insulin should be scheduled every 4 hours as EN is provided via continuous infusion. For instances where regular insulin is used, the administration frequency should be extended to every 6 hours because regular insulin has a longer duration of action than rapid-acting agents. Higher doses of intermediate- or long-acting insulin can be used to provide both basal and nutrition coverage, although this approach is not commonly used because the effects of such an insulin regimen will persist if the enteral feedings are discontinued, placing the patient at increased risk for hypoglycemia.

A 2009 retrospective study of 156 medical, surgical, and ICU patients compared 3 different insulin regimens (NPH every 4 hours, NPH every 6 hours, or aspart insulin) used to obtain glycemic control in hospitalized patients receiving continuous

EN. Improved glycemic control was noted in both NPH groups compared with the group receiving insulin aspart (P <0.001). Mean glucose levels were also significantly lower in the NPH groups (134.7 mg/dL for NPH every 4 hours, 133.7 mg/dL for NPH every 6 hours, and 156.8 mg/dL for insulin aspart). Hypoglycemic episodes occurred less often in the insulin aspart group (P = 0.03) compared with the group receiving NPH every 4 hours. No significant difference was found between the insulin aspart group and the group receiving NPH every 6 hours.[94] These findings are consistent with those from Campbell and Braithwaite, who proposed using small, frequent doses of intermediate-acting insulin to reduce the potential for hypoglycemia when EN is unnecessarily interrupted or stopped.[95] Regardless of the regimen used to manage hyperglycemia in the hospital, appropriate monitoring is needed to provide safe and effective insulin therapy (see Practice Scenario 34-1).[23]

Practice Scenario 34-1

Question: What is the optimal management for a patient with type 2 diabetes requiring enteral nutrition (EN)?

Scenario: A 65-year-old man weighing 75 kg and with a body mass index of 27 reported decreased oral intake, early satiety, nausea, and vomiting for the past 5 days and was admitted to the hospital for uncontrolled diabetes. Shortly after admission, he decompensated and was transferred to the intensive care unit (ICU) for management. Shortly after ICU admission, he was intubated for respiratory failure. His previous medical history included hypertension, hyperlipidemia, and type 2 diabetes, which he managed at home with 15 units of glargine at night and 10 units of insulin aspart before each meal. Review of medical records indicated that his diabetes was poorly controlled, with the most recent A1C being 8.2%. A 12-French gastric feeding tube was placed and a diabetes-specific enteral formula composed of 36% carbohydrate, 20% protein, 44% fat, and 15.2 g of fiber/L was initiated within 24 hours at 20 mL/h, providing 1.2 kcal/mL. Water flushes were programmed on the enteral feeding pump for 30 mL every 4 hours, and additional water was given before and after medications. Laboratory data suggested dehydration (sodium, 153 mEq/L; chloride, 121 mEq/L; and blood urea nitrogen, 38 mg/dL) and a 5% dextrose in water (D5W) infusion was started at 100 mL/h to replenish the calculated free water deficit. The patient's abdomen became distended and EN was held. Gastroparesis was suspected. Point-of-care finger-stick glucose measurements were obtained every 4 hours, and the levels fluctuated between 225 and 350 mg/dL before EN was stopped.

Intervention: Metoclopramide was prescribed, and a continuous intravenous (IV) insulin infusion was started. A trial of lower fat, lower fiber enteral formula was also initiated. If abdominal distension persisted, the team planned to divert the level of feeding infusion to the jejunum.

Answer: With gastroparesis, obtaining glucose control is imperative to improving outcome. Continuous IV insulin infusions are recommended over subcutaneous insulin regimens for uncontrolled glucose in critically ill patients.[23] Use of a prokinetic agent is also recommended to enhance gastric emptying.[23] Finally, EN regimens for critically ill patients and those with gastroparesis should be changed to a lower fat, lower fiber product because fat delays gastric emptying and fiber is poorly digested. A 5% dextrose in water infusion, while necessary for treating hypernatremia, provides additional carbohydrate, which should be considered when managing hyperglycemia.

Rationale: Nutrition needs for patients with diabetes can be met with either a standard or diabetes-specific enteral formula. While diabetes-specific enteral formulas are beneficial in some populations, their routine use has no clear benefit. Clinical judgment and an overall cost-benefit analysis should influence enteral formula selection. In patients with gastroparesis, formulas higher in fat and fiber may be poorly tolerated. Because most diabetes-specific enteral formulas contain higher percentages of fat (42% to 49% of energy) and a considerable amount of fiber (14.4 to 16.1 g/L), a standard formula may be more clinically useful for this situation. Hyperglycemia can also adversely impact the rate of gastric emptying. In the ICU, glycemic control can quickly be achieved by using a continuous IV insulin infusion. Additional sources of dextrose (such as the D5W) should be identified and discontinued if possible. Changing the level of feeding infusions to the jejunum is another strategy to employ if gastric feeding is poorly tolerated since jejunal feedings bypass the stomach. In such cases, the EN formula would no longer need to be low in fat.

Parenteral Nutrition

PN support is indicated for individuals who have alterations in the GI tract that preclude safe enteral or oral intake. Two parameters that help determine when PN should be started include the degree of nutrition risk and the severity of malnutrition. When a patient's nutrition risk is high or malnutrition is severe, PN should be started as soon as possible. Supplemental PN may also be indicated in patients who are unable to meet more than 60% of their energy and protein needs after 7 to 10 days of EN.[23]

Hyperglycemia is the most common metabolic complication of PN, even for those without diabetes, and maintaining glucose levels within recommended range of 140 to 180 mg/dL is vital to promoting the best outcomes. Studies of hospitalized critically ill and noncritically ill patients receiving PN found that hyperglycemia was associated with increased risk for renal and cardiac dysfunction, infection, sepsis, pneumonia, and death.[42,44,92-98] For every 10 mg/dL increase in blood glucose greater than 250 mg/dL, the mortality risk increases by a factor of 1.3,[98] and the risk of infection or organ dysfunction increases 7% to 9% for every 10 mg/dL increase in mean blood glucose beyond 114 mg/dL.[42] For more in-depth information on PN, refer to Chapter 14.

Parenteral Nutrition Composition, Initiation, and Advancement

The macronutrient composition of PN can exacerbate hyperglycemia because carbohydrate is provided intravenously in the form of dextrose. Ideally, carbohydrate should be provided in the amount necessary to spare the use of protein for energy while avoiding hyperglycemia. Minimum requirements for carbohydrate delivery are 1 mg dextrose per kg/min; maximum requirements of 4 to 7 mg/kg/min are individualized for the patient.

In patients with hyperglycemia and those who are at risk for refeeding syndrome, dextrose should be limited to 100 g per 24 hours in the first bag of PN. PN should not be advanced until glucose levels are well controlled and within target range. At this time, PN may be advanced over the next 1 to 3 days toward nutrition goal while focusing on maintaining glycemic control and electrolyte balance. During the first week of PN, hypocaloric feeding is recommended for critically ill patients to reduce potential of hyperglycemia and refeeding syndrome; targets are (1) equal to or less than 20 kcal/kg/d or 80% of estimated energy needs and (2) at least 1.2 g protein per kg per day.[23]

In a prospective, randomized controlled trial (N = 50), PN regimens providing either 20 nonprotein kcal/kg/d (n = 20) or 30 nonprotein kcal/kg/d (n = 30) were compared.[94] Severity of hyperglycemia was lower in the 20 kcal/kg group (mean glucose area under the curve 118 ± 22 vs 172 ± 44 mg/dL), reducing the average daily insulin requirement (0 vs 10.9 units; $P <0.001$) and resulting in $6047 in healthcare cost savings. Dextrose infusion rate exceeding 4 mg/kg/min was identified as a predictor of hyperglycemia.

Currently, the maximum dextrose infusion recommended for critically ill patients or those with diabetes is 4 mg/kg/min.[99] Equations for calculating the dextrose infusion rate to achieve target level of administration and avoid excessive dextrose in PN are found in Table 34-10.

TABLE 34-10 Calculating Dextrose Infusion Rates in Parenteral Nutrition (PN)

Formula 1:

    Maximum Daily Dextrose Infusion Rate for Patient
    = Desired Glucose Infusion Rate (mg/kg/min)
    × Weight (kg) × 1440 (min/24 h) ÷ 1000

Example: Calculate the maximum daily dextrose infusion rate for a 70-kg critically ill patient:

    4 mg/kg/min × 70 kg × 1440 min/24 h ÷ 1000
    = 403 g dextrose

Formula 2:

    Dextrose Infusion Rate of PN = [Dextrose (g/d) in PN]
    ÷ Weight (kg) ÷1440 (min/24 h) × 1000

Example: Patient is receiving 500 g dextrose per day in PN. Does this rate exceed the recommended maximum of 4 mg/kg/min in a 70-kg patient?

    500 g/d ÷ 70 kg ÷ 1440 minutes × 1000 = 4.96 mg/kg/min

Therefore, current PN exceeds the maximum for dextrose in PN and the dextrose in the PN should be decreased to provide a rate of ≤4 mg/kg/min as determined using formula 1.

Adjusting the macronutrient composition of the PN by increasing the percentage of energy from fat may help prevent hyperglycemia. However, most lipid injectable emulsions (ILEs) available in the United States are soybean oil–based and composed primarily of long-chain triglycerides, which may promote proinflammatory mediators, hyperlipidemia, cholestasis, and immunosuppression. The use of ILE during the first week of PN in the ICU remains controversial. The 2016 guidelines from ASPEN and SCCM for the provision and assessment of nutrition support therapy in the adult critically ill patient suggest withholding soybean oil–based ILE or limiting it to 100 g/wk if there is concern for essential fatty acid deficiency during the first week of PN (quality of evidence: very low).[23] The recommended maximum dose of ILE is 2.5 g/ kg/d,[100] with equal to or less than 1 g/kg/d commonly employed for critically ill patients and those PN-associated liver disease.[100,101]

Monitoring

Bedside point-of-care finger-stick glucose monitoring should be initiated in patients on PN with a history of diabetes and in those without a diagnosis of diabetes whose blood glucose levels are elevated. The frequency of point-of-care finger-stick glucose monitoring varies depending on facility protocols, insulin dosing, and the patient's clinical condition. Generally, glucose monitoring is recommended every 4 to 6 hours, with more frequent monitoring (every 30 minutes to 2 hours) indicated when IV insulin is used.[3,11] (Approaches to insulin therapy during PN are discussed in the next section of this chapter.) Clinicians should use standard protocols for monitoring all aspects of PN, as discussed in Chapter 14. Special attention should be paid to the patient's magnesium, phosphorus, and potassium levels because requirements for these electrolytes increase as patients convert from a catabolic to anabolic state, and circulating levels can be reduced by carbohydrate infusion and insulin therapy. Patients may require supplementation of these minerals outside of the PN bag during the first few days of PN. Advancement of PN should not occur until glucose control and desired electrolyte levels are achieved.

Hypoglycemia may occur with abrupt cessation of PN, regardless of whether the patient is receiving insulin. This is referred to as "rebound hypoglycemia." If the PN infusion must be interrupted, 10% dextrose in water infusion should be initiated at the same rate as the PN until PN infusion resumes. This situation may occur if the central venous access is removed, the new bag of PN infusion is unavailable, or its delivery has been delayed. Another method to avoid rebound hypoglycemia associated with PN is to taper the infusion during the last 1 to 2 hours prior to discontinuation.

Insulin Therapy During Parenteral Nutrition

Hyperglycemia is common among patients receiving PN. Use of PN has been found to be an independent risk factor for the occurrence or worsening of hyperglycemia, regardless of previous diabetes diagnosis.[39] Risk factors associated with PN-associated hyperglycemia include increasing age, severity of illness, dextrose infusion rate, and previous history of diabetes diagnosis.[102] Park and colleagues found that in patients with diabetes not previously treated with insulin, 77% required insulin to control hyperglycemia during PN, with average insulin doses of 100 ± 8 units/d.[103] Adverse consequences related to PN-induced hyperglycemia include increased infections, sepsis, acute kidney injury, cardiac complications, and death.[49]

Patients receiving PN often need insulin therapy because infusion of carbohydrate into the systemic circulation bypasses regulators of glucose metabolism in the intestine. There are several different methods for insulin administration during PN therapy, including continuous IV insulin infusions, addition of insulin to PN, and subcutaneous insulin administration. The choice of insulin regimen depends on multiple factors, including patient location in the hospital, current medical condition of the patient, amount of carbohydrate administered, diabetes type, presence and degree of insulin resistance, obesity, and organ function. IV administration of insulin is the primary route of insulin administration for PN patients, with subcutaneous administration of rapid- or short-acting insulin used to correct any remaining hyperglycemia. In critically ill patients, continuous IV insulin infusion is preferred because the clinical condition of the patient and pharmacotherapy can lead to significant fluctuations in glucose values. IV insulin infusion is highly effective in reducing hyperglycemia to goal levels within 24 hours in most patients. Facilities should have protocols directing the use of insulin to ensure the best standard of care.

As a patient's critical illness resolves and transfer out of the ICU is planned, the patient must be transitioned off the continuous IV insulin infusion. For many patients on PN, the requirement for insulin therapy persists to some degree after ICU discharge. In these situations, the addition of insulin to the PN bag is frequently employed. Regular insulin is the only insulin product appropriate to add to PN formulations. To prevent potential hypoglycemia, which could lead to the interruption in parenteral feeding and insufficient energy provision, only a portion (60% to 80%) of the patient's daily insulin requirements from IV insulin infusion should be added to the PN bag.[49] Point-of-care finger-stick glucose monitoring is recommended every 4 to 6 hours to determine whether to administer correction coverage using subcutaneous rapid-acting or short-acting insulin. To make appropriate adjustments to PN insulin doses, clinicians should assess daily the patient's glucose values and the amount of correction insulin required. Reaching glycemic targets in such situations may require several days of insulin-dosing adjustments.

In patients outside of the ICU, continuous IV insulin infusion is not standard of care. To determine initial insulin dosing to add to PN, clinicians usually calculate 0.1 unit of regular insulin for every gram of dextrose in the PN infusion (eg, 200 g dextrose × 0.1 unit/g = 20 units of regular insulin).[100,104] For patients with obesity or significant insulin resistance, a higher ratio of insulin to infused carbohydrate may be required (0.1 unit of regular insulin per 0.5 g dextrose).[100] During PN advancement, dextrose should not be increased in the PN infusion until blood glucose concentrations are consistently less than 200 mg/dL; regular glucose monitoring with correction insulin is required.[100] Adjustments to the PN insulin dose can be made by adding two-thirds of the correction insulin

needed from the previous 24 hours to the dose. Use of continuous IV insulin infusion and/or reduction in the carbohydrate dose is required if the patient does not achieve glycemic control within several days or if a dose of 0.3 units of insulin per gram of PN dextrose is administerd.[100]

A modified basal-bolus insulin regimen may be preferred for patients with preexisting diabetes. For this method, the patient's basal dose of long- or intermediate-acting insulin is administered subcutaneously and the daily dose of bolus insulin to cover PN carbohydrates is added to the PN bag. In either case, if PN is discontinued, patient safety is maintained. Correction insulin and glucose monitoring every 4 to 6 hours is recommended as described earlier. Patients with type 1 diabetes require basal insulin to prevent hyperglycemic complications such as diabetic ketoacidosis. Successful glycemic management of these patients can be accomplished through the sole addition of insulin to the PN bag; however, there is a risk of hyperglycemic complications if PN is discontinued and basal insulin needs are not met. Patients with type 2 diabetes and high preadmission insulin requirements may also be ideal candidates for a modified basal-bolus insulin regimen because it provides baseline insulin delivery, preventing the need for the addition of high doses of insulin to the PN bag, which some clinicians consider to be unsafe.

Due to the complexity of care and need for continued insulin therapy on discharge, coordination of care with diabetes specialists is recommended. See Practice Scenario 34-2 for an example of managing a patient receiving PN who has hyperglycemia.[99]

Practice Scenario 34-2

Question: What is the optimal management for a patient with hyperglycemia requiring parenteral nutrition (PN)?

Scenario: A 59-year old woman who is postoperative Day 7 from exploratory laparotomy for elective resection of sigmoid colon mass requires a nutrition support consult for initiation of PN. Her nasogastric tube was removed on postoperative Day 5 with diet advancement. Subsequently, multiple episodes of vomiting ensued, the patient was made nothing by mouth, and the nasogastric tube was replaced for decompression. The patient's past medical history indicates hypertension and hypothyroidism have both been controlled with medications and the patient has had stage 1 colon cancer. Patient is hemodynamically stable with blood pressure of 138/68 mmHg and heart rate of 80 beats per minute. Serum laboratory data from this morning are sodium 138 mEq/L, potassium 4.2 mEq/L, chloride 102 mEq/L, blood urea nitrogen 15 mg/dL, serum creatinine 0.9 mg/dL, glucose 128 mg/dL, and liver function tests within normal limits. Preoperative A1C was 6.2%. Admission height and weight were recorded as 64 inches (162.6 cm) and 158 pounds (71.8 kg), meaning the body mass index was 27.1. Weight 6 months ago was noted as 165 pounds (75 kg). Findings from the physical examination are unremarkable except for positive abdominal distension, tenderness, and lack of bowel sounds. An abdominal x-ray reveals distended, gas-filled loops of small bowel consistent with ileus.

PN is initiated that evening to provide 1000 kcal and 100 g dextrose. PN is then increased over the next 2 days to provide 1920 kcal, 100 g protein, 300 g carbohydrate, and 50 g fat. When the PN goal is reached, hyperglycemia is noted. Point-of-care finger-stick glucose monitoring is initiated and reveals 2 readings greater than 180 mg/dL.

Intervention: To address observed hyperglycemia, the simple formula of 1 unit of regular insulin per 10 g infused carbohydrate is used, and it is determined that 30 units of regular insulin (300 g dextrose ÷ 10 = 30 units) should be added to the PN bag. Point-of-care finger-stick glucose monitoring is continued and correction insulin is administered according to the subcutaneous insulin protocol.

Answer: Glycemic control can be managed in patients receiving PN by continuous IV insulin infusion, by adding insulin to the PN formula, or with a subcutaneous insulin regimen containing basal, nutrition, and correction components. The addition of insulin to the PN formulation is an appropriate measure to manage hyperglycemia in this patient because she is in a nonintensive care unit where continuous IV insulin infusions are not typically allowed. Subcutaneous correction insulin using a standardized protocol allows for administration of additional insulin requirements and provides a basis for insulin dose titration. Adding two-thirds of the amount of correction insulin used in the past 24 hours to the current PN insulin dose is an appropriate titration measure. Medication adjustments and changes in patient condition should be monitored daily in addition to point-of-care glucose measurements. Energy goals for this patient were estimated at 25 to 30 kcal/kg (1795 to 2154 kcal/d) using her admission weight. PN is initiated at 1000 kcal and 100 g dextrose to reduce the risk of hyperglycemia and prevent large electrolyte shifts because the patient has not received significant oral intake for a week, placing her at risk for refeeding syndrome. As glucose and electrolyte levels remain stable, the PN order is increased to the goal amount, at which time hyperglycemia occurs.

Rationale: Regarding the use of PN itself, it is appropriate to use PN therapy in this patient because her prolonged postoperative ileus precluded oral diet or enteral feeding for 7 days. PN should be continued until at least 60% to 70% of estimated energy needs are met via the oral and/or enteral route. For glycemic control, a continuous IV insulin infusion is typically only administered in the ICU setting because this method requires frequent monitoring and specially trained staff. When patients are not being treated with an IV insulin infusion, insulin can be added to the PN solution or provided through scheduled subcutaneous administration with basal, nutrition, and correctional components.[11] Prevention of overfeeding and excess glucose infusion rates are crucial to reduce the risk of hyperglycemia associated with PN (Table 34-10). Dextrose infusion rates should be limited to equal to or less than 4 mg/kg/min.[99] In this patient scenario, a maximum of 414 g dextrose per day should be administered. Patients with diabetes or hyperglycemia requiring PN require frequent assessments of glucose levels and close monitoring of total carbohydrate and energy intake, electrolyte values, and medication adjustments to provide safe and effective care.

Nutrition and Diabetes Treatment During Transitions in Care

Inpatient Transitions of Care

Glycemic control often deteriorates when patients transition from IV to subcutaneous insulin therapy in the ICU or when transferring to lower acuity–care floors. Effective transition of insulin therapy requires accurate determination of daily IV insulin usage (from which subcutaneous insulin dosages are determined) and appropriate timing of the transitional regimen.

A retrospective analysis found that a total daily subcutaneous insulin dose equal to 60% to 78% of the 24-hour IV insulin dose achieved glucose levels within an 80 to 150 mg/dL target range 70% of the time.[59] Another retrospective study determined that a total daily subcutaneous insulin dose equal to 50% to 59% of the 24-hour IV insulin dose achieved target glucose levels of 70 to 150 mg/dL within 48 hours after ICU discharge.[58] Therefore, while variability exists, 50% to 70% of the IV dose requirement is a reasonable estimation of the total daily subcutaneous insulin dose. The basal-bolus regimen can then be established with 50% of total daily subcutaneous insulin dose given as basal insulin and 50% administered in bolus injections as described previously.

However, when patients are advancing through diet progressions, they are unlikely to consume full isocaloric meals until the goal diet is obtained. Therefore, the bolus doses (nutrition component) should be decreased to match actual food intake without substantial alteration in the basal insulin dose. Based on carbohydrate-counting principles, 1 unit of rapid- or short-acting insulin could be given for every 10 g carbohydrate in the meal to be consumed. The bolus insulin doses at meals can be increased as the diet advances until full bolus doses (approximately 50% of the estimated total daily insulin dose) are used when the patient advances to regular isocaloric meals. In hospitals, insulin is often not administered to consistently achieve full therapeutic effectiveness. Regular insulin should be administered 30 minutes before the meal and rapid-acting insulin administered either with the first bite of the meal or 5 to 15 minutes before the meal.

When a patient is transitioning from the ICU to another unit in the hospital, subcutaneous injections should be provided 1 to 2 hours before continuous IV insulin is discontinued.[3] In addition, the patient should not miss the bolus insulin injection before the next meal, even if the dose must be decreased in patients on advancing diets. (See Practice Scenario 34-3.[2,3,23,49])

Practice Scenario 34-3

Question: How is glycemic control managed during transitions in hospital care?

Scenario: A 63-year-old male patient was admitted to the intensive care unit (ICU) 6 days ago for sepsis related to pneumonia. Upon ICU admission, fluid resuscitation and antimicrobial therapy were initiated, and the patient required intubation for respiratory failure. A nutrition consult was obtained at that time. Continuous enteral nutrition (EN) was started on Day 1 of ICU admission with advancement to goal by ICU Day 3. Because the patient had persistent hyperglycemia, a continuous intravenous (IV) insulin infusion was initiated.

Today, plans for discharge to the general medicine floor were discussed on ICU rounds. Continuous EN is to be continued at the current macronutrient regimen because the patient failed swallow evaluation. Transition off the continuous IV insulin infusion to a subcutaneous insulin regimen is desired. Insulin requirements from the continuous IV insulin infusion for the previous 24 hours were recorded as 60 units (average 2.5 units/h). Point-of-care finger-stick glucose readings during this time ranged from 150 to 170 mg/dL. Laboratory test data and renal function are within normal limits. The patient's past medical history is unremarkable, except for type 2 diabetes. His admission height and weight were recorded as 70 inches (177.8 cm) and 200 pounds (90.9 kg), and his body mass index was calculated to be 28.6.

Intervention: To address insulin requirements for continued glucose control on transfer to the general medicine floor, a subcutaneous insulin-dosing regimen using insulin requirements from the insulin infusion protocol is developed. The patient required 60 units of regular insulin during the previous 24 hours, and two-thirds of this amount (40 units) is calculated as the total daily subcutaneous insulin dose. A subcutaneous basal-bolus regimen is constructed as follows: 20 units of subcutaneous insulin glargine daily (40 units × 0.5 = 20 units) and 5 units subcutaneous regular insulin every 6 hours (20 units ÷ 4 doses/d = 5 units). The continuous IV insulin infusion is discontinued 1 hour after the first dose of insulin glargine is administered. The subcutaneous correction insulin protocol is initiated with point-of-care finger-stick glucose monitoring every 6 hours.

Answer: Close attention to insulin requirements during transitions of care is imperative to prevent complications associated with both hyper- and hypoglycemia, particularly in patients transitioning off continuous IV insulin infusions to subcutaneous insulin regimens. The use of a basal-bolus insulin regimen is an appropriate measure for hyperglycemia management for this patient, and the total daily subcutaneous insulin dose calculated is within the recommended range of 60% to 80% of his previous 24-hour IV insulin requirements.[49] The care team follows recommendations to provide 50% of the total daily subcutaneous insulin dose as long-acting insulin (basal component) and 50% as short-acting regular insulin (bolus component). Since regular insulin has been chosen, the bolus component is divided into 4 equal doses administered every 6 hours. Subcutaneous correction insulin using a standardized protocol is employed, which allows for administration of additional insulin to meet requirements and provides a basis for insulin dose titration. If the EN regimen is changed to bolus administration or the patient transitions to an oral diet, the bolus insulin dose will need to be adjusted for carbohydrate intake, with insulin administration and glucose monitoring rescheduled to occur prior

to meals. Medication adjustments and changes in patient condition should also be monitored daily and insulin doses adjusted as warranted.

Rationale: The use of early EN in this critically ill patient is supported by current guideline recommendations.[23] Continued use of EN after discharge from the ICU is appropriate for this patient because the swallow evaluation indicated that an oral diet would be unsafe. A standard enteral formula can be used as long as overfeeding is prevented.

This patient was admitted to the ICU for sepsis secondary to pneumonia, which placed him at risk for stress-induced hyperglycemia. EN therapy and his history of type 2 diabetes further added to the development of hyperglycemia for which insulin therapy was required. Because critical illness can lead to fluctuating glucose values and unreliable responses to standard subcutaneous insulin regimens, use of continuous IV insulin infusion is recommended to control glucose in critically ill patients.[2,3]

Transition off continuous IV insulin infusions to less-intensive subcutaneous insulin regimens is desired once the patient's condition improves and he no longer needs ICU monitoring. Frequently, the requirement for continued insulin therapy persists in patients with a history of type 2 diabetes after ICU discharge. Providing a safe and effective insulin regimen can help prevent unexpected adverse events. The most common and effective method used to maintain glycemic control in EN patients upon transfer is a subcutaneous insulin regimen containing basal, bolus, and correctional components.[2,3]

Communication between the ICU and medical/surgical teams regarding the patient care plan should occur at the time of patient transfer, with the nutrition care plan including insulin therapy documented in the medical record. A pharmacist should complete a comprehensive medication review to identify duplicate, omitted, or unnecessary medication therapy at the time of the patient transfer. Including patients in their own diabetes care early during the hospital admission can help them achieve glycemic targets and prevent complications. Comprehensive diabetes education should begin as soon as possible and continue through discharge.

Transition to Postdischarge Care

A critical transition occurs during hospital discharge. According to the Centers for Disease Control and Prevention, in 2009, 5.5 million patients with diabetes were discharged from hospitals.[105] Poorly controlled diabetes following discharge is associated with a marked increase in rates of rehospitalization.[106] Determining the appropriate insulin-dosing regimen at discharge is often difficult because multiple factors, such as activity, diet, medication compliance, and stress levels, vary from patient to patient. A telephone survey evaluating postdischarge glycemia found hypoglycemia (blood glucose less than 70 mg/dL) and hyperglycemia (blood glucose greater than 300 mg/dL) occurred in 30% and 49% of discharged patients, respectively.[107] Patients reported problems using resources from discharge for self-management and indicated that they prioritized other events over the need to control glucose levels.[107] Patients who are discharged on insulin therapy should be given very specific instructions about which types of insulin to take, dosing, and the timing of insulin administration. Particular care should be taken if the patient's home insulin regimen was converted in the hospital to a different insulin product due to formulary restrictions. The patient's blood glucose levels may need to be monitored closely when switching between insulin products.

Diabetes education with the patient should start in the hospital, and a plan for follow-up care should be clearly communicated to outpatient providers prior to patient discharge. The patient should be actively involved in self-care and understand the dietary prescription, how to perform home glucose monitoring, and how to take insulin and other medications. The patient should also know what actions to take at various glucose levels, and how to respond to hypoglycemia. Discharge instructions should include follow-up appointments and contacts for clinicians who can provide medical advice prior to the first appointments, as well as prescriptions and access to all medications, glucometers and strips, and insulin syringes as needed.

References

1. Penn EL, Thijssen S, Raimann JG, et al. Correction of serum sodium for glucose concentrations in hemodialysis patients with poor glucose control. *Diabetes Care.* 2010;33:e91–e91.
2. Moghissi ES, Korytkowski MT, DiNardo M, et al; American Association of Clinical Endocrinologists; American Diabetes Association. American Association of Clinical Endocrinologists and American Diabetes Association consensus statement on inpatient glycemic control. *Endocr Pract.* 2009;15(4):353–369.
3. American Diabetes Association. Standards of medical care in diabetes—2016. *Diabetes Care.* 2016;39(Suppl 1):S51–S112.
4. American Diabetes Association. Statistics about diabetes. http://www.diabetes.org/diabetes-basics/statistics. Accessed June 6, 2016.
5. American Association of Clinical Endocrinologists, American College of Endocrinology. Consensus statement by the American Association of Clinical Endocrinologists and American College of Endocrinology on the comprehensive type 2 diabetes management algorithm: 2016 executive summary. *Endocr Pract.* 2016;22:84–113.
6. American Diabetes Association. Diagnosis and classification of diabetes mellitus. *Diabetes Care.* 2010;33(Suppl 1):S62–S69. doi:10.2337/dc10-S062.
7. Stenström G, Gottsäter A, Bakhtadze E, Berger B, Sundkvist G. Latent autoimmune diabetes in adults. *Diabetes.* 2005;54(Suppl 2):S68–S72. doi:10.2337/diabetes.54.suppl_2.S.
8. Schmitz O, Brock B, Rungby J. Amylin agonists: a novel approach in the treatment of diabetes. *Diabetes.* 2004;53(Suppl 3):S233–S238. doi:10.2337/diabetes.53.suppl_3.S233.
9. American Diabetes Association. Hyperglycemic crisis in diabetes. Diabetes Care. 2009;32(7):1335–1343. doi:10.2337/dc09-9032.
10. National Heart, Lung, and Blood Institute. ATP III At-A-Glance: Quick Desk Reference. 2001. https://www.nhlbi.nih.gov/health-pro/guidelines/current/cholesterol-guidelines/quick-desk-reference-html. Accessed January 17, 2017.
11. International Diabetes Federation. The IDF consensus worldwide definition of the metabolic syndrome. http://www.idf.org/webdata/docs/IDF_Meta_def_final.pdf. Accessed July 10, 2016.
12. World Health Organization. Definition, diagnosis, and classification of diabetes mellitus and its complications. Part 1: diagnosis and classification of diabetes mellitus. 1999. http://apps.who.int/iris/bitstream/10665/66040/1/WHO_NCD_NCS_99.2.pdf. Accessed January 17, 2017.
13. Handelsman Y, Bloomgarden ZT, Grunberger G, et al. American Association of Clinical Endocrinologists and American College of Endocrinology clinical practice guidelines for developing a diabetes mellitus comprehensive care plan 2015. *Endocr Pract.* 2015;21(suppl1):1S–87S.
14. Barbour LA, McCurdy CE, Hernandez TL, et al. Cellular mechanisms for insulin resistance in normal pregnancy and gestational diabetes. *Diabetes Care.* 2007;30(Suppl 2):S112–S119.
15. Metzger BE, Gabbe SG, Persson B, et al; International Association of Diabetes and Pregnancy Study Groups Consensus Panel. International Association of Diabetes and Pregnancy Study Groups recommendations on the diagnosis and classification of hyperglycemia in pregnancy. *Diabetes Care.* 2010;33:676–682.
16. Nathan DM, Davidson MB, DeFronzon RA, et al; American Diabetes Association. Impaired fasting glucose and impaired glucose tolerance: implications for care. *Diabetes Care.* 2007;30:753–759.
17. Committee on Practice Bulletins—Obstetrics. Practice bulletin no. 137: gestational diabetes mellitus. *Obstet Gynecol.* 2013;122:406–416.
18. Carpenter MW, Coustan DR. Criteria for screening tests for gestational diabetes. *Am J Obstet Gynecol.* 1982;144:768–773.
19. National Diabetes Data Group. Classification and diagnosis of diabetes mellitus and other categories of glucose intolerance. *Diabetes.* 1979;28:1039–1057.
20. Mizock BA. Alterations in fuel metabolism in critical illness hyperglycemia. *Best Pract Res Clin Endocrinol Metab.* 2001;15:533–551.
21. Das S, Misra B, Roul L, et al. Insulin resistance and β cell function as prognostic indicator in multi-organ dysfunction syndrome. *Metab Syndr Relat Disord.* 2009;7:47–51.
22. Rosmarin DK, Wardlaw GM, Mirtallo J. Hyperglycemia associated with high, continuous infusion rates of total parenteral nutrition dextrose. *Nutr Clin Pract.* 1996;11:151–156.
23. McClave SA, Taylor BE, Martindale RG, et al. Guidelines for the provision and assessment of nutrition support therapy in the adult critically ill patient: Society of Critical Care Medicine (SCCM) and American Society for Parenteral and Enteral Nutrition (A.S.P.E.N.). *JPEN J Parenter Enteral Nutr.* 2016;40:159–211.
24. Rehman A, Setter SM, Vue MH. Drug-induced glucose alterations part 2: drug-induced hyperglycemia. *Diabetes Spectrum.* 2011;24:234–238.
25. Monnier L, Lapinski H, Colette C. Contributions of fasting and postprandial plasma glucose increments to the overall diurnal hyperglycemia of type 2 diabetic patients: variations with increasing levels of HbA(1c). *Diabetes Care.* 2003;26:881–885.
26. Ceriello A, Kilpatrick ES. Glycemic variability: both sides of the story. *Diabetes Care.* 2013;36(Suppl 2):S272–S275.
27. Diabetes Control and Complications Trial Research Group. The effect of intensive treatment of diabetes on the development and progression of long-term complications in insulin-dependent diabetes mellitus. *N Engl J Med.* 1993;329: 977–986.
28. Stratton IM, Adler AI, Neil HA, et al. Association of glycaemia with macrovascular and microvascular complications of type 2 diabetes (UKPDS 35): prospective observational study. *BMJ.* 2000;321:405–412.
29. Diabetes Control and Complications Trial/Epidemiology of Diabetes Interventions and Complications (DCCT/EDIC) Study Research Group. Intensive diabetes treatment and cardiovascular disease in patients with type 1 diabetes. *N Engl J Med.* 2005;353:2643–2653. doi:10.1056/NEJMoa052187.
30. Diabetes Control and Complications Trial/Epidemiology of Diabetes Interventions and Complications (DCCT/EDIC) Study Research Group. Intensive diabetes treatment and cardiovascular outcomes in type 1 diabetes: The DCCT/EDIC study 30-

Year follow-up. *Diabetes Care.* 2016;39(5):686–93. doi:10.2337/dc15-1990.

31. Holman RR, Sanjoy KP, Bethel MA, Matthews DR, Neil HAW. 10-Year follow-up of intensive glucose control in type 2 diabetes. *N Engl J Med.* 2008;359:1577–1589. doi:10.1056/NEJMoa0806470.

32. ADVANCE Collaborative Group. Intensive blood glucose control and vascular outcomes in patients with type 2 diabetes. *N Engl J Med.* 2008;358(24):2560–2572. doi:10.1056/NEJMoa0802987. Epub 2008 Jun 6.

33. Duckworth W, Abraira C, Moritz T, et al. Glucose control and vascular complications in veterans with type 2 diabetes. *N Engl J Med.* 2009;360:129–139. doi:10.1056/NEJMoa0808431.

34. Action to Control Cardiovascular Risk in Diabetes Study Group. Effects of intensive glucose lowering in type 2 diabetes. *N Engl J Med.* 2008;358(24):2545–2559. doi:10.1056/NEJMoa0802743.

35. McMahon MM, Bistrian BR. Host defenses and susceptibility to infection in patients with diabetes mellitus. *Infect Dis Clin North Am.* 1995;9:1–9.

36. Pomposelli JJ, Baxter JK, Babineau TJ, et al. Early post-operative glucose control predicts nosocomial infection rate in diabetic patients. *JPEN J Parenter Enteral Nutr.* 1998;22:77–81.

37. Van den Berghe G, Wouters P, Weekers F, et al. Intensive insulin therapy in critically ill patients. *N Engl J Med.* 2001;345:1359–1367.

38. Van den Berghe G, Wilmer A, Hermans G, et al. Intensive insulin therapy in the medical ICU. *N Engl J Med.* 2006;354:449–461.

39. Ziegler TR. Parenteral nutrition in the critically ill patient. *N Engl J Med.* 2009;361:1088–1097.

40. Pancorbo-Hidalgo PL, García-Fernandez FP, Ramírez-Pérez C. Complications associated with enteral nutrition by nasogastric tube in an internal medicine unit. *J Clin Nurs.* 2001;10:482–490.

41. Umpierrez GE. Basal versus sliding-scale regular insulin in hospitalized patients with hyperglycemia during enteral nutrition therapy. *Diabetes Care.* 2009;32:751–753.

42. Olveira G, Tapia MJ, Ocon J, et al. Parenteral nutrition–associated hyperglycemia in non-critically ill inpatients increases the risk of in-hospital mortality (multicenter study). *Diabetes Care.* 2013;36:1061–1066.

43. Pittas AG, Siegel RD, Lau J. Insulin therapy for critically ill hospitalized patients: a meta-analysis of randomized controlled trials. *Arch Intern Med.* 2004;164(18):2005–2011.

44. Lin LY, Lin HC, Lee PC, et al. Hyperglycemia correlates with outcomes in patients receiving total parenteral nutrition. *Am J Med Sci.* 2007;333(5):261–265.

45. Cheung NW, Zaccaria Z, Napier B, Fletcher JP. Hyperglycemia is associated with adverse outcomes in patients receiving total parenteral nutrition. *Diabetes Care.* 2005;28:2367–2371.

46. Dossett LA, Cao H, Mowery NT, et al. Blood glucose variability is associated with mortality in the surgical intensive care unit. *Am Surg.* 2008;74(8):679–685.

47. Finfer S, Chittock DR, Su SY, et al. Intensive versus conventional glucose control in critically ill patients. *N Engl J Med.* 2009;360:1283–1297.

48. Kansagara D, Fu R, Freeman M, et al. Intensive insulin therapy in hospitalized patients: a systematic review. *Ann Intern Med.* 2011;154(4):268–282.

49. Umpierrez GE, Hallman R, Korytkowski MT, et al. Management of hyperglycemia in hospitalized patients in non-critical care setting: an Endocrine Society clinical practice guideline. *J Clin Endocrinol Metab.* 2012;97:16–38.

50. McMahon MM, Nystrom E, Branschweig C, Miles J, Compher C. A.S.P.E.N. clinical guidelines: nutrition support of adult patients with hyperglycemia. *JPEN J Parenter Enteral Nutr.* 2013;37:23–36.

51. Curkendall SM, Natoli JL, Alexander CM, et al. Economic and clinical impact of inpatient diabetic hypoglycemia. *Endocr Pract.* 2009;15:302–312.

52. Turchin A, Matheny ME, Shubina M, et al. Hypoglycemia and clinical outcomes in patients with diabetes hospitalized in the general ward. *Diabetes Care.* 2009;32:1153–1157.

53. Dendy JA, Chockalingam V, Tirumalasetty NN, et al. Identifying risk factors for severe hypoglycemia in hospitalized patients with diabetes. *Endocr Pract.* 2014;20:1051–1056.

54. Tomky D. Detection, prevention, and treatment of hypoglycemia in the hospital. *Diabetes Spectrum.* 2005;18:39–44.

55. Hulkower RD, Pollack RM, Zonszein J. Understanding hypoglycemia in hospitalized patients. *Diabetes Manag (Lond).* 2014;4(2):165–176.

56. Humalog prescribing information. http://www.accessdata.fda.gov/drugsatfda_docs/label/2015/020563s163lbl.pdf. Accessed December 11, 2016.

57. Goldberg PA, Kedves A, Walter K, Groszmann A, Belous A, Inzucchi SE. "Waste not, want not": determining the optimal priming volume for intravenous insulin infusions. *Diabetes Technol Ther.* 2006;8:598–601.

58. Doolin MK, Walroth TA, Harris SA, Whitten JA, Fritschle-Hilliard AC. Transition from intravenous to subcutaneous insulin in critically ill adults. *J Diabetes Sci Technol.* 2016;10(4):932–938.

59. Weant KA, Ladha A. Conversion for continuous insulin infusions to subcutaneous insulin in critically-ill patients. *Ann Pharmacother.* 2009;43:629–634.

60. A.S.P.E.N definition of terms, style, and conventions used in A.S.P.E.N. Board of Directors–approved documents. 2015. http://www.nutritioncare.org/Guidelines_and_Clinical_Resources/Clinical_Practice_Library/Special_Reports. Accessed January 18, 2017.

61. Baltzis D, Eleftheriadou I, Veves A. Pathogenesis and treatment of impaired wound healing in diabetes mellitus: new insights. *Adv Ther.* 2014;31:817–836.

62. Davis CJ, Sowa D, Keim KS. The use of prealbumin and c-reactive protein for monitoring nutrition support in adult patients receiving enteral nutrition in an urban medical center. *JPEN J Parenter Enteral Nutr.* 2012;36:197–204.

63. Frankenfield DC, Coleman A, Alam S, et al. Analysis of estimation methods for resting metabolic rate in critically ill adults. *JPEN J Parenter Enteral Nutr.* 2009;33(1):27–36.

64. Rubinson L, Diette GB, Song X, et al. Low caloric intake is associated with nosocomial bloodstream infections in patients in the medical intensive care unit. *Crit Care Med.* 2004;32:350–357.

65. National Kidney Foundation. NKF KDOQI Guidelines. 2007. http://www2.kidney.org/professionals/KDOQI/guideline_diabetes/guide5.htm. Accessed June 11, 2016.

66. National Institutes of Health Office of Dietary Supplements. Dietary Reference Intakes for energy, carbohydrate, fiber, fat, fatty acids, cholesterol, protein and amino acids (2002/2005). https://ods.od.nih.gov/Health_Information/Dietary_Reference_Intakes.aspx. Accessed June 13, 2016.

67. Layman DK, Clifton P, Gannon MC, Krauss RM, Nuttall FQ. Protein in optimal health: heart disease and type 2 diabetes. *Am J Clin Nutr.* 2008;87(Suppl):1571S–1575S.

68. US Department of Health and Human Services, US Department of Agriculture, 2015–2020 Dietary Guidelines for Americans, 8th ed. http://health.gov/dietaryguidelines/2015. Accessed June 12, 2016.

69. Sacks FM, Bray GA, Carey VJ, et al. Comparison of weight-loss diets with different compositions of fat, protein, and carbohydrates. *N Engl J Med.* 2009;360:859–873.

70. deSouza RJ, Bray GA, Carey VJ, et al. Effects of 4 weight-loss diets differing in fat, protein, and carbohydrate on fat mass, lean mass, visceral adipose tissue, and hepatic fat: results from the POUNDS LOST trial. *Am J Clin Nutr.* 2012;95:614–625.

71. Johnston BC, Kanters S, Bandayrel K, et al. Comparison of weight loss among named diet programs in overweight and obese adults: a meta-analysis. *JAMA.* 2014;312:923–933.

72. Jensen MD, Ryan DH, Apovian CM, et al; American College of Cardiology/American Heart Association Task Force on Practice Guidelines; Obesity Society. 2013 AHA/ACC/TOS guideline for the management of overweight and obesity in adults: a report of the American College of Cardiology/American Heart Association Task Force on Practice Guidelines and the Obesity Society. *J Am Coll Cardiol.* 2014;63(25 Pt B):2985–3023.

73. Franz MJ, Bantle JP, Beebe CA, et al. The evidence for medical nutrition therapy for type 1 and type 2 diabetes in adults. *J Am Diet Assoc.* 2010;110(12):1852–1889.

74. Masaoka T, Tack J. Gastroparesis: current concepts and management. *Gut Liver.* 2009;3:166–193.

75. Parkman HP, Yates KP, Hasler WL. Dietary intake and nutritional deficiencies in patients with diabetic or idiopathic gastroparesis. *Gastroenterology.* 2011;14:486–498.

76. Parrish CR, McCray S. Gastroparesis and nutrition: the art. *Pract Gastroenterol.* 2011;35(9):26–41.

77. Brown B, Roehl K, Betz M. Enteral nutrition formula selection: current evidence and implications for practice. *Nutr Clin Pract.* 2015:30:72–85.

78. Ming M, Joang B, Cui SW, Jin Z. Slowly digestible starch—a review. *Crit Rev Food Sci Nutr.* 2013;55(12):1642–1657. doi:10.1080/10408398.2012.704434.

79. Vanschoonbeek K, Lansink M, venLaere KM, et al. Slowly digestible carbohydrate sources can be used to attenuate the postprandial glycemic response to the ingestion of diabetes-specific enteral formulas. *Diabetes Educ.* 2009;35(4):631–640.

80. Elia M, Ceriello A, Laube H, et al. Enteral nutrition support and use of diabetes-specific formulas for patients with diabetes. *Diabetes Care.* 2005;28:2267–2279.

81. Pohl M, Mayr P, Mertl-Roetzer M, et al. Glycemic control in patients with type 2 diabetes mellitus with a disease-specific enteral formula: stage 2 of a randomized, controlled multicenter trial. *JPEN J Parenter Enteral Nutr.* 2009;33(1):37–49.

82. Alish CA, Garvey WT, Maki KC, et al. A diabetes-specific enteral formula improves glycemic variability in patients with type 2 diabetes. *Diabetes Technol Ther.* 2010;12(6):419–425.

83. Voss AC, Maki KC, Garvey WT, et al. Effect of two carbohydrate-modified tube-feeding formulas on metabolic responses in patients with type 2 diabetes. *Nutrition.* 2008;24:990–997.

84. Lansink M, Hofman Z, Genovese S, et al. Improved glucose profile in patients with type 2 diabetes with a new, high-protein, diabetes-specific tube feed during 4 hours of continuous feeding. *JPEN J Parenter Enteral Nutr.* 2016(Jan 29). Epub ahead of print. doi:0148607115625635.

85. Mesejo A, Montejo-Gonzalez JC, Vaquerizo-Alonso C, et al. Diabetes-specific enteral nutrition formula in hyperglycemic, mechanically ventilated critically ill patients: a prospective, open-label, blind-randomized, multicenter study. *Crit Care.* 2015;19:390.

86. Abbott Laboratories. 2015–2016 Abbott Nutrition Product References. August 2015.

87. Nestlé Health Science. 2015–2016 Product Guide. 2015.

88. US Department of Agriculture. USDA National Nutrient Database for Standard Reference Release. https://ndb.nal.usda.gov/ndb/foods?format=&sort=&fgcd=&manu=&offset=630&order=desc. Accessed July 3, 2016.

89. Ghosh D, Bhattacharya B, Mukherjee B, et al. Role of chromium supplementation in Indians with type 2 diabetes mellitus. *J Nutr Biochem.* 2002;13:690–697.

90. Robinovitz H, Friendensohn A, Leibovitz A, et al. Effects of chromium supplementation on blood glucose and lipid levels in type 2 diabetes mellitus elderly patients. *Int J Vitam Nutr Res.* 2004;74:178–182.

91. Hamdy O, Ernst FR, Baumer D, et al. Differences in resource utilization between patients with diabetes receiving glycemia-targeted specialized nutrition vs standard nutrition formulas in U.S. hospitals. *JPEN J Parenter Enteral Nutr.* 2014;38(Suppl 2):86S–91S.

92. Critical Care Nutrition. Canadian Clinical Practice Guidelines. www.criticalcarenutrition.com. Accessed May 25, 2016.

93. Baldwin D, Zander J, Munoz C, et al. A randomized trial of two weight-based doses of insulin glargine and glulisine in hospitalized subjects with type 2 diabetes and renal insufficiency. *Diabetes Care.* 2012;35:1970–1974.

94. Cook A, Burkitt D, McDonald L, Sublett L. Evaluation of glycemic control using NPH insulin sliding scale versus insulin aspart sliding scale in continuously tube-fed patients. *Nutr Clin Pract.* 2009;24(6):718–722.

95. Campbell KR, Braithwaite SS. Hospital management of hyperglycemia. *Clin Diabetes.* 2004;22:81–88.

96. Gosmanov AR, Umpierrez GE. Management of hyperglycemia during enteral and parenteral nutrition therapy. *Curr Diab Rep.* 2013;13:155–162.

97. Pasquel FJ, Spiegelman R, McCauley M, et al. Hyperglycemia during total parenteral nutrition: an important marker of poor outcome and mortality in hospitalized patients. *Diabetes Care.* 2010;33(4):739–741.

98. Yan CL, Huang YB, Chen CY, et al. Hyperglycemia is associated with poor outcomes in surgical critically ill patients receiving parenteral nutrition. *Acta Anaesthesiol Taiwanica.* 2013;5:67–72.

99. Ahrens CL, Barletta JF, Kanji S, et al. Effect of low calorie parenteral nutrition on the incidence and severity of hyperglycemia in surgical patients: a randomized, controlled trial. *Crit Care Med.* 2005;33:2507–2512.

100. Mirtallo J, Canada TW, Johnson D, et al. Safe practices for parenteral nutrition. *JPEN J Parenter Enteral Nutr.* 2004;28(6 Suppl):S39–S70.

101. Dietitians in Nutrition Support. Intravenous fat emulsion guide. *Support Line.* 2014;36(5):27–29.

102. Clement S, Braithwaite SS, Magee MF, et al. Management of diabetes and hyperglycemia in hospitals. *Diabetes Care.* 2004;27:553–591.

103. Park HR, Hansell DT, Davidson LE, et al. Management of diabetic patients requiring nutritional support. *Nutrition.* 1992;8:316.

104. Donner TW, Flammer KM. Diabetes management in the hospital. *Med Clin N Am.* 2008;92:407–425.

105. Centers for Disease Control and Prevention. Number (in thousands) of hospital discharges with diabetes as any-listed diagnosis, United States, 1988–2009. http://www.cdc.gov/diabetes/statistics/dmany/fig1.htm. Accessed July 19, 2016.

106. Robbins JM, Webb DA. Diagnosing diabetes and preventing rehospitalizations: the urban diabetes study. *Med Care.* 2006;44:292–296.

107. Kimmel B, Sullivan MM, Rushakoff RJ. Survey on transition from inpatient to outpatient for patients on insulin: what really goes on at home? *Endocr Pract.* 2010;16:785–791.

35 Obesity

Jayshil J. Patel, MD, Manpreet S. Mundi, MD, Robert G. Martindale, MD, PhD, and Ryan T. Hurt, MD, PhD

CONTENTS

Acknowledgment: Thomas H. Frazier, MD, was a coauthor for this chapter in the second edition.

Objectives

1. Define the current classification of overweight and obesity for adults.
2. Determine treatment options for obese patients in the ambulatory setting.
3. Understand bariatric surgery indications, procedures, outcomes, and complications.
4. Discuss the complexity of nutrition support in obese patients in the intensive care unit (ICU).
5. Determine the optimal enteral nutrition (EN) support for obese patients in the ICU.

Test Your Knowledge Questions

1. Which of the following statements regarding the current World Health Organization (WHO) and National Institutes of Health (NIH) classification of overweight and obesity is true?
   A. Overweight is defined as a body mass index (BMI) of 25 to 29.9, and obesity is defined as BMI equal to or greater than 30.
   B. Obesity is defined as equal to or greater than 120% ideal body weight (IBW).
   C. Obesity is defined as body fat equal to or greater than 20% of body weight for men and equal to or greater than 30% for women.
   D. Obesity is defined as a BMI greater than 25, and morbid obesity is defined as a BMI greater than 30.
2. Which of the following is a criterion for selecting patients to undergo gastric bypass surgery?
   A. BMI greater than 35 and no history of substance abuse or psychiatric disorders
   B. BMI equal to or greater than 35 and obesity-associated comorbidities
   C. BMI equal to or greater than 30 and obesity-associated comorbidities
   D. BMI equal to or greater than 30 and inability to achieve weight control with low-calorie diets
3. According to the most recent (2016) American Society for Parenteral and Enteral Nutrition (ASPEN) and Society of Critical Care Medicine (SCCM) guidelines, what is the enteral feeding strategy based on energy requirements for obese patients?
   A. Hypocaloric with normal protein
   B. Hypocaloric with low protein
   C. Hypocaloric with high protein
   D. Hypercaloric with high protein
4. What is the most accurate way to determine energy requirements for obese patients in the ICU requiring EN support?
   A. The Harris-Benedict equation
   B. Indirect calorimetry (IC)
   C. The Mifflin–St. Jeor equation
   D. The Penn State equation

Test Your Knowledge Answers

1. The correct answer is **A**. WHO and NIH currently use BMI to classify overweight and obesity in adults, in contrast to prior use of IBW or percent body fat. Use of BMI is encouraged because it provides a standardized method for expressing weight relatively independent of height and correlates reasonably well with body fat as well as mortality. Although BMI does not always accurately reflect excess body fat (eg, when ascites or edema is present), it represents a simple and reproducible method for categorizing weight.

2. The correct answer is **B**. Patients are candidates for gastric bypass surgery if they have a BMI equal to or greater than 40. Individuals are also candidates if their BMI is equal to or greater than 35 and they have weight-related comorbidities and more conservative efforts have not resulted in adequate weight control. Patients without weight-related comorbid conditions may be candidates for surgery; indeed, some advocates of surgical treatment suggest that surgery is best performed before lasting health problems or surgical risks are present. Patients with active bulimia, active substance abuse, or major disturbances of thought or mood should be evaluated carefully and treated for these issues before surgery.

3. The correct answer is **C**. The ASPEN/SCCM guidelines recommend high-protein, hypocaloric feeding (grade D). The guidelines suggest that for obese patients (BMI greater than 30), the goal of the EN regimen should not exceed 60% to 70% of target energy requirements. Estimated protein requirements may be 2.0 g/kg IBW/d for patients with class I or class II obesity, and 2.5 g/kg IBW/d for patients with class III obesity.

4. The correct answer is **B**. Various equations (Harris-Benedict, Penn State, and Mifflin–St. Jeor) have been widely used to predict resting metabolic rate, but most predictive equations were validated in patients without extremes of weight or age. Overestimation of total energy requirements when using actual body weight (ABW) and underestimation when using the IBW lead to inadvertent overfeeding and underfeeding, respectively. Efforts to account for altered body composition with these equations by using corrections for ABW have led to even more confusion. For these reasons, IC should be used, when available, to determine the energy requirements of critically ill obese patients.

Introduction

Obesity is becoming the leading cause of preventable death in the United States. The incidence of obesity in adults in the United States has doubled over the past 30 years. Approximately 70% of adults in the United States are considered overweight, and more than 35% are considered obese.[1,2] The overall healthcare burden for obesity in the United States is conservatively estimated to be approximately $150 billion per year.[2,3] In addition, obesity is emerging as a global epidemic with worldwide health consequences. Obesity has more than 60 associated comorbid medical conditions, including 12 different types of cancer.[4] Obesity-associated medical conditions, such as type 2 diabetes mellitus, hypertension, coronary artery disease, nonalcoholic fatty liver disease (NAFLD), and obstructive sleep apnea, can complicate management in both the ambulatory and the ICU settings.

Both clinical settings present unique challenges for nutrition specialists treating obesity and its associated comorbidities.

Defining Obesity

The WHO and NIH use BMI to classify obesity. The recommended classifications are as follows:[5]
- Underweight: BMI equal to or less than 18.49
- Normal weight: BMI from 18.5 to 24.9
- Overweight: BMI from 25 to 29.9
- Obesity class I: BMI from 30 to 34.9
- Obesity class II: BMI from 35 to 39.9
- Obesity class III: BMI equal to or greater than 40

Furthermore, BMI equal to or greater than 50 is considered *superobesity*.

Waist circumference (WC) is another variable that can predict risk associated with adiposity and is a surrogate for organ fat (visceral). Assessment of WC is most useful when performed in individuals with a BMI between 25 and 35. Elevated WC (women: greater than 88 cm; men: greater than 102 cm) in these BMI classifications increases health risk when compared with BMI alone.[6]

Obesity Epidemiology

As noted earlier, the number of overweight and obese adults has steadily increased in the past 30 years.[2,7,8] The percentage of US adults classified as obese or overweight has risen from 45% in 1962 to almost 70% in 2014.[2,7–9] This increase is predominately associated with the rise in prevalence of obesity, as the number of overweight (but not obese) individuals remained relatively stable during this period.[2] The prevalence of adult obesity rose rapidly between 1980 and 2004 (from 15% to 33% of the US population), doubling the prevalence in 25 years.[2] In the past 10 years, the overall adult prevalence of obesity has been estimated to be 37.7%, which suggests that the rate of increase in the prevalence of overweight and obesity has recently leveled off.[7,9] These data might lead some to conclude that the epidemic is stabilizing. However, one needs to consider that with 70% of the adult population being classified as overweight, only a limited number of individuals are left. Furthermore, recent animal and human evidence involving the genetics of obesity suggest that a proportion of the population may be resistant to obesity and its related complications.[10,11]

Although the overall prevalence of obesity has leveled off, the prevalence of obesity class III has increased disproportionately, from 0.9% in 1960 to 7.7% in 2014.[2,9] Within obesity class III, the percentage of individuals with a BMI equal to or greater than 50 has increased at a faster rate than all other obesity groups. Approximately 1.5 million adults in the United States have a BMI equal to or greater than 50.

Obesity is clearly a global epidemic. The WHO has recognized the increased worldwide prevalence of obesity and the global implications caused by this trend. Obesity and overweight are among the top 10 leading causes of global mortality.[12] In North America, Central America, South America, Western Europe, the Middle East, and Eastern Europe, the combined prevalence of overweight (BMI between 25 and

29.9) and obesity (BMI equal to or greater than 30) is 40% or greater among individuals ages 45 to 59 years.[13] Asian nations have reported lower rates of obesity using the WHO classification, but the use of this classification in Asian populations may be problematic because of cultural and ethnic variability in the relationship between BMI and the amount of body fat as well as in adipose distribution.[14] In these Asian nations, rates of type 2 diabetes mellitus and cardiovascular disease (CVD) are increased at BMIs less than the WHO cutoff for overweight (BMI equal to or greater than 25), which is most likely related to proportionate increases in body fat percentage compared with other ethnicities and races.[15,16]

Obesity Genetics

The variation in prevalence of obesity observed among different races suggests a genetic role. Many diseases and medical conditions involve a complex interplay of genetic, developmental, environmental, and behavioral factors. The most commonly recognized heterogeneous disease is cancer. There are many different types of cancer, different environmental influences, various mechanisms of action, and variable responses to a wide range of treatments. Like cancer, obesity is a complex, heterogeneous disease that is associated with many conditions and involves numerous subtypes. Obese individuals often have associated conditions such as diabetes, atherosclerosis, hypertension, hyperlipidemia, and obstructive sleep apnea, to name only a few. The body sites where obese individuals carry the extra adiposity, such as around the abdomen, hips, buttocks, and organs, are highly variable. Some obese individuals have strong food cravings, but others do not—which suggests differences in the neuroendocrine control over appetite regulation.[17,18] This complex, heterogeneous nature of obesity makes finding treatments difficult and often frustrating for healthcare professionals and patients alike. Interactions between gene environment and gene behavior are critical to understanding the heterogeneity of obesity and developing potential targeted therapies.[19,20]

There are some rare monogenic causes of obesity. For example, 25 genetic syndromes (such as Prader Willi and Alstrom syndromes) have obesity as a central feature of the disorder.[21] Furthermore, a number of mutations in genes cause nonsyndromic monogenic forms of obesity.[21,22] These mutations are located in genes that affect leptin and leptin receptors and in the hypothalamic proopiomelanocortin (POMC) and melanocortin-4 receptor (MC4R) genes.[22] Mutations in these genes have been well studied in rodent models, and the phenotypes compared with humans are similar in most cases.[21] Leptin deficiency has been successfully addressed with directed therapy, specifically recombinant leptin.[22] In children treated with recombinant leptin, food ingestion ceased to be the focus of daily activity, and weight loss was significant. These monogenic diseases account for only a small fraction of the obesity cases. Most cases are polygenic.[23]

Polygenic obesity is the result of a group of a gene variants (alleles) that have an influence on body weight.[23] These polygenic variants are presumably associated with most cases of obesity.[23] More than 30 polygenic variants are currently recognized as potential contributors to weight regulation.[24,25] Recent advances in molecular techniques have provided the tools to perform genome-wide association studies (GWASs). These GWASs have a greater ability to detect polygenic variants, and advances in chip technology have made high-density, single-nucleotide polymorphism GWASs possible.[23,24] The first 2 gene variants to be discovered using GWASs were the MC4R and fat mass– and obesity-associated (FTO) genes.[26,27] One GWAS evaluated the combined contribution of MC4R and FTO in a European population and found the combined polymorphisms were additive in obesity and type 2 diabetes mellitus.[24] Another GWAS correlating single-nucleotide polymorphisms of 249,796 subjects with BMI confirmed 14 previous known loci and 18 new loci associated with elevated BMI.[25] Many genes associated with obesity have undoubtedly not yet been identified.

Environmental Factors

Genetics alone cannot explain the recent obesity epidemic. Our "obesogenic" environment provides increased opportunities for obtaining low-cost, energy-dense foods and decreased opportunity and need for physical activity. Access to energy-dense foods (as opposed to access to food in general) has likely contributed to the increased obesity rates observed during the past 30 years. The genetic predisposition toward obesity combined with the exposure to energy-dense foods could be one of the major driving factors of the current obesity epidemic.[28] Numerous factors have led to increased availability of energy-dense foods and decreased opportunity for physical activity. A 4-year large prospective cohort analysis (120,877 patients) found that, on average, participants gained 3.35 pounds. Based on daily servings, this 4-year weight gain was most associated with intake of potato chips, potatoes, fries, processed meats, and sugar-sweetened beverages. Consumption of vegetables, fruits, nuts, whole grains, and yogurt, and increased physical activity were inversely associated with weight gain.[29] Energy-dense foods, such as potato chips, potatoes, fries, processed meats, and sugar-sweetened beverages, provide "empty calories" with little nutritional value. Food additives such as high-fructose corn syrup and *trans* fatty acids have been linked with obesity-associated conditions such as metabolic syndrome, dyslipidemia, and NAFLD.[30–34] However, the role of these additives in the development of the obesity epidemic is debated, and clinicians should therefore focus on overall reduction of fats and excess sugars from diets.[35–46]

Decreased physical activity is the other major component of the obesogenic environment. Williamson and colleagues evaluated self-reported levels of physical activity and weight change in a 10-year study of a US cohort.[47] Individuals who reported low physical activity at the follow-up (10 years) were more likely to have had a major weight gain (greater than 13 kg) than other individuals who reported medium or high levels of physical activity.[47] A prospective study measured 24-hour energy expenditure and subsequent weight gain in 95 adult subjects.[48] In a 2-year period, subjects with low 24-hour energy expenditure (200 kcal below predicted values) were 4 times more likely to gain significant weight (equal to or greater than 7.5 kg) than subjects with high 24-hour energy expenditure (200 kcal above predicted values).[48] These studies support the notion that elements of the recent obesogenic environment

(including energy-dense food and decreased physical activity) combined with the genetic predisposition to develop obesity have been major factors in the obesity epidemic.

Obesity Neuroendocrine Pathophysiology

The pathophysiology of obesity is complex because of the heterogeneous nature of the disease. The laws of thermodynamics as applied to obesity dictate that energy intake must be greater than energy expenditure to increase body fat. The neuroendocrine response and obesity-induced inflammation and its metabolic consequences (eg, NAFLD, type 2 diabetes mellitus, dyslipidemia) further complicate our understanding of obesity and its treatment and consequences.

The central nervous system (CNS) receives information from several regulatory loops that help control energy balance.[17,18] The brain gets information about metabolic need from the most metabolically active tissues, including adipose tissue, liver, stomach, muscle, and bone. Furthermore, the CNS gets information about current energy availability in the environment through the sensory organs and primarily through the stomach, small intestine, pancreas, and liver.

Central controls influence food intake, and energy expenditure can be divided into satiation/satiety signals and "adiposity" hormones.[18] Satiety signals such as cholecystokinin (CCK), ghrelin, peptide tyrosine-tyrosine (PYY), and glucagon-like peptide-1 (GLP-1) result in feelings of fullness, which contribute to cessation of food intake (satiation) and suppression of appetite after meal intake (satiety).[18] "Adiposity" hormones are secreted not in response to a meal, but instead as a result of the amount of adipose tissue present in the host organism. Both satiety/satiation signals and adiposity hormones represent a complex messaging system between the CNS and peripheral nervous system that influence energy homeostasis and intake. In addition to the aforementioned mechanisms, many of these molecules (eg, leptin) are also important to the maladaptive obesity-induced inflammation and its resultant complications.[49]

As macronutrients are consumed, satiety/satiation signals result in a message delivered to the CNS. CCK is secreted from I cells (mucosal epithelial cells in the small intestine) in response to fat and protein as they pass into the duodenum. CCK then influences various gastrointestinal (GI) mechanisms, such as motility, gastric acid secretion, pancreatic enzyme secretion, and contraction of the gallbladder.[50] However, CCK produces satiation signaling through a paracrine mechanism via vagal sensory nerves.[51] These signals are relayed to the dorsal medial hindbrain and result in CCK-induced satiation.[52]

Another satiation signal, PYY, is released by intestinal L cells lining the distal small intestine and colon.[53] PYY is released in response to meals, and serum levels rise rapidly even before the meal reaches the distal small intestine or colon, suggesting an indirect neuronal reflex.[54,55] Subsequent sustained circulating levels of PYY are thought to be caused by direct stimulation of L cells by dietary fat.[56] The anorexigenic activity of PYY has been attributed to the expression of neuropeptide Y_2 receptors in neurons of the arcuate nucleus in the hypothalamus.[53,57] In addition, PYY can decrease motility and influence electrolyte absorption in the colon.[58]

In opposition to CCK and PYY, ghrelin is a potent orexigenic agent that stimulates food intake.[59] In response to fasting, specific endocrine cells in the stomach and duodenum release ghrelin, which seems to have several actions, including acting directly on receptors in the hypothalamus to increase hunger. Actions in the hypothalamus then result in compensatory stimulation of appetite.[59,60] Another major effect of ghrelin is its stimulation of growth hormone release.[61] Following diet and exercise-induced weight loss, serum concentrations of ghrelin increase.[62,63] These compensatory changes may partially explain why weight loss is difficult to maintain over the long term.

Intestinal L cells located predominantly in the ileum and colon are triggered to produce GLP-1. While our understanding of this process is not complete, there seems to be neural, nutrient, and endocrine control of GLP-1 release.[64] The peripheral actions of GLP-1 are numerous and include stimulation of insulin release, glucagon secretion inhibition, inhibition of GI motility and secretions, anorectic actions, and others. Central actions of GLP-1 include reducing food intake via energy-homeostatic circuits in the hypothalamus and eliciting symptoms of stress in the amygdala.[65-68] Both animal models and human studies have shown the satiation actions of GLP-1 stemming from the variety of aforementioned mechanisms.[65,69,70] These actions are further demonstrated with long-acting GLP-1 pharmacotherapy for diabetes mellitus, which not only results in improvement in glucose control but can also lead to meaningful weight loss.[71]

Several other satiation-/satiety-signaling molecules, such as glicentin, glucagon-like peptide-2 (GLP-2), glucagon, and enterostatin, have been described.[17] Whereas satiation signals depend on the intake of nutrients, "adiposity" signals are directly related to the amount of body fat present in the host organism.[17] As a result of these contrasting control mechanisms, satiation signaling is a phasic response, whereas "adiposity" signaling is a tonic phenomenon. Both insulin and leptin are classically recognized as "adiposity" signals.[17] Pancreatic beta cells and white adipose tissue release insulin and leptin, respectively, in response to the amount of body fat present. These hormones then act centrally on the hypothalamus to influence energy homeostasis, resulting in decreased food intake and weight loss. The use of hormones such as leptin for the treatment of obesity is confounded by the development of resistance, as well as by their multiple, often intolerable actions that are not directly related to weight loss.[17] In addition to controlling appetite, leptin plays a role in both innate and adaptive inflammatory responses. Leptin increases the production of proinflammatory cytokines from macrophages.[49] The neuroendocrine pathophysiology is complex, incompletely understood, and further complicated when the more than 60 recognized obesity-associated conditions are considered. See Chapter 1 for further discussion of nutrient intake, digestion, absorption, and excretion.

Comorbidities of Obesity

Numerous epidemiologic studies have identified a clear association between obesity and various diseases and comorbidities. The Third National Health and Nutrition Examination survey (NHANES III) studied 16,884 adults, age 25 years and older with BMI equal to or greater than 25, and it revealed a graded increase in prevalence ratio of type 2 diabetes, gallbladder disease, high blood pressure, and osteoarthritis with increasing severity of overweight and obesity.[72] When comparing patients with class III obesity with normal weight individuals, the prevalence ratio of type 2 diabetes was 18.1 (95% confidence interval [CI], 6.7–46.8) in men and 12.9 (CI, 5.7–28.1) in women. Furthermore, obesity is associated with at least 12 types of cancers, including postmenopausal breast cancer, colon cancer, esophageal cancer, and renal cancer.[73] See Chapter 33 for additional information on cancer rates and etiologies.

The relationship between obesity and mortality is striking.[46,73-75] Numerous large epidemiologic studies have found that obesity is associated with increased all-cause mortality,[73,74] as well as cause-specific mortality, including ischemic heart disease, diabetes, and respiratory disease.[76] In the Prospective Studies Collaboration, 57 prospective studies with approximately 900,000 subjects were analyzed for all-cause and cause-specific mortality according to BMI.[76] All-cause mortality was increased by approximately 30% in obese subjects compared with normal weight individuals.[76] Cause-specific mortality for increased BMI included 40% for vascular mortality; 60% to 120% for diabetic, renal, and hepatic mortality; and 20% for respiratory causes.[76] Median survival for subjects with class I obesity was reduced by 2 to 4 years. In subjects with class III obesity, median survival was reduced by 8 to 10 years, which is similar to the reduction of median survival observed in smokers.[76]

Although data clearly demonstrate that obesity is generally associated with increased prevalence of comorbidities and mortality, some individuals who are obese have normal to high levels of insulin sensitivity and favorable cardiovascular risk profiles, including low triglyceride and elevated high-density lipoprotein levels, and some individuals are metabolically unhealthy but of normal weight (MUNW).[77] Individuals in the metabolically healthy obese (MHO) group tend to share certain phenotypes, including distribution of body fat that favors decreased visceral fat.[78,79] In fact, Messier et al has noted that MHO postmenopausal women tended to have approximately 50% less visceral fat when compared with metabolically unhealthy obese (MUO) women with equivalent BMI, WC, and fat mass.[80] On the other hand, MUNW individuals tend to have a larger visceral fat area, higher triglyceride levels, lower high-density lipoprotein levels, and greater insulin resistance.[78,81]

In addition to increased visceral fat, other factors being evaluated to explain the relationship between obesity and comorbidities include adipose tissue hypertrophy and ectopic fat distribution. Hypertrophic obesity is associated with an increased size of existing adipocytes (as opposed to hyperplastic obesity, which involves an increased number of adipocytes). Hypertrophic obesity has been associated with increased inflammation, adipokine dysregulation, and insulin resistance and type 2 diabetes.[82] MUNW individuals tend to have increased adipocyte hypertrophy, especially in visceral adipose tissue; in contrast, MHO individuals were noted to have approximately 15% smaller adipocytes than their MUO counterparts.[83,84] Ectopic fat (the accumulation of fat in tissue such as the liver, skeletal muscle, and pancreas) may also contribute obesity-related comorbidities. Studies have found that MHO individuals tend to have lower ectopic fat accumulation compared with their MUO counterparts.[85]

Ambulatory Obese Patients

Initial Clinical Evaluation

The initial steps in diagnosing and treating an overweight or obese patient are to calculate BMI, measure WC in those whose BMI is between 25 and 35, and classify the patient's weight status.[86] Further assessment of obesity should address the presence of comorbid conditions, such as CVD, hypertension, dyslipidemia, and sleep apnea, as well as tobacco use. Patients are candidates for weight loss if they are classified as obese, or if they are overweight with increased WC (greater than 88 cm for women, greater than 102 cm for men) and have 2 or more risk factors for CVD or diabetes. Overweight patients without associated risk are also candidates for weight loss if they are motivated, whereas those who are not motivated to lose weight can be counseled to maintain weight. Assessment of motivation is important because patients who are not self-motivated sometimes request obesity treatment in response to family or health care provider concern.

The goals of obesity treatment are to achieve and sustain weight loss and to reduce health risk. A reasonable initial goal is loss of 10% of initial weight within 6 months. The rationale for this recommendation is based on multiple trials of weight loss in which participants lost an average of 6% to 8% of their initial weight within approximately 6 months, after which weight loss became more difficult.[87] In obese adults with cardiovascular risk factors, sustained weight loss of just 3% can produce meaningful health benefits.[2] Patients may possibly lose more than 10% of initial weight, but these larger weight losses are less likely to be sustained. After a patient loses 10% of initial weight, efforts should focus on weight maintenance. If more than 10% weight loss is desired, motivated patients can restart the process of losing weight after a 6-month period of weight maintenance.

Many patients will want to lose more than 10% of their initial weight, and they may want to achieve their goal in less than 6 months. Such goals are often unrealistic and may lead to patients failing in their attempts to sustain weight loss over the long term. Patients should be counseled about the benefits of smaller amounts of weight loss that are realistic to maintain. Modest weight loss (eg, 5% to 15% of initial weight) improves glucose tolerance, decreases fasting blood glucose levels and hyperinsulinemia, improves serum lipid concentrations, reduces blood pressure, and improves sleep apnea.[88-91] Gradual weight loss is more likely to promote development of skills that improve long-term weight maintenance, whereas rapid weight loss is less likely to be maintained. Repeated cycles of weight loss and gain are associated with negative health and psychological effects, and the effort, time, and expense of these cycles further justify modest goals for weight loss and maintenance.[87,92] Furthermore, recidivism and cycling of weight loss with weight gain may alter body composition,

ultimately decreasing lean body mass (LBM) and increasing body fat mass.

Weight Loss Methods

An essential part of weight loss is negative energy balance—energy expenditure exceeds energy intake. Thus, effective weight loss strategies must address decreasing intake of food, increasing output of energy, or both. Other factors involved in effective weight loss include behavioral factors. Combining behavior strategies with decreased intake of food and increased activity will lead to the most effective weight loss strategy. This combined strategy is called *lifestyle intervention* and has been used successfully in patients with diabetes and/or obesity.[93-95]

Diet

Diets popularly promoted for weight loss number in the hundreds or more, and Americans spend close to $40 billion annually on weight loss products.[96] No specific weight loss strategy has consistently been shown to both safely reduce weight and result in long-term weight maintenance for most participants. Regardless of the composition of the diet, negative energy balance induced by decreases in intake will reduce weight, and the differences in lost weight and body composition associated with specific diets are generally small compared with the overall effect of reducing intake.[97] In one study, 811 overweight and obese subjects were randomly assigned for 2 years to 1 of 4 energy-reduction strategies that varied in percentages of energy derived from fat, protein, and carbohydrate. After 6 months, the amount of weight lost by participants was comparable in all groups. The average weight loss at 2 years was 4 kg, and measurements of satiety, hunger, and satisfaction with the diet were the same for the 4 groups.[97] This study emphasizes the importance of reduced energy intake to help create a negative energy balance, regardless of the diet strategy and macronutrient composition used.

Low-Calorie Diets

Energy intake to a lower limit of 800 kcal/d is considered a low-calorie diet. Weight loss on a low-calorie diet is typically 0.5 to 1 kg/wk, although the relationship between the level of energy intake and weight lost depends on multiple factors, including the individual's degree of obesity, level of activity, gender, and age. Most obese patients will lose weight when consuming between 1000 and 1500 kcal/d.[98]

The ideal macronutrient composition and meal pattern of a low-calorie diet remains controversial. Patients who limit dietary fat without also decreasing energy intake are unlikely to lose weight. There is no scientific evidence that low-calorie diets should routinely be very low in fat (less than 20% of energy from fat), very low in carbohydrate (less than 100 g/d), or very high in protein (more than 130 g/d). Studies comparing diets with variable carbohydrate and fat content have found minor differences in weight loss at 6 months, but no significant weight differences at 12 to 24 months.[99,100]

Diets can be structured around portion size, energy or fat intake, or other constructs. Structuring a diet and lifestyle plan must be a joint effort between the patient and the clinician. An inflexible, clinician-driven plan that is not developed with consideration of the patient's lifestyle and psychology may result in short-term weight loss but is unlikely to be effective long term. Low-calorie diets offer the advantage of sustainability over longer periods of time and can be adapted to a wide range of lifestyles. Low-calorie diets based on commonly consumed foods may be preferable to specialized or commercial diets because the former are less expensive and easier to obtain. However, commercial plans and prepared foods may offer structure and convenience, decrease the need for planning, and limit choice in high-risk situations.

Energy intake on a low-calorie diet is theoretically at a level where the food consumed can provide adequate micronutrients without need for supplementation. However, the consumption of micronutrient-rich foods will vary from individual to individual, and micronutrient reference intakes are not established specifically for those who are consuming hypocaloric diets. Therefore, it is reasonable to recommend a standard multivitamin to patients who use a low-calorie or very-low-calorie diet. Individuals consuming few dairy products may require calcium supplementation.

Patients on low-calorie diets generally require minimal medical monitoring because the rate of weight loss and diet quality do not predispose them to serious complications. However, patients on medications for hypertension, diabetes, and other conditions should be monitored to assess the need for medication adjustments with reduced energy intake and weight loss.

Very-Low-Calorie Diets

Very-low-calorie diets typically contain 400 to 800 kcal/d, but decreases in energy intake below 800 kcal/d are associated with little additional weight loss, perhaps because of diminished compliance and/or decreased resting energy expenditure. Protein intake usually ranges from 70 to 100 g/d. Very-low-calorie diets can be based on liquid products or on consumption of lean meat, fish, or poultry supplemented with micronutrients. Weight losses are in the range of 2 kg/wk. Weight lost by very-low-calorie diets is more rapid and can be greater over time than that achieved by low-calorie diets. Long-term maintenance of weight lost by very-low-calorie diets has not been superior to that of low-calorie diets,[101] although a meta-analysis suggests that very-low-calorie diets may have a modest long-term advantage.[102] Medical monitoring (preferably weekly and not less frequently than every 2 weeks) is necessary because of risks of electrolyte abnormalities, dehydration, gallstone formation, cardiac arrhythmia, and other complications.[101]

Because low-calorie diets promote a similar longer-term outcome without the health risks and necessary monitoring of very-low-calorie diets, low-calorie diets are preferred for most patients. However, a very-low-calorie diet might be considered in several circumstances. Poorly controlled comorbid conditions may respond favorably to a period of rapid weight loss. Patients who are unable to achieve weight goals on a low-calorie-diet may benefit from a very-low-calorie diet, perhaps because of the increased structure of the diet and frequency of clinical monitoring, which both promote compliance.

Weight loss before semielective or elective surgery is often recommended to reduce postoperative morbidity, and a very-low-calorie diet can be considered if a 10% reduction over 6 months is consistent with need for surgery.[103-105]

Physical Activity

Physical activity expends energy, promotes a sense of well-being, maintains or increases LBM, and improves several obesity-related comorbid conditions. However, increasing physical activity is unlikely to result in significant weight loss without a concomitant decrease in energy intake. A meta-analysis of weight loss trials suggests that a hypocaloric diet plus exercise does not lead to significantly more weight loss than the diet alone.[106] However, exercising during weight loss promotes preservation of LBM,[107] and exercise can help prevent weight gain after successful weight loss from dieting. A meta-analysis compared exercise, exercise plus diet, and diet alone on weight gain.[108] Over the course of 15 weeks, weight loss in the exercise-only group was 2.9 kg, compared with weight loss of 10.7 kg in the diet-only group. The weight loss that occurred by combining diet with exercise was not significantly different from that seen with diet alone. At 1-year follow-up, however, the diet-plus-exercise group had maintained the weight loss better than the diet-only group (mean 8.6 ± 0.8 kg vs 6.6 ± 0.5 kg total weight lost).[108] Other studies have confirmed that use of exercise alone usually leads to only a small amount of weight loss and that the more important role of physical activity is maintaining the weight loss after a successful diet program.[109,110]

A plea for patients to increase activity without specific objectives is often met with little and short-lived success. Thus, a realistic and detailed exercise prescription is often useful. An exercise plan should start very slowly, with consideration of the patient's existing capacity for activity. For example, individuals with a BMI exceeding 40 may have severely limited capacities and may experience fatigue dyspnea or joint pain after walking short distances. For such patients, an effective plan might focus on increasing the frequency of small amounts of physical activity, allow for frequent breaks, and find creative ways to promote movement. Creative exercise regimens include chair exercises, water aerobics, and walking in the shallow end of a pool, all of which facilitate exercise among those with pain in weight-bearing joints.

Structured exercise programs offer education, some degree of supervision, and a social environment. However, time constraints, cost, and other factors can discourage patients from participation in structured programs. Two recent trials have evaluated the effects of structured exercise compared with increases in lifestyle-based activity and have reported that both interventions were associated with comparable beneficial effects on blood pressure, blood lipids, and fitness.[111,112] Thus, patients who do not participate in structured exercise should be encouraged to incorporate physical activity as part of a lifestyle intervention.

Self-Monitoring

Self-monitoring of activity and energy intake can be part of a behavioral weight loss program. Historically, self-monitoring techniques have included written food and activity diaries.[113] With the introduction of the Internet, personal computers, wearable devices, and smart phone applications, the process of recording nutrition and activity data has become less time-consuming. A meta-analysis of 22 studies (1993–2009) that evaluated the relationship between self-monitoring and weight loss found a significant association between self-monitoring and weight loss; however, the authors noted the limited demographics (most participants were white women) and reliance on self-report as significant limitations of the studies.[113]

A recent randomized clinical trial (RCT) evaluated a wearable technology–enhanced intervention vs a standard behavioral intervention for weight loss.[114] The 471 adult participants (BMI 25 to 40) were placed on an energy-restricted diet, given an increased physical activity prescription, and offered group counseling sessions. After 6 months, phone counseling, text message prompts, and access to online resources were added.[114] At the end of 12 months, participants were randomly assigned to receive continued support through self-monitoring of diet and physical activity online (standard intervention; n = 233) vs being provided with a wearable device with online interface to self-monitor diet and physical activity (enhanced intervention; n = 237).[114] Participants were followed for another 12 months (24 months total from baseline), with the primary outcome being changes in weight at the end of the study period. The participants in the standard group had more weight loss (2.4 kg; 95% CI, 1.0–3.7; $P = 0.02$) than the enhanced group. Both groups had significant improvements in body composition, physical activity, fitness, and diet from baseline, with no differences between the groups.[114] Notably, both groups were able to self-monitor but used different methods (wearable device vs online).[114] We continue to recommend that overweight and obese patients self-monitor with the method of their choice and that these logs be reviewed with clinicians on a regular basis.

Behavioral Treatment

Eating and exercising are ultimately behaviors. Many patients have excellent knowledge of good dietary choices and the need for activity, and yet they cannot put this knowledge into practice. Several trials have demonstrated that behavioral treatment increases efficacy of dietary and pharmacological interventions.[93,115] The first step in behavioral treatment is to set realistic goals for the proposed lifestyle intervention (eg, lose 5% to 10% of initial weight in the first year). The patient should set a specific date to initiate the lifestyle intervention. Counselors and clinicians can help the patient realize that excessive weight is usually gained over a period of years and will require extended time and commitment to lose; this guidance may help prevent patients from having unrealistic weight loss expectations. Despite these discussions at the beginning of a lifestyle intervention, many patients will have unrealistic expectations. In a trial of sibutramine reported in 2003, 53 obese subjects were told they could expect to lose 5% to 15% of their initial weight in the first year.[116] However, the subjects expected to lose 28% of their initial weight and they continued to hold this unrealistic weight loss expectation during the trial. (In 2010, the US Food and Drug Administration [FDA] withdrew approval for sibutramine due to concerns about serious adverse effects.[117]) Patients who do not meet their expectations during a lifestyle intervention may feel frustrated and become discouraged about pursuing future interventions.

Ongoing behavioral treatment focuses on several key issues, including self-monitoring, stimulus control, and relapse prevention.[94] Self-monitoring is necessary to identify maladaptive behaviors and elevate the patient's level of awareness about behaviors. Food diaries and activity records should be used as part of behavioral treatment. Patients should record everything they eat, noting the calories consumed and the situations in which they are eating. Numerous smart phone and computer applications make these tasks simple. *Stimulus control* refers to identifying and restructuring environmental factors (such as television, phones, and reading materials) associated with maladaptive behavior and providing alternative responses to these stimuli. Patients should be encouraged to turn off the television and phones during mealtimes. Placing fresh fruits, vegetables, and low-calorie foods in prominent positions, such as in the front of the refrigerator or on the counter, can help control stimuli that contribute to overeating. Relapse control entails development of strategies to prevent relapse or limit the extent of relapse when it occurs. Frequent reinforcement of the lifestyle intervention and encouragement from the clinician can help when relapse occurs.[94]

In an RCT of 390 obese adults, Wadden and colleagues found that an enhanced lifestyle intervention helped approximately one-third of the subjects maintain meaningful weight loss at 2 years.[118] The enhanced lifestyle consisted of quarterly visits with a primary care physician as well as brief monthly sessions with lifestyle coaches who instructed participants about behavioral weight control. In addition, patients in the enhanced lifestyle group were given meal replacements or weight loss medications (orlistat or sibutramine). Enhanced lifestyle counseling was superior to usual care for both short- and long-term weight loss.

Behavioral treatment can be provided to individual patients (as in the RCT reported by Wadden et al[118]) or in groups. Group interventions may be more cost-effective and provide additional social support.

Pharmacological Treatment

Obese individuals should initially attempt to lose weight by nonpharmacological means. If they do not achieve weight goals, the use of medication in addition to diet and lifestyle changes may be an option. Drug therapy can be considered in those with a BMI equal to or greater than 30, or in those with existing comorbid conditions and BMI equal to or greater than 27.[119] These criteria reflect the increased risk of weight-related disease associated with these BMIs.

Medications currently available for the treatment of obesity have a demonstrated favorable impact on weight loss and weight maintenance after weight loss. Use of these medications is associated with greater average losses and greater maintenance of lost weight, and patients who take them are more likely to lose 5%, 10%, 15%, or more of their initial weight. Pharmacological therapy may augment weight loss in patients who responded partially to dietary and lifestyle interventions, and it may also help those who did not respond at all to nonpharmacological treatment. The use of medications does not generally alter weight loss goals, which remain between 5% and 10% of initial weight. Patients need to understand that medications serve only as an adjunct to dietary and lifestyle changes.

Several pharmacotherapy agents are currently approved by the FDA for long-term (12 weeks or longer) weight loss (Table 35-1). In a 2016 meta-analysis, Khera and coauthors evaluated the effectiveness of these long-term medications in 29,018 patients from 28 RCTs.[120] The meta-analysis found that orlistat—a GI lipase inhibitor available in both prescription and over-the-counter formulas that prevents absorption of dietary triglycerides and eventual utilization of free fatty acids—had a 2.6 kg weight loss (95% CI, –3.04 to –2.16 kg) compared with placebo at 1 year. Phentermine-topiramate and naltrexone-bupropion are combinations of older medications. In the meta-analysis by Khera and colleagues, subjects who took phentermine-topiramate had the greatest weight loss compared with placebo at 1 year (–8.8 kg; 95% CI, –10.2 to –7.42 kg), but it also had the highest odds of adverse event–related discontinuation.[120] The meta-analysis concluded that naltrexone-bupropion was associated with less weight loss compared with placebo at 1 year (–5.0 kg; 95% CI, –5.94 to –3.96 kg), as well as fewer adverse effects. Liraglutide is a GLP-1 agonist that leads to increased insulin secretion. It has been used in patients with diabetes and was recently approved for weight loss in obesity. In the meta-analysis by Khera et al, weight loss in subjects who took liraglutide was greater at 1 year compared with placebo (–5.6 kg; 95% CI, –6.06 to –4.52 kg), but, like naltrexone-bupropion, liraglutide was associated with higher rates of adverse event–related discontinuation. The final long-term, FDA-approved drug for obesity is lorcaserin, a serotonin receptor (selective 5HT$_2$c) agonist. Khera and associates found that the weight loss for this monotherapy was 3.2 kg (95% CI, –3.97 to –2.46 kg) at 1 year compared with placebo.[120]

Phentermine monotherapy has been approved for short-term weight loss (12 weeks or less) and was half of the medication phentermine-fenfluramine, which was removed from the market because of cardiovascular side effects. Fenfluramine enhances serotonin production, which has been shown to induce fibrogenesis and is associated with underlying valvular dysfunction, such as aortic and/or pulmonary regurgitation.[121] Unlike fenfluramine, phentermine has not been associated with valvular dysfunction.[119] Phentermine is an adrenergic agent that promotes weight loss by activation of the sympathetic nervous system to increase resting energy expenditure and decrease food intake. This sympathetic activation can lead to tachycardia and high blood pressure; therefore, use of phentermine in patients with cardiovascular conditions, including hypertension, may be contraindicated. A 2005 meta-analysis demonstrated weight loss at 6 months for phentermine was 3.6 kg compared with placebo.[122]

Several pharmacological agents have been associated with significant weight loss when used for other indications. The antidepressants bupropion and fluoxetine are associated with modest but significant weight loss. When bupropion is combined with naltrexone, weight loss is greater than the when the single agents are used.[123] The antidiabetic agents metformin, exenatide, pramlintide, and liraglutide are all associated with weight loss in obese patients with type 2 diabetes mellitus.[119] The seizure medication zonisamide have been associated with mild to moderate weight loss.[119]

Multiple dietary supplements given in pharmacological doses (pharmaconutrition) have also been associated with weight loss. Some examples include green tea, L-carnitine, L-arginine, L-leucine, soy and whey protein, and St. John's wort.[49,124,125] Most of these agents have not been shown to produce long-term, meaningful (greater than 5% of baseline) weight loss, and long-term safety has not been assessed; therefore, we do not recommend their routine use in the ambulatory obese patient. Nutrition specialists should review all supplements a patient uses for weight loss (or other purposes), counsel the patient on potential risks, and dispel the purported claims of such agents. See Chapter 19 for additional information on dietary supplements.

Endoscopic Bariatric Procedures

With recent FDA approval of 2 intragastric balloons and the AspireAssist by Aspire Bariatrics, endoscopic bariatric procedures have reemerged as a treatment modality for obesity.

TABLE 35-1 Pharmacotherapy for Long-Term^a Weight Loss in Obesity

Agent	Year Approved by FDA	Weight Loss Mechanism	Common Adverse Effects
Orlistat	2006	Lipase inhibitor to reduce energy intake	GI problems, including steatorrhea
Naltrexone-bupropion	2010	CNS-mediated satiety	Mood and behavioral changes
Liraglutide	2010	GLP-1 agonist	Edema, weight gain, nausea, vomiting, pancreatitis
Phentermine-topiramate	2012	Unknown mechanism	Paresthesia, dizziness, altered taste, constipation
Lorcaserin	2012	Serotonin receptor agonist produces satiety	Headache, respiratory tract infection, nausea

CNS, central nervous system; FDA, US Food and Drug Administration; GI, gastrointestinal; GLP-1, glucagon-like peptide-1.
^{a}≥12 weeks.

Work with intragastric balloons dates back to the early 1980s, when Nieben and colleagues revealed that a free-floating rubber balloon could remain in stomach for 7 to 21 days and produce an average of 5 kg of weight loss.[126] This work culminated in the 1985 FDA approval of the Garren-Edwards gastric bubble (GEGB) as an adjunct to diet and exercise for obesity. Early GEGB trials showed approximately 5% to 10% weight loss at 24 weeks; however, GEGB continued to cause complications related to early deflation and small bowel obstructions, and it was therefore removed from the market.[127,128]

After GEGB was pulled from the US market, work on intragastric balloons continued in Europe and South America, leading to the development and FDA approval of 2 intragastric balloons (Orbera by Apollo Endosurgery and ReShape Duo by ReShape Medical). Orbera is an elastic, spherical balloon made of silicone and filled with 400 to 700 mL of saline that can be left in the stomach for 6 months. A meta-analysis by the Bariatric Endoscopic Task Force found that Orbera was associated with total body weight loss of 13.2% (95% CI, 12.4%–14.0%) at 6 months; 11.3% (95% CI, 8.2%–14.4%) at 12 months; and 6.0% (95% CI, 2.4%–9.7%) at 36 months.[129] Adverse effects included pain, which was reported by 33% of patients, as well as nausea (29%), gastroesophageal reflux disease (18.3%), erosion (12%), and small bowel obstruction (0.3%). Early removal occurred in 7.5% of subjects.

ReShape Duo features 2 intragastric balloons that are attached to each other through a flexible tube, with each balloon being able to be filled with 450 mL of saline. The dual chamber system allows the device to stay in the stomach even if 1 of the balloons deflates early. In the REDUCE pivotal trial—a prospective trial that randomly assigned 326 subjects to either the dual balloon system with lifestyle intervention or a sham procedure with lifestyle intervention—total weight loss in the dual balloon group was 7.6% ± 5.5% vs 3.6% ± 6.3% in the sham group.[130] Early in the trial, 9.1% of subjects had the device removed early. The percentage of early removals was reduced to 7.7% once adjustment of fill volume was based on height of the patient. Similarly, gastric ulcerations were noted in approximately 35% of patients early in the study, but they were reduced by 74% with a redesign of the system to include a softer, smaller, and smoother tip.

The FDA has also recently approved the AspireAssist aspiration therapy system (Aspire Bariatrics), which consists of an endoscopically placed gastrostomy tube along with an external device that allows aspiration of approximately 30% of energy consumed in a meal.[131] Thompson and colleagues randomly assigned 207 participants (BMI 35 to 55) in a 2:1 fashion to either the AspireAssist plus lifestyle intervention or lifestyle intervention alone.[131] At 52 weeks, the AspireAssist group lost 12.1% ± 9.6% of their total weight vs 3.5% ± 6.0% for the lifestyle group. Most of the adverse events were those commonly associated with percutaneous gastrostomy (PEG) tubes, including abdominal pain (37.8%), peristomal granulation tissue (40.5%), as well as peristomal irritation (17.1%). Serious adverse events were noted in the AspireAssist group including peritonitis (0.9%), severe abdominal pain requiring overnight hospitalization (0.9%), prepyloric ulcer (0.9%), and tube replacement due to skin-port malfunction (0.9%).

Bariatric Surgery

The frequency of surgical treatment for intractable extreme obesity has dramatically increased. Since the inception of surgical treatment more than 5 decades ago, several surgical procedures have been developed to promote weight loss. To be considered for bariatric surgery, patients must have a BMI greater than 40, or have a BMI greater than 35 and at least 1 severe obesity-associated comorbidity, such as type 2 diabetes mellitus, obstructive sleep apnea, cardiomyopathy, NAFLD, or severe joint disease.[132,133] This guideline was given a grade A recommendation in the recent perioperative guidelines approved by the American Association of Clinical Endocrinologists, the Obesity Society, and the American Society for Metabolic and Bariatric Surgery.[133] In early 2011, the FDA approved expanding the indication for laparoscopic adjustable gastric band (LAGB) to include patients with a BMI between 30 to 35 and at the highest risk of obesity-related complications; however, medical societies have not made similar recommendations as of yet. All potential candidates for bariatric surgery should have a history of repeated failed attempts to control weight by medical means, including supervised lifestyle intervention programs. Patients should also be acceptable surgical candidates and well informed of the risks of surgery.

The choice of which procedure is best for a patient should be based on risk and full disclosure to the patient. Most bariatric surgery is now performed laparoscopically to minimize wound complications, postoperative pain, and recovery time.

Types of Procedures

Bariatric surgery broadly defines 3 types of procedures: restrictive, malabsorptive, or a mixture of both. Restrictive procedures reduce oral intake by limiting gastric volume, which produces early satiety. The alimentary canal remains intact, minimizing metabolic complications. Laparoscopic banding and sleeve gastrectomy (SG) are examples of purely restrictive procedures, which reduce the stomach's reservoir capacity and restrict energy intake.

The LAGB is a gastric restrictive procedure that produces early satiety and limits food intake.[133] The band is positioned on the upper stomach, just below the gastroesophageal junction, where it limits food intake by constricting the stomach to a shape similar to an hourglass. The upper chamber is a 15- to 20-mL gastric pouch. Short-term complications include band slippage, erosion, balloon failure, port malposition, and band infections; such complication are rare (overall complication rate is less than 10%).[134] LAGB is associated with better weight loss maintenance than lifestyle intervention alone.[133] A study published in 2006 evaluated the long-term complications with LAGB in 317 obese adults.[135] The failure rate increased from 13.2% at 18 months to 36.9% at 7 years. Approximately 22% of patients required a major reoperation (band removal) at some point during the 7-year study.[135] In addition, only 43% of patients had weight loss of greater than 50% during 7 years.[135] LABG has recently fallen out of favor, secondary to its associated long-term complications and the positive results seen with SG.

As of 2015, SG was the most common procedure performed in the United States.[136] In SG, the greater curvature of the stomach is laparoscopically removed and a tubular stomach is created, leading to surgically induced early satiety. Juodeikis and associates conducted a systematic review of 20 studies of SG outcomes and found the mean percentage weight loss 11 years after SG was greater than 50%.[137] The review also concluded that 78% of subjects had resolution or improvement in type 2 diabetes 5 years after SG, and more than 50% had improvement or resolution of hypertension, obstructive sleep apnea, dyslipidemia, and degenerative joint disease at 5 years post SG.[137] This review suggests that SG can lead to substantial and sustained weight loss and improvement in comorbidities.[137]

In Roux-en-Y gastric bypass (RYGB), the upper portion of the stomach is transected and a small proximal gastric pouch is created. The gastric pouch is connected to a proximal jejunum segment (Roux limb), bypassing the rest of the stomach, duodenum, and a portion of the jejunum.[133] The Roux limb length can be variable, ranging from 75 cm to more than 200 cm; malabsorption increases as limb length is increased. The traditional thinking is that weight loss is accomplished by both restriction and malabsorption, although this hypothesis has come into question as other metabolic mechanisms have been elucidated. RYGB limits food intake and can induce some nutrient malabsorption. Longer Roux limbs (as in distal RYGB) are associated with greater macronutrient malabsorption and thus the potential for greater weight loss. However, these procedures have not shown to have significant benefit and are associated with increased risk for micronutrient deficiencies.[138]

Biliopancreatic diversion (BPD) also causes weight loss by a combination of gastric restriction and malabsorption and is generally reserved for individuals with a BMI equal to or greater than 50.[133] A subtotal gastrectomy is performed, and a proximal gastric pouch is created (200 to 500 mL). A common channel is created using the distal small intestine, which is anastomosed to the gastric remnant and the ileum. As compared with RYGB, the common channel in BPD is much shorter, reduced to approximately 100 to 150 cm. Because this common channel is where most macronutrients and micronutrients are absorbed, BPD induces much more malabsorption than RYGB and has a higher risk for postoperative nutrition complications, such as fat-soluble vitamin deficiencies.[139] These factors have limited BPD as an option for weight loss. Adverse effects include steatorrhea, flatus, and metabolic bone disease.[140]

BPD is also performed with a duodenal switch. In this procedure, the stomach is partially removed, creating a gastric sleeve (as opposed to a pouch), and the pylorus is preserved with the food bypass limb anastomosed to the duodenum. The purpose of the "switch" is to avoid dumping syndrome associated with removal of the pylorus.[141]

Purely malabsorptive procedures reduce the alimentary tract, thus reducing nutrient absorption. The jejunoileal bypass, which was among the first bariatric procedures, was a purely malabsorptive procedure and was first performed in 1953.[142] The procedure remained popular into the early 1970s, but it is no longer recommended because it is associated with numerous complications, including bacterial overgrowth, diarrhea, and severe nutrition deficiencies.[142]

Preoperative Assessment and Lifestyle Modification

Clinical nutrition specialists are often a part of a multidisciplinary team whose goal is to provide comprehensive care to obese patients before and after bariatric surgery. The *NIH Consensus Statement on Bariatric Surgery* recommends using a team approach involving a physician obesity specialist, bariatric surgeon, psychologist, primary care physician, and nutrition specialist.[132] The preoperative evaluation should include a comprehensive medical history, physical examination, and appropriate laboratory testing.[115] Patient commitment for compliance with follow-up appointments and medical requirements following surgery should be assessed. Patients with uncontrolled severe psychiatric illness or current alcohol or drug abuse should be excluded from surgical candidacy.[133] To optimize management and reduce postoperative complications, patients should undergo a preoperative psychiatric assessment to determine whether they can make necessary lifestyle changes for sustained weight loss and to identify disorders such as major depression, bipolar disorder, and antisocial personality disorder.

The nutrition specialist should perform a preoperative nutrition assessment that includes the patient's weight history, previous weight loss strategies, alcohol intake, vitamin and supplement use, physical activity, and motivation to make long-term lifestyle modifications.[143] Importantly, the patient should be assessed for malnutrition, particularly for micronutrient deficiencies. Vitamin D is the most common micronutrient deficiency identified in the preoperative obese patient.[144] See Chapters 8 and 9 for further discussion of micronutrient deficiencies and malnutrition assessment, respectively.

The lifestyle modification program should include losing 5% to 10% of preoperative weight in the months prior to surgery. Some studies have shown that patients who lose 5% to 10% of preoperative weight are less likely to have surgical complications, have shorter hospital stays, have reduced need for conversion to open surgical technique, and have improved long-term weight loss.[145-147] A preoperative anesthesia evaluation should follow current guidelines and identify those at increased cardiovascular risk.[148]

Postoperative Nutrition Care

Early Postoperative Nutrition Care

Nutrition specialists who are part of a bariatric surgery team should be involved in the postoperative nutrition assessment. In general, bariatric patients are advanced to clear liquids on postoperative Day 1. In RYGB and BPD, patients will often undergo a swallow test to evaluate for leaks before a liquid diet is started. On postoperative Day 3, patients are advanced to full liquids that are protein-rich, noncarbonated, and low in sugar (no more than 15 g per serving).[133] On postoperative Days 3 to 10, patients should consume a minimum of 48 to 64 oz of fluid per day (at least 24 to 32 oz of clear liquids plus 24 to 32 oz of full liquids). Full liquid options include nonfat milk, lactose-free milk, soy milk, blended light yogurt, or blended plain nonfat yogurt.

At postoperative Weeks 2 to 4, clear liquids can be increased to 48 to 64 oz or more, and full liquids should be replaced with low-fat, high-protein, pureed soft solid foods, such as eggs, ground lean meats, low-fat cottage cheese, yogurt, and moist fish.[133,147] During this period, patients should be encouraged to eat 4 to 6 small meals per day of these protein sources without fluids (waiting 30 minutes after meals before resuming fluid intake); patients must chew foods thoroughly before swallowing them.[133,147] The protein goal should be 60 to 80 g/d, and protein foods should be consumed first.

During postoperative Weeks 4 to 6, patients who have tolerated the protein foods may eat well-cooked soft vegetables and fruits after daily protein goals are met. Fluid goals are maintained at 48 to 64 oz of clear, noncarbonated, caffeine-free, noncaloric liquids.

For Week 7 postoperatively and beyond, daily energy needs should be based on height, weight, and age. Patients should consume a healthy, balanced diet of low-fat protein foods, well-cooked vegetables, fruits, and whole grains as part of 3 meals with 2 snacks each day. Patients should avoid rice, bread, and pasta until protein goals are met.[133] Fluids should be continued at 48 to 64 oz of clear noncarbonated, caffeine-free, noncaloric liquids. Follow-up with nutrition specialists should be recommended if patients are having difficulty maintaining dietary goals or regain weight.

Nutrition Complications

Multiple nutrition complications can arise following bariatric surgery. Many LAGB patients experience vomiting, but it is less common in RYGB and BPD patients. Usually, vomiting is related to eating habits, such as eating too quickly, not chewing food well enough, or overeating.[149] If vomiting persists after eating habits are corrected, it should be evaluated by the bariatric surgeon who is familiar with the patient's procedure. In rare cases, nausea and vomiting following bariatric surgery are symptoms of the syndrome of acute postgastric reduction surgery neuropathy. Acute postgastric reduction surgery neuropathy is a polynutrition (vitamin B_{12} and/or thiamin deficiency), multisystem disorder characterized by protracted postoperative vomiting, hyporeflexia, and muscular weakness.[150] Stenosis and ulcers (frequently caused by nonsteroidal anti-inflammatory drug use) are occasional causes of vomiting in RYGB, BPD, and SG. In LAGB, nausea and vomiting can be caused by the band being too tight, having slipped out of position, or having eroded.[149]

Dumping syndrome is common in the first few months after RYGB because of the inability of the pylorus to regulate gastric emptying of simple carbohydrates. This problem is rarely clinically significant. Dumping can occur early (10 to 30 minutes after eating), causing nausea, bloating, abdominal cramps, or explosive diarrhea, or it can occur late (1 to 3 hours after eating), causing flushing, dizziness, or lightheadedness.[147] Most patients affected by dumping syndrome experience early dumping, which may be resolved by reducing carbohydrate intake, eating smaller portions, and avoiding liquids for at least 30 minutes after meals.[147]

Other long-term complications associated with rapid weight loss following bariatric surgery include gallstone formation and NAFLD.

Nutrition Deficiencies

Bariatric surgery can lead to profound protein, macronutrient, and micronutrient deficiencies.[133] Nutrition deficiencies are usually more severe in malabsorptive surgical procedures, such as RYGB and BPD.[151] Current recommendations for routine vitamin and mineral supplementation in RYGB and BPD include a standard adult or prenatal multivitamin twice a day, calcium citrate, vitamin D_3, vitamin B_{12}, folic acid, and elemental iron (Table 35-2).[133] LAGB patients should take a multivitamin twice a day, calcium citrate, and vitamin D_3, but they do not require routine folic acid, vitamin B_{12}, or iron supplements.[134,148] Deficiencies of the fat-soluble vitamins A, E, and K are rare in RYGB patients who routinely take 2 multivitamins a day; however, they are common in BPD patients, who may need additional supplements of these micronutrients.

The current recommended biochemical surveillance of nutrition status for malabsorptive surgical procedures depends on the surgical procedure (see Table 35-3).[133] BPD patients should have the recommended biochemical surveillance every 3 months following surgery during the first year and every 3 to 6 months thereafter (see Practice Scenario 35-1).[145] RYGB patients should be evaluated every 3 to 6 months during the first year and then annually thereafter. Depending on symptoms, bariatric patients should have biochemical evaluation when clinically indicated outside of the usual surveillance schedule.

Nutrition Support

Complications of bariatric surgery requiring nutrition support have been reported. In a study of patients receiving parenteral nutrition (PN) at home after bariatric surgery, Van Gossum and colleagues reported that early complications included anastomotic leakage and fistula, and late complications included vitamin and trace element deficiencies and hypoalbuminemia.[152] In the same report, 29 of 77 patients who required home PN (HPN) were weaned from PN, 16 required surgical reintervention, and 6 died. Mundi et al[153] reported failure to thrive and malnutrition as the most common indications for HPN. In this report, 45 of 54 patients required revision surgery, and the authors concluded that HPN was a useful bridge to the same.

TABLE 35-2 Nutrient Supplementation After Bariatric Surgery

Supplement	Dose
Multivitamin	2 multivitamins/d
Calcium citrate	1200–2000 mg/d
Vitamin D	400–800 IU/d
Folic acid	400 mcg/d
Elemental iron (premenopausal women)	40–65 mg/d
Vitamin B_{12}	≥350 mcg/d (po) or 1000 mcg/mo (im) or 3000 mcg every 6 months (im)

im, intramuscularly; po, by mouth.

TABLE 35-3 **Recommended Routine Biochemical Surveillance of Nutrition Status After Bariatric Surgery**

Recommended Test	RYGB	BPD
CBC	X	X
Electrolytes	X	X
Glucose	X	X
Lipid profile	X	X
Albumin, prealbumin		X
Liver function (AST, ALT)	X	X
Intact PTH	Optional	X
Vitamin B$_{12}$	X	X
Thiamin	Optional	X
Folate	Optional	X
25(OH)D	X	X
Vitamin E		X
Vitamin K, INR		X
24-hour calcium		X
Iron studies, ferritin	X	X
Zinc		X
Selenium		X

25(OH)D, 25-hydroxyvitamin D; ALT, alanine aminotransferase; AST, aspartate aminotransferase; BPD, biliopancreatic diversion; CBC, complete blood count; INR, international normalized ratio; PTH, parathyroid hormone; RYGB, Roux-en-Y-gastric bypass.
Source: Data are from reference 133.

Practice Scenario 35-1

Question: Which micronutrient deficiencies are common after bariatric surgery?

Scenario: A 35-year-old obese woman (body mass index, 52; actual body weight, 160 kg; ideal body weight, 65 kg; height, 175 cm) with a history of hypertension underwent an elective biliopancreatic diversion (BPD). She lost 70 kg over the next 2 years. At 2-year follow-up, she complained of nonspecific joint pain, fatigue, lower extremity numbness with tingling, losing her balance, and difficulty seeing at night.

Intervention: A physical examination and laboratory evaluation were performed. Serum retinol level (for vitamin A), serum 25-hydroxyvitamin D (for vitamin D), vitamin B$_{12}$, and copper levels were all below reference range. Methylmalonic acid (for vitamin B$_{12}$ deficiency) was above reference range.

Answer: Micronutrient deficiencies are common after bariatric surgery. Deficiencies of fat-soluble vitamins (eg, vitamin A and D), water-soluble vitamins (eg, vitamin B$_{12}$) and trace minerals (eg, copper) may occur.

Rationale: Of the bariatric procedures, the mixed restrictive-malabsorptive BPD procedure is associated with significant

malabsorption because of the creation of a short common channel. Numerous micronutrient deficiencies may develop months to years after BPD. Vitamins A and D are the most common fat-soluble vitamin deficiencies and can lead to night blindness and acne (vitamin A) and fatigue and muscle pain (vitamin D). Laboratory findings include low serum retinol and 25-hydroxyvitamin D levels. Vitamin B$_{12}$ deficiency is the most common water-soluble vitamin deficiency after BPD and Roux-en-Y gastric bypass (RYGB) and presents with a myriad of symptoms, including lower extremity numbness, sensory loss, loss of taste, and glossitis.[145] Laboratory findings include macrocytic anemia (mean corpuscular volume [MCV] greater than 96 femtoliters), low vitamin B$_{12}$ level, and elevated serum methylmalonic acid level. Iron, zinc, and copper are the most common trace mineral deficiencies after BPD and RYGB.[144] Zinc deficiency can cause frontal hair loss, dermatitis, and altered taste. Iron and copper deficiencies can cause a microcytic anemia (MCV less than 80 femtoliters). Iron deficiency is identified by low serum ferritin, and copper deficiency by low serum copper.

In 2014, Isom and associates[154] reviewed nutrition and metabolic support (including nutrition support) for bariatric patients. The authors recommended EN when complications did not preclude its use, although care must be taken to account for surgical alterations to anatomy when inserting feeding tube devices. The appropriate enteral feeding method (bolus, intermittent, or continuous) is determined by the access device and site. Small-volume bolus feeding may be done into a remnant stomach; continuous or slow intermittent feeding may be administered into the small bowel. When the GI tract cannot absorb adequately because of complications (fistula, obstruction, ileus, ischemia, or malabsorption), PN is indicated if nutrition support is required for more than 7 days. The energy and protein prescription is the same as the prescription recommended for overweight and obese patients (see Chapters 2, 23, and 24).

Reports of the use of HPN in patients after bariatric surgery are anecdotal and indicate that it is safe and effective. Hamilton and colleagues[155] reported that hypocaloric HPN in 34 post–bariatric procedure patients was safe and effective in terms of weight reduction and complications. Others have reported that some patients receiving HPN after bariatric surgery successfully weaned from PN and transitioned to oral diets; however, other recipients of HPN after bariatric surgery later required bowel transplantation because of extensive complications.[156,157]

Critically Ill Obese Patients

Effect of Obesity on Intensive Care Unit Mortality

Obesity in general is associated with increased all-cause mortality.[74,158,159] Furthermore, obesity is also associated with increased cause-specific mortality, as mentioned previously.[76] One-third of critically ill patients are obese. When the obese patient becomes critically ill, the ICU team is faced with additional physical and nonphysical challenges. Physical challenges include potentially difficult airway and ventilator management, difficulties with positioning, limited testing options because of weight restrictions, and difficulty with intravenous access. Nonphysical issues include challenges with ICU drug dosing.[160] Despite higher pre-ICU risk for morbidity and mortality and ICU-specific challenges, obesity has been associated in clinical studies and 3 meta-analyses[161-163] with improved ICU outcomes, a phenomenon known as the critical care "obesity paradox." The reason for improved ICU outcomes is not clear and seems to be counterintuitive.

A meta-analysis of 14 studies on the effect of obesity in critically ill patients demonstrated no difference overall in ICU mortality between lean and obese patients. However, ICU length of stay and duration of mechanical ventilation were significantly longer in obese patients compared with nonobese controls.[161] Improved survival was observed in patients with class I and class II obesity, compared with their lean counterparts.[161] Another meta-analysis, which evaluated 22 studies, found no significant difference in ICU or hospital mortality between obese patients and normal weight controls.[162] There were also no differences in ICU length of stay or duration of mechanical ventilation. In a third meta-analysis, individuals with a BMI in a range of 30 to 40 had a lower mortality rate than normal weight controls.[163] ICU length of stay was significantly increased for patients who were underweight or had class III obesity when compared with normal weight individuals.[163]

The critical care obesity paradox has several potential explanations. One hypothesis is that obese individuals have a survival benefit because these patients have nutrition "reserves," which provide substrate during critical illness. A second hypothesis suggests that anti-inflammatory adipokines favorably modulate the inflammatory response. In contrast, leptin and resistin are proinflammatory cytokines, which activate macrophages and induced hepatic tumor necrosis factor–α and interleukin-6, further perpetuating the inflammatory response. Obesity may result in a form of "inflammatory preconditioning," as is seen with ischemic preconditioning in the setting of acute on chronic vasculopathy. In obesity, the baseline inflammation is somehow advantageous in the setting of an acute insult.[160] Furthermore, BMI may not be the best way to estimate obesity-associated ICU mortality. For patients with obesity class I or II, WC and presence of central adiposity (which are predictors of visceral adiposity) may be better anthropometric measures of risk. A recent prospective study in 2 general ICUs evaluated mortality in obese subjects by comparing abdominal adiposity.[164] Subjects with increased abdominal adiposity had higher Acute Physiology and Chronic Health Evaluation (APACHE) II scores and increased mortality compared with obese controls without central adiposity (44% vs 25%, respectively; $P < 0.01$). Furthermore, after adjustment for age and APACHE II scores, abdominal obesity was associated with an increased risk of mortality. BMI greater than 30 was not an independent risk factor for increased mortality.[164]

The methodologic limitations of studies evaluating obesity outcomes must be noted. The 3 aforementioned meta-analyses[161-163] did not differentiate the type of ICU (trauma or surgical vs medical) to which patients were admitted. Clinical outcomes seem to be different in the trauma ICU studies vs medical or mixed ICU studies. Studies with a higher percentage of trauma patients demonstrate an increased hospital or

ICU mortality in obese patients compared with normal weight subjects.[160] Medical ICU studies have shown either the opposite trend or no significant differences in mortality.[161] Trauma and medical ICU patient populations have different pathophysiological consequences, and thus obesity may affect their outcomes differently.[165]

The best explanation for the critical care obesity paradox may be that the overall curve for mortality across all categories of BMI is U-shaped. Mortality may be lowest for patients with overweight or class I or II obesity. Mortality, in turn, may be higher for underweight individuals (BMI less than 20) and patients with class III obesity.

Impact of Obesity on Critical Care

Regardless of differences in mortality, obesity in the critically ill patient can present unique challenges to the overall management of the patient. The presence of any of the more than 60 comorbidities can complicate the assessment and treatment of obese patients, requiring very individualized management. Intubation as indicated by the Mallampati score (standard anesthesia airway assessment) can be difficult when the neck circumference is large, especially in patients with class III obesity.[166] Furthermore, patients with class III obesity have severely reduced functional residual capacity and heavy noncompliant chest walls, making mechanical ventilation difficult.[167] Placement of central venous and arterial catheters for monitoring and vascular access can be extremely difficult because of the lack of defined anatomical landmarks. Repositioning and mobilizing obese ICU patients is difficult but essential in preventing skin breakdown. Obese patients need specialized beds, lifts, and dedicated teams to move them, to ensure that both staff and patients are protected from injury.

Obesity and Intensive Care Unit Nutrition Assessment

Initial Nutrition Assessment

With the rising prevalence of obesity in the ICU population, healthcare providers must be prepared to address the specific nutrition needs of these patients. Although obese patients may have different metabolic responses to stress (obesity-associated inflammation, hyperglycemia, and dyslipidemia) compared with lean patients, the basic principles of ICU care for obese patients, such as the need for and benefit from early EN, are much the same as those for their lean counterparts.[28,168] However, the ability of the healthcare team to address the patient's needs is often adversely affected by the physical and functional limitations induced by obesity.[169]

Obese patients admitted to the ICU should have a detailed nutrition assessment performed by a clinical nutrition specialist. This assessment should include a detailed history, physical examination, and determination of energy and protein requirements. Nutrition assessment of the critically ill obese patient includes evaluating the presence of preexisting protein-energy malnutrition or micronutrient deficiencies, oral intake prior to hospitalization, recent weight change, and the details of any obesity-related surgeries. In addition, the presence, treatment, and control of any preexisting or evolving comorbidities, such as obstructive sleep apnea, CVD, type 2 diabetes mellitus, and NAFLD, must be addressed. Finally, recent use of any weight loss pharmacotherapies, including complementary and alternative medicines, should be ascertained.

A thorough physical examination of the obese patient must include accurate measures of BMI and initial and subsequent body weights, which are crucial in determining a patient's protein and energy requirements. Usual body weight and IBW should be determined. Abnormalities discovered on a complete skin examination, such as *acanthosis nigricans,* can provide clues about undiagnosed or poorly controlled comorbidities, such as insulin resistance. A record of any skin wounds on admission to the ICU and throughout the course of hospitalization should be recorded; obese patients are at increased risk for complex wound injuries and related complications.[170] (See Chapter 21 for more information on wound care.) Finally, because central adiposity often better reflects visceral fat deposition and obesity-induced inflammation, determination of waist-to-hip ratio and WC should be obtained in patients with class I or class II obesity.[158,164,171-173]

Determining Energy Expenditure in Obesity

Determining energy requirements for obese patients can be challenging, and the optimal way to predict energy and protein requirements for the critically ill obese patient remains a topic of much debate and controversy. Predictive equations, such as the Harris-Benedict equation, have been widely used to estimate resting metabolic rate, but we lack the evidence of their accuracy in critically ill patients.[174,175] In addition, most predictive equations were validated in patients without extremes of weight or age. Overestimation of total energy requirements when using ABW and underestimation when using the IBW lead to inadvertent overfeeding and underfeeding, respectively.[172] Attempts to account for altered body composition by using corrections for adjusted body weight with these equations has led to even more confusion.

For these reasons, when IC is available, it should be used to determine the energy requirements of the critically ill obese patient. When IC is not available, predictive equations such as the Mifflin–St. Jeor equation[176-178] or the Penn State 1998 equation[179] can be used. Alternatively, energy requirements have been estimated with simpler weight-based equations.[170,180,181] With these equations, nutrition specialists must be aware of the frequent inaccuracies that may occur and apply clinical judgment to assess the appropriateness of nutrition therapy derived from their use. See Chapter 2 for further information on energy requirements, IC, and predictive equations.

High-Protein, Hypocaloric Feeding

The observation in the 1970s of negative consequences of "hyperalimentation" led to the idea of a possible benefit of hypocaloric feeding in obesity. Researchers and clinicians have noted that (1) the metabolic rate may not be markedly increased in patients with critical illness; (2) weight gain during nutrition support in critical illness usually involves an increase in fat mass out of proportion to LBM; (3) provision of glucose in excess of needs causes increased lipogenesis and

fatty liver; and (4) hyperglycemia increases the risk of infectious complications. For example, in a controlled trial of preoperative nutrition, patients who received 1000 kcal more than the metabolic rate had increased infectious complications.[182]

High-protein, hypocaloric feeding (ie, providing adequate or increased protein while delivering less energy) must be distinguished from permissive underfeeding (delivering inadequate amounts of all macronutrients). High-protein, hypocaloric feeding is thought to maintain nitrogen balance and LBM while facilitating the mobilization of adipose tissue for fuel utilization. Six studies have examined high-protein, hypocaloric nutrition in critically ill obese patients.[183-186] Major findings of these studies include lower insulin requirements, shorter ICU stays, decreased number of days receiving antibiotics, improved wound healing, better closure of fistulas, and a trend toward reduced duration of mechanical ventilation in subjects receiving high-protein, hypocaloric feeding strategies. Only 1 of these studies involved EN.[183] Notably, none of these studies demonstrated inferior outcomes when compared with eucaloric feeding.[187] Further RCTs are needed to evaluate major outcomes, such as mortality, in the ICU.

The joint ASPEN/SCCM 2016 guidelines provide a specific recommendation for nutrition support in critically ill obese patients.[188] The guidelines recommend that goal feeding should not exceed 65% to 70% of energy requirements, calculated using 11 to 14 kcal per kg ABW for patients whose BMI is between 30 and 50, or 22 to 25 kcal per kg of IBW for patients with a BMI greater than 50. For obese patients receiving PN, the protein and energy goals should follow the same recommendations as those given for EN.[188]

Protein Requirements

RCTs of hypocaloric, high-protein vs eucaloric feeding in critically ill, obese patients have not be done. Data from small, nonrandomized studies of trauma patients receiving mostly PN[183-186] led to a grade D recommendation from ASPEN/SCCM[188] for high-protein, hypocaloric nutrition for critically ill obese patients. The 2016 ASPEN/SCCM guidelines recommend a protein goal of 2.0 to 2.5 g per kg IBW for the critically ill obese patient.[188] A 24-hour urine collection for urinary urea nitrogen may be used to subsequently adjust the prescription for protein delivery.[183] Given the dynamic changes that can occur in the ICU and the inaccuracy of predictive measures, nutrition specialists should routinely monitor nitrogen balance and cumulative protein balance throughout a patient's hospital course.

The Impact of Obesity on the Delivery of Nutrition

Enteral Access

Obesity is associated with increased abdominal pressure, which promotes gastroesophageal reflux and aspiration.[189,190] Comorbidities such as diabetes mellitus and its associated enteric neuropathy are more prevalent in obesity. Delayed gastric emptying and poor tolerance to gastric feeding because of diabetic gastroparesis can further complicate enteral access. Limitations in weight for fluoroscopy tables may preclude or complicate methods of feeding tube placement that require imaging for guidance and/or confirmation. For these reasons, selective postpyloric feeding and use of prokinetics may be needed more frequently in critically ill obese patients.

Placement of a PEG tube may be relatively contraindicated in morbidly obese patients.[160] Surgical and endoscopic placements of PEG tubes in this population are associated with increased rates of complications, including postprocedure ileus, wound infection, and possibly mortality.[191,192] Because a large pannus increases risk for displacement of the PEG tube, the authors recommend that efforts should be made to secure the stomach against the abdominal wall with multiple T-fasteners; movement of the pannus may be further reduced by using an abdominal binder.

Monitoring the Delivery of Nutrition

Obese patients may be more prone to increased morbidity in the ICU compared with lean patients.[170] All critically ill patients, regardless of the presence or absence of obesity, should be evaluated for the level of enteral feeding within the GI tract, the appropriate access device, and whether simultaneous gastric decompression of the stomach is required. Also, to reduce the likelihood for bowel ischemia, all critically ill patients should be fully resuscitated before EN is initiated.

Clinicians may need to use IC periodically to reassess energy requirements as the patient's clinical condition improves or deteriorates. Cumulative energy balance should be followed to confirm that patients are maintained at 60% to 70% of expenditure throughout the provision of the nutrition regimen. Monitoring nitrogen balance periodically with serial 24-hour collections of urinary urea nitrogen assists in confirming the adequacy of protein provision.[193] In high-protein, hypocaloric feeding, excess protein load should also be monitored with measurements of blood urea nitrogen and creatinine and daily physical assessments for asterixis.

Because fluid status can be difficult to assess in patients with morbid obesity, strict records of intake and output should be followed to ensure delivery of the nutrition regimen. Volume-based feeds may help ensure delivery of the prescribed EN. Patients should be monitored to maintain moderate glucose control, keeping glucose levels less than 180 mg/dL (10 mmol/L).[188] See Practice Scenario 35-2 for an example of the use of EN in a critically ill obese patient.[188,194]

Practice Scenario 35-2

Question: What are the enteral nutrition (EN) recommendations for a critically ill, obese trauma patient?

Scenario: A 46-year-old obese man (body mass index [BMI], 36; actual body weight, 121 kg; ideal body weight [IBW], 81 kg; height, 183 cm) with a history of nonalcoholic fatty liver disease was admitted to the trauma service following a motor vehicle collision; he required mechanical ventilation. The trauma team predicted that the patient would require at least 1 week of mechanical ventilation and consulted the nutrition support service for recommendations for EN.

Intervention: A physical examination was performed, and history was obtained from the family. The trauma team placed a nasoenteric feeding tube, and indirect calorimetry (IC) was performed to determine the patient's energy requirements. Energy expenditure measured by IC was 2985 kcal/d. Protein requirements were estimated by the equation for obesity class II.

Answer: Obese patients should receive a high-protein, hypocaloric feeding regimen via a nasoenteric feeding tube (which allows for concurrent nasogastric decompression, if required). Using IBW, the feeding should provide 162 g protein per day (81 kg × 2.0 g/kg/d). Goal energy delivery should be approximately 2089 kcal/d (70% of the resting energy expenditure, 2985 kcal/d, as estimated by IC).

Rationale: High-protein, hypocaloric feeding has been recommended (grade D) by the most recent guidelines for the provision and assessment of nutrition support therapy in the adult critically ill patient from the Society of Critical Care Medicine and American Society for Parenteral and Enteral Nutrition. The guidelines suggest that for patients with BMI greater than 30, the energy goal of the EN regimen should not exceed 60% to 70% of target energy requirements.[188] Protein requirements can be predicted with simple weight-based equations. Protein requirements may be estimated by the equation 2.0 g/kg IBW/d for patients with class I or class II obesity, and 2.5 g/kg IBW/d for patients with class III obesity.[188,194]

Practicality of Enteral Nutrition Delivery

The availability of tube feeding formulations suited for achieving the recommendations of high-protein, hypocaloric feeding for obese patients in the ICU is evolving. The addition of various protein modules to current formulations represents the best available method of meeting these recommendations. However, it may be challenging to add to available enteral formulas the large amount of protein powder required to achieve the daily goal of 2.0 to 2.5 g protein per kg IBW (while remaining hypocaloric). An excessive volume of fluid may be required to dissolve the protein powder, and the consistency of such a mixture is often unsuitable for delivery through smaller caliber enteral tubes. The addition of such quantities of protein several times per day also requires a large amount of time and effort from an already busy ICU nursing staff. These issues of practicality frequently lead to inadequate delivery of protein and underscore the need for an enteral formula specifically designed to meet the recommendations for protein for obese patients receiving EN.

References

1. Ogden CL, Carroll MD, Flegal KM. Epidemiologic trends in overweight and obesity. *Endocrinol Metab Clin North Am.* 2003;32(4):741–760.
2. Ogden CL, Yanovski SZ, Carroll MD, Flegal KM. The epidemiology of obesity. *Gastroenterology.* 2007;132(6):2087–2102.
3. Finkelstein EA, Ruhm CJ, Kosa KM. Economic causes and consequences of obesity. *Annu Rev Public Health.* 2005;26:239–257.

4. Calle EE, Rodriguez C, Walker-Thurmond K, Thun MJ. Overweight, obesity, and mortality from cancer in a prospectively studied cohort of U.S. adults. *N Engl J Med.* 2003;348(17):1625-1638.

5. Kuczmarski RJ, Flegal KM. Criteria for definition of overweight in transition: background and recommendations for the United States. *Am J Clin Nutr.* 2000;72(5):1074-1081.

6. Balkau B, Deanfield JE, Després JP, et al. International Day for the Evaluation of Abdominal Obesity (IDEA): a study of waist circumference, cardiovascular disease, and diabetes mellitus in 168,000 primary care patients in 63 countries. *Circulation.* 2007;116(17):1942-1951. doi:10.1161/CIRCULATIONAHA.106.676379.

7. Ogden CL, Carroll MD, McDowell MA, Flegal KM. Obesity among adults in the United States—no statistically significant change since 2003-2004. *NCHS Data Brief.* 2007;1:1-8.

8. Ogden CL, Kuczmarski RJ, Flegal KM, et al. Centers for Disease Control and Prevention 2000 growth charts for the United States: improvements to the 1977 National Center for Health Statistics version. *Pediatrics.* 2002;109(1):45-60.

9. Ogden CL, Carroll MD, Flegal KM. Prevalence of obesity in the United States. *JAMA.* 2014;312(2):189-190.

10. Choi JW, Wang X, Joo JI, et al. Plasma proteome analysis in diet-induced obesity-prone and obesity-resistant rats. *Proteomics.* 2010;10(24):4386-4400.

11. Fawcett KA, Barroso I. The genetics of obesity: FTO leads the way. *Trends Genet.* 2010;26(6):266-274.

12. Lopez AD, Mathers CD, Ezzati M, Jamison DT, Murray CJ. Global and regional burden of disease and risk factors, 2001: systematic analysis of population health data. *Lancet.* 2006;367(9524):1747-1757.

13. James PT. Obesity: the worldwide epidemic. *Clin. Dermatol.* 2004;22(4):276-280.

14. Goh VH, Tain CF, Tong TY, Mok HP, Wong MT. Are BMI and other anthropometric measures appropriate as indices for obesity? A study in an Asian population. *J Lipid Res.* 2004;45(10):1892-1898.

15. World Health Organization Expert Consultation. Appropriate body-mass index for Asian populations and its implications for policy and intervention strategies. *Lancet.* 2004;363(9403):157-163.

16. Stevens J, Nowicki EM. Body mass index and mortality in Asian populations: implications for obesity cut-points. *Nutr Rev.* 2003;61(3):104-107.

17. Woods SC, D'Alessio DA. Central control of body weight and appetite. *J Clin Endocrinol Metab.* 2008;93(11 Suppl 1):S37-S50.

18. Woods SC, Seeley RJ, Cota D. Regulation of food intake through hypothalamic signaling networks involving mTOR. *Annu Rev Nutr.* 2008;28:295-311.

19. Agurs-Collins T, Bouchard C. Gene-nutrition and gene-physical activity interactions in the etiology of obesity. Introduction. *Obesity (Silver Spring).* 2008;16(Suppl 3):S2-S4.

20. Bouchard C. Gene-environment interactions in the etiology of obesity: defining the fundamentals. *Obesity (Silver Spring).* 2008;16(Suppl 3):S5-S10.

21. Chung WK, Leibel RL. Considerations regarding the genetics of obesity. *Obesity (Silver Spring).* 2008;16(Suppl 3):S33-S39.

22. Farooqi S, O'Rahilly S. Genetics of obesity in humans. *Endocr Rev.* 2006;27(7):710-718.

23. Hinney A, Hebebrand J. Polygenic obesity in humans. *Obes Facts.* 2008;1(1):35-42.

24. Hinney A, Vogel CI, Hebebrand J. From monogenic to polygenic obesity: recent advances. *Eur Child Adolesc Psychiatry.* 2010;19(3):297-310.

25. Speliotes EK, Willer CJ, Berndt SI, et al. Association analyses of 249,796 individuals reveal 18 new loci associated with body mass index. *Nat Genet.* 2010;42(11):937-948.

26. Cauchi S, Stutzmann F, Cavalcanti-Proenca C, et al. Combined effects of MC4R and FTO common genetic variants on obesity in European general populations. *J Mol Med.* 2009;87(5):537-546.

27. Stutzmann F, Cauchi S, Durand E, et al. Common genetic variation near MC4R is associated with eating behaviour patterns in European populations. *Int J Obes (Lond).* 2009;33(3):373-378.

28. Hurt RT, Frazier TH, McClave SA, Kaplan LM. Obesity epidemic: overview, pathophysiology, and the intensive care unit conundrum. *JPEN J Parenter Enteral Nutr.* 2011;35(5 Suppl):4S-13S.

29. Mozaffarian D, Hao T, Rimm EB, Willett WC, Hu FB. Changes in diet and lifestyle and long-term weight gain in women and men. *N Engl J Med.* 2011;364(25):2392-2404.

30. Bantle JP. Dietary fructose and metabolic syndrome and diabetes. *J Nutr.* 2009;139(6 Suppl):1263S-1268S.

31. Bantle JP, Raatz SK, Thomas W, Georgopoulos A. Effects of dietary fructose on plasma lipids in healthy subjects. *Am J Clin Nutr.* 2000;72(5):1128-1134.

32. Bray GA, Nielsen SJ, Popkin BM. Consumption of high-fructose corn syrup in beverages may play a role in the epidemic of obesity. *Am J Clin Nutr.* 2004;79(4):537-543.

33. Vos MB, McClain CJ. Fructose takes a toll. *Hepatology.* 2009;50(4):1004-1006.

34. Vos MB, Weber MB, Welsh J, et al. Fructose and oxidized low-density lipoprotein in pediatric nonalcoholic fatty liver disease: a pilot study. *Arch Pediatr Adolesc Med.* 2009;163(7):674-675.

35. Bray GA. The epidemic of obesity and changes in food intake: the fluoride hypothesis. *Physiol Behav.* 2004;82(1):115-121.

36. Choi HK, Curhan G. Soft drinks, fructose consumption, and the risk of gout in men: prospective cohort study. *BMJ.* 2008;336(7639):309-312.

37. Vos MB, Kimmons JE, Gillespie C, Welsh J, Blanck HM. Dietary fructose consumption among US children and adults: the Third National Health and Nutrition Examination Survey. *Medscape J Med.* 2008;10(7):160.

38. Stender S, Dyerberg J. Influence of trans fatty acids on health. *Ann Nutr Metab.* 2004;48(2):61-66.

39. Stender S, Dyerberg J, Astrup A. High levels of industrially produced trans fat in popular fast foods. *N Engl J Med.* 2006;354(15):1650-1652.

40. Stender S, Dyerberg J, Astrup A. Fast food: unfriendly and unhealthy. *Int J Obes (Lond).* 2007;31(6):887-890.

41. Stender S, Dyerberg J, Bysted A, Leth T, Astrup A. A trans world journey. *Atheroscler Suppl.* 2006;7(2):47-52.

42. Dansinger M. Ban trans fats in 2007. *Med Gen Med.* 2006;8(4):58.

43. Mozaffarian D, Katan MB, Ascherio A, Stampfer MJ, Willett WC. Trans fatty acids and cardiovascular disease. *N Engl J Med.* 2006;354(15):1601-1613.

44. Mozaffarian D, Willett WC. Trans fatty acids and cardiovascular risk: a unique cardiometabolic imprint? *Curr Atheroscler Rep.* 2007;9(6):486-493.

45. Pietinen P, Ascherio A, Korhonen P, et al. Intake of fatty acids and risk of coronary heart disease in a cohort of Finnish men. The Alpha-Tocopherol, Beta-Carotene Cancer Prevention Study. *Am J Epidemiol.* 1997;145(10):876-887.

46. Hurt RT, Kulisek C, Buchanan LA, McClave SA. The obesity epidemic: challenges, health initiatives, and implications for gastroenterologists. *Gastroenterol Hepatol.* 2010;6(12):780-792.

47. Williamson DF, Madans J, Anda RF, et al. Recreational physical activity and ten-year weight change in a US national cohort. *Int J Obes Relat Metab Disord.* 1993;17(5):279-286.

48. Ravussin E, Lillioja S, Knowler WC, et al. Reduced rate of energy expenditure as a risk factor for body-weight gain. *N Engl J Med.* 1988;318(8):467-472.

49. Cave MC, Hurt RT, Frazier TH, et al. Obesity, inflammation, and the potential application of pharmaconutrition. *Nutr Clin Pract.* 2008;23(1):16-34.

50. Chandra R, Liddle RA. Cholecystokinin. *Curr Opin Endocrinol Diabetes Obes.* 2007;14(1):63–67.

51. Lorenz DN, Goldman SA. Vagal mediation of the cholecystokinin satiety effect in rats. *Physiol Behav.* 1982;29(4):599–604.

52. Edwards GL, Ladenheim EE, Ritter RC. Dorsomedial hindbrain participation in cholecystokinin-induced satiety. *Am J Physiol.* 1986;251(5 Pt 2):R971–R977.

53. Kirchner H, Tong J, Tschop MH, Pfluger PT. Ghrelin and PYY in the regulation of energy balance and metabolism: lessons from mouse mutants. *Am J Physiol Endocrinol Metab.* 2010;298(5):E909–E919.

54. le Roux CW, Batterham RL, Aylwin SJ, et al. Attenuated peptide YY release in obese subjects is associated with reduced satiety. *Endocrinology.* 2006;147(1):3–8.

55. Renshaw D, Batterham RL. Peptide YY: a potential therapy for obesity. *Curr Drug Targets.* 2005;6(2):171–179.

56. Onaga T, Zabielski R, Kato S. Multiple regulation of peptide YY secretion in the digestive tract. *Peptides.* 2002;23(2):279–290.

57. Batterham RL, Bloom SR. The gut hormone peptide YY regulates appetite. *Ann N Y Acad Sci.* 2003;994:162–168.

58. Liu CD, Aloia T, Adrian TE, et al. Peptide YY: a potential proabsorptive hormone for the treatment of malabsorptive disorders. *Am Surg.* 1996;62(3):232–236.

59. Wiedmer P, Nogueiras R, Broglio F, D'Alessio D, Tschop MH. Ghrelin, obesity and diabetes. *Nat Clin Pract Endocrinol Metab.* 2007;3(10):705–712.

60. Asakawa A, Inui A, Kaga T, et al. Ghrelin is an appetite-stimulatory signal from stomach with structural resemblance to motilin. *Gastroenterology.* 2001;120(2):337–345.

61. Kreitschmann-Andermahr I, Suarez P, Jennings R, Evers N, Brabant G. GH/IGF-I regulation in obesity—mechanisms and practical consequences in children and adults. *Horm Res Paediatr.* 2010;73(3):153–160.

62. Cummings DE, Weigle DS, Frayo RS, et al. Plasma ghrelin levels after diet-induced weight loss or gastric bypass surgery. *N Engl J Med.* 2002;346(21):1623–1630.

63. Foster-Schubert KE, McTiernan A, Frayo RS, et al. Human plasma ghrelin levels increase during a one-year exercise program. *J Clin Endocrinol Metab.* 2005;90(2):820–825.

64. Dubé PE, Brubaker PL. Nutrient, neural and endocrine control of glucagon-like peptide secretion. *Horm Metab Res.* 2004;36(11–12):755–760.

65. Gutzwiller JP, Drewe J, Goke B, et al. Glucagon-like peptide-1 promotes satiety and reduces food intake in patients with diabetes mellitus type 2. *Am J Physiol.* 1999;276(5 Pt 2):R1541–R1544.

66. Kinzig KP, D'Alessio DA, Seeley RJ. The diverse roles of specific GLP-1 receptors in the control of food intake and the response to visceral illness. *J Neurosci.* 2002;22(23):10470–10476.

67. Larsen PJ, Tang-Christensen M, Holst JJ, Orskov C. Distribution of glucagon-like peptide-1 and other preproglucagon-derived peptides in the rat hypothalamus and brainstem. *Neuroscience.* 1997;77(1):257–270.

68. Larsen PJ, Tang-Christensen M, Jessop DS. Central administration of glucagon-like peptide-1 activates hypothalamic neuroendocrine neurons in the rat. *Endocrinology.* 1997;138(10):4445–4455.

69. McMahon LR, Wellman PJ. Decreased intake of a liquid diet in nonfood-deprived rats following intra-PVN injections of GLP-1 (7-36) amide. *Pharmacol Biochem Behav.* 1997;58(3):673–677.

70. Naslund E, Bogefors J, Skogar S, et al. GLP-1 slows solid gastric emptying and inhibits insulin, glucagon, and PYY release in humans. *Am J Physiol.* 1999;277(3 Pt 2):R910–R916.

71. Mafong DD, Henry RR. Exenatide as a treatment for diabetes and obesity: implications for cardiovascular risk reduction. *Curr Atheroscler Rep.* 2008;10(1):55–60.

72. Must A, Spadano J, Coakley EH, et al. The disease burden associated with overweight and obesity. *JAMA.* 1999;282(16):1523–1529.

73. Pischon T, Nothlings U, Boeing H. Obesity and cancer. *Proc Nutr Soc.* 2008;67(2):128–145.

74. Adams KF, Schatzkin A, Harris TB, et al. Overweight, obesity, and mortality in a large prospective cohort of persons 50 to 71 years old. *N Engl J Med.* 2006;355(8):763–778.

75. Hu FB, Manson JE, Stampfer MJ, et al. Diet, lifestyle, and the risk of type 2 diabetes mellitus in women. *N Engl J Med.* 2001;345(11):790–797. doi:10.1056/NEJMoa010492.

76. Whitlock G, Lewington S, Sherliker P, et al. Body-mass index and cause-specific mortality in 900,000 adults: collaborative analyses of 57 prospective studies. *Lancet.* 2009;373(9669):1083–1096.

77. Karelis AD, St-Pierre DH, Conus F, Rabasa-Lhoret R, Poehlman ET. Metabolic and body composition factors in subgroups of obesity: what do we know? *J Clin Endocrinol Metab.* 2004;89(6):2569–2575. doi:10.1210/jc.2004-0165.

78. Brochu M, Poehlman ET, Ades PA. Obesity, body fat distribution, and coronary artery disease. *J Cardiopulm Rehabil.* 2000;20(2):96–108.

79. Matsuzawa Y. Pathophysiology and molecular mechanisms of visceral fat syndrome: the Japanese experience. *Diabetes Metab Rev.* 1997;13(1):3–13.

80. Messier V, Karelis AD, Robillard MÈ, et al. Metabolically healthy but obese individuals: relationship with hepatic enzymes. *Metabolism.* 2010;59(1):20–24. doi:10.1016/j.metabol.2009.06.020.

81. Katsuki A, Sumida Y, Urakawa H, et al. Increased visceral fat and serum levels of triglyceride are associated with insulin resistance in Japanese metabolically obese, normal weight subjects with normal glucose tolerance. *Diabetes Care.* 2003;26(8):2341–2344.

82. Badoud F, Perreault M, Zulyniak MA, Mutch DM. Molecular insights into the role of white adipose tissue in metabolically unhealthy normal weight and metabolically healthy obese individuals. *FASEB J.* 2015;29(3):748–758. doi:10.1096/fj.14-263913.

83. Srdić B, Stokić E, Korać A, et al. Morphological characteristics of abdominal adipose tissue in normal-weight and obese women of different metabolic profiles. *Exp Clin Endocrinol Diabetes.* 2010;118(10):713–718. doi:10.1055/s-0030-1254165.

84. O'Connell J, Lynch L, Cawood TJ, et al. The relationship of omental and subcutaneous adipocyte size to metabolic disease in severe obesity. *PLoS One.* 2010;5(4). doi:10.1371/journal.pone.0009997.

85. Stefan N, Kantartzis K, Machann J, et al. Identification and characterization of metabolically benign obesity in humans. *Arch Intern Med.* 2008;168(15):1609–1616. doi:10.1001/archinte.168.15.1609.

86. Jensen MD, Ryan DH, Apovian CM, et al. 2013 AHA/ACC/TOS guideline for the management of overweight and obesity in adults: a report of the American College of Cardiology/American Heart Association Task Force on Practice Guidelines and the Obesity Society. *J Am Coll Cardiol.* 2014;63(25 Pt B):2985–3023.

87. Kiernan M, Winkleby MA. Identifying patients for weight-loss treatment: an empirical evaluation of the NHLBI obesity education initiative expert panel treatment recommendations. *Arch Intern Med.* 2000;160(14):2169–2176.

88. Kelley DE. The regulation of glucose uptake and oxidation during exercise. *Int J Obes Relat Metab Disord.* 1995;19(Suppl 4):S14–S17.

89. Wadden TA, Anderson DA, Foster GD. Two-year changes in lipids and lipoproteins associated with the maintenance of a 5% to 10% reduction in initial weight: some findings and some questions. *Obes Res.* 1999;7(2):170–178.

90. McCarron DA, Reusser ME. Body weight and blood pressure regulation. *Am J Clin Nutr.* 1996;63(3 Suppl):423S–425S.

91. Strobel RJ, Rosen RC. Obesity and weight loss in obstructive sleep apnea: a critical review. *Sleep.* 1996;19(2):104–115.

92. Weight cycling. National Task Force on the Prevention and Treatment of Obesity. *JAMA*. 1994;272(15):1196–1202.

93. Wadden TA, Berkowitz RI, Womble LG, et al. Randomized trial of lifestyle modification and pharmacotherapy for obesity. *N Engl J Med*. 2005;353(20):2111–2120.

94. Wadden TA, Crerand CE, Brock J. Behavioral treatment of obesity. *Psychiatr Clin North Am*. 2005;28(1):151–170, ix.

95. Rubin RR, Fujimoto WY, Marrero DG, et al. The Diabetes Prevention Program: recruitment methods and results. *Control Clin Trials*. 2002;23(2):157–171.

96. Kruger J, Galuska DA, Serdula MK, Jones DA. Attempting to lose weight: specific practices among U.S. adults. *Am J Prev Med*. 2004;26(5):402–406.

97. Sacks FM, Bray GA, Carey VJ, et al. Comparison of weight-loss diets with different compositions of fat, protein, and carbohydrates. *N Engl J Med*. 2009;360(9):859–873.

98. National Institutes of Health. Clinical guidelines on the identification, evaluation, and treatment of overweight and obesity in adults—the evidence report. *Obes Res*. 1998;6(Suppl 2):51S–209S.

99. Stern L, Iqbal N, Seshadri P, et al. The effects of low-carbohydrate versus conventional weight loss diets in severely obese adults: one-year follow-up of a randomized trial. *Ann Intern Med*. 2004;140(10):778–785.

100. Foster GD, Wyatt HR, Hill JO, et al. A randomized trial of a low-carbohydrate diet for obesity. *N Engl J Med*. 2003;348(21):2082–2090.

101. National Task Force on the Prevention and Treatment of Obesity, National Institutes of Health. Very low-calorie diets. *JAMA*. 1993;270(8):967–974.

102. Anderson JW, Konz EC, Frederich RC, Wood CL. Long-term weight-loss maintenance: a meta-analysis of US studies. *Am J Clin Nutr*. 2001;74(5):579–584.

103. Benotti PN, Still CD, Wood GC, et al. Preoperative weight loss before bariatric surgery. *Arch Surg*. 2009;144(12):1150–1155.

104. Wiezer M, Jansen I, Thorell A. Preoperative weight loss: a component of the preoperative program in bariatric surgery. *Obes Surg*. 2010;20(1):130; author reply 131.

105. Solomon H, Liu GY, Alami R, Morton J, Curet MJ. Benefits to patients choosing preoperative weight loss in gastric bypass surgery: new results of a randomized trial. *J Am Coll Surg*. 2009;208(2):241–245.

106. Ballor DL, Keesey RE. A meta-analysis of the factors affecting exercise-induced changes in body mass, fat mass and fat-free mass in males and females. *Int J Obes*. 1991;15(11):717–726.

107. Ballor DL, Poehlman ET. Exercise-training enhances fat-free mass preservation during diet-induced weight loss: a meta-analytical finding. *Int J Obes Relat Metab Disord*. 1994;18(1):35–40.

108. Miller WC, Koceja DM, Hamilton EJ. A meta-analysis of the past 25 years of weight loss research using diet, exercise or diet plus exercise intervention. *Int J Obes Relat Metab Disord*. 1997;21(10):941–947.

109. Slentz CA, Duscha BD, Johnson JL, et al. Effects of the amount of exercise on body weight, body composition, and measures of central obesity: STRRIDE—a randomized controlled study. *Arch Intern Med*. 2004;164(1):31–39.

110. Curioni CC, Lourenco PM. Long-term weight loss after diet and exercise: a systematic review. *Int J Obes (Lond)*. 2005;29(10):1168–1174.

111. Andersen RE, Wadden TA, Bartlett SJ, et al. Effects of lifestyle activity vs structured aerobic exercise in obese women: a randomized trial. *JAMA*. 1999;281(4):335–340.

112. Dunn AL, Marcus BH, Kampert JB, et al. Comparison of lifestyle and structured interventions to increase physical activity and cardiorespiratory fitness: a randomized trial. *JAMA*. 1999; 281(4):327–334.

113. Burke LE, Wang J, Sevick MA. Self-monitoring in weight loss: a systematic review of the literature. *J Am Diet Assoc*. 2011;111(1):92–102.

114. Jakicic JM, Davis KK, Rogers RJ, et al. Effect of wearable technology combined with a lifestyle intervention on long-term weight loss: The IDEA randomized clinical trial. *JAMA*. 2016; 316(11):1161–1171.

115. Phelan S, Wadden TA. Combining behavioral and pharmacological treatments for obesity. *Obes Res*. 2002;10(6):560–574.

116. Wadden TA, Womble LG, Sarwer DB, et al. Great expectations: "I'm losing 25% of my weight no matter what you say." *J Consult Clin Psychol*. 2003;71(6):1084–1089.

117. Sibutramine (Meridia) withdrawn. *Med Lett Drugs Ther*. 2010; 52(1350):88.

118. Wadden TA, Volger S, Sarwer DB, et al. A two-year randomized trial of obesity treatment in primary care practice. *N Engl J Med*. 2011;365(21):1969–1979.

119. Kaplan LM. Pharmacologic therapies for obesity. *Gastroenterol Clin North Am*. 2010;39(1):69–79.

120. Khera R, Murad MH, Chandar AK, et al. Association of pharmacological treatments for obesity with weight loss and adverse events: a systematic review and meta-analysis. *JAMA*. 2016; 315(22):2424–2434.

121. Robiolio PA, Rigolin VH, Wilson JS, et al. Carcinoid heart disease. correlation of high serotonin levels with valvular abnormalities detected by cardiac catheterization and echocardiography. *Circulation*. 1995;92(4):790–795.

122. Li Z, Maglione M, Tu W, et al. Meta-analysis: pharmacologic treatment of obesity. *Ann Intern Med*. 2005;142(7):532–546.

123. Greenway FL, Fujioka K, Plodkowski RA, et al. Effect of naltrexone plus bupropion on weight loss in overweight and obese adults (COR-I): a multicentre, randomised, double-blind, placebo-controlled, phase 3 trial. *Lancet*. 2010;376(9741):595–605.

124. Blanck HM, Serdula MK, Gillespie C, et al. Use of nonprescription dietary supplements for weight loss is common among Americans. *J Am Diet Assoc*. 2007;107(3):441–447.

125. Saper RB, Eisenberg DM, Phillips RS. Common dietary supplements for weight loss. *Am Fam Physician*. 2004;70(9):1731–1738.

126. Gyring Nieben O, Harboe H. Intragastric balloon as an artificial bezoar for treatment of obesity. *Lancet*. 1982;319(8265):198–199. doi:10.1016/S0140-6736(82)90762-0.

127. Benjamin SB, Maher KA, Cattau EL, et al. Double-blind controlled trial of the Garren-Edwards gastric bubble: an adjunctive treatment for exogenous obesity. *Gastroenterology*. 1988; 95(3):581–588.

128. Benjamin SB. Small bowel obstruction and the Garren-Edwards gastric bubble: an iatrogenic bezoar. *Gastrointest Endosc*. 1988; 34(6):463–467.

129. Abu Dayyeh BK, Kumar N, Edmundowicz SA, et al. ASGE Bariatric Endoscopy Task Force systematic review and meta-analysis assessing the ASGE PIVI thresholds for adopting endoscopic bariatric therapies. *Gastrointest Endosc*. 2015;82(3):425–438.e5. doi:10.1016/j.gie.2015.03.1964.

130. Ponce J, Woodman G, Swain J, et al. The REDUCE pivotal trial: a prospective, randomized controlled pivotal trial of a dual intragastric balloon for the treatment of obesity. *Surg Obes Relat Dis*. 2015;11(4):874–881. doi:10.1016/j.soard.2014.12.006.

131. Thompson CC, Abu Dayyeh BK, Kushner R, et al. Percutaneous gastrostomy device for the treatment of class II and class III obesity: results of a randomized controlled trial. *Am J Gastroenterol*. 2017;112(3):447–457. doi:10.1038/ajg.2016.500.

132. National Institutes of Health Conference. Gastrointestinal surgery for severe obesity. Consensus Development Conference Panel. *Ann Intern Med*. 1991;115(12):956–961.

133. Mechanick JI, Kushner RF, Sugerman HJ, et al. American Association of Clinical Endocrinologists, the Obesity Society, and

American Society for Metabolic and Bariatric Surgery medical guidelines for clinical practice for the perioperative nutritional, metabolic, and nonsurgical support of the bariatric surgery patient. *Obesity (Silver Spring).* 2009;17(Suppl 1):S1–S70.

134. Buchwald H, Oien DM. Metabolic/bariatric surgery worldwide. *Obes Surg.* 2013;23(4):427–436.

135. Suter M, Calmes JM, Paroz A, Giusti V. A 10-year experience with laparoscopic gastric banding for morbid obesity: high long-term complication and failure rates. *Obes Surg.* 2006;16(7):829–835.

136. American Society for Metabolic and Bariatric Surgery. Estimate of bariatric surgery numbers, 2011–2015. Updated 2016. https://asmbs.org/resources/estimate-of-bariatric-surgery-numbers. Accessed December 7, 2016.

137. Juodeikis Z, Brimas G. Long-term results after sleeve gastrectomy: a systematic review. *Surg Obes Relat Dis.* 2016(Oct 17). Epub ahead of print. doi:10.1016/j.soard.2016.10.006.

138. Brolin RE, LaMarca LB, Kenler HA, Cody RP. Malabsorptive gastric bypass in patients with superobesity. *J Gastrointest Surg.* 2002;6(2):195–205.

139. Slater GH, Ren CJ, Siegel N, et al. Serum fat-soluble vitamin deficiency and abnormal calcium metabolism after malabsorptive bariatric surgery. *J Gastrointest Surg.* 2004;8(1):48–55.

140. Prachand VN, Ward M, Alverdy JC. Duodenal switch provides superior resolution of metabolic comorbidities independent of weight loss in the super-obese (BMI > or = 50 kg/m^2) compared with gastric bypass. *J Gastrointest Surg.* 2010;14(2):211–220.

141. Weiner RA, Blanco-Engert R, Weiner S, Pomhoff I, Schramm M. Duodenal switch: three different duodeno-ileal anastomotic techniques and initial experience. *Obes Surg.* 2004;14(3):334–340.

142. Celio AC, Pories WJ. A history of bariatric surgery: the maturation of a medical discipline. *Surg Clin North Am.* 2016;96(4):655–667.

143. Cunningham E. What is the registered dietitian's role in the preoperative assessment of a client contemplating bariatric surgery? *J Am Diet Assoc.* 2006;106(1):163.

144. Strohmayer E, Via MA, Yanagisawa R. Metabolic management following bariatric surgery. *Mt Sinai J Med.* 2010;77(5):431–445.

145. Alvarado R, Alami RS, Hsu G, et al. The impact of preoperative weight loss in patients undergoing laparoscopic Roux-en-Y gastric bypass. *Obes Surg.* 2005;15(9):1282–1286.

146. Still CD, Benotti P, Wood GC, et al. Outcomes of preoperative weight loss in high-risk patients undergoing gastric bypass surgery. *Arch Surg.* 2007;142(10):994–999.

147. Kulick D, Hark L, Deen D. The bariatric surgery patient: a growing role for registered dietitians. *J Am Diet Assoc.* 2010;110(4):593–599.

148. Fleisher LA, Beckman JA, Brown KA, et al. ACC/AHA 2007 guidelines on perioperative cardiovascular evaluation and care for noncardiac surgery: a report of the American College of Cardiology/American Heart Association Task Force on Practice Guidelines (Writing Committee to Revise the 2002 Guidelines on Perioperative Cardiovascular Evaluation for Noncardiac Surgery). *Circulation.* 2007;116(17):e418–e499.

149. McMahon MM, Sarr MG, Clark MM, et al. Clinical management after bariatric surgery: value of a multidisciplinary approach. *Mayo Clin Proc.* 2006;81(10 Suppl):S34–S45.

150. Chang CG, Adams-Huet B, Provost DA. Acute post-gastric reduction surgery (APGARS) neuropathy. *Obes Surg.* 2004;14(2):182–189.

151. Davies DJ, Baxter JM, Baxter JN. Nutritional deficiencies after bariatric surgery. *Obes Surg.* 2007;17(9):1150–1158.

152. Van Gossum A, Pironi L, Chambrier C, et al. Home parenteral nutrition (HPN) in patients with post-bariatric surgery complications. *Clin Nutr.* 2016(Sept 8). Epub. doi:10.1016/j.clnu.2016.08.025.

153. Mundi MS, Vallumsetia N, Davidson JB, et al. Use of home parenteral nutrition in post-bariatric surgery-related malnutrition. *JPEN J Parenter Enteral Nutr.* 2016(May 13). Epub ahead of print.

154. Isom KA, Andromalos L, Ariagno M, et al. Nutrition and metabolic support recommendations for he bariatric patient. *Nutr Clin Pract.* 2014;29(6):718–739.

155. Hamilton C, Dasari V, Shatnawei A. Hypocaloric home parenteral nutrition and nutrition parameters in patients following bariatric surgery. *Nutr Clin Pract.* 2011;26:577–582.

156. Genton L, Nardo P. Huber O, Pichard C. Parenteral nutrition independence in a patient left with 25 cm of ileum and jejunum: a case report. *Obes Surg.* 2010;20:666–671.

157. Raheem SA, Deen OJ, Corrigan ML. Bariatric surgery complications leading to small bowel transplant: a report of 4 cases. *JPEN J Parenter Enteral Nutr.* 2104;38(4):513–517.

158. McTigue K, Larson JC, Valoski A, et al. Mortality and cardiac and vascular outcomes in extremely obese women. *JAMA.* 2006; 296(1):79–86.

159. Pischon T, Boeing H, Hoffmann K, et al. General and abdominal adiposity and risk of death in Europe. *N Engl J Med.* 2008;359(20):2105–2120.

160. Patel JJ, Rosenthal MD, Miller KR, et al. The critical care obesity paradox and implications for nutrition support. *Curr Gastroenterol Rep.* 2016;18(9):45.

161. Akinnusi ME, Pineda LA, El Solh AA. Effect of obesity on intensive care morbidity and mortality: a meta-analysis. *Crit Care Med.* 2008;36(1):151–158.

162. Hogue CW Jr, Stearns JD, Colantuoni E, et al. The impact of obesity on outcomes after critical illness: a meta-analysis. *Intensive Care Med.* 2009;35(7):1152–1170.

163. Oliveros H, Villamor E. Obesity and mortality in critically ill adults: a systematic review and meta-analysis. *Obesity (Silver Spring).* 2008;16(3):515–521.

164. Paolini JB, Mancini J, Genestal M, et al. Predictive value of abdominal obesity vs. body mass index for determining risk of intensive care unit mortality. *Crit Care Med.* 2010;38(5):1308–1314.

165. Matheson PJ, Hurt RT, Franklin GA, McClain CJ, Garrison RN. Obesity-induced hepatic hypoperfusion primes for hepatic dysfunction after resuscitated hemorrhagic shock. *Surgery.* 2009; 146(4):739–748.

166. Brodsky JB, Lemmens HJ, Brock-Utne JG, Vierra M, Saidman LJ. Morbid obesity and tracheal intubation. *Anesth Analg.* 2002;94(3):732–736.

167. Ladosky W, Botelho MA, Albuquerque JP. Chest mechanics in morbidly obese non-hypoventilated patients. *Respir Med.* 2001; 95(4):281–286.

168. McClave SA, Kushner R, Van Way CW, et al. Nutrition therapy of the severely obese, critically ill patient: summation of conclusions and recommendations. *JPEN J Parenter Enteral Nutr.* 2011;35(5 Suppl):88S–96S.

169. Kiraly L, Hurt RT, Van Way CW. The outcomes of obese patients in critical care. *JPEN J Parenter Enteral Nutr.* 2011;35(5 Suppl):29S–35S.

170. Port AM, Apovian C. Metabolic support of the obese intensive care unit patient: a current perspective. *Curr Opin Clin Nutr Metab Care.* 2010;13(2):184–191.

171. Schneider HJ, Friedrich N, Klotsche J, et al. The predictive value of different measures of obesity for incident cardiovascular events and mortality. *J Clin Endocrinol Metab.* 2010;95(4):1777–1785.

172. Testa G, Cacciatore F, Galizia G, et al. Waist circumference but not body mass index predicts long-term mortality in elderly subjects with chronic heart failure. *J Am Geriatr Soc.* 2010; 58(8):1433–1440.

173. Welborn TA, Dhaliwal SS. Preferred clinical measures of central obesity for predicting mortality. *Eur J Clin Nutr.* 2007; 61(12):1373–1379.

174. Walker RN, Heuberger RA. Predictive equations for energy needs for the critically ill. *Respir Care.* 2009;54(4):509–521.

175. Boullata J, Williams J, Cottrell F, Hudson L, Compher C. Accurate determination of energy needs in hospitalized patients. *J Am Diet Assoc.* 2007;107(3):393–401.

176. Frankenfield D, Roth-Yousey L, Compher C. Comparison of predictive equations for resting metabolic rate in healthy nonobese and obese adults: a systematic review. *J Am Diet Assoc.* 2005; 105(5):775–789.

177. Carrasco F, Papapietro K, Csendes A, et al. Changes in resting energy expenditure and body composition after weight loss following Roux-en-Y gastric bypass. *Obes Surg.* 2007;17(5):608–616.

178. Dobratz JR, Sibley SD, Beckman TR, et al. Predicting energy expenditure in extremely obese women. *JPEN J Parenter Enteral Nutr.* 2007;31(3):217–227.

179. Anderegg BA, Worrall C, Barbour E, Simpson KN, Delegge M. Comparison of resting energy expenditure prediction methods with measured resting energy expenditure in obese, hospitalized adults. *JPEN J Parenter Enteral Nutr.* 2009;33(2):168–175.

180. Stucky CC, Moncure M, Hise M, Gossage CM, Northrop D. How accurate are resting energy expenditure prediction equations in obese trauma and burn patients? *JPEN J Parenter Enteral Nutr.* 2008;32(4):420–426.

181. Zauner A, Schneeweiss B, Kneidinger N, Lindner G, Zauner C. Weight-adjusted resting energy expenditure is not constant in critically ill patients. *Intensive Care Med.* 2006;32(3):428–434.

182. Jeejeebhoy KN. Permissive underfeeding of the critically ill patient. *Nutr Clin Pract.* 2004;19(5):477–480.

183. Dickerson RN, Boschert KJ, Kudsk KA, Brown RO. Hypocaloric enteral tube feeding in critically ill obese patients. *Nutrition.* 2002;18(3):241–246.

184. Dickerson RN, Rosato EF, Mullen JL. Net protein anabolism with hypocaloric parenteral nutrition in obese stressed patients. *Am J Clin Nutr.* 1986;44(6):747–755.

185. Burge JC, Goon A, Choban PS, Flancbaum L. Efficacy of hypocaloric total parenteral nutrition in hospitalized obese patients: a prospective, double-blind randomized trial. *JPEN J Parenter Enteral Nutr.* 1994;18(3):203–207.

186. Choban PS, Burge JC, Scales D, Flancbaum L. Hypoenergetic nutrition support in hospitalized obese patients: a simplified method for clinical application. *Am J Clin Nutr.* 1997;66(3):546–550.

187. Joffe A, Wood K. Obesity in critical care. *Curr Opin Anaesthesiol.* 2007;20(2):113–118.

188. McClave SA, Taylor BE, Martindale RG, et al. Guidelines for the provision and assessment of nutrition support therapy in the adult critically ill patient: Society of Critical Care Medicine (SCCM) and American Society for Parenteral and Enteral Nutrition (A.S.P.E.N.). *JPEN J Parenter Enteral Nutr.* 2016;40(2): 159–211.

189. Honiden S, McArdle JR. Obesity in the intensive care unit. *Clin Chest Med.* 2009;30(3):581–599.

190. Pieracci FM, Hydo L, Pomp A, et al. The relationship between body mass index and postoperative mortality from critical illness. *Obes Surg.* 2008;18(5):501–507.

191. Alexander JW. Wound infections in the morbidly obese. *Obes Surg.* 2005;15(9):1276–1277.

192. Calton WC, Martindale RG, Gooden SM. Complications of percutaneous endoscopic gastrostomy. *Mil Med.* 1992;157(7): 358–360.

193. Dickerson RN. Hypocaloric feeding of obese patients in the intensive care unit. *Curr Opin Clin Nutr Metab Care.* 2005; 8(2):189–196.

194. Choban PS, Dickerson RN. Morbid obesity and nutrition support: is bigger different? *Nutr Clin Pract.* 2005;20(4):480–487.

36 Nutrition Support for Older Adults

Rena Zelig, DCN, RD, CDE, CSG, Phyllis J. Famularo, DCN, RD, LDN, CSG, FAND, and Maria Szeto, MS, RD

CONTENTS

Acknowledgments: Charles Mueller, PhD, RD, CNSC, was coauthor of this chapter for the second edition.

Objectives

1. Review the theoretical and known causes of aging and factors that affect the nutrition status of older adults.
2. Describe and differentiate the conditions of sarcopenia, frailty, and advanced dementia.
3. Understand the process of nutrition screening and assessment of older adults as well as the determination of nutrient requirements for members of this population.
4. Distinguish the roles of dietary and dining interventions and nutrition support interventions used in healthcare for older adults.

Test Your Knowledge Questions

1. Of the following, which is the best currently known nutrition intervention to minimize negative outcomes associated with sarcopenia?
   A. Protein supplementation
   B. Amino acid supplementation
   C. Protein adequacy
   D. ω-3 fatty acid adequacy
2. What is the most reasonable justification to initiate enteral nutrition (EN) in an individual with advanced dementia?
   A. Decreased morbidity
   B. Specific and limited goal
   C. Improved mortality
   D. Improved quality of life
3. Which of the following nutrition support interventions has demonstrated the best outcomes in frail, community-dwelling older adults and in postoperative orthopedic surgery populations?
   A. Oral nutritional supplement
   B. Intravenous (IV) hydration
   C. EN
   D. Parenteral nutrition (PN)
4. Which of the following nutrition interventions have been shown to improve clinical outcomes and quality of life in institutionalized older adults?
   A. Diet modification and liberalization
   B. Modification of dining environment
   C. Provision of aides to improve functional status and increase independence at meals
   D. Honoring food preferences and providing snacks and fortified foods
   E. All of the above

Test Your Knowledge Answers

1. The correct answer is **C**. Adequacy of protein intake seems to be the most important nutrition-related factor in preserving lean body mass (LBM) in older adults. The type of protein, essential amino acid supplementation, and ω-3 fatty acid supplementation may all play roles in preventing sarcopenia.
2. The correct answer is **B**. EN has not been shown to be an effective intervention to decrease mortality, improve morbidity outcomes, or improve quality of life in patients with advanced dementia. However, according to the Academy of Nutrition and Dietetics (AND), a specific and realistically achievable goal may be a reason to initiate tube feeding in an older adult with advanced dementia.
3. The correct answer is **A**. Oral nutritional supplements have demonstrated the best outcome in frail, community-dwelling older adults and in post–orthopedic surgery populations. EN, PN, and IV hydration have demonstrated limited success in achieving positive outcomes in older adults.
4. The correct answer is **E**. This chapter explores food and dining interventions to increase intake and improve nutrition status of older adults. Interventions range from individualizing a diet and liberalizing restrictions or altering food

and fluid consistencies where appropriate, to providing food preferences at and between meals and fortifying foods with supplemental protein and energy. Dining-related interventions can include use of a social dining environment, restorative dining, and provision of adaptive feeding aides to increase the older adult's functional independence at meals.

Background

The number of adults aged 65 years and older worldwide has increased almost 50% from 420 million in 2000 to approximately 617 million in 2015 and is projected to increase to 1.6 billion by 2050, which would represent nearly 17% of the world's population.[1] In the United States, the population 65 years and older grew from 35 million in 2000 to 48 million in 2015 and is expected to nearly double to 88 million by 2050.[1] Life expectancy also continues to rise—in the United States, it is projected to increase from 68.6 years in 2015 to 76.2 years by 2050.[1] This chapter focuses on nutrition-related concerns in older adults, with an emphasis on selection of appropriate nutrition interventions including nutrition support.

The Aging Process

The process of aging can be attributed in part to *senescence*, the irreversible process of cellular aging that causes decreased function, morbidity, and even death. Multiple theories have been proposed to explain senescence and the aging process on the cellular level. A review of organ system senescence is beyond the scope of this chapter and can be reviewed in detail elsewhere.[2] Regardless, aging is a process associated with a natural decline or slowing in most body systems, which affects sensory, functional, and physiological well-being independent of any given disease state. Almost all organ system senescence contributes to malnutrition. Assessing nutrition status and treating nutrition-related problems of older adults requires consideration of the aging process and the effects of acute and chronic disease.

Acute and Chronic Conditions Associated with Aging

Healthcare and medical treatment have led to a decrease in fatal infectious disease and an increase in life expectancy, although chronic disease remains a constant challenge to older adults living longer.[3] Chronic health care problems most associated with morbidity and mortality in older adults include heart disease, cancer, stroke, diabetes, and Alzheimer's disease.[3] Acute and chronic infections, including influenza, pneumonia, bronchitis, and urinary tract infections, as well as pressure injuries (see Chapter 21), are also substantial risks for older adults and can lead to prolonged hospitalizations, debility, malnutrition, and death.[3] Given the inevitable outcome of aging, treatment goals for older adults generally focus less on definitive treatment of disease and more on maximizing functional status and quality of life. These essential primary outcomes in geriatric health thus shape all interventions, including nutrition interventions.

Factors Affecting the Nutrition Status of Older Adults

Physiological, psychological, socioeconomic, and functional changes associated with aging can all alter appetite, intake, and nutrition status. Sarcopenia, frailty, dementia, and related functional decline compromise one's ability to procure and prepare food, which may lead to inadequate intake and unintended weight loss. Older adults in functional decline are also more likely to encounter chewing and swallowing difficulty and diminished hydration (which is compounded by age-associated loss of thirst sensation). The net result is an increased risk for malnutrition, exacerbated sarcopenia and frailty, and, eventually, disability, institutional placement, and mortality.[4,5]

This chapter focuses on issues related to this decline typically seen in older adults, including a review of sarcopenia, frailty, and dementia as causative factors. Nutrition screening and assessment are discussed as they relate to healthy older adults as well as those with or at risk for malnutrition. Nutrient requirements for this population; nutrition interventions, including dietary approaches, EN, and PN; and end-of-life ethical decisions regarding artificial nutrition and hydration are also covered.

Sarcopenia

Sarcopenia is age-related decline in skeletal muscle mass, strength, and function and usually begins in the fifth decade of life.[6–9] Its prevalence more than doubles in individuals 80 years of age and older.[9,10] It can predict disability when a decrease in muscle mass is adjusted for height and fat mass.[11] Sarcopenia increases the risk of immobility, falls, fractures, cognitive impairment, and institutionalization.[9,10,12,13] When sarcopenia is present with elevated inflammatory cytokines, low serum albumin concentrations characteristic of inflammatory conditions, or abnormal carbohydrate, protein, and lipid metabolism, it is associated with cachexia, a severe wasting condition that is common in many chronic diseases and often irreversible unless the underlying disease is improved.[14–17]

Numerous factors—including a sedentary lifestyle, myofiber degeneration caused by myocyte apoptosis or "cell death" mediated by mitochondrial DNA mutations, oxidative stress, endocrinosenescence, altered muscle protein metabolism in the context of anabolic resistance, proinflammatory mediators, and reduced 25-hydroxyvitamin D (25[OH]D) levels—seem to be the mechanisms of sarcopenia. Inadequate nutrition and inadequate protein intake in particular have also been implicated in the development and progression of sarcopenia. However, the precise relationships among these factors, including their interactions with nutrition status, are not clear.[9,11,18–22]

Professional sarcopenia working groups have suggested that various tools to measure muscle mass, such as bioelectrical impedance analysis (BIA), computed tomography (CT), magnetic resonance imaging, and dual x-ray absorptiometry (DXA), may be used to quantify and diagnose sarcopenia. However, none of these tools have been validated for diagnosing sarcopenia and no consensus exists as to which measurement(s) provide the best estimation of body composition. CT holds the most promise because of its precision, and when a CT scan of a cross-sectional area is taken at the third lumbar vertebra (L3) region, it strongly correlates to total body muscle distribution.[23]

Sarcopenic obesity, a subgroup of sarcopenia, has become prevalent as obesity rates in older adults have risen. These individuals commonly have sarcopenia and a high percentage of body fat.[12,17,24] Adults with sarcopenic obesity have worse functional outcomes; more disabilities; and a higher risk of metabolic syndrome, cardiovascular disease, and mortality when compared with sarcopenic lean or sarcopenic normal individuals.[22,24] When examined by abdominal CT using the L3 region, sarcopenic obese individuals have lower estimated total LBM than their nonsarcopenic obese counterparts with the same body mass index (BMI).[23] Central adiposity in relation to loss of LBM underpins sarcopenic obesity and disease risks but is not identifiable by BMI alone.[23,24] In fact, a study by Janssen et al found that BMI and waist circumference (WC) together better predict all-cause mortality in older adults than BMI only. In this same study, higher BMI was associated with decreased mortality for those with low and moderate WC whereas mortality rates increased as BMI increased in those with high WC (equal to or greater than 102 cm for men, equal to or greater than 88 cm for women).[25] More accurate assessment of sarcopenic obesity requires direct measurements of body composition such as the use of BIA, DXA, and abdominal CT scans.[23,24] Since simple anthropometric measures are not reliable indicators of sarcopenic obesity, individuals with this condition may be overlooked clinically and interventions may be delayed.[23]

The principal intervention for sarcopenia is exercise and a minimum daily protein intake of 1 g per kg body weight.[26–28] Higher protein intake in community-dwelling older adults has been associated with slower loss of skeletal muscle mass,[29] but the primary role of nutrition in the management of sarcopenia continues to be adequate overall intake.[30,31] Weight management strategies with the aim to preserve LBM can be a possible goal for those with sarcopenic obesity.[24] The type and timing of protein intake,[28,32] essential amino acid content,[33] and ω-3 fatty acids[34] may also have roles in the management of sarcopenia.

Endurance or aerobic training enhances oxidative metabolism and mitochondrial density. This type of activity improves body composition by increasing the ratio of lean to fat mass, and it down-regulates inflammatory mediators and results in lower circulating interleukin-6 and C-reactive protein levels.[13] Resistance or strength training seems to reverse the inability of skeletal muscle to accumulate protein, perhaps by reversing age-related insensitivity to insulin-like growth factor 1.[35]

In a randomized clinical trial with 48 participants, Pennings and colleagues found that whey protein ("fast" protein) stimulated postprandial muscle protein synthesis more effectively than casein ("slow" protein) and casein hydrolysate in older men (ages 74 ± 1 year); this finding was attributed to a combination of faster digestion and absorption kinetics and the higher leucine content of whey.[32] For optimum muscle protein synthesis, older adults may require meals containing more than 25 g high-quality protein or at least 10 g essential amino acids.[36-38] Consuming protein soon after exercise brings the most benefits from exercise-sensitizing muscle-to-insulin or amino acid–dependent anabolic effects.[28] Exercise and protein supplementation together enhance net muscle protein synthesis the most.[28] Essential amino acid supplementation resulted in improved LBM at 6 and 18 months in a randomized open-label crossover study (treatment vs placebo) of older adults with sarcopenia.[39] Additionally, essential amino acid supplementation was associated with improved muscle protein fractional synthesis rate and increased LBM, but not improved strength, at 3 months in a clinical trial with older women participants.[40] ω-3 fatty acid supplementation stimulated muscle protein synthesis (compared with a corn oil control) in older adults, although subjects in the study did not have sarcopenia.[34]

Frailty

Frailty is described as a multifactorial syndrome that has various phenotypes and leads to significant changes in quality of life, vulnerability, and disability in the older adult population.[13,17,41] Loss of muscle mass and strength, typical of sarcopenia, is also a hallmark of frailty.[41] In a study of 341 older subjects, Jung et al found that, in a 5-year period, those who were determined to be frail sustained a significant loss in LBM that was almost 3 times greater than those who were determined to be healthy.[41] The most widely cited index used to establish frailty proposes a diagnosis of frailty if 3 or more of the following criteria are met: unintentional weight loss (10 pounds in the last year), self-reported exhaustion, weakness (grip strength), slow walking speed, and low physical activity.[42] Older adults with at least 3 of these characteristics are at increased risk for adverse clinical outcomes. Frailty may also have cognitive, social, and psychological components.[13,17] Although inflammation (and chronic disease) probably plays a causative role in frailty,[43] oxidative stress and organ system senescence also play a role. In this view of causation, frailty is the result of an aggregate of abnormalities rather than a single cause.[44]

Nutrition status is thought to play a role in frailty, and early identification of nutrition-related problems may help manage frailty.[17,22] Although evidence has not supported the role of nutrition interventions in improving outcomes associated with frailty, individual nutrients seem to have a potential impact in the treatment of frailty. Low daily intake of energy; protein; vitamins D, E, and C; and folate were significantly and independently associated with frailty in an older adult European cohort[45] and high Mini Nutritional Assessment (MNA) scores (which indicate normal nutrition status) were inversely associated with a neuropsychiatric score in a population of older adults with dementia living at home.[46]

Clinical trials involving diet and/or exercise interventions for frailty have produced mixed results. A systematic review of clinical trials[47] that included community-dwelling frail older adults found no evidence for the effectiveness of nutrition interventions on disability measures. According to the same review, 3 of 9 physical exercise intervention trials showed positive outcomes for disability: (1) less functional decline at 12 months in participants with moderate frailty; (2) larger

increase in functional ability; and (3) less difficulty reported with activities of daily living (ADLs) and instrumental activities of daily living (IADLs) after a 9-month program when compared with the control group.[47] A study by Tieland et al showed that protein supplementation with a protein distribution of at least 25 g with each meal (equivalent to 1.4 g/kg/d) did not increase total or appendicular muscle mass in frail older adults; however, compared with a placebo, it significantly increased muscle strength and physical performance.[38] A 3-month multicomponent exercise program increased LBM and strength in a small sample of obese, frail older adults, and diet and exercise together produced the best results in the preservation of LBM and improvement in strength, gait, and balance.[48]

Data from the Third National Health and Nutrition Examination Survey indicated that serum 25(OH)D levels less than 15 ng/mL were associated with increased risk for frailty after adjusting for the season of the year and latitude to account for sunlight exposure.[49] Serum 25(OH)D levels below 20 ng/mL and above 30 ng/mL were associated with the greatest odds for frailty in older women.[50] A similar study of older men found the odds for frailty increased with serum 25(OH)D levels less than 20 ng/mL.[51]

Along with vitamin D, carotenoids, creatine, dehydroepiandrosterone, and beta-hydroxy beta-methylbutyrate (HMB) have been identified as potentially therapies to treat frailty in older adults,[52] although few clinical trials in frail or sarcopenic older subjects have been published. Creatine is naturally synthesized by the body and generally stored in skeletal muscle.[28] In some studies, creatine supplementation, depending on the dosage and timing, was associated with an increase in muscle strength.[28] Whether creatine can be treated as an essential nutrient in the older adult is the subject of ongoing research.[28] HMB is a leucine metabolite and is believed to enhance physical performance in young athletes.[28] Although there are only a paucity of HMB studies, results suggest supplementation may preserve muscle mass in older adults. One study randomly assigned bedridden nursing home subjects receiving EN to either HMB supplement (n = 40) or control (n = 39) and found higher blood urea nitrogen levels in the control group and lower urinary urea nitrogen excretion in the HMB group at 2 to 4 weeks.[53] The investigators concluded that HMB supplementation may reduce muscle breakdown in the population.[53]

Despite the effort of multiple studies in shedding light on the nutrition-related aspects of frailty, we lack a systematic and comprehensive approach to address these issues. Given the complex nature of frailty, additional research is required to help define the conceptual framework of frailty and its key components, including nutrition. The best possible strategies can then be determined to assist clinicians in recognizing the conditions that, if not treated in a timely fashion, might ultimately lead to significant compromised quality of life for older adults.[17]

Dysphagia

Dysphagia, or difficulty swallowing, is a common problem in the older adult population.[54] Although dysphagia is more commonly associated with neurologic conditions such as stroke and Parkinson's disease, it is also linked to other age-related illnesses, such as congestive heart failure and frailty.[54] The loss of muscle strength that signifies sarcopenia may affect the smaller striated muscles in the head and neck, thereby contributing to dysphagia.[54]

Dementia and Delirium

Dementia and delirium are conditions that involve cognitive and behavioral problems and are frequently experienced by older adults. Table 36-1 highlights the differences between them.

Dementia

Dementia often accompanies frailty, but it can occur earlier in old age. It is particularly relevant to nutrition support because patients with dementia comprise one of the largest homogeneous populations using EN in the United States.[55] Advanced dementia is a state of chronic, progressive, and usually irreversible deterioration of cognition, including memory, which eventually renders patients mute, dysphagic, unable to walk, and unable to perform ADLs. Other features of dementia include an inability to recognize family members, minimal verbal communication, total functional dependence, incontinence of urine and stool, and inability to ambulate independently.

Dementia is caused by primary neurodegenerative diseases such as Alzheimer's disease, vascular cognitive impairment/vascular dementia, and Lewy body dementia, which encompasses both dementia with Lewy bodies and Parkinson's disease dementia.[56,57] Dementia in older adults is rarely explained by a single pathology.[57] For example, Alzheimer's disease and vascular dementia often coexist as a type of "mixed dementia."[58]

Risk factors for dementia include old age; genetic predisposition; genetic mutations; Down syndrome; modifiable risk factors such as hypertension, obesity, dyslipidemia, and diabetes; and lifestyle factors such as smoking and physical activity.[57] Strategies that help prevent vascular disease risks also help to some extent prevent dementia.[58]

Symptoms of dementia vary from mild cognitive impairment to severe loss of memory and function. Dementia can progress in stages where further decline is preceded by a period of relative stability.[58] Behavioral and psychological disturbances inevitably occur in most people with dementia and can be difficult to manage even in an institutionalized setting.

Nonpharmacological interventions are encouraged as first-line measures to address nutrition-related problems, constipation, and sleep and sensory deficits.[57] Delirium also needs to be ruled out before the patient with behavioral or psychological disturbances is treated.[57]

Various nutrient deficiencies, including vitamins B_{12}, B_6, folate, and ω-3 fatty acids, have been associated with dementia, including Alzheimer's dementia. A systematic review concluded that evidence is not yet sufficient to draw definitive conclusions about the associations between these nutrients and dementia or cognitive decline.[59]

As dementia progresses, it is accompanied almost inevitably by weight loss, decreased appetite and eating difficulties.[60] Oral apraxia, chewing and swallowing difficulties, pocketing and spitting of food, lack of desire for food, and altered sense of smell and taste due to cerebral degeneration contribute to the constellation of problems associated with eating.[60,61] Weight loss ensues even when oral supplements and appropriate texture modification are used.[60] An 18-month prospective study found 86% of an advanced dementia cohort had eating problems and that survival was poor after the onset of this problem. Advanced dementia patients have a 6-month mortality rate of 25% and a median survival of 1.3 years, which is a life expectancy similar to that of commonly recognized end-of-life conditions such as end-stage congestive heart failure.[62]

Dysphagia can be a temporary result of an acute illness; however, in advanced dementia, it is usually a sign of poor prognosis.[61] Furthermore, aspiration pneumonia predicts high risk of mortality within a 6- to 12-month period.[63]

Delirium

Delirium is a state of acute confusion with concomitant changes in level of consciousness, attention, perception, and cognition. Onset is often abrupt, and its course fluctuates throughout the day.[64,65] Its presence may suggest an underlying medical emergency such as dehydration, infection, or fracture.[65]

There are 3 types of delirium: hyperactive, hypoactive and mixed. Hypoactive delirium is characterized by at least 4 of the following behaviors: decreased level of alertness, decreased awareness, decreased speech output or slow speech, staring, lethargy, or apathy. Hyperactive delirium can have the following traits: restlessness, irritability, combativeness, uncooperativeness, distractibility, wandering, hypervigilance, or loud speech. Mixed delirium involves hypoactive and

TABLE 36-1 Differences Between Dementia and Delirium

	Dementia	Delirium
Onset	Insidious	Acute and abrupt
Course	Progressive with deterioration in cognition including memory, physical function, and ability to perform activities of daily living	Fluctuating throughout the day, with altered levels of consciousness, attention, perception, and cognition
Etiology and likely outcome	Neurodegenerative disease; usually irreversible	Underlying medical illness; reversible when treated
Features	Multiple symptoms, which may vary depending on specific pathology	Hyperactive, hypoactive, and mixed forms

hyperactive traits and is the most common subtype in hospitalized patients.[65]

Although the prevalence of delirium in long-term care facilities is not known, residents in these facilities are at high risk when they have cognitive and functional impairments, and they generally present with hypoactive delirium.[65] Hypoactive delirium is also common in hospice and palliative care settings.[65] Delirium has many predisposing factors, including dementia, depression, malnutrition, polypharmacy, sensory impairment, and chronic pain.[65] It has multiple precipitating factors including but not limited to dehydration, poor nutrition, metabolic abnormalities, fracture, infection, surgery, uncontrolled pain, medications, urinary and stool retention, and sleep deprivation.[65]

Early identification of at-risk individuals can minimize delirium in older adults admitted to the hospital. Preventive and treatment strategies are multimodal. Once diagnosed, the underlying causes should be treated. Nonpharmacological treatment of delirium addresses the environment, communication, sensory stimulation, nutrition and hydration, mobility, and sleep.[66] A malnutrition screening tool should be used on a routine basis, and a full nutrition assessment should be completed for individuals at higher nutrition risk.[66]

Nutrition Screening and Assessment

Nutrition screening is the process of identifying patients, clients, or groups who may be at elevated nutrition risk and benefit from nutrition assessment and intervention.[67] Nutrition screening has been further defined by the American Society for Parenteral and Enteral Nutrition (ASPEN) as "a process to identify an individual who is malnourished or who is at risk for malnutrition to determine if a detailed nutrition assessment is indicated."[68] A positive nutrition screen leads to a more comprehensive nutrition assessment, which encompasses evaluation of patient/client history; food and nutrition-related history; anthropometric measurements; biochemical data; medical tests and procedures; and nutrition-focused physical findings.[68–70]

Nutrition screening may be carried out by any member of the interdisciplinary health care team who has been trained to do so. The timing of nutrition screening varies among settings. In acute care settings, nutrition screening is typically completed within 24 hours of admission, as required by the Joint Commission.[71] In long-term care, rehabilitation, and extended care settings, the Centers for Medicare and Medicaid Services (CMS) require a complete nutrition assessment within 14 days;[72] however, according to usual standards of practice, clinicians typically complete the nutrition screening—and nutrition assessment where appropriate—within 3 to 5 days. Efforts are being made to enhance nutrition screening in community-dwelling older adults, but currently no standard has been established; therefore, the timing of screening is inconsistent, and, in many cases, screening and assessment do not occur in this setting.

Screening and Assessment Tools

Nutrition screening tools should be quick (take less than 10 minutes to complete), easy to use, and valid and reliable for the patient population or setting.[67] The AND Nutrition Screening Workgroup evaluated 11 nutrition screening tools for their validity and reliability to identify nutrition problems in acute care and hospital-based ambulatory care settings. Grade I evidence was available to support the use of the Nutritional Risk Screening 2002 (NRS-2002). Grade II evidence was available to support the use of 4 tools: the Simple Two-Part Tool, Malnutrition Screening Tool (MST), Mini Nutritional Assessment–Short Form (MNA-SF), and the Malnutrition Universal Screening Tool (MUST).[67] The tools with the highest sensitivity included the MNA-SF and the MST. Based on the available evidence, the MST has been shown to be both valid and reliable for identifying nutrition problems in acute care and hospital-based ambulatory care settings.[67] The MNA-SF and the Nutrition Screening Initiative (NSI DETERMINE checklist) are the most widely studied and validated nutrition screening tools specific to older adults.[73]

The most effective tools to assist nutrition screening and assessment of older adults capture not only the individual's anthropometric and clinical status but also his or her functional ability to maintain or achieve adequate intake. With the possible exception of a thorough assessment by a qualified clinician, evidence suggests that the MNA is the most valid tool for malnutrition assessment in ambulatory, community-living older adults and those residing in long-term care facilities.[74] As both a nutrition screening and assessment tool, the MNA-SF, which is the current version of MNA, has been validated to identify older adults who are malnourished or at risk for malnutrition and has been used extensively in different settings, both institutional and community, and around the world.[75–77] Kaiser et al pooled analyses from multinational studies that used the MNA to evaluate malnutrition prevalence and risk and reported that 22.8% of older adults studied were malnourished and 46.2% were at risk for malnutrition; however, the prevalence of malnutrition differed among settings. Among community-dwelling older adults, 5.8% were identified as being malnourished and 31.9% were at risk for malnutrition; by comparison, in institutionalized settings, 13.8% of older adults were malnourished and 53.4% were at risk for malnutrition.[78]

More recently, Huhmann et al validated a self-administered version of the MNA called the Self-MNA to determine malnutrition risk in community-dwelling older adults.[79] Using the Self-MNA, the investigators found that 27% of subjects were malnourished, 38% were at risk for malnutrition, and 35% had normal nutrition status. The Self-MNA can be completed by trained or untrained individuals in a community or ambulatory setting, and the results can be used by individuals to seek further care and by healthcare professionals to provide the appropriate guidance and referrals for further nutrition assessment and interventions. The MNA-SF and Self-MNA were developed by Nestlé and are available online.[80]

CMS mandates that Medicare- and Medicaid-certified long-term care facilities use the Resident Assessment Instrument (RAI). The RAI provides an interprofessional framework for resident assessment and the identification of problems, which are addressed with appropriate interventions through an individualized care plan. The RAI consists of the Minimum Data

Set (MDS) and the Care Area Assessment (CAA). The MDS is completed by the members of the interprofessional team who use it to assess all aspects of clinical status and facilitate problem identification ("triggers"). As part of this assessment, the MDS also collects information about the individual resident's perception of his or her health, well-being, and activity preferences. CAA is the investigation of "trigger" areas from the MDS to determine whether further interventions and care planning are required. The nutrition assessment component of MDS, section K, assesses a resident's ability to maintain adequate nutrition and hydration and covers swallowing disorders, height and weight, weight changes, and nutrition approaches. Nutrition approaches include the use of mechanically altered and therapeutic diets and artificial nutrition and hydration (nutrition support, including PN and EN), specifically documenting the mode and percentage of required intake by the artificial route.[81]

Malnutrition Definitions and Assessment

Malnutrition develops from an imbalance of nutrients and has been defined as "an acute, subacute or chronic state of nutrition, in which varying degrees of overnutrition or undernutrition with or without inflammatory activity have led to a change in body composition and diminished function."[68] Table 36-2 lists common causes of malnutrition in older adults. In 2010, a consensus group proposed new definitions for malnutrition that are based on the etiology of inflammatory metabolism in the pathogenesis of malnutrition.[82] The definitions include uncomplicated starvation, chronic disease–related malnutrition, and acute disease– or trauma-related malnutrition (see Chapter 9). In 2012, AND and ASPEN published a joint consensus statement identifying the characteristics recommended for the identification and documentation of adult malnutrition.[83] The diagnosis of malnutrition is based on the presence of at least 2 of the following 6 criteria: insufficient energy intake, weight loss, loss of muscle mass, loss of subcutaneous fat, localized or generalized fluid accumulation, and diminished functional status as measured by handgrip strength.[83]

TABLE 36-2 Causes of Malnutrition in Older Adults

- Chronic disease
- Poor oral health
- Loss of taste and smell
- Polypharmacy
- Social isolation
- Dementia
- Obesity
- Sarcopenia/frailty
- Loss of functional capacity; inability to procure, prepare, and consume food

According to ASPEN, the purpose of nutrition assessment relative to malnutrition is "to identify any specific nutrition risk(s) or clear existence of malnutrition" so that nutrition interventions may be put into place to improve nutrition status and prevent or treat malnutrition.[68] (These interventions will be further described in the following sections.) Comprehensive individualized nutrition assessment is the gold standard. Table 36-3 lists criteria that are essential to comprehensive nutrition assessment of the older adult.[84] Historically, nutrition assessment has encompassed 5 domains of evaluation: patient/client

TABLE 36-3 Components of a Comprehensive Nutrition Assessment for the Older Adult

1. *Food and nutrition history*—assessment of food choices and the adequacy of oral intake and/or nutrition support and comparison to estimated requirements.

2. *Medical status/history and pertinent medication use*—assessment of the contribution of acute and chronic disease to current clinical status and any medication-nutrient interactions.

3. *Social environmental history*—assessment of food security and availability, and other social, behavioral, cultural, and economic influences on intake and nutrition status.

4. *Anthropometrics*—assessment of height and weight, comparison of current weight with usual body weight to assess weight changes, and BMI to assess weight status. Other measures of body composition and/or body compartment estimates *may* be assessed as appropriate or as available.

5. *Laboratory*—assessment of the pertinent and available laboratory values, which *may* include measures of hydration and kidney function, electrolytes, glycemic control, nutrition anemias, liver function, lipid profile, and inflammation and transport proteins as appropriate. Other laboratory values and medical tests may be appropriate to assess based on clinical presentation.

6. *Nutrition-focused physical examination*—assessment of physical appearance, wasting, muscle and subcutaneous fat mass, sarcopenia, dentition status and function, swallowing function, GI function, skin, hair and nails, edema, and vital signs to assess for barriers to adequate nutrient intake and to assess overall and specific nutrient deficiencies and toxicities and the effects of altered function of nutrient metabolism.

7. *Cognitive function*—assessment of cognitive function and its influence on nutrition status; may include measures of depression and delirium.

8. *Functional status*—assessment of functional status, including physical strength (measured via handgrip strength) and performance (mobility/physical activity level), and ability to perform ADLs, such as feeding, ambulation and toileting, and IADLs, such as shopping and food preparation.

ADL, activity of day living; BMI, body mass index; GI, gastrointestinal; IADL, instrumental activity of daily living.
Source: Data are from reference 84.

history; food and nutrition-related history; anthropometric measurements; biochemical data, medical tests, and procedures; and nutrition-focused physical findings.[69] In addition to these domains, nutrition assessment of the older adult should specifically focus on the effects of chronic diseases and include social, functional, and cognitive assessments. The nutrition assessment of older adults and subsequent interventions can be complicated because challenges related to the procurement and preparation of food (food security) are common among older adults and, can independent of the inflammatory complications of aging, lead to starvation-related malnutrition.[85] An assessment of functional capacity can assist in determining an older individual's ability to provide for his or her food security. Evaluation of an individual's ADLs and IADLs helps determine whether he or she needs assistance to procure, prepare, or eat food. A decline in cognitive function also affects the ability of the older adult to purchase and prepare adequate food and to meet their nutrition needs.

Nutrient Requirements

Nutrition requirements to achieve nutrient adequacy in older adults are generally the same as in younger adults, although there are some modifications associated with physiological and functional decline (eg, organ/system senescence, sarcopenia, chronic disease, and diminished physical activity). Tables 36-4 and 36-5 summarize these nutrient requirements for healthy older adults.[86–92]

As with all patients, nutrition requirements of older adults will vary considerably depending on the individual clinical condition and circumstances. Therefore, nutrition recommendations should always be individualized. Adequacy of fluid and energy, and perhaps a higher protein intake than that for younger adults, are the principal nutrition priorities in older adults.

Fluid

Fluid needs may be slightly lower in older adults than younger ones because of changes in body composition. However, older adults tend to drink less and have a higher risk of dehydration than younger adults. The risk of dehydration may be related to multiple overlapping factors, including delayed or diminished thirst sensation, decreased ability of kidneys to concentrate fluid, polypharmacy (specifically diuretics and laxatives), loss of cognitive and communication skills, loss of mobility, and fear of having "accidents" and thus restricting fluid intake to limit bathroom dependence. As a result, the need for adequate hydration becomes greater. It has been estimated that 20% to 30% of older adults are dehydrated.[93–95] Signs and symptoms of dehydration observed in older adults include decreased skin elasticity/turgor, sunken eyes, dry mucous membranes, confusion, headache, lethargy, and dizziness, as well as abnormal laboratory values indicative of dehydration.[93–95]

Estimation of fluid requirements in older adults is complicated by endocrinosenescence and the inability of the aging kidneys to concentrate urine and conserve fluid in conditions of dehydration. Therefore, although the absolute requirement for fluid in older adults may be less than that in younger adults, the decreased ability to conserve fluid means the focus is on the need to meet the minimal rather than absolute requirement. Based on expert opinion, minimal fluid requirements have been set for older adults at 1500 mL/d.[86] Multiple methods to calculate fluid needs of healthy older adults are proposed in Table 36-4. It is important to note that in the case of acute and chronic disease, fluid needs may change. Fluid recommendations are lower than 30 mL/kg/d in those with heart failure (25 mL/kg/d) and end-stage renal disease (may be as low as 1 L/d), and higher fluid requirements are noted in the presence of infection and draining wounds (~35 mL/kg/d) among others.[86]

TABLE 36-4 Fluid, Energy, Protein, and Fiber Requirements for Healthy Older Adults

	Daily Requirements
Fluid[a]	• 30 mL/kg (≥1500 mL/d) • 1 mL/kcal • 100 mL for the first 10 kg actual weight + 50 mL for the next 10 kg actual weight + 25 mL per kg actual weight thereafter

Energy	• 25–30 kcal/kg is most commonly used for weight maintenance in healthy older adults (values ranging from 18 to 40 kcal/kg have been suggested depending on weight status and illness)
	• The Mifflin–St. Jeor predictive equations[b] can be used to estimate basal metabolic rate (BMR):
	  – Men: BMR = (10 × Weight) + (6.25 × Height) − (5 × Age) + 5
	  – Women: BMR = (10 × Weight) + (6.25 × Height) − (5 × Age) − 161
	  – Where weight is measured in kg, height in cm, and age in years.
	• BMR can then be multiplied by an activity, stress, or injury factor, or the estimated energy requirement may be adjusted to promote weight loss or gain.

Protein	• 1.0–1.2 g/kg
Dietary fiber	• 25–35 g

[a]Refer to Chapter 7 and reference 86 for additional information on fluid requirements.
[b]See Chapter 2 for more detailed information on estimating energy requirements.

TABLE 36-5 Micronutrient Requirements for Healthy Older Adults: Recommended Dietary Allowances and Adequate Intakes

Nutrient	Women Age 51–70 y	Women Age >70 y	Men Age 51–70 y	Men Age >70 y
Vitamin A, mcg	700	700	900	900
Vitamin C, mg	75	75	90	90
Vitamin D,ᵃ mcg (IU)	15 (600)	20 (800)	15 (600)	20 (800)
Vitamin E, mg	15	15	15	15
Vitamin K, mcg	90*	90*	120*	120*
Thiamin, mg	1.1	1.1	1.2	1.2
Riboflavin, mg	1.1	1.1	1.3	1.3
Niacin, mg	14	14	16	16
Vitamin B₆,ᵃ mg	1.5	1.5	1.7	1.7
Folate, mcg	400	400	400	400
Vitamin B₁₂, mcg	2.4	2.4	2.4	2.4
Pantothenic acid, mg	5*	5*	5*	5*
Biotin, mcg	30*	30*	30*	30*
Choline, mg	425*	425*	550*	550*
Calcium,ᵃ mg	1200	1200	1000	1200
Chromium, mcg	20*	20*	30*	30*
Copper, mcg	900	900	900	900
Fluoride, mg	3*	3*	4*	4*
Iodine, mcg	150	150	150	150
Iron, mg	8	8	8	8
Magnesium, mg	320	320	420	420
Manganese, mg	1.8*	1.8*	2.3*	2.3*
Molybdenum, mcg	45	45	45	45
Phosphorus, mg	700	700	700	700
Selenium, mcg	55	55	55	55
Zinc, mg	8	8	11	11
Potassium, g	4.7*	4.7*	4.7*	4.7*
Sodium, g	1.3*	1.2*	1.3*	1.2*
Chloride, g	2.0*	1.8*	2.0*	1.8*

Recommended Dietary Allowances (RDAs) are in **bold** type and Adequate Intakes (AIs) are in ordinary type followed by an asterisk (*).
ᵃDietary Reference Intakes are higher than those for adults younger than 50 years.
Source: Data are from references 87–92.

Energy and Macronutrients

Energy

In comparison to younger adults, older adults generally have slightly decreased requirements for energy. The decrease in basal energy requirements for older adults is mostly related to the decline in LBM, coupled with decreases in overall activity and energy expenditure. If energy intake is not adjusted as requirements decrease, weight gain can result and contribute to a greater reduction in activity. In fact, as previously noted, the phenomenon of sarcopenic obesity and subsequent frailty

is increasing among the older adults[12,48] and, along with unintended weight loss, is associated with increased morbidity and mortality.[4,7,96]

Energy requirements for all older adults should be estimated after a thorough evaluation of an individual's clinical status, activity level, and body habitus. (See Chapters 3 and 9 for more information on energy requirements and nutrition assessment, respectively.) To promote weight gain, approximately 500 kcal/d above estimated requirements may be needed. To promote weight loss, 500 kcal/d less than the calculated requirements is recommended.[97]

Macronutrient Distribution

Macronutrient distribution for healthy older adults is similar to that suggested for younger adults: 45% to 65% of energy from carbohydrate, 20% to 35% from fat, and 10% to 35% from protein.[98,99] General recommendations for fiber intake are 14g per 1000 kcal or 20 to 30 g/d,[86,98,99] but individual requirements may be slightly higher to address gastrointestinal (GI) irregularities, which occur more frequently in older adults. Most experts advise a dietary fiber intake of 25 to 35 g/d.[86] The Dietary Guidelines for Americans encourage all individuals to make at least half of the grains consumed whole grains and limit the intake of refined grains and added sugars.[99] Recommendations for dietary fat focus on evidence supporting the benefits of reducing cardiovascular disease risk by replacing dietary saturated fatty acid and *trans* fatty acids with monounsaturated and polyunsaturated fatty acids as well as ω-3 fatty acids.[99]

Protein

The Dietary Reference Intake (DRI) for protein for all adults (age 19 years and older), including older men and women, is 0.8 g/kg/d.[98] However, anabolic resistance associated with aging may support higher protein intake to maintain health in adults older than age 65 years. The decrease in anabolic hormones coupled with insulin resistance result in a blunted response of dietary protein availability and utilization, and the net effect of decreased muscle uptake of amino acids and protein synthesis.[28,100] In addition, most experts recommend slightly higher intakes of protein based on nitrogen balance (NB) studies and, more recently, concerns related to sarcopenia and the risk for chronic disease conditions (inflammatory metabolism) associated with old age.[29,101,102] NB studies over time (to allow the quantification of muscle mass change and potential equilibration of intake and nitrogen loss) have demonstrated that 0.8 g dietary protein per kg per day may be inadequate to maintain muscle mass and strength in older men and women.[101] A cross-sectional study found that hospitalized older adults in rehabilitation required a minimum of 1.06 ± 0.28 g/kg/d to maintain NB.[103] A 3-year prospective study of protein intake and LBM in community-dwelling older men and women concluded that those in the highest quintile of protein intake lost the least amount of LBM over 3 years. Mean protein intake at the highest quintile was 1.2 g/kg/d.[29] Others have suggested that higher rates of nonmuscle protein turnover (eg, hepatic acute-phase proteins associated with inflammatory metabolic adaptation) justify slightly higher protein requirements (1 to 1.3 g/kg/d) in frail older adults.[102] The European Union Geriatric Medicine Society (the PROT-AGE Study Group) recommends average protein intake of 1 to 1.2 g/kg/d for healthy older adults and 1.2 to 1.5 g/kg/d for those who have acute or chronic diseases. For those with critical illness or injury, the study group advises that protein requirements may be as high as 2 g/kg/d.[28]

Micronutrients

Table 36-5 lists the micronutrient DRIs (Recommended Dietary Allowances and Adequate Intakes) for older adults.[87–98] The micronutrient requirements for calcium, vitamin D, and vitamin B_6 are slightly higher in older adults than in younger adults. In 2011, DRIs for vitamin D and calcium were increased because of evidence supporting the importance of these nutrients in bone and skeletal health.[92] Vitamin D in particular has been noted for a potential role in frailty, as previously discussed, and its requirement may be even greater than the suggested DRI. The role of vitamin D in health and disease is still emerging.[92,104]

The need for calcium is perhaps greater in women than men because women have a higher risk for osteoporosis. Most older adults cannot achieve the recommended intake (1200 mg/d) without supplementation.[105] It is estimated that more than 50% of women and men older than 50 years have inadequate intake of calcium and vitamin D; more than 40% of older adults consume vitamin D supplements; and more than 50% of men and more than 65% of women older than 50 years take calcium supplements to meet their needs.[106]

Vitamin B_6 requirements are higher in older adults because of age-associated changes in metabolism and bioavailability.[107] The DRI for vitamin B_{12} is not increased for older adults; however, older adults are more likely than younger adults to be deficient,[108–110] because of malabsorptive disorders related to aging and the prolonged use of certain medications such as proton pump inhibitors and metformin.[109,110] While experts propose that B_{12}, folate, B_6, and homocysteine metabolism play a role in prevention of cognitive decline, cardiovascular disease, and cancer (conditions prevalent in older adults), no consistent evidence indicates that supplementing these nutrients benefits populations at risk for these conditions. Further research is warranted in these areas.[111,112]

Finally, limiting sodium to less than 2300 mg/d is recommended as part of a heart-healthy eating pattern.[99]

Nutrition Interventions

Figure 36-1 presents a continuum of nutrition care interventions for older adults. While a healthy diet may be the ideal intervention for the community-living older adult, the medically compromised person may be able to achieve adequate intake only through a series of interventions. When desired nutrition-related goals cannot be met despite these efforts, EN or PN support can be considered. In some circumstances, palliative care or comfort measures may also be a realistic option.

Healthy Diet

The 2015–2020 Dietary Guidelines for Americans offer current recommendations for all Americans, including older adults.[99] Ideally, the consumption of a healthy diet, which can be characterized as a diet comprised of relatively high amounts of whole vegetables and fruits, whole grains, lean meats, low-fat dairy products, legumes, and nuts, should be the initial intervention in the nutrition care of the older adult. Adherence to this type of diet has been associated with optimal nutrition status, quality of life, and reduced mortality in older community-dwelling adults as compared with diets with high amounts of saturated animal fats, processed foods, sodium, and simple carbohydrates.[113] To achieve a healthy diet, older adults must have access to healthy food items and be able to obtain, prepare, and consume them. Community-dwelling older adults are at particular risk for food insecurity, defined as the "state of being without reliable access to a sufficient quantity of affordable, nutritious food."[114] Home-delivered meals is one intervention that may address this problem.[115] However, the challenge to clinicians and public health professionals is to not only address issues universally associated with food insecurity but also those that are specifically problematic for older adults, including sarcopenia, obesity, frailty, dementia, and food safety, among others.[85] Table 36-6 lists federal and state food and nutrition programs geared toward helping community-dwelling older adults meet their nutrition needs.[116]

Individualized Diet

In acute care and long-term care settings, dietary interventions should be guided by individualized nutrition assessment and goals for nutrition care. In general, liberalized diets may both improve a patient's quality of life and aid in preserving nutrition status, particularly in frail older adults. Therapeutic diets may be less palatable and acceptable to older individuals, thus compromising intake; therefore, the costs and benefits should be weighed when considering whether to implement them for specific patients. In addition, including older adults in decisions about food may enhance their desire to eat and improve their perceived quality of life.[117,118] Because of the potential for adverse health outcomes, the decision to liberalize a diet restriction should be made by a qualified clinician. (See Practice Scenario 36-1.)

FIGURE 36-1 Nutrition Intervention Algorithm for Older Adults

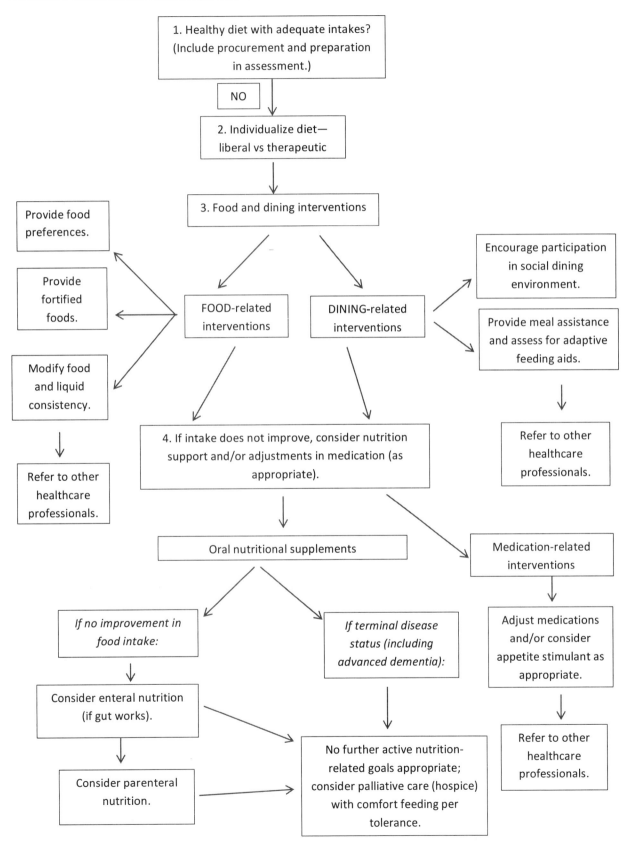

TABLE 36-6 Federal and State Food and Nutrition Programs for Community-Dwelling Older Adults

Program	Purpose	Services	Eligibility
US Department of Health and Human Services Administration on Aging			
Older Americans Act Title I–VII	Grants to state, tribal, and community programs on aging.	Nutrition and other supportive and health services.	Age is the sole requirement. There are no income requirements. Targets older adults with economic/social needs.
	Title III Nutrition services to older adults.	Congregate and home-delivered meals. Nutrition screening, assessment, education, counseling.	Age is the sole requirement. There are no income requirements. Targets older adults with economic/social needs. Only home-bound individuals qualify for home-delivered meals.
	Title VI Support for tribal and native organizations' aging-related programs and services.	Congregate and home-delivered meals. Nutrition screening, assessment, education, counseling and other supportive and health services.	There are no income requirements. Age is the sole requirement. Age requirement is determined by tribal organizations or native Hawaiian program.
Nutrition Services Incentive Program	Provides grants to states, territories and eligible tribal organizations to support the congregate and home-delivered nutrition programs by providing an incentive to serve more meals. States, territories and eligible tribal organizations can choose to receive their grant as cash, commodities (food) or a combination of cash and commodities.		
US Department of Agriculture Food and Nutrition Service			
Supplemental Nutrition Assistance Program	Authorizes low-income families to buy food that is nutritionally adequate.	Coupons or electronic benefits to purchase bread, cereal, fruit, vegetables, meat, fish, poultry, dairy products, or seeds or plants that produce food for households.	US citizens or legal residents who are in need, gross income ≤130% of federal poverty level; up to $2000 countable resources, $3000 if aged ≥60 y and/or disabled.
Food Distribution Program on Indian Reservations	Provides US Department of Agriculture foods to low-income households living on or near Indian reservations; an alternative for households that do not have access to Supplemental Nutrition Assistance Program offices or authorized food stores.	Provides US Department of Agriculture–purchased foods and nutrition education to recipients.	Low-income American Indian and non-Indian households living on a reservation and families living in approved areas near a reservation. Also includes homes in Oklahoma that have at least 1 person who is a member of a federally recognized tribe. Participants are certified based on income. Recertification occurs every 12 mo; however, elderly and disabled applicants may be qualified for up to 24 mo. Participants cannot participate in Supplemental Nutrition Assistance Program and Food Distribution Program on Indian Reservations during the same month.

TABLE 36-6 Federal and State Food and Nutrition Programs for Community-Dwelling Older Adults (continued)

Program	Purpose	Services	Eligibility
US Department of Agriculture Food and Nutrition Service			
Commodity Supplemental Food Program	Food and administrative funds to states and tribes to supplement diets. Available in 23 states and 2 tribes.	Pregnant and breastfeeding women, mothers up to 1 y postpartum, infants, children aged ≤6 y.	Adults aged ≥60 y, ≤130% of federal poverty guidelines. Women, infants, children, ≤185% of federal poverty guidelines.
Seniors' Farmers Market Nutrition Program	Grants to states and tribes to provide fresh foods and nutrition services while providing an opportunity for farmers to boost their business.	Coupons or vouchers to be exchanged for fresh fruits and vegetables at local farmers markets.	Low-income adults aged ≥60 y with household income ≤185% of federal poverty guidelines.
Child and Adult Care Food Program	Healthy, nutritious meals for children and adults in day care.	Nutritionally adequate meals and snacks.	≤185% of federal poverty guidelines. Children aged ≤12 y; homeless children; migrant children aged ≤15 y; adults aged ≥60 y; adults, regardless of age, who are functionally impaired to an extent that limits their independence and ability to carry out activities of daily living.

Source: Adapted from reference 116: Academy of Nutrition and Dietetics. Position of the Academy of Nutrition and Dietetics. Food and nutrition for older adults: promoting health and wellness. *J Acad Nutr Diet*. 2012;112:1255-1277. Used with permission from Elsevier.

Practice Scenario 36-1

Question: How can a diet be liberalized in a frail older adult with end-stage renal disease on hemodialysis?

Scenario: An 87-year-old, frail woman, a resident of a skilled nursing center, started hemodialysis because her glomerular filtration rate was 10 mL/min/1.73 m^2. The renal dietitian at the dialysis center recommended implementing an 80 g protein, 2 g sodium, 2 g potassium, 1 g phosphorous diet with a fluid restriction of 1200 mL/d. As her kidney disease worsened, the woman was eating poorly and had a significant 5% weight loss in 30 days. During the first month of dialysis, the resident's weight declined further and her oral intake remained poor. The resident asked for a few of her favorite foods, such as chocolate milk, but the physician did not elect to liberalize the diet. Despite patient's impaired renal function, serum potassium and phosphorous levels were within normal limits.

Intervention: Recognizing that malnutrition and a low albumin level increases mortality in dialysis patients, the registered dietitians (RDs) from the dialysis center and the nursing facility collaborated to determine the best plan for this resident. The individualized approach was to allow the resident to have her favorite foods, such as chocolate milk and mashed potatoes, and monitor her laboratory test values to determine the effects on her serum potassium and phosphorus levels. As a result of the diet changes, the resident improved her intake and had a significant 5% weight

gain. The patient's phosphorous level increased because of the increased phosphorous in her diet; however, phosphate binders could be added as needed to control the level.

Answer: By collaborating with the renal RD and monitoring laboratory test values, the resident's food preferences were incorporated into her diet, with a resultant increase in intake and body weight and no compromise to renal status.

Rationale: This resident's poor intake and weight loss increased her risk for malnutrition. Collaboration with the health care team and individualizing the resident's diet helped to improve both nutrition status and renal function.

A sodium-restricted diet for patients with heart failure, hypertension, or cardiovascular disease is one example of a therapeutic diet commonly prescribed for older adults. The American Heart Association's current guidelines recommend limiting daily sodium intake in all population groups to 1500 mg to prevent and control hypertension and cardiovascular disease.[119] However, in adults with heart failure, a meta-analysis found a U-shaped relation between sodium intake and all-cause mortality, noting higher mortality rates not only in subjects with excessive sodium intakes (greater than 4900 mg/d) but also in those with low sodium intakes (less than 2700 mg/d).[120] As with most clinical conditions, heart failure management comprises of medication management as well as nutrition management of sodium and fluid intake. The interprofessional healthcare team should individualize interventions for optimal care based on the patient's clinical condition and goals.

Food and Dining Interventions

Once the older adult's diet has been individualized to address his or her nutrition requirements and disease management, additional interventions may be useful for maintaining or improving nutrition status. The patient's preferred foods and beverages should be provided at and in between meals (snacks) to maximize intake and quality of life. Providing meals at alternate times and adjusting meal/snack frequency (such as 6 small meals per day) may increase intake. Fortified foods can increase energy and protein intake without adding volume to meals and snacks. Altering food textures and fluid consistencies may also be appropriate, especially for those older adults with dysphagia or difficulty chewing due to impaired dentition. Individuals with difficulty chewing or swallowing may consume more food and fluid when their diet is modified to facilitate easier mastication and safer swallowing of liquids. The individual's food and fluid intake must be monitored for acceptance of mechanically altered foods and thickened fluids to ensure that he or she receives the highest level of diet tolerated for safe swallowing and chewing. In these situations, referral to a speech language pathologist or dentist may also be indicated.

Assisting and/or cueing patients with eating, serving meals in a socially stimulating environment, improved dining ambiance, and creative dining programs have all be reported to increase food intake of older adults in long-term care communities.[73] Providing adaptive feeding devices, including special flatware and cups may promote independence in feeding and help the older adult consume adequate food and fluid intake. Serving foods that can be held with the hands (finger foods), including quarter sandwiches and raw vegetable sticks, may also promote eating independence. Referrals to the physical and occupational therapy teams may be appropriate to increase functional ability and ability to self-feed.

Oral Nutritional Supplements and Medication-Related Interventions

When nutrition requirements are not met despite food and dining modifications, oral nutritional supplements should be considered. They will be discussed in more detail in the next section on nutrition support.

The medication regimen of the older adult should be reviewed as part of the nutrition assessment. Medications can cause loss or increase of appetite, nausea, diarrhea, weight changes, taste alterations, drug-nutrient interactions, and reduction in saliva, among other nutrition-related effects.[121] Potential changes in medication regimen to improve nutrition status, such as appetite stimulants, should be discussed with the primary prescribing healthcare provider. Although the evidence supporting the use of appetite stimulant in older adults is limited, they can be considered. Megestrol acetate (Megace) has been used as an appetite stimulant in older adults with inadequate intakes and anorexia resulting in weight loss and malnutrition. Benefits should be weighed against risks before using in older adults.[122] Mirtazapine (Remeron), an antidepressant that has also been shown to stimulate appetite, has also been used as an approach to improve appetite in older adults. Further clinical investigation has been recommended to better determine its role in appetite stimulation.[123]

At times, the nutrition status of the older adult may fail to stabilize even with multiple interventions. In this situation, the need for EN or PN may need to be broached. These interventions, along with palliative care and comfort feeding, are reviewed in the following sections.

Nutrition Support

Evidence-based guidelines on the use of nutrition support for older adults come from both the ASPEN and the European Society for Clinical Nutrition and Metabolism (ESPEN).[124-126] Nutrition support encompasses oral nutritional supplements, EN, and PN.[124] PN refers to central and peripheral vein administration of fluid and nutrients as well as the subcutaneous administration of fluid and electrolytes or hypodermoclysis. The latter is a potential intervention for moderate dehydration in older adults; however, it is a more common practice in Europe than in the United States, where it is used infrequently for reasons that are undetermined.[127]

Oral nutritional supplementation is recommended as the initial form of nutrition support for older adults with multiple morbidities, for the frail, and for those following orthopedic surgical procedures. EN is recommended for individuals with neurologic dysphagia but is not indicated in end-stage disease, including advanced dementia. PN is used to provide nutrition when GI function is compromised.[124] Even if GI function is intact, PN is a safe and effective alternative for some patients who cannot meet nutrition requirements enterally, and it should not be withheld as a treatment because of a patient's older age. The decision to use EN or PN should be considered in the context of the individual's clinically feasible chances of survival, as well as factors such as age-related physiological changes; drug interactions; and susceptibility to glycemic, fluid, electrolyte, and micronutrient complications associated with older age.[124-126] Both hydration and PN are appropriate in terminal illness when they are consistent with the goals of palliative treatment and in concert with the wishes of the patient or surrogate decision maker.[125,126] (See Chapter 39 for additional information on the ethics of nutrition support.)

The use of nutrition support to improve the nutrition status of malnourished older adults and those with sarcopenia differs between acute care and long-term care settings. In the acute environment, oral nutritional supplements are often the intervention of choice because the patient's length of stay is limited and it is imperative to achieve maximum energy and protein intake in a short time frame. A comprehensive review on the use of oral nutritional supplements in acute care has reported decreased lengths of stay, episode cost, and 30-day readmission risk, which may result from improvement in nutrition status.[128] For patients at risk for unintended weight loss and malnutrition in the long-term care setting, current recommendations are to provide "real food first" before oral nutritional supplements because patients tend to dislike/refuse the supplements and because of the costs associated with supplement waste.[118]

A systematic review reports that oral nutritional supplement interventions are effective in the treatment of sarcopenia in older adults.[129] A meta-analysis concluded that the use of oral nutritional supplements may also facilitate physical rehabilitation and reduce complications in older women after a hip fracture; however, there was no difference in mortality between the intervention and control groups.[130]

While the use of oral nutritional supplements and assisted oral feeding can be resource-intensive and costly, the initiation of EN should not be considered as an immediate alternative when a patient can eat orally. In older adults, EN via percutaneous endoscopic gastrostomy is preferred over nasogastric feeding for patient comfort, ease of use, and long-term durability.[131] Nasogastric tubes (NGTs) are not recommended for older adults because of the increased risk of aspiration and the potential of NGTs to impede swallowing in those who may still be eating some foods and fluids orally.[132] A percutaneous endoscopic jejunostomy may be considered in older adults with gastroparesis, severe gastroesophageal reflux, upper GI tract obstruction, or a high risk for aspiration.[131]

Short-term EN may be indicated for older adults who have had surgery or an acute critical illness and temporarily cannot meet the metabolic demands of the illness or trauma. In cases where rehabilitation is a realistic goal, tube feeding to provide adequate nutrition can be a prerequisite for recovery or functional improvement.[125,133] The interdisciplinary healthcare team, including the speech language pathologist and the registered dietitian, should be work together to reintroduce foods and fluids to patients who may be able to resume oral feedings. (See Practice Scenario 36-2.) Long-term EN may be required by individuals with dysphagia caused by a vascular disease such as cerebrovascular accident (CVA), Parkinson's disease, alcoholism, or damage to the GI tract.[131] EN has been noted to improve quality of life or survival in the following conditions: cancers of the head and neck, acute CVA with dysphagia, neuromuscular dystrophy, and growth failure (in children), No improvement in nutrition-related or functional status was found in patients with cachexia, anorexia, aspiration (and aspiration pneumonia), or cancer with a poor prognosis.[134]

Practice Scenario 36-2

Question: Can an enteral nutrition regimen be planned to enable participation in activities (including rehabilitation)?

Scenario: A 79-year-old long-term care resident has recently been hospitalized for aspiration pneumonia. Prior to hospitalization, she had been on a dysphagia diet with puree consistency and nectar-thickened liquids. A percutaneous endoscopic gastrostomy tube was placed in the hospital, and the resident is to be allowed no food or fluids by mouth. Her prior medical history includes diabetes, hypertension, coronary artery disease, depression, and mild dementia. She has been a relatively active member of the nursing home and enjoys socializing at meals and attending activities. Following her hospital stay, she will require 1 hour each of physical and occupational therapy for the next 30 days.

The resident is 63 inches tall and weighs 135 pounds. In the past 6 months, her weight gradually decreased from her usual body weight of 150 pounds, a significant unintended weight loss of 10% in 6 months. On physical examination, her skin is warm and dry with good turgor, no edema, and a reddened sacrum. She owns upper and lower dentures but does not wear them, as they do not fit properly since she lost weight. Blood pressure is 130/90 mmHg. Recent laboratory values outside of normal limits include an albumin level of 3.0 g/dL and a blood glucose level of 146 mg/dL. In the hospital, she was receiving Glucerna at a continuous rate of 70 mL/h, providing a total volume of 1680 mL of Glucerna, 1680 kcal, and 70 g protein, which met 100% of her nutrition needs. In the long-term care facility, the feeding has been turned off during care and while she is at therapy, resulting in a total daily volume of 1260 mL, which meets 75% of her estimated nutrition needs.

Intervention: The enteral feeding order is changed to Glucerna 1.2 at 80 mL/h to provide a total volume of 1400 mL, 1680 kcal, and 84 g protein. Feeding starts at 4:00 PM and runs for approximately 17.5 hours, until 9:30 AM, so that she can partake in her morning therapy session and the daily afternoon activity. Water flushes are given before feeding begins and when feeding is completed. Extra water flushes are done at scheduled times during the day to coincide with times when medications are administered. A speech language pathologist is consulted to reassess the ability to swallow and initiate oral intake.

Answer: By providing a more energy-dense formula, the infusion time is shortened, which allows the resident to participate in rehabilitation and therapeutic recreation. Fluid requirements are met by giving water flushes throughout the day. Scheduling these flushes around medication times decreases omission errors. Extra water can also be given when necessary as part of the feeding schedule. A feeding pump with flushing capability can provide water without disturbing the resident during the night. If the swallowing assessment fails, attempts can be further made to consolidate the tube feeding schedule to a bolus daytime regimen to mimic an oral feeding pattern.

Rationale: While in the hospital, patients can meet their nutrition needs through a 24-hour continuous enteral feeding regimen; however, such a regimen is difficult to manage in a long-term care facility, especially if the feeding needs to be turned off during rehabilitation and therapeutic recreation. The resident's nutrition goals can be achieved by providing a nurse-driven, volume-based protocol to adjust the rate of infusion and fluid schedule.

Guidance on PN use in older adults is limited. When older adults cannot meet nutrition requirements via the enteral route, PN is an option. PN is infused through peripheral catheters, peripherally inserted central catheters, or central catheters (usually tunneled catheters for long-term administration).[126] (See Chapter 16 for more information on PN access and devices.) PN is safe when managed correctly, although the chances for clinical improvement and the increased likelihood of complications in older adults should be considered.[126] Compared with younger adults, older adults are more susceptible to metabolic complications associated with PN because insulin resistance and impaired cardiac and renal functions are more common in this population. They are also more likely than younger adults to have micronutrient deficiencies. In addition, the repletion of LBM is slower in older adults than in those who are younger.[126]

A retrospective Taiwanese study reported the most common indications for PN in older adults was for perioperative status, severe GI tract hemorrhage, ileus, and persistent vomiting.[135] Anecdotally, reluctance to use PN is perhaps due to clinicians' perceptions that the risks, such as catheter-associated sepsis and metabolic complications associated with refeeding syndrome especially at the end of life, outweigh the benefits.[124] In addition, the fragility of older adults' skin and veins, the required expertise of clinicians in management and compounding solutions, and the cost of PN may moderate its use. According to ESPEN guidelines, parenteral delivery with the catheter tip in a peripheral vein is discouraged in older adults because the fragility of peripheral veins and the need for a frequent change of site cause understandable distress to older patients; however, more advanced peripheral catheters, such as polyurethane and silicon catheters, including midline catheters, can remain in place longer than the standard peripheral catheter.[126] Even if PN is indicated, short-term infusion may be clinically meaningless, and every effort should be made to accommodate patient comfort.

Neither the ESPEN guidelines[125,126] nor the ASPEN ethics position[136] recommend the use of EN or PN in end-stage disease or terminal illness, including advanced stages of dementia and neurologic conditions, such as persistent vegetative state. Chapter 39 reviews this issue and related ethical considerations in detail.

Advanced Dementia, Ethics, and End-of-Life Care

Patients with advanced dementia may develop neurologic dysphagia similar to the dysphagia that affects patients with CVA, Parkinson's disease, or multiple sclerosis.[137,138] Older adults with advanced dementia who cannot meet nutrition requirements orally are potential candidates for artificial nutrition and hydration, which is usually in the form of EN because GI function remains intact. Before nutrition support is considered, steps should be taken to examine reversible causes of poor nutrition intake first and foremost. For example, oversedation from medications, dehydration leading to changes in level of consciousness, and oral fungal infection leading to odynophagia are problems that should be corrected.[60]

The use of EN in older adults with advanced dementia is controversial. A Cochrane Database evaluation[139] of the outcome of tube feeding in older adults with advanced dementia did not identify any randomized controlled trials for use in the evaluation. Controlled observational studies offered no evidence that EN increases survival, improves nutrition status, decreases the prevalence of pressure injuries, prevents aspiration pneumonia, reduces the risk of infection, or improves the comfort of the patient.[133,134,140] In addition, none of the studies in the Cochrane review evaluated quality of life.[139] Studies have consistently demonstrated a high rate of mortality in older adults with advanced dementia who have feeding tubes, and up to 34% of United States nursing home residents with advanced dementia are enterally fed.[138] Advanced dementia is a terminal illness, and EN is therefore not indicated unless a specific and limited goal is realistically attainable.[140] A specific goal might be the improvement in physical function, which, according to a 6-month review of medical records, did improve among patients with advanced dementia who received adequate EN support.[133]

End-of-life discussions and decisions about medical treatment such as nutrition support for patients with dementia are often wrought with emotion, especially under the pressure of a medical crisis.[63] Clinicians and families may not recognize that advanced dementia is a terminal disease.[61,63] Because these patients are usually incapable of actively participating in health care decisions, they must rely on family or surrogate decision makers who may already be frustrated or anxious and naturally see food as an essential aspect of life.[141,142] Nutrition support is not without risks and burdens when given at the end of life. There are risks associated with feeding tube placement. Patients may experience discomfort from the maintenance and changing of angiocatheter sites, increased oropharyngeal and pulmonary secretions, fluid overload, cough, constipation, frequent urination, the need for chemical or physical restraints, and prodding to monitor for possible treatment-related metabolic complications.[60,143,144]

When oral consumption is still feasible, comfort feeding has been found to sufficiently satisfy hunger and thirst. *Comfort feeding* (Figure 36-1) is the medical terminology used for giving foods and fluids orally as tolerated even if intake is not adequate to meet nutrition requirements. Comfort feeding involves feeding by hand small amounts of food or sips of liquids frequently as long as undue pressure to the patient is avoided.[60,143] This allows patients to eat orally based on what they are able to safely tolerate.[145] Patients' behaviors are taken into consideration and refusal of food is regarded as an act of will that should be respected.[61,142] Mouth care consists of cleaning and lubrication of the oral cavity, when regularly performed, mitigates symptoms of dry mouth and increases comfort.[60] Knowing that a patient with advanced disease will continue to receive some foods and fluids by mouth can reassure families that their loved one is not starving.

Many factors affect the family's perceptions and preference about treatment: the perceived patient's quality of life, the invasiveness of treatment, their cultural and religious values, and their trust in the healthcare team.[63] Central to any clinical decision-making process is the patient's best interests, and a patient's values and preferences may seem more relevant and at times challenging to determine when the patient lacks capacity to make decisions and end-of-life goals and wishes have not been expressed.[63,140] An advance directive documenting a person's previously stated goals of care, can be of tremendous value in guiding family members and the healthcare team in the decision-making process in the event the patient is unable to participate.[63] However, when a patient's explicit wishes are not known, collaboration among the healthcare team is crucial to formulate an accurate clinical picture whereby ethical discussions can follow. The decision-making process with all interested parties involved is dynamic and may require multiple discussions before any common ground or goals of care can be reached. The healthcare team needs to communicate risks, burdens, benefits, and options clearly in an open and compassionate fashion to ultimately assist and support surrogate decision makers as they make decisions that are informed and most reflective of the values of the patient.[140,142,146] (See Chapter 39.)

References

1. He W, Goodkind D, Kowal P. An aging world: 2015. US Census Bureau, International Population Report P95/16-1. 2016. http://www.census.gov/library/publications/2016/demo/P95-16-1.html. Accessed January 2, 2017.

2. Chernoff R. *Geriatric Nutrition: The Health Professional's Handbook.* 4th ed. Burlington, MA: Jones & Bartlett Learning; 2014.

3. Centers for Disease Control and Prevention. *The State of Aging and Health in America 2013.* Atlanta, GA: Centers for Disease Control and Prevention; 2013. https://www.cdc.gov/aging/agingdata/data-portal/state-aging-health.html. Accessed January 2, 2017.

4. Morley JE. Undernutrition in older adults. *Family Pract.* 2012; 29(Suppl 1):i89–i93.

5. Chapman IM. The anorexia of aging. *Clin Geriatr Med.* 2007; 23(4):735–756.

6. Waters DL, Baumgartner RN, Garry PJ, et al. Advantages of dietary, exercise-related, and therapeutic interventions to prevent and treat sarcopenia in adult patients: an update. *Clin Interv Aging.* 2010;5:259–270.

7. Cruz-Jenthoft AJ, Baeyens JP, Bauer JM, et al. European Working Group on Sarcopenia in Older People. Sarcopenia: European consensus on definition and diagnosis: report of the European Working Group on Sarcopenia in Older People. *Age Ageing.* 2010;39(4):412–423.

8. Fielding RA, Vellas B, Evans WJ, et al. Sarcopenia: an undiagnosed condition in older adults. Current consensus definition: prevalence, etiology, and consequences. International Working Group on Sarcopenia. *J Am Med Dir Assoc.* 2011;12(4):249–256.

9. Rondanelli M, Faliva M, Monteferrario F, et al. Novel insights on nutrient management of sarcopenia in elderly. *Biomed Res Int.* 2015; 524948. doi:10.1155/2015/524948.

10. Cooper C, Dere W, Evans W, et al. Frailty and sarcopenia: definitions and outcome parameters. *Osteoporos Int.* 2012;23(7):1839–1848.

11. Delmonico MJ, Harris TB, Lee JS, et al. Alternative definitions of sarcopenia, lower extremity performance, and functional impairment with aging in older men and women. *Am Geriatr Soc.* 2007;55:769–774.

12. Batsis JA, Mackenzie TA, Barre LK, et al. Sarcopenia, sarcopenic obesity and mortality in older adults: results from the National Health and Nutrition Examination Survey III. *Eur J Clin Nutr.* 2014(68):1001–1007.

13. Landi F, Abbatecola AM, Provinciali M, et al. Moving against frailty: does physical activity matter? *Biogerontology.* 2010;11(5): 537–545.

14. Visser M, Kritchevsky SB, Newman AB, et al. Lower serum albumin concentration and change in muscle mass: the Health Aging and Body Composition Study. *Am J Clin Nutr.* 2005;82:531–537.

15. Argiles JM, Busquets S, Felipe A, Lopez-Soriano FJ. Muscle wasting in cancer and ageing: cachexia versus sarcopenia. *Adv Gerontol.* 2006;18:39–54.

16. Thomas DR. Loss of skeletal muscle mass in aging: examining the relationship of starvation, sarcopenia, and cachexia. *Clin Nutr.* 2007;26:389–399.

17. Rizzoli R, Reginster JY, Arnal JF, et al. Quality of life in sarcopenia and frailty. *Calcif Tissue Int.* 2013;93(2):101–120.

18. Marzetti E, Leeuwenburgh C. Skeletal muscle apoptosis, sarcopenia, and frailty at old age. *Exp Gerontol.* 2006;41:1234–1238.

19. Hiona A, Leeuwenburgh C. The role of mitochondrial DNA mutations in aging and sarcopenia: implications for the mitochondrial vicious cycle theory at old age. *Exp Gerontol.* 2008;43(1):24–33.

20. Lee CE, McArdle A, Griffiths RD. The role of hormones, cytokines and heat shock proteins during age-related muscle loss. *Clin Nutr.* 2007;26:524–534.

21. Gianoudis J, Bailey CA, Daly RM. Associations between sedentary behavior and body composition, muscle function and sarcopenia in community-dwelling older adults. *Osteoporos Int.* 2015(26):571–579.

22. Bales CW, Ritchie CS. Sarcopenia, weight loss, and nutritional frailty in the elderly. *Annu Rev Nutr.* 2002;22(1):309–323.

23. Peterson SJ, Braunschweig CA. Prevalence of sarcopenia and associated outcomes in the clinical setting. *Nutr Clin Pract.* 2016; 31(1):40–48.

24. Li A, Heber D. Sarcopenic obesity in the elderly and strategies for weight management. *Nutr Clin Care.* 2011;70(1):57–64.

25. Janssen I, Katzmarzyk PT, Ross R. Body mass index is inversely related to mortality in older people after adjustment for waist circumference. *J Am Geriatr Soc.* 2005;53:2112–2118.

26. Mangione KK, Miller AH, Naughton IV. Cochrane review: Improving physical function and performance with progressive resistance strength training in older adults. *Phys Ther.* 2010;90(12): 1711–1715.

27. Burton LA, Sumukadas D. Optimal management of sarcopenia. *Clin Interv Aging.* 2010;5:217–228.

28. Bauer J, Biolo G, Cederholm T, et al. Evidence-based recommendations for optimal dietary protein intake in older people: a position paper from the PROT-AGE Study Group. *J Am Med Dir Assoc.* 2013;14:542–559.

29. Houston DK, Nicklas BJ, Ding J, et al. Dietary protein intake is associated with lean mass change in older, community-dwelling adults: the Health, Aging, and Body Composition (Health ABC) Study. *Am J Clin Nutr.* 2008;87(1):150–155.

30. Paddon-Jones D, Short KR, Campbell WW, et al. Role of dietary protein in the sarcopenia of aging. *Am J Clin Nutr.* 2008;87(5 Suppl):1562S–1566S.

31. Campbell WW. Synergistic use of higher-protein diets or nutritional supplements with resistance training to counter sarcopenia. *Nutr Rev.* 2007;65(9);416–422.

32. Pennings B, Boire Y, Senden JM, et al. Whey protein stimulates postprandial protein accretion more effectively than do casein and casein hydrolysate in older men. *Am J Clin Nutr.* 2011;93(5): 997–1005.

33. Morley JE, Argiles JM, Evans WJ, et al. Nutritional recommendations for the management of sarcopenia. *J Am Med Dir Assoc.* 2010;11(6):391–396.

34. Smith GI, Atherton P, Reeds DN, et al. Dietary omega-3 fatty acid supplementation increases the rate of muscle protein synthesis in older adults: a randomized controlled trial. *Am J Clin Nutr.* 2011;93(2):402–412.

35. Adamo ML, Farrar RP. Resistance training, and IGF involvement in the maintenance of muscle mass during the aging process. *Ageing Res Rev.* 2006;5(3):310–331.

36. Pennings B, Groen B, de Lange A, et al. Amino acid absorption and subsequent muscle protein accretion following graded intakes of whey protein in elderly men. *Am J Physiol Endocrinol Metab.* 2012;302 (8):E992–E999.

37. Paddon-Jones D, Rasmussen BB. Dietary protein recommendations and the prevention of sarcopenia. *Curr Opin Clin Nutr Metab Care.* 2009;12(1):86–90.

38. Tieland M, van de Rest O, Dirks ML, et al. Protein supplementation improves physical performance in frail elderly people: a randomized, double-blind, placebo-controlled trial. *J Am Med Dir Assoc.* 2012;13(8):720–726.

39. Solerte SB, Gassaruso C, Bonacasa R, et al. Nutritional supplements with oral amino acid mixtures increases whole-body lean mass and insulin sensitivity in elderly subjects with sarcopenia. *Am J Cardiol.* 2008;101(11A):69E–77E.

40. Dillon EL, Sheffield-Moore M, Paddon-Jones D, et al. Amino acid supplementation increases lean body mass, basal muscle protein synthesis, and insulin-like growth factor-1 expression in older women. *J Clin Endocrinol Metab.* 2009;94(5):1630–1637.

41. Jung HW, Kim SW, Lim JY, et al. Frailty status can predict further lean body mass decline in older adults. *J Am Geriatr Soc.* 2014;62(11):2110–2117.

42. Fried LP, Tangen CM, Watson J, et al. Frailty in older adults: evidence for a phenotype. *J Gerontol A Biol Sci Med Sci.* 2001;56;M146–M157.

43. Hubbard RE, O'Mahony MS, Calver BL, Woodhouse KW. Nutrition, inflammation, and leptin levels in aging and frailty. *J Am Geriatr Soc.* 2008;56(2):279–284.

44. Hubbard RE, Woodhouse KW. Frailty, inflammation and the elderly. *Biogerontology.* 2010;11(5):635–641.

45. Bartali B, Frongillo EA, Bandinelli S, et al. Low nutrient intake is an essential component of frailty in older persons. *J Gerontol A Biol Sci Med Sci.* 2006;61(6):589–593.

46. Isaia G, Mondino S, Germinara C, et al. Malnutrition in an elderly demented population living at home. *Arch Gerontol Geriatr.* 2011;53(3):249–251.

47. Daniels R, van Rossum E, de Witte L, et al. Interventions to prevent disability in frail community-dwelling elderly: a systematic review. *BMC Health Serv Res.* 2008;8:278.

48. Villareal DT, Smith GI, Sinacore DR, et al. Regular multicomponent exercise increases physical fitness and muscle protein anabolism in frail, obese, older adults. *Obesity.* 2011;19(2):312–318.

49. Wilhelm-Leen ER, Hall YN, DeBoer IH, Chertow GM. Vitamin D deficiency and frailty in older Americans. *J Intern Med.* 2010;268(2):171–180.

50. Ensrud KE, Ewing SK, Fredman L, et al. Circulating 25–hydroxyvitamin D levels and frailty status in older women. *J Clin Endocrinol Metab.* 2010;95(12):5266–5273.

51. Ensrud KE, Blackwell TL, Cauley JA, et al. Circulating 25–hydroxyvitamin D levels and frailty in older men: the osteoporotic fractures in men study. *J Am Geriatr Soc.* 2011;59(1):101–106.

52. Cherniack EP, Florex HJ, Troen BR. Emerging therapies to treat frailty syndrome in the elderly. *Altern Med Rev.* 2007:12(3):246–258.

53. Hsieh LC, Chow CJ, Chang WC, Liu TH, Chang CK. Effect of beta-hydroxy-beta-methylbutyrate on protein metabolism in bed-ridden elderly receiving tube feeding. *Asia Pac J Clin Nutr.* 2010;19(2):200–208.

54. Robbins J, Gangnon RE, Theis SM, et al. The effects of lingual exercise on swallowing in older adults. *J Am Geriatr Soc.* 2005;53(9):1483–1489.

55. Braun UK, Rabeneck L, McCullough LB, et al. Decreasing use of percutaneous endoscopic gastrostomy tube feeding for veterans with dementia—racial differences remain. *J Am Geriatr Soc.* 2005;53(2):242–248.

56. Beers MH, ed. *The Merck Manual,* 18th ed. Whitehouse Station, NJ: Merck; 2006:1811–1821.

57. LoGiudice D, Watson R. Dementia in older people: an update. *J Intern Med.* 2014;44:1066–1073.

58. Heart and Stroke Foundation. Stroke Report 2016. Mind the Connection: Preventing Stroke and Dementia. http://www.heartandstroke.com/site/c.ikIQLcMWJtE/b.9341045/k.64B5/Understanding_stroke.htm#strokedementia-tab. Accessed July 15, 2016.

59. Dangour AD, Whitehouse PJ, Rafferty K, et al. B vitamins and fatty acids in the prevention and treatment of Alzheimer's disease and dementia: a systematic review. *J Alzheimers Dis.* 2010;22(1):205–224.

60. Arcand M. End-of-life issues in advanced dementia: part 2: management of poor nutritional intake, dehydration, and pneumonia. *Can Fam Physician.* 2015;61(4):337–341.

61. Congedo M, Causarano RI, Alberti F, et al. Ethical issues in end of life treatments for patients with dementia. *Eur J Neurol.* 2010;17:774–779.

62. Mitchell SL, Teno JM, Kiely DK, et al. The clinical course of advanced dementia. *N Engl J Med.* 2009;361(16):1529–1537.

63. Arcand M. End-of-life issues in advanced dementia: part 1: goals of care, decision-making process, and family education. *Can Fam Physician.* 2015;61:330–334.

64. Radinovic KS, Markovic-Denic L, Dubljanin-Raspopovic E, et al. Effect of the overlap syndrome of depressive symptoms and delirium on outcomes in elderly adults with hip fracture: a prospective cohort study. *J Am Geriatr Soc.* 2014;62(9):1640–1648.

65. Kalish VB, Gillham JE, Unwin BK. Delirium in older persons: evaluation and management. *Am Fam Physician.* 2014;90(3):150–158.

66. McLafferty E, Farley A. Delirium part two: nursing management. *Nurs Stand.* 2007;21(30):42–46.

67. Academy of Nutrition and Dietetics. Evidence Analysis Library: nutrition screening project. 2009–2010. https://www.andeal.org/topic.cfm?menu=3584&cat=3958. Accessed July 19, 2016.

68. Mueller C, Compher C, Druyan ME; American Society for Parenteral and Enteral Nutrition (A.S.P.E.N.) Board of Directors. A.S.P.E.N. clinical guidelines: nutrition screening, assessment, and intervention in adults. *JPEN J Parenter Enteral Nutr.* 2011;35(1):16–24.

69. Academy of Nutrition and Dietetics. eNCPT Nutrition Terminology Reference Manual. http://ncpt.webauthor.com. Accessed January 2, 2017.

70. Academy of Nutrition and Dietetics. Nutrition Care Manual. https://www.nutritioncaremanual.org. Accessed August 23, 2016.

71. The Joint Commission. Standards FAQ: nutritional and functional screening—requirement. Updated April 11, 2016. https://www.jointcommission.org/standards_information/jcfaqdetails.aspx?StandardsFaqId=872&ProgramId=46. Accessed January 2, 2017.

72. Centers for Medicare and Medicaid Services. CMS State Operations Manual Appendix PP—Guidance to Surveyors for Long Term Care Facilities (Rev. 157, 06-10-16). https://www.cms.gov/Regulations-and-Guidance/Guidance/Manuals/downloads/som107ap_pp_guidelines_ltcf.pdf. Accessed January 2, 2017.

73. Academy of Nutrition and Dietetics. Evidence Analysis Library: Unintended weight loss in older adults. 2009. http://www.andeal.org/template.cfm?template=guide_summary&key=2710. Accessed July 19, 2016.

74. Sieber CC. Nutritional screening tools--how does the MNA compare? Proceedings of the session held in Chicago May 2–3, 2006 (15 Years of Mini Nutritional Assessment). *J Nutr Health Aging.* 2006;10(6):488–492.

75. Guigoz Y. The Mini Nutritional Assessment (MNA) review of the literature—What does it tell us? *J Nutr Health Aging.* 2006;10(6):466–485.

76. Kaiser MJ, Bauer JM, Ramsch C, et al. Validation of the Mini Nutritional Assessment Short-Form (MNA-SF): a practical tool for identification of nutritional status. *J Nutr Health Aging.* 2009;13(9):782–788.

77. Kaiser MJ, Bauer JM, Uter W, et al. Prospective validation of the modified Mini Nutritional Assessment Short-Forms in the community, nursing home, and rehabilitation setting. *J Am Geriatr Soc.* 2011;59(11):2124–2128.

78. Kaiser MJ, Bauer JM, Ramsch C, et al. Frequency of malnutrition in older adults: a multinational perspective using the Mini Nutritional Assessment. *J Am Geriatr Soc.* 2010;58(9):1734–1738.

79. Huhmann MB, Perez V, Alexander DD, Thomas DR. A self-completed nutrition screening tool for community-dwelling older adults with high reliability: a comparison study. *J Nutr Health Aging.* 2013;17(4):339–344.

80 Nestlé Nutrition Institute. MNA Mini Nutrition Assessment. http://www.mna-elderly.com/mna_forms.html. Accessed January 19, 2017.

81. Centers for Medicare and Medicaid Services. Long-Term Care Facility Resident Assessment Instrument 3.0 User's Manual Version 1.14. Updated October 2016. Section K. https://downloads.cms.gov/files/MDS-30-RAI-Manual-V114-October-2016.pdf. Accessed November 17, 2016.

82. Jensen GL, Mirtallo J, Compher C, et al. Adult starvation and disease-related malnutrition: a proposal for etiology-based diagnosis in the clinical practice setting from the International Consensus Guideline Committee. *JPEN J Parenter Enteral Nutr.* 2010; 34(2):156–159.

83. White JV, Guenter P, Jensen G, et al. Consensus statement of the Academy of Nutrition and Dietetics/American Society for Parenteral and Enteral Nutrition: characteristics recommended for the identification and documentation of adult malnutrition (undernutrition). *JPEN J Parenter Enteral Nutr.* 2012; 36:275–283.

84. Mueller C. Nutrition assessment and older adults. *Top Clin Nutr.* 2015;30(1):95–102.

85. Johnson MA, Dwyer JT, Jensen GL, et al. Challenges and new opportunities for clinical nutrition interventions in the aged. *J Nutr.* 2011;141(3):535–541.

86. Chernoff R. Carbohydrate, fat and fluid requirements in older adults. In: Chernoff R, ed. *Geriatric Nutrition.* 4th ed. Burlington, MA: Jones & Bartlett Publishers; 2014.

87. Institute of Medicine. *Dietary Reference Intakes for Vitamin A, Vitamin K, Arsenic, Boron, Chromium, Copper, Iodine, Iron, Manganese, Molybdenum, Nickel, Silicon, Vanadium, and Zinc.* Washington, DC: National Academies Press; 2001. https://www.nap.edu/catalog/10026/dietary-reference-intakes-for-vitamin-a-vitamin-k-arsenic-boron-chromium-copper-iodine-iron-manganese-molybdenum-nickel-silicon-vanadium-and-zinc. Accessed January 13, 2017.

88. Institute of Medicine. *Dietary Reference Intakes for Vitamin C, Vitamin E, Selenium, and Carotenoids.* Washington, DC: National Academies Press; 2000. https://www.nap.edu/catalog/9810/dietary-reference-intakes-for-vitamin-c-vitamin-e-selenium-and-carotenoids. Accessed January 13, 2017.

89. Institute of Medicine. *Dietary Reference Intakes for Calcium, Phosphorus, Magnesium, Vitamin D, and Fluoride.* Washington, DC: National Academies Press; 1997. https://www.nap.edu/catalog/5776/dietary-reference-intakes-for-calcium-phosphorus-magnesium-vitamin-d-and-fluoride. Accessed January 13, 2017.

90. Institute of Medicine. *Dietary Reference Intakes for Water, Potassium, Sodium, Chloride, and Sulfate.* Washington, DC: National Academies Press; 2005. https://www.nap.edu/catalog/10925/dietary-reference-intakes-for-water-potassium-sodium-chloride-and-sulfate. Accessed January 13, 2017.

91. Institute of Medicine. *Dietary Reference Intakes for Thiamin, Riboflavin, Niacin, Vitamin B6, Folate, Vitamin B12, Pantothenic Acid, Biotin, and Choline.* Washington, DC: National Academies Press; 1998. https://www.nap.edu/catalog/6015/dietary-reference-intakes-for-thiamin-riboflavin-niacin-vitamin-b6-folate-vitamin-b12-pantothenic-acid-biotin-and-choline. Accessed January 13, 2017.

92. Institute of Medicine. *Dietary Reference Intakes for Vitamin D and Calcium.* Washington, DC: National Academies Press; 2011. https://www.nap.edu/catalog/13050/dietary-reference-intakes-for-calcium-and-vitamin-d. Accessed January 2, 2017.

93. Dorner B. Friedrich EK, Posthauer ME. Practice paper of the American Dietetic Association: individualized nutrition approaches for older adults in healthcare communities. *J Am Diet Assoc.* 2010;110(10):1554–1563.

94. Hooper L, Bunn D, Jimoh FO, Fairweather-Tait SJ. Water-loss dehydration and aging. *Mech Ageing Dev.* 2014;136–137:50–58.

95. Morley JE. Dehydration, hypernatremia, and hyponatremia. *Clin Geriatr Med.* 2015;31(3):389–399.

96. Zajacova A, Ailshire J. Body mass trajectories and mortality among older adults: a joint growth mixture-discrete-time survival analysis. *Gerontologist.* 2014;54(2):221–231.

97. Academy of Nutrition and Dietetics. Nutrition Care Manual. Overweight and obesity: nutrition intervention. https://www.nutritioncaremanual.org/topic.cfm?ncm_toc_id=267967. Accessed November 20, 2016.

98. Institute of Medicine. *Dietary Reference Intakes for Energy, Carbohydrate, Fiber, Fat, Fatty Acids, Cholesterol, Protein, and Amino Acids.* Washington, DC: National Academies Press; 2002.

99. US Department of Health and Human Services, US Department of Agriculture. 2015–2020 Dietary Guidelines for Americans. 8th ed. December 2015. http://health.gov/dietaryguidelines/2015/guidelines. Accessed November 20, 2016.

100. Deutz NEP, Bauer JM, Barazzoni R, et al. Protein intake and exercise for optimal muscle function with aging: recommendations from the ESPEN Expert Group. *Clin Nutr.* 2014;33(6):929–936.

101. Campbell WW, Carnell NS, Thalacker AE. Protein metabolism and requirements. In: Chernoff R, ed. *Geriatric Nutrition.* 3rd ed. Sudbury, MA: Jones & Bartlett Publishers; 2006:15–22.

102. Morais JA, Chevalier S, Gougeon R. Protein turnover and requirements in the healthy and frail elderly. *J Nutr Health Aging.* 2006;10(4):272–283.

103. Gaillard C, Alix E, Boirie Y, et al. Are elderly hospitalized patients getting enough protein? *J Am Geriatr Soc.* 2008;56:1045–1049.

104. Chung M, Balk EM, Brendel M, et al. *Vitamin D and Calcium: Systematic Review of Health Outcomes.* Rockville, MD: Agency for Healthcare Research and Quality; 2009.

105. Lindeman RD, Johnson MA. Mineral requirements. In: Chernoff R, ed. *Geriatric Nutrition.* 4th ed. Burlington, MA: Jones & Bartlett Learning; 2014:79–94.

106. Bailey RL, Dodd KW, Goldman JA, et al. Estimation of total usual calcium and vitamin D intakes in the United States. *J Nutr.* 2010;140(4):817–822.

107. Suter PM. Vitamin metabolism and requirements in the elderly: selected aspects. In: Chernoff R, ed. *Geriatric Nutrition.* 4th ed. Burlington, MA: Jones & Bartlett Learning; 2014:35–77.

108. Dangour AD, Allen E, Clarke R, et al. A randomized controlled trial investigating the effect of vitamin B_{12} supplementation on neurological function in healthy older adults: the Older People and Enhanced Neurological function (OPEN) study protocol. *Nutr J.* 2011;10:22.

109. Langan RC, Zawistoski KJ. Update on vitamin B_{12} deficiency. *Am Fam Physician.* 2011;83(12):1425–1430.

110. den Elzen WP, van der Weele GM, Gussekloo J, Westendorp RG, Assendelft WJ. Subnormal vitamin B_{12} concentrations and anaemia in older people: a systematic review. *BMC Geriatr.* 2010;10:42.

111. Malouf R, Grimley Evans J. Folic acid with or without vitamin B_{12} for the prevention and treatment of healthy elderly and demented people. *Cochrane Database Syst Rev.* 2008;(4): CD004514. doi:10.1002/14651858.CD004514.pub2.

112. Martí-Carvajal AJ, Solà I, Lathyris D. Homocysteine-lowering interventions for preventing cardiovascular events. *Cochrane Database Syst Rev.* 2015;(1):CD006612. doi:10.1002/14651858.CD006612.pub4.

113. Ford DW, Jensen GL, Hartman TJ, Wray L, Smiciklas-Wright H. Association between dietary quality and mortality in older adults: a review of the epidemiological evidence. *J Nutr Gerontol Geriatr.* 2013;32(2):85–105.

114. Franklin B, Jones A, Love D, et al. Exploring mediators of food insecurity and obesity: a review of recent literature. *J Community Health.* 2012;37(1):253–264.

115. Zhu H, Ruopeng A. Impact of home-delivered meal program on diet and nutrition among older adults: a review. *Nutr Health.* 2013;22(2):89–103.

116. Academy of Nutrition and Dietetics. Position of the Academy of Nutrition and Dietetics. Food and nutrition for older adults: promoting health and wellness. *J Acad Nutr Diet.* 2012;112:1255–1277.

117. Dorner B, Friedrich EK, Posthauer ME. Position of the American Dietetic Association: individualized nutrition approaches for older adults in health care communities. *J Am Diet Assoc.* 2010;110(10);1549–1553.

118. Pioneer Network Food and Clinical Standards Task Force. New Dining Practice Standards. August 2011. http://www.pioneernetwork.net/Data/Documents/NewDiningPracticeStandards.pdf. Accessed August 16, 2016.

119. Lloyd-Jones DM, Hong Y, Labarthe D, et al; American Heart Association Strategic Planning Task Force and Statistics Committee. Defining and setting national goals for cardiovascular health promotion and disease reduction: the American Heart Association's strategic impact goal through 2020 and beyond. *Circulation.* 2010;121:586–613.

120. Graudal N, Gesche J, Baslund B, Alderman, MH. Compared with usual sodium intake, low- and excessive-sodium diets are associated with increased mortality: a meta-analysis. *Am J Hypertens.* 2014;27(9):1129–1137.

121. Jyrkkä J, Mursu J, Hannes E, Lönnroos E. Polypharmacy and nutritional status in elderly people. *Curr Opin Clin Nutr Metab Care.* 2012;15(1):1–6.

122. American Geriatrics Society. 2015 updated Beers criteria for potentially inappropriate medication use in older adults. *J Am Geriatr Soc.* 2015;63:2227–2246.

123. Hilas O, Avena-Woods C. Potential role of mirtazapine in underweight older adults. *J Am Soc Consult Pharm.* 2014;29(2):124–130.

124. ASPEN Board of Directors; Clinical Guidelines Task Force. Guidelines for the use of parenteral and enteral nutrition in adult and pediatric patients. *JPEN J Parenter Enteral Nutr.* 2002;26(1 Suppl):1SA–138SA. http://pen.sagepub.com/content/17/4_suppl/1SA.long. Accessed December 3, 2016.

125. Volkert D, Berner YN, Berry E, et al. ESPEN guidelines on enteral nutrition: geriatrics. *Clin Nutr.* 2006;25(2):330–360.

126. Sobotka L, Schneider SM, Berner YN, et al. ESPEN guidelines on parenteral nutrition: geriatrics. *Clin Nutr.* 2009;28(4):461–466.

127. Remington R, Hultman T. Hypodermoclysis to treat dehydration: a review of the evidence. *J Am Geriatr Soc.* 2007;55(12):2051–2055.

128. Philipson TJ, Snider JT, Lakdawalla DN, Stryckman B, Goldman DP. Impact of oral nutritional supplementation on hospital outcomes. *Am J Manag Care.* 2013;19(2):121–128.

129. Malafarina V, Uriz-Otano F, Iniesta R, Gil-Guerrero L. Effectiveness of nutritional supplementation on muscle mass in treatment of sarcopenia in old age. *J Am Med Dir Assoc.* 2013;14(1):10–17.

130. Liu M, Yang J, Yu X, Huang X., et al. The role of perioperative oral nutritional supplementation in elderly patients after hip surgery. *Clin Interv Aging.* 2015;10:849–858.

131. Posthauer ME, Dorner B, Friedrich EK. Enteral nutrition for older adults in healthcare communities. *Nutr Clin Pract.* 2014;29(4):445–458.

132. Pryor LN, Ward EC, Petrea L, et al. Impact of nasogastric tubes on swallowing physiology in older, healthy subjects: a randomized controlled crossover trial. *Clin Nutr.* 2015;34(4):572–578.

133. Mueller C, Gilbride J. Nestle M. Enteral support in elderly residents of long-term care facilities. *Top Clin Nutr.* 2003;18(1):13–20.

134. Niv Y, Abuksis G. Indications for percutaneous endoscopic gastrostomy insertion: ethical aspects. *Dig Dis.* 2002;20(3–4):253–256.

135. Feng YL, Lee CS, Chiu CC, Chao CM, Lai CC. Appropriateness of parenteral nutrition in elderly adults. *J Am Geriatr Soc.* 2015;63(7):1478–1479.

136. Barrocas A, Geppert C, Durfee SM, et al. A.S.P.E.N. ethics position paper. *Nutr Clin Pract.* 2010;25(6):672–679.

137. Teno JM, Gozalo PL, Mitchell SL, et al. Does feeding tube insertion and its timing improve survival? *J Am Geriatr Soc.* 2012;60(10):1918–1921.

138. Daniel K, Rhodes R, Vitale C, Shega J. American Geriatrics Society feeding tubes in advanced dementia position statement. *J Am Geriatr Soc.* 2014;62(8):1590–1593.

139. Sampson EL, Candy B, Jones L. Enteral tube feeding for older people with advanced dementia. *Cochrane Database Syst Rev.* 2009;15(2):CD007209.

140. O'Sullivan Maillet, J, Baird Schwartz D, Posthauer ME. Position of the Academy of Nutrition and Dietetics: ethical and legal issues in feeding and hydration. *J Acad Nutr Diet.* 2013;113:828–833.

141. Lobbe VA. Nutrition in the last days of life. *Curr Opin Support Palliat Care.* 2009;3:195–202.

142. Clarke G, Galbraith S, Woodward J, et al. Eating and drinking interventions for people at risk of lacking decision-making capacity: who decides and how? *BMC Med Ethics.* 2015;16:41.

143. American Dietetic Association. Position of the American Dietetic Association: ethical and legal issues in nutrition, hydration, and feeding. *J Am Diet Assoc.* 2008;108:873–882.

144. Ferris FD, Gunten CF, Emanuel LL. Competency in end-of-life care: last hours of life. *J Palliat Med.* 2003;6:605–613.

145. Palecek EJ, Teno JM, Casarett DJ, et al. Comfort feeding only: a proposal to bring clarity to decision-making regarding difficulty with eating for persons with advanced dementia. *J Am Geriatr Soc.* 2010;58(3):580–584.

146. Monod S, Chiolero R, Bula C, et al. Ethical issues in nutrition support of severely disabled elderly persons: a guide for health professionals. *JPEN J Parenter Enteral Nutr.* 2011;35(3):295–302. https://www.nutritioncare.org/Guidelines_and_Clinical_Resources/Toolkits/Nutrition_Support_and_Ethics_Toolkit/JPEN_and_NCP_Papers. Accessed December 3, 2016.

37 Surgical Alteration of the Gastrointestinal Tract

Neal Bhutiani, MD, Matthew V. Benns, MD, Sam Pappas, MD, Lena B. Palmer, MD, MSCR, and Keith R. Miller, MD

CONTENTS

Objectives

1. Understand unique challenges involved in the care of patients with surgically reconstructed anatomy.
2. Recognize pathologies specific to patients who have undergone common abdominal and pelvic operations.
3. Understand principles of surgical reconstruction and diversion and the impact of these interventions on postoperative nutrition.

Test Your Knowledge Questions

1. Which of the following does *not* represent a potential complication following gastric resection and anastomosis?
   A. Anastomotic stricture
   B. Anastomotic ulcer
   C. Acid hyposecretion
   D. Biliary limb obstruction
2. Which of the following is an example of a malabsorptive procedure for weight loss?
   A. Gastric band
   B. Sleeve gastrectomy
   C. Biliopancreatic diversion with duodenal switch
   D. Gastric balloon
3. For patients with colitis or proctitis after colon resection and proximal diversion of the fecal stream, which of the following represents an effective first-line treatment?
   A. Short-chain fatty acid (SCFA) enemas
   B. Hydrocortisone enemas
   C. Topical 5-aminosalicylic acid
   D. Fecal microbiota transplant

Test Your Knowledge Answers

1. The correct answer is C. The remnant stomach continues to secrete acid in sufficient amounts to maintain an acidic stomach pH. Persistent secretion of acid is one of the contributing factors to development of anastomotic ulcers (answer B) and, ultimately, anastomotic strictures (answer A). Biliary limb obstruction (answer D) can occur for a number of reasons, including torsion of said limb around adhesive bands or at the point of its distal anastomosis to the jejunum.
2. The correct answer is C. A duodenal bypasses the functional small bowel (duodenum and a portion of the jejunum), thereby inhibiting absorption of water and nutrients from an ingested food bolus by these portions of the small bowel. Answers A, B, and D represent restrictive procedures for weight loss.
3. The correct answer is A. SCFAs are the treatment of choice for patients with diversion proctitis or colitis, because a deficiency in SCFAs has been implicated in the etiology of this disease process. Answers B, C, and D represent alternative treatments for patients who have persistent symptoms after 2 to 4 weeks of treatment with SCFAs.

Introduction

Patients who have undergone surgical alteration of the gastrointestinal (GI) tract present unique challenges to clinicians. Anatomical alterations can directly impact nutrition support strategies related to associated physiological changes and impaired micro- and macronutrient absorption. A fundamental understanding regarding the indications for the intervention and resultant anatomy is necessary for those involved in the care of these patients. Here, we review distinct subsets of patients commonly encountered in clinical practice. For each group, we describe common operations, the most common postoperative complications, and the optimal treatment for each of these complications.

Enteral Access Procedures

Surgical enteral access most often involves placement of either a gastrostomy or a jejunostomy tube. Gastrostomy tubes can allow for either feeding or, in the case of a downstream obstruction or poor gastric emptying, gastric decompression. Indeed, should the patient's condition change, the same tube can be used for both purposes. Jejunostomy tubes allow for direct feeding of the small bowel, but they are not used for decompression. They are often useful in cases where a more proximal anastomosis or suture line is present, or in cases of poor gastric emptying.

Not all gastrostomy and jejunostomy tubes are equivalent. The method of creation directly influences the complications that arise in the setting of these tubes as well as management of these issues. The Stamm technique, first described in 1894, involves placement of a double purse-string suture circumferentially around a gastrostomy or jejunostomy tube and subsequently securing that area of either the stomach or jejunum to the anterior abdominal wall (Figure 37-1).[1] The Witzel technique involves creation of a seromuscular tunnel through which a jejunostomy or gastrostomy tube travels retrograde with respect to the site of insertion into the jejunum or stomach (Figure 37-2).[2] In general, gastrostomies are most often created using the Stamm technique, whereas jejunostomies are done using the Witzel technique. Stammed tubes allow for easier replacement at the bedside should the tube become dislodged, and Witzeled tubes allow for greater freedom of movement of the target organ (stomach, jejunum), which can prevent rotation around a fixed point and subsequent obstruction and ischemia.[1,2] However, the Stamm approach can result in ischemia around the gastrostomy/jejunostomy because of mucosal compression by the intravisceral portion of the tube. Meanwhile, the Witzel approach can result in visceral narrowing, leading to stenosis or obstruction. More generally, complications of gastrostomy tubes include extravasation of contents into the abdomen due to enlargement of the gastrostomy or slippage of the intragastric portion of the tube out of the stomach and, over time, small bowel obstruction due to intra-abdominal adhesions.[1] Similarly, jejunostomy tubes can result in bowel obstruction either as a result of adhesions or, more acutely, as a result of tubal obstruction of the intestinal lumen preventing upstream contents from flowing distally.[2]

FIGURE 37-1 Stamm Gastrostomy with Mushroom-Tipped Catheter

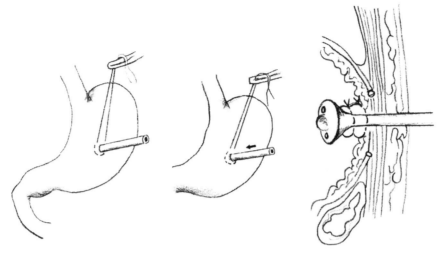

Source: Reprinted with permission from reference 1: Vanek VW. Ins and outs of enteral access: part 2—long term access—esophagostomy and gastrostomy. *Nutr Clin Pract.* 2003;18(1):50–74.

Foregut (Esophagus, Stomach, and Pancreas) Interventions

Surgical alteration of the foregut including the esophagus, stomach, and pancreaticobiliary system can have significant implications for nutrition support. These operations (eg, esophagogastrectomy, Roux-en-Y gastric bypass [RYGB], and pancreaticoduodenectomy) are performed commonly in the setting of malignancy and as bariatric weight loss procedures.

Oncologic Resections

Improvements in diagnostics, surgical techniques, neoadjuvant therapy, and anesthesia have allowed for a larger number of patients with abdominal and esophageal solid tumors to be candidates for surgical resection. Here, we discuss the anatomical alterations that occur as a result of tumor resection, their impact on nutrition, and approaches to postoperative patients presenting with GI complaints. Refer to Chapter 33 for a detailed discussion of the effects of malignancy on patients' nutrition status and means of nutritional supplementation.

Esophagogastrectomy

Most patients undergoing esophagectomy do so in the setting of malignant and premalignant conditions. Esophagogastrectomy involves an abdominal incision and either a right thoracotomy (Ivor Lewis esophagectomy) or neck incision (transhiatal esophagectomy), with resection of the esophagus to normal tissue as well as the proximal portion of the stomach.[3] In performing the gastrectomy, the remaining stomach is fashioned into a tubular conduit subsequently anastomosed to the remnant esophagus either in the right chest or neck. Should the gastric conduit fail to reach the remnant esophagus, a segment of colon (with mesenteric pedicle attached)

can be interposed between the esophagus and the remaining stomach or small bowel.[3]

The substitution of gastric or colonic tissue for the distal esophagus presents nutrition challenges. Coordinated peristalsis is lost and food boluses travel the length of the conduit largely by gravity. Furthermore, as with restrictive bariatric procedures, the remaining stomach has restricted capacity to act as an alimentary reservoir.[4] This combination requires that patients limit themselves to softer foods and eat smaller, more frequent meals. Despite these dietary modifications, many patients obtain insufficient nutrition in the perioperative period and require simultaneous jejunostomy tube placement at the time of esophagogastrectomy for prolonged enteral nutrition (EN) support.[4,5]

Potential complications of an esophagogastrectomy include anastomotic leaks, anastomotic strictures, chylothorax, and bowel obstructions.[6] Leaks can manifest as respiratory symptoms and/or tachycardia, while strictures often manifest as dysphagia and reflux. Management usually involves drainage as well as endoscopic stenting or operative anastomotic revision in the case of leaks and endoscopic dilation or, in severe cases, resection of the stenotic segment and reanastomosis. In the setting of esophageal leak, distal enteral access is the preferred conduit.

Partial/Subtotal/Total Gastrectomy

Patients undergoing either a partial or total gastrectomy for gastric cancer experience anatomical and physiological alterations akin to patients undergoing RYGB both with respect to decreased gastric storage capacity and the presence of gastric anastomosis. Following total gastrectomy, restoration of continuity via an esophagojejunostomy leaves patients without an alimentary reservoir or pylorus, further limiting the size of meals patients can tolerate and decreasing protein and

FIGURE 37-2 Witzel Jejunostomy

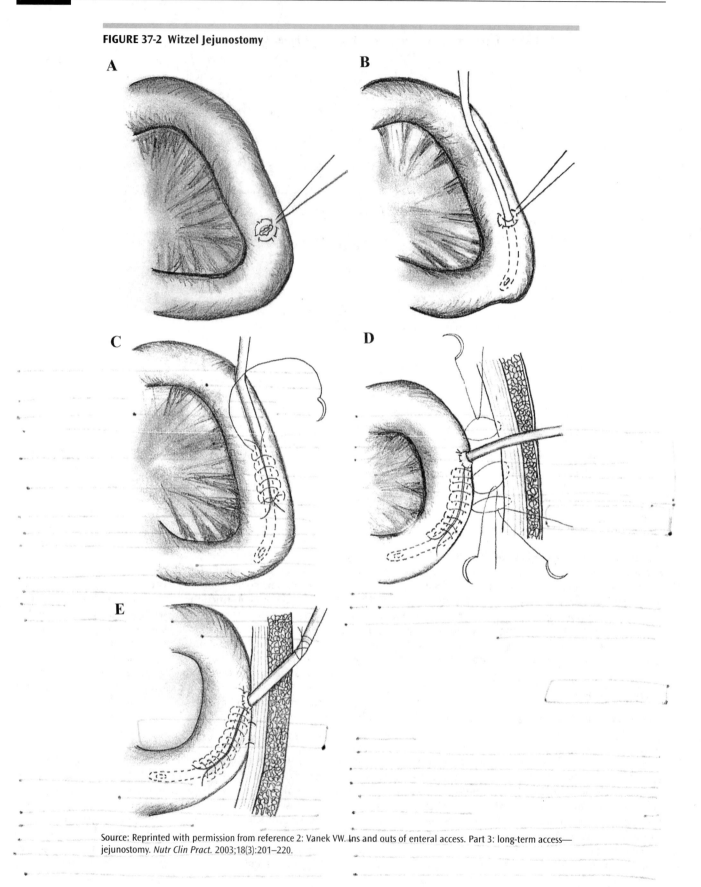

Source: Reprinted with permission from reference 2: Vanek VW. Ins and outs of enteral access. Part 3: long-term access—
jejunostomy. *Nutr Clin Pract.* 2003;18(3):201–220.

carbohydrate digestion that usually occurs in the presence of gastric acid and pepsin.[7,8]

Gastric surgery is accompanied by a host of potential complications, including anastomotic stricture, anastomotic ulcer, and small bowel obstruction. Additionally, patients can experience vitamin deficiencies, particularly vitamins B_{12}, C, and D, owing to the lack of gastric tissue. Deficiencies can result in anemia, delayed wound healing, and osteopenia or osteoporosis, respectively.[8,9] Furthermore, because of increased water in the small bowel resulting from undigested carbohydrates, patients can develop dumping syndrome. As with bariatric patients, treatment of dumping syndrome in this patient population often involves avoiding simple carbohydrates, increasing dietary fiber, and eating smaller, more frequent meals. Finally, as a result of transection of the vagus nerve during gastrectomy, along with increased osmolarity of intestinal contents, patients may experience debilitating watery diarrhea.[8] In many cases, antimotility agents such as loperamide, in addition to dietary alterations, can ameliorate these symptoms.

Pancreaticoduodenectomy and Distal Pancreatectomy

Pancreatic resection may be performed in the setting of trauma or chronic pancreatitis, but most pancreatic resections are performed for malignancy. Although patients with pancreatic cancer often present with unresectable or widely metastatic disease, surgery represents a mainstay of therapy in those who are candidates. The nature of resection depends on the anatomical location of the tumor within the pancreas. Patients with tumors in the head of the pancreas undergo a pancreaticoduodenectomy, referred to as a *Whipple procedure*, which involves resection of the head of the pancreas, duodenum, and part of the stomach. Additionally, following resection, significant reconstruction is necessary—a gastrojejunostomy (GJ), hepaticojejunostomy (HJ), and pancreaticojejunostomy (PJ) to restore pancreato-biliary-enteric continuity, as well as potential placement of a jejunostomy tube for prolonged EN support (Figure 37-3).[10,11] Importantly, gastric resection can include the pylorus or spare the pylorus, the implications of which will subsequently be discussed. Additionally, the GJ can be performed in an antecolic (anastomosis in front of the transverse colon) or retrocolic (anastomosis behind the transverse colon) fashion. Generally, an antecolic anastomosis is preferred in the setting of malignancy and has been shown to decrease the incidence of postoperative delayed gastric emptying.[12]

Given the complexity of resection and reconstruction involved in a pancreaticoduodenectomy, patients can have complications stemming from each anastomosis. Patients can develop marginal ulcers or strictures at the GJ and are generally maintained on proton pump inhibitors (PPIs). Strictures, should they occur, can often be managed with endoscopic dilation. With respect to both the HJ and PJ, leaks represent the most common complication and can manifest

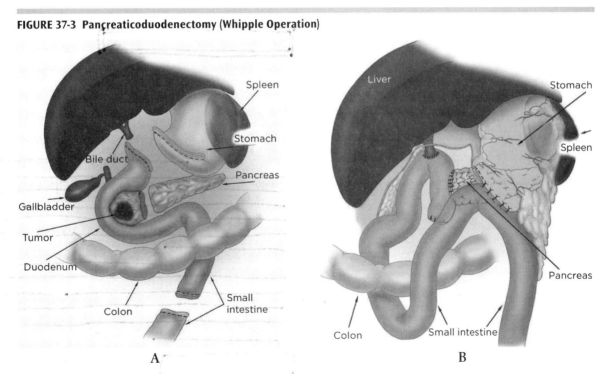

FIGURE 37-3 Pancreaticoduodenectomy (Whipple Operation)

(A) Normal extent of resection, including a portion of the stomach, head of the pancreas, distal common bile duct, gallbladder, and duodenum.
(B) Reconstruction after pancreaticoduodenectomy, namely (1) pancreaticojejunostomy, (2) hepaticojejunostomy, and (3) loop gastrojejunostomy.
Source: Reprinted from reference 11: Reynolds RB, Folloder JJ. Clinical management of pancreatic cancer. *Adv Pract Oncol.* 2014;5(5):356–364.
Copyright © 2008, M.D. Anderson.

as jaundice (biliary leak), abdominal pain, and change in character of surgical drain output in addition to signs of a systemic inflammatory response (fever, tachycardia, etc).[13] Biliary leaks that do not resolve spontaneously may require endoscopic retrograde pancreatography (ERCP) with stent placement, whereas high-volume or persistent pancreatic leaks may require prolonged *nil per os* (NPO) status with parenteral nutrition (PN) support.[14] Particularly severe biliary or pancreatic leaks or those that have failed nonoperative management may require reoperation and anastomotic revision. Finally, between 10% and 20% of patients experience delayed gastric emptying after undergoing pancreaticoduodenectomy. Although the etiology remains unclear, risk factors include pancreatic and biliary fistulas. Management includes prokinetic agents such as erythromycin and metoclopramide together with dietary changes (small meals spaced 2 to 3 hours apart with avoidance of foods that cause constipation or abdominal pain).[10,12,13] See Practice Scenario 37-1 for more information on interventions for delayed gastric emptying.

Practice Scenario 37-1

Question: How does delayed gastric emptying manifest after a pancreaticoduodenectomy and how should it be managed?

Scenario: A 56-year-old man presented to the emergency department after noting new-onset scleral icterus and unintentional 20-pound weight loss over the past 2 months. A computed tomography (CT) scan of the abdomen and pelvis with intravenous (IV) contrast showed evidence of a mass in the pancreatic head. He was subsequently referred to surgical oncology and repeat pancreatic protocol CT demonstrated a 4-cm lesion in the head of the pancreas. The patient was taken to the operating room for a pancreaticoduodenectomy with jejunostomy tube placement, which he tolerated well. He enjoyed an unremarkable postoperative course and was discharged on postoperative Day 5 in good condition. He was admitted 2 days later with persistent nausea, vomiting, and abdominal pain without radiographic evidence of obstruction.

Intervention: The patient was treated with IV fluid resuscitation, metoclopramide, and ondansetron. His diet was slowly advanced, and he was discharged home on a full liquid diet with jejunostomy tube feeds for nutritional supplementation.

Answer: Patients with nausea, vomiting, or abdominal pain after pancreaticoduodenectomy who do not have evidence of obstruction on imaging likely have some degree of delayed gastric emptying. Treatment includes correcting fluid and electrolyte imbalances resulting from poor oral intake and emesis as well as symptomatic treatment with antiemetics and prokinetic agents (eg, ondansetron and metoclopramide or erythromycin).

Rationale: Delayed gastric emptying occurs in approximately 15% of patients undergoing pancreaticoduodenectomy. These patients often experience nausea, vomiting, and poor oral intake for several days before they are seen by a clinician. Initial evaluation and

treatment should involve confirmation of a lack of peritoneal signs or obstruction; IV fluid administration; and close monitoring of urine output. Subsequently, patients should have their nausea treated with antiemetics and their decreased GI motility treated with prokinetic agents. Diet should be advanced slowly over the course of several days. Postpyloric enteral nutrition supplementation should be initiated with jejunal tube feeding (through the jejunostomy tube placed at time of pancreaticoduodenectomy) to prevent excessive energy deficits and dehydration.

For tumors in the distal pancreatic body or tail, the procedure of choice is a distal pancreatectomy and splenectomy. The procedure entails no reconstruction, but pancreatic duct leaks can occur from the transected end of the pancreas.[15] High-volume leaks can be managed similarly to pancreatic leaks in the setting of a pancreaticoduodenectomy.[15,16]

Finally, a small subset of patients will require subtotal or total pancreatectomy for multifocal malignancy or malignancy that requires pancreatic resection beyond the level of the portal vein. Patients who lose all endocrine and exocrine pancreatic tissue will experience hyperglycemia as a result of insulin insufficiency, hypoglycemia as a result of glucagon insufficiency, and fat malabsorption with concomitant steatorrhea and fat-soluble vitamin deficiencies; patients who lose most of endocrine and exocrine pancreatic tissue may experience these complications.[17] Treatment consists of exogenous insulin and pancreatic enzyme (pancrelipase) supplementation titrated based upon the individual's dietary fat content and the persistence of steatorrhea.

Bariatric Weight Loss Procedures

As discussed in Chapter 35, the incidence and prevalence of both obesity (body mass index [BMI] greater than 30) and morbid obesity (BMI greater than 40 or greater than 35 with an associated obesity-related health condition such as hypertension or diabetes mellitus) in the United States and throughout the industrialized world have increased significantly over the last 25 to 30 years. Diet and lifestyle modification are first-line therapies, but many patients fail to effectively incorporate or respond to these interventions. Existing adjunctive pharmacological agents for weight loss have severe limitations, and surgical intervention has been associated with achieving weight loss and secondary prevention of associated components of the metabolic syndrome (diabetes, hypertension, and coronary artery disease). The objective of bariatric surgery is to anatomically decrease intake capacity and/or decrease absorptive capacity, thereby contributing to weight loss. Bariatric surgery is the only therapy for weight loss repeatedly shown to result in sustained, substantial weight loss in obese patients, but it is complicated by a host of issues.[18]

Roux-en-Y Gastric Bypass

Bariatric operations either restrict food intake or decrease macronutrient absorption, or both. Historically, beginning in the 1950s, procedures focused primarily on inducing malabsorption in the GI tract. Early procedures, most notably the jejunoileal bypass (JIB) left the stomach intact while bypassing most of the small bowel.[19] Patients experienced weight loss but also experienced numerous complications related to vitamin and mineral deficiencies and protein-energy malnutrition. Focus subsequently shifted to combining restrictive and malabsorptive principles with the introduction of the gastric bypass. Over time, this operation has evolved into its current form, the RYGB. The procedure essentially divides the stomach into a remnant (nonfunctional) stomach and a gastric pouch that remains in continuity. The remnant stomach, together with the duodenum and a portion of the jejunum (the biliary, or Y, limb), is attached to the distal jejunum, which is anastomosed to the gastric pouch (Roux limb) (Figure 37-4).[19] This procedure allows for maintenance of GI continuity, and the biliary limb establishes downstream pancreaticobiliary continuity. The gastric pouch acts as a much smaller reservoir (approximately 5% of a normal stomach) for food, while food passing through the Roux limb bypasses the duodenum and a portion of the jejunum, thereby decreasing nutrient absorption. This intervention results in effective weight loss with a lower rate of vitamin and mineral deficiency than that seen in JIB patients.

As with any operation involving a significant anatomical alteration, the RYGB can result in multiple types of complications.[20,21] Gastric division and construction of a GJ creates an inherently ulcerogenic environment because of the alteration of acid secretion, disruption of vagal innervation to the stomach, and direct exposure of small bowel mucosa to the gastric contents. Ulceration can cause epigastric pain as well as hematemesis or melanotic stool. Pain and bleeding usually occur in the setting of active ulcer disease. However, even after resolution, patients can be left with an anastomotic stricture resulting from scarring at the previous ulcer site. Treatment for ulcers usually involves high-dose PPI therapy and endoscopic intervention to cauterize bleeding vessels. Anastomotic strictures may be dilated endoscopically. In both cases, however, persistent symptoms after medical or endoscopic interventions usually require operative intervention with anastomotic revision.[22] Anastomotic revision is inherently unsatisfying, as the existing anastomosis is excised and reestablished without eliminating any of the elements that initially contributed to the issue.

Normally, gastric contents achieve iso-osmolarity prior to leaving the stomach. However, the absence of a pylorus in the gastric pouch as well as the bypassing of the duodenum and a portion of the jejunum results in reduced digestion of carbohydrates, making the food bolus passing from the gastric pouch down the Roux limb more osmotically active, which causes approximately 85% of patients to experience a constellation of symptoms including abdominal pain, nausea, vomiting, fatigue, dizziness, and diarrhea known as *dumping syndrome*.[23,24] As a result of nausea, vomiting, and diarrhea, patients can also experience dehydration; additionally, hypoglycemia can occur as a result of increased pancreatic insulin secretion in response to rapid transit of food boluses. Treatment, which will subsequently be discussed in greater detail, includes dietary changes (smaller meals spaced 2 to 3 hours apart), avoidance of simple carbohydrates, and increased fiber consumption or fiber supplementation.

Bowel obstruction in the setting of prior RYGB can be particularly devastating when not managed appropriately. Computed tomography (CT) should be performed to evaluate the location of the obstruction (in the Roux limb, biliary limb, or distal small bowel) in all cases.[25,26] Although adhesive small bowel obstruction is a possibility following gastric bypass, more pressing concerns include the presence of an internal hernia and obstruction involving the biliary limb.[27] Gastric bypass patients are particularly prone to internal hernia because of the mesenteric defects created, and the accelerated weight loss following surgery can increase the size of these defects because of the loss of mesenteric fat. In general, conservative management of a bowel obstruction in a gastric bypass patient with intravenous fluid resuscitation and nasogastric tube decompression should be undertaken with caution because the complication could possibly progress to irreversible ischemia and loss of significant bowel length.

Analogously, management of symptomatic choledocholithiasis and cholangitis in post-RYGB patients presents a particular challenge, given that accessing the biliary limb and common bile duct endoscopically with ERCP may be difficult to impossible, depending on the skill of the endoscopist and the patient's anatomy.[28] In these cases, surgical common duct exploration and decompression is appropriate and can be accomplished with either a laparoscopic or open approach. Alternatively, ERCP may be done with surgical assistance. The remnant stomach can be accessed surgically (laparoscopic or open) and a gastrostomy can be made to accommodate an endoscope.[29]

FIGURE 37-4 Roux-en-Y Gastric Bypass

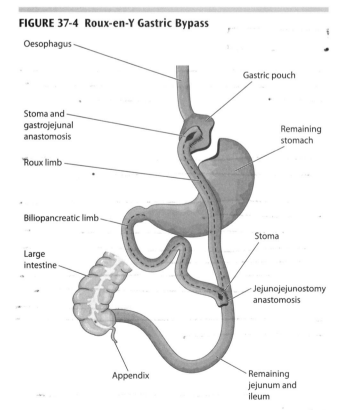

Oesophagus

Gastric pouch

Stoma and gastrojejunal anastomosis

Remaining stomach

Roux limb

Biliopancreatic limb

Stoma

Large intestine

Jejunojejunostomy anastomosis

Appendix

Remaining jejunum and ileum

Source: Blamb/Shutterstock.com.

Gastric Banding

Given the fluid, electrolyte, and nutrition issues associated with malabsorptive procedures, current practice in weight loss surgery has shifted toward strictly restrictive procedures—namely, gastric banding and sleeve gastrectomy. Gastric banding, first reported in 1978, involves placement of an adjustable band around the stomach to limit its capacity for food storage without transecting or resecting any portion of the stomach (Figure 37-5).[19] Insertion of the band is usually performed laparoscopically, and the tightness of the band can be adjusted in the clinic with aspiration or injection of saline into a subcutaneous port located on the patient's anterior abdomen.

Band slippage and band erosion are the most common complications resulting from the procedure.[20,30,31] Band slippage occurs when the band migrates distally and the gastric fundus and body move upward; if left untreated, it can lead to gastric necrosis.[30] Patients usually present with acute nausea and vomiting, and diagnosis is made with abdominal plain film. On these radiographs, a phi angle formed by the band and the vertical spinal axis greater than 58° confirms the diagnosis (Figure 37-6).[32] Treatment generally requires band removal, but many patients can be temporized with band deflation and nasogastric tube placement if bariatric surgical consultation is not immediately available. Patients presenting with peritonitis or shock require immediate abdominal exploration, as they likely have gastric necrosis.[30]

Patients experiencing band erosion usually present with epigastric pain, although of a more subacute or chronic variety than is common with band slippage. Esophagoduodenoscopy (EGD) demonstrates visualization of the eroded band from within the stomach. Definitive treatment for most cases requires band removal, but this intervention is usually not required in urgent fashion. Laparoscopic, open surgical, or endoscopic approaches to band removal are frequently employed.[33]

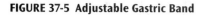

FIGURE 37-5 Adjustable Gastric Band

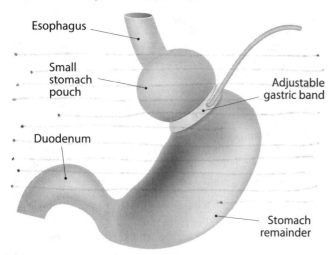

Source: Designua/Shutterstock.com.

FIGURE 37-6 Abdominal Plain Film Demonstrating a Slipped Gastric Band

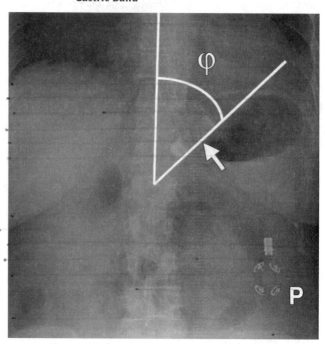

Note the angle (φ) between the gastric band and the vertical axis of the spine.
Source: Reprinted with permission from Figure 4b in reference 32: Sonavane SK, Menias CO, Kantawala KP, et al. Laparoscopic adjustable gastric banding: what radiologists need to know. *Radiographics*. 2012;32(4):1168–1171.

Sleeve Gastrectomy

Sleeve gastrectomy represents a purely restrictive bariatric procedure and is presently the preferred surgical treatment for obesity. Usually performed laparoscopically, the procedure involves cranio-caudal resection of the stomach along the greater curvature, thereby resulting in restriction alone without bypassing any portion of the GI tract (Figure 37-7).[19] Because sleeve gastrectomy does not involve bypass, patients experience fewer micronutrient deficiencies. Furthermore, because a sleeve gastrectomy does not involve an anastomosis, it avoids the anastomotic ulcer and anastomotic stricture that is a risk with RYGB. Patients can, however, experience gastroesophageal reflux because of the removal of the fundus and body of the stomach as well as disruption of vagal fibers during gastric transection; the reflux often can be managed with PPI therapy. More significantly, leakage of gastric contents may develop from the gastric transection line. This complication often first manifests as tachycardia and mild abdominal tenderness and leukocytosis before proceeding to septic shock and peritonitis. Treatment involves prolonged nasogastric decompression to promote spontaneous resolution of the gastric leak or reoperation to reinforce the transection line.[34] This complication generally necessitates either distal enteric access for EN support or PN if distal routes are not achievable.

FIGURE 37-7 Sleeve Gastrectomy

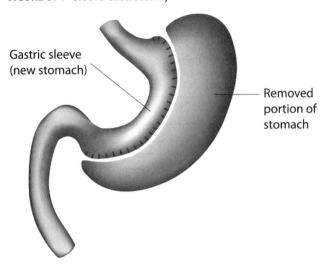

Gastric sleeve
(new stomach)

Removed
portion of
stomach

Source: Alila Medical Media/Shutterstock.com.

Midgut and Hindgut Interventions

Patients undergoing small bowel and colonic interventions can be categorized into 3 groups: those being treated for malignancy, those being treated for inflammatory bowel disease, and those being treated for benign disease (obstruction, diverticulitis, blunt or penetrating trauma, etc).

Segmental Enterectomy/Colectomy

The primary difference between bowel resection for malignancy and enterectomies performed for benign or traumatic pathology is the extent of lymphadenectomy. Short-segment enterectomies are generally well tolerated and result in little anatomical or physiological perturbation. While patients lose the absorptive capacity of a portion of their colon or small bowel, they rarely experience clinically significant dehydration unless extended enterectomies are performed (see Chapter 30). As with any enteric anastomosis, patients can develop anastomotic leakage or stricture leading to obstruction.

Low Anterior Resection and Abdominoperineal Resection

Depending on the location of the tumor along the rectum from the anal verge, patients with resectable rectal cancer undergo 1 of 2 operations: a low anterior resection (LAR) or an abdominoperineal resection (APR). LAR involves removal of the sigmoid colon and upper rectum along with a regional lymphadenectomy.[35] In many cases, it also includes creation of a temporary diverting loop ileostomy. APR entails removal of the sigmoid colon, the entire rectum, anus, and regional lymph nodes with creation of an end colostomy.[35] In general, LAR is the treatment of choice for tumors located in the upper and middle third of the rectum, while APR is reserved

for tumors in the distal third of the rectum.[35] Of note, APR is also employed in treatment of patients with anal squamous cell cancer who have persistent disease after first-line chemoradiation.

The most significant differences between the 2 operations lies in the preservation of the anal sphincter complex with LAR and preservation of continence. Various factors affect continence after LAR, including injury to the sphincter complex and innervating nerves, previous pelvic floor muscle damage (including that induced by preoperative external beam radiation therapy [XRT]), and decreased rectal compliance and capacity as a fecal reservoir.[36] Treatment includes pelvic floor rehabilitation and biofeedback, dietary modification, antimotility agents, and topical phenylephrine. In addition, patients undergoing XRT can develop radiation colitis/proctitis, which can present as diarrhea, rectal bleeding, and tenesmus in the weeks following XRT.[37] Radiation proctitis can often be treated with SCFAs (eg, butyrate) enemas for improved delivery of SCFAs to the radiation-damaged colorectal epithelium.[38] As patients are further removed from radiation therapy, radiation-induced fibrosis and ischemia can manifest as strictures and fistulas between radiated tissue and adjacent organs.[37,38] Choosing the optimal treatment in the case of stricture and fistulas often proves challenging and must account for the patient's overall nutrition status, the organs involved, and the morbidity associated with reoperation.[39]

Inflammatory Bowel Disease and Enterectomy/Colectomy

For patients with inflammatory bowel disease refractory to medical management, surgical treatment allows for symptom relief or, in the case of ulcerative colitis, cure of their disease. Chapter 26 discusses the details of both Crohn's disease and ulcerative colitis. Here, we focus on situations requiring surgical intervention in patients with these colitides and the issues arising in the postsurgical period.

Ulcerative colitis generally represents continuous inflammation beginning at the rectum and extending proximally to the ileocecal valve (and, in cases of backwash ileitis, the terminal ileum). Surgery in the form of a total proctocolectomy (removal of the entire colon and rectum) offers patients definitive treatment of their disease. Depending on patient considerations, maintaining GI continuity involves either creation of an end ileostomy or an ileal pouch anal anastomosis (IPAA), where a segment of distal ileum is fashioned into a pouch and anastomosed directly to the anus (Figure 37-8).[40] An IPAA allows patients to avoid an ileostomy and the associated issues. However, it can often result in problems with continence in a situation analogous to that following an LAR; other possible complications of IPAA include anastomotic strictures, which can often be managed with endoscopic dilation, and malignancy within the ileal pouch.[40] Pouchitis represents an additional pathological entity unique to patients with ileal pouch reconstruction.[41] Causes of inflammation of the ileal pouch are poorly understood but thought to be related to bacterial overgrowth in the pouch. Treatment includes antibiotics with either metronidazole or ciprofloxacin for 7

FIGURE 37-8 Ileal Pouch Reconstruction (Here, J-Pouch) and Ileal Pouch–Anal Anastomosis

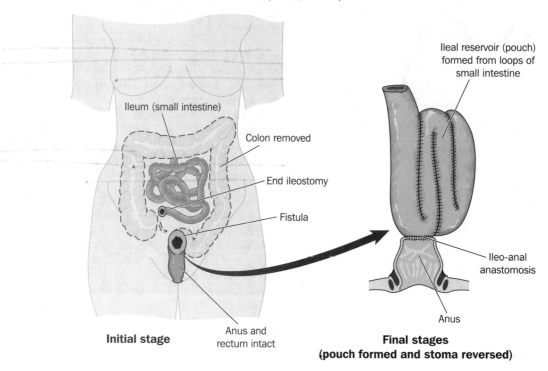

Source: Blamb/Shutterstock.com.

to 10 days, with administration of 5-acetylsalicylic acid, azathioprine, 6-mercaptopurine, or steroids in cases of persistent symptoms.[42–44]

Unlike ulcerative colitis, Crohn's disease can affect the entire length of the GI tract from mouth to anus. Therefore, surgery can only offer symptom relief from structures, obstructions, and fistulas. Given the issues stemming from extensive small bowel resection (see Chapter 30), surgery in patients with Crohn's disease usually aims to preserve as much small bowel as possible. In general, patients require more than 200 cm (50%) of small bowel to avoid short bowel syndrome. In patients without a colon, 110 to 150 cm are required to avoid dependence on PN; if the colon is present, only 50 to 70 cm are necessary.[45–48] Techniques for addressing Crohn's strictures or obstructions include ileocecectomy or segmental small bowel resection as well as strictureplasty, which involves longitudinal transection of the stricture and transverse closure of the segment to maximize lumenal diameter.[49] Of note, even with efforts to preserve small bowel length, patients may experience macro- and micronutrient deficiencies and thus may require EN or PN supplementation, or both, to optimize their overall nutrition status.

The pan-gastrointestinal and, in some cases, cutaneous involvement in patients with Crohn's disease renders them particularly susceptible to developing fistulas in various locations over the course of their disease. Possibilities include enterocutaneous, enterovaginal, enterovesicular, and enterocolonic fistulas with significant associated functional and lifestyle limitations.[45,49–52] Enterocutaneous fistulas and their

nutrition implications are discussed in greater detail later in this chapter. Practice Scenario 37-2 considers interventions for a malnourished patient with Crohn's disease.

Practice Scenario 37-2

Question: What preoperative nutrition support regimen and operative intervention would be appropriate for a patient with Crohn's disease admitted with failure to thrive and physical signs of severe acute malnutrition in the setting of radiographic evidence of a bowel obstruction?

Scenario: A 21-year-old woman with a history of Crohn's disease refractory to adalimumab was admitted for failure to thrive. The patient reported a 2-month history of nausea, abdominal pain, and anorexia. Past surgical history was significant for a previous ileocecectomy for Crohn's disease of the terminal ileum. On physical examination, the patient showed signs of muscle wasting and fat loss consistent with malnutrition. The patient was given parenteral nutrition (PN) supplementation for 10 days, with a resultant improvement in her global appearance and laboratory parameters. Computed tomography scan with oral contrast demonstrated an obstruction at her ileocolic anastomosis.

Intervention: The patient was taken to the operating room for a segmental resection of 8 to 10 cm, including her previous anastomosis, and creation of a new ileocolic anastomosis. Pathology was consistent for recurrent Crohn's disease.

Answer: This patient presents signs of obstruction and has a history of medically refractory Crohn's disease as well as ileocecectomy with an obstruction at her ileocolic anastomosis; therefore, she likely has recurrent Crohn's disease at this site. After initial augmentation of her nutrition status, she requires resection of the diseased segment of bowel to address her obstruction.

Rationale: Patients with inadequately treated or medically refractory inflammatory bowel disease can develop bowel obstruction from persistent enteric inflammation or stricture. In patients who have undergone previous segmental resection with primary anastomosis, these pathologies often occur at the anastomosis. These patients generally require an operation to address their pathophysiology and, by extension, their poor nutrition status. Because these patients usually present with global malnutrition, short-term total partial PN can sufficiently improve their nutrition status and thus their ability to tolerate and recover well from an operation. Operative intervention consists of segmental resection.

Principles of Fecal Diversion

Surgeons use various techniques to divert GI contents, including bile, pancreatic secretions, and stool, to (1) prevent intra-abdominal contamination and, if continuity can be restored, (2) preserve/protect an anastomosis. Stomas of the small bowel and colonic variety can be constructed in 1 of 2 conformations: end or loop. An end ostomy provides complete GI content diversion at the level of the abdominal wall with no downstream intestinal or colonic continuity or flow. Loop ostomy maintains continuity of the GI tract from stomach to anus and diverts most, but not all, GI contents from flowing downstream.[35] Indications for ileostomy include, but are not limited to, emergent subtotal colectomy (of any etiology), anastomotic protection after distal bowel resection, and anastomotic avoidance in a patient with distal small bowel injuries.[35] Indications for colostomy generally include injuries or perforations of the colon in patients thought to be at high risk for reanastomosis.[35] In patients with obstruction caused by unresectable intra-abdominal malignancy, diverting ostomies can palliate their symptoms and allow for improved EN tolerance. In some cases, this intervention can allow patients to undergo systemic chemotherapy in hopes of downstaging their tumor and rendering it resectable.

In cases of malignant distal colonic obstruction, a diverting colostomy is generally the treatment of choice over a diverting ileostomy. In general, ileostomies carry more potential complications than colostomies owing to their more proximal location along the GI tract. Both interventions can result in fluid and electrolyte imbalances and dehydration, ileostomies more so than colostomies. Thus, clinicians caring for patients with ostomies should carefully monitor their fluid and electrolyte status and ostomy output. Particularly with ileostomies, output should be less than approximately 1 liter per 24 hours. Treatment for high ostomy output in hemodynamically normal patients consists of fiber supplementation to thicken output and antimotility agents such as loperamide or diphenoxylate/atropine to decrease GI transit time and increase water absorption.

The inability to achieve a good seal around the ostomy pouch can result in skin irritation and breakdown. This phenomenon is far more common with ileostomies than colostomies because of the high concentration of active digestive enzymes and acidic pH of ileal contents. In the elective setting, the optimal location for an ostomy given the patient's abdominal anatomy and body habitus can be identified and marked preoperatively. Changes with sitting and other common postures can be considered. The inability to preoperatively assess these factors in the emergent setting frequently predisposes these patients to future issues in managing ostomy effluent.

Nutrition Assessment

Given the frequency of nutrition compromise in patients undergoing gastric and upper intestinal surgeries, careful nutrition assessment both pre- and postoperatively is important in this patient population. Malnutrition affects wound healing, infection risk, length of stay postoperatively, morbidity and possibly mortality.[53] Studies of patients with gastric cancer have shown that patients with a BMI less than 18.5 and low preoperative levels of serum albumin are at higher risk of complications and have decreased survival.[53] Numerous nutrition screening algorithms exist, including the Nutrition Risk Score 2002, Short Nutritional Assessment Questionnaire, Prognostic Nutrition Index, and Nutrition Risk Index. Screening algorithms can help identify those patients who will benefit from perioperative nutrition support via EN or PN.[54]

Weight loss of 10% to 30% of preoperative weight is not uncommon following partial gastrectomy, total gastrectomy, and pancreaticoduodenectomy.[55] Reasons for this weight loss are multifactorial and are often attributed to insufficient oral intake, malabsorption, rapid intestinal transit time, and bacterial overgrowth.[56] In patients with malignant disease, cancer cachexia can also play a role. Nevertheless, weight gain after surgery is possible.[57] Nutrition assessment should focus on actual dietary intake and weight history. Specifically, the clinician should ask about postprandial complaints, including early satiety, epigastric fullness, nausea, vomiting, symptoms of dumping syndrome, diarrhea (steatorrhea), or lactose intolerance.

Nutrition Management

Although diet therapy may be beneficial in treating nutrition intolerances, it is important to minimize diet restrictions and encourage frequent tolerable meals. Undue restrictions can further aggravate weight loss. If weight loss persists despite dietary management, enteral feedings for supplemental nutrition should be initiated. In cases where a small gastric remnant precludes gastrostomy tube placement, a surgically or endoscopically placed jejunostomy tube may be considered. PN should be used only as a last resort.

Table 37-1 provides a summary of nutrition management guidelines following gastric resection.[58] Many of these points are further explored in this chapter, and a more comprehensive review on managing the nutrition consequences following gastrectomy is available elsewhere.[58]

TABLE 37-1 Summary of Nutrition Management Guidelines Following Gastric Resection

Maintain optimal nutrition status:
- Determine cause(s) of weight loss through careful diet history.
- Provide diet education to minimize symptoms of dumping syndrome and lactose intolerance, if present.
- Administer a daily multivitamin with minerals.
- Use additional calcium and vitamin D supplementation as warranted.
- Individualize nutrition interventions for at-risk patients.

Treat fat malabsorption:
- Determine whether steatorrhea is present (ensure that patient consumes ≥100 g fat per day when checking qualitative or quantitative fecal fat).
- Consider use of pancreatic enzymes.
- Use gut-slowing agents if needed.
- Treat bacterial overgrowth if present.
- Monitor and supplement fat-soluble vitamins as needed.
- Administer a daily multivitamin with minerals.

Prevent nutrition anemias:
- Monitor:
  — Vitamin B$_{12}$
  — Red blood cell folate
  — Ferritin
- Supplement as needed.

Prevent and treat metabolic bone disease:
- Monitor 25-hydroxyvitamin D.[a]
- Supplement with 1500 mg of calcium: 500 mg doses 3 times a day.
- Supplement with 800 IU vitamin D daily.
- Monitor bone mineral density (dual-energy x-ray absorptiometry scan).
- Evaluate need for antiresorptive and bone-formation agents.

Manage gastric stasis:
- Treat bezoars.
- Treat bacterial overgrowth.
- Treat gastroparesis.

[a]1,25-dihydroxyvitamin D is not a good indicator of vitamin D status (it can be normal, high, or low in vitamin D deficiency; the most commonly used and most sensitive index is 25-hydroxyvitamin D).
Source: Adapted with permission from reference 58: Radigan A. Post-gastrectomy: managing the nutrition fall-out. *Pract Gastroenterol.* 2004;28(6):63–75.

Oral Nutrition Therapy

Physiological and anatomical alterations after surgery create unique barriers to optimal nutrition support. Early satiety, decreased appetite, bloating, nausea, and sometimes vomiting are possible problems. Oral nutrition therapy can be used to manage many of the complications of upper GI surgeries. Clinicians should counsel the patient to consume multiple small meals throughout the day and separate beverage intake from food intake to decrease fullness and early satiety. Patients should focus on protein and complex carbohydrate intake at every meal, and avoid concentrated sweets. Dietary manipulation is the primary intervention for complications such as gastric stasis and dumping syndrome, which are discussed in more detail later in the chapter.

Enteral Nutrition

Many patients need EN before and after gastric or pancreatic resections. Indeed, perioperative EN alone or as part of a group

of interventions can reduce postoperative complications, the length of the hospital stay, and costs.[59-61] Preoperative carbohydrate loading with a 12.5% carbohydrate drink is also recommended by some surgical consortia; however, this practice is more common in Europe than in the United States.[53]

Immunonutrition

Immunonutrition refers to the use of oral or enteral formulas specifically enhanced with elements that support immune function, including ω-3 fatty acids, nucleotides, and arginine. Meta-analyses of immunonutrition in patients undergoing elective GI procedures show that immune-modulating formulas may improve inflammatory markers, decrease postoperative complications, and reduce the length of hospital stay, and their use is recommended by some surgical societies to improve postoperative outcomes.[62-64] See Chapter 11 for further discussion of immune-modulating enteral formulations.

Parenteral Nutrition

Patients who fail EN or develop severe complications such as postsurgical strictures, motility disorders, anastomotic leaks, or fistulas may require PN. Studies are conflicting regarding outcomes when EN and PN are compared, but initiation of PN prevents further nutrition decline in instances where patients lack a functioning GI tract or are unable to tolerate oral intake or EN (see Chapter 14).[65–67]

Complications

Many complications associated with abdominal surgery have been discussed. Here, we will discuss specific consequences of GI and pancreatobiliary surgery, including chylothorax and enterocutaneous fistula (ECF), that result in significant macro- or micronutrient deficiencies.

Anemias

Nutrition anemias, resulting from vitamin B$_{12}$, folate, or iron deficiency, are common in patients with gastric resections. Because consequences of anemia can be severe, baseline and periodic monitoring of anemia-related laboratory data are important. Patients with a distant history of gastric resection may be at greater risk of nutrition anemia because it often presents as a late complication.

Iron Deficiency Anemia

Iron deficiency, a microcytic anemia, is the most common anemia following gastric resection.[68] The reported incidence varies tremendously. Alterations in digestion and absorption are thought to be responsible for iron deficiency in patients with total and partial gastrectomy. Except in Billroth I reconstructions, the gastrectomy bypasses the primary site for iron absorption, the duodenum, and reduced gastric acidity impairs the conversion of ferric iron to the more absorbable ferrous form (see Chapter 8).[68] Poor iron intake may also play a role in iron deficiency. In a multistudy review, 5% to 62% of patients with Billroth II reconstructions were found to be iron deficient.[69] Indeed, at 10 years post gastrectomy, iron deficiency was noted to be the most frequent nutrient deficiency.[55] Ferritin levels in the nonacute-phase setting are an accurate indicator of iron stores.[70] Guidelines for iron repletion are available elsewhere.[58]

Vitamin B$_{12}$ Deficiency and Anemia

Megaloblastic anemia results from either vitamin B$_{12}$ or folate deficiency. B$_{12}$ deficiency (sometimes referred to as *pernicious anemia*) can occur in patients with a history of gastric resection for several reasons. In the patient with unaltered anatomy, intrinsic factor is complexed to B$_{12}$ and facilitates its absorption by the terminal ileum. A lack of intrinsic factor from the stomach and overall reduced gastric acidity in postgastrectomy patients impairs cleavage of protein-bound B$_{12}$ and its attachment to intrinsic factor.[71] Bacterial overgrowth and reduced intake of B$_{12}$-rich foods may also contribute to a deficiency.

The incidence of B$_{12}$ deficiency has been reported in patients with partial (10% to 43%) and total gastrectomy (theoretically, 100%). Although deficiencies have been found as early as 1 year postoperatively, they are more common in the late postoperative state.[55] Clinical features, while useful in the diagnosis of megaloblastic anemia, can often be nonspecific or absent in some patients;[70] therefore, periodic serum monitoring and supplementation of B$_{12}$ is prudent. Measuring metabolic intermediaries such as methylmalonic acid and homocysteine concurrently with B$_{12}$ monitoring may lead to higher sensitivity in detecting early deficiency.[72] A study investigating the effects of either oral or intramuscular B$_{12}$ supplementation in patients with total gastrectomy found that enteral B$_{12}$ treatment increased serum concentration rapidly.[72] Symptom resolution was comparable in patients who received enteral or parenteral supplementation. It is possible that the body adapts after total gastrectomy and may produce intrinsic factor in the duodenum and jejunum.[72] The decision to supplement B$_{12}$ orally or via intramuscular injection should be based on expected patient compliance. It may be prudent to start with intramuscular injections initially when neurologic function is impaired or until compliance has been established. See Chapter 8 for further information on vitamin B$_{12}$.

Folate Deficiency

Folate deficiency may develop after gastric surgery. Causes of folate deficiency likely include malabsorption and impaired digestion.[68] Folate is absorbed in the proximal small bowel. Tests for serum folate indicate the short-term balance and fluctuate according to meals. Red blood cell folate represents long-term balance and more accurately reflects body stores. A daily dose of 5 mg folate is recommended in deficiency states. The 100-mcg dose supplied in a daily multivitamin should be sufficient for maintenance.[73] See Chapter 8 for further discussion of folate.

Metabolic Bone Disease

Metabolic bone disease, such as osteoporosis, osteopenia, or osteomalacia, is commonly reported in patients with gastric resections. The prevalence of metabolic bone disease, defined as having a low bone mineral density (BMD), is approximately 27% to 44%.[74,75] The etiology of metabolic bone disease in gastrectomy patients is poorly understood. Bone remodeling occurs throughout a patient's lifetime, and appropriate bone mass and strength are maintained through a closely regulated homeostatic relationship between bone reabsorption and formation.[25] Bone disease is usually attributed to decreased formation of new bone, often as a result of vitamin and mineral deficiencies. However, an increased rate of bone reabsorption can also result in net bone loss. For example, a study found that osteomalacia was present in up to 18% of patients with partial gastrectomy despite the finding that most of these patients had normal serum calcium, alkaline phosphatase, and 25-hydroxyvitamin D (25-OHD) levels.[76] Homeostatic dysregulation, in addition to impaired mineral and vitamin absorption, may play an important role in the development of metabolic bone disease after gastric resection.[77] Because of these findings, it has been postulated that older studies relying solely on laboratory values have underestimated the prevalence of osteomalacia in gastric resection patients.[74] Klein and colleagues found that vertebral body fractures were 3 times as common in men who had undergone a Billroth II procedure than in controls.[76] Notably, age and bone status at the time of surgery play roles in overall bone disease independent of gastric resection, and most patients who undergo gastric resection are older.

Patients who have undergone gastric resection are at higher risk of malabsorption despite their age. The loss of the duodenal surface area, an increased transit time, and alterations in diet all contribute to the development of malnutrition after gastrectomy.[78] Some patients may require dietary supplementation to overcome the effects of malnutrition. One study demonstrated an increase in 25-OHD when patients with total gastrectomy and partial gastrectomy were supplemented with 400 IU of vitamin D daily.[78] Another study found statistically significant increases in 25-OHD in patients with partial gastrectomy supplemented with 400 to 600 IU of vitamin D$_2$.[74] Currently, there are no accepted supplementation guidelines for calcium and vitamin D in postgastrectomy states. For patients with bone disease, 1500 mg of calcium and 800 IU of vitamin D daily are recommended. Patients should be encouraged to include calcium-rich foods in their diet as tolerated.

Dual-energy x-ray absorptiometry provides an inexpensive, reproducible method to determine BMD.[79] It is reasonable to monitor BMD, even in the setting of normal laboratory values, at baseline and then every 1 to 2 years. Prompt initiation of antiresorptive agents (calcium, vitamin D, calcitonin, and bisphosphonates) and bone-formation agents (recombinant parathyroid hormone) may need to be considered in severe cases. Continuous nutrition assessment and intervention is an effective tool to prevent or minimize dietary intolerances and manifestations of nutrient deficiencies. See Chapter 8 for additional information on calcium and vitamin D supplementation.

Postgastrectomy Syndrome

Postgastrectomy syndrome encompasses nutrition intolerances and deficiencies. The most common intolerances include early satiety, dumping syndrome, fat maldigestion, gastric stasis, and lactose intolerance. Specific nutrient deficiencies develop months to years after gastric resections, often resulting in serious consequences. Anemia and bone disease are the most common manifestations of nutrient deficiencies seen in patients who have undergone gastric resections. Less common postgastrectomy symptoms include afferent and efferent limb syndrome, alkaline reflux gastritis, and postvagotomy diarrhea.

Stasis and Delayed Gastric Emptying

Among patients with a truncal vagotomy, 3% to 5% are reported to experience problems with gastric stasis. Poor emptying may manifest as postprandial bloating, discomfort, or fullness lasting many hours. Emesis of undigested food consumed hours to days before may also be present. These patients are at a higher risk of bezoar formation, bacterial overgrowth, and intolerance to solid food. Liquids may be processed normally or rapidly.[68] Diet manipulation and/or prokinetic drugs may be effective to varying degrees (see section on gastroparesis).

Delayed gastric emptying is the most common complication after a Whipple procedure, but weight loss, dumping syndrome, diabetes mellitus, and malabsorption due to pancreatic exocrine insufficiency may also occur.[80] The pathophysiological mechanisms that are involved in gastric stagnation are multifactorial and not fully understood. Patients experiencing delayed gastric emptying often require a nasogastric tube because of intractable nausea and vomiting. Treating acid hypersecretion with a PPI (vs an H$_2$-receptor antagonist) postoperatively can significantly improve gastric stagnation.[81] Pharmacological treatment with prokinetic agents is also common.

Dumping Syndrome

As previously described, multiple factors—including loss of the gastric reservoir, altered secretion of GI hormones, and accelerated gastric emptying of hyperosmolar contents into the proximal small bowel resulting in release of vasoactive hormones—contribute to dumping syndrome.[82] Dumping syndrome can be divided into early and late symptoms. Early dumping occurs within approximately 30 minutes of eating when hyperosmotic fluids enter the small bowel and cause rapid fluid shifts.[83] Symptoms associated with early dumping include abdominal cramping, nausea, diarrhea, and palpitations. In contrast, late dumping occurs up to 3 hours after eating and is characterized by symptoms typically associated with hypoglycemia. Late dumping syndrome results from rapid absorption of simple sugars in the small bowel, which triggers an exaggerated release of insulin that results in a reactive hypoglycemia. Patients complain of sweating, dizziness, tachycardia, irritability, hunger, and syncopal symptoms. The percentage of patients who develop dumping syndrome after gastrectomy has been reported to range from 1% to 75%.[55] Dumping syndrome symptoms are more prevalent in the immediate postoperative period and frequently resolve over time.[84] Approximately 1% of patients will develop persistent, debilitating symptoms.[85] Dumping syndrome unresponsive to diet manipulation may require use of gut-slowing medication.[84] Table 37-2 presents guidelines for an antidumping diet.[58,86]

Fat Maldigestion and Exocrine Pancreatic Insufficiency

Exocrine pancreatic insufficiency (EPI) and increased fecal fat excretion (steatorrhea) have been demonstrated following both partial and total gastrectomy, and they are quite common after pancreatic resections.[56] The etiology of fat malabsorption is multifactorial. First, an accelerated transit time or dumping syndrome and the surgically altered anatomy prevent sufficient mixing of food with digestive enzymes and bile salts. Second, decreased enzyme production reduces the ratio of enzymes to food.[87] Unattached bile salts can irritate the colon and compound the effects of diarrhea. Finally, before loss of the distal stomach, and hence its sieving function, larger-than-normal food particles empty into the jejunum, making their degradation by enzymes more difficult.[68] Measurements of fecal elastase and fecal fat can aid in the diagnosis. Fecal elastase is a pancreatic enzyme that is not degraded in the intestinal

TABLE 37-2 Antidumping Diet Guidelines

- Eat 6 or more small meals a day.

- Eat slowly, and chew all foods thoroughly.

- Sit upright while eating.

- Avoid or limit high-sugar foods and beverages including the following: fruit-flavored drinks, juice, soda, Ensure (Abbott Nutrition, Abbott Park, IL), Boost (Novartis, Basel, Switzerland), cakes, pies, candy, doughnuts, cookies, etc.

- Limit fluid consumption at meals. Drink liquids 30 to 60 minutes either before or after meals.

- Eat a protein-containing food with each meal. High-protein foods include the following: eggs, meat, poultry, fish, lunch meat, nuts, milk, yogurt, cottage cheese, cheese, peanut butter, dried beans, lentils, and tofu.

- If you have difficulty maintaining your weight, you may need to drink a nutritional supplement for extra calories. You can try low-sugar, over-the-counter supplements, such as no-sugar-added Carnation Instant Breakfast (Nestlé Health Science, Fremont, MI), sugar-free Nutrishakes (Neolife, Freemont, CA), or Glucerna weight loss shakes (Abbott Nutrition, Abbott Park, IL); lactose-free products are also available.

- Choose high-fiber foods when possible. These include whole wheat bread, fruits, vegetables, and beans (pinto, black, brown, kidney).

Source: Adapted from reference 86: University of Virginia Health System. Anti-dumping diet. https://med.virginia.edu/ginutrition/wp-content/uploads/sites/199/2014/04/Post_Gastrectomy_and_Dumping_Diet_12.5.14.pdf. Accessed June 7, 2017. Used with permission from the University of Virginia Health System GI Nutrition Website: www.ginutrition.virginia.edu.

lumen and is not affected by exogenous pancreatic enzyme use, which makes it a convenient measure of exocrine pancreatic function. A common cutoff for the diagnosis of EPI is a fecal elastase level less than 200 mcg/g. However, fecal elastase levels must be interpreted carefully—diarrhea or intestinal inflammation of any kind can cause false-positive tests.[88,89]

Fecal fat can be measured in 2 ways: as a *qualitative* measure where only the presence or absence of fat is noted, or as a *quantitative* measure that requires a timed stool collection. Traditionally, a 72-hour stool collection has been used because it can provide a more accurate accounting of the actual grams of fecal fat lost per day; however, given patient distaste for the procedure and difficulty in laboratory handling, the 72-hour collection is often replaced with a 24-hour collection. Both qualitative and quantitative measures can be helpful in monitoring pancreatic enzyme replacement therapy. Prolonged steatorrhea may necessitate monitoring and replacement of fat-soluble vitamins.[84]

Patients with a partial or total gastrectomy usually have normal fecal elastase levels because pancreatic exocrine function and secretion are maintained. However, given the altered anatomy, the secreted pancreatic enzymes may not mix with ingested food at the proper time to cause digestion, thus leading to fat malabsorption and steatorrhea. A fecal fat level is particularly helpful in diagnosing and managing this situation. Patients with a partial or total gastrectomy may benefit from pancreatic enzyme replacement therapy; the addition of exogenous pancreatic enzymes has been shown to reduce fecal fat excretion in some patients.[90]

Lactose Intolerance

Lactase, the enzyme required for lactose absorption, is found primarily on villi in the jejunum.[91] Most gastrectomized patients have an intact jejunum. Patients who experience abdominal cramping or pain, bloating, diarrhea, flatulence, and distention after consumption of lactose may benefit from decreasing or avoiding lactose-containing foods. Tolerance to lactose is typically dose-dependent and may improve over time.[91]

Afferent Limb Syndrome, Alkaline Reflux Gastritis, and Postvagotomy Diarrhea

GJ reconstruction with a Billroth II reconstruction results in the formation of an afferent limb and an efferent limb of the small bowel attached to the gastric remnant. In rare cases, the afferent limb, which drains the biliary system, can become obstructed from malpositioning, stricture, radiation enteritis, or adhesions.[92] Afferent limb syndrome is a late-term complication of partial gastrectomy where the afferent limb is positioned in a dependent position, allowing it to fill with food during a meal. A dilated afferent limb on imaging is diagnostic, and symptoms of pain and cramping are attributed to limb distension. Patients describe relief with vomiting, which temporarily clears or decompresses the afferent limb. Surgical revision is the usual treatment.

Alkaline reflux gastritis can occur after Billroth II reconstruction because the bile stream must pass through the anastomosis of GJ to reach the efferent limb. Bile salts are irritating to the gastric and esophageal mucosa. Patients often experience dyspepsia and bile reflux. Evidence of gastritis and esophagitis are seen on endoscopic examination. Treatment is generally conservative, as with other cases of gastritis, and should include an empiric trial of cholestyramine, which binds bile salts. Surgical reconstruction could be considered in refractory cases.[93]

Postvagotomy diarrhea results from unclear mechanisms in patients who have undergone a truncal vagotomy. A study looking at patients who had undergone vagotomy found an increased incidence of diarrhea after fluid meals and a significant decrease in intestinal motility in response to dry meals.[87] Treatment is conservative.

Chylothorax and Chylous Ascites

Chylothorax and chylous ascites can be classified as primary (a result of lymphangiectasis/malignant obstruction of the lymphatic outflow) or secondary (iatrogenic injury, complications from thoracic/esophageal surgery) in nature. Simply put, *chylothorax* is the presence of chyle (composed of lymphatic fluids and chylomicrons) within the pleural space and *chylous ascites* is the presence of chyle within the peritoneal cavity. The abdominal lymphatic system coalesces into a single duct structure that traverses the aortic hiatus, travels within the posterior mediastinum, and empties into the confluence of the left subclavian and internal jugular vein and can be disrupted at any point.

Chyle contains approximately 70% of dietary fat in addition to protein and lymphocytes. Thus, several immunological and nutrition consequences are observed when a chyle leak is present. Electrolyte abnormalities, profound protein/lean body mass loss, and fat-soluble vitamin deficiencies are commonly observed. In addition, because the cellular content of chyle is predominately lymphocytes, T cell depletion can occur, resulting in impaired cell-mediated immunity and increased infectious risk.

Surgical or conservative measures may be employed in the treatment of chylothorax and chylous ascites, with decisions made on a case-by-case basis. In the setting of conservative management, nutrition support strategies play a significant role. Following adequate drainage of the affected space, management becomes focused on the reduction of chyle flow to facilitate closure. Oral diets consist of high-protein and very-low-fat foods with medium-chain triglyceride supplementation. In patients who are unable to tolerate oral feeding, EN can be administered via a nasogastric, gastrostomy, nasojejunal, or jejunostomy tube. In the setting of enteral intolerance, PN can be used. It is important to note that essential fatty acid deficiency can become an issue if long-chain fatty acids are restricted for more than 2 weeks. Postprandial chyle flow rates of 225 mL/min can be reduced to fasting rates of 0.93 mL/min in the setting of long-term PN administration.[64]

The Open Abdomen

The open abdomen refers to situations where the abdominal fascia is not definitively closed at the index operation and temporizing measures such as negative pressure dressings are applied during the interval prior to return to the operating room. This approach is most commonly used in the setting of trauma in the presence of the lethal triad of acidosis, hypothermia, and coagulopathy. Additional indications include planned re-exploration in the setting of patchy bowel ischemia, and this approach has become increasingly prevalent in the acute care surgical patient population.

EN has been extensively examined in the setting of the open abdomen and found to be safe and potentially reduce time to definitive abdominal closure, ECF rates, and infectious complications.[59,60] EN can be delivered within the first 24 to 48 hours following resuscitation through either nasoenteric access or surgically placed access points. Because of the overall complexity and physiological alteration in these patients, enteral access is often placed at the time of definitive abdominal closure. Ongoing concern for bowel ischemia and excessive vasopressor requirements may be suitable reasons to avoid EN; however, in most patients, early EN is beneficial and appropriate.[61-63]

Enterocutaneous Fistulas

Fistulas are defined as communications between any 2 epithelialized surfaces and are described with the higher-pressure component listed first (ie, enterocutaneous, aortoduodenal, etc). Ostomies are an example of an intended ECF. ECFs are characterized as either high output (greater than 500 mL) or low output; high-output fistulas have significantly higher mortality. Most ECFs (75% to 80%) are complications of surgery (unrecognized enterotomy, anastomotic leaks), with the minority developing spontaneously as a result of ongoing inflammatory processes (Crohn's disease). Metabolic complications include fluid and electrolyte abnormalities, D-lactic acidosis, micronutrient deficiencies, and osteoporosis and osteomalacia.

The cornerstones of management of ECFs include resuscitation, source control, wound care, and nutrition support. PN has dramatically decreased the mortality associated with ECFs. During initial presentation, most patients with suspected or confirmed ECF should be kept NPO, and PN should be considered. Most low-output ECFs will close and do so within 4 weeks of presentation. Enteral feeding via a tube placed directly into the fistula (fistuloclysis) should be considered in patients with a proximal ECF. Unfortunately, these tubes are often difficult to secure, which may lead to frequent feeding interruptions, making supplemental PN necessary. Goals are to maintain fluid and electrolyte homeostasis, minimize the loss of lean body mass, and prevent micronutrient deficiency through appropriate trace mineral, zinc, copper, and vitamin supplementation.

Often, these patients require prolonged periods of PN. Bowel rest with PN will allow for the best hope of spontaneous closure in low-output fistulas. Initially, strict NPO with PN will decrease output and allow for correction of fluid and electrolyte losses. If feeding via the GI tract is then started, it should be done in a controlled fashion with antimotility agents and monitoring of electrolyte status. Regardless of indication, surgical procedures leading to significant anatomical alterations will require specific nutrition support strategies to address the patient's potential nutrition deficiencies. Recovery and long-term improvement in functional status and quality of life require the coordinated effort of surgeons, gastroenterologists, dietitians, and physical and occupational therapists as well as the patient and his or her family members. Practice Scenario 37-3 further explores interventions to manage ECF.

Summary

Regardless of indication, surgical procedures involve significant alterations of normal anatomy and physiology that affect

Practice Scenario 37-3

Question: What is the appropriate initial management of a newly diagnosed enterocutaneous fistula (ECF)?

Scenario: A 56-year-old woman with a history of Roux-en-Y gastric bypass presented with a small bowel obstruction. She was taken emergently to the operating room and found to have an internal hernia. The surgical team resected 50 cm of bowel with a primary anastomosis. The patient initially did well; however, on postoperative Day 14, she had copious bilious drainage from her midline incision, tachycardia, and orthostatic hypotension.

Intervention: The patient underwent an abdominal computed tomography scan and was not found to have any drainable fluid collections. A fascial defect in close proximity to proximal jejunum was demonstrated. An ostomy appliance was fitted over the area of drainage and the effluent was controlled. She was admitted to the hospital, resuscitated with crystalloids, and provided parenteral electrolyte. Parenteral nutrition (PN) was initiated following placement of a peripherally inserted central catheter. Over the next several days, her output decreased to approximately 100 mL/d. Full liquids were then trialed with subsequent increases in ECF output to 750 mL/d. Elemental tube feeds and antimotility agents were initiated, which decreased ECF output to 500 mL/d. She was subsequently made *nil per os* and discharged on long-term PN.

Answer: Initial management of ECF involves resuscitation, source control if necessary in the event of intra-abdominal fluid collection, skin protection, and nutrition support.

Rationale: In this scenario, a proximal portion of small bowel seems to be involved, suggesting that initial attempts at enteral nutrition (EN) would prove unsuccessful. Following maturation of the fistula, either direct measures to deliver EN via the fistula or fistuloclysis (readministration of enteric output via the fistula) could be attempted.

nutrition support strategies. Care of postsurgical patients should entail a review of operative reports, pre- and postoperative records, and, in complex cases, a discussion with either the operative surgeon or a surgeon experienced in the procedure(s) in question. Given the multidisciplinary nature of care with regard to nutrition support, all clinicians involved need to understand the most salient anatomical and physiological considerations contributing to the patient's overall status and, in the case of acute or subacute illness, their underlying pathophysiology.

References

1. Vanek VW. Ins and outs of enteral access: part 2—long term access—esophagostomy and gastrostomy. *Nutr Clin Pract.* 2003; 18(1):50–74.
2. Vanek VW. Ins and outs of enteral access. Part 3: long-term access—jejunostomy. *Nutr Clin Pract.* 2003;18(3):201–220.
3. Lada MJ, Peters JH. The management of esophageal cancer. In: Cameron JL, Cameron AM, eds. *Current Surgical Therapy.* 11 ed. Philadelphia, PA: Elsevier; 2014.
4. Kight CE. Nutrition considerations in esophagectomy patients. *Nutr Clin Pract.* 2008;23(5):521–528.
5. Elshaer M, Gravante G, White J, et al. Routes of early enteral nutrition following oesophagectomy. *Ann R Coll Surg Engl.* 2016; 98(7):1–7.
6. Hanyu T, Kosugi S, Ishikawa T, Ichikawa H, Wakai T. Incidence and risk factors for anastomotic stricture after esophagectomy with gastric tube reconstruction. *Hepato-gastroenterology.* 2015;62 (140):892–897.
7. Oh SY, Lee HJ, Yang HK. Pylorus-preserving gastrectomy for gastric cancer. *J Gastric Canc.* 2016;16(2):63–71.
8. Konishi H, Nakada K, Kawamura M, et al. Impaired gastrointestinal function affects symptoms and alimentary status in patients after gastrectomy. *World J Surg.* 2016;40(11):2713–2718.
9. Dias Rodrigues V, Barroso de Pinho N, Abdelhay E, et al. Nutrition and immune-modulatory intervention in surgical patients with gastric cancer. *Nutr Clin Pract.* 2017;32(1):122–129.
10. Pappas S, Krzywda E, McDowell N. Nutrition and pancreatico-duodenectomy. *Nutr Clin Pract.* 2010;25(3):234–243.
11. Reynolds RB, Folloder JJ. Clinical management of pancreatic cancer. *Adv Pract Oncol.* 2014;5(5):356–364.
12. Bell R, Pandanaboyana S, Shah N, et al. Meta-analysis of antecolic versus retrocolic gastric reconstruction after a pylorus-preserving pancreatoduodenectomy. *HPB (Oxford).* 2015;17(3):202–208.
13. Kapoor VK. Complications of pancreato-duodenectomy. *Rozhl Chir.* 2016;95(2):53–59.
14. Girard E, Messager M, Sauvanet A, et al. Anastomotic leakage after gastrointestinal surgery: diagnosis and management. *J Visc Surg.* 2014;151(6):441–450.
15. Pannegeon V, Pessaux P, Sauvanet A, et al. Pancreatic fistula after distal pancreatectomy: predictive risk factors and value of conservative treatment. *Arch Surg.* 2006;141(11):1071–1076.
16. de Rooij T, Tol JA, van Eijck CH, et al. Outcomes of distal pancreatectomy for pancreatic ductal adenocarcinoma in the Netherlands: a nationwide retrospective analysis. *Ann Surg Oncol.* 2016; 23(2):585–591.
17. Suzuki S, Miura J, Shimizu K, et al. Clinicophysiological outcomes after total pancreatectomy. *Scan J Gastroenterol.* 2016; 51(12):1526–1531.
18. Chang SH, Stoll CR, Song J, et al. The effectiveness and risks of bariatric surgery: an updated systematic review and meta-analysis, 2003–2012. *JAMA Surg.* 2014;149(3):275–287.
19. Thomas S, Schauer P. Bariatric surgery and the gut hormone response. *Nutr Clin Pract.* 2010;25(2):175–182.
20. Aman MW, Stem M, Schweitzer MA, Magnuson TH, Lidor AO. Early hospital readmission after bariatric surgery. *Surg Endosc.* 2016;30(6):2231–2238.
21. Finks JF, Kole KL, Yenumula PR, et al. Predicting risk for serious complications with bariatric surgery: results from the Michigan Bariatric Surgery Collaborative. *Ann Surg.* Oct 2011;254(4): 633–640.
22. de Moura EG, Orso IR, Aurelio EF, et al. Factors associated with complications or failure of endoscopic balloon dilation of anastomotic stricture secondary to Roux-en-Y gastric bypass surgery. *Surg Obes Relat Dis.* 2016;12(3):582–586.
23. Concors SJ, Ecker BL, Maduka R, et al. Complications and surveillance after bariatric surgery. *Curr Treat Options Neurol.* 2016; 18(1):5.
24. Ramadan M, Loureiro M. Risk of dumping syndrome after sleeve gastrectomy and Roux-en-Y gastric bypass: early results of a multi-centre prospective study. *Gastroenterol Res Pract.* 2016;2016:2570237.

25. Nimeri AA, Maasher A, Al Shaban T, Salim E, Gamaleldin MM. Internal hernia following laparoscopic Roux-en-Y Gastric bypass: prevention and tips for intra-operative management. *Obes Surg.* 2016;26(9):2255-2256.

26. Park J, Chung M, Teixeira J, Baer J, Frager D. Computed tomography findings of internal hernia after gastric bypass that may precede small bowel obstruction. *Hernia.* 2016;20(3):471-477.

27. Hwang RF, Swartz DE, Felix EL. Causes of small bowel obstruction after laparoscopic gastric bypass. *Surgical Endosc.* 2004;18(11):1631-1635.

28. Brockmeyer JR, Grover BT, Kallies KJ, Kothari SN. Management of biliary symptoms after bariatric surgery. *Am J Surg.* 2015;210(6):1010-1017.

29. Greuter T, Frey DM, Magdeburg B. Is ERCP after Roux-en-Y gastric bypass possible with a standard gastroscope? A new but simple technique to solve many problems. *J Clin Gastroenterol.* 2016;50(10):895-896.

30. Abdelbaki TN, Abdelsalam WN, ElKayal S. Management modalities in slipped gastric band. *Surg Obes Relat Dis.* 2016;12(3):714-716.

31. Belachew M, Belva PH, Desaive C. Long-term results of laparoscopic adjustable gastric banding for the treatment of morbid obesity. *Obes Surg.* 2002;12(4):564-568.

32. Sonavane SK, Menias CO, Kantawala KP, et al. Laparoscopic adjustable gastric banding: what radiologists need to know. *Radiographics.* 2012;32(4):1168-1171.

33. Quadri P, Gonzalez-Heredia R, Masrur M, Sanchez-Johnsen L, Elli EF. Management of laparoscopic adjustable gastric band erosion. *Surg Endosc.* August 23, 2016 [Epub ahead of print].

34. Corona M, Zini C, Allegritti M, et al. Minimally invasive treatment of gastric leak after sleeve gastrectomy. *Radiol Med.* 2013;118(6):962-970.

35. Bullard Dunn KM, Rothenberger DA. Colon, rectum, and anus. In: Brunicardi FC, ed. *Schwartz's Principles of Surgery.* 10th ed. New York: McGraw-Hill Education; 2015.

36. Batignani G, Monaci I, Ficari F, Tonelli F. What affects continence after anterior resection of the rectum? *Dis Colon Rectum.* 1991;34(4):329-335.

37. Ashburn JH, Kalady MF. Radiation-induced problems in colorectal surgery. *Clin Colon Rectal Surg.* 2016;29(2):85-91.

38. Bansal N, Soni A, Kaur P, Chauhan AK, Kaushal V. Exploring the management of radiation proctitis in current clinical practice. *J Clin Diagn Res.* 2016;10(6):xe01-xe06.

39. Yuan ZX, Ma TH, Wang HM, et al. Colostomy is a simple and effective procedure for severe chronic radiation proctitis. *World J Gastroenterol.* 2016;22(24):5598-5608.

40. Buckman SA, Heise CP. Nutrition considerations surrounding restorative proctocolectomy. *Nutr Clin Pract.* 2010;25(3):250-256.

41. Schieffer KM, Williams ED, Yochum GS, Koltun WA. Review article: the pathogenesis of pouchitis. *Aliment Pharmacol Ther.* 2016;44(8):817-835.

42. Nitzan O, Elias M, Peretz A, Saliba W. Role of antibiotics for treatment of inflammatory bowel disease. *World J Gastroenterol.* 2016;22(3):1078-1087.

43. Shen B. Problems after restorative proctocolectomy: assessment and therapy. *Curr Opin Gastroenterol.* 2016;32(1):49-54.

44. Singh S, Stroud AM, Holubar SD, Sandborn WJ, Pardi DS. Treatment and prevention of pouchitis after ileal pouch-anal anastomosis for chronic ulcerative colitis. *Cochrane Database Syst Rev.* 2015;(11):CD001176.

45. Bailey EH, Glasgow SC. Challenges in the medical and surgical management of chronic inflammatory bowel disease. *Surg Clin N Am.* 2015;95(6):1233-1244.

46. Carroll RE, Benedetti E, Schowalter JP, Buchman AL. Management and complications of short bowel syndrome: an updated review. *Curr Gastroenterol Rep.* 2016;18(7):40.

47. Pironi L. Definitions of intestinal failure and the short bowel syndrome. *Best Pract Res Clin Gastroenterol.* 2016;30(2):173-185.

48. Pironi L, Arends J, Bozzetti F, et al. ESPEN guidelines on chronic intestinal failure in adults. *Clin Nutrition (Edinburgh).* 2016;35(2):247-307.

49. Tonelli F, Alemanno G, Di Martino C, et al. Results of surgical treatment for jejunal Crohn's disease: choice between resection, strictureplasty, and combined treatment. *Langenbecks Arch Surg.* August 17, 2016 [Epub ahead of print].

50. Akiba RT, Rodrigues FG, da Silva G. Management of complex perineal fistula disease. *Clin Colon Rectal Surg.* 2016;29(2):92-100.

51. Gribovskaja-Rupp I, Melton GB. enterocutaneous fistula: proven strategies and updates. *Clin Colon Rectal Surg.* 2016;29(2):130-137.

52. Kaimakliotis P, Simillis C, Harbord M, et al. A systematic review assessing medical treatment for rectovaginal and enterovesical fistulae in Crohn's disease. *J Clin Gastroenterol.* 2016;50(9):714-721.

53. Rosania R, Chiapponi C, Malfertheiner P, Venerito M. Nutrition in patients with gastric cancer: an update. *Gastrointest Tumors.* 2016;2(4):178-187.

54. Veterans Affairs Total Parenteral Nutrition Cooperative Study Group. Perioperative total parenteral nutrition in surgical patients. *N Engl J Med.* 1991;325(8):525-532.

55. Tovey FI, Godfrey JE, Lewin MR. A gastrectomy population: 25-30 years on. *Postgrad Med J.* 1990;66(776):450-456.

56. Grant JP, Chapman G, Russell MK. Malabsorption associated with surgical procedures and its treatment. *Nutr Clin Pract.* 1996;11(2):43-52.

57. Braga M, Zuliani W, Foppa L, Di Carlo V, Cristallo M. Food intake and nutritional status after total gastrectomy: results of a nutritional follow-up. *Br J Surg.* 1988;75(5):477-480.

58. Radigan A. Post-gastrectomy: managing the nutrition fall-out. *Pract Gastroenterol.* 2004;28(6):63-75.

59. Bond-Smith G, Belgaumkar AP, Davidson BR, Gurusamy KS. Enhanced recovery protocols for major upper gastrointestinal, liver and pancreatic surgery. *Cochrane Database Syst Rev.* 2016;(2):CD011382.

60. Ding D, Feng Y, Song B, Gao S, Zhao J. Effects of preoperative and postoperative enteral nutrition on postoperative nutritional status and immune function of gastric cancer patients. *Turk J Gastroenterol.* 2015;26(2):181-185.

61. Li B, Liu HY, Guo SH, et al. Impact of early postoperative enteral nutrition on clinical outcomes in patients with gastric cancer. *Genet Mol Res.* 2015;14(2):7136-7141.

62. Song GM, Tian X, Liang H, et al. Role of enteral immunonutrition in patients undergoing surgery for gastric cancer: a systematic review and meta-analysis of randomized controlled trials. *Medicine.* 2015;94(31):e1311.

63. Heyland DK, Novak F, Drover JW, et al. Should immunonutrition become routine in critically ill patients? A systematic review of the evidence. *JAMA.* 2001;286(8):944-953.

64. Gianotti L, Braga M, Nespoli L, et al. A randomized controlled trial of preoperative oral supplementation with a specialized diet in patients with gastrointestinal cancer. *Gastroenterology.* 2002;122(7):1763-1770.

65. Li G, Gu R, Wen X, et al. The effect of early enteral nutrition on hyperthermic intraoperative intraperitoneal chemotherapy-induced mucosal permeability following gastrectomy. *JPEN J Parenter Enteral Nutr.* 2012;36(2):213-218.

66. Kim HU, Chung JB, Kim CB. [The comparison between early enteral nutrition and total parenteral nutrition after total gastrectomy in patients with gastric cancer: the randomized prospective study]. *Korean J Gastroenterol.* 2012;59(6):407-413.

67. Li J, Ji Z, Yuan C, et al. Limited efficacy of early enteral nutrition in patients after total gastrectomy. *J Invest Surg.* 2011;24(3):103-108.

68. Meyer J. Chronic morbidity after ulcer surgery. In: Sleisenger MI, Fordtran JS, eds. *Gastrointestinal Diseases.* 5th ed. Philadelphia, PA: Saunders; 1994:731–744.

69. Fischer AB. Twenty-five years after Billroth II gastrectomy for duodenal ulcer. *World J Surg.* 1984;8(3):293–302.

70. Pawson R, Mehta A. Review article: the diagnosis and treatment of haematinic deficiency in gastrointestinal disease. *Aliment Pharmacol Ther.* 1998;12(8):687–698.

71. Rege RV, Jones DB. Current role of surgery in peptic ulcer disease. In: Feldman MD, Friedman LS, Sleisenger MI, eds. *Gastrointestinal and Liver Disease.* New York: Elsevier Science; 2002.

72. Lindenbaum J, Savage DG, Stabler SP, Allen RH. Diagnosis of cobalamin deficiency: II. Relative sensitivities of serum cobalamin, methylmalonic acid, and total homocysteine concentrations. *Am J Hematol.* 1990;34(2):99–107.

73. Adachi S, Kawamoto T, Otsuka M, Todoroki T, Fukao K. Enteral vitamin B12 supplements reverse postgastrectomy B12 deficiency. *Ann Surg.* 2000;232(2):199–201.

74. Bisballe S, Eriksen EF, Melsen F, et al. Osteopenia and osteomalacia after gastrectomy: interrelations between biochemical markers of bone remodelling, vitamin D metabolites, and bone histomorphometry. *Gut.* 1991;32(11):1303–1307.

75. Vestergaard P. Bone loss associated with gastrointestinal disease: prevalence and pathogenesis. *Eur J Gastroenterol Hepatol.* 2003;15(8):851–856.

76. Klein KB, Orwoll ES, Lieberman DA, et al. Metabolic bone disease in asymptomatic men after partial gastrectomy with Billroth II anastomosis. *Gastroenterology.* 1987;92(3):608–616.

77. Bisballe S, Buus S, Lund B, Hessov I. Food intake and nutritional status after gastrectomy. *Hum Nutr Clin Nutr.* 1986;40(4):301–308.

78. Bernstein CN, Leslie WD. The pathophysiology of bone disease in gastrointestinal disease. *Eur J Gastroenterol Hepatol.* 2003;15(8):857–864.

79. Arden NK, Cooper C. Assessment of the risk of fracture in patients with gastrointestinal disease. *Eur J Gastroenterol Hepatol.* 2003;15(8):865–868.

80. Redlick PN, Steven AA, Pitt HA. Tumors of the pancreas, gallbladder, and bile ducts. In: Lenhard RF, Osteen RT, Gansler T, eds. *Clinical Oncology.* Atlanta, GA: American Cancer Society; 2001: 373–394.

81. Toyota N, Takada T, Yasuda H, et al. The effects of omeprazole, a proton pump inhibitor, on early gastric stagnation after a pylorus-preserving pancreaticoduodenectomy: results of a randomized study. *Hepato-gastroenterology.* 1998;45(22):1005–1010.

82. Ukleja A. Dumping syndrome: pathophysiology and treatment. *Nutr Clin Pract.* 2005;20(5):517–525.

83. Abell TL, Minocha A. Gastrointestinal complications of bariatric surgery: diagnosis and therapy. *Am J Med Sci.* 2006;331(4): 214–218.

84. Harju E. Metabolic problems after gastric surgery. *Int Surg.* 1990; 75(1):27–35.

85. Gray JL, Debas HT, Mulvihill SJ. Control of dumping symptoms by somatostatin analogue in patients after gastric surgery. *Arch Surg.* 1991;126(10):1231–1236.

86. University of Virginia Health System. Anti-dumping diet. https:// med.virginia.edu/ginutrition/wp-content/uploads/sites/199 /2014/04/Post_Gastrectomy_and_Dumping_Diet_12.5.14.pdf. Accessed June 7, 2017.

87. McKelvey ST. Gastric incontinence and post-vagotomy diarrhoea. *Br J Surg.* 1970;57(10):741–747.

88. Daftary A, Acton J, Heubi J, Amin R. Fecal elastase-1: utility in pancreatic function in cystic fibrosis. *J Cystic Fibrosis.* 2006;5(2): 71–76.

89. Beharry S, Ellis L, Corey M, Marcon M, Durie P. How useful is fecal pancreatic elastase 1 as a marker of exocrine pancreatic disease? *J Pediatr.* 2002;141(1):84–90.

90. Bae JM, Park JW, Yang HK, Kim JP. Nutritional status of gastric cancer patients after total gastrectomy. *World J Surg.* 1998;22(3): 254–261.

91. McCray S. Lactose intolerance: considerations for the clinician. *Pract Gastroenterol.* 2003;27(2).

92. Pannala R, Brandabur JJ, Gan SI, et al. Afferent limb syndrome and delayed GI problems after pancreaticoduodenectomy for pancreatic cancer: single-center, 14-year experience. *Gastrointest Endosc.* 2011;74(2):295–302.

93. Yamada T, Alpers DH. *Textbook of Gastroenterology.* 5th ed. Hoboken, NJ: Blackwell Publishing; 2009.

PART IV

MANAGEMENT AND PROFESSIONAL ISSUES

38 Home Nutrition Support

Denise Konrad, RD, CNSC, Ronelle Mitchell, MA, RD, CNSC, and Eileen Hendrickson, RPh, PharmD, MBA

CONTENTS

Acknowledgments: Marion Winkler, PhD, RD, CNSC, Elizabeth Hagan, RN, CNSC, BSN, and Jorge E. Albina, MD, were the authors of this chapter for the second edition.

Objectives

1. Describe the process for establishing a safe and appropriate discharge plan for the patient beginning home enteral nutrition (HEN) or home parenteral nutrition (HPN).
2. List the elements involved in developing treatment goals for home nutrition support.
3. Identify teaching strategies for effective patient education.
4. Summarize the role of nutrition support clinicians in caring for patients receiving HEN or HPN.
5. Review monitoring protocols and interpret clinical data to prevent complications of HEN or HPN.

Test Your Knowledge Questions

1. Medicare coverage for HPN is possible with adequate documentation in which of the following conditions?
   A. Anorexia nervosa
   B. Massive small bowel resection resulting in short bowel syndrome with less than 150 cm bowel remaining
   C. Six weeks of bowel rest for severe pancreatitis
   D. Swallowing disorder with history of aspiration pneumonia
2. Which of the following is a primary reason for administering HPN as a cyclic infusion?
   A. To provide a more normal lifestyle
   B. To reduce complications of parenteral nutrition–associated liver disease (PNALD)
   C. Because cyclic infusion allows for administration of intravenous (IV) medications that are incompatible with parenteral nutrition (PN)
   D. All of the above
3. The success of home nutrition support depends on which of the following strategies?
   A. Facilitating insurance reimbursement for nutrition support
   B. Providing individualized care to the patient at home
   C. Educating the patient and/or caregiver in managing enteral nutrition (EN) or PN at home
   D. Providing comfort to the families caring for the patient
4. Which of the following should clinicians do to support patients who are dealing with lifelong dependency on home nutrition support?
   A. Include the patient in decision-making regarding the choice of access device and administration schedule.
   B. Recognize symptoms of depression, and refer patients with those symptoms for additional evaluation and care.
   C. Promote the benefit of patient support groups.
   D. All of the above.
5. Patient adherence to the nutrition support regimen is key to achieving goals of therapy. Which of the following are indications of nonadherence?
   A. Unwillingness to review a product inventory or report of excess supplies
   B. Unintentional weight loss despite adequate energy being prescribed
   C. Good communication between the patient and healthcare team
   D. Answers A and B

Test Your Knowledge Answers

1. The correct answer is **B**. Coverage for HPN under Medicare is available for patients who have undergone massive small bowel resection leaving less than 150 cm residual bowel. Operative notes must include documentation of intestinal length. Patients with anorexia nervosa would not meet Medicare criteria for permanent severe pathology of the alimentary tract. A patient requiring bowel rest for 6 weeks for severe acute pancreatitis may have an appropriate clinical indication for HPN; however, per Medicare guidelines, bowel rest must be required for 3 months or longer and the patient must have evidence that EN is contraindicated. A patient who has a swallowing disorder with or without evidence of aspiration pneumonia would be a candidate for EN.
2. The correct answer is **D**. The primary reason to administer HPN using a cyclic or overnight infusion is to allow the patient freedom during the day and thereby improve quality of life (QOL). Cyclic infusions allow a period of rest and may decrease the incidence of fatty liver. Off-cycle time allows for administration of other IV medications (eg, vancomycin) that are incompatible with PN. Cyclic infusions are appropriate if a patient can tolerate the volume of PN over a shorter period of time as evidenced by frequency of urination, blood glucose control, and absence of cardiopulmonary distress.
3. The correct answer is **C**. Home nutrition support uses complex technical equipment. Ensuring that the patient or caregiver is willing and able to safely manage this equipment as well as all related procedures reduces the risk for complications. Short-term goals for the new home nutrition support patient or caregiver are to optimize the organization and safety of the home environment and identify risks related to potential complications. Long-term goals are to promote patient independence and adherence, and prevent hospital readmission.
4. The correct answer is **D**. Patients who receive long-term HEN or HPN are at high risk for depression, social isolation, and poor QOL. Patients and their caregivers should have an active role in determining the appropriate access device and infusion therapy plan to fit their lifestyle. Home care professionals should help patients adapt and cope with the required lifestyle adjustments by painting a realistic picture of what will occur at home, providing education on HEN/HPN procedures and technology, and designing a care plan consistent with the patients' desired goals. Patients should be introduced to the many organizations that provide important outreach services, educational materials, and emotional support.
5. The correct answer is **D**. The physician managing HEN or HPN patients will need assistance from other providers to monitor patient adherence to therapy. A multidisciplinary approach involving the dietitian, home health nurse, and infusion pharmacist is crucial. Patients or caregivers who are unwilling to review the product inventory or report of excess supplies, or who are not responding appropriately to treatment (ie, experience unintentional weight loss or unresolved electrolyte imbalances), may not be adhering to the

nutrition support plan. Infusion pump reports may be useful for verifying infusion history for patients receiving PN.

Overview

Home-based healthcare provides skilled health-related services to a patient in a familiar and comfortable environment with support from family members and trained healthcare professionals. According to the Home Health Chart Book, published by the research firm Avalere Health in 2015, 3.3 million Medicare beneficiaries in the United States receive home healthcare each year.[1] In 2013, the Centers for Medicare and Medicaid Services (CMS) reported 12,500 home health agencies participated in providing home care.[2] Spending for home healthcare in 2014 was estimated to be $83.2 billion.[2] Episodes of care billed to Medicare and Medicaid combined accounted for nearly 77% of the total expenditures for home healthcare and hospice care in 2014.[3]

Home nutrition support allows many patients with chronic diseases to be managed successfully outside the hospital for the correction of nutrition disorders. The discharge of the first patient on HPN in 1968 established a model for other "high-tech" home infusion therapies. Approximately 56,000 people receive HPN and another 344,000 receive HEN annually.[2] In 2014, CMS noted $594 million in allowable charges for HEN and HPN.[2]

Advantages and Benefits of Home Nutrition Support

The advantages of HEN and HPN relate to survival, economic, and QOL outcomes.[4-6] Home care services are cost effective when compared with typical per-day charges in a hospital or skilled nursing facility.[7] Technological advances for home care now allow patients to avoid prolonged hospital stays, skilled nursing facility admissions, or repeated hospitalizations for nutrition therapies. Home infusion enables patients and their family members to take an active role in the nutrition therapy.

Patient Selection and Indications for Home Nutrition Support

Standards of practice from the American Society for Parenteral and Enteral Nutrition (ASPEN) specify that home nutrition support should be used in adult patients who cannot meet their nutrient requirements orally and who can receive the therapy safely outside of an acute care facility.[8] Prior to the initiation of home nutrition support, the candidate's primary disease and clinical condition should be stable.

Clinical Indications

Clinical indications for HEN and HPN encompass more disease states than those specified as eligible for reimbursement under the Medicare coverage guidelines and by other public or private insurers. Tables 38-1 and 38-2 list common indications for HEN and HPN, respectively. For patients with stroke, objective predictors for the need for EN include a wet voice after swallowing water, National Institutes of Health stroke

TABLE 38-1 Indications for Home Enteral Nutrition

- Mechanical GI tract dysfunction
- Motility disorders
- Malabsorptive syndromes
- Malignancies of the head, neck, or digestive system
- Dysphagia and swallowing disorders
- Pancreatitis
- GI fistula—feeding distal to upper GI fistula
- Bowel obstruction—feeding distal to obstruction
- Acute and progressive neurologic conditions
- Hyperemesis gravidarum
- Failure to thrive
- Inborn errors of metabolism

GI, gastrointestinal.

TABLE 38-2 Indications for Home Parenteral Nutrition

- Intestinal failure or dysfunction
- Short bowel syndrome
- Malabsorptive disorders
- Acute or chronic bowel obstruction
- Crohn's disease
- Radiation enteritis
- Intestinal ischemia
- Intestinal and pancreatic fistulas
- Pancreatitis
- Severe, life-threatening malnutrition

scale score, abnormal laryngeal elevation, abnormal gag reflex, incomplete oral labial closure, and coughing during or after swallowing.[9] Table 38-3 lists codes from the *International Classification of Diseases, 10th Revision, Clinical Modifications* (ICD-10-CM) for common diagnoses related to the need for EN and PN.[10] ICD-10-CM codes provide substantially increased specificity compared with codes from the ninth revision (ICD-9-CM). The ICD-10-CM codes in Table 38-3 represent the most simplified versions of the diagnoses. ICD-10-CM codes must be thoroughly reviewed to meet the documentation standards of insurers.

Other Considerations

In some situations, the burden of home nutrition support management may outweigh the benefits. Clinicians should evaluate the risks and benefits of home nutrition support on an individual basis. This assessment should reflect any relevant cultural and religious values of the patient as well as other pertinent patient and family preferences.[11] The ability of the patient or caregiver to comprehend and perform the necessary technical tasks and organize their daily care must be evaluated. If the cognitive abilities of the patient decline or caregiver's capacity to give support becomes more limited, the nutrition support team should reassess whether home care is appropriate.

TABLE 38-3 International Classification of Diseases, 10th Revision, Clinical Modification Codes for Common Diagnoses Related to Home Enteral and Parenteral Nutrition

Code	Diagnosis
Anatomical Conditions	
C02.-	Malignant neoplasm of tongue
C06.-	Malignant neoplasm of other and unspecified parts of mouth
C16.-	Malignant neoplasm of stomach
C76.0	Malignant neoplasm of head, face, and neck
D00.0	Carcinoma in situ of lip, oral cavity, and pharynx
D00.1	Carcinoma in situ of esophagus
D00.2	Carcinoma in situ of stomach
D01.-	Carcinoma in situ of other and unspecified digestive organs (includes colon, other parts of the intestine)
J86.0	Tracheoesophageal fistula
K22.2	Esophageal stricture or stenosis
K31.5	Duodenal obstruction
K31.6	Gastrojejunocolic fistula
K63.2	Intestinal fistula
S02.6	Mandible fracture
Motility Disorders	
J38.0-	Vocal cord paralysis
J69.0	Aspiration pneumonia
K21.9	Esophageal reflux
K31.84	Gastroparesis
K31.89	Other functional disorder of the intestine
K56.6-	Other and unspecified intestinal obstruction
K91.1	Postgastrectomy dumping syndrome
O21.0–O21.1	Hyperemesis gravidarum
R13.1-	Dysphagia
Intestinal Disease and Malabsorptive Disorders	
C25.-	Malignant neoplasm of pancreas
E84.-	Cystic fibrosis
K50.-	Regional enteritis (Crohn's disease)
K52.-	Other and unspecified noninfective gastroenteritis and colitis
K55.0	Acute vascular insufficiency of intestine (ischemia)
K56.60	Unspecified intestinal obstruction
K63.9	Intestinal disorder (unspecified)
K85.-	Acute pancreatitis
K86.1	Chronic pancreatitis
K90.3	Pancreatic steatorrhea
K90.4	Malabsorption: other specified intestinal
K90.9	Intestinal malabsorption, unspecified
K91.1	Postvagotomy syndrome
K91.2	Short bowel syndrome
Nutrition Disorders	
D50.8	Iron deficiency anemia (dietary)
D64.9	Anemia, unspecified
E43	Malnutrition: unspecified severe protein-calorie
E44.0	Malnutrition: moderate protein-calorie
E44.1	Malnutrition: mild protein-calorie
E66.-	Overweight and obesity
E78.-	Disorders of lipoprotein metabolism and other lipidemias
E83.4-	Magnesium disorder
E83.51	Hypocalcemia
E86.-	Volume depletion
E87.-	Other disorders of fluid, electrolyte, and acid-base balance
R63.4	Abnormal weight loss

Source: Data are from reference 10.

To identify appropriate candidates for HEN, one factor to consider is whether the patient is expected to recover or have a limited life expectancy. The issue of whether gastrostomy feedings in patients with advanced dementia afford a survival benefit is controversial.[11-15] When a patient has advanced dementia or another end-stage terminal illness, the benefits and burdens associated with the use of artificial nutrition and hydration should be carefully evaluated.[11,16] In these situations, loss of the desire to eat and drink is a natural part of the dying process.[17] See Chapter 39 for further discussion of the ethics of artificial nutrition and hydration and end-of-life care.

Discharge Planning

Patients receiving home nutrition support usually are discharged from an acute care or rehabilitation care facility; however, a small percentage of patients may initiate nutrition support in the home.[18] It is never too early to begin the discharge planning process. Table 38-4 lists ways that the hospital personnel can facilitate the transition to home. In addition to nutrition needs, factors to assess as part of the discharge planning process include financial resources and insurance coverage; home safety; the patient's physical, psychological, and learning needs; and any cultural or religious considerations.

Reimbursement Eligibility Criteria

If a patient seems to be a candidate for home nutrition support, his or her insurance coverage must be investigated to determine whether home care will be reimbursed. Understanding the reimbursement process includes knowledge of restrictions or limitations for services, equipment, and supplies. In situations of limited, pending, or no insurance coverage, discharge may be delayed until sufficient home health benefits are available.

Patients and caregivers, as well as the care team, need to understand the details of the coverage benefits. Often, patients will be responsible for a percentage of the charges. They may have a secondary or supplemental insurance that will consider the changes unpaid by the primary insurer.

Insurance coverage for HEN and HPN varies by type of program as well as individual plans. Government programs (eg, Medicare and Medicaid) have strict coverage criteria and require detailed history, tests, and nutrition data to determine eligibility at the initiation of therapy. Coverage policies and reimbursement for HEN and HPN also vary among private payers and managed care organizations and frequently require preauthorization or precertification. Most insurance companies require that the therapy be medically necessary and the sole source of nutrition. Many insurance policies have their own criteria for EN and PN, but others follow the guidelines for coverage set forth by Medicare.[19] Case-by-case review is often required. Regardless of the type of insurance, the care team needs to determine whether the patient has home health benefits of sufficient scope for a therapy that may be needed lifelong. Government payers and insurers who follow the Medicare coverage criteria may require substantiation of need over time. As more insurers default their coverage criteria to the Medicare standard, this trend is likely to increase in frequency. Insurance may or may not also cover home nursing visits for reasons other than nutrition support, or care of non–nutrition-related needs such as wound care, tracheostomy care, ostomy care, or disease and medication management.

Although not all patients are insured by Medicare, the detailed Medicare coverage guidelines significantly affect the standards for the care of all EN and PN patients in the United States. Furthermore, many patients who are initially insured by commercial plans will eventually require reconsideration of eligibility under government plans secondary to disability or age. EN and PN are primarily covered under the "prosthetic device" benefit under the Medicare Part B program.[19] This provision requires a permanent dysfunction of a body organ. Medicare reimbursement for EN or PN requires the therapy be "reasonable and necessary for the diagnosis or treatment of illness or injury or to improve the functioning of a malformed body part."[19] For reimbursement for either EN or PN, the therapy must provide "sufficient nutrients to maintain weight and strength commensurate with the patient's overall health status." Additionally, the condition must have a "permanent impairment of long and indefinite duration" (ie, at least 3 months).[19] Coverage under Medicare Part D depends

TABLE 38-4 Tips to Facilitate Discharge of Patients Who Will Receive Home Nutrition Support

- Obtain required diagnostic tests and procedures to demonstrate medical necessity and verify insurance coverage.
- Document the diagnosis requiring enteral or parenteral nutrition for treatment.
- Establish feeding access.
- Determine the patient's tolerance to the enteral or parenteral formulation.
- Explain to the patient and caregiver the risks and benefits of home nutrition support.
- Assess the patient's or caregiver's ability to perform activities of daily living, enteral and parenteral nutrition–related tasks.
- Assess the learning needs of the patient and caregivers and provide appropriate patient education. If necessary, develop patient-specific learning materials to address literacy or language barriers.
- Engage the patient and family in a discussion about their expectations of involvement in daily care; include social workers or interpreters as needed in this discussion.
- Conduct psychosocial assessment of the patient.
- Identify caregiver(s).
- Determine the home infusion and/or home care provider(s).
- Identify all necessary home infusion therapies and the follow-up communication required by each provider (blood samples for laboratory tests, wound care, etc).
- Identify who will prescribe the home enteral or parenteral nutrition orders after discharge.
- Establish the type and amount of communication desired by the physician and nutrition support team after discharge.
- Educate the patient and family on how to contact the nutrition support team and reasons for urgent after-hours contact.

on the insurer. Increasingly, Medicare D plans exclude IV pharmaceuticals from their formulary. If a Medicare D plan covers the PN formulation, it technically pays for PN for all situations that are not covered under Part B; however, Part D does not pay for the equipment, supplies, or professional services associated with the provision of PN or any other Part D–covered infusion therapy.[20]

Table 38-5 outlines key elements for eligibility and documentation of medical necessity for HEN.[19] Eligible conditions typically include anatomical disorders, such as obstruction due to head and neck cancer or reconstructive surgery, as well as conditions resulting from a motility disorder, such as severe dysphagia following a stroke or gastroparesis (see Practice Scenario 38-1). EN is not covered for individuals who have a functional GI tract or for patients whose need for EN is related to anorexia or nausea associated with end-stage disease. Under Medicare guidelines, standard polymeric formulas are considered appropriate for most patients requiring HEN. Additional documentation of medical necessity is required for specialty products. Clinicians should be aware that not all formulas within a Medicare coverage category are clinically equivalent or interchangeable, even though they may be reimbursed at the same rate. If coverage requirements for EN are met, administration supplies and equipment (replacement feeding tubes, tube anchoring devices) are covered, but the quantity and frequency are specified. Enteral infusion pumps are covered only with documentation that gravity feeding is not tolerated or is contraindicated for situations such as reflux, aspiration, dumping syndrome, glycemic control, circulatory overload, slow infusion rate, or jejunal feeding.

Practice Scenario 38-1

Question: What clinical documentation is necessary to support eligibility for reimbursement under Medicare for a patient who has a swallowing disorder and requires home enteral nutrition?

Scenario: A 70-year-old man with a complicated medical history was hospitalized with bilateral cerebral infarcts, left-upper and right-lower extremity paralysis, and aspiration pneumonia. On physical examination, he was alert, oriented, and not short of breath. His nostrils and oral cavity were clear and neurocranial nerves II through XII were intact. His voice was hoarse; he produced a poor cough; and he was observed to be choking with oral intake. A speech-language pathologist evaluated him and conducted a bedside swallow study. Findings included an inability to initiate a dry swallow, regurgitation with trials of pureed and thin liquids, coughing, choking, and an absent pharyngeal swallow. A percutaneous endoscopic gastrostomy (PEG) tube was placed for an anticipated prolonged course of enteral nutrition (EN) therapy. The patient agreed to the discharge plan that included going home with his wife who would provide care for the PEG tube and administer tube feedings with the assistance of a daughter who lived nearby. The patient and caregiver's education needs were identified, and a care plan was developed. An intermittent feeding schedule was designed to accommodate the patient's lifestyle and caregiver considerations. The patient had Medicare as his primary insurance. Visiting nurse services were arranged for training and monitoring of EN. A durable medical equipment (DME) company was contacted to provide the enteral formula, equipment, and supplies. The DME provider requested documentation of the medical necessity for EN and for the infusion pump.

Intervention: The hospital-based nutrition support team, working in collaboration with the discharge planner, provided documentation that the patient's condition involved dysphagia and that adequate nutrition was not safe by oral means. Diagnostic studies to document dysphagia and aspiration pneumonia along with the dietitian's nutrition assessment were submitted to the DME company as documentation of medical necessity.

Answer: EN products are covered under the prosthetic device benefit under the Medicare Part B program. Required documentation for medical necessity includes a diagnosis pertinent to the need for EN (dysphagia), history and physical examination (bilateral cerebral infarcts, left-upper and right-lower extremity paralysis, aspiration pneumonia, hoarse voice, poor cough, choking with oral intake), swallowing study (speech-language pathologist notes), diagnostic tests (chest x-ray demonstrating aspiration pneumonia), nutrition assessment (weight and weight history, pertinent laboratory test results), and documentation from clinician that a pump is required because of known aspiration.

Rationale: Documentation of medical necessity includes evidence that the patient's diagnosis and clinical condition fit into a

---

TABLE 38-5 Elements for Documentation of Medical Necessity for Home Enteral Nutrition

- Condition that will require EN for >3 months
- Condition that involves permanent nonfunction or disease of the GI tract or impaired digestion or absorption (anatomical disorders; motility disorders)
- Evidence that adequate nutrition is not possible by dietary adjustment or oral nutrition supplementation
- Diagnosis (ICD-10-CM code) pertinent to need for EN[a]
- Radiographic evidence of obstruction
- Motility studies
- Swallowing studies
- Operative notes
- Weight and weight history
- Nutrition assessment
- Justification for specialty enteral formulation, if applicable
- Energy prescription expressed in kcal/kg/d (usually between 20 and 35 kcal/kg/d)
- Site of feeding tube
- If a feeding pump is requested, evidence that gravity feeding causes reflux, aspiration, severe diarrhea or dumping syndrome or blood glucose fluctuations, circulatory overload, or need for jejunostomy feeding

EN, enteral nutrition; GI, gastrointestinal; ICD-10-CM, *International Classification of Disease, 10th Revision, Clinical Modification.*
[a]See Table 38-3.
Source: Data are from reference 19.

defined Medicare benefit category and the therapy is reasonable and necessary for the diagnosis or treatment of illness or injury or to improve the functioning of a malformed body part. In this case, the patient was unable to swallow or eat food because of dysphagia and there was evidence of aspiration pneumonia. Medical necessity was demonstrated by inclusion of the speech-language pathologist's swallow evaluation recommending *nil per os* (nothing by mouth) status and radiographic evidence of aspiration pneumonia. The medical necessity for a pump was met with preexisting diagnosis of aspiration pneumonia.

Table 38-6 lists the requirements for eligibility and documentation of PN.[19] Medicare requires that the patient have permanent dysfunction of the alimentary tract to qualify for payment of PN; therefore, conditions such as swallowing disorders, psychological disorders, anorexia, dyspnea of severe pulmonary or cardiac disease, medication side effects, or renal failure are not routinely covered.[19] The PN prescription must meet specified calorie and protein guidelines,[21] and reimbursement for lipids is also limited by Medicare guidelines. Medicare covers the rental of infusion pumps and the cost of supplies for patients who meet PN eligibility criteria. Generally, Medicare does not pay for nursing care for administration of feedings; however, it offers limited coverage for teaching the patient and family how to administer infusions.

Safety Evaluation

Once the criteria for medical necessity and benefit coverage are met, the next step is to evaluate the safety of the home environment and whether the patient or caregiver can manage the necessary equipment. The following questions should be explored to determine the safety of the home environment:[8]

- Is there access to home care agencies (infusion pharmacy and home care nursing as needed) with appropriate skill competencies to serve the patient's needs?
- Are there any geography or transportation challenges that may prevent access to care?
- Is the environment clean with reliable utilities (sanitary water, electricity, refrigeration, storage space, electrical outlets, telephone)?
- Can the patient move safely around the house and to the bathroom (are there obstacles such as stairs or carpeting)?
- Is the patient or caregiver willing and able to learn the home infusion procedures and operation of the equipment?
- Is the caregiver willing and able to provide additional needed assistance for care within the home?
- Can the patient or caregiver learn to recognize problems and contact the home healthcare provider or emergency services for assistance?
- Is laboratory monitoring available as frequently as needed to prevent fluid and electrolyte complications?

Needs Assessment

Assessment of home care suitability includes evaluation of the patient's skilled nursing needs, capacity to perform activities of daily living, medication management, wound and skin care, and ability to recognize when to seek medical attention.

When beginning home nutrition support, the patient and caregiver should also be assessed for their ability to learn to reliably monitor weight, hydration status, and blood or urine glucose levels, recognize early signs of infection, and care for the EN or PN access device and site.

The nutrition support team should prepare patients and caregivers for the necessary time they will need to dedicate to the administration of EN or PN (see Practice Scenario 38-2). While the tasks will become easier with repetition, the responsibility may initially be overwhelming. Reassurance and patience on the part of the home healthcare professionals will inspire confidence.

Home nutrition support requires use of complex technical equipment. When possible, demonstration of the equipment prior to discharge will provide both an opportunity for teaching and insight into the patient's and caregiver's ability to learn. If the patient or caregiver cannot master the use of equipment and learn procedures in the acute care or rehabilitation setting, extra teaching time should be allotted for the initial home visits. Ensuring that the patient or caregiver can safely manage special equipment and procedures will prevent complications and hospital readmission.[22] Patient satisfaction and adherence to the care plan increase when extra time is spent on one-on-one teaching of care and management of nutrition support.[23]

Social changes related to the loss of a job, shifting family roles, disconnection from friends, and physical limitations (eg, decreased stamina) all contribute to a patient's stress on hospital discharge. The new responsibility of home nutrition support can also increase stress or contribute to feelings of depression. Depression is a common response to chronic illness and may increase risk of home nutrition support–related complications. Signs of depression should prompt referral for additional evaluation and care.

As noted earlier, culture and religious beliefs that influence health-related practices should be considered in the overall patient assessment. The patient's perception of health and illness will affect behaviors, tolerance of discomfort, knowledge of options, and expectations of change and outcome. The home care team should provide appropriate follow-up in the form of appointments and telephone numbers of providers. Providing information on available local or national organizations for peer support and education has been shown to improve outcomes associated with home nutrition support.[24]

Selection of Home Care and Infusion Provider Services

The process of choosing providers to meet the patient's home care needs should include the patient. Medicare conditions of participation ensure that patients have a right to choose their home care agencies and participate in the decisions that affect their care. Successful outcomes of home nutrition support require highly skilled home care nursing and home infusion providers. When assessing home care, infusion, and durable medical equipment (DME) providers consider the following:

- How is home care nursing and home infusion pharmacy coordinated?
- Do various providers have established working relationships that will ensure communication?

TABLE 38-6 Elements for Documentation of Medical Necessity for Home Parenteral Nutrition

All patients:
- Condition that requires PN for >3 months
- Condition that is severe enough that patient cannot maintain weight and strength on oral intake or a combination of oral nutrition and EN
- Diagnosis (ICD-10-CM code) pertinent to need for PN[a]
- Weight and weight history
- Serum albumin within 1 week of home PN

Disease-specific criteria and supporting documentation:
- Massive small bowel resection within 3 months, leaving ≤5 feet of small bowel beyond the ligament of Treitz:
  - Operative report with evidence of ≤5 feet of small bowel
  - Radiographic reports
- Short bowel syndrome with net GI fluid and electrolyte malabsorption on an oral diet of 2.5–3 L/d, enteral losses >50% of the oral/enteral intake, and urine output of <1 L/d:
  - Operative report indicating extent of resection
  - Radiographic reports
  - Motility studies
  - I/O records demonstrating net fluid loss
  - Signs of dehydration and electrolyte imbalance
  - Results of 72-h fecal fat test[b]
  - List of medications used to control diarrhea
  - Documentation of nutrient modification and/or failed tube trial
- Severe exacerbation of regional enteritis requiring bowel rest for ≥3 months:
  - Operative report
  - Pathology report
  - Radiographic reports
  - Indication for bowel rest
- Pancreatitis with or without pseudocyst requiring bowel rest for ≥months:
  - Operative report
  - Radiographic report
  - Indication for bowel rest
- Enterocutaneous fistula requiring bowel rest for ≥3 months where feeding distal to the fistula is not possible:
  - Operative report
  - Radiographic report
  - Motility studies
  - Contraindication to EN
  - Evidence of inability to place tube distal to fistula
- Complete mechanical small bowel obstruction where surgery is not an option:
  - Operative report that confirms obstruction
  - Radiographic report that confirms obstruction
  - Evidence of inability to place tube distal to obstruction
- Severe fat malabsorption and malnutrition where fecal fat is >50% of oral/enteral intake on a diet of ≥50 g fat per day as measured by a 72-h fecal fat test:
  - Results of 72-h fecal fat test[b]
  - Operative report
  - Radiographic report
  - Pharmacological approaches tried
  - Evidence of EN failure
  - Nutrition assessment with evidence of malnutrition[c]
- Severe motility disorder that is unresponsive to prokinetic medication:
  - Radiographic report
  - Motility studies
  - Medications attempted to improve motility
  - Result of tube trial or contraindication to tube feeding
  - Nutrition assessment with evidence of malnutrition[c]

EN, enteral nutrition; GI, gastrointestinal; ICD-10-CM, *International Classification of Disease, 10th Revision, Clinical Modification*; I/O, input/output; PN, parenteral nutrition.
[a]See Table 38-3.
[b]The fecal fat test requires significant coordination by the nursing, laboratory and nutrition support teams.
[c]Defined as >10% weight loss within ≤3 months and serum albumin ≤3.4 g/dL.
Source: Data are from reference 19.

- Are the home care nursing provider and the pharmacy fully accredited by an agency such as the Joint Commission or Community Health Accreditation Partner?
- Can the pharmacy provide sterile compounding services that are consistent with the federal US Pharmacopeia <797> guidelines?
- Do the providers have skill competencies in nutrition, vascular access, or wound/ostomy care?
- If patient will be receiving HPN, does the pharmacy have consistent access to the pharmaceuticals and solutions required to compound the PN?
- Is there on-call support available for patients?
- Are the providers willing and able to support the outcomes data collection initiatives of the nutrition support team?
- Has the patient's insurer designated preferred providers?

A variety of organizations may participate in the delivery and management of home nutrition services, including DME companies, home infusion providers, and home care agencies. Clinical liaisons or representatives of home care agencies specializing in nutrition support are available either in person or via telephone support to assist with the transition from the hospital to home. These agencies will either provide all home care needs or coordinate with another community agency for home nursing visits and medical equipment, nutrition formulations, and supplies. A predischarge teaching visit provides insight for the patient as to what he or she is expected to learn and a chance for the home care clinician to assess the patient's receptiveness and ability to manage at home.

Practice Scenario 38-2

Question: How do you evaluate a patient's ability to learn the skills and procedures associated with safe and effective home care therapy?

Scenario: A 62-year-old woman with Crohn's disease was identified as a potential home parenteral nutrition (HPN) candidate after multiple admissions for dehydration. Training for HPN began in the hospital several days before discharge. The home care clinician demonstrated the various procedures for HPN using the actual equipment on models with vascular access devices. The patient correctly return-demonstrated use of sterile gloves, use of needle and syringe, and priming of intravenous tubing. Because of her desire to maintain independence, all education focused on the patient. After discharge, the home care nurse reported that the patient was having difficulty performing the techniques of the infusion protocol and was not likely to be safe alone.

Intervention: A caregiver was identified and, with the patient's approval, home care teaching continued. The home care nurse negotiated that the patient and caregiver would have different roles and each would learn and manage separate aspects of HPN procedures.

Answer: The transition from hospital to home can be an overwhelming experience for any patient, especially for one who needs to become independent in self-care. Even when a patient or caregiver is technically capable of performing tasks, the individual's ability to carry out home nutrition support procedures can only be effectively evaluated in the real home setting. The home care clinician is in a key position to assess education needs and abilities, investigate family dynamics, and identify alternate caregivers among the patient's family and friends. A patient's anxiety and fear about the home care experience can be lessened by painting a realistic picture of what will occur at home and adequately portraying the complexity of the technology. Conducting a thorough patient assessment helps identify the patient's emotional and experiential readiness to learn. Establishing a teaching plan with short- and long-term objectives helps prioritize the learning steps. Engaging the patient in active participation by demonstrating each procedure and requesting a return demonstration enhances training. Use of checklists, illustrations, and other materials matched to the patient's style of learning, intelligence, and comprehension improves the teaching and learning experiences. The instructor should encourage the patient to ask questions, address individual concerns, and provide encouragement.

Rationale: The patient may have the cognitive and physical ability to learn, but learning may be influenced by the emotional and experiential readiness to learn. By recognizing that the patient lives alone, has minimal support systems, and has a substantial medical history with frequent hospitalizations, the nutrition support team is better prepared to develop a realistic care plan. Although patients may receive training in many aspects of HPN management before they leave the hospital, they should be reassured that additional training and retraining will occur after they go home.

Nutrition Care Plan

Short- and Long-Term Goals

Short-term goals of the nutrition care plan are to provide patient education and ensure safety. The care team should provide patients and caregivers with information about how to contact all home care providers; which providers to call for each concern; reasons to call for help; how to decrease risk of infectious, metabolic, or mechanical complications; and how to promote comfort.

Long-term goals are to promote the patient's independence and prevent rehospitalization. Independence is achieved through comprehensive patient and family education that addresses care of the enteral or vascular access device, troubleshooting high-tech equipment, and adherence to diet and activity. Optimizing the organization and safety of the home environment will decrease therapy-related anxiety, facilitate learning, and promote independence. At the start of therapy, the team providing care and the patient or caregiver should discuss the anticipated length of time that nutrition support will be needed and when it will end. The projected end of therapy may be when the patient is ready for future surgery or when the GI condition (eg, bowel obstruction, fistula) resolves; in some cases, lifelong nutrition support may be the goal.

Barriers to achieving short- and long-term nutrition support goals can be overcome with intensive patient and family teaching, assessment of adherence, and monitoring for early signs and symptoms of problems. By identifying individual patient risks and communicating about them, the members of the healthcare team who are managing the patient can anticipate special needs. Any information regarding safety, community resources, and ways to improve care management within the home environment will promote good QOL and reduce complications. Well-educated HEN and HPN patients will also be likely to experience less stress.

Route and Access for Home Nutrition Support

The appropriate route and access device for infusion of HEN or HPN should be addressed early in the discharge planning process. The access device chosen should be one that the patient/caregiver can safely manage with minimal risk for complications (see Chapters 12 and 16). Information on device insertion date, diameter, style, location, length, patency, and site condition should be made available to the home care provider.

Long-term enteral access devices include percutaneous gastrostomy or jejunostomy tubes. These may be placed in an endoscopic, laparoscopic, radiologic, or open surgical procedure. The device should be positioned so that it does not interfere with daily activities such as bathing and clothing changes. The external tubing should be anchored securely to the skin to minimize irritation during movement. Gastric feeding is preferred over small bowel feeding for several practical reasons. Compared with jejunal tubes, most gastric tubes are easier to place and replace, and they are larger gauge with lower incidence of occlusion. Gastric feedings can be administered as bolus feedings at meal times or spaced throughout the day. In cases of gastroparesis, ileus, gastric outlet obstruction, or significant gastric reflux, small bowel feedings are a good alternative. If needed, a combination gastrojejunostomy tube can be considered to simultaneously provide gastric decompression and small bowel feeding, or to provide medications through the gastric port and feedings through the jejunal port.

Long-term PN requires a central venous access device. Peripheral and mid lines should not be used for HPN because they can easily become dislodged, need to be changed routinely, and cannot handle high-osmolarity solutions. Central venous catheter placement is defined by the final catheter tip location in the superior or inferior vena cava. HPN catheters may be placed into either a large peripheral vein, such as the basilic or cephalic, or into the subclavian or internal jugular vein. The catheter is then advanced to the distal portion of the superior vena cava. A peripherally inserted central catheter (PICC) is readily placed, replaced, or removed, and has low risk for insertion complications. PICCs should only be used for short-term therapy (less than 3 months) because the risks of displacement, loss of patency, and thrombosis increase with longer term use.[25] A caregiver or home care nurse must change the PICC catheter dressing; the patient cannot change it because of its location in the arm. Extension tubing can be provided to allow the patient to perform the infusion procedures independently. Subclavian or internal jugular catheters are either tunneled or implanted. Tunneled catheters—known as Hickman, Broviac, PowerLine, Hohn, or Groshong catheters—enter the vein and are then tunneled subcutaneously to exit lower on the

chest wall. The purpose of the tunnel is to decrease the risks of infection and accidental removal. Ethanol lock can be used in silicone-based catheters as another level of protection to help offset infection risk.[26] Catheter names may contain the word "power" (eg, PowerHickman), which means they are power injection and allow for injections of contrast media among other medications. The entire external portion of PICCs and tunneled catheters, including the end caps, should be covered when bathing to protect against infection.

An implanted device, or port, is a disk with a self-sealing silicone septum and rigid titanium or plastic base. It is surgically placed into a subcutaneous pocket and connected to a catheter that is inserted into a vein using a medical wire and advanced into the central venous system. The most common location of an implanted port is on the chest wall, but, in some situations the upper arm may be the site of choice. Because the entire port is under the skin, unrestricted bathing is permitted, after the incision heals, when the port is deaccessed. However, the port would need to be covered for bathing or swimming if it is accessed. The port is accessed using a specially designed right-angle tapered needle with a side opening known as a Huber needle. Tunneled or implanted devices on the chest wall are usually not visible under clothing and allow a full range of arm and hand movement.

External or tunneled catheters require regular, direct nursing care or patient/caregiver training for proper catheter and site care. Catheter dressings and tubing should be clean and dry at all times. Implanted ports require professional care or training for needle placement, site care, and catheter flushing. Tunneled catheters and implanted ports that are located on the chest wall allow patients to be independent with catheter care.

Swimming with enteral and central venous access devices is controversial because exposure to contaminated waters can cause catheter-related bloodstream, site, or tunnel infections. Enteral tubes should be kept dry, have the cap and/or clamp closed, taped to the abdomen with waterproof tape, and tucked into the bathing suit to prevent accidental dislodgement.[27] In 2013, Miller et al conducted a survey among HPN programs in the United States to identify current swimming recommendations and found that the 16 programs that responded followed varying practices.[28] The survey asked if patients were permitted to swim, which bodies of water were allowed (eg, ocean, lake, pool, hot tub), and if specific dressings were required. The 13 programs that allowed swimming agreed that pools were safe and patients with deaccessed ports could swim. Most programs allowed those with tunneled catheters to swim and recommended covering the catheter with various products and changing the catheter dressing immediately afterward.[28] The nutrition support physician should be consulted for advice for the individual patient interested in swimming.

Requirements

Nutrient requirements are developed following a nutrition assessment (see Chapter 10). Energy requirements are measured using indirect calorimetry, if available, or determined by predictive equations (see Chapter 2). Nutrient and total fluid requirements should reflect whether the EN or PN therapy is providing total or partial nutrition support. In patients receiving EN, recommended macro- and micronutrient goals may be higher than estimated requirements to account for poor absorptive capacity. Goals of therapy should be determined with the patient and caregiver and individualized based on assessment of nutrition status, body composition, fluid status, performance status and function, and any preexisting nutrition deficits. A nutrition-focused physical exam should be performed on all patients to identify areas of muscle and fat wasting as well as physical signs of vitamin, mineral, and essential fatty acid deficiencies. Laboratory tests can be done to confirm deficiencies. The overall goals of nutrition therapy are to provide adequate amounts of macro- and micronutrients, replete and maintain normal serum electrolyte levels, maintain euglycemia and euvolemia, and improve or maintain lean body mass, performance status, and function. In situations where a patient's body weight is either above or below the preferred weight, a maximum or minimum weight goal may be set.

Patients who are on *nil per os* (nothing by mouth) status or have abnormal fluid losses will likely need additional fluids. For the HEN patient, water can either be delivered through the routine tube flushes (by dividing the desired daily volume between the flushes) or additional water boluses, by diluting the enteral formula, or by adding IV fluids via a central catheter. For the HPN patient, the PN volume is based on the desired total daily fluid volume, inclusive of fluid losses. A period of evaluation to assess tolerance of EN or PN and fluid and electrolyte stability is invaluable for determining the home nutrition support prescription. Signs of tolerance include achieving normal blood glucose, acceptable chemistry values, patient tolerance to infusion rate, absence of edema or shortness of breath, and acceptable urine output. Careful supervision of changes to the formula in the inpatient setting may minimize changes and maximize uncomplicated delivery in the home setting for what may be an indeterminate period of time.

Administration Schedule

The patient's and caregiver's preferences should be carefully considered when determining the infusion cycle. Gastric feedings may be delivered as bolus, intermittent drip, or continuous infusion. Bolus or intermittent drip feedings are typically done is 3 to 5 times per day, but some patients may tolerate fewer feedings or require more. Small bowel feedings require controlled delivery through an electronic pump for continuous feeding. Based on individual patient situations, continuous feeding may be delivered over less than 24 hours if EN is used to supplement an oral diet, or to allow the patient to have time off the pump and resume a more normal lifestyle. An ambulatory, battery-operated pump can hang from an IV pole or be situated in a backpack, which allows movement within the home as well as the ability to go out of the home with the infusion, if needed. A cycled schedule may be used to infuse EN over 8 to 14 hours per day to allow freedom from connections. The decision to adopt a cycled schedule for EN is based on total volume of feeding, the patient's demonstrated tolerance of a high infusion rate (determined by GI symptoms), and the patient's or caregiver's ability to manage the equipment.

PN always requires controlled pump delivery. While most PN regimens begin as a 24-hour infusion, decreasing the number of hours of infusion allows for freedom to resume normal activities. By increasing the flow rate, the total infusion time is decreased. This is referred to as a *cyclic infusion*. Monitoring urine volume and frequency can assess the fluid tolerance. The convenience of a shorter infusion cycle is balanced against the higher volume delivered over a shorter period of time. The cycle should include a tapered rate at the end of the infusion to minimize risk of hypoglycemia.[29] The tapers may include 1 hour at the beginning and 1 to 2 hours at the end of the infusion. Careful monitoring of blood glucose is needed as the infusion rate is increased. The glucose utilization rate is between 4 and 7 mg/kg/min,[30] with the generally accepted rate of glucose infusion being 5 mg/kg/min.[31] However, these recommendations are based on studies of critically ill, hospitalized patients; no studies of this kind have been conducted in home patients. Most HPN patients will tolerate higher glucose infusion rates because they are usually on cycled infusions.

For patients at risk for hyperglycemia, blood glucose checks should be scheduled prior to infusion, within the first 2 hours, 4 to 6 hours later, and 1 hour after the cycle ends. Insulin therapy should be initiated and advanced cautiously to avoid hypoglycemia, especially postinfusion. Blood glucose monitoring should be continued until acceptable blood glucose levels are achieved. Regimens for home insulin administration may be either a sliding scale (ie, correction insulin) or addition of regular insulin to the PN solution. Insulin is a high-risk medication that is prone to administration error.[30] It cannot be added by the infusion pharmacy during compounding; therefore, patients and caregivers must receive adequate education on the dose, proper syringe and needle size, and technique for adding insulin to the PN bag. Patients with diabetes may have basal insulin requirements met by insulin in the PN solution, while breakthrough elevations in blood glucose are covered with subcutaneous injections.

Prevention of Rehospitalization

Because hospital readmission is discouraging, disruptive, and costly, the home care plan should stress prevention of complications and early intervention when complications occur. Clearly, not all complications can be prevented, but there are known strategies that minimize risk.[32] Reasons for complications within the first 90 days of home nutrition support include inadequate training, patient and caregiver nonadherence, prescription error, healthcare worker error, and equipment malfunction.[33]

Early recognition of the signs and symptoms of complications promotes early treatment intervention. Regular measurement of weight before and after infusion (eg, in the morning and evening) and awareness of output help detect dehydration or volume overload. If possible, patients leaving an inpatient facility should be provided with the equipment to measure urine output as well as instructions for use. Dehydration can be treated at home by providing IV fluid for HPN patients to have on-hand to infuse when early signs are noted. Standard treatment is 1 liter IV fluid for 3 consecutive days in addition to scheduled PN infusions.[34] Additionally, some institutions have implemented outpatient hydration clinics where patients can go to receive IV fluid with an order from their healthcare provider as an alternative to emergency department or inpatient treatment.

A standardized protocol for diagnosis and management of common complications helps ensure that the home care clinician has the vital information needed for treatment decisions. One example of such a protocol is the use of standing orders to obtain blood cultures and complete blood count in the event of body temperature greater than 101.5° Fahrenheit.

Good communication between the patient and healthcare team reduces the risk of rehospitalization. Most nutrition support teams, infusion pharmacies, and nursing agencies provide 24/7 access to patients and their caregivers to troubleshoot issues. Patients should inform their healthcare team to changes in medications that could affect electrolyte balance, glucose levels, and hydration status.

Community resources provide peer support to enhance independence and promote a sense of well-being.[35] Patients who participate in peer support groups report less depression, anxiety, and worry, fewer rehospitalizations, and increased self-care and satisfaction with the care by their healthcare professionals.[24]

Patient Education

Patient education provides information patients need to be responsible for their own therapy, including skilled procedures such as dressing changes, catheter access, feeding tube flushes, and medication administration. Education is the foundation for success and avoids procedure- and therapy-related complications.[36] Verbal instruction and written resources empower patients to recognize signs and symptoms of serious complications such as fever, thirst, cramping, or bleeding and act appropriately if such problems occur. When possible, caregivers should be included in education sessions as they can provide a backup, a second set of hands, and reinforcement for administration of nutrition support.

Educational Materials

According to the National Assessment of Health Literacy in the United States, at least one-third of Americans have limited reading comprehension.[37] Ideally, patient education should be written at a fifth to sixth reading grade level—all words should be familiar and shorter than 3 syllables, and medical and technical terms should be limited or avoided altogether.[38] If complex or medical language is used, concepts should be explained using familiar words. Despite the availability of methods to calculate health literacy, the Institute of Medicine reported that more than 300 studies found printed health-related materials exceed the average reading ability of Americans.[39]

The care team should select printed patient education material written in a simple, casual, and conversational style. The materials should bridge language barriers or be printed in the patient's primary language, and provide content relevant to the age and culture of patient. All information should focus on the specific type of nutrition support the patient will

TABLE 38-7 Components of Patient-Specific Education for Home Nutrition Support

- Why the therapy is being recommended
- How the type of nutrition support is expected to work in the body
- Step-by-step directions for skilled procedures
- Common pitfalls to avoid
- Signs and symptoms of complications and actions to take
- Telephone numbers of all healthcare providers

receive and reflect current standards of practice.[40] Well-written materials highlight the most important information or otherwise make it easy to locate, and repeat key points as a means of reinforcement. The document should use terms consistently. Although an educational guide may identify medical equipment by the manufacturer's names or abbreviations, it should use only 1 term per type of equipment.

Effective patient education material presents all steps for any skilled procedures in a manner that is organized, precise, and easy to read. When content is complex or detailed, most people understand and retain less of the information. Documents should use active verbs when listing directions and avoid any excess words or information. Table 38-7 provides suggested content for printed education materials.

Lists and graphics in patient education can help clarify written text, emphasize skills presented, and provide the patient with cues for future reference. Drawings and photographs can illustrate important points of information. All graphics should focus on patient action and be simple, realistic, and relevant.[41] Attractive and friendly illustrations will keep the patient's attention and motivate patients to read the information.[42] Use of mnemonics will reinforce learning new concepts.

Learning Assessment

By engaging the patient and family in the belief that the nutrition support will improve the patient's health, the patient education instructor can facilitate the patient's and caregiver's desire to learn. Patients can be motivated to achieve a goal or outcome expected from home nutrition support. The instructor can influence the patient's attitude by conveying enthusiasm and providing encouragement that the outcome will be successful. When learning a new skill, positive reinforcement provides motivation to continue. When a person succeeds at a task, he or she is usually motivated to continue learning. Other helpful strategies are to create a friendly environment and to convey respect for patient needs, desires, and limitations.

A patient's readiness to learn is affected by physical or emotional conditions. When scheduling teaching sessions, the patient's physical limitations, such as pain, fatigue, immobility, or vision or hearing impairments, will need to be considered and accommodations provided. A caregiver may be needed to participate in the session. A one-on-one session conducted in a private and quiet environment may enhance learning readiness and help the patient concentrate without feeling stressed or anxious. If possible, education completed during hospitalization should occur outside of the patient's hospital room to limit interruptions. Teaching sessions should be scheduled at the patient's convenience and during a time of day free from other family obligations.

After an initial demonstration, the instructor should assess learning by asking the patient or caregiver to perform the required procedure. New learners will likely require repeated demonstrations. The goal is to have the patient become capable of independently managing the home nutrition support; this independence can improve QOL and make living with HEN or HPN as normal as possible.[43]

Teaching and Evaluation Strategies

High-tech home care equipment contributes to nutrition support delivery, but, at the same time, it imposes significant constraints on patients' lives.[44,45] A patient's perception of how this technology affects his or her life will influence acceptance.[46] Factors such as motor noise, light, misunderstood digital messages, alarms, and tubing attachment are physical barriers to acceptance. Fear of exposure to illness, anxiety over equipment malfunction, and altered body image interfere with usual family and social activities.[47] Use of appropriate technology and proper education on the use of equipment will increase adherence and acceptance of home therapy.[48]

The objectives of the initial home visit are to teach or reinforce correct technique for EN or PN infusion, help patients and caregivers feel comfortable with all aspects of home nutrition support and ensure that the appropriate supplies are available in the home. The home care nurse can also use this training period to assess knowledge and explain reasons behind the procedures and techniques. Issues such as storage of supplies, refrigeration of formulas, and disposal of medical waste can be addressed efficiently within the home. The home care nurse can immediately correct the patient's technique while observing the patient and caregiver within the home environment. Selection of an appropriate work area with adequate lighting, proper hand hygiene, use of clean or disposable toweling, and restriction of access by small children and pets are issues that should be addressed. Preparation of PN may require the patient/caregiver to demonstrate competence in the use of needles and syringes. Management of a vascular access device may require sterile technique for flushing or dressing changes.

Objectives for subsequent home visits are to ensure adherence to the regimen and adherence with procedure and handling techniques. The repeated demonstration of procedures should be consistently and carefully done. Follow-up home visits provide reassurance to the patient and caregiver that continued assistance and support are available. A printed guide of steps for new procedures can serve as a reference after the visit, thereby helping the patient reduce procedure-related anxiety and feel more confident while working toward independence. Every effort should be made to anticipate and respond to the patient's physical and emotional needs through interdisciplinary communication among the prescribing provider, members of the nutrition support team (if applicable), the home infusion provider, and home nursing agencies.

The home care team can use telephone contact to consistently reassess the patient's status at regular intervals. Focused questions should target known issues or problems. Special needs can also be addressed on an individual and ongoing basis to eliminate barriers to achieving goals of therapy. Other means of ongoing education include newsletters and interactive webinars for patients and their caregivers.[49] Developing a relationship with the patient and family will reduce therapy-related anxiety and result in increased satisfaction and enhanced adherence with nutrition support–related procedures. Table 38-8 describes strategies for relationship building.

TABLE 38-8 Strategies for Building Patient Trust

- Consistently reinforce goals.
- Make regular and frequent contact.
- Provide encouragement.
- Demonstrate respect for others and their concerns.
- Express understanding of circumstances.
- Anticipate needs.
- Deal with limitations.
- Ensure that services are available for all needs.

Clinical Monitoring in the Home

During home care visits, providers can obtain the patient's vital signs, record weight, assess hydration status, note any pertinent physical examination findings, observe and assess the enteral or vascular access device site, review medication use, and, if applicable, evaluate the patient's readiness to transition to oral nutrition. Blood pressure, pulse, temperature, and weight are easily obtained, objective physical assessment criteria. Keeping a record of these data in the home facilitates communication among various home care providers. Additionally, this record can be brought to office visits or referenced during telephone calls to the primary care provider. Dehydration can be recognized by blood pressure and pulse changes, especially when measured in both lying and standing positions (orthostatic vital sign measurement). Elevations of temperature and pulse may be early signs of infection. Rapid weight loss or gain may reflect a change in fluid status and should be assessed in the context of other symptoms of dehydration (low urine output, dry mouth, excessive thirst, dizziness, headaches) or fluid retention (edema, shortness of breath). Recording of output (emesis, urine, and stool) can be difficult in the home and should be limited to special situations requiring evaluation of formula volume or significant electrolyte imbalance, or as a means to prevent rehospitalization. Patients and caregivers should be educated about reporting significant changes in character or volume of outputs.

Home care providers should assess the enteral or vascular access device site at each home visit. Early signs and symptoms of infectious problems may be recognized by visual inspection of the insertion site, dressing, and surrounding skin for inflammation, swelling, tenderness, and drainage. Signs of mechanical malfunction of the device include leaking, difficulty flushing, or frequent pump alarms. Pain or swelling may also indicate vascular access catheter damage and subcutaneous infiltration.

Adequacy and tolerance of therapy is assessed through functional status, physical examination, and laboratory values. Functional status is how well a patient performs activities of daily living, such as ambulation, bathing, dressing, and meal preparation. Other performance indicators include independence with household chores, hobbies, and recreational activities. Physical examination will reveal changes in weight, anthropometrics, presence of edema, or signs of nutrient deficiencies.

There is no widely accepted standard for laboratory monitoring in the home nutrition support patient population, but experienced home nutrition support programs have created their own guidelines. All laboratory results should be documented at "baseline" (on discharge or at the beginning of home nutrition support) and then regularly recorded throughout the course of therapy (see Practice Scenario 38-3[8]). Long-term patients with tunneled or implanted catheters may be trained on how to draw their own blood specimens when home care nursing is no longer needed; patients with PICCs are not eligible to draw their own blood because of the risk of catheter dislodgement. Blood draw kits and shipping containers can be provided by laboratories, saving patients a trip to a clinic to get blood work done.[49] Suggested laboratory parameters to evaluate include basic metabolic panel, hepatic function panel, plasma proteins (eg, albumin, prealbumin), complete blood count, magnesium, and phosphorus. Initially, laboratory tests should be done on a weekly basis for 4 weeks or until values are stable. Once they are deemed stable, laboratory monitoring may be incrementally shifted to once a month, or a less-frequent schedule may be used depending on patient situation and plan of care. Ongoing monthly to bimonthly follow-up should continue unless there is a change in clinical condition necessitating more frequent monitoring on an individual, case-by-case basis.[8] Trace elements, vitamins, and the phospholipid fatty acid profile (triene:tetraene ratio) should be checked every 3 to 12 months, with more frequent monitoring for patients with known deficiencies or toxicities, or when national shortages of IV trace elements, vitamins, or lipids occur.[50,51] Triene:tetraene ratio is the gold standard for essential fatty acid deficiency assessment, and the ratio should be evaluated for patients receiving lipid-free or lipid-minimized HPN, or lipids with decreased levels of ω-6 fatty acids. Table 38-9 lists laboratory parameters and frequency of assessment for PN. To facilitate processing and correct billing, it is helpful to inform the laboratory of the diagnosis, clinical condition, or ICD-10-CM codes that correlate with the requested diagnostic test (Table 38-3). Table 38-10 provides examples of clinical monitoring parameters for EN.

Practice Scenario 38-3

Question: What is the appropriate clinical monitoring plan to ensure a successful transition from the hospital to home for a newly discharged patient receiving parenteral nutrition (PN) therapy?

Scenario: A 59-year-old woman suffered a mesenteric thrombosis resulting in loss of all but 60 cm of small bowel, an end jejunostomy, and a mucous fistula. PN was initiated in the

hospital and, after an extended hospitalization, the patient was discharged home with a large-volume PN solution designed to provide total daily fluid requirements and meet energy and nutrient goals. The patient advanced to an oral diet appropriate for short bowel syndrome and was receiving medication to decrease gastric hypersecretion, slow motility, and reduce ostomy output. The macro- and micronutrient components of her PN solution were established during hospitalization, and she was stable on the regimen prior to discharge. The patient discharge instructions included documentation of weight, measuring urine output volume, and blood work weekly for the first 4 weeks.

Intervention: Laboratory data were obtained within 48 hours prior to discharge and initiation of PN at home, as specified in the American Society for Parenteral and Enteral Nutrition (ASPEN) standards of practice for home care patients.[8] A protocol specified the frequency of laboratory testing for complete blood count, basic metabolic profile (sodium, potassium, chloride, bicarbonate, blood urea nitrogen, creatinine, glucose, calcium), magnesium, phosphorus, liver function tests, iron studies, and trace elements. Home visits were scheduled to provide education on how to monitor weight, intake and output, and temperature, as well as who to contact for reports and problems. Inspection of the access device site and assessment of the patient's psychosocial and functional status were also part of home visits.

Answer: According to the ASPEN standards for specialized nutrition support of home care patients,[8] the process of patient monitoring must ensure that the nutrition goals are achieved and that risks of complications related to nutrition therapy are reduced. Laboratory parameters are assessed at baseline, at least weekly for 4 weeks, and then monthly unless there is a change in clinical condition necessitating more frequent monitoring on an individual, case-by-case basis. Review of systems and inspection of the access device and site should occur at each home care visit. Periodic review of the patient's acceptance of the therapy, adherence to procedures, psychosocial adjustment, and general well-being is necessary.

Rationale: The patient's nutrition status is monitored and documented regularly. The assessment includes observation for signs and symptoms of intolerance to therapy, evaluation of weight change, evaluation of hydration status, review of systems and physical examination, periodic review of biochemical and other pertinent laboratory data, assessment for clinical signs of nutrient deficiencies or excesses, assessment of other disease states that may affect the nutrition therapy, consideration of any potential nutrition therapy and medication interactions, evaluation of functional status and performance, inspection of access device and site, and evaluation of patient adherence to techniques and procedures. Ongoing review of the appropriateness of the nutrition therapy and the need for continued nutrition support is conducted. Additionally, the psychosocial status of the patient and caregiver is periodically reviewed and the patient's home environment is reassessed. Patients who are eating or will be transitioning to oral intake or enteral nutrition require monitoring of fluid, nutrient, and oral intake as well as monitoring of urine, stool, and other gastrointestinal losses or output.

TABLE 38-9 Laboratory Monitoring for Home Parenteral Nutrition

Parameter	New Patients		Stable Patients	
	Baseline	Weeks 1, 2, 3, and 4	Monthly	Every 3–12 Months[a]
Basic metabolic panel: sodium, chloride, carbon dioxide, potassium, glucose, blood urea nitrogen, creatinine, calcium	X	X	X	
Hepatic function panel: total protein, albumin, total bilirubin, AST, ALT, alkaline phosphatase	X	X	X	
Magnesium	X	X	X	
Phosphorus	X	X	X	
CBC with differential	X	X	X	
Trace elements: zinc, copper, chromium, selenium, whole blood manganese	X			X
Phospholipid fatty acid profile	X			X
Water-soluble vitamins B$_6$, B$_{12}$, MMA, RBC folate	X[b]			X
Fat-soluble vitamins A, 25(OH)D, and E	X[b]			X
Iron indices: iron, ferritin, transferrin saturation, TIBC	X[c]			X

25(OH)D, 25- hydroxy vitamin D; ALT, alanine aminotransferase; AST, aspartate aminotransferase; CBC, complete blood count; MMA, methylmalonic acid; RBC, red blood cell; TIBC, total iron-binding capacity.

[a]Repeat blood work as warranted based on previous results, nutrition-focused physical exam (NFPE) findings, and national IV shortages. Repeat less frequently if results are normal (eg, 12 months).

[b]Check other micronutrients (eg, vitamin C, vitamin K, thiamin, biotin, niacin, riboflavin, and parathyroid hormone) if deficiencies are suspected based on NFPE findings. MMA is necessary for vitamin B$_{12}$ metabolism and used to help diagnose deficiency.

[c]Only check at baseline in the absence of recent surgery, blood transfusion, or major blood loss.

Source: Adapted with permission from guidelines used by Cleveland Clinic Home Nutrition Support Service.

TABLE 38-10 Clinical Monitoring of Home Enteral Nutrition

- Medical progress
- Weight
- Hydration
- Elimination
- Laboratory values as clinically indicated to assess for vitamin deficiencies, hydration, and electrolyte abnormalities
- Enteral nutrition tolerance
- Medication and water administration
- Drug-nutrient interaction
- Access device and site care
- Medical equipment and supplies
- Achievement of nutrition goals
- Readiness to transition to oral diet, including ability to chew and swallow safely, and need for modification of food consistency and texture

Patient Adherence

Assessment of patient adherence to the nutrition regimen is critical in the provision of home nutrition support. The patient interview may offer the clinician insight into the ability of the patient or caregiver to provide independent care. Additionally, feedback from the home nursing provider or home infusion provider is helpful. Members of the team should consider whether reports of excess supply inventory or unwillingness to review the inventory may indicate poor adherence. Moreover, if the usage of medical supplies and the nutrition formula do not coincide, patients may be having trouble with adherence. Clinical evidence, such as no response to treatment, weight loss, or unresolved electrolyte imbalances despite ordered interventions, may also suggest adherence issues. Technical evidence such as obtaining the infusion history from the patient's infusion pump can also provide insight into adherence.[52]

Prevention of Complications

Complications related to nutrition support can be categorized as mechanical, infectious, or metabolic.[5] Mechanical complications include occlusion, leakage, malposition, or accidental removal of the access device, as well as equipment failure or malfunction. Infectious complications relate to the access device, exit site, and surrounding skin. Metabolic complications include blood glucose or fluid and electrolyte abnormalities, GI intolerance, organ system dysfunction, and vitamin, mineral, and trace element deficiencies or toxicities (see Chapters 10 and 17 for more information on EN and PN complications, respectively).

HEN is relatively safe, and complications can usually be avoided or corrected.[5,8,53] Frequent tube surveillance, proper skin care, prevention of excessive traction on the tube, and routine tube flushing with water can prevent mechanical complications associated with the feeding tube. GI intolerance may occur in patients receiving HEN.[5] The potential causes of diarrhea should be evaluated before antidiarrheal agents are prescribed, as diarrhea may be related to new medications, infection, underlying disease, preparation and sanitation of the formula, change in rate or method of administration, or presence or absence of fiber. Patients on HEN may also experience constipation that may be related to hydration, physical activity level, medications, or laxative use. Patients with nausea, bloating, or abdominal distention should be evaluated for changes in clinical condition, medications, or method of feeding administration. Periodic evaluation of routine serum chemistries helps to monitor patients for metabolic complications associated with fluid, electrolyte, or mineral abnormalities.

In patients receiving HPN, catheter infection is the most common complication of PN therapy and the most common reason for hospital readmission.[54,55] Signs and symptoms of a catheter-related bloodstream infection may include fever, lethargy, chills, rigors, elevated leukocytes, and hyperglycemia. Redness, tenderness, or discharge from the skin at the access site may indicate catheter exit–site infection. A suspected or actual infection requires immediate evaluation and intervention.[56] If a patient experiences a catheter-related bloodstream infection, follow-up monitoring should include a home visit for reassessment of the patient's or caregiver's adherence with procedures. During this visit, proper handling of EN or PN access and equipment can be reviewed and the home environment can be evaluated.

Catheter occlusion may occur because of a kink in the catheter or from thrombus or precipitation of PN components. Diagnostic studies may be indicated when catheter flushing or aspiration is difficult. Patients requiring long-term HPN and those who have had multiple catheters are at increased risk of catheter-related venous thrombosis, and some patients may require anticoagulation therapy for prevention.[25]

Abnormal liver function may occur in patients requiring long-term HPN.[57] The mechanism for liver dysfunction is not completely understood and is thought to be multifactorial.[5] Potential causes of PN-associated liver dysfunction include overfeeding, excessive glucose or IV lipid dosage, lack of enteral stimulation, infection, choline or carnitine deficiency, and aluminum toxicity from contamination of PN components.[58] If signs of cholestasis occur, ultrasonography should be done to rule out extrahepatic causes. The PN solution should routinely be evaluated to confirm that the patient is not receiving excessive energy or excess lipids.[59] Soybean oil–based lipid injectable emulsions (ILEs) should provide less than 1g fat per kg body weight per day.[58] Smoflipid, an alternative ILE recently approved in the United States, has been shown in European clinical trials to provide an acceptable lipid source at levels of 1 to 1.5 g/kg/d with no deleterious effects on liver function tests or triglyceride levels.[60–64] If the patient is receiving continuous therapy, changing to a cyclic PN infusion may be beneficial.[65] Every attempt should also be made to encourage oral intake or transition to or inclusion of EN. If a patient experiences multiple HPN complications, referral for evaluation of intestinal or multivisceral transplantation should be considered.

Patients receiving long-term HPN may develop metabolic bone disease.[66] The causes of osteopenia and osteoporosis are multifactorial and may include preexisting disease, malabsorption, metabolic acidosis, use of steroids, inactivity, mineral deficiency (calcium, phosphorus, magnesium), or vitamin D deficiency or excess.[67] Bone mineral density testing should be done annually.

Micronutrient deficiencies are uncommon in patients receiving long-term PN because multivitamin and trace element additives are routinely added to PN formulations.[51] Patients should be monitored for iron deficiency because iron is not routinely added to PN. Serum levels of trace elements should be monitored every 3 to 12 months to prevent deficiency and toxicity. Because serum values are not always representative of deficiency and toxicity, patients should also be examined for physical signs of nutrient-related problems.

Role of Nutrition Support Clinicians

Continuity of care and communication within and among all organizations participating in the care of the patient receiving HEN or HPN should be frequent, structured, in-depth, and ongoing.[8] Ideally, the communication process starts during the transition from hospital-based care to home care. The communication should include the reason for nutrition support, goals of therapy, and follow-up plan.[68] Office visits should be scheduled for 1 month after start of therapy with the physician and nutrition support clinician and then every 3 to 6 months while nutrition support continues. More frequent office visits may be needed if complications arise. The home care agency should coordinate EN or PN therapy with care from other professional services providing wound care, ostomy care, respiratory care, physical therapy, or home health aide services.

Frequently, the hospital-based nutrition support team or home infusion provider takes responsibility for monitoring safe delivery of EN or PN; however, these activities should be coordinated with the patient's primary care physician (if he or she is not the prescribing physician) and all other medical specialists. It is not uncommon for a patient who is receiving HEN or HPN to receive regular follow-up care from a gastroenterologist, endocrinologist, or oncologist. A psychologist or psychiatrist may also be involved for treatment of anxiety or depression. Regular communication with the primary care physician is essential for new or ongoing cardiac, respiratory, renal, or neurologic concerns. Collaboration by all specialists, including the home nutrition support team or provider, can be achieved through active communication and documentation.

The ASPEN home care standards recommend interdisciplinary collaboration by the referring physician, nutrition support practitioners, and home care agencies.[8] Ideally, a physician with expertise in HEN and HPN is available for the management of the patient's nutrition care plan, interpretation of diagnostic testing, and evaluation of changes in medical condition. The roles and responsibilities and required competencies of the home care pharmacist, nurse, and dietitian are detailed in the ASPEN discipline-specific standards of professional practice and may overlap depending on the availability of each professional in the home care setting.[69–72]

The home care pharmacist has an essential role in evaluating the nutrition therapy prescription, compounding of PN formulations, evaluating drug-nutrient interactions, dispensing medical supplies and equipment, and monitoring laboratory results. The home care nurse has an active role in teaching the patient and caregiver, conducting in-home patient physical and psychosocial assessment, performing dressing changes and access site care, collecting blood or other specimens, medication oversight, evaluating adherence, and monitoring the response to nutrition support. The home care dietitian assists in the development of the nutrition care plan; recommends nutrition therapy based on energy, macronutrient, and micronutrient requirements; performs and evaluates the nutrition-focused physical examination; assesses adequacy and appropriateness of nutrient delivery and intake; evaluates adherence and response to nutrition support; and monitors the transition to tube feeding and/or oral diet.

A process for timely communication among the physician, nutrition support practitioners, home care agencies, patient, caregiver, and any other healthcare professionals is essential. There is a national shortage of nutrition support physicians, but dietitians, nurses, nurse practitioners, physician assistants, and pharmacists with specialized training have successfully assumed the lead in providing protocol-driven nutrition support care.[73] In a pilot study to prevent EN access–device complications, a nutrition support clinic trained dietitians and set care standards that would allow the dietitian to order specific interventions, laboratory tests, and other tests relevant to the practice of the clinic.[74] This program demonstrated a reduction in tube reinsertions and other complications.

Quality of Life, Outcomes Management, and Resources

Tools to Monitor Quality of Life

QOL is a multidimensional concept that includes evaluation of physical health status, psychological well-being, social and cognitive function, and illness and treatment. Because expectations regarding health and the ability to cope with limitations and disability can greatly affect a person's perception of health and satisfaction with life, people with the same objective health status may have very different QOLs. The World Health Organization defines QOL as "an individual's perception of their position in life in the context of the culture and value system in which they live and in relation to their goals, expectations, standards, and concerns."[75] Good QOL is generally accepted as a "state of complete physical, mental, and social well-being and not merely the absence of disease."[75] QOL may also be defined as the subjective perception of satisfaction or happiness with life in domains of importance to an individual. HPN-dependent adults have defined QOL as "how much one enjoys life, being happy and satisfied with life, and being able to do what you want to do when you want to do it."[76]

There is no gold standard measure of QOL, and, until recently, no therapy-specific QOL instrument for home nutrition support had been validated. Consequently, most published studies use generic measures of health status or disease-specific questionnaires to study the QOL of HEN and HPN patients.[77,78] In patients just starting PN, 2 studies using either the Functional Assessment of Cancer Therapy-General

questionnaire or the European Organization for the Research and Treatment of Cancer Quality of Life Questionnaire, the Karnofsky Performance Status, and Subjective Global Assessment found improvement in QOL in cancer patients after as little as 1 month of HPN therapy.[79,80] Published research demonstrates that poor QOL in patients receiving HEN and HPN is influenced by age, self-esteem, drug and narcotic use, depression, coping skills, family and peer support systems, financial insecurity, and underlying disease.[77,78,81-83] Qualitative reviews of HEN- and HPN-dependent adults identify disturbed social life, inability to eat normally, diarrhea, pain, polyuria, sleep disruption, and a need for psychosocial support as factors influencing QOL.[76,84-89] Despite technological inconveniences associated with infusion therapy, patients recognize and report the benefit of being kept alive with HEN or HPN.[76,81,89]

Baxter and colleagues[90] designed the first patient-based treatment-specific QOL questionnaire for HPN (HPN-QOL). The instrument includes 8 functional scales (general health, travel, physical function, coping, ability to eat and drink, employment, sexual function, and emotional function), 2 HPN items, and 9 symptom scales (body image, weight, immobility, fatigue, sleep pattern, GI symptoms, pain, presence of stoma, and financial issues). The HPN-QOL differentiates between how HPN therapy vs the underlying illness or disease affects QOL. Although this tool still requires validation in the United States, benefits of using a therapy-specific QOL instrument for individual patient care include providing information for therapy management and identifying problems requiring intervention.[90]

Clinicians and patients should discuss QOL at routine intervals whether a validated instrument is used or not. We know from studies and discussion with individuals requiring long-term HEN or HPN that patients benefit from knowing one can live a "normal" life even with HEN or HPN dependency.[76,89] Patients desire information to help them better understand the prognosis of their condition and the rationale for the therapy.[91-94] Because these individuals face potentially long-term therapies requiring substantial lifestyle adaptations with known risks and complications, a frank and open conversation about goals and expectations is necessary. Open communication between clinician and patient can help identify how a patient defines QOL and what makes QOL poor or good. When introducing these therapies, the clinician is obligated to paint a realistic picture for the patient of what will occur at home and adequately portray the complexity of the technology.[45] Continued dialogue with the patient will help him or her adapt and adequately cope with the lifestyle adjustments associated with HEN or HPN.

Improving Care and Tracking Outcomes

Tracking outcomes can easily identify how well nutrition support is provided and the benefit to the patient in terms of avoidance of complications, improved nutrition parameters, and enhanced performance status and function.[95] ASPEN has a prospective, longitudinal nutrition therapy patient registry, Sustain: ASPEN's National Patient Registry for Nutrition Care, which covers the period from January 2011 to January 2015 and information on approximately 1600 patients. Data collection for the registry is complete, and the current focus is to encourage public use and analysis of the information to improve outcomes and quality of care for people receiving PN.[96]

Patient Support

Many organizations provide important outreach services, free educational materials, and emotional support to patients, families, and caregivers.[45,97] The nonprofit Oley Foundation, established in 1983, is a national education, self-help, and research organization for consumers of HEN and HPN.[98] Networking occurs through communication with volunteer regional coordinators, who provide inspiration, support, and information via a toll-free hotline. Some of the educational resources available through the Oley Foundation include a video library, equipment and formula exchange, bimonthly newsletters with articles about medical advances and personal experiences, the My HPN online education modules (Take Charge, Catheter-Associated Infection, Fluid Balance, Glucose Control), and an annual summer conference. The website also provides links to other national and international organizations related to HEN and HPN, GI societies, disease- and condition-specific societies and foundations, home care agencies, equipment and products, infection control and safety, insurance and disability benefits, discount and free prescription services, government agencies, and parenting and caregiver resources.[98] Table 38-11 lists selected online resources for HEN and HPN patients and their families.

TABLE 38-11 Selected Online Resources for Home Enteral Nutrition and Home Parenteral Nutrition Consumers

- *Inspire* (www.inspire.com/groups/oley-foundation): The Oley Foundation Support Community connects patients, families, friends, and caregivers for support and inspiration.

- *Coping Well* (www.copingwell.com/copingwell): A self-help manual for adults living with home enteral nutrition seeking to learn to cope more effectively with the therapy-related challenges they face.

- *Feeding Tube Awareness Foundation* (www.feedingtubeawareness.com): A parent organization whose mission is to share information about the day-to-day care of infants and young children with feeding tubes.

- *Short Bowel Syndrome Foundation* (www.shortbowelfoundation.org): A nationally based foundation providing education, support, and advocacy services to patients, families, and healthcare providers who deal with short bowel syndrome or similar medical conditions.

- *Living Life on Total Parenteral Nutrition (TPN)—Facebook* group (https://www.facebook.com/groups/299634454491/?ref=ts&__adt=2&__att=iframe): A social media site for parents of children receiving parenteral nutrition and patients living on parenteral nutrition to share tips and ideas and discuss problems.

Summary

Home nutrition support involves more than simply transferring nutrition support from the hospital to the home. Home care agencies need to be prepared to teach therapy-related skills and provide education to ensure the technology used is safe and effective. Ongoing clinical monitoring can prevent complications, ensure adherence to nutrition support, and promote successful achievement of nutrition outcomes, as well as patient satisfaction and comfort. Multidisciplinary collaboration among the prescribing physician, hospital-based nutrition support team, home infusion provider, and home care nursing agencies along with the patient and caregiver facilitates the successful transition from an inpatient setting to home.

References

1. Avalere Health. Prepared for the alliance for home health quality and innovation. Updated 2015. www.ahhqi.org. Accessed September 1, 2016.

2. Centers for Medicare and Medicaid Services. 2014 CMS Statistics. https://www.cms.gov/Research-Statistics-Data-and-Systems/Statistics-Trends-and-Reports/CMS-Statistics-Reference-Booklet/Downloads/CMS_Stats_2014_final.pdf. Accessed September 12, 2016.

3. Cubanski J, Neuman T. The facts on Medicare spending and financing. Henry J. Kaiser Family Foundation. July 20, 2016. http://kff.org/medicare/issue-brief/the-facts-on-medicare-spending-and-financing/. Accessed September 21, 2016.

4. Howard L, Ament M, Fleming CR, et al. Current use and clinical outcome of home parenteral and enteral nutrition therapies in the United States. *Gastroenterology*. 1995;109:355–365.

5. DiBaise JK, Scolapio JS. Home parenteral and enteral nutrition. *Gastroenterol Clin N Am*. 2007;36:123–144.

6. Howard L. Home parenteral nutrition: survival, cost, and quality of life. *Gastroenterology*. 2006;130(Suppl):S52–S59.

7. National Association for Home Care. Basic statistics about home care. Updated 2010. www.nahc.org. Accessed May 1, 2011.

8. Kovacevich DS, Frederick A, Kelly D, et al. Standards for specialized nutrition support: home care patients. *Nutr Clin Pract*. 2005;20:579–590.

9. Wojner AW, Alexandrov AV. Predictors of tube feeding in acute stroke patients with dysphagia. *AACN Clin Issues*. 2000;11(4):531–540.

10. Centers for Disease Control and Protection. International Classification of Diseases, Tenth Revision, Clinical Modification (ICD-10-CM). Updated February 2, 2017. https://www.cdc.gov/nchs/icd/icd10cm.htm. Accessed April 6, 2017.

11. Barrocas A, Geppert C, Durfee S, et al. A.S.P.E.N. ethics position paper. *Nutr Clin Pract*. 2010;25:672–679.

12. Finucane TE, Christmas C, Travis K. Tube feeding in patients with advanced dementia: a review of the evidence. *JAMA*. 1999;282:1365–1370.

13. Gillick MR. Rethinking the role of tube feeding in patients with advanced dementia. *N Engl J Med*. 2000;342:206–210.

14. Sampson EL, Candy B, Jones L. Enteral tube feeding for older people with advanced dementia. *Cochrane Database Syst Rev*. 2009:CD007209.

15. Teno JM, Mitchell SL, Kuo SK, et al. Decision-making and outcomes of feeding tube insertion: a five-state study. *J Am Geriatr Soc*. 2011;49:881–886.

16. Monturo C. The artificial nutrition debate: still an issue . . . after all these years. *Nutr Clin Pract*. 2009;24:206–213.

17. Palecek EJ, Teno JM, Casarett DJ, et al. Comfort feeding only: a proposal to bring clarity to decision-making regarding difficulty with eating for persons with advanced dementia. *J Am Geriatr Soc.* 2010;58:580–584.

18. Newton AF, DeLegge MH. Home initiation of parenteral nutrition. *Nutr Clin Pract.* 2007;22:57–65.

19. Centers for Medicare and Medicaid Services. National Coverage Determination section180.2: enteral and parenteral nutritional therapy. Medicare Coverage Database. https://www.cms.gov/medicare-coverage-database/overview-and-quick-search.aspx. Accessed September 12, 2016.

20. Centers for Medicare and Medicaid Services. Medicare Parts B/D coverage issues. www.cms.gov/pharmacy/downloads/partsbd coverageissues.pdf. Accessed September 12, 2016.

21. Centers for Medicare and Medicaid Services. Medicare coverage database. https://www.cms.gov/medicare-coverage-database. Accessed October 17, 2016.

22. Bonifacio R, Alfonsi L, Santarpia L, et al. Clinical outcome of long-term home parenteral nutrition in non-oncological patients: a report from two specialised centres. *Intern Emerg Med.* 2007;2:188–195.

23. Shepperd S, Doll H, Angus RM, et al. Avoiding hospital admission through provision of hospital care at home: a systematic review and meta-analysis of individual patient data. *CMAJ.* 2009;180:175–182.

24. Smith CE, Curtas S, Werkowitch M, et al. Home parenteral nutrition: does affiliation with a national support and educational organization improve patient outcomes? *JPEN J Parenter Enteral Nutr.* 2002;26:159–163.

25. Steiger E. Dysfunction and thrombotic complications of vascular access devices. *JPEN J Parenter Enteral Nutr.* 2006;20(Suppl):S70–S72.

26. John BK, Khan MA, Speerhas R, et al. Ethanol lock therapy in reducing catheter-related infections in adult home parenteral nutrition patients: results of a retrospective study. *JPEN J Parenter Enteral Nutr.* 2012;36:603–610.

27. Gura KM. Swimming with lines and tubes: it's a team effort. *LifelineLetter.* 2014(Jul–Aug).

28. Miller J, Dalton MK, Duggan C, et al. Going with the flow or swimming against the tide: should children with central venous catheters be allowed to go swimming? *Nutr Clin Pract.* 2014;29:97–109.

29. Metheny NM. Parenteral nutrition. In: Metheny NM, ed. *Fluid & Electrolyte Balance: Nursing Considerations.* Sudbury, MA: Jones & Bartlett Learning; 2012:169–178.

30. Mirtallo J, Canada T, Johnson D, et al. A.S.P.E.N. safe practices for parenteral nutrition. *JPEN J Parenter Enteral Nutr.* 2004;28(Suppl):S39–S70.

31. A.S.P.E.N. Board of Directors and the Clinical Guidelines Task Force. Guidelines for the use of parenteral and enteral nutrition in adult and pediatric patients. *JPEN J Parenter Enteral Nutr.* 2002;26(Suppl):1SA–138SA. Errata in *JPEN J Parenter Enteral Nutr.* 2002;26:144.

32. Smith CE, Curtas S, Kleinbeck SVM, et al. Clinical trial of interactive and videotaped educational interventions reduce infection, reactive depression, and rehospitalizations for sepsis in patients on home parenteral nutrition. *JPEN J Parenter Enteral Nutr.* 2003;27:137–145.

33. de Burgoa LJ, Seidner D, Hamilton C, et al. Examination of factors that lead to complications for new home parenteral nutrition patients. *J Infusion Nurs.* 2006;29:74–80.

34. Konrad D, Corrigan ML, Hamilton C, et al. Identification and early treatment of dehydration in home parenteral nutrition and home intravenous fluid patients prevents hospital admissions. *Nutr Clin Pract.* 2012;27:802–807.

35. Dakof GA, Taylor SE. Victim's perceptions of social support: what is helpful from whom? *J Pers Soc Psychol.* 1990;58:80–89.

36. Cox JA, Westbrook LJ. Home infusion therapy. Essential characteristics of a successful education process—a grounded theory study. *J Infusion Nurs.* 2005;28:99–107.

37. National Center for Education Statistics. *National Assessment of Adult Literacy of America's Adults in the 21st Century.* Washington, DC: National Center for Education Statistics. http://nces.ed.gov/naal/pdf/2006470.pdf. Accessed May 1, 2011.

38. Sand-Jecklin K. The impact of medical terminology on readability of patient education materials. *J Community Health Nurs.* 2007;24:119–129.

39. Nielsen-Bohlman L, Panzer AM, Hamlin B, et al., eds. *Health Literacy: A Prescription to End Confusion.* Washington DC: National Academies Press; 2004.

40. Clayton LH. Strategies for selecting effective patient nutrition education materials. *Nutr Clin Pract.* 2010;25:436–442.

41. Doak LG, Doak CC, Meade CD. Strategies to improve cancer education materials. *Oncol Nurs Forum.* 1996;23:1305–1312.

42. Doak C, Doak L, Root J. *Teaching Patients with Low Literacy Levels.* 2nd ed. Philadelphia, PA: Lippincott; 1996.

43. Gifford H, DeLegge M, Epperson LA. Education methods and techniques for training home parenteral nutrition patients. *Nutr Clin Pract.* 2010;25:443–450.

44. Marden SF. Technology dependence and health-related quality of life: a model. *J Adv Nurs.* 2005;50:187–195.

45. Winkler MF, Ross VM, Piamjariyakul U, et al. Technology dependence in home care: impact on patients and their family caregivers. *Nutr Clin Pract.* 2006;21:544–556.

46. Lehoux P. Patients' perspectives on high-tech home care: a qualitative inquiry into the user-friendliness of four technologies. *BMC Health Serv Res.* 2004;4:28–36.

47. Lehoux P, Saint-Arnaud J, Richard L. The use of technology at home: what patient manuals say and sell vs. what patients face and fear. *Sociol Health Illn.* 2004;26;617–644.

48. Huisman-de Waal G, van Achterberg T, Jansen J, et al. "Hightech" home care: overview of professional care in patients on home parenteral nutrition and implications for nursing care. *J Clin Nurs.* 2011;20:2125–2134.

49. Gifford H, DeLegge M, Epperson LA. Education methods and techniques for training home parenteral nutrition patients. *Nutr Clin Pract.* 2010;25:443–450.

50. Staun M, Pironi L, Bozzetti F, et al. ESPEN guidelines on parenteral nutrition: home parenteral nutrition (HPN) in adults. *Clin Nutr.* 2009;28:467–479.

51. Howard L, Ashley C, Lyon D, Shenkin A. Autopsy tissue trace elements in 8 long-term parenteral nutrition patients who received U.S. Food and Drug Administration formulation. *JPEN J Parenter Enteral Nutr.* 2007;31:388–396.

52. Austhof SI, Mitchell R, Konrad D, et al. Management of nonadherence in the home parenteral nutrition patient. *Support Line.* 2016;38:7–9.

53. Siepler J. Principles and strategies for monitoring home parenteral nutrition. *Nutr Clin Pract.* 2007;22:340–350.

54. Bozzetti F, Mariani L, Bertinet DB, et al. Central venous catheter complications in 447 patients on home parenteral nutrition: an analysis of over 100,000 catheter days. *Clin Nutr.* 2002;21:475–485.

55. Ghabril MS, Aranda-Michel J, Scolapio JS. Metabolic and catheter complications of parenteral nutrition. *Curr Gastroenterol Rep.* 2004;6:327–334.

56. Mermel LA, Farr BM, Sherertz RJ, et al. Guidelines for the management of intravascular catheter-related infections. *Clin Infect Dis.* 2011;32:1249–1272.

57. Dray X, Joly F, Reijasse D, et al. Incidence, risk factors, and complications of cholelithiasis in patients with home parenteral nutrition. *J Am Coll Surg.* 2007;204:13–21.

58. Cavicchi M, Beau P, Crenn P, et al. Prevalence of liver disease and contributing factors in patients receiving home parenteral nutrition for permanent intestinal failure. *Ann Intern Med.* 2000;132:525–532.

59. Fulford A, Scolapio JS, Aranda-Michel J. Parenteral nutrition-associated hepatotoxicity. *Nutr Clin Pract.* 2004;19:274–283.

60. Wu MH, Wang MY, Yang CY, et al. Randomized clinical trial of new intravenous lipid (Smoflipid 20%) versus medium-chain triglycerides/long-chain triglycerides in adult patients undergoing gastrointestinal surgery. *JPEN J Parenter Enteral Nutr.* 2014; 38(7):800–808.

61. Antébi H, Mansoor O, Ferrier C, et al. Liver function and plasma antioxidant status in intensive care unit patients requiring total parenteral nutrition: comparison of 2 fat emulsions. *JPEN J Parenter Enteral Nutr.* 2004;28(3):142–148.

62. Mertes N, Grimm H, Furst P, et al. Safety and efficacy of a new parenteral lipid emulsion (Smoflipid) in surgical patients. *Ann Nutr Metab.* 2006;50(3):253–259.

63. Klek S, et al. Four-week parenteral nutrition using a third generation lipid emulsion (Smoflipid): a double-blind, randomised, multicentre study in adults. *Clin Nutr.* 2013;32(2):224–231.

64. Ma CJ, Sun LC, Chen FM, et al. A double-blind randomized study comparing the efficacy and safety of a composite vs a conventional intravenous fat emulsions in postsurgical gastrointestinal tumor patients. *Nutr Clin Pract.* 2012;27:410–415.

65. Maini B, Blackburn G, Bristrian BR, et al. Cyclic hyperalimentation: an optimal technique for preservation of visceral protein. *J Surg Res.* 1976;20:515–525.

66. Seidner DL. Parenteral nutrition-associated metabolic bone disease. *JPEN J Parenter Enteral Nutr.* 2002;26(5 suppl):S37–S42.

67. Pironi L, Tjellesen L, DeFrancesco A, et al. Bone mineral density in patients on home parenteral nutrition: a follow-up study. *Clin Nutr.* 2004;23:1288–1302.

68. Holst M, Rasmussen HH. Nutrition therapy in the transition between hospital and home: an investigation of barriers. *J Nutr Metab.* 2013;2013:1–8.

69. Mascarenhas MR, August DA, DeLegge MH, et al. Standards of practice for nutrition support physicians. *Nutr Clin Pract.* 2012;27(2):295–299.

70. Tucker A, Ybarra J, Bingham A, et al. American Society for Parenteral and Enteral Nutrition (A.S.P.E.N.): standards of practice for nutrition support pharmacists. *Nutr Clin Pract.* 2015;30(1):139–146.

71. DiMaria-Ghalili RA, Gilbert K, Lord L, et al. Standards of nutrition care practice and professional performance for nutrition support and generalist nurses. *Nutr Clin Pract.* 2016;4:527–547.

72. Brantley SL, Russell MK, Morgensen KM, et al. American Society for Parenteral and Enteral Nutrition and Academy of Nutrition and Dietetics: revised 2014 standards of practice and standards of professional performance for registered dietitian nutritionists (competent, proficient, and expert) in nutrition support. *Nutr Clin Pract.* 2014;29(6):792–828.

73. Kiraly LN, McClave SA, Neel D, et al. Physician nutrition education. *Nutr Clin Pract.* 2014;29(3):332–337.

74. Hall BT, Englehart MS, Blaseg K, et al. Implementation of a dietitian-led enteral nutrition support clinic resulted in quality improvement, reduced readmissions, and cost savings. *Nutr Clin Pract.* 2014;29:649–655.

75. Orley J. The World Health Organization (WHO) quality of life project. In: Trimble MR, Dodson WE, eds. *Epilepsy and Quality of Life.* New York: Raven; 1994:99–133.

76. Winkler MF, Hagan E, Wetle T, et al. An exploration of quality of life and the experience of living with home parenteral nutrition. *JPEN J Parenter Enteral Nutr.* 2010;34:395–407.

77. Baxter JP, Fayers PM, McKinlay AW. A review of the instruments used to assess the quality of life of adult patients with chronic

78. Winkler MF. Quality of life in adult home parenteral nutrition patients. *JPEN J Parenter Enteral Nutr.* 2005;29:162–170.

79. Culine S, Chambrier C, Tadmouri A, et al. Home parenteral nutrition improves quality of life and nutritional status in patients with cancer: a French observational multicenter study. *Support Care Cancer.* 2014;22:1867–1874.

80. Vashi PG, Dahlk S, Popiel B, et al. A longitudinal study investigating quality of life and nutritional outcomes in advanced cancer patients receiving home parenteral nutrition. *BMJ Cancer.* 2014;14:593–602.

81. Baxter JP, Fayers PM, McKinlay AW. A review of the quality of life of adult patients treated with long-term parenteral nutrition. *Clin Nutr.* 2006;25:543–554.

82. Fortune DG, Varden J, Parker S, et al. Illness beliefs of patients on home parenteral nutrition (HPN) and their relation to emotional distress. *Clin Nutr.* 2005;24:896–903.

83. Persoon A, Huisman-de Waal G, Naber TA, et al. Impact of home parenteral nutrition on daily life—a review. *Clin Nutr.* 2005;24:304–313.

84. Silver HJ. The lived experience of home total parenteral nutrition: an online qualitative inquiry with adults, children, and mothers. *Nutr Clin Pract.* 2004;19:297–304.

85. Brotherton AM, Judd PA. Quality of life in adult enteral tube feeding patients. *J Hum Nutr Diet.* 2007;20:513–525.

86. Brotherton A, Abbott J. Clinical decision making and the provision of information in PEG feeding: an exploration of patients and their carers' perceptions. *J Hum Nutr Diet.* 2009;22:302–309.

87. Walker A. In the absence of food: a case of rhythmic loss and spoiled identity for patients with percutaneous endoscopic gastrostomy feeding tubes. *Food, Culture Soc.* 2005;8:161–180.

88. Huisman-de Waal G, Naber T, Schoonhoven L, et al. Problems experienced by patients receiving parenteral nutrition at home: results of an open interview study. *JPEN J Parenter Enteral Nutr.* 2006;30:215–221.

89. Thompson CW, Durrant L, Barusch A, et al. Fostering coping skills and resilience in home enteral nutrition (HEN) consumers. *Nutr Clin Pract.* 2006;21:557–565.

90. Baxter JP, Fayers PM, McKinlay AW. The clinical and psychometric validation of a questionnaire to assess the quality of life of adult patients treated with long-term parenteral nutrition. *JPEN J Parenter Enteral Nutr.* 2010;34:131–142.

91. Mansilla ME. Benefits from artificial nutritional support: a testimonial. *Nutrition.* 2003;19:78–80.

92. Kindle R. Life with Fred: 12 years of home parenteral nutrition. *Nutr Clin Pract.* 2003;18:235–237.

93. Ireton-Jones C, Lang RK, Gravenstein ME, et al. Home nutrition support from the patient's perspective: the real reality story! *Nutr Clin Pract.* 2006;21:542–543.

94. Fairman J, Compher C, Morris J, et al. Living long with short bowel syndrome: a historical case of twenty-nine years of living with home parenteral nutrition. *JPEN J Parenter Enteral Nutr.* 2007;31:127–134.

95. Ireton-Jones C, DeLegge M. Home parenteral nutrition registry: a five-year retrospective evaluation of outcomes of patients receiving home parenteral nutrition support. *Nutrition.* 2005; 21:156–160.

96. American Society for Parenteral and Enteral Nutrition. Sustain: ASPEN's National Patient Registry for Nutrition Care. www .nutritioncare.org/sustain. Accessed March 14, 2017.

97. Kovacevich DS. Parenteral and enteral nutrition support groups. *Nutr Clin Pract.* 2003;18:238–239.

98. Oley Foundation. http://oley.org. Accessed March 14, 2017.

intestinal failure receiving parenteral nutrition at home. *Br J Nutr.* 2005;94:633–638.

39 Ethics and Law

*Denise Baird Schwartz, MS, RD, FADA, FAND, FASPEN,
and Albert Barrocas, MD, FACS, FASPEN*

CONTENTS

Acknowledgments: Cynthia M.A. Geppert, MD, MA, PhD, MPH, FAMP, DAAPM, was a coauthor for this chapter in the second edition.

Objectives

1. Understand how ethical principles, reasoning, and guidelines can be used to prevent or resolve ethical and legal dilemmas encountered in clinical nutrition practice.
2. Analyze clinical ethics arguments related to the use of artificial nutrition and hydration (ANH) for patients with a terminal illness or advanced dementia and those in a persistent vegetative state (PVS).
3. Reflect sensitivity to cultural values and religious beliefs in approaching ethical issues related to nutrition and end-of-life care.
4. Review the legal framework and precedent cases for decision making in nutrition support.

Test Your Knowledge Questions

1. What is the definition of ANH?
   A. A medical treatment that allows a person to receive nutrition and hydration when he or she is no longer able to consume them by mouth.
   B. Provision of specialized nutrients orally, enterally, or parenterally with therapeutic intent.
   C. Nutrition provided through the gastrointestinal (GI) tract via a tube, catheter, or stoma that delivers nutrients distal to the oral cavity.
   D. Administration of nutrients and fluid intravenously to maintain the patient's nutrition status during acute illness.

2. Which of the following core ethical principles is the predominant value in American bioethics?
   A. Respect for autonomy: The patient has a right to self-determination in healthcare decision making.
   B. Beneficence: The healthcare professional is fundamentally obligated to seek the good of the patient above all other priorities.
   C. Nonmaleficence: The prime directive of medicine is to prevent, minimize, and relieve needless suffering and pain.
   D. Justice: When treating patients, healthcare providers should consider only clinically relevant factors and provide equitable care to clinically similar patients.

3. Which of the following statements is true about the decision to withhold or withdraw ANH?
   A. There is an ethical distinction between withholding and withdrawing treatment.
   B. Decisions to withhold ANH tend to be more psychologically and emotionally charged for families than decisions to withdraw ANH.
   C. There is a legal distinction between withholding and withdrawing any treatment.
   D. The term *forgoing* refers to both withholding and withdrawing ANH.

4. Which of the following would be a reason to not place a long-term feeding tube in a patient with advanced dementia?
   A. A swallow evaluation was not recently completed.
   B. During the hospitalization, the healthcare team did not have a meeting where the family could ask questions about the rationale for the tube placement.
   C. The patient's expected survival post feeding tube placement is less than 30 days.
   D. The patient does not have an advance directive indicating a designated decision maker and specific healthcare wishes.

Test Your Knowledge Answers

1. The correct answer is A. ANH involves technology-assisted administration of nutrients when a patient is unable to swallow or unable to absorb nutrients through the GI tract.[1] ANH is considered a medical intervention.[2]

2. The correct answer is A. In the US ethico-legal framework, the primary goal is to provide medical therapies based on the individual's quality-of-life goals, as determined by the patient with decision-making capacity or an authorized surrogate. Completion of advance directives for individuals is encouraged. Beneficence is the fundamental obligation of a healthcare professional to seek the good of the patient above all other priorities, and nonmaleficence addresses the aspect of "do no harm." The justice principle deals with fairness and requires that nutrition support clinicians equitably treat similar patients similarly and consider only clinically relevant information.[1]

3. The correct answer is D. The term *forgoing* refers to both withholding and withdrawing ANH. There is no ethical or legal distinction between withholding and withdrawing treatment. However, decisions to withdraw ANH may be more psychologically and emotionally charged for clinicians, patients, and families than decisions to withhold intervention.[3]

4. The correct answer is C. A patient's expected survival time affects the evaluation of the benefits vs burdens and risks of the procedure. A swallow evaluation, family meeting, and presence of an advance directive are not limiting factors for placement of a long-term feeding tube.[4]

Background

Healthcare professionals often confront clinical dilemmas at the intersection of technology, ethics, culture, and law. Technology can provide the physiological support to keep selected organs functioning; however, for some patients, this support may come with burdens, risks, and discomfort that outweigh any benefits of the intervention. As individuals, family members, and professionals, we are often conflicted by the challenges presented as we try to reconcile what the available technology can do with our obligations to the individuals under our care and our respect for state and federal laws. Barrocas has used the term *troubling trichotomy* to describe this milieu of technology (what "can" be done), ethics (what "should" be done), and law (what "must" be done).[5–7]

In the context of nutrition care, the troubling trichotomy often involves ANH. Certainly, in many cases, patients and clinicians can agree that the benefits of ANH outweigh the risks. For example, ANH can enable a patient with head and neck cancer to receive adequate nutrition so she can successfully complete chemotherapy. However, the decision whether to administer ANH to an elderly patient with end-stage dementia poses ethical challenges—ANH may extend his physical survival but not provide any benefit that outweighs the burdens and risks of the intervention. Patients and families have a right to informed consent or refusal of ANH, but relatively few people express their wishes with a clarity and consistency sufficient to guide healthcare decision making or satisfy the dictates of the law.[8]

This chapter reviews ethical and legal principles of importance to nutrition support clinicians. In particular, it addresses how these principles apply to controversies over the provision of ANH to patients with 3 clinical conditions, terminal illness, advanced dementia, and PVS, in light of the empirical evidence regarding the clinical benefits, burdens, and risks of this intervention. The chapter also identifies the most important legal precedents and rulings on ANH and discusses their relevance to clinical practice.

Basics of Ethics in Nutrition Practice

Principles and Terminology

The term *ethics* originates from the Greek word *ethos*, which refers to establishing acceptable behavior. Ethics provide the basic structure for putting morals or rules of conduct into practice. In a professional context, ethics involve the rules and standards that govern the actions of members of the profession. Thus, *medical ethics* or *bioethics* refers to a set of moral values that govern the behavior of healthcare professionals.[9] Although some bioethical principles have evolved with changes in medical technology, many remain immutable and offer basic guidelines for patient care.

Core ethical principles relevant to nutrition support therapy include autonomy, beneficence, nonmaleficence, and justice. *Autonomy* refers to individual self-determination. In US healthcare, a decisionally capable patient is authorized to make decisions about his or her treatment and care. Like other life-sustaining interventions, such as cardiopulmonary resuscitation and intubation/mechanical ventilation, nutrition support is a medical treatment. Thus, autonomy means that a patient with intact decisional capacity can determine whether he or she will receive ANH, regardless of the clinician's recommendation for or against the medical therapy. If the patient is unable to make decisions about treatment, an informed surrogate represents the patient for healthcare decisions. When respect for the patient's autonomy is fundamental, the care is patient-centered. Such care is facilitated by good communication among all relevant parties (eg, interdisciplinary members of the healthcare team, the patient/surrogate, and loved ones), who share a commitment to the best interest of the patient.[1]

Respect for autonomy of the patient in decision making is as paramount in the legal sphere as autonomy is in the ethical arena. As discussed in greater detail later in this chapter, in the case of the decisionally incapable individual, the patient's wishes as expressed in an advance directive and/or by a surrogate decision maker ideally would be respected in a similar fashion. Many state statutes provide immunity from legal recourse to providers who follow the stipulations of the advance directive.

Although patient autonomy is the preeminent value in the ethical and legal framework for US healthcare, the clinician may sometimes find it challenging to uphold this value if the patient or surrogate seeks treatment that the clinician regards as harmful. In these cases, clinicians should seek guidance from an ethics committee and/or legal counsel about the appropriate course of action.

Beneficence implies that the healthcare professional's primary goal is to seek the good of the patient. *Nonmaleficence* refers to the clinician's goal to do no harm. Together, beneficence and nonmaleficence support the goal of achieving maximum benefit with minimum harm or burden. There are times when ANH meets this goal, and other times when it does not. For example, a nutrition support clinician demonstrates beneficence by following evidence-based guidelines for ANH

when a patient undergoing medical treatment would become malnourished without nutrition support. However, like other medical interventions, ANH may potentially cause complications that harm the patient (see Chapters 13 and 17). Also, in some cases, ANH may not achieve the intended benefits of comfort or prolonged survival. Withholding or withdrawing ANH is ethically appropriate, based on the ethical principles of beneficence and nonmaleficence, when the burdens and risks of ANH outweigh its benefits, provided there is appropriate consent from a patient with decisional capacity.

Justice deals with fairness. This principle guides nutrition support clinicians to treat all patients with similar clinical status equitably without regard to nonclinical factors, such as the patient's ability to pay for treatment. In the United States, medical ethics has traditionally focused on treatment decisions and advocacy for the individual patient. However, economic pressures related to the cost of healthcare, the advent of managed care systems, and the number of uninsured patients have underscored issues of social and distributive justice in public health and population health debates.[1] Nutrition support professionals are obligated to responsibly and wisely utilize scarce resources, and the financial cost of treatment may be a consideration in a patient's care plan. However, most ethicists would caution providers against employing bedside rationing when deciding on the appropriateness of ANH. Treatment decisions ideally would be based on the clinical standard of care, evidence-based medicine, patient and family preferences, and institutional policy. Nutrition support professionals can work through their professional organizations to influence the public policy debate on controversial questions involving ANH in a direction that balances the needs of individual patients with the duty to equitably use healthcare resources.[1]

In addition to the key ethical principles of autonomy, beneficence, nonmaleficence, and justice, a discussion of ethics in nutrition support requires understanding of several other important terms. Table 39-1 provides definitions of additional notable terms.[1,2,79,21]

Ethical Theory

An *ethical theory* is a general philosophical source of many ethical standards and the guide for how these standards are applied through ethical reasoning in specific situations. Ethical theories are schools of thinking that form our moral decisions. A working familiarity with these theories can provide methods of analysis within which nutrition support professionals can contribute to the identification and resolution of ethical dilemmas.[22] Among the most common ethical theories used in contemporary bioethics are principlism, deontology, utilitarianism, and virtue ethics.

Beauchamp and Childress have developed principlism into one of the most widely employed modes of ethical analysis in contemporary bioethics.[23] Principlism bases ethical decisions on general rules and principles that express broad moral considerations applied to particular situations. Dilemmas are resolved through the weighing, balancing, and specification of the basic principles of autonomy, beneficence, nonmaleficence, and justice.

TABLE 39-1 Selected Ethics Terms Related to Nutrition Support

Term	Definition
Advance directive	• General term for any document that gives instructions about a patient's healthcare and/or appoints someone to make medical treatment decisions for the patient if he or she cannot make them. • Living wills and durable powers of attorney for healthcare are types of healthcare advance directives.
Agent, proxy, representative, or surrogate	• A person appointed to make healthcare decisions for a decisionally incapable patient.
Autonomy	• The individual's right to self-determination in healthcare decision making. • The predominant value in American bioethics and law.
Beneficence	• The fundamental obligation of a healthcare professional to seek the good of the patient above all other priorities.
Bioethics or medical ethics	• The set of moral values that governs the professional behavior of healthcare providers.
Clinical ethics	• The type of ethics that guides daily clinical practice by healthcare providers in their care for patients. • Clinical ethics are firmly grounded in medical science, law, and policy and demonstrate respect for the autonomy of each patient.
Durable power of attorney for healthcare	• A document that appoints someone else to make all medical treatment decisions for the patient if he or she cannot make them. Instructions for decision making can also be included.
Ethical decision making	• A decision-making approach in which every stakeholder in the decision participates and focuses on the best interests of the patient.
Ethical dilemma	• Tension or conflict between and among ethical principles or obligations. • In an ethical dilemma, an act can be seen as both morally justified and unjustified.
Health literacy	• The degree to which an individual can obtain, process, and understand health information needed to make informed health decisions. • Communication that does not reflect a patient's level of health literacy may undermine the individual's autonomy.
Justice	• Fairness. • In healthcare, justice involves the equitable treatment of clinically similar patients with a sole focus on clinically relevant factors.
Living will	• A document in which the patient states his or her wishes about life-sustaining medical treatment.
Morality	• Often used interchangeably with *ethics* to refer to standards of right and wrong behavior. • Usually refers to conduct that conforms to widely accepted customs, values, or beliefs of a group of people. • Sources of moral guidance include parental and family values, cultural traditions, and religious beliefs. • A person's moral values create a disposition to make the right choices; however, a clinician cannot rely on personal morals as the only guidance in clinical ethics.
Nonmaleficence	• The "do no harm" *(primum non nocere)* principle. • In medicine, the prime directive to prevent, minimize, and relieve needless suffering and pain.
Palliative care	• An approach to care for patients with serious, life-threatening, or terminal illnesses that aims to ease pain and discomfort, alleviate or control symptoms, improve or sustain quality of life, and meet the psychosocial, and spiritual needs of the patient and family. • Not a curative treatment.

Term	Definition
Patient-centered care	• Care that is respectful of and responsive to individual patient preferences, needs, and values. • Ensures that the patient's values guide all clinical decisions and patients or their surrogates are actively engaged when healthcare decisions must be made. • Recognizes the health literacy level of the patient and provides healthcare information that is understandable at that level.
Patient Self-Determination Act	• US law that ensures that a patient's right to self-determination in healthcare decisions is communicated and protected.
Physician Orders for Life-Sustaining Treatment (POLST)	• POLST forms translate an individual's treatment preferences into medical orders, including for cardiopulmonary resuscitation, scope of treatment, artificial nutrition by tube, and, in some states, antibiotic use. • An approach to end-of-life planning based on conversations between patients, loved ones, and medical providers. • Designed to ensure that seriously ill patients can choose the treatments they want and that their wishes are honored by medical providers.
Preventive ethics	• Activities performed by an individual or group on behalf of a healthcare organization to identify, prioritize, and address systemic ethics issues, rather than approaching ethics on a case-by-case basis. • Proposes that ethical conflict is largely preventable if common triggers are identified and proactively managed by interventions aimed at the organization, unit, and individual levels.
Shared decision making	• A patient-centered approach to healthcare decision making in which clinicians relinquish their traditional authoritative role and train to become more effective coaches or partners to patients, who are educated about the essential role they play in decision making and given effective tools to help them understand their options and the consequences of their decisions. • Patients also receive the emotional support they need to express their values and preferences and ask questions without censure from their clinicians.
Teach-back method	• Approach to patient education in which patients are asked to explain or demonstrate what they have been taught to ensure that they understand. • If patients do not understand, they are retaught using a different method and then asked again to explain or demonstrate what they have been taught.
Team approach	• The view that ethics is a group effort involving all stakeholders and not the action of a single agent.
Transdisciplinary care	• A holistic, collaborative approach that minimizes traditional boundaries between healthcare disciplines as clinicians across disciplines continually collaborate to provide patient-centered care. • The team collectively determines what functions are to be performed and who is the most appropriate individual available to do them at a particular time and in a given environment. • When providing transdisciplinary care, each individual acts within limits of his/her state or federal certificate or license.

Source: Data are from references 1, 2, 7, and 9 through 21.

Deontology, or the ethics of duty, assumes the existence of absolute duties or judgments that are nearly unconditional in their application to particular circumstances. The philosopher Immanuel Kant is one of the most significant figures in deontological ethics.[24] For a decision to be ethical under the rubric of deontology, the decision would be universal, as expressed in Kant's famous categorical imperative as a philosophical formulation of the golden rule. The rightness or wrongness of decisions from the deontological perspective depends on the intentions of the agent, not on the consequences of the act. Deontological reasoning is the basis of the sanctity-of-life claims that ANH must be provided to all human beings, including those who are potentially in PVS.

Utilitarianism is an ethical theory that begins from the opposite premise as deontology. Utilitarians posit that it is the consequences, not the intentions, of decisions that determine their ethical valence. This ethical theory is most often associated with the English philosopher John Stuart Mill, and it frequently informs debates over healthcare economics, resource allocation, and policy.[25] Many utilitarians contend that actions and obligations that maximize the good or benefit for the largest number of people are the most ethical.

Virtue ethics is the theory that finds the locus of right and wrong in the character of the individual. Deriving from Aristotle,[26] virtue ethics is among the oldest theories used in professional ethics, and one that many practitioners find the most natural. It suggests that a clinician whose conduct displays habits of compassion, honesty, integrity, fidelity, and courage will develop a virtuous character from which will spring good clinical decisions. For example, a good clinical decision for a patient in a PVS might be to provide a time-limited trial of ANH as an expression of the fiduciary commitment to the patient and his or her family.

Key Ethico-Legal Concepts

The ethics of principlism, deontology, utilitarianism, and virtue provide the structure for decision making, but the process of these decisions is operationalized in clinical practice and law (regulatory or policy) through a series of interrelated key ethico-legal concepts: informed consent and refusal; decisional capacity; surrogates; standards of surrogate decision making; and withholding and withdrawing treatment.

Informed Consent

The legal and ethical doctrine of informed consent expresses the high valence of autonomy and respect for persons in Western bioethics. Informed consent is not the mere signing of a form but the outcome of a shared decision-making process between patient and/or surrogate and the healthcare professionals caring for the patient. Authentic informed consent has 3 main components. First, the patient or surrogate is provided adequate information regarding the proposed treatment or procedure in understandable language. At a minimum, the information includes the following: the diagnosis for which the treatment is clinically indicated; the prognosis (both short and long term) with and without the proposed intervention; the benefits, burdens, and risks of the procedures; and alternatives to the proposed intervention, including no treatment. Second, the patient or surrogate has intact decision-making capacity. Third, the patient possesses *voluntarism*, the ability to make a choice free of excessive internal or external coercion.[27,28]

Competence and Decisional Capacity

Advance directives are pivotal in the legal and ethical arena related to ANH and exemplify the intersection of law and bioethics in medical decision making. Our discussion in this chapter of the purpose of advance directives requires a brief explanation of the terms *competence* and *decisional capacity*. Only a court can determine competence, but such determinations are often materially based on healthcare providers' judgments regarding the patient's decisional capacity—that is, the ability of the individual to comprehend and communicate health information, reason regarding aspects of treatment, appreciate the consequences of medical decisions for his or her life and values, and freely choose a course of action.[27]

Decisional capacity is task-specific and not global in nature. For example, a person may be able to make medical decisions but not manage his or her finances, or the reverse. Decisional

capacity can fluctuate, particularly when an impairment is secondary to physical or mental illness. A patient may thus be more or less capable of making specific decisions at different times and under varying conditions.[29]

Surrogate

According to 2009–2010 survey data, about 26% of Americans have completed an advance directive.[30] All 50 states have legislation granting an order of priority in making decisions for patients who lack both capacity and an advance directive. Generally, the hierarchy or priority for surrogacy is as follows: spouse, adult children, siblings, other relatives, and, in some states, friends. Divorce or legal separation may void the first-order rank of the spouse as surrogate. Significant others, including same-sex partners who are in long-standing relationships, are considered the legal surrogate in some states, but not in others. The legal limitations on types of decisions that surrogates can make also vary from state to state.[31] Because of differences in the state laws, nutrition support professionals should be familiar with the content of the statutes in their own jurisdiction and seek expert legal advice as questions arise. Disputes among self-presumed surrogates, especially in the absence of formal directives, are common and troubling. Such problems can be referred to the ethics committee or ethics consultant, hospital risk management, a hospital attorney, or professional mediators.[32]

Standards of Surrogate Decision Making

The surrogate is obligated to render decisions that are in accordance with legal criteria. When a patient's values and wishes are known, decisions are to be made in accordance with the standard called *substituted judgment*.[33] The 1985 Conroy case[34] presented guidelines for the exercise of substituted judgment for incompetent patients according to the following 3 levels of credibility:

- A *subjective test* provides clear and unequivocal evidence of the patient's wishes as expressed in an advance directive or oral instructions to a healthcare professional, family, or friend. It is the most trustworthy test.
- A *limited-objective* test may be used when a subjective test is unavailable. It is based on other evidence of the patient's best interests, such trustworthy testimony that he or she would have refused treatment or had informally or casually expressed preferences in reaction to news reports or knowledge of the condition of another person.
- A *pure objective test* may be appropriate when there is no trustworthy evidence of the patient's wishes, but it is the least credible form of substituted judgment. When the patient's wishes are not ascertainable, then the surrogate optimally would make decisions in accordance with a best interest standard.

Withholding vs Withdrawing Treatment

In 1983, the President's Commission for the Study of Ethical Problems in Medicine and Biomedical Research published *Deciding to Forego Life-Sustaining Treatment*.[35] This document remains useful today when dealing with ethical decisions related to withholding and withdrawing therapies. Conclusions of the report include the following:

- The competent patient's voluntary and informed choice should determine whether a life-sustaining therapy is initiated, withheld, or withdrawn.
- The patient's best interests are served by healthcare professionals who maintain a presumption in favor of sustaining life while also recognizing that patients with decision-making capacity are entitled to choose to forgo any treatments, including those that sustain life.
- Whether individualized treatment is warranted depends on the balance of its usefulness or benefits for a particular patient and consideration of the burdens and risks that the treatment would impose.
- An appropriate surrogate, often a family member, can make decisions for patients who have insufficient capacity to make their own decisions.

There is no ethical distinction between withholding and withdrawing life-sustaining therapies, including ANH. However, decisions to actively withdraw ANH can be more psychologically and emotionally charged for practitioners, patients, and families than decisions to passively withhold intervention. The potential benefits of a limited trial of ANH ought not be eschewed in an effort to avoid the difficult emotional interactions of withdrawing nutrition support if those benefits are not realized.[9] A decisionally capable patient or authorized surrogate may refuse any form of medical care, including lifesaving treatments, even if the inevitable result of that refusal is death.

Cultural Values and Religious Beliefs

Failure to appreciate the way in which the cultural values and religious beliefs of patients, families, and even other healthcare professionals impact healthcare decisions, including end-of-life choices, can trigger or amplify ethical conflicts. In particular, food, even nutrient solutions delivered through tubes, remains a symbol of caring and a social bond with family and friends. Thus, decisions about nutrition care can involve cultural values and religious beliefs to a greater degree than other medical therapy decisions.[36]

Nutrition support professionals and other clinicians cannot realistically become experts in every culture and religion of our increasingly ethnically and spiritually diverse society. Also, within a religion or culture, different individuals may not adhere to the same beliefs.[28,37] Therefore, practitioners may inquire to what degree any particular patient's wishes adhere to religious or cultural views. Table 39-2 presents examples of religious, ethnic, and cultural perspectives on end-of-life care.[37–46]

Healthcare professionals and even institutions have their own religious and ethical beliefs and values that influence their decision making regarding ANH. A clinician who imposes personal values on the patient or family violates the fundamental ethical principle of respect for persons. However, there may be times in which a nutrition support professional or other practitioner feels he or she cannot participate in the care of a patient due to moral or religious objections. Federal, state, and institutional policies have "conscience clause" provisions to define

the clinician's options in such situations. In general, an orderly transfer of care is completed, the clinician continues to be responsible for the care of the patient. If the clinician does not fulfill this responsibility, he or she could be accused of abandonment. *Abandonment* refers to the unilateral severance of the professional relationship without reasonable notice, under the circumstances when continued attention is required.[6]

Ethical Aspects of Artificial Nutrition and Hydration in Different Conditions

Recent medical history is a story of exponential technological innovation and scientific discovery that have outstripped the pace of jurisprudence and ethical analysis regarding these new developments. As a result, healthcare providers today may face unprecedented ethical dilemmas related to ANH. As the technology has evolved, the use of ANH in advanced disease states may in some circumstances be legal but, arguably, not truly ethical.

Terminal Illness

The central ethical question to ask about the use of ANH at the end of life is whether it is palliative or painful to not have access to food and water when dying. Common sense moral intuitions may create a distressing contradiction in which healthcare professionals, families, and patients alike are caught. On the one hand, patients who are terminally ill often experience a decreased hunger and thirst drive. Physiologically, patients with end-stage disease processes, such as cancer or heart failure, will become dehydrated and malnourished. The ethical issue is whether omission of nutrition and hydration causes suffering. Some people will instinctually answer that, of course, it does, and anyone who has such a response will naturally be repulsed by the inhumanity and cruelty of the idea of depriving sick and dying loved ones of the basic necessities of food and water.

On the other hand, hospice and palliative care professionals have long clinically recognized that dying patients stop eating and drinking as a matter of course and comfort. The term *terminal dehydration* is used to indicate a process in which the dying patient's condition naturally results in a decrease in fluid intake.[47] Several theories have been advanced for the ameliorative effect of terminal dehydration. The analgesic theory proposes that starvation boosts the production of ketones, thereby having an anesthetic effect. Synergistically, dehydration may increase the production of endogenous opioids.[48] Providing hydration in this situation has the potential to increase fluid accumulation and may lead to uncomfortable symptoms, including edema, ascites, nausea, vomiting, and pulmonary congestion.[47]

Patients experiencing terminal dehydration may have dysphagia, nausea, and fatigue and gradually withdraw from activities of daily living. These individuals may report thirst; however, data show no correlation between thirst and hydration, and the use of artificial hydration to relieve thirst may be futile.[49] Fortunately, the sensation of a dry mouth, a distressing symptom often reported with dehydration, can be easily treated. Sips of water or beverages, ice chips, hard candy and spraying normal saline into the mouth, as well as, meticulous mouth care have all been reported to be of benefit.[47]

TABLE 39-2 Religious, Ethnic, and Cultural Perspectives on End-of-Life Care

Identity	Perspective[a]
African-American/black	• Compared with white patients, more likely to prefer life-sustaining treatment. • Feel that the patient should be primary decision maker in end-of-life care. • Perceive suffering as spiritually meaningful, and life as always having some value. • May equate the cessation of aggressive therapies with "giving up." • Believe that the end of life is in God's hands.
Asian (specific national/ethnic group not designated)	• Give special status to older adults, believing they should not be burdened with bad news. • Consider illness to be a family event rather than something that primarily affects an individual. • Expect that family members and physicians will share decisional duties.
Bosnian	• Prefer that a physician, due to expert knowledge, make independent decisions to reduce burden on individuals and families. • Expect the physician to maintain the patient's optimism by not revealing a terminal diagnosis.
Buddhist	• Do not believe in a mandatory or moral obligation to preserve life at all costs. • Lack specific teachings on artificial nutrition and hydration for individuals in persistent vegetative state. • Support availability of terminal care and hospice movement.
Catholic	• Believe the individual has a moral obligation to use ordinary or proportionate means of preserving his or her life but may forgo extraordinary or disproportionate means of sustaining life. • Assert that medically assisted nutrition and hydration become morally optional when they cannot reasonably be expected to prolong life; when they would be excessively burdensome for an individual; or when they would cause significant physical discomfort (eg, resulting from complications of the intervention method). • Advocate that free and informed judgment made by a competent adult concerning use or withdrawal of life-sustaining procedures should always be respected and normally complied with, unless the choice is contrary to Catholic moral teaching.
Chinese	• Stress importance of hope in care of people who are dying, as hope prevents suffering by avoiding despair. • Prefer family-centered decision making. • Believe food represents more than a source of energy; it embodies family, love, and caring. • Expect family members to protect terminally ill individuals by withholding knowledge of condition. • Prefer to not discuss possibility of death due to belief that direct acknowledgment of mortality may be self-fulfilling.
Confucian	• Believe that death is good if one has fulfilled one's moral duties in life, whereas resistance to accepting terminal illness or insisting on futile treatment may reflect an individual's perception of unfinished business.
Eastern European	• Have tradition of physician-centered, paternalistic decision making. • May expect physician, rather than patient or family, to determine a person's level of life support.
Filipino	• May not want to discuss end-of-life care because these exchanges demonstrate a lack of respect for belief that an individual's fate is determined by God.
Greek Orthodox	• Do not allow artificial nutrition to be withheld or withdrawn, even if there is no prospect of recovery.
Hindu and Sikh	• Believe in karma, a causal law where all acts and human thoughts have consequences. • Understand choices to be duty-based rather than rights-based. • View death as a passage to a new life; the way a person dies is important factor in determining what new life will be like. • Usually accept or desire a do-not-attempt-resuscitation order because death should be peaceful.

TABLE 39-2 Religious, Ethnic, and Cultural Perspectives on End-of-Life Care *(continued)*

Identity	Perspective[a]
Hispanic	• Prefer less-aggressive, comfort-focused end-of-life care. • Favor family-centered decision making over individual patient autonomy. • Expect family members to actively protect a terminally ill person from knowledge of his or her condition. • Consider family members, rather than individual alone, as holding decision-making power regarding life support. • May be reluctant to formally appoint a specific family member to be in charge because of concerns about isolating that person or offending other relatives. • May value a consensus-oriented decision-making approach.
Islamic	• Believe that premature death should be prevented, but treatments can be withheld or withdrawn in terminally ill individuals when physicians are certain about the inevitability of death, and that treatment will not improve condition or quality of life. • Assert that the intention of end-of-life care must never be to hasten death.
Jewish	• May not allow withdrawal of continuous life-sustaining therapy, but withholding further treatment is allowed as part of dying process if the intervention is an intermittent life-sustaining treatment, and if withholding treatment was the clear wish of patient. • May consider food and fluid to be basic needs and not treatment. • Can permit the withholding of food and fluid, if that is the individual's expressed wishes, when individual approaches final days of life, when food or fluids may cause suffering and complications.
Korean	• Believe that family members, rather than individual alone, hold the decision-making power regarding life support.
Lebanese	• Stress the role of the family in every interaction at the end of life. • Prioritize loyalty to family even before religion, nationality, or ethnicity. • Expect family to be included in communication protocol.
Native American	• Believe that words should be chosen carefully because, once spoken, they may become a reality. • Worry that negative words and thoughts about health can become self-fulfilling. • Value thinking and speaking in a positive way.
North American	• Emphasize patient autonomy and open discussion of treatment decisions; norm is for individual to take lead in healthcare decision making.
Pakistani	• Expect family members to protect terminally ill individuals from knowledge of their condition. • May "adopt" physicians into the family unit and address them as parent, aunt, uncle, or sibling; this family status sanctions the physician's involvement in intimate discussions.
Protestant	• If there is little hope of recovery, will usually accept and understand the withholding or withdrawal of therapy.
Taoist	• Philosophical Taoism: Believe that acceptance is the only appropriate response when facing death, and artificial measures contradict natural events. • Religious Taoism: Fear that death may lead to an afterlife of torture in endless hell; may therefore cling to any means of extending life to postpone that possibility.
White (non-Hispanic)	• Compared with black patients, less likely to prefer life-sustaining interventions. • Feel that patient should be primary decision maker for end-of-life care. • Have concerns about dying individuals undergoing needless suffering.

[a]These descriptions are generalizations; individuals who identify with a religion, ethnicity, or culture may not hold the perspective described.
Source: Adapted by permission of Taylor and Francis Group, LLC, a division of Informa plc, from reference 38: Schwartz DB. Ethical considerations in the critically ill patient. In: Cresci G, ed. *Nutrition Support for the Critically Ill Patient: A Guide to Practice.* 2nd ed. Boca Raton, FL: Taylor & Francis; 2015:635–652. Data are from references 37 and 39 through 46.

Advanced Dementia

In 2014, the International Clinical Ethics Section of the American Society for Parenteral and Enteral Nutrition published a special report on gastrostomy tube placement in patients with advanced dementia or near end of life. It advocates for weighing the potential benefits derived from a mode of nutrition support therapy against inherent burdens and risks within a patient-centered framework that recognizes the individual's culture, religion, ethical principles, and personal values.[4]

Advanced dementia is a terminal illness.[50] Patients with the most prevalent form of dementia, Alzheimer's disease, have an average life expectancy of 5 to 7 years after diagnosis.[51] Dysphagia, anorexia, apraxia with utensils, inability to self-feed, resistance to feeding by caregivers, and poor oral intake are all aspects of the natural course of progressive dementia.[52] These dysfunctions frequently result in malnutrition and substantial weight loss, which are upsetting to the family members and practitioners alike.

The efficacy and effectiveness of enteral nutrition (EN) in patients with advanced dementia is controversial. Among the justifications for percutaneous endoscopic gastrostomy (PEG) tube placement for EN are that EN prevents or reduces symptoms, improves functional and nutrition status, enhances comfort, or prolongs survival.[53] However, PEG tube use in advanced dementia does not reduce aspiration or prevent the pneumonia to which patients with dementia so often succumb; aspiration from oral and gastric secretions continues unabated.[53] In addition, PEG tube placement requires concomitant use of physical or chemical restraints, exacerbating discomfort, increasing the risk of pressure sores, and further compromising patient comfort and human dignity.[54,55] Short-term survival may be reduced after placement of the feeding tube, especially in hospitalized patients, who often have acute delirium superimposed on chronic dementia.[55-57] Chapter 36 reviews the evidence-based literature on the effectiveness of EN in end-stage dementia.

Given the evidence that PEG tubes may cause more harm than good in patients with end-stage dementia, why are they often placed? Brody and colleagues[8] underscore that family, physician, and administrative factors serve as a force contravening the empirical data about ANH in both terminal illness and advanced dementia. Surveys suggest that the physicians who ultimately order feeding tubes believe they reduce morbidity and mortality.[58,59] Nutrition support professionals can constructively educate clinicians regarding the data on the effect of feeding tubes on short- and long-term survival. As practitioners, nutrition support professionals can also be aware and attuned to the complex and conflicting emotions of denial, guilt, fear, and responsibility that accompany ANH decisions. Figure 39-1 presents a suggested sample checklist to facilitate the decision-making process for initiating EN in patients with advanced dementia. Practice Scenario 39-1 illustrates the use of the sample checklist.[4]

Vegetative and Minimally Conscious States

Improvements in intensive care have led to an increase in the number of patients who survive severe brain injury, and, regardless of the etiology (traumatic, metabolic, degenerative,

Practice Scenario 39-1

Question: What factors would a clinician ideally consider before recommending a gastrostomy tube placement in a patient with advanced dementia?

Scenario: An 85-year-old man with advanced dementia was admitted to the hospital for the third time in a month with aspiration pneumonia. A video fluoroscopic swallowing exam revealed the patient was aspirating. The speech language pathologist recommended that the patient be considered for a long-term feeding tube.

Intervention: The primary care physician reviewed the Checklist for Use Prior to Long-Term Enteral Access Device Placement (Figure 39-1) and decided to order a palliative care and nutrition consult to help the family make the most appropriate decision about enteral nutrition on behalf of the patient. In the family meeting, the family expressed that they did not want to "starve the patient" during the end stage of life. The palliative care team and the nutrition support clinician explained the benefits, burdens, and risks for the patient of the long-term feeding tube. The family met together after the clinician-family meeting and decided against tube placement. They were comforted by knowing that the patient would continue to be offered food. They all agreed that their loved one would not want to be sustained on a feeding tube for the rest of his life. For this patient, food represented family meals and the enjoyment of being together, not nutrients artificially administered through a tube.

Answer: The factors to consider before recommending a gastrostomy tube placement in a patient with dementia include the patient's prior wishes for medical therapies (if known before the advanced dementia), the length of time that the tube feeding may be required, the patient's medical condition, and his expected survival time.

Rationale: There is a lack of evidence that enteral nutrition improves morbidity or decreases mortality in advanced dementia.[4]

and so on), the spectrum of consciousness and awareness conditions after such an injury ranges from normal to brain death (see Figure 39-2). Some patients recover completely. Others live in a vegetative or minimally conscious state—they may awaken from an acute comatose state but do not show any signs of awareness, or they may exhibit no evidence of a sustained, reproducible, purposeful, or voluntary behavioral response to visual, auditory, tactile, or noxious stimuli. Some patients remain in a vegetative state permanently. Others eventually show inconsistent but reproducible signs of awareness, including the ability to follow commands, but they remain unable to communicate interactively.[60]

PVS was first described by the Scottish neurosurgeon Bryan Jennett and the American neurologist Fred Plum in a landmark 1972 article.[61] The authors characterized PVS as a condition of wakefulness without awareness, in which the eyes are open but there is no awareness of self, others, or the surrounding environment. In contract, a coma is "eyes-closed" unconsciousness. In 1994, the Multi-Society Task Force in the

FIGURE 39-1 Sample Checklist for Use Prior to Long-Term Enteral Access Device Placement

Clinical indications	Presumed oral intake will provide insufficient nutrition and/or is unsafe due to possible aspiration for a period greater than 4 weeks on nasogastric tube feeding? ☐ Yes ☐ No Life expectancy, specify: _____
Swallow evaluation	Was a video swallow study completed? ☐ Yes ☐ No If yes, when? _____ Were results abnormal? Specify: _____
Consistent with patient's wishes?	Is use of G-tube consistent with patient's preferences, as supported by patient's quality-of-life goals? ☐ Yes ☐ No
Preferences obtained	How have patient's preferences, goals, and values been obtained? Check all that apply: ☐ Discussed directly with patient ☐ Discussed with patient's surrogate (for patient lacking decision-making capacity) ☐ Documented in patient's advance directive and/or POLST form ☐ Surrogate committee formed to make decision on patient's behalf ☐ Other (specify): _____
Preferences documented	Are patient's preferences, goals and values formally documented in medical record or surrogate committee? ☐ Yes (date): _____ ☐ No
Stability of medical condition	Is patient's medical condition expected to remain stable to discharge? ☐ Yes ☐ No
Expected survival time	Is patient expected to survive for at least 30 days post G-tube placement? ☐ Yes ☐ No
Recommendation	Based on above answers is patient an appropriate candidate for G-tube? ☐ Yes ☐ No If no, recommend consults for discussion/decision-making with patient, family, caregiver, surrogate decision maker for feeding option needs by: ☐ Ethics ☐ Registered dietitian ☐ Physician ☐ Palliative care ☐ Pharmacist ☐ Speech-language pathologist

G-tube, gastrostomy tube; POLST, physician orders for life-sustaining treatment.
Source: Adapted with permission from reference 4: Schwartz DB, Barrocas A, Wesley JR, et al. A.S.P.E.N. special report: gastrostomy tube placement in patients with advanced dementia or near end of life. *Nutr Clin Pract.* 2014;29:829–840.

FIGURE 39-2 Levels of Consciousness After Brain Injury[a]

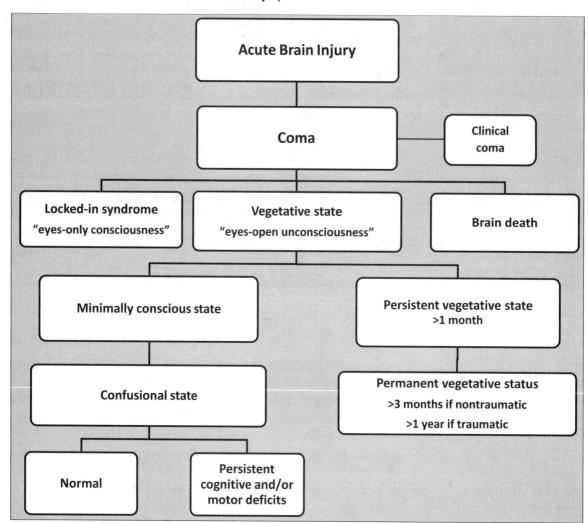

[a]Patients with certain chronic clinical conditions, such as severe/advanced dementia, may also exhibit minimally conscious or confusional states.

Persistent Vegetative State reported on degrees of vegetative state. Patients whose brain injury was not caused by trauma are deemed to be in a PVS if they continue to exhibit the same conditions of unconsciousness and unawareness beyond 3 months. For patients whose brain injury was caused by trauma, PVS is defined as at least 1 year of eyes-open unconsciousness.[62,63] In 2002, the Aspen Neurobehavioral Conference Work Group created the term *minimally conscious state* (MCS) to describe a subgroup of patients with severe alteration in consciousness who do not meet diagnostic criteria for coma or the vegetative state, adding a new clinical diagnosis to the spectrum of disorders of consciousness.[64]

In the early stages of the vegetative state or coma, patients have the potential for regaining some or all consciousness and awareness. For this reason, clinicians are cautioned against the premature forgoing of ANH in these patients based solely on their neurologic status. The importance of accurate diagnosis and reassessment of the patient's neurologic status throughout this period of potential recovery cannot be overemphasized.

The question of whether patients in a PVS suffer is a common concern of surrogates and healthcare professionals. Evidence of the absence of suffering in patients in a PVS has been provided through sophisticated functional neuroimaging techniques such as position emission tomography scans.[65] These techniques have established the disconnect between the thalamic and cortical areas necessary to experience pain in patients in a PVS compared to conscious patients. Neuroimaging has also demonstrated a return to normal functional imagery when the clinical picture demonstrates return of consciousness.[66]

In a functional magnetic resonance imaging (MRI) study of 54 patients initially classified as in a PVS, Monti and colleagues demonstrated brain activation reflecting some awareness and cognition in 1 patient, and only imaging activation in another.[60] The clinical significance of such neuroimaging findings has been questioned by Ropper[67] as well as Billings and colleagues.[68] The study by Monti et al stressed the importance of accurate evaluation, classification, and reassessment of these patients because 3 of them (approximately 6%) were found to be in an MCS rather than in a PVS.[60]

Schnakers and colleagues[69] suggest that some patients who are in a MCS may be misdiagnosed as being in a vegetative state. The results of the study indicate that the systematic use of a sensitive standardized neurobehavioral assessment scale may help decrease diagnostic error in differentiating vegetative state vs MCS. A 2015 systematic review and meta-analysis of 20 clinical studies of 906 patients with either PVS or MCS revealed a sensitivity of 44% and a specificity of 67% for functional MRI-based techniques. Furthermore, the study demonstrated that 10% to 24% of PVS patients can regain consciousness with significant functional impairment, sometimes years after the event.[70]

One of the most difficult decisions facing healthcare professionals and surrogates of patients in a PVS is whether to use a PEG tube to provide nutrition. Clinicians should optimally provide information to the surrogate decision maker about likely long-term outcomes for the patient in a PVS. Decisions to forgo PEG tubes in the early phase of the vegetative state may be premature, particularly if the diagnosis of PVS is not confirmed. In these cases, a time-limited trial of EN may be warranted, along with frank discussions with the surrogate decision maker, other family members, and significant others regarding specific goals and expectations.

Legal Framework for Decision Making

The duty of a healthcare professional to provide the most appropriate care with the most appropriate available technology is governed by the legal system—the third component of the "troubling trichotomy." The US legal system (Figure 39-3) has its foundation in the federal and state constitutions, statutes, regulations, court decisions, and opinions of attorneys general.[9]

The 2 major branches of the law are criminal and civil. Civil law applies to most cases involving healthcare professionals. Contract and tort (harm) are the most notable components of civil law. Although contract law may be occasionally implicated in cases of alleged abandonment, tort law dominates the legal concerns for the healthcare professional. Tort law includes intentional and unintentional harm as well as strict liability. The latter is often associated with product liability, which does not usually involve healthcare professionals.

Intentional tort includes allegations of assault (attempt or threat to touch another without justification), battery (actual act of touching another), invasion of privacy, defamation, misinterpretation, fraud, and false imprisonment. Violation

FIGURE 39-3 The "Must": The US Legal System

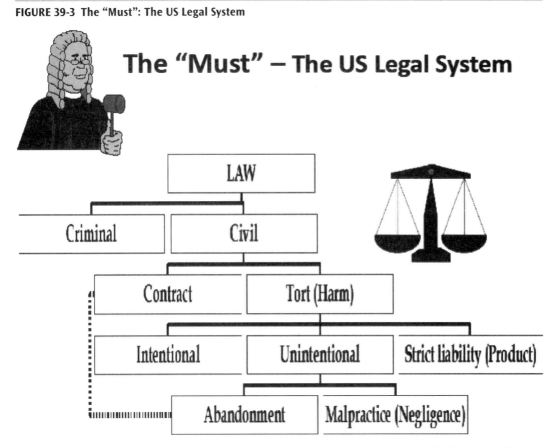

Source: Reprinted with permission from reference 9: Barrocas A, Yarbrough G, Becnel PA, et al. Ethical and legal issues in nutrition support of the geriatric patient: the can, should, and must of nutrition support. *Nutr Clin Pract.* 2003;18(1):37–47.

of privacy rights and the potential for alleged defamation may occur secondary to inattention to a person, place, or type of communications. Assault and battery charges against healthcare professionals can be precipitated by the absence of appropriate informed consent when any of the following occurs:

- Consent is not for the specific procedure performed (eg, PEG tube).
- The patient is not provided with the information needed to give informed consent (eg, the risks of bleeding and peritonitis and long-range morbidity and mortality outcomes with PEG tube insertion).
- Consent is not obtained for the individual(s) who perform the procedure (eg, the partner of gastroenterologists who obtained consent the previous day is the one to place the PEG tube).
- Consent is obtained from a patient with decisional incapacity (eg, a patient with dementia or a patient who recently received an intramuscular and intravenous narcotic).

Abandonment, an unintentional tort, refers to the termination of the professional relationship without reasonable notice in situations when continued attention is required. Refusal to treat, insufficient or delayed treatment, withdrawal without adequate notice, and premature discharge are potential triggers for allegations of abandonment.

Malpractice (negligence) is another unintentional tort that may confront healthcare professionals. Palmisano's quick guide, known as the *ABCD (accept, breach, cause, damage) rule*, may be used to characterize what constitutes a credible malpractice claim: the healthcare practitioner must accept the patient, establishing a legal relationship between the 2 parties; provide less than the reasonable standard of care, indicating a breach of duty that leads to a cause, which results in a specific alleged damage.[71] Appropriate communications and documentation provide useful prophylaxis against charges of abandonment and/or malpractice (negligence).

Patient Self-Determination Act and Advance Directives

The Patient Self-Determination Act (PSDA) was passed by the US Congress in 1990 and became effective in 1991. This law requires hospitals, skilled nursing facilities, home health agencies, hospice programs, and health maintenance organizations to do the following: (1) inform patients of their rights under state law to make decisions concerning their medical care; (2) periodically inquire as to whether a patient executed an advance directive and document the patient's wishes regarding his or her medical care; (3) not discriminate against persons who have executed an advance directive; (4) ensure that legally valid advance directives and documented medical care wishes are implemented to the extent permitted by state law; and (5) provide educational programs for staff, patients, and the community on ethical issues concerning patient self-determination and advance directives.[18]

Under the PSDA, advance directives are documents that allow individuals to document their treatment preferences and identify a surrogate or proxy decision maker to act in the patient's stead when he or she loses the ability to make decisions. Use or nonuse of ANH is a component of some advance directives. An advance directive is effectuated only if and when the patient loses the capacity to make his or her own decisions.[72] In all states, court-appointed guardians for persons adjudicated as incompetent can make healthcare decisions for their wards. Increasingly, states and institutions are combining various types of directives onto a single comprehensive form.

Advance directives that specify limitations on end-of-life care have been associated with significantly lower levels of Medicare spending, reduced likelihood of in-hospital deaths, and higher use of hospice care in regions characterized by higher levels of end-of-life spending. Advance directives may be especially important for ensuring medical treatment that is consistent with patients' preferences for those individuals who prefer less aggressive treatment at the end of life but live in areas with a healthcare system that is characterized by high intensity of treatment.[73]

Unfortunately, in the United States, end-of-life care often does not reflect patients' values and preferences.[74] However, observational and interventional studies in selected patients suggest that advance directives substantially improve the patient-centered aspect of end-of-life care.[75,76] Surrogate decision makers may be reluctant to not provide aggressive medical therapies for patients and might experience substantial distress unless they are acting in accordance with an advance directive or an understanding of the patient's values. Perhaps the goal of advance care planning is not only to document the individual's treatment preferences for specific medical scenarios but also to prepare surrogates for in-the-moment decision making. The focus of such planning should include giving family members and physicians the legal tools they need to make appropriate treatment decisions for patients who lack decision-making capacity.[74]

National Healthcare Decisions Day (NHDD) is an initiative to encourage advance care planning and completion of advance directives. NHDD exists as a 50-state annual initiative to provide clear, concise, and consistent information on healthcare decision making to both the public and providers/facilities through the widespread availability and dissemination of simple, free, and uniform tools (not just forms) to guide the process. NHDD entails 50 independent, but coordinated, state and local events (necessitated by the differences in state laws and dynamics) supported by a national media and public education campaign. Additional information is available on the NHDD website, along with access to specific state advance directives.[77]

Precedent Cases

Karen Ann Quinlan

ANH has been the focus of a litany of legal decisions during recent decades. The seminal case of Karen Ann Quinlan[78] in 1976 set the stage for a cascade of additional cases, legal decisions, and statutes. Quinlan, who was 21 years old at the time of her brain injury, was in a PVS as a result of anoxic encephalopathy, rendering her ventilator dependent. Her parents, attempting to honor her previously expressed wishes, requested removal of the ventilator. The physicians caring for her were reluctant to comply, fearing criminal repercussions. The New Jersey Supreme Court ruled that the ventilator, a life-sustaining measure, could be removed if a prognosis existed of "no reasonable possibility of a patient returning to a cognitive, sapient state" and a hospital ethics committee could confirm such a conclusion. Additionally, the court provided for criminal and civil legal protection for all involved parties in the decision-making process. Interestingly, Quinlan lived without ventilator support for many years while receiving enteral feedings, which were never challenged by the healthcare team or family. The Quinlan case served as a stimulus for the establishment of hospital ethics committees and enactment of states' living will legislation.

Awareness of the vegetative state came to international prominence in this case. Fred Plum, a neurologist, served as a court-appointed expert witness and confirmed the vegetative state diagnosis. Based on his testimony, the court allowed for the removal the ventilator. Plum had done an apnea test as part of his court-sanctioned neurologic exam to assess brain stem function and differentiate the vegetative state from whole brain death. When the ventilator was removed, Quinlan survived for several years, maintaining respiration with an intact brain stem. Her survival was unexpected by individuals outside of the medical profession and points out the ethical and clinical relevance of clinicians' efforts to help manage family members' expectations about outcomes for loved ones in PVS.[79]

Nancy Cruzan

In 1983, 25-year-old Nancy Cruzan experienced an anoxic brain injury in an automobile accident.[80] A feeding tube was placed because she was unable to swallow. After she spent several years in a PVS, her parents requested permission from the courts to remove her feeding tube. The Missouri Supreme Court determined that the tube could lawfully be removed only if there was "clear and convincing evidence" that such removal was in accordance with Cruzan's wishes. Without the documentation in an advance directive, the court concluded that the relatively stringent evidential standard it had set was not met by the family's testimony that Cruzan would prefer to not receive ANH. The court required such evidence to override the state's compelling interest in preserving the life of a patient who lacked decisional capacity to make her own choices.[81]

The Cruzan family appealed the decision to the US Supreme Court, which upheld the right of states to set their own evidential standards for withdrawal of feeding tubes. Within a year of the US Supreme Court decision, additional testimony from friends of Cruzan was presented in another Missouri court, which ruled that this evidence met the Missouri criteria for clear and convincing evidence. The feeding tube was legally removed in 1990, with Cruzan dying shortly after the tube was removed.[81] Among the notable outcomes of the US Supreme Court decision are the following:

- Affirmation of the authority of individual states to establish their own standards of evidence for withdrawal of ANH
- Establishment of ANH as life-sustaining medical treatment comparable to ventilators and hemodialysis
- Greater use of healthcare proxies or durable powers of attorney for healthcare decisions and the enactment of the PDSA mandating advance directives[18,82]

Theresa Marie Schiavo

In 1990, 26-year-old Theresa Marie Schiavo went into cardiac arrest; she was given cardiopulmonary resuscitation but sustained severe brain damage. The hospital inserted a PEG tube in Schiavo, who was subsequently diagnosed as being in a PVS, and her husband, Michael, was appointed guardian. In 1998, he filed a petition to have the feeding tube removed because his wife would not wish to be maintained in a PVS. Her parents argued the opposite position, resulting in a contentious debate that spanned 2 removals and reinsertions of the feeding tube, 4 rejected appeals to the US Supreme Court, and the unprecedented intervention of the Florida legislature and governor, the US Congress, and the president. Finally, in March 2005, the federal district court refused to order reinsertion of the PEG tube for a third time, and Schiavo died soon afterward.[83]

In several states, political reaction to the Schiavo case led to the refinement of living will legislation with regards to ANH. In many instances, the forgoing of ANH in decisionally incapable patients requires clearly expressed wishes in an advance directive. This trend goes against decades of legal and ethical opinion regarding the authority of a surrogate, even without an advance directive, to make decisions about ANH.[84]

Empirical Ethics Research

Empirical research suggests that shared decision making regarding ANH, especially PEG tube placement, may not consistently meet the ethical and legal criteria discussed previously. A retrospective study of 154 hospital patients receiving PEG tubes for serious illness found that only 1 patient had a documented discussion of benefits, burdens, and risks of the tube placement, and 12 of 33 patients providing signed consent had questionable or unclear decisional capacity.[85] Callahan analyzed the decisional process in 100 patients who received PEG tubes and physicians caring for these patients.[86] Patients or surrogates reported discussing placement with multiple providers, but being given incomplete information, and physicians, patients, and families experienced considerable distress around the ANH decision. In this study, many of the people involved in the process experienced it as one of "nondecision" because alternatives were not presented, and discussion seemed to focus on short-term acuity rather than long-term functional outcomes. Physicians perceived pressures both from families and other providers to place PEG tubes.[86] In an interview-based study, 21 hospital nurses caring for patients with dementia reported that they experienced considerable moral distress related to ANH. The nurses felt conflicted because they considered the provision of nutrition, including food and water, to be part of their role, but they were often limited in their ability to influence ANH decisions.[87]

In a systematic review of the empirical evidence linking patient outcomes and shared decision making, 39 studies met the inclusion criteria. Because the number of studies was small, meta-analysis could not be done. Most of the included studies were observational in design. The patient perception that shared decision making had occurred was associated with improved affective-cognitive outcomes; however, evidence was lacking for the association between empirical measures of shared decision making and patient behavioral and health outcomes.[88]

The opinions and choices of patients about ANH have been studied. O'Brien and colleagues presented 379 randomly selected decisionally capable residents of 49 randomly selected nursing homes with a hypothetical scenario in which brain injury had damaged their ability to take oral nutrition. Initially, 33% of the participants chose ANH and approximately 5% were unsure what they would choose. After being educated that restraint might be necessary to keep the feeding tube in place, 25% of those who chose ANH or were unsure changed their preference to refuse ANH. Factors associated with desiring a feeding tube were the belief that nursing home staff would respect the choice, never having completed an advance directive or discussing healthcare preferences with family or providers, and being African-American.[89] Hoefler's 2000 review of numerous public opinion polls and scholarly studies found that most Americans did not want a feeding tube at the end of life.[90]

Ethics Committees

The Joint Commission requires that every US hospital must have an ethics committee. The composition and functions of these committees vary among institutions and states. Their composition is multidisciplinary and often includes community members and/or patient and family representatives. They may function in a transdisciplinary fashion; in other words, they may employ a strategy of healthcare providers collaborating beyond the boundaries of traditional job descriptions while remaining within their scopes of practice, licensures, or certifications.[28] The committee is responsible for promoting patient rights; developing policies and procedures and ensuring their implementation; offering continuing education to the hospital and medical staffs; integrating ethics from the bedside to the boardroom; and providing a consultation process. Usually, a referral to the committee is open to anyone in the institution, including patients and families. Referrals can be solicited whenever there is any question regarding potential conflicts in values, patient rights, shared decision making, policies and procedures, or questions of fair treatment.

Translating Ethical Decision Making for Artificial Nutrition and Hydration into Clinical Practice

Although numerous articles, book chapters, recommendations, and guidelines have been published on ethical decision making for ANH,[28,38,91-94] the application of ethical decision making to clinical practice is not optimum, in part because there is a lack of communication among patients, families, and clinicians. In some cultures, discussion of healthcare decisions during a critical illness or end of life is discouraged; sometimes, families are unable to broach the subject with the patient before the illness severity and therapies escalate. At that point, the patient may be unable to speak and express his or her wishes regarding medical interventions and a surrogate may be needed. If the subject of the patient's preferences

is not addressed before the individual reaches the hospital, healthcare providers must be prepared to advocate for patient-centered decision making in the increasingly technology-driven healthcare environment.[28]

Palliative Care as a Treatment Option

When a patient has a life-threatening illness, palliative care may be beneficial well before the end of life. Formal palliative care consults are used for situations when complex aspects of depression, anxiety, grief, or hopelessness are present.[95] Practice Scenario 39-2 provides an example of the relevance of palliative care during the decision-making process about ANH.

Practice Scenario 39-2

Question: If a decision were made to withhold enteral nutrition when a patient is unable to eat or only consume a small amount of food, is a palliative care consult still useful?

Scenario: A 75-year-old man was admitted with a massive stroke. Prior to his current illness, he had not indicated his wishes for medical therapies in an advance directive. He had a large family with children and grandchildren, and many of the family members disagreed over whether a tracheostomy should be done and a long-term enteral feeding device placed, so that he could be transferred to a long-term care facility. His oldest son decided to not move forward with the tracheostomy and percutaneous endoscopic gastrostomy tube placement.

Intervention: The primary care physician recognized early in the patient's hospitalization that the family needed extensive assistance to sift through the complex healthcare options and come to consensus about the patient's best interest. A palliative care consult was ordered.

Answer: The primary care team can provide basic palliative care for all patients or their family members so they can participate in shared decision making to identify treatment goals; however, family members may disagree with each other or with healthcare team members regarding the best options for the patient. Seamless transition to the palliative care team, if the family accepts its guidance, can help resolve conflicts regarding goals or methods of treatment within families and between staff and families.

Rationale: The palliative care team can devote the time needed for family members to come to agreement about the patient's care.

Family Meetings Regarding Nutrition Support

In complex healthcare situations, effective communication between the patient or surrogate and healthcare professionals is needed to choose therapies based on the patient's quality-of-life goals. Decisions about nutrition, even when administered through tubes, are integral and emotional issues for patients and their families. Family meetings can clarify goals of care, advance open communication with healthcare providers and other decision makers, and foster shared decision making. Sensitive discussions about benefits vs burdens and risks of the nutrition therapy can be included in these meetings. Table 39-3 provides a process for conducting fruitful family meetings that facilitate decision making about nutrition support.[95-99]

TABLE 39-3 Preparing and Conducting a Family Meeting Involving Nutrition Support

Family Meeting Sections	Meeting Components and Considerations
Premeeting with healthcare clinicians only	1. Clarify conference goals in advance; agree on medical facts and a facilitator. 2. Determine who to invite: decision maker, family members, physicians, the patient's nurse, social worker, chaplain, nutrition support clinician, and others. 3. Arrange for teleconferencing or other technology to increase participation. 4. Choose a private meeting space—ideally, a comfortable room with circular seating. 5. Plan a strategy for disclosing information.
Family meeting introduction	1. Seat participants. If possible, intersperse healthcare providers among family members. 2. Introduce all participants, discuss goals for the meeting, and assign a recorder. 3. Ask the family members to describe the patient prior to the illness/hospitalization as well as the patient's values. 4. Initiate discussion of the family's concerns, questions, and understanding of current medical status.
Main elements of family meeting	1. Provide family-centered communication: 　a. Elicit surrogates' perceptions first. 　b. Use active listening skills, and deliver information in small chunks, free of medical jargon. 　c. Respond to questions and check for understanding of key facts using the teach-back method. 　d. Assess how much the patient or family wants to know. 　e. Acknowledge and address emotion and respond empathetically to the patient's or family's feelings. 　f. Assess the patient's or family's ability to discuss bad news. 　g. Detect whether the patient or family is angry from verbal and nonverbal cues. 　h. Support religious/spiritual needs and concerns. 2. Foster shared decision making: 　a. Discuss the clinical prognosis and its degree of certainty. 　b. Evaluate surrogate preferences for decision-making responsibility. 　c. Elicit the patient's treatment preferences and health-related values. 3. Communicate evidence-based information on benefits vs risks and burdens for nutrition support therapies, as applicable. 4. Differentiate emotions about food from feelings about nutrition support as a medical therapy. 5. Affirm nonabandonment and support the patient's and family's decisions about treatment. 6. Reinforce and clarify information. Emphasize that while treatments may be modified or withdrawn, compassionate care will always be provided.
Summation of family meeting	1. Summarize consensus, disagreements, decisions, and resulting plan. 2. Explain what is going to happen next, to minimize surprises. 3. Identify a family member and a spokesperson for the transdisciplinary team who will partner for ongoing communication; exchange contact information. 4. Schedule follow-up meetings as needed. 5. Whenever possible, have the family representative sign the written plan.
Postmeeting follow-up with healthcare clinicians only	1. Evaluate the ongoing process from each clinician's perspective. 2. Determine whether changes are needed for future interactions with the patient and family. 3. Document in the chart who was present at the family meeting, decisions made, and the follow-up plan.

Source: Adapted with permission from reference 95: Schwartz DB, Olfson K, Babak B, Barrocas A, Wesley JR. Incorporating palliative care concepts into nutrition practice: across the age spectrum. *Nutr Clin Pract*. 2016;31:305–315.

FIGURE 39-4 Managing the Troubling Trichotomy

The Troubling Trichotomy

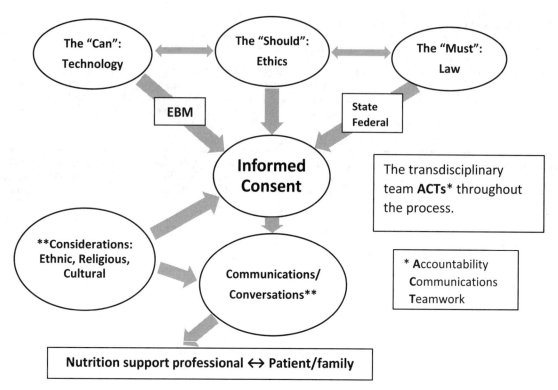

EBM, evidence-based medicine.

Summary

The focus of the chapter has been to provide nutrition support clinicians with ethically and legally sound information on the issues surrounding decision making related to ANH and how ethical conflicts might be resolved. The authors want to emphasize that optimum application of clinical ethics requires that clinicians operate according to the ACT principle (accountability, communication, and transdisciplinary teamwork) as they manage the troubling trichotomy (Figure 39-4).

References

1. Fine RL. Ethical issues in artificial nutrition and hydration. *Nutr Clin Pract.* 2006;21:118–125.
2. Schwartz DB, Posthauer ME, O'Sullivan Maillet. J. Practice paper of Academy of Nutrition and Dietetics: ethical and legal issues of feeding and hydration. June 2013. http://www.eatrightpro.org/resource/practice/position-and-practice-papers/practice-papers/practice-paper-ethical-and-legal-issues-in-feeding-and-hydration. Accessed February 4, 2017.
3. Geppert CMA, Andrews MR, Druyan ME. Ethical issues in artificial nutrition and hydration: a review. *JPEN J Parenter Enteral Nutr.* 2010;34:79–88.
4. Schwartz DB, Barrocas A, Wesley JR, et al. A.S.P.E.N. special report: gastrostomy tube placement in patients with advanced dementia or near end of life. *Nutr Clin Pract.* 2014;29:829–840.
5. Barrocas A. Nutrition support and the troubling trichotomy: a call to action. *Nutr Clin Pract.* 2006;21(2):109–112.
6. Barrocas A, Cohen ML. Have the answers to the common legal questions concerning nutrition support changed over the past decade? 10 questions for 10 years. *Nutr Clin Pract.* 2016;31(3):285–294.
7. Barrocas A. The troubling trichotomy 10 years later: where are we now? *Nutr Clin Pract.* 2016;31(3):295–304.
8. Brody H, Hermer LD, Scott LD, et al. Artificial nutrition and hydration: the evolution of ethics, evidence, and policy. *J Gen Intern Med.* 2011;26(9):1053–1058.
9. Barrocas A, Yarbrough G, Becnel PA, et al. Ethical and legal issues in nutrition support of the geriatric patient: the can, should, and must of nutrition support. *Nutr Clin Pract.* 2003;18(1):37–47.
10. Sabatino C. Myths and facts about health care advance directives. *Bifocal.* 2015;37(1):19–21. www.americanbar.org/publications/bifocal/vol_37/issue_1_october2015/myths_and_facts_advance_directives.html. Accessed February 2, 2017.
11. O'Sullivan Maillet J, Schwartz DB, Posthauer ME. Position of the Academy of Nutrition and Dietetics: ethical and legal issues of feeding and hydration. *J Acad Nutr Diet.* 2013;113;828–833.
12. Ethical foundations of clinical practice. In: Post LF, Blustein J, Dubler NN, eds. *Handbook for Health Care Ethics Committees.* Baltimore, MD: Johns Hopkins University Press; 2007:11–22.

13. Carbone ET, Zoellner JM. Nutrition and health literacy: a systematic review to inform nutrition research and practice. *J Acad Nutr Diet.* 2012;112:254–265.

14. Lo B. An approach to ethical dilemmas in patient care. In: *Resolving Ethical Dilemmas: A Guide for Clinicians.* 4th ed. Philadelphia, PA: Lippincott Williams & Wilkins; 2010:3–10.

15. Mirel M, Hartjes T. Bringing palliative care to the surgical intensive care unit. *Crit Care Nurs.* 2013;33:71–74.

16. Ruben DB, Tinetti ME. Goal-oriented patient care–an alternative health outcomes paradigm. *New Engl J Med.* 2012;366:777–779.

17. Barry MJ, Edgman-Levitan S. Shared decision making–the pinnacle of patient-centered care. *N Engl J Med.* 2012;366:780–781.

18. H.R.4449: Patient Self-Determination Act of 1990. www.congress .gov/bill/101st-congress/house-bill/4449. Accessed February 2, 2017.

19. National POLST Paradigm. www.polst.org. Accessed February 2, 2017.

20. Epstein EG. Preventive ethics in the intensive care unit. *AACN Adv Crit Care.* 2012;23:217–224.

21. Weiss BD. *Health Literacy and Patient Safety: Help Patients Understand—Manual for Clinicians.* 2nd ed. American Medical Association Foundation. May 2007. med.fsu.edu/userFiles/file/ahec _health_clinicians_manual.pdf. Accessed February 2, 2017.

22. Ferrie S. A quick guide to ethical theory in healthcare: solving ethical dilemmas in nutrition support situations. *Nutr Clin Pract.* 2006;21(2):113–117.

23. Beauchamp TL, Childress JF. *Principles of Biomedical Ethics.* 6th ed. New York: Oxford University Press; 2009.

24. Kant I. The Philosophy of Kant: Immanuel Kant's Moral and Political Writings. Friedrich CJ, ed. New York: Modern Library; 1949.

25. Burtt EA, ed. *The English Philosophers from Bacon to Mill.* New York: Random House; 1939.

26. Aristotle. *The Ethics of Aristotle: The Nicomachean Ethics.* Thomson JAK, trans. New York: Penguin Books; 1976.

27. Appelbaum PS. Clinical practice. Assessment of patients' competence to consent to treatment. *N Engl J Med.* 2007;357(18): 1834–1840.

28. Barrocas A, Schwartz DB. Ethical considerations in nutrition support in critical care. In: Seres DS, Van Way CW, eds. *Nutrition Support for the Critically Ill.* Basel, Switzerland: Springer International; 2016:195–227.

29. Ganzini L, Volicer L, Nelson WA, et al. Ten myths about decision-making capacity. *J Am Med Dir Assoc.* 2004;5(4):263–267.

30. Rao JK, Anderson LA, Lin FC, Laux JP. Completion of advance directives among U.S. consumers. *Am J Prev Med.* 2014;46(1):65–70. doi:10.1016/j.amepre.2013.09.008.

31. Default Surrogate Consent Statues. http://www.americanbar .org/content/dam/aba/administrative/law_aging/2014_default _surrogate_consent_statutes.authcheckdam.pdf. Accessed February 4, 2017.

32. DuVal G, Sartorius L, Clarridge B, et al. What triggers requests for ethics consultations? *J Med Ethics.* 2001;27(Suppl 1):i24–i29.

33. Sulmasy DP, Snyder L. Substituted interests and best judgments: an integrated model of surrogate decision making. *JAMA.* 2010;304(17):1946–1947.

34. *In re Conroy,* 486 A. 2d 1209 (1985).

35. President's Commission for the Study of Ethical Problems in Medicine and Biomedical and Behavioral Research. *Deciding to Forego Life-Sustaining Treatment: Ethical, Medical and Legal Issues in Treatment Decisions.* Washington, DC: US Government Printing Office; 1983.

36. Monturo C. The artificial nutrition debate: still an issue... after all these years. *Nutr Clin Pract.* 2009;24(2):206–213.

37. Bayer W, Mallinger JB, Krishman A, Shields CG. Attitudes toward life-sustaining interventions among ambulatory black and white patients. *Ethn Dis.* 2006;16:914–919.

38. Schwartz DB. Ethical considerations in the critically ill patient. In: Cresci G, ed. *Nutrition Support for the Critically Ill Patient: A Guide to Practice.* 2nd ed. Boca Raton, FL: Taylor & Francis; 2015:635–652.

39. Gebara J, Tashjian H. End-of-life practices at a Lebanese hospital: courage or knowledge? *J Transcultural Nurs.* 2006;17:381–388.

40. Phipps E, True G, Harris D, et al. Approaching the end of life: attitudes, preferences, and behaviors of African-American and white patients and their family caregivers. *J Clin Oncol.* 2003;21:549–554.

41. Torke AM, Garas NS, Sexson W, Branch WT. Medical care at the end of life: views of African American patients in an urban hospital. *J Palliat Med.* 2005;8:593–602.

42. Volandes AE, Paasche-Orlow M, Gillick MR, et al. Health literacy not race predicts end-of-life care preferences. *J Palliat Med.* 2008;11:754–762.

43. Searight HR, Gafford J. Cultural diversity at the end of life: issues and guidelines for family physicians. *Am Fam Physician.* 2005; 71:515–522.

44. Preedy VR, ed. *Diet and Nutrition in Palliative Care.* Boca Raton, FL: CRC Press; 2011.

45. United States Conference of Catholic Bishops. *Ethical and Religious Directives.* 5th ed. 2009. http://www.usccb.org/issues-and -action/human-life-and-dignity/health-care/upload/Ethical -Religious-Directives-Catholic-Health-Care-Services-fifth-edition -2009.pdf. Accessed May 6, 2017.

46. Kelley AS, Wenger NS, Sarkisian CA. Opiniones: end-of-life care preferences and planning of older Latinos. *J Am Geratr Soc.* 2010;58:1109–1116.

47. Berry P, Griffie J. Planning for the actual death. In: Ferrell BR, Coyle N, Paice JA, eds. *Oxford Textbook of Palliative Nursing.* 4th ed. New York: Oxford University Press; 2015:515–530.

48. Printz LA. Is withholding hydration a valid comfort measure in the terminally ill: *Geriatrics.* 1988;43(11):84–88.

49. Raijmakers NJH, van Zuylen L, Costantini M, et al. Artificial nutrition and hydration in the last week of life in cancer patients: a systematic literature review of practices and effects. *Ann Oncol.* 2011;22(7):1478–1486. doi:10.1093/annonc/mdq620.

50. Curtis JR, Levine S, Rocker G, et al, eds. *The Hospice and Palliative Medicine Approach to Selected Chronic Illnesses: Dementia, COPD, and CHF.* 3rd ed. Glenview, IL: American Academy of Hospice and Palliative Medicine; 2008.

51. Wolfson C, Wolfson DB, Asgharian M, et al. A reevaluation of the duration of survival after the onset of dementia. *N Engl J Med.* 2001;344(15):1111–1116.

52. Chernoff R. Tube feeding patients with dementia. *Nutr Clin Pract.* 2006;21(2):142–146.

53. Li I. Feeding tubes in patients with severe dementia. *Am Fam Physician.* 2002;65(8):1605–1610,1615.

54. Cervo FA, Bryan L, Farber S. To PEG or not to PEG: a review of evidence for placing feeding tubes in advanced dementia and the decision-making process. *Geriatrics.* 2006;61(6):30–35.

55. Gillick MR. Rethinking the role of tube feeding in patients with advanced dementia. *N Engl J Med.* 2000;342(3):206–210.

56. Meier DE, Ahronheim JC, Morris J, et al. High short-term mortality in hospitalized patients with advanced dementia: lack of benefit of tube feeding. *Arch Intern Med.* 2001;161(4):594–599.

57. Murphy LM, Lipman TO. Percutaneous endoscopic gastrostomy does not prolong survival in patients with dementia. *Arch Intern Med.* 2003;163(11):1351–1353.

58. Shega JW, Hougham GW, Stocking CB, et al. Barriers to limiting the practice of feeding tube placement in advanced dementia. *J Palliat Med.* 2003;6(6):885–893.

59. Vitale CA, Hiner T, Ury WA, et al. Tube feeding in advanced dementia: an exploratory survey of physician knowledge. *Care Manag J.* 2006;7(2):79–85.

60. Monti MM, Vanhaudenhuyse A, Coleman MR, et al. Willful modulation of brain activity in disorders of consciousness. *N Engl J Med.* 2010;362(7):579–589.

61. Jennett B, Plum F. Persistent vegetative state after brain damage. A syndrome in search of a name. *Lancet.* 1972;1(7753):734.

62. The Multi-Society Task Force on PVS. Medical aspects of the persistent vegetative state (1). *N Engl J Med.* 1994;330(21):1499–1508.

63. The Multi-Society Task Force on PVS. Medical aspects of the persistent vegetative state (2). *N Engl J Med.* 1994;330(22):1572–1579.

64. Giacino JT, Ashwal S, Childs N, et al. The minimally conscious state: definition and diagnostic criteria. *Neurology.* 2002;58:349–353.

65. Laureys S, Faymonville ME, Peigneux P, et al. Cortical processing of noxious somatosensory stimuli in the persistent vegetative state. *Neuroimage.* 2002;17(2):732–741.

66. Laureys S. Functional neuroimaging in the vegetative state. *Neurorehabilitation.* 2004;19(4):335–341.

67. Ropper AH. Cogito ergo sum by MRI. *N Engl J Med.* 2010;362(7):648–649.

68. Billings JA, Churchill LR, Payne R. Severe brain injury and the subjective life. *Hastings Cent Rep.* 2010;40(3):17–21.

69. Schnakers C, Vanhaudenhuyse A, Giacino J, et al. Diagnostic accuracy of the vegetative and minimally conscious state: clinical consensus versus standardized neurobehavioral assessment. *BMC Neurology.* 2009;9:35. doi:10.1186/1471-2377-9-35.

70. Bender A, Jox RJ, Grill E, Straube A, Lulé D. Persistent vegetative state and minimally conscious state—a systematic review and meta-analysis of diagnostic procedures. *Dtsch Arztebl Int.* 2015;112:235–242. doi:10.3238/arztebl.2015.0235.

71. Palmisano DJ. Malpractice prophylaxis: overview of the law and definitions. *Capsules.* 1983;6:2–5.

72. Tulsky JA. Beyond advance directives: importance of communication skills at the end of life. *JAMA.* 2005;294(3):359–365.

73. Nicholas LH, Langa KM, Iwashyna TJ, et al. Regional variation in the association between advance directives and end-of-life Medicare expenditures. *JAMA.* 2011;306(13);1447–1453.

74. White DB, Arnold RM. The evolution of advance directives. *JAMA.* 2011;306(13):1485–1486.

75. Silveira MJ, Kim SY, Langa KM. Advance directives and outcomes of surrogate decision making before death. *N Engl J Med.* 2010;362(13);1211–1218.

76. Detering KM, Hancock AD, Reade MC, et al. The impact of advance care planning on end of life care in elderly patients: randomised controlled trial. *BMJ.* 2010;340:c1345.

77. National Healthcare Decisions Day website: http://www.nhdd.org. Accessed May 6, 2017.

78. In re Quinlan, 355 A.2d 647(70 N.J. 10 1976).

79. Fins JJ. Neuroethics and disorders of consciousness: discerning brain states in clinical practice and research. *AMA J Ethics.* 2016;18(12):1182–1191. doi:10.1001/journalofethics.2016.18.12.ecas2-1612.

80. Cruzan v. Director Missouri Department of Health, 497 261 (1990).

81. Pence GE. *Classic Cases in Medical Ethics.* 5th ed. Boston, MA: McGraw-Hill; 2008.

82. Omnibus Reconciliation Act of 1990. Vol 101-508: Pub. L; 1990.

83. Barrocas A, Bivona B, Schwartz DB. Medical, ethical, legal aspects. In: Buchman AL, ed. *Clinical Nutrition in Gastrointestinal Disease.* Thorofare, NJ: Slack; 2006.

84. Jonsen AR, Seigler M, Winslade WJ. *Clinical Ethics: A Practical Approach to Ethical Decisions in Clinical Medicine.* 7th ed. New York: McGraw-Hill; 2010.

85. Brett AS, Rosenberg JC. The adequacy of informed consent for placement of gastrostomy tubes. *Arch Intern Med.* 2001;161(5):745–748.

86. Callahan CM, Haag KM, Buchanan NN, et al. Decision-making for percutaneous endoscopic gastrostomy among older adults in a community setting. *J Am Geriatr Soc.* 1999;47(9):1105–1109.

87. Bryon E, Dierckx DECB, Gastmans C. "Because we see them naked"— nurses' experiences in caring for hospitalized patients with dementia: considering artificial nutrition or hydration (ANH). *Bioethics.* 2012;26(6):285–295. doi:10.1111/j.1467-8519.2010.01875.x.

88. Shay LA, Lafata JE. Where is the evidence? A systematic review of shared decision making and patient outcomes. *Med Decis Making.* 2015;35(1):114–131. doi:10.1177/0272989X14551638.

89. O'Brien LA, Siegert EA, Grisso JA, et al. Tube feeding preferences among nursing home residents. *J Gen Intern Med.* 1997;12(6):364–371.

90. Hoefler JM. Making decisions about tube feeding for severely demented patients at the end of life: clinical, legal, and ethical considerations. *Death Stud.* 2000;24(3):233–254.

91. Barrocas A, Geppert C, Durfee SM, et al. A.S.P.E.N. ethics position paper. *Nutr Clin Pract.* 2010;25(6):672–679.

92. Schwartz DB. Ethical and legal issues in gastrointestinal nutrition interventions. In: Matarese LE, Mullin G, Raymond J, eds. *The Health Professional's Guide to Gastrointestinal Nutrition.* Chicago, IL: Academy of Nutrition and Dietetics; 2014:333–344.

93. Schwartz DB. Applying dietetics practitioner's code of ethics to ethical decisions for withholding/withdrawing medically assisted nutrition and hydration. *J Acad Nutr Diet.* 2015;115:440–443.

94. Schwartz DB, Armanios N, Cheryl M, et al. Clinical ethics and nutrition support practice: implications for practice change and curriculum development. *J Acad Nutr Diet.* 2016;116:1738–1746.

95. Schwartz DB, Olfson K, Babak B, Barrocas A, Wesley JR. Incorporating palliative care concepts into nutrition practice: across the age spectrum. *Nutr Clin Pract.* 2016;31:305–315.

96. Lang F, Quill T. Making decisions with families at the end of life. *Am Fam Physician.* 2004;70(4):719–723.

97. Shaw DJ, Davidson JE, Smilde RI, Sondoozi T, Agan D. Multidisciplinary team training to enhance family communication in the ICU. *Crit Care Med.* 2014;42:265–271.

98. Oncotalk. Conducting a family conference. Medical Oncology Communication Skills Training Learning Modules. 2002. depts.washington.edu/oncotalk/learn/modules/Modules_06.pdf. Accessed February 4, 2017.

99. Bosslet GR, Pope TM, Rubenfeld GD, et al; American Thoracic Society Ad Hoc Committee on Futile and Potentially Inappropriate Treatment. An official ATS/AACN/ACCP/ESICM/SCCM policy statement: responding to requests for potentially inappropriate treatments in intensive care units. *Am J Respir Crit Care Med.* 2015;191:1318–1330.

40 Quality Improvement in Clinical Practice

Kristen Mathieson, MBA, RD, CDN, and E. Annelie M. Vogt, DCN, RD, LDN, CSO, CNSC

CONTENTS

Acknowledgment: Naomi E. Cahill, RD, MSc, was the author of this chapter for the second edition.

Objectives

1. Define quality improvement (QI) and its importance in healthcare.
2. Identify quality standards developed and governed by interdisciplinary organizations and regulatory agencies.
3. Discuss quality indicators and the necessity of benchmarking practices in today's healthcare environment.
4. Describe methods for improving nutrition outcomes in the clinical setting.

Test Your Knowledge Questions

1. What is the main difference between a QI project and a clinical outcomes research project?
   A. QI intends to improve generalizable knowledge, whereas outcomes research aims to improve clinical performance.
   B. QI intends to answer a clinical question, whereas outcomes research aims to improve a procedure.
   C. QI intends to improve a process, whereas outcomes research aims to test a hypothesis.
   D. QI intends to produce a publishable manuscript, whereas outcomes research aims to improve system performance.

2. Which of the following is the best example of a QI project?
   A. A randomized controlled trial to evaluate the impact of an enteral nutrition (EN) protocol
   B. A clinical audit to assess the appropriateness of parenteral nutrition (PN) ordering
   C. A needs assessment of patients' compliance with home PN guidelines
   D. A prospective study to assess hold times for EN caused by high gastric residual volumes in enterally fed patients

3. Which of the following best represents a quality indicator for assessing the appropriateness of ordering PN?
   A. The prevalence of central line infections in the study population
   B. The total number of patients who received PN
   C. The mortality rate in the population
   D. The proportion of patients with a contraindication to EN

Test Your Knowledge Answers

1. The correct answer is **C**. The goal of QI is to improve a process, a program, a system, or the performance of an individual practitioner by comparing current processes, programs, systems, or performances with a set of published standards for use within that facility or system. Clinical outcomes research, on the other hand, aims to answer a clinical question and test hypotheses to improve knowledge and produce a peer-reviewed publication.

2. The correct answer is **B**. Randomized controlled trials and prospective studies aim to test hypotheses to produce generalizable knowledge and are clinical outcomes research. A needs assessment can be a quality or research project. A clinical audit may be completed before and during a QI project to assess the baseline and progress with the change measure.

3. The correct answer is **D**. Quality indicators are objective metrics by which quality of care and professional performance can be assessed. These indicators allow for continuous improvement of processes, procedures, and clinical outcomes. Nutrition indicators can be derived from published guidelines and standards, the Joint Commission's National Patient Safety Goals (NPSGs); the Institute of Medicine (IOM; now known as Health and Medicine Division of the National Academies of Science) quality aims; treatment or patient outcomes; or by facility consensus. All answers to the question could be used as quality indicators, but, in this scenario, the most appropriate metric to measure appropriate ordering of PN would align with guidelines stating that PN is indicated when EN is contraindicated.

Background

Modern monitoring of quality of healthcare developed out of business and industrial initiatives during the 20th century that recognized that unexplained variation diminishes quality; and streamlined production and continuous improvement lead to systems change.[1,2] To develop strategies to improve patient safety and quality in US healthcare facilities, the National Coalition on Health Care commissioned the IOM in the late 1990s to evaluate the status quo of quality in healthcare on a national level. The result was a series of government reports[3-5] detailing the current state of healthcare quality and the need for healthcare reform. Reporting of quality measures has become an integral component of today's healthcare to increase transparency, demonstrate favorable patient outcomes with medical interventions, and receive ratings of services that are tied to payer systems; however, defining quality of care remains inherently difficult due to the intricacy of its parts. Selected definitions of quality are presented in Table 40-1.[4,6-8] Ultimately, providing high-quality care involves incorporating

TABLE 40-1 Selected Definitions of Quality

Source	Definition
Institute of Medicine[4]	The degree to which health services for individuals and population increase the likelihood of desired health outcomes and are consistent with current professional knowledge
Academy of Nutrition and Dietetics[6]	A systematic process with identified leadership, accountability, and dedicated resources for the purpose of meeting or exceeding established professional standards
Lynn et al[7]	Systematic, data-guided activities designed to bring about immediate improvements in healthcare delivery in particular settings
Batalden and Davidoff[8]	The combined and unceasing efforts of everyone—healthcare professionals, patients and their families, researchers, payers, planners and educators—to make the changes that will lead to better patient outcomes (health), better system performance (care), and better professional development (learning)

FIGURE 40-1 Donabedian Model of the Dimensions of Quality Relating to Nutrition Care

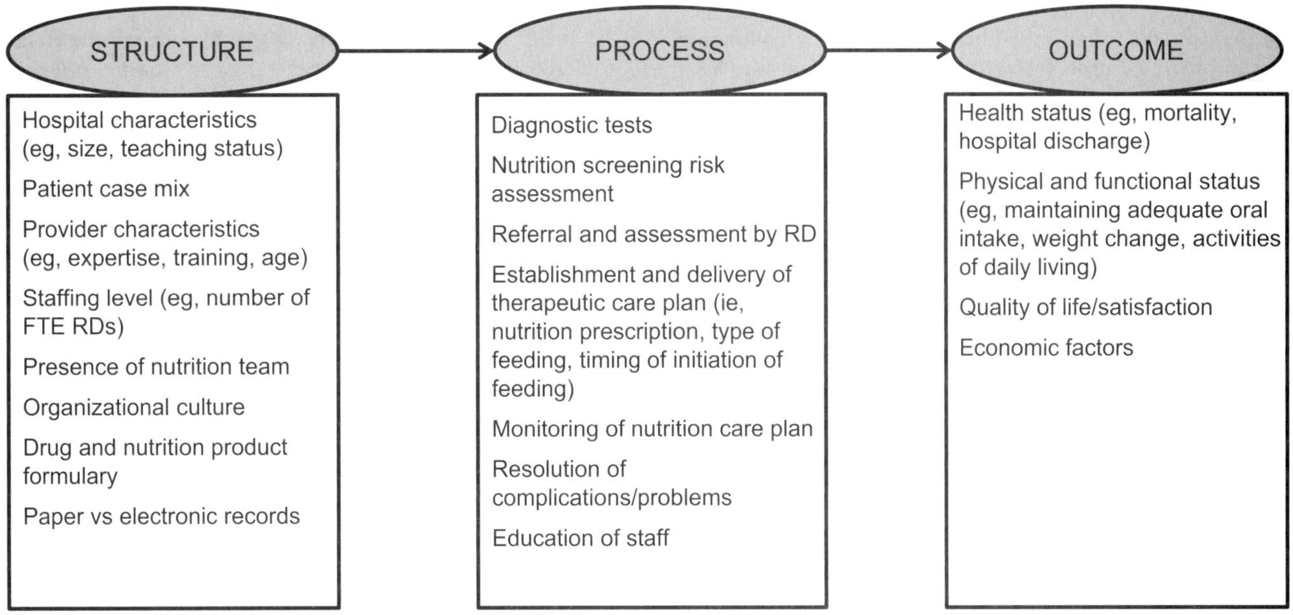

FTE, full-time equivalent; RD, registered dietitian.

the 6 dimensions of care: safety, timeliness, effectiveness, efficiency, equitability, and patient-centeredness.[4]

A framework for describing the dimensions of quality of healthcare first presented by Donabedian[9] involves 3 interdependent dimensions: structure, process, and outcomes (Figure 40-1). This framework represents the most basic model for accomplishing QI. Applied to clinical nutrition, *structure* can be described as providers, facilities and technology; *process* as nutrition screening, assessment, and follow up; and *outcome* as the end result of care.

QI projects can be initiated when clinical audits demonstrate trends or practice gaps, and they often rely on a clinician's experience to interpret or implement practice changes.[7] Chelluri,[2] Lynn et al,[7] and McDowell[10] suggest that QI projects be incorporated into policies, procedures, and performance evaluations to demonstrate their importance to healthcare professionals while involving the appropriate stakeholders and providing support for successful completion.[2,7] The incorporation of continuous QI measures into practice can improve patient outcomes, practitioner performance, and systems function, resulting in enhanced quality of care.[8] Examples of QI projects include implementation of evidence-based protocols, the use of care bundles and order sets to increase quality of care and reduce cost, refinement of practices and procedures to reduce patient admissions, and execution of strategies to improve patients' quality of life.[11]

Importance of Improving Quality of Care

QI is an essential component of healthcare that can result in delivery of consistent, effective, safe, and patient-centered care.[12] Despite significant national resources devoted to QI,

quality of healthcare remains inconsistent across the United States.[13-15] The IOM reports[3,4] and subsequent research have compiled an increasing amount of evidence of the serious national shortcomings regarding quality and safety, such as incidents of vascular and enteral tube misconnections, avoidable surgeries, inadequate disease and infection prevention strategies, avoidable exacerbations of chronic conditions, and long delays in the translation of evidence into practice.[4,7] Inconsistencies in quality are in part related to the complexity of healthcare, which reflects a wide diversity of values and beliefs and involves interactions among patients, families, and clinicians; logistical coordination among communities, healthcare facilities, and insurer and payer organizations; and legal and technological challenges. Bridging the gap between analytic frameworks and clinical practice is important to optimize patient outcomes, control cost, and achieve improvements in quality of care.[16] Publicly available reports detailing the quality of healthcare in local facilities help consumers make informed decisions about where to access healthcare. Objective metrics regarding healthcare quality are also necessary for local and national policy decisions, to prevent or reduce errors, and to identify the most cost-effective care as well as areas needing improvement.[17,18] Practitioner competence governed by healthcare facilities and accreditation organizations is further measured within the continuum of QI.[7]

Quality Improvement vs Outcomes Research

QI projects are an increasingly accepted part of healthcare, and clarification of the differences between quality management and outcomes research is warranted.[11,12] Two major differences are their goals and the processes of ethical review.

Goals

The goal of QI is to improve a process, a program, a system, or the performance of an individual practitioner by comparing current processes, programs, systems, or performances to a set of published standards for use within the facility or system. In contrast, clinical research aims to answer a clinical question and test hypotheses to improve knowledge and produce a peer-reviewed publication. According to the Common Rule,[19] clinical research is defined as "a systematic investigation, including research development, testing, and evaluation, designed to develop or contribute to generalizable knowledge."

Ethical Review Process

There is currently no established framework or process for ethical review of QI projects comparable to the federally mandated institutional review board (IRB) that reviews and approves formally submitted research projects. The IRB process through which research projects gain generalizable knowledge is rigid, time-consuming and ill-fitted for the continuously changing quality management process designed to produce immediate improvements locally.[7] However, because QI projects can include vulnerable populations, it is reasonable to expect that the ethical implications regarding such efforts will be carefully considered, especially when research and quality projects overlap.[12] For example, a project that involves an assessment of practices to improve care at a local facility is QI, whereas a comparison of delivery of nutrition support with and without a protocol could be both QI and research and might require IRB approval.[7,12] Refer to Practice Scenario 40-1 for an example of a QI project regarding nutrition support in a hospital setting.[20,21]

Practice Scenario 40-1

Question: How can we improve the appropriateness of referrals of parenteral nutrition (PN) in our hospital?

Scenario: The clinical nutrition manager noticed an increase in the number of referrals for PN that did not meet criteria provided in the American Society for Parenteral and Enteral Nutrition (ASPEN) guidelines.

Intervention: A clinical audit of current practices for initiating PN and comparison of those practices to the ASPEN clinical guidelines was conducted.

Answer: The clinical nutrition manager completed a retrospective chart review of 30 patients who received PN during the previous 3 months to evaluate decisions to initiate PN. The results were compared to guidelines about when it is appropriate to initiate PN from the ASPEN standards for nutrition support in adult hospitalized patients[20] and the Joint ASPEN/Society of Critical Care Medicine (SCCM) guidelines for the provision and assessment of nutrition support therapy in the adult critically ill patient.[21] According to the ASPEN standards,[20] PN is appropriately ordered when enteral nutrition (EN) is contraindicated, or the patient is receiving inadequate nutrition from EN. Furthermore, the joint ASPEN/

SCCM guidelines[21] state that PN should be initiated early in high-risk or poorly nourished patients when EN is not feasible or adequate. Of the 30 patients in the chart review who received PN, 10 orders (33%) were inappropriate because the patients (1) had a functioning gastrointestinal tract, (2) were receiving adequate nutrition from EN, (3) were well nourished, or (4) were assessed to be at moderate or low nutrition risk. The results were presented to the pharmacy manager and the Pharmacy and Therapeutics committee members, along with recommendations to revise current policies, train the pertinent staff on appropriate ordering of PN, and initiate twice weekly interdisciplinary rounds to discuss cases. As a result, the PN order form and policies regarding initiation of PN were revised, medical staff was trained, and twice weekly interdisciplinary rounds were initiated. During a postintervention clinical audit of 30 patients' charts, the clinical nutrition manager demonstrated that PN was appropriately ordered in 100% of patients. To continuously monitor this process, the team decided to conducts clinical audits of ordering practices on a quarterly basis.

Rationale: Inappropriate use of PN can result in increased costs. By comparing current practices to published guidelines, a gap in practice and need for improvement was established. The ASPEN Standards for Nutrition Support in Adult Hospitalized Patients[20] state that the route selected to provide nutrition support must be appropriate to the patient's medical condition, and PN should only be used if there is a contraindication to EN (eg, intestinal, obstruction, ileus, peritonitis, bowel ischemia, or intractable vomiting and diarrhea), or if the provision of EN is inadequate due to intolerance. The joint ASPEN/SCCM guidelines[21] state that PN should be initiated early for high-risk or poorly nourished patients when EN is not a viable or adequate option. Comparing these standards to current practices is an accepted way to improve quality of care.

To adequately address ethical issues of QI projects, Lynn et al[7] and Ogrinc et al[12] suggest forming local QI IRBs, using checklists to differentiate between research and QI, and obtaining informed consent for participation in routine, minimal risk activities; these procedures can allow flexibility and immediate integration of changes into practice and address the ethical implications of patient participation. Lynn et al[7] argue that informed consent should acknowledge that participation is less risky than introducing changes without monitoring effects or allowing safety or quality deficits to remain in place. These authors further suggest that patients have a responsibility to participate in QI efforts if they are to reap the benefits of improvements.[7] However, introducing more bureaucracy into the QI process is likely to reduce timeliness of implementation while increasing cost.[7]

When considering whether to seek IRB approval of a QI project, project leaders must consider whether they want to publish the results. Journals may require IRB approval for publication, or editors unfamiliar with the QI process may reject manuscripts about QI projects that were not ethically or legally required to have IRB approval.[7] The result may be decreased dissemination of knowledge regarding QI processes for the benefit of other facilities, and diminished healthcare quality as a whole.

Quality Standards and Regulatory Considerations

Standards of Professional Practice

Standards of professional practice developed by national and international professional groups and associations clarify the specific roles, responsibilities, and scope of practice for various practitioners at every level of experience and expertise. These standards are not to be used as a substitute for the use of ethical and clinical judgment by the healthcare professional; rather, they are used in conjunction with the practitioner's judgment. To continually drive growth, both clinically and professionally, standards of professional practice are updated on a regular basis as new research is released.

ASPEN and the Academy of Nutrition and Dietetics (AND) jointly published the Standards of Practice and the Standards of Professional Performance for Registered Dietitians in Nutrition Support.[22] Last updated in 2014, these guidelines (Table 40-2) are to be used by dietitians in daily practice to consistently improve and appropriately provide safe, efficient, and effective nutrition support therapy. Several organizations, such as the Health and Medical Division (formerly IOM) of the National Academies of Sciences, have taken standards of professional practice to the next level by creating clinical practice guidelines to help translate the complexity of scientific research into clear recommendations for practice that can potentially enhance healthcare quality and outcomes.[23]

All healthcare professionals should regularly take part in outcomes monitoring and QI projects. Clinicians at any level of expertise may take the lead to initiate quality monitoring, and every professional should understand how his or her practice fits into ongoing QI at the institutional level.

ASPEN Nutrition Care Process

The ASPEN Nutrition Care Process is designed to improve the consistency and quality of patient's nutrition care.[22] The Nutrition Care Process is comprised of 4 steps: nutrition assessment; diagnosis; intervention; and monitoring and evaluation. Nutrition assessment is a systematic process of obtaining, verifying, and interpreting data to make decisions about the nature of nutrition-related problems a patient may be experiencing. Typically, nutrition assessments are initiated either by referral or by screening for potential nutrition risk factors. Through assessing a patient's nutrition status and history, a specific nutrition problem becomes evident and, from here, a plan of care, including a proposed nutrition intervention and the desired outcome, is developed by the interdisciplinary team to appropriately address the current issue. Nutrition interventions should be individualized to the patient and developed with the intent to change a specific nutrition-related behavior, risk factor, or environmental condition. Through monitoring and evaluating whether the interventions produced desired outcomes, nutrition support clinicians can decide to continue or revise the plan of care.

The 4 steps of the Nutrition Care Process can be initiated and implemented by any qualified nutrition support professional, including a registered dietitian, pharmacist, nurse, physician, or another licensed practitioner. An interdisciplinary team approach has been shown to enhance the overall quality of care, improve patient safety and patient outcomes, and reduce healthcare costs, and, as testimony to the continued high quality of nutrition interventions provided by nutrition support teams, the American Medical Association has announced and recognized the value of their role for positive patient outcomes.[24,25] The ASPEN Nutrition Care Process outlines the basic steps for providing nutrition care to the hospitalized patient; however, the process should ultimately be used in conjunction with other institution and regulatory standards for documentation. In monitoring the effectiveness of the nutrition interventions provided, nutrition support clinicians may need to participate and implement process improvement strategies to improve their practice in a continuous effort to provide optimal patient care.

TABLE 40-2 ASPEN/AND Standards of Practice and Standards of Professional Performance for the Registered Dietitians in Nutrition Support

- RDs electing to practice in nutrition support are to achieve at least three of the following qualifications: (1) Certification by NBNSC, (2) formal education/training/continuing professional education in nutrition support, (3) minimum of 30% professional practice time devoted to the practice of nutrition support, (4) participation in health care institution's nutrition support activities, or (5) membership in professional societies devoted to nutrition support.
- RDs in nutrition support are also expected do the following:
  - Conduct a self-assessment of appropriate skills and knowledge to provide safe and effective nutrition support therapy for their level of practice (competent, proficient, or expert).
  - Identify the competencies needed (education/knowledge, experience, and abilities) to provide nutrition support therapy to patients in a variety of settings.
  - Provide a foundation for public accountability.
  - Assist management in the planning of services and resources.
  - Enhance professional identity and communicate the nature of dietetics.
  - Guide the development of nutrition support therapy–related dietetics education programs, job descriptions, and career pathways.

AND, Academy of Nutrition and Dietetics; ASPEN, American Society for Parenteral and Enteral Nutrition; NBNSC, National Board of Nutrition Support Certification; RD, registered dietitian.
Source: Data are from reference 22.

Federal, State, and Local Regulations

Nutrition care, like all healthcare, is governed by specific laws and regulations set in place to help ensure the best and safest care for all patients. At a federal level, the Centers for Medicare and Medicaid Services (CMS) has developed conditions of participation and provides interpretive guidelines as instructions for areas that require compliance. States and some localities also regulate nutrition care. Therefore, although a specific institution may have protocols and procedures in place, clinicians must remember to follow the most stringent applicable regulation. This point is particularly important for clinicians practicing in multiple states where licensing and credentialing laws may vary.

Joint Commission Standards

Standards set by CMS, the Joint Commission, and other organizations define the parameters of compliance within the hospital setting. Regular monitoring and evaluation are encouraged to ensure compliance.

Provisions of Care and Elements of Performance

In 1995, the Joint Commission, ASPEN, the American Society of Nutrition, and AND came together to develop survey accreditation standards that emphasize the interdisciplinary delivery of nutrition care and require that all patients have a nutrition screening completed within 24 hours of admission.[26] The following Joint Commission provisions of care (PCs) and elements of performance (EPs) were developed as a result:[27]

- PC.01.02.01: "The hospital assesses and reassesses its patients."
  - EP 2: "The hospital defines, in writing, criteria that identify when additional, specialized, or more in-depth assessments are performed."
  - EP 3: "The hospital has defined criteria that identify when nutritional plans are developed."
- PC.01.02.03: "The hospital assesses and reassesses the patient and his or her condition according to defined time frames."
  - EP 7: "The hospital completes a nutritional screening (when warranted by the patient's needs or condition) within 24 hours after inpatient admission."

When regular monitoring and evaluation indicate that a certain quality measure (such as nutrition screening) is below benchmark for the institution, QI/performance improvement programs should be initiated to analyze and change processes to provide the best and safest care for all patients.

The Joint Commission periodically evaluates the necessity of the numerous standards it governs. As of July 1, 2016, the Joint Commission had deemed that 131 EPs were no longer necessary to assess quality and patient safety because they (1) had become a routine part of hospital operations and clinical care processes, (2) duplicated other existing EPs, or (3) are adequately addressed by external laws or regulations.[28] With this change, PC 01.02.03 EP 7, related to nutrition screening,

was removed as it has been widely adopted by practitioners and has become a part of routine patient care.

National Patient Safety Goals

In 2002, the Joint Commission established NPSGs to help accredited organizations address specific areas of concern regarding patient safety through the various stages of care (ambulatory, behavioral health, critical access, hospital, and home care).[29] The NPSGs for hospitals (Table 40-3) include 15 measures on such topics as accurate patient identification, medication use, surgery, and infections.[30] Evidence-based rationales and Joint Commission EPs to be monitored are provided for each NPSG to ensure that standardized quality care is provided.

In institutions where anti-coagulation therapy (specifically warfarin) is provided to patients, nutrition support clinicians appointed to provide patient education on drug-nutrient interactions should pay special attention to NPSG 03.05.01. As a regulatory requirement, all patients initiated on warfarin are to be provided with the appropriate education in a timely manner. From a clinical standpoint, poor international normalized ratio (INR) control has a variety of negative health outcomes and providing drug-nutrient interaction education to a patient may help prevent or ameliorate those negative outcomes. When provision of drug-nutrient education falls below the compliance benchmark, implementing QI strategies is imperative and action plans should be reported through your institution's quality department.

In October 2015, ASPEN petitioned the Patient Safety Advisory Group of the Joint Commission to consider malnutrition prevention and treatment as an NPSG. This call to action proposes 3 priority actions and 12 supplementary actions to support the improvement of nutrition care within the hospital (Table 40-4).[31] Although the proper identification, treatment, coding, and subsequent reimbursement of malnutrition continues to show a direct positive impact on patient outcomes, prevents readmissions, and reduces costs; the NPSG petition remains with the Patient Safety Advisory Group for review and final determination. In the meantime, nutrition support clinicians can use the points outlined in Table 40-4 to educate other members of the interdisciplinary team and promote the importance of caring for malnourished patients.

Order-Writing Privileges

To develop dedicated nutrition support teams, hospitals need to identify who is qualified and authorized to issue nutrition orders, including therapeutic diet orders, EN, and PN, orders for medical foods or vitamin and mineral supplementation, and ordering nutrition-related laboratory work. Dietitians and other clinicians in hospital settings interested in petitioning for order-writing privileges at their institution should review state practices (licensure, certification, title protection) and state healthcare facility regulations to determine potential barriers that may need to be addressed.[32] Monitoring and analyzing the accuracy and timeliness of prescribed diets can be used

TABLE 40-3 National Patient Safety Goals for Hospitals (Effective January 1, 2017)

Improve the accuracy of patient identification.
- *NPSG 01.01.01:* Use at least two patient identifiers when providing care, treatment, and services.
- *NPSG 01.03.01:* Eliminate transfusion errors related to patient misidentification.

Improve the effectiveness of communication among caregivers.
- *NPSG 02.03.01:* Report critical results of tests and diagnostic procedures in a timely basis.

Improve the safety of using medications.
- *NPSG 03.04.01:* Label all medications, medication containers, and other solutions on and off the sterile field in perioperative and other procedural settings.
- *NPSG 03.05.01:* Reduce the likelihood of patient harm associated with the use of anticoagulant therapy. *(Includes provision of drug/nutrient interaction education.)*
- *NPSG 03.06.01:* Maintain and communicate accurate patient medication information.

Reduce the harm associated with clinical alarm systems.
- *NPSG 06.01.01:* Improve the safety of clinical alarm systems.

Reduce the risk of healthcare-associated infections.
- *NPSG 07.01.01:* Comply with either the current Centers for Disease Control and Prevention (CDC) hand hygiene guidelines or the current World Health Organization (WHO) hand hygiene guidelines.
- *NPSG 07.03.01:* Implement evidence-based practices to prevent healthcare-associated infections due to multidrug-resistant organisms in acute care hospitals.
- *NPSG 07.04.01:* Implement evidence-based practices to prevent central line–associated bloodstream infections.
- *NPSG 07.05.01:* Implement evidence-based practices for preventing surgical site infections.
- *NPSG 07.06.01:* Implement evidence-based practices to prevent indwelling catheter-associated urinary tract infections (CAUTI).

The hospital identifies safety risks inherent in its patient population.
- *NPSG 15.01.01:* Identify patients at risk for suicide.

Introduction to the Universal Protocol for Preventing Wrong Site, Wrong Procedure, and Wrong Person Surgery™
- *UP 01.01.01:* Conduct a preprocedure verification process.
- *UP 01.02.01:* Mark the procedure site.
- *UP 01.03.01:* A time-out is performed before the procedure.

NPSG, National Patient Safety Goal; UP, Universal Protocol.
Source: Excerpted from reference 30: The Joint Commission. Hospital: 2017 National Patient Safety Goals effective January 1, 2017: hospital accreditation program. https://www.jointcommission.org/hap_2017_npsgs. © The Joint Commission, 2017. Reprinted with permission.

TABLE 40-4 Actions to Support Improvement in Nutrition Care Quality in Hospitals

Priority actions:
1. Each clinician on the interdisciplinary care team should participate in the execution of the nutrition care.
2. Develop systems to quickly diagnose all malnourished patients and those at risk.
3. Develop nutrition care plans in a timely fashion and implement comprehensive nutrition interventions (optimally within 48 hours of identification of the malnourished patient).

Additional actions:
1. Each clinician should include nutrition as part of his or her daily patient care.
2. Use consistent definitions and validated nutrition screening and assessment tools so that all stakeholders are using consistent language.
3. Develop a comprehensive nutrition plan for the transition of care settings, including a repeat nutrition screening completed just before discharge to assess if risk has elevated during the hospital stay and needs to be addressed in the discharge plan.
4. Analyze hospital systems to determine what resources would be required to complete a nutrition assessment and have each patient who is malnourished or at nutrition risk have a plan of care implemented within 48 hours of admission.
5. Acceptable staffing levels should be evidence-based to provide sound nutrition care.
6. Hospitals should assess and enhance their electronic health record systems to allow for better organization of nutrition care parameters and interventions, and link this to diagnostic coding systems.
7. Hospitals should develop safety checklists for each patient to make sure clinicians are completing all the steps of nutrition screening, assessment, rescreening, and intervention using the algorithm of care above.
8. Use of restricted diets should be periodically evaluated.
9. Supportive mealtime environments should be built into care processes.
10. Hospitals should support development of dedicated teams for protocol development and management of enteral or parenteral nutrition as appropriate to facilitate timely initiation of the prescribed nutrition support therapy.
11. Institutions should develop a system to track nutrition care and its relation to outcome indicators.
12. Institutions should facilitate nutrition care across the healthcare transitions to provide continuity of therapy.

Source: Adapted with permission from reference 31: Guenter P, Jensen G, Patel V, et al. Addressing disease-related malnutrition in hospitalized patients: a call for a national goal. *Jt Comm J Qual Patient Saf.* 2015;41(10):469–473. Copyright © Elsevier 2015.

as the beginning of a QI program in which petitioning for order-writing privileges for the various qualified professionals as the action that will create the desired improvement (refer to Practice Scenario 40-2).

Practice Scenario 40-2

Question: How do you determine staff competency for diet order–writing privileges?

Scenario: The clinical nutrition manager of a 650-bed academic medical center was notified that the state practice guidelines have been changed to allow dietitians to write therapeutic diet orders, including enteral nutrition (EN) and parenteral nutrition (PN); nutrition-related laboratory work; and vitamin and mineral supplementation. Of the 15 dietitians on staff:

- Five of the 15 staff members had the certified nutrition support clinician (CNSC) credential administered by the National Board of Nutrition Support Certification.
- Four of the 15 staff members were new to the field, with less than 3 years of experience mostly covering medical surgical populations and without any advanced degrees or credentials.
- Four of the 15 staff members were more experienced dietitians, with 5 to 15 years of experience, and regularly covered oncology and other patient populations with higher rates of nutrition support.
- Two of the 15 staff members are experienced dietitians, with more than 15 years of experience covering pediatrics and cardiac service lines; both of these dietitians had advanced degrees.

Intervention: The nutrition support team developed a competency assessment tool addressing the criteria and skills associated with diet order–writing privileges, and developed a continuous learning plan to maintain competency.

Answer: Both education and experience level of a staff member were among the first factors considered by the institution when granting diet order–writing privileges. The clinical nutrition manager created a detailed outline with various levels to document what it means to a qualified nutrition professional and determine which staff members would be eligible to write orders. Basic qualifications to order therapeutic diets included that a registered dietitian must hold current registration and be certified or licensed in the state. Qualifications to order EN, PN, laboratory tests, and vitamin/mineral supplementation required additional years of experience, advanced degrees, and CNSC advanced certification. An education module and evaluation were developed to test staff competency at the level of both basic and advanced order writing. Yearly assessment of this skill would be required for all staff members to maintain competency in the area, and professional development plans were developed to help move practitioners from basic to advanced levels. Regular monitoring and evaluation through chart reviews and clinical audits were used to help determine adequate clinical judgment and the need for additional training.

Rationale: If therapeutic diet order–writing privileges are approved by Centers for Medicare and Medicaid Services and the state, the institution's medical board also must approve them. Depending on acuity, patient population, and staffing profile at the institution, the competency assessment model of basic and advanced order-writing privileges may vary.

Quality Improvement Methodologies

Several monitoring methodologies have been developed to improve the quality and safety of healthcare. Each methodology uses different strategies, but all involve an analysis, an intervention, and an evaluation. The Plan-Do-Study-Act (PDSA) method and Six Sigma are commonly used and effective process improvement methodologies. The selection of a methodology depends on the nature of the institution and the outcomes to be measured. No single method is best for every situation. Principles from several methodologies may be employed in a single outcomes study, especially in large-scale studies with various measures to be addressed.

Plan-Do-Study-Act Cycle

The PDSA cycle is one of the most common improvement strategies used in healthcare quality initiatives.[33] This method involves defining a problem, proposing a solution, and then testing the proposal by following the PDSA cycle (Figure 40-2[33] and Table 40-5[34]). When defining the problem and proposed solution, the following questions are explored:

- *What are we trying to accomplish?* Aims or goals of performance improvement should be time-specific and measurable, and should clearly define the specific patient population to be affected. Aims that are clearly defined and relentlessly pursued increase the chance of success in QI initiatives.[35]
- *How will we know that a change is an improvement?* It is important to select measures that are regulatory- or outcome-driven. Any positive results qualify as improvement.
- *What changes can we make that will result in improvement?* Although all improvements require making changes, not all changes result in improvement.[36] An effective action plan is developed by determining changes that are most likely to result in a desired improvement within a team's scope of practice, realizing barriers to changing current practice, and selecting strategies to overcome barriers.

The implementation results are used to decide whether to continue, modify, or abandon the proposed solution. If the tested solution does not achieve the desired results, an additional change is made, implemented, and evaluated. If the results are achieved, the solution is implemented on a larger scale and monitored over time for continuous improvement. When spreading the success of process improvement to other departments or more complex areas, the PDSA cycle often needs to be restarted, with current processes modified to apply to the new issue (Figure 40-3).[33]

FIGURE 40-2 The Plan-Do-Study-Act Cycle for Change

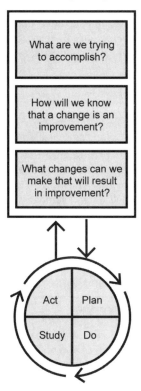

Source: Reprinted with permission from reference 33: Langley GJ, Moen RM, Nolan KM, Nolan TW, Norman CL, Provost LP. *The Improvement Guide: A Practical Approach to Enhancing Organizational Performance.* 2nd ed. San Francisco, CA: Jossey-Bass; 2009. Copyright ©2009, John Wiley and Sons.

TABLE 40-5 Specifics of the Plan-Do-Study-Act Method of Benchmarking and Quality Improvement

Step	Objectives
Plan	Create a plan: • Formulate specific aims. • Plan for data collection and analyses. • Determine project timelines.
Do	Test the change: • Execute the plan. • Document problems, challenges, and barriers. • Track progress against timeline benchmarks.
Study	Review the plan: • Analyze data. • Compare results to project aims. • Summarize and present data.
Act	Implement the changes: • Go through the cycle again or implement what you learned.

Source: Adapted from reference 34: Health Resources and Services Administration. US Department of Health and Human Services. Managing data for performance improvement. http://www.hrsa.gov/quality/toolbox /methodology/performanceimprovement/part2.html.

FIGURE 40-3 The Ramp of Improvement: Spreading Change by Repeating the Plan-Do-Study-Act (PDSA) Cycle

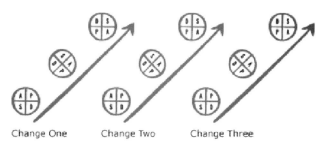

Change One   Change Two   Change Three

Source: Reprinted with permission from reference 33: Langley GJ, Moen RM, Nolan KM, Nolan TW, Norman CL, Provost LP. *The Improvement Guide: A Practical Approach to Enhancing Organizational Performance.* 2nd ed. San Francisco, CA: Jossey-Bass; 2009. Copyright ©2009, John Wiley and Sons.

Six Sigma

The Six Sigma model is a disciplined, data-driven QI methodology adapted from techniques used by Motorola and other companies in the manufacturing and production industries to eliminate defects in any process.[37] The term *Six Sigma* comes from the use in statistics of the Greek letter *sigma* to denote a standard deviation from the mean. *Six sigma* is equivalent to 3.4 defects or errors per million.[38] The goal of Six Sigma is not to eliminate all failures of quality but to reduce them until it is no longer cost-effective to pursue any further reduction.[39] The following DMAIC model is used to this end:[40]

- *D:* Define the goals to be reached.
- *M:* Measure the current performance levels to establish a baseline for comparison.
- *A:* Analyze the current performance, focusing on which factors affect quality.
- *I:* Improve these factors through the implementation of appropriate performance improvement strategies.
- *C:* Control mechanisms are implemented to prevent errors before they occur.

Use of the Six Sigma model is expanding in all industries, including healthcare. Refer to Practice Scenario 40-3 for an applied example of using the Six Sigma DMAIC methodology.

Practice Scenario 40-3

Question: How do you ensure that all patients are screened for nutrition risk on admission to the hospital?

Scenario: To comply with the Joint Commission standards for nutrition care, the nutrition services department of a 550-bed, non-teaching hospital developed a policy document stating that nutrition risk screening should be conducted on all hospital patients within 24 hours of admission, and any high-risk patients should be referred to the dietitian for nutrition assessment. To support the policy, a care pathway coupled with a paper-based nutrition screening tool was developed and completed by nursing on admission. However, since its implementation, use of the tool has not been monitored and, anecdotally, it has been observed that nutrition screening is not routinely completed on admission to the hospital.

Intervention: The Six Sigma define, measure, analyze, improve, control (DMAIC) methodology is used to update the care pathway so that the nutrition screening tool can be used more effectively at the bedside and noncompliance rates can be reduced.

Answer:
- *Define:* A literature review is conducted so that the team clearly understands the evidence that supports nutrition screening and can update the tools accordingly.
- *Measure:* A chart review is conducted on 50 inpatients on the medical floor to audit the current provision of nutrition screening.
- *Analyze:* As suspected, nutrition screening was not completed within 24 hours of admission for 45 out of the 50 charts reviewed (10% completion rate). It is identified that very few paper-based forms have been used since the introduction of the electronic health record in 2010; therefore, the care pathway and tool are no longer easily accessible to nursing staff and are not part of the routine admission assessment.
- *Improve:* A project steering group is established to identify the root causes of the problem, and an action plan is developed to integrate the care pathway and nutrition screening tool into the electronic patient admission assessment form completed by nursing on admission of all patients. Training modules to educate nursing on the use of the tool are created. The action plan is first implemented on the medical floor on which the baseline audit was conducted. After a 3-month implementation and education phase, the chart review is repeated. Adherence to the care pathway and completion of the nutrition screening tool is now 92%.
- *Control:* A monitoring component is incorporated into the electronic health record to produce monthly reports of the proportion of admitted patients who are screened daily for nutrition risk factors to determine the need for additional process changes. The steering group plans to review the evidence for nutrition screening and regulatory guidelines to maintain compliance. With success on the medical floor, the electronic tool is implemented hospital-wide.

Rationale: Quality monitoring is important; however, if improvement strategies are not implemented when indicators fall below the benchmark, the root cause of the problem is never fixed. Over time, care pathways and screening tools and the implementation of the electronic health record created major changes in current processes but also ultimately allowed for greater automation and ease of monitoring. Using the Six Sigma DMAIC model, the project steering group successfully increases compliance of nutrition screening on admission. Notably, another QI methodology could have been used to achieve the same goal.

Healthcare Informatics

In recent years, healthcare researchers and policymakers have proposed that healthcare informatics—the application of computer-related technologies within the healthcare setting—can improve healthcare outcomes. For example, a systematic review of the effects of electronic health records and computerized order entry systems on the quality, efficiency, and costs of medical care concluded that these technologies improve quality by increasing adherence to guidelines, enhancing disease surveillance, and decreasing medication errors.[41]

Measuring Quality

Quality Indicators

Quality indicators are objective metrics by which quality of care and professional performance can be assessed. Use of such metrics allows for continuous improvement of processes, procedures, and outcomes. Nutrition indicators can be derived from published guidelines and standards, the Joint Commission's NPSGs, the IOM quality aims, or treatment or patient outcomes, or by facility consensus. Table 40-6 outlines quality

TABLE 40-6 Nutrition Support Quality Indicators Based on Institute of Medicine Metrics

Indicator	Sample Quality Monitor
Patient safety	• Correct permanent feeding tube selection • Avoidance of central line placement if therapy duration is less than 7 to 10 days • Tight glycemic control (serum glucose: 90 to 140 mg/dL) • Criteria for therapy use
Patient-centeredness	• Home enteral nutrition patient satisfaction survey • Consideration of patient wishes and ethical issues prior to permanent tube feeding placement • Creation of patient-friendly schedules for specialized nutrition support delivery
Effectiveness	• Evidence-based practice • Glycemic protocols • Criteria for enteral nutrition specialty formula use
Efficiency	• Protocol pathways for providing specialized nutrition support • Order sets for multivitamin and trace element therapy • Wound care protocols
Timeliness	• Consult response time within 48 hours • Early enteral feeding to prevent malnutrition • Preoperative oral supplementation when poor nutrition status identified by physician
Equity	• Consistent care to all patients • Age-specific competencies defined and measured

Reprinted from reference 10: McDowell L. Clinical nutrition quality indicators and patient outcomes. *Support Line*. 2007;29(4):3–9. ©2017 Support Line, Dietitians in Nutrition Support, a dietetic practice group of the Academy of Nutrition and Dietetics. Used with permission.

indicators in nutrition support based on the 6 IOM quality goals—patient safety, patient-centeredness, effectiveness, efficiency, timeliness, and equity.[10]

Quality indicators are derived by dividing the number of times a measure has been met (numerator) by the number of opportunities that were present to measure the particular objective (denominator).[42] For example, to track how many ambulatory oncology patients with a newly placed percutaneous endoscopic gastrostomy (PEG) tube received a nutrition consult with a goal of 100%, the number of nutrition consults would be divided by the number of ambulatory oncology patients with a new PEG tube. If you are measuring the percentage of positive responses on a patient satisfaction questionnaire, the number of patients that answered in a positive manner would be divided by the number of patients surveyed.

Further examples of quality indicators include appropriate initiation, access, and use of EN and PN; care of EN and PN access sites; accuracy of blood glucose draws in PN patients or the frequency of incorrect draws; frequency and management of occlusion of feeding tubes and venous access lines; frequency of EN hold times due to high gastric residual volume; number of days at EN goal; frequency of diversion from EN goal; the gap between prescribed and administered EN; complications of EN and PN; initiation of and staff compliance with existing and new protocols and procedures; and discharge education of patients with EN and PN to prevent complications.[10,43] Careful selection of the denominator is essential to avoid over- or underestimation of responses or performance metrics. Specifying subgroup populations to include age, gender, race or ethnicity groups, treatment status, or disease severity can provide additional valuable information.[42]

FIGURE 40-4 Example of a Parenteral Nutrition Quality Survey

PN QUALITY SURVEY

RD ____________________ Date____________________

Service recommending PN ____________________

1. PN is being started on ____________________
   Therapy ended on __________ for a total duration of ________ days
2. PN is indicated because:
3. Was the enteral route tried?
   If yes, what happened?
   Oral versus stomach versus bowel feeding?
4. Known disposition of patient: Discharged with PN
   Discharged without PN
   Died

	Yes	No	Comments
5. Were you involved in the decision to start PN?			
6. Is PN appropriate for this patient per our standards of care?			
7. If central PN was ordered, did the patient have an existing clean line for infusion?			
8. Did the patient receive a central line ONLY for PN?			
9. Did the patient receive a PICC line ONLY for PN?			
10. Did you prevent therapy that was not indicated?			

PICC, peripherally inserted central catheter; PN, parenteral nutrition; RD, registered dietitian.

Source: Reprinted from reference 10: McDowell L. Clinical nutrition quality indicators and patient outcomes. *Support Line*. 2007;29(4):3–9. ©2017 Support Line, Dietitians in Nutrition Support, a dietetic practice group of the Academy of Nutrition and Dietetics. Used with permission.

Data Collection

Data collection for QI can be accomplished using multiple methods, including observation, electronic health record and registry review, surveys, interviews, focus groups, audits, and the use of clinical data collection tools originating from scientific publications, accreditation organizations, payers, healthcare facilities, or professional societies. The type of data to collect depends on the goals of the QI project, which could, for example, involve problem solving using clinician experience, monitoring of adherence to evidence-based guidelines, or surveying patient outcomes after a systems change is implemented.[44] Using a standardized and validated tool increases the likelihood that accurate, reliable and consistent data are collected. Figures 40-4 and 40-5 display examples of EN and PN quality surveys.[10]

When planning the data collection period, investigators must allow sufficient time between an intervention and a new behavior for change to occur, and decide how frequently data will be collected to identify any deviation from the implemented change over time. The Health Resources and Services Administration of the US Department of Health and Human Services[34] suggests that, after establishing a baseline process, monthly frequency may be adequate while active changes are undertaken; quarterly collection should be implemented after a goal is achieved; and yearly monitoring after performance is stable may be sufficient.

Benchmarking

Benchmarking is a continuous QI process that is built on comparison of performance, identification of practice gaps, and process change.[45] During benchmarking, organizations measure their performance against best-practice organizations internal or external to their industry, and improve their performance by implementing processes associated with high performance.[46] According to the American Society for Quality,[47] an organization can benchmark their procedures and policies to improve their performance. Benchmarking can provide an understanding of an organization's strengths and weaknesses, the level of performance needed to compete with best-practice organizations, and how to better satisfy customer's needs for quality, cost, products, and services.[45]

Benchmarking is imperative in today's healthcare because of increasing financial and competitive pressures, and it is mandated by organizations such as CMS, the Joint Commission, and the American College of Surgeons Commission on Cancer. Facilities are required to meet national accountability measures and provide performance data to receive reimbursement of services, avoid penalties, and receive accreditation status.[48,49] Benchmarking also occurs on a voluntary basis.

Examples of benchmarking programs include the ASPEN Sustain registry,[50] which was established to determine

FIGURE 40-5 Example of an Enteral Nutrition Quality Survey

Permanent Feeding Tube Quality Survey

Name _____   Date_____

Type of tube placed (please circle one below):

	GI:	PEG
		PEG-J
	Radiology:	PG
		PG-J, single lumen
		PG-J, double lumen
	Surgery:	G-tube
		G-J tube
		J tube

Date of tube placement _____

Service/attending who placed tube_____

	Yes	No	Comments
Were you involved with the decision as to the type of tube placed?			
Was the type of tube placed appropriate given the patient's medical condition?			
Were any ethical issues (e.g., end of life, futile care) present? If so, how was it addressed?			
Were there any complications associated with the feeding tube? If yes, please circle from the list below and provide comments			
Major complications • Peritonitis • Hemorrhage necessitating transfusion • External catheter leak necessitating catheter removal or repeat gastric puncture for new site • Other complication necessitating catheter removal (severe infection, ruptured viscus, repeat aspiration)			
Minor complications • Tube malfunction requiring catheter exchange • Site infection—superficial stoma infection • Bleeding from tube site—no transfusion required • External leak required catheter exchange • Pneumonia • New-onset aspiration or worsening of aspiration not requiring tube removal			
Other • Tube dislodgement with catheter revision not requiring repeat gastric puncture (include reason for dislodgement) • Clogged tube requiring revision with repeat gastric puncture			
Note: Confer with medical staff regarding determination of tube-related complication(s). *Physician's name* _____			
If there were complications associated with the tube, was it:			
• Repositioned • Replaced without new gastric puncture • Replaced with new gastric puncture			

G, gastronomy; GI, gastrointestinal; J, jejunostomy; PEG, percutaneous endoscopic gastrostomy. PEG/J, percutaneous enterocutaneous gastrostomy/jejunostomy.
Reprinted from reference 10: McDowell L. Clinical nutrition quality indicators and patient outcomes. *Support Line*. 2007;29(4):3–9. ©2017 Support Line, Dietitians in Nutrition Support, a dietetic practice group of the Academy of Nutrition and Dietetics. Used with permission.

performance outcome metrics and standards of care for patients receiving PN at home. The International Nutrition Survey by Critical Care Nutrition at the Clinical Evaluation Research Unit[51] is a voluntary benchmarking study, where intensive care units can compare their practices to other facilities with the aim to improve practice. Local benchmarking efforts headed by nutrition support clinicians have included programs to reduce the number of hours of *nil per os* (NPO) status prior to surgery to reduce malnutrition rates,[48] and

efforts to reduce weight loss among ambulatory oncology patients by implementing a malnutrition screening tool (unpublished research).

Benchmarking should be a continuous process because best practices change with implementation of new evidence. To be successful, benchmarking requires continuous surveillance of key processes, a committed leadership team, adequate resources, preparation of the organization, and experience with implementation of continuous QI.[47] However, benchmarking as originally defined by the industrial sector with continuous gathering of indicators for long-term monitoring is rarely practiced in healthcare.[49] Lack of time, cost, resistance to change, poor planning, and short term expectations are regarded as main barriers to achieving benchmarking goals.[45] In nutrition support, the ASPEN standards[21] represent benchmarks for providing competent, safe, and efficacious nutrition care, and can be utilized to improve care. Refer to Practice Scenario 40-4 for an example of a benchmarking QI project.[21,34,45,47,49]

Practice Scenario 40-4

Question: How can clinicians improve timeliness of initiation of enteral nutrition (EN) in mechanically ventilated intensive care unit (ICU) patients to comply with published standards suggesting initiation within 24 to 48 hours of ICU admission?

Scenario: When performing a clinical audit, a nutrition support clinician noticed a gap between actual practice and the American Society for Parenteral and Enteral Nutrition (ASPEN) standards[21] regarding initiation of EN. The ASPEN standards state that EN should be initiated within 24 to 48 hours of ICU admission. The audit showed that mean time to initiation of EN in the medical ICU was more than 48 hours, and the guidelines were followed in only 40% of cases.

Intervention: The quality improvement (QI) team chose the plan-do-study-act (PDSA) cycle to help achieve the desired goal of improving the timeliness of EN initiation.

Answer:
- *Plan:* The QI team identified that EN was not routinely addressed in rounds from Day 1 of admission. A plan was developed as follows:
  - An EN initiation order was added to the electronic ICU admission order set.
  - A nutrition category was added to the bedside daily rounds checklist.
  - Staff was educated on the importance of nutrition during critical illness and the advantages of early initiation of EN.
- *Do:* The appropriate staff members and committees approved the order set, and the nutrition support clinician completed staff education.
- *Study:* After 2 months, the nutrition support clinician reviewed the implementation data relating to the checklist and the admission order set. The clinician determined that the nutrition category was completed in less than 60% of cases, and that the admission order sets were used in 90% of cases.

- *Act:* The benchmarking team decides to complete another PDSA cycle, and to add staff education regarding the importance of completing the checklist. After a subsequent clinical audit, the nutrition support clinician found that the mean time to the initiation of EN has been reduced to 49 hours and 60% of patients were receiving EN within the window of 24 to 48 hours. Additional cycles were added until the desired benchmarks were reached.

Rationale: The PDSA model is often used to in QI projects to guide clinical performance because of its simplicity, cost-effectiveness, and ability to assess a change prior to implementation, while sustaining the continuous performance improvement process.[34,45,49] The PDSA methodology includes selecting a process *(plan)*, characterizing the process using available metrics and practices *(do)*, performing a gap analysis to identify where improvements are needed *(study)*, and determining what strategies should be implemented *(act)*[34,47] (Table 40-5). The "study" part of the cycle is fundamental to determine whether the desired aims are obtainable and if the study can proceed to the "act" phase, or should return to the "planning" phase for another round in the PDSA cycle.[34]

Data Management

Effective data management is essential to improve practice and achieve desired outcomes in QI projects. Data management is a systematic approach that includes collection of data related to the QI project; analyses, interpretation, reporting, and acting on the results; and ongoing monitoring.[34] This process allows for identification of gaps in practice, identification of opportunities for improvement, and monitoring of progress as changes are implemented.[34]

Data analysis and interpretation of results are processes by which meaning is assigned to the procedure under review. Data analyses are initiated by a review of current practice, and comparisons of data to baseline, benchmarks, and QI aims. QI data can be analyzed using spreadsheets or statistical software, such as Statistical Package for the Social Science (SPSS) (IBM, Armonk, NY), and Statistical Analysis System (SAS) (SAS Institute, Cary, NC), and, at a minimum, the analysis should include frequencies.

Data are often presented using graphs and charts, which allows the reader to get a snapshot of the most important findings and visualize differences at defined time frames. Progress toward or steadiness with a benchmark can be displayed using a dashboard table to display an overview of the compliance with a specific metric. Dashboards are often accompanied by separate action plans detailing the study particulars as well as any necessary changes to the QI methodology.[34]

Summary

It is imperative that nutrition support clinicians participate in the measurement of quality outcomes at their institutions so they can continue to advocate for the best, safest and most effective care possible for their patients. QI strategies help healthcare providers to identify the root causes of problems and develop successful solutions. While there are many variations of quality and outcomes monitoring, the chosen method should be individualized to address the specific needs and barriers of a situation and to achieve the goal at hand.

References

1. Chassin MR, O'Kane ME. History of the quality improvement movement. In: March of Dimes. *Toward Improving the Outcome of Pregnancy: Enhancing Perinatal Health Through Quality, Safety and Performance Initiatives.* 2010:1–8. http://www.marchofdimes.org/materials/toward-improving-the-outcome-of-pregnancy-iii.pdf. Accessed December 22, 2016.
2. Chelluri LP. Quality and performance improvement in critical care. *Indian J Crit Care Med.* 2006;12(2):67–76.
3. Institute of Medicine. *To Err Is Human: Building a Safer Health System.* Washington, DC: National Academies Press; 1999.
4. Institute of Medicine. *Crossing the Quality Chasm: A New Health System for the 21st Century.* Washington, DC: National Academies Press; 2001.
5. Agency for Healthcare Research and Quality. National healthcare quality report. http://www.ahrq.gov/qual/nhqr05/nhqr05.htm. Accessed August 8, 2016.
6. Academy of Nutrition and Dietetics. Definition of terms list. http://www.eatrightpro.org/~/media/eatrightpro%20files/advocacy/definitionofterms.ashx. Accessed August 8, 2016.
7. Lynn J, Bailty MA, Bottrell M, et al. The ethics of using quality improvement methods in health care. *Ann Intern Med.* 2007; 146:666–673.
8. Batalden PB, Davidoff F. What is "quality improvement" and how can it transform healthcare? *Qual Saf Health Care.* 2007;16:2–3.
9. Donabedian A. Evaluating the quality of medical care. *Milbank Q.* 2005;83(4):691–729.
10. McDowell L. Clinical nutrition quality indicators and patient outcomes. *Support Line.* 2007;29(4):3–9.
11. Stanford University. Quality assessment and quality improvement (QA/QI) FAQ. http://humansubjects.stanford.edu/research/documents/qa_qi_faqs_AID03H16.pdf. Accessed August 6, 2016.
12. Ogrinc G, Nelson WA, Adams SM, O'Hara AE. An instrument to differentiate between clinical research and quality improvement. *IRB.* 2013;35(5):1–8.
13. Institute of Medicine. *Best Care at Lower Cost: The Path to Continuously Learning Health Care in America.* Washington, DC: National Academies Press; 2012.
14. Mangione-Smith R, DeCristofaro AH, Setodji CM, et al. The quality of ambulatory care delivered to children in the United States. *N Engl J Med.* 2007;11;357(15):1515–1523.
15. McGlynn EA, Asch SM, Adams J, et al. The quality of health care delivered to adults in the United States. *N Engl J Med.* 2003; 348(26):2635–2645.
16. McDonald KM, Chang C, Schultz E. Through the quality kaleidoscope: reflections on the science and practice of improving health care quality. In: *Closing the Quality Gap: Revisiting the State of the Science.* Rockville, MD: Agency for Healthcare Research and Quality; 2013. http://www.ncbi.nlm.nih.gov/books/NBK126724. Accessed August 8, 2016.
17. National Committee for Quality Assurance. Quality measurement products. http://www.ncqa.org/hedis-quality-measurement/quality-measurement-products. Accessed August 6, 2016.
18. Claxton G, Cox C, Gonzales S, Kamal R, Levitt L. Measuring the quality of healthcare in the U.S. Kaiser Family Foundation Insight Brief. September 10, 2015. http://www.healthsystemtracker

.org/insight/measuring-the-quality-of-healthcare-in-the-u-s. Accessed August 6, 2016.

19. US Department of Health and Human Services. Protection of human subjects. 45 CFR 46.102. 2011.

20. Ukleja A, Freeman KL, Gilbert K, et al. Standards for nutrition support: adult hospitalized patients. *Nutr Clin Pract.* 2010;25(4): 403–414.

21. McClave SA, Taylor BE, Martindale RG, et al. Guidelines for the provision and assessment of nutrition support therapy in the adult critically ill patient: Society of Critical Care Medicine (SCCM) and American Society for Parenteral and Enteral Nutrition (ASPEN). *JPEN J Parenter Enteral Nutr.* 2016;40(2): 159–211.

22. Brantley S, Russell MK, Mogensen KM, et al. American Society for Parenteral and Enteral Nutrition and Academy of Nutrition and Dietetics: revised 2014 Standards of Practice and Standards of Professional Performance for registered dietitian nutritionists (competent, proficient, and expert) in nutrition support. *Nutr Clin Pract.* 2014;29(6):792–828.

23. Institute of Medicine. *Clinical Practice Guidelines We Can Trust.* Washington, DC: National Academies Press; 2011.

24. American Medical Association. Proceedings of the 2014 annual meeting of the house of delegates: resolution 705 payment for nutrition support services. Approved resolution June 9–10, 2014. Now policy H-150.931. https://www.ama-assn.org/about-us /proceedings-2014-annual-meeting-house-delegates.

25. DeLegge M, Kelley A. State of nutrition support teams. *Nutr Clin Pract.* 2013;28(6):691–697.

26. Dougherty D, Bankhead R, Kushner R, Mirtallo J, Winkler M. Nutrition care given new importance in JCAHO standards. *Nutr Clin Pract.* 1995;10(1):26–31.

27. The Joint Commission. *2016 Comprehensive Accreditation Manual for Hospitals.* Oak Brook, IL: Joint Commission Resources; 2015.

28. EP review project: The Joint Commission deletes 225 hospital requirements. *Jt Comm Perspect.* 2016;36(5):5–14.

29. The Joint Commission. 2017 National Patient Safety Goals. https://www.jointcommission.org/standards_information/npsgs .aspx. Accessed January 30, 2017.

30. The Joint Commission. Hospital: 2017 National Patient Safety Goals effective January 1, 2017: hospital accreditation program. https://www.jointcommission.org/hap_2017_npsgs. Accessed January 30, 2017.

31. Guenter P, Jensen G, Patel V, et al. Addressing disease-related malnutrition in hospitalized patients: a call for a national goal. *Jt Comm J Qual Patient Saf.* 2015;41(10):469–473.

32. Academy of Nutrition and Dietetics. Therapeutic diet orders: state status and regulation. http://www.eatright.org/dietorders. Accessed July 31, 2016.

33. Langley GJ, Nolan KM, Nolan TW, et al. *The Improvement Guide: A Practical Approach to Enhancing Organizational Performance.* San Francisco, CA: Jossey-Bass; 1996.

34. US Department of Health and Human Services. Managing data for performance improvement. http://www.hrsa.gov/quality /toolbox/methodology/performanceimprovement/part2.html. Accessed August 8, 2016.

35. Leape L, Kabcenell AI, Gandhi TK, et al. Reducing adverse drug events: lessons from a breakthrough collaborative. *Jt Comm J Qual Improv.* 2000;26(6):321–331.

36. Berwick DM. Harvesting knowledge from improvement. *JAMA.* 1996;275(11):877–878.

37. Chassin MR. Is healthcare ready for Six Sigma quality? *Millbank Q.* 1998;76(4):565–591.

38. Varkey P, Reller MK, Resar RK. Basics of quality improvement in healthcare. *Mayo Clin Proc.* 2007;82(6):735–739.

39. Vonderheide-Liem DN, Pate B. *Applying Quality Methodologies to Improve Healthcare: Six Sigma, Lean Thinking, Balanced Scorecard, and More.* Marblehead, MA: HCPro; 2004.

40. Barry R, Murcko AC, Brubaker CE. *The Six Sigma Book for Healthcare: Improving Outcomes by Reducing Errors.* Chicago, IL: Health Administration Press; 2003.

41. Chaudry B, Wang J, Wu S, et al. Systematic review: impact of health information technology on quality, efficiency, and costs of medical care. *Ann Intern Med.* 2010;144(10):742–752.

42. Agency for Healthcare Research and Quality. Practice Facilitation Handbook. Module 7. Measuring and benchmarking clinical performance. http://www.ahrq.gov/professionals/prevention -chronic-care/improve/system/pfhandbook/mod7.html. Accessed on August 6, 2016.

43. Gimenez Verotti CC, de Miranda Torrinhas RS, Pires Corona L, Waitzberg DL. Design of quality indicators for oral nutrition therapy. *Nutr Hosp.* 2015;1;31(6):2692–2695.

44. American Society for Quality. Quality glossary: B. http://asq.org /glossary/b.html. Accessed August 6, 2016.

45. Kay JFL. Health care benchmarking. *Hong Kong Medical Diary.* 2007;12(2):22–27.

46. Sower VE. Benchmarking in hospitals: more than a scorecard. *Quality Progress.* 2007;40(8):58–60.

47. Amerinet. The benefits of healthcare benchmarking. how to measure and beat the competition (white paper). http://www.intalere .com/Amerinet%20Documents/Amerinet-Benchmarking -Whitepaper.pdf. Accessed August 6, 2016.

48. Phillips W. The value of benchmarking. *Today's Dietitian.* 2015; 17(2):44.

49. Ettorchi-Tardy A, Levif M, Michel P. Benchmarking: a method for continuous quality improvement in health. *Healthcare Policy.* 2012;7(4):e101–e119.

50. American Society for Parenteral and Enteral Nutrition. A.S.P.E.N.'s National Patient Registry for Nutrition Care. https:// www.nutritioncare.org/sustain. Accessed January 21, 2017.

51. Critical Care Nutrition at the Clinical Evaluation Research Unit (CERU). http://www.criticalcarenutrition.com/index.php?option =com_content&view=article&id=146&Itemid=50. Accessed January 21, 2017.

41 Evidence-Based Medicine and Derivation of Clinical Guidelines

Stephen A. McClave, MD, FASPEN, FASGE, FACN, AGAF, and Jayshil J. Patel, MD

CONTENTS

Acknowledgment: Kelly A. Tappenden, PhD, RD, was the author of this chapter for the second edition.

Objectives

1. Recognize the hierarchy of levels of evidence in the literature, and understand that strengths and weaknesses occur at every level.
2. Appreciate the value of the Grading of Recommendations, Assessment, Development, and Evaluation (GRADE) classification system and how it is used to interpret clinical trials.
3. Learn what information may be gleaned from a Forest plot in a meta-analysis.
4. Understand how medical societies derive clinical guidelines.

Test Your Knowledge Questions

1. Which of the following represents the highest grade of evidence for interpreting clinical trials in the literature?
   A. A well-written editorial piece by a recognized expert in the field
   B. A large observational trial of critically ill patients in hospitals around the world
   C. A prospective cohort study with nonrandomized contemporaneous controls
   D. A large, multicenter randomized controlled trial (RCT)
2. Which of the following best describes clinical guidelines issued by a scientific or medical society?
   A. Clinical recommendations to guide clinicians
   B. Medical legal benchmarks by which to gauge clinical competency
   C. Practice parameters to guarantee the best patient outcomes in clinical practice
   D. A well-organized list of clinical topics that can be used to gauge future research
3. Which of the following is true concerning the Forest plots from a meta-analysis?
   A. The test of heterogeneity evaluates similarity between patients in a study.
   B. The test of overall treatment effect indicates whether the quality of the meta-analysis is high or low.
   C. Relative risk tends to overestimate the treatment effect.
   D. Absolute risk reduction is determined by counting the number of positive studies divided by the total number of studies in the meta-analysis.

Test Your Knowledge Answers

1. The correct answer is **D**. A large, well-conducted RCT, particularly if it is multicenter, provides the highest level of evidence. Even if an editorial is well written by a recognized expert, it is the lowest grade of evidence and is considered expert opinion. Nonrandomized cohort studies mean that the study group is compared in a nonrandomized fashion with either contemporaneous patients who were in the hospital or being treated at the same time or historical controls who were treated at some time in the past. Such trials provide a low level of evidence. A large observational trial may represent practice at different institutions around the world, but the absence of a prospectively randomized control group renders the study a lower level of evidence than a large RCT.

2. The correct answer is **A**. Clinical guidelines represent a set of recommendations for practicing clinicians that are derived from a vigorous review of the literature. Adherence to the guidelines does not guarantee clinical outcome. Guidelines are not rules or laws and do not distinguish whether someone's clinical practice is legal or illegal. Guidelines organize the literature into topics that can direct further study, but they are not designed to be a rigorous guide for future research.

3. The correct answer is **C**. Relative risk is calculated in the meta-analysis and does tend to overestimate the treatment effect. The absolute risk reduction is calculated by the number of events in both the treatment and control groups divided by the denominator in each group. The absolute risk reduction is usually lower than the relative risk reduction. The test for heterogeneity looks at the similarities between studies, not between patients in an individual study. The overall treatment effect tells whether the outcome parameter being evaluated by the meta-analysis was significantly different in the study group compared to controls.

Introduction

Although clinical trials have been conducted for decades, interest in evidence-based medicine (EBM) has grown exponentially since its formal introduction in 1992.[1] Clinical practice was historically viewed as the "art of medicine." Expert opinion, experience, and authoritarian judgment comprised the foundation for decision-making. The uses of scientific methodology, as in biomedical research, and statistical analysis, as in epidemiology, were rare in the world of medicine.[2] EBM requires integration of the best research evidence with clinical expertise and the patient's unique values and circumstances.[3] EBM not only stresses the importance of examining evidence from clinical research trials but, at the same time, also discourages clinicians from using methods that rely on intuition, unsystematic clinical experience, and pathophysiological rationale as sufficient grounds for clinical decision-making.[4] EBM is a process by which to improve patient outcomes by providing clinicians with the highest grade of evidence available, which facilitates informed decisions regarding the distribution of limited resources and the application of clinical practice techniques.[4] The consistent flow of new research into the clinical setting allows for the application of new therapies to patients and reduces the reliance on long-standing, but sometimes suboptimal, treatment methods. Therefore, EBM helps clinicians maximize their *effectiveness* (adequacy to accomplish a purpose) and *efficiency* (production of the desired effect with minimal waste of time, effort, or skill) both clinically and economically. The advantages garnered by using EBM have increased the demand for high-quality research, online databases, and Internet search engines that provide access to quality evidence libraries for the convenient incorporation of EBM into clinicians' daily routines.

EBM has strongly influenced the science and practice of clinical nutrition. The American Society for Parenteral and Enteral Nutrition (ASPEN) and other societies have developed an array of evidence-based clinical practice guidelines for the provision of nutrition support. ASPEN guidelines, as well as selected guidelines from other societies, are published in the *Journal of Parenteral and Enteral Nutrition*.

A 2004 report evaluating the impact of routine administration of evidence-based clinical guidelines indicates that intensive care units (ICUs) that adhered more consistently to the Canadian clinical practice guidelines were more likely to feed patients successfully with enteral nutrition (EN).[5] The prevalence of using EBM in specialized nutrition therapy is not well studied. Among pediatric dietitians working in Australian teaching hospitals, survey results indicate that most of the dietitians strongly believed in the philosophy of EBM, but almost three-quarters of them failed to integrate the principles into their practice.[6] Within the field of clinical nutrition, leadership is needed to enhance the teaching and implementation of EBM.

Derivation of Clinical Guidelines

Although guidelines in some fashion have been available for decades, dramatic improvements in their brevity, clarity, and evidence-based support have occurred just in the last 10 years. Clinicians have come to realize guidelines have value because they are compiled by a committee of experts in the field who have comprehensively reviewed the clinical trials in the literature. Theoretically, the recommendations should represent the best current advice, which should result in better outcomes for patient management than would be achieved with approaches that were not evidence-based.

Clinical guidelines are simply a basic list of recommendations derived through various forms of evidence and do not represent absolute requirements. They do not project or guarantee outcome or mortality benefits, and they are never a substitute for clinical judgment.

The clinician's judgment at the bedside always takes precedence of any guideline recommendation. Nonetheless, the support of evidence behind the recommendations can be incredibly comprehensive, taking into consideration data from prospective RCTs and observational trials from the literature, evaluation of other national and international guidelines, polling of expert opinion, and, always, issues of clinical practicality. The process of generating clinical guidelines can have a surprisingly long "gestation period" from the assembly of the guidelines committee to the publication of the final journal article. The gestation periods for the 2009 and 2016 guidelines from the ASPEN and the Society for Critical Care Medicine (SCCM) were 4 to 5 years.[7,8] The review of the literature can take up to 2 years and now requires input into an electronic database. The manuscript can take 1 to 2 years to complete, and then a review process is done by external journal reviewers and executive boards for the sponsoring society.

Despite this exhaustive process, guidelines are surprisingly prone to criticism. Following publication of the 2009 ASPEN/ SCCM guidelines, an opinion paper published in the *Journal of Parenteral and Enteral Nutrition* criticized the guidelines for their poor definition of malnutrition and underappreciation of protein.[9] The committee was criticized for using expert opinion as a category of evidence. The authors of the article summarized their point by saying that guidelines "just don't make sense."[9] Following publication of the 2016 ASPEN/ SCCM guidelines, an opinion piece published in the *Journal of Parenteral and Enteral Nutrition* focused on the December 2013 cutoff for articles included in the literature review, claiming that the gap between that inclusion date and the date when the guidelines were published (February 2016) rendered the guidelines obsolete.[10] The author of that paper concluded that the guidelines should be retracted![10]

GRADE Classification System

Immediately following the publication of the 2009 ASPEN/ SCCM guidelines, the ASPEN Board of Directors voted to adopt the GRADE classification system for evaluating the literature.[11,12] GRADE standardizes evaluation of the literature on RCTs and observational studies. Training programs have been developed to educate GRADE experts, who then can serve on a guidelines committee and help direct the derivation of the strength and quality of the recommendations. The

entire process starts when the sponsoring organization invites a group of experts to form the guidelines committee. Importantly, the committee members should first clearly define their target patient population. Such a definition may be difficult in a heterogeneous population, such as all patients with critical illness, or relatively easier in a homogeneous group, such as patients with acute pancreatitis. The experts on the committee are directed to put together a list of proposed recommendations (action statements) on the pertinent issues. An example of a proposed recommendation or action statement might be "We recommend that the use of gastric residual volume as a monitor should be avoided in the ICU." The compiled list organizes the guidelines process and facilitates the review of the literature for supporting evidence that follows.

The process of reviewing the literature is complex and time-consuming and begins by analyzing each of the individual trials published on a topic or recommendation. Committee members complete a data abstraction form (DAF) for each trial to extract the main clinical results and then perform an evaluation of study design using a standardized scoring system. Several aspects of study design and methodological quality are addressed in the evaluation process, each being scored as 0, 1, or 2 points (See Table 41-1).[13] These parameters include randomization (concealed), analysis (intention to treat), blinding, patient selection (selected or consecutive eligible), comparability of groups at baseline, extent of follow-up, treatment protocol, co-interventions, and outcomes.[13]

The GRADE expert then takes the individual DAF evaluations by committee members on all the trials that pertain to a topic and uses the GRADE process to summarize the evidence in a table.[11,12] The basic principle of GRADE is to start by assigning an RCT the highest level of evidence (++++). An observational study starts out at the lowest level (+). The score then can be adjusted based on issues of methodological

TABLE 41-1 Canadian Nutrition Support Clinical Practice Guidelines: Methodology for Scoring Randomized Controlled Trials[a]

	Score		
	0	1	2
Randomization	—	Not concealed or not sure	Concealed randomization
Analysis	Other	—	Intention to treat
Blinding	Not blinded	Single blinded	Double blinded
Patient selection	Selected patients or unable to tell	Consecutive eligible patients	—
Comparability of groups at baseline	No or not sure	Yes	—
Extent of follow-up	<100%	100%	—
Treatment protocol	Poorly described	Reproducibly described	—
Co-interventions	Not described	Described but not equal or not sure	Well described and all equal
Outcomes	Not described	Partially described	Objectively defined

[a]Maximum total score for a trial is 14. Meta-analyses are scored separately.
Source: Data are from reference 13.

quality discovered in the DAF analysis by the committee members. For RCTs, the score may be decreased because of problems with bias, consistency, precision, or directness. With trials performed in clinical nutrition, *bias* most likely stems from failure to blind the process or failure to analyze results on an intent-to-treat basis. *Consistency* is diminished if other RCTs show differing results. *Imprecision* occurs if the trial enrolled a small number of patients, and *directness* is a measure of the degree to which the methodological design and the results of the trial can be applied directly to patient care. The score for an observational trial may be increased if the therapy and the outcome effects are strongly associated, if the unmeasured factors that could interfere with the treatment effect are minimal, or if there is a dose-response gradient such that the outcome improves as the amount or dose of therapy increases.[11,12] Expert opinion is the lowest level of evidence, the details of which would not be included in the final GRADE table.

The GRADE table constructed by the GRADE expert summarizes the evaluation of the individual trials and their methodological issues. If the evaluation indicates strong support from the literature, then the terminology "we recommend" prefaces the recommendation. If the data are weak, the recommendation may be prefaced with "we suggest." If the literature includes an insufficient number of trials and/or the results from several trials are contradictory, the guideline statement may indicate "no recommendation at this time."[11,12]

Previous scoring systems for evaluating quality of evidence in the literature focused on large vs small RCTs, and whether controls were contemporaneous or historical in nonrandomized trials (see Table 41-2).[14] These elements are built into the GRADE process, but they may be less evident because of newer terminology (eg, large vs small size is incorporated into "imprecision") and because nonrandomized "observational" trials are evaluated by different criteria than RCTs.[11,12] For observational trials, GRADE focuses less on the overall size of the trial and more on the association between therapy and outcome, the dose-response gradient, and the lack of confounding factors. All the issues incorporated in the evaluation

TABLE 41-2 Example of Scoring System to Grade the Quality of Evidence

Levels of Evidence	Type of Evidence
I	Large randomized trials with clear-cut results; low risk of false-positive and/or false-negative error
II	Small randomized trials with uncertain results; moderate risk of false-positive and/or false-negative error
III	Nonrandomized cohort with contemporaneous controls
IV	Nonrandomized cohort with historical controls
V	Case series, uncontrolled studies, and expert opinion

Source: Data are from reference 14.

process are summarized in the GRADE table, which is usually included in an online appendix. However, GRADE tables are not self-explanatory to individuals who do not have a working knowledge of GRADE, and the entire process may therefore seem to lack transparency.

Several nuances in the literature reflect efforts to improve either quality of evidence or the generalizability of study results to patient care. *Propensity scoring* of observational trials emphasizes analysis of covariants or potential confounding factors, so that comparative groups (eg, patients who get treatments vs those who do not) may be better stratified by these factors, thereby yielding higher quality study results.[15] *Pragmatic trials* are designed to reflect "real world conditions" of clinical practice, and, after designating the conditions for randomization (eg, enteral vs parenteral route of feeding), such trials leave other treatment decisions (eg, choice of formula or amount of energy or protein) and co-interventions (eg, details of glycemic control or choice of antibiotics) up to the discretion of the attending physician or primary team.[16] *Comparative effectiveness research* involves the generation and synthesis of evidence that compares the benefits and harms of alternative methods to prevent, diagnose, treat, and monitor a clinical condition or to improve the delivery of care. All 3 of these elements would be captured in the GRADE analysis process.[17]

Interpreting Meta-Analyses

The information compiled in the GRADE table allows the GRADE expert to perform a meta-analysis and create a Forest plot that visually displays the information. The Forest plot is a valuable tool that gives the clinician a quick sense of the strength and consistency of the message from the literature (see Figure 41-1).[8] Horizontal lines on the Forest plot represent confidence intervals. If those lines do not touch or cross the vertical line of unity, then the difference in outcome between the study and control groups has reached statistical significance to a level $P <0.05$. Narrow confidence intervals indicate tighter results and suggest that the results would be similar if the test were repeated. Heterogeneity measures consistency from one study to the next regarding the patient population and therapy applied. For example, a meta-analysis of a group of studies performed in acute pancreatitis patients might show very low heterogeneity, with an I^2 value less than 40%, whereas a different compilation of trials in a wide range of different ICU patient populations might show moderate to marked heterogeneity with an I^2 value greater than 50%.[18] Each of the trials are listed on the Forest plot in vertical fashion by date of publication, with the patients with an outcome parameter (an event) tallied and the total denominator of patients displayed for both the treatment group and controls. The relative risk ratio shows the likelihood of the outcome effect (eg, infection) in the study group compared with controls. In a study comparing EN with parenteral nutrition (PN) where the outcome (incidence of infection) between the 2 groups was equal, the relative risk would be 1.00 (the group receiving EN is 100% as likely to get infection as those receiving PN). If the relative risk of infection in the study group receiving EN was 0.74, that would indicate a 26% reduction in infection compared with the control group receiving PN (1.00 − 0.74 = 0.26). Relative risk or odds

FIGURE 41-1 Forest Plot from GRADE Meta-analysis of Early vs Delayed Enteral Nutrition for the Outcome of Infection

Study or Subgroup	Early EN Events	Total	Delayed/None Events	Total	Weight	Risk Ratio M-H, Random, 95% CI	Year	Risk Ratio M-H, Random, 95% CI
Sagar 1979	3	15	5	15	3.1%	0.60 [0.17, 2.07]	1979	
Moore 1986	3	32	9	31	3.3%	0.32 [0.10, 1.08]	1986	
Schroeder 1991	1	16	0	16	0.5%	3.00 [0.13, 68.57]	1991	
Carr 1996	0	14	3	14	0.6%	0.14 [0.01, 2.53]	1996	
Beier-Holgersen 1996	2	30	14	30	2.5%	0.14 [0.04, 0.57]	1996	
Singh 1998	7	21	12	22	7.6%	0.61 [0.30, 1.25]	1998	
Minard 2000	6	12	7	15	6.6%	1.07 [0.49, 2.34]	2000	
Malhotra 2004	54	100	67	100	20.9%	0.81 [0.64, 1.01]	2004	
Kompan 2004	9	27	16	25	9.4%	0.52 [0.28, 0.96]	2004	
Peck 2004	12	14	11	13	17.7%	1.01 [0.74, 1.39]	2004	
Nguyen 2008	3	14	6	14	3.5%	0.50 [0.15, 1.61]	2008	
Moses 2009	17	29	19	30	14.5%	0.93 [0.61, 1.39]	2009	
Chourdakis 2012	13	34	12	25	9.8%	0.80 [0.44, 1.44]	2012	
Total (95% CI)		**358**		**350**	**100.0%**	**0.74 [0.58, 0.93]**		
Total events	130		181					

Heterogeneity: Tau² = 0.05; Chi² = 19.58, df = 12 (P = 0.08); I² = 39%
Test for overall effect: Z = 2.54 (P = 0.01)

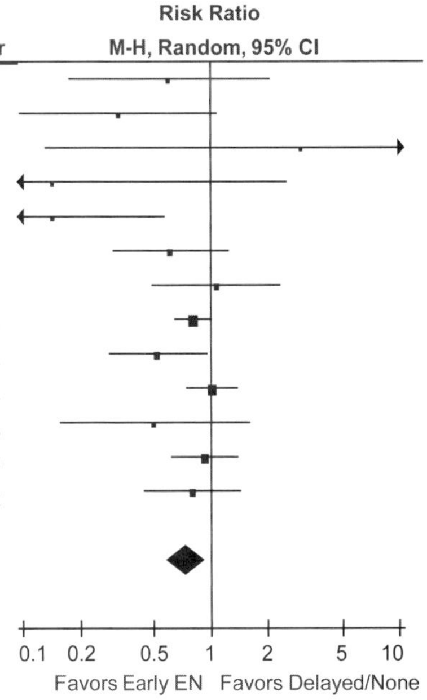

0.1 0.2   0.5   1   2   5   10
Favors Early EN   Favors Delayed/None

CI, confidence interval; EN, enteral nutrition; GRADE, Grading of Recommendations, Assessment, Development, and Evaluation.
Source: Data are from reference 8.

ratio statistics always tend to overestimate the treatment effect. Looking at the events (patients who had an infection) divided by the denominator or total number of patients in each group (EN vs PN), allows the reader to determine the absolute risk reduction. The absolute risk reduction is usually lower and probably gives clinicians a more accurate assessment of the treatment effect. The test for overall effect is given at the bottom of the Forest plot, with P <0.05 indicating that the difference in outcome between 2 two groups in response to treatment was statistically significant.

Style Issues for Guidelines Committees

The styles and philosophies of different guideline committees are evident when various societies' guidelines are compared. The guidelines processes for the 2009 and 2016 ASPEN/SCCM guidelines were as scientifically rigorous as the processes for other major guidelines published, but the philosophy of the ASPEN/SCCM committee was different.[7,8] In the absence of RCTs for any given topic, the committee chose to take advantage of the experts involved and provide guidelines based on expert opinion. In the 2016 ASPEN/SCCM guidelines, an anonymous vote of committee members was taken regarding the level of support for each recommendation, with all but one recommendation receiving greater than 70% affirmation by committee members.[8] Guidelines also differ in their terminology of the final recommendations. Some committees use GRADE methodological terminology to preface each recommendation, based on size, blinding, precision, and bias (eg, "Based on unblinded pseudorandomized small studies with high likelihood of bias, we suggest. . . ."). The ASPEN/

SCCM guidelines committee included this information in the GRADE tables but chose to exclude this terminology from each recommendation to provide the greatest clinical value to practitioners. At some point, the committee must establish a cutoff date for trials to be included in the analysis upon which support of the recommendations is based. In the situation of the 2016 ASPEN/SCCM guidelines, there was a 2-year gap between the cutoff of December 31, 2013, and the publication of the guidelines in early February 2016. The rationale for the cutoff date was that the inclusion of even a single trial following that date would require a literature search of every section in the entire manuscript to avoid bias. Several important RCTs were published in the interim period. Committee members, peer reviewers for the journal, and the societal board of directors reviewing the manuscript were all aware of these studies. Committee members made great effort to ensure that the guidelines were not obsolete at the time of publication and that trials published after the cutoff did not contradict the final recommendations.[8]

Levels of Evidence in the Literature

Various schemes to provide a hierarchy of evidence for evaluating the literature have been published.[19] Although the hierarchies used by different guideline committees may vary, large RCTs are usually considered to be at the highest level of evidence, nonrandomized cohort studies in the middle, and case series or expert opinion at the lowest level (see Table 41-2).[14] In the past, there was controversy as to where meta-analysis ranked in the hierarchy of levels of evidence (ie, whether meta-analysis should be at the highest level or be omitted entirely).[14] Recent adaptation of GRADE by most medical societies has elevated meta-analysis to the highest level.[11,12] Notably, strengths and weaknesses exist at every level of evidence. While the GRADE classification system has helped objectify the evaluation process, conflict and discrepancies still exist.

Observational studies are a popular mode of scientific evaluation because they can evaluate large patient populations and the results intuitively seem to reflect patient care in the real world. However, the results of observational trials can only show an association between treatment and outcome; they cannot infer cause and effect. Also, confounding factors can influence study results in observational trials. Failure to adjust for those confounding factors can generate conflicting or erroneous conclusions. In an observational trial by Arabi and colleagues evaluating the outcome effects by the percentage of goal energy delivered to critically ill patients, results associated delivery of a greater percentage of the energy goal with increased infection, hospital and ICU mortality, and incidence of ventilator-associated pneumonia.[20] The top tertile of patients who received the most energy had a hospital mortality that was nearly twice that of the lowest tertile (odds ratio, 1.99; $P = 0.02$).[20] A year later, Heyland and associates reproduced the same methodology in an observational trial looking at the same endpoints but in a different ICU population.[21] Initially, their results were identical to those of Arabi et al. However, Heyland et al then corrected for a confounding factor, advancement to all oral days (where a patient on tube feeding is advanced to oral diet and the number of calories from tube feeding is counted as zero). After adjusting for this confounding factor, Heyland and colleagues showed that hospital mortality actually went down when the amount of energy that patients were fed was closer to the goal, such that the highest tertile of patients experienced a 27% reduction in hospital mortality compared with the lowest tertile.[21] A separate study compared observational trials with intervention trials on the effect of beta-carotene on cardiovascular disease.[22] Six observational trials showed an overall beneficial treatment effect of beta-carotene on reduction of cardiovascular disease, whereas aggregation of the data from 4 RCTs showed the exact opposite—that ingestion of beta-carotene increased the incidence of cardiovascular disease. These examples show that larger numbers of participants in observational trials may amplify confounding factors, in which case study results may be further from the true scientific answer. In contrast, for RCTs, larger numbers of participants should get closer to the true science.[23]

Meta-analyses have their strengths and weaknesses. If the RCTs included are of high quality and low bias, the quality of the meta-analysis created by aggregating their data approaches that of a large well-designed RCT.[24] However, a well-done meta-analysis of poor studies is still a poor meta-analysis. While the GRADE process helps standardize the quality of evidence and the way an individual trial is evaluated, it does not influence or objectify the selection criteria by which studies are included in a meta-analysis. LeLorier and colleagues evaluated 12 instances where a meta-analysis published in the literature was subsequently followed by a large RCT on the same subject.[25] Results showed that the meta-analyses failed 35% of the time to predict the results of the large subsequent RCT.[25]

Evidence from large RCTs should trump findings from smaller trials, observational studies, and nonrandomized studies, as well as expert opinion. Large, prospective RCTs should carry weight in directing therapy. However, no study is flawless and supersedes all other trials—the totality of evidence should ultimately direct management.[19]

Large RCTs can have a number of potential flaws. Generalizability may be diminished in a trial with good internal validity and sound methodological design, but the external validity may be reduced when the results are generalized to patient care.[19] For example, the Early Parenteral Nutrition Completing Enteral Nutrition in Adult Critically Ill Patients (EPaNIC) trial from Europe evaluating the timing of supplemental PN had excellent internal validity and study design, such that the investigators were given the international 2009 Stoutenbeek award for study design.[26] However, details related to patient management (infusion of large doses of intravenous glucose prior to initiation of PN, and a strategy of tight glucose control) reduced the external validity and the application of EPaNIC study results to general patient care.[26] Practice Scenario 41-1 considers the relevance of evidence from EPaNIC and another trial to the case of a patient at high nutrition risk.[8,26,27]

Practice Scenario 41-1

Question: How does an interpretation of levels of evidence in the literature help guide clinical practice for a patient requiring supplemental parenteral nutrition (PN)?

Scenario: A 65-year-old man with type 2 diabetes mellitus, obesity, and metabolic syndrome was admitted to the intensive care unit with community-acquired pneumonia. The patient's clinical condition deteriorated to the point that he required intubation and placement on mechanical ventilation. A nasoenteric tube was placed initially, but early attempts at enteral nutrition (EN) were unsuccessful in delivering more than 20% of the energy goal. Using 2 separate scoring systems for nutrition risk, the patient was determined to be at high nutrition risk. The nutrition support team was consulted and recommended that supplemental PN be added to the insufficient EN toward the end of the first week of hospitalization. The primary team was reluctant to initiate supplementary PN, citing a large trial from Europe regarding the danger of early supplemental PN in critically ill patients.

Intervention: A review of the literature was conducted, and the discussion focused on the difference in implications from the Early Parenteral Nutrition Completing Enteral Nutrition in Adult Critically Ill Patients (EPaNIC) trial[26] of early vs late supplemental PN and a Swiss supplemental PN trial by Heidegger.[27]

Answer: The discussion clearly identified both the EPaNIC trial and the Swiss supplemental PN trial as large, multicenter, randomized controlled trials. The EPaNIC trial was the larger study (4,600 patients) and had strong internal validity in its rigorous methodology. However, the external validity, or generalizability to clinical practice, is diminished somewhat by the fact that a large intravenous glucose load was given to the early supplemental PN group before PN was initiated, and tight glucose control was used to manage the patients throughout the study. Such practice is not routine at medical centers outside of the research study center that was performing the trial. The results of the EPaNIC trial would suggest that the early addition of supplemental PN to insufficient tube feeding in this patient would be deleterious and should be avoided for at least 8 days. In contrast, the Swiss supplemental PN trial was smaller (300 patients), but it concluded that patients who received supplemental PN were given it in a safe manner and were not at greater risk compared with the control group that received EN alone. The treatment regimen used in the Swiss study better reflected common practice for providing PN, indicating better external validity and generalizability. The 2016 guidelines from the American Society for Parenteral and Enteral Nutrition (ASPEN) and the Society of Critical Care Medicine (SCCM) provide a full discussion of these 2 trials.[8] The key issue for this case relates to the nutrition risk of the patient. Because he was a high-risk patient, efforts to provide sufficient nutrition therapy might be needed sooner rather than later. Assurance of the safety of supplemental PN and recognition that a high-risk patient needed sufficient nutrition therapy as close to goal as possible became the 2 leading concerns that led the primary team to change management.

Rationale: An examination of the levels of evidence of the trials discussed in this scenario in combination with recommendations from ASPEN/SCCM guidelines encouraged the clinicians to add supplemental PN to the insufficient EN.

An assessment of harms can be an issue with RCTs, as RCTs tend to be short in duration and are less likely than observational trials to identify uncommon harms of therapy. Recent RCTs have tried to account for this weakness. The Acute Respiratory Distress Syndrome Network (ARDSNet) trial of trophic vs full feeds in patients with acute respiratory distress syndrome completed a 12-month follow-up to confirm that the trophic feeding in the first week of ICU stay did not have adverse effects on discharge status or long-term mortality.[28]

Multiplicity can be an issue with large RCTs. Repeated tests of statistical significance (looking for subsets of patients or additional study endpoints) are likely to produce at least 1 significant result if enough examples are evaluated.[19] In general, statisticians would expect 1 positive result for every 20 endpoints evaluated. Finding a significant result out of 20 endpoints would be interpreted to suggest that the treatment strategy provided to study patients was superior to that given to controls, whereas the positive result might simply be an example of multiplicity (and the 2 treatment strategies are truly no different).

Large RCTs also suffer from rigidity about the P value.[19] Clinicians focus on $P < 0.05$ to indicate whether results are statistically significant (a perspective that can be compared to the analogy that "someone is either pregnant or not"). However, such rigidity toward the P value is appropriate only for the initial study trial where the investigators are attempting to reject the null hypothesis (which implies that both treatments are equal). Once positive data are obtained in the initial trial, $P < 0.05$ is less relevant. For trials where there are previous positive studies published on the same subject or for trials

designed to show equivalence or noninferiority, rigid adherence to the value $P < 0.05$ may not be appropriate.[19] In other words, a trend that just misses statistical significance in such trials may still be clinically important and should not be discounted because the P value did not reach the level of <0.05. Large RCTs can suffer from a type 1 α error. This flaw suggests that an early significant difference would disappear if more subjects were entered in the trial. In a single-center RCT comparing underfeeding with full feeding in 240 patients, Arabi and colleagues showed a significant decrease in mortality in the patients who were underfed.[29] However, when the same lead author used nearly the same methodology in a larger multicenter trial of 885 patients, that difference disappeared and there was no difference in mortality between the 2 groups.[30] A type 2 β error suggests that no difference is seen early, but a difference would emerge with the inclusion of more subjects. When investigators were comparing permissive underfeeding with full feeding in a group of trauma patients, a study that was powered to 164 patients was stopped early because of poor patient recruitment following the inclusion of only 84 patients.[31] There was no difference in outcome between the 2 groups, but concern for type 2 β error is suggested by reduced patient entry rendering the study underpowered.

Clinicians vs Epidemiologists

As clinical guidelines have evolved in the era of GRADE evaluation, an important balance has emerged between the clinicians and the GRADE experts on the committee itself.[23] Most guideline committee members are expert clinicians who likely performed the RCTs. These individuals have expertise in the field, but they can sometimes be too close to the subject or have too much invested interest in the topic and, therefore, they may minimize methodological flaws in evaluation of the literature. GRADE experts, on the other hand, tend to be epidemiologists. Typically, they are the ones who do the meta-analyses, and they may not be experts in the particular field. They may miss clinical issues, but they are led in their thinking by close attention to methodological quality. A balance of both perspectives is of tremendous value to a guidelines committee in deriving the final recommendations, but conflict can arise between the 2 camps when interpreting study results.[23]

For the 2016 ASPEN/SCCM guidelines committee, such a conflict arose on a recommendation for EN vs PN in traumatic brain injury (TBI).[8] A 2005 meta-analysis by Simpson and Doig evaluating EN vs PN excluded 5 out of 14 RCTs based on flawed methodology and showed a statistically significant reduction in mortality with use of PN compared with EN ($P = 0.04$).[32] In a revised and updated meta-analysis (2014) on the same topic, Harvey and associates, prior to the initiation of the CALORIES trial, showed similar results with a tendency toward reduced mortality with PN compared with EN that did not reach statistical significance ($P = 0.278$).[33] Both of these meta-analyses were driven by a single trial by Rapp et al in 1983 that showed a statistically significant reduction in mortality with use of PN compared with EN.[34] Notably, this 1983 study was the first of 3 trials published by a single group of clinical neurosurgeons. The first trial, which showed a reduction in mortality from 44% to 0% ($P < 0.05$) with the use of PN compared with EN, was misleading.[34] The EN group really received standard therapy (advancement to oral diet with no tube feeding), and received very little nutrition therapy. When the trial was repeated 4 years later and the control group now received intragastric EN, the results flipped and the incidence of mortality was higher in the group receiving PN compared with the EN group (43.5% vs 35.7%; P = nonsignificant).[35] However, problems with tolerance of the gastric feeds resulted in the EN group getting less protein and energy. When the trial was repeated a third time and the group receiving EN was fed into the jejunum, both groups received equal amounts of energy and protein and results showed that mortality in the PN group was significantly greater than the EN group (50% vs 18%; P <0.05).[36] In reviewing the literature on route of feeding for patients with TBI, there was clearly a discrepancy or conflict between conclusions drawn by the epidemiologist (Doig) and that drawn by the clinicians (neurosurgeons). In the Simpson and Doig meta-analysis, the second trial was omitted because 4% of patients were lost to follow-up.[32] The third trial was published only in abstract form and was therefore excluded because a full manuscript could not be peer reviewed.[36] As the 2016 ASPEN/SCCM guidelines committee evaluated this experience in the literature, committee members voted to exclude any discussion of the study published in abstract form. Although the resulting GRADE meta-analysis suggested a nonsignificant clinical trend toward better outcome with PN, the ultimate recommendation by the committee was to use EN preferably over PN in TBI patients.[8]

Should All Guidelines Agree?

Clinicians often express frustration that guidelines from one society to the next (or from one nation to the next) do not always agree in their recommendations on a subject. In an initiative by the European Society for Parenteral and Enteral Nutrition to address this issue, the suggestion was made to form a pilot global guidelines committee that would look specifically at one topic (acute pancreatitis was chosen) and, instead of writing new guidelines, develop a process to compare previously published recommendations across multiple societal guidelines.[32] Seven separate guidelines from Europe and North America were compared, and a process of evaluation was designed based on level of evidence in the literature and the degree of consensus agreement between the societies. Surprisingly, the results showed incredible consensus on multiple recommendations for nutritional therapy in acute pancreatitis, with little or no disagreement.[37] No further projects were pursued, and the pilot committee was disbanded. See Practice Scenario 41-2 for an example of how clinical guidelines on nutrition care might be applied to a patient with acute pancreatitis.[8]

In a second effort to promote cooperation and agreement among societal guidelines, a "harmonization process" was developed by the leaders of the Canadian Critical Care Guidelines.[8] Designed to unify the ASPEN and Canadian guideline groups, meetings were held to set up a formal evaluation of the literature. Committee members from ASPEN/SCCM and the Canadian group spent 2 years evaluating the literature and entering data from RCTs into an electronic database.[8] However, when the entry process was completed, the groups separated to derive their own recommendations and ultimate guidelines.

Practice Scenario 41-2

Question: How can guidelines help in the management of a patient with severe acute pancreatitis?

Scenario: A 46-year-old white man is admitted 24 hours after an endoscopic retrograde cholangiopancreatogram (ERCP) with fever, elevated white count, abdominal pain, nausea, and vomiting. Laboratory test results show elevated amylase and lipase, and a computed tomography scan shows evidence of acute pancreatitis. Although the patient is relatively young and athletic and is considered to have post-ERCP pancreatitis, further laboratory tests indicate that he has 5 Ransom criteria, which would predict a 40% mortality rate. The attending staff on the case orders parenteral nutrition (PN), commenting that the need to put the pancreas to rest is an automatic and traditional indication for PN. Nonetheless, a consult to the nutrition support team is placed, and it recommends early enteral feeding. The question is raised as to whether clinical guidelines published by the nutrition societies would help resolve this apparent conflict in strategies of management.

Intervention: A review of the most recent (2016) American Society for Parenteral and Enteral Nutrition (ASPEN) and Society of Critical Care Medicine (SCCM) clinical guidelines[8] is conducted and discussed between the primary medicine and consulting nutrition teams.

Answer: The ASPEN/SCCM clinical guidelines provide an excellent discussion of the physiological principles behind the nutrition management for acute pancreatitis. While it is important to provide feeding that lowers the degree of stimulation of the pancreas, the review of the literature shows that enteral nutrition (EN) can put the pancreas to rest and is preferred over PN because EN maintains gut integrity and can reduce the risk for systemic inflammatory response syndrome. The guidelines provide clear-cut recommendations for monitoring the patient with pancreatitis who is receiving EN, as well as recommendations for when to use PN. The transparency of the guidelines allows both the physicians and the nutrition support clinicians to follow the thread of evidence back to the studies in the literature that support each of the recommendations.

Rationale: After discussing the guidelines, the primary medicine team and the nutrition support team agree to initiate early EN and delineate the monitoring parameters to gauge the patient's tolerance of EN. The guidelines support the view espoused by the nutrition support team and allay fears on the part of the medicine team for how the therapy might influence the patient's ultimate outcome.

Ensuring that all guidelines agree is not practical or feasible, and really may not be that important in the long run. The guidelines of each society or nation reflect distinctive values, culture, and financing for medical therapy. Getting these disparate groups to decide or agree on a list of recommendations is unnecessary. What may be appropriate for a group in North America (such as leaving off immunosuppressive ω-6 lipids in

PN the first week after admission to the ICU) may be inappropriate in Europe (where clinicians have multiple choices for parenteral lipids that are less immunosuppressive).

Conclusion

Several strategies may help improve EBM and the value that guidelines offer to clinicians in the future. Agreeing on a standard by which to evaluate the literature (such as GRADE) is an important step toward agreement among societies. Measures to direct which trials should or should not be included in a meta-analysis are needed. In addition, results of individual trials may be improved by making data available in the public domain.[23] In other words, researchers should start with a clearly defined question, register the study at the onset, identify primary and secondary endpoints, complete the study, analyze the data, and publish the results. Then, the data should be turned over to the public domain so separate and independent groups may independently analyze the data and possibly draw different conclusions.

When using guideline recommendations in an era of EBM, clinicians need to remain flexible. Findings from large RCTs should be carefully interpreted and, where appropriate, should carry weight in directing therapy. However, management and treatment decisions should be based on the totality of information. As others have noted, the notion that evidence from the literature can be placed into rigid hierarchies is "illusionary" or, at best, a difficult endeavor.[19] Guidelines are rigorous and evidence-based, but their recommendations should never take priority over clinical judgment. Guidelines should always be interpreted in the context of the institutional setting. The most important contributions of guidelines are that they organize information, transparently connect recommendations to the supporting trials in the literature, and provide the clinician with a good place to start when managing patients.

References

1. Evidence-Based Medicine Working Group. Evidence-based medicine. A new approach to teaching the practice of medicine. *JAMA.* 1992;268:2420–2425.

2. Sur R, Dahm P. The history of evidence based medicine. *Indian J Urol.* 2011;27(4):487–489.

3. Straus S, Richardson WS, Glasziou P, Haynes RB. *Evidence-Based Medicine: How to Practice and Teach EBM.* 3rd ed. London, UK: Elsevier Churchill Livingstone; 2005.

4. Jennings BM, Loan LA. Misconceptions among nurses about evidence-based practice. *J Nurs Scholarsh.* 2001;33:121–127.

5. Heyland DK, Dhaliwal R, Day A, et al. Validation of the Canadian clinical practice guidelines for nutrition support in mechanically ventilated, critically ill adult patients: results of a prospective observational study. *Crit Care Med.* 2004;32:2260–2206.

6. Thomas DE, Kukuruzovic R, Martino B, et al. Knowledge and use of evidence-based nutrition: a survey of paediatric dietitians. *J Hum Nutr Diet.* 2003;16:315–322.

7. McClave SA, Martindale RG, Vanek VW, et al. Guidelines for the provision and assessment of nutrition support therapy in the adult critically ill patient: Society of Critical Care Medicine (SCCM) and American Society for Parenteral and Enteral Nutrition (A.S.P.E.N.). *JPEN J Parenter Enteral Nutr.* 2009;33(3):277–316.

8. McClave SA, Taylor BE, Martindale RG, et al. Guidelines for the provision and assessment of nutrition support therapy in the adult critically ill patient: Society of Critical Care Medicine (SCCM) and American Society for Parenteral and Enteral Nutrition (A.S.P.E.N.). *JPEN J Parenter Enteral Nutr.* 2016;40(2):159–211.

9. Hoffer LJ, Bistrian BR. Why critically ill patients are protein deprived. *JPEN J Parenter Enteral Nutr.* 2013;37(3):300–309.

10. Koretz RL. Is the guideline already out of date? *JPEN J Parenter Enteral Nutr.* 2016;40(5):611–614.

11. Atkins D, Best D, Briss PA, et al. Grading quality of evidence and strength of recommendations. *BMJ.* 2004;328(7454):1490.

12. Balshem H, Helfand M, Schünemann HJ, et al. GRADE guidelines: 3. Rating the quality of evidence. *J Clin Epidemiol.* 2011;64(4):401–406.

13. Heyland DK, Dhaliwal R, Drover JW, et al. Canadian clinical practice guidelines for nutrition support in mechanically ventilated, critically ill adult patients. *JPEN J Parenter Enteral Nutr.* 2003;27(5):355–373.

14. Dellinger RP, Carlet JM, Masur H, et al. Surviving Sepsis Campaign guidelines for management of severe sepsis and septic shock. *Intensive Care Med.* 2004;30(4):536–555.

15. Kitsios GD, Dahabreh IJ, Callahan S, et al. Can we trust observational studies using propensity scores in the critical care literature? A systematic comparison with randomized clinical trials. *Crit Care Med.* 2015;43(9):1870–1879.

16. Roland M, Torgerson DJ. What are pragmatic trials? *BMJ.* 1998;316(7127):285.

17. Fiore LD, Lavori PW. Integrating randomized comparative effectiveness research with patient care. *N Engl J Med.* 2016;374(22):2152–2158.

18. Higgins JPT, Green S, eds. *Cochrane Handbook for Systematic Reviews of Interventions.* Version 5.1.0 (updated March 2011). www.handbook.cochrane.org. Accessed March 16, 2017.

19. Rawlins M. *De testimonio:* on the evidence for decisions about the use of therapeutic interventions. *Clin Med (Lond).* 2008;8(6):579–588.

20. Arabi YM, Haddad SH, Tamim HM, et al. Near-target caloric intake in critically ill medical-surgical patients is associated with adverse outcomes. *JPEN J Parenter Enteral Nutr.* 2010;34(3):280–288.

21. Heyland DK, Cahill N, Day AG. Optimal amount of calories for critically ill patients: depends on how you slice the cake! *Crit Care Med.* 2011;39(12):2619–2626.

22. Egger M. *Systematic Review of Health Care.* London, UK: BMJ Books; 2001:218.

23. Bier DM. Dragged kicking and screaming into the evidence-based century. ASPEN Rhoads Lecture, Clinical Nutrition Week, February 11, 2013, Phoenix, AZ.

24. Ioannidis JP. Why most published research findings are false. *PLoS Med.* 2005;2(8):e124.

25. LeLorier J, Grégoire G, Benhaddad A, LaPierre J, Derderian F. Discrepancies between meta-analyses and subsequent large randomized, controlled trials. *N Engl J Med.* 1997;337(8):536–542.

26. Casaer MP, Mesotten D, Hermans G, et al. Early versus late parenteral nutrition in critically ill adults. *N Engl J Med.* 2011;365(6):506–517.

27. Heidegger CP, Berger MM, Graf S, et al. Optimisation of energy provision with supplemental parenteral nutrition in critically ill patients: a randomised controlled clinical trial. *Lancet.* 2012;381(9864):385–393. doi:10.1016/S0140-6736(12)61351-8.

28. Rice TW, Wheeler AP, Thompson BT, et al. Initial trophic vs full enteral feeding in patients with acute lung injury: the EDEN randomized trial. *JAMA.* 2012;307(8):795–803.

29. Arabi YM, Tamim HM, Dhar GS, et al. Permissive underfeeding and intensive insulin therapy in critically ill patients: a randomized controlled trial. *Am J Clin Nutr*. 2011;93(3):569–577.

30. Arabi YM, Aldawood AS, Solaiman O. Permissive underfeeding or standard enteral feeding in critical illness. *N Engl J Med*. 2015;373(12):1175–1176.

31. Charles EJ, Petroze RT, Metzger R, et al. Hypocaloric compared with eucaloric nutritional support and its effect on infection rates in a surgical intensive care unit: a randomized controlled trial. *Am J Clin Nutr*. 2014;100(5):1337–1343.

32. Simpson F, Doig GS. Parenteral vs. enteral nutrition in the critically ill patient: a meta-analysis of trials using the intention to treat principle. *Intensive Care Med*. 2005;31(1):12–23.

33. Harvey SE, Parrott F, Harrison DA, et al. Trial of the route of early nutritional support in critically ill adults. *N Engl J Med*. 2014;371(18):1673–1684.

34. Rapp RP, Young B, Twyman D, et al. The favorable effect of early parenteral feeding on survival in head-injured patients. *J Neurosurg*. 1983;58(6):906–912.

35. Young B, Ott L, Haack D, et al. Effect of total parenteral nutrition upon intracranial pressure in severe head injury. *J Neurosurg*. 1987;67(1):76–80.

36. Charash WE, Kearney PA, Annus KA, et al. Early enteral feeding is associated with an attenuation of the acute phase/cytokine response and improved outcome following multiple trauma. *J Trauma*. 1994;37:1015.

37. Mirtallo J, Forbes A, Jensen GI, McClave SA. International consensus guidelines for nutrition therapy in pancreatitis. *JPEN J Parenter Enteral Nutr*. 2012;36(3):284–291.

Index

Page numbers followed by *f* or *t* indicate figures and tables, respectively.